ENDOCRINOLOGY

VOLUME 2

ENDOCRINOLOGY

VOLUME 2

Edited by

Leslie J. DeGroot

George F. Cahill, Jr.   William D. Odell

Luciano Martini   John T. Potts, Jr.

Don H. Nelson   Emil Steinberger

Albert I. Winegrad

GRUNE & STRATTON

A Subsidiary of Harcourt Brace Jovanovich, Publishers

New York   London   Toronto   Sydney   San Francisco

Library of Congress Cataloging in Publication Data
Main entry under title:

Endocrinology.

    Bibliography
    Includes index.
    1.   Endocrine glands—Diseases. 2. Endocrinology.
I. DeGroot, Leslie J. [DNLM: 1. Endocrine diseases.
2. Endocrine glands. 3. Hormones. WK100.3 E56]
RC648.E458   616.4   78-24043
ISBN 0-8089-1168-6 (v. 2)

Grune & Stratton, Inc.
111 Fifth Avenue
New York, New York 10003

Distributed in the United Kingdom by
Academic Press, Inc. (London) Ltd.
24/28 Oval Road, London NW 1

Library of Congress Catalog Number 78-24043
International Standard Book Number 0-8089-1168-6

Printed in the United States of America

Contents
Volume 2

Contents
Volume 1

Preface

Contributors

Contents
Volume 3

Preface

Contributors

ENDOCRINOLOGY OF CONCEPTION, PREGNANCY, AND PARTURITION

DIFFUSE HORMONAL SYSTEMS

INTEGRATED HORMONAL CONTROL SYSTEMS

GENERAL PRINCIPLES OF ENDOCRINE PATHOPHYSIOLOGY

Preface

This new text is intended to provide a complete contemporary source of basic and clinical aspects of endocrinology. Our book is directed to serious students of endocrinology; the authors believe that this encompasses undergraduates, house officers, fellows, and physicians practicing in the field. We hope to provide a source to which these serious students can turn in order to find an answer to all of their questions.

It is obvious that there is no dearth of endocrine texts, but, in surveying the field, we have not found a volume which presents "molecular" or "metabolic" endocrinology with the emphasis that we feel is appropriate, or which has adequately attempted a synthesis into a coherent whole data available from basic science and the clinic.

In the past years, endocrinology and metabolism have gone through stages of development that may be arbitrarily characterized as descriptive, anatomic, physiologic, and biochemical. Current endocrinology is featured by (1) a great increase in knowledge of the biochemical basis of endocrine function and dysfunction, (2) development of sensitive techniques for the measurement of hormones, their precursors and metabolites, and (3) a flood of information on integrated endocrine responses in various physiologic states. It is now possible to characterize many endocrinologic events in molecular terms and to integrate isolated observations into meaningful and unifying concepts. This additional information has called for a new approach to the teaching of endocrinology.

Our book is written with a physiologic and biochemical interpretive bias, indicating the change in endocrinology from a largely descriptive discipline to one integrating basic science. Because the book is meant to be used by practicing physicians, however, we have made it just as comprehensive in its clinical presentation, which we consider crucial. We have stressed the relation of clinical endocrinology to physiology, genetics, biochemistry, and immunology. We have used basic science data to add to clinical data to aid in interpretation, and have indicated areas in which problems exist or where ignorance remains.

While the editors philosophically would have preferred to develop a book totally integrated around "processes" or "functions" controlled by coincident endocrine stimuli, the proper peda-gogic approach demands a more traditional introduction to the field. Thus our work is divided into two complementary sections. In the first, a typically organ-oriented section of about 1400 pages, basic endocrine physiology and clinical problems are thoroughly covered. Clinical problems that confront the practicing physician are emphasized. The second section, of about 700 pages, integrates, in a series of chapters, contemporary endocrinologic knowledge in relation to important processes or problems. Here, for example, we consider growth, puberty, the response to starvation, obesity, and so forth. In these areas there are normal and abnormal homeostatic processes that involve multifactorial endocrine control, and concepts that can now be seen to unify endocrine physiology.

Volumes of this size suffer from the delay between writing and publication. In an effort to counteract this problem, we have given authors the opportunity to add important new material during proofing of the final galleys. New references have simply been inserted in the appropriate sequence by letter designation, e.g. 10a, 10b, etc. We believe this small departure from custom offers an important improvement in our text.

The proliferation of abbreviations in medical writings is in one way a benefit, and in another a curse. Abbreviations surely accelerate the transmission of information, but only if one understands the key. We have attempted to standardize all abbreviations to conform with those used by *Endocrinology,* a style familiar to most of our readers. Variations from these standards are, we hope, adequately explained.

This book is, in every sense, the joint effort of eight editors and nearly two hundred authors. To these distinguished scientists, teachers, and clinicians, the chief editor expresses his sincere thanks and great respect. It is the broad knowledge and hard work of these collaborators which makes the volume unique in its contribution.

Sincere appreciation is also offered to our co-workers at Grune and Stratton, to the secretaries across the nation who came to recognize my voice quite easily, to Ms. Myrna Zimberg for a vast amount of help, and to Helen DeGroot for patiently page-proofing a mountain of text.

Leslie J. DeGroot, M.D.

Contributors

Paul Aiginger, M.D.
II Medical University Klinik
Abt. f. Nuclearmedizin
University of Vienna
Vienna, Austria

Thomas T. Aoki, M.D.
Assistant Professor of Medicine
Harvard Medical School
and Associate, Peter Bent Brigham
    Hospital
and Investigator, Howard Hughes Medical
    Institute
Boston, Massachusetts

Cesare Aragona
Senior Research Fellow
Department of Physiology
University of Manitoba
Winnipeg, Manitoba

Ronald A. Arky, M.D.
Professor of Medicine
Harvard Medical School
and Chief of Medicine
Mount Auburn Hospital
Cambridge, Massachusetts

Claude D. Arnaud, M.D.
Professor of Medicine and Physiology
University of California School of
    Medicine
and Chief, Endocrine Unit
San Francisco Veterans Administration
    Hospital
San Francisco, California

Jurgen Aschoff, Dr. Med.
Director at the Institute
Max-Planck-Institut fur
    Verhaltensphysiologie
Erling-Andechs, Germany

Louis V. Avioli, M.D.
Schoenberg Professor of Medicine
Washington University School of Medicine
and the Jewish Hospital of St. Louis
St. Louis, Missouri

Lester Baker, M.D.
Director, Clinical Research Center
Children's Hospital of Philadelphia
and Professor of Pediatrics
University of Pennsylvania School of
    Medicine
Philadelphia, Pennsylvania

Susanne Barton, Ph.D.
Associate Professor, Department of
    Physiology
University of Alberta
Edmonton, Alberta

Tomas Berl, M.D.
Assistant Professor of Medicine
University of Colorado Medical Center
Denver, Colorado

M. Bonnyns, M.D.
Charge de Clinique
University of Brussels
and Adjoint in the Department of Medicine
Saint-Pierre Hospital
Brussels, Belgium

Philippe J. Bordier, M.D. (deceased)
Metre de Researche
I.N.S.E.R.M.
Paris, France

Cyril Y. Bowers, M.D.
Professor of Medicine
Tulane University Medical School
New Orleans, Louisiana

F. R. Bringhurst, M.D.
Clinical and Research Fellow in Medicine
Massachusetts General Hospital
and Research Fellow in Medicine
Harvard Medical School
Boston, Massachusetts

John E. Buster, M.D.
Assistant Professor of Obstetrics and
    Gynecology
University of California at Los Angeles
    School of Medicine
Los Angeles, California

George F. Cahill, Jr., M.D.
Professor of Medicine
Harvard Medical School
and Physician, Peter Bent Brigham
    Hospital
and Director of Research, Howard Hughes
    Medical Institute
Boston, Massachusetts

Vito M. Campese, M.D.
Assistant Professor of Medicine
University of Southern California School of
    Medicine
Division of Nephrology
Los Angeles County–University of South-
    ern California Medical Center
Los Angeles, California

Fabio Celotti, M.D.
Department of Endocrinology
University of Milano
Milano, Italy

Ding Chang, Ph.D.
Institute for Biomedical Research
The University of Texas at Austin
Austin, Texas

Alan Cherrington, Ph.D.
Assistant Professor of Physiology
Vanderbilt University Medical School
Nashville, Tennessee

Jean-Louis Chiasson, M.D.
Assistant Professor of Medicine
Vanderbilt University Medical School
Nashville, Tennessee

Nicholas P. Christy, M. D.
Professor of Medicine
Columbia University College of Physicians
    and Surgeons
and Director, Medical Service
The Roosevelt Hospital
New York, New York

Felix A. Conte, M.D.
Associate Professor of Pediatrics
University of California
San Francisco, California

Cary W. Cooper, Ph.D.
Professor of Pharmacology
Department of Pharmacology
University of North Carolina School of
    Medicine
Chapel Hill, North Carolina

**D. Harold Copp, M.D., Ph.D.,
    F.R.C.P.(c), F.R.S.C., F.R.S.**
Professor of Physiology
University of British Columbia
Vancouver, British Columbia

Marilyn C. Crim, Ph.D.
Research Associate, Department of
Nutrition and Food Science
Massachusetts Institute of Technology
Cambridge, Massachusetts

Val Davajan, M.D.
Professor of Obstetrics and Gynecology
University of Southern California School of
Medicine
Los Angeles, California

Leonard J. Deftos, M.D.
Professor of Medicine
University of California
San Diego School of Medicine
and Chief, Endocrinology
San Diego Veterans Administration
Hospital
La Jolla, California

Leslie J. DeGroot, M.D.
Professor of Medicine and Head,
Endocrine Section
University of Chicago School of Medicine
Chicago, Illinois

Hector F. DeLuca, Ph.D.
Professor of Biochemistry
College of Agricultural and Life Sciences
University of Wisconsin
Madison, Wisconsin

Vincent DeQuattro, M.D.
Professor of Medicine
University of Southern California School of
Medicine
Los Angeles, California

Eugene R. DeSombre, Ph.D.
Associate Professor, Ben May Laboratory
for Cancer Research
and Research Associate, Biomedical
Computation Facilities
The University of Chicago
Chicago, Illinois

Francis P. DiBella, Ph.D.
Upjohn Company
Kalamazoo, Michigan

Jacques E. Dumont, M.D.
Professor and Head of Institute of
Interdisciplinary Research
Institut de Recherche Interdisciplinaire en
Biologie Humaine et Nucléaire
Brussels University
Brussels, Belgium

Edward N. Ehrlich, M.D.
Professor of Medicine
University of Wisconsin
and Head, Endocrine Section
and Associate Chairman, Department of
Medicine
University of Wisconsin
Madison, Wisconsin

Harvey Eisenberg, M.D.
Associate Professor
University of California Medical Center
Department of Radiology
Orange, California

Ragnar Ekholm, M.D., Ph.D.
Professor of Anatomy
Department of Anatomy
University of Göteborg
Göteborg, Sweden

Andre M. Ermans, M.D.
Associate Professor of Experimental
Medicine
Head of the Department of Nuclear
Medicine
St. Peter Hospital
Free University of Brussels
Brussels, Belgium

Imogen M. A. Evans, M.D., F.R.C.P.
Research Fellow, Endocrine Unit
Royal Postgraduate Medical School
London, England

David C. Evered, B.Sc., M.D., F.R.C.P.
Physician, Royal Victoria Infirmary
Newcastle Upon Tyne, England

**Calvin Ezrin, M.D., F.R.C.P.-C.,
F.A.C.P.**
Professor of Medicine and Associate
Professor of Pathology
University of Toronto School of Medicine
Toronto, Ontario

Stefan S. Fajans, M.D.
Professor of Internal Medicine
Head, Division of Endocrinology and
Metabolism
and Director, Metabolism Research Unit
The University of Michigan Medical
School
Ann Arbor, Michigan

Freddy Febres, M.D.
Director, Laboratory of Endocrinology
Maternidad Concepcion Palacios
Caracas, Venezuela

Philip Felig, M.D.
C.N.H. Long Professor and Vice
Chairman, Department of Internal
Medicine
Yale University School of Medicine
New Haven, Connecticut

Gianfranco Fenzi, M.D.
Assistant Professor of Medicine
Cattedra di Patologia Speciale Medica II
University of Pisa
Pisa, Italy

James B. Field, M.D.
Rutherford Professor of Medicine
Head, Division of Endocrinology and
Metabolism
Baylor University
Houston, Texas

Delbert A. Fisher, M.D.
Professor of Pediatrics
University of California at Los Angeles
School of Medicine
Torrance, California

Jeffrey S. Flier, M.D.
Assistant Professor of Medicine
Harvard Medical School
and Chief, Diabetes and Metabolism Unit
Beth Israel Hospital
Boston, Massachusetts

Karl Folkers, Ph.D.
Institute for Biomedical Research
University of Texas at Austin
Austin, Texas

Daniel W. Foster, M.D.
Professor of Internal Medicine
University of Texas Southwestern Medical
School
Dallas, Texas

Paul Henry Frank, M.D.
Assistant Professor, Department of
Radiology
Pritzker School of Medicine
The University of Chicago
Chicago, Illinois

Andrew G. Frantz, M.D.
Professor of Medicine and Chief, Division
of Endocrinology
Columbia University College of Physicians
and Surgeons
and Attending Physician, Presbyterian
Hospital
New York, New York

Donald Fraser, M.D.
Departments of Pediatrics and Physiology
University of Toronto
The Research Institute
The Hospital for Sick Children
Toronto, Ontario

Norbert Freinkel, M.D.
Kettering Professor of Medicine
and Director, Center for Endocrinology,
Metabolism, and Nutrition
Northwestern University Medical School
and Attending Physician, Northwestern
Memorial Hospital
and Consultant, Veterans Administration
Lakeside Hospital
Chicago, Illinois

Henry G. Friesen, M.D.
Professor and Head, Department of
  Physiology
University of Manitoba
Winnipeg, Manitoba

Lawrence A. Frohman, M.D., Ph.D.
Professor of Medicine
University of Chicago Pritzker School of
  Medicine
and Director, Division of Endocrinology
  and Metabolism
Michael Reese Medical Center
Chicago, Illinois

Steven R. Goldring, M.D.
Instructor in Medicine
Massachusetts General Hospital
and Assistant to the Chief of Medicine
Department of Medicine
New England Deaconess Hospital
Boston, Massachusetts

Donald P. Goldstein, M.D.
Assistant Clinical Professor, Department of
  Obstetrics and Gynecology
Harvard Medical School
Boston, Massachusetts

Samuel Goldstein, M.D.
Associate Professor of Medicine and
  Associate in Biochemistry
McMaster University Medical School
and Attending Physician, McMaster
  University Medical Center
Hamilton, Ontario

David Goltzman, M.D.
Assistant Professor of Experimental
  Medicine
McGill University
and Assistant Physician
Royal Victoria Hospital
Montreal, Quebec

Victor E. Gould, M.D.
Professor of Pathology
Rush Medical School
Chicago, Illinois

**David G. Grahame-Smith, M.B., B.S.,
  F.R.C.P.**
Rhodes Professor of Clinical Pharmacology
and Honorary Director, M.R.C. Unit of
  Clinical Pharmacology
University of Oxford
Oxford, England

Douglas A. Greene, M.D.
Assistant Professor of Medicine
University of Pennsylvania School of
  Medicine
Philadelphia, Pennsylvania

Monte A. Greer, M.D.
Professor of Medicine
Head of the Department of Endocrinology
University of Oregon Medical School
Portland, Oregon

Marie H. Greider, Ph.D.
Associate Professor of Pathology
Washington University School of Medicine
St. Louis, Missouri

Melvin M. Grumbach, M.D.
Professor of Pediatrics
University of California
and Director, Pediatric Services
University of California Hospitals
San Francisco, California

Erlio Gurpide, Ph.D.
Professor of Obstetrics and Gynecology
  and of Biochemistry
Mount Sinai School of Medicine
New York, New York

Joel F. Habener, M.D.
Associate Professor of Medicine
Harvard Medical School
Endocrine Unit, Massachusetts General
  Hospital
Boston, Massachusetts

Theodore J. Hahn, M.D.
Assistant Professor of Medicine
Washington University School of Medicine
and the Jewish Hospital of St. Louis
St. Louis, Missouri

Peter F. Hall, M.D., Ph.D.
Professor and Chairman, Department of
  Physiology
California College of Medicine
University of California
Irvine, California

Reginald Hall, B.Sc., M.D., F.R.C.P.
Professor of Medicine
University of Newcastle Upon Tyne
and Physician, Royal Victoria Infirmary
Newcastle Upon Tyne, England

Madeleine Harbison, M.D.
Department of Medicine
Division of Medical Genetics
The Johns Hopkins Hospital
Baltimore, Maryland

Boyd W. Harding, M.D., Ph.D.
Professor of Medicine and Biochemistry
University of Southern California School of
  Medicine
Los Angeles, California

Morey W. Haymond, M.D.
Assistant Professor of Pediatrics
Mayo Clinic
Rochester, Minnesota

Eileen Higham, Ph.D.
Assistant Professor in Medical Psychology
and Adjunct Professor of Psychology
Department of Psychiatry and Behavioral
  Sciences
and Department of Pediatrics
The Johns Hopkins University
Baltimore, Maryland

Raymond L. Hintz, M.D.
Associate Professor of Pediatrics
Stanford University School of Medicine
Palo Alto, California

Michael F. Holick, Ph.D., M.D.
Assistant Professor of Medicine
Harvard Medical School
and Clinical Assistant in Medicine
Massachusetts General Hospital
Boston, Massachusetts

Richard Horton, M.D.
Professor of Medicine
and Chief, Endocrinology Section
University of Southern California Medical
  Center
Los Angeles, California

Eva Horvath, Ph.D.
Assistant Professor of Pathology
Department of Pathology
University of Toronto
Toronto, Ontario

John Humphries, Ph.D.
Institute for Biomedical Research
The University of Texas at Austin
Austin, Texas

Robert Israel, M.D.
Associate Professor, Department of
  Obstetrics and Gynecology
University of Southern California School of
  Medicine
Los Angeles, California

Bernard H. Jaffe, M.D.
Professor of Surgery
Washington University School of Medicine
St. Louis, Missouri

Elwood V. Jensen, Ph.D.
Professor, Departments of Biophysics and
  Theoretical Biology
and Director, Ben May Laboratories
The University of Chicago
Chicago, Illinois

Ulrich Keller, M.D.
Instructor in Medicine
Vanderbilt University Medical School
Nashville, Tennessee

Henry T. Keutmann, M.D.
Principal Research Associate in Medicine
Harvard Medical School
and Associate in Biochemistry (Medicine)
Massachusetts General Hospital
Boston, Massachusetts

John M. Kinney, M.D.
Professor of Surgery
Columbia University College of Physicians
  and Surgeons
and Attending Surgeon
Presbyterian Hospital
New York, New York

Charles R. Kleeman, M.D.
Professor of Medicine and Chief, Division
  of Nephrology
University of California at Los Angeles
  School of Medicine
Los Angeles, California

Ronald Knudsen, Ph.D.
Institute for Biomedical Research
The University of Texas at Austin
Austin, Texas

**Kalman Kovacs, M.D., Ph.D., D.Sc.,
  F.R.C.P.(c), F.A.C.P., M.R.C. (Path.)**
Associate Professor
Department of Pathology
University of Toronto
and Pathologist, St. Michael's Hospital
Toronto, Ontario

Stephen M. Krane, M.D.
Professor of Medicine
Harvard Medical School
Chief, Arthritis Unit and Physician,
  Medical Services
Massachusetts General Hospital
Boston, Massachusetts

Dorothy T. Krieger, M.D.
Professor of Medicine
Mount Sinai School of Medicine
and Director, Division of Endocrinology
  and Metabolism
Mount Sinai Hospital
New York, New York

Paul E. Lacy, M.D.
Mallinckrodt Professor and Chairman
Department of Pathology
Washington University School of Medicine
St. Louis, Missouri

Yiu-Kuen Lam, Ph.D.
Institute for Biomedical Research
The University of Texas at Austin
Austin, Texas

Richard L. Landau, M.D.
Professor of Medicine
The University of Chicago School of
  Medicine
Chicago, Illinois

Elizabeth M. K. Leovey
Postdoctoral Fellow
Georgetown University School of Medicine
Washington, D.C.

John F. Liljenquist, M.D.
Assistant Professor of Medicine
Vanderbilt University Medical School
Nashville, Tennessee

Mortimer B. Lipsett, M.D.
Director, The Clinical Center
National Institutes of Health
Bethesda, Maryland

Iain MacIntyre
Director, Endocrine Unit
Royal Postgraduate Medical School
London, England

Jane E. Mahaffey, M.D.
Instructor in Medicine
Harvard Medical School
and Clinical Assistant in Medicine
Massachusetts General Hospital
Boston, Massachusetts

John R. Marshall, M.D.
Professor of Obstetrics and Gynecology
University of California at Los Angeles
  School of Medicine
Los Angeles, California

Robert W. Marshall, B.Sc., Ph.D.
M.R.C. Mineral Metabolism Unit
The General Infirmary, Leeds
Leeds, England

Luciano Martini, M.D.
Professor of Pharmacology and
  Endocrinology
University of Milano
Milan, Italy

Renato Massa, M.D.
Department of Endocrinology
University of Milano
Milan, Italy

Franz M. Matschinsky, M.D.
Professor of Biochemistry and Biophysics
University of Pennsylvania School of
  Medicine
Philadelphia, Pennsylvania

G. P. Mayer, D.V.M., M.Sc. (Med.)
Professor of Physiology
College of Veterinary Medicine
Oklahoma State University
Stillwater, Oklahoma

Samuel M. McCann, M.D.
Professor and Chairman, Department of
  Physiology
Southwestern Medical School
University of Texas Health Science Center
  at Dallas
Dallas, Texas

Bruce S. McEwen, Ph.D.
Associate Professor
The Rockefeller University
New York, New York

John D. McGarry, M.D.
Professor of Internal Medicine and
  Biochemistry
University of Texas Southwestern Medical
  School
Dallas, Texas

J. M. McKenzie, M.D.
Professor of Medicine
McGill University School of Medicine
and Senior Physician and Director
Endocrinology and Metabolism Division
Royal Victoria Hospital
Montreal, Quebec

A. Wayne Meikle, M.D.
Associate Professor of Medicine
University of Utah School of Medicine
and Department of Medicine
Veterans Administration Hospital
Salt Lake City, Utah

James C. Melby, M.D.
Professor of Medicine
Boston University School of Medicine
and Visiting Physician and Head, Section
  of Endocrinology and Metabolism
University Hospital
Boston, Massachusetts

Thomas J. Merimee, M.D.
Professor of Medicine, and Head, Endocri-
  nology and Metabolism
University of Florida School of Medicine
University of Florida Hospital
Gainesville, Florida

Béla Mess, M.D., D. Med. Sci.
Professor of Anatomy
University Medical School
Pecs, Hungary

Boyd E. Metzger, M.D.
Professor of Medicine
Northwestern University Medical School
and Attending Physician
Northwestern Memorial Hospital
Chicago, Illinois

Claude J. Migeon, M.D.
Professor of Pediatrics
Johns Hopkins University School of
  Medicine
Baltimore, Maryland

Daniel R. Mishell, Jr., M.D.
Professor and Chairman, Department of
  Obstetrics and Gynecology
University of Southern California School of
  Medicine
Los Angeles, California

John Money, Ph.D.
Professor of Medical Psychology
and Associate Professor of Pediatrics
Department of Psychiatry and Behavioral
    Sciences
and Department of Pediatrics
The Johns Hopkins University
Baltimore, Maryland

Anthony D. Morrison, M.D.
Research Associate Professor of Medicine
University of Pennsylvania School of
    Medicine
Philadelphia, Pennsylvania

Marcella Motta, M.D.
Department of Endocrinology and
    Pharmacology
University of Milano
Milano, Italy

Hamish N. Munro, Ph.D., M.B.
Department of Nutrition and Food Science
Massachusetts Institute of Technology
Cambridge, Massachusetts

Mark R. Myers, B.S.
Research Assistant, Hypertension Service
Department of Medicine
Los Angeles County–University of
    Southern California Medical Center
Los Angeles, California

Robert M. Neer, M.D.
Associate Professor of Medicine
Harvard Medical School
and Associate Physician
Massachusetts General Hospital
Boston, Massachusetts

Don H. Nelson, M.D.
Professor of Medicine
University of Utah College of Medicine
Salt Lake City, Utah

William D. Odell, M.D., Ph.D.
Professor of Medicine and Physiology
University of California Medical School at
    Los Angeles
and Chairman, Department of Medicine
Harbor General Hospital
Torrance, California

Sergio R. Ojeda, D.V.M.
Department of Physiology
Southwestern Medical School
University of Texas Health Science Center
    at Dallas
Dallas, Texas

Jack H. Oppenheimer, M.D.
Professor of Medicine and Physiology
and Head, Section of Endocrinology and
    Metabolism
Department of Medicine
University of Minnesota School of
    Medicine
Minneapolis, Minnesota

Lelio Orci, M.D.
Director, Institut d'Histologie et
    d'Embryologie
Ecole de Medecine
Universite de Geneva
Geneva, Switzerland

Anthony S. Pagliara, M.D.
Associate Professor of Pediatrics
Assistant Professor of Medicine
Co-Director, Pediatric Endocrinology and
    Metabolism
Washington University School of Medicine
and Associate Pediatrician
St. Louis Children's Hospital
and Assistant Physician
Barnes Hospital
St. Louis, Missouri

Johanna A. Pallotta, M.D.
Assistant Professor of Medicine
Harvard Medical School
and Assistant Physician, Department of
    Medicine
Beth Israel Hospital
Boston, Massachusetts

A. Michael Parfitt, M.B., B. Chir.,
M.R.C.P., F.R.A.C.P., F.A.C.P.
Clinical Associate Professor of Medicine
University of Michigan Medical School
and Physician, Fifth Medical Division
and Director, Mineral Metabolism
    Laboratory
Ann Arbor, Michigan

J. A. Parsons
Head: Laboratory for Endocrine
    Physiology and Pharmacology
National Institute for Medical Research
London, England

Munro Peacock, M.B., Ch.B., M.R.C.P.
Honorary Consultant Physician
General Infirmary, Leeds
and Assistant Director, M.R.C. Mineral
    Metabolism Unit
General Infirmary, Leeds
Leeds, England

Richard L. Phelps, M.D.
Assistant Professor of Medicine
and Assistant Professor of Obstetrics &
    Gynecology
Northwestern University Medical School
and Attending Physician
Prentice Women's Hospital and Maternity
    Center
Chicago, Illinois

Aldo Pinchera, M.D.
Associate Professor of Medicine
Cattedra di Patologia Speciale Medica II
University of Pisa
Pisa, Italy

Constance S. Pittman, M.D.
Professor of Medicine
University of Alabama School of Medicine
and Endocrinology Section
Veterans Administration Hospital
Birmingham, Alabama

Flavio Piva, M.D.
Departments of Endocrinology and
    Pharmacology
University of Milano
Milan, Italy

Allan Pont, M.D.
Assistant Professor of Medicine
Stanford University School of Medicine
and Chief of Endocrinology
Santa Clara Valley Medical Center
San Jose, California

John T. Potts, Jr., M.D.
Professor of Medicine
Harvard Medical School
and Chief, Endocrine Unit
Massachusetts General Hospital
Boston, Massachusetts

Peter W. Ramwell, Ph.D.
Professor of Physiology
Georgetown University School of Medicine
Washington, D.C.

Samuel Refetoff, M.D.
Professor of Medicine
Pritzker School of Medicine
University of Chicago
Director of Thyroid Function Laboratory
Billings Hospital
Chicago, Illinois

Eric Reiss, M.D.
Professor and Vice Chairman
Department of Medicine
University of Miami School of Medicine
Miami, Florida

M. Markus Riek, M.D.
Chief Resident in Internal Medicine
University of Bern Medical School
Bern, Switzerland

William G. Robertson, B.Sc., Ph.D.
M.R.C. Mineral Metabolism Unit
The General Infirmary, Leeds
Leeds, England

Luis J. Rodriguez-Rigau, M.D.
Assistant Professor, Department of
    Reproductive Medicine and Biology
University of Texas Medical School at
    Houston
and Active Medical Staff
Hermann Hospital
Houston, Texas

Robert L. Rosenfield, M.D.
Associate Professor of Pediatrics
University of Chicago Pritzker School of
  Medicine
and Wyler Children's Hospital
Chicago, Illinois

Griff T. Ross, M.D., Ph.D.
Deputy Director, The Clinical Center
National Institutes of Health
Bethesda, Maryland

Aldo A. Rossini, M.D.
Associate in Medicine
Joslin Research Laboratory
and Assistant Professor of Medicine
Harvard Medical School
Boston, Massachusetts

Jesse Roth, M.D.
Chief, Diabetes Section
National Institute of Arthritis, Metabolism,
  and Digestive Diseases
National Institutes of Health
Bethesda, Maryland

S. I. Roth, M.D.
Professor and Chairman
Department of Pathology
University of Arkansas Medical Center
Little Rock, Arkansas

Corbin P. Roubebush, M.D.
Pritzker School of Medicine
The University of Chicago
Chicago, Illinois

Arthur H. Rubenstein, M.D.
Professor and Associate Chairman
Department of Medicine
University of Chicago School of Medicine
and Attending Physician, Billings Hospital
Chicago, Illinois

R. G. G. Russell, Ph.D., M.D., M.R.C.P.
Professor of Chemical Pathology
and Honorary Consultant in Human Me-
  tabolism to Sheffield Area Health
  Authority
University of Sheffield Medical School
Sheffield, England

Charles H. Sawyer, Ph.D.
Professor of Anatomy
University of California at Los Angeles
  School of Medicine
and Brain Research Institute
Los Angeles, California

Melville Schachter, Ph.D.
Professor and Chairman, Department of
  Physiology
University of Alberta
Edmonton, Alberta

Alan L. Schiller, M.D.
Assistant Professor of Pathology
Harvard Medical School
and Chief, Autopsy Pathology and Bone
  Laboratory
Department of Pathology
Massachusetts General Hospital
Boston, Massachusetts

Gustav Schonfeld, M.D.
Professor of Preventative Medicine and
  Medicine
Washington University School of Medicine
St. Louis, Missouri

Charles R. Scriver, M.D.
The deBelle Laboratory for Biochemical
  Genetics
Departments of Pediatrics and Biology
McGill University–Montreal Children's
  Hospital Research Institute
Montreal, Quebec

Robert E. Scully, M.D.
Professor of Pathology
Massachusetts General Hospital
and Harvard Medical School
Boston, Massachusetts

Gino V. Segre, M.D.
Assistant Professor of Medicine
Harvard Medical School
and Assistant Physician
Massachusetts General Hospital
Boston, Massachusetts

Robert Sherwin, M.D.
Assistant Professor of Medicine
Yale University School of Medicine
New Haven, Connecticut

Louis M. Sherwood, M.D.
Professor of Medicine
University of Chicago
and Physician-in-Chief and Chairman, De-
  partment of Medicine
Michael Reese Hospital and Medical
  Center
Chicago, Illinois

Pentti Siiteri, M.D.
Professor of Obstetrics
Department of Obstetrics-Gynecology and
  Reproductive Sciences
University of California School of
  Medicine
San Francisco, California

Ethan A. H. Sims, M.D.
Professor of Medicine, Department of
  Medicine and Metabolic Unit
University of Vermont College of Medicine
and Attending Physician, Medical Center
  Hospital of Vermont
Burlington, Vermont

Eduardo Slatopolsky, M.D.
Professor of Medicine
Department of Medicine
Washington University School of Medicine
St. Louis, Missouri

Keith D. Smith, M.D.
Professor, Department of Reproductive
  Medicine and Biology
University of Texas Medical School at
  Houston
and Active Medical Staff, Hermann
  Hospital
Department of Internal Medicine
Houston, Texas

John B. Stanbury, M.D.
Professor of Experimental Medicine
Massachusetts Institute of Technology
Cambridge, Massachusetts

Charles A. Stanley, M.D.
Assistant Professor of Pediatrics
University of Pennsylvania
and Division of Endocrinology
Children's Hospital of Philadelphia
Philadelphia, Pennsylvania

Emil Steinberger, M.D.
Professor and Chairman, Department of
  Reproductive Medicine and Biology
The University of Texas Health Science
  Center at Houston
Houston, Texas

Donald F. Steiner, M.D.
Professor of Biochemistry and Medicine
Pritzker School of Medicine
The University of Chicago
Chicago, Illinois

Hugo Studer, M.D.
Professor of Medicine
Head of the Department of Medicine
University of Bern Medical School
Berne, Switzerland

Howard S. Tager, Ph.D.
Assistant Professor of Biochemistry
Pritzker School of Medicine
The University of Chicago
Chicago, Illinois

Roy V. Talmage, Ph.D.
Professor of Surgery and Pharmacology
Director of Orthopedic Research
Departments of Surgery and Pharmacology
University of North Carolina
Chapel Hill, North Carolina

Alvin Taurog, Ph.D.
Professor of Pharmacology
University of Texas Health Science Center
Dallas, Texas

Michael D. Trus
Postdoctoral Fellow in Biochemistry and
    Biophysics
School of Medicine
University of Pennsylvania
Philadelphia, Pennsylvania

Roger H. Unger, M.D.
Veterans Administration Hospital
and Professor of Internal Medicine
University of Texas Southwestern Medical
    School
Dallas, Texas

Robert D. Utiger, M.D.
Professor of Medicine
Endocrine Section
University of Pennsylvania
Philadelphia, Pennsylvania

Judson J. Van Wyk, M.D.
Kenan Professor of Pediatrics
University of North Carolina School of
    Medicine
Chapel Hill, North Carolina

Gilbert Vassart, M.D.
Charge de Recherche F.N.R.S.
Institute of Interdisciplinary Research
Brussels University Medical School
Brussels, Belgium

Helmuth Vorherr, M.D.
Professor of Obstetrics and Gynecology
    and Pharmacology
University of New Mexico School of
    Medicine
Albuquerque, New Mexico

John Wahren, M.D.
Professor of Clinical Physiology
Karolinska Institute and Huddinge
    Hospital
Huddinge, Sweden

Yieh-Ping Wan, Ph.D.
Institute for Biomedical Research
The University of Texas at Austin
Austin, Texas

Chiu-an Wang, M.D., F.A.C.S.
Associate Clinical Professor of Surgery
Harvard Medical School
and Visiting Surgeon
Massachusetts General Hospital
Boston, Massachusetts

Michelle P. Warren, M.D.
Assistant Professor of Medicine and
    Obstetrics and Gynecology
Columbia University College of Physicians
    and Surgeons
Associate Attending Physician,
    Departments of Medicine and Obstetrics/
    Gynecology
The Roosevelt Hospital
New York, New York

Ann Ruhmann-Wennhold, M.D.
Associate Research Professor
University of Utah College of Medicine
Salt Lake City, Utah

Charles D. West, M.D.
Professor of Medicine and Biochemistry
University of Utah College of Medicine
Salt Lake City, Utah

John F. Wilber, M.D.
Chief of Endocrinology and Professor of
    Medicine
Louisiana State University Medical
    Sciences Center
New Orleans, Louisiana

E. D. Williams
Professor of Pathology
Department of Pathology
Welsh National School of Medicine
Cardiff, Wales

H. G. Williams-Ashman, Ph.D.
Professor of Biochemistry
Ben May Laboratory for Cancer Research
University of Chicago
Chicago, Illinois

Albert I. Winegrad, M.D.
Professor of Medicine
University of Pennsylvania School of
    Medicine
Philadelphia, Pennsylvania

Richard J. Wurtman, M.D.
Professor of Endocrinology and
    Metabolism
Laboratory of Neuroendocrine Regulation
Department of Nutrition and Food Science
Massachusetts Institute of Technology
Cambridge, Massachusetts

Margita Zakarija, M.D.
Assistant Professor
McGill University School of Medicine
and Assistant Physician
Royal Victoria Hospital
Montreal, Quebec

Walter S. Zawalich, Ph.D.
Assistant Professor of Physiology
School of Medicine
University of Pennsylvania
Philadelphia, Pennsylvania

Disorders of Bone and Bone Mineral Metabolism: Relation to Parathyroid Hormone, Calcitonin, and Vitamin D

Calcium and Phosphate Distribution, Turnover, and Metabolic Actions

F. R. Bringhurst
John T. Potts, Jr.

The purpose of this chapter is to review essential details of the metabolic role of calcium and phosphate present in blood and tissue fluids. Although most of the calcium and phosphate of the body occurs in an insoluble form in the skeleton, soluble, extraskeletal calcium and phosphate are involved in varied and crucial regulatory and energy-related body functions. An understanding of these concentration-dependent metabolic functions requires knowledge of the distribution, absorption, and excretion of these mineral ions. As a result, apparently, of the metabolic importance of the extraskeletal calcium and phosphate and the varied availability of these ions from external sources (influenced by diet and sunlight under different environment circumstances), considerable precision of regulation of extracellular fluid calcium and phosphate is found. This is accomplished through endocrine control by PTH and vitamin D and through other hormonal and nonhormonal regulatory influences affecting transcellular transport of calcium and phosphate by the kidney and intestine and exchange between bone reservoirs and extracellular fluid.

Adequate concentration and satisfactory throughput of extracellular fluid calcium and phosphate are needed to support bone mineral formation; conversely, both ions are released together with dissolution of bone mineral. Extremes in variation of concentration of one ion affect the distribution of the other through reciprocal physiochemical effects. The solubility product, calcium ion concentration multiplied by phosphate ion concentration, is normally close to a solubility maximum.

Despite these closely linked biological roles, there are many differences between calcium and phosphate with regard to extraskeletal distribution, precision of regulation of hour-by-hour concentration in extracellular fluid, direction of change induced by

regulatory hormones, and, finally, the nature of Ca^{2+} and P_i extraskeletal metabolic and regulatory actions. Details of the distribution and turnover of calcium and phosphate; a description of the action of hormones, drugs, and other factors on absorption and renal excretions of Ca^{2+} and P_i; and the metabolic actions of these two mineral ions, including the adverse consequences of excessive or deficient extracellular fluid content, are reviewed in this chapter. Chapter 52 deals with the intricate process of mineral ion homeostasis per se. Chapter 69 reviews central features in the exchange between extracellular-fluid calcium and phosphate and the mineral phase of bone.

CALCIUM

DISTRIBUTION

Less than 1 percent of the body calcium is found in blood, in extracellular fluid, and intracellularly in various soft tissues. In addition, about 1 percent of skeletal calcium is freely exchangeable with extracellular fluid. Together, these fractions are termed the miscible pool of calcium (Fig. 40-1).

The concentration of calcium in bone is relatively constant from one species of mammal to another, although the total amount per unit of body mass varies in relation to the relative size of the skeleton. Table 40-1 indicates the relative distribution of calcium (and also phosphorus) in body tissues.[1-3]

Calcium in Plasma and Extracellular Fluid

Table 40-2 lists the various forms in which calcium and phosphate circulate in normal plasma. Slightly less than half the circulating calcium is in the form of free calcium ions; it is this fraction that is important physiologically. Changes in ionized calcium bring about the dramatic changes in neuromuscular activity and the various biochemical processes in which calcium plays an important role. The remainder of plasma calcium is bound to serum proteins, but a small portion circulates in the form of complexes with citrate and phosphate. The normal range of blood calcium is 8.8–10.4 mg/100 ml of blood.[2]

Albumin is the principal calcium-binding factor in plasma, but other proteins, including globulins, also bind significant quantities of the ion.[1,2] Calcium binding by proteins is pH-dependent; decreased binding occurs at acid pH.[2] Significant changes in plasma

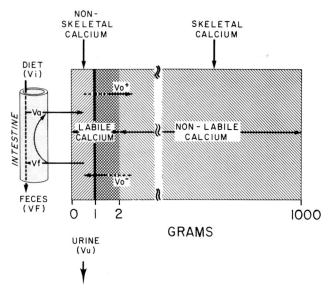

Fig. 40-1. Schematic representation of the distribution of calcium in the body and its exchange among the different compartments that have been inferred through calcium kinetic studies. Double cross-hatched area shown in skeletal calcium compartment just to right of heavy vertical line is the small skeletal component of labile calcium, the surface, freely diffusible component. Not represented in this diagram is the nonlabile, nonskeletal pool of calcium that is found in sites such as renal stones. See text for full discussion and definition of symbols. Vi, dietary calcium intake; VF, fecal calcium; Va, calcium absorption; Vf, endogenous fecal calcium; Vo+, bone calcium accretion; Vo−, bone calcium release; Vu, urinary calcium excretion. (Modified after Potts and Deftos.[28])

protein concentration can be associated with abnormalities in total blood calcium concentration.

Attempts to measure ionized calcium have presented some formidable experimental difficulties,[4,5] but recent methods have shown promise. Two basic methods are currently employed: one using a solid state, dip electrode with calcium-sensitive components (details of the latter not yet reported); and a second (improved through several models), featuring a flow-through electrode. Corrections are required for postcollection changes in pH and CO_2 unless samples are collected anaerobically (such as by completely filling a vacuum tube).[6–10] The principal difficulties hampering widespread application of the technique have involved the stability of the electrodes. These issues may now be or shortly will be improved. Physiological and clinical correlations have already suggested the usefulness of the approach as more discriminant of disturbances in blood or serum calcium than total calcium measurement.

Table 40-1. Distribution of Calcium and Phosphate in Body Tissues

	Calcium	Phosphorus
Total body content (g/kg fat-free tissue)	20–25	11–14
Specific tissue	Relative distribution	
	(Percentage of total body content)	
Skeleton	99	85
Muscle	0.3	6
Other tissue	0.7	9

Adapted from S. M. Krane: Calcium, phosphate and magnesium, in, H. Rasmussen (ed.): The International Encyclopedia of Pharmacology and Therapeutics. London, Pergamon Press, Ltd., 1970, p 19 (reference 94).

Table 40-2. Distribution of Calcium and Phosphate in Normal Human Plasma

State	Concentration		Percentage of Total
	mM/l	mg/100 ml	
Phosphorus			
Free $HPO_4^=$	0.50	1.55	44%
Free $H_2PO_4^-$	0.11	0.34	10
Protein-bound	0.14	0.43	12
$NaHPO_4^-$	0.33	1.02	28
$CaHPO_4$	0.04	0.12	3
$MgHPO_4$	0.03	0.10	3
Total	1.15	3.56	
Calcium			
Free Ca^{2+}	1.18	4.72	48%
Protein-bound	1.14	4.56	46
Complexed	0.08	0.32	3
Unidentified	0.08	0.32	3
Total	2.48	9.92	

Adapted from M. Walser: Ion association VI. Interaction between calcium, magnesium, inorganic phosphate, citrate and protein in normal human plasma. *J Clin Invest 40:* 723, 1961.[95]

Calcium in the Skeleton

Greater than 99 percent of the body calcium occurs in the skeleton.[1,2] Calcium in bone exists primarily in the form of small crystals presumed to be identical to hydroxyapatite, a precise crystalline structure of calcium, phosphate, and hydroxyl ions (see Chapter 69).[1,2,11] Some calcium in bone also exists in more amorphous crystals in combination with phosphate. The normal calcium-to-phosphate ratio in bone is 1.5:1, slightly lower than that found in pure hydroxyapatite.[1,2,11]

Bone is a cellular tissue undergoing constant remodeling;[12,13] a variety of hormones, vitamins, and other less well understood factors, in addition to parathyroid hormone and calcitonin, influence the metabolism and the turnover of bone. (These aspects of the metabolism of bone are reviewed in Chapter 69.)

Calcium in Extraskeletal Cells

The concentration of extracellular-fluid calcium (Table 40-2) is 2.5×10^{-3} M (1.2×10^{-3} M of free calcium); the concentration of intracellular calcium, specifically in the cytosol, although difficult to measure, has been estimated to be much lower than that present in extracellular fluid, less than 10^{-6} M.[14–16] Rasmussen et al.[14] have emphasized, however, that the total cellular content of calcium, much of it sequestered within mitochondria and other cellular membranes and particles, is sufficient, if uniformly distributed, to raise the cellular calcium concentration considerably, to 2×10^{-3} M, close to that of extracellular fluid.

Details of factors controlling shifts in intracellular calcium distribution and increased cellular uptake of calcium and the magnitude (as well as biological role) of such transcellular and intracellular fluxes of calcium are not well understood.[14,15] It is presumed that cells contain an active calcium pump, analogous to other cellular ion transport pumps, that maintains the estimated 1000-fold concentration gradient between cytosolic and extracellular-fluid calcium content by extrusion of calcium. Alternatively, part of the regulation of cellular calcium content may involve membrane permeability. It is known that the permeability of the plasma membrane to calcium does change dramatically with various tropic influences, such as the action of hormones on target cells.[14]

Recent studies in squid axons attest to the complexity of

regulation of intracellular calcium,[14,17] especially the nature of the cellular membrane permeability, Ca^{2+} pump interactions, linkage of Na^+ transport with Ca^{2+} transport, metabolic results of changes in intracellular and extracellular Ca^{2+} content, and the activation of the energy-dependent calcium extrusion system by ATP. The results seen in nerve cells[17] are similar to earlier findings in erythrocytes[18] and point to a specific Ca^{2+}/ATPase pump mechanism.

Many of the widespread physiological actions of calcium (discussed below) will be undoubtedly understood ultimately in terms of metabolic consequences of rapid compartmental shifts and specific interactions involving this critical but minute (<<1 percent) fraction of total body calcium (Fig. 40-2).

ABSORPTION

General

A fuller appreciation of the complex process of calcium absorption and of the factors that influence it have come from a variety of studies of calcium absorption in mammalian and vertebrate species: in vitro experiments using inverted gut sacs and intestinal slices; detailed analysis of the mode of action of vitamin D metabolites in vivo and in vitro; and, finally, in vivo studies in humans as well as in animals using metabolic balance techniques and radioactive calcium.[1,2,19–24]

The normal dietary intake of human subjects varies greatly but is usually within the range of 0.5–1.0 g/day.[3] From 25 to 70 percent of the ingested calcium is absorbed. A variety of factors, including the actual dietary intake, previous dietary history, age, general state of overall calcium balance, and intake of vitamin D, influence the efficiency of absorption.[1,2,23–26] The fecal calcium not only consists of the fraction of the ingested calcium that was not absorbed, but some portion also reflects secretion into the gastrointestinal tract of calcium contained in the digestive juices. Calcium secreted but not resorbed is termed "endogenous fecal calcium." Differing estimates of the quantities have been reported; conservative estimates indicate the amount of endogenous fecal calcium to be 60–150 mg/day.[2,26] Under most conditions, even for example in experimentally induced hypercalcemia, this endogenous fecal secretion of calcium is maintained at a constant rate.[2]

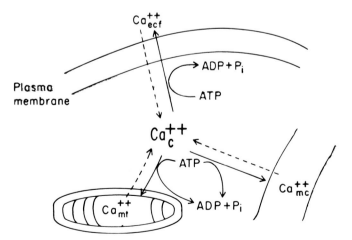

Fig. 40-2. Calcium entry into and loss from the cytosol occur via three sites: extracellular fluid, Ca^{++}_{ecf}; mitochondria, Ca^{++}_{mt}; and microsomes, Ca^{++}_{mc}. Entry rates (dotted lines) are thought to be passive, and the controlling influences uncertain; exit rates (solid lines) are believed to occur by active transport involving ATP and a calcium-dependent ATPase. (Modified after Rasmussen et al.)[14]

Hence variations in endogenous secretion are probably not important in overall calcium balance.

Mechanisms of Intestinal Calcium Absorption

Extensive studies[23,24] have established two general mechanisms in intestinal calcium absorption; both active transport and a passive or diffusion-related process are involved. In the presence of adequate concentrations of vitamin D, calcium is transported from mucosa to serosa against a concentration gradient.[23,24,27,28] The ratio of calcium concentration on the serosal to the mucosal side of everted gut sacs can reach a concentration difference of six fold.[19,29] Similar studies involving in situ perfusion studies[23] have also shown concentration gradients indicating active calcium transport. A requirement for metabolic energy in this mechanism of calcium transport has been shown as expected for an active transport process.[23,28] Calcium transport is depressed whenever aerobic metabolism is interfered with, for example, by anaerobic conditions, addition of metabolic inhibitors, or lowering of the ambient temperature.[2,19,23,24,28] The overall data indicate that intestinal cells must contain a "pump mechanism" capable of moving calcium against an electrochemical gradient from mucosal to serosal surfaces.

There is abundant evidence, however, indicating that passive permeability or simple diffusion also plays a quantitatively important role in the absorption of calcium and that this process is also influenced or regulated by vitamin D, as is active transport. The existence of this diffusion-limited or passive absorption process is deduced from several lines of evidence. Study of calcium absorption as a function of calcium concentration in the intestinal fluid indicates that the rate of mucosal to serosal flux of calcium varies as the calcium concentration increases, even to very high levels, without evidence of saturation in the intestinal lumen. An active transport process would, of course, be saturable (Fig. 40-3). Studies employing calcium transport in intestinal slices from rat intestine[30] indicated a curvilinear function, similar to that in Fig. 40-3, as calcium concentration is increased in the bathing medium. Inclusion of metabolic inhibitors such as dinitrophenol abolishes the two-phase process, leaving a purely linear function corresponding to the presumed passive permeability mechanism. Several workers have extensively reviewed the theoretical aspects of this facet of calcium transport.[23,31] Theoretical treatments of the active transport and passive diffusion mechanism have led to equations describing the net flux or calcium absorption as a complex function relating the maximum transport ratio of the active transport or saturable process, the diffusional coefficient or transport rate equivalent of the passive diffusion mechanism, and the calcium-ion concentration available for transport. The equation describing the process, as derived by Wilkinson[31] is

$$J = \frac{J \max [Ca]}{[Ca] + K_t} + D[Ca] - J_0$$

where J = net flux or absorption, $J \max$ = maximum flux rate due to the active transport process, K_t = transport constant, D = diffusional constant, or flux rate, due to passive permeability, and $[Ca]$ = calcium concentration in the lumen. J_0 (unidirectional flux back from blood to lumen) is added to correct for back diffusion. Studies using intubation methods[31] have confirmed the two-component kinetic model as applicable to humans as well as to chicks and rats. Wasserman and Taylor[23] studied the concentration of calcium in the intestinal lumen required to equal the electrochemical potential difference between the concentration of calcium in the

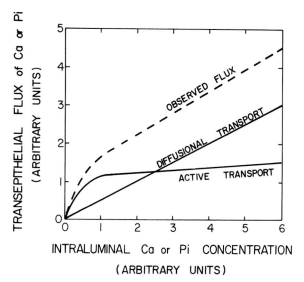

Fig. 40-3. The active and passive components of intestinal mineral ion transport. The experimentally observed mucosal-to-serosal flux, *Jms* (dashed line), is resolved into its active and diffusional components. The active transport mechanism is responsible for most of the flux at low intraluminal ion concentrations, while the diffusional mechanism acquires greater quantitative importance at high ion concentrations that saturate the active transport system. By subtraction of the outward flux, J_0 (not shown) from *Jms* (dashed line), one may obtain the net inward flux (net mineral ion absorption).

lumen and in blood. They estimated that above a luminal calcium concentration of 6.7 millimolar, calcium is transported primarily by the diffusional process. Stated in other terms, this analysis leads to the conclusion that under conditions of calcium intake or in regions of the intestine where calcium concentration is high, absorption is diffusion-limited, and the passive permeability process predominates; in other regions of the intestine or at times when luminal calcium concentration is lower than approximately 6 millimolar, the active transport process assumes a preponderant role.

Intestinal Sites Involved in Calcium Absorption

The actual sites at which the bulk of calcium is absorbed in humans and in other species require an examination of a variety of issues, including the microscopic anatomy of the intestinal epithelial cells, the cellular mechanisms involved that influence the rate of absorption in any particular intestinal segment, and the residence time of calcium in that region of the intestine.[23,24]

Recent studies in which efforts have been made to analyze the mechanisms of calcium absorption in detail have led necessarily to careful consideration of the microscopic anatomy. The epithelial cells of the intestine contain multiple specialized structures important in the special function of controlled absorption of calcium and other nutrients. The external luminal surface is covered with microvilli, and adjacent epithelial cells have tight junctions that presumably hinder the movement of calcium between cells and restrict absorption to direct transcellular transport.[23] Recent studies,[23,32] however, employing lanthanum (La³⁺) have suggested that there may be a paracellular path for calcium absorption. In some sites or under some conditions the tight junctions may be leaky. On the surface of the microvilli is a mucopolysaccharide (glycocalyx) coat. The transcellular transport of calcium involves movement through this mucopolysaccharide coat and then through the microvilli on the luminal membrane surface. Multiple subcellular organelles and finally a pump mechanism operating at the lateral or basal membranes of the cells adjacent to the capillary bed represent additional components in the pathway of overall transepithelial transport of calcium from lumen to blood. Detailed analyses of the uptake of calcium by the intestine[33,34] have led to detection of several phases of calcium uptake corresponding to uptake by the outer coat (rapid) and actual transmembrane passage (slower).

With regard to specific regions of the small intestine, duodenum, jejunum, or ileum, most important for accomplishing the bulk of calcium absorption in humans and other species, several issues must be considered. Estimates of intraluminal calcium concentration in animal species have indicated a much higher concentration of calcium in the ileum than in the duodenum and jejunum; the concentration in the ileum exceeds that needed for predominant absorption via passive permeability.[35] These observations have led to reexamination of the regions of the intestine most important for bulk calcium absorption. Although it had been known that the duodenum is the region of most efficient calcium absorption, a variety of lines of evidence[35,36] suggest that the greatest proportion of intestinal calcium absorption is accomplished in the ileum, especially under natural conditions when calcium is ingested along with solid food. The active transport process seems to predominate in the duodenum and the jejunum. The importance of the duodenum and upper regions of the jejunum becomes greatest when the calcium content of the diet is low.

Controlling Influences in Calcium Absorption

Vitamin D, Calcium Transport Proteins, and Adaptation of Absorption. The major controlling influence on the efficiency of intestinal calcium absorption is 1,25-(OH)₂-D₃, the presumed sole active metabolite of vitamin D acting on intestinal transport mechanisms. The critical role of vitamin D in the enhancement of intestinal absorption of calcium has been extensively studied by many workers for many years, since the original observation of Mellanby in 1919.[37] The dependency of the active transport mechanism on the presence of adequate vitamin D metabolites has been abundantly demonstrated.[23,27,38] At the same time, other studies have indicated that vitamin D plays an important role in the second process, or diffusional-permeability absorptive pathway for calcium.[23,38] It is not clear whether vitamin D *independently* affects both the calcium pump mechanism involved in active transport and some critical component(s) involved in passive diffusional absorption of calcium.

In any event, it is clear that both mechanisms of intestinal calcium absorption are severely depressed in vitamin D-deficient animals. One speculation by Harrison and Harrison[38] is that the defect in the absence of vitamin D could be simply a decreased passive entry of calcium into the intestinal cell from the lumen; such a defect would then show up as a limitation in both diffusion-limited absorption and active transport, since the latter is dependent upon an adequate cellular uptake of calcium. On the other hand, as discussed below, there is evidence that the synthesis of certain proteins that may constitute part of the active transport mechanism may be absolutely dependent on vitamin D action; hence the issue of a unitary versus a dual action of vitamin D on intestinal calcium absorption remains unresolved.

One issue is especially confusing in regard to vitamin D action and synthesis of proteins believed to be part of the active transport chain. Although the synthesis of these specific intestinal tissue proteins is absolutely dependent on vitamin D, stimulation of intestinal calcium transport after administration of vitamin D, as

1,25-$(OH)_2$-D, to rachitic chicks occurs prior to synthesis of all but trivial amounts of the proteins.[39] Further interest in regard to the critical role of vitamin D and vitamin D metabolites on intestinal calcium absorption resides in (1) the remarkable physiological process of adaptation of calcium absorption in states of calcium deficiency, and (2) the confusing but intriguing role of the specific proteins, believed to be important in cellular transport, whose synthesis is under the control of vitamin D.

Much evidence has accumulated regarding the nature of the intestinal components involved in the active transport process as well as the effects of vitamin D through effects on protein synthesis.[21-23,40-43] Wasserman et al. have shown vitamin D-directed synthesis of a calcium-binding protein in intestinal mucosa.[21,23,44-46] This protein may play an important role in the active transport mechanism. The protein has been isolated from several animal species including humans; the sequences of several forms have been determined.[47-51] The concentration of the binding protein changes in response to physiological and nutritional variables.[21,23,44,45] A second protein, a calcium-dependent ATPase present in intestinal brush borders, has been described and linked in function to the calcium-binding protein.[42,43] Synthesis of the ATPase is also under control of vitamin D.[42,43] Other studies have pointed to a third protein involved in calcium transport, a brush-border alkaline phosphatase.[40,41] Certain studies indicate that the ATPase and the alkaline phosphatase may be the same protein.[23,40,52]

Good correlations have been established between the calcium-binding protein (CaBP) and intestinal calcium transport. Synthesis of the protein appears to be dependent on vitamin D action, as is efficient calcium absorption.[23] When calcium absorption rates are high, as in vitamin D-treated animals or in animals given a low-calcium or low-phosphate diet, the content of calcium-binding protein is high.[23,53] When calcium absorption is depressed, as in strontium-induced rickets, anticonvulsant therapy, or diabetes, the content of binding protein in intestine falls.[23,53] CaBP has a high and relatively selective affinity for calcium, consistent with a postulated role at some step in the transepithelial transport of calcium, but a specific role for CaBP has not been clarified. Continuing uncertainty persists, in fact, as to whether any of the three proteins, CaBP, brush-border alkaline phosphatase, or Ca^{2+}-dependent ATPase (or two proteins if the latter two are identical), plays a rate-limiting as distinct from a facilitative role in calcium absorption. Studies of the early phases of restoration toward normal of intestinal calcium absorption in vitamin D-deficient animals, after dosing with vitamin D or vitamin D metabolites, have shown enhanced absorption prior to appearance of the activity of the brush-border alkaline phosphatase[23] or prior to the detection of synthesis of the CaBP (the latter based on detection of CaBP-specific messenger RNA in intestinal tissues).[39]

The impressive adaptation of dietary absorption under stress of calcium deficiency has received wide attention both as a physiological process and in terms of control mechanisms. Under chronic deprivation of calcium intake, a remarkable adaptation occurs in the efficiency of absorption of calcium in the intestine.[23-26] This process was initially identified by Nicolaysen et al.[25] When rats were deprived of dietary calcium until about a 5 percent calculated reduction of total calcium content in the body had been achieved, and then again given diets adequate in calcium, the efficiency of calcium absorption increased from control values prior to calcium deprivation of 10 to 20 percent to values of 35 to 50 percent or greater.

Extensive studies[23,54,55] confirmed that adaptation occurs in humans as well. Nicolaysen et al.[25] postulated an endogenous

factor believed to arise from the calcium-deficient skeleton as responsible for the adaptation process. Considerable effort has been made to define the mediator of adaptation. Vitamin D is clearly needed for adaptation to operate. In parallel experiments performed in rats on a diet free of vitamin D, there was no adaptation.[23,25]

Although it is clear that vitamin D is an absolute requirement for the adaptive mechanism to be expressed, it has not been clear that vitamin D is responsible for directly mediating the adaptation response. A potential role for other factors has been investigated, but the results have merely served to eliminate many possibilities. It has been shown that the adaptation of dietary absorption will occur after hypophysectomy, thyroparathyroidectomy, or adrenalectomy.[56]

Synthesis of the 1,25-dihydroxy metabolite is controlled by blood calcium in parathyroid-intact animals, synthesis rising with feeding of a low-calcium diet and falling with intake of diets high in calcium. (See Chapter 51 for details.) This has led to the speculation[57] that 1,25-dihydroxycholecalciferol made by the kidney (not a hormone made by bone) could be the adaptation factor of Nicolaysen et al.[25] Wasserman and Taylor[23] have reviewed carefully much of the still confusing data in regard to specific aspects of the adaptation phenomenon, especially the proposed link between adaptation and 1,25-$(OH)_2$-D production. It has been reported to be difficult to detect a correlation between adaptation and increased synthesis of CaBP induced by a calcium-deficient diet in rats on the one hand and a decline in blood calcium on the other; the lack of correlation led to the view that the mechanism of adaptation cannot be a sequence of events involving increased parathyroid hormone secretion (since hypocalcemia was not seen), which in turn caused increased production of 1,25-$(OH)_2$-D.[58] Without direct measurements of parathyroid hormone secretion, however, it is difficult to exclude an increased secretion of PTH, since a new steady state could be envisioned in which increased PTH corrects hypocalcemia (see Chapter 52).

A more serious apparent objection to a role for 1,25-$(OH)_2$-D production as the exclusive mediator of adaptation derives from experiments with phosphate deficiency. In addition to adaptation induced by calcium-deficient diets, phosphate deficiency leads to enhanced calcium absorption.[23,59] Severe phosphate deficiency, it is generally agreed (see Chapter 51), also leads to increased 1,25-$(OH)_2$-D synthesis so that, per se, adaptation induced by phosphate deficiency need not eliminate a central role for altered D metabolism in adaptation. Wasserman and Taylor,[23] however, in a detailed test of the hypothesis that 1,25-$(OH)_2$-D serves as endogenous factor, studied animals on either calcium- or phosphate-deficient diets. The animals' only source of vitamin D was dihydrotachysterol (DHT).[23,60] The latter compound, already having a hydroxyl group in a pseudo 1-position (see Chapter 51), would not be a substrate for the renal 1-hydroxylase. As consistent with the postulated role for 1,25-$(OH)_2$-D synthesis in adaptation, calcium-deficient diets did not evoke adaptation or increased synthesis of CaBP, inasmuch as with DHT as sole vitamin D, there can be no increased 1,25-$(OH)_2$-D. A comparable group fed vitamin D_3 showed both increased efficiency of calcium absorption and CaBP synthesis. In phosphate deficiency, CaBP synthesis increased even in the presence of dihydrotachysterol as the sole source of vitamin D, and there was a definite increase in intestinal calcium absorption (although less striking than when D_3 itself was provided to the phosphate-deficient animals). This type of experiment, if confirmed and extended, may lead, as Wasserman and Taylor suggest, to detection of factors other than 1,25-$(OH)_2$-D as mediating adaptation of calcium absorption.

At present, it must be concluded that it is unclear whether the signal to adaptation originates in the skeleton, as originally proposed, or rather, as many recent observations suggest, through changes in vitamin D metabolism brought about by changes in blood phosphate or blood calcium. Likewise, it is still unsettled whether 1,25-dihydroxycholecalciferol is the mediator, and sole mediator, of the adaptation process or whether other mechanisms are involved.

A separate issue is what specific steps in the active transport or diffusion process are altered during adaptation. Earlier work[61,62] led to the conclusion that adaptation reflected an increased affinity for calcium of some carrier in the transport chain, rather than an increased quantity of the carrier. Studies using in vivo techniques in humans, however, led to a different conclusion, namely that the amount of carrier in intestinal tissue is actually increased in amount without a change in affinity for calcium. As discussed by Wasserman and Taylor,[23] the latter observation suggests by analogy with Michaelis–Menton kinetics, that the V_{max}, or absolute transport rate, is increased during adaptation to calcium deprivation and is consistent with studies in animals, indicating a considerable increase in the concentration of calcium-binding protein during the process of adaptation. There is no evidence of a change in the intrinsic binding affinity (K_m) for calcium by the calcium-binding protein.

It must be concluded that much remains to be clarified about the important process of physiological adaptation of intestinal calcium absorption in the face of calcium deprivation. Neither the precise humoral mediating mechanism responsible for adaptation nor the critical rate-limiting step affected in the transport process has yet been defined.

Other Factors Influencing Intestinal Calcium Absorption. Parathyroid hormone, calcitonin, phosphate, certain cations, cortisol, several drugs, and certain sugars and amino acids have all been shown to influence intestinal calcium absorption. With the probable exception of parathyroid hormone, however, and, to a certain extent, phosphate, most of the factors identified as influencing intestinal calcium absorption do not seem to represent physiologically important controlling influences. As discussed extensively in Chapter 52, in animals[63] and in humans,[28] parathyroid hormone markedly increases the efficiency of intestinal calcium absorption. The bulk of evidence (Chapters 51 and 52) indicates that the effect of parathyroid hormone is indirect through the stimulation of increased synthesis of 1,25-dihydroxyvitamin D. In most studies,[23,28,64] it is clear that effects of parathyroid hormone are not rapidly mediated but require 24 hours or more to be expressed, consistent with an indirect action through changes in the rate of 1,25-dihydroxyvitamin D production. There is considerable evidence that the action of parathyroid hormone on intestinal calcium absorption, even though indirect, i.e., stimulation of 1,25-(OH)$_2$-D, may be the most important factor physiologically in regulation of intestinal calcium absorption.

In addition to evidence discussed above concerning adaptation of intestinal calcium absorption induced by prolonged phosphate deficiency, it is clear that high intakes of phosphate depress intestinal calcium absorption. Since there is abundant evidence that the calcium absorptive and phosphate absorptive pathways or transport systems are separate (see discussion of phosphate absorption in this chapter), the most likely explanation of the effect of high-phosphate diets on intestinal calcium absorption is that relatively insoluble calcium-phosphate complexes are formed, thereby rendering the calcium less available for transepithelial uptake.[23]

Sodium, potassium, and strontium can all be shown to inhibit calcium absorption when present in high concentrations;[65,67] alternatively, low concentrations of sodium increase intestinal calcium transepithelial uptake in vitro. It is not clear that the effects attributable to sodium and potassium are normally operative at physiological concentrations of these two ions. The effect of strontium is seen only in experimental studies featuring high intakes of strontium. Recent work using high intakes of strontium[68,69] suggests that the cause of the severe rickets seen in association with high strontium intake is an inhibition of the formation of 1,25-dihydroxyvitamin D.

Cortisone or other glucocorticoids in high doses has been known for many years to inhibit the efficiency of calcium absorption.[23,28] The blockade of intestinal calcium absorption brought about by cortisone has led to its therapeutic use in the management of disorders associated with hypercalcemia due to excessive intake of or excessive sensitivity to vitamin D (see Chapters 54 and 57). Cortisone might (1) interfere with the metabolism of vitamin D, (2) block the action of vitamin D at the receptor level, or (3) inhibit calcium absorption at some site separate from that directly influenced by vitamin D. Recent evidence[70,71] suggests that the synthesis of calcium-binding protein may be normal during cortisone-induced blockade of intestinal calcium absorption and that the rate of formation of 1,25-dihydroxyvitamin D also remains unaltered. The overall results are interpreted to suggest that cortisone acts independently of vitamin D metabolism or the site of 1,25-(OH)$_2$-D action, at some independent site in the calcium absorptive pathway.

Lactose and other sugars such as mannose, xylose, and related compounds (but not glucose) exert an inhibitory effect on intestinal calcium absorption. Most studies have involved special experimental circumstances in which high doses of the effective sugars are given.[23] It is not clear that under normal environmental circumstances these effects are important in limiting intestinal calcium absorption. Certain amino acids such as the highly basic compounds lysine and arginine can be shown experimentally[72,73] to inhibit intestinal calcium absorption. The mechanism of the amino acid effect, like that of lactose and sugars, is not settled, but certain evidence suggests that both the sugars and the amino acids may act to chelate calcium.[23] Ethanol in high doses both in animals and in humans[74,75] can be shown to inhibit intestinal calcium absorption, but only in chronic alcoholism in humans is there evidence that the effect is quantitatively significant. Recent studies in diabetic animals[76] that calcium-binding protein is depressed in content in intestinal tissue correlates with earlier observations[77] that calcium absorption is reduced in diabetic animals.

Extensive studies both in patients and in experimental animal models have indicated that the anticonvulsant diphenylhydantoin in pharmacologic doses severely impairs intestinal calcium absorption. There remains controversy about both the frequency of the process and the mechanism (see Chapter 67). The principal relevance of the reported actions of anticonvulsant agents and the impairment of the intestinal calcium absorption with continuous high ethanol intake and in diabetes may ultimately be found in the clinical reports of osteopenia in epileptic subjects and those with long histories of chronic alcoholism or diabetes. The genesis of osteopenia in these patients may be deficient calcium absorption (see Chapter 71).

EXCRETION

There seems to be little variation in intestinal secretion of calcium; hence endogenous fecal calcium excretion does not seem to be an important route of calcium excretion that can be modified in response to an excess or deficiency of calcium. Losses of calcium in sweat are usually minor. Only with deliberately induced, heavy, sustained loss of sweat does excretion via the skin become significant, reaching values of 100–200 mg/day. The principal route of excretion is therefore renal. Excretion via the kidneys in a normal subject may be as great as 400 mg/24 hours, although it is usually lower.[3,78,79]

It is difficult to deal quantitatively with renal calcium handling for several reasons. First, the concentration of calcium in the glomerular filtrate is considerably less than that in serum because the approximately 50 percent of serum calcium that is bound to proteins is not filtered. Micropuncture studies in rats have suggested that the actual content of glomerular calcium is best approximated by the ultrafiltrable calcium.[80] The ultrafiltrable and ionized calciums of serum (which are similar but not identical to one another) are difficult to measure accurately because of the changes induced by changes in serum pH or Pco_2. Secondly, the physical state of filtered calcium in urine is itself complex. Urinary calcium is bound, in part, by anions which are present at much higher concentrations than in plasma because of high rates of renal clearance; much of the calcium is complexed to citrate and other organic ions. The reabsorption of different calcium complexes must differ.[79] Finally, even after correction for the extent of complex formation, it is evident that the concentration of calcium and phosphate in urine considerably exceeds the solubility product of the free ions.[78] Hence, it is believed, as discussed elsewhere in this chapter, that substances such as pyrophosphate or other, as yet unidentified, endogenous substances may play an important role in inhibiting precipitation of calcium salts that should otherwise occur.[81] It is not clear to what extent inhibitors of precipitation influence reabsorption.

Clearly one of the important factors controlling renal excretion of calcium is simply the total quantity of filtered calcium.[78] When calculations are made of the amount of non-protein-bound calcium filtered daily by the glomerulus, it is seen that 7–10 g/24 hours may be filtered. Since urinary calcium excretion normally ranges only between 135 and 400 mg/24 hours, it is clear that approximately 96 to 99 percent of the filtered calcium is normally resorbed. Theoretical treatments of calcium excretion lead to the conclusion that below 9.5 mg/100 ml of total serum calcium or 5.8 mg/100 ml of ultrafiltrable calcium, reabsorption exceeds 99 percent.[79] If blood calcium concentration falls to hypocalcemic levels, this efficiency of resorption can rise to essentially 100 percent; when serum protein concentration is normal, this disappearance of calcium from the urine occurs when blood calcium concentration falls below 7.5 mg/100 ml.[78,79]

A detailed and critical review of renal tubular calcium transport has recently been published by Bijvoet,[79] with emphasis on controlling influences, differences between proximal and distal nephron calcium handling, and the overall homeostatic effects of renal calcium excretion. A variety of lines of evidence suggests that approximately two-thirds of calcium reabsorption, like that of sodium, takes place in the proximal tubule.[78,79] The remaining third is presumed to be absorbed in the loop of Henle, the distal convolution, and the collecting ducts.[78,79] It appears that calcium and sodium ions share a common pathway of active transport in the proximal tubule.[79,80,82,83] Rapid infusion of saline increases the excretion of calcium as well as sodium.[78,79] Also, it has been shown that a reduction of sodium intake leads to a reduction in urinary calcium excretion; conversely, high intakes of sodium can lead to large increases in urinary calcium excretion.[78,79] Diuretics such as furosemide which lead to increased sodium excretion cause striking increases in urinary calcium excretion.[79,84]

Proximal tubular calcium reabsorption is probably concentra-

tion-dependent without a Tm, or maximal reabsorptive rate. Although there is some evidence to suggest that parathyroid hormone (PTH) may inhibit proximal tubular calcium transport,[83] most evidence suggests that parathyroid hormone does not affect proximal calcium absorption;[79,85] if there is under any circumstances an effect of PTH, it seems indirect, related to actions of the hormone on proximal sodium reabsorption.[79] Hence the principal modifying influence on proximal tubular calcium transport is the rate of sodium transport.

By contrast, the reabsorption of calcium in distal tubular sites does have a maximal rate, or Tm, and is under homeostatic control. Parathyroid hormone acts directly to increase distal tubular calcium reabsorption.[79,80,83] This action, qualitatively at least, is homeostatic in that any tendency to hypocalcemia is counteracted by an increased PTH secretion, which in turn leads to renal calcium conservation by distal nephron action. The relative quantitative homeostatic importance of this renal action of parathyroid hormone and its relation to intestinal and bone actions of the hormone have been thoroughly reviewed by Nordin and Peacock,[87] by Bijvoet,[79] and by Neer (see Chapter 52).

Bijvoet has estimated that the rate of concentration-dependent proximal tubular reabsorption is best approximated by the expression $0.5 \times$ filtered calcium,[79] and the reabsorption process in the distal nephron, by the number 2.9 mg/100 ml, representing Tm_{Ca}/GFR.

Considered overall, the implications concerning calcium excretion are several. First, as serum calcium falls below the threshold value (9.5 mg/100 ml), urinary calcium excretion falls rapidly, which, as discussed above, is homeostatic; conversely, when serum calcium rises, calcium is rapidly excreted, since the maximum capacity of distal reabsorption is overwhelmed, and the filtered calcium not reabsorbed proximally and passed to distal nephrons is largely excreted (Fig. 40-4). The mechanisms summarized in Fig. 40-4, relating calcium excretion to total serum calcium, apply only when renal function is normal, serum protein concentration is normal, and sodium reabsorption is not greatly altered (by dietary changes or drugs). Changes in the previous parameters alter glomerular or tubular delivery rates, reduce fil-

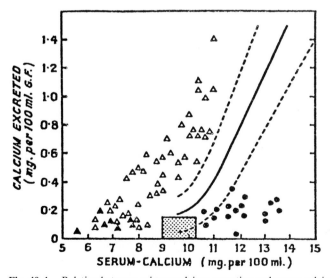

Fig. 40-4. Relation between urinary calcium excretion and serum calcium during calcium loading in normal subjects and in normal subjects and in patients with hypoparathyroidism (Δ) and hyperparathyroidism (•). The solid and broken lines show the mean values (±2 SD) obtained in normal subjects, and the shaded area represents the normal basal range. (From Nordin and Peacock, 1969, by courtesy of the authors and the publishers.)[86]

tered load, or greatly alter proximal reabsorption rates, respectively, any of which alter overall calcium excretion.

Several hormones, as well as minerals, nutrients, and drugs (especially diuretic agents) affect urinary calcium excretion. Of the hormones acting on renal tubular calcium transport, only PTH has clear physiological significance.

Parathyroid hormone directly reduces the urinary clearance of calcium. Under controlled conditions a twofold to threefold reduction in urinary calcium clearance in humans can be achieved by parathyroid hormone administration.[89] In other species such as the hamster, the effect of parathyroid hormone on urinary calcium clearance is even more striking; much of the hypocalcemia in hamsters that follows parathyroidectomy can be attributed directly to excessive urinary calcium excretion.[90]

As discussed extensively in Chapters 52, 53, and 62 and by Bijvoet,[79] the action of parathyroid hormone on distal tubular calcium reabsorption in humans is of great homeostatic importance; the excessive urinary calcium loss seen in hypoparathyroidism reflects loss of the distal renal tubular action of PTH (Fig. 40-4). Conversely, the hypercalcemia of hyperparathyroidism is largely attributable to the renal action of pathologically elevated levels of PTH (Fig. 40-4).

Growth hormone leads to hypercalciuria, apparently by a direct renal effect.[78,79] Calcitonin, at least in most species including humans, causes hypercalciuria even in hypoparathyroid subjects.[79] Chronically, as in the therapy of Paget's disease, the intrinsic action of calcitonin to lower urinary calcium reabsorption may be masked by skeletal effects, and urinary calcium excretion may even fall.[79] The physiological significance, if any, of this effect of calcitonin, as with many other actions of the hormone, has not been defined. The direct actions, if any, of vitamin D metabolites on renal calcium handling remain uncertain.

Estrogens lower urinary calcium excretion; estrogen deprivation after oophorectomy causes a rise in urine (and serum) calcium.[88] The effects, confirmed in other studies,[79] suggest that the estrogen effect is indirect; the hormone antagonizes parathyroid hormone action. Urinary calcium falls because the reduction in filtered load of calcium is a more predominant action than any interference with renal actions of PTH.[79,88] Another aspect of the hypocalciuric effect of estrogens is the well-known antagonism by estrogens of growth-hormone action, since the latter is hypercalciuric.

Administration of large quantities of cortisone or other glucocorticoids increases urinary calcium excretion as well as bringing about a wide range of other effects on calcium turnover. The effect of glucocorticoids seems not to be a direct action on the kidney but rather an increase in bone mineral release.[78,79] Furosemide and ethacrynic acid, potent natriuretic agents, by interference with sodium reabsorption, cause striking increases in urinary calcium in excess of 1000 mg/day (an effect that has recently been used therapeutically in control of hypercalcemia[79,84] (see Chapter 57). One diuretic group, the benzothiadiazines, such as chlorothiazide, unlike most natriuretic agents, does not cause increased calcium excretion. Administration of the benzothiadiazines leads to substantial reduction in urine calcium and has been used for control of stone formation in patients with idiopathic hypercalciuria.[91] There is evidence of a complex action of thiazides on calcium metabolism, including possible potentiating effects on parathyroid hormone action[79] (see Chapter 54).

Certain aspects of the diuretic-induced effects on renal calcium transport deserve emphasis. Although, as discussed later in the chapter (phosphate reabsorption), extracellular-fluid volume expansion and contraction affect mineral ion reabsorption, there is

a clear direct involvement of the calciuric action of furosemide through interference with sodium transport; whether volume is expanded or contracted, calcium excretion follows sodium excretion.[79]

Increased oral intakes of inorganic phosphate lead to a reduction in urinary calcium excretion.[89] It was believed that this action reflected the effects of phosphate in lowering blood calcium concentration by enhancing the deposition of calcium in the bone. Studies by Eisenberg,[89] however, have conclusively demonstrated that increased oral intake of phosphate has a direct effect on reduction of renal calcium clearance. Conversely, hypercalciuria is noted in severe phosphate depletion.[116] A high intake of magnesium leads to increased urinary excretion of calcium. Metabolic acidosis leads to hypercalciuria; the explanation of the mechanism is not clear,[78] but it may be an indirect effect, with an increased filtered load secondary to increased bone resorption.

METABOLIC ACTIONS AND CONSEQUENCES OF HYPERCALCEMIA AND HYPOCALCEMIA

The critical role of calcium ions in determining the excitability of nerve function and neural transmission as well as the contractibility of cardiac and skeletal muscle has been appreciated since the classic studies of Ringer in the nineteenth century.[14] However, great attention has been drawn over the last decade to a wide variety of previously unappreciated and subtle metabolic actions of calcium. Calcium in extracellular fluids and critical cellular translocations of calcium (Fig. 40-2) seem to play important roles in the structure and function of cell plasma membranes and cell organelles and in numerous cellular metabolic events. Intracellular calcium, acting with or independent of cyclic AMP, may play a critical role[14] in (1) transfer of other inorganic ions across cell membranes; (2) the release of neurotransmitters at synaptic junctions; (3) the secretion of numerous hormones such as parathyroid hormone, calcitonin, vasopressin, and various pituitary hormones; (4) the release of cellular enzymes such as amylase from the parotid, and protein secretions from leukocytes; (5) the level of activity of intracellular enzymes such as isocitric dehydrogenase, phosphorylase-b kinase, and phosphofructokinase; and (6) the action of numerous hormones on their respective target tissues, for example, vasopressin, MSH, and ACTH.[2,14,92] Extensive reviews of the general metabolic and cellular actions of calcium have been recently published.[14,516]

These findings emphasize the diverse metabolic actions of calcium. It is clear that the symptoms associated with clinical disturbances in calcium concentration (hypercalcemia or hypocalcemia), although readily recognized and described clinically, are not easily explained in terms of specific effects of calcium. Derangements in cellular metabolic activity may account for some symptoms associated with abnormal calcium levels; the relative effectiveness or failure of adaptive cellular responses that modify results of changes in cellular calcium content may help explain why it is often difficult to establish precise correlations between the presence or severity of symptoms versus the absolute degree of hypercalcemia in any given patient.

Finally, it must be emphasized that the majority of clinically recognized symptoms associated with hypercalcemia and hypocalcemia (Chapters 53 and 62) reflect either the well-established, physiologically significant actions of calcium on the central nervous system, as well as nerve and muscle function, or chronic harmful actions such as deposition of calcium and phosphate in normally noncalcified organ tissue. The multiple intracellular effects ascribed to calcium action are not presently well understood physiologically or pathophysiologically, since the concentrations present intracellularly are difficult to estimate (as discussed under calcium distribution, above), both per se and in relation to concentrations used in in vitro experiments in which actions on hormone release and enzyme activity are shown.[14] With the growing attention to the widespread intracellular actions of calcium, however, the in vivo metabolic role of calcium intracellularly may be clarified, thereby permitting an understanding of still-poorly-understood symptoms associated with calcium deficiency or excess.

PHOSPHATE

DISTRIBUTION

In contrast to calcium, phosphate is widely distributed in nonosseous tissues in both inorganic form and as a component of various structural, genomic, and functional macromolecules, including phospholipids, phosphoproteins, nucleic acids, glycogen, and other intermediates of carbohydrate metabolism.[93] These soft-tissue phosphates nevertheless comprise only about 15 percent of the total body content (Table 40-1), the remainder of which is deposited as inorganic phosphate in the mineral phase of bone, primarily as hydroxyapatite but also as more loosely complexed, amorphous forms of bone crystal.[94]

In serum (Table 40-2), phosphate exists almost exclusively as the free ion or in association with cations, and, unlike calcium, only a small fraction (12 percent) is protein-bound.[95] Serum phosphate concentrations may exhibit a daily variation of as much as 50 percent, which suggests that the evolution of the hormonal regulation of phosphate metabolism has not been driven by a need to confine within narrow limits the level of this mineral in blood. Indeed, as discussed later, carbohydrate ingestion provokes a significant decline in serum phosphate concentration as a result, not of negative phosphate balance, but of an internal redistribution of phosphate from serum into cells. Moreover, serum phosphate undergoes a diurnal variation of as much as 1.5 mg/100 ml (Fig. 40-5), with the nadir between 8 AM and 11 AM.[96-99] Although nocturnal feeding reverses this rhythm,[100] evenly spaced feedings do not

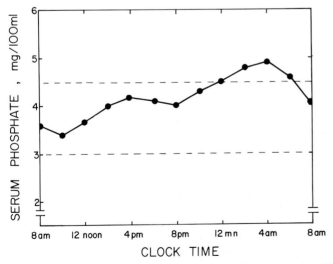

Fig. 40-5. The diurnal variation in serum phosphate concentration. The curve shows the average values at 2-hour intervals for 10 nonfasting normal humans with nocturnal sleep patterns and self-selected diets ●. The dashed lines indicate the normal limits of fasting serum phosphate concentration. (Adapted from data of Jubiz et al.)[103]

abolish it,[101] so that the timing of meals seems not to be entirely responsible for this variation. A similar circadian rhythm of PTH secretion has been described, with peak levels between 2 AM and 6 AM,[102,103] although it is not certain that such fluctuations in immunoreactive PTH directly reflect changes in bioactive hormone, given the heterogeneity of plasma PTH (Chapter 45). The possible role of PTH-induced phosphaturia in this phosphate rhythm remains intriguing and is strengthened by the finding that most of the individual variation in fasting serum phosphate concentration may be ascribed to fluctuations in the renal threshold for phosphate.[104] Others have suggested that the well-known diurnal rhythm of plasma cortisol may underlie that of phosphate, since cortisol may lower renal phosphate threshold (see below). Direct evidence for this postulate is lacking, however. The fasting serum concentration of phosphate is modified by other factors, including age and hormonal status, with higher levels during childhood and adolescence[105] and in postmenopausal females.[106,107]

ABSORPTION

The average dietary intake of phosphate, derived largely from dairy products, cereals, and meats, is 800–900 mg/day,[94] roughly twice the estimated minimum requirement of 400 mg/day.[108] Absorptive efficiency averages about 70 percent but may increase up to 90 percent if dietary phosphate falls below 2 mg/kg/day.[94]

Because of the abundance of phosphate in the normal diet and the efficient absorptive adaptation to dietary restriction, phosphate deficiency is rarely attributable to inadequate absorption. Prolonged fasting does not cause phosphate depletion, since the release of phosphate by catabolized tissues provides more than adequate compensation for obligate phosphate losses.[109,110] In contrast to fasting, experimental diets selectively deficient in phosphate (<0.1 percent) lead to a syndrome of phosphate deficiency in growing animals.[111-113] A similar study in human volunteers[114] produced significant hypophosphatemia in adult females, but not in males, after 3 weeks on a synthetic diet containing only 0.12 percent phosphate. Clinically and experimentally, inadequate dietary phosphate absorption has been observed in subjects consuming excessive quantities (300 ml/day) of nonabsorbable calcium or magnesium hydroxide antacids.[115,116] In these individuals, whose diets were already only marginally adequate in phosphate, the addition of antacids precipitated the development of symptomatic hypophosphatemia and florid osteomalacia. Finally, defective intestinal phosphate absorption has been described in patients with familial hypophosphatemic rickets, although others have not confirmed this finding.[117-119]

The mechanism of intestinal phosphate transport has not been investigated as intensely as has that of calcium. In vitro studies in rats and chicks, employing the standard everted-gut-sac technique, have shown phosphate absorption to occur via a saturable process against a lumenal-to-intracellular electrochemical gradient at lumenal phosphate concentrations below 2 mM, above which transport proceeds mainly by passive diffusion[120-123] (see Fig. 40-3)). Mucosal uptake requires adequate glucose[120] and intralumenal sodium[122] and is enhanced by higher concentrations of potassium.[120] Recent studies by Berner et al.[124] of phosphate accumulation by isolated rat intestinal brush-border vesicles demonstrated a biphasic response to alterations in intralumenal pH. At physiologic pH (7.4), phosphate uptake was strongly dependent upon available sodium and unaffected by manipulation of the transmembrane potential, which is consistent with an electroneutral cotransport of sodium and monovalent phosphate ($H_2PO_4^-$), whereas accelerated uptake at lower pH (6.0) was independent of intralumenal sodium concentration and appeared to involve transfer of a net negative charge. Sodium-dependent active cotransport of phosphate by the intestine is thus analogous to similar mechanisms described for neural and renal tubular cells.[124]

In rats and chicks, phosphate absorption is maximal in the jejunum (in contrast to the preferential duodenal absorption of calcium),[122,123,125–127] although studies of ponies and calves implicate a more distal small intestinal and/or colonic site and are also suggestive of net phosphate secretion by the proximal bowel in these species.[128,129] Similar data in humans are not available.

The precise role that vitamin D and vitamin D-stimulated calcium transport play in intestinal phosphate absorption is unclear. Harrison and Harrison[120] first reported stimulation of phosphate transport in vitro after in vivo administration of vitamin D to deficient rats, but they noted that this effect required adequate concentrations of intralumenal calcium and therefore postulated that vitamin D-stimulated phosphate absorption was linked to that of calcium. Subsequent studies in rats,[125] chicks,[123,130] hens,[126] and humans[131] confirmed the beneficial effect of vitamin D on phosphate absorption but not the requirement for calcium, with the exception of one recent study by Chen et al.[132] Using everted gut sacs from vitamin D-deficient rats, these workers demonstrated moderate enhancement of jejunal phosphate transport after in vivo vitamin D therapy when calcium was excluded from the lumenal fluid but found acceleration of duodenal as well as jejunal transport in the presence of calcium, in which case the percentage stimulation and absolute rate of transport were considerably greater in the more proximal segment. These findings contrast with the results of two studies[123,126] in chicks which demonstrated that phosphate transport in the jejunum, although exceeded by that in the duodenum in untreated rachitic birds, was selectively enhanced by vitamin D treatment in vivo.

It seems reasonable at present to postulate that vitamin D may stimulate two mechanisms for phosphate absorption—a calcium-dependent duodenal process and a calcium-independent (? sodium dependent) jejunal system. While translocation of phosphate may occur passively in response to active Ca transport in the duodenum, additional evidence provides further support for the existence of the calcium-independent mechanism. First, Harrison et al.[133] found that stimulation of phosphate transport by everted gut sacs from parathyroidectomized rats was greater after treatment in vivo with dihydrotachysterol (a conformational analog of 1,25-(OH)₂-D₃,the active form of vitamin D) than with vitamin D₂, despite the use of doses providing comparable stimulation of calcium absorption. Moreover, it has recently been shown by Ferrar et al.[134] that treatment of normal rats with actinomycin D or cyclohexamide blocked absorption of phosphate but not calcium from both intact intestines and ligated loops, whereas corticosteroids blocked both processes. They concluded that the phosphate mechanism may be dependent upon proteins that turn over more rapidly than do those responsible for calcium absorption and that, in any event, the transport systems are probably different.

Finally, although pharmacologic doses of vitamin D have been shown to increase phosphate absorption when administered in vitro, Chen et al.[132] have demonstrated that physiologic doses of vitamin D₃ or 25-hydroxyvitamin D₃ act only after a delay of many hours and, unlike 1,25-(OH)₂-D₃, are ineffective in nephrectomized animals. As in the case for calcium absorption, it therefore appears that the active principle responsible for the stimulation of phosphate transport is the dihydroxy metabolite 1,25-(OH)₂-D. This metabolite has been shown to increase both calcium and phosphate transport in deficient rats within 3 to 6 hours of administration, and similar effects have been demonstrated for the 1,25-(OH)₂-D₃-like conjugated secosteroids present in extracts of the tropical plants

Cestrum diurnum and *Solanum glaucophyllum*.[135–137]

The extent to which 1,25-(OH)₂-D₃ is responsible for the adaptive increase in phosphate absorption following dietary phosphate restriction is unclear. It is probably true that vitamin D-deficient animals are unable to perform this adaptation,[127] so that the role of the vitamin in this process is at least a permissive one. The more recent discovery that phosphate deficiency per se enhances formation of 1,25(OH)₂D₃ (Chapter 52), however, suggests that this metabolite may play a more active role in the maintenance of adequate phosphate absorption than was hitherto fully appreciated.

Surprisingly enough, the possible influence of parathyroid hormone on phosphate absorption has received little recent attention. Older studies utilizing in vivo administration of the hormone must now be reinterpreted in the light of the known physiologic role of parathyroid hormone in the stimulation of renal 1-hydroxylation of 25-hydroxyvitamin D, since previously observed effects of parathyroid hormone (or parathyroidectomy) may have been mediated by changes in levels of 1,25-(OH)₂-D₃. Borle et al.[138] found a 70 percent increase in mucosal phosphate uptake by perfused rat duodena 1 hour after the administration of PTH in vitro, but net phosphate absorption was not measured. Others[139] have observed no effects of PTH in vivo on phosphate transport.

Definition of the effects, if any, of calcitonin on phosphate absorption has been similarly elusive. Cramer et al.[140] found no effect of porcine calcitonin following in vivo treatment of young dogs, Tanzer and Navia[141] adduced indirect evidence for inhibition of absorption in rats in vivo, and Caniggia et al.[142] noted a significant increase in blood ³²P levels in human volunteers after administration of porcine calcitonin compared with self-controls. Juan et al.[143] have recently studied jejunal electrolyte transport with triple-lumen catheters during calcitonin infusion in normal volunteers. They confirmed the induction of net secretion of water and all electrolytes except calcium and phosphate. Net absorption of these ions decreased, but not significantly, and their results might be interpreted as evidence for enhanced relative absorption of both calcium and phosphate. The interpretation of these studies is particularly difficult, however, in view of the uncertainty of any physiologic role of calcitonin in humans.

Phosphate absorption increases with intralumenal pH over the range 3.3–7.9,[122,144] although more alkaline pH's are believed to interfere with absorption through the promotion of insoluble phosphate salts.[145] Ammonium chloride has also been shown to interfere with phosphate transport in the chick intestine.[146]

EXCRETION

Phosphate losses in sweat are negligible (<25 mg/day), even at estimated maximum rates of sweating.[147] Studies in fasting humans have identified an obligate daily fecal phosphate loss of 200–300 mg/day in normophosphatemic volunteers,[110] but the major site of phosphate excretion and regulation is clearly the kidney.

Although about 12 percent of serum phosphate is protein-bound (Table 40-2), considerations of the technique of serum phosphate measurement and of Donnan membrane equilibria[95,148] predict that the concentration of phosphate in the glomerular filtrate is equal to that measured in serum. Thus the filtered load at any moment is simply the product of the serum inorganic phosphate concentration (P_i) and the glomerular filtration rate (GFR). Daily urinary phosphate excretion approximates net intestinal absorption in the absence of ongoing tissue catabolism or anabolism or of excessive fecal losses,[108] and tubular reabsorption normally exceeds 85 percent of the filtered load.[149]

Renal tubular phosphate reabsorption occurs via a saturable active transport mechanism.[150,151] Although the transport sites were initially localized to the proximal tubule on the basis of micropuncture studies in animals,[150,152-154] ample evidence now supports the existence of one or more distal tubular reabsorptive sites as well.[153,155-161] Clinical studies of the hyperphosphaturic disorder, familial X-linked hypophosphatemic rickets, have provided additional evidence in humans for multiple sites or mechanisms for phosphate reabsorption.[162-165] The phenomenon of tubular secretion has been demonstrated in chickens,[166] certain fishes,[167-169] snakes,[170] and alligators;[171] although suggestive evidence exists for rats[172] and humans,[163] definite proof of such a mechanism in mammals is lacking. Tubular secretion at high filtered-phosphate loads may be partly responsible for the failure of some investigators to observe a tubular reabsorptive maximum in the rat.[173] In rats, proximal tubular reabsorption manifests an absolute requirement for intralumenal sodium ions[174] and, in rabbits, is blocked by ouabain,[175] which may be indicative of a sodium-dependent cotransport phenomenon analogous to that postulated for intestinal phosphate absorption.[124] Dennis et al.[175] have emphasized that the dissociation of net proximal tubular sodium and phosphate reabsorption under several experimental conditions[160,161] does not weaken the case for sodium-driven phosphate reabsorption, since back-diffusion of reabsorbed sodium may greatly exceed that of phosphate. Moreover, sodium may be reabsorbed independently of phosphate and under separate hormonal control. Like the intestinal mechanism, proximal tubular reabsorption is saturated at physiologic concentrations (2 mM) of intralumenal phosphate,[175] and the monovalent ion ($H_2PO_4^-$) is the predominant transported species.[176]

The overall net renal reabsorption of phosphate with respect to the filtered load is characterized in humans by a transport maximum, or threshold (Tm_{P_i}, in milligrams per minute), which, when exceeded, leads to quantitative excretion of additional filtered phosphate.[104,177,180] Were the kidney to behave in such a way that all amounts of filtered phosphate below threshold were completely reabsorbed (Fig. 40-6, broken line), a threshold concentration (($P_i)_{Th}$, in milligrams per 100 milliliters) of serum or of glomerular-filtrate phosphate could be defined, above which all filtered phosphate over that amount corresponding to the transport maximum would be excreted. Thus

$$Tm_{P_i} = (P_i)_{Th} \times GFR \qquad (1)$$
$$(P_i)_{Th} = Tm_{P_i}/GFR \qquad (2)$$

It has been shown[177-179] that the Tm_{Pi}, apart from responding to numerous ionic and hormonal influences, varies linearly with GFR, tending to increase or decrease with similar changes in GFR. The mechanism underlying this form of "glomerulotubular balance" is unclear, but it operates so as to minimize perturbations of $(P_i)_{Th}$ in the face of fluctuations in GFR (Equation 2). For this reason, the use of $(P_i)_{Th}$, and not Tm_{P_i}, permits better definition of renal phosphate handling in relation to physiologic and pathologic alterations in tubular reabsorptive capacity. Indeed, Bijvoet[104] found that changes in $(P_i)_{Th}$ accounted for nearly 80 percent of the variation in fasting serum phosphate concentration among patients and normal human subjects, the remainder of which was attributable to differences in GFR and filtered load of phosphate. The normal range of $(P_i)_{Th}$ among 100 individuals was found to be 2.5–4.2 mg/100 ml.[104,177,180]

In reality, of course, the discontinuous linear function used to define $(P_i)_{Th}$ does not pertain when measured urinary phosphate is related to the simultaneous serum concentration or filtered load. Rather (Fig. 40-6, unbroken curve), net phosphate excretion ac-

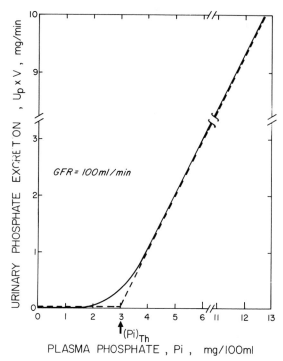

Fig. 40-6. The relationship between plasma concentration and urinary excretion of phosphate for a normal (solid line) and idealized (broken line) kidney with a glomerular filtration rate of 100 ml/min. Since total plasma and ultrafiltrable phosphate concentrations are nearly equal (see text), the filtered load at any plasma concentration, P_i, is $P_i \times GFR$, and the slope of the excretion curve in the region well above $(P_i)_{Th}$ is equal to the GFR. The Tm_{P_i}; for the idealized kidney is defined by the filtered load at which the reabsorptive mechanism becomes saturated and phosphate begins to appear in the urine, or (see text, Equation 1) by $GFR \times (P_i)_{Th}$. (Modified from Bijvoet.)[79]

tually occurs at serum levels well below $(P_i)_{Th}$ and gradually rises as serum phosphate approaches the theoretical threshold from below.[104,151] This curvilinear region of the phosphate excretion curve is termed "splay" and may reflect nephron heterogeneity with regard to GFR and/or phosphate reabsorption or simply the saturation kinetics expected of a single transport mechanism possessing a finite affinity for phosphate.[104] At any rate, because of this splay, $(P_i)_{Th}$ cannot be measured directly but, instead, must be estimated by back-extrapolation of the linear portion of the excretion curve to its imaginary intercept with the abscissa. This necessitates elevation of serum phosphate well above $(P_i)_{Th}$, which is traditionally achieved by infusion of phosphate at progressively greater rates, with simultaneous measurements of urinary phosphate excretion.[180] Thus, at serum levels above threshold, phosphate excretion becomes a linear function of serum phosphate (Fig. 40-1) with a slope equal to the GFR:

$$U_{P_i} \times V = GFR[P_i - (P_i)_{Th}] \qquad (3)$$

or

$$(P_i)_{Th} = P_i - \frac{U_{P_i} \times V}{GFR} \qquad (4)$$

If simultaneous serum and urine samples are then analyzed for phosphate and creatinine, the clearance ratio may be calculated:

$$\frac{C_{P_i}}{C_{Cr}} = \frac{U_{P_i}}{P_i} \times \frac{Cr}{U_{Cr}} \qquad (5)$$

Equation 4 then becomes

$$(P_i)_{Th} = P_i\left(1 - \frac{C_{P_i}}{C_{Cr}}\right) = P_i \times TRP \qquad (6)$$

where TRP is the tubular reabsorption of phosphate as used by Bernstein.[181]

In this way, phosphate infusion may be employed to allow indirect determination of $(P_i)_{Th}$, although the method is tedious. More important, there is evidence that phosphate infusion may itself lower $(P_i)_{Th}$, either indirectly via parathyroid stimulation or extracellular-fluid volume expansion (see below) or by a direct effect of high serum phosphate levels.[173,182,183] Unfortunately, measurement of $(P_i)_{Th}$ at basal levels of serum phosphate, conditions of more physiologic relevance, cannot usually be performed directly, since renal excretion then almost invariably occurs in the splay region of the curve. Estimation of the $(P_i)_{Th}$ from measurements of filtered, excreted, and serum phosphate would then require some knowledge of the shape and position of the excretion curve operative in the individual under study. Bijvoet has shown, however, that the wide variation in this curve observed during phosphate infusion of both normals and patients with certain disorders of renal phosphate reabsorption may be reduced, through appropriate normalization techniques, to a single curve (Fig. 40-7) relating $P_i/(P_i)_{Th}$ to C_{P_i}/C_{Cr} (or TRP).[184] Use of this curve has been extended to the determination of $(P_i)_{Th}$ from simultaneous measurements of fasting serum and urinary phosphate and creatinine in a wide variety of disorders affecting the renal phosphate threshold. Moreover, in the definition of renal phosphate handling in the splay region (TRP > 0.80), the use of $(P_i)_{Th}$ seems preferable to TRP or C_{P_i}/C_{Cr} alone (which depend upon both P_i and $(P_i)_{Th}$) or such empirically derived estimates as the "phosphate excretion index" of Nordin and Fraser,[185,186] which, as a linear approximation of a curvilinear function, tends to overestimate normal phosphate excretion at low serum phosphate concentrations (< 2.5 mg/100 ml) and to underestimate it at high levels (> 4.5 mg/100 ml). It is important to note that Bijvoet's normalized excretion curve (Fig. 40-6) was generated from data obtained in normal humans and in patients with a limited number of disorders associated with abnormal renal phosphate excretion (hyperparathyroidism and hypoparathyroidism, thyrotoxicosis).[104] Although his results suggest that these disorders lead to predictable changes in both $(P_i)_{Th}$ and the size of the splay region (which is proportional to the magnitude of $(P_i)_{Th}$), the relationships observed may not be generally applica-ble to all disorders of phosphate excretion. Thus a condition that produces a major distortion of the splay region might alter renal phosphate handling significantly in the basal state without affecting the absolute Tm_{P_i} or $(P_i)_{Th}$ as determined during phosphate infusion. Moreover, as will soon become apparent, the renal tubular mechanisms for phosphate reabsorption are in fact quite heterogeneous, both in their location within the nephron and in their responsiveness to ionic and hormonal regulatory influences. Thus, despite its operational utility, the characterization of overall renal phosphate reabsorption by a single parameter like $(P_i)_{Th}$ is at best a useful oversimplification of a complex, multifactorial renal function.

With these stipulations in mind, the observed effects of a variety of agents on phosphate excretion (Table 40-3) will be discussed in the following sections in terms of changes in $(P_i)_{Th}$ alone (with the associated changes in splay as predicted by Bijvoet's normalized curve), despite the fact that even this parameter has only rarely been measured directly.

Parathyroid Hormone

The importance of parathyroid hormone (PTH) in the determination of renal phosphate disposal was suggested by early observations that parathyroidectomy led to a dramatic decline in urinary phosphate excretion[187] and that parathyroid extract produced acute phosphaturia in normals and patients with hypoparathyroidism.[188-190] That this phosphaturic response is largely attributable to a decrease in the renal threshold $((P_i)_{Th})$ was convincingly demonstrated in studies using direct selective intrarenal arterial PTH infusion in the dog[191] and subsequently confirmed by other means in dogs,[152,153,159,161] rats,[157,171,183] and humans.[104,192,193] The phosphaturic response to PTH is accompanied by a rise in urinary cyclic AMP both in vivo and in isolated tubules in vitro,[194-198] and administration of dibutyryl cyclic adenosine nucleotides mimics the effects of PTH itself upon phosphate excretion,[152,153,199-201] which suggests that cyclic AMP may directly mediate the effects of membrane-receptor-bound PTH on the renal tubules.

The tubular site and mechanism of PTH action have been intensively studied, originally by stop-flow techniques and, more recently, by direct tubular micropuncture. Such studies have

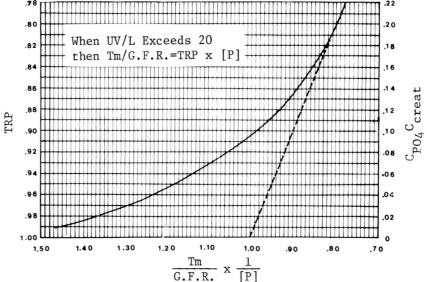

Fig. 40-7. Nomogram of Bijvoet for the estimation of renal $(P_i)_{Th}$ (Tm/GFR) from simultaneous measurements of TRP (or C_{P_i}/C_{Cr}) and P_i, generated by phosphate infusion in normal humans and patients with thyrotoxicosis, hyperparathyroidism, and hypoparathyroidism. This relationship between $(P_i)_{Th}$ and the shape of the splay region may have been influenced by the direct and indirect phosphaturic effects of phosphate infusion and, in addition, may not apply to all disorders of renal phosphate handling (see text). When TRP is below 0.80 (above splay), $(P_i)_{Th} = TRP \times P_i$. (Reproduced from Bijvoet and Morgan, with permission.)[517]

shown that, at least in rats and dogs, PTH induces a dramatic inhibition of the proximal tubular reabsorption of phosphate, as well as of sodium, calcium, and bicarbonate.[152,153,161,176] The relatively selective phosphaturia usually observed in the final urine results from preferential reabsorption of the other ions in nephron segments beyond the proximal tubule.[152]

The close correlation typically found between the proximal tubular rejection of phosphate and that of sodium following either PTH administration or parathyroidectomy has fostered the hypothesis[152] that the primary effect of PTH, perhaps via cyclic AMP, may be a reduction of proximal tubular sodium reabsorption, with only secondary inhibition of sodium-coupled phosphate reabsorption. Although, as discussed previously, proximal phosphate reabsorption in the rat is dependent upon the presence of the sodium ion,[174] several studies in the dog have demonstrated that the magnitude of the tubule-to-plasma sodium gradient is not the sole determinant of the rate of phosphate reabsorption[153,156,161] and that PTH, in addition to decreasing the sodium gradient, also reduces the ratio of phosphate to sodium in the reabsorbed fluid.[156] Thus, if the sodium gradient provides the driving force for phosphate reabsorption, PTH may inhibit the ability of the phosphate mechanism to respond to that gradient, perhaps by selectively reducing the tubular permeability to phosphate.

Since, in addition to its effect on sodium reabsorption, PTH induces a proximal tubular rejection of calcium and bicarbonate, each of which may be independently phosphaturic (see below), it has been proposed that these ions may participate in the reduction of phosphate reabsorption after PTH administration.[176,202,203] In the rat, Bank et al.[176] have shown in micropuncture studies that the bicarbonaturia induced by PTH is associated with an increase in the pH of proximal tubular fluid and a shift from monovalent to divalent acid phosphate. Since the monobasic form is preferentially reabsorbed, this alkalinization could account for some reduction of proximal phosphate reabsorption. Studies of prolonged PTH infusion in humans, however, have shown an unmitigated phosphaturia despite the disappearance of the initial, transient bicarbonaturia and the development of a systemic hyperchloremic acidosis.[204] This study thus argues against a major role of proximal tubular fluid alkalinity in the genesis of PTH-induced phosphaturia. There has been no direct study of the contribution of tubular fluid calcium to the phosphaturia of PTH infusion.

Under ordinary circumstances, the phosphaturic effect of PTH may be quantitatively ascribed to the action of the hormone on the proximal tubule.[150,153,156,205,206] Nevertheless, numerous micropuncture studies have established the existence of a more distal site of PTH-responsive phosphate reabsorption in both rats[155,157,199] and dogs,[159-161,207] which, in rats, has been localized to the loop of Henle.[157,208]

The most convincing evidence for this distal PTH-responsive reabsorptive site derives from studies of urinary phosphate excretion following saline infusion into parathyroidectomized dogs.[159-161,207] As discussed below, saline infusion causes a reduction in proximal tubular phosphate reabsorption that is partly independent of PTH effects. In all these studies, the parathyroidectomized animals displayed a blunted phosphaturia compared with intact animals, despite similarly high rates of phosphate delivery out of the late proximal tubule in the two groups. This suggests that removal of the parathyroid glands unmasks a phosphate reabsorptive mechanism in the distal tubule which is normally tonically inhibited by low levels of PTH. Similar results followed administration of acetazolamide,[161,207] a diuretic that also inhibits proximal tubular phosphate reabsorption. In both types of studies, simultaneous treatment with PTH restored the phosphaturia without significantly affecting proximal delivery of phosphate, which again points to inhibition by PTH of a distal reabsorptive site.

Calcitonin

Calcitonin is acutely phosphaturic and natriuretic in rats,[209-215] sheep,[216] and humans.[217-222] In normal humans, this phosphaturia has been related to a reduction of the measured phosphate threshold, $(P_i)_{Th}$.[223] The equivocal or absent phosphaturia seen in dogs[221,224-226] given calcitonin is of interest in light of the absence of a calcitonin-induced natriuresis in that species,[224] although the mechanism of the phosphaturia associated with calcitonin has not yet been shown in any species to result from a primary alteration in tubular sodium reabsorption. The phosphaturia may result partly from calcitonin-induced hypocalcemia and secondary stimulation of the parathyroids. In addition, a direct effect of the hormone on the renal tubule is suggested by the fact that urinary calcium is increased (not decreased) by calcitonin in humans[217,220,221,227,228] and sheep[216] and that the phosphaturic effect persists in hypoparathyroid rats,[209,214,215] sheep,[216] and human patients.[221,222,227,228] Independent evidence for a direct renal action of calcitonin has been gathered in the dog by Puschett et al.,[226] who found that pretreatment with calcitonin blocked the antiphosphaturic effect of 25-hydroxyvitamin D_3 (25-OH-D_3) in thyroparathyroidectomized animals, although calcitonin alone did not effect phosphate excretion. The mechanism of the renal effect of calcitonin remains obscure, although high-affinity receptors for the hormone have been found in renal tissue[229] and increased renal tubular cyclic AMP levels have been found in vitro after calcitonin administration.[196]

Interpretation of the physiologic significance of calcitonin-induced phosphaturia in humans or of the observed species heterogeneity in renal responsiveness is difficult, however, since the calcitonins used in these studies were obtained from a variety of species and were administered in doses that far exceed the endogenous secretory rate of the hormone.

Vitamin D

The possibility of a direct effect of vitamin D or its metabolites on renal phosphate excretion has been the subject of enormous controversy since the early work of Harrison and Harrison,[230] who showed that the marked phosphaturia of rachitic dogs was ameliorated by treatment with vitamin D. Interpretation of that study, as well as of subsequent reports in rats[231] and in humans,[232,233] however, has been complicated by the possibility that in the presence of intact parathyroid glands, the observed antiphosphaturia might merely reflect the suppression of parathyroid overactivity by the rising serum calcium induced by vitamin D therapy. Studies of vitamin D effects in parathyroidectomized animals have yielded apparently conflicting results. Chronic administration of large doses of vitamin D over several days to rats[234] or dogs[235] has usually led to increased renal phosphate excretion, although in another rat study, employing lower but still-pharmacologic doses of vitamin D, phosphate reabsorption apparently increased.[236]

Such inconsistencies may be explained in part by secondary changes in serum calcium and phosphate resulting from the vitamin D treatment, since, as described below, these ions may exert independent effects on renal phosphate handling and thereby obscure those of vitamin D. Studies in parathyroidectomized animals are also hampered by the already low phosphate excretion associated with the hypoparathyroid state, which may have contributed to the failure of early investigators to detect acute effects of vitamin D.[234,235] By enhancing phosphate excretion with intravenous saline infusion, however, Puschett et al. were able to detect a significant acute stimulation of renal phosphate reabsorption (increased $(P_i)_{Th}$) by vitamin D, 25-OH-D, and 1,25-$(OH)_2$-D, given intravenously in supraphysiologic doses to thyroparathyroidectomized dogs.[226,237,238] This effect was maximal within 1 or 2 hours and was produced most rapidly by 1,25-$(OH)_2$-D, which was also the most potent of the vitamin D metabolites in this respect. Similar results have been obtained in the rat, except that in this species, unlike in the dog, the vitamin D metabolites are only effective in the presence of low, permissive levels of PTH.[231,239,240] The vitamin D-induced phosphate reabsorption is reversed by large doses of infused PTH and blocked by pretreatment of thyroparathyroidectomized dogs with intravenous calcium, dibutyryl cyclic AMP, or calcitonin.[226]

The issue of the possible dependence of PTH upon adequate levels of vitamin D or its metabolites for the generation of phosphaturia has also been hotly debated in the literature for over 10 years. The original observation by Harrison and Harrison[241] of a blunted phosphaturia after PTH administration to intact vitamin D-deficient rats is probably best explained by the presence of already maximal parathyroid stimulation engendered by the hypocalcemia of vitamin D deficiency. However, subsequent studies have confirmed a diminished renal phosphaturic response to PTH in vitamin D-deficient rats, even in the absence of the parathyroid glands.[242-244] Although some have found this response to be normal,[245] these latter studies have been criticized for a failure to achieve sufficient vitamin D deficiency. Further support for the importance of vitamin D in the expression of the renal phosphaturic effects of PTH has appeared in the studies of parathyroidectomized dogs by Puschett et al.,[240] who found that infusion of PTH alone at a relatively high dose (2 U/hr) caused no change in urinary phosphate excretion, but addition of 25-OH-D at 25 ng/hr produced significant phosphaturia. Higher doses of PTH (5 U/hr), however, were effective even without added 25-OH-D. With regard to this blunted phosphaturic response to PTH in vitamin D deficiency, Arnaud et al.[242] reported that correction of the hypocalcemia of parathyroidectomized, vitamin D-deficient rats by calcium infusion nearly normalized the phosphaturic effect of PTH, which suggests that the synergy between vitamin D and PTH may operate through the calcemic effect of the vitamin and that the true permissive factor for the renal action of PTH on phosphate excretion is an adequate level of serum calcium. A similar dependence of PTH effects on calcium has been observed in hypoparathyroid dogs.[246] On the other hand, the synergy observed between PTH and 25-OH-D by Puschett et al.[240] occurred without a significant rise in serum calcium, so the mechanism of the apparent vitamin D permissiveness remains unsettled. In a recent study of thyroparathyroidectomized rats, Forte et al.[244] reported a significant inhibition of the cyclic AMP response to PTH in vitamin D-deficient animals, both in vivo and in vitro, although the total (NaF-stimulated) adenylate cyclase activity was normal. These workers concluded that vitamin D deficiency somehow interferes with the transmission of the PTH signal, via the membrane receptors, to the cyclase system. Others, however, have found normal renal cyclic AMP responses to PTH in vitamin D deficiency.[247]

The large body of experimental data thus provides a somewhat confusing picture with regard to the possible direct, independent effects of vitamin D metabolites on renal phosphate threshold and the potential synergy or antagonism between PTH and vitamin D metabolites with respect to phosphate reabsorption. It is particularly difficult to separate direct from indirect effects of vitamin D action. Thus, high-dose vitamin D therapy or low doses of 1,25-$(OH)_2$-D_3 clearly reverse the hyperphosphatemia and subnormal phosphate clearance of hypoparathyroidism (Chapter 62), but the relative role of direct vitamin D action versus the indirect consequence of normalizing blood calcium remains unsettled, as mentioned above. It seems possible that PTH and vitamin D metabolites are directly synergistic with respect to their effects on renal phosphate handling; thus, at low levels of PTH, the net effect on $(P_i)_{Th}$ is determined by the relative balance between the two hormones. High levels of PTH alone, on the other hand, are clearly phosphaturic even in the face of vitamin D deficiency, although the response may be diminished when compared to that in vitamin D-sufficient subjects.[242-244]

Growth Hormone

Administration of growth hormone to human subjects causes an acute fall in urinary phosphate excretion, an elevation of fasting serum phosphate, and an increase in the renal phosphate threshold, $(P_i)_{Th}$.[248-252] Since growth hormone may stimulate intestinal calcium absorption[250] and thereby suppress parathyroid hormone release and, secondarily, renal phosphate reabsorption, however, the observed rise in $(P_i)_{Th}$ may be indirect. The persistence of the growth hormone effect in thyroparathyroidectomized dogs,[253] on the other hand, argues for a direct renal action of the hormone. This effect of growth hormone probably accounts for the elevation of fasting serum phosphate commonly observed in patients with active acromegaly.[105] Although normal children have higher fasting serum phosphate concentrations and $(P_i)_{Th}$'s than adults,[254] the same is true of children with pituitary dwarfism,[105] so that it is not certain whether the relative hyperphosphatemia of childhood results from hypersecretion of growth hormone or from other factors that play upon the renal tubule at younger ages.

Estrogen

Serum phosphate rises significantly after the menopause or oophorectomy[106,107] and may be lowered again by estrogen treatment,[107,255] which suggests that estrogens may decrease $(P_i)_{Th}$. Indeed, treatment of normal humans with stilbestrol for several weeks led to a measurable decline in $(P_i)_{Th}$ in one study.[256] Since estrogens may stimulate PTH secretion,[257,258] however, it is possible that the observed fall in $(P_i)_{Th}$ was merely secondary to higher levels of PTH. A portion of the estrogen effect on $(P_i)_{Th}$ may also result from direct antagonism by estrogens of growth hormone action in the kidney, since, for example, estrogen lowers the elevated serum phosphate in acromegaly[259,260] without altering serum growth hormone levels. Growth hormone levels are probably unchanged or only slightly lower after menopause,[107,261] which would tend to lower serum phosphate were it not that the effect of the fall in estrogen levels is proportionately greater. Thus, menopause may be accompanied by a loss of tonic estrogen opposition to the growth hormone-dependent phosphate reabsorptive stimulus, which would elevate $(P_i)_{Th}$ and account for the increase in fasting serum phosphate. Estrogen replacement would then lower $(P_i)_{Th}$ again by antagonizing the renal tubular effect of growth hormone, since growth hormone levels actually rise with estrogen therapy and would otherwise tend to raise $(P_i)_{Th}$.[107] Appropriate studies of the direct effects of estrogen, if any, on tubular phosphate reabsorption are unfortunately not available at present, despite the obvious potential clinical implications of this question.

Thyroxine

Hyperthyroidism produces a marked elevation of daily urinary phosphate excretion,[262-265] which indicates an acceleration of intestinal phosphate absorption or of net tissue catabolism; such observations, however, provide no information regarding possible effects on $(P_i)_{Th}$. In fact, though, fasting serum phosphate is often elevated in hyperthyroid patients or rats,[266–268] which is suggestive of a high $(P_i)_{Th}$. This has been confirmed by direct measurements of $(P_i)_{Th}$[264,267,269] and, indirectly, by earlier reports of elevated tubular reabsorption of phosphate[270] or depressed "phosphate excretion index"[262] in hyperthyroidism,[268,271] which reverts to normal after successful treatment. This observed elevation of $(P_i)_{Th}$ contrasts with the acutely phosphaturic effect of pharmacologic doses of triiodothyronine found in one study in dogs and shown to result from an acute reduction in $(P_i)_{Th}$.[272] A possible explanation for this paradox is that the enhanced bone resorption and hypercalcemic tendency associated with hyperthyroidism[268,273] leads to slight parathyroid suppression[274] and a reversal of the tonic PTH inhibition of phosphate reabsorption,[262,268] an effect that overshadows the direct renal action of thyroxine. One study of thyroidectomized rats, however, has demonstrated the occurrence of thyroxine-stimulated phosphate reabsorption even in chronically parathyroidectomized animals,[272] so that secondary hypoparathyroidism is probably not the only explanation for the enhanced phosphate reabsorption seen in hyperthyroidism.

Cortisol

Corticosteroids have been reported to increase[275] or decrease[276–278] phosphate reabsorption in humans, and further study is needed to clearly define the direct effects, if any, of cortisol on $(P_i)_{Th}$. Cortisol has been implicated in the genesis of the circadian rhythm of phosphate excretion[103,275] and, in one study, correlated inversely with the increase in fractional phosphate excretion which occurs between 8 AM and 12 noon.

Other Hormones

Glucagon lowers $(P_i)_{Th}$ in humans and animals,[279,280] although it is not known whether this results from a direct renal effect of the hormone. Insulin typically causes transient hypophosphaturia, the probable result of acute relative hypophosphatemia and reduced filtered load of phosphate, although one recent study, employing the glucose-clamp technique, suggests that insulin also raises $(P_i)_{Th}$ directly.[281] Vasopressin,[282] norepinephrine,[283] dopamine,[284] acetylcholine,[285] prostaglandin E,[285] and angiotensin I [286] have all been shown to acutely inhibit phosphate reabsorption, but the mechanisms and possible physiologic significance, if any, of these effects in humans remains speculative.

Phosphate

The level of dietary phosphate, in addition to determining the quantity of urinary phosphate excreted, engenders appropriate alterations in $(P_i)_{Th}$, so that filtered phosphate is either conserved or rejected more readily by the kidney during periods of low or high phosphate intake, respectively. Diets rich in phosphate lead to inhibition of renal tubular phosphate reabsorption in dogs, rats, and humans.[179,287,288] High dietary phosphate also causes low urinary calcium excretion, occasional hypocalcemia, parathyroid gland hyperplasia, and histologic evidence of hyperparathyroidism.[289–294] While the low $(P_i)_{Th}$ associated with phosphate loading may therefore result primarily from concomitant mild secondary hyperparathyroidism, observations supporting its occurrence in phosphate-loaded thyroparathyroidectomized rats[259,288,295] suggest that PTH may not be the sole factor responsible for this renal adaptation. Such studies in rats must be interpreted cautiously, however, in view of the uncertainty regarding the existence of a tubular maximum for phosphate reabsorption and/or of tubular phosphate secretion in that species.[173,288] Nevertheless, the finding of Cuche et al.[246] that phosphate infusion decreases $(P_i)_{Th}$ in parathyroidectomized dogs, even in those given "physiologic" infu-

sions of parathyroid extract, provides further evidence, as do the studies of Eisenberg in hypoparathyroid humans,[89] that hyperphosphatemia lowers $(P_i)_{Th}$ independently of changes in serum PTH levels.

Phosphate restriction, with or without accompanying hypophosphatemia, engenders a dramatic elevation of $(P_i)_{Th}$ within 24 to 48 hours.[114,161,288,295–299] This accelerated phosphate reabsorption is probably not the result of the functional hypoparathyroidism associated with phosphate depletion (see below), since it also occurs in parathyroidectomized animals.[161,288,298,299] Moreover, the magnitude of the change in $(P_i)_{Th}$ is greater than that associated with variations in PTH levels,[298] and the phosphaturic effect of infused PTH is greatly diminished in phosphate-deprived animals despite normal stimulation of cyclic AMP.[299–302] This renal resistance to PTH extends to the effects of the hormone on calcium reabsorption as well, so that the renal tubule displays a generalized inability to respond normally to PTH during periods of severe dietary phosphate restriction.[299] Finally, the elevation of $(P_i)_{Th}$ during phosphate deprivation is not attributable to acid-base disturbances, extracellular volume depletion,[267] enhanced vitamin D activity,[297] or fluctuations in serum calcium[288,298] or potassium.[303] The available evidence therefore suggests that intrarenal-cell phosphate concentration or some unrecognized factor triggered by phosphate depletion operates in response to low levels of dietary phosphate to adjust $(P_i)_{Th}$ upward and thereby provide avid renal conservation of this ion.

Calcium

Studies of the effect of the calcium ion on renal phosphate handling have yielded a confusing and incomplete picture. In normal humans, calcium infusion usually leads to a fall in phosphate excretion, despite an acute rise (60 to 90 min) in serum phosphate and little change in GFR, which is indicative of a net rise in $(P_i)_{Th}$.[304–307] This decline in fractional phosphate excretion is typically delayed, its nadir often occurring after the end of the calcium infusion,[305] and, in fact, a more acute increase in phosphate excretion has occasionally been detected, particularly at higher initial rates of calcium infusion.[308,309] Since the delayed rise in $(P_i)_{Th}$ is most pronounced in subjects with stimulated levels of PTH (normals on low-calcium–high-phosphate diets, patients with osteomalacia)[309,310] and can be prevented in normals by exogenous PTH administration,[307] it is thought to result from parathyroid suppression induced by the hypercalcemia. This possibility is further supported by the finding that hypoparathyroid patients display an increase, not a decrease, in fractional phosphate excretion during calcium infusion.[203,307,309–312]

Although this last finding would appear to implicate a direct phosphaturic action of hypercalcemia, this interpretation is clouded by the substantial rise in serum phosphate that attends calcium infusion, even in hypoparathyroid patients. The etiology of this phosphatemia remains unclear, but since, as just noted, it is clearly not entirely the result of parathyroid suppression and is also not attributable to an acute change in renal clearance of phosphate,[310,313,314] it presumably represents a calcium-induced shift of phosphate from the intracellular to the extracellular pool. Since elevations of serum phosphate may directly decrease $(P_i)_{Th}$, however (see previous section), it is unclear whether the phosphaturic response of hypoparathyroid subjects results directly from the hypercalcemia or from the induced rise in serum phosphate concentration.

A variety of animal studies attempting to elucidate the effects of calcium on phosphate excretion have been reported. That of Lavender and Pullman in the dog[315] has been interpreted as evidence for a direct antiphosphaturic effect of calcium, since infusion of calcium into one renal artery of normal dogs produced a greater depression of fractional phosphate excretion in the infused than in the contralateral kidney. Two considerations obviate such an interpretation, however. First, the GFR decreased significantly, as has been observed by others in the hypercalcemic dog,[161,246] and this decrease was greater on the infused side. Since tubular phosphate reabsorption varies directly with changes in GFR (discussed previously), it is possible that a disproportionate reduction in GFR of the infused kidney partly accounted for the observed relative fall in fractional phosphate excretion. Second, although total and ultrafiltrable serum phosphate concentration both rise during calcium infusion, the fraction of total phosphate that is ultrafiltrable actually declines significantly, perhaps as a result of the formation of calcium–phosphate complexes.[161,246,316] Since total serum phosphate was used to calculate the filtered load, the formation of complexes in the calcium-infused kidney may have led to an underestimation of the fractional phosphate excretion. Indeed, more recent studies, in which ultrafiltrable phosphate concentrations were directly measured, have confirmed the phosphaturic effect of acute hypercalcemia in thyroparathyroidectomized dogs. Thus, Cuche et al.[246] observed a significant (25 percent) increase in fractional phosphate excretion after intravenous or unilateral intrarenal arterial calcium infusion in thyroparathyroidectomized dogs provided with "physiologic" levels of exogenous PTH by constant infusion. In a micropuncture study, Wen[161] noted an increase in proximal tubular phosphate reabsorption in calcium-infused normal dogs, consistent with secondary parathyroid suppression, but a decrease in distal tubular reabsorption. In parathyroidectomized animals, proximal reabsorption was unaffected by hypercalcemia, but the reduction of distal reabsorption was again observed. Unfortunately, serum ultrafiltrable phosphate increased substantially in both studies, so that the phosphaturic effect of the calcium infusion, the apparent result of inhibition of distal tubular reabsorption, was not clearly ascribable to the hypercalcemia alone.

Studies in rats would appear to favor the view that the phosphaturic effect of acute hypercalcemia is solely attributable to the secondary elevation of serum phosphate. Thus, Beck et al.[317] and Popovtzer et al.[318] could detect no change in fractional phosphate excretion or serum phosphate during induction of hypercalcemia in thyroparathyroidectomized rats. The failure of calcium infusion to elevate serum phosphate in these rats may relate to their already high basal levels (10–12 mg/100 ml), which contrast with the lower levels (5–6 mg/100 ml) in the thyroparathyroidectomized dogs mentioned above. Additional species differences have been noted, as in the effect of normalization of the serum calcium of hypocalcemic thyroparathyroidectomized animals, which leads to an increase in $(P_i)_{Th}$ in rats[319] but no change in dogs,[246] so the extent to which the conclusions of these studies can be compared is unclear.

These animal studies have also identified a number of indirect effects of calcium on phosphate excretion. Thus, it is of interest that normalization of serum calcium in parathyroidectomized dogs leads to an enhancement of the phosphaturic response to PTH,[246] whereas in rats, on the other hand, both in vivo and in vitro evidence suggest that calcium inhibits the renal adenylate cyclase and its response to PTH. Moreover, Popovtzer et al.[318] observed that calcium infusion diminished the phosphaturic effect of volume expansion in parathyroidectomized rats, although, unlike Beck et al.,[317] they were unable to detect any inhibition of the PTH effect by the hypercalcemia. This discrepancy may relate to the fact that the animals in the study of Popovtzer et al. were volume-expanded compared with those of Beck et al., since preexisting volume expansion may blunt the cyclic AMP response to PTH[320] and thereby obscure any further inhibitory effect of hypercalcemia on

the cyclase enzyme. Additional studies are clearly needed before a full understanding of the possible direct and indirect effects of calcium on renal phosphate excretion, including species differences and their relation to the responses observed in humans, is achieved.

With regard to a possible direct effect of calcium on $(P_i)_{Th}$, it should be noted that several studies in humans and dogs have documented a persistent elevation in fractional phosphate excretion by parathyroidectomized subjects during chronic (several days) calcium infusion, by which time serum phosphate has returned to normal.[203,321] Such data are strongly suggestive of a direct phosphaturic effect of hypercalcemia. Moreover, Schussler et al.[322] showed that the fractional phosphate excretion of a group of 29 chronically hypercalcemic, nonazotemic, breast-cancer patients was greatly elevated (46 percent) by comparison with normocalcemic breast-cancer and other patients or hospital controls, despite a lower GFR and serum phosphate level. While this reduction in $(P_i)_{Th}$ may have been due to ectopic PTH secretion (iPTH levels were not measured), the possibility remains that hypercalcemia, acute or chronic, may directly depress $(P_i)_{Th}$.

Hypocalcemia, on the other hand, has also been associated with a reduction in $(P_i)_{Th}$ during studies of the effects of infused chelators of calcium (EDTA, EGTA).[210,308,323] While such a response would be predictable on the basis of secondary parathyroid stimulation, similar results are obtained in thyroparathyroidectomized rats in which urinary phosphate excretion rises despite a fall in serum phosphate and no change in GFR.[210] These changes implicate a reduction in $(P_i)_{Th}$, although the possible roles of a direct effect of the chelating agent itself on the tubule, of the increased phosphate load from induced bone resorption, or of other hormonal influences on the $(P_i)_{Th}$ remain unclear.

In summary, studies in humans and animals of the effects of calcium on renal phosphate excretion have been plagued by a variety of secondary influences, including parathyroid suppression, volume expansion, independent reductions in GFR, and disproportionate elevations in total and ultrafiltrable serum phosphate concentrations, as well as by important species differences and variations among studies in diet, hydration, hormonal status, and duration of hypercalcemia. The major difficulty has been the distinction of the possible phosphaturic effect of hypercalcemia from that of the induced relative hyperphosphatemia. Incomplete evidence suggests that elevation of the serum calcium may directly lower $(P_i)_{Th}$, although this has been observed only in situations of relatively chronic hypercalcemia.

Potassium

There have been several reports of hypophosphatemia, hyperphosphaturia, and reduced TRP accompanying severe hypokalemia in humans.[324–326] In a study of hypokalemic potassium-starved rats, Beck and Davis[327] found that the phosphaturic and cyclic AMP responses to PTH were impaired, but so was the phosphaturic response to dibutyryl cyclic AMP, which suggests that the defect in phosphate reabsorption may represent a nonspecific tubular toxicity of severe hypokalemia.

Magnesium

Although experimental magnesium depletion causes phosphaturia, frank hypophosphatemia in this setting is uncommon.[328–332] A reduction in Tm_{P_i} has been reported in magnesium-depleted rats,[333] but changes in GFR were not controlled in that study, and the ultimate effect on $(P_i)_{Th}$ thus remains obscure. Severe hypomagnesemia does inhibit PTH release,[334–336] but its possible inhibition of the renal response to PTH is controversial.[334,335,337–339] Magnesium infusion transiently reduces urinary phosphate in dogs, despite an increase in serum phosphate, but this increase in $(P_i)_{Th}$ is apparently mediated by or dependent upon PTH, since it is not observed in parathyroidectomized animals.[340] Thus, although available data are meager, it seems doubtful that ordinary fluctuations in magnesium status directly affect renal phosphate handling.

Extracellular Fluid Volume

Acute expansion of the extracellular fluid volume with saline provokes a dramatic phosphaturia in normal rats,[205,341-343] dogs,[152,160,344-348] and humans.[349] This results from a reduction in $(P_i)_{Th}$ which, on the basis of micropuncture studies in rats[343] and dogs,[160,152,350] has been localized mainly to the proximal tubule. The mechanism of this phenomenon is obscure, but since saline infusion of parathyroidectomized animals induces little or no phosphaturia,[159,160,340-343,348,351] much attention has been focused upon the possible etiologic role of PTH. In this regard, several studies have established that saline infusion acutely lowers the serum concentration of total and, to a lesser extent, ionized calcium.[340,341,346,348,349,352] Moreover, degranulation of rat parathyroid cells[352] and significant elevations of serum immunoreactive PTH in dogs[348] have been documented after acute extracellular volume expansion, which suggests that PTH may be wholly or partly responsible, by virtue of its direct effect to lower renal tubular $(P_i)_{Th}$, for the phosphaturia observed during volume expansion. However, attempts to prevent the fall in serum total and ionized calcium (and hence the rise in PTH) during volume expansion by infusion of electrolyte solutions enriched in calcium have not been consistently successful. In volume-expanded rats[342] and dogs,[353] addition to the infusate of sufficient calcium to maintain a normal total serum calcium has been reported to diminish or prevent the phosphaturia observed in controls, although several other studies have found no effect of calcium infusion on volume-induced phosphaturia in dogs[346,348] or humans.[349] Moreover, since volume expansion with saline dilutes serum proteins, maintenance of a "normal" serum *total* calcium in the former studies may actually have induced an elevation of *ionized* calcium, suppression of PTH release, and a secondary elevation of $(P_i)_{Th}$ sufficient to cause the observed reduction in the magnitude of the phosphaturia. Nevertheless, it seems clear that the phosphaturic effect of volume expansion depends in some way upon PTH, since it is greatly reduced in parathyroidectomized animals (even those with relatively normal serum levels of calcium and phosphate) and is partially or completely restored in such animals by infusion of exogenous PTH.[342,348]

The role of PTH has been greatly clarified by a series of micropuncture studies in rats[343] and dogs,[152,159,160] which have demonstrated that in parathyroidectomized animals, volume expansion significantly depresses proximal tubular phosphate reabsorption, despite the fact that little or no augmentation of overall fractional phosphate excretion is seen in the final urine. This has been interpreted as evidence for a distal tubular phosphate reabsorptive site which must normally be inhibited by PTH. Further evidence for such a mechanism was provided by Knox and Lechene,[159] who found a much greater urinary phosphate excretion in intact dogs treated with PTH than in acutely parathyroidectomized dogs whose proximal phosphate reabsorption had been comparably suppressed by saline infusion.

The reason for the failure of early investigators to observe a normal rise in phosphate clearance during volume expansion of parathyroidectomized animals, therefore, may not have been a lack of direct inhibition of proximal phosphate reabsorption by volume expansion per se but rather the unmasking by parathyroidectomy of a potent reabsorptive mechanism in the distal tubule capable of accommodating almost all of the increased phosphate

delivery from the inhibited proximal segment. If this distal mechanism were maximally inhibited at normal serum levels of PTH, and if saline infusion alone were a maximally potent inhibitor of proximal phosphate reabsorption, then the rise in serum PTH known to occur during saline infusion might not further augment phosphate excretion. This would explain the failure of calcium infusion to consistently abolish the phosphaturia of volume expansion, since such animals would retain the normal levels of PTH necessary to inhibit distal tubular reabsorption and allow excretion of proximally rejected phosphate. It is not clear, however, that stimulation of PTH plays no role in the proximal rejection of phosphate, since at least one micropuncture study[343] has shown a blunted fall in proximal tubular phosphate reabsorption in thyroparathyroidectomized compared to normal rats. On the other hand, Beck and Goldberg[231] found the magnitude of the fall in proximal tubular fractional phosphate reabsorption to be the same in volume-expanded parathyroidectomized and normal dogs, although the former displayed a predictably higher initial rate of reabsorption.

That extracellular fluid volume expansion can directly reduce proximal tubular $(P_i)_{Th}$ independently of PTH was shown by Suki et al.,[351] who demonstrated a significant increase in urinary fractional phosphate excretion after release of inferior vena caval constriction in acutely volume-expanded parathyroidectomized dogs. The ability to detect phosphaturia in parathyroidectomized animals after volume expansion has varied from one study to the next but seems more typical of those employing animals parathyroidectomized several days, as opposed to hours, before study. This suggests that some downward adaptation of the distal tubular $(P_i)_{Th}$ may occur with time following parathyroidectomy.

Finally, the work of Knox et al.[354] supports the concept that the phosphaturic effect of saline infusion is related more to expansion of the interstitial fluid compartment than of the intravascular volume. These workers infused into dogs salt-poor albumin, which expands plasma volume acutely at the expense of interstitial fluid volume, and observed a phosphaturia in association with a rise in total serum calcium, a fall in ionized calcium, and an elevation of immunoreactive PTH levels. In their study, however, addition of calcium to the albumin in quantities sufficient to prevent the fall of ionized calcium (and the rise in iPTH) completely abolished the phosphaturia, as well as the reduction in proximal tubular sodium reabsorption, which contrasts with the results of most studies employing saline infusions[346,348,349] and demonstrates, in the case of albumin infusion, a strong dependence of proximal tubular reabsorption on changes in PTH alone. Moreover, administration of albumin to parathyroidectomized animals given constant infusions of exogenous PTH (to approximate normal levels of iPTH) also failed to induce phosphaturia, in contrast to earlier studies using saline[342,348] in which PTH restored the phosphaturia. This study suggests that interstitial fluid volume expansion is the responsible factor in the reduction of proximal tubular $(P_i)_{Th}$ and that plasma expansion alone with hyperoncotic albumin, which actually dehydrates the interstitial space, affects $(P_i)_{Th}$ only through secondary changes in PTH secretion.

In summary, the phosphaturia induced by volume expansion results from an apparently direct inhibition by increased extracellular (? interstitial) fluid volume of proximal tubular phosphate reabsorption which, in subjects with intact parathyroids, becomes apparent in the final urine as an increase in overall fractional phosphate excretion. The expression of this phenomenon is PTH-dependent, since in the absence of adequate serum PTH levels, tonic inhibition of a potent distal tubular phosphate reabsorptive site is lost and the increased distal phosphate load is then rapidly reabsorbed, resulting in little or no increase in urinary phosphate excretion. The extent to which the increase in PTH secretion known to accompany saline infusion contributes to the reduction in proximal tubular $(P_i)_{Th}$ remains an unsettled issue.

Hydrogen Ion

The administration of sodium bicarbonate to humans, dogs, or rats produces phosphaturia despite a fall in serum phosphate, which is indicative of a decrease in $(P_i)_{Th}$.[355,359] Since, as just discussed, extracellular fluid volume expansion decreases $(P_i)_{Th}$, it is likely that this result is at least partly attributable to the associated sodium load. It has been shown in dogs[320] and humans,[358] however, that infused sodium bicarbonate leads to a greater phosphaturia than does sodium chloride at comparable rates of natriuresis. Mercado et al.[320] have recently shown in dogs that the infusion of sodium bicarbonate is associated with a greater reduction in ionized than in total calcium and with a fivefold increase in immunoreactive PTH levels. Elimination of the PTH rise during bicarbonate administration by simultaneous calcium infusion or by the use of parathyroidectomized dogs abolished all but 10 percent of the previously observed increase in fractional phosphate excretion. This small residual phosphaturia may have resulted from the extracellular fluid volume expansion, since, as noted above, this effect is at least partly PTH-independent. Alternatively, it may have been due to a slight but significant increase in serum phosphate or a direct effect of alkalosis to decrease $(P_i)_{Th}$. These workers did show that the phosphaturia accompanying bicarbonate infusion, whether or not it is mediated by PTH, does not depend mainly upon alkalinization of the blood or urine, since infusion of hydrochloric acid with bicarbonate in quantities sufficient to normalize serum and urinary pH blunted the rise in fractional phosphate excretion by only 25 percent. Thus, sodium bicarbonate administration lowers $(P_i)_{Th}$ both directly, via extracellular fluid volume expansion, and indirectly, by parathyroid stimulation consequent to the fall in the level of ionized calcium induced by the alkalosis. Although the additional contributions of alkalosis per se and of elevated levels of tubular fluid bicarbonate ion have not been carefully defined, it is clear that these factors do not influence $(P_i)_{Th}$ in a major way.

Relatively little is known of the mechanism of the phosphaturia that accompanies metabolic acidosis.[360,361] Data recently obtained by micropuncture study in dogs[362] indicate that ammonium chloride acidosis leads to inhibition of proximal tubular phosphate reabsorption, although another study demonstrated inhibition by acidosis of the phosphaturic effect of PTH.[363] In acute respiratory acidosis, both serum and urinary phosphate levels rise.[364–368] Although this situation is complicated by the occurrence of changes in PTH secretion, extracellular fluid volume, plasma bicarbonate concentration, and serum and urinary pH, it has been recently shown in the rat that the phosphaturia in acute hypercapnia is mainly attributable to a decrease in $(P_i)_{Th}$ induced by the hypercapnia per se.[359] Whether this effect contributes to the phosphaturia that accompanies acute metabolic alkalosis, discussed above, is unclear, but the findings of Webb et al. would predict that the associated compensatory respiratory acidosis might directly lower $(P_i)_{Th}$ in this situation. Acute respiratory alkalosis may be associated with profound hypophosphatemia, but, as discussed later, this is not thought to involve a change in renal phosphate handling.

Drugs

A variety of drugs and chemicals have been found to alter renal phosphate excretion. Early renal physiologists recognized that sodium aminohippurate[369] and acetoacetate[151] induce phosphaturia, possibly through competition for the same tubular reabsorptive site. The induction of glycosuria with intravenous dextrose lowers $(P_i)_{Th}$ by as much as 20 percent,[370] probably by the

same mechanism. The neutral amino acids alanine, glycine, valine, and tryptophan, when infused at a rate of several grams per hour, directly increase fractional phosphate excretion in dogs without a consistent change in serum phosphate concentrations.[371] This reduction in $(P_i)_{Th}$ is independent of PTH, specific for the L-enantiomers, not seen with basic amino acids, and may result from direct inhibition of tubular cell phosphate uptake.[372] The extent to which this effect may participate in the clinically significant hypophosphatemia during prolonged intravenous hyperalimentation is unknown but probably minimal, particularly since the amino acid dosage rates in this situation rarely approach those shown to be effective experimentally.

The diuretic acetazolamide, a carbonic anhydrase inhibitor, produces phosphaturia and bicarbonaturia[355] in a manner qualitatively similar to that of PTH.[152,156] The effects of acetazolamide and PTH appear to be intimately related, since PTH has been shown to inhibit canine renal carbonic anhydrase in vitro,[373] and, conversely, acetazolamide stimulates renal adenylate cyclase in the rat, an effect that is enhanced in the presence of PTH in vivo but that persists in hypoparathyroid animals.[374] Nevertheless, the mechanisms of action of these two agents have been shown to differ through application of micropuncture analysis in dogs.[207] In this study, acetazolamide greatly inhibited proximal, but not distal, tubular phosphate reabsorption in thyroparathyroidectomized dogs. Administration of PTH to animals already receiving maximal phosphaturic doses of acetazolamide produced a slight but significant further reduction in proximal phosphate reabsorption and a dramatic inhibition of distal reabsorption, as expressed in the ultimate urinary fractional phosphate excretion. It is thus clear that if both PTH and acetazolamide produce phosphaturia through stimulation of adenylate cyclase or inhibition of carbonic anhydrase or both, they must affect the enzyme(s) by different mechanisms and/or at different sites along the nephron.

In contrast to acetazolamide, surprisingly little is known of the effects of other diuretics on renal phosphate excretion.[375] The conclusions of studies in humans and animals have varied regarding the possible phosphaturic effects of mercurials,[376–378] thiazides,[378–380] and the "loop" diuretics furosemide and ethacrynic acid,[378,379,381,382] although a decrease in phosphate excretion has not been reported for any of these. Eknoyan et al.[378] have emphasized that a failure to control for extracellular volume depletion and/or secondary parathyroid stimulation induced by the calciuric response to some diuretics may have partly accounted for this confusion. They studied thyroparathyroidectomized dogs whose urinary losses were continuously replaced and found that the fractional excretion of phosphate was increased by all the diuretics, most profoundly by acetazolamide and chlorothiazide. Although changes in serum phosphate concentration were not discussed, these findings suggest that most diuretics cause an acute depression of $(P_i)_{Th}$ independent of PTH, GFR, or extracellular fluid volume. The relative phosphaturic potency of chlorothiazide over furosemide and ethacrynic acid may relate to its greater carbonic anhydrase inhibitory activity, as measured in vitro.[381]

Osmotic diuresis with mannitol or urea has long been held not to produce phosphaturia in mammals.[383–385] Maesaka et al.,[386] however, recently reexamined this issue in intact and thyroparathyroidectomized rats and demonstrated a clear-cut inhibition of phosphate reabsorption during hypertonic mannitol diuresis. This effect appeared to result indirectly from secondary parathyroid stimulation, however, since the mannitol infusion significantly lowered serum ionized-calcium levels and the phosphaturia could be prevented by maintenance of a normal serum calcium or by parathyroidectomy, in which case it was restored by the simultaneous infusion of parathyroid extract. The failure of earlier studies to identify these effects may have resulted from the use of inadequate amounts of mannitol[385] or from interference by mannitol in the chemical determination of phosphate.[384,387]

In summary, almost all the commonly used diuretics produce phosphaturia acutely, although a sustained alteration in $(P_i)_{Th}$ during chronic diuretic therapy is rare, probably because of normal compensatory hormonal adjustments.

The uricosuric agent probenecid lowers the serum phosphate concentration transiently over several days in patients with hypoparathyroidism,[305,388] idiopathic hypercalciuria,[389] and in some unusual disorders with abnormally accelerated renal tubular phosphate reabsorption.[305,390] Since urinary phosphate is either slightly elevated or unchanged by probenecid administration, the drug appears to lower $(P_i)_{Th}$, although this effect has not been observed in normal humans, in whom it may be obscured by a compensatory reduction in parathyroid activity.

Serum phosphate often rises dramatically during prolonged therapy of humans or animals with disodium ethane-1-hydroxy-1,1 diphosphonate (EHDP) as a result of an upward alteration in $(P_i)_{Th}$ which is dose- and time-dependent.[391–394] This drug does not inhibit the phosphaturic response to infused PTH in normal humans[391] but may, in addition to its effects on $(P_i)_{Th}$, limit the intracellular translocation of infused phosphate.[394]

Prolonged therapy with heparin leads to mild hyperphosphatemia attributable to an elevation of $(P_i)_{Th}$.[395] Digitalis glycosides have been shown to reduce $(P_i)_{Th}$ in dogs following direct renal arterial infusion.[396] Finally, it is of interest that dogs given large doses of lithium, which has been postulated to cause a generalized inhibition of adenylate cyclase activity,[397] display a blunted phosphaturic response to PTH, as well as to cyclic AMP, acetazolamide, and bicarbonate, although basal phosphate handling is normal.[398] Since the PTH response is normal in humans given usual therapeutic doses of lithium,[399] however, the clinical importance of this effect remains unresolved.

METABOLIC EFFECTS OF PHOSPHATE

Because of the wide distribution of phosphate in organic form, as a component of structural and functional macromolecules as well as of smaller metabolic intermediates, a complete discussion of the role of phosphate in cellular metabolism and physiology is beyond the scope of this chapter. In contrast to calcium, inorganic phosphate does not participate critically in membrane electrophysiology or other processes necessitating strict control of extracellular fluid ion concentration, and this is reflected in the rather substantial daily variation in serum phosphate levels, as discussed previously. The inorganic phosphate pool does represent a reservoir of substrate for intracellular phosphorylases and kinases, however, and, as such, may become critical to the maintenance of cellular energy metabolism in states of phosphate depletion and/or hypophosphatemia. Thus the normal physiologic role of inorganic phosphate has largely been deduced indirectly by study of the dysfunction that attends clinically significant depletion or excess of this mineral ion. In the following sections, we will examine the pathophysiology of common clinical disorders of phosphate metabolism from the standpoint of the mechanisms responsible for alterations in the level of serum phosphate and the resulting dysfunction of vital organ systems.

Hyperphosphatemia

Hyperphosphatemia is a characteristic feature of hypoparathyroidism, whether idiopathic, postsurgical, or pseudohypoparathyroidism (see Chapters 62 and 63), and results from an elevation of $(P_i)_{Th}$ as a result of the absence of tonic PTH effects on the renal tubule. As previously discussed, elevation of $(P_i)_{Th}$ is also at least

partly responsible for the mild hyperphosphatemia of acromegaly, as well as that occasionally associated with Paget's disease,[400] prolonged heparin or diphosphonate therapy, hyperthyroidism, and vitamin D intoxication, although the underlying mechanisms in these latter conditions are poorly understood.

A familial disorder has been described that is characterized by episodes of hyperphosphatemia, polyuria, and seizures,[401] although the cause of the hyperphosphatemia has not been determined.

In acute or chronic renal failure, alterations in $(P_i)_{Th}$ play only a minor role in the genesis of hyperphosphatemia.[402,403] Thus, in the setting of a greatly reduced GFR, serum phosphate becomes primarily dependent upon the magnitude of the net delivery of phosphate to the kidney from dietary and endogenous sources, since glomerular filtration, and not tubular rejection, is then the limiting factor in urinary phosphate excretion. Under such circumstances, a small increment in phosphate delivery may so overwhelm the renal excretory capacity that a substantial elevation of plasma phosphate must occur to provide, in the new steady state, a filtered load high enough to allow excretion of the daily phosphate throughput:

$$\text{Phosphate turnover} = U_{P_i} \times V = \text{GFR} \times P_i - Tm_{P_i}$$

When GFR is severely impaired, therefore, the problem faced by the kidney is no longer one of reclaiming 80 percent or more of a large quantity of filtered phosphate but is rather the opposite one of filtering enough phosphate to accommodate the requisite excretion of the daily phosphate turnover. Although compensatory reductions in Tm_{P_i} may occur to allow excretion of the established phosphate throughput at a slightly lower filtered load (or P_i), major reductions in serum phosphate are ordinarily achieved only by reduction of the phosphate turnover, whether by dietary restriction, therapy with phosphate-binding antacids, or both.

The pathologic situation in renal failure, therefore, represents an exception to the usual rule that fasting serum phosphate concentrations are established not by the magnitude of the phosphate throughput but mainly by the level of the renal threshold, $(P_i)_{Th}$. Thus the hyperphosphatemia seen in multiple myeloma, vitamin D intoxication, and the milk–alkali syndrome probably results from enhanced phosphate throughput in the face of a simultaneous reduction in renal function. The interplay between phosphate turnover, renal function, and hormonal adjustments in $(P_i)_{Th}$ is best illustrated by the situation of advancing chronic renal failure with secondary hyperparathyroidism, which is discussed more fully in Chapter 59. In this condition, excessive PTH secretion should blunt the rise in serum phosphate by lowering $(P_i)_{Th}$, except that the enhanced phosphate load from PTH-stimulated osteolysis may ultimately become the dominant influence over serum phosphate levels. This agrees with clinical observations that serum phosphate may actually fall after parathyroidectomy in renal failure.[404]

A second departure from the usual preponderance of intrarenal effects on the determination of serum phosphate occurs during phosphate infusion, with excessive laxative use in infants,[405,406] or in situations of massive tissue destruction, such as severe hypothermia, acute myelogenous leukemia, fulminant hepatitis, osteolytic tumor metastases in bone, or chemotherapy of hematologic malignancies, where an acutely exaggerated phosphate load may overwhelm the filtration capacity of even normal kidneys.[407–410] The potential magnitude of this problem was dramatically illustrated by a recent report of 2 patients with Burkitt's lymphoma and normal renal function who developed serum phosphate concentrations of 16 and 28 mg/100 ml with serum calcium levels of 2.6 and 4.5 mg/100 ml, respectively, during initial treatment with cyclophosphamide.[410]

The major clinical consequences of severe hyperphosphatemia relate to the associated propensity for soft-tissue deposition of calcium-phosphate salts and to the sequelae of hypocalcemia,[411] although the potential consequences of interference with the renal 1-hydroxylation of 25-OH-D in chronic hyperphosphatemic states has not been carefully examined.

Hypophosphatemia

Chronic. As previously discussed, inadequate phosphate intake is a very rare cause of clinically significant hypophosphatemia. It is worth reemphasizing that starvation causes phosphate depletion but not hypophosphatemia, since the resultant tissue catabolism provides more than enough free phosphate to maintain a normal serum concentration. Hypophosphatemia may result from diets selectively deficient in phosphate, particularly in growing subjects, but such severe phosphate restriction can be achieved only with experimental diets or, clinically, in patients on marginally adequate phosphate intakes who simultaneously consume excessive quantities of nonabsorbable antacids. Antacid-induced hypophosphatemia may be particularly troublesome among uremic patients on dialysis[412] who may already have an underlying defect in intestinal phosphate absorption,[413] possibly related to 1,25-$(OH)_2$-D_3 deficiency,[120,131-133] in addition to the phosphate drain imposed by hemodialysis (see below). As discussed below, in the absence of selective dietary phosphate deficiency (i.e., antacid abuse), the major manifestation of total body phosphate deficiency caused by malnutrition or starvation is not hypophosphatemia per se but a predisposition to the development of iatrogenic hypophosphatemia.

In the usual situation of adequate dietary phosphate input, the fasting serum level is set largely by the renal phosphate threshold, $(P_i)_{Th}$, so that chronic hypophosphatemia may nearly always be traced to an ongoing excess of factors negatively affecting $(P_i)_{Th}$. The hypophosphatemia of hyperparathyroidism (Chapter 53) is thus explicable by the known action of PTH to lower $(P_i)_{Th}$ and, perhaps, by a directionally similar effect of hypercalcemia. Vitamin D deficiency, of whatever cause (Chapters 66 and 67), leads to hypophosphatemia via hypocalcemia and secondary hyperparathyroidism,[414] although, as discussed earlier, the possibility exists that declining levels of active vitamin D metabolites may directly reduce $(P_i)_{Th}$.[226,238-240] Hypokalemia, metabolic alkalosis, and chronic intravascular volume expansion, as in primary hyperaldosteronism, may all cause mild hypophosphatemia, probably by a direct effect of these disturbances to lower $(P_i)_{Th}$.[324-326]

A primary renal defect has been postulated as the cause of the low $(P_i)_{Th}$ and hypophosphatemia variably expressed in a heterogeneous group of disorders classified as "phosphate diabetes" and/or "renal rickets." These include sex-linked and sporadic hypophosphatemia, the childhood and adult Fanconi syndromes, and a variety of heritable and acquired renal "tubulopathies" characterized by defects in the secretion of hydrogen ion and/or in the reabsorption of sodium, potassium, phosphate, glucose, and amino acids, either alone or in combination (Chapters 66 and 67). While the reduction in $(P_i)_{Th}$ seems likely to be a primary renal abnormality in some of these (i.e., Fanconi syndromes), this is less clearly so for others, particularly the sex-linked variety (Chapter 66). although recent evidence does suggest an abnormality of renal tubular sensitivity to PTH in that condition.[164]

The recently recognized association of hypophosphatemia with Reye's syndrome[415,416] may represent yet another form of acquired renal phosphate wasting, since proximal tubular dysfunction is thought to occur in this syndrome.[417] The $(P_i)_{Th}$ has not been

directly measured in these cases, however, so that the pathogenesis of the hypophosphatemia remains speculative, especially as other factors known to affect serum phosphate acutely (respiratory alkalosis, intravenous glucose—see below) may be operative in these very ill patients. An unusual syndrome of hypophosphatemia in association with benign tumors, especially of bone (sclerosing hemangioma, giant cell tumor, nonossifying fibroma), has been described[418-420] and is characterized by a low $(P_i)_{Th}$ and restoration of normophosphatemia following extirpation of the tumor. Radiologically, such tumors may resemble brown tumors of hyperparathyroidism, causing diagnostic confusion. A humoral factor has been postulated[418] but not proven. Finally, chronic hemodialysis with phosphate-free dialysate may lead to profound hypophosphatemia and phosphate depletion and has been implicated as a cause of osteomalacia in uremia.[421-423]

Acute. Most instances of severe hypophosphatemia result not from a reduction in $(P_i)_{Th}$ but from an acute redistribution of phosphate from the extracellular to the intracellular space. This intracellular shift underlies the frequently profound hypophosphatemia that may accompany acute respiratory alkalosis, treatment of diabetic ketoacidosis, hyperalimentation, glucose administration to alcoholics, or treatment of hypomagnesemia with coexistent hypocalcemia.

The hypophosphatemic effect of acute respiratory alkalosis was first identified by Haldane in 1924.[364] Subsequent studies have demonstrated that serum phosphate may fall 2–3 mg/100 ml during hyperventilation to a P_{CO_2} of about 15 mm Hg in association with a simultaneous disappearance of phosphate from the urine.[356,424,425] Induction of metabolic alkalosis with intravenous sodium bicarbonate also effects a significant, though less dramatic, hypophosphatemia. In this case, urinary phosphate excretion does increase slightly but not enough to account for the mass of phosphate lost from the extracellular fluid.[356] In both forms of acute alkalosis, then, the drop in serum phosphate probably results mostly from the rapid intracellular migration of phosphate salts in exchange for organic acids destined to buffer the extracellular alkalosis,[356] although accelerated synthesis of intracellular organophosphate compounds may also contribute, especially as this is known to occur during acute alkalosis.[364,426] The reason for the more rapid disappearance of serum phosphate in respiratory as opposed to metabolic alkalosis is not known, particularly since urinary phosphate actually increases in the latter. The fact that a respiratory alkalosis is more rapidly transmitted intracellularly may be important, as may competition for intracellular translocation between phosphate and elevated levels of extracellular bicarbonate during metabolic alkalosis.[356] At any rate, this effect of respiratory alkalosis is felt to be responsible for the hypophosphatemia observed occasionally in salicylate intoxication and frequently in gram-negative sepsis.[427]

Hypophosphatemia is a frequent concomitant of large carbohydrate loads, provided that insulin is present. The relationship of transient hypophosphatemia to meals was actually first described by Fiske in 1921,[428] and subsequent investigators have demonstrated that the magnitude of the phosphate drop after acute oral or intravenous glucose loads is roughly proportional to the amount of glucose given (Table 40-4A). A meal containing 100–200 g of carbohydrate may, therefore, lead to a 1.0–1.5 mg/100 ml fall in serum phosphate which is maximal at 2 to 2½ hours after eating. This decrement in serum phosphate appears to be blunted in diabetics,[429,433,434] and, since insulin treatment of diabetic ketoacidosis has long been known to result frequently in dramatic hypophosphatemia,[435-438] the likelihood is that insulin lack and not

Table 40-3. Summary of Factors Known to Influence Phosphate Metabolism

Intestinal Absorption	
Stimulatory	Inhibitory
Dietary phosphate restriction	Nonabsorbable antacids
1,25-Dihydroxyvitamin D	Glucocorticoids
Calcitonin	

Renal Tubular Reabsorption	
Stimulatory	Inhibitory
Intrarenal	
Intratubular sodium ions	Cyclic AMP
	Extracellular-fluid volume expansion*
	Glycosuria, Amino acid infusion
Dietary and Ionic	
Phosphate restriction*	Phosphate loading,* Acute hyperphosphatemia
Acute hypercalcemia (normals)*	Acute or chronic hypercalcemia
	(hypoparathyroidism)*
Acute hypermagnesemia*	Acute hypocalcemia
	Hypokalemia, Hypomagnesemia*
	Bicarbonate infusion*
	Ammonium chloride acidosis,* Acute
	hypercapnia*
Hormonal	
Growth hormone	Parathyroid hormone
Vitamin D metabolites*	Calcitonin
Insulin*	Estrogens*
Hyperthyroidism*	Triiodothyronine
? Glucocorticoids	Others (Glucagon,* Vasopressin,*
	Angiotensin I,* Norepinephrine,*
	Dopamine,* Acetylcholine,*
	Prostaglandins E)
Pharmacologic	
Diphosphonates (humans)*	Acetazolamide, Mannitol,* other diuretics*
Prolonged heparin therapy*	Probenecid*
	Digitalis glycosides
	Acetoacetate, Aminohippurate

*Effect likely to be wholly or partly indirect.

tissue resistance to phosphate uptake is the responsible factor. Studies in pancreatectomized animals have, in fact, shown the hypophosphatemic response to glucose to be an insulin-dependent phenomenon,[439,440] and this concept is supported by the observation that a dramatic hypophosphatemia attends the administration to diabetics of fructose, the cellular uptake of which is not insulin-dependent.[441,442] Insulin promotes hepatic glucose uptake by stimulation of glucokinase activity and, in both liver and muscle, enhances phosphofructokinase.[443] Both enzymes utilize inorganic phosphate, although hepatic uptake of glucose disposes of the bulk of an administered load. Even so, much evidence obtained in animals and humans suggests that the fall in serum phosphate following glucose is largely attributable to the uptake and organification of phosphate in peripheral tissues (muscle, bone) as opposed to the liver.[429,440,443-448]

This insulin- and glucose-stimulated cellular phosphate uptake presumably underlies the rapid development of hypophosphatemia observed in a significant fraction of all patients treated with insulin for diabetic ketoacidosis.[435-438] This complication is probably often intensified by preexisting phosphate depletion, the result of intense tissue catabolism,[449-451] osmotic electrolyte diuresis, and an independent effect of acidosis per se. The role of acidosis in the genesis of phosphate depletion resides in its stimulation of the catabolism of intracellular organophosphates,[426,452,453] its potential for direct reduction of $(P_i)_{Th}$ (discussed previously), and in ketoacidosis, the probable competition between phosphate and acetoacetate for a common tubular reabsorptive site,[151,454] which further lowers the apparent $(P_i)_{Th}$. The magnitude of the phosphate deficit in diabetic ketoacidosis is on the order of several grams,[436,449,450] and at least part of the hypophosphatemia observed during treatment probably reflects reconstruction of previously catabolized soft tissue and bone. Severe hypophosphatemia during the treatment of diabetic ketoacidosis may actually inhibit the utilization of glucose, since hypophosphatemic dogs display impaired glucose disposal despite enhanced insulin reserve,[455] and, in diabetic ketoacidosis, phosphate supplementation may accelerate the return to normoglycemia.[436]

For a variety of reasons, the development of hypophosphatemia is particularly common among hospitalized alcoholics during the first several days following admission.[456] First, although hypophosphatemia upon admission is uncommon,[456] alcoholics, like poorly controlled diabetics, may have preexisting phosphate depletion to the extent that they are malnourished, abuse antacids, or display malabsorption,[457] vitamin D deficiency, hypomagnesemia (see below), or hypokalemia. Second, cirrhotics exhibit an element of glucose intolerance,[443] which permits a greater fraction of administered glucose to bypass the liver, reach the peripheral tissues, and thereby produce an exaggerated hypophosphatemia.[429,443] Third, malnutrition or fasting causes an exaggerated fall in phosphate after glucose because of additional abnormal shunting of glucose from the liver to peripheral tissues, which further stimulates phosphate uptake.[448,458] This phenomenon results from reduced activity of hepatic glucokinase during periods of low carbohydrate intake and is also observed in fasting normal subjects.[443,458]

Fourth, alcoholics commonly develop respiratory alkalosis, a potent hypophosphatemic stimulus, in conjunction with infection or the alcohol withdrawal syndrome. Finally, alcoholics are frequently magnesium deficient,[459-461] and, as discussed below, correction of hypomagnesemia may lead to acute hypophosphatemia in the presence of coexisting hypocalcemia. Given the imposition of these hypophosphatemic stresses upon an alcoholic who may already be marginally phosphate deficient, it is perhaps not surprising that a serum phosphate level of 1–2 mg/100 ml is frequently observed by the third or fourth hospital day in alcoholics given intravenous glucose.[456]

The increasingly frequent use of total parenteral nutrition has led to the recognition of severe hypophosphatemia as a common complication of this therapy. A series of studies in animals and patients has shown (Table 40-4B) that continuous infusion of glucose at the usual rates of 10–30 g/hr, with or without accompanying amino acids or protein, predictably leads to profound hypophosphatemia after 4 or 5 days in the absence of adequate phosphate supplements. The hypophosphatemic stress of glucose infusion is frequently compounded in these patients by severe malnutrition or starvation, which leads to phosphate deficiency and, as shown experimentally in rats, to a greatly aggravated hypophosphatemia during the early phase of hyperalimentation.[462] Moreover, this hypophosphatemia and underlying phosphate depletion impair the utilization of administered nutrients in the formation of new tissue.[455,463] The amount of phosphate supplementation necessary to avert progressive hypophosphatemia during hyperalimentation has been empirically determined by Sheldon and Grzyb[464] to be 700 mg of elemental phosphorus per 1000 kcal of carbohydrate.

Experimental magnesium deficiency causes phosphaturia and phosphate depletion in animals and humans,[328-332] but hypophosphatemia is quite rare. Because of the inhibition of PTH secretion

Table 40-4. The Hypophosphatemic Effect of Glucose Loads

A. Acute Administration

Dose*	Route	Decrement in Pi (mg/100 ml)	Time to Nadir in Pi (min)	Ref. No.
60 g	oral	0.2	45	431
100 g	oral	0.5	120	428
200 g	oral	1.6	150	430
40 g	iv push	0.2	90	444
35 g	iv over 30 mins	0.9	90–120	434
35 g	iv over 30 mins	1.1	90–120	429
70 g	iv over 60 mins	1.1	60	433
50–80 g/hr	iv over sev. hrs	1.6	150	446
140 g/hr	iv over sev. hrs	2.6	120	440†

B. Prolonged Intravenous Infusion or Hyperalimentation

Dose (g/hr)*	Decrement in Pi (mg/100 ml)	Time to Nadir in Pi (days)	Ref. No.
6	1.8	2	432
10 + N**	1.5	4	464
18 + N	1.8	5	463
20	3.0	4	446
28 + N	3.0	4	468
100 + N	3.0	4	470†

*Normalized for a 70-kg man.
**"+ N" signifies concomitant administration of protein during hyperalimentation.
†Study performed in dogs.

engendered by severe hypomagnesemia[336] (see also Chapters 57 and 62), hypocalcemia frequently coexists. In this setting, rapid correction of hypomagnesemia unleashes a surge of PTH in response to the prevalent hypocalcemia,[336] and phosphaturia occurs, which, in concert with the preexisting phosphate depletion, may result in dramatic hypophosphatemia.[331,365] The phosphaturia is probably the major factor responsible for the fall in phosphate, although rapid phosphate uptake into soft tissues or bone has not been excluded in this situation.

METABOLIC EFFECTS OF HYPOPHOSPHATEMIA

Phosphate is fundamentally involved in a variety of cellular metabolic activities, including gene replication, enzyme regulation, carbohydrate and purine metabolism, and membrane integrity, in addition to its critical role in skeletal mineralization and resorption, vitamin D metabolism, and renal acid and electrolyte excretion. A recent rekindling of interest in this area has been sparked by a wider appreciation of the protean manifestations of severe phosphate deficiency, the following discussion of which will serve to illustrate the importance of this ion in the broad context of normal mammalian physiology.

Hematologic

The effects of hypophosphatemia on the erythrocyte may be considered in terms of two key phosphorylated compounds, adenosine triphosphate (ATP) and 2,3-diphosphoglycerate (2,3-DPG), both of which are products of glycolysis (Fig. 40-8A). In 1966, Rose and Warms[466] showed that the erythrocyte glycolytic rate varies directly with the concentration of phosphate in the medium in vitro, and, not surprisingly, several studies in dogs and humans have identified a linear correlation of red-cell ATP and 2,3-DPG levels with serum phosphate concentration.[452,467-470] The erythrocyte membrane is not freely permeable to inorganic phosphate,[426] and red-cell phosphate uptake probably proceeds via its incorporation into 1,3-DPG by membrane-bound glyceraldehyde-3-phosphate dehydrogenase, with subsequent rapid equilibration with ATP and 2,3-DPG.[471] Hypophosphatemia should therefore cause a glycolytic blockade at the level of the dehydrogenase, low levels of ATP and 2,3-DPG, and elevations of precursor triose phosphates. This has been confirmed by direct measurement and shown to become significant at serum phosphates below 1.0 mg/100 ml[468] (Fig. 40-8B).

Deficiencies of red-cell ATP and 2,3-DPG are expressed clinically by an increased erythrocyte fragility and a leftward shift of the oxyhemoglobin dissociation curve. Hemolysis, with membrane rigidity and microspherocytosis, has been described at serum phosphate concentrations of 0.5 mg/100 ml or less and simultaneous red-cell ATP contents at or below 50 percent of normal,[469,472,473] which agrees with in vitro studies of the deleterious effect of reductions in red-cell ATP levels on membrane deformability.[474,475] Erythrocytes from patients with hypophosphatemic hemolysis have been found to have an unusually high membrane lipid content,[473] and their abnormal fragility has been corrected by incubation in vitro with adenosine.[472] With regard to oxyhemoglobin dissociation, both ATP and 2,3-DPG lower the affinity of hemoglobin for oxygen,[476] so that hypophosphatemia would be expected to enhance this attraction. Indeed, direct measurements of blood samples with serum phosphate concentrations below 1.0 mg/100 ml have confirmed a significant reduction in the P_{50} (P_{O_2} causing 50 percent saturation) of hemoglobin to levels known to provoke a doubling of cardiac output.[468,473,477,480] Although impaired hepatic oxygen extraction has been described in hypophos-

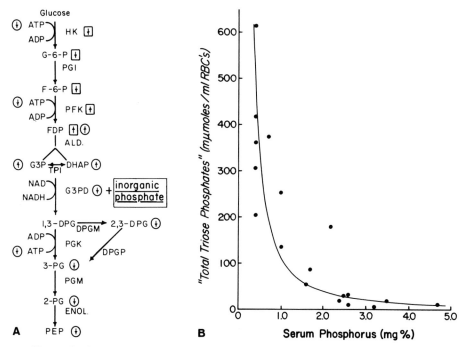

Fig. 40-8. The importance of inorganic phosphate in intracellular carbohydrate and energy metabolism. (A) Inorganic phosphate enters the glycolytic pathway as a substrate for glyceraldehyde-3-phosphate dehydrogenase. This phosphorylation yields the precursor (1,3-DPG) for the key high-energy compounds ATP and 2,3-DPG (see text). The arrows within circles (○) indicate changes postulated to result directly from hypophosphatemia, whereas those in squares (□) depict alterations secondary to lowered ATP concentrations. Abbreviations are as defined in the original publication. (B) Severe hypophosphatemia induced by hyperalimentation in humans blocks the formation of erythrocyte 1,3-DPG, ATP, and 2,3-DPG (data not shown) and leads to an accumulation of precursor triose phosphates. As shown, this blockade becomes significant at serum phosphate levels below 1.0 mg/100 ml. (Reprinted from Travis et al.,[468] with permission.)

phatemic alcoholics,[177] the relative importance of tissue hypoxia from altered oxyhemoglobin dissociation as opposed to glycolytic arrest due to deficiency of phosphorylated intermediates remains unclear.[473]

Dysfunction of leukocytes and platelets in hypophosphatemia has been investigated mainly in animals, although, in one patient with a serum phosphate level of 0.5 mg/100 ml during hyperalimentation, impaired in vitro leukocyte chemotaxis was found and shown to be reversible by preincubation with adenosine.[479] Similar levels of serum phosphate were associated with a significantly increased rate of major infection among hyperalimented dogs, compared with phosphate-supplemented controls, as well as with marked reductions in leukocyte ATP content, and significant impairment of in vitro chemotaxis, phagocytosis and bacterial killing.[479] Garner et al., studying experimental salmonella sepsis in guinea pigs, found that phosphate supplements significantly improved mortality,[480] which is particularly intriguing in view of the association of gram-negative sepsis, respiratory alkalosis, and hypophosphatemia mentioned earlier. Finally, another study of hyperalimented dogs demonstrated a 50 percent lowering of platelet ATP levels, an 80 percent reduction in platelet count and survival, significantly impaired clot retraction, and visible gastrointestinal and cutaneous hemorrhages at a serum phosphate concentration of 0.2 mg/100 ml.[470]

In summary, erythrocytes, leukocytes, and platelets all display serious functional abnormalities at serum phosphate levels below 1.0 mg/100 ml, levels that may be associated with an increased risk of hemolysis, tissue hypoxia, infection, and hemorrhage. The available evidence supports the view that severe hypophosphatemia, when found, should be treated aggressively, especially in the usual setting of coexistent major illness.

Skeletal

In addition to weakness, bone pain was a prominent complaint of the phosphate-depleted patients reported by Lotz et al.,[116] and skeletal involvement in hypophosphatemia is further emphasized by reports of classic osteomalacia, including waddling gait, bone tenderness and pseudofractures, accompanying hypophosphatemic rickets (Chapter 66), and antacid abuse.[115,481,482] Early studies of growing animals documented the occurrence of rickets and measurable bone loss after severe dietary phosphate deprivation.[112,113,483] In these animals, phosphate levels in bone and blood were lower than in other tissues, which, together with the observed hypercalcemia and hypercalciuria, suggested that bone was preferentially catabolized to provide phosphate needed for the growth of nonosseous tissues. Thus, net osteolysis seems to occur, in addition to osteomalacia, in phosphate-starved subjects, and this has been confirmed by kinetic studies with bone-seeking radionuclides in hypophosphatemic humans[481] and rats.[484,485] Increased urinary hydroxyproline excretion has also been observed,[485] and histologic studies of phosphate-deprived growing rats have documented accelerated endosteal bone resorption, wide osteoid seams, and depressed mineralization and collagen matrix formation.[486]

Young rats, within 48 hours of the institution of dietary phosphate restriction, display enhanced bone resorption, which may be preceded by an even earlier inhibition of mineralization.[487] Interestingly enough, sustained hypercalcemia, a typical feature of phosphate-depleted young animals,[112,113,484,485] is not observed in adults similarly stressed,[114,488,489] which may relate to the lower rate of preexisting bone turnover in the latter.

The osteolysis induced by dietary phosphate restriction is not mediated by PTH, as underscored by Lotz et al.,[116] who documented a dramatic rise in serum calcium during phosphate depletion in hypoparathyroid patients. This phenomenon has been observed repeatedly in animal studies.[295,485,490] Moreover, phosphate deficiency, with or without hypophosphatemia, has been designated a state of functional hypoparathyroidism on the basis of its association with histologic parathyroid hypoplasia[485] despite hypercalciuria and frequent hypercalcemia,[112,113,295,483,485,488,489] a strong dependence of serum calcium on levels of serum phosphate,[295,488,490] the lack of effect of parathyroidectomy on serum or urinary calcium and phosphate,[295,488,490] and measurably lower levels of PTH compared with those before phosphate restriction.[114] Accordingly, Baylink et al.[396] found no effect of thyroparathyroidectomy on the histologic changes of bone resorption in phosphate-restricted rats.

Overall, these results suggest that the direct and indirect effects of hypophosphatemia to elevate extracellular-fluid calcium concentrations are experienced by the parathyroid glands as a suppressive influence, which results in a reduction of PTH secretion and chronic parathyroid suppression. Such evidence for parathyroid suppression argues strongly against the possibility that the osteolysis that occurs during phosphate depletion may be merely secondary to a renal calcium leak, even though the latter does occur in hypophosphatemia (see below); such a leak would tend to lower rather than raise serum calcium and to stimulate, not suppress, parathyroid activity.

The potential role of $1,25\text{-}(OH)_2\text{-}D_3$ in this enhancement of bone resorption must be considered, especially since phosphate depletion has been shown to be a powerful stimulus for the renal 1-hydroxylation of $25\text{-}OH\text{-}D_3$, even in the absence of PTH[491,492] (Chapter 51).

In phosphate-deprived chicks[493] and rats,[494] increased tissue levels of $1,25\text{-}(OH)_2\text{-}D_3$ have been found, and the intestinal calcium absorption of these animals is stimulated over controls.[495-497] Although it is not known whether the levels of $1,25\text{-}(OH)_2\text{-}D_3$ in the bones of these animals are high enough to directly resorb bone, it is possible to produce net bone resorption by administration of exogenous $1,25\text{-}(OH)_2\text{-}D_3$ in parathyroidectomized, phosphate-depleted rats.[498,499] Vitamin D deficiency does prevent the development of hypercalcemia in phosphate-depleted rats[297] and, more important, blunts the histologic resorptive responses in such animals.[482] This inhibition is only partial, however, which suggests that other factors participate in the genesis of the osteolysis. In support of this conclusion, it has been demonstrated that the enhancement of intestinal calcium absorption in response to phosphate deprivation is also only partly attributable to stimulation of $1,25\text{-}(OH)_2\text{-}D_3$ production. Thus, administration of supraphysiologic doses of $1,25\text{-}(OH)_2\text{-}D_3$ or dihydrotachysterol (sufficient to saturate the vitamin D-dependent mechanism) does not prevent a further increase in calcium absorption during phosphate deprivation, whereas such treatment results in no residual enhancement of calcium absorption in response to calcium deprivation.[497,499]

It is thus likely that active vitamin D metabolites are partly responsible for the adaptive increase in bone resorption and intestinal calcium absorption during phosphate depletion, but other factors must also play a significant role. One of these is likely to be the hypophosphatemia per se, since lowering medium phosphate concentration below 1 mg/100 ml directly stimulates bone resorption, regardless of the calcium-phosphate product, and inhibits collagen matrix synthesis in bone organ cultures.[500,501] In addition, it is possible that an unknown humoral mechanism operates to increase phosphate throughput in response to phosphate depletion or, more likely, to lowered intracellular phosphate concentrations.

In summary, chronic dietary phosphate restriction leads to an osteodystrophy characterized both by osteomalacia, the probable consequence of phosphate levels too low for effective matrix mineralization, and by accelerated net bone resorption, despite a state of "functional hypoparathyroidism." The osteolysis presumably occurs in response to a perceived deficiency of soft tissue or dietary phosphate, is mediated by $1,25\text{-}(OH)_2\text{-}D_3$, hypophosphatemia, per se and, possibly, additional humoral factors, and provides for the mobilization of skeletal mineral stores to compensate for this deficit. It explains the propensity of phosphate-deficient subjects for hypercalcemia, hypercalciuria, and negative calcium balance, although the adaptive increase in intestinal calcium absorption is clearly important in the determination of net calcium balance, there being recent evidence that adult males may perform this adjustment more effectively than females.[114]

The mechanism and time course of this skeletal response are incompletely understood, as is the relative importance, in its genesis, of absolute hypophosphatemia as opposed to dietary phosphate deficiency alone. It is unlikely that clinically significant skeletal effects occur in the setting of the acute hypophosphatemia of diabetic ketoacidosis, alcoholism, or hyperalimentation, although adequate data are unavailable. Moreover, in many situations of chronic hypophosphatemia, additional influences on skeletal metabolism are operative, so that the extent to which the osteodystrophy of primary dietary phosphate deprivation contributes to that found in these disorders remains unknown.

Renal

In addition to the rapid and dramatic PTH-independent stimulation of phosphate reabsorption previously discussed, dietary phosphate depletion to the point of hypophosphatemia evokes significant alterations in many other aspects of renal function. Although a 25 percent reduction in GFR has been reported in profoundly hypophosphatemic rats and dogs,[300,301,488] this is not a consistent finding in these species[299,303] or in humans.[300] The discrepancies may reflect variations in the severity of the hypophosphatemia achieved. Studies of glucose reabsorption have also yielded discordant results. Harter et al. reported a significant elevation of the glucose threshold (Tm_{Glu}/GFR) in phosphate-deprived dogs, which occurred by virtue of a large fall in GFR with only a slight increase in Tm_{Glu}.[300] On the other hand, Gold et al., also studying dogs, found that Tm_{Glu} and Tm_{Glu}/GFR both decreased significantly.[502] Since glucose and phosphate are believed to compete for a similar reabsorptive mechanism,[503] the low intralumenal levels of phosphate in hypophosphatemia should enhance Tm_{Glu}/GFR, unless profound hypophosphatemia were to so interfere with cellular energy availability that renal transport mechanisms become generally depressed, offsetting the stimulatory effect of hypophosphaturia. Such an effect might explain the disagreement in the above observations, as the phosphate depletion was more prolonged and the hypophosphatemia more severe, in the study of Gold et al.[502]

Chronically phosphate-depleted dogs acquire a systemic acidosis and a reduction in the renal bicarbonate threshold (Tm_{HCO_3}/GFR).[503] Serum bicarbonate becomes linearly related to serum phosphate concentration, and bicarbonaturia appears at lower levels of filtered bicarbonate in phosphate-depleted dogs than in controls. This probably represents a direct effect of low serum or intracellular phosphate concentration and not PTH, since, as discussed earlier, hypophosphatemia causes functional hypoparathyroidism. The renal bicarbonate leak has been indirectly confirmed in rats by Emmett et al.[303] who showed that the metabolic acidosis resulting from phosphate depletion is initially offset by a greatly accelerated liberation of fixed bone-mineral alkali. With further depletion, however, metabolic acidosis does develop as a result of an apparent decline in the rate of bone-alkali mobilization in the face of a persistent renal bicarbonate leak. While studying the etiology of the lowered Tm_{HCO_3}/GFR, Gold et al. found an elevated intracellular pH in the muscles of phosphate-depleted dogs, as compared with normophosphatemic controls, and postulated that a relative intracellular alkalosis in hypophosphatemia might impair the renal tubular secretion of hydrogen ion necessary for bicarbonate reabsorption.[504] On the other hand, impaired sodium reabsorption in hypophosphatemia (see below) might also inhibit bicarbonate reabsorption.[299] Hypophosphatemia may also cause metabolic acidosis by an independent inhibition of renal tubular production of ammonia,[505] although this has not been directly studied.

Convincing evidence for a depression of proximal tubular sodium and water reabsorption has recently been obtained in the hypophosphatemic dog[299] and, for reasons given above, cannot be readily ascribed to a PTH effect. The potential role of this natriuresis in the genesis of the variable reductions in GFR, Tm_{Glu}/GFR,[300] and Tm_{HCO_3}/GFR[299] requires further exploration, since it is equally possible that these defects all result from a fundamental generalized metabolic derangement of tubular transport induced by hypophosphatemia.

Hypercalciuria is a prominent feature of hypophosphatemia induced by phosphate deprivation[116,483,488] and, as previously discussed, may result mainly from an increase in the filtered load of calcium caused by accelerated intestinal absorption and bone breakdown. In addition, however, a defect in renal tubular calcium reabsorption has been documented in phosphate-depleted rats[297] and dogs.[299,494] That this is not a manifestation of functional hypoparathyroidism has been shown by the failure of PTH infusions to normalize calcium reabsorption.[299,488] This finding is more consistent with the previously described resistance of renal phosphate and calcium handling to the action of PTH in hypophosphatemia. Interestingly enough, infusion of phosphate does acutely normalize urinary calcium excretion, even in parathyroidectomized animals,[297,299,488] and micropuncture studies in dogs have localized this phenomenon to a correction of defective calcium uptake in the distal tubules.[299] Even with phosphate infusion, however, proximal tubular calcium reabsorption remains subnormal, so that defects in calcium reabsorption may exist in both proximal and distal tubules, which is again consistent with a generalized derangement of proximal tubular function in hypophosphatemia.

Neuromuscular

Early studies of phosphate-deprived growing animals led to the recognition of weakness as a prominent manifestation of hypophosphatemia.[111–113] Weakness was also a common symptom of the phosphate-depleted patients reported by Lotz et al., as were anorexia, malaise, and tremor.[116] Subsequent reports of patients with hypophosphatemia due to hyperalimentation, alcoholism, dialysis with antacid abuse, and other causes have disclosed a panorama of associated neuromuscular findings, including paresthesias; lethargy; confusion; cranial-nerve palsies; nystagmus; anisocoria; myalgia; muscle weakness, paralysis, and sensory deficits (predominantly distal); cerebellar tremor; ballismus; depressed muscle tone and deep tendon reflexes; a Guillain–Barré type of ascending paralysis; respiratory paralysis; seizures; coma; and death.[506–516] The flaccid paralysis, arreflexia, complete anesthesia, confusion, and seizures are typically associated with serum phosphates below 0.8 mg/100 ml. The electroencephalogram and nerve-conduction studies may be abnormal, and prompt objective and symptomatic improvement has followed the institution of vigorous phosphate repletion in some cases.[509–513] The neuromuscular symptoms have been ascribed to the presumed widespread derangement of cellular energy production engendered by hypophosphatemia. Thus, erythrocyte glucose utilization and lactate production,[469] forearm lactate production during exercise,[473] and the hyperglycemic response to glucagon[473] have all been shown to be subnormal in patients with severe hypophosphatemia, which is consistent with impaired glycolysis in red cells, muscle, and liver, respectively. The dependence of muscular contraction on stored high-energy organophosphate compounds should render muscle especially sensitive to this effect of hypophosphatemia, although interference with intracellular calcium uptake and distribution has also been postulated,[510] given the fundamental role of calcium in excitation–contraction coupling. In addition, Fuller et al.[512] have recently reported that the skeletal muscle of adult dogs rendered hypophosphatemic (1.5–2.0 mg/100 ml) by dietary phosphate restriction and oral antacids displayed an increased sodium, chloride, and water content; a decreased phosphate and potassium content; and a 16 percent drop (15 mV) in the magnitude of the resting-membrane potential, all of which was slowly reversible with phosphate repletion. These abnormalities would be expected to cause weakness through a reduction in sarcolemmal excitability and are a predictable consequence of inhibition of the ATP-dependent ion pump responsible for the maintenance of intracellular electronegativity,[516] although an increase in resting-membrane ion permeability induced by hypophosphatemia would explain these findings equally well. These investigators had earlier reported similar muscle-cell abnormalities in hospitalized alcoholics who developed weakness, elevated muscle enzymes in serum, and a reduction in resting-membrane potential during glucose-induced hypophosphatemia,[514] although these abnormalities had not been clearly shown to be due to the hypophosphatemia in these patients.

In summary, the neuromuscular manifestations of hypophosphatemia are diverse and appear to result from impaired cellular glycolysis and energy availability for contraction and impulse transmission, although further study is needed to better define the pathogenetic mechanisms involved.

Cardiac

Although the dramatic effects of severe hypophosphatemia on skeletal muscle function might be expected to extend to myocardial performance as well, little investigation of this issue has been undertaken. It has recently been reported, however, that within a group of critically ill patients with severe hypophosphatemia of diverse etiology, correction of serum phosphate concentration from an average of 1.0 mg/100 ml before therapy to 2.9 mg/100 ml led to a highly significant improvement in left ventricular contractility, as reflected by elevations of stroke volume and stroke work at the same or slightly lower preload and by higher mean arterial blood pressure.[515]

Therapeutic Considerations

The accumulated evidence suggests the need to detect more carefully and routinely the occurrence of acute hypophosphatemia in susceptible individuals (hospitalized alcoholics, diabetics in ketoacidosis, etc.) and, in view of the deleterious and widespread metabolic consequences of severe hypophosphatemia, to consider parenteral phosphate supplementation for serum levels below 1.5–2.0 mg/100 ml.

REFERENCES

1. Bronner, F.: Dynamics in function of calcium, in Comar, L. C., Bronner, F. (ed): Mineral Metabolism, vol 2, pt A. New York, Academic Press, 1964, pp 342–447.

2. Krane, S. M.: Calcium, phosphate and magnesium, in Rasmussen, H. (ed): The International Encyclopedia of Pharmacology and Therapeutics, sect 51, vol I. London, Pergamon Press, 1970, pp 19–59.

3. Neer, R., Berman, M., Fisher, L., et al: Multicompartmental analysis of calcium kinetics in normal adult males. *J Clin Invest 46:* 1364–1379, 1967.

4. Ross, J. W.: Calcium-selective electrode with liquid ion exchanger. *Science 156:* 1378–1379, 1967.

5. Romero, P. J., Whittam, R.: The control by internal calcium of membrane permeability to sodium and potassium. *J Physiol 214:* 481–507, 1971.

6. Wybenga, D. R., Ibbott, F. A., Cannon, D. C.: Determination of ionized calcium in serum that has been exposed to air. *Clin Chem 22:* 1009–1011, 1976.

7. Ladenson, J. H., Bowers, G. N. Jr.: Free calcium in serum. I. Determination with the ion-specific electrode, and factors affecting the results. *Clin Chem 19:* 565–574, 1973.

8. Fuchs, C., Dorn, D., McIntosh, C., et al: Comparative calcium ion determinations in plasma and whole blood with a new calcium ion analyzer. *Clin Chim Acta 67:* 99–102, 1976.

9. Schwartz, H. D.: New techniques for ion-selective measurements of ionized calcium in serum after pH adjustment of aerobically handled sera. *Clin Chem 22:* 461–467, 1976.

10. Burman, K. D., Monchik, J. M., Earll, J. M., et al: Ionized and total serum calcium and parathyroid hormone in hyperthyroidism. *Ann Intern Med 84:* 668–671, 1976.

11. Glimcher, M. K., Krane, S. M.: Organization and structure of bone and the mechanism of calcification, in Gould, B. S., Ramachandran, G. N. (ed): Treatise on Collagen. New York, Academic Press, 1968, pp 68–241, Part B.

12. Johnson, L. C.: Morphologic analysis in pathology: Kinetics of disease and general biology of bone, in Frost, H. M. (ed): Bone Biodynamics, Henry Ford Hospital International Symposium. Boston, Little, Brown, 1964, pp 543–654.

13. Johnson, L. C.: Kinetics of skeletal remodeling, in Bergsma, D. (ed): Structural Organization of the Skeleton: A Symposium. (Birth Defects Original Article Series.) vol 2. New York, The National Foundation, 1966, pp 66–142.

14. Rasmussen, H., Goodman, D. B. P., Friedmann, N., et al: Ionic control of metabolism, in Aurbach, G. D. (vol ed), Greep, R. O., Astwood, E. B. (sec ed), Geiger, S. R. (bk ed): Handbook of Physiology, sec. 7, Endocrinology, vol. VII, Parathyroid Gland. Washington, D.C., The American Physiological Society, 1976, pp 225–264.

15. Raisz, L. G.: Mechanisms of bone resorption, in Aurbach, G. D. (vol ed), Greep, R. O., Astwood, E. B. (sec ed), Geiger, S. R. (bk ed): Handbook of Physiology, sec. 7, Endocrinology, vol. VII, Parathyroid Gland. Washington, D.C., The American Physiological Society, 1976, pp 117–136.

16. Borle, A. B.: Membrane transfer of calcium. *Clin Orthop Relat Res 52:* 267–291. 1967.

17. DiPolo, R.: The influence of nucleotides on calcium fluxes. *Fed Proc 35:* 2579–2582, 1976.

18. Schatzmann, H. J., Vincenzi, F. F.: Calcium movements across the membrane of human red cells. *J Physiol (Lond) 201:* 369–395, 1969.

19. Schacter, D.: Vitamin D and the active transport of calcium by the small intestine, in: Transfer of Calcium and Strontium Across Biological Membranes. New York, Academic Press, 1963, pp 197–210.

20. Wasserman, R. H., Corradino, R. A., Taylor, A. N., et al: Intestinal calcium absorption, vitamin D adaptation, and the calcium-binding protein, in Nichols, G. Jr., Wasserman, R. H. (ed): Cellular Mechanisms for Calcium Transfer and Homeostasis. New York, Academic Press, 1971, pp 293–307.

21. Wasserman, R. H.: The vitamin D-dependent calcium-binding protein, in DeLuca, H. F., Suttie, J. W. (ed): The Fat Soluble Vitamins. Madison, University of Wisconsin Press, 1969, p 21.

22. DeLuca, H. F.: 1,25-Dihydroxycholecalciferol: Isolation, identification, regulation and mechanism of action, in Taylor S. (ed): Endocrinology, 1971. London, W. Heinemann, 1972, pp 452–467.

23. Wasserman, R. H., Taylor, A. N.: Gastrointestinal absorption of calcium and phosphorus, in Aurbach, G. D. (vol ed), Greep, R. O., Astwood, E. B. (sec ed), Geiger, S. R. (bk ed): Handbook of Physiology, sec. 7, Endocrinology, vol. VII, Parathyroid Gland. Washington, D.C., The American Physiological Society, 1976, pp. 137–155.

24. Berger, E. Y.: Techniques for studying ion transfer across the alimentary tract, in Wasserman, R. H. (ed): Transfer of Calcium and Strontium Across Biological Membranes. New York, Academic Press, 1963, pp 57–74.

25. Nicolaysen, R., Eeg-Larsen, N., Malm, O. J.: Physiology of calcium metabolism. *Physiol Rev 33:* 425–444, 1953.

26. Malm, O. J.: Adaptation to alterations in calcium intake, in Wasserman, R. H. (ed): Transfer of Calcium and Strontium Across Biological Membranes. New York, Academic Press, 1963, pp 143–173.

27. Schachter, D., Rosen, S. M.: Active transport of Ca^{45} by the small intestine and its dependence on vitamin D. *Am J Physiol 196:* 357–362, 1959.

28. Potts, J. T. Jr., Deftos, L. J.: Parathyroid hormone, thyrocalcitonin, vitamin D, bone and bone mineral metabolism, in Bondy, P. K., Rosenberg, L. E. (ed): Duncan's Diseases of Metabolism (ed 7). Philadelphia, Saunders, 1974, chap 20, pp 1225–1430.

29. Schachter, D., Kimberg, D. V., Schenker, H.: Active transport of calcium by intestine: Action and bio-assay of vitamin D. *Am J Physiol 200:* 1263–1271, 1961.

30. Papworth, D. G., Patrick, G.: The kinetics of influx of calcium and strontium into rat intestine in vitro. *J Physiol 210:* 999–1020, 1970.

31. Wilkinson, R.: Studies of calcium absorption by the small intestine of rat and man. (PhD thesis.) Leeds, Great Britain, M.R.C. Mineral Metabolism Unit, Univ. of Leeds, 1971.

32. Wasserman, R. H., Taylor, A. N., Lippiello, L.: Effect of vitamin D_3 on lanthanum (La^{+3}) translocation: Evidence for a shunt path. *Fed Proc 32:* 918, 1973.

33. O'Donnell, J. M., Smith, M. W.: Influence of cholecalciferol (vitamin D_3) on the intitial kinetics of the uptake of calcium by rat small intestinal mucosa. *Biochem J 134:* 667–669, 1973.

34. O'Donnell, J. M., Smith, M. W.: Uptake of calcium and magnesium by rat duodenal mucosa analyzed by means of competing metals. *J Physiol (Lond) 229:* 733–749, 1973.

35. Cramer, C. F.: Sites of calcium absorption and the calcium concentration of gut contents in the dog. *Can J Physiol Pharmacol 43:* 75–78, 1965.

36. Cramer, C. F., Copp, D. H.: Progress and rate of absorption of radiostrontium through the intestinal tracts of rats. *Proc Soc Exp Biol Med 102:* 514–517, 1959.

37. Mellanby, E.: An experimental investigation on rickets. *Lancet 1:* 407–412, 1919.

38. Harrison, H. E., Harrison, H. C.: Transfer of Ca^{45} across intestinal wall in vitro in relation to action of vitamin D and cortisol. *Am J Physiol 199:* 265–271, 1960.

39. Spencer, R., Charman, M., Wilson, P., et al: Vitamin D-stimulated intestinal calcium absorption may not involve calcium-binding protein directly. *Nature 263:* 161–163, 1976.

40. Holdsworth, E. S.: The effect of vitamin D on enzymes activities in the mucosal cells of the chick small intestine. *J Membr Biol 3:* 43–53, 1970.

41. Norman, A. W., Mircheff, A. K., Adams, T. H., et al: Studies on the mechanism of action of calciferol. III. Vitamin D-mediated increase of intestinal brush border alkaline phosphatase activity. *Biochim Biophys Acta 215:* 348–359, 1970.

42. Kowarski, S., Schachter, D.: Vitamin D and adenosine triphosphatase dependent on divalent cations in rat intestinal mucosa. *J Clin Invest 52:* 2765–2773, 1973.

43. Melancon, M. J., Jr., DeLuca, H. F.: Vitamin D stimulation of calcium-dependent adenosine triphosphatase in chick intestinal brush borders. *Biochemistry 9:* 1658–1664, 1970.

44. Wasserman, R. H., Corradino, R. A., Taylor, A. N.: Vitamin D-dependent calcium-binding protein: Purification and some properties. *J Biol Chem 243:* 3978–3986, 1968.

45. Wasserman, R. H., Taylor, A. N.: Vitamin D-dependent calcium-binding protein: Response to some physiological variables. *J Biol Chem 243:* 3987–3993, 1968.

46. Wasserman, R. H., Taylor, A. N.: Vitamin D_3-induced calcium binding protein in chick intestinal mucosa. *Science 152:* 791–793, 1966.

47. Hitchman, A. J. W., Hui, A., Hoffmann, T., et al: Studies of human and pig CaBP, in Drabikowski, W., Strzelecka-Golaszewska, H., Carofoli, E. (ed): Calcium Binding Proteins. Amsterdam, Elsevier Scientific Publishing Company, 1974, pp 771–790.

48. Kallfelz, F. A., Taylor, A. N., Wasserman, R. H.: Vitamin D-induced calcium binding factor in rat intestinal mucosa. *Proc Soc Exp Biol Med 125:* 54–58, 1967.

49. Hitchman, A. J. W., Harrison, J. E.: Calcium binding proteins in the duodenal mucosa of the chick, rat, pig, and human. *Can J Biochem 50:* 758–765, 1972.

50. Hitchman, A. J. W., Kerr, M-K., Harrison, J. E.: The purification of pig vitamin D-induced intestinal calcium binding protein. *Arch Biochem Biophys 155:* 221–222, 1973.

51. Wasserman, R. H., Taylor, A. N.: Vitamin D_3-induced calcium-binding protein in chick intestinal mucosa. *Science 152:* 791–793, 1966.

52. Russell, R. G. G., Monod, A., Bonjour, J-P., et al: Relation between alkaline phosphatase and Ca^{2+}-ATPase in calcium transport. *Nature 240:* 126–127, 1972.

53. Wasserman, R. H., Corradino, R. A.: Vitamin D, calcium and protein synthesis. *Vit Horm 31:* 43–103, 1973.

54. Fourman, P., Royer, P., Levell, M. J., et al: Calcium Metabolism and the Bone. Philadelphia, FA Davis Company, 1968.

55. Ireland, P., Fordtran, J. S.: Effect of dietary calcium and age on jejunal calcium absorption in humans studied by intestinal perfusion. *J Clin Invest 52:* 2672–2681, 1973.

56. Kimberg, D. V., Schachter, D., Schenker, H.: Active transport of calcium by intestine: Effects of dietary calcium. *Am J Physiol 200:* 1256–1262, 1961.

57. DeLuca, H. F.: The functional metabolism of vitamin D_3, in Talmage, R. V., Munson, P. L. (ed): Calcium, Parathyroid Hormone, and the Calcitonins. New York, Academic Press, 1972, pp 221–235.

58. Kemm, J. R.: The effect of previous dietary intake of calcium on calcium absorption in rats. *J Physiol 223:* 321–332, 1972.

59. Morrissey, R. L., Wasserman, R. H.: Calcium absorption and calcium binding protein (CaBP) in chicks on differing calcium and phosphorus intakes. *Am J Physiol 220:* 1509–1519, 1971.

60. Bar, A., Wasserman, R. H.: Control of calcium absorption and intestinal calcium-binding protein synthesis. *Biochem Biophys Res Commun 54:* 191–196, 1973.

61. Kimberg, D. V., Schachter, D., Schenker, H.: Active transport of calcium by intestine: Effects of dietary calcium. *Am J Physiol 200:* 1256–1262, 1961.

62. Walling, M. W., Rothman, S. S.: Apparent increase in carrier affinity for intestinal calcium transport following dietary calcium restriction. *J Biol Chem 245:* 5007–5011, 1970.

63. Shah, B. G., Draper, H. H.: Depression of calcium absorption in parathyroidectomized rats. *Am J Physio 211:* 963–966, 1966.

64. Wasserman, R. H., Comar, C. L.: The parathyroids and the intestinal absorption of calcium, strontium and phosphate ions in the rat. *Endocrinology 69:* 1074–1079, 1961.

65. Martin, D. L., DeLuca, H. F.: Influence of sodium on calcium transport by the rat small intestine. *Am J Physiol 216:* 1351–1359, 1969.

66. Schachter, D., Dowdle, E. B., Schenker, H.: Accumulation of Ca^{45} by slices of the small intestine. *Am J Physiol 198:* 275–279, 1960.

67. Shipley, P. G., Park, E. A., McCollum, E. V., et al: Studies on experimental rickets. xx. The effects of strontium administration on the histological structure of the growing bones. *Bull Johns Hopkins Hosp 33:* 216–220, 1922.

68. Omdahl, J. L., DeLuca, H. F.: Strontium induced rickets: Metabolic basis. *Science 174:* 949–951, 1971.

69. Omdahl, J. L., DeLuca, H. F.: Rachitogenic activity of dietary strontium. I. Inhibition of intestinal calcium absorption and 1,25-dihydroxycholecalciferol synthesis. *J Biol Chem 247:* 5520–5526, 1972.

70. Kimberg, D. V., Baerg, R. D., Gershon, E., et al: Effect of cortisone treatment on the active transport of calcium by the small intestine. *J Clin Invest 50:* 1309–1321, 1971.

71. Lukert, B. P., Stanbury, S. W., Mawer, E. B.: Vitamin D and intestinal transport of calcium: Effects of prednisolone. *Endocrinology 93:* 718–722, 1973.

72. Penzes, L., Adam, A., Boross, M.: Effect of L-lysine in the intestinal absorption of radiocalcium in aging rats. *Acta Gerontol 3:* 531–535, 1973.

73. Wasserman, R. H., Comar, C. L., Nold, M. M.: The influence of amino acids and other organic compounds on the gastrointestinal absorption of calcium-45 and strontium-89 in the rat. *J Nutr 59:* 371–383, 1956.

74. Krawitt, E. L.: Ethanol inhibits intestinal calcium transport in rats. *Nature 243:* 88–89, 1973.

75. Verdy, M., Caron, D.: Ethanol et absorption du calcium chez l'humain. *Biol Gastroenterol (Paris) 6:* 157–160, 1973.

76. Schneider, L. E., Wilson, H. D., Schedl, H. P.: Intestinal calcium binding protein in the diabetic rat. *Nature 245:* 327–328, 1973.

77. Schneider, L. E., Schedl, H. P.: Diabetes and intestinal calcium absorption in the rat. *Am J Physiol 223:* 1319–1323, 1972.

78. Epstein, F. H.: Calcium and the kidney. *Am J Med 45:* 700–715, 1968.

79. Bijvoet, O. L. M.: Kidney function in calcium and phosphate metabolism, in Avioli, L. V., Krane, S. M. (ed): Metabolic Bone Disease, vol. I. New York, Academic Press, 1977, pp 49–140.

80. Lassiter, W. E., Gottschalk, C. W., Mylle, M.: Micropuncture study of renal tubular reabsorption of calcium in normal rodents. *Am J Physiol 204:* 771–775, 1963.

81. Nichols, G.: Introductory remarks, in Talmage, R. V., Munson, P. L. (ed): Calcium, Parathyroid Hormone, and the Calcitonins. Amsterdam, Excerpta Medica, 1972, p 445.

82. Beck, L. H., Goldberg, M.: Effects of acetazolamide and parathyroidectomy on renal transport of sodium, calcium, and phosphate. *Am J Physiol 224:* 1136–1142, 1973.

83. Agus, Z. S., Gardner, L. B., Beck, L. H., et al: Effects of parathyroid hormone on renal tubular reabsorption of calcium, sodium, and phosphate. *Am J Physiol 224:* 1143–1148, 1973.

84. Lamberg, B. A., Kuhlbach, B.: Effect of chlorothiazide on the excretion of calcium in urine. *Scand J Clin Lab Invest 11:* 351–357, 1959.

85. Frick, A., Rumrich, G., Ullrich, K. J., et al: Microperfusion study of calcium transport in the proximal tubule of the rat kidney. *Pfluegers Archiv Gesamte Physiol Menschen Tiere 286:* 109–117, 1965.

86. Nordon, B. E. C., Peacock, M.: Role of kidney in regulation of plasma-calcium. *Lancet 2:* 1280–1283. 1969.

87. Peacock, M., Robertson, W. G., Nordin, B. E. C.: Relation between serum and urinary calcium with particular reference to parathyroid activity. *Lancet 1:* 384–386, 1969.

88. Gallagher, J. C., Nordin, B. E. C.: in van Keep, P. A., Lauritzen, C. (ed): Ageing and Estrogens: Frontiers of Hormone Research. Basel, Karger, 1973, p 98.

89. Eisenberg, E.: Renal effects of parathyroid hormone, in Talmage, R. V., Bélanger, L. F. (ed): Parathyroid Hormone and Thyrocalcitonin (Calcitonin). Amsterdam, Excerpta Medica, 1968, pp 465–475.

90. Biddulph, D. M., Hirsch, P. F., Munson, P. L.: Thyrocalcitonin and parathyroid hormone in the hamster, in Calcitonin, 1969, Proceedings of the Second International Symposium. New York, Springer-Verlag, 1970, pp 392–399.

91. Yendt, E.: Personal communications.

92. Rasmussen, H., Tenenhouse, A.: Cyclic adenosine monophosphate, calcium and membranes. *Proc Natl Acad Sci 59:* 1364–1370, 1965.

93. Irving, J. T.: Dynamics and function of phosphorus, in Comar, C. L., Bronner, F., (eds): Mineral Metabolism, vol. 2, pt. A. New York, Academic Press, 1964, pp 249–297.

94. Krane, S. M.: Calcium, phosphate and magnesium, in Rasmussen, H. (ed): The International Encyclopedia of Pharmacology and Therapeutics. London, Pergamon Press, 1970, p 19.

95. Walser, M.: Ion association VI. Interaction between calcium, magnesium, inorganic phosphate, citrate and protein in normal human plasma. *J Clin Invest 40:* 723, 1961.

96. Wesson, L. G.: Electrolyte excretion in relation to diurnal cycles of renal function. *Medicine 43:* 547, 1964.

97. Carruthers, B. M., et al: Diurnal variation in urinary excretion of calcium and phosphate and its relation to blood levels. *J Lab Clin Med 63:* 959, 1964.

98. Mills, J. N.: Human circadian rhythms. *Physiol Rev 46:* 128, 1966.

99. Somell, A., Alveryd, A.: Diurnal variation in the urinary excretion of calcium and phosphate in hyperparathyroidism. *Acta Chir Scand 142:* 357, 1976.

100. Dossetor, J. B., Gorman, H. M., Beck, J. C.: The diurnal rhythm of urinary electrolyte excretion I. Observations in normal subjects. *Metabolism 12:* 1083, 1963.

101. Birkenhager, W. H., Hellendoorn, H. B. A., Gerbrandy, J.: Enkle aspecten van de calcium-en fosfaatstofwisseling, in het bijzonder na intraveneuze injectie van calcium-levulinaat. *Ned Tijdschr Geneesk 101:* 1294, 1957.

102. Sinha, T. K., et al: Demonstration of a diurnal variation in serum parathyroid hormone in primary and secondary hyperparathyroidism. *J Clin Endocrinol Metab 41:* 1009, 1975.

103. Jubiz, W., et al: Circadian rhythm in serum parathyroid hormone concentration in human subjects: Correlation with serum calcium, phosphate, albumin and growth hormone levels. *J Clin Invest 51:* 2040, 1972.

104. Bijvoet, O. L. M.: Relation of plasma phosphate concentration to renal tubular reabsorption of phosphate. *Clin Sci 37:* 23, 1969.

105. Corvilain, J., Abramow, M.: Growth and renal control of plasma phosphate. *J Clin Endocrinol Metab 34:* 452, 1972.

106. Young, M. M., Nordin, B. E. C.: The effect of the natural and the artificial menopause on plasma and urinary calcium and phosphorus. *Lancet 2:* 118, 1967.

107. Aitken, J. M., et al: Plasma growth hormone and serum phosphorus concentration in relation to the menopause and to oestrogen therapy. *J Endocrinol 59:* 593, 1973.

108. Marshall, D. H., et al: Calcium, phosphorus and magnesium requirements. *Proc Nutr Soc 35:* 163, 1976.

109. Spencer, H., et al: Changes in metabolism in obese persons during starvation. *Am J Med 40:* 27, 1966.

110. Bell, N. H.: Observation concerning the effects of fasting on collagen metabolism in man. *J Clin Endocrinol Metab 29:* 338, 1969.

111. Aubel, C. E., et al: The effects of low-phosphorus rations on growing pigs. *J Agric Res 52:* 149, 1936.

112. Schneider, H., Steenbock, H.: A low phosphorus diet and the response of rats to vitamin D₂. *J Biol Chem 128:* 159, 1939.

113. Freeman, S., McLean, F. C.: Experimental rickets. Blood and tissue changes in puppies receiving a diet very low in phosphorus, with and without vitamin D. *Arch Pathol 32:* 387, 1941.

114. Dominguez, J. H., et al: Dietary phosphate deprivation in women and men: Effects on mineral and acid balances, parathyroid hormone and the metabolism of 25-OH-vitamin D. *J Clin Endocrinol Metab 43:* 1056, 1976.

115. Bloom, W. L., Flinchum, D.: Osteomalacia with pseudofractures caused by ingestion of aluminum hydroxide. *JAMA 174:* 1327, 1960.

116. Lotz, M., et al: Evidence for a phosphorus-depletion syndrome in man. *N Engl J Med 278:* 409, 1968.

117. Condon, J. R., et al: Defective intestinal phosphate absorption in familial and non-familial hypophosphatemia. *Br Med J 3:* 138, 1970.

118. Short, E. M., et al: Familial hypophosphatemic rickets: Defective transport of inorganic phosphate by intestinal mucosa. *Science 179:* 700, 1973.

119. Glorieux, F., et al: Intestinal phosphate transport in familial hypophosphatemic rickets. *Pediatr Res 10:* 691, 1976.

120. Harrison, H. E., Harrison, H. C.: Intestinal transport of phosphate: Action of vitamin D, calcium and potassium. *Am J Physiol 201:* 1007, 1961.

121. Lifshitz, F. H., et al: Intestinal transport of calcium and phosphate in experimental magnesium deficiency. *Proc Soc Exp Biol Med 125:* 19, 1967.

122. McHardy, G. J. R., Parsons, D. S.: The absorption of inorganic phosphate from the small intestine of the rat. *Q J Exp Psychol 41:* 398, 1956.

123. Wasserman, R. H., Taylor, A. N.: Intestinal absorption of phosphate in the chick: Effect of vitamin D and other parameters. *J Nutr 103:* 586, 1973.

124. Berner, W., et al: Phosphate transport into brush-border membrane vesicles isolated from rat small intestine. *Biochem J 160:* 467, 1976.

125. Kowarski, S., Schachter, D.: Effects of vitamin D on phosphate transport and incorporation into mucosal constituents of rat intestinal mucosa. *J Biol Chem 244:* 211, 1969.

126. Hurwitz, S., Bar, A.: Absorption of calcium and phosphorus along the gastrointestinal tract of the laying fowl as influenced by dietary calcium and egg shell formation. *J Nutr 86:* 433, 1965.

127. Walling, M. W.: Effects of 1α,25-dihydroxyvitamin D₃ on active intestinal inorganic phosphate absorption, in Norman, A. W., Schaefer, K., Coburn, J. W., et al (eds): Vitamin D: Biochemical, Chemical and Clinical Aspects Related to Calcium Metabolism. Berlin—New York, Walter de Gruyter, 1977, pp 321–330.

128. Schryver, H. F., et al: Site of phosphorus absorption from the intestine of the horse. *J Nutr 102:* 143, 1972.

129. Yang, M. G., Thomas, J. W.: Absorption and secretion of some organic and inorganic constituents throughout the alimentary tract of young calves. *J Nutr 87:* 444, 1965.

130. Corradino, R. A.: Embryonic chick intestine in organ culture. A unique system for the study of the intestinal calcium absorptive mechanism. *J Cell Biol 58:* 64, 1973.

131. Caniggia, A., Gennari, C., Benchini, M., Palazzuoli, V.: Intestinal absorption of radiophosphate in osteomalacia before and after vitamin D treatment. *Calcif Tissue Res 2:* 299, 1968.

132. Chen, T. C., et al: Role of vitamin D metabolites in phosphate transport of rat intestine. *J Nutr 104:* 1056, 1974.

133. Harrison, H. E., Harrison, H. C., Lifshitz, F.: Interrelation of vitamin D and parathyroid hormone: The responses of vitamin D depleted and of thyroparathyroidectomized rats to ergocalciferol and dihydrotachysterol, in Talmage, R. V., Bélanger, L. F. (eds): Parathyroid Hormone and Thyrocalcitonin. Amsterdam, Excerpta Medica, 1968, p 455.

134. Ferraro, C., et al: Intestinal absorption of phosphate: Action of protein synthesis inhibitors and glucocorticoids in the rat. *J Nutr 106:* 1752, 1976.

135. Walling, M. W., et al: Duodenal active transport of calcium and phosphate in vitamin D-deficient rats: Effect of nephrectomy, *Cestrum diurnum* and 1α,25-dihydroxyvitamin D₃. *Endocrinology 98:* 1130, 1976.

136. Walling, M. W., Kimberg, D. V.: Effects of 1α,25-dihydroxyvitamin D₃ and *Solanum glaucophyllum* on intestinal calcium and phosphate transport and on plasma Ca, Mg and P levels in the rat. *Endocrinology 97:* 1567, 1975.

137. Matualen, C. A.: Mechanism of action of *Solanum malacoxylon* upon calcium and phosphate metabolism in the rabbit. *Endocrinology 90:* 563, 1972.

138. Borle, A. B., Keutmann, H. T., Neumann, W. F.: Role of parathyroid hormone in phosphate transport across rat duodenum. *Am J Physiol 204:* 705, 1963.

139. Clark, I., Rivera-Cordero, F.: Effect of parathyroid function on absorption and excretion of calcium, magnesium and phosphate by rats. *Endocrinology 88:* 302, 1971.

140. Cramer, C. F., Parks, C. O., Copp, D. H.: The effect of chicken and hog calcitonin on some parameters of Ca, P and Mg metabolism in dogs. *Can J Physiol Pharmacol 47:* 181, 1969.

141. Tanzer, F. S., Navia, J. M.: Calcitonin inhibition of intestinal phosphate absorption. *Nature New Biol 242:* 221, 1973.

142. Caniggia, A., Genari, C., Bencini, M., et al: Action of thyrocalcitonin on intestinal absorption of radiophosphate in man. *J Nucl Biol Med 12:* 83, 1968.

143. Juan, D., et al: Absorption of inorganic phosphate in the human jejunum and its inhibition by salmon calcitonin. *J Clin Endocrinol Metab 43:* 517, 1976.

144. Cramer, C. F.: Effect of Ca/P ratio and pH on calcium and phosphorus absorption from dog gut loops in vivo. *Can J Physiol Pharmacol 43:* 75, 1965.

145. Street, H. R. Influence of aluminum sulfate and aluminum hydroxide upon the absorption of dietary phosphorus by the rat. *J Nutr 24:* 111, 1942.

146. Chow, K. W., Pond, W. G., Lengemann, F. W.: Effects of ammonia on the absorption and accumulation of glucose, ⁴⁵Ca and ³²P from the ligated intestinal loop of the chick. *J Nutr 102:* 1513, 1972.

147. Altman, P. L., Dittmer, D. S. (eds): Excretion products in sweat: Man. *Metabolism—Biol Handbook,* 1968, p 519.

148. Treschsel, U., et al: A new device for ultrafiltration. The ultrafiltrability of calcium and inorganic phosphate in human serum. *Clin Chim Acta 69:* 367, 1976.

149. Aurbach, G. D., Potts, J. T.: The parathyroids. *Adv Metab Dis 1:* 45, 1964.

150. Strickler, J. C., et al: Micropuncture study of inorganic phosphate excretion in the rat. *J Clin Invest 43:* 1596, 1964.

151. Pitts, R. F., Alexander, R. S.: The renal reabsorptive mechanism for inorganic phosphate in normal and acidotic dogs. *Am J Physiol 42:* 648, 1944.

152. Agus ZS, et al: Mode of action of parathyroid hormone and cyclic adenosine-5-monophosphate on renal tubular phosphate reabsorption in the dog. *J Clin Invest 50:* 617, 1971.

153. Agus ZS, et al: Effects of parathyroid hormone on renal tubular

reabsorption of calcium, sodium and phosphate. *Am J Physiol 224:* 1143, 1973.

154. Staum, B. B., et al: Tracer microinjection study of renal tubular phosphate reabsorption in the rat. *J Clin Invest 51:* 2271, 1972.

155. Amiel, C., et al: Micropuncture study of handling of phosphate by proximal and distal nephron in normal and parathyroidectomized rats. Evidence for distal absorption. *Pflugers Arch Eur J Physiol 317:* 93, 1970.

156. Beck, L. H., Goldberg, M.: Effect of acetazolamide and parathyroidectomy on renal transport of sodium, calcium and phosphate. *Am J Physiol 224:* 1136, 1973.

157. Brunette, M. G., et al: Effect of parathyroid hormone on phosphate reabsorption along the nephron of the rat. *Am J Physiol 225:* 1071, 1973.

158. Le Grimellac, C., et al: Simultaneous Mg, Ca, P, K, Na and Cl analysis in rat tubular fluid. *Pflugers Arch 346:* 171, 1974.

159. Knox, F. G., Lechene, C.: Distal site of action of parathyroid hormone on phosphate reabsorption. *Am J Physiol 229:* 1556, 1975.

160. Beck, L. H., Goldberg, M.: Mechanism of the blunted phosphaturia in saline-loaded thyroparathyroidectomized dogs. *Kidney Int 6:* 18, 1974.

161. Wen, S. F.: Micropuncture studies of phosphate transport in the proximal tubule of the dog. The relationship to sodium reabsorption. *J Clin Invest 53:* 143, 1974.

162. Barbour, B. H., et al: Studies on the mechanism of phosphorus excretion in vitamin D-resistant rickets. *Nephron 3:* 40, 1966.

163. Glorieux, F., Scriver, C. R.: Loss of a parathyroid hormone-sensitive component of phosphate transport in X-linked hypophosphatemia. *Science 175:* 997, 1972.

164. Short, E., et al: Exaggerated phosphaturic response to circulating parathyroid hormone in patients with familial X-linked hypophosphatemic rickets. *J Clin Invest 58:* 152, 1976.

165. Hahn, T. J., et al: Parathyroid hormone status and renal responsiveness in familial hypophosphatemic rickets. *J Clin Endocrinol Metab 41:* 926, 1975.

166. Levinsky, N. G., Davidson, D. G.: Renal action of parathyroid extract in the chicken. *Am J Physiol 191:* 530, 1957.

167. Marshall, E. K. Jr., Grafflin, A. L.: Excretion of inorganic phosphate by the aglomerular kidney. *Proc Soc Exp Biol Med 31:* 44, 1933.

168. Wolbach, R. A.: Phlorizin and renal phosphate secretion in the spinydogfish *Squalus acanthias. Am J Physiol 219:* 886, 1970.

169. Grafflin, A. L.: Renal function in marine teleosts. *Biol Bull 71:* 360, 1936.

170. Clark, N. B., Dantzler, W. H.: Renal tubular transport of calcium and phosphate in snakes: A role of parathyroid hormone. *Am J Physiol 223:* 1455, 1972.

171. Hernandez, T., Coulson, R. A.: Renal clearance in the alligator. *Fed Proc 15:* 91, 1956.

172. Boudry, J. F., et al: Secretion of inorganic phosphate in the rat nephron. *Clin Sci 48:* 475, 1975.

173. Frick, A.: Reabsorption of inorganic phosphate in the rat kidney. *Pflugers Arch 304:* 351, 1968.

174. Baumann, K., et al: Renal phosphate transport inhomogeneity of local proximal transport rates and sodium dependence. *Pflugers Arch 356:* 287, 1975.

175. Dennis, V. W., et al: Characteristics of phosphate transport in isolated proximal tubule. *Am J Physiol 231:* 979, 1976.

176. Bank, N., et al: A microperfusion study of phosphate reabsorption by the rat proximal renal tubule. Effect of parathyroid hormone. *J Clin Invest 54:* 1040, 1974.

177. Bijvoet, O. L. M., et al: The assessment of phosphate reabsorption. *Clin Chim Acta 26:* 15, 1969.

178. Anderson, J., Parsons, V.: The tubular maximal resorptive rate for inorganic phosphate in normal subjects. *Clin Sci 25:* 431, 1963.

179. Hellman, D., et al: Relationship of maximal tubular phosphate reabsorption to dietary phosphate in the dog. *Am J Physiol 207:* 97, 1964.

180. Stamp, T. C., Stacey, T. E.: Measurement of the theoretical renal phosphorus threshold in the investigation and treatment of osteomalacia. *Clin Sci 38:* 34P, 1970.

181. Bernstein, M., Yamahiro, H. S., Reynolds, T. B.: Phosphorus excretion tests in hyperparathyroidism with controlled phosphorus intake. *J Clin Endocrinol 25:* 895, 1965.

182. Foulks, J. G.: Homeostatic adjustment in the renal tubular transport of inorganic phosphate in the dog. *Can J Biochem Physiol 33:* 638, 1955.

183. Engle, J. E., Steele, T. H.: Renal phosphate reabsorption in the rat: Effect of inhibitors. *Kidney Int 8:* 98, 1975.

184. Bijvoet, O. L. M.: Renal phosphate excretion in man. *Folia Med Neerl 15:* 84, 1972.

185. Nordin, B. E. C., Fraser, R.: Assessment of urinary phosphate excretion. *Lancet 1:* 947, 1960.

186. Nordin, B. E. C., Bulusu: A modified index of phosphate excretion. *Postgrad Med J 44:* 93, 1968.

187. Collip, J. B.: The excretion of a parathyroid hormone which will prevent or control parathyroid tetany and which regulates the level of blood calcium. *J Biol Chem 63:* 395, 1925.

188. Greenwald, I., Gross, J.: The effect of the administration of a potent parathyroid extract upon the excretion of nitrogen, phosphorus, calcium and magnesium, with some remarks on the solubility of calcium phosphate in serum and on the pathogenesis of tetany. *J Biol Chem 66:* 217, 1925.

189. Albright, F., et al: Studies of calcium and phosphorus metabolism IV. The effect of the parathyroid hormone. *J Clin Invest 7:* 139, 1929.

190. Ellsworth, R., Howard, J. E.: Studies on the physiology of parathyroid glands VII. Some responses of normal human kidneys and blood to intravenous parathyroid extract. *Bull Johns Hopkins Hosp 55:* 296, 1934.

191. Pullman, T. N., et al: Direct renal action of a purified parathyroid extract. *Endocrinology 67:* 570, 1960.

192. Hyde, R. D., et al: Investigation of hyperparathyroidism in the absence of bone disease. *Lancet 1:* 250, 1960.

193. Hiatt, H. H., Thompson, D. D.: The effects of parathyroid extract on renal function in man. *J Clin Invest 36:* 557, 1956.

194. Chase, L. R., Aurbach, G. D.: Parathyroid function and the renal excretion of 3',5'-adenylic acid. *Proc Natl Acad Sci USA 58:* 518, 1967.

195. Rasmussen, H., et al: Effect of dibutyryl cyclic adenosine-3',5'-monophosphate, theophyline, and other nucleotides upon calcium and phosphate metabolism. *J Clin Invest 47:* 1843, 1968.

196. Melson, G. L., et al: Parathyroid hormone-sensitive adenyl cyclase in isolated renal tubules. *Endocrinology 86:* 511, 1970.

197. Kaminsky, N. I., et al: Effects of parathyroid hormone on plasma and urinary adenosine 3', 5'-monophosphate in man. *J Clin Invest 49:* 2387, 1970.

198. Gill, J. R., Jr., Casper, A. G. T.: Renal effects of adenosine 3',5'-cyclic monophosphate. Evidence for a role for adenosine 3',5'-cyclic monophosphate in the regulation of proximal tubular sodium reabsorption. *J Clin Invest 50:* 1231, 1971.

199. Kuntziger, H., et al: Effects of parathyroidectomy and cyclic AMP on renal transport of phosphate, calcium and magnesium. *Am J Physiol 227:* 905, 1974.

200. Wells, H., Lloyd, W.: Hypercalcemic and hypophosphatemic effects of dibutyryl cyclic AMP in rats after parathyroidectomy. *Endocrinology 84:* 861, 1969.

201. Bell, N. H., et al: Effects of dibutyryl cyclic adenosine 3',5'-monophosphate and parathyroid extract on calcium and phosphorus metabolism in hypoparathyroidism and pseudohypoparathyroidism. *J Clin Invest 51:* 816, 1972.

202. Puschett, J. B., Goldberg, M.: The relationship between the renal handling of phosphate and bicarbonate in man. *J Lab Clin Med 73:* 956, 1969.

203. Eisenberg, E.: Effects of serum calcium level and parathyroid extracts on phosphate and calcium excretion in hypoparathyroid patients. *J Clin Invest 44:* 942, 1965.

204. Froeling, P. G. A. M., Bijvoet, O. L. M.: Kidney-mediated effects of parathyroid hormone on extracellular homeostasis of calcium, phosphate and acid-base balance in man. *Neth J Med 17:* 174, 1974.

205. Frick, A.: Proximal tubular reabsorption of inorganic phosphate during saline infusion in the rat. *Am J Physiol 223:* 1034, 1972.

206. Lambert, P. P.: Study of phosphate excretion by the stop-flow technique. Effects of parathyroid hormone. *Nephron 1:* 103, 1964.

207. Knox, F. G., et al: Effect of parathyroid hormone on phosphate reabsorption in the presence of acetazolamide. *Kidney Int 10:* 211, 1976.

208. Colindres, R. E., et al: Effect of extracellular volume expansion on phosphate reabsorption along the nephron in acutely thyroparathyroidectomized rats. *Kidney Int 10:* 488, 1976.

209. Robinson, C. J., et al: Phosphaturic effect of thyrocalcitonin. *Lancet 2:* 83, 1966.

210. Rasmussen, H., et al: Thyrocalcitonin, EGTA and urinary electrolyte excretion. *J Clin Invest 46:* 746, 1967.

211. Bijvoet, O. L. M., Van der Sluys Veer, J., Jansen, A. P.: Effects of calcitonin on patients with Paget's disease, thyrotoxicosis, or hypercalcaemia. *Lancet 1:* 876, 1968.

212. Aldred, J. P., et al: Effects of porcine calcitonin on some urine electrolytes in the rat. *Acta Endocrinol 65:* 737, 1970.

213. Keller, R., et al: Natriuretic and diuretic effects of salmon calcitonin in rats. *Can J Physiol Pharmacol 48:* 838, 1970.

214. Nielson, S. P., et al: Acute effects of synthetic porcine calcitonins on the renal excretion of magnesium, inorganic phosphate, sodium and potassium. *J Endocrinol 51:* 455, 1971.

215. Sorensen, D. H., Hindberg, I.: The acute and prolonged effect of porcine calcitonin on urine electrolyte excretion in intact and parathyroidectomized rats. *Acta Endocrinol 70:* 295, 1972.

216. Barlet, J. P.: Effect of porcine, salmon and human calcitonin on urinary excretion of some electrolytes in sheep. *J Endocrinol 55:* 153, 1972.

217. Ardaillou, R., et al: Renal excretion of phosphate, calcium and sodium during and after a prolonged thyrocalcitonin infusion in man. *Proc Soc Exp Biol Med 131:* 56, 1969.

218. Martin, T. J., Melick, R. A.: The acute effects of porcine calcitonin in man. *Australas Ann Med 18:* 258, 1969.

219. Singer, F. R., et al: Some acute effects of administered porcine calcitonin in man. *Clin Sci 37:* 181, 1969.

220. Bijvoet, O. L. M., et al: Natriuretic effect of calcitonin in man. *N Engl J Med 284:* 681, 1971.

221. Paillard, F., et al: Renal effects of salmon calcitonin in man. *J Lab Clin Med 80:* 202, 1972.

222. Bijvoet, O. L. M., Van de Sluys Veer J.: The interpretation of laboratory tests in bone disease. *J Clin Endocrinol Metab 1:* 217, 1972.

223. Bijvoet, O. L. M., Froeling, P. G. A. M.: In Frame, B., Parfitt, A. M., Duncan, H. (eds): Clinical Aspects of Metabolic Bone Disease, Int Con Ser No 270. Amsterdam, Excerpta Medica, 1973, p 184.

224. Clark, J. D., Kenny, A. D.: Hog thyrocalcitonin in the dog: Urinary calcium, phosphorus, magnesium and sodium responses. *Endocrinology 84:* 1199, 1969.

225. Pak, C. Y. C., et al: Renal effects of porcine thyrocalcitonin in the dog. *Endocrinology 87:* 262, 1970.

226. Puschett, J. B., et al: Study of the renal tubular interaction of thyrocalcitonin, cyclic adenosine 3',5'-monophosphate, 25-hydroxycholecalciferol and calcium ion. *J Clin Invest 53:* 756, 1974.

227. Haas, H. G., et al: Renal effects of calcitonin and parathyroid extract in man. *J Clin Invest 50:* 2689, 1971.

228. Sorensen, O. H., et al: The renal effect of calcitonin in hypoparathyroid patients. *Acta Med Scand 191:* 103, 1972.

229. Marx, S. J., et al: Renal receptors for calcitonin, binding and degradation of the hormone. *J Biol Chem 248:* 4797, 1973.

230. Harrison, E. E., Harrison, H. C.: The renal excretion of inorganic phosphate in relation to the action of vitamin D and the parathyroid hormone. *J Clin Invest 20:* 47, 1941.

231. Gerkle, D., et al: The effect of vitamin D on renal inorganic phosphate reabsorption of normal rats, parathyroidectomized rats, and rats with rickets. *Pediatr Res 5:* 40, 1971.

232. Klein, R., Gow, R. C.: Interaction of parathyroid hormone and vitamin D on the renal excretion of phosphate. *J Clin Exp Med 13:* 271, 1953.

233. Morgan, D. B., et al: Osteomalacia after gastrectomy: A response to very small doses of vitamin D. *Lancet 2:* 1089, 1965.

234. Crawford, J. D., et al: Mechanism of renal tubular phosphate reabsorption and the influence thereon of vitamin D in completely parathyroidectomized rats. *Am J Physiol 180:* 156, 1955.

235. Ney, R. L., et al: Actions of vitamin D independent of the parathyroid glands. *Endocrinology 82:* 760, 1968.

236. Clark, I., Rivera-Cordero, F.: Effect of parathyroid function on absorption and excretion of calcium, magnesium and phosphate by rats. *Endocrinology 88:* 302, 1971.

237. Puschett, J. B., et al: Evidence for a direct action of cholecalciferol and 25 hydroxycholecalciferol on the renal transport of phosphate, sodium and calcium. *J Clin Invest 51:* 373, 1972.

238. Puschett, J. B., et al: The acute renal tubular effects of 1,25 dihydroxycholecalciferol. *Proc Soc Exp Biol Med 141:* 379, 1972.

239. Popvtzer, M. M., et al: The acute effect of 25 hydroxycholecalciferol on renal handling of phosphorus. *J Clin Invest 53:* 913, 1974.

240. Puschett, J. B., et al: Parathyroid hormone and 25 hydroxyvitamin D₃: Synergistic and antagonistic effects on renal phosphate transport. *Science 190:* 473, 1975.

241. Harrison, H. E., Harrison, H. C.: The interaction of vitamin D and parathyroid hormone on calcium, phosphorus and magnesium homeostasis. *Metabolism 13:* 952, 1964.

242. Arnaud, C., et al: Further studies on the interrelationship between parathyroid hormone and vitamin D. *J Clin Invest 45:* 1955, 1966.

243. Rasmussen, H., Feinblatt, J.: The relationship between the actions of vitamin D, parathyroid hormone and calcitonin. *Calcif Tissue Res 6:* 265, 1971.

244. Forte, L. R., et al: Renal adenylate cyclase and the interrelationship between parathyroid hormone and vitamin D in the regulation of urinary phosphate and adenosine cyclic 3', 5'-monophosphate excretion. *J Clin Invest 57:* 559, 1976.

245. Ney, R. L., et al: Action of parathyroid hormone in the vitamin D-deficient dog. *J Clin Invest 44:* 2003, 1965.

246. Cuche, J. L., et al: Intrarenal calcium in phosphate handling. *Am J Physiol 230:* 790, 1976.

247. Nagata, N., Rasmussen, H.: Parathyroid hormone and renal cell metabolism. *Biochemistry 7:* 3728, 1968.

248. Ikkos, D., et al: The effects of human growth hormone in man. *Acta Endocrinol 32:* 341, 1959.

249. Beck, J. C., et al: Primate growth hormone studies in man. *J Clin Invest 39:* 1223, 1960.

250. Henneman, P., et al: Effects of human growth hormone in man. *J Clin Invest 39:* 1223, 1960.

251. Corvilain, J., Abramow, M.: Some effects of human growth hormone on renal hemodynamics and on tubular phosphate transport in man. *J Clin Invest 41:* 1230, 1962.

252. Schwartz, E., et al: Estrogenic antagonism of metabolic effects of administered growth hormone. *J Clin Endocrinol Metab 29:* 1176, 1969.

253. Corvilain, J., Abramow, M.: Effect of growth hormone on tubular transport of phosphate in normal and parathyroidectomized dogs. *J Clin Invest 43:* 1608, 1964.

254. Dean, R. F. A., McCance, R. A.: Phosphate clearances in infants and adults. *J Physiol 107:* 182, 1948.

255. Donaldson, I. A., Nassim, J. R.: The artificial menopause with particular reference to the occurrence of spinal porosis. *Br Med J 1:* 1228, 1954.

256. Nassim, J. R., Saville, P. D., Mulligan, L.: The effect of stilbestrol on urinary phosphate excretion. *Clin Sci 15:* 367, 1956.

257. Aitken, J. M., et al: The effect of long-term mestranol administration on calcium and phosphorus homeostasis in oophorectomized women. *Clin Sci 41:* 233, 1971.

258. Riggs, B. L., et al: Quantitative evaluation of treatment for primary osteoporosis, in: International Symposium on Clinical Aspects of Metabolic Bone Disease. Amsterdam, Excerpta Medica, 1973.

259. Reifenstein, E. C., et al: Observations on the use of the serum phosphorus level as an index of pituitary growth hormone activity; the effect of estrogen therapy in acromegaly. *Endocrinology 39:* 71, 1946.

260. Schwartz, E., et al: Mechanism of estrogenic action in acromegaly. *J Clin Invest 48:* 260, 1969.

261. Frantz, A. G., Rabkin, M. T.: Effects of estrogen and sex difference on secretion of human growth hormone. *J Clin Endocrinol Metab 25:* 1470, 1965.

262. Aub, J. C., et al: Studies of calcium and phosphorus metabolism. III. Effects of thyroid hormone and thyroid disease. *J Clin Invest 7:* 97, 1929.

263. Robertson, J. D.: Calcium and phosphorus excretion in thyrotoxicosis and myxoedema. *Lancet 1:* 672, 1942.

264. Malamos, B., et al: The renal handling of phosphate in thyroid disease. *J Endocrinol 45:* 269, 1969.

265. Brommer, J., et al: Parathyroid activity in hyperthyroidism. *Cell Tissue Res 21 (Supp):* 288, 1976.

266. Cook, P. B., et al: Effect of thyrotoxicosis upon the metabolism of calcium, phosphorus and nitrogen. *Q J Med 28:* 505, 1959.

267. Parsons, V., Anderson, J.: The maximum renal tubular reabsorptive rate for inorganic phosphate in thyrotoxicosis. *Clin Sci 27:* 313, 1964.

268. Adams, P. H., et al: Effects of hyperthyroidism on bone and mineral metabolism in man. *Q J Med 36:* 1, 1967.

269. Bijvoet, O. L. M., et al (eds): Water and Electrolyte Metabolism II. Amsterdam, Elsevier, 1964, p 151.

270. Bortz, N., et al: Differentiation between thyroid and parathyroid causes of hypercalcemia. *Ann Intern Med 54:* 610, 1961.

271. Haden, R. M. G., et al: Phosphate excretion and parathyroid function in thyrotoxicosis. *J Endocrinol 28:* 281, 1964.

272. Beisel, W. R., et al: Phosphaturesis: A direct renal effect of triiodothyronine. *Am J Physiol 195:* 357, 1958.

273. Smith, D. A., Fraser, S. A., Wilson, G. M.: Hyperthyroidism and calcium metabolism. *J Clin Endocrinol Metab 2:* 33, 1973.

274. Bouillon, R., Demoor, P.: Parathyroid function in patients with hyper- or hypothyroidism. *J Clin Endocrinol Metab 38:* 999, 1974.

275. Goldsmith, R. S., et al: Primary role of plasma hydrocortisone concentration in the regulation of the normal forenoon pattern of urinary phosphate excretion. *J Clin Endocrinol Metab 25:* 1649, 1965.

276. Ingbar, S. H., et al: The effects of ACTH and cortisone on the renal tubular transport of uric acid, phosphorus and electrolytes in patients with normal renal and adrenal function. *J Lab Clin Med 38:* 533, 1951.

277. Roberts, R. E., Pitts, R. F.: The effects of cortisone and desoxycorticosterone on the renal tubular reabsorption of phosphate and the excretion of titratable acid and potassium in dogs. *Endocrinology 52:* 324, 1953.

278. Anderson, J., Foster, J. B.: The effect of cortisone on urinary phosphate excretion in man. *Clin Sci 18:* 437, 1959.

279. Elrick, H., et al: Effects of glucagon on renal function in man. *J Clin Endocrinol Metab 18:* 813, 1958.

280. Staub, A., et al: A renal action of glucagon. *Proc Soc Exp Biol Med 94:* 57, 1957.

281. DeFronzo, R. A., et al: The effect of insulin on renal handling of sodium, potassium, calcium and phosphate in man. *J Clin Invest 55:* 845, 1975.

282. Eisinger, A. J., et al: Effect of vasopressin on the renal excretion of phosphate in man. *Clin Sci 39:* 687, 1970.

283. Morey, E. R., Kenney, A. D.: Effects of catecholamines on urinary calcium and phosphorus in intact and parathyroidectomized rats. *Endocrinology 75:* 78, 1964.

284. Cuche, J., et al: Phosphaturic effect of dopamine in dogs. Possible role of intrarenally produced dopamine in phosphate regulation. *J Clin Invest 58:* 71, 1976.

285. Schneider, E. G., et al: Relationship between proximal sodium reabsorption and excretion of calcium, magnesium and phosphate. *Kidney Int 4:* 369, 1973.

286. Brodehl, J., Gellissen, K.: Die einfluss des angiotensins II auf die tubulare phosphatruck resorption beim Menschen. Ein beitrag zum wirkungsmechanismus des angiotensins. *Klin Wochenschr 44:* 1171, 1966.

287. Crawford, J. D., et al: The parathyroid glands and phosphate homeostasis. *J Clin Invest 29:* 1448, 1950.

288. Trohler, U., et al: Inorganic phosphate homeostasis. Renal adaptation to the dietary intake in intact and thyroparathyroidectomized rats. *J Clin Invest 57:* 264, 1976.

289. Drake, T. G., Albright, F., Castleman, B.: Parathyroid hyperplasia in rabbits produced by parenteral phosphate administration. *J Clin Invest 16:* 203, 1937.

290. Engfelt, B., et al: The parathyroid function in long-term dietary experiments. *Acta Endocrinol 15:* 119, 1954.

291. Malm, O. J.: On phosphates and phosphoric acid as dietary factors in the calcium balance of man. *Scand J Clin Lab Invest 5:* 75, 1957.

292. Edwards, N. A., Hodgkinson, A.: Metabolic studies in patients with idiopathic hypercalciuria. *Clin Sci 29:* 143, 1965.

293. Reiss, E., et al: The role of phosphate in the secretion of parathyroid hormone in man. *J Clin Invest 49:* 2146, 1970.

294. Jowsey, J., Balasubramaniam, P.: Effect of phosphate supplements on soft-tissue calcification and bone turnover. *Clin Sci 42:* 289, 1972.

295. Steele, T. H., DeLuca, H. F.: Influence of dietary phosphorus on renal phosphate reabsorption in the parathyroidectomized rat. *J Clin Invest 57:* 867, 1976.

296. McCrory, W. W., et al: Renal excretion of inorganic phosphate in newborn infants. *J Clin Invest 31:* 357, 1952.

297. Steele, T. H., et al: On the phosphatemic action of 1,25-dihydroxyvitamin D_3. *Am J Physiol 229:* 489, 1975.

298. Trohler, U., et al: Renal tubular adaptation to dietary phosphorus. *Nature 261:* 145, 1976.

299. Goldfarb, S., et al: Renal tubular effects of chronic phosphate depletion. *J Clin Invest 59:* 770, 1977.

300. Harter, H. R., et al: Effects of phosphate depletion and parathyroid hormone on renal glucose reabsorption. *Am J Physiol 227:* 1422, 1974.

301. Steele, T. H., et al: Renal resistance to parathyroid hormone during phosphorus deprivation. *J Clin Invest 58:* 1461, 1976.

302. Beck, N.: Effect of dietary phosphorus intake on renal actions of parathyroid hormone and cyclic AMP. (Abstr) *Kidney Int 10:* 487, 1976.

303. Emmett, M., et al: The pathophysiology of acid-base changes in chronically phosphate-depleted rats. *J Clin Invest 59:* 291, 1977.

304. Baylor, C. H., et al: The fate of intravenously administered calcium. Effect on urinary calcium and calcium–phosphorus balance. *J Clin Invest 29:* 1167, 1950.

305. Jackson, W. P. U., et al: Syndrome of steatorrhea, pseudohypoparathyroidism and amenorrhea. *J Clin Endocrinol Metab 16:* 1043, 1956.

306. Chambers, E. L., Jr. et al: Tests for hyperparathyroidism: Tubular reabsorption of phosphate, phosphate deprivation, and calcium infusion. *J Clin Endocrinol Metab 16:* 1517, 1956.

307. Hiatt, H. H., Thompson, D. D.: Some effects of intravenously administered calcium on inorganic phosphate metabolism. *J Clin Invest 36:* 573, 1957.

308. Levitt, M. F., et al: The effect of abrupt changes in plasma calcium concentration on renal function and electrolyte excretion in man and monkey. *J Clin Invest 37:* 294, 1958.

309. Bernstein, D., et al: Studies of the renal clearance of phosphate and the role of parathyroid glands in its regulation. *J Clin Endocrinol Metab 22:* 641, 1962.

310. Nordin, B. E. C., Fraser, R.: The effect of intravenous calcium on phosphate excretion. *Clin Sci 13:* 477, 1954.

311. Goldman, R., Bassett, S. H.: Effects of intravenous calcium gluconate upon the excretion of calcium and phosphorus in patients with idiopathic hypoparathyroidism. *J Clin Endocrinol Metab 14:* 278, 1954.

312. Verbanck, M., Toppet, N.: Study of the regulation of phosphorus metabolism in a hypoparathyroid patient. Effect of calcemia on the urinary excretion of phosphorus and on the variation in serum phosphorus. *Rev Fr Etud Clin Biol 6:* 239, 1961.

313. Howard, J. E., et al: On certain physiologic responses to intravenous injection of calcium salts into normal, hyperparathyroid and hypoparathyroid persons. *J Clin Endocrinol Metab 13:* 1, 1953.

314. Kyle, L. H., Schaaf, M., Erdman, L. A.: The metabolic effects of intravenous administration of calcium. *J Lab Clin Med 43:* 123, 1954.

315. Lavender, A. R., Pullman, T. N.: Changes in inorganic phosphate excretion induced by renal arterial infusion of calcium. *Am J Physiol 205:* 1025, 1963.

316. Hopkins, T., Howard, J. E., Eisenberg, H.: Ultrafiltration studies on calcium and phosphorus in human serum. *Bull J Hopkins Hosp 91:* 1, 1952.

317. Beck, N., et al: Direct inhibitory effect of hypercalcemia on renal actions of parathyroid hormone. *J Clin Invest 53:* 717, 1974.

318. Popovtzer, M. I., et al: Effect of Ca^{++} on renal handling of PO_4^+: Evidence for two reabsorptive mechanisms. *Am J Physiol 229:* 901, 1975.

319. Amiel, C., et al: Evidence for a parathyroid hormone-independent calcium modulation of phosphate transport along the nephron. *J Clin Invest 57:* 256, 1976.

320. Mercado, A., et al: On the mechanisms responsible for the phosphaturia of bicarbonate administration. *J Clin Invest 56:* 1386, 1975.

321. Pak, C. Y. C.: Parathyroid hormone and thyrocalcitonin: Their mode of action and regulation. *Ann NY Acad Sci 179:* 450, 1971.

322. Schussler, G. C., Verso, M. A., Nemoto, T.: Phosphaturia in hypercalcemic heart cancer patients. *J Clin Endocrinol Metab 35:* 497, 1972.

323. Estep, H. L., et al: Phosphate excretion patterns following intravenous injections of ethylenediaminetetraacetate (EDTA). *J Clin Endocrinol Metab 25:* 1385, 1965.

324. Black, D. A. K., Milne, M. D.: Experimental potassium depletion in man. *Clin Sci 11:* 397, 1952.

325. Mahler, R. F., Stanbury, S. W.: Potassium-losing renal disease. *Q J Med 25:* 21, 1956.

326. Anderson, D. C., et al: Association of hypokalemia and hypophosphatemia. *Br Med J 4:* 402, 1969.

327. Beck, N., Davis, B. B.: Impaired renal response to parathyroid hormone in potassium depletion. *Am J Physiol 228:* 179, 1975.

328. Smith, W., et al: Effect of magnesium depletion on renal function in the rat. *J Lab Clin Med 59:* 211, 1962.

329. Peterson, V. P.: Metabolic studies in clinical magnesium deficiency. *Acta Med Scand 173:* 285, 1963.

330. Whang, R., Welt, L. G.: Observation in experimental magnesium depletion. *J Clin Invest 42:* 305, 1963.

331. Shils, M. E.: Experimental human magnesium depletion. *Medicine 48:* 61, 1969.

332. Levi, J., et al: Hypocalcemia in magnesium depleted dogs. Evidence for reduced responsiveness to parathyroid hormone and relative failure of parathyroid gland function. *Metabolism 23:* 323, 1974.

333. Ginn, H. E., Shanbour, L. L.: Phosphaturia in magnesium-deficient rats. *Am J Physiol 212:* 1347, 1967.

334. Suh, S. M., et al: Pathogenesis of hypocalcemia and primary hypomagnesemia: Normal end-organ responsiveness to parathyroid hormone, impaired parathyroid gland function. *J Clin Invest 52:* 153, 1973.

335. Anast, C. S., et al: Impaired release of parathyroid hormone in magnesium deficiency. *J Clin Endocrinol Metab 42:* 707, 1976.

336. Rude, R. K., Oldham, S. B., Singer, F. R.: Functional hypoparathyroidism and parathyroid hormone end-organ resistance in human magnesium deficiency. *Clin Endocrinol 5:* 209, 1976.

337. Estep, H., et al: Hypocalcemia due to hypomagnesemia and reversible parathyroid hormone unresponsiveness. *J Clin Endocrinol Metab 29:* 812, 1969.

338. Hahn, T. J., et al: Effect of magnesium depletion and responsiveness to parathyroid hormone in parathyroidectomized rats. *J Clin Invest 51:* 886, 1972.

339. Chase, L. R., Slatopolsky, E.: Secretion and metabolic efficacy of parathyroid hormone in patients with severe hypomagnesemia. *J Clin Endocrinol Metab 38:* 363, 1974.

340. Massry, S. G., Coburn, J. W., Kleeman, C. R.: Evidence for suppression of parathyroid gland activity by hypermagnesemia. *J Clin Invest 49:* 1619–1629, 1970.

341. Frick, A.: Mechanism of inorganic phosphate diuresis secondary to saline infusions in the rat. *Pflugers Arch 313:* 106, 1969.

342. Frick, A.: Parathormone as a mediator of inorganic phosphate diuresis during saline infusion in the rat. *Pflugers Arch Eur J Physiol 325:* 1, 1971.

343. Maesaka, J. K., Levitt, M. F., Abramson, R. G.: Effect of saline infusion on phosphate transport in intact and thyroparathyroidectomized rats. *Am J Physiol 225:* 1421, 1973.

344. Blythe, W. B., Gittleman, H. J., Welt, L. G.: Effect of expansion of the extracellular space on the rate of urinary excretion of calcium. *Am J Physiol 214:* 52, 1968.

345. Massry, S. G., et al: The influence of extracellular volume expansion on renal phosphate reabsorption in the dog. *J Clin Invest 48:* 1237, 1969.

346. Hebert, C. S., et al: Decreased phosphate reabsorption by volume expansion in the dog. *Kidney Int 2:* 247, 1972.

347. Schneider, E. G., et al: Relationship between proximal sodium reabsorption and excretion of calcium, magnesium and phosphate. *Kidney Int 4:* 369, 1973.

348. Schneider, E. G., et al: Role of parathyroid hormone in the phosphaturia of extracellular fluid volume expansion. *Kidney Int 7:* 317, 1975.

349. Steele, T. H.: Increased urinary phosphate excretion following volume expansion in normal man. *Metabolism 19:* 128, 1970.

350. Kuntziger, H., et al: Phosphate handling by the rat nephron during saline diuresis. *Kidney Int 2:* 318, 1972.

351. Suki, W. N., et al: Effect of expansion of extracellular fluid volume on renal phosphate handling. *J Clin Invest 48:* 1888, 1969.

352. Spornitz, U. N., Frick, A.: Effects of saline infusion on calcium concentration in plasma ultrafiltrate and on the ultrastructure of the parathyroid glands of the rat. *Pflugers Arch Eur J Physiol 340:* 161, 1973.

353. Gradowska, L., et al: On the mechanism of the phosphaturia of extracellular fluid volume expansion in the dog. *Kidney Int 3:* 230, 1973.

354. Knox, F. G., et al: Proximal tubule reabsorption after hyperoncotic albumin infusion. *J Clin Invest 53:* 501, 1974.

355. Malvin, R. L., Lotspeich, W. D.: Relation between tubular transport of inorganic phosphate and bicarbonate in the dog. *Am J Physiol 187:* 51, 1956.

356. Mostellar, M. E., Tuttle, E. P. Jr.: The effects of alkalosis on plasma concentration and urinary excretion of inorganic phosphate in man. *J Clin Invest 43:* 138, 1964.

357. Fulop, M., Brazeau, P.: The phosphaturic effect of sodium bicarbonate and acetazolamide in dogs. *J Clin Invest 47:* 983, 1968.

358. Puschett, J. F., Goldberg, M.: The relationship between the renal handling of phosphate and bicarbonate in man. *J Lab Clin Med 73:* 956, 1969.

359. Webb, R. K., et al: Relationship between phosphaturia and acute hypercapnia in the rat. *J Clin Invest 60:* 829, 1977.

360. Haldane, J. B. S., Hill, R., Luck, J. M.: Calcium chloride acidosis. *J Physiol 57:* 301, 1923.

361. Martin, H. E., Jones, R.: The effect of ammonium chloride and sodium bicarbonate on the urinary excretion of magnesium, calcium and phosphate. *Am Heart J 62:* 206, 1961.

362. Glassman, V. P., et al: Effects of metabolic acidosis on proximal tubule ion reabsorption in dog kidney. *Am J Physiol 227:* 759, 1974.

363. Beck, N., et al: Effect of metabolic acidosis on renal action of parathyroid hormone. *Am J Physiol 228:* 1483, 1975.

364. Haldane, J. B. S., Wigglesworth, V. B., Woodrow, C. E.: The effect of reaction changes on human inorganic metabolism. *Proc R. Soc Med 96:* 1, 1924.

365. Giebisch, G., Berger, L., Pitts, R. F.: The extrarenal response to acute acid-base disturbances of respiratory origin. *J Clin Invest 34:* 231, 1955.

366. Freeman, S., Jacobson, A. B., Williamson, B. J.: Acid-base balance and removal of injected calcium from the circulation. *Am J Physiol 191:* 377, 1957.

367. Schwartz, W. B., Brackett, N. C. Jr., Cohen, J. J.: The response of extracellular hydrogen ion concentration to graded degrees of chronic hypercapnia: The physiologic limits of the defense of pH. *J Clin Invest 44:* 291, 1965.

368. Gray, S. P., Morris, J. E. W., Brooks, C. J.: Renal handling of calcium, magnesium, inorganic phosphate and hydrogen ions during prolonged exposure to elevated carbon dioxide concentrations. *Clin Sci Mol Med 45:* 751, 1973.

369. West, C. D., Rapaport, S.: Urinary excretion of phosphate following injection of sodium amino hippurate. *Proc Soc Exp Biol Med 71:* 322, 1949.

370. Gershberg, H.: Renal effects of parathyroid extract. *Trans NY Acad Sci 24:* 273, 1962.

371. Michael, A. F., Drammond, K. N.: Inhibitory effect of certain amino acids on renal tubular absorption of phosphate. *Can J Physiol Pharmacol 45:* 103, 1967.

372. Drammond, K. N., Michael, A. F.: Specificity of the inhibition of tubular phosphate reabsorption by certain amino acids. *Nature 201:* 1333, 1964.

373. Beck, N., et al: Inhibition of carbonic anhydrase by parathyroid hormone and cyclic AMP in rat renal cortex in vitro. *J Clin Invest 55:* 149, 1975.

374. Rodriguez, H. J., et al: Effects of acetazolamide on the urinary excretion of cyclic AMP and on the activity of renal adenyl cyclase. *J Clin Invest 55:* 122, 1974.

375. Massry, S. G., Friedler, R. M., Coburn, J. W.: Excretion of phosphate and calcium. *Arch Intern Med 131:* 828, 1973.

376. Barber, E. S., Elkington, J. R., Clark, J. K.: Studies on the renal excretion of magnesium in man. *J Clin Invest 38:* 1733, 1959.

377. Wesson, L. G.: Organic mercurial effects on renal tubular reabsorption of calcium and magnesium and on phosphate excretion in the dog. *J Lab Clin Med 59:* 630, 1962.

378. Eknoyan, G., Suki, W. N., Martinez-Maldonado, M.: Effect of diuretics on urinary excretion of phosphate, calcium and magnesium in thyroparathyroidectomized dogs. *J Lab Clin Med 76:* 257, 1970.

379. Duarte, C. G.: Effects of ethacrynic acid and furosemide on urinary calcium, phosphate and magnesium. *Metabolism 17:* 867, 1968.

380. Steinmuller, S. R., Puschett, J. B.: Effects of metolazone in man. *Kidney Int 1:* 169, 1972.

381. Puschett, J. B., Goldberg, M.: The acute effects of furosemide on acid and electrolyte excretion in man. *J Lab Clin Med 71:* 666, 1968.

382. Steele, T. H.: Dual effect of potent diuretics on renal handling of phosphate in man. *Metabolism 20:* 749, 1971.

383. Mudge, G. H., Foulks, J., Gilman, A.: Effect of urea diuresis on renal excretion of electrolytes. *Am J Physiol 158:* 218, 1949.

384. Seldin, D. W., Tarail, R.: Effect of hypertonic solutions on metabolism and excretion of electrolytes. *Am J Physiol 159:* 160, 1949.

385. Wesson, L. G. Jr.: Magnesium, calcium and phosphate excretion during osmotic diuresis in the dog. *J Lab Clin Med 60:* 422, 1962.

386. Maesaka, J. K., et al: Effect of mannitol on phosphate transport in intact and acutely thyroparathyroidectomized rats. *J Lab Clin Med 87:* 680, 1976.

387. Cook, B. S., Simmons, D. H.: Mannitol interference in phosphate determination: Method of correction. *J Lab Clin Med 60:* 160, 1962.

388. Pascale, L. R., Dubin, A., Hoffman, W. S.: Influence of Benemid on urinary excretion of phosphate in hypoparathyroidism. *Metabolism 3:* 462, 1954.

389. Garcia, D. A., Yendt, E. R.: The effects of probenecid and thiazides and their combination on the urinary excretion of electrolytes and on acid-base equilibrium. *Can Med Assoc J 103:* 473, 1970.

390. Schneider, R. W., Corcoran, A. C.: Familial nephrogenic osteopathy due to excessive tubular reabsorption of inorganic phosphate: A new syndrome and a novel mode of relief. *J Lab Clin Med 36:* 985, 1950.

391. Recker, R. R., et al: The hyperphosphatemic effect of disodium ethane-1-hydroxy-1,1-diphosphonate (EHDP): Renal handling of phosphorus and the renal response to parathyroid hormone. *J Lab Clin Invest 81:* 258, 1973.

392. Bijvoet, O. L. M., et al: Effect of a diphosphonate on para-articular ossification after total hip replacement. *Acta Orthop Scand 45:* 926, 1974.

393. Rosenblum, I. Y.: The effect of disodium ethane-1-hydroxy-1,1-diphosphonate (EHDP) on bone and serum chemistry in rabbits. *Calcif Tissue Res 16:* 145, 1974.

394. Walton, R. J., et al: Changes in the renal and extrarenal handling of phosphate induced by disodium etidronate (EHDP) in man. *Clin Sci Mol Med 49:* 45, 1975.

395. Bijvoet, O. L. M., et al: The renal phosphate threshold: Its evaluation and application in different clinical conditions, in de Graeff, J., Leynse, B. (eds): Water and Electrolyte Metabolism II. Amsterdam, Elsevier, 1974.

396. Kupfer, S., Kosovsky, J. D.: Effects of cardiac glycosides on renal tubular transport of calcium, magnesium, inorganic phosphate and glucose in the dog. *J Clin Invest 44:* 1132, 1965.

397. Singer, I., Rotenberg, D.: Mechanism of lithium action. *N Engl J Med 2389:* 254, 1973.

398. Arruda, J. A. L., et al: Lithium administration and phosphate excretion. *Am J Physiol 231:* 1140, 1976.

399. Spiegel, A. M., et al: Lithium does not inhibit the parathyroid hormone-mediated rise in urinary cyclic AMP and phosphate in humans. *J Clin Endocrinol Metab 43:* 1390, 1976.

400. DeVries, H. R., Bijvoet, O. L. M.: Results of prolonged treatment of Paget's disease of bone with disodium ethane-1-hydroxy-1,1-diphosphonate (EHDP). *Neth J Med 17:* 281, 1974.

401. Miller, W. L., Meyer, W. J., Bartter, F. C.: Intermittent hyperphosphatemia, polyuria and seizures—a new familial disorder. *J Pediatr 86:* 233, 1975.

402. Slatopolsky, E., et al: Control of phosphate excretion in uremic man. *J Clin Invest 47:* 1865, 1968.

403. Kleeman, C. R., et al: Calcium and phosphorus metabolism and bone disease in uremia. *Clin Orthop Relat Res 68:* 210, 1970.

404. Stanbury, S. W., et al: Elective subtotal parathyroidectomy for renal hyperparathyroidism. *Lancet 1:* 793, 1960.

405. Smith, M. S., Feldman, K. W., Furukawa, C. T.: Coma in an infant due to hypertonic sodium phosphate medication. *J Pediatr 82:* 481, 1973.

406. Levitt, M., Gessert, C., Finberg, L.: Inorganic phosphate (laxative) poisoning resulting in tetany in an infant. *J Pediatr 82:* 479, 1973.

407. Beaton, J. R., Orme, T.: Phosphorus and lactic acid metabolism in the hypothermic rat. *Can J Biochem Physiol 39:* 1267, 1961.

408. Zusman, J., Brown, D. M., Nesbit, M. E.: Hyperphosphatemia, hyperphosphaturia and hypocalcemia in acute lymphoblastic leukemia. *N Engl J Med 289:* 1335, 1973.

409. Armata, J., Depowska, T.: Hyperphosphatemia and hypocalcemia in neoplastic disorders. *N Engl J Med 290:* 858, 1974.

410. Brereton, H. D., et al: Hyperphosphatemia and hypocalcemia in Burkitt's lymphoma. *Arch Intern Med 135:* 307, 1975.

411. Alfrey, A. C., et al: Extraosseous calcification. Evidence for abnormal pyrophosphate metabolism in uremia. *J Clin Invest 57:* 692, 1976.

412. Baker, L. R. I., et al: Iatrogenic osteomalacia and myopathy due to phosphate depletion. *Br Med J 3:* 150, 1974.

413. Stanbury, S. W., Lumb, G. A.: Calcium, phosphorus and nitrogen metabolism in rickets, osteomalacia, and hyperparathyroidism complicating chronic uremia and in the osteomalacia of the adult Fanconi syndrome. *Medicine 41:* 1, 1962.

414. Scriver, C.R.: Rickets and the pathogenesis of impaired tubular transport of phosphate and other solutes. *Am J Med 57:* 43, 1974.

415. Keating, J. P., et al: Hypophosphatemia in Reye's syndrome. *Lancet 2:* 39, 1975.

416. Cooperstock, M. S., et al: Possible pathogenic role of endotoxin in Reye's syndrome. *Lancet 1:* 1272, 1975.

417. Reye, R. D. K., et al: Encephalopathy and fatty degeneration of the viscera. A disease entity in childhood. *Lancet 2:* 749, 1963.

418. Salassa, R. M., et al: Hypophosphatemic osteomalacia associated with "nonendocrine" tumors. *N Engl J Med 283:* 65, 1970.

419. Stanbury, S. W.: Osteomalacia. *Clin Endocrinol Metab 1:* 239, 1972.

420. Linovitz, R. J., et al: Tumor-induced osteomalacia and rickets: A surgically curable syndrome. *J Bone Joint Surg 58A:* 419, 1976.

421. Bishop, M. C., Ledingham, J. G. C., Oliver, D. O.: Phosphate deficiency in hemodialyzed patients. *Proc Eur Dial Transplant Assoc 8:* 106.

422. Ahmed, K. Y., et al: Persistent hypophosphatemia and osteomalacia in dialysis patients not on oral phosphate-binders: Response to dihydrotachysterol therapy. *Lancet 2:* 439, 1976.

423. Pierides, A. M., et al: Phosphate-deficiency osteomalacia during regular hemodialysis. *Lancet 2:* 746, 1976.

424. Rapaport, S., et al: The effect of voluntary overbreathing on the electrolyte equilibrium of arterial blood in man. *J Biol Chem 163:* 411, 1946.

425. Okel, B. B., Hurst, J. W.: Prolonged hyperventilation in man. Associated electrolyte changes and subjective symptoms. *Arch Intern Med 108:* 757, 1961.

426. Tulin, M., et al: The distribution and movements of inorganic phosphate between cells and serum of human blood. *Am J Physiol 149:* 678, 1947.

427. Reidler, G. F., Scheitlin, W. A.: Hypophosphatemia in septicemia: Higher incidence in gram-negative than in gram-positive infections. *Br Med J 1:* 753, 1969.

428. Fiske, C. H.: Inorganic phosphate and acid excretion in the postabsorptive period. *J Biol Chem 49:* 171, 1921.

429. Forsham, P. H., Thorn, G. W.: Changes in inorganic serum phosphorus during the intravenous glucose tolerance test as an adjunct to the diagnosis of early diabetes mellitus. *Proc Am Diab Assoc 9:* 101, 1949.

430. Harrold, G. A. Jr., Benedict, E. M.: The participation of the inorganic substances in carbohydrate metabolism. *J Biol Chem 59:* 683, 1924.

431. Annino, J. S., Relman, A. S.: The effect of eating on some of the clinically important chemical constituents of the blood. *Am J Clin Pathol 31:* 155, 1959.

432. Guillou, P. J., et al: Hypophosphatemia: A complication of "innocuous dextrose-saline." *Lancet 2:* 710, 1976.

433. Miller, M., et al: Metabolism of intravenous fructose and glucose in normal and diabetic subjects. *J Clin Invest 31:* 115, 1952.

434. Gunderson, K., et al: Serum phosphorus and potassium levels after intravenous administration of glucose. *N Engl J Med 250:* 547, 1954.

435. Danowski, T. S., et al: Sodium, potassium and phosphate in the cell and serum of blood in diabetic acidosis. *Am J Physiol 149:* 667, 1947.

436. Franks, M., et al: Metabolic studies in diabetic acidosis: II. The effect of the administration of sodium phosphate. *Arch Intern Med 81:* 42, 1948.

437. Nabarro, J. D., et al: Metabolic studies in severe diabetic ketosis. *Q J Med 21:* 225, 1952.

438. Alberti, K. G. M. M., et al: 2,3-Diphosphoglycerate and tissue oxygenation in uncontrolled diabetes mellitus. *Lancet 2:* 391, 1972.

439. Bolliger, A., Hartman, F. W.: Observations on blood phosphates as related to carbohydrate metabolism. *J Biol Chem 64:* 91, 1925.

440. Pollack, H., et al: Serum phosphate changes induced by injections of glucose into dogs under various conditions. *Am J Physiol 110:* 117, 1934.

441. Cori, C. F., Cori, G. T.: Fate of glucose and other sugars in the eviscerated animal. *Proc Soc Exp Biol Med 26:* 432, 1928–1929.

442. Smith, L. H., et al: A comparison of the metabolism of fructose and glucose in hepatic disease and diabetes mellitus. *J Clin Invest 32:* 273, 1953.

443. Danowski, T. S., et al: Significance of blood sugar and serum

electrolyte changes in cirrhosis following glucose, insulin, glucagon, or epinephrine. *Yale J Biol Med 29:* 361, 1956–1957.

444. Danowski, T. S., et al: Muscular dystrophy V. Blood sugar and serum electrolytes following insulin and dextrose, alone or in combination. *Am J Dis Child 91:* 429, 1956.

445. McArdle, B.: Myopathy due to a defect in muscle glycogen breakdown. *Clin Sci 10:* 13, 1951.

446. Groen, J., et al: Effects of glucose administration on the potassium and inorganic phosphate content of the blood serum and the electrocardiogram in normal individuals and in nondiabetic patients. *Acta Med Scand 141:* 352, 1952.

447. Kay, H. D., Robison, R.: Role of phosphates in carbohydrate metabolism. *Biochem J 18:* 1139, 1924.

448. Hill, G. L., et al: Phosphorus distribution in hyperalimentation-induced hypophosphatemia. *J Surg Res 20:* 527, 1976.

449. Atchley, D. W., et al: On diabetic acidosis: A detailed study of electrolyte balances following the withdrawal and reestablishment of insulin therapy. *J Clin Invest 12:* 297, 1933.

450. Butler, A. M., et al: Metabolic studies on diabetic coma. *Trans Assoc Am Physiol 40:* 102, 1947.

451. Guest, G. M., Rapoport, S.: Electrolytes of blood plasma and cells in diabetic acidosis and during recovery. *Proc Am Diab Assoc 7:* 95, 1947.

452. Guest, G. M., Rapoport, S.: Role of acid-soluble phosphorus compounds in red blood cells. *Am J Dis Child 58:* 1072, 1939.

453. Guest, G. M., Rapoport, S.: Clinical studies of the organic acid-soluble phosphorus of red blood cells in different acidotic states. *J Lab Clin Med 26:* 190, 1940.

454. Cohen, J. J., et al: Renal tubular reabsorption of acetoacetate, inorganic sulfate and inorganic phosphate in the dog as affected by glucose and phlorizin. *Am J Physiol 184:* 91, 1956.

455. Harter, H. R., et al: The relative roles of calcium, phosphorus, and parathyroid hormone in glucose- and tolbutamide-mediated insulin release. *J Clin Invest 58:* 359, 1976.

456. Stein, J. N., et al: Hypophosphatemia in acute alcoholism. *Am J Med Sci 252:* 78, 1966.

457. Oberhauser, E., et al: Further studies on intestinal absorption in liver cirrhosis, using an intraintestinal reference substance. *Am J Dig Dis 7:* 699, 1962.

458. Corredor, D. G., et al: Enhanced post glucose hypophosphatemia during starvation therapy of obesity. *Metabolism 18:* 754, 1969.

459. Wallach, S., et al: Plasma and erythrocyte magnesium in health and disease. *J Lab Clin Med 59:* 195, 1962.

460. Lim, P., Jacob, E.: Magnesium status of alcoholic patients. *Metabolism 21:* 1045, 1972.

461. Matter, B. J., et al: Effect of ethanol on phosphate excretion in man. *Clin Res 12:* 255, 1965.

462. Derr, R., Zieve, L.: Intracellular distribution of phosphate in the underfed rat developing weakness and coma following total parenteral nutrition. *J Nutr 106:* 1398, 1976.

463. Rudman, D., et al: Elemental balances during intravenous hyperalimentation of underweight adult subjects. *J Clin Invest 55:* 94, 1974.

464. Sheldon, G. F., Grzyb, S.: Phosphate depletion and repletion: Relation to parenteral nutrition and oxygen transport. *Ann Surg 182:* 683, 1975.

465. Muldowney, F. P., et al: Parathormone-like effect of magnesium replenishment in steatorrhea. *N Engl J Med 282:* 61, 1970.

466. Rose, I. A., Warms, J. V. B.: Control of glycolysis in the human red blood cell. *J Biol Chem 241:* 4848, 1966.

467. Lichtman, M. A., et al: Erythrocyte adenosine triphosphate depletion during hypophosphatemia in a uremic subject. *N Engl J Med 280:* 240, 1969.

468. Travis, S. F., et al: Alterations of red-cell glycolytic intermediates and oxygen transport as a consequence of hypophosphatemia in patients receiving intravenous hyperalimentation. *N Engl J Med 285:* 763, 1971.

469. Lichtman, M. A., et al: Reduced red cell glycolysis, 2,3-diphosphoglycerate and adenosine triphosphate concentration and increased hemoglobin oxygen affinity caused by hypophosphatemia. *Ann Intern Med 74:* 562, 1971.

470. Yawata, Y., et al: Blood cell abnormalities complicating the hypophosphatemia of hyperalimentation: Erythrocyte and platelet ATP deficiency associated with hemolytic anemia and bleeding in hyperalimented dogs. *J Lab Clin Med 84:* 643, 1974.

471. Niehaus, W. G.: Mode of orthophosphate uptake and ATP labelling by mammalian cells. *Biochim Biophys Acta 443:* 515, 1976.

472. Jacob, H. S., Amsden, P.: Acute hemolytic anemia with rigid red cells in hypophosphatemia. *N Engl J Med 285:* 1446, 1971.

473. Klock, J. C., et al: Hemolytic anemia and somatic cell dysfunction in severe hypophosphatemia. *Arch Intern Med 134:* 360, 1974.

474. Nakao, M., et al: Adenosine triphosphate and shape of erythrocytes. *J Biochem 49:* 487, 1961.

475. Weed, R. I., et al: Metabolic dependence of red cell deformability. *J Clin Invest 48:* 795, 1969.

476. Benesch, R., Benesch, R. E.: Intracellular organic phosphates as regulators of oxygen release by hemoglobin. *Nature 221:* 618, 1969.

477. Rajan, K. S., et al: Hepatic hypoxia secondary to hypophosphatemia. *Clin Res 23(3):* 521, 1973.

478. Oski, F. A., et al: The role of the left-shifted or right-shifted oxygen-hemoglobin equilibrium curve. *Ann Intern Med 74:* 44, 1971.

479. Craddock, P. R., et al: Acquired phagocyte dysfunction. A complication of the hypophosphatemia of parenteral hyperalimentation. *N Engl J Med 290:* 1403, 1974.

480. Garner, G. B., et al: Dietary phosphorus and salmonellosis in guinea pigs. *Fed Proc 26:* 799, 1967.

481. Lotz, M., et al: Osteomalacia and debility resulting from phosphorus depletion. *Trans Assoc Am Physiol 77:* 281, 1964.

482. Dent, C. E., Winter, C. S.: Osteomalacia due to phosphate depletion from excessive aluminium hydroxide ingestion. *Br Med J 1:* 551, 1974.

483. Day, H. J., McCollum, E. V.: Mineral metabolism, growth and symptomatology of rats on a diet extremely deficient in phosphorus. *J Biol Chem 130:* 269, 1939.

484. Thomasset, M., et al: Bone resorption measurement with unusual bone markers: Critical evaluation of the method in phosphorus-deficient and calcium-deficient growing rats. *Calcif Tissue Res 21:* 1, 1976.

485. Cuisinier-Gleizes, P., et al: Phosphorus deficiency, parathyroid hormone and bone resorption in the growing rat. *Calcif Tissue Res 20:* 235, 1976.

486. Baylink, D., et al: Formation, mineralization and resorption of bone in hypophosphatemic rats. *J Clin Invest 50:* 2519, 1971.

487. Bruin, W. J., et al: Acute inhibition of mineralization and stimulation of bone resorption mediated by hypophosphatemia. *Endocrinology 96:* 394, 1975.

488. Coburn, J. W., Massry, S. G.: Changes in serum and urinary calcium during phosphate deprivation: Studies on mechanisms. *J Clin Invest 49:* 1073, 1970.

489. Eisenberg, E.: Effects of varying phosphate intake in primary hyperparathyroidism. *J Clin Endocrinol Metab 23:* 651, 1968.

490. Stoerk, H. C., Carnes, W. H.: The relation of the dietary Ca:P ratio to serum calcium and to parathyroid volume. *J Nutr 29:* 43, 1945.

491. Baxter, L. E., DeLuca, H. F.: Stimulation of 25-hydroxyvitamin D_3-1α-hydroxylase by phosphate depletion. *J Biol Chem 251:* 3158, 1976.

492. Hughes, M. R., et al: Regulation of serum 1α,25-dihydroxyvitamin D_3 by calcium and phosphate in the rat. *Science 190:* 578, 1975.

493. Edelstein, S., et al: The functional metabolism of vitamin D in chicks fed low-calcium and low-phosphorus diets. *Biochim Biophys Acta 385:* 438, 1975.

494. Tanaka, Y., DeLuca, H. F.: The control of 25-hyroxyvitamin D_3 metabolism by inorganic phosphate. *Arch Biochem Biophys 154:* 566, 1973.

495. Morrissey, R. L., Wasserman, R. H.: Calcium absorption and calcium-binding protein in chicks on differing calcium and phosphorus intakes. *Am J Physiol 220:* 1509, 1971.

496. Tanaka, Y., Frank, H., DeLuca, H. F.: Intestinal calcium transport: Stimulation by low phosphorus diets. *Science 181:* 564, 1973.

497. Bar, A., Wasserman, R. H.: Control of calcium absorption and intestinal calcium-binding protein synthesis. *Biochem Biophys Res Commun 54:* 191, 1973.

498. Castillo, L., et al: The mobilization of bone mineral by 1,25-dihydroxyvitamin D_3 in hypophosphatemic rats. *Endocrinology 97:* 995, 1975.

499. Ribovich, M. L., DeLuca, H. F.: The influence of dietary calcium and phosphorus on intestinal calcium transport in rats given vitamin D metabolities. *Arch Biochem Biophys 170:* 529, 1975.

500. Raisz, L. G., Niemann, I.: Effect of phosphate, calcium and magnesium on bone resorption and hormonal responses in tissue culture. *Endocrinology 85:* 446, 1969.

501. Asher, M. A., et al: The effect of inorganic phosphate on the rates

of collagen formation and degradation in bone and cartilage in tissue culture. *J Clin Endocrinol Metab 38:* 376, 1974.

502. Gold, L., Massry, S. G., Friedler, R. M.: Effect of phosphate depletion on renal glucose reabsorption (Abstr) *Clin Res 24:* 400A, 1976.

503. Ginsburg, J. M.: Effect of glucose and free fatty acid on phosphate transport in dog kidney. *Am J Physiol 222:* 1153, 1972.

504. Gold, L. W., et al: Renal bicarbonate wasting during phosphate depletion. A possible cause of altered acid base homeostasis in hyperthyroidism. *J Clin Invest 52:* 2256, 1973.

505. O'Donovan, D. J., Lotspeich, W. D.: Activation of kidney mitochondrial glutaminase by inorganic phosphate and organic acids. *Nature 212:* 930, 1966.

506. Boelens, P. A., et al: Hypophosphatemia with muscle weakness due to antacids and hemodialysis. *Am J Dis Child 120:* 350, 1970.

507. Silvis, S. E., Paragas, P. U., Jr.: Paresthesias, weakness, seizures and hypophosphatemia in patients receiving hyperalimentation. *Gastroenterology 62:* 513, 1972.

508. Prins, J. G., Schrijver, H., Staghouwer, J. H.: Hyperalimentation, hypophosphatemia and coma. *Lancet 1:* 1253, 1973.

509. Weintraub, M. I., Chakravorty, H. P.: Nutrient deficiencies after intensive parenteral alimentation. *N Engl J Med 291:* 799, 1974.

510. Moser, C. R., Fessel, W. J.: Rheumatic manifestations of hypophosphatemia. *Arch Intern Med 134:* 674, 1974.

511. Furlan, A. J., et al: Acute areflexic paralysis. Association with hyperalimentation and hypophosphatemia. *Arch Neurol 32:* 706, 1975.

512. Fuller, T. J., et al: Reversible changes of the muscle cell in experimental phosphorus deficiency. *J Clin Invest 57:* 1019, 1976.

513. Newman, J. H., Neff, T. A., Ziporin, P.: Acute respiratory failure associated with hypophosphatemia. *N Engl J Med 296:* 1101, 1977.

514. Knochel, J. R., et al: The muscle cell in chronic alcoholism. The possible role of phosphate depletion in alcoholic myopathy. *Ann NY Acad Sci 252:* 274, 1975.

515. O'Connor, L. R., Wheeler, W. S., Bethune, J. E.: Effect of hypophosphatemia on myocardial performance in man. *N Engl J Med 297:* 901, 1977.516.

516. Scarpa, A., Carafoli, E. (eds): Calcium transport and cell function. *Ann NY Acad Sci 307:* 1–655, 1978.

517. Bijvoet, O. L. M., Morgan, D. B.: In Hioco, D. J. (ed): Phosphate et Métabolisme Phosphocalcique. Paris, L'Expansion Scientifique Française, 1971, p. 153.

41

Anatomy of the Parathyroid Glands

S. I. Roth

Though Askanazy and Virchow recognized the parathyroid glands in humans, the first thorough description of the parathyroid glands was by Sandström.[1] Weller's[2] first studies of human embryonic parathyroid glands were followed by Norris's[3] extensive, complete, and well-documented study. Norris divided the embryonic development of the parathyroid glands into five overlapping stages; preprimordial, early primordial, branchial complex, isolation, and definitive-form stages.

During the time between the development of the foregut and the earliest appearance of the parathyroid anlage (the preprimordial stage), the third and fourth gill pouches develop in the embryo with a crown-rump length (C-R) of 4–9 mm. After the pouches contact the ectoderm of the branchial cleft they extend ventrally. In the 8–9 mm (C-R) embryo, the early primordial stage is defined when the parathyroid anlage is clearly recognizable. Parathyroid III* begins as a localized proliferation of large (7–12 mμ in diameter) polyhedral cells with well-defined borders and clear cytoplasm within the wall of the cephalic portion of the third pouch. Parathyroid IV begins as a solid nodule of similar cells on the dorsal part of the fourth pouch extending laterally and anteroposteriorly. This stage ends when the parathyroid glands are elongate columnar bodies similar to the developing thyroid in size and form.

In the 13 mm (C-R) embryo, the branchial complex stage occurs when the third and fourth gill pouches sever their connection to the pharynx but still remain joined to one another as bilobed bodies representing thymus III, parathyroid III, parathyroid IV, and what Norris[3] called the lateral thyroid or ultimobranchial body. Branchial complex III is more lateral and cranial than complex IV. At this point the medial thyroid extends laterally and craniocaudad as a flat plate between branchial complexes III and IV. Thymus III grows more rapidly and extends more caudally than parathyroid III. As the heart descends into the thorax, it pulls the thymus and parathyroid III caudally. In the 15 mm (C-R) embryo the reticulo-cellular pattern characteristic of the parathyroid gland begins to develop and the closely packed cells separate into islands. Parathyroid III usually separates from thymus III and frequently ceases its migration near the lower pole of the thyroid in the 18 mm (C-R) embryo. In some cases the parathyroid remains joined with the thymus and is found in the adult in the cephalad tongue of thymus or as a mediastinal structure embedded in the thymus. Parathyroid IV remains almost stationary and attached to the ultimobranchial body by a thin stalk which finally separates

after the incorporation into the thyroid gland of the ultimobranchial body in the 18–20 mm embryo.

The isolation stage represents the period when the paired components of the branchial complexes separate from each other and the parathyroid glands are in their adult position: parathyroid III at the level of the lower pole of the thyroid, and parathyroid IV at the dorsal or dorsomedial aspect of the lateral lobe of the thyroid posteriorly. The definitive-form stage essentially covers alteration in the shape and size of the glands from a globular form to the ultimate form determined by the adjacent structures, a flattened ellipsoid.

The gland grows linearly in volume by an increase in the number of cells until birth (Fig. 41-1). Norris[4] felt that histologic changes seen during fetal life were consistent with evidence of prenatal function. Ultrastructural studies[5,6] have also supported this contention. After birth the growth of the glands continues briskly until the third or fourth decade when it levels off (Fig. 41-2).

Although between two and eight parathyroid glands have been reported in humans, [3,9–14] Norris[3] noted at least four glands in all embryos studied and Zoli and Morase[14] noted four or more glands in all but one of 31 patients studied. Accessory glands arising from division of the four main glands were seen in 2 percent of embryos studied by Norris.[3] Accessory glands were found by Boyd[9] in 2 to 6.5 percent of embryos, by Gilmour[10] in 3 of 14 fetuses serially sectioned, and by Millzner[12] in 36 of 42 cases of adult neck dissections. Thus, evidence suggests that almost all humans have at least four parathyroid glands.

The upper, or superior, gland (parathyroid IV) is usually located at or near the point where the middle thyroid artery crosses the recurrent laryngeal nerve, and is supplied by the inferior thyroid artery or more rarely by the superior thyroid artery. The gland may be attached to the posterior thyroid capsule or, on rare occasions, embedded in the thyroid. It may lie as medial as the laryngeal-esophageal groove or it may lie posterior to the esophagus.

The lower or inferior gland (parathyroid III) usually lies just below the lower pole of the thyroid gland in the interstitial tissue lateral to the trachea and is supplied by the inferior thyroid artery. Parathyroid III is almost invariably associated with thymic remnants. The location of parathyroid III is more variable than that of parathyroid IV and may be anywhere from cephalad and lateral to parathyroid IV, in the carotid sheath or in the anterior mediastinum as low as the pericardium.

The adult glands measure approximately 6 × 4 × 2 mm each, are flattened ellipsoids, and vary from a dark tan to a yellow-grey-tan depending upon fat content.

In children the parathyroid glands are composed of uniform sheets and cords of chief cells, with few mature fat cells in the

These studies were supported in part by U.S.P.H.S. grant CA-18616.

*The Roman numerals indicate the branchial pouch of origin of a particular parathyroid gland. Because the parathyroid glands are usually bilaterally symmetrical, only the singular will be used.

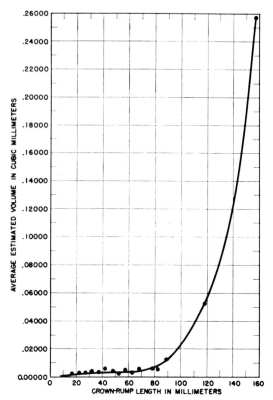

Fig. 41-1. Growth curve based upon the average estimated volume in cubic millimeters of the parathyroid tissue of 374 human embryos and fetuses plotted against body length in millimeters. The averages were determined for all of the individuals included within groups corresponding to an increase of 5 mm in body length. (From Norris.[4])

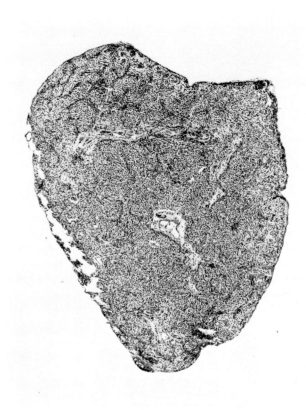

Fig. 41-3. Normal parathyroid from a 9-day-old infant. A moderate amount of fat-free stroma is present between uniform sheets and cords of chief cells. Hematoxylin and eosin. X55.

stroma (Fig. 41-3). The chief cells are divided by capillaries into cords. The only alterations in histology of the parathyroid glands in infants and children is at puberty, when an increase in the highly vascular reticular connective tissues isolates the chief cells into nests and cords. Increasing numbers of stromal fat cells appear, the number increasing throughout life (Figs. 41-2, 41-4, 41-5, and 41-6) until in older persons fat cells may occupy 60 to 70 percent of the volume of the parathyroid gland.[15-17] The numbers of fat cells may also be modified by the nutritional status of the patient. The most common cell is the chief cell, which is responsible for the synthesis and secretion of parathyroid hormone.[18] It is 4–8 μm in diameter, with an easily identifiable cell membrane, a centrally located small nucleus with dark dense chromatin, and an ampho-

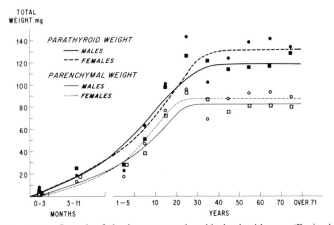

Fig. 41-2. Growth of the human parathyroid gland with age. (Derived from data of Gilmour and Martin.[7])

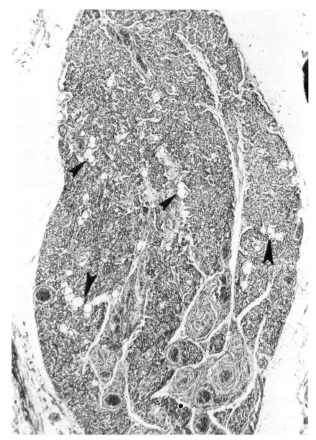

Fig. 41-4. Normal parathyroid gland from a 27-year-old man with a few stromal fat cells (arrows). Hematoxylin and eosin. X46.

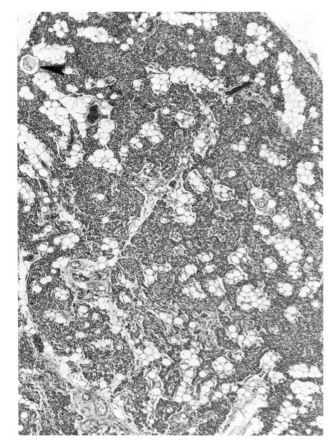

Fig. 41-5. Normal parathyroid gland from a 58-year-old man. The stromal fat cells are abundant. Hematoxylin and eosin. X46.

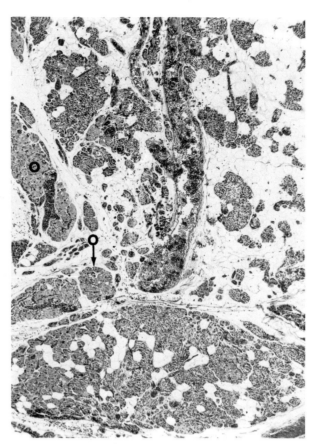

Fig. 41-7. Photomicrograph of groups of oxyphil cells (O) with brightly eosinophilic granular cytoplasm and small pyknotic nuclei in a 79-year-old woman. Hematoxylin and eosin. X46.

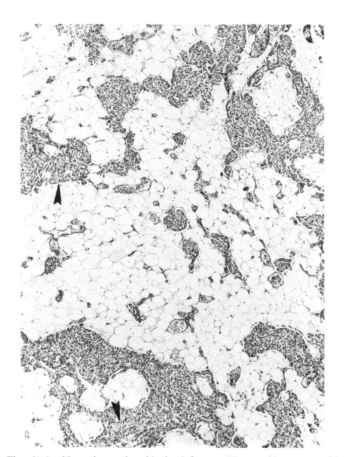

Fig. 41-6. Normal parathyroid gland from a 79-year-old woman with abundant stromal fat occupying more than 50 percent of the gland volume. Oxyphil cells (arrows) are present in nodules. Hematoxylin and eosin. X46.

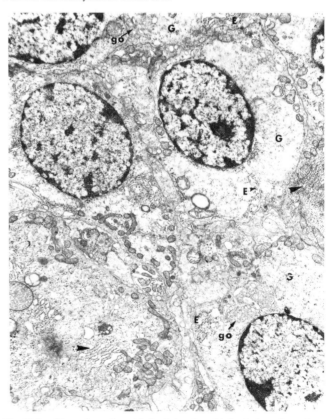

Fig. 41-8. Normal parathyroid gland showing chief cells in various phases of activity. There are inactive cells with abundant glycogen (G), and dispersed granular endoplasmic reticulum (E). Other cells entering the active phase show enlarging Golgi apparatuses (go). Aggregates of granular endoplasmic reticulum (arrows) indicate synthesis of hormone. Lead citrate and uranyl acetate. X10,000. (From Roth.[8])

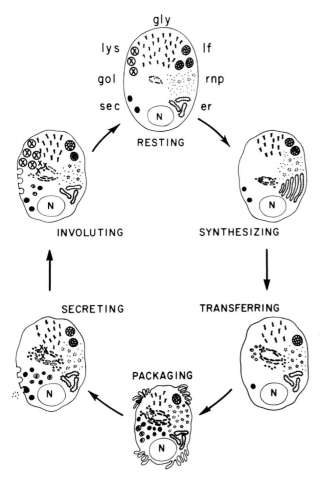

Fig. 41-9. Diagram of the chief cell cycle of the parathyroid gland.

Resting phase: The chief cells are large with relatively straight cell membranes, abundant glycogen (gly) and lipid and lipofuscin bodies (lf). The profiles of granular endoplasmic reticulum (er) are dispersed. The free ribonucleoprotein particles (rnp) are largely dispersed. The Golgi apparatus (gol) is small, with few vesicles and vacuoles, and free of acid phosphatase. There are relatively few peripherally located secretory granules (s) and acid-phosphatase-positive ($\bigotimes$) lysosomes (lys).

Synthesizing phase: The chief cells are somewhat reduced in size, with somewhat increased tortuosity of the cell membranes due to a mild reduction in glycogen and lipid content. The Golgi apparatus begins to enlarge, with a few vacuoles and vesicles. Lysosomes are absent. The granular endoplasmic reticulum aggregates into parallel arrays and stacks.

Transferring phase: The chief cells further decrease in size, with a further increase in cell membrane tortuosity. The glycogen and lipid are further decreased. The ribosomes are more frequently in aggregates. The granular endoplasmic reticulum disperses, and the Golgi apparatus further increases in size, with more vacuoles and vesicles. Secretory granules are further decreased.

Packaging phase: The cells are at a minimum dimension, with maximum tortuosity of the cell membranes. The glycogen and lipid are at a minimum, and the Golgi apparatus is at its maximum size and complexity, with numerous vacuoles and vesicles and numerous prosecretory granules. The free ribonucleoprotein particles have their maximum aggregation into spirals and rosettes.

Secreting phase: The cells begin to increase in size, with reaccumulation of glycogen and lipid. The ribonucleoprotein particles begin to disperse. With the involution of the Golgi apparatus, acid phosphatase ($\bigotimes$) begins to appear in the Golgi profiles. The mature secretory granules move away from the Golgi toward the cell periphery, where their membranes fuse with the cell membranes and empty the hormone into the extracellular space.

Involuting phase: The cells continued to enlarge with further accumulation of lipid and glycogen. The free ribonucleoprotein particles continue

philic cytoplasm (Fig. 41-7). Except in the most ideally fixed preparations the light and dark varieties are difficult to distinguish. The cells sometimes take on a follicular arrangement with eosinophilic colloidlike material in the lumens in old age; this colloidlike material has been shown to contain amyloid. Lymphatics have been described in the human parathyroid gland.

Two ultrastructural types of chief cells have been described in the normal human parathyroid gland. The active chief cells[18] contain large prominent Golgi apparatuses composed of parallel arrays of agranular membranes with numerous vesicles, vacuoles, and small membrane-limited granules, which might be prosecretory granules. Rare secretory granules and lysosomelike bodies are present. The endoplasmic reticulum consisted of parallel arrays of granular membranes. Inactive or resting chief cells (Fig. 41-8) had abundant glycogen, lipofuscin, and Golgi apparatuses with few vacuoles and vesicles, and a few clusters or individual membrane-limited secretory granules. Inactive or resting cells outnumber cells in the active stages by a ratio of 3–5:1 in the normal human parathyroid gland, and a ratio of 10:1 under chronic calcium suppression.[19] These two stages have been found to correspond to a continuum of stages of synthesis and secretory activity (Fig. 41-9) seen in animal glands.[20,21] The dispersed sacs of granular endoplasmic reticulum aggregate into the large arrays of flattened sacs. It is presumed that it is during this first active phase that large quantities of proparathyroid hormone are synthesized. Transfer of the hormone to the Golgi region then occurs, where it is packaged into the secretory granules. The sacs of granular endoplasmic reticulum concomitantly disperse and the Golgi complex enlarges. The number of membranous arrays as well as the numbers of vesicles, vacuoles, prosecretory granules, and mature secretory granules increases, while the glycogen content decreases and the aggregation of free ribosomes increases at the termination of this phase. A gradual involution of the Golgi apparatus and reaccumulation of glycogen and lipofuscin bodies accompany a return to the resting phase. The cell membranes of the chief cells of normal parathyroid glands appear to undergo a minimal increase in tortuosity from the resting to the secretory phase, possibly due to a decrease in glycogen and cell volume.

The mature membrane-limited secretory granules and the lysosomelike bodies move toward the periphery of the cell, where their limiting membranes appear to fuse with the cell membranes. This is similar to the process of emiocytosis described by Lacy et al.[22,23] in pancreatic beta cells. Another method of secretion has been suggested[24-26] in the chief cells of pigs whereby the secretory granules are extruded from chief cells within cytoplasmic projections into the perivascular space. Secretion by this mechanism has not been noted in the human parathyroid gland.

The role of the microtubules and the peripheral microfilaments has not been established in the chief cell of the parathyroid glands of human beings. It is presumed that they play a role in secretion similar to that reported in pancreatic beta cells.[22,23]

Each individual chief cell appears to undergo its cycle independently of adjacent chief cells, as adjacent chief cells often are in different phases of the cell cycle. The ambient serum calcium controls the length of the resting phase of the chief cell[19] and the rate of secretion of preformed secretory granules.

———————————

to disperse. The acid-phosphatase-rich lysosomes increase in number, condensing from the Golgi apparatus, which continues to decrease in size and complexity, with decreasing amounts of acid phosphatase. Secretory granules continue their movement toward the cell periphery with secretion of their contents as the cells return to the resting phase. (From Shannon and Roth.[20])

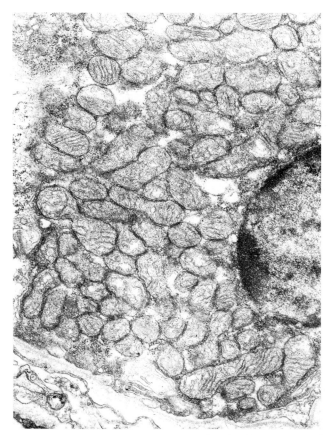

Fig. 41-10. Electromicrograph of an oxyphil cell with numerous mitochondria filling the cytoplasm. Lead citrate and uranyl acetate. X34,000.

A second cell type, the oxyphil cell, appears in the normal human parathyroid gland around the time of puberty.[27-30] After puberty the oxyphil cells continue to increase, either individually scattered among the chief cells or in nodules, cords, sheets, or follicles. The oxyphil cell is 6–10 μm in diameter with an easily identifiable cell membrane, a small dark, pyknotic, centrally located nucleus, and a brightly eosinophilic granular cytoplasm (Fig. 41-6). The cytoplasm stains positively with Bensley's acid aniline fuchsin or phosphotungstic acid/hematoxylin for mitochondria,[29] and is histochemically rich in mitochondrial, oxidative, and other enzymes.[31-35] The nucleus is generally smaller than that of the chief cell, while the cytoplasm is filled with numerous, often bizarre mitochondria (Fig. 41-10). Sacs of granular endoplasmic reticulum and small atrophic Golgi apparatuses are rare. Cytoplasmic glycogen is abundant. It has been suggested that the oxyphil cells of normal parathyroid glands do not synthesize and secrete parathyroid hormone.

In contrast, the oxyphil cells of adenomas and the chief cells in hyperplasias of the parathyroid glands in patients with primary hyperparathyroidism may contain abundant granular endoplasmic reticulum, large Golgi apparatuses, and secretory granules, indicating a capability for parathyroid hormone synthesis and secretion. This explains the rare hyperfunctioning adenoma or chief-cell hyperplasia composed almost entirely of oxyphil cells.[36]

REFERENCES

1. Sandström, I. Om en ny Körtel hos menniska och atskilliga däggdjur. Upsala Läkareförenings Förh. *15:* 441, 1880. (Translated by C. M. Seipel with biographical notes by J. H. Hammar in Bull. Hist. Med. *6:* 179, 1938.)

2. Weller, G. L. Development of the Thyroid, Parathyroid and Thymus Glands in Man. Carnegie Inst. Wash. Contrib. Embryol. *24:* 93, 1933.

3. Norris, E. H. The Parathyroid Glands and the Lateral Thyroid in Man: Their Morphogenesis, Histogenesis, Topographic Anatomy and Prenatal Growth. Carnegie Inst. Wash. Contrib. Embryol. *159:* 249, 1937.

4. Norris, E. H. Embryology: Anatomic Evidence of Prenatal Function of Human Glands. Anat. Record *96:* 129, 1946.

5. Altenähr, E., and Wöhler, J. Ultrastrukturelle Untersuchungen zur funktionellen Epithelkörperchen differenzierung während der Embryonal-, Fetal- und Neonatal-periode. Verhandl. Deut. Ges. Pathol. *55:* 160, 1971.

6. Nakagami, K., Yamazaki, Y., and Tsunoda, Y. An Electron Microscopic Study of the Human Fetal Parathyroid Gland. Z. Zellforsch. Mikrosk. Anat. *85:* 89, 1968.

7. Gilmour, J. R., and Martin, W. J. The Weight of Parathyroid Glands. J. Pathol. Bacteriol. *44:* 431, 1937.

8. Roth, S. I. Recent Advances in Parathyroid Gland Pathology. Am. J. Med. *50:* 612, 1971.

9. Boyd, J. D. Development of Thyroid and Parathyroid Glands and Thymus. Ann. R. Coll. Surg. Eng. *7:* 455, 1960.

10. Gilmour, J. R. The Embryology of the Parathyroid Glands, Thymus and Associated Rudiments. J. Pathol. Bacteriol. *45:* 507, 1937.

11. Gilmour, J. R. Gross Anatomy of Parathyroid Glands. J. Pathol. Bacteriol. *46:* 133, 1938.

12. Millzner, R. J. The Normal Variations in the Position of the Human Parathyroid Glands. Anat. Record. *48:* 399, 1931.

13. Vail, A. D., and Coller, F. C. The Number and Location of Parathyroid Glands Recovered from 202 Routine Autopsies. Mo. Med. *63:* 347, 1966.

14. Zoli, A., and Morase, G. Contributo alla Conoscenza dell Aspetto Morphologica delle Paratiroidi del Verchio. Rass. Neurol. Veg. *17:* 109, 1963.

15. Allara, E. Lo Stroma delle Paratiroida nelle varie eta. Anat. Anz. *80:* 401, 1935.

16. Gilmour, J. R. The Normal Histology of the Parathyroid Glands. J. Pathol. Bacteriol. *48:* 187, 1939.

17. Roth, S. I., and Schiller, A. L. Comparative Anatomy of the Parathyroid Glands, in *Handbook of Physiology,* Section 7, vol. 7, Chapter 12, *Endocrinology,* Section Eds. R. O. Greep and E. B. Astwood, Vol. Ed. G. D. Aurbach. American Physiological Society, Washington, D.C., 1976, pp. 281–311.

18. Munger, B. L., and Roth, S. I. The Cytology of the Normal Parathyroid Glands of Man and Virginia Deer. A Light and Electron Microscopic Study with Morphologic Evidence of Secretory Activity. J. Cell Biol. *16:* 379, 1963.

19. Roth, S. I., and Gallagher, M. J. The Rapid Identification of "Normal" Parathyroid Glands by the Presence of Intracellular Fat. Amer. J. Path. *84:* 521, 1976.

20. Shannon, W. A., Jr., and Roth, S. I. An Ultrastructural Study of Acid Phosphatase Activity in Normal, Adenomatous and Hyperplastic (Chief Cell Type) Human Parathyroid Glands. Amer. J. Path. *77:* 493, 1974.

21. Roth, S. I., and Raisz, L. G. The Course and Reversibility of Calcium Effect on the Ultrastructure of the Rat Parathyroid Gland in Organ Culture. Lab. Invest. *15:* 1187, 1966.

22. Lacy, P. E. The Pancreatic Beta Cell: Structure and Function. New Engl. J. Med. *276:* 187, 1967.

23. Lacy, P. E., Howell, S. L., Young, D. A., and Fink, C. J. New Hypothesis of Insulin Secretion (Letter to the Editor). Nature *219:* 1177, 1968.

24. Fetter, A. W., and Capen, C. C. The Ultrastructure of the Parathyroid Glands of Young Pigs. Acta Anat. *75:* 359, 1970.

25. Capen, C. C., and Fetter, A. W. Scanning and Transmission Electron Microscopic Evaluation of Parathyroid Glands. *Proceedings of the Electron Microscopy Society of America,* 29th Annual Meeting, Boston, Mass. Claitor's Publishing Division, Baton Rouge, 1971, pp. 500–501.

26. Capen, C. C., and Roth, S. I. Ultrastructural and Functional Relationships of Normal and Pathological Parathyroid Cells, in *Pathobiology Annual*, edited by H. L. Ioachim. Appleton-Century-Crofts, New York, 1973, pp. 129–175.

27. Hamperl, H. Über das Vorkammen von Onkocyten in verschiedenen Organen und ihren Geschwülsten (Mundspeicheldrüsen, Epithelkörperchen, Hypophyse, Schilddrüse, Eileiter). Virchows Arch. Abt. A. Pathol. Anat. *298:* 327, 1936.

28. Hamperl, H. Onkocyten and Onkocytome. Virchows Arch. Abt. A. Pathol. Anat. *335:* 452, 1962.

29. Roth, S. I., Olen, E., and Hansen, L. S. The Eosinophilic Cells of the Parathyroid (Oxyphil Cells), Salivary (Oncocytes), and Thyroid (Hürthle Cells) Glands. Light and Electron Microscopic Observations. Lab. Invest. *11:* 933, 1962.

30. Rother, P. Über Vorkommen und Funktion der oxyphilen welshschen Zellen in Glandulae parathyreoideae. Z. Mikroskop. Anat. Forsch. *79:* 533, 1969.

31. Balogh, K., Jr., and Cohen, R. B. Oxidative Enzymes in the Epithelial Cells of Normal and Pathological Human Parathyroid Glands. Lab. Invest. *10:* 354, 1961.

32. Christie, A. C. Histochemical Property of Oxyphil Cells of Human Parathyroid Glands. J. Clin. Pathol. *8:* 302, 1955.

33. Harcourt-Webster, J. N., and Truman, R. F. Histochemical Study of Oxidative and Hydrolytic Enzymes in the Abnormal Human Parathyroid. J. Pathol. *97:* 687, 1969.

34. Tremblay, G. The Oncocytes. Methods Achievements Exp. Pathol. *4:* 121, 1969.

35. Tremblay, G., and Pearse, A. G. E. A Cytochemical Study of Oxidative Enzymes in the Parathyroid Oxyphil Cell and Their Functional Significance. Brit. J. Exp. Pathol. *40:* 66, 1959.

36. Roth, S. I., and Capen, C. C. Ultrastructural and Functional Correlations of the Parathyroid Gland, in *International Review of Experimental Pathology,* edited by G. W. Richter and M. A. Epstein. Academic Press, New York, 1973, vol. 13, pp. 161–221.

42

Chemistry of Parathyroid Hormone

Henry T. Keutmann

An active principle, capable of correcting hypercalcemia when injected into dogs, was first extracted from bovine parathyroid glands by Collip in 1925.[1] These original extractions were carried out with hot hydrochloric acid, a procedure still used in preparation of the commercial bovine parathyroid extract (Parathormone, Eli Lilly and Co.). Evidence accumulated, however, that preparations obtained in this way contained multiple active fragments of the hormone, prompting a search for milder extraction reagents. The most successful of these proved to be phenol[2] and urea/cysteine/cold HCl.[3] The crude extracts were further processed by ether precipitation, salt fractionation, and precipitation with trichloroacetic acid.[2]

Among effective procedures subsequently introduced for further purification were countercurrent distribution[2,4] or gel filtration on columns of Sephadex G50 or G100.[3,5,6] Gel filtration followed by ion exchange chromatography on carboxymethylcellulose[7] is now in widespread use as a rapid, efficient means for preparing hormone of ample purity for most purposes. Ion exchange chromatography in urea buffers[8] provided even more homogeneous preparations for use in structural analyses and also resolved the hormone into three distinct but closely related variants, or isohormones: the predominant form (bPTH I) and two lower-yield forms—bPTH II, differing from bPTH I in composition by two amino acids (Table 42-1), and bPTH III, differing by several additional residues.

The same procedures have been employed in the purification of porcine parathyroid hormone (pPTH). For the isolation of the human hormone, however, supplies of starting material have been limited to tumor tissue removed at surgery. Because of the very small quantities available as a result, certain modifications have been introduced to the purification scheme aimed at improving yield.[9]

The structures of the major form of bovine,[10,11] the porcine,[12] and the completed portion of the human hormone[13–16] are shown in Figure 42-1, and their amino acid compositions are summarized in Table 42-1. The sequences in each case have been determined by automated Edman degradation of the intact molecule plus further degradations using peptides representing the middle and carboxyl regions of the hormone obtained by cleavage with specific proteolytic enzymes including trypsin, chymotrypsin, and staphylococcal protease.

Bovine parathyroid hormone is a single-chain polypeptide of 84 amino acids, molecular weight 9300, with no cysteine residues and, hence, no disulfide bridges. There is a preponderance of basic residues (arginine, lysine) conferring an overall positive charge to the molecule. A distinctly hydrophobic region is found through the central portion of the sequence (residues 31–43) including the single tyrosine residue, site of radioiodine labeling for immunoassay procedures.

There is extensive sequence homology among all three species of hormone. The porcine peptide differs from the bovine at seven sequence positions (Fig. 42-1). These include substitution of histidine for tyrosine at position 43, and presence of an amino-terminal serine instead of alanine.

Investigation of the human hormone structure has relied upon several newly refined techniques[17] for high-sensitivity sequence determination; analysis of peptide extracted from pooled tumor tissue has been supplemented by use of hormone labeled biosynthetically by incubation with radioactive amino acids in vitro. The human sequence differs from each of the other species at eleven positions[16] (Fig. 42-1). The most extensive substitutions occur in the middle portion, including six of eight residues between positions 40 and 47. Notable is the high content of proline in this region of hPTH. Tyrosine, found at position 43 of the bovine hormone, is absent from the human. The amino-terminal residue is serine (as in the porcine), and the human polypeptide is the only one of the three to contain a threonine residue (position 79).

There is, however, a discrepancy between the findings of two laboratories involving three residues at the amino terminus of the human hormone. Our own proposed structure[14] contains glutamic acid at position 22, leucine at 28, and aspartic acid at 30; these are identical with the bovine and porcine hormones. By contrast, Brewer et al.[13] have proposed these residues to be glutamine, lysine, and leucine, respectively; they have also found glutamine at position 22 of the bovine and porcine hormones.[19] The reason for these differences is not readily apparent, but because of their extent (the Brewer structure contains three-more positive charges than our own), both groups have reexamined and reported reconfirmation of their findings.[18,20] Studies in our own laboratory[18] have used both the biosynthetic-labeling approach and repeat degradations of fresh lots of hormone. The results at all positions consistently reconfirm our original findings (Niall et al.[14]) shown in Figure 42-1.

Despite the lack of cysteine disulfide bridges, the parathyroid hormone molecule does appear to have elements of secondary and tertiary structure which may influence its activity and metabolism. Circular-dichroism studies by Brewer et al.[21] showed that the bovine peptide in aqueous solution is predominantly a random coil, with only 10 to 15 percent alpha helix. In some nonpolar solvents, the percent helix is markedly higher, suggesting that interaction with hydrophobic membrane receptor sites could be associated with an increase in helical content of the molecule. More recently, using computer techniques and electron microscopy, Cohn et al.[22] have developed a model for the hormone showing extensive, tightly

Table 42-1. Amino Acid Composition of the Parathyroid Hormones[a]

Amino Acid	Bovine I	Bovine II	Porcine	Human
Aspartic acid[b]	9	9	8	10
Threonine	0	1	0	1
Serine	8	8	8	7
Glutamic acid[c]	11	11	11	11
Proline	2	2	2	3
Glycine	4	4	5	4
Alanine	7	7	6	7
Valine	8	7	9	8
Methionine	2	2	1	2
Isoleucine	3	3	3	1
Leucine	8	8	10	10
Tyrosine	1	1	0	0
Phenylalanine	2	2	1	1
Lysine	9	9	9	9
Histidine	4	4	5	4
Arginine	5	5	5	5
Tryptophan	1	1	1	1
Total	84	84	84	84

[a] All values expressed as moles amino acid per mole peptide.
[b] Includes asparagine plus aspartic acid.
[c] Includes glutamine plus glutamic acid.

folded alpha helices in the N- and C-terminal regions; these are joined by predominantly random-coil and beta-turn structures through the hydrophobic middle region, which includes several sites of metabolic cleavage in vivo[23] (Chapter 45).

The close homology found among the respective species of hormone accounts for their generally good immunological cross-reactivity and has permitted measurement of human hormone by use of bovine antisera and tracer (Chapter 45). However, through application of more precisely characterized region-specific assay systems, made possible through the availability of a variety of synthetic fragments, immunological differences between hPTH and bPTH may be discerned. At the carboxyl terminus, for example, the substitutions at 79 and 83 may account for the different reactivity found with at least one antiserum directed toward this region.[24] The sequence differences among the species are also sufficient to confer certain differences in biological potency, a finding that has served as one point of departure in a wide-ranging series of structure/function analyses of the hormone.

Opportunity to study the effects of alteration of structure on biological activity came with the introduction during the 1950s of satisfactory assay methods for parathyroid hormone. Among the number of useful systems that are now available,[25,26] two have been employed extensively. One is an in vitro system utilizing the activation of the enzyme adenyl cyclase in homogenates of rat renal cortex,[27] and the other is an in vivo assay measuring the hypercalcemic response to the intravenous injection of hormone into intact chicks.[28] Despite differences in activity found in certain cases between measurements made by the two systems, there is general agreement, and a number of quite precise and meaningful conclusions have been reached concerning the structural features of the molecule that are important for activity.

In the course of earlier efforts to purify bovine parathyroid hormone extracted with hot hydrochloric acid, evidence accumulated indicating that shorter fragments or cleavage products might retain biological activity. It became clear during initial work with the structural analysis that such fragments originated from the amino terminus of the molecule.[29] Ultimately, a peptide was isolated, after treatment with dilute HCl under controlled conditions, which was active by both in vivo rat hypercalcemic assay and in

vitro adenyl cyclase assays; this fragment was found to comprise residues 1–29 of the native bovine molecule.[30]

Further investigations to define the minimum sequence necessary for biological activity have been greatly facilitated by the rapid refinement of techniques for solid-phase peptide synthesis.[31–33] The use of synthetic fragments for structure/function analysis offers, among other advantages, much more flexibility than is possible with natural products, where the choice of peptides is usually dictated by the location of residues susceptible to enzymatic or chemical cleavage. The first synthetic biologically active parathyroid peptide was a fragment consisting of the amino-terminal 34 residues of the bovine hormone.[34] It was shown to have all the effects of the native hormone on both renal and skeletal tissue in vivo and in vitro. Recent preparations of the 1–34 peptide have full biological activity when compared on a molar basis with native bovine parathyroid hormone by either renal adenyl cyclase or chick hypercalcemia assay (Table 42-2).

Systematic evaluation of fragments successively shortened at both the C-terminal and N-terminal ends has defined the minimum sequence required for biological activity of the bovine hormone (Table 42-3).[35] This fragment must comprise a continuous sequence from residue 2 extending to at least residue 27 (Fig. 42-2). Recently, even shorter fragments have been found to elicit responses in the adenyl cyclase assay under certain conditions. The dose-response curves of these differ qualitatively from those of the longer fragments, however, and the meaning of these findings requires further investigation.

The influence of the amino-terminal residue on biological activity was suggested by the finding that the porcine and human native hormones, both of which have amino-terminal serine in-

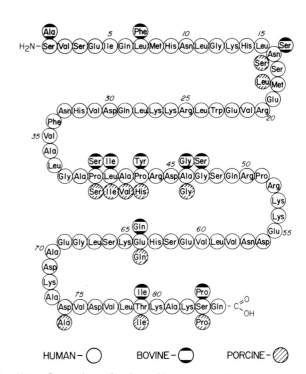

Fig. 42-1. Comparison of amino acid sequences of bovine, porcine, and human parathyroid hormone. The backbone sequence represents the human structure. Added residues indicate sequence changes found in the porcine hormone and in the bovine hormone. Dashes indicate those residues that are identical to the human. Residues 22, 28, and 30 of the human have also been reported[13,20] to be Gln, Lys, and Leu, respectively.

Table 42-2. Comparison of Biological Activity of Parathyroid Peptides from Different Species

	Potency, MRC U/mg[a]	
Peptide	In Vitro Rat Renal Adenyl Cyclase Assay	In Vivo Chick Hypercalcemia Assay
Native hormones:		
Bovine 1–84	3000 (2500–4000)	2500 (2100–4000)
Porcine 1–84	1000 (850–1250)	4800 (3300–7000)
Human 1–84	350 (275–425)	—
Synthetic fragments:		
Bovine 1–34	5400 (3900–8000)	7700 (5200–11100)
Human 1–34	1700 (1400–2150)	7400 (5200–9700)
[Ala¹]-Human 1–34	4300 (3400–5400)	—

[a]Values expressed as mean potency with 95% confidence limits, based on Medical Research Council research standard A for parathyroid hormone.[25] Data from Tregear et al.[37] and Keutmann et al.[9]

stead of alanine, are considerably lower in potency than the bovine hormone by in vitro renal adenyl cyclase assay[9] (Table 42-2). Commensurately the human-(1–34) synthetic fragment is lower in potency (1700 U/mg) than the bovine fragment (5400 U/mg).[36] This prompted the study of several analogues of the bovine-(1–34) peptide containing substitutions at the amino terminus (Table 42-4). Replacement of the N-terminal alanine residue invariably results in diminution of activity as measured by the in vitro assay.[37] Conversely, replacement of the N-terminal serine in the human-(1–34) fragment by an alanine elevates the biological activity to levels approaching that of the bovine fragment (Table 42-2). The very low activity of the sarcosine and desamino analogues of bovine-(1–34) indicates, furthermore, that a free amino group is essential for in vitro activity. The deletion or alteration of the amino-terminal residue has little effect, however, on the biological potency when assessed by in vivo chick hypercalcemic assay. Hence the human and bovine 1–34 fragments are comparably active in this system (Table 42-2) and even the 2–34 fragment retains most of its biological activity.[37] Additional experiments employing still other types of assay systems will be needed to fully evaluate the significance of these contrasting results.

Extension of the chain at the amino terminus has been found through assays of several such analogues of the bovine 1–34 peptide to result in a loss of biological activity.[38] These findings are helpful in interpreting biological studies of the nature of the cleav-

age of proparathyroid hormone into native PTH,[39] using fragment −6 through +34 which contains the prohormone-specific hexapeptide sequence attached to the amino terminus (Chapter 43).

A large number of synthetic peptides have also been prepared to explore the effect of substitutions affecting the amino acids within the 1–34 region. Among the most important of these residues are the methionines, found at positions 8 and 18 of the bovine hormone. It has long been appreciated[5,7,40] that oxidation of the methionines to the sulfoxide form causes complete loss of biological activity, although immunological activity is for the most part preserved. A synthetic analogue of the bovine 1–34 peptide with the methionines replaced by sterically similar norleucine residues is resistant to oxidation, and highly active by both in vivo and in vitro assay.[41] It would thus appear that the methionine residues may be replaced outright with retention of biological activity, in contrast to the inactivation resulting from oxidation to the more negatively charged sulfoxide form. This inactivation occurs when the natural hormone is radiolabeled by conventional iodination procedures which employ an oxidation step. The methionine-free analogue has thus been prepared with a tyrosine residue in place of phenylalanine at position 34, creating a peptide (Fig. 42-3) which may be readily iodinated without loss of activity, for use in studies of hormone-receptor interactions where biologically active labeled preparations of high specific activity are required.

Also an example of a labile residue within the active region is the tryptophan at position 23. Analogues of the bovine 1–34 fragment with tryptophan modified by an N-formyl or N-phenylsulfonyl group on the side chain retain high potency in the in vitro renal adenyl cyclase system.[42] Substitution of glutamine for glutamic acid at position 22 likewise has little effect on activity. Hence, alterations in this region of the molecule appear not to influence biological potency by this particular assay system. However, a synthetic human 1–34 fragment incorporating the more extensive changes called for by the sequence of Brewer et al.[13] including lysine at 28 and leucine at 30, as well as glutamine at 22, shows markedly reduced potency by both in vivo adenyl cyclase and in vitro chick hypercalcemia assay.[43–45]

Another phase of structure/function analysis concerns efforts to produce peptides with enhanced biological potency. This has led to synthesis of a series of analogues which are protected against metabolic degradation at either or both ends, by substitution of the "D" enantiomer of alanine at the N-terminus or by provision of an amide moiety in place of the free carboxyl group at position 34.

Table 42-3. Effect of Chain Length on Biological Activity of Synthetic Bovine Parathyroid Hormone Fragments

	In Vitro Rat Renal Cortical Adenylate Cyclase Assay		In Vivo Chick Hypercalcemia Assay	
Peptide	Potency, MRC U/mg[a]	Potency, mole percent[b]	Potency, MRC U/mg[a]	Potency, mole percent[b]
1–84 (native)	3000 (2500–4000)	100	2500 (2100–4000)	100
1–34	5400 (3900–8000)	77	7700 (5200–11100)	132
2–34	200[c]	3	3800 (2700–5400)	64
3–34	<10	<0.3	<5	<0.2
1–26	<10	<0.3	—	—
1–27	200[c]	2	—	—
1–28	440[c]	5	<10	<0.3
1–31	740 (610–980)	10	4800 (2500–9300)	74
1–12 + 13–34	<10	<0.3	<5	<0.2

[a]Values expressed as mean potency with 95% confidence limits. Data from Tregear et al.[35]

[b]Activity per mole peptide/activity per mole purified native bPTH

[c]Response curve nonparallel to the standard. Potency estimated by comparing activity at half-maximal response.

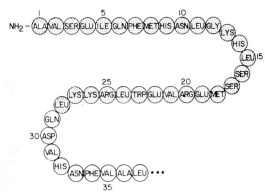

Fig. 42-2. Amino-terminal 37 residues of bovine parathyroid hormone, showing (shaded circles) the minimum sequence length required for biological activity by in vitro adenyl cyclase assay. Peptides lacking residue 1 or 28 (cross-hatched) are active but give a dose-response that is nonparallel to the native hormone standard. (From Tregear et al.[35]).

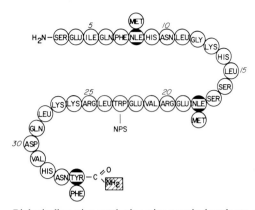

Fig. 42-3. Biologically active synthetic amino-terminal analogue of bovine parathyroid hormone. It is stable to oxidation by virtue of substitution of norleucine for methionine at positions 8 and 18. A tyrosine residue has been substituted at position 34 to provide a site for labeling with radioiodine, the tyrosine residue is amidated for greater resistance to degradation. (From Rosenblatt et al.)[41,47]

These preparations show potencies up to threefold that of the unmodified bovine 1–34 sequence by both in vivo and in vitro assays.[37] Amidation of the C-terminus appears particularly effective, especially when tyrosine is provided in place of phenylalanine at position 34 (Fig. 42-3). Although the ultimate biological usefulness of these high-potency analogues remains to be determined, they already are proving of great interest in recent studies of peptide analogues as inhibitors of hormone action.

To act as an inhibitor, an analogue must bind to the appropriate cell membrane receptor without eliciting a response, such as adenyl cyclase activation. Such compounds, despite extensive study of analogues of peptide hormones, are still comparatively rare. In seeking a possible inhibitor to PTH action, numerous partially active or even inactive analogues have been tested for their ability to block the adenyl cyclase response of native or 1–34 bPTH. This is necessarily an indirect approach, since satisfactory assays for direct measurement of receptor binding of parathyroid hormone are still not available. Nonetheless, distinct inhibitory properties were found with two bovine analogues: bPTH-(3–34) and [desamino-Ala^1]bPTH-(1–34).[46] The K_i, or receptor binding avidity, of these was still far below that of bPTH-(1–34) itself, a 50- to 300-fold molar excess of analogue relative to active hormone (agonist) being required to achieve half-maximal inhibition of agonist.

To design more-potent inhibitors, these results have been combined with the structure/activity conclusions arising from studies of the "protected" analogues with enhanced biological potency. The peptide [Nle^8,Nle^{18},Tyr^{34}]bPTH-(3–34)amide, representing potency-enhancing modifications on bPTH-(1–34) combined with the inhibitor nucleus 3–34, shows greatly increased

antagonist properties;[47] half-maximal inhibition of native hormone or bPTH-(1–34) is produced at equimolar concentrations of agonist and antagonist. Detailed pharmacokinetic analysis confirms that this peptide is a competitive inhibitor.[47] These peptides have not as yet been evaluated for inhibition of parathyroid hormone action in vivo, but it is anticipated that their unique properties will greatly benefit studies of the mode of hormone action (Chapter 47).

Although it is clear from the foregoing that synthetic work has concentrated on the active region, peptides from other portions of the native molecule as well as biosynthetic precursors have also been prepared to serve a variety of special investigations covered in further detail elsewhere in this volume. Several fragments have been utilized in the development and characterization of region-specific immunoassays for PTH; the human 53–84 fragment should be especially useful in providing highly sensitive carboxyl-terminal hPTH antisera (Chapter 45). Fragment 28–48 from the bovine hormone is being used in further definition of the nature and significance of the peripheral cleavage of the hormone in vivo[23,48] (Chapter 45). In the area of hormone biosynthesis (Chapter 43), use of the prohormone fragment, ProPTH-(−6−+34), in biological studies of proparathyroid hormone[39] has already been mentioned. Finally, synthetic peptides comprising the structure of the ribosomal precursor of bPTH (pre-proparathyroid hormone)[49] (Chapter 43) are providing the basis for a number of important studies of this form of the hormone.

Table 42-4. Effect of Amino-Terminal Substitutions on Biological Activity of Synthetic Bovine Parathyroid Hormone Fragment 1–34

N-Terminal Residue	Potency, MRC U/mg[a]
Alanine	5400 (3900–8000)
D-Alanine	3100 (2200–4550)
Desamino-Alanine	<10[b]
Serine	1200 (1000–1600)
Sarcosine	500 (410–660)
Tyrosine	520 (430–690)

[a]Values expressed as mean potency with 95% confidence limits, assessed by in vitro rat renal adenyl cyclase assay.
[b]Inhibits in vitro action of native hormone.
Data from Tregear et al.[37]

REFERENCES

1. Collip, J. B. Extraction of a Parathyroid Hormone Which Will Prevent or Control Parathyroid Tetany and Which Regulates the Level of Blood Calcium. J. Biol. Chem.*63:* 395, 1925.
2. Aurbach, G. D. Isolation of Parathyroid Hormone After Extraction with Phenol. J. Biol. Chem. *234:* 3179, 1959.
3. Rasmussen, H., Sze, Y. L., and Young, R. Further Studies on the Isolation and Characterization of Parathyroid Polypeptides. J. Biol. Chem. *239:* 2852, 1964.
4. Rasmussen, H., and Craig, L. C. Purification of Parathyroid Hormone by Use of Counter-current Distribution. J. Amer. Chem. Soc. *81:* 5003, 1959.
5. Rasmussen, H., and Craig, L. C. The Parathyroid Polypeptides. Rec. Prog. Horm. Res. *18:* 269, 1962.
6. Aurbach, G. D., and Potts, J. T., Jr. Partition of Parathyroid Hormone on Sephadex G-100. Endocrinology *75:* 290, 1964.
7. Potts, J. T., Jr., Aurbach, G. D., and Sherwood, L. M. Parathyroid Hormone: Chemical Properties and Structural Requirements for Bio-

logical and Immunological Activity. Rec. Prog. Horm. Res. *22:* 101, 1966.

8. Keutmann, H. T., Aurbach, G. D., Dawson, B. F., Niall, H. D., Deftos, L. J., and Potts, J. T., Jr. Isolation and Characterization of the Bovine Parathyroid Isohormones. Biochemistry *10:* 2779, 1971.

9. Keutmann, H. T., Barling, P. M., Hendy, G. N., Segre, G. V., Niall, H. D., Aurbach, G. D., et al. Isolation of Human Parathyroid Hormone. Biochemistry *13:* 1646, 1974.

10. Brewer, H. B., Jr., and Ronan, R. Bovine Parathyroid Hormone: Amino Acid Sequence. Proc. Nat. Acad. Sci. *67:* 1862, 1970.

11. Niall, H. D., Keutmann, H. T., Sauer, R., Hogan, M. L., Dawson, B. F., Aurbach, G. D., and Potts, J. T., Jr. The Amino Acid Sequence of Bovine Parathyroid Hormone I. Hoppe-Seyler's Z. Physiol. Chem. *351:* 1586, 1970.

12. Sauer, R. T., Niall, H. D., Hogan, M. L., Keutmann, H. T., O'Riordan, J. L. H., and Potts, J. T., Jr. The Amino Acid Sequence of Porcine Parathyroid Hormone. Biochem. *13:* 1994, 1974.

13. Brewer, H. B., Jr., Fairwell, T., Ronan, R., Sizemore, G. W., and Arnaud, C. D. Human Parathyroid Hormone: Amino Acid Sequence of the Amino-Terminal Residues 1–34. Proc. Nat. Acad. Sci. *69:* 3585, 1972.

14. Niall, H. D., Sauer, R. T., Jacobs, J. W., Keutmann, H. T., Segre, G. V., O'Riordan, J. L. H., et al. The Amino Acid Sequence of the Amino-Terminal 37 Residues of Human Parathyroid Hormone. Proc. Nat. Acad. Sci. *71:* 384, 1974.

15. Keutmann, H. T., Niall, H. D., Jacobs, J. W., et al. A Reinvestigation of the Amino-Terminal Sequence of Human Parathyroid Hormone and Analysis of the Sequence of Residues 44–69, in *Calcium-Regulating Hormones: Proceedings of the Fifth Parathyroid Conference,* edited by R. Talmage, M. Owen, and J. A. Parsons. Excerpta Medica, Amsterdam, 1975, pp. 9–14.

16. Keutmann, H. T., Sauer, M. M., Hendy, G. N., O'Riordan, J. L. H. and Potts, J. T., Jr., The Complete Amino Acid Sequence of Human Parathyroid Hormone. Biochemistry (in press).

17. Jacobs, J. W., and Niall, H. D. High Sensitivity Automated Sequence Determination of Polypeptides. J. Biol. Chem. *250:* 3629, 1975.

18. Keutmann, H. T., Niall, H. D., O'Riordan, J. L. H., et al. A Reinvestigation of the Amino-Terminal Sequence of Human Parathyroid Hormone. Biochem. *14:* 1842, 1975.

19. Brewer, H. B., Jr., Fairwell, T., Rittel, W., et al. Recent Studies on the Chemistry of Human, Bovine and Porcine Parathyroid Hormone. Amer. J. Med. *56:* 17, 1974.

20. Brewer, H. B., Jr., Fairwell, T., Ronan, R., et al. Human Parathyroid Hormone, in *Calcium-Regulating Hormones: Proceedings of the Fifth Parathyroid Conference,* edited by R. V. Talmage, M. Owen, and J. A. Parsons. Excerpta Medica, Amsterdam, 1975, pp. 23–32.

21. Brewer, H. B., Jr. Chemistry and Conformation of Bovine Parathyroid Hormone, in *Endocrinology 1971: Proceedings of the Third International Symposium,* edited by S. Taylor. Heinemann Press, London, 1972, pp. 324–332.

22. Cohn, D. V., Hamilton, J. M., MacGregor, R. R., et al. Parathyroid Hormone: Biosynthesis and Metabolism, in *Endocrinology: Proceedings of the Fifth International Congress of Endocrinology,* edited by V. H. T. James. Excerpta Medica, Amsterdam, vol. 2, 1977, pp. 248–255.

23. Segre, G. V., Niall, H. D., Habener, J. F., and Potts, J. T., Jr. Metabolism of Parathyroid Hormone. Physiologic and Clinical Significance, in *Proceedings of the Third F. Raymond Keating, Jr., Memorial Symposium - Parathyroid Hormone, Calcitonin and Vitamin D: Clinical Considerations* (Part I) Am. J. Med. *56:* 774, 1974.

24. Hendy, G. N., Barling, P. M., and O'Riordan, J. L. H. Human Parathyroid Hormone: Immunological Properties of the Amino Terminus and of Synthetic Fragments. Clin. Sci. Molec. Med. *47:* 567, 1974.

25. Parsons, J. A., and Potts, J. T., Jr. Physiology and Chemistry of Parathyroid Hormone, in *Clinics in Endocrinology and Metabolism,* edited by I. MacIntyre. Saunders, London, 1972, vol. 1, no. 1, pp. 33–78.

26. Zanelli, J. M., and Parsons, J. A. Bioassay of Parathyroid Hormone, in *Hormones and Their Assays.* Springer-Verlag, Berlin (in press).

27. Marcus, R., and Aurbach, G. D. Bioassay of Parathyroid Hormone in Vitro with a Stable Preparation of Adenyl Cyclase from Rat Kidney. Endocrinology *85:* 801, 1969.

28. Parsons, J. A. Reit, B., and Robinson C. J. A Bioassay for Parathyroid Hormone Using Chicks. Endocrinology *92:* 454, 1973.

29. Potts, J. T., Jr., Keutmann, H. T., Niall, H. D., Deftos, L. J., Brewer, H. B., Jr., and Aurbach, G. D. Covalent Structure of Bovine

Parathyroid Hormone in Relation to Biological and Immunological Activity, in *Parathyroid Hormone and Thyrocalcitonin (Calcitonin),* edited by R. V. Talmage and L. F. Bélanger. Amsterdam, Excerpta Medica, 1968, pp. 44–53.

30. Keutmann, H. T., Dawson, B. F., Aurbach, G. D., and Potts, J. T., Jr. A Biologically Active Amino-Terminal Fragment of Bovine Parathyroid Hormone Prepared by Dilute Acid Hydrolysis. Biochemistry *11:* 1973, 1972.

31. Merrifield, R. B. New Approaches to the Chemical Synthesis of Peptides. Rec. Prog. Horm. Res. *23:* 451, 1967.

32. Meienhofer, Jr. Peptide Synthesis: A Review of the Solid-Phase Method, in *Hormonal Proteins and Peptides,* edited by C. H. Li. New York, Academic Press, 1973, vol. II pp. 45–267.

33. Tregear, G. W., van Rietschoten, J., Greene, E., et al. Principles and Recent Applications of the Solid-Phase Synthesis of Peptide Hormones, in *Endocrinology 1973: Proceedings of the Fourth International Symposium,* edited by S. Taylor. Heinemann Press, London, 1974, pp. 1–15.

34. Potts, J. T., Jr., Tregear, G. W., Keutmann, H. T., Niall, H. D., Sauer, R., Deftos, L. J., et al. Synthesis of a Biologically Active N-Terminal Tetratriacontapeptide of Parathyroid Hormone. Proc. Nat. Acad. Sci. *68:* 63, 1971.

35. Tregear, G. W., van Rietschoten, J., Greene, E., Keutmann, H. T., Niall, H. D., Reit, B., et al. Bovine Parathyroid Hormone: Minimum Chain Length of Synthetic Peptide Required for Biological Activity. Endocrinology *93:* 1349, 1973.

36. Tregear, G. W., van Rietschoten, J., Greene, E., Niall, H. D., Keutmann, H. T., Parsons, J. A., et al. Solid-Phase Synthesis of the Biologically Active N-Terminal 1–34 Peptide of Human Parathyroid Hormone. Hoppe-Seyler's Z. Physiol. Chem. *355:* 415, 1974.

37. Parsons, J. A., Rafferty, B., Gray, D., et al. Pharmacology of Parathyroid Hormone and Some of Its Fragments and Analogues, in *Calcium-Regulating Hormones: Proceedings of the Fifth Parathyroid Conference,* edited by R. V. Talmage, M. Owen, and J. A. Parsons. Excerpta Medica, Amsterdam, 1975, pp. 33–39.

38. Potts, J. T., Jr., Keutmann, H. T., Niall, H. D., Tregear, G. W., Habener, J. F., O'Riordan, J. L. H., et al. Parathyroid Hormone: Chemical and Immunochemical Studies of the Active Molecular Species, in *Endocrinology 1971: Proceedings of the Third International Symposium,* edited by S. Taylor. London: Heinemann Medical, 1972, pp. 333–349.

39. Peytremann, A., Goltzman, D., Callahan, E., et al. Metabolism and Biological Activity of Proparathyroid Hormone and Synthetic Analogues in Renal Cortical Membranes. Endocrinology *97:* 1270, 1975.

40. Tashjian, A. H., Jr., Ontjes, D. A., and Munson, P. L. Alkylation and Oxidation of Methionine in Bovine Parathyroid Hormone: Effects on Hormonal Activity and Antigenicity. Biochemistry *3:* 1175, 1964.

41. Rosenblatt, M., Goltzman, D., Keutmann, H. T., Tregear, G. W., and Potts, J. T., Jr. Chemical and Biological Properties of Synthetic, Sulfur-free Analogues of Parathyroid Hormone. J. Biol. Chem. *251:* 159, 1977.

42. Rosenblatt, M. (in preparation).

43. Di Bella, F. P., Arnaud, C. D., and Brewer, H. B., Jr. Relative Biological Activities of Human and Bovine Parathyroid Hormones and Their Synthetic, NH₂-Terminal (1–34) Peptides, as Evaluated in Vitro with Renal Cortical Adenylate Cyclase Obtained from Three Different Species. Endocrinology *99:* 429, 1976.

44. Bader, C. A., Monet, J. D., Rivaille, P., et al. Comparison of in Vitro Biological Activity of 1–34 Amino-Terminal Synthetic Fragments of Human Parathyroid Hormone on Bovine and Porcine Kidney Membranes. Endocrine Res. Comm. *3:* 167, 1976.

45. Parsons, J. A., Keutmann, H. T., Rosenblatt, M. R., and Potts, J. T., Jr. Unpublished observations.

46. Goltzman, D., Peytremann, A., Callahan, E., et al. Interaction of Parathyroid Hormone with Membranes of Renal Target Cells: Analysis of Intrinsic Prohormone Activity and Actions of Peptide Analogs with Inhibitory Effects, in *Calcium-Regulating Hormones: Proceedings of the Fifth Parathyroid Conference,* edited by R. Talmage, M. Owen, and J. A. Parsons. Excerpta Medica, Amsterdam, 1975, pp. 172–176.

47. Rosenblatt, M., Callahan, E. N., Mahaffey, J. E., et al. Parathyroid Hormone Inhibitors: Design, Synthesis and Biological Evaluation of Hormone Analogues. J. Biol. Chem. *252:* 5847, 1977.

48. Rosenblatt, M., Segre, G. V., and Potts, J. T., Jr. Synthesis of a Fragment of Parathyroid Hormone, bPTH-(28–48): An Inhibitor of Hormone Cleavage in Vivo. Biochemistry *16:* 2811, 1977.

49. Habener, J. F., Kemper, B. W., Rich, A., et al. Biosynthesis of Parathyroid Hormone. Rec. Prog. Horm. Res. *33:* 249, 1977.

43

Parathyroid Hormone Biosynthesis

Joel F. Habener

A substantial body of information is now available concerning the processes involved in the cellular formation of parathyroid hormone. In many respects, studies of the biosynthesis of parathyroid hormone have provided insights into the biosynthetic processes that take place on many specialized "secretory" cells whose functions are to produce proteins for export. Just a few years have elapsed since the earliest successful demonstrations of the biosynthesis of radiolabeled PTH by parathyroid gland slices incubated in vitro with radioactive amino acids.[1] As a result of continued studies of hormone synthesis in vitro using intact cell preparations as well as cell-free systems, it has been possible to identify and to characterize a biosynthetic pathway for the formation of PTH involving successive proteolytic cleavages of the hormone from a larger polypeptide precursor, to identify the subcellular locations where the proteolytic processing of the precursors takes place, to isolate and to characterize the messenger RNA for the hormone, and finally to synthesize a functionally active gene copy of the parathyroid mRNA.[2] These observations emphasized the general fact that biosynthetic precursors and their post-translational modifications by proteolytic cleavages are characteristic of the biosynthetic processes involved in the formation of most if not all secretory proteins, not only parathyroid hormone and other polypeptide and protein hormones, but such diverse proteins as immunoglobulins, enzymes, and albumin. Furthermore, it is now evident by several criteria that these biosynthetic precursors belong to two distinct classes, preproteins and proproteins. These criteria include (1) the time that elapses between synthesis of the precursor and the proteolytic conversion to the product; (2) the subcellular site at which the cleavages occur; (3) the specificity of the enzymic cleavage; and (4) the characteristics of the primary structures of the precursors.[2]

In addition to the information obtained regarding the biosynthetic pathways for PTH, studies in vitro have also led to considerable new information concerning the regulation of hormone production by the parathyroid gland. Several reviews of parathyroid hormone biosynthesis are available.[2–5]

After the initial discovery of a biosynthetic precursor to insulin, proinsulin,[6] it was expected that similar biosynthetic precursors eventually would be identified for other polypeptide and protein hormones. The first indication that a precursor to PTH existed came from the finding that, when analyzed by chromatographic techniques, the hypercalcemic activity in extracts of parathyroid glands resided in more than a single fraction.[7] In addition to a fraction containing PTH, a second fraction containing hypercalcemic activity, calcemic fraction A (CF-A), was observed. Subsequently, pulse and pulse-chase labeling studies using parathyroid gland slices incubated for short periods in the presence of radioactive amino acids demonstrated that CF-A was a precursor,

or prohormone, of parathyroid hormone. It was consequently designated proparathyroid hormone (ProPTH) (Fig. 43-1).[8,9] It was soon recognized by analyses of the products resulting from the translation of parathyroid messenger RNA in heterologous cell-free systems (wheat-germ extract),[10] and by more detailed analyses of hormone synthesis in parathyroid gland slices,[11] that an even larger precursor of parathyroid hormone existed, a preproparathyroid hormone (Fig. 43-2). ProPTH was therefore identified as an intermediate product in the synthesis of PTH.

The primary amino acid sequence of bovine ProPTH was determined with 1–2 mg of prohormone by automated, sequential Edman degradation using [³⁵S]methionine-labeled phenylthioisocyanate to identify the phenylthiohydantoin derivatives of the amino acids at each cycle of degradation.[12] Subsequently, the primary sequences of the corresponding hormones from human[13] and other species[5] were determined by more sensitive radioimmunosequencing methods in which biosynthetically incorporated radioactive amino acids are sequentially removed and identified by the Edman reaction.

Through the use of these same highly sensitive radiomicrosequencing techniques it has been possible to determine the complete primary structure of Pre-ProPTH (Fig. 43-2). Pre-ProPTH is a polypeptide of 115 amino acids and contains within its amino acid sequence the sequences of both ProPTH (90 amino acids) and PTH (84 amino acids). Pre-ProPTH is believed to be the initial hormonal product synthesized in the parathyroid cell and to represent all of the structural information encoded in the gene for PTH. This conclusion is based on studies of the translation of parathyroid messenger RNA in heterologous cell-free systems where it was shown that Pre-ProPTH, not ProPTH or PTH, is the major product synthesized.[10,14–17] Moreover, studies in cell-free systems using initiator methionyl tRNA (from wheat germ) showed that the N-terminal methionine (position −31) is incorporated into the sequence of Pre-ProPTH specifically in response to the initiator AUG codon of the parathyroid mRNA.[17] In addition, when the C-terminal tetrapeptide produced by digestion of Pre-ProPTH with pancreatic trypsin was analyzed by chromatography and electrophoresis, it was shown to be indistinguishable from its counterpart in both ProPTH and PTH.[17] These data strongly indicate that Pre-ProPTH represents the total polypeptide sequence translated from the parathyroid mRNA between the initiation (AUG) codon at the 5′ region and the termination (UAG or UAA) codon at the 3′ region of the mRNA.

Recently, use of RNA-dependent DNA polymerase (reverse transcriptase) made it possible to synthesize a functionally active DNA transcript of parathyroid messenger RNA.[18] The major product synthesized in a linked transcriptional/translational system in response to the complementary DNA was shown to be a polypep-

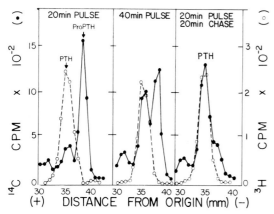

Fig. 43-1. Conversion of newly synthesized ProPTH to PTH in parathyroid gland slices during pulse and pulse/chase labeling studies in vitro. Gland slices were incubated for times indicated with [¹⁴C]leucine. In the right-hand panel, a 20-minute incubation with [¹⁴C]leucine was followed by a 20-minute chase incubation with unlabeled leucine. Patterns shown are from electrophoresis of the gland extracts on 10 percent urea-acetate polyacrylamide gels. [³H]Leucine-labeled PTH was electrophoresed with the extracts as a marker of PTH. (Habener.³ Courtesy of Elsevier/Excerpta Medica.)

tide indistinguishable from Pre-ProPTH. These observations gave further support to the evidence that Pre-ProPTH is the authentic and complete representation of the gene for PTH.

Kinetic analyses of the appearance and disappearance of Pre-ProPTH, ProPTH, and PTH, as determined by electrophoretic characterizations of the polypeptides labeled during short pulse and pulse-chase incubations of parathyroid gland slices with radioactive amino acids (Fig. 43-3),¹¹ and studies both of the distributions of the hormonal polypeptides in subcellular fractions¹⁹,²⁰ and of radioautographic analyses of protein migration in parathyroid cells²¹ have provided insights into the subcellular sites where cleavages of the hormonal precursors occur and the possible functions of the precursors in the biosynthetic pathway for the hormone. The details of the transport pathway for PTH can be appreciated better in conjunction with a brief description of the pathway for the transport of secretory proteins proposed by Palade and co-workers²² based on their studies of protein synthesis in pancreatic exocrine cells. The work of Palade et al. indicates that the synthesis of exportable proteins, as opposed to proteins that remain in the cell, takes place on ribosomes bound to the membrane (rough) of the endoplasmic reticulum (RER). Newly synthesized polypeptide chains are vectorially discharged into the cisternal space of the endoplasmic reticulum, and thus the proteins that are to be secreted are segregated from other proteins whose functions are fulfilled within the cell (e.g., structural proteins). The secretory proteins are then transported either in continuous channels of the reticulum or discontinuously within membrane-limited vesicles to the Golgi region of the cell where they are incorporated into secretory vesicles or granules. The protein within granules is then either stored within the cell or transported to the cytoplasmic membrane and released by an exocytotic process into the extracellular fluid in response to the appropriate stimulus.

In light of this background of the secretion processes delineated by Palade et al., the results of studies of the biosynthesis of parathyroid hormone have provided the model shown in Figure 43-4 for the synthesis, transport, and sequential proteolytic processing of the parathyroid hormonal precursors.

The initiation of the synthesis of Pre-ProPTH occurs on polyribosomes located within the cell matrix. When the growing poly-

peptide chain is approximately 20 to 30 amino acids in length, the N-terminus of the chain first emerges from the large subunit of the ribosome, and, at this time, the two N-terminal methionines of Pre-ProPTH are removed by a putative methionyl amino peptidase. As the nascent chain continues to grow, the hydrophobic amino-terminal sequence of Pre-ProPTH emerges and associates with the membrane of the endoplasmic reticulum in accord with the "signal" hypothesis originally proposed by Blobel and co-workers.²³,²⁴ In this regard, Pre-ProPTH is believed to be representative of a distinct class of biosynthetic precursors that probably exist for many, if not all, exportable, or secretory, proteins, all of which share the common property of having a hydrophobic amino-terminal sequence of 20 to 25 amino acids in length. Such initial biosynthetic precursors or "presecretory" forms of exportable proteins have been identified for proinsulin,²⁵,²⁶ growth hormone,²⁷ placental lactogen,²⁸ prolactin, ²⁹,³⁰ immunoglobulins, ³¹⁻³³ albumin,³⁴ and pancreatic enzymes.³⁵ The function of the amino-terminal "pre"-sequence is believed to be one of attachment of the polyribosome/nascent-chain complex to the reticular membrane, thus ensuring access of the protein to the cisternal space of the endoplasmic reticulum. This process results in the specific segregation and distinction of just the exportable cellular proteins within the transport pathway. Either during or immediately after completion of synthesis of the polypeptide chain, the "pre"-sequence of 23 amino acids of Pre-ProPTH is removed by cleavage of the glycyl–lysyl bond by enzymic activity located in or near the reticular membrane.¹¹

Evidence that the enzymic activity responsible for the conversion of Pre-ProPTH to ProPTH resides in the membranes of the endoplasmic reticulum has come from comparisons of the products resulting from the translations of parathyroid messenger RNA in cell-free systems devoid of reticular membranes (wheat germ extract) compared with those containing reticular membranes (Krebs ascites extract).¹⁶,²⁴,³³,³⁶ Pre-ProPTH is the only hormonal product synthesized in a cell-free system derived from extracts of wheat germ,¹⁰,¹⁴ whereas both Pre-ProPTH and ProPTH appear as products of synthesis (ProPTH predominates) in the Krebs ascites cell-free system. Additional evidence indicates that the responsible enzyme is highly localized within the membrane, inasmuch as only polypeptide chains undergoing synthesis and vectorial discharge through the membrane are cleaved to form ProPTH.¹⁶ Pre-ProPTH

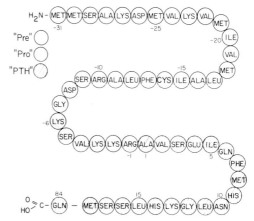

Fig. 43-2. Complete amino acid sequence of bovine pre-proparathyroid hormone as determined by microsequencing technique. The radiolabeled prehormone was synthesized in the cell-free extract of wheat germ by addition of parathyroid messenger RNA and radioactive amino acids. The NH₂-terminal methionine (residue −31) is the initiator amino acid not removed in the wheat germ system.

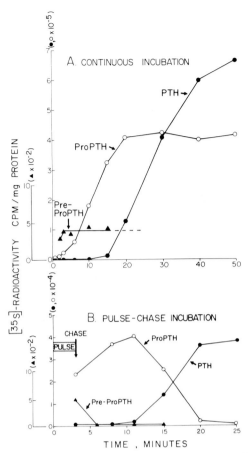

Fig. 43-3. Kinetics of incorporation by slices of parathyroid glands of [³⁵S]methionine into Pre-ProPTH, ProPTH, and PTH during (a) a continuous incubation with [³⁵S]methionine and (b) a 3-minute pulse incubation with [³⁵S]methionine followed by a chase incubation with unlabeled methionine. Amounts of radioactive ProPTH and PTH were determined by electrophoresis on urea–acetate gels. Amounts of Pre-ProPTH were determined by reelectrophoresis on urea–sodium dodecyl sulfate gels of the material corresponding to Pre-ProPTH isolated from urea–acetate gels. (Habener et al.[11] Courtesy of American Society of Biological Chemists.)

added to cell-free extracts of parathyroid glands remains intact and is not converted either to ProPTH or to PTH under conditions in which ProPTH is readily converted to PTH.[37] Moreover, addition of exogenous Pre-ProPTH to biosynthetically active heterologous cell-free translation systems containing reticular membranes (e.g., Krebs ascites extract), which readily process the endogenous newly synthesized Pre-ProPTH to ProPTH, does not result in the formation of ProPTH from the exogenous Pre-ProPTH.[16]

At present, the enzymic process(es) that converts Pre-ProPTH to PTH is poorly understood. It has not been possible to identify either in parathyroid cells or in cell-free systems a peptide corresponding to the first 23 amino acids of Pre-ProPTH. Clearly, such a peptide, if removed from Pre-ProPTH by an endopeptidase, should be present in the protein-synthesizing systems. The failure to detect the peptide suggests that other enzymic mechanisms may be at play—such as removal of the peptide by sequential action of exopeptidase activity or enzymic destruction of the peptide immediately after its removal by endopeptidase. The specificity of the endopeptidase (if such exists) is unusual inasmuch as it is directed toward a glycyl-lysyl bond—a bond not known to be susceptible to any of the commonly recognized cellular enzymes.

After a delay of approximately 15 minutes from the time of its initial formation from Pre-ProPTH in the rough endoplasmic retic-

ulum, ProPTH arrives at the Golgi apparatus where it is converted to PTH by the proteolytic removal of the N-terminal sequence of six amino acids from ProPTH. Evidence that the conversion of ProPTH to PTH occurs in the Golgi elements of the cell was given by radioautographic analyses of the migration of newly synthesized protein and by the use of pharmacologic agents that specifically disrupt the Golgi complex. Radioautographic grains, observed by electronmicroscopy in parathyroid cells pulse-labeled with [³H]leucine, first appear in the Golgi region after 15 minutes, corresponding to the time at which conversion of ProPTH to PTH is first observed by electrophoretic analyses of the newly synthesized proteins in extracts of the cells.[21] Both amine compounds[38] and the ionophore X537A[39] have been shown to be potent and selective inhibitors of the conversion of ProPTH to PTH and both of these agents have been shown by electronmicroscopy to produce corresponding disruptive alterations in the Golgi complex. The process of translocation of ProPTH from the rough ER to the Golgi apparatus was shown to require energy[40] and, quite likely, to be mediated by the action of microtubules;[40,41] inhibitors of oxidative phosphorylation (dinitrophenol, antimycin A) and of microtubular function (vinblastine, colchicine) impair the conversion of ProPTH.

More is known about the nature of the enzymic activities that convert ProPTH to PTH than about the enzymic activity that converts Pre-ProPTH to ProPTH. Incubation of ProPTH with dilute pancreatic trypsin[4,9,42] or with subcellular fractions prepared from homogenates of parathyroid glands[37,43] readily and selectively results in the formation of PTH without other cleavages in the sequence of PTH. The arginyl–alanyl bond (or arginyl–seryl in human ProPTH) (Fig. 43-2) is preferentially susceptible to cleavage by trypsinlike activities. The trypticlike activity in the parathyroid cell that accomplishes the conversion of ProPTH to PTH, however, does not appear to be identical to pancreatic trypsin, inas-

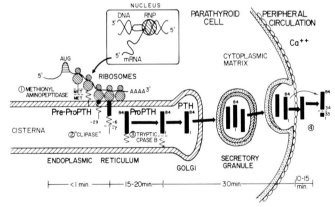

BIOSYNTHETIC PATHWAY FOR PARATHYROID HORMONE
SEQUENTIAL PROTEOLYTIC CLEAVAGES

Fig. 43-4. Schema depicting the proposed intracellular pathway of the biosynthesis of parathyroid hormone. Pre-proparathyroid hormone (Pre-ProPTH), the initial product of synthesis on the ribosomes, is converted into proparathyroid hormone (ProPTH) by removal of (1) the NH₂-terminal methionyl residues and (2) the NH₂-terminal sequence (-29 thru -7) of 23 amino acids during or within seconds after synthesis, respectively. The conversion of Pre-ProPTH probably occurs during transport of the polypeptide into the cisterna of the rough endoplasmic reticulum. By 20 minutes after synthesis, ProPTH reaches the Golgi region and is converted into PTH by (3) removal of the NH₂-terminal hexapeptide. PTH is stored in the secretory granule until released into the circulation in response to a fall in the blood concentration of calcium. The time needed for these events is given below the schema. (Habener et al.[2] Courtesy of Academic Press.)

much as it is not inhibited by TLCK or by soybean trypsin inhibitor (but is inhibited by addition of EDTA).[37,43] Recently, it was shown that the hexapeptide at the N-terminal sequence of the ProPTH removed by the trypticlike cleavage is further modified in the cell by sequential actions of carboxypeptidase-B-like activity.[37] Although the trypticlike activity is sufficient by itself to convert ProPTH to PTH, the observation that the hexapeptide cleaved from ProPTH is further modified by the action of an exopeptidase is relevant because it indicates that such combined endopeptidase and exopeptidase activities may be involved in the proteolytic processing of many if not all prohormones or proproteins (Fig. 43-5). It was shown that the conversion of proinsulin to insulin was accomplished by the actions of both trypticlike and carboxypeptidase-B-like enzymes[44,45] and that the primary amino acid sequences of other polypeptides thought to be prohormones or proproteins (e.g., the proglucagon fragment, big gastrins, betalipotropic hormone, proalbumin) contain sequences of two to three basic amino acids (lysines and/or arginines) at the sites of cleavage, which, predictably, would be preferred sites of cleavages by enzymes with specificities similar to trypsin and carboxypeptidase B.[45]

The efficiency of the conversion of ProPTH to PTH, at least as observed in studies of normal parathyroid tissues, is high. Radioactive ProPTH reaches a constant specific activity in the tissue within 20 minutes after a pulse label of [³H]leucine has been introduced into the media bathing the parathyroid gland slices.[11] Moreover, analyses by specific radioimmunoassays of the amounts of ProPTH and PTH in normal parathyroid glands indicate that PTH is the predominant form of the hormone stored in the gland; ProPTH comprises only 7 percent of the total immunoreactive hormone.[46,47] This quantity of prohormone can be attributed to the amount of precursor in transit within the cisternal space of the endoplasmic reticulum to the site of cleavage in the Golgi complex. Attempts to detect ProPTH in the media of parathyroid gland slices incubated in vitro or in parathyroid effluent blood collected from calves or patients undergoing surgical removal of parathyroid adenomas have been unsuccessful. Thus, it seems probable that little, if any, ProPTH is stored within the secretory granules of the parathyroid gland and that, in contrast to pancreatic islet cells, which secrete up to 10 percent proinsulin with respect to insulin, the parathyroid gland does not normally secrete ProPTH.

Transport of PTH to the site of release at the plasma membrane presumably occurs via the secretion granules. Analyses by electron microscopy of parathyroid cells, however, have shown that mature, membrane-limited secretion granules are few in number compared, for example, with pancreatic islet cells or pituitary somatotropes.[21] At the same time, numbers of "immature" vesicles derived from the Golgi elements are abundant, suggesting that some fraction of PTH may be transported directly to the periphery of the cell without prior incorporation into mature secretion granules. Indeed, some evidence has been reported suggesting that there may exist two separate pathways for the secretion of PTH, one utilized by stored, or "mature," hormone, and the other preferentially used by newly synthesized hormone.[48] The evidence was obtained from studies of PTH secretion from parathyroid gland slices in vitro where comparisons were made of the specific activities (ratios of radioactively labeled to total immunoreactive PTH) of hormone in the tissue compared with those released from the tissue into the media.

More is known about the pathways of PTH biosynthesis (described above) than about the precise cellular mechanisms involved in the regulation of PTH biosynthesis. Based on results of studies in vitro of the effects of extracellular calcium on rates of ProPTH synthesis and formation of PTH, some general statements can be made regarding the regulation of hormone synthesis. Calcium is the principal factor known to regulate the biosynthetic activity of the parathyroid gland (see Chapter 44). The rates of secretion, and ultimately the synthesis, of PTH vary inversely with the concentration of extracellular calcium ion. In Figure 43-6, the proposed steps in the biosynthetic pathway of PTH where calcium or other agents may exert a regulatory influence are schematically summarized. At present, information about the actions of calcium at these specific control points is incomplete, but some general conclusions can be stated. The overall regulation of the rates of hormone biosynthesis most likely occurs at the level of transcriptional (step 2 of Fig. 43-6) rather than translational (step 3, Fig. 43-6) events.

Studies of hormone biosynthesis in vitro have shown that changes in the rates of ProPTH formation in response to changes in concentrations of calcium in extracellular fluid require hours to become apparent.[49,50] Such observations are more consistent with a regulatory system in which changes in the intracellular concentrations or distributions of calcium ions, or alternatively, intracellular events invoked by calcium-mediated alterations in hormone secretion, influence rates of mRNA synthesis (transcriptional events that take hours to become manifest) rather than protein

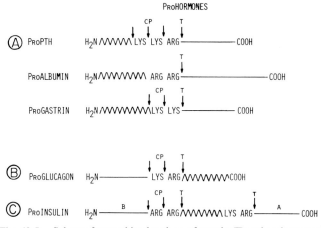

Fig. 43-5. Schema for combined actions of tryptic (T) and carboxypeptidase-B-like (CP) activities in the conversion of proproteins (prohormones) to the authentic products. (a) Mechanism whereby tryptic cleavage alone results in formation of final product; (b) combined action of the two enzymes is necessary for production of glucagon; (c) proinsulin is an example of the existence of both cleavage mechanisms. (Habener et al.[37] Courtesy of the American Chemical Society.)

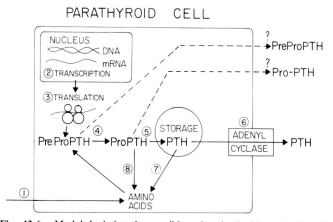

Fig. 43-6. Model depicting the possible points in the biosynthetic pathways of a parathyroid cell where calcium may exert regulatory effects. PSP, parathyroid secretory protein (Habener.[3] Courtesy of Elsevier/Excerpta Medica.)

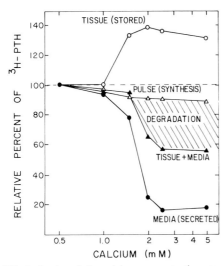

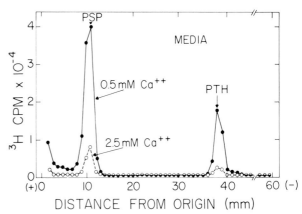

Fig. 43-7. Effect of extracellular calcium concentrations on synthesis (△), secretion (●), and storage (○) of PTH. The calcium-dependent degradation of PTH (▲) is also shown. Slices of parathyroid glands were incubated in vitro for 4 hours in MEM media containing [³H]leucine and various concentrations of calcium. Amounts of ³H-labeled PTH were determined by polyacrylamide gel electrophoresis of extracts of tissue (○) and media (●) at the end of the incubation as described previously. Rates of PTH synthesis (△)were determined by preincubating tissue slices for 3 hours in various concentrations of calcium and then adding [³H]leucine for an additional 35 minutes of incubation (pulse-label). Extracts of tissues were analyzed for their content of ³H-labeled ProPTH and PTH by gel electrophoresis. In the higher concentrations of calcium, up to 40 percent of the [³H]PTH is neither secreted from nor stored in the tissue but, instead, is degraded within the tissue (shaded area). Data are expressed as percent of [³H]PTH in extracts from tissues and media incubated at lowest concentration of calcium (0.5 mM of calcium = 100 percent [³H]PTH). (Habener.[3] Courtesy of Elsevier/ Excerpta Medica.)

(Pre-ProPTH) synthesis in response to preexisting mRNA (translational events that would be expressed in synthesis of protein immediately). Calcium, at least through changes in its concentration in extracellular fluid, does not appear to affect directly the activity of the enzymic process that converts ProPTH to PTH (step 5, Fig. 43-6).[49,50]

There is evidence, however, that intracellular stores of PTH may be regulated through a pathway of intracellular turnover of PTH or of ProPTH (steps 7 and 8 of Fig. 43-6).[50,51] High concentrations of extracellular calcium stimulate, and low concentrations inhibit, intracellular degradation of hormone (Fig. 43-7). It has been suggested that inhibition of this degradative pathway, mediated by a lowering of extracellular calcium concentrations may, in addition to drawing on preformed stores of hormone, provide a means for a rapid increase of the amounts of hormone available for secretion before the rates of hormone biosynthesis have time to increase to the extent required to meet secretory demands. Conversely, stimulation of the degradative pathway by elevations of extracellular calcium may be a mechanism used by the cell to dispose of excess of hormone that is synthesized during the rather long time (hours) required for the suppression of rates of biosynthesis to take place.

The studies of PTH biosynthesis that have led to the discovery of precursor forms of PTH indicate that products other than PTH may be secreted from the parathyroid gland (Figs. 43-8 and 43-9). At least one protein distinct from PTH is secreted from parathyroid tissue during studies in vitro. The protein, termed parathyroid secretory protein, or PSP,[52] is a high-molecular-weight protein (mol wt 150,000) that is released from the parathyroid gland in response to changes in calcium concentration in the medium.

Fig. 43-8. Products secreted by bovine parathyroid gland slices during 4-hour incubation in vitro with [³H]leucine and low (0.5 mM) versus high (2.5 mM) levels of calcium chloride. A major protein of mol wt 150,000, parathyroid secretory protein (PSP) accompanies the secretion of PTH. Patterns shown were obtained by electrophoresis of incubation media on 10 percent ureaacetate gels. Patterns are coplotted for ease of comparison. (Kemper et al.[52] Courtesy of American Association for the Advancement of Science.)

The fractional stimulation or inhibition of release of PSP, due to lowering or raising of ambient calcium concentrations, shows precisely the same pattern as that of PTH itself (Fig. 43-8). At present, the biological function of PSP is unknown. Clearly, it is not a biosynthetic precursor of PTH, but it may be a transport protein for PTH, analogous to the neurophysins, the proteins involved in the intracellular transport of oxytocin and vasopressin in the posterior pituitary gland.[53,54] The eventual development of an immunoassay specific for the detection of PSP could prove to be particularly useful for monitoring the secretory activity of the parathyroids.

Radioimmunoassays for the detection of ProPTH have been developed with antisera produced by immunization with synthetic peptides containing the prohormone-specific hexapeptide sequence.[47,55] The recognition site of two of the antisera involves the region of hormone sequence at the site of attachment of the prohormone hexapeptide to PTH. Assays based on these antisera

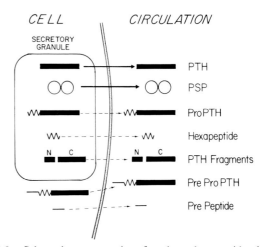

Fig. 43-9. Schematic representation of products that are either known to be released (solid arrows) or potentially could be released (interrupted arrows) from the storage granules in the parathyroid cell. PSP, parathyroid secretory protein. (Habener.[3] Courtesy of Elsevier/Excerpta Medica.)

readily detect intact, natural ProPTH and synthetic peptides of the prohormone but not PTH or the prohormone hexapeptide sequence alone. In preliminary applications, the prohormone assay readily detects prohormone in extracts of parathyroid tissue but not in blood. Initially, it was thought that proteolytic enzymes in blood that rapidly degrade ProPTH prevented the detection of the prohormone.[46] Subsequent studies, however, with inhibitors of proteinases in conditions in which degradation of ProPTH was prevented also failed to detect the prohormone, even when it was searched for directly in parathyroid effluent blood of calves and patients with primary hyperparathyroidism.[47] Within the detection limits of the assays, ProPTH at a concentration of less than 1 to 2 percent of the PTH in the blood samples would not have been detected.

Thus, no final conclusion has yet been reached about secretion of prohormone. Pre-ProPTH has not been isolated in amounts sufficient for immunization of animals, and therefore no immunoassay for its detection is available. If specific and sensitive radioimmunoassays can be developed to detect the presence of ProPTH or of Pre-ProPTH in the circulation, then evidence of the release of the precursors might serve as a useful marker of abnormal parathyroid gland function or of ectopic hormone production (secretion of PTH by nonparathyroid tumors). It is believed that nonparathyroid tissue, as a consequence of neoplastic transformation, initiates uncontrolled production and release of PTH as a result of what may be abnormalities in the intracellular transport and cleavage of the hormone. Hence, defects such as release of predominantly pre-prohormone or prohormone (lack of specific cleavage enzymes) or predominantly fragments of hormone (excessive proteolytic degradation) might be found in states of uncontrolled parathyroid secretory activity.

Although no direct evidence has yet been obtained to indicate that ProPTH, Pre-ProPTH, or the peptide fragments of the precursors that are removed from ProPTH and PTH in the cell are secreted into the circulation (Fig. 43-9), indirect evidence suggests that malignant tumors (not of parathyroid origin) and adenomas of the parathyroids may secrete a precursor along with the hormone. Material of high molecular weight that reacts with antisera to parathyroid hormone has been observed in the blood of patients with the syndrome of pseudohyperparathyroidism—i.e., the secretion of PTH-like material by nonparathyroid cancer and hyperparathyroidism due to parathyroid adenomas.[55] It is not known whether this high-molecular-weight material contains PTH covalently linked or whether PTH is noncovalently bound to some larger macromolecule.

Obviously, additional information is needed about the normal control processes within the parathyroid cell involved in regulation between the initial steps of ProPTH synthesis and eventual release of PTH from storage granules. Such information will be of great fundamental interest and may eventually serve as a model with which to evaluate the defects in cellular control that are characteristic of the excessive secretion of PTH seen in primary and ectopic hyperparathyroidism.

REFERENCES

1. Hamilton, J. W., and Cohn, D. V. Studies on the Biosynthesis *in vitro* of Parathyroid Hormone. I. Synthesis of Parathyroid Hormone by Bovine Parathyroid Gland Slices and Its Control by Calcium. J. Biol. Chem. *244:* 5421, 1969.
2. Habener, J. F., Kemper, B. W., Rich, A., et al. Biosynthesis of Parathyroid Hormone. Rec. Prog. Horm. Res. *33:* 249, 1977.
3. Habener, J. F. New Concepts in the Formation, Regulation of Release, and Metabolism of Parathyroid Hormone, in *Polypeptide Hormones: Molecular and Cellular Aspects* (Ciba Foundation Symposium 41). Elsevier/Excerpta Medica/North-Holland, Amsterdam, 1976, p 197.
4. Habener, J. F., and Potts, J. T., Jr. Chemistry, Biosynthesis, Secretion, and Metabolism of Parathyroid Hormone, in *Handbook of Physiology, Endocrinology VII*, edited by E. B. Astwood and R. O. Greep. American Physiological Society, Washington, D.C., 1976, p 313.
5. Cohn, D. V., and Hamilton, J. W. Newer Aspects of Parathyroid Chemistry and Physiology. Cornell Vet. *66:* 271, 1976.
6. Steiner, D. F., and Oyer, P. E. The Biosynthesis of Insulin and a Probable Precursor of Insulin by a Human Islet Cell Adenoma. Proc. Nat. Acad. Sci. *57:* 473, 1967.
7. Hamilton, J. W., MacGregor, R. R., Chu, L. L. H., et al. The Isolation and Partial Purification of a Non-parathyroid Hormone Calcemic Fraction from Bovine Parathyroid Gland. Endocrinology *89:* 1440, 1971.
8. Kemper, B., Habener, J. F., Potts, J. T., Jr., et al. Proparathyroid Hormone: Identification of a Biosynthetic Precursor to Parathyroid Hormone. Proc. Nat. Acad. Sci. USA *69:* 643, 1972.
9. Cohn, D. V., MacGregor, R. R., Chu, L. L. H., et al. Calcemic Fraction-A: Biosynthetic Peptide Precursor of Parathyroid Hormone. Proc. Nat. Acad. Sci. USA *69:* 1521, 1972.
10. Kemper, B., Habener, J. F., Mulligan, R. C., et al. Pre-proparathyroid Hormone: A Direct Translation Product of Parathyroid Messenger RNA. Proc. Nat. Acad. Sci. USA *71:* 3731, 1974.
11. Habener, J. F., Potts, J. T., Jr., and Rich, A. Pre-preparathyroid Hormone: Evidence for an Early Biosynthetic Precursor of Proparathyroid Hormone. J. Biol. Chem. *251:* 3893, 1976.
12. Hamilton, J. W., Niall, H. D., Jacobs, J. W., et al. The N-Terminal Amino-Acid Sequence of Bovine Proparathyroid Hormone. Proc. Nat. Acad. Sci. USA *71:* 653, 1974.
13. Jacobs, J. W., Kemper, B., Niall, H. D., et al. Structural Analysis of Human Proparathyroid Hormone by a New Microsequencing Approach. Nature *249:* 155, 1974.
14. Kemper, B. [W.], Habener, J. F., Ernst, M. D., et al. Pre-proparathyroid Hormone: Analysis of Radioactive Tryptic Peptides and Amino Acid Sequence. Biochemistry *15:* 15, 1976.
15. Habener, J. F., Kemper, B., Potts, J. T., Jr., et al. Pre-proparathyroid Hormone Identified by Cell-free Translation of Messenger RNA from Hyperplastic Human Parathyroid Tissue. J. Clin. Invest. *56:* 1328, 1975.
16. Habener, J. F., Kemper, B., Potts, J. T., Jr., et al. Parathyroid mRNA Directs the Synthesis of Pre-proparathyroid Hormone and Proparathyroid Hormone in the Krebs Ascites Cell-free System. Biochem. Biophys. Res. Commun. *67:* 1114, 1975.
17. Kemper, B. [W.], Habener, J. F., Potts, J. T., Jr., et al. Pre-proparathyroid Hormone: Fidelity of the Translation of Parathyroid Messenger RNA by Extracts of Wheat Germ. Biochemistry *15:* 20, 1976.
18. Kronenberg, H. M., Roberts, B. E., Habener, J. F., et al. DNA Complementary to Parathyroid mRNA Directs the Synthesis of Pre-proparathyroid Hormone in a Linked Transcription–Translation System. Nature *267:* 804, 1977.
19. MacGregor, R. R., Chu, L. L. H., Hamilton, J. W., et al. Studies on the Subcellular Localization of Proparathyroid Hormone and Parathyroid Hormone in the Bovine Parathyroid Gland: Separation of Newly Synthesized from Mature Forms. Endocrinology *93:* 1387, 1973.
20. Habener, J. F., and Potts, J. T., Jr. Subcellular Distributions of Parathyroid Hormone, Hormonal Precursors, and Parathyroid Secretory Protein. Endocrinology (in press).
21. Habener, J. F., Amherdt, M., and Orci, L. Subcellular Organelles Involved in the Conversion of Biosynthetic Precursors of Parathyroid Hormone. Trans. Assoc. Am. Physicians *90:* 366, 1977.
22. Palade, G. Intracellular Aspects of the Process of Protein Synthesis. Science *189:* 347, 1975.
23. Blobel, G., Sabatini, D. D. Ribosome-Membrane Interaction in Eukaryotic Cells. Biomembranes *2:* 193, 1971.
24. Blobel, G., and Dobberstein, B.: Transfer of Proteins Across Membranes. I. Presence of Proteolytically Processed and Unprocessed Nascent Immunoglobulin Light Chains on Membrane-Bound Ribosomes of Murine Myeloma. J. Cell Biol. *67:* 835, 1975.
25. Permutt, M. A., Biesbroeck, J., Chyn, R., et al. Isolation of a Biologically Active Messenger RNA: Preparation from Fish Pancreatic Islets by Oligo (2'-Deoxythymidylic Acid) Affinity Chromatography, in *Polypeptide Hormones: Molecular and Cellular Aspects* (Ciba Foundation Symposium 41), 1976, p. 97.

26. Chan, S. J., Keim, P., and Steiner, D. F. Cell-free Synthesis of Rat Preproinsulins: Characterization and Partial Amino Acid Sequence Determination. Proc. Nat. Acad. Sci. USA 73: 1964, 1976.

27. Sussman, P. M., Tushinski, R. J., and Bancroft, F. C. Pregrowth Hormone: Product of the Translation in vitro of Messenger RNA Coding for Growth Hormone. Proc. Natl. Acad. Sci. USA 73: 29, 1976.

28. Boime, I., Boguslawski, S., and Caine, J. The Translation of a Human Placental Lactogen mRNA Fraction in Heterologous Cell-free Systems: The Synthesis of a Possible Precursor. Biochem. Biophys. Res. Commun. 62: 103, 1975.

29. Maurer, R. A., Stone, R., and Gorski, J. Cell-free Synthesis of a Large Translation Product of Prolactin Messenger RNA. J. Biol. Chem. 251: 2801, 1976.

30. Evans, G. A., and Rosenfeld, M. G. Cell-free Synthesis of a Prolactin Precursor Directed by mRNA from Cultured Rat Pituitary Cells. J. Biol. Chem. 251: 2842, 1976.

31. Milstein, C., Brownlee, G. G., Harrison, T. M., et al. A Possible Precursor of Immunoglobulin Light Chains. Nature New Biol. 239: 117, 1972.

32. Burstein, Y., Kantor, F., and Schechter, I. Partial Amino-Acid Sequence of the Precursor of an Immunoglobulin Light Chain Containing NH$_2$-Terminal Pyroglutamic Acid. Proc. Natl. Acad. Sci. USA 73: 2604, 1976.

33. Blobel, G., and Dobberstein, B. Transfer of Proteins Across Membranes. II. Reconstitution of Functional Rough Microsomes from Heterologous Components. J. Cell Biol. 67: 852, 1975.

34. Strauss, A. W., Bennett, C. D., Donohue, A. M., et al. Rat Liver Preproalbumin: Complete Amino Acid Sequence of the Pre-Piece. Analysis of the Direct Translation Product of Albumin Messenger RNA. J. Biol. Chem. 252: 6846, 1977.

35. Devillers-Thiery, A., Kindt, T., Scheele, G., et al. Homology in Amino-Terminal Sequence of Precursors to Pancreatic Secretory Proteins. Proc. Natl. Acad. Sci. USA 72: 5016, 1975.

36. Szczesna, E., and Boime, I. mRNA-Dependent Synthesis of Authentic Precursor to Human Placental Lactogen: Conversion to Its Mature Hormone Form in Ascites Cell-free Extracts. Proc. Natl. Acad. Sci. 73: 1179, 1976.

37. Habener, J. F., Chang, H., and Potts, J. T., Jr. Enzymic Processing of Proparathyroid Hormone by Cell-free Extracts of Parathyroid Glands. Biochemistry 16: 3910, 1977.

38. Chu, L. H., MacGregor, R. R., Hamilton, J. W., et al. Conversion of Proparathyroid Hormone to Parathyroid Hormone: The Use of Amines as Specific Inhibitors. Endocrinology 95: 1431, 1974.

39. Habener, J. F., Stevens, T. D., Ravazzola, M., et al. Effects of Calcium Ionophores on the Synthesis and Release of Parathyroid Hormone. Endocrinology 101: 1524,, 1977.

40. Chu, L. L. H., MacGregor, R. R., and Cohn, D. V.: Energy-Dependent Intracellular Translocation of Proparathormone. J. Cell Biol. 72: 1, 1977.

41. Kemper, B. [W.], Habener, J. F., Rich, A., et al. Microtubules and the Intracellular Conversion of Proparathyroid Hormone to Parathyroid Hormone. Endocrinology 96: 903, 1975.

42. Goltzman, D., Callahan, E.N., Tregear, G. W., et al. Conversion of Proparathyroid Hormone to Parathyroid Hormone: Studies in Vitro with Trypsin. Biochemistry 15: 5076, 1976.

43. MacGregor, R. R., Chu, L. L. H., and Cohn, D. V. Conversion of Proparathyroid Hormone to Parathyroid Hormone by a Particulate Enzyme of the Parathyroid Gland. J. Biol. Chem. 251: 6711, 1976.

44. Kemmler, W., Steiner, D. F., and Borg, J. Studies on the Conversion of Proinsulin to Insulin. III: Studies in Vitro with a Crude Secretion Granule Fraction Isolated from Rat Islets of Langerhans. J. Biol. Chem. 248: 4544, 1973.

45. Steiner, D. F. Peptide Hormone Precursors: Biosynthesis, Processing and Significance, in Peptide Hormones, edited by J. A. Parsons. Macmillan, London, 1976, p 49.

46. Habener, J. F., Tregear, G. W., Stevens, T. S., et al. Radioimmunoassay for Proparathyroid Hormone. Endocrine Res. Commun. 1: 1, 1974.

47. Habener, J. F., Stevens, T. D., Tregear, G. W., et al. Radioimmunoassay of Human Proparathyroid Hormone: Analysis of Hormone Content in Tissue Extracts and in Plasma. J. Clin. Endocrinol. Metab. 42: 520, 1976.

48. MacGregor, R. R., Hamilton, J. W., and Cohn, D. V. The By-pass of Tissue Hormone Stores During Secretion of Newly Synthesized Parathyroid Hormone. Endocrinology 97: 178, 1975.

49. Habener, J. F., Kemper, B. W., Potts, J. T., Jr., et al. Calcium-independent Intracellular Conversion of Proparathyroid Hormone to Parathyroid Hormone. Endocrine Res. Commun. 1: 239, 1974.

50. Habener, J. F., Kemper, B., and Potts, J. T., Jr. Calcium-dependent Intracellular Degradation of Parathyroid Hormone: A Possible Mechanism for the Regulation of Hormone Stores. Endocrinology 97: 431, 1975.

51. Chu, L. L. H., MacGregor, R. R., Anast, C. S., et al. Studies on the Biosynthesis of Rat Parathyroid Hormone and Proparathyroid Hormone: Adaptation of the Parathyroid Gland to Dietary Restriction of Calcium. Endocrinology 93: 915, 1973.

52. Kemper, B. [W.], Habener, J. F., Rich, A., et al. Parathyroid Secretion: Discovery of a Major Calcium-dependent Protein. Science 184: 167, 1974.

53. Cheng, K. W., and Friesen, H. G.: A Radioimmunoassay for Vasopressin Binding Proteins—Neurophysin. Endocrinology 88: 608, 1971.

54. Martin, M. J., Chard, T., and Landon, J. The Development of a Radioimmunoassay for Bovine Neurophysin. J. Endocrinol. 52: 481, 1972.

55. Benson, R. C., Jr., Riggs, B. L., Pickard, B. M., et al. Immunoreactive Forms of Circulating Parathyroid Hormone in Primary and Ectopic Hyperparathyroidism. J. Clin. Invest. 54: 175, 1974.

44

Parathyroid Hormone Secretion

G. P. Mayer

CONTROL OF SECRETION

CALCIUM

Despite recent indications of changes in parathyroid secretory rate in response to other factors (see below), plasma calcium concentration retains a predominant role in the regulation of parathyroid hormone secretion. It is generally agreed that the ionized portion is responsible for effects on the parathyroids, although most experiments report results in terms of total plasma calcium concentration. In simple terms, the parathyroid gland is stimulated by a subnormal plasma calcium concentration and suppressed by hypercalcemia. The existence of this relationship was first demonstrated by experiments in which effluent from parathyroid glands perfused with decalcified blood produced a rise in serum calcium of recipient dogs.[1] Later experiments involving radioimmunoassay of parathyroid hormone concentration in plasma collected from cows before and during induced hypocalcemia[2,3] confirmed the validity of interpretations drawn from the earlier experiments. Recent investigations indicate that the regulation of parathyroid secretion by plasma calcium concentration is more complex than a simple inverse relationship. Analyses of approximately 600 plasma samples collected from cows during the onset of hypocalcemia at parturition and after intravenous calcium therapy suggest that the relation between plasma immunoreactive parathyroid hormone concentration and plasma calcium concentration is sigmoid in nature.[4] A similiar relationship between parathyroid hormone secretion rate (determined by collection and radioimmunoassay of parathyroid effluent blood) and plasma calcium concentration (Fig. 44-1) was demonstrated using calves.[5] Thus, while in a general sense the concept that the parathyroid is stimulated by hypocalcemia and suppressed by hypercalcemia is correct, it is evident from Figure 44-1 that this response occurs over a very narrow range of plasma calcium concentration (i.e., 7.5–10.5 mg/100 ml). Changes in plasma calcium concentration above and below this range elicit only minor changes in hormone secretion rate. The continued secretion of parathyroid hormone despite hypercalcemia appears to represent a basal rate of secretion which is independent of plasma calcium concentration, while the absence of

a progressive increase in secretion rate in response to severe hypocalcemia (below 7.5 mg/100 ml) probably represents attainment of a maximal secretory output early in the development of hypocalcemia.

The sigmoid nature of the parathyroid secretory response to changes of plasma calcium concentration appears appropriate for the performance of the function of the parathyroid glands, i.e., the prevention of hypocalcemia. When the threat of hypocalcemia is remote, as during hypercalcemia, secretion rate is unresponsive to changes in plasma calcium concentration and is suppressed to a minimal rate. Within the normocalcemic range (9–11 mg/100 ml), the threat of hypocalcemia is more of a possibility, and the gland is more responsive to changes in plasma calcium concentration. When plasma calcium concentration declines below the normocalcemic range and hypocalcemia becomes a reality, the parathyroid response is pronounced, and a maximal secretory output is attained in response to only a mild hypocalcemia. This response appears appropriate to forestall the development of life-endangering, severe hypocalcemia.

PHOSPHATE

In the past, elevated plasma inorganic phosphate was thought to stimulate the parathyroids directly;[6] subsequent experiments have disproved this contention. Resolution of the question as to whether low calcium or high phosphate provided the stimulus for parathyroid secretion was complicated by the tendency toward a reciprocal relationship between concentrations of calcium and phosphorus in the blood. In other words, in the presence of a concurrent high phosphorus and low calcium concentration of the plasma, which is the stimulus for increased parathyroid secretion? Indirect evidence for the control of parathyroid activity by plasma calcium and not plasma phosphorus concentration was provided by experiments in rats using bone osteoclast count to assess changes in parathyroid activity associated with alterations in plasma concentrations of the ions induced by peritoneal lavage with solution of varying calcium and phosphate concentration.[6] More direct evidence for lack of a direct effect of phosphorus on parathyroid secretory rate was provided by radioimmunoassay of parathyroid hormone concentration in plasma collected from cows given intravenous infusions of sodium phosphate solution.[7] In these experiments the rise in plasma immunoreactive hormone concentration coincided with the decline in plasma calcium concentration rather than the rise in plasma inorganic phosphorus concentration which preceded the decrease in plasma calcium. During phosphate infusions not accompanied by a decline in plasma calcium concentration, plasma immunoreactive hormone concentration was not increased despite a fourfold increase in plasma inorganic phosphorus concentration.[7] In other experiments with cows, intravenous infusion of phosphate was associated with a rapid rise in plasma parathyroid hormone concentration, unac-

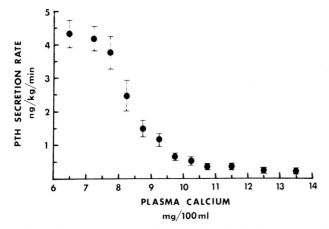

Fig. 44-1. Secretory response of the parathyroid glands to changes in plasma calcium concentration. The data represent results of experiments on three anesthetized calves. The secretion rate of a superior parathyroid gland was measured by quantitative collection (flow rate measured) and radioimmunoassay of its venous effluent. The solid symbols indicate the mean secretion rate for either 1.0 or 0.5 mg/100 ml range of plasma calcium concentration, and the vertical bars indicate the S.E. Alterations in plasma calcium concentration were induced by intravenous infusion of solutions of either Na₂EDTA or calcium chloride. The figure is a composite of measurements made during periods of declining plasma calcium concentration as well as periods of increasing concentration. (From G. P. Mayer in *Calcium-Regulating Hormones,* edited by R. V. Talmage, M. Owen, and J. A. Parsons. Excerpta Medica, Amsterdam, 1975.)

companied by a decline of total plasma calcium concentration; however, measurement of calcium ion concentration revealed that the rise in plasma hormone concentration coincided with a decline in calcium ion concentration of the plasma.[8] The results of all of the foregoing experiments indicate that plasma inorganic phosphorus concentration does not have a direct effect on parathyroid secretory rate, but rather influences secretion rate secondarily through an effect on plasma calcium concentration.

MAGNESIUM

Magnesium has been shown to affect parathyroid secretory rate both in vitro and in vivo. The release of immunoreactive parathyroid hormone into the medium bathing slices of parathyroid glands increased as the concentration of magnesium in the medium was decreased, provided that the calcium concentration was held constant.[9,10] Likewise, during in situ perfusion of the parathyroid glands of sheep and goats with blood of varying magnesium concentration, the concentrations of magnesium and parathyroid hormone in the effluent blood were inversely related.[11,12] Intravenous infusion of magnesium chloride decreased parathyroid secretory rate in calves (assessed by collection and radioimmunoassay of parathyroid effluent blood), but when disodium ethylenediamine tetraacetate (Na₂EDTA) was infused concurrently so that the rise in plasma magnesium concentration was offset by an equimolar decline in plasma calcium concentration, hormone secretion was increased,[5] suggesting that the effect of magnesium is not equipotent to that of calcium. On a molar basis, the effect of magnesium appeared to be approximately one-third to one-half that of calcium.[5] This finding agrees closely with results of recent in vitro experiments,[12a] but is contrary to results of previous in vitro experiments in which the effect of magnesium was determined to be equal to that of calcium.[10] Although an explanation for the different results obtained in these experiments is not readily apparent, the majority of the evidence favors the view that magnesium

does influence parathyroid secretory rate, but its effect is not equipotent to that of calcium. In view of the lesser effect and lower plasma concentration of magnesium relative to calcium, it seems unlikely that plasma magnesium concentration will play a major role in the control of parathyroid secretory rate except in those conditions involving pathological alterations of blood magnesium concentration.

During chronic magnesium depletion, the normal inverse relationship between plasma magnesium concentration and parathyroid secretory rate documented in the preceding paragraph may be altered. In studies in man[13,14] and dogs,[15] hypomagnesemia was associated with hypocalcemia and an inappropriately low concentration of immunoreactive parathyroid hormone in the plasma. Elevation of plasma magnesium concentration by intravenous administration of magnesium was accompanied by an increase in plasma immunoreactive parathyroid hormone concentration.[13] These observations suggest that the secretion of parathyroid hormone may be impaired during chronic magnesium depletion. This interpretation is supported by in vitro experiments demonstrating diminished secretion by parathyroid slices during incubation in a medium of extremely low magnesium concentration.[10]

EPINEPHRINE

Experiments both in vitro and in vivo indicate that epinephrine stimulates increased secretion of parathyroid hormone. The addition of epinephrine to the incubation medium of parathyroid slices in vitro increased the release of hormone into the medium,[16] suggesting that the increase of plasma immunoreactive parathyroid hormone concentration associated with epinephrine administration to cows[17] and man[18] is the result of a direct effect of epinephrine on the parathyroid gland. The following observations suggest that the effect of epinephrine is mediated via beta-adrenergic receptors: (1) administration of phenylephrine, an alpha-adrenergic agent, did not affect plasma immunoreactive parathyroid hormone concentration;[18] (2) administration of isoproterenol, a specific beta agent, was accompanied by a rise in plasma immunoreactive hormone concentration;[17,18] and (3) the epinephrine-induced increase of plasma hormone concentration was inhibited by a beta blocking agent, propranolol.[17,18] Since beta-adrenergic influences can increase intracellular levels of adenosine 3',5'-monophosphate (cAMP) in many types of cells,[19] it seems plausible that a similiar effect on the parathyroid cell may be involved in the mediation of the effect of beta-adrenergic stimulation upon parathyroid hormone secretion rate (see Mediation of the Secretory Response, in this chapter).

The foregoing observations raise the possibility that epinephrine may play a significant role in the regulation of parathyroid hormone secretion under pathological as well as physiological conditions. The suppression of basal plasma immunoreactive parathyroid hormone concentration by the administration of propranolol[18] suggests that beta-adrenergic influences may be playing a role in the regulation of parathyroid secretion, and hence calcium homeostasis, under normal physiological conditions. In regard to pathological conditions, the suggestion of an increased incidence of hyperparathyroidism in patients with bronchial asthma[20] may be explained as an effect of the beta-adrenergic agents used to treat asthma, since therapeutic doses of these agents appear to stimulate the parathyroid glands.[18] Furthermore, the hypercalcemia associated with pheochromocytoma appears to involve parathyroid stimulation by excessive catecholamine secretion, since removal of the tumor is followed by a decrease in plasma parathyroid hormone concentration and disappearance of the hypercalcemia.[21]

Recent observations in the author's laboratory have established in greater detail the response in parathyroid hormone secretion to graded infusions of epinephrine (Fig. 44-2). Of particular significance was the finding that a point in the dose-response curve relating parathyroid hormone secretion rate to dose of infused catechol occurred at a dose of epinephrine close to estimates of circulating endogenous epinephrine (Fig. 44-2). Essential details of the role of epinephrine in secretion of parathyroid hormone, especially the physiological role, if any, of epinephrine as a secretagogue and its relation to regulation by calcium remain to be established.

METABOLITES OF VITAMIN D

The pronounced effect of vitamin D (cholecalciferol) upon calcium metabolism is dependent upon conversion to more active metabolites by hydroxylation, first in the liver and subsequently in the kidney. Parathyroid hormone acts on the kidney to enhance the conversion of 25-hydroxycholecalciferol, the metabolite produced in the liver, to 1,25-dihydroxycholecalciferol,[22] a metabolite that is active in both intestinal mucosa and bone.[22] In parathyroidectomized animals or in the absence of parathyroid stimulation as during normocalcemia or hypercalcemia, the production of 1,25-dihydroxycholecalciferol is diminished, and production of 24,25-dihydroxycholecalciferol, a metabolite without effect on bone, is increased.[22] In view of the important roles of both parathyroid hormone and vitamin D in blood calcium homeostasis, the demonstration of a regulatory role of parathyroid hormone in the activation of vitamin D has stimulated interest in the possibility of a feedback control of parathyroid secretion by vitamin D metabolites. Preliminary experiments involving in situ perfusion of the superior parathyroid gland of goats have demonstrated suppression of parathyroid secretory rate by 24,25-dihydroxycholecalciferol (24,25-DHCC).[23] The concentration of 24,25-DHCC in the perfusing solution was similiar to that found in normocalcemic human plasma. The authors suggest that a low plasma concentration of 24,25-DHCC might explain the hypersecretion of parathyroid hormone associated with the normocalcemic phase of vitamin-D-deficiency rickets. However, an appreciation of the full significance of their findings and the role of other vitamin D metabolites in parathyroid regulation will await further investigation.

CIRCADIAN RHYTHM

The existence of circadian changes in the blood concentration of several hormones has been documented.[24] Recent investigations have been conducted to determine whether the parathyroid glands may respond in this manner also. A peak of plasma immunoreactive parathyroid hormone concentration, occurring between 2 and 4 A.M., was a consistent feature in a group of 10 human patients sampled every 2 hours throughout a 24-hour period.[25] Although the peak hormone concentration coincided with a nadir in total plasma calcium concentration, several items of evidence suggest that the rise in hormone concentration was not dependent upon a fall in plasma ionized calcium concentration. The decrease in calcium concentration was paralleled by a decline in plasma albumin concentration, suggesting that the decrease in total calcium concentration may have been due to a decrease in the protein-bound portion. Furthermore, the nocturnal hypocalcemia, but not the immunoreactive hormone peak, was abolished by either continuous intravenous infusion of calcium or confinement to bed throughout the 24-hour period. Another group of investigators collected blood from normal human subjects at 10- to 20-minute intervals and found three to five episodes of increased plasma immunoreactive parathyroid hormone concentration during a 24-hour period.[26] In these studies, the changes in hormone concentration could not be related to changes in plasma calcium concentration. From the foregoing observations, it appears that further investigation will be required to convincingly establish patterns of circadian rhythm for parathyroid secretion. Nevertheless, the above experiments draw attention to another situation in which changes in parathyroid secretory rate appear to be independent of changes in plasma calcium concentration.

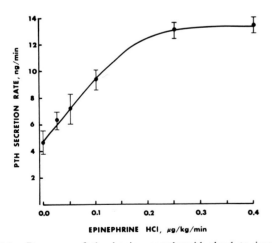

Fig. 44-2. Response of the bovine parathyroid gland to increasing amounts of epinephrine. Secretion rate of a superior parathyroid gland of an anesthetized calf was determined by radioimmunoassay of parathyroid venous blood which was collected over timed intervals and measured volumetrically. Epinephrine was infused intravenously at each rate for a period of 40 minutes. Each point indicates the mean (±S.E.) of four determinations of secretion rate made during the 40-minute period. Note that the smallest infusion rate of epinephrine elicited a response and that the maximum response was about 2.5 times the secretion rate obtained prior to the infusion of epinephrine. Also note that the range of infusion rates employed encompasses the endogenous secretion rate of epinephrine in calves (0.35 μg/kg/min); hence, it appears that the infusion rates employed are likely to have produced physiologic concentrations of epinephrine in the blood perfusing the parathyroid gland.

MEDIATION OF THE SECRETORY RESPONSE

Various experimental evidence suggests that the effect of cations and other factors on the release of hormone by the parathyroid cells may be mediated through cAMP. Theophylline[27] and aminophylline,[16] which are inhibitors of phosphodiesterase, an enzyme involved in the degradation of cAMP, caused increased secretion by parathyroid slices maintained in vitro. Likewise, dibutyryl cAMP (which mimics the effect of cAMP and also inhibits phosphodiesterase) increased the release of hormone by gland slices.[16,27] In other experiments, the quantity of parathyroid hormone secreted by gland slices varied in parallel with the amount of cAMP released into the medium.[27] Results from experiments conducted in vivo also substantiate the contention that cAMP is a mediator of parathyroid hormone secretion. The administration of aminophylline to rats was associated with an increase in plasma immunoreactive parathyroid hormone concentration,[28] and similar results were obtained in cows in response to the administration of epinephrine,[17] which is known to promote cAMP formation.

cAMP mediation of the effect of a stimulus on hormone secretion by endocrine glands is thought to involve activation of adenyl cyclase, an enzyme that is bound to the cell membrane and catalyzes the formation of cAMP from adenosine triphosphate. The demonstration of adenyl cyclase activity in homogenates of dog parathyroid glands[29] is complementary to other evidence suggesting that cAMP may be involved in the secretion of parathyroid hormone. Compared to adenyl cyclase of other tissues, the enzyme present in parathyroid tissue was much more sensitive to inhibition by calcium.[29] This finding is particularly significant, in view of the inhibitory effect of calcium on parathyroid secretion rate. Collectively, the evidence cited in this and the foregoing paragraph makes a strong case for the involvement of cAMP in the mediation of changes in parathyroid secretory rate induced by various stimuli.

RATE OF SECRETION

Collection of parathyroid effluent blood from calves and subsequent measurement of its hormone concentration using a homologous radioimmunoassay have provided a technique for direct measurement of parathyroid secretory rate. The secretory rate of normocalcemic calves is approximately 0.5–1.0 ng/kg/min (Fig. 44-1). These figures agree closely with estimates of secretion rate based upon the quantity of hormone required to maintain normocalcemia in the acutely parathyroidectomized dog,[30] i.e., 0.1 USP U/kg/hr, which is equivalent to 0.67 ng/kg/min. The secretion rate during maximal stimulation induced by hypocalcemia is of the order of 4–5 ng/kg/min, whereas acute hypercalcemia is attended by a basal secretion rate of about 0.3 ng/kg/min (Fig. 44-1).

In view of the foregoing measurements of secretion rate, the quantity of hormone stored in the parathyroid glands can now be viewed as having greater significance than previously thought. Each milligram of bovine parathyroid tissue (wet weight) contains approximately 0.2 μg of extractable hormone,[31] and cattle have approximately 2 mg of parathyroid tissue per kilogram of body weight (G. P. M., unpublished observations). Based on these data and the foregoing measurements of secretory rate, stored hormone can be expected to sustain secretion at hypercalcemic, normocalcemic, and hypocalcemic rates for approximately 22, 7, and 1.5 hours, respectively. Thus, the quantity of stored hormone appears sufficient for maintenance of secretory output until the biosynthetic rate of the hormone can be appropriately adjusted to meet changing needs.

RELATION OF SECRETORY RATE TO PLASMA CONCENTRATION

Plasma immunoreactive parathyroid hormone concentration can now be conveniently measured in several species. Since direct measurement of secretion rate as described in the preceding sections is usually inconvenient or infeasible, plasma immunoreactive hormone concentration is routinely used as an index of parathyroid secretory rate. However, this practice is attended by some uncertainty since plasma immunoreactive hormone concentration is dependent upon other factors in addition to secretion rate: e.g., volume of distribution within the body and the rate of removal from the blood. The latter involves equilibration between the blood and interstitial fluid as well as removal by degradation and metabolism of the hormone. Recently, the relation between secretion rate

and plasma immunoreactive hormone concentration* has been assessed in calves by continuous intravenous infusion of purified bovine parathyroid hormone until a steady state of plasma concentration was attained.[32] By employing several different rates of infusion in each animal, the relation between infusion rate and plasma concentration was defined in each of three calves. On the average, an increase of 1 ng/kg/min in the infusion rate resulted in a rise in plasma immunoreactive hormone concentration of 0.1 ng/ml.[32] In view of this observation and the rates of endogenous parathyroid hormone secretion mentioned previously, it appears that rather slight changes in plasma immunoreactive hormone concentration are indicative of significant changes in secretory rate. On the other hand, it appears unlikely that small changes in secretion rate will be discernible through measurement of plasma immunoreactive hormone concentration. The latter offers one possible explanation for the failure, in many instances, to find the expected correlation between plasma calcium and immunoreactive parathyroid hormone concentration in studies involving normocalcemic subjects, since secretory rate varies only slightly within the normocalcemic range (Fig. 44-1).

SUMMARY

Recent findings indicate that the regulation of parathyroid secretory rate is more complex than suggested by the concept of a simple negative feedback system between the parathyroid glands and plasma calcium concentration. Although plasma calcium concentration may be regarded as the principal regulator of parathyroid secretion, it now appears that other agents, which have been shown to affect parathyroid secretion, may participate with calcium in the control of secretory rate. Even the control exerted by plasma calcium is more complex than initially suspected. The essential feature of the negative feedback concept, an inverse relationship between parathyroid secretion rate and plasma calcium concentration, is present over a narrow range of plasma calcium concentration (7.5–10.5 mg/100 ml), which encompasses only the normocalcemic and mildly hypocalcemic ranges. Moreover, changes in secretion rate occurring in response to alterations in calcium concentration are much more pronounced in the mildly hypocalcemic range than in the normocalcemic range. During hypercalcemia and severe hypocalcemia, secretion rate appears to be independent of changes in plasma calcium concentration. Hypercalcemia is characterized by a basal nonsuppressible secretory rate, and severe hypocalcemia (<7.0 mg/100 ml) is accompanied by a maximal rate. Regarding the effects of other ions on parathyroid secretory rate, the predominance of calcium is supported by evidence demonstrating that phosphate affects parathyroid secretion only indirectly through suppression of calcium ion concentra-

---

*As a result of heterogeneity of the immunoreactivity in plasma,[33–35] the concentration of immunoreactivity measured depends, in part, upon the antiserum used and the location of its antigenic recognition sites on the hormone molecule. Since a carboxyl fragment of the hormone molecule comprises a major portion of the immunoreactivity in peripheral blood,[34] the use of antisera having recognition sites on this region of the hormone molecule results in the measurement of a greater concentration of immunoreactivity than when antisera having solely amino-terminal recognition sites are used.[35] The antiserum (GP-133) used in these studies recognizes the large carboxyl hormonal fragment[35] present in the peripheral circulation. Presumably, the use of an antiserum having only amino-terminal recognition sites would diminish the increase in plasma immunoreactive hormone concentration obtained in response to an increase in the infusion rate.

tion and by experiments suggesting that the effects of acute changes of plasma magnesium concentration are less potent, although similiar in nature to those of calcium. However, chronic magnesium depletion may impair rather than stimulate parathyroid secretion. Epinephrine and other beta-adrenergic agents have a stimulatory effect upon parathyroid secretion, while 24,25-dihydroxycholecalciferol, a metabolite of vitamin D, is inhibitory. The effects of calcium and epinephrine, and presumably other agents as well, upon parathyroid secretion rate appear to be mediated through changes in the intracellular concentration of cAMP. Variations in the secretory rate of normal calves range from a nonsuppressible rate of 0.3 ng/kg/min during hypercalcemia to a maximal rate of 4–5 ng/kg/min during hypocalcemia. Large changes in secretion rate may be conveniently assessed by measurement of plasma immunoreactive parathyroid hormone concentration; however, the detection of small changes in secretory rate is impaired as a result of attenuation of the secretory response in blood as a result of postsecretory distribution of immunoreactivity within and removal from the extracellular fluid.

REFERENCES

1. Patt, H. M., and Luckhardt, A. B. Relationship of Low Blood Calcium to Parathyroid Secretion. Endocrinology 31: 384, 1942.
2. Sherwood, L. M., Potts, J. T., Jr., Care, A. D., et al. Evaluation by Radioimmunoassay of Factors Controlling the Secretion of Parathyroid Hormone. 1. Intravenous Infusion of Calcium and EDTA in the Cow and Goat. Nature 209: 52, 1966.
3. Ramberg, C. F., Jr., Mayer, G. P., Kronfeld, D. S., et al. Plasma Calcium and Parathyroid Hormone Response to EDTA Infusion in the Cow. Am. J. Physiol. 213: 878, 1967.
4. Blum, J. W., Mayer, G. P., and Potts, J. T., Jr. Parathyroid Hormone Response During Spontaneous Hypocalcemia and Induced Hypercalcemia in Cows. Endocrinology 95: 84, 1974.
5. Mayer, G. P. Effect of Calcium and Magnesium on Parathyroid Secretion Rate in Calves, in Proceedings of the 5th Parathyroid Hormone Conference, Calcium-Regulating Hormones, edited by R. V. Talmage, M. Owen, and J. A. Parsons. Excerpta Medica, Amsterdam, 1975, p. 122.
6. Talmage, R. V., and Toft, R. J. The Problem of the Control of Parathyroid Secretion, in The Parathyroids, edited by R. O. Greep and R. V. Talmage. Thomas, Springfield, 1961, p. 224.
7. Sherwood, L. M., Mayer, G. P., Ramberg, C. F., Jr., et al. Regulation of Parathyroid Hormone Secretion: Proportional Control by Calcium, Lack of Effect of Phosphate. Endocrinology 83: 1043, 1968.
8. Fisher, J. A., Binswanger, U., and Blum, J. W. The Acute Parathyroid Hormone Response to Changes in Ionized Calcium During Phosphate Infusions in the Cow. Europ. J. Clin. Invest. 3: 151, 1973.
9. Sherwood, L. M., Herrman, I., and Bassett, C. A. Parathyroid Hormone Secretion in Vitro: Regulation by Calcium and Magnesium Ions. Nature 225: 1056, 1970.
10. Targovnik, J. H., Rodman, J. S., and Sherwood, L. M. Regulation of Parathyroid Hormone Secretion in Vitro: Quantitative Aspects of Calcium and Magnesium Ion Control. Endocrinology 88: 1477, 1971.
11. Care, A. D., Sherwood, L. M., Potts, J. T., Jr., et al. Evaluation by Radioimmunoassay of Factors Controlling the Secretion of Parathyroid Hormone: Perfusion of the Isolated Parathyroid Gland of the Goat and Sheep. Nature 209: 55, 1966.
12. Buckle, R. M., Care, A. D., Cooper, C. W., et al. The Influence of Plasma Magnesium Concentration on Parathyroid Hormone Secretion. J. Endocr. 42: 529, 1968.
12a. Habener, J. F., and Potts, J. T., Jr. Relative Effectiveness of Magnesium and Calcium on the Secretion and Biosynthesis of Parathyroid Hormone in Vitro. Endocrinology 98: 197, 1976.
13. Anast, C. S., Mohs, J. M., Kaplan, S. L., et al. Evidence for Parathyroid Failure in Magnesium Deficiency. Science 177: 606, 1972.
14. Suh, S. M., Tashjian, A. H., Jr., Matsuo, N., et al. Pathogenesis of Hypocalcemia in Primary Hypomagnesemia: Normal End-organ Responsiveness to Parathyroid Hormone, Impaired Parathyroid Gland Function. J. Clin. Invest. 52: 153, 1973.
15. Levi, J., Massry, S. G., Coburn, J. W., et al. Hypocalcemia in Magnesium-depleted Dogs: Evidence for Reduced Responsiveness to Parathyroid Hormone and Relative Failure of Parathyroid Gland Function. Metabolism 23: 323, 1974.
16. Williams, G. A., Hargis, G. K., Bowser, E. N., et al. Evidence for a Role of Adenosine 3′,5′-Monophosphate in Parathyroid Hormone Release. Endocrinology 92: 687, 1973.
17. Fischer, J. A., Blum, J. W., and Binswanger, U. Acute Parathyroid Hormone Response to Epinephrine in Vivo. J. Clin. Invest. 52: 2434, 1973.
18. Kukreja, S. C., Hargis, G. K., Bowser, E. N., et al. Role of Adrenergic Stimuli in Parathyroid Hormone Secretion in Man. J. Clin. Endocrinol. Metab. 40: 478, 1975.
19. Robison, G. A., Butcher, R. W., and Sutherland, E. W.: Adenyl Cyclase as an Adrenergic Receptor. Ann. NY Acad. Sci. 139: 703, 1967.
20. Aberg, H., Johansson, H., and Werner, L. Hyperparathyroidism and Asthma. Lancet II: 381, 1972.
21. Kukreja, S. C., Hargis, G. K., Rosenthal, I. M., et al. Pheochromocytoma Causing Excessive Parathyroid Hormone Production and Hypercalcemia. Ann. Intern. Med. 79: 838, 1973.
22. DeLuca, H. F. Vitamin D: The Vitamin and the Hormone. Fed. Proc. 33: 2211, 1974.
23. Bates, R. F. L., Care, A. D., Peacock, M., et al. Inhibitory Effect of 24,25-Dihydroxycholecalciferol on Parathyroid Hormone Secretion in the Goat. J. Endocrinol. 64: 6P, 1975.
24. Mills, J. N. Human Circadian Rhythms. Physiol. Rev. 46: 128, 1966.
25. Jubiz, W., Canterbury, J. M., Reiss, E., et al. Circadian Rhythm in Serum Parathyroid Hormone Concentration in Human Subjects: Correlations with Serum Calcium, Phosphate, Albumin and Growth Hormone Levels. J. Clin. Invest. 51: 2040, 1972.
26. Deftos, L. J., Kripke, D., Miller, E., et al. Pulsatile Secretory Pattern of Parathyroid Hormone. Program of the 57th Annual Meeting of the Endocrine Society, New York, 1975, p 72 (abstract).
27. Abe, M., and Sherwood, L. M.: Regulation of Parathyroid Hormone Secretion by Adenyl Cyclase. Biochem. Biophys. Res. Commun. 48: 396, 1972.
28. Bowser, E. N., Hargis, G. K., Henderson, W. J., et al. Parathyroid Hormone Secretion in the Rat: Effect of Aminophylline. Proc. Soc. Exp. Biol. Med. 148: 344, 1975.
29. Dufresne, L. R., and Gitelman, H. J. A Possible Role of Adenyl Cyclase in the Regulation of Parathyroid Activity by Calcium, in Calcium, Parathyroid Hormone and the Calcitonins, edited by R. V. Talmage and P. L. Munson. Proceedings of the Fourth Parathyroid Conference. Excerpta Medica, Amsterdam, 1972, p 202.
30. Copp, D. H., Moghadam, H., Mensen, E. D., et al. The Parathyroids and Calcium Homeostasis, in The Parathyroids, edited by R. O. Greep and R. V. Talmage. Thomas, Springfield, 1961, p 203.
31. Habener, J. F., Stevens, T. D., Tregear, G. W., et al. Radioimmunoassay of Proparathyroid Hormone: Analysis of Hormone Content in Tissue Extracts and in Plasma. J. Clin. Endocrinol. Metab. 42: 520, 1976.
32. Mayer, G. P., Staley, J. A. S., Keaton, J. A., et al. Relation Between Intravenous Infusion Rate of PTH and Its Plasma Concentration. Program of the 57th Annual Meeting of the Endocrine Society, New York, 1975, p 73 (abstract).
33. Berson, S. A., and Yalow, R. S. Immunochemical Heterogeneity of Parathyroid Hormone in Plasma. J. Clin. Endocr. 28: 1037, 1968.
34. Habener, J. F., Powell, D., Murray, T. M., et al. Parathyroid Hormone: Secretion and Metabolism in Vivo. Proc. Nat. Acad. Sci. USA 68: 2986, 1971.
35. Segre, G. V., Habener, J. F., Powell, D., et al. Parathyroid Hormone in Human Plasma: Immunochemical Characterization and Biological Implications. J. Clin. Invest. 51: 3163, 1972.

Heterogeneity and Metabolism of Parathyroid Hormone

Gino V. Segre

The term "heterogeneity," with respect to peptide hormones, has been used to describe the existence of more than one form of the hormone in blood or tissue extracts. These forms often appear to be larger in molecular size than the "intact hormone" and contain either the entire structure of the intact hormone or a sufficiently large portion of the structure to react, immunologically, with the intact hormone. In the case of insulin,[1,2] ACTH,[3] and gastrin,[4] one of the "big" forms of the circulating hormone appears to be a "prohormone." The identity of other "big" and "big-big" forms is not clear; noncovalent hormone aggregation, binding of the hormone to large proteins, disulfide interchange, and covalent linkages[5-8] of other types have all been suggested.

Several examples of heterogeneity also exist in which the apparent explanation is the presence of forms of the hormone that are smaller than the intact hormone. Circulating α-subunits of LH and TSH[9-11] and β-subunits of TSH[9] have been described; small forms of ACTH,[12,13] calcitonin,[14] growth hormone,[6] and parathyroid hormone,[15-21] which appear to be fragments of the parent hormone, have been described.

Various techniques have been used to demonstrate heterogeneity of peptide hormones. Historically, the presence of heterogeneous forms of the hormone was first suggested by finding that when measured by radioimmunoassay, the slope of tracer displacement given by serial dilutions of the sample of unknown serum or plasma containing circulating hormone is different from that given by appropriately prepared hormonal standard (hormone extracted from the gland).[22] This provides firm evidence that the sample contains one or more immunoreactive entities that are different from those present in the hormonal standard. In most instances, heterogeneity has been appreciated by detecting hormonal activity, usually by radioimmunoassay, in multiple regions after fractionation by one or more physicochemical methods.

HETEROGENEITY OF PARATHYROID HORMONE

Berson and Yalow[22] made the earliest observations concerning heterogeneity of parathyroid hormone, demonstrating that the plasma parathyroid hormone differed immunologically from hormone extracted from human parathyroid glands and suggesting the presence of more than one circulating immunoreactive form of

the hormone. Immunologic differences between plasma parathyroid hormone in patients with primary hyperparathyroidism and hormone extracted from glands were established. The slope of inhibition of tracer binding given by successively increasing aliquots of plasma differed from that given by the extracted hormone when assayed using one of several antisera. Berson and Yalow also showed that, following surgical correction of hyperparathyroidism, the disappearance of immunoreactive parathyroid hormone seemed to vary as a function of the antisera used in the assay[22] (Fig. 45-1). Although little was known at that time concerning the immunologic recognition sites of the antisera used, the data indicated that the antisera were reacting with antigens having more than one clearance rate from plasma. This suggested that the sample contained more than one immunoreactive hormonal form.

Studies subsequently performed in several laboratories have confirmed the prediction from the work of Berson and Yalow. These studies, which have applied radioimmunoassays to examine fractions after gel filtration of plasma samples from patients with hyperparathyroidism, have consistently shown that in addition to a peak of immunoreactivity which elutes at a position corresponding to intact hormone (mol wt 9500) and which accounts for 5 to 25 percent of the total immunoreactivity, there is a major peak of immunoreactive hormone which elutes later, corresponding to a molecular weight of approximately 6000. In addition, data from some groups[16,19,20,21,23] suggest that still smaller forms of the hormone circulate.

It is as yet unresolved whether forms of parathyroid hormone that are larger than the intact hormone circulate. No evidence has been found based on examination of blood samples taken from the parathyroid gland effluent in calves or in patients with hyperparathyroidism (the latter during venous catheterization; see Chapter 56) that proparathyroid hormone or the prohormone hexapeptide are secreted. However, it should be noted that both prohormone and the hexapeptide may undergo such rapid catabolism in plasma that necessary conditions to permit their detection may not yet have been satisfied. A form of parathyroid hormone that is presumably larger than prohormone has been reported to circulate in patients with ectopic hyperparathyroidism.[24] The chemical nature of this peptide has not yet been established; the possibility remains to be tested that pre-proparathyroid hormone might circulate.

ORIGIN OF CIRCULATING FRAGMENTS

The origin of the late-eluting immunoreactive form(s) of parathyroid hormone is uncertain. The studies of Habener et al.[15,17] and Segre et al.[18] have shown that most of the parathyroid hormone in

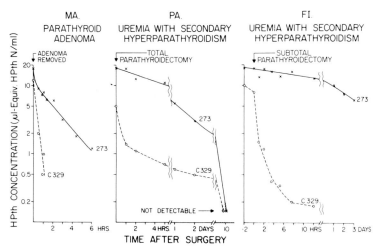

Fig. 45-1. Disappearance of immunoreactive parathyroid hormone from plasma following parathyroidectomy in patients with primary or secondary hyperparathyroidism. Samples were assayed using antisera C329 and 273. ^{125}I-BPTH and an extract of normal human parathyroid gland were used as tracer and standard, respectively. (From Berson and Yalow,[22] by permission of the author and the *Journal of Clinical Endocrinology and Metabolism.*)

the venous effluent draining normal parathyroid glands in cows and parathyroid adenomas in humans is indistinguishable from hormone extracted from parathyroid glands in cows and humans, respectively, both immunochemically and in regard to molecular size (elution position upon gel filtration). Immunoreactive parathyroid hormone in the general circulation, however, consisted largely of hormonal fragments that were immunochemically distinct from hormone extracted from glands. These fragments had an estimated molecular weight of approximately 3000 less than that of intact hormone. These results, in vivo, indicated that cleavage of intact hormone was a postsecretory event and most likely did not occur at the time of hormone release as had been suggested by earlier organ culture studies.[25,26] Hormone secreted by human parathyroid monolayer cell cultures also appeared to be intact hormone,[27] thus confirming the findings observed in vivo.

Subsequent studies in which the metabolism of intact hormone has been studied in vitro and after exogenous administration to test animals (see below)[28–34] leave no doubt that postsecretory proteolysis of parathyroid hormone occurs, resulting in the appearance of circulating fragments that cannot be distinguished by immunological or physicochemical characteristics from the fragments seen in studies of endogenous hormone.

However, recent studies have challenged the concept that postsecretory proteolysis is the exclusive or even the major source of circulating hormonal fragments. Silverman and Yalow showed that multiple immunoreactive peaks seen after gel filtration of both hormone from crude human parathyroid gland extracts and from human peripheral plasma were similar.[20] They also showed that, at least in the presence of renal failure, the hormonal fragments persisted in circulation for an extraordinarily long time ($t_{1/2}$ greater than 100 times longer than that of the intact hormone). From these observations, they concluded that because of their prolonged survival in circulation, these smaller immunoreactive forms of parathyroid hormone might become the dominant form found in plasma, even if their secretion rate was a very small fraction of that of intact hormone. Based on these considerations, they suggested that all circulating immunoreactive forms of the hormone may be secreted by the parathyroid glands.[20]

Flueck et al[35] have more directly addressed the question of secretion of hormonal fragments by reexamining the immunoreactive forms of hormone present in parathyroid venous effluent in patients with hyperparathyroidism. These workers report that approximately half of the immunoreactivity in the parathyroid ve-

nous effluent is associated with fragments of smaller molecular size than intact hormone.

Because of the differences reported[15,17,18,35] concerning the forms of immunoreactive parathyroid hormone in the parathyroid venous effluent blood, it is impossible to decide at this time the extent to which secretion of hormonal fragments contributes to the heterogeneity of circulating parathyroid hormone. If fragments are secreted, their contribution to this heterogeneity versus the contribution made by metabolism of intact hormone after secretion will require quantitation.

CHARACTERIZATION AND SIGNIFICANCE OF CIRCULATING FRAGMENTS

Three general methods—immunochemical, chemical, and biologic—have been used to further our understanding of the nature and significance of circulating fragments of parathyroid hormone.

The immunochemical properties of the molecular entities eluting later than intact hormone upon gel filtration of plasma samples could be determined only by applying radioimmunoassays with antisera which specifically recognize defined regions of the hormonal molecule (Fig. 45-2). There have been two general approaches. First, antisera to intact bovine parathyroid hormone have been used that either recognize defined portions of the sequence[19–21,23,29,30,32,35] or have been made specific by blocking some of the antibodies within the antisera by addition of saturating concentrations of selected hormonal fragments.[17,18,28,29,34] In general, either bovine hormonal fragment 1–34 or 53–84 has been used to saturate these antisera (Fig. 45-3). Second, antisera produced in response to immunization with synthetic hormonal fragments have been used. Assays with antisera that recognize determinants in the NH$_2$-terminal portions of the sequence ("NH$_2$- or N-terminal specific") and COOH-terminal portions of the sequence ("COOH- or C-terminal specific") have been employed in many laboratories.

Results from our laboratory[17,18] and others[21,35] have shown that there are 3- to 20-fold higher concentrations of immunoreactive parathyroid hormone in plasma from the general circulation of patients with hyperparathyroidism when a COOH-terminal specific, rather than an NH$_2$-terminal specific, assay system is used. Assay of fractions after gel filtration of these plasma samples has shown that, in addition to a small peak of intact hormone which is

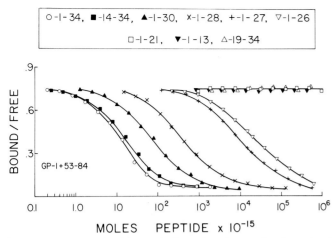

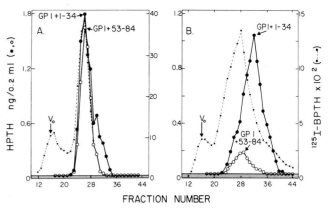

Fig. 45-2. An example of the methods used to characterize the antigenic recognition sites of antisera. The NH$_2$-terminal recognition site of GP-1 has been defined by assessing the inhibition of binding of ^{125}I-bovine parathyroid hormone to GP-1 preincubated with bovine hormone fragment 53–84 by increasing concentrations of several synthetic NH$_2$-terminal fragments. (From Segre et al.[53] by permission from Academic Press, Inc.)

Fig. 45-4. Immunoreactive parathyroid hormone in gel filtration fractions. (a) Parathyroid effluent sample; (b) peripheral venous sample. Assays used GP-1 preincubated with excess bovine fragment 1–34 (●—●) and GP-1 preincubated with bovine fragment 53–84 (○—○), COOH-terminal and NH$_2$-terminal assays, respectively. Broken line represents ^{125}I-labeled bovine parathyroid hormone cochromatographed as marker. V$_0$ marks the void volume; the cross-hatched area represents the detection limits of the assays. (From Segre et al.,[18] by permission of the *Journal of Clinical Investigation*.)

recognized equally well in both assays, there is a large peak of immunoreactive material which elutes later than intact hormone (mol wt approximately 6000) and which is measured only in assays using COOH-terminal specific antisera and is not recognized by NH$_2$-terminal specific antisera[17,18,21] (Fig. 45-4). This late eluting peak is the dominant form of immunoreactivity. Inasmuch as studies of the structure/function relationships of bovine parathyroid hormone have shown that the minimal sequence required for biologic activity must include the valine at position 2 and extend to the lysine at position 27,[36] it can be concluded that the dominant form of immunoreactive parathyroid hormone in human plasma is biologically inactive. Studies of endogenous immunoreactive parathyroid hormone in the bovine have been confirmatory.[15] Use of COOH-terminal specific antisera in clinical studies is analyzed in Chapter 55.

Some laboratories have also reported peaks of immunoreactive parathyroid hormone in human plasma which elute upon gel filtration with molecular weights of approximately 2500[16,19] and 4500.[16,19–21]

When sequence-specific assays are used to measure immunoreactive parathyroid hormone in fractions after gel filtration of plasma samples collected from dogs and cows given exogenous bovine parathyroid hormone, fragments of the hormone are seen which are indistinguishable from those present endogenously with

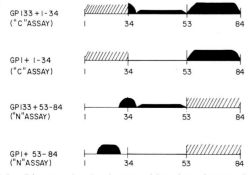

Fig. 45-3. Diagram of antigenic recognition sites of two antisera, GP-133 and GP-1, after each was blocked by bovine parathyroid fragment 1–34 or 53–84. Blocked regions of the molecule are indicated by hatched areas; the recognition sites are indicated by the heavily shaded areas. (From Segre et al.,[28] by permission of the *American Journal of Medicine*.)

respect to both their immunologic properties and their physicochemical properties; that is, proteolysis of intact hormone results in rapid disappearance of intact hormone and appearance of circulating COOH-terminal fragments with a molecular size of approximately 6000[28,30–34,37] (Figs. 45-5 and 45-6). At present, there is no agreement as to whether NH$_2$-terminal fragments, molecular size of approximately 4500,[30] are seen in the circulation as well as COOH-terminal fragments.

We have also used chemical methods to define the late-eluting peak by studying the metabolism of radioiodinated bovine hormone in dogs and rats. The immunochemical studies indicated that the single tyrosyl residue at position 43 in the bovine molecule should be contained within the late-eluting immunoreactive hormonal peak and that the immunoreactive hormone in this peak should be missing some of the amino-terminal portion present in the intact hormone. Therefore, we injected ^{125}I-bovine PTH into dogs and rats; collected the labeled, late-eluting peak; subjected the material in this peak to automated sequence analysis using the Edman reaction; and identified the cycles at which radioactive iodotyrosyl residues appeared. These studies showed that cleavage of the originally secreted hormone occurs principally between residues 33 and 34 and, in addition, at other sites that all are carboxyl terminal to position 34, mostly between residues 36 and 37. This finding provides direct evidence that the heterogeneity of plasma immunoreactive hormone reflects true cleavage of intact hormone after its release into circulation, not intact hormone with an altered conformation, and it also suggested that since the cleavage occurs carboxyl terminal to the critical sequence required for biological activity, hormonal fragments that are biologically active might be generated (Fig. 45-7). In addition, since incubation of either labeled or unlabeled bovine PTH in plasma in vitro did not result in cleavage of intact hormone at rates remotely comparable to those of hormonal cleavage in vivo, the findings indicate that at least the initial cleavage does not occur in plasma.[28,33,34]

The similarities found in the molecular sites at which hormone is cleaved in rats and dogs, as determined by these chemical techniques, coupled with evidence from immunochemical studies indicating that similar cleavages occur in hormone in humans and cows, are consistent with the concept that proteolysis of parathyroid hormone in peripheral tissues is specific, at least in several

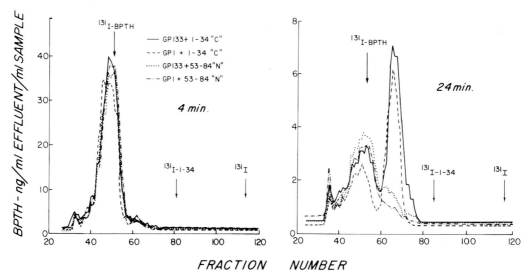

Fig. 45-5. Immunoreactive parathyroid hormone in gel filtration fractions of plasma samples collected from a dog 4 and 24 minutes after intravenous injection of intact bovine parathyroid hormone. Fractions were assayed using GP-1 and GP-133, alternately preincubated with either bovine fragment 1–34 (COOH-terminal assays) or with bovine fragment 53–84 (NH$_2$-terminal assays).

mammalian species, and may be a critical step in controlling the availability of biologically active hormone for interaction with receptors.

Canterbury et al.[38] have attempted to examine whether any of the small immunoreactive forms of circulating human parathyroid hormone are biologically active. Using the in vitro rat renal cortical adenyl cyclase assay, pools of concentrated human plasma were subjected to bioassay after these concentrates were separated by gel filtration. Biologic activity was associated with two regions of the elution profile, the intact hormonal peak and a peak having an estimated molecular size of 4500. No biologic activity was associated with the larger fragment. These results have been challenged by Silverman and Yalow,[20] who deduced that the NH$_2$-terminal fragment they identified as having a molecular size of 4500 must be biologically inactive.[20]

In summary, studies indicate that the dominant forms of parathyroid hormone in human plasma are fragments that contain about 60 percent (middle and COOH-terminal portions) of the intact hormone. Chemically, they appear to consist mostly of peptides whose NH$_2$-terminal residues are those at positions 34

and 37 of the intact hormone sequence. Since these fragments do not contain the NH$_2$-terminal region, they must be biologically inactive. There is a lack of consensus concerning the presence of NH$_2$-terminal fragments in circulation, but clearly if NH$_2$-terminal fragments do circulate, they do not constitute more than perhaps 10 percent of the immunoreactivity in plasma. In addition, among those laboratories that have detected the latter fragments in plasma, opinion is divided concerning biological activity of the endogenous NH$_2$-terminal fragment.

The fate of the NH$_2$-terminal portion of the hormonal sequence is critical to understanding the physiology of parathyroid hormone. Regardless of whether NH$_2$-terminal fragments circulate, if they are produced during peripheral metabolism and are biologically active within organs in which they are produced, such as kidney or other sites, they may constitute the dominant active molecular species of hormone or alternatively a form of the hormone with a spectrum of activities different from that of intact hormone.

METABOLISM OF PARATHYROID HORMONE

Several lines of evidence suggest that the liver and kidneys are the principal organs involved in the metabolism of parathyroid hormone. Davis et al.[39] showed that rats with parathyroid glands transplanted to their spleen could not maintain their serum calcium

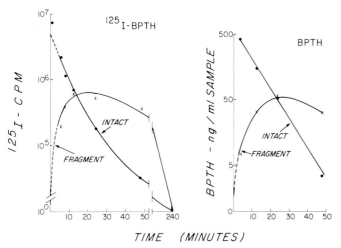

Fig. 45-6. Disappearance of intact parathyroid hormone and appearance and disappearance of hormonal fragments after intravenous injection of ^{125}I-labeled and unlabeled bovine parathyroid hormone into dogs. (From Segre et al.,[28] by permission of the *American Journal of Medicine*.)

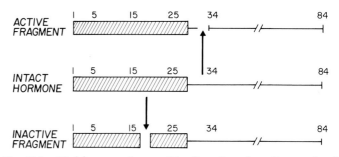

Fig. 45-7. Model representing possible alternatives depending on site of hormonal cleavage. Region required for biologic activity is represented by the hatched area. (From Segre et al.,[28] by permission of the *American Journal of Medicine*.)

levels under the stress of calcium removal by peritoneal lavage as well as did rats with parathyroid glands transplanted to their testes. This suggested that the liver was inactivating PTH, presumably by removing it. Longer half-lives of PTH have also been seen in partially hepatectomized rats,[40] nephrectomized rats and dogs,[41] and in humans with renal failure.[22,42,43] Studies in our laboratory have shown that after infusion of bovine PTH to dogs, arteriovenous differences of 23 percent and 19 percent were seen across the liver and kidney, respectively.[44] A more detailed analysis by Hruska et al.[30] showed that 61 percent of the metabolic clearance of immunoreactive PTH could be accounted for by the kidneys in normal dogs. Induced renal failure prolonged the disappearance of PTH from plasma of all immunoreactive components, but particularly the COOH-terminal fragment. The decrease in clearance rate appeared to be due to decreases in renal plasma flow without compensation by extrarenal sites. Uremia reduced both renal and extrarenal clearance. These results indicate that the kidneys are important in removing immunoreactive PTH from the circulation and that the critical determinant is renal plasma flow. However, perhaps, of equal importance, a significant effect on extrarenal clearance resulted from the uremic state.

Recently, Martin et al.[32] studied hepatic and renal extraction of immunoreactive parathyroid hormone in dogs with explanted kidneys and chronic indwelling hepatic vein catheters. The livers selectively extracted intact hormone, but not fragments of the hormone, suggesting that the liver did not appear to have a role in the catabolism of parathyroid fragments. The kidney, however, extracted the intact hormone and both COOH- and NH$_2$-terminal fragments.

METABOLISM OF PARATHYROID HORMONE IN VITRO AND ITS RELATIONSHIP TO BIOLOGIC ACTIVITY OF THE HORMONE

The enzyme(s) responsible for proteolysis of parathyroid hormone have not yet been isolated. Therefore, in vitro studies concerned with metabolism of the hormone thus far performed provide, at best, only a partial understanding of the pertinent events.

Inactivation of the bioactivity of bovine PTH or degradation of the radioiodinated hormone has been demonstrated by liver homogenates,[40] kidney slices,[45] kidney homogenates,[46] and kidney cell fractions.[47-50] Catherwood and Singer[49] described a carboxyl-terminal fragment which resembled the circulating carboxyl-terminal fragment in molecular size that was generated by incubating radioiodinated bovine parathyroid hormone with canine renal plasma membranes. Chu et al.[50] showed that the breakdown of intact hormone by rat renal cortical plasma membranes was related to a decrease and not an increase in the parathyroid hormone-dependent adenyl cyclase response. Inasmuch as degradative activity was also found in plasma membranes from renal medulla and liver, they concluded that, most likely, the enzyme(s) active in membrane preparations was nonspecific, i.e., was not a specific or single enzyme active in intact tissue in vivo.

Studies in our laboratory have examined whether proteolysis of parathyroid hormone is a requisite initial step before the hormone could stimulate parathyroid hormone-dependent rat renal cortical adenyl cyclase. In experiments using plasma membranes prepared from canine renal cortex, we demonstrated that activation of adenyl cyclase by intact hormone occurred without evidence that the hormone had undergone proteolysis.[51]

This indicated that, at least within the limitations of the methods employed, this biologic expression of parathyroid hormone activity—stimulation of adenyl cyclase—does not require proteolysis of the hormone. It does not exclude the possibility, however, that proteolysis is necessary for other biologic expressions of the hormone, or that fragments resulting from hormonal metabolism may be more active than the intact hormone in stimulating the renal adenyl cyclase reaction. These experiments did permit the conclusion that the receptors are probably linked to activation of adenyl cyclase and those responsible for hormonal cleavage are probably not in close proximity.[51]

Some in vitro studies have attempted to determine the significance of proteolysis of PTH by examining the relationship between hormonal cleavage and the calcium concentration of the media. Fischer et al.[52] found a calcium-dependent peptidase in homogenates from various tissues, including liver, kidney, and parathyroid glands. Activity of this peptidase resulted in the generation of a biologically active fragment. This fragment, however, appears to have a molecular weight of 6000–7000. Inasmuch as structure/activity studies require the presence of the amino-terminal portion of the hormone in any active fragment, the counterpart of this tissue fragment in blood would have to differ from the 6000–7000 molecular-weight fragment that lacks the amino terminus. No circulating fragment corresponding to the fragment reported in vitro by Fischer et al.[52] has been reported. Inasmuch as the fragment described by Fischer et al. also differs appreciably in size from the biologically active circulating fragment described by Canterbury et al.[38] and the studies of Arnaud and Fischer and associates[19,21,23,35] indicate that the circulating form of hormone in the 6000–7000 molecular-weight class lacks NH$_2$-terminal reactivity, one must conclude that the physiologic significance of the calcium-dependent peptidase of Fischer et al.[52] is not clear, at present.

Using the perfused rat liver, Canterbury et al.[29] have made the observation that proteolysis of PTH results in the release of fragments into the circulating media which are indistinguishable from those they have previously described in the circulation of humans.[38] One of these fragments consists of the amino-terminal portion of the sequence and is biologically active. Hormone proteolysis is calcium-dependent; increased concentration of calcium in the medium results in less conversion, and, conversely, lower calcium results in more conversion. This is consistent with the hypothesis that cleavage may be related to the production of a biologically active form of PTH. The relevancy of these observations to in vivo events has not yet been demonstrated, nor has it been ascertained that the fragments generated in this in vitro system are the same as those seen in vivo. Nevertheless, these observations are quite provocative and suggest that metabolism of PTH may be a carefully regulated step that modulates the availability of biologically active hormone.

Obviously, many issues must yet be resolved before the heterogeneity of circulating parathyroid hormone is completely understood. Although earlier studies indicated that postsecretory metabolism of the intact hormone was the major, if not the only, source of circulating hormonal fragments, more recent studies have suggested that identical fragments, or very similar fragments, are secreted also by the parathyroid glands. The chemical and immunochemical properties of the circulating fragments appear to be very similar, if not identical, in several mammalian species, indicating that the mechanisms responsible for hormonal proteolysis are closely related. The lack of evolutionary divergence in this proteolytic process is consistent with the concept that hormonal cleavage may be an important regulatory process in controlling the concentration of circulating biologically active hormone. This control could be accomplished merely as a catabolic process; that is, cleavage of the intact hormone with release of the smaller amino-terminal fragment could merely accelerate the catabolism of the biologically active portions. Alternatively, metabolism could be an activation process; however, although several lines of evidence suggest that fragments of parathyroid hormone may be active, this is not sufficiently well resolved. In addition, it is not yet known whether alterations in the physiological status of the animal influence the rate of peripheral metabolism or the amount of fragments produced.

Furthermore, the mechanisms responsible for metabolism of intact hormone appear to differ from those of its fragments. This indicates that a complex mechanism for clearance of intact hormone and hormonal fragments may be required to efficiently and effectively control the concentration of circulating biologically active hormone. However, all these issues remain to be better defined.

A more thorough understanding of issues relating to the heterogeneity and metabolism of parathyroid hormone may lead to uncovering disease processes which result from aberrations or deficiencies in the mechanisms responsible for parathyroid hormone proteolysis. In addition, since differential diagnosis of the various hypercalcemic and hyperparathyroid states has been significantly improved by use of present assays for the hormone, one might foresee still more significant developments in this field as advances are made in our understanding of the nature and importance of the complex circulating forms of the hormone.

The overall results suggest that present immunoassays for parathyroid hormone provide, at best, an index of glandular activity. Assays based on COOH-terminal specific antisera, if properly interpreted, seem highly useful in distinguishing patients with chronically abnormal states of parathyroid overactivity from patients with normal rates of parathyroid activity or hypercalcemic disorders due to causes other than hyperparathyroidism, primary or ectopic (Chapter 55). However, present assays do not measure exclusively, or even principally, biologically active hormone. As studies continue to define (1) details of hormone biosynthesis and release of precursor or other glandular products (Chapter 43) and (2) the nature and origin of circulating, heterogeneous forms of hormone, new types of immunoassays may be developed that are more useful in analysis of hormone secretory rate and states of parathyroid glandular activity. Such "second-generation" assays, which should permit a more accurate definition of pathophysiological defects in states of abnormal parathyroid function, may be based on assays of requisite sensitivity to detect exclusively intact hormone, NH_2-terminal immunoreactive hormonal forms, or glandular products other than intact hormone (see Chapter 43).

REFERENCES

1. Sherman, B., Gorden, P., Roth, J., et al. Circulating Insulin: The Proinsulin-like Properties of "Big" Insulin in Patients without Islet Cell Tumors. J. Clin. Invest. 50: 849, 1971.
2. Gorden, P., Freychet, P., and Nankin, H. A Unique Form of Circulating Insulin in Human Islet Cell Carcinoma. J. Clin. Endocrinol. Metab. 33: 983, 1971.
3. Yalow, R. S., and Berson, S. A. Size Heterogeneity of Immunoreactive Human ACTH in Plasma and in Extracts of Pituitary Glands and ACTH-producing Thymoma. Biochem. Biophys. Res. Commun. 44: 439, 1971.
4. Yalow, R. S., and Berson, S. A. Size and Charge Distinctions between Endogenous Human Plasma Gastrin in Peripheral Blood and Heptadecapeptide Gastrins. Gastroenterology 58: 609, 1970.
5. Antoniades, H. N., Simon, J. D., and Stathakos, D. Conversion of [^{125}I]Insulin and [^{121}I]Proinsulin into High Molecular Weight Forms in Vivo. Endocrinology 95: 1543, 1974.

6. Antoniades, H. N. Conversion of [^{125}I]Growth Hormone into High Molecular Weight Forms in Vivo. Endocrinology 96: 799, 1975.
7. Antoniades, H. N. Metabolism of Single-Component and High-Molecular Weight Radioactive Insulin in Rats. Endocrinology 99: 481, 1976.
8. Gorden, P., Hendricks, C. M., and Roth, J. Evidence for "Big" and "Little" Components of Human Plasma and Pituitary Growth Hormone. Endocrinology 36: 178, 1973.
9. Kourides, I. A., Weintraub, B. D., Ridgway, E. C., and Maloof, F. Pituitary Secretion of Free Alpha and Beta Subunit of Human Thyrotropin in Patients with Thyroid Disorders. J. Clin. Endocrinol. Metab. 40: 872, 1975.
10. Benveniste, R., Bell, J., Koeppel, J., and Rabinowitz, D. Alpha Chain of Glycoprotein Hormones: Presence in Human Serum after Thyroid Stimulating Hormone Releasing Hormone. J. Clin. Endocrinol. Metab. 37: 822, 1973.
11. Rabinowitz, D., Benveniste, R., and Bell, J. Heterogeneity of Human Luteinizing Hormone: Behavior in Radioimmunoassay and Radio-Ligand-Receptor Assay Systems and Evidence for the Presence of α-Subunit in Serum, in Heterogeneity of Polypeptide Hormones, New York, 1974, p 90.
12. Besser, G. M., Orth, D. N., Nicholson, W. E., et al. Dissociation of the Disappearance of Bioactive and Radioimmunoactive ACTH from Plasma in Man. J. Clin. Endocrinol. Metab. 32: 595, 1971.
13. Orth, D. N., Nicholson, W. E., Mitchell, W. M., et al. Biologic and Immunologic Characterization and Physical Separation of ACTH and ACTH Fragments in the Ectopic ACTH Syndrome. J. Clin. Invest. 52: 1756, 1973.
14. Deftos, L. H., Roos, B. A., Bronzert, D., et al. Immunochemical Heterogeneity of Calcitonin in Plasma. J. Clin. Endocrinol. Metab. 40: 409, 1975.
15. Habener, J. F., Powell, D., Murray, T. M., et al. Parathyroid Hormone: Secretion and Metabolism in Vivo. Proc. Natl. Acad. Sci. USA 68: 2986, 1971.
16. Canterbury, J. M., and Reiss, E. Multiple Immunoreactive Molecular Forms of Parathyroid Hormone in Human Serum. Proc. Soc. Exper. Biol. Med. 140: 1393, 1972.
17. Habener, J. F., Segre, G. N., Powell, D., et al. Immunoreactive Parathyroid Hormone in Circulation of Man. Nature New Biol. 238: 152, 1972.
18. Segre, G. V., Habener, J. F., Powell, D., et al. Parathyroid Hormone in Human Plasma: Immunochemical Characterization and Biological Implications. J. Clin. Invest. 51: 3163, 1972.
19. Goldsmith, R. S., Furszyfer, J., Johnson, W. J., et al. Etiology of Hyperparathyroidism and Bone Disease during Chronic Hemodialysis. III. Evaluation of Parathyroid Suppressibility. J. Clin. Invest. 52: 173, 1973.
20. Silverman, R., and Yalow, R. S.: Heterogeneity of Parathyroid Hormone: Clinical and Physiologic Implications. J. Clin. Invest. 52: 1958, 1973.
21. Fischer, J. A., Binswanger, U., and Dietrich, F. M. Human Parathyroid Hormone: Immunological Characterization of Antibodies against a Glandular Extract and the Synthetic Amino-Terminal Fragments 1–22 and 1–34 and Their Use in the Determination of Immunoreactive Hormone in Human Sera. J. Clin. Invest. 54: 1382, 1974.
22. Berson, S. A., and Yalow, R. S. Immunochemical Heterogeneity of Parathyroid Hormone in Plasma. J. Clin. Endocrinol. Metab. 28: 1037, 1968.
23. Arnaud, C. D., Goldsmith, R. S., Bordier, P. J., et al. Influence of Immunoheterogeneity of Circulating Parathyroid Hormone on Results of Radioimmunoassays of Serum in Man. Am. J. Med. 56: 785, 1974.
24. Benson, R. C., Jr., Riggs, B. L., Pickard, B. M., et al. Immunoreactive Forms of Circulating Parathyroid Hormone in Primary and Ectopic Hyperparathyroidism. J. Clin. Invest. 54: 175, 1974.
25. Sherwood, L. M., Rodman, J. S., and Lundberg, W. B. Evidence for a Precursor to Circulating Parathyroid Hormone. Proc. Natl. Acad. Sci. USA 67: 1631, 1970.
26. Arnaud, C. D., Sizemore, G. W., Oldham, S. B., et al. Human Parathyroid Hormone: Glandular and Secreted Molecular Species. Am. J. Med. 50: 630, 1971.
27. Martin, T. J., Greenberg, P. B., and Melick, R. A. Nature of Human Parathyroid Hormone Secreted by Monolayer Cell Cultures. J. Clin. Endocrinol. Metab. 34: 437, 1972.
28. Segre, G. V., Niall, H. D., Habener, J. F., et al. Metabolism of Parathyroid Hormone: Physiological and Clinical Significance. Am. J. Med. 56: 774, 1974.

29. Canterbury, J. M., Bricker, L. A., Levey, G. S., et al. Metabolism of Bovine Parathyroid Hormone: Immunological and Biological Characteristics of Fragments Generated by Liver Perfusion. J. Clin. Invest. 55: 1245, 1975.

30. Hruska, K. A., Kopelman, R., Rutherford, W. E., et al. Metabolism of Immunoreactive Parathyroid Hormone in the Dog: The Role of the Kidney and the Effects of Chronic Renal Disease. J. Clin. Invest. 56: 39, 1975.

31. Neuman, W. F., Neuman, M. W., Sammon, P. J., et al. The Metabolism of Labeled Parathyroid Hormone. III: Studies in Rats. Calcif. Tissue Res. 18: 251, 1975.

32. Martin, K., Hruska, K. A., Greenwalt, A., et al. Selective Uptake of Intact Parathyroid Hormone by the Liver. Differences between Hepatic and Renal Uptake. J. Clin. Invest. 58: 781, 1976.

33. Segre, G. V., D'Amour, P., and Potts, J. T., Jr. Metabolism of Radioiodinated Bovine Parathyroid Hormone in the Rat. Endocrinology 99: 1645, 1976.

34. Segre, G. V., Niall, H. D., Sauer, R. T., et al. Edman Degradation of Radioiodinated Parathyroid Hormone: Application to Sequence Analysis and Hormone Metabolism in Vivo. Biochemistry 16: 2417, 1977.

35. Flueck, J., Edis, A., McMahon, J., et al. Direct Secretion of COOH-Terminal Fragments of Human Parathyroid Hormone by Parathyroid Tumors in Vivo: Contribution to Immunoheterogeneity of Serum PTH in Hyperparathyroid Man. 58th Annual Meeting, Endocrine Society, San Francisco, June 1976, p 64.

36. Tregear, G. W., van Rietschoten, J., Greene, E., et al. Bovine Parathyroid Hormone: Minimum Chain Length of Synthetic Peptide Required for Biological Activity. Endocrinology 93: 1349, 1973.

37. Habener, J. F., Mayer, G. P., Dee, P. C., et al. Metabolism of Amino- and Carboxyl-Sequence Immunoreactive Parathyroid Hormone in the Bovine: Evidence for Peripheral Cleavage of Hormone. Metabolism 25: 385, 1976.

38. Canterbury, J. M., Levey, G. S., and Reiss, E. Activation of Renal Cortical Adenylate Cyclase by Circulating Immunoreactive Parathyroid Hormone Fragments. J. Clin. Invest. 52: 524, 1973.

39. Davis, R., and Talmage, R. V. Evidence for Liver Inactivation of Parathyroid Hormone. Endocrinology 66: 312, 1960.

40. Fang, V. S., and Tashjian, A. H., Jr. Studies on the Role of the Liver in the Metabolism of Parathyroid Hormone: I. Effects of Partial Hepatectomy and Inactivation of the Hormone with Tissue Homogenates. Endocrinology 90: 1177, 1972.

41. Martin, T. J., Melick, R. A., and de Luise, M.: The Effect of Nephrectomy on the Metabolism of Labeled Parathyroid Hormone. Clin. Sci. 37: 137, 1969.

42. Melick, R. A., and Martin, T. J. Parathyroid Hormone Metabolism in Man: Effect of Nephrectomy. Clin. Sci. 37: 677, 1969.

43. Potts, J. T., Jr., Murray, T. M., Peacock, M., et al. Parathyroid Hormone: Sequences, Synthesis, and Immunoassay Studies. Am. J. Med. 50: 639, 1971.

44. Singer, F. R., Segre, G. V., Habener, J. F., et al. Peripheral Metabolism of Bovine Parathyroid Hormone in the Dog. Metabolism 24: 139, 1975.

45. Orimo, H., Fujita, T., Morii, H., et al. Inactivation in Vitro of Parathyroid Hormone Activity in Kidney Slices. Endocrinology 76: 255, 1965.

46. Vajda, F. J. E., Martin, T. J., and Melick, R. A. Destruction of Bovine Parathyroid Hormone Labeled with ^{131}I by Rat Kidney Tissue. Endocrinology 84: 162, 1969.

47. Fujita, T., Orimo, H., Ohata, M., et al. Enzymatic Inactivation of Parathyroid Hormone by Rat Kidney Homogenate. Endocrinology 86: 42, 1970.

48. Martin, T. J., Melick, R. A., and de Luise, M. Metabolism of Parathyroid Hormone: Degradation of ^{125}I-Labeled Hormone by a Kidney Enzyme. Biochem. J. 111: 509, 1969.

49. Catherwood, B., and Singer, F. R. Generation of a Carboxyl-Terminal Fragment of Bovine Parathyroid Hormone by Canine Renal Plasma Membranes. Biochem. Biophys. Res. Commun. 57: 469, 1974.

50. Chu, L. L. H., Forte, L. R., Anast, C. S., et al. Interaction of Parathyroid Hormone with Membranes of Kidney Cortex: Degradation of Hormone and Activation of Adenylate Cyclase. Endocrinology 97: 1014, 1975.

51. Goltzman, D., Petyremann, A., Callahan, E. N., et al. Metabolism and Biological Activity of Parathyroid Hormone in Renal Cortical Membranes. J. Clin. Invest. 57: 8, 1976.

52. Fischer, J. A., Oldham, S. B., Sizemore, G. W., et al. Calcium-regulated Parathyroid Hormone Peptidase. Proc. Natl. Acad. Sci. USA 69: 2341, 1972.

53. Segre, G. V., Tregear, G. W., and Potts, J. T., Jr. Development and Application of Sequence-Specific Radioimmunoassays for Analysis of the Metabolism of Parathyroid Hormone. Methods Enzymol. 37: 38, 1975.

46

Physiology of Parathyroid Hormone

J. A. Parsons

INTRODUCTION

Modern methods of protein chemistry and immunoassay have led during the last decade to extremely rapid advances in understanding all the major endocrine systems that utilize peptide chains as their specific messengers. Among these systems, that comprising the parathyroid glands, the short-lived product of their secretion, and target cells in the kidney and skeleton is perhaps unique in the extent to which its apparent biological significance has been changed by recent quantitative studies.

Classic descriptions of the physiology of parathyroid hormone (PTH), based largely on the results of injecting massive doses and on studies of overt clinical hyperparathyroidism, emphasized its character as principally an agent of bone destruction. Several earlier reviews of parathyroid physiology that share this general emphasis are still particularly worth consulting for their individual viewpoints and as guides to the massive literature.[1-5] However, a review of in vitro and in vivo evidence indicates that the concentrations of PTH required to significantly increase bone breakdown lie between 10^{-10} and 10^{-17} molar or $10^{-9} - 10^{-6}$ g/ml of bPTH 1–84, the exact value depending on the species and method of measurement[6-10] (for further discussion and references, see ref. 11).

No bioassay method yet published is sensitive enough to measure normal circulating levels of biologically active parathyroid hormone (bioPTH). However, many methods capable of detecting circulating *immunoactive* PTH (iPTH) in the majority of normal subjects have been published in recent years. As described by Segre (Chapter 45), extensive cross-comparison and calibration with chemically defined fragments have lowered estimates of the normal level of iPTH to about 10^{-10} g/ml (10^{-11} molar), but this must overestimate the concentration of biologically active hor-mone, since material measured by existing sensitive immunoassays is heterogeneous, much of it probably devoid of biological activity. Thus, as discussed more fully below, all the evidence is compatible with indirect estimates that the normal circulating level of bioPTH is of the order of 10^{-11} g/ml (10^{-12} molar) or about 2 orders of magnitude below the significantly osteolytic level.

Particular interest is therefore attached to consideration of the relative sensitivity of other responses to PTH, three of which do not directly involve the skeleton. The early evidence for these extraskeletal actions was summarized by Parsons and Potts.[12] As discussed below, they are more sensitive than the osteolytic response and combine to enhance calcium absorption and retention by the organism.

PTH is also well known to stimulate bone *formation* under some circumstances by a mechanism that is probably direct. The long history of this relatively neglected action is given elsewhere, in a review which concludes that, at near-normal rates of secretion, the overall action of the parathyroids is predominantly anabolic rather than catabolic to the skeleton.[13]

ORIGIN OF THE PARATHYROIDS

Recent work has tantalizingly reopened the issue of the evolutionary and embryological origin of the PTH molecule. Evidence was published in 1976 that the parathyroid cells are not, as had long been thought, of endodermal origin, but arise from a specialized region, or placode, of the neuroectoderm.[14] At almost exactly the same time, Drs. Snell and Smythe of the National Institute for Medical Research (London) pointed out the existence of strong homology between a region in the bioactive part of parathyroid hormone (residues 15–25) and the amino-terminal 11 residues of corticotropin (Fig. 46-1).

The homology is indicated by four identities and an additional five one-step mutations, and its significance (which would appear striking on purely statistical grounds) is greatly increased by the fact that the regions include the highly unusual tryptophan and methionine residues of the two molecules. These two pieces of evidence, taken together, should cause us to consider the possibility that parathyroid hormone may have evolved from a hypercalcemic factor in the fish pituitary, evidence for the existence of which has appeared in at least five papers in the last 20 years[15-19] (for discussion, see ref. 20). Because of the relatively late evolution of bone in fish[21] and the fact that few species have developed the cellular apparatus to use bone as a calcium reservoir,[22,23] this theory would imply that the primitive hypercalcemic factor evolved primarily in association with calcium regulation by the kidneys and gills.

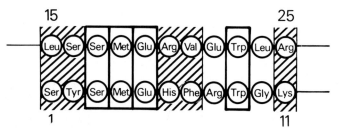

Fig. 46-1. Comparison of a portion of the sequence of the biologically active region of bovine parathyroid hormone (bPTH 15–25) with the amino-terminal 11 residues of corticotropin from the same species. This contains the heptapeptide core region (ACTH 4–10) which is common to corticotropin, lipotropin, and the melanocyte-stimulating hormones and is essential for their biological activity.[14a] Identical residues are enclosed in solid lines; residues related by the criteria of Barker and Dayhoff[14b] are joined by cross-hatching. (Reproduced from ref. 13 by permission.)

MULTIPLE ACTIONS OF PARATHYROID HORMONE

The secretion of the parathyroids has five major established effects. We cannot hope to understand its overall pattern of action without considering them all in the context of their widely differing dose and time relationships, and it is perhaps most interesting to do this in the historical order of their discovery.

RENAL PHOSPHATE EXCRETION

Largely for technical reasons, the induction of phosphaturia was identified before any other effect of injecting parathyroid extracts. PTH simultaneously reduces reabsorption of sodium, calcium, phosphate, and bicarbonate in the proximal renal tubule.[24,25] Most of the sodium rejected proximally is absorbed distally, and PTH causes only a minor natriuresis. However, the rejected anions are not reabsorbed, and the net result is a substantial phosphaturia, accompanied by increased bicarbonate excretion.

The exact significance of this complex PTH-induced rearrangement of ion fluxes is still not understood. However, it can be viewed, at least in part, as an adaptation to the function of bone as an emergency calcium reservoir[26] because bicarbonate, like phosphate, is liberated as a counter ion during the mobilization of calcium from bone. It is interesting in this regard that PTH does not cause phosphaturia in amphibia.[27]

The sensitivity and magnitude of the phosphaturic response is perhaps best illustrated by the result of graded infusions of highly purified bovine PTH in two patients with normal calcium metabolism[28] (Fig. 46-2). The linear log dose-response regressions calculated for the two subjects intersect the baseline at points suggesting endogenous secretion rates of 0.04 and 0.07 U/kg/hr, respectively. These figures are virtually identical with other published estimates of the endogenous secretion rate of PTH (for references, see ref. 11), confirming that the parathyroids almost certainly play a role in modulating phosphate excretion under conditions of normal life, as has long been indicated by the reduced phosphate excretion and hyperphosphatemia caused by PTH deficiency or parathyroidectomy.[29]

BONE RESORPTION (BONE CATABOLISM)

The second action of PTH to be established was the acceleration of bone breakdown. This is still the hormone's best-known effect, but it forms only part of a remarkably complex bone response, which affects all cell types and thus contains not only

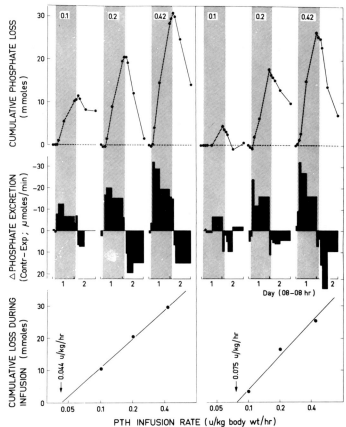

Fig. 46-2. Diagram showing the dose-related effects on phosphate excretion of infusing bovine parathyroid hormone (2,500 U/mg) to 2 patients with normal calcium and phosphate metabolism. Each infusion lasted 24 hours (hatched areas) at the rates shown on logarithmic scales at the bottom of the two halves of the figure.

Each center panel shows the difference between measured phosphate excretion and the excretion during a corresponding period on the previous day, when the patient was given a control infusion. Since the experiments were conducted on diets of constant phosphate content (37 and 55 mmol/day, respectively), these differences in excretion are also the differences in phosphate balance.

Each upper panel shows the same measurements replotted as a cumulative phosphate loss and each lower panel shows the regression of the cumulative loss figures on the log dose-rate. The latter points fall on straight lines intersecting the baseline at the calculated rates shown by arrows, indicating the levels of endogenous PTH secretion as discussed in the text. The phosphate measurements were continued during a second 24 hours after termination of each infusion, showing that the induced phosphate losses were largely made up during this recovery period. (From ref. 28, by courtesy of the authors and publisher.)

catabolic but also anabolic elements. The latter will be discussed in more detail below, but even the osteolytic part of the bone response is complex. It can be subdivided into a fast component, which presumably depends on the activation of existing cellular apparatus, and a slow component, which clearly involves enzyme synthesis and cellular proliferation and destroys all constituents of bone, including the organic matrix. This slow component is abolished by inhibitors of protein synthesis (e.g., actinomycin D), whereas the rapid component of PTH-induced calcium mobilization is actinomycin-D-resistant.[30]

The complex cellular relationships involved in these actions on bone can be well seen in the very informative study of the time course of changes in synthesis of cytoplasmic and nuclear RNA following injection of large doses of parathyroid extract (PTE) to rabbits by Bingham and co-workers[31] (Fig. 46-3). Increased uridine incorporation into existing osteoclasts was already well marked 1½ hours after the dose but was even more obvious at 15 to 20 hours, the time at which increased proliferation was first seen in the preosteoclast population.

The mechanism of the rapid component of the calcium mobilization response is still the subject of intensive investigation, reviewed in detail elsewhere.[32] Talmage[33] believes that it involves movement of calcium already in solution, coming from a bone fluid compartment with specific activity identical to the plasma and extracellular fluid (ECF) and markedly different from the specific activity of bone mineral. This explanation is in good agreement with evidence that calcium is mobilized without phosphate in the early phases of the hypercalcemic response.[34,35]

RENAL CALCIUM RETENTION

The fundamentally important calcium-retaining action of PTH on the kidney was the third major effect of the hormone to be established, probably because it depends on an increase in tubular

reabsorption and can be studied only by controlling or correcting for any rise in plasma calcium level which increases the filtered load. As mentioned in connection with the phosphaturic response, calcium is one of the elements whose reabsorption is reduced by parathyroid hormone acting on the proximal tubule. However, its reabsorption by the distal tubule is markedly enhanced by PTH, and, under normal circumstances, this is the effect that predominates.

The fundamentally important calcium-retaining action of PTH on the kidney was the third major effect of the hormone to be established, probably because it depends on an increase in tubular reabsorption and can be studied only by controlling or correcting for any rise in plasma calcium level which increases the filtered load. As mentioned in connection with the phosphaturic response, calcium is one of the elements whose reabsorption is reduced by parathyroid hormone acting on the proximal tubule. However, its reabsorption by the distal tubule is markedly enhanced by PTH, and, under normal circumstances, this is the effect that predominates.

Perhaps the clearest illustration of the magnitude of parathyroid hormone's effect on renal calcium handling under normal physiological and clinical conditions is provided by the work of Nordin and Peacock[37] (Fig. 46-4). They studied the relationship between urinary calcium excretion and the serum calcium level, giving calcium infusions to normal subjects and patients with disturbed parathyroid function. All the hypoparathyroid subjects lost large quantities of calcium in the urine even at subnormal serum levels, while the hyperparathyroid subjects retained calcium even in the face of quite severe hypercalcemia.

INTESTINAL CALCIUM ABSORPTION

The fourth major way in which the parathyroids have been shown to affect mineral metabolism is by modulating the fractional absorption of dietary calcium and phosphate. For reasons re-

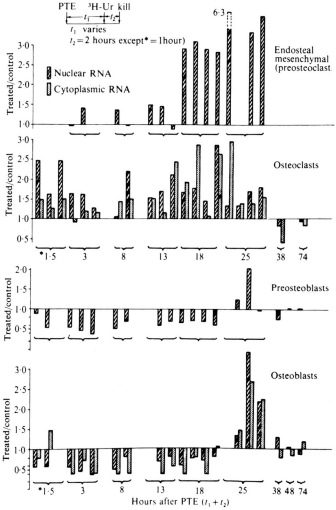

Fig. 46-3. Effects of PTE on incorporation of ³H-uridine in different bone cell types of the midshaft of the femur in young rabbits. The amount of ³H-uridine incorporated into nuclear and cytoplasmic RNA over a short period of time in different cell types was measured at various times after injection of PTE. Results were compared between PTE-treated and paired control animals in the same litter. Each bar or pair of bars in the histogram represents the ratio of the results from each pair of animals. (Reproduced from ref. 31 by courtesy of the authors and publisher.)

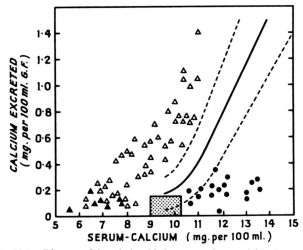

Fig. 46-4. Diagram of the relationship between urinary calcium (as mg/100 ml glomerular filtrate (G.F.)) and serum calcium concentration, comparing hyperparathyroid (●) with hypoparathyroid (▲) patients and illustrating the effects of infusing calcium to the latter (△). The solid and broken lines show the mean values (±2 S.D.) obtained in normal subjects, and the shaded area represents the normal basal range. Methods used are described by Peacock et al.[36]

All the hypoparathyroid subjects lost large quantities of calcium in the urine even at subnormal serum levels, whereas the hyperparathyroids retained calcium even in the face of quite severe hypercalcemia. (From ref. 37, by courtesy of the authors and the publishers.)

viewed elsewhere, this effect was long regarded as controversial,[12] but its reality can no longer be doubted, and there is much evidence that it is mediated by changes in the rate at which the active metabolite of vitamin D is formed in the kidney (for reviews, see refs. 38 and 39). Clinically, this mechanism is supported by measurements of circulating 1,25-dihydroxycholecalciferol (DHCC) in 20 cases of primary hyperparathyroidism.[40] Although levels in the group were somewhat scattered, they were significantly higher than those of a control group, and, most important, individual values were closely correlated with corresponding measurements of the calcium absorption coefficient (α).[41]

Although the modulation of calcium absorption by the parathyroids is indirect and slow (requiring 24 to 48 hours for the full induction of major changes), it is sensitive and specific, and the long-term balance between intestinal absorption and excretion in the urine and feces is vitally important in determining the mineralization of the skeleton. In vivo measurements of α by a double-isotope method have been shown to be practicable in mature rats and are being used to investigate various aspects of the pharmacology of calcium absorption.[42] Both bovine PTH and the synthetic amino-terminal fragment of human PTH[43] have been shown to induce large increases in α when given by repeated subcutaneous injection. The effect of bovine PTH was not additive to that of maximal doses of 1,25-DHCC, which is fully consistent with the mechanism discussed above (Fig. 46-5).

BONE FORMATION (BONE ANABOLISM)

Finally, we come to the anabolic effect of parathyroid hormone on bone. This has been listed as the fifth major effect to be established because skepticism regarding its reality and significance dies hard, but a recent literature survey[44] produced what seems an incontrovertible body of evidence for PTH-induced increases in bone mass going back to x-ray observations of Bauer et al.,[45] which even preceded the classic experiments of Selye and Pugsley[46-48] and the strangely neglected bone-weight measurements of Shelling et al.[49] Subsequent work has eliminated the possibility that the increased bone formation was due to impure hormone or compensatory secretion of calcitonin.[50,51]

The mechanism of the anabolic effect of PTH is still under active investigation, but there is much evidence that it involves a direct cellular response. Two of the actions of PTH already discussed, those that increase calcium absorption and retention by the body, are clearly capable of providing the extra mineral required for increased bone formation, and there is evidence that during continuous administration of small doses of PTH, these

actions can even cause hypercalcemia which does not depend on a significant increase in bone breakdown.[52] However, hypercalcemia does not stimulate osteoblasts.[51,53] Neither does administration of vitamin D or its active metabolites (in doses sufficient to markedly enhance calcium absorption) maintain a positive calcium balance or increase the incorporation of calcium into bone for any longer than can be accounted for by mineralization of preexisting osteoid.[54-56] Although in the Danish trial,[54] histochemical measurements of alkaline phosphatase activity were thought to indicate stimulation of osteoblasts, such data are notoriously difficult to quantitate. The more reliable serum level of alkaline phosphatase activity, in fact, fell or was unchanged in 6 patients, rising only in 1. The strongest evidence that the anabolic effect of PTH on bone represents a direct peripheral response comes from studies by Herrmann-Erlee et al.[57] on bone in tissue culture. They incubated 15-day embryonic mouse radii in the system of Gaillard[58] and found that synthetic bovine PTH 1–34 at a concentration of 5 × 10⁻⁹ M induced a striking increase in the number of active osteoblasts, together with increased maturation of the cartilage, and osteoid formation within the bone shaft (Fig. 46-6).

Other evidence on the mechanism and character of the anabolic effect can be found in the work of Bingham et al. already cited[31] (Fig. 46-3). Uridine incorporation into both preosteoblasts and osteoblasts was markedly stimulated by PTH but not for at least 24 hours after administration of the hormone.

BALANCE OF ACTIONS: DOSE DEPENDENCE OF THE OVERALL EFFECT

The actions of parathyroid hormone on bone thus affect directly or indirectly every process involved in formation and destruction of the skeleton. In order to understand the overall balance of its effects under various circumstances, it is most helpful to classify individual actions according to their apparent significance as *anabolic* (contributing to the formation and mineralization of bone) or *catabolic* (leading to bone demineralization and destruction). In making such a classification, one is immediately confronted by the fact that the action of the parathyroids on bone formation is biphasic. As can be seen in Figure 46-3, the incorporation of uridine into osteoblasts was initially depressed for many hours, and marked stimulation appeared only on the second day. This time lag before bone formation could be seen to be stimulated was first pointed out by Selye in 1932,[46] and the initial depression of formation by high doses is in agreement with the findings of many other authors, not all of whom have studied the subsequent stimulation.

On reflection, the biphasic nature of the effect on formation is seen to increase the value of distinguishing between anabolic and catabolic responses because depressed formation is only seen in association with enhanced destruction and should correctly be classified as a catabolic effect. The simple generalization then emerges that anabolic actions of PTH, which have a latent period of several hours, are favored by near-normal blood levels and chronic exposure, whereas high blood concentrations elicit catabolic effects that have a short latency and may overwhelm the anabolic response.

In the tissue culture experiments of Herrmann-Erlee et al. already cited,[57] both the hormone and its fragment elicited the well-known osteolytic response at the high concentration of 5 × 10⁻⁷ M. At no concentration did the intact hormone cause the same anabolic effect that was shown in those experiments with the amino-terminal fragment at 5 × 10⁻⁹ M. This observation, together with the studies of peripheral metabolism of PTH discussed in

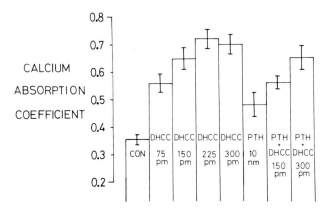

Fig. 46-5. Calcium absorption coefficients measured by a double-isotope method in control rats and in rats receiving daily injections for 3 days of various doses of dihydroxycholecalciferol, with and without PTH. (From ref. 42 by courtesy of the publishers.)

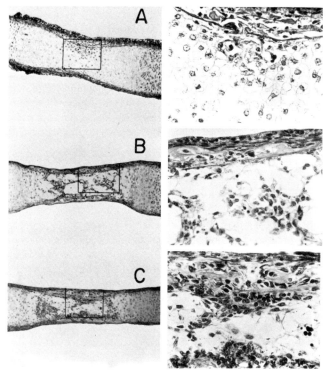

Fig. 46-6. Photomicrographs from radii of 15-day-old Swiss albino mouse embryos (azan stained; magnification 120 × to the left; further enlargement of rectangular area to the right). (*a*) Noncultivated. (*b*) Cultivated for 48 hours in Hanks' balanced salt solution containing 15 percent heat-inactivated human serum, showing development of a bone collar and replacement of most of the hypertrophic cartilage cells by reticular connective tissue in the primitive marrow cavity. (*c*) Sister radius of that depicted in (*b*) but with addition to the culture medium of 0.2 µg/ml of hPTH 1–34 (≃50 nanomolar). The increased bone-collar volume and extensions of the osteoid into the marrow cavity are clearly visible. (Illustrations kindly provided by Professor P. J. Gaillard. For further details and extension of dose–response relationship, see Gaillard et al. *Proc. Kon. Ned. Akad. Wetensch., C80, 267–280,* 1977.)

Chapter 45, raise the interesting possibility that anabolic responses to the intact hormone in vivo may depend on its prior cleavage—a suggestion that clearly requires and is receiving further investigation.

A similar biological significance of near-normal blood levels can be made out in the dose dependence of extraskeletal actions of parathyroid hormone. The evidence presented above on PTH-induced intestinal absorption and renal retention of calcium strongly implies that both play a part in regulating mineral metabolism under normal conditions of life and are diminished after parathyroidectomy. These considerations suggested that under normal physiological conditions, all the calcium-regulating effects of the parathyroids have a predominantly anabolic effect on the skeleton and that the catabolic mobilization of calcium from bone should be seen as an emergency response, likely to be important only under conditions of severe calcium stress (e.g., dietary deficiency, pregnancy, and lactation).

EVIDENCE FOR A PREDOMINANTLY ANABOLIC EFFECT AT NEAR-NORMAL RATES OF SECRETION OR DOSAGE

The validity of this altered concept of the biological significance of the parathyroids has been tested in three principal ways. One line of evidence comes from the effects of exogenous parathy-

roid hormone given to dogs by continuous infusion to determine the dosage rate needed to cause hypercalcemia when major peaks and troughs in the blood level were avoided. It was found that as little as 100 ng (0.2 U)/kg/hr caused moderately severe hypercalcemia under these conditions and that its mechanisms owed little to bone breakdown but involved primarily the extraskeletal actions of enhanced calcium absorption and retention.[52] These experiments by infusion incidentally provided strong support for other indirect estimates that the normal rate of secretion of endogenous PTH cannot much exceed 50 ng/kg/hr because the infusions caused marked hypercalcemia, while activity of the animal's own parathyroids must have been almost entirely suppressed.

Second, small subcutaneous injections of the synthetic amino-terminal fragment of human parathyroid hormone (hPTH 1–34) were tested in patients with postmenopausal osteoporosis. As described in a preliminary report,[59] this treatment caused a remarkable acceleration of bone turnover, an effect now demonstrated by isotopic tracer and/or histological methods in 14 of 15 patients. However, calcium balances still significantly positive at the end of 6 months' treatment were observed in only 4 of the 15. The fact that the majority of balances remained unchanged indicates that in most subjects treated with this simple regimen, the increase in bone formation was matched by increased resorption of bone. Within an hour of the 100-µg subcutaneous doses initially used, amino-terminal radioimmunoassay revealed plasma levels of hPTH 1–34 several-hundred-times higher than the normal circulating level of iPTH, but the peptide became unmeasurable again within 4 hours. With regard to the therapeutic possibilities, encouragement can be found in the fact that despite these unphysiological blood PTH levels, such increases in bone turnover can be produced in elderly people without side effects and without producing a net negative calcium balance. As already discussed, pulsatile administration of PTH induces long-lasting waves of bone breakdown, and one can reasonably hope that modifications of the protocol will improve the ratio of anabolic to catabolic responses. The hPTH 1–34 is therefore being tested in combination with calcitonin and other agents to inhibit bone breakdown, and, at the same time, other efforts are being made to develop controlled-release preparations of the hormone fragment.

Finally, it is possible to reassess the relationship between anabolic and catabolic effects in published clinical studies of hyperparathyroidism. As discussed in fuller detail elsewhere, this reassessment also provided strong support for the view that mild parathyroid hyperactivity has a predominantly anabolic effect on the skeleton, the well-known signs of net bone destruction occurring only in severe forms of the disease or in association with concurrent deficiency in calcium or vitamin D.[60]

The radiological findings in hyperparathyroidism are remarkably variable, but there are a number of reports of localized increases in bone density in both primary and secondary forms of the disease. More recently, a few cases of generalized osteosclerosis have been described in the primary form.[61,62] In each of the latter, the radiological appearance of increased bone density was confirmed by microradiography of iliac-crest biopsy samples. Osteosclerosis rarely gives rise to symptoms, and in any case the recognition of overall increases in density is a far more difficult technical problem than the detection of patchy sclerosis; Connor has suggested that the finding will become more common with the availability of more precise methods of quantitating bone density measurements.

There are five published series of calcium balance studies in patients with primary hyperparathyroidism, data from which are summarized in Figure 46-7. In each case, the net calcium balance is plotted against the plasma calcium level as a rough measure of the

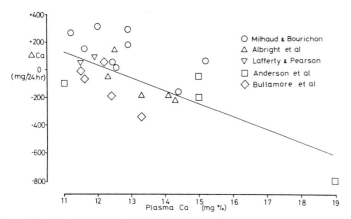

Fig. 46-7. Net calcium balance plotted as a function of plasma calcium level in 25 patients with primary hyperparathyroidism studied by Albright et al.[85] Lafferty and Pearson,[62a] Anderson et al.,[62b] Milhaud and Bourichon,[62c] and Bullamore et al.[62d] Albright's cases were restudied during ingestion of large doses of sodium phosphate. In two of them this produced a new steady state, with lower values of serum calcium and a more positive balance, and both sets of values are shown. Four cases from Anderson's series and one from Milhaud's are omitted because they were hyperthyroid, cushingoid, in renal failure, or receiving an abnormal diet. The data are strongly correlated ($r = 0.67$, $p = 0.001$), and the regression line calculated by the method of least squares is drawn in. As discussed in the text, the data strongly support the view that patients with mild degrees of hyperparathyroidism are in zero or positive balance, demineralization occurring only in severe forms of the disease. (From ref. 13 by permission.)

severity of the disease. A strong negative correlation is seen, and although there is considerable scatter among the points, this appears largely to result from methodological differences between investigators, because roughly parallel regression lines can be made out among the data in several of the individual series. Taken as a whole, the measurements suggest that hyperparathyroid patients are unlikely to be in negative calcium balance unless their plasma calcium concentrations exceed 12 mg/100 mg (assuming adequate dietary supplies of calcium, phosphate, and vitamin D). In other clinical studies, demineralization of the skeleton has similarly been found to be correlated with the size of the parathyroid tumor[63,64] and the plasma level of iPTH.[65,68]

COMPLEX PATHOPHYSIOLOGY OF CLINICAL HYPERPARATHYROIDISM

All the above studies are therefore compatible with the view that it is only patients with severe degrees of parathyroid hyperfunction or those affected by concurrent functional deficiencies who show net loss of bone. In milder cases of uncomplicated hyperparathyroidism, there is invariably evidence of increased bone breakdown, but formation is increased in parallel, resulting only in increased turnover. Such patients may remain in zero or positive calcium balance for years, with abnormally high calcium absorption keeping pace with any increased urinary loss which may result from the hypercalcemia and abnormal filtered load. For example, patients in whom parathyroidectomy was unsuccessful have been followed by repeated neutron activation analysis for years and have maintained constant figures for total body calcium content in spite of persistent hypercalcemia and hypercalciuria.[66,67] Prospective studies of the type conducted by R. M. Neer and associates at the Massachusetts General Hospital also agree that patients with biochemically well-established mild hyperparathyroidism may not show any reduction in bone density over several years of continuous observation.[67]

However, the pathological appearances in bone tissue from patients with hyperparathyroidism are varied (Chapter 53), and in addition to fully developed osteitis fibrosa cystica, a simpler generalized osteopenia is common in many series. What is not clear in such cases is the pattern of evolution of the pathological processes that have led to this condition. Two fundamentally important questions bearing on this issue are (1) the magnitude of the parathyroid hyperfunction required to produce net bone destruction and (2) the nature of other factors predisposing to the net destruction of bone.

DEGREES OF PARATHYROID HYPERFUNCTION

Purnell et al.[68] and O'Riordan et al.[65] agree that in those hyperparathyroid patients that develop osteitis fibrosa, iPTH levels are commonly 10 to 20 times normal. However, the heterogeneity of circulating PTH and the dissociation between immunological and biological activity in this molecule imply that current radioimmunoassays may severely underestimate the degree of hypersecretion[69-76] (for discussion, see ref. 77). If one can judge from Mayer's important experiments on the relationship between peripheral iPTH and direct measurements of parathyroid secretion in the calf,[78,79] the measurements of Purnell and O'Riordan and their colleagues may reflect 100- to 200-fold increases in circulating bioPTH in patients with osteitis fibrosa.

OTHER PREDISPOSING FACTORS

There are several types of clinical observation indicating that one of the factors predisposing hyperparathyroid patients to the development of osteitis fibrosa is a relative deficiency of vitamin D. Woodhouse et al.[80] and Bordier et al.[81] have expressed the view that the vitamin D requirement is increased in hyperparathyroidism, and Bordier et al. did note an increased calcium absorption coefficient and an improvement in histological indexes of calcification after administering only 500 IU per day of calciferol to four hyperparathyroid patients receiving a standard hospital diet. However, a properly controlled series of observations to support the suggestion of increased vitamin D requirement in this condition is still lacking.

Peacock[82] has investigated the old clinical observation that although bone disease and renal stone disease are both common in primary hyperparathyroidism, they rarely occur together in the same patient. Measuring the calcium absorption coefficient by a double-isotope method in 111 cases of the disease, he showed that it was raised in virtually all those with a history of stone formation and normal or depressed in the majority of those without. Other correlations confirmed the generalization that patients with hyperabsorption of calcium and stone disease had a lower rate of bone resorption than those with normal or low calcium absorption and no stone formation. The reason that this study suggests the importance of the vitamin D status of patients in protecting the skeleton is that the PTH-induced intestinal calcium absorption is presumably mediated by formation of the active metabolite 1,25-dihydroxycholecalciferol. Further support is lent to this interpretation by preliminary measurements of the circulating precursor metabolite 25-hydroxycholecalciferol, reported by O'Riordan.[83] Levels of this precursor were significantly lower in those hyperparathyroid patients who had raised serum levels of alkaline phosphatase, which almost invariably accompanied radiologically clear-cut bone disease.

Another important variable that may affect the likelihood that a hyperparathyroid patient will develop bone disease is the adequacy of dietary supplies of phosphate or, more probably, the phosphate balance. Albright and Reifenstein[3] believed that a diet deficient in calcium played an important role in increasing the likelihood of net bone destruction in such patients. It seems self-evident that this must be true in cases of extreme calcium deprivation, but Dent et al.[84] were unable to find any difference in mean dietary calcium content between groups of their hyperparathyroid patients with and without bone involvement. However, this paper also provided data on the mean phosphate intake of those patients with and without bone disease. Although no statistically significant difference was found, mean phosphate ingestion was in fact 20 percent higher among patients free from bone involvement. An earlier paper of Albright et al.[85] had already shown convincingly that dietary supplementation with sodium phosphate greatly reduced demineralization in three hyperparathyroid patients and led in one case to a positive calcium balance. Similar remineralization on a high-phosphate diet was documented by whole-body neutron irradiation in one case discussed by Hosking et al.[66] In the series of 50 cases discussed by Hodgkinson,[63] the mean serum level of inorganic phosphate was 9 percent higher in the patients without bone disease. Again, this was not statistically significant, but the 7 patients with levels below 2 mg/100 ml were all in the "with bone disease" group.

In addition to this clinical data, rat experiments of Baylink et al.[86] showed an inverse relationship between serum phosphorus and the percentage of endosteal surface involved in resorption. It is also clear from many in vitro experiments on bone metabolism by Raisz and his colleagues that a relatively high phosphate concentration enhances bone formation and inhibits osteoclastic resorption.[9,87,88]

Thus the weight of the suggestive evidence that adequate plasma levels of phosphate may be essential to support the anabolic component of the response to PTH and to protect the skeleton against net loss of bone in hyperparathyroidism is clearly sufficient to warrant further intensive investigation. The variability of phosphate excretion is well known, and it is most probably phosphate balance rather than dietary content which is the factor affecting the ratio between skeletal anabolism and catabolism.

It is worth pointing out that the probable protective role of phosphate on the hyperparathyroid skeleton, just discussed, may in fact be interrelated with that of vitamin D. Both PTH[89] and vitamin D[90,91] enhance intestinal phosphate absorption by a mechanism apparently independent of that for calcium transport, and vitamin D probably enhances renal tubular reabsorption of phosphate.[92] The general interrelationship between vitamin D and phosphate metabolism has been reviewed by DeLuca et al.,[93] and indeed MacIntyre et al.[94] have proposed that mobilization of phosphate rather than that of calcium may represent the primitive role of 1,25-dihydroxycholecalciferol.

CONCLUSION

The overall evidence thus indicates that under normal physiological circumstances, parathyroid hormone directly stimulates osteoblasts as well as osteoclasts, exerting on balance a predominantly anabolic effect on the skeleton, which is supported at a systemic level by enhanced calcium absorption and retention.

The apparent paradox between this view and the long-standing clinical impression that hyperparathyroidism leads to bone destruction may be resolved if future work confirms present indications that hyperparathyroid patients with overt bone disease are afflicted with either intercurrent deficiencies that prevent the acceleration of bone formation or simply an extreme degree of hypersecretion of the hormone.

This altered view of the biological role of the parathyroids has

suggested a new approach to the therapy of osteoporosis and reemphasizes the clinical wisdom of correcting dietary deficiencies of calcium, phosphate, and vitamin D in mild cases of parathyroid hyperactivity.

REFERENCES

1. Thomson, D. L. and Collip, J. B. The parathyroid glands. *Physiol. Rev., 12,* 309–383, 1932.
2. Greep, R. O. The physiology and chemistry of the parathyroid hormone. *In* The Hormones (ed.) G. Pincus and K. V. Thimann. Academic Press, New York, Vol. 1, 1948, pp. 255–299.
3. Albright, F. and Reifenstein, E. C. The Parathyroid Glands and Metabolic Bone Disease. Williams and Wilkins, Baltimore, 1948.
4. McLean, F. C. The parathyroid glands and bone. *In* The Biochemistry and Physiology of Bone, 1st edition (ed.) G. H. Bourne. Academic Press, New York, 1956, p. 705.
5. Munson, P. L., Hirsch, P. F., and Tashjian, A. H. Parathyroid gland. *Ann. Rev. Physiol., 25,* 325–360, 1963.
6. Gaillard, P. J. Parathyroid and bone in tissue culture. *In* The Parathyroids (ed.) R. O. Greep and R. V. Talmage. Thomas, Springfield, Ill., 1961, pp. 20–45.
7. Gaillard, P. J. Observations on the effect of parathyroid products on explanted mouse limb-bone rudiments. *In* The Parathyroid Glands; Ultrastructure, Secretion and Function (ed.) P. J. Gaillard, R. V. Talmage and A. M. Budy. Chicago University Press, Chicago, 1965, pp. 145–152.
8. Gaillard, P. J. The physiology and biochemistry of parathyroid function. *In* Parathyroid Hormone and Thyrocalcitonin (Calcitonin) (ed.) R. V. Talmage, L. F. Bélanger and I. Clark. Excerpta Medica, Amsterdam, 1968, pp. 18–24.
9. Raisz, L. G. Physiologic and pharmacologic regulation of bone resorption. *N. Engl. J. Med., 282,* 909–916, 1970.
10. Hekkelman, J. W., Herrmann-Erlee, M. P. M., and Heersche, J. N. M. et al. Studies on the mechanism of parathyroid hormone action on embryonic bone in vitro. *In* Calcium-Regulating Hormones (ed.) R. V. Talmage, M. Owen and J. A. Parsons. Excerpta Medica, Amsterdam, 1975, pp. 185–194.
11. Parsons, J. A., Rafferty, B., Gray, D. et al. Pharmacology of parathyroid hormone and some of its fragments and analogues. *In* Calcium-Regulating Hormones (ed.) R. V. Talmage, M. Owen and J. A. Parsons. Excerpta Medica, Amsterdam, 1975, pp. 33–39.
12. Parsons, J. A. and Potts, J. T. Jr. Physiology and chemistry of parathyroid hormone. *Clin. Endocrinol. Metab., 1,* 33–78, 1972.
13. Parsons, J. A. Parathyroid physiology and the skeleton. *In* Biochemistry and Physiology of Bone (ed.) G. H. Bourne. Academic Press, New York, Vol. IV, 1976, pp. 159–225.
14. Pearse, A. G. E. and Takor, T. T. Neuroendocrine embryology and the APUD concept. *Clin. Endocrinol, 5* Suppl, 229–244, 1976.
14a. Scott, A. P., Bloomfield, G. A., and Lowry, P. et al. Pituitary adrenocorticotrophin and the melanocyte stimulating hormones. *In* Peptide Hormones (ed.) J. A. Parsons. Macmillan, London, 1976, pp. 247–271.
14b. Barker, W. C. and Dayhoff, M. O. Detecting distant relationships; computer methods and results. *In* Atlas of Protein Sequence and Structure (ed.) M. O. Dayhoff. National Biomedical Research Foundation, Washington, 1972, pp. 101–110.
15. Pickford, G. E. A study of the hypophysectomised male killifish, Fundulus heteroclitus. *Bull. Bingham Oceanogr. Coll, 14,* 5–41, 1953.
16. Fontaine, M. The hormonal control of water and salt-electrolyte metabolism in fish. *Mem. Soc. Endocrinol, 5,* 69–82, 1956.
17. Fontaine, M. and Lopez, E. Comparative endocrine aspects of calcium homeostasis. *In* Endocrinology (ed.) V. H. T. James. Vol. II. Excerpta Medica, Amsterdam, ICS 403, 277–281, 1977.
18. Stanley, J. G. and Fleming, W. R. The effect of hypophysectomy on the electrolyte content of Fundulus kansae held in fresh water and in sea water. *Comp. Biochem. Physiol, 20,* 489–497, 1967.
19. Pang, P. K. T., Griffith, R. W., and Pickford, G. E. Hypocalcaemia and tetanic seizures in hypophysectomized killifish. *Proc. Soc. Exp. Biol. Med., 136,* 85–87, 1971.
20. Reference 13, pp. 172–174.
21. Urist, M. Biogenesis of bone. *In* Handbook of Physiology, Section 7: Endocrinology, Vol VII (ed.) G. D. Aurbach, E. Astwood and R. O. Greep. American Physiological Society, Williams and Wilkins, Baltimore, pp. 183–213, 1976.

22. Moss, M. L The biology of acellular teleost bone. *Ann. N.Y. Acad. Sci., 109,* 337–350, 1963.

23. Simmons, D. J. Calcium and skeletal tissue physiology in teleost fishes. *Clin. Orthop., 76,* 244–280, 1971.

24. Hellman, D., Au, W. Y. W., and Bartter, F. C. Evidence for a direct effect of parathyroid hormone on urinary acidification. *Amer. J. Physiol., 209,* 643–650, 1965.

25. Agus, Z. S., Puschett, J. B., and Senesky, D., et al. Mode of action of parathyroid hormone and cyclic adenosine 3′, 5′-monophosphate on renal tubular phosphate reabsorption in the dog. *J. Clin. Invest., 50,* 617–626, 1971.

26. Froeling, P. G. A. M. and Bijvoet, O. L. M. Kidney-mediated effects of parathyroid hormone on extracellular homeostasis of calcium, phosphate and acid-base balance in man. *Neth. J. Med., 17,* 174–183, 1974.

27. Cortelyou, J. R. and McWhinnie, D. J. Parathyroid glands of amphibians, I; parathyroid structure and function in the amphibian, with emphasis on regulation of mineral ions in body fluids. *Amer. Zool., 7,* 843–855, 1967.

28. Bijvoet, O. L. M., Will, E. J., and Van Aken, J. et al. Renal physiology and the phosphate ion. *In* Proc. 1st Int. Sympos. Urolithiasis Research (ed.) H. Fleisch (in press).

29. Albright, F. and Ellsworth, R. Studies on the physiology of the parathyroid glands. I. Calcium and phosphorus studies on a case of idiopathic hypoparathyroidism. *J. Clin. Invest., 7,* 183–201, 1929.

30. Rasmussen, H., Arnaud, C. D., and Hawker, C. Actinomycin D and the response to parathyroid hormone. *Science, 144,* 1019–1021, 1964.

31. Bingham, P., Brazell, I., and Owen, M. The effect of parathyroid extract on cellular activity and plasma calcium levels in vivo. *J. Endocrinol., 45,* 387–400. 1969.

32. Reference 13, pp. 205–215.

33. Talmage, R. V. Effect of fasting and parathyroid hormone injection on plasma 45Ca concentrations in rats. *Calcif. Tiss. Res., 17,* 103–112, 1975.

34. Parsons, J. A., Neer, R. M., and Potts, J. T. Jr. Initial fall of plasma calcium after intravenous injection of parathyroid hormone. *Endocrinology, 89,* 735–740. 1971.

35. Meyer, R. A. and Talmage, R. V. Effects of parathyroid hormone on bone calcium without concurrent effects on phosphate. *In* Calcium, Parathyroid Hormone and the Calcitonins (ed.) R. V. Talmage and P. L. Munson. Excerpta Medica, Amsterdam, 1972, pp. 416–421.

36. Peacock, M., Robertson, W. G., and Nordin, B. E. C. Relation between serum and urinary calcium with particular reference to parathyroid activity. *Lancet, 1,* 384–386, 1969.

37. Nordin, B. E. C. and Peacock, M. Role of kidney in regulation of plasma-calcium. *Lancet, ii,* 1280–1283, 1969.

38. DeLuca, H. F. Regulation of functional vitamin D metabolism; a new endocrine system involved in calcium homeostasis. *In* Metabolism and Function of Vitamin D (ed.) D. R. Fraser. Biochem. Soc., London, Spec. Publ. No. 3. 1974, pp. 5–26.

39. Wasserman, R. H., Corradino, R. A., and Fullmer, C. S. et al. Some aspects of vitamin D action; calcium absorption and the vitamin D-dependent calcium-binding protein. *Vit. Horm., 32,* 299–324, 1974.

40. Haussler, M. R., Baylink, D. J., and Hughes, M. R. et al. The assay of 1α,25-dihydroxyvitamin D₃: Physiologic and pathologic modulation of circulating hormone levels. *Clin. Endocrinol., 5,* Suppl., 151s–165s, 1976.

41. Haussler, M. R., Bursac, K. M., and Bone, H. et al. Increased circulating 1α,25-dihydroxy vitamin D₃ in patients with primary hyperparathyroidism. *Clin. Res., 23,* 322A, 1975.

42. Parsons, J. A., Zanelli, J. M., and Gray, D. et al. Double isotope estimates of intestinal calcium absorption in rats; enhancement by parathyroid hormone and 1,25-dihydroxycholecalciferol. *Calcif. Tissues Res. 22 Suppl.:* 127–132, 1977.

43. Tregear, G. W., Rietschoten, J. van, and Greene, E. et al. Bovine parathyroid hormone: Minimum chain length of synthetic peptide required for biological activity. *Endocrinology, 93,* 1349–1353, 1973.

44. Reference 13, pp. 181–198.

45. Bauer, W., Aub, J. C., and Albright, F. A study of the bone trabeculae as a readily available reserve supply of calcium. *J. Exp. Med., 49,* 145–162, 1929.

46. Selye, H. On the stimulation of new bone-formation with parathyroid extract and irradiated ergosterol. *Endocrinology, 16,* 547–558, 1932.

47. Pugsley, L. I. The effect of parathyroid hormone and of irradiated ergosterol on calcium and phosphorus metabolism in the rat. *J. Physiol. (Lond.), 76,* 315–328, 1932.

48. Pugsley, L. I. and Selye, H. The histological changes in the bone responsible for the action of parathyroid hormone on the calcium metabolism of the rat. *J. Physiol., 79,* 113–117, 1933.

49. Shelling, D. H., Asher, D. E., and Jackson, D. A. Calcium and phosphorus studies; (vii) the effects of variations in dosage of parathormone and of calcium and phosphorus in the diet on the concentration of calcium and inorganic phosphorus in the serum and on the histology and chemical composition of the bones of rats. *Bull. Johns Hopkins Hosp., 53,* 348–389, 1933.

50. Kalu, D. N., Pennock, J., and Doyle, F. H. et al. Parathyroid hormone and experimental osteosclerosis. *Lancet, 1,* 1363–1366, 1970.

51. Walker, D. G. The induction of osteopetrotic changes in hypophysectomized, thyroparathyroidectomized, and intact rats of various ages. *Endocrinology, 89,* 1389–1406, 1971.

52. Parsons, J. A. and Reit, B. Chronic response of dogs to parathyroid hormone infusion. *Nature (Lond.), 250,* 254–257, 1974.

53. McGuire, J. L. and Marks, S. C. Jr. The effects of parathyroid hormone on bone cell structure and function. *Clin. Orthop. Rel. Res., 100,* 392–405, 1974.

54. Lund, B., Kjaer, I., and Friis, T. et al. Treatment of osteoporosis of ageing with 1α-hydroxycholecalciferol. *Lancet, ii,* 1168–1171, 1975.

55. Riggs, B. L., Jowsey, J., and Kelly, P. J. et al. Effects of oral therapy with calcium and vitamin D in primary osteoporosis. *J. Clin. Endocrinol. Metab., 42,* 1139–1144.

56. Davies, M., Mawer, E. B., and Adams, P. H. Vitamin D metabolism and the response to 1,25-dihydroxycholecalciferol in osteoporosis. *Calcif. Tissues Res. 22 Suppl.:* 74, 1977.

57. Herrmann-Erlee, M. P. M., Heersche, J. N. M., and Hekkelman, J. W. et al. Effects on bone in vitro of bovine parathyroid hormone and synthetic fragments representing residues 1–34, 2–34 and 3–34. *Endocrine. Res. Comm., 3,* 21–35, 1976.

58. Gaillard, P. J. The influence of ascorbic acid on the effect of parathyroid extract on the histology of explanted mouse radius rudiments. *Proc. Kon. Akad. Wetensch., C77,* 101–115, 1974.

59. Reeve, J., Hesp, R., and Williams, D. et al. The anabolic effect of low doses of human parathyroid hormone fragment on the skeleton in postmenopausal osteoporosis. *Lancet, 1,* 1035–1038, 1976.

60. Reference 13, pp. 187–192.

61. Connor, T. B., Freijanes, J., and Stoner, R. E. et al. Generalized osteosclerosis in primary hyperparathyroidism. *Trans. Amer. Clin. Climatol. Assoc. 85,* 185–201, 1973.

62. Genant, H. K., Baron, J. M., and Paloyan, E. et al. Osteosclerosis in primary hyperparathyroidism. *Amer. J. Med., 59,* 104–113, 1975.

62a. Lafferty, F. W. and Pearson, O. H. Skeletal, intestinal and renal calcium dynamics in hyperparathyroidism. *J. Clin. Endocrinol. Metab., 23,* 891–902, 1963.

62b. Anderson, J., Osborn, S. B., and Tomlinson, R. W. S. et al. Calcium dynamics of the gastrointestinal tract and bone in primary hyperparathyroidism. *Q. J. Med, 33,* 421–438, 1964.

62c. Milhaud, G. and Bourichon, J. Etude du métabolisme du calcium chez l'homme à l'aide de calcium 45. L'hyperparathyroidie et l'hypoparathyroidie. *C. R. Acad. Sci. (Paris), 258,* 3398–3401, 1964.

62d. Bullamore, J. R., Wilkinson, R., and Marshall, D. H. Radiocalcium measurement of bone turnover in disorders of calcium metabolism using a model based on an expanding pool. *In* Dynamic Studies with Radioisotopes in Medicine. Int. Atomic Energy Agency, Vienna, Va., 1971, pp. 519–538.

63. Hodgkinson, A. Biochemical aspects of primary hyperparathyroidism: an analysis of 50 cases. *Clin. Sci., 25,* 231–242, 1963.

64. Lloyd, H. M. Primary hyperparathyroidism: An analysis of the role of the parathyroid tumor. *Medicine, 47,* 53–71, 1968.

65. O'Riordan, J. L. H., Watson, L., and Woodhead, J. S. Secretion of parathyroid hormone in primary hyperparathyroidism. *Clin. Endocrinol., 1,* 149–155, 1972.

66. Hosking, D. J., Chamberlain, M. J., and Fremlin, J. H. Changes in total body calcium content in primary hyperparathyroidism. *Clin. Sci, 43,* 627–637, 1972.

67. Neer, R. M. Massachusetts General Hospital. (Personal communication.)

68. Purnell, D. C., Smith, L. H., and Scholz, D. A. Primary hyperparathyroidism: a prospective clinical study. *Amer. J. Med., 50,* 670–678, 1971.

69. Berson, S. A. and Yalow, R. S. Immunochemical heterogeneity of parathyroid hormone in plasma. *J. Clin. Endocrinol. 28,* 1037–1047, 1968.

70. Habener, J. F., Powell, D., and Murray, T. M. Parathyroid hormone: Secretion and metabolism in vivo. *Proc. Nat. Acad. Sci., (Wash), 68,* 2986–2991, 1971.

71. Habener, J. F., Segre, G. V., and Powell, D. et al. Immunoreactive parathyroid hormone in the circulation of man. *Nature New Biol., 238,* 152–154, 1972.

72. Segre, G. V., Habener, J. F., and Powell, D. et al. Parathyroid hormone in human plasma; immunochemical characterization and biological implications. *J. Clin. Invest, 51,* 3163–3172, 1972.

73. Segre, G. V., Niall, H. D., and Habener, J. F. et al. Metabolism of parathyroid hormone: Physiologic and clinical significance. *Amer. J. Med., 56,* 774–784, 1974.

74. Canterbury, J. M. and Reiss, E. Multiple immunoreactive molecular forms of parathyroid hormone in human serum. *Proc. Soc. Exp. Biol. Med, 140,* 1393–1398, 1972.

75. Silverman, R. and Yalow, R. S. Heterogeneity of parathyroid hormone; clinical and physiologic implications. *J. Clin. Invest., 52,* 1958–1971, 1973.

76. Arnaud, C. D., Goldsmith, R. S., and Bordier, P. J. et al. Influence of immunoheterogeneity of circulating parathyroid hormone on results of radioimmunoassays of serum in man. *Amer. J. Med., 56,* 785–793, 1974.

77. Reference 13, pp. 164–170.

78. Mayer, G. P. Effect of calcium and magnesium on parathyroid hormone secretion rate in calves. *In* Calcium-Regulating Hormones (ed.) R. V. Talmage, M. Owen, and J. A. Parsons. Excerpta Medica, Amsterdam, 1975, pp. 122–124.

79. Mayer, G. P., Staley, J. A. S., and Keaton, J. A. et al. Relation between intravenous infusion rate of PTH and its plasma concentration. Proc. Endocr. Soc. 57th Ann. Mtg., *Endocrinology, 96,* Suppl., 73, 1975.

80. Woodhouse, N. J. Y., Doyle, F. H., and Joplin, G. F. Vitamin D deficiency and primary hyperparathyroidism, *Lancet, ii,* 283–287, 1971.

81. Bordier, J., Woodhouse, N. J. Y., and Sigurdsson, G. et al. Osteoid mineralization defect in primary hyperparathyroidism. *Clin. Endocrinol., 2,* 377–386, 1973.

82. Peacock, M. Renal stone disease and bone disease in primary hyperparathyroidism and their relationship to the action of parathyroid hormone on calcium absorption. *In* Calcium-Regulating Hormones (ed.) R. V. Talmage, M. Owen, and J. A. Parsons. Excerpta Medica, Amsterdam, 1975, pp. 78–81.

83. O'Riordan, J. L. H. Discussion of paper by A. W. Norman and H. Henry, *Recent Prog. Horm. Res., 30,* 479–480, 1974.

84. Dent, C. E., Hartland, B. V., and Hicks, J. et al. Calcium intake in patients with primary hyperparathyroidism. *Lancet, 2,* 336–338, 1961.

85. Albright, F., Bauer, W., and Claflin, D. et al. Studies in parathyroid physiology;(iii) the effect of phosphate ingestion in clinical hyperparathyroidism. *J. Clin. Invest., 11,* 411–435, 1932.

86. Baylink, D., Wergedal, J. and Stauffer, M. Formation, mineralization and resorption of bone in hypo-phosphataemic rats. *J. Clin. Invest, 50,* 2519–2530, 1971.

87. Raisz, L. G. and Niemann, I. Effect of phosphate, calcium and magnesium on bone resorption and hormonal responses in tissue culture. *Endocrinology, 85,* 446–452, 1969.

88. Bingham, P. J. and Raisz, L. G. Bone growth in organ culture: effects of phosphate and other nutrients on bone and cartilage. *Calc. Tiss. Res., 14,* 31–48. 1974.

89. Borle, A. B., Keutmann, H. T., and Neuman, W. F. Role of parathyroid hormone in phosphate transport across rat duodenum. *Amer. J. Physiol., 204,* 705–709, 1963.

90. Harrison, H. E. and Harrison, H. C. Intestinal transport of phosphate: action of vitamin D, calcium and potassium. *Amer. J. Physiol, 201,* 1007–1012, 1961.

91. Wasserman, R. H. and Taylor, A. N. Intestinal absorption of phosphate in the chick: Effect of vitamin D_3 and other parameters, *J. Nutr., 103,* 586–599, 1973.

92. Puschett, J. B., Moranz, J., and Kurnick, W. S. Evidence for a direct action of cholecalciferol and 25-hydroxycholecalciferol on the renal transport of phosphate, sodium and calcium. *J. Clin. Invest., 51,* 373–385. 1972.

93. Deluca, H. F., Tanaka, Y., and Castillo, L. Interrelationships between vitamin D and phosphate metabolism. *In* Calcium-Regulating Hormones (ed.) R. V. Talmage, M. Owen and J. A. Parsons. Excerpta Medica, Amsterdam, 1975, pp. 305–317.

94. MacIntyre, I., Colston, K. W., and Evans, I. M. A. et al. Regulation of vitamin D: An evolutionary view. *Clin. Endocrinol., 5* Suppl., 85s–95s, 1976.

47

Biochemical Mode of Action of Parathyroid Hormone

David Goltzman

The hormonal activation of target tissue represents two discrete phases: (1) the biosynthetic, secretory, or metabolic events generated in tissue fluids adjacent to receptor sites in target organs by the specific chemical structure of the hormone that is the active species, and (2) the special differentiating processes occurring within the target cells following acceptance of the hormonal "message" by the binding sites or receptors. Consideration of the biochemical mode of action of parathyroid hormone (PTH) must therefore take into account both the chemical characteristics of the activating form of the hormone and the special features of the target tissue, as well as the nature of the interaction between the two.

ACTIVATING MOIETY OF PTH

Considerable effort has been expended in attempting to unravel the "message" or code contained within the structure of the PTH molecule to which the target cell responds. This has been aided by information evolving from the design and synthesis of analogues of PTH, yet confused by discovery of the complexity of hormonal metabolism and the heterogeneity of circulating PTH (see Chapters 42 and 45).

The discovery[1-4] of intraglandular biosynthetic precursors, which are composed of the NH_2-terminal extensions of the intact native 84-amino-acid form of parathyroid hormone, raised the additional possibility that, at least in some circumstances, release of these larger precursors from the gland might occur (Chapter 43).

Information employing in vitro techniques suggests that the 90-amino-acid prohormone, the immediate precursor to the hormone, has little, if any, inherent activity.[5] It is dependent for most, if not all, of its biopotency on conversion to the hormone by a trypticlike cleavage,[6] removing the prohormone hexapeptide extension and exposing the free hormonal NH_2-terminal region. Consequently, although release of this entity into the circulation would increase the concentration of potentially active circulating moie-

ties, the molecule probably would have to be proteolytically modified before it could act.

In addition to the possibility that larger PTH moieties might reach the target cell, recent evidence suggests that fragments of the intact hormone might be important, biologically active hormone species. A systematic analysis of the structural requirements of parathyroid hormone for biological activity employing synthetic bovine hormonal analogues has demonstrated[7,8] that virtually the full requirements for biological activity in assays, both in vivo and in vitro, reside in the NH_2-terminal 34 residues of the 84-amino-acid hormone and that certain types of activity are retained by considerably shorter sequences (Chapter 42). In view of these findings, the demonstration of circulating fragments[9-14] generated by peripheral metabolism in vivo led to the possibility that some of these smaller hormonal fragments might be physiologically important. One study has, in fact, suggested that an NH_2-terminal fragment capable of stimulating renal adenylyl cyclase may exist in the circulation of man.[14] A cleavage process capable of generating such a fragment in the periphery has been demonstrated[15] (Chapter 45).

These findings support the possibility that the native 84-amino-acid form might itself be inactive and be only a precursor form, which is subjected to postsecretory proteolysis resulting in a bioactive NH_2-terminal fragment.

In more recent studies using in vitro techniques,[16] however, it has been possible to demonstrate that the intact hormone, without proteolytic modification, does stimulate adenylyl cyclase in renal cortical membranes. To the extent that these in vitro studies reflect the overall action of PTH in vivo, they suggest that the 84-amino-acid form of the hormone, rather than being only an inert precursor, is indeed biologically active. Further investigation of the molecular entity active in kidney and also in bone, the other major target tissue, is continuing.

However, even if it is definitively substantiated that the intact 84-amino-acid molecular form is active uncleaved in all target tissues, the apparently specific metabolic pathway might still be of importance either in generating fragments of biological significance with a spectrum or duration of activity different from the intact hormone or in regulating the quantity of circulating bioactive hormone available for interaction with target tissues (Chapter 45).

Before resolution of these issues concerning the exact number and nature of active forms of the hormone in tissue fluids, analysis of hormone action must be based on knowledge of the results of interaction between the receptor and the native hormone of 84 amino acids and/or the synthetic analogues based on the NH_2-terminal 34 residues that seem to emulate closely the actions of the native hormone.

TISSUE RESPONSES

Considerable information has accumulated regarding the interaction of the target tissues with native PTH and synthetic fragments and some of the events occurring as a consequence thereafter. Nevertheless, large gaps in our knowledge persist.

PTH BINDING TO RECEPTORS

In common with other peptide hormones, the action of PTH is believed to be initiated by binding to specific receptor sites on the surfaces of cell membranes in target tissues.[17,18] There is as yet no good evidence that either the intact 84-amino-acid form of the hormone or a potentially active NH_2-terminal fragment ever requires cell entry to exert its action. Although the character of the receptor, at least in the kidney, is believed to be partly protein,[19] there is little other direct information about the nature, numbers, distribution, or regulation of PTH receptors. Characterization of the PTH receptor has lagged behind that of other hormone receptors because of the difficulties in developing a highly radioactive, biologically active, PTH ligand required for such studies.[20]

However, studies correlating hormone structure with function (outlined in detail in Chapter 42) have provided considerable insight into the nature of the molecular requirements for interaction between the receptor and the active NH_2-terminal region of the hormone. The demonstration[21] that the fragment bPTH-(3–34), although inactive, antagonizes the stimulating effect of native PTH or bPTH-(1–34) on adenylyl cyclase in vitro suggests that this entity still contains sufficient sequential and/or conformational requirements for binding to renal-membrane receptors but lacks the requirements for stimulating the enzyme. Therefore, residues within the first two sequence positions seem necessary for agonist activity.

In contrast, if substantial deletions at the C-terminus of the tetratriacontapeptide are made, the resulting peptide (shorter than bPTH-(1–26)) lacks both agonist and antagonist activity,[21] suggesting that important recognition sites for the membrane receptor may reside in the region between residues 25 and 34.

TRANSDUCERS—cAMP

Adenylyl Cyclase System

Much evidence suggests that most of the effects of PTH are mediated by cyclic adenosine 3':5'-monophosphate (cAMP),[22,23] in basic agreement with the general model of Sutherland.[24] This "second messenger" was demonstrated to accumulate in response to PTH stimulation of the membrane-bound enzyme adenylyl cyclase in vivo in both blood and urine[25] and in vitro in both bone[26] and kidney cells.[27] Direct adenylyl cyclase stimulation in response to PTH was demonstrated in homogenates[28,29] or cell membranes[30] prepared from the major target tissues, bone and kidney.

The demonstration that proteases will diminish the PTH-specific adenylyl cyclase response in vitro but permit continued responses to the fluoride ion indicates that the catalytic portion of the adenylyl system is an entity discrete from the membrane receptor.[19] Similarly, the identification of antagonists of PTH-stimulated adenylyl cyclase that are themselves inert[21] also points to a distinction between hormonal binding to receptors and adenylyl cyclase activation.

Augmentation of urinary cAMP is the most rapid response seen in vivo after infusion of PTH.[23] Either cAMP or its dibutyryl analogues will, after infusion into thyroparathyroidectomized animals, at least qualitatively mimic the effect of PTH.[31,32] Plasma calcium rises, plasma phosphate falls, and urinary phosphate ex-

cretion increases. Furthermore, concentrations of PTH achieved in vivo in physiological and pathological states have been reported to noticeably alter cAMP concentrations; thus, urinary cAMP excretion, particularly of renal origin, has been reported to increase in hyperparathyroidism and diminish in hypoparathyroidism.[33,34]

PTH-sensitive adenylyl cyclase has been localized in vitro to the renal cortex[35] and within the nephron to the proximal convoluted tubule, pars recta, cortical portion of the thick ascending limb, distal convoluted tubule, and first, branched portion of the collecting tubule.[36] The multiplicity of sites of PTH generation of cAMP is consistent with the apparent mediation of solute transport in both proximal (e.g., inhibition of phosphate reabsorption)[37] and distal (e.g., enhancement of calcium reabsorption)[38] portions of the nephron.

Studies of the interaction of PTH and synthetic analogues with adenylyl cyclase in vitro have not always been consistent with actions of the hormone in vivo. Discrepancies of both sensitivity and, to some extent, specificity have occasionally been observed. With respect to sensitivity, the concentrations of highly active PTH agonists required to elicit significant renal adenylyl cyclase activity in vitro are generally of the order of 10^{-9} to 10^{-10} M,[16] whereas circulating PTH concentrations in vivo, which are presumably capable of stimulating the enzyme in vivo, are estimated to be of the order of 10^{-12} M.[39] Concentrations of PTH that stimulate cAMP in isolated bone cells are generally closer to those found in vivo.[39]

With respect to specificity, certain discrepancies exist between the activity of analogues of PTH observed in vitro with those seen in vivo. For example, the in vitro renal adenylyl cyclase assay appears to be much more influenced by alterations in position 1[40] (Chapter 42) of the hormone than is the in vivo chick bioassay, even though the effects measured are also presumably mediated through adenylyl cyclase. One could perhaps explain the latter discrepancies by the requirement in vivo for generation of only minimal amounts of cAMP for the triggering of intracellular events; the distinctions in physiological potency in vivo of these position-1 analogues would then be minimized, although they might be readily evident in the in vitro assay.

Another possible source of discrepancies between the characteristics of adenylyl cyclase in vivo and in vitro is the potential loss of physiological cofactors during in vitro preparation of suspensions with adenylyl cyclase activity. Such cofactors may include guanyl nucleotides.

It was originally postulated that guanyl nucleotides, especially guanosine triphosphate (GTP), might play an important role in the activation of adenylyl cyclase in liver membranes.[41] With the introduction of the synthetic, apparently nonhydrolyzable analogue of GTP, guanylyl imidodiphosphate (GMP-PNP), to analysis of adenylyl cyclase activity, many studies demonstrated that adenylyl cyclase activity in virtually all eukaryotic cells is markedly enhanced by the guanyl nucleotide analogue, which presumably interacts with a nucleotide regulatory site on the enzyme.[42] In the case of PTH, this effect is demonstrable in the PTH-responsive adenylyl cyclase found in preparations of renal cortical membranes[40–43] in vitro. The effect of the nucleotide analogue on enzyme activity appears to proceed independently of any hormone receptor and to be preceded by a dose-dependent latent period.

Hormone-mediated adenylyl cyclase activation may be considerably augmented in the presence of guanyl nucleotides, and intrinsic activity of apparently inert materials expressed. Thus the analogue [desamino-Ala-1]bPTH-(1–34) is converted from an inert material with antagonist properties to a definite partial agonist in

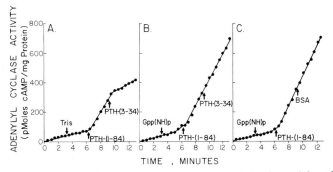

Fig. 47-1. Effect of addition of bovine PTH-(3–34) on the activity of adenylyl cyclase after prior exposure to bovine PTH-(1–84) with and without Gpp(NH)p. Addition of Gpp(NH)p plus agonist prior to antagonist (b) prevents inhibition seen in absence of Gpp(NH)p (a).

the presence of the nucleotide,[40] more in agreement with its in vivo effects. Furthermore, competitive hormonal antagonists appear to lose their effectiveness when added after guanyl nucleotide-enhanced hormonal stimulation of adenylyl cyclase activity has been initiated (Fig. 47-1).[43] The physiological role if any, of naturally occurring guanyl nucleotides, such as GTP, in the stimulation of adenylyl cyclase by PTH is unknown. The nonhydrolyzable analogues may serve only as artificial models. The irreversibility of the effects of GMP-PNP seems to reflect the unusual stability of the guanyl nucleotide; effects of naturally occurring guanyl nucleotides would presumably be reversible, consistent with rapidly modulated effects of PTH operating physiologically. In any event, studies with analogues of guanyl nucleotides have introduced new concepts of the intricacies of the adenylyl cyclase system in eukaryotic cells and afford an interesting tool for further dissection of this system.

Events Distal to cAMP Generation

The sequence of events occurring distal to the PTH-mediated generation of cAMP in the kidney, and culminating ultimately in PTH-stimulated ion transport, is unknown. In analogy with the action of cAMP in other tissues, it has been suggested that a cAMP-dependent protein kinase (or kinases) is activated by combination of the nucleotide with a regulatory subunit of the enzyme, releasing the catalytic component. The nonsuppressed catalytic moiety is then capable of phosphorylating one or more specific cell proteins required for succeeding intracellular PTH-mediated events.

PTH-sensitive adenylyl cyclase was localized preferentially in the contraluminal region of the plasma membrane of responsive renal cortical epithelial cells.[44] In contrast, an intrinsic self-phosphorylating system consisting of a cAMP-dependent protein kinase, a phosphoprotein phosphatase, and the substrate(s) of these enzymes was localized primarily at the brush border of the cells.[44] If this preferential phosphorylation of luminal membrane-associated protein kinase(s) plays a role in the PTH-mediated alteration of solute transport in the renal tubule, it indicates that the mechanism of action of PTH on the responsive renal tubule cell involves intracellular transport of cAMP produced at the antiluminal surface to the phosphorylase located at the luminal border.

Whether PTH-mediated conversion in the kidney[45] of 25-hydroxyvitamin D to the active 1α-25, dihydroxy derivative occurs directly, and whether the activity of the renal 1α-hydroxylase enzyme is regulated directly or indirectly by cAMP is presently unclear. However, this intramitochondrial enzyme may be a significant intermediary in the eventual expression of a variety of apparent PTH effects on solute transport in the intestine and perhaps in the kidney as well.

The sequence of PTH-mediated events in bone occurring after the generation of cAMP is even less well understood than in kidney. The net bone-resorbing activity of PTH occurs in at least two distinct forms. An early (response occurring within minutes) effect,[46,47] predominantly upon resorption of bone mineral, is probably mediated mainly via "osteocytic osteolysis," i.e., by enhancing the lytic activity of osteocytes. A more delayed bone-remodelling effect[46] (response occurring within hours) involves primarily osteoclastic osteolysis with an accompanying but less pronounced osteoblast-induced new bone synthesis. Consequently, if cAMP is the sole mediator of PTH effects, it must directly or indirectly (1) stimulate the activity of existing or newly formed osteocytes, osteoclasts, and osteoblasts either in the early or delayed phases of PTH action, respectively; (2) stimulate cell differentiation and proliferation to account for the increased osteoclast and osteoblast pools occurring in the delayed phase; and (3) mediate, although perhaps indirectly, the destruction of both matrix and bone mineral. The demonstration that the infusion of the cyclic nucleotide or its dibutyryl analogue into thyroparathyroidectomized animals can increase plasma calcium and increase urinary excretion of hydroxyproline-containing peptide[48] suggests that the cyclic nucleotide may well mediate the enhanced activity of bone cells, resulting ultimately in net increased bone resorption. Although cAMP has not as yet been demonstrated to enhance cell differentiation and proliferation from progenitor cells in bone tissue, it is well known to alter phases of cell growth in other tissues.[49]

TRANSDUCERS—OTHER

Whether cAMP mediates all of the effects of PTH or only some is at present unknown—the effect of PTH on cyclic GMP levels, for example, has been little studied.

Calcium has been advocated as an additional "second messenger" for the action of peptide hormones[50–52] (Fig. 47-2). There is some evidence that calcium may be a mediator of PTH action in bone. Thus, it has been demonstrated that (1) PTH, in vitro, independently augments cAMP accumulation in bone cells and increases calcium transport into bone cells, although exogenous cAMP or dibutyryl cAMP does not enhance calcium transport;[53] and (2) rapid hypocalcemia precedes the hypercalcemia consequent upon infusion of PTH into animals in vivo[54,55] (i.e., the PTH-induced hypocalcemia is a rapid event). Exogenous cAMP in vivo will induce an increase in bone resorption but will not stimulate calcium uptake by bone cells. Consequently, it was postulated that facilitation of calcium uptake is a rapid early action of PTH independent of cAMP generation and perhaps of equal importance.[50,52] The increased cytosol calcium might then modulate cAMP accumulation in response to PTH by inhibiting adenylyl cyclase, an action demonstrable in vitro.[56] Calcium might also influence net cAMP levels by altering the activity of phosphodiesterase.[57] Administration of supplemental calcium in vivo (insufficient by itself to produce hypercalcemia) evokes greater PTH-induced hypercalcemia in animals than does the administration of the hormone without supplemental calcium,[51] but there is no evidence that calcium per se will enhance bone resorption independent of PTH, as does the cyclic nucleotide. Conceivably then, the divalent cation may play only a modulating role in the action of PTH in bone via cAMP.

With respect to kidney, calcium infusion in vivo affects PO_4 clearance,[58] thereby in a sense mimicking the effect of PTH in the kidney. Studies with kidney tubules and isolated kidney cells in

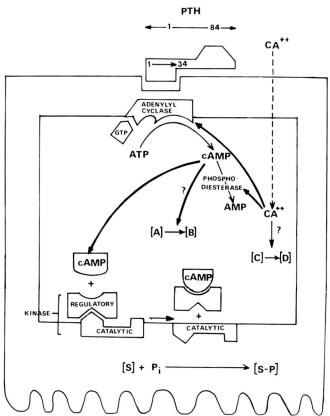

Fig. 47-2. Hypothetical scheme of parathyroid hormone (PTH) action on its target cell (renal cell). The active NH₂-terminal portion of the PTH molecule binds to the specific membrane receptor and stimulates adenylyl cyclase (whose activity can be influenced by nucleotide, e.g., GTP, interaction), resulting in cAMP accumulation. Concomitantly, calcium (Ca⁺⁺) influx is enhanced by the hormone. Cyclic AMP may activate a kinase (presumably on the luminal surface of the renal cell) to phosphorylate a protein [S] participating in solute transport. Other intracellular reactions ([A] → [B]) may be mediated as well. The cytosol calcium levels may, in turn, influence net cAMP concentrations by effects on the activity of the cyclase and the esterase and may perhaps independently alter intracellular enzyme sequences ([C] → [D]) involved in hormonal action.

vitro have also shown that PTH independently activates adenylyl cyclase and stimulates calcium influx into cells.[59–61]

Consequently, the initial hormone/target-cell interaction may evoke several responses. The primary one is apparently cAMP generation, but other responses are possibly independent and important in the modulation of events leading to the ultimate actions of the hormone in the target tissue. Whether the responses evoked by the membrane/hormone interaction in target cells are mediated by several specific receptors, each perhaps binding different sequential and/or conformational regions of the PTH molecule, or whether a simultaneous widespread membrane pertubation occurs consequent to hormone/membrane interaction is a subject for future investigation.

INFLUENCE OF VITAMIN D ON PTH ACTION

Several studies have demonstrated that the overall effects of PTH on bone and, to some extent, on kidney, are impaired in vitamin-D-deficient animals.[62–66] Thus PTH-induced calcium mobilization from bone may be severely reduced or absent,[62–64] and PTH-induced renal phosphaturia may be depressed.[65] The molecular basis of the interaction of vitamin D with PTH is unknown.

Inasmuch as protein synthesis may be stimulated during the course of action of the vitamin, it is conceivable that the influence of vitamin D on PTH is via the regulation of the concentration or structure of a vital protein(s) located somewhere in the sequence of action of the hormone from surface membrane receptor to final solute transport protein. Alternatively, the sterol or more likely one of its metabolites could be a cofactor directly involved in the sequence of reactions mediated by PTH. Several studies examined the characteristics of the PTH-sensitive adenylyl cyclase system in vivo and in vitro in bone and kidney. In both tissues it was demonstrated that PTH-stimulated cAMP generation in vitamin D-deficient animals is present. Quantitative dose/response relationships have not been reported in bone, whereas activation of adenylyl cyclase by PTH is apparently quantitatively reduced[69] in kidney, although still present. The pathway by which the quantitative reduction of cyclic nucleotide generation occurs and the significance of the reduction remain to be elucidated.

An alternative mechanism of influence of the sterol on the peptide hormone might be via its action on the gut, by which it provides adequate levels of calcium either as a mediator in the cellular action of PTH or as a substrate for the bone-mineral resorbing activity enhanced by PTH.

Irrespective of the precise biochemical nature of the interaction, it appears certain that as the biochemical mode of action of the peptide hormone is disclosed, the role of the sterol hormone will be found to be intimately intertwined.

REFERENCES

1. Cohn, D. V., MacGregor, R. R., Chu, L. L. H., et al. Studies on the Biosynthesis in Vitro of Parathyroid Hormone and Other Calcemic Polypeptides of the Parathyroid Gland, in *Calcium, Parathyroid Hormone and the Calcitonins,* edited by R. V. Talmage and P. L. Munson. Proceedings of the Fourth Parathyroid Conference. Excerpta Medica, Amsterdam, 1972, pp. 173–182.
2. Kemper, B., Habener, J. F., Potts, J. T., Jr., et al. Proparathyroid Hormone: Identification of a Biosynthetic Precursor to Parathyroid Hormone. Proc. Natl. Acad. Sci. USA 59: 643, 1972.
3. Hamilton, J. W., Niall, H. D., Jacobs, J. W., et al. The N-Terminal Amino-Acid Sequence of Bovine Proparathyroid Hormone. Proc. Natl. Acad. Sci. USA 71: 653, 1974.
4. Kemper, B., Habener, J. F., Mulligan, R. C., et al. Preproparathyroid Hormone: A Direct Translation Product of Parathyroid Messenger RNA. Proc. Natl. Acad. Sci. USA 71: 3731, 1974.
5. Peytremann, A., Goltzman, D., Callahan, E. N., et al. Metabolism and Biological Activity of Proparathyroid Hormone and Synthetic Analogues in Renal Cortical Membranes. Endocrinology 97: 1270, 1975.
6. Goltzman, D., Callahan, E. N., Tregear, G. W., et al. Conversion of Proparathyroid Hormone to Parathyroid Hormone: Studies in Vitro with Trypsin. Biochemistry 15: 5076, 1976.
7. Potts, J. T., Jr., Tregear, G. W., Keutmann, H. T., et al. Synthesis of a Biologically Active N-Terminal Tetratriacontapeptide of Parathyroid Hormone. Proc. Natl. Acad. Sci. USA 68: 63, 1971.
8. Tregear, G. W., van Rietschoten, J., Greene, E., et al. Bovine Parathyroid Hormone: Minimum Chain Length of Synthetic Peptide Required for Biological Activity. Endocrinology 93: 1349, 1973.
9. Berson, S. A., and Yalow, R. S. Immunochemical Heterogeneity of Parathyroid Hormone in Plasma. J. Clin. Endocrinol. Metab. 28: 1037, 1968.
10. Habener, J. F., Powell, D., Murray, T. M., et al. Parathyroid Hormone: Secretion and Metabolism in Vivo. Proc. Natl. Acad. Sci. USA: 68: 2986, 1971.
11. Canterbury, J. M., and Reiss, E. Multiple Immunoreactive Molecular Forms of Parathyroid Hormone in Human Serum. Proc. Soc. Exp. Biol. Med. 140: 1393, 1972.
12. Silverman, R., and Yalow, R. S. Heterogeneity of Parathyroid Hormone: Clinical and Physiologic Implications. J. Clin. Invest. 52: 1958, 1973.

13. Arnaud, C. D., Goldsmith, R. S., Bordier, P. G., et al. Influence of Immunoheterogeneity of Circulating Parathyroid Hormone on Results of Radioimmunoassays of Serum in Man. Am. J. Med. *56:* 785, 1974.

14. Canterbury, J. M., Levey, G. S., and Reiss, E. Activation of Renal Cortical Adenylate Cyclase by Circulating Immunoreactive Parathyroid Hormone Fragments. J. Clin. Invest. *52:* 524, 1973.

15. Segre, G. V., Niall, H. D., Habener, J. F., et al. Metabolism of Parathyroid Hormone: Physiologic and Clinical Significance. Am. J. Med. *56:* 774, 1974.

16. Goltzman, D., Peytremann, A., Callahan, E. N., et al. Metabolism and Biological Activity of Parathyroid Hormone in Renal Cortical Membranes. J. Clin. Invest. *57:* 8, 1976.

17. Sutcliffe, H. S., Martin, T. J., Eisman, J. A., et al. Binding of Parathyroid Hormone to Bovine Kidney-Cortex Plasma Membranes. Biochem. J. *134:* 913, 1973.

18. Di Bella, F. P., Dousa, T. P., Miller, S., et al. Parathyroid Hormone Receptors of Renal Cortex: Specific Binding of Biologically Active, ^{125}I-labeled Hormone and Relationship to Adenylate Cyclase Activation. Proc. Natl. Acad. Sci. USA *71:* 723, 1974.

19. Chase, L. Selective Proteolysis of the Receptor for Parathyroid Hormone in Renal Cortex. Endocrinology *96:* 70, 1975.

20. Rosenblatt, M., Goltzman, D., Keutmann, H. T., Tregear, G. W., and Potts, J. T., Jr. Chemical and Biological Properties of Synthetic, Sulfur-free Analogues of Parathyroid Hormone. J. Biol. Chem. *251:* 159, 1976.

21. Goltzman, D., Peytremann, A., Callahan, E. N., et al. Analysis of the Requirements for Parathyroid Hormone Action in Renal Membranes with the Use of Inhibiting Analogues. J. Biol. Chem. *250:* 3199, 1975.

22. Chase, L. R., and Aurbach, G. D. Parathyroid Function and the Renal Excretion of 3′5′-Adenylic Acid. Proc. Natl. Acad. Sci. USA *58:* 518, 1967.

23. Aurbach, G. D., and Chase, L. R. Cyclic 3′5′-Adenylic Acid in Bone and the Mechanism of Action of Parathyroid Hormone. Fed. Proc. *29:* 1179, 1970.

24. Sutherland, E. W. Studies on the Mechanism of Hormone Action. Science *177:* 401, 1972.

25. Kaminsky, N. I., Broadus, A. E., Hardman, J. G., et al. Effects of Parathyroid Hormone on Plasma and Urinary Adenosine 3′5′-Monophosphate in Man. J. Clin. Invest. *49:* 2387, 1970.

26. Peck, W. A., Carpenter, J., Messinger, K., et al. Cyclic 3′5′Adenosine Monophosphate in Isolated Bone Cells: Response to Low Concentrations of Parathyroid Hormone. Endocrinology *92:* 692, 1973.

27. Melson, G. L., Chase, L. R., and Aurbach, G. D. Parathyroid Hormone-Sensitive Adenyl Cyclase in Isolated Renal Tubules. Endocrinology *86:* 511, 1970.

28. Marcus, R., and Aurbach, G. D. Bioassay of Parathyroid Hormone *in Vitro* with a Stable Preparation of Adenyl Cyclase from Rat Kidney. Endocrinology *85:* 801, 1969.

29. Chase, L., Fedak, S. A., and Aurbach, G. D. Activation of Skeletal Adenyl Cyclase by Parathyroid Hormone in Vitro. Endocrinology *84:* 761, 1969.

30. Marx, S. J., Fedak, S. A., and Aurbach, G. D. Preparation and Characterization of a Hormone-responsive Renal Plasma Membrane Fraction. J. Biol. Chem. *247:* 6913, 1972.

31. Wells, H., and Lloyd, W. Hypercalcemic and Hypophosphatemic Effects of Dibutyryl Cyclic AMP in Rats after Parathyroidectomy. Endocrinology *84:* 861, 1969.

32. Rasmussen, H., Pechet, M., and Fast, D. Effect of Dibutyryl Cyclic Adenosine 3′5′-Monophosphate, Theophylline, and Other Nucleotides upon Calcium and Phosphate Metabolism. J. Clin. Invest. *47:* 1843, 1968.

33. Murad, F., and Pak, C. Y. C. Urinary Excretion of Adenosine 3′5′-Monophosphate and Guanosine 3′5′-Monophosphate. N. Engl. J. Med. *286:* 1382, 1972.

34. Shaw, J. W., Oldham, S. B., Rosoff, L., et al. Urinary Cyclic AMP Analyzed as a Function of the Serum Calcium and Parathyroid Hormone in the Differential Diagnosis of Hypercalcemia. J. Clin. Invest. *59:* 14, 1977.

35. Chase, L. R., and Aurbach, G. D. Renal Adenyl Cyclase: Anatomically Separate Sites for Parathyroid Hormone and Vasopressin. Science *159:* 547, 1968.

36. Chabardès, D., Imbert, M., Clique, A., et al. PTH Sensitive Adenyl Cyclase Activity in Different Segments of the Rabbit Nephron. Pflugers Arch. *354:* 229, 1975.

37. Agus, Z. S., Gardner, L. B., Beck, L. H., et al. Effects of Parathyroid Hormone on Renal Tubular Reabsorption of Calcium, Sodium, and Phosphate. Amer. J. Physiol. *224:* 1143, 1973.

38. Windrow, S. H., and Levinsky, N. G. The Effect of Parathyroid Extract on Renal Tubular Calcium Reabsorption in the Dog. J. Clin. Invest. *41:* 2151, 1962.

39. Parsons, J. A., Rafferty, B., Gray, D., et al. Pharmacology of Parathyroid Hormone and Some of Its Fragments and Analogues, in *Calcium-Regulating Hormones,* edited by R. V. Talmage, M. Owen, and J. A. Parsons. Excerpta Medica, Amsterdam, 1975, pp. 33–39.

40. Goltzman, D., Callahan, E. N., Tregear, G. W., et al. Studies of Bioactive Analogs of Parathyroid Hormone, in *Peptides: Chemistry, Structure and Biology,* edited by R. Walter and J. Meienhofer. Ann Arbor Science, Ann Arbor, 1975, pp. 571–577.

41. Rodbell, M., Birnbaumer, L., Pohl, S. L., et al. The Glucagon-sensitive Adenyl Cyclase System in Plasma Membranes of Rat Liver. V. An Obligatory Role of Guanyl Nucleotides in Glucagon Action. J. Biol. Chem. *246:* 1877, 1971.

42. Londos, C., Salomon, Y., Lin, M. C., et al. 5′-Guanylylimidodiphosphate, a Potent Activator of Adenylate Cyclase Systems in Eukaryotic Cells. Proc. Nat. Acad. Sci. USA *71:* 3087, 1974.

43. Goltzman, D., Callahan, E. N., Tregear, G. W., et al. Role of 5′-Guanylylimidodiphosphate in the Activation of Adenylyl Cyclase by Parathyroid Hormone. Endo. Res. Commun. *3:* 407, 1976.

44. Kinne, R., Shlatz, L. J., Kinne-Saffran, E., et al. Distribution of Membrane Bound Cyclic AMP-dependent Protein Kinase in Plasma Membranes of Cells of the Kidney Cortex. J. Membrane Biol. *24:* 145, 1975.

45. Garabedian, M., Holick, M. F., DeLuca, H. F., et al. Control of 25-Hydroxycholecalciferol Metabolism by Parathyroid Glands. Proc. Natl. Acad. Sci. USA *69:* 1673, 1972.

46. Talmage, R. V. A Study of the Effect of Parathyroid Hormone on Bone Remodelling and on Calcium Homeostasis. Clin. Orthop. Relat. Res. *54:* 163, 1967.

47. Bélanger, L. F. Osteolysis: An Outlook on Its Mechanism and Causation, in *Parathyroid Glands: Ultrastructure, Secretion, and Function,* edited by P. J. Gaillard, R. V. Talmage, and A. M. Budy. University of Chicago Press, Chicago, 1965. p. 137–143.

48. Rasmussen, H. Ionic and Hormonal Control of Calcium Homeostasis. Am. J. Med. *50:* 567, 1971.

49. Whitfield, J. F., MacManns, J. P., and Rixon, R. H. The Possible Mediation by Cyclic AMP of Parathyroid Hormone-induced Stimulation of Mitotic Activity and Deoxyribonucleic Acid Synthesis in Rat Thymic Lymphocytes. J. Cell. Physiol. *75:* 213, 1970.

50. Rasmussen, H. Cell Communication, Calcium Ion and Cyclic Adenosine Monophosphate. Science *170:* 404, 1970.

51. Parsons, J. A., and Potts, J. T., Jr. Physiology and Chemistry of Parathyroid Hormone, in *Calcium Metabolism and Bone Disease, Clinics in Endocrinology and Metabolism,* edited by I. MacIntyre. London and Philadelphia, W. B. Saunders, Philadelphia, 1972, vol. I, p. 33–78.

52. Berridge, M. The Interaction of Cyclic Nucleotides and Calcium in the Control of Cellular Activity, P. Greengard and G. A. Robinson (eds.). Adv. Cyclic Nucleotide Res. *6:* 1, 1975.

53. Dziak, R., and Stern, P. H. Calcium Transport in Isolated Bone Cells III. Effects of Parathyroid Hormone and Cyclic 3′5′-AMP. Endocrinology *97:* 1281, 1975.

54. Copp, D. H., and Cameron, E. C. Demonstration of a Hypocalcemic Factor (Calcitonin) in Commercial Parathyroid Extract. Science *134:* 2038, 1961.

55. Parsons, J. A., Neer, R. M., Potts, J. T., Jr. Initial Fall of Plasma Calcium after Intravenous Injection of Parathyroid Hormone. Endocrinology *89:* 735, 1971.

56. Streeto, J. M. Renal Cortical Adenyl Cyclase: Effect of Parathyroid Hormone and Calcium Metabolism *18:* 968, 1969.

57. Weiss, B. Differential Activation Inhibition of the Multiple Forms of Cyclic Nucleotide Phosphodiesterase, G. I. Drummond, P. Greengard, and G. A. Robinson (eds.). Adv. Cyclic Nucleotide Res. *5:* 195, 1975.

58. Eisenberg, E. Effects of Serum Calcium Level and Parathyroid Extracts on Phosphate and Calcium Excretion in Hypoparathyroid Patients. J. Clin. Invest. *44:* 942, 1965.

59. Borle, A. B. Effects of Purified Parathyroid Hormone on the Calcium Metabolism of Monkey Kidney Cells. Endocrinology *83:* 1316, 1968.

60. Borle, A. B. Calcium Metabolism at the Cellular Level. Fed. Proc. *32:* 1944, 1973.

61. Borle, A. B. Regulation of the Mitochondrial Control of Cellular Calcium Homeostasis and Calcium Transport by Phosphate, Parathyroid Hormone, Calcitonin, Vitamin D and Cyclic AMP, in *Calcium-Regulating Hormones,* edited by R. V. Talmage, M. Owen, and J. A. Parsons. Excerpta Medica, Amsterdam, 1975, pp. 217–228.

62. Harrison, H. C., Harrison, H. E., and Park, E. A. Vitamin D and Citrate Metabolism: Effect of Vitamin D in Rats Fed Diets Adequate in Both Calcium and Phosphorus. Am. J. Physiol. *192:* 432, 1958.

63. Morii, H., and DeLuca, H. F. Relationship Between Vitamin D Deficiency, Thyrocalcitonin and Parathyroid Hormone. Am. J. Physiol. *213:* 358, 1967.

64. Au, W. Y. W., and Raisz, L. Restoration of Parathyroid Responsiveness in Vitamin D-Deficient Rats by Parenteral Calcium or Dietary Lactose. J. Clin. Invest. *46:* 1572, 1967.

65. Harrison, H. E., and Harrison, H. C.: The Interaction of Vitamin D and Parathyroid Hormone on Calcium, Phosphorus, and Magnesium Homeostasis in the Rat. Metab. Clin. Exp. *13:* 952, 1964.

66. Rasmussen, H., and Feinblatt, J. The Relationship Between the Actions of Vitamin D, Parathyroid Hormone, and Calcitonin. Calcif. Tiss. Res. *6:* 265, 1971.

67. Tsai, H. C., and Norman, A. W.: Studies on the Mode of Action of Calciferol. VI. Effect of 1,25-Dihydroxy-Vitamin D_3 on RNA Synthesis in the Intestinal Mucosa. Biochem. Biophys. Res. Commun. *54:* 622, 1973.

68. Kakuta, S., Suda, T., Sasaki, S., et al. Effects of Parathyroid Hormone on the Accumulation of Cyclic AMP in Bone of Vitamin D-Deficient Rats. Endocrinology *97:* 1288, 1975.

69. Forte, L., Nichols, G. A., and Anast, C. S.: Renal Adenylate Cyclase and the Interrelationship Between Parathyroid Hormone and Vitamin D in the Regulation of Urinary Phosphate and Adenosine Cyclic 3′5′-Monophosphate Excretion. J. Clin. Invest. *57:* 559, 1976.

48

Calcitonin: Comparative Endocrinology

D. Harold Copp

In common with other homeostatic controls, all vertebrates are able to regulate the concentration of calcium in the body fluids with remarkable precision.[1] In mammals, this depends upon the vast reservoir of calcium in bone, absorption of calcium from the gut, and excretion of calcium from the kidney.[2] These organ systems are modulated by three hormones: calcitonin (CT) from the ultimobranchial C cells in the thyroid and parathyroids; parathyroid hormone (PTH) from the parathyroid glands; and 1,25-dihydroxycholecalciferol (1,25-DHCC), the metabolite of vitamin D_3 produced in the kidney. However, as shown in Table 48-1, marine cyclostomes (lampreys and hagfish) are able to maintain and regulate a level of calcium in plasma that is substantially lower than that in the sea and, in the case of the lamprey, is very similar to that in mammals.[3] This occurs in spite of the fact that cyclostomes do not have the calcium-regulating peptide hormones CT and PTH, nor do they have a calcified skeleton.

According to Romer,[4] primitive vertebrates evolved in freshwater lakes, rivers, and estuaries during the late Ordovician period and developed rapidly through the Silurian and Devonian periods. The fossil records indicate that they had an exoskeleton and often an endoskeleton which had many of the features of mammalian bone, including lamellae, trabeculae, and what appear to be osteocytic lacunae. However, when our vertebrate ancestors migrated into the sea with its high calcium concentration (40 mg/100 ml), the need for such a calcium reservoir had disappeared, and both the cyclostomes and elasmobranchs reverted to a cartilaginous skeleton rather than to mineralized bone. Even the teleosts (bony fishes) in many cases reverted to acellular bone. It may be significant that during this period of high calcium exposure in the sea, the ultimobranchial glands and calcitonin first appeared. Thus, although it was not discovered until 1961,[5] calcitonin is one of the earliest vertebrate hormones.

The next major transition was when the vertebrate moved onto land. It was at this point that the parathyroid glands developed to provide the primary calcium-regulating hormone for air-breathing tetrapods. It may be significant that this migration in-

Table 48-1. Calcium and Phosphate in Serum and in the Environment

Environment and Representative Species	Total Ca, mg/100 ml	Ionic Ca, mmol/liter	Total P, mg/100 ml
Environment			
Pacific Ocean	40.0 ± 0.4	10.0	
Brackish water	8–20		0.001
Lake Huron	3.6 ± 0.4	0.9 ± 0.1	0.01
Marine invertebrate			
Spiny lobster (*Palinurus vulgaris*)	46		0.7
Cyclostomes			
Hagfish (*Eptatretus stoutii*)	21.6 ± 0.4	3.0 ± 0.4	4.5 ± 0.6
Lamprey (*Petromyzon marinus*)	10.40 ± 0.4	1.74 ± 0.2	3.9 ± 0.3
Chimaerid			
Ratfish (*Hydrolagus colliei*)	17.2 ± 1.2		6.6 ± 1.2
Elasmobranchs			
Marine shark (*Carcharhinus leucas*)	18.0 ± 3.6	3.10 ± 0.4	6.0 ± 1.8
Freshwater shark (*Carcharhinus leucas nicaraguensis*)	12.0 ± 0.8	1.7 ± 0.1	4.8 ± 5.1
Teleost			
Marine (*Paralabrax clathratus*)	12.8 ± 3.2	2.0 ± 0.9	6.0 ± 0.6
Freshwater (*Megalops atlantica*)	10.0 ± 0.8	1.8 ± 0.2	3.6 ± 1.2
Mammal			
Man (*Homo sapiens*)	9.3 ± 0.3	1.15	3–4

From Copp.[3] Reprinted through the courtesy of Academic Press.

volved a change from the high-calcium, low-phosphate environment of the sea to a condition in which calcium was generally in low supply and phosphate was plentiful. In spite of the very exciting recent work on the role of the vitamin D metabolites in calcium regulation in birds and mammals,[6] little is known of their role in lower vertebrates, and this promises to be a very exciting field for future investigation.

ULTIMOBRANCHIAL EMBRYOLOGY

The term "ultimobranchialen Körper" was suggested by Greil in 1905[7] because they develop around the most posterior branchial pouch, and this is true in the embryos of higher vertebrates, as shown in Figure 48-1. It is interesting that the parathyroid, aortic, and carotid glands also develop in the vicinity of specific branchial (gill) pouches, since they are also involved in the regulation of the

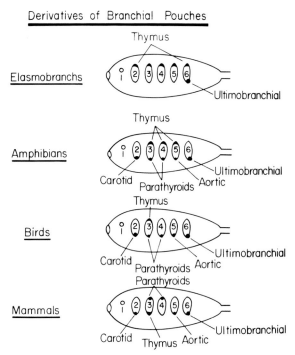

Fig. 48-1. Endocrine glands that develop around the embryonic branchial pouches.

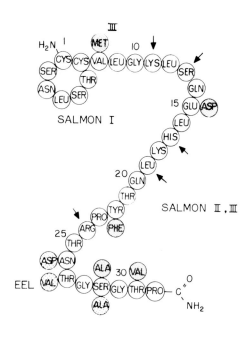

Structure of Fish Calcitonins

Fig. 48-2. Amino acid sequences of salmon and eel calcitonins. (From Copp[10] and after Potts and Aurbach.[11] Reproduced through the courtesy of Excerpta Medica Foundation and the American Physiological Society.)

ionic composition of body fluids. In fish, the gills are of great importance in ion regulation.

In a brilliant series of experiments Le Douarain and Le Lièvre[8] transplanted the neural crest from the embryo of a Japanese quail (10-somite stage) into a corresponding chick embryo and found that the quail cells, which could be distinguished by a chromatin marker, migrated to the region of the posterior branchial pouch to form the ultimobranchial gland. Pearse and Polak[9] confirmed the neural-crest origin of the calcitonin-producing cells of mouse thyroid, using histochemical techniques.

CHEMISTRY

Much is now known of the comparative biochemistry of calcitonin.[10] The amino acid sequences of nine calcitonins have now been determined. These include five mammalian species— porcine, bovine, ovine, human[11] and rat[12]—and four nonmammalian species—salmon I, II, III, and eel.[13] All have a similar structure consisting of a straight-chain peptide of 32 amino acids with a seven-membered disulphide ring at the N-terminal and prolinamide at the C-terminal. Compared to the mammalian calcitonins, the nonmammalian hormones are more stable and have a potency 10 to 50 times greater in the standard hypocalcemic rat bioassay. This may reflect a basic difference in stability and in function. The similar structures of the four fish calcitonins are shown in Figure 48-2, with arrows indicating the amino acids present in all four fish hormones which differ from those present in the mammalian hormones. It is possible that these differences may account for the differences in potency and stability. From the point of view of cross-reactivity in the radioimmunoassay, there appear to be three main hormone groups. First are the nonmammalian hormones, all of which react with our antibodies to the salmon I calcitonin. This group includes Pacific salmon (all species), rainbow trout, cod, tuna, Japanese and American eels, domestic fowl, pigeons, turkey,

and Japanese quail. The next group includes the artiodactyls (sheep, pigs, and cows), and all have a very similar structure and cross-react very well. The antibodies to porcine calcitonin also cross-react with dog calcitonin. In the third group, rat and human calcitonin differ by only two amino acids, at positions 16 and 26.[12] The evolution of calcitonin has been discussed by Potts and Aurbach,[11] Staehelin,[14] and Copp.[10] A possible schema is shown in Figure 48-3. It is suggested that the elasmobranchs may have diverged early from the ancestral hormone, since we found no cross-reactivity between calcitonin from the dogfish shark and antibodies to salmon or porcine hormone. A further split occurs between nonmammals and mammals and between the rat and human and the artiodactyls. It is of interest that human and porcine calcitonin differ by 18 amino acids, while there is only a single amino acid difference between human and porcine insulin.

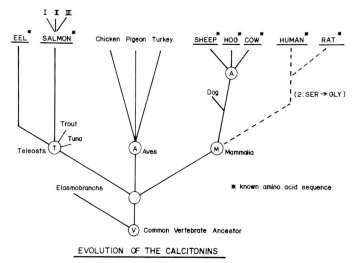

EVOLUTION OF THE CALCITONINS

Fig. 48-3. Schema for the evolution of the calcitonins. (After Copp.[10] Reproduced through the courtesy of Excerpta Medica Foundation.)

FUNCTION

ELASMOBRANCHS (SHARKS AND RAYS)

The elasmobranchs have well-developed ultimobranchial glands from which calcitonin has been isolated. Highly purified hormone prepared from the dogfish (*Squalus acanthus*)[15] has a very potent natriuretic effect in the rat. It is similar to salmon calcitonin but with a lower specific activity. Injection of salmon or porcine calcitonin had no significant effect on the plasma calcium or phosphate of the dogfish.

TELEOSTS (BONY FISH)

In 1954, Rasquin and Rosenbloom[16] reported that the ultimobranchial glands hypertrophied when Mexican cavefish (*Astyanax mexicanus*) were maintained for long periods in total darkness. This was associated with bony changes, and they suggested that the ultimobranchials might be homologues of the parathyroid. It now appears that there are at least two other glands involved in calcium regulation in teleosts—the pituitaries and the corpuscles of Stannius.[1] Purified extracts of the corpuscles contain a peptide hormone that inhibits gill uptake of calcium in the eel and lowers plasma calcium, while Pang et al.[17] observed a profound fall in plasma calcium when hypophysectomized killifish (*Fundulus heteroclitus*) were maintained in a low-calcium environment. Lopez et al.[18] produced hypercalcemia in the European eel (*Anguilla anguilla*) by injecting carp pituitary extracts or by removing the corpuscles of Stannius. In each case, the hypercalcemia led to hypertrophy of the ultimobranchials.

In most laboratories, including our own, injection of calcitonin has failed to produce any significant change in plasma calcium in fish. This is not too surprising, since the marked hypocalcemic effect of the hormone in young mammals is due to inhibition of bone resorption, which is minimal in fish. However, there is some evidence that it may reduce calcium loss during low-calcium stress, as it does in other vertebrates. Lopez et al.[19] maintained young 20–30-g rainbow trout (*Salmo gairdnerii*) in calcium-free water for 3 weeks and injected 50 mU of porcine calcitonin every 2 days into the treated fish. In the untreated controls, there was a significant reduction in plasma calcium and bone mineral density which was prevented by the administration of the hormone, suggesting that it may function to protect the skeleton from mineral loss during calcium deprivation.

LUNGFISH

Lungfish represent an interesting bridge between teleosts and amphibians. They possess an ultimobranchial gland, but the parathyroids have not yet been demonstrated. Pang and Sawyer[20] found that injection of salmon calcitonin (1 MRC U) or 5 U bovine PTH into the South American lungfish (*Lepidosiren paradoxa*) had no significant effect on plasma calcium. However, the salmon calcitonin elicited a marked diuresis (sixfold), while bovine PTH (including the synthetic 1–34 sequence) had an antidiuretic effect.

AMPHIBIANS

Much of the work in this field has been done by Robertson. He observed hypercalcemia and increased ultimobranchial activity in both frog and tadpoles (*Rana catesbeiana*) maintained for 3 to 6 weeks in a high-calcium environment of 50 mEq/liter.[21] He was also able to produce reversible hypertrophy in the ultimobranchial glands in adult green frogs (*Rana pipiens*) by maintaining them for 2 weeks in a high-calcium water (0.8 percent $CaCl_2$) with weekly injections of 100,000 U of vitamin D_2.[22] This resulted in a 50 percent increase in the concentration of plasma calcium. Removal of the ultimobranchial glands in adult *R. pipiens* resulted in an elevation of plasma calcium and a depletion of the calcium stores in the paravertebral lime sacs.[23] Histological examination of the bones revealed a shift from osteoblastic to osteoclast and chondroclast activity.

REPTILES

Calcitonin has been extracted from the ultimobranchial glands of a number of reptiles, but there is no clear-cut evidence of its function in these animals, and injection of the hormone does not cause hypocalcemia.[24] However, Bélanger and co-workers[25] have shown that the chronic administration of salmon calcitonin to growing turtles fed a low-calcium diet did result in better growth and higher calcium levels and substantially denser bone.

BIRDS

In the developing chick embryo, activity in the ultimobranchial gland appears after 11 days of incubation and corresponds to the beginning of calcification in the skeleton.[26] Highest levels of calcitonin occurred at the pipping stage just prior to hatching[27] and fell shortly thereafter. In chickens fed a high-calcium diet, the ultimobranchial glands hypertrophy, and there is depletion of the secretory apparatus along with ultrastructural evidence of increased secretory activity.[28] However, most investigators have been unable to demonstrate any significant fall in plasma calcium after injection of the hormone. Ultimobranchialectomized hens have been carried through several months of egg laying without serious effects, although they do tend to eat less and lay smaller and thinner-shelled eggs.[29] Bélanger and Copp[30] studied the effect of chronic administration of salmon calcitonin into growing chicks and found that after 4 months, the cortical bone in the mid-diaphyseal region of the tibia was much denser than the controls and there was little or no evidence of bone resorption.

MAMMALS

Much of the work concerning calcitonin function has been carried out in mammals. Hypercalcemia is clearly associated with stimulation of the calcitonin-producing C cells of the thyroid, with an increase in secretion of calcitonin that is proportionally related to the rise of plasma calcium. The hormone has a rapid inhibitory effect on osteolysis and on release of calcium from the skeleton both in tissue culture[31] and in vivo. In young mammals, this results in a rapid fall in plasma calcium and phosphate, but in adults in which skeletal turnover is slow, this hypocalcemic effect is minimal.[32]

The following have been proposed as possible functions of calcitonin in mammals.[33]

1. Control of hypercalcemia, particularly in young mammals.
2. Protection of the skeleton from loss of calcium during periods of calcium stress such as pregnancy and lactation[34] and prolonged calcium deprivation.[35]
3. Control of hypercalcemia following ingestion of a high-calcium meal. Gray and Munson[36] showed that significant hypercalcemia occurred under these circumstances if the thyroids had been removed from rats, but no significant changes in the calcium level occurred in intact rats. Calcitonin levels in plasma were elevated under these circumstances, and it has been suggested that this may have

been mediated by secretion of gastrin, which is a potent calcitonin secretagogue.

SUMMARY

Although calcitonin appeared early in vertebrate evolution, understanding of its function is still limited. In fish, frogs, and birds the ultimobranchial glands respond to hypercalcemia by hypertrophy and increased secretory activity, as do the C cells of the mammalian thyroid. With few exceptions, injection of the hormone failed to produce any significant fall in plasma calcium, but this was also true in adult mammals. However, chronic administration of calcitonin in trout, turtles, chickens, and cats reduced osteolytic activity and loss of calcium from bone and counteracted some of the effects of a low-calcium diet. Thus, it appears that the hormone has effects on calcium metabolism in lower vertebrates similar to those in mammals. There is also some indication that it may be involved in osmotic regulation in fish.

REFERENCES

1. Copp, D. H. Evolution of Calcium Regulation in Vertebrates. Clinics Endocrinol. Metabol. *1:* 21, 1972.

2. Copp, D. H. Endocrine Control of Calcium Homeostasis. J. Endocrinol. *43:* 137, 1969.

3. Copp, D. H. The Ultimobranchial Glands and Calcium Regulation, in *Fish Physiology,* edited by W. S. Hoar and D. J. Randall. Academic Press, New York, 1969, vol II, pp. 377–398.

4. Romer, A. S. Bone in Early Vertebrates, in *Bone Biodynamics,* edited by H. M. Frost. Little, Brown, Boston, 1964, pp. 13–17.

5. Copp, D. H., Cameron, E. C., Cheney, B. A., et al. Evidence for Calcitonin—a New Hormone from the Parathyroid That Lowers Blood Calcium. Endocrinology 70: 638, 1972.

6. DeLuca, H. F. Vitamin D: the Vitamin and the Hormone. Fed. Proc. *33:* 2211, 1974.

7. Greil, A. Über die Anlage der Lungen sowie der ultimobranchialen (postbranchialen, suprapericordialen) Körper bei anuren Amphibien. Arb. Anat. Inst. (Wiesbaden) 29: 447, 1905.

8. Le Douarain, H., and Le Lièvre, C. Demonstration de l'Origine Neurales des Cellules à Calcitonine du Corps Ultimobranchial chez l'Embryon de Poulet. Compt. Rend. 270: 2857, 1970.

9. Pearse, A. G. E., and Polack, J. M. Cytochemical Evidence for the Neural Crest Origin of Mammalian Ultimobranchial C cells. Histochemie 27: 96, 1971.

10. Copp, D. H. Endocrine Regulation of Calcium Metabolism. Ann. Rev. Physiol. 32: 61, 1970.

11. Potts, J. T., and Aurbach, G. D. Chemistry of the Calcitonins, in *Handbook of Physiology,* Section 7, *Endocrinology,* vol. 7 *Parathyroid Gland,* edited by G. D. Aurbach. American Physiological Society, Washington, 1976, pp. 423–430.

12. Raulais, D., Hagaman, J., Onties, D. A., et al. The Complete Amino-Acid Sequence of Rat Thyrocalcitonin. Eur. J. Biochem. 64: 607,- 1976.

13. Otani, M., Noda, T., Yamauchi, H., et al. Isolation, Chemical Structure and Biological Properties of Ultimobranchial Calcitonin of the Eel, in *Calcium-Regulating Hormones,* edited by R. V. Talmage, M. Owen, and J. A. Parsons. Excerpta Medica, Amsterdam, 1975, pp. 111–115.

14. Staehelin, M. The Calcitonin: An Example of Unusual Evolution. J. Mol. Evolution *1:* 258, 1972.

15. MacIntyre, I., Byfield, P. G. H., Galante, L., et al. Studies of the Effects of Human Synthetic Calcitonin in Experimental Animals and Man, in *Endocrinology 1971,* edited by S. Taylor. Heinemann, London, 1972, pp. 21–26.

16. Rasquin, P., and Rosenbloom, L. Endocrine Imbalance and Tissue Hyperplasia in Teleosts Maintained in Darkness. Bull. Am. Museum Nat. Hist. *104:* 363, 1954.

17. Pang, P. K. T., Griffith, R. W., and Pickford, G. E. Hypocalcemia and Tetanic Seizures in Hypophysectomized Killifish *Fundulus heteroclitus.* Proc. Soc. Exp. Biol. Med. 136: 85, 1970.

18. Lopez, E., Deville, J., and Bagot, E. Etude Histophysiologique d'un Téléostéen "*Anguilla anguilla L.*" au cours d'Hypercalcémie Experimentale. Compt. Rend. (D) *267:* 1531, 1968.

19. Lopez, E., Chartier-Baraduc, M. M., and Deville, J. Mise en Évidence de l'Action de la Calcitonine Porcine sur l'Os de la Truite *Salmo gairdnerii* Soumise à un Traitement Déminéralisant. Compt. Rend. (D) *272:* 2600, 1971.

20. Pang, P. K. T., and Sawyer, W. H. Parathyroid Hormone, Salmon Calcitonin, and Urine Flow in the South American Lungfish, *Lepidosiren paradoxa.* J. Exp. Zool. *193:* 407, 1975.

21. Robertson, D. R. Cytological and Physiological Activity of the Ultimobranchial Glands in the Premetamorphic Anuran *Rana Catesbeiana.* Gen. Comp. Endocrinol. *16:* 329, 1971.

22. Robertson, D. R. The Ultimobranchial Gland in *Rana pipiens.* IV. Hypercalcemia and Glandular Hypertrophy. Z. Zellforsch. *85:* 453, 1968.

23. Robertson, D. R. The Ultimobranchial Body of *Rana pipiens.* VIII. Effects of Extirpation Upon Calcium Distribution and Bone Cell Types. Gen. Comp. Endocrinol. *12:* 479, 1969.

24. Clark, N. B. Calcium Regulation in Reptiles. Gen. Comp. Endocrinol. Suppl. 3, 430–440, 1972.

25. Bélanger, L. F., Dimond, M. T., and Copp, D. H. Histological Observations on Bone and Cartilage of Growing Turtles Treated with Calcitonin. Gen. Comp. Endocrinol. *20:* 297, 1973.

26. Stoeckel, M. E., and Porte, A. Etude Ultrastructural des Corps Ultimobranchiaux du Poulet. I. Aspect Normal et Développement Embryonaire. Z. Zellforsch. *94:* 495, 1969.

27. Baimbridge, K. G., and Taylor, T. L. Effects of Salmon Calcitonin in Chick Embryos. J. Endocr. *68:* 17P, 1976.

28. Bélanger, L. F. The Ultimobranchial Gland of Birds and the Effects of Nutritional Variations. J. Exp. Zool. *178:* 125, 1971.

29. Speers, G. M., Perey, D. Y. E., and Brown, D. M. Effect of Ultimobranchialectomy in the Laying Hen. Endocrinol. *87:* 1291, 1970.

30. Bélanger, L. F., and Copp, D. H. The Skeletal Effects of Prolonged Calcitonin Administration in Birds, Under Various Conditions, in *Calcium, Parathyroid Hormone and the Calcitonins,* edited by R. V. Talmage and P. L. Munson. Excerpta Medica, Amsterdam, 1972, pp. 41–50.

31. Minkin, C., Reynolds, J. J., and Copp, D. H. Inhibitory Effect of Salmon and Other Calcitonins on Calcium Release from Mouse Bone in Vitro. Can. J. Physiol. Pharmac. *49:* 263, 1971.

32. Copp, D. H., and Kuczerpa, A. V. A New Bioassay for Calcitonin and the Effect of Age and Dietary Ca on the Response, in *Calcitonin. Proc. Sympos. Thyrocalcitonin and the C Cells,* edited by S. Taylor. Heinemann, London, 1968, pp. 18–24.

33. Munson, P. L. Physiology and Pharmacology of Thyrocalcitonin, *Handbook of Physiology,* Section 7, *Endocrinology,* vol. 7, *Parathyroid Gland,* edited by G. D. Aurbach. American Physiological Society, Washington, 1976, pp. 443–464.

34. Taylor, T. G., Lewis, P. E., and Balderstone, O. Role of Calcitonin in Protecting the Skeleton During Pregnancy and Lactation. J. Endocr. *66:* 297, 1975.

35. Jowsey, J. Effect of Long-term Administration of Porcine Calcitonin in the Development of Dietary Osteoporosis in Cats. Endocrinology *85:* 1196, 1969.

36. Gray, T. K., and Munson, P. L. Thyrocalcitonin: Evidence for a Physiological Function. Science *166:* 512, 1969.

49

Secretion and Metabolism of Calcitonin in Man

Allan Pont

Calcitonin is a 32-amino-acid polypeptide synthesized and secreted by cells located in the adult in glands derived embryologically from the last two pharyngeal pouches of the primitive foregut.[1] These cells are referred to as parafollicular, C cells, light cells, or argyrophilic cells. In lower species, C cells are the major constituents of a distinct organ, the ultimobranchial body, while in mammals they are distributed throughout the thyroid. As discussed in Chapter 64, present evidence indicates that C cells are actually of neural-crest origin and that they migrate widely during embryogenesis.

Immunofluorescent studies have demonstrated that C cells are concentrated in the central portions of the lateral lobes of the thyroid at the junction of upper and middle one third of the lobes.[2] In 1966, Williams noted that a tumor, medullary carcinoma of the thyroid gland, was composed chiefly of C cells and suggested that the tumor might secrete calcitonin.[3] This was confirmed by a number of investigators in 1968[4,4a,4b] Recently, several authors have reported elevated calcitonin blood levels in patients with a variety of nonthyroid tumors,[5-7] and Ellison and co-workers have demonstrated calcitonin secretion by human lung carcinoma in culture.[8] Therefore, the usual source of calcitonin secretion (thyroid C cells) and the production of calcitonin in a variety of pathological conditions are established, but there is still much to learn about the control of secretion in both physiological and pathological states.

A major barrier to the understanding of calcitonin secretion in man has been the problem of measuring the hormone at circulating concentrations. Biological assays, based on the hypocalcemic effect of the hormone in rats, are relatively insensitive and cannot be used to detect calcitonin at physiological levels.[9] Bioassays occasionally demonstrate elevated calcitonin in patients with medullary carcinoma of the thyroid.[49] A radioimmunoassay for porcine calcitonin was developed in 1968.[10] Although useful in studying porcine (as well as ovine and bovine) calcitonin secretion, the porcine assay did not detect the human hormone. Subsequently, several workers developed antisera specifically directed against human calcitonin.[4,11] Although lower levels of human calcitonin could be measured with the radioimmunoassay than with the bioassay, the hormone could not be detected in normal subjects.

Since no clear physiological function of calcitonin in humans had been demonstrated, it was hypothesized that calcitonin may not circulate under physiological circumstances. However, the assays did permit extensive study of control of calcitonin secretion in patients with medullary carcinoma of the thyroid. Subsequent improvements in the radioimmunoassay have permitted detection of circulating calcitonin in normals.[50,51] Parthemore and Deftos used immunoextraction and concentration to show that calcitonin normally circulates at levels of 5–100 pg/ml.[12] Most workers would now agree that human calcitonin does indeed circulate basically in that concentration range. However, the assay improvements needed to achieve that degree of detection sensitivity are very recent. Subsequently, most of our knowledge about control of secretion of calcitonin is derived from study of patients with medullary carcinoma of the thyroid and from in vivo and in vitro animal data.

REGULATION OF CALCITONIN SECRETION

As suggested above, there is still uncertainty about control of calcitonin secretion under physiological circumstances. There is only minimal evidence that calcitonin can inhibit its own secretion. Evidence for a trophic hormone with primary function being calcitonin regulation analogous to hypothalamic/pituitary/peripheral endocrine organ system has not been presented. It is generally agreed that TSH, the normal regulator of thyroid secretion, has no significant effect on calcitonin secretion.[48] The main candidates for regulators of calcitonin secretion include calcium and gastrointestinal hormones.

EFFECT OF CALCIUM

In 1962, Copp discovered calcitonin by perfusing hypercalcemic plasma through the thyroid/parathyroid complex of a dog and noting that this resulted in a small but significant fall in peripheral calcium concentration greater than that based on suppression of parathyroid hormone secretion, thus suggesting a hypocalcemic hormone liberated in response to hypercalcemia.[13] Hirsh et al. demonstrated that calcitonin was derived from the thyroid.[14] It is well established that acute hypercalcemia, such as occurs with calcium infusion, results in increase in peripheral calcium levels in certain situations. In patients with medullary carcinoma of the thyroid, calcium infusion causes a dramatic rise in calcitonin, often from undetectable to levels greater than 1 ng/ml[15] (see Fig. 49-1). In hypocalcemic states, such as pseudohypoparathyroidism, Deftos and co-workers showed that calcium infusion caused a significant rise in calcitonin, suggesting that the

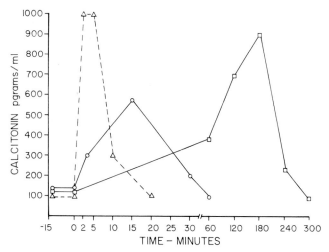

Fig. 49-1. Schematic illustrating typical calcitonin responses to secreta-gogues in patients with early medullary carcinoma of the thyroid gland. Δ = pentagastrin, 0.5 μg/kg IV at time 0; ○ = alcohol, 2 ounces PO at time 0; □ = calcium, 5 mg/kg/hr for 3 hours.

hypocalcemia had resulted in increased stores of calcitonin which were released upon calcium infusion.[16] This represented the first data concerning calcitonin production from other than medullary carcinoma. That hypocalcemia could result in decreased calcitonin secretion was shown by using EDTA to lower serum calcium in patients with medullary carcinoma of the thyroid.[11] Thus, it seemed that calcitonin secretion would rise with increased calcium and fall with decreased calcium and that gland content in normal thyroids rose with chronic hypocalcemia.[16] However, this only applied to pharmacological alterations in serum calcium and only in patients with calcitonin-secreting tumors or long-standing hypo-calcemia. To demonstrate that alterations in serum calcium could affect normal patients, Parthemore and Deftos used immunoex-traction combined with radioimmunoassay to show that calcium infusions caused a change in calcitonin levels in normal patients from 12 ± 3 pg/ml to 113.8 ± 21 pg/ml. However, the calcium infusions resulted in very large changes in peripheral calcium concentrations. It has yet to be demonstrated that daily, physiolog-ical fluctuations in serum calcium concentration, such as might result from food intake or overnight fasting, would result in signifi-cant alteration in calcitonin secretion in humans. Cooper and co-workers did show in animals that minor changes in serum calcium would result in increased calcitonin secretion.[17]

Studies on calcitonin secretion in vitro have yielded some interesting albeit contradictory results. Bell and Queener in 1970 showed that calcium enhanced calcitonin secretion by porcine thyroid slices.[18] However, Selawry and Becker could not demon-strate a significant effect of calcium alone in human thyroid slices, although they did show that calcium had a permissive effect on calcitonin response to other secretagogues.[19] Similarly, Roos et al. could not show a significant effect of calcium on calcitonin release in cultured trout C cells.[20] However, they could demonstrate a calcitonin rise in cultured medullary carcinoma cells in response to calcium.

In summary, it is clear that large changes in serum calcium can elicit changes in peripheral calcitonin in normal humans and that smaller changes in calcium affect calcitonin release in animals. However, since the effect of small, physiological alterations of calcium in humans is unknown, it is not clear that calcium concen-tration in blood per se is by any means the major regulator of calcitonin secretion in normal humans. In this regard, however, it

is of interest that Cooper et al. showed that oral calcium would cause an elevation of calcitonin in pigs without altering serum calcium. They therefore suggested that calcium exerts a physiolog-ical effect on calcitonin secretion via alteration of gut hormone.[21] Hence, calcium might be involved physiologically via indirect effects. The effect of gastrointestinal hormones is discussed below.

The effects of cations other than calcium on calcitonin secre-tion are small, if present at all. In vitro data have shown that extremely high concentrations of magnesium are required to elicit changes in calcitonin secretion and that no changes are seen when magnesium is varied within a physiological range. Similar results have been obtained in animal experiments.[52] In contrast, Anast and co-workers have shown that magnesium infusion results in lowered plasma calcitonin in patients with medullary carcinoma of the thyroid.[22] No consistent physiological effect for potassium or phosphate on calcitonin secretion has been demonstrated. Heynen and Franchiment have reported a single case in which phosphate infusion resulted in a large increase in calcitonin.[23]

CYCLIC NUCLEOTIDES AND CALCITONIN SECRETION

The role of cyclic nucleotides in calcitonin secretion is under active investigation. Ziegler et al. in 1969 showed that dibutyryl cAMP with theophylline could enhance calcitonin secretion in the perfused hen ultimobranchial gland.[24] Care and co-workers re-ported similar results in perfused porcine thyroids and showed that the effect could be inhibited by beta-adrenergic blockade.[25] Hsu and Cooper demonstrated increased calcitonin in response to cate-cholamines in the rat.[26] As many substances may exert their effect via adenylyl cyclase, it is possible that calcitonin secretion is regulated by local changes in cAMP; however, a definite function for either circulating catecholamines or local cyclic nucleotide alterations in the physiological control of human calcitonin has yet to be demonstrated.

GASTROINTESTINAL HORMONES AND CALCITONIN SECRETION

As suggested above, a major focus of investigation has been the role of gastrointestinal hormones in calcitonin regulation. In 1971, Cooper and co-workers[28] and Care et al.[27] independently reported significantly increased calcitonin secretion induced by gastrin infusion. Both groups of workers did their experiments in the pig, where calcitonin was shown to increase rapidly (within 2 to 5 minutes) in response to various gastrin species or synthetic pentagastrin.[27,28] The quantities of gastrin used were sufficiently low to suggest that physiological levels of gastrin may stimulate calcitonin secretion. This work also led to the use of pentagastrin as a stimulus for calcitonin secretion in patients with suspected medullary carcinoma of the thyroid (see Fig. 49-1). Results to date indicate that gastrin is at least as potent a stimulus for calcitonin secretion as is calcium. Sizemore et al. reported elevated calci-tonin in 4 of 7 patients with Zollinger-Ellison syndrome, a state of endogenous hypergastrinemia.[29] It is thus clear that gastrin can be a potent secretagogue for calcitonin in animals and in humans with medullary carcinoma of the thyroid. What effect physiological variations of gastrin have on calcitonin in normal humans is un-known and awaits applications of the recently improved radioim-munoassays.

Other gastrointestinal hormones have also proven to be potent secretagogues. Care and co-workers[30] showed that both pancreo-zymin and the structurally related compound cerulein stimulated calcitonin secretion in isolated pig thyroid glands. Bell[47] demonstrated that glucagon stimulated calcitonin in vitro. Tashjian et al.[31] showed that glucagon infusion could increase calcitonin in patients with medullary carcinoma of the thyroid. However, the glucagon response is not consistent. Therefore the role of glucagon (and specifically pancreatic versus gut glucagon) as a calcitonin secretagogue remains unresolved. Similar conflicting data with secretin have been reported.[32] Thus, a variety of gastrointestinal hormones can influence calcitonin secretion. Gastrin would appear to be the most potent stimulus so far tested. Gastrin, as pentagastrin, is one of the more useful tools in the investigation of calcitonin secretion by medullary carcinoma of the thyroid, but the defined role of gastrointestinal hormones in the physiological regulation of calcitonin secretion awaits further investigation.

ALCOHOL AND CALCITONIN SECRETION

In 1973, Cohen et al.[33] reported that alcohol caused a significant rise in calcitonin in a patient with medullary carcinoma of the thyroid (see Fig. 49-1). Wells and co-workers[34] extended this work and demonstrated that the rise in calcitonin in response to ethanol is mediated by neither calcium nor gastrin. Heynen and Gaspar[35] have recently shown that the effect of ethanol could be blocked by the beta-adrenergic antagonist propranolol.

HETEROGENEITY OF CALCITONIN

Peripheral levels of calcitonin are elevated in a variety of disease states, including medullary carcinoma of the thyroid, islet-cell tumors, malignant tumors (especially breast, lung and prostate) renal failure, pyknodysostosis, and Zollinger–Ellison syndrome. Increased levels have also been reported in maternal and fetal plasma at term.[5,31,36,37]

The high levels of both plasma and tissue calcitonin in the above-mentioned conditions have permitted several groups to evaluate the chromatographic appearance of immunochemically detectable hormone.[38–40] Typically, plasma or tumor extract is submitted to gel filtration on a column. The fractions obtained are analyzed by radioimmunoassay for calcitonin. Singer and Habener[38] reported four distinct peaks (Fig. 49-2) on gel filtration. Peak 1 was in the void volume. Peak 4 coeluted with labeled human calcitonin. Peak 3 was near the dimer form of calcitonin. They concluded that peak 3 was probably not the dimer by showing that its elution position did not alter after exposure to mercaptoethanol. Since monomeric calcitonin when added to human plasma eluted only in peaks 1 and 4, Singer and Habener suggested that the heterogeneity demonstrated was not a function of artifact of column chromatography.

Deftos et al.[39] and Sizemore and Heath[40] similarly demonstrated four to six immunoreactive peaks of calcitonin on gel filtration. Deftos et al.[39] showed a peak eluting after calcitonin, suggesting that a fragment of the hormone may have been present. The nature of the peaks remained unresolved. Specifically, it is as yet unknown whether the larger immunoreactive peaks represent precursors of human calcitonin, aggregated fragments, or other polypeptides with immunochemical resemblance to calcitonin. However, the issue of hormone heterogeneity has great significance for both calcitonin measurement and for our understanding of secretory events. Parthemore and Roos[41] analyzed plasma and tumor extracts from patients with medullary carcinoma of the thyroid and showed that secreted calcitonin is more heterogeneous than the glandular form, suggesting that some of the heterogeneity may represent a postsecretory event. However, the presence of multiple tumor peaks in gland extracts implies that at least some of the heterogeneity represents a presecretory event. Roos et al.[42] investigated calcitonin secreted by trout C cells in culture. Using incorporation of ^{14}C-leucine as a marker they demonstrated two distinct calcitonin species, one with a molecular weight of approximately 6000, the other coeluting with trout monomeric calcitonin, molecular weight 3400. Based on pulse/chase experiments, they

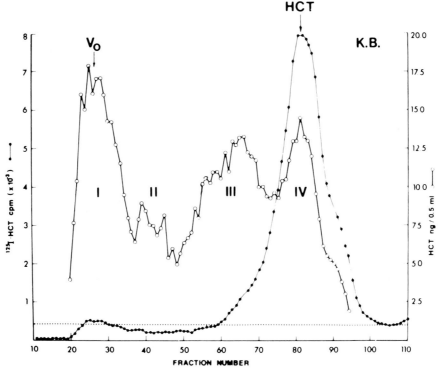

Fig. 49-2. Gel filtration and radioimmunoassay of calcitonin in the plasma of a patient with medullary carcinoma of the thyroid. Arrows mark the void volume (Vo) of the column and the elution position of synthetic monomer human calcitonin (HCT). The detection limits of the assay are indicated by dotted lines.[38]

were able to propose that the larger species represented a precursor form of calcitonin. Moya and co-workers[43] studied calcitonin biosynthesis in chick ultimobranchial glands in the presence of radioactive amino acids. With pulse/chase, they were able to show a large-molecular-weight form (13,000), which gradually resolved into a form coeluting on gel electrophoresis with monomeric chicken calcitonin. An intermediate form was also demonstrated. They suggested that the large form was a precursor of calcitonin with minimal biological activity which was then cleaved to give an intermediate-size peptide plus calcitonin. Alternatively, they postulated that the intermediate form may represent the first step in cleavage of the prohormone. The issue of calcitonin heterogeneity and the extent to which it represents biosynthetic or intraglandular events, metabolism after secretion, or artifacts during sample processing remain unresolved. However, the possibility of a prohormone for calcitonin is becoming more plausible.

METABOLISM OF CALCITONIN

The metabolic fate of human calcitonin is still being investigated. There are considerable data on the metabolism of injected calcitonin in various animal species. Conclusions about human calcitonin metabolism cannot be directly inferred from these data, as it is clear that different calcitonin species are handled variably in different species. Clark and co-workers[44] infused human calcitonin into dogs and analyzed arteriovenous differences across the kidney and liver by immunoassay. They concluded that the majority of human calcitonin was cleared by the kidney and that most of it was removed by enzymatic degradation. They also concluded that there were two half-times of disappearance, one of 3 minutes and the other of 40 minutes. However, some calcitonin may pass through the kidney unaltered; Voelkel and Tashjian were able to demonstrate biologically active calcitonin in the urine of a patient with medullary carcinoma of the thyroid.[45] The fact that the kidney plays a major role in metabolism of calcitonin is in agreement with recent data suggesting high levels of calcitonin in both acute and chronic renal failure.[36] However, whether renal failure results in decreased catabolism by the kidney, alteration of degradation by other organs (e.g., liver), or modification of secretion remains unresolved.[46]

CONCLUSION

Species variation, uncovered with respect to calcitonin physiology, makes inference to secretion and metabolism of human calcitonin difficult.

Calcitonin circulates in most animals at higher concentrations than in man (see Table 49-1); therefore, radioimmunoassays for these calcitonins have detected the hormone in the blood of these species. However, until recently, available assays for human calcitonin have not been sufficiently sensitive to detect the hormone present in blood of man. Therefore, alterations in calcitonin secretion, if any, could not be analzyed under physiologic conditions. With improved radioimmunoassays, we may soon know whether the effect of calcium, gut hormones, and/or cyclic nucleotides pertains to physiologic variations of secretion in humans. Indeed, it still remains to be proven that physiologic variations in normal humans exist at all, although it is widely believed that the hormone is secreted under basal conditions. The issue of a human calcitonin prohormone is unresolved. The relative importance of secretory versus postsecretory events in the immunochemical heterogeneity of the hormone is being actively investigated.

The existing assay methods, however, properly applied and interpreted, are highly useful and reliable in the major clinical application of the assay, detection, and improved management of medullary carcinoma of the thyroid (Chapter 65). New developments in assay sensitivity and specificity based on resolution of the nature and significance of circulating calcitonin may in future years help to clarify the physiology and biologic role of this hormone, whose function in humans remains largely unsettled.

REFERENCES

1. Langman, J. *Medical Embryology*. Williams and Wilkins, Baltimore, 1952, p. 194.
2. Wolfe, H. J., Melvin, K. E. W., Cervi-Skinner, S. J. et al. C-Cell Hyperplasia Preceding Medullary Thyroid Carcinoma. N. Engl. J. Med. *289:* 437, 1973.
3. Williams, E. D. Histogenesis of Medullary Carcinoma of the Thyroid. J. Clin. Path. *19:* 114, 1966.
4. Clark, M. B., Byfield, P. G. H., Boyd, G. W., and Foster, G. U. A Radioimmunoassay for Human Calcitonin. Lancet *2:* 74, 1969.
4a. Melvin, K. E. W., and Tashjian, A. J., Jr. The Syndrome of Excessive Thyrocalcitonin Produced by Medullary Carcinoma of the Thyroid. Proc. Nat. Acad. Sci. *59:* 1216, 1968.
4b. Milhaud, G., Tubiana, M., Paramentier, C., and Contris, G. Epithelioma de la Thyroide Sécretant de la Thyrocalcitonine. CR Acad. Sci. (D) (Paris) *266:* 608, 1968.
5. Coombes, R. C., Greenberg, P. B., Hillyard, C., and MacIntyre, J. Plasma-Immunoreactive-Calcitonin in Patients with Non-thyroid Tumors. Lancet 2: 1080, 1974.
6. Silva, O. L., Becker, K. L., Primrack, A., et al. Hypercalcitonemia in Bronchogenic Cancer. J.A.M.A. *234:* 183, 1975.
7. Deftos, L. J., McMillan, P. J., Sartiano, G. P., et al. Simultaneous Ectopic Production of Parathyroid Hormone and Calcitonin. Metabolism 25: 543, 1976.
8. Ellison, M., Woodhouse, D., Hillyard, C., et al. Immunoreactive Calcitonin Production by Human Lung Carcinoma Cells in Culture. Br. J. Cancer *32:* 373, 1975.
9. Cooper, C. W., Hirsch, P. F., and Munson, P. L. Calcitropic Hormones. Calcitonin. Measurement-Bioassay, in *Methods in Investigative and Diagnostic Endocrinology. Peptide Hormones,* edited by S. A. Berson and R. Yalow. North Holland, Amsterdam, 1973, vol 2B, pp. 1003–1010.
10. Deftos, L. J., Lee, M. R., and Potts, J. T., Jr. A Radioimmunoassay for Thyrocalcitonin. Proc. Nat. Acad. Sci. (US) *60:* 293, 1968.
11. Deftos, L. J. Immunoassay for Human Calcitonin. I. Method. Metabolism *20:* 1122, 1971.
12. Parthemore, J. G., and Deftos, L. G. The Regulation of Calcitonin in Normal Human Plasma as Assessed by Immuno Extraction and Immunoprecipitation. J. Clin. Inv. *56:* 835, 1975.
13. Copp, D. H., Cameron, E. C., Chaney, B. A., et al. Evidence for Calcitonin—A New Hormone from the Parathyroid That Lowers Blood Calcium. Endocrinology *70:* 638, 1962.
14. Hirsh, P. F., Gauthier, G. F., and Munson, P. L. Thyroid Hypocalcemic Principle and Recurrent Laryngeal Nerve Injury as Factors Affecting the Response to Parathyroidectomy in Rats. Endocrinology *79:* 655, 1966.

Table 49-1.   Calcitonin Levels in Various Animal Species

Species	Blood Calcitonin Level	Antisera Used	References
1. Human	10–50 pg/ml	Antihuman	12
2. Chicken	3400 ± 1100 pg/ml	Antisalmon	53
20-day-old embryo			
3. Salmon		Antisalmon	54
Female—seawater	2,230 ± 920 pg/ml		
Female—freshwater	2,000 ± 380 pg/ml		
Female—spawning	20,000 ± 4600 pg/ml		
4. Bovine			
Cow	100–220 pg/ml	Antiporcine	55
Bull	240–550 pg/ml	Antiporcine	55
5. Porcine	20,000 pg/ml	Antiporcine	56
6. Rabbit	140 ± 50 pg/ml	Antiporcine	57

15. Melvin, K. E., Miller, H. H., and Tashjian, A. H., Jr. Early Diagnosis of Medullary Carcinoma of the Thyroid Gland by Means of Calcitonin Assay. N. Engl. J. Med. *285:* 1115, 1971.

16. Deftos, L. J., Powell, D., Parthemore, J. G., and Potts, J. T., Jr. Secretion of Calcitonin in Hypocalcemia States in Man. J. Clin. Inv. *52:* 3109, 1973.

17. Cooper, C. W., Deftos, L. J., and Potts, J. T., Jr. Direct Measurement of in Vivo Secretion of Pig Thyrocalcitonin by Radioimmunoassay. Endocrinology *88:* 747, 1971.

18. Bell, N. H., and Queener, S. Stimulation of Calcitonin Synthesis and Release in Vitro by Calcium and Dibutyryl Cyclic AMP. Nature *248:* 343, 1974.

19. Selawry, H. P., Becker, K. L., Bivins, R. H., et al. In Vitro Studies of Calcitonin Release in Man. Hormone Metab. Res. *7:* 432, 1975.

20. Roos, B. A., Bundy, C. L., and Deftos, L. J. Calcitonin Secretion in Vitro. Endocrinology *95:* 1144, 1974.

21. Cooper, C. W., Schwesing, A. M., Mahgoub, D. A., et al. Regulation of Secretion of Thyrocalcitonin, in *Calcium, Parathyroid Hormone and the Calcitonins,* edited by R. V. Talmage and P. L. Munson. Excerpta Medica, Amsterdam, 1972, p 128.

22. Anast, C., David, L., Winnacker, J., et al. Serum Calcitonin-lowering Effect of Magnesium in Patients with Medullary Carcinoma of the Thyroid. J. Clin. Inv. *56:* 1615, 1975.

23. Heynen, G., and Franchiment, P. Human Calcitonin and Serum Phosphate. Lancet *2:* 627, 1974.

24. Ziegler, R., Delling, M., and Pfeiffer, E. F. The Secretion of Calcitonin by the Perfused Ultimobranchial Gland of the Hen. *Calcitonin. Proceedings of the Second International Symposium.* William Heinemann, London, 1969.

25. Care, A. D., Bates, R. F. L., and Gitelman, H. J. A Possible Role for Adenyl Cyclase System in Calcitonin Release. J. Endocr. *48:* 1, 1970.

26. Hsu, W. H., and Cooper, C. W. Hypercalcemic Effect of Catecholamines and Its Prevention by Thyrocalcitonin. Calcif. Tiss. Res. *19:* 125, 1975.

27. Care, A. D., Bates, R. F. L., Swaminathan, R., and Ganguli, P. C. The Role of Gastrin as a Calcitonin Secretagogue. J. Endocrin. *51:* 735, 1971.

28. Cooper, C. W., Schwesinger, W. H., Malgoub, A. M., and Ontjes, D. A. Thyrocalcitonin: Stimulation of Secretion by Gastrin. Science *172:* 1238, 1971.

29. Sizemore, G. W., Go, V. L. W., Kaplan, E. L., et al. Relations of Calcitonin and Gastrin in the Zollinger–Ellison Syndrome and Medullary Carcinoma of the Thyroid. N. Engl. J. Med. *288:* 641, 1973.

30. Care, A. D., Bruce, J. B., Boelkins, J., et al. Role of Pancreozymin-Choleystokinin and Structurally Related Compounds as Calcitonin Secretagogues. Endocrinology *89:* 262, 1971.

31. Tashjian, A. H., Haviland, B. G., Melvin, K. E. W., and Hill, C. S., Jr. Immuno-assay of Human Calcitonin in Normal and Disease States. New Eng. J. Med. *283:* 890, 1970.

32. Roos, B. A., and Deftos, L. J. Calcitonin Secretion in Vitro. II. Regulatory Effects of Enteric Mammalian Polypeptide Hormones on Trout C-Cell Cultures. Endocrinology *98:* 1286, 1976.

33. Cohen, S. L., Grahane-Smith, D., MacIntyre, J., and Walker, J. G. Alcohol-Stimulated Calcitonin Release in Medullary Thyroid Carcinoma. Lancet *4:* 472, 1973.

34. Wells, S. A., Cooper, C. W., and Ontjes, D. A. Stimulation of Thyrocalcitonin Secretion by Ethanol in Patients with Medullary Thyroid Carcinoma—an Effect Apparently Not Mediated by Gastrin. Metabolism *24:* 1215, 1975.

35. Heynen, G., and Gaspar, S. Calcitonin, Parathyroid Hormone and the Autonomic Nervous System. Abs. XII European Symposium on Calcified Tissue, York, England, 1976. p. 31.

36. Ardaillou, R., Beaufils, M., Nivez, M. P., et al. Increased Plasma Calcitonin in Early Acute Renal Failure. Clin. Sci. Mol. Med. *49:* 301, 1975.

37. Tashjian, A. H., Jr., Wolfe, H. J., and Voelkel, E. F. Human Calcitonin Immunologic Assay, Cytological Localization and Studies in Medullary Thyroid Carcinoma. A.J.M. *56:* 840, 1974.

38. Singer, F. R., and Habener, J. F. Multiple Immunoreactive Forms of Calcitonin in Human Plasma. Bioch. Biophys. Res. Commun. *61:* 660, 1974.

39. Deftos, L. J., Roos, B. A., Bronzert, D., and Parthemore, J. G. Immunochemical Heterogeneity of Calcitonin in Plasma. J. Clin. Endo. Met. *40:* 410, 1975.

40. Sizemore, G. W., and Heath, H., III. Immunochemical Heterogeneity of Calcitonin in Plasma of Patients with Medullary Thyroid Carcinoma. J. Clin. Inv. *55:* IIII, 1975.

41. Parthemore, J. G., and Roos, B. A. Calcitonin Heterogeneity in Vivo and in Vitro Studies. 58th Annual Meeting of the Endocrine Society, 1976, p. 65. (abstract)

42. Roos, B. A., Okano, K., and Deftos, L. J. Evidence for a Procalcitonin. Biochem. Biophy. Res. Commun. *60*(3): 1134, 1974.

43. Moya, F., Nieto, A., and Candela, J. L. R. Calcitonin Biosynthesis: Evidence for a Precursor. Eur. J. Biochem. *55:* 407, 1975.

44. Clark, M. B., William, C. C., Nathanson, B. M., et al. Metabolic Fate of Human Calcitonin in the Dog. J. Endoc. *61:* 199, 1974.

45. Voelkel, E. F., and Tashjian, A. H., Jr. Measurement of Thyrocalcitonin-like Activity in Urine of Patients with Medullary Thyroid Carcinoma. J. Clin. Endo. *32:* 102, 1971.

46. Deftos, L. J., Gogo, A., Lee, J., and Parthemore, J. G. Hypercalcitoninism and Hyperparathyroidism in Chronic Renal Disease. Immuno-chemical Heterogeneity. 58th Annual Meeting of the Endocrine Society, 1976, p. 264 (abstract).

47. Bell, N. H. Effects of Glucagon, Dibutyryl Cyclic 3'5'-Adenosine Monophosphate and Theophylline on Calcitonin Secretion in Vitro. J. Clin. Inv. *49:* 1368, 1970.

48. Goltzman, M. D., Potts, J. T., Jr., Ridgway, E. C., and Maloof, F. Calcitonin as a Tumor Marker. N. Engl. J. Med. *290:* 1035, 1974.

49. Tashjian, A. H., Jr. Calcitropic Hormones: Calcitonin: Measurement; Radioimmunoassay, in *Methods of Investigative and Diagnostic Endocrinology: Part III: Peptide Hormones,* edited by S. A. Berson and R. Yalow. North Holland, Amsterdam, 1973, vol. 2B, p. 1010–1019.

50. Silva, O. L., Snider, R. H., and Beeker, K. L. Radioimmunoassay of Calcitonin in Human Plasma. Clin. Chem. *20:* 337, 1974.

51. Samaan, N. A., Hill, C. S., Jr., Beceiro, Jr., et al. Immunoreactive Calcitonin in Medullary Carcinoma of the Thyroid and in Maternal and Cord Serum. J. Lab. Clin. Med. *81:* 671, 1973.

52. Care, A. D., Bell, N. H., and Bates, R. F. L. The Effect of Hypermagnesemia on Calcitonin Secretion in Vivo. J. Endocrinol. *51:* 381, 1971.

53. Cutler, G. B., Habener, J. F., Dee, P. C., and Potts, J. T., Jr. Radioimmunoassay for Chicken Calcitonin. FEBS Letters *38:* 209, 1974.

54. Wahs, E. G., Copp, D. H., and Deftos, L. J. Changes in Plasma Calcium and Calcitonin in the Spawning Cycle of Sockeye Salmon. Proc. Can. Fed. Biol. Soc. *15:* 406, 1972 (abstract).

55. Deftos, L. J., Murray, T. M., Powell, D., et al. Radioimmunoassays for Parathyroid Hormones and Calcitonins, in *Calcium, Parathyroid Hormone and the Calcitonins,* edited by R. V. Talmage and P. L. Munson. Excerpta Medica, Amsterdam, 1972, p. 140.

56. Cooper, C. W., and Deftos, L. J. Evaluation of Thyrocalcitonin in Pig Thyroid Vein Blood Following Oral Administration of Calcium. Fed. Proc. *29:* 253, 1970.

57. Deftos, L. J., Lee, M. R., and Potts, J. T., Jr. A Radioimmunoassay for Thyrocalcitonin. P.N.A.S. *60:* 293, 1968.

50

Physiology and Mode of Action of Calcitonin

Roy V. Talmage
Cary W. Cooper

Calcitonin (thyrocalcitonin) is recognized as a hypocalcemic agent in mammals, its secretion being controlled by feedback between the ionic calcium concentration of plasma and the so-called C cells of the thyroid. It was in this relationship that the first active extract was characterized by Hirsch and Munson.[1] However, in naming the hormone, Copp[2] suggested that it played a role in the minute-to-minute maintenance of normal plasma calcium concentrations in mammals. One of the primary problems in conclusively establishing maintenance of normocalcemia as the primary physiological function of the hormone has been the fact that both in man and in experimental mammals, plasma calcium values appear to remain within normal limits for long periods of time following total thyroidectomy even without supplementation with calcitonin.[3]

The ability of calcitonin to lower plasma phosphate concentrations was also recognized from the outset of the discovery of the hormone.[4] However, only recently has it become apparent that the hypocalcemic and hypophosphatemic effects occur by independent mechanisms and, therefore, are probably produced by different physiological processes.[5] It has even been suggested that the effects of calcitonin on phosphate or on ions other than calcium may be the key to eventually understanding fully the physiological role of the hormone.

It is quite possible that the most important function of calcitonin in man has not yet been discovered, for it is difficult to believe that a hormone known to circulate in blood does not have an easily demonstrable physiological role to play. It is with these thoughts in mind that this brief review of the physiology and biochemical action of calcitonin is written.

ROLE OF CALCITONIN IN CALCIUM HOMEOSTASIS

SECRETION IN RESPONSE TO HYPERCALCEMIC CHALLENGE

If the plasma calcium level is raised artificially, there is an immediate increase in the circulating level of calcitonin.[3,6] This response has been thoroughly tested in many mammalian species including man. For the most part, calcium salt has been administered intravenously or intraperitoneally, but the same result has been achieved when calcium in solution has been given orally by gavage on an empty stomach. When calcium is injected intravenously, the amount of circulating calcitonin increases in accordance with the extent of the rise in the plasma calcium concentration.

Equally well established is the finding that when calcium is administered to mammals, the rise in plasma calcium concentrations is smaller and the return to normal more rapid in animals with intact thyroid glands than in thyroidectomized animals.[6] This, of course, has been the basis for the belief that the major role of the hormone is to protect against hypercalcemia. Since even short periods of hypercalcemia, especially those approaching or exceeding 15 mg Ca/100 ml, are extremely dangerous and may be life-threatening to man, this antihypercalcemic role for calcitonin is a very attractive hypothesis.

OCCURRENCE OF HYPERCALCEMIA IN NORMAL INDIVIDUALS

The normal range for plasma calcium levels in man is considered to be between 9.5 and 10.5 mg/100 ml. At these concentrations of total plasma calcium, the ionized portion is slightly over 50 percent. In rats adapted to a regular standardized feeding schedule, plasma calcium fluctuates rhythmically; the highest daily plasma calcium concentrations occur during the fasting portion of the cycle and may rise to above 11 mg/100 ml.[7,8] In neither animals nor man is it possible to significantly elevate plasma calcium levels by addition of calcium to the diet, unless the calcium-to-phosphate ratio is extremely high, and this is true regardless of whether or not the thyroid gland is present. In contrast, hyperparathyroidism (primary) in man can be accompanied by high plasma calcium concentrations even in the presence of the thyroid gland. In this latter case, therefore, calcitonin obviously cannot completely protect the individual against hypercalcemia, at least not on a long-term basis.

The point to be emphasized is that under normal dietary conditions, calcitonin would not seem to be needed in man to prevent hypercalcemia, since hypercalcemia ordinarily does not occur. Even in pathological conditions in which hypercalcemia tends to occur, plasma calcium concentrations can rise dangerously even in the presence of normal thyroid glands and an increase in calcitonin secretion.

RELATIVE ROLES OF PARATHYROID HORMONE AND CALCITONIN

It is very likely that the daily maintenance of plasma calcium concentrations within the normal range is primarily the responsibility of parathyroid hormone. Removal of these glands causes an obvious, drastic and life-threatening fall in plasma calcium levels, while continued excessive secretion of the hormone raises the blood calcium above normal. The participation of calcitonin in this regulation appears to be limited. While calcitonin can produce a temporary acute fall in plasma calcium and can help restrict experimentally produced hypercalcemia, it appears that one might profit by looking elsewhere for a physiological role of this hormone in man.

ROLE OF CALCITONIN IN BONE PHYSIOLOGY

SUPPRESSION OF BONE RESORPTION—ACTION ON OSTEOCLASTS

The aspect of calcitonin action on bone that has been most thoroughly studied has been the ability of the hormone to reduce bone resorptive processes. In this discussion, we define bone "resorption" as the simultaneous breakdown of all components of bone, both organic and inorganic. In extensive tissue culture studies by several different groups of investigators, it has been established that rates of bone resorption can be reduced by addition of calcitonin to the incubation media.[3,6] These studies have included gross anatomical and ultrastructural studies, measurement of rates of release of ^{45}Ca from prelabeled bone, and evaluation of rates of hydroxyproline release from bone collagen. The in vivo evaluation of this action of the hormone has been developed primarily through studies involving calcitonin administration regularly over long periods of time. In experimental animals, including vertebrates other than mammals, such treatment has resulted in more-dense bones with fewer resorption centers. Both in vitro and in vivo, calcitonin has been found to alter the morphology of osteoclasts. This ability of calcitonin to reduce bone resorptive rates is the basis for its use in clinical treatment of certain metabolic bone diseases, particularly Paget's disease.[3,6]

Because of the striking effects of calcitonin on bone resorption, and the ability of the hormone to oppose skeletal effects produced by parathyroid hormone, the concept that calcitonin produces hypocalcemia by suppressing bone resorptive rates has been widely held for many years.

RAPID EFFECTS OF CALCITONIN ON THE OSTEOCYTE/OSTEOBLAST COMPLEX OF COMPACT BONE

There is continuously mounting evidence that cells of compact bone, osteocytes and bone surface cells (lining cells, or osteoblasts), play the major role in the control of plasma calcium concentrations.[9] A model illustrating the anatomical relationships among the cells of this area and the fluid spaces surrounding them is shown in Figure 50-1. This model has been developed primarily from a realization that calcium fluxes between body fluids and bone are many orders of magnitude greater with regard to the total amount of calcium transported than can be accounted for by the amount of calcium normally made available through bone resorptive rates.[10] Both morphological and physiological data have provided evidence that the osteocyte/osteoblast complex responds rapidly to both parathyroid hormone and calcitonin and that the sequence of morphological changes produced, as observed with

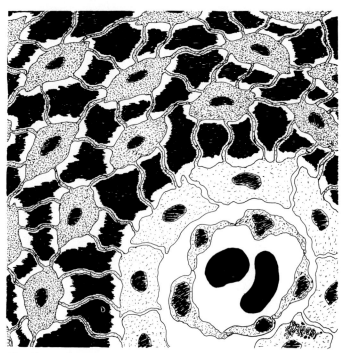

Fig. 50-1. *The Osteocyte–Lining-Cell (Osteoblast) Complex of Bone.* A diagrammatic representation of a portion of a Haversian system modified to show the location of the bone fluid compartment, and to demonstrate the relationship of osteocytes to the cells on the surface of bone.

the electron microscope, can be correlated closely with the changes in plasma calcium concentrations.[9] Both hormones act within minutes on these cells—parathyroid hormone increasing the rate of calcium transfer back to the primary extracellular fluid (ECF) compartment and calcitonin interfering with the source of calcium for transfer out of bone into the ECF. Since these cells in the osteocyte/osteoblast complex outnumber osteoclasts many thousands to one, and since total calcium in the ECF is only a small fraction of that in bone, small changes in flux rates of calcium can be accomplished, at least temporarily, with no appreciable effect on the total calcium content of bone but at the same time producing large changes in plasma calcium concentrations.

POSTULATED ROLES OF CALCITONIN IN BONE PHYSIOLOGY

A number of years ago, it was postulated that parathyroid hormone had two different roles in bone, one involving bone remodeling and the other involving maintenance of plasma calcium concentrations.[11] A similar dual role is now postulated for calcitonin. One role is to suppress bone resorption, and the second is to produce a temporary hypocalcemia. The first action is mediated through osteoclasts and through effects on bone progenitor cell populations and is relatively slow; large amounts of calcitonin chronically will produce morphological changes in bone. The second action, mediated through established Haversian systems in bone, is rapid and produces a temporary hypocalcemia by reducing calcium efflux from bone into ECF.[11a] Since most studies on the action of calcitonin have involved exogenous hormone given in large doses to experimental animals, the general applicability of these principles to the normal bone physiology of man is not clear. As pointed out later in this chapter, changes in calcitonin secretion in laboratory animals appear to be related more to feeding and digestive events than to changes in the plasma calcium level. It is possible that calcitonin, in concert with digestive factors, may play a role in the proper distribution of absorbed calcium and other digestive products to bone.

POSSIBLE MODES OF ACTION OF CALCITONIN

STIMULATION OF ADENYLATE CYCLASE ACTIVITY

Calcitonin is one of the many peptide hormones that stimulate adenylate cyclase activity in known target tissues.[3] While the magnitude of the response of skeletal and renal tissues to calcitonin is less than that to parathyroid hormone, levels of cAMP (the "second messenger") increase in all primary cell types of bone following calcitonin administration.[12] This finding has been reported from both in vivo and tissue culture studies. In addition, calcitonin also increases both the activity of adenylate cyclase and the intracellular levels of cAMP in several other tissues, the most notable being the renal cortex. Specific receptor sites in cell membranes prepared from renal tissue have been identified.[13] Since calcitonin is a peptide hormone, it is not surprising that the hormone reacts with cell membranes. It must, therefore, be concluded that cAMP serves as a messenger mediating at least a portion of the activity of calcitonin.

RELATIONSHIP OF CALCITONIN TO PHOSPHATE

Studies utilizing radiophosphorus as a tracer strongly suggest that calcitonin promotes phosphate movement out of the ECF and that it is through this action that the hormone produces its hypophosphatemia.[5,13a] The tissue or tissues into which this phosphate moves have not been definitely identified. The primary tissue implicated is bone. Increased renal excretion of phosphate following calcitonin administration in large doses, particularly in thyroparathyroidectomized animals, has been reported but has never been shown conclusively. For review of this issue and related effects of calcitonin, see the review by Munson.[20] It is not surprising that it has been difficult to trace the phosphate moved out of the ECF by calcitonin. The total inorganic phosphate in the ECF can be measured in micromoles, while that in soft tissues such as liver, bone, and, particularly, muscle exists in millimolar quantities. In addition, even much larger amounts of phosphate are bound organically in each of these tissues. Since tissue phosphate pools exceed the ECF pool so greatly, even major losses from the ECF are difficult to trace.

It is well known that the action of calcitonin is characterized by changes in phosphate homeostasis. In fact, an independence of calcitonin effects on phosphate from those on calcium has been demonstrated.[13c] To go one step further, it is even possible that changes in phosphate mediate or, in turn, regulate the hypocalcemic effect of calcitonin. Many years ago, Hirsch demonstrated that the hypocalcemia following calcitonin injection was augmented by concurrent phosphate administration,[14] and this has been confirmed.[11a] More recently, a relationship of phosphate to the effect of calcitonin on the osteocyte/osteoblast complex in compact bone has been reported; supplemental phosphate increases the amount of the metastable calcium/phosphate complex found in bone fluid following calcitonin injection.[15]

RELATIONSHIP OF CALCITONIN TO CALCIUM MOVEMENT

One of the most widely accepted physiological effects of calcitonin is a decrease in the movement of calcium from bone into blood and ECF. The original conclusion that this was due entirely to reduced rates of bone resorption (which do occur) gradually is being superseded by the concept that hypocalcemia is achieved rapidly by a reduction in the calcium flux from the bone fluid compartment through the osteoblast/osteocyte bone cell layer and into the ECF. In both the old and the new concepts, however, the action of calcitonin must involve net changes in intracellular calcium movements.

Based on his work in vitro with isolated cell cultures, Borle has evolved a model explaining calcitonin influences on intracellular calcium movement.[16] He concludes that calcitonin increases mitochondrial calcium uptake (binding), thereby reducing the amount of "active" or "free" calcium in the cytosol; this secondarily reduces the calcium efflux out of the cell cytosol to the exterior of the cell. According to his model, phosphate aids by complexing calcium in mitochondria, thereby augmenting the calcitonin effect. While this is an extremely plausible explanation, physiological and morphological evidence related to the osteoblast/osteocyte complex as a cellular interface between two fluid compartments suggests that the interference with net calcium release from bone occurs both intracellularly and extracellularly and includes movement of material, containing phosphate, from osteocytes into the bone fluid compartment (where calcium also could be complexed).

RELATIONSHIP OF CALCITONIN TO DIGESTIVE PROCESSES

CONTROL OF SECRETION OF CALCITONIN

Extensive studies have been reported demonstrating that one or more hormones of the digestive tract have the ability to elicit increased calcitonin secretion.[3] The most widely tested hormone in this regard has been gastrin and its synthetic analogue, pentagastrin. It is known to stimulate calcitonin secretion in a variety of experimental animals and in man. Gastrin injection can be used as a rapid and convenient provocative test for C-cell function, especially for uncovering suspected subclinical cases of medullary carcinoma of the thyroid.[17]

Our own search for a role for calcitonin has resulted in recent studies demonstrating that calcitonin secretion increases following feeding. In rats maintained on a standardized feeding and light schedule, calcitonin secretion, as measured by radioimmunoassay, rose markedly in serum 1 to 2 hours after the start of the feeding period and remained elevated for 4 to 5 hours.[18] At all other times, serum concentrations were below the limits of the assay. In these rats, plasma calcium concentrations fall prior to the start of the feeding period and remain at their lowest daily level during the first part of the active eating period. Therefore, the stimulus for secretion of calcitonin had to be derived from the digestive tract following entry of food and could not be attributed to a rise in plasma calcium levels. This is illustrated in Figure 50-2. Other animal studies also have shown that stimulation of gastrin or oral calcium administration can increase calcitonin secretion without raising plasma calcium.[3] These studies suggest that under normal physiological conditions, the primary control of calcitonin secretion may reside with feeding, the release of intestinal hormones, or other as yet unidentified gastrointestinal factors. Similar findings in the rat have been reported by Milhaud et al.[7]

INVOLVEMENT OF CALCITONIN IN DIGESTIVE PROCESSES

Not only can gastrin and other hormones from the intestinal tract influence calcitonin secretion but also the reverse can occur:

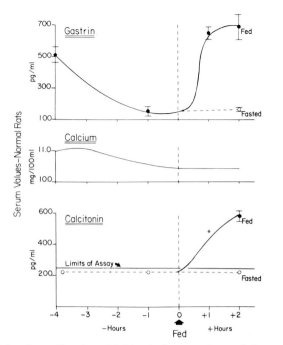

Fig. 50-2. *Serum Gastrin and Calcitonin Concentrations as Influenced by the Availability of Food. (Taken from Reference 18.)*

Notes: 1) Points on graphs are means ± S.E. of serum samples taken from 12–16 rats (calcium values are for plasma)
2) Fasted = not fed at regular feeding time.
3) *Calcitonin values, 1 hr after food became available, ranged from non-detectable to >600 pg/ml

namely, calcitonin can affect secretion of gastrointestinal hormones.[3] Data obtained from studies with rats have suggested that gastrin secretion, normally elevated immediately after eating, is suppressed by thyroparathyroidectomy even when accompanied by thyroxine maintenance. Bolman[19] found that PTH stimulated gastrin secretion without causing hypocalcemia. Calcitonin alone did not influence gastrin.

The important conclusion to be drawn from these various findings is that calcitonin is a hormone that appears to be closely involved with digestive processes. Whether this involvement pertains only to calcium and phosphate metabolism or whether it has other physiological ramifications remains to be determined. While studies to date have been limited to experimental animals, the known effect of gastrin on calcitonin secretion in man suggests that it may be in relationship to feeding and digestion that an important role of calcitonin in man may be found.

MISCELLANEOUS EFFECTS OF CALCITONIN

POSSIBLE EFFECT ON RENAL 1-HYDROXYLASE ACTIVITY

The role of the kidney cortex in the final hydroxylation of vitamin D is now well established. While some disagreements persist as to the relative importance of various factors that have been found to influence rates of formation of 1,25-dihydroxycholecalciferol, both parathyroid hormone and phosphate appear to exert major influences on the activity of the enzyme. The possible role of calcitonin is more controversial. Both augmentation and reduction in the activity of the hydroxylating enzyme have been reported. At present, most workers in the field agree that calcitonin is not a major factor in controlling hydroxylation of the

vitamin and that its role, if any, is to decrease enzyme activity and thus restrict formation of 1,25-dihydroxycholecalciferol.[3]

CALCITONIN IN PREGNANCY AND LACTATION

Several recent reports have shown that circulating levels of calcitonin are high both in pregnancy and in lactation, at least in experimental animals. There appears to be a rise in serum calcitonin, particularly near the end of pregnancy. A similar rise has been found in embryonic birds. In suckling pups and their lactating mothers, serum calcitonin concentrations are elevated. The elevated calcitonin in lactating rats is related to the fact that the daily consumption of food is increased many times above normal and that the rats eat almost continuously. In suckling rat pups, calcitonin remains high unless animals are prevented from nursing for 8 hours or more, at which time it falls to very low levels. Allowing fasted pups to nurse results in a rapid release of calcitonin.

CALCITONIN IN THE AGING ANIMAL

It has been established that the hypocalcemic action of exogenously administered calcitonin decreases with age, at least in experimental mammals.[6] However, recent studies suggest that its proposed role in protecting man and other animals from hypercalcemia may be more pronounced as the animal ages. Based on studies in rats, the number of calcitonin-secreting cells also are greatly increased in the older animal, plasma calcitonin levels are raised, and thyroparathyroidectomy has been reported to produce a temporary hypercalcemia only in older rats. There is no information available at present to indicate whether a similar situation exists in man. However, one must keep in mind that the laboratory rat, unlike man, throughout life feeds on a diet with a high calcium/phosphate ratio and with a dietary calcium content of greater than 1 percent by weight.

SUMMARY

Calcitonin is a peptide hormone known to be synthesized and secreted endogenously in man, in mammals, and in every submammalian vertebrate tested. Because of this wide distribution and evolutionary preservation, it is logical to assume that the hormone serves an important role in normal physiology. What this role is in mammals has not as yet been established with certainty. The rapid increase in plasma calcitonin that occurs in man and experimental mammals when the ionic plasma calcium level is artificially raised logically led to the assumption that calcitonin plays an important role in the maintenance of plasma calcium concentrations. This role is questionable because thyroidectomy in man does not seem to produce hypercalcemia and because hypercalcemic events rarely occur in man as an environmental stress (as distinct from disease states).

Further questioning of the postulated calcium homeostatic role of calcitonin has been developed from experiments demonstrating that calcitonin concentrations rise following ingestion of a meal. This rise occurs when plasma calcium levels are in the low-normal range. It is suggested, therefore, that calcitonin is involved in digestive events, that its primary function may be related to ions other than calcium, and that it may be secreted primarily in response to intestinal hormones.

Calcitonin's effect on plasma phosphate was shown to be independent of its effect on calcium, and it may, therefore, be concerned with the homeostatic control of phosphate. Teleologically, there is a good rationale for this suggestion. The highest concentrations of calcitonin are found in marine fish in which the conservation of phosphate is of major importance and in which the hormone has no hypocalcemic action.

In experimental mammals, calcitonin produces rapid (in minutes) changes in the osteocyte/osteoblast complex of compact bone. By this action, it interferes with calcium fluxes from bone into the ECF. Its ability to decrease calcium release from these areas of bone is augmented by phosphate. This has led to the suggestion that the hypocalcemia produced by the hormone is mediated through intracellular and extracellular effects on phosphate.

Based on the observations that (1) secretion of calcitonin can be regulated by intestinal hormones and that (2) the hormone rapidly affects calcium fluxes between blood and compact bone, one function of calcitonin in man may be to help regulate and facilitate absorption and distribution of calcium and other digestive products to bone or other tissues.

REFERENCES

1. Hirsch, P. F., Gauthier, G. F., and Munson, P. L. Thyroid Hypocalcemic Principle and Recurrent Laryngeal Nerve Injury as Factors Affecting the Response to Parathyroidectomy in Rats. Endocrinology *73:* 244, 1963.

2. Copp, D. H., Davidson, A. G. F., and Cheney, B. Evidence for a New Parathyroid Hormone Which Lowers Blood Calcium. Proc. Can. Fed. Biol. Soc. *4:* 17, 1961.

3. Gray, T. K., Cooper, C. W., and Munson, P. L. Parathyroid Hormone, Thyrocalcitonin and the Control of Mineral Metabolism, in *Endocrine Physiology, Physiology* Series 1, edited by S. M. McCann. University Park Press, Baltimore, 1974, vol. 5. p. 239.

4. Hirsch, P. F., Voelkel, E. F., and Munson, P. L. Thyrocalcitonin: Hypocalcemic Hypophosphatemic Principle of the Thyroid Gland. Science *146:* 412, 1964.

5. Talmage, R. V., Anderson, J. J. B., and Cooper, C. W. The Influence of Calcitonins on the Disappearance of Radiocalcium and Radiophosphorus from Plasma. Endocrinology *90:* 1185, 1972.

6. Hirsch, P. F., and Munson, P. L. Thyrocalcitonin. Physiol. Rev. *49:* 548, 1969.

7. Milhaud, G., Perault-Staub, A. M., and Staub, J. -F. Diurnal Variation of Plasma Calcium and Calcitonin Function in the Rat. J. Physiol. *222:* 559, 1972.

8. Talmage, R. V., Roycroft, J. H., and Anderson, J. J. B. Daily Fluctuations in Plasma Calcium, Phosphate, and Their Radionuclide Concentrations in the Rat. Calcif. Tiss. Res. *17:* 91, 1975.

9. Davis, W. L., Matthews, J. L., Martin, J. H., et al. The Endosteum as a Functional Membrane, in *Calcium-Regulating Hormones,* edited by R. V. Talmage, M. Owen, and J. A. Parsons. Excerpta Medica, Amsterdam, 1975, p. 275.

10. Neuman, W. F. The Bone:Blood Equilibrium: A Possible System for Its Study in Vitro in *Calcium, Parathyroid Hormone and the Calcitonins,* edited by R. V. Talmage and P. L. Munson. Excerpta Medica, Amsterdam, 1972, p. 389.

11. Talmage, R. V. Morphological and Physiological Considerations in a New Concept of Calcium Transport in Bone. Am. J. Anat. *129:* 467, 1970.

11a. Grubb, S. A., Markham, T. C., and Talmage, R. V. Effect of Calcitonin Infusion on Plasma Concentrations of Recently Administered [45]Ca. Calcif. Tiss. *24:* 201, 1977.

12. Smith, D. M., and Johnston, C. C., III. Cyclic 3',5' Adenosine Monophosphate Levels in Separated Bone Cells. Endocrinology *96:* 1261, 1975.

13. Heersche, J. N. M., Marcus, R., and Aurbach, G. D. Calcitonin and the Formation of 3',5'-AMP in Bone and Kidney. Endocrinology *94:* 241, 1974.

13a. Talmage, R. V., Whitehurst, L. A., and Anderson, J. J. B. Effect of Calcitonin and Calcium Infusion on Plasma Phosphate. Endocrinology *92:* 792, 1973.

13b. Talmage, R. V., Doppelt, S. H., and Postma, J. H., Jr. Observations on the Relationship of Parathyroid Hormone and Calcitonin to Plasma and Liver Phosphate. Proc. Soc. Exp. Biol. Med. *153:* 131, 1976.

13c. Talmage, R. V., Anderson, J. J. B., and Kennedy, J. W. III. Separation of the Hypocalcemic and Hypophosphatemic Actions of Calcitonin with Disodium Ethane-1-Hydroxy-1,1-Diphosphonate. Endocrinology *94:* 413, 1974.

14. Hirsch, P. F. Enhancement of Hypocalcemic Activity of Thyrocalcitonin by Inorganic Phosphate, in *Calcitonin,* edited by S. Taylor. Springer, New York, 1968, p. 11.

15. Talmage, R. V., Matthews, J. L., Martin, J. H., et al. Calcitonin, Phosphate and the Osteocyte-Osteoblast Bone Cell Unit, in *Calcium-Regulating Hormones* edited by R. V. Talmage, M. Owen, and J. A. Parsons. Excerpta Medica, Amsterdam, 1975, p. 297.

16. Borle, A. B. Regulation of the Mitochondrial Control of Cellular Calcium Homeostasis and Calcium Transport by Phosphate, Parathyroid Hormone, Calcitonin, Vitamin D and Cyclic AMP, in *Calcium-Regulating Hormones,* edited by R. V. Talmage, M. Owen, and J. A. Parsons. Excerpta Medica, Amsterdam, 1975, p. 217.

17. Hennessy, J. F., Wells, S. A., Jr., Ontjes, D. A., et al. A Comparison of Pentagastrin Injection and Calcium Infusion as Provocative Agents for the Detection of Medullary Carcinoma of the Thyroid. J. Clin. Endocrinol. Metab. *39:* 487, 1974.

18. Talmage, R. V., Doppelt, S. H., and Cooper, C. W. Relationship of Blood Concentrations of Calcium, Phosphate, Gastrin and Calcitonin to the Onset of Feeding in the Rat. Proc. Soc. Exp. Biol. Med. *149:* 855, 1975.

19. Bolman, R. M., III, Cooper, C. W., Garner, S. C., Munson, P. L., and Wells, S. A., Jr. Stimulation of Gastrin Secretion in the Pig by Parathyroid Hormone and Its Inhibition by Thyrocalcitonin. Endocrinology *100:* 1014, 1977.

20. Munson, P. L. Physiology and Pharmacology of Thyrocalcitoning, in *Handbook of Physiology,* Section 7, *Endocrinology,* edited by E. B. Astwood and R. O. Greep. American Physiological Society, Washington, D.C., 1976, vol. 7, pp. 443–464.

51

Vitamin D: Biosynthesis, Metabolism, and Mode of Action

Hector F. DeLuca
Michael F. Holick

The disease rickets was recognized even in antiquity and was described in detail in 1645.[1] However, it was not until 1919 that the disease was related to nutritional deficiency. At that time, Sir Edward Mellanby was able to produce the disease in dogs by dietary means and was able to prevent or cure the disease with cod liver oil.[2] Although he ascribed the activity to newly discovered vitamin A, it soon became clear that this activity was due to a new substance which McCollum and his colleagues designated as a new fat-soluble vitamin D.[3] Confusion existed at that particular time, inasmuch as clinical investigators could demonstrate that rickets

Some of the original investigations in this review were supported by the Harry Steenbock Research Fund of the Wisconsin Alumni Research Foundation and a program-project grant from the National Institutes of Health No. AM-14881.

could also be cured in children by exposure to ultraviolet light from the sun or from artificial sources.[4] Steenbock and collaborators, and later Hess and collaborators, resolved the question when they demonstrated that irradiation of food and in particular the sterol fractions with ultraviolet light produced antirachitic activity.[5,6] This led ultimately to the isolation and identification of vitamin D_2 from irradiation mixtures of plant sterols by Askew et al.[7] and somewhat later by Windaus and collaborators.[8] It was not until 1937, however, that the natural form of the vitamin was isolated from irradiation mixtures of 7-dehydrocholesterol and identified.[9] Although other forms of vitamin D have been described or identified, there is little doubt that vitamin D_2 and vitamin D_3 represent the only significant forms of vitamin D.

From a physiologic point of view, it is well recognized that the vitamin performs three basic functions. First, it causes mineralization of bone, thus preventing osteomalacia in the adult and rickets in the young; second, it plays a role in the prevention of low-calcium tetany (although this was at first ascribed entirely to parathyroid hormone, it is now clear that the vitamin D system plays a role as important as that of parathyroid hormone); and third, in the muscle, the vitamin plays some role that has not yet been described from either a biochemical or a physiologic point of view. In all but the muscle function, it will become apparent in this contribution that the vitamin does not act directly but must be metabolically altered before it can carry out the functions that ultimately result in the alleviation of low-calcium tetany and of the bone lesions of rickets and osteomalacia. Besides these obvious relationships, it may be possible that derangements in vitamin D metabolism or function may contribute to other bone disorders being described in this volume.

The primary focus of this chapter is on the new advances in the metabolism of vitamin D, the regulation of the metabolism, and the mechanism of action of the active form of vitamin D in the target tissues.

BIOSYNTHESIS OF VITAMIN D

It is well recognized that if man were to receive sufficient exposure to ultraviolet light, he would not require dietary sources of vitamin D.[10] However, in the temperate zones of the earth and considering the habits by which man has chosen to live, there is a limitation on ultraviolet exposure of the skin and presumably the ability to synthesize vitamin D. As a result, especially during winter months, there is a clear dependence of man on dietary sources of the vitamin.

There are two major sources of the vitamin available to man through diet. Vitamin D is not widely distributed and is not found to any significant extent in the plant world. It is, however, found in large amounts in the livers of certain fish, sharks, and other sea animals, which have in the past provided therapeutic forms of the vitamin.[11] In addition, man has learned to artificially convert the plant sterol, ergosterol, to vitamin D_2 by ultraviolet irradiation. Thus the fortification of foods in many countries is from vitamin D_2, which historically has been the more readily available and least expensive. Although this has changed in recent years, vitamin D_2 still remains a significant and major source of the vitamin.

The biosynthesis of vitamin D in skin has not been a well-studied process. At present, it is recognized that skin taken from rachitic animals possesses no antirachitic activity but attains antirachitic activity upon exposure to ultraviolet light. A major sterol component of skin is 7-dehydrocholesterol,[10,12] and the biosynthesis of this substance has been well studied, although it is beyond the scope of this chapter. Interested readers are directed elsewhere for a discussion of biosynthesis of 7-dehydrocholesterol in skin and other organs.[10] The 7-dehydrocholesterol of skin is found in the epidermis, a site to which ultraviolet light is known to penetrate easily. From a chemical point of view, it is known that 7-dehydrocholesterol exposed to 280–320 nm of ultraviolet light will undergo a photolysis yielding not only a substance known as previtamin D_3 but also other closely related isomers that do not possess vitamin D activity. The previtamin D_3 then undergoes spontaneous but temperature-dependent conversion to vitamin D_3. Although vitamin D_3 is the suspected product from the skin process, it has never been satisfactorily isolated and identified. Furthermore, it is unknown whether or not the side-reaction products of irradiation are found in skin tissue following exposure to ultraviolet light. It is indeed possible that the 7-dehydrocholesterol is bound to some protein or template that would help provide specificity of conversion to the vitamin D structure rather than to the inactive photoisomers. However, this remains to be clarified. It is believed that the product of the irradiation of skin, therefore, is vitamin D_3, whose structure is shown in Figure 51-1. For a comparison, the structure of vitamin D_2 is also shown, as are their precursors, 7-dehydrocholesterol and ergosterol.

Although the process of irradiation of skin and conversion of 7-dehydrocholesterol to vitamin D_3 has never been studied from a biochemical point of view, recently it has been shown that sunbathers exposed to large amounts of ultraviolet irradiation show increased circulating levels of 25-hydroxyvitamin D_3 (25-OH-D_3),[13] the major metabolite of the vitamin, thus providing additional evidence for the idea that vitamin D_3 is the product of skin irradiation.

The only other known biosynthetic source of vitamin D is that found in fish livers.[11] There has been much controversy about whether the vitamin D found in shark and fish liver oils originates from the food they ingest or from the production of vitamin D by a nonphotochemical process. In the authors' view, this question has not been settled, despite experiments reported to the contrary. In the most definitive experiments carried out, Bills[14] studied the production of vitamin D_3 in the oils of catfish grown in the absence of light and on a regulated and defined diet. He demonstrated that these fish accumulate vitamin D during this time, and he therefore suggested that there must be a nonphotochemical production of vitamin D_3 in the animals. Unfortunately, small amounts of vitamin D in the diet provided could have easily been accumulated in these fish if they have no mechanism whereby this sterol could be degraded and excreted. Thus, this experiment is not conclusive.

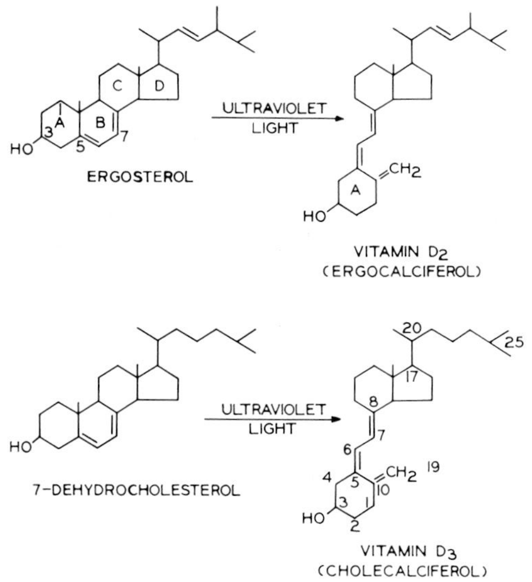

Fig. 51-1. Vitamin D_2 and vitamin D_3 production by irradiation of their respective sterol precursors.

More recently, attempts with livers from Atlantic striped bass have been made to demonstrate a nonphotochemical process whereby vitamin D_3 might be produced. Again, as Blondin et al.[14a] point out, the experiments were inconclusive. Therefore, the question of whether sharks and fish can produce vitamin D by a nonphotochemical process remains unanswered.

Finally, it should be recognized that there are other forms and sources of vitamin D that have not yet been identified and that may considerably alter the considerations of whether there is biosynthesis of vitamin D in other species. Of particular importance is the plant *Solanum malacoxylon,* which produces a calcification toxicity in cattle that ingest the leaves.[15] Present evidence suggests that this plant and its relatives produce a substance that acts very similarly to the active metabolite of vitamin D, 1,25-dihydroxyvitamin D_3 (1,25-$(OH)_2D_3$), and it was suggested that the active component is a $1\alpha,25$-$(OH)_2D_3$-glycoside.[15A]

ABSORPTION OF VITAMIN D

Naturally, vitamin D is found in high concentrations in the livers of fish and sharks.[14] In addition, man now provides large amounts of vitamin D_2 and vitamin D_3 as food supplements or as additives of such foods as milk, bread, and butter. It is, therefore, important to consider the route whereby vitamin D is absorbed. Unfortunately, little information is available. It seems clear that the absorption of vitamin D requires the presence of bile salts.[16,17] The site of vitamin D absorption has not been settled and in fact remains controversial. Using in vitro preparations Schachter and colleagues[17] have concluded that vitamin D is absorbed more rapidly in the upper segments of small intestine. Using indirect in vivo studies, other investigators have concluded that vitamin D dissolved in oil is absorbed in the distal small intestine.[18,19] Obviously, more definitive work will have to be done before this issue can be settled. Because of its lipid-soluble nature, it seems quite likely that vitamin D is absorbed through the lymphatic system.[20] It is therefore apparent that patients suffering from malabsorption disorders may well show a malabsorption of vitamin D. Also, patients suffering from a defect in bile salt secretion or manufacture will likely have difficulty in absorbing sufficient quantities of vitamin D. Therefore, calcium metabolic abnormalities in diseases of the small intestine such as celiac disease, blind-loop syndrome, and Whipple's disease may in part be related to failure of vitamin D absorption.

METABOLISM OF VITAMIN D₃ (FIGURE 51-2)

CONVERSION OF VITAMIN D₃ TO 25-OH-D₃, THE MAJOR CIRCULATING FORM OF THE VITAMIN

It is well accepted that upon administration of vitamin D from a variety of sources, it accumulates in the liver within the first hour.[21,22] The degree of this accumulation has been set at between 40 and 80 percent, depending upon the study and investigator. It nevertheless seems certain that the liver is the major initial site of appearance of the vitamin molecule after its entry into the systemic circulation. In the liver the vitamin undergoes 25-hydroxylation.[22–24] The site of this hydroxylation is believed to be the endoplasmic reticulum or microsomal fraction and this reaction requires NADPH, molecular oxygen, and magnesium ions.[24,25] There has been a report that 25-hydroxylation of vitamin D also occurs in intestine and kidney.[26] This work was carried out in chicks in which in vitro preparations of these organs can be shown to carry out vitamin D-25-hydroxylation. However, comparable rat and human tissues do not show this capability, which suggests that this peculiarity may only be related to avian species. Furthermore, the fact that vitamin D₃ accumulates largely in the liver suggests that even if the kidney and intestine possess 25-hydroxylation activity, they probably provide quantitatively insignificant amounts of 25-hydroxylation.[21]

The vitamin D-25-hydroxylase in the liver appears to be regulated by the product of the reaction.[25] It seems that the hepatic level of 25-OH-D₃ in some way suppresses vitamin D-25-hydroxylase activity. It is certain that vitamin-D-deficient rats or chicks given a dose of vitamin D will show markedly reduced vitamin D-25-hydroxylase activity when measured in vitro, and this suppression could not have been due to dilution of the radioactive sub-

strate. The degree and length of this suppression are related to the dose of the vitamin given to the deficient animals.

To what extent regulation of 25-hydroxylation occurs in vivo is a matter of considerable debate. It seems certain that, in the near-physiologic range, regulation does occur. It is also well known that, if large amounts of vitamin D are given, increased amounts of 25-OH-D₃ can be found in the plasma,[27,28] suggesting that the regulatory system is of limited capacity and ability. The mechanism of overcoming the suppression remains unknown, but it may be related to the existence of a nonspecific cholesterol 25-hydroxylase found in liver tissue. This enzyme will act on vitamin D if provided in sufficient quantities. Thus, this enzyme, which is not subject to feedback inhibition or regulation, may produce large amounts of 25-OH-D₃ once the substrate concentration is high enough to permit activity. Whatever the mechanism, the 25-hydroxylation regulation must be regarded as one that does function in the physiologic range but that can be overcome by large and pharmacological amounts of vitamin D.

The 25-OH-D₃ is two to five times more active than vitamin D₃ itself in curing rickets, in the elevation of intestinal calcium absorption, in intestinal phosphorus absorption, and in the mobilization of calcium from bone in rats.[29] It is more rapidly turned over than vitamin D₃ itself, which means its biological activity is more short-lived than that of the vitamin itself. Although the 25-OH-D₃ can be shown to cause bone resorption when added to cultures in vitro,[30] it seems that at physiologic doses, 25-OH-D₃ does not participate in any of the known functions of the vitamin and must be further metabolically altered before it can carry out its functions.[31,32] As far as is known at present, 25-OH-D₃ is an essential intermediate for the production of all other known metabolites. One can, therefore, consider that the 25-hydroxylation is the primary conversion point and the last point beyond which the metabolism of vitamin D branches to different pathways.

METABOLISM OF 25-OH-D₃ TO 1,25-(OH)₂D₃

In the nephrectomized animal, 25-OH-D₃ will not stimulate intestinal calcium transport, mobilization of calcium from bone, or intestinal phosphate transport, at least when given at physiologic doses.[31,32] It is now known that the 25-OH-D₃ must be metabolized

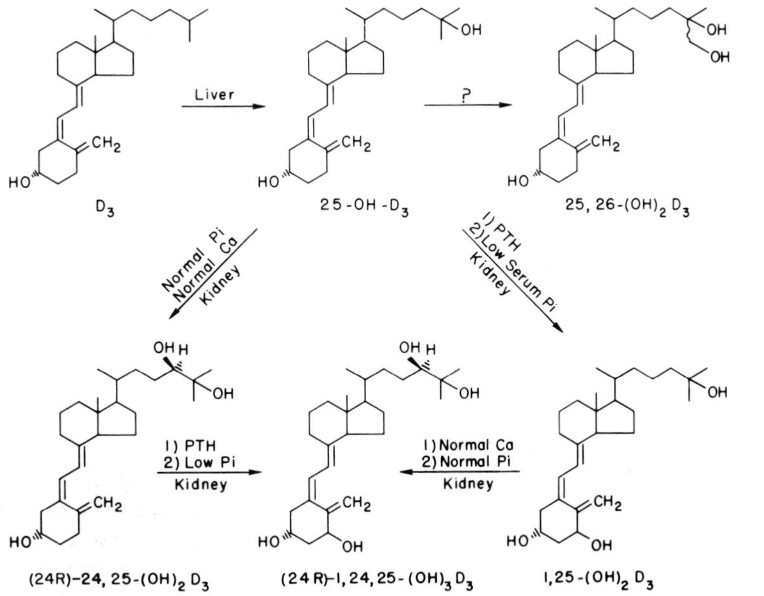

Fig. 51-2. Summary of the known metabolic reactions involving vitamin D and their points of regulation.

further before it can carry out these functions. 25-OH-D$_3$ is transported to the kidney, where it undergoes conversion to 1,25-(OH)$_2$D$_3$, the most potent form of vitamin D known.[33,34] This reaction is presumed to occur in the proximal convoluted tubules, but this has not yet been established. Nevertheless, it is known to occur in the mitochondria, and much is known concerning the biochemistry of this reaction.[35] The reaction requires reducing equivalents generated from Krebs-cycle substrates, molecular oxygen, and magnesium ions. It has been demonstrated that NADPH is the specific reducing substance needed[36] and, furthermore, that oxygen derived from molecular oxygen is activated and incorporated into the 25-OH-D$_3$ molecule to form 1,25-(OH)$_2$D$_3$, demonstrating this to be a mixed-function oxidase.[37] The reaction is dependent upon a cytochrome P-450, as demonstrated by its extreme carbon monoxide sensitivity and by the fact that carbon monoxide inhibition is alleviated by white light or, preferably, by 450-nm wavelength light.[36,38] It is also inhibited by glutethimide and metyrapone, all suggesting dependence on cytochrome P-450.[39] More recent work has shown that isolated chick kidney mitochondria contain significant amounts of a cytochrome P-450, which is reducible by malate. This cytochrome P-450 has now been solubilized from mitochondrial membrane and has been combined with both beef adrenal ferredoxin and beef adrenal ferredoxin reductase to reconstruct an active 25-OH-D$_3$-1-hydroxylase system.[39,40] More recently, an iron-sulphur protein called renal ferredoxin has been isolated in pure form from rachitic chick mitochondria and shown to be a component of this hydroxylase. In continuing reconstruction experiments, it has now been demonstrated that this system contains a flavoprotein (an iron-sulfur protein), called renal ferredoxin, and a cytochrome P-450, which function, as shown in Figure 51-3, in converting 25-OH-D$_3$ to the 1,25-(OH)$_2$D$_3$. Exactly where in isolated mitochondria this system exists is not yet clear.

Although the estimates of biological activity of 1,25-(OH)$_2$D$_3$ range anywhere from 2 times that of vitamin D$_3$ to 33 times, if it is administered daily in a careful log/dose study, it seems clear that its biological activity is somewhere between 8 to 10 times that of vitamin D$_3$.[29] Of great importance is the fact that 1,25-(OH)$_2$D$_3$ stimulates intestinal calcium transport,[31] intestinal phosphate transport,[41] and bone calcium mobilization[32] in nephrectomized animals as well as it does in normals.

Since nephrectomized animals cannot produce 1,25-(OH)$_2$D$_3$, it is apparent that the kidney is the sole site of 1-hydroxylation and, therefore, since nephrectomized animals cannot respond to 25-

OH-D$_3$ but do respond to 1,25-(OH)$_2$D$_3$, it is clear that 1,25-(OH$_2$D$_3$ and not its precursors represents the metabolically active form of the vitamin. Furthermore, since the renal 25-OH-D-1α-hydroxylase does not hydroxylate vitamin D$_3$ but will act only on a vitamin that contains the hydroxyl in the 25 position, it is evident that 25-hydroxylation is also essential for the function of vitamin D. Since 1,25-(OH)$_2$D$_3$ originates in the kidney and stimulates intestine and bone, this substance can be regarded as a hormone.[42]

BIOSYNTHESIS OF 24,25-DIHYDROXYVITAMIN D$_3$

When animals are vitamin D deficient and are given a source of radioactive vitamin D, they convert the vitamin D to 25-OH-D$_3$ and subsequently to 1,25-(OH)$_2$D$_3$.[43] However, when they are given diets high in calcium and a source of vitamin D, vitamin D$_3$ is converted to 25-OH-D$_3$ and predominantly to another metabolite, which has been isolated and identified as 24,25-dihydroxyvitamin D$_3$ (24,25-(OH)$_2$D$_3$)[44]. The site of this metabolism is the kidney, inasmuch as nephrectomy will reduce the conversion of 25-OH-D$_3$ in vivo to the 24,25-(OH)$_2$D$_3$. There is some evidence that the 24-hydroxylase is not confined to the kidney, although a major site of this reaction is in renal tissue.[45] In vitamin-D-deficient animals, there is virtually no 25-OH-D$_3$-24-hydroxylase, and it is now known that 1,25-(OH)$_2$D$_3$ induces or causes the formation of the 25-OH-D$_3$-24-hydroxylase in renal tissue.

The 24-hydroxylase has been studied extensively in chick kidney mitochondria, and shows a requirement for NADPH, molecular oxygen, and magnesium ions.[46] This hydroxylase is not sensitive to carbon monoxide and other inhibitors of the cytochrome P-450 series of reactions. Little is known beyond that, and much work remains to be carried out.

There are two possible isomers of 24,25-(OH)$_2$D$_3$, as shown in Figure 51-4; they are the 24R and 24S isomers. Both isomers have been chemically synthesized.[47-49] The availability of the synthetic compounds permitted an examination of the natural product, and by means of cochromatography of the isomeric mixture with the radioactive natural product, it was possible to demonstrate conclusively that the natural form of the 24,25-(OH)$_2$D$_3$ has the R configuration.[50]

The role of the 24-hydroxylation reaction in general and the role of the 24,25-(OH)$_2$D$_3$ have not been settled. However, it is important to realize that the 24-hydroxylase will hydroxylate not only the 25-OH-D$_3$ but also 1,25-(OH)$_2$D$_3$ to give either the 24,25-(OH)$_2$D$_3$ or the 1,24,25-trihydroxyvitamin D$_3$ (1,24,25-(OH)$_3$D$_3$).[51] Inasmuch as the 24-hydroxylase appears whenever there is a

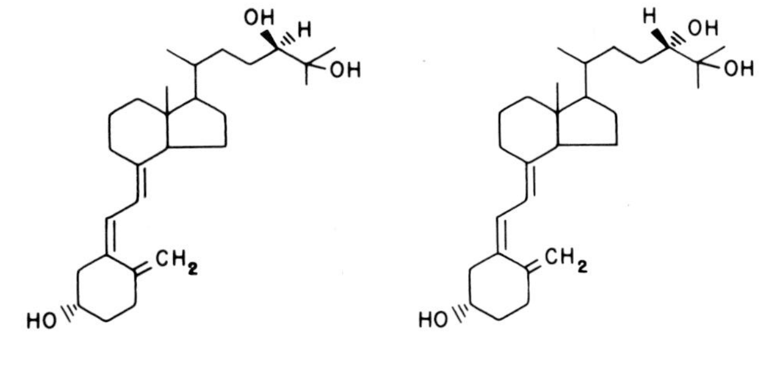

COMPONENTS OF 25-OH-D$_3$-1α-HYDROXYLASE

OF CHICK KIDNEY

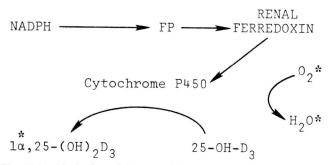

NADPH ⟶ FP ⟶ RENAL FERREDOXIN

Cytochrome P450

O$_2$*

H$_2$O*

1α,25-(OH)$_2$D$_3$ 25-OH-D$_3$

Fig. 51-3. Mechanism of 1-hydroxylation of 25-OH-D$_3$ by the renal 1-hydroxylase system.

24 R 24,25-(OH)$_2$D$_3$ 24 S 24,25-(OH)$_2$D$_3$

Fig. 51-4. Stereoisomers of 24,25-(OH)$_2$D$_3$. The natural form of this compound has the R configuration.

suppression of the 25-OH-D$_3$-1-hydroxylase, it could be suggested that the 24-hydroxylase is intimately associated with the regulatory phenomenon that will be described in a subsequent section. Alternatively, one can ask what might be the possible metabolic or target-tissue function of 24,25-(OH)$_2$D$_3$. An examination of biological activity of the 24,25-(OH)$_2$D$_3$ in vitamin-D-deficient rats revealed the striking observation that the 24-hydroxylated vitamin D's have marked biological activity approaching that of their non-24-hydroxylated counterparts.[50,52,53] However, inasmuch as this compound is not made in the vitamin-D-deficient animal, the testing of its biological activity in a deficient animal would appear to be inappropriate. Unfortunately it is not possible to test clearly its biological activity in a normal animal. However, an examination of the biological effectiveness of the 24-hydroxylated compounds in the vitamin-D-deficient chick gives quite a different picture. It is quite apparent that in this species the 24-hydroxylated vitamins are much less active than their non-24-hydroxylated analogs. This suggests that 24-hydroxylation may represent the initial step in the subsequent metabolism and elimination of the vitamin D molecule.[54] In support of this concept, an examination of the metabolism of the 24-hydroxylated vitamin D's has revealed that it is very rapidly metabolized and excreted in the chicken.[54] Although alternate suggestions have been made that the 24,25-(OH)$_2$D$_3$ plays some role in the mineralization process or that it plays some role in suppression of parathyroid hormone secretion, this has not as yet been supported by experimental evidence. The current view, therefore, is that 24-hydroxylation is the first metabolic reaction leading to inactivation of the vitamin D molecule.

This concept has led to the suggestion that the discrimination against vitamin D$_2$ by the chicken and other fowl is because the vitamin D$_2$ molecule, which possesses a methyl group on carbon 24, resembles structurally a 24-hydroxylated vitamin, which is earmarked for rapid metabolism and elimination. However, much additional work is required in the area of 24-hydroxylation, the nature of the reaction, and biological meaning of its product.

1,24,25-TRIHYDROXYVITAMIN D$_3$

During the course of an examination of the biological activity of 24,25-(OH)$_2$D$_3$, it was learned that in the rachitic or vitamin-D-deficient rat, 24,25-(OH)$_2$D$_3$ could not exert its biological effectiveness when the animals were nephrectomized.[53] This suggested that to be effective in the vitamin-D-deficient animal, the 24,25-(OH)$_2$D$_3$ must be hydroxylated on carbon 1. With radioactive 24,25-(OH)$_2$D$_3$, it was possible to demonstrate that it is converted to a more polar compound.[53] This compound could be produced by in vitro incubation with rachitic chick kidney mitochondria, which led ultimately to the isolation and identification of its structure as 1,24,25-(OH)$_3$D$_3$.[55] Its structure has subsequently been confirmed by chemical synthesis. Furthermore, the production of this compound could also be demonstrated by the incubation of 1,25-(OH)$_2$D$_3$ with kidney mitochondria from rats given high calcium diets plus vitamin D.[51] In experiments in which vitamin D$_3$ or 25-OH-D$_3$ has been given to vitamin-D-deficient animals, however, very little 1,24-25-(OH)$_3$D$_3$ has been demonstrated, raising the question of whether it is a physiologically important metabolite. However, more recent work with chronically administered radioactive vitamin D$_3$ has demonstrated that it is a significant metabolite of vitamin D but that its role remains unknown (Ribovich and DeLuca, unpublished results).

The biological activity of 1,24,25-(OH)$_3$D$_3$ has revealed that it

is less active than 1,25-(OH)$_2$D$_3$.[55] In the rat, its activity on intestine is approximately 60 percent that of 1,25-(OH)$_2$D$_3$, whereas in the chick it is less than 10 percent.[54] There is no doubt, therefore, that the 1,24,25-(OH)$_3$D$_3$ is less biologically active than its non-24-hydroxylated counterpart, suggesting that it could actually be the initial reaction for inactivation and elimination.

METABOLISM OF 1,25-(OH)$_2$D$_3$

Inasmuch as 1,25-(OH)$_2$D$_3$ must be regarded as the most potent metabolite of vitamin D and as the most likely metabolically active form of the vitamin, its metabolism is of great interest. Following the demonstration that 1,25-(OH)$_2$D$_3$ is fully active in anephric animals, while its precursor is not, the conclusion could be made that 1,25-(OH)$_2$D$_3$ or a further metabolite is the metabolically active form in the target tissue. To determine whether there was further metabolism, radioactive 1,25-(OH)$_2$D$_3$ was prepared with the radioactive label in either the terminal part of side chain or in ring A, and at the time the intestine and bone responded maximally to this radioactive 1,25-(OH)$_2$D$_3$, the tissues were removed, extracted, and chromatographed to reveal only one peak of radioactivity corresponding to 1,25-(OH)$_2$D$_3$.[56-58] However, only 80 percent of the tissue radioactivity could be accounted for even at 6 hours after dosage, which suggests that an additional 20 percent of radioactivity was located elsewhere. In addition, poor recoveries of total tritium from tritiated 1,25-(OH)$_2$D$_3$ were experienced when it was given to either rats or chicks. Because the label for these studies was primarily the 1,25-(OH)$_2$-[26,27-^{3}H]D$_3$, it was considered that possibly some of the label was lost as a result of the metabolism of the side chain. Consequently, 25-OH-[26,27-^{14}C]D$_3$ was prepared chemically and injected into vitamin-D-deficient animals. Surprisingly, it was found that 7 percent of the administered ^{14}C on C-26 and C-27 appeared in the expired carbon dioxide. Nephrectomy eliminated the evolution of carbon dioxide from the 25-OH-D$_3$, suggesting that this compound must undergo 1-hydroxylation before it is subsequently subjected to side-chain oxidation.[59,60] The preparation of 26,27-^{14}C-labeled 1,25-(OH)$_2$D$_3$ revealed that as much as 30 percent of the injected 1,25-(OH)$_2$D$_3$ yielded its terminal 26 and 27 carbons as expired ^{14}CO$_2$, illustrating that side-chain oxidation represents a major path of 1,25-(OH)$_2$D$_3$ metabolism. Inasmuch as the metabolism as 1,25-(OH)$_2$D$_3$ to carbon dioxide occurred at 4 hours after administration, it seemed plausible that a side-chain oxidation may have functional significance. It certainly may have significance as an inactivation mechanism of this very potent hormone. In any case, this metabolic sequence should be of considerable importance to our understanding of the metabolism and function of vitamin D.

Besides being metabolized to the 1,24,25-(OH)$_3$D$_3$ and to the compound that results from side-chain oxidation, little is known concerning the further metabolism of 1,25-(OH)$_2$D$_3$. Of great interest is the fact that 1,25-(OH)$_2$D$_3$ given to rats will cause the intestine to transport calcium for at least 96 hours after dosage.[55] However, there remains in the intestine at that time significant amounts of 1,25-(OH)$_2$D$_3$, so that it may still remain as the active principle in the maintenance of this metabolic function. The turnover of 1,25-(OH)$_2$D$_3$ is much more rapid than that of 25-OH-D$_3$. Although $t_{1/2}$'s have been estimated for plasma in man at about 1 day, the $t_{1/2}$'s for tissues that are functional in response to the 1,25-(OH)$_2$D$_3$ have not been estimated. It seems certain, however, that 1,25-(OH)$_2$D$_3$ is metabolized much more rapidly than either 25-OH-D$_3$ or vitamin D$_3$.

OTHER METABOLITES OF VITAMIN D

The only other known metabolite of vitamin D is 25,26-dihydroxyvitamin D_3 (25,26-$(OH)_2D_3$).[61] Although it has been isolated, identified, and synthesized, the site of its synthesis is unknown, and its biological function, if any, remains unknown. In terms of biological activity, 25,26-$(OH)_2D_3$ is the least active of the isolated and identified metabolites, showing activity only in intestinal calcium transport but at a level much lower than that of 25-OH-D_3. Because of its low biological activity, it has received little attention and may represent either an excretory product or a biochemical curiosity.

EXCRETION OF VITAMIN D AND ITS METABOLITES

The primary excretion route for vitamin D is the bile, with less than 4 percent of the radioactivity from vitamin D appearing in urinary products.[18,20] So far, no excretory products have been identified from a chemical point of view, although the presence of vitamin D sulfates has been shown to occur after large doses of vitamin D.[62] A vitamin D sulfate has been postulated to represent the form of vitamin D that is found in normal milk,[63] but so far little work on this has appeared, and no confirmation has yet been forthcoming. In the case of bile, there is some evidence for glucuronide conjugates of vitamin D and its metabolites, but so far chemical evidence is lacking.[20,64]

VITAMIN D_2

Throughout the course of the investigation of vitamin D metabolism, vitamin D_3 has been the major substance studied because of the availability of labeled compounds and because vitamin D_3 probably represents the natural form of the vitamin. However, vitamin D_2 was the first labeled vitamin D to be prepared. Recent work with ^{14}C-vitamin D_2 and ^{3}H-vitamin D_2 has appeared, demonstrating that vitamin D_2 is metabolized normally both in mammals and in birds to 25-hydroxyvitamin D_2 (25-OH-D_2).[65,66] Furthermore, 25-OH-D_2 is converted to 1,25-dihydroxyvitamin D_2 (1,25-$(OH)_2D_2$) in both rats and chicks.[67] In fact, chicken preparations in vitro carry out the 25- and the 1-hydroxylation reactions at approximately the same rate as they hydroxylate the vitamin D_3 derivatives.[66] 25-OH-D_2 and 1,25-$(OH)_2D_2$ have both been isolated and their structures unequivocally demonstrated. These substances in the rat are equal to their vitamin D_3 counterparts in biopotency, but in the chicken they are approximately one-tenth as active as their vitamin D_3 analogues.[67,68] More recent work has demonstrated that chick tissues will also carry out 24-hydroxylation of vitamin D_2, which does indicate that the substitution on carbon 24 does not interfere with this hydroxylation reaction (Jones and DeLuca, unpublished results).

A major biological problem has been an understanding of the biochemical basis of discrimination by birds against vitamin D_2. It is well known that vitamin-D-deficient chicks show only one-tenth the biological response to vitamin D_2 that they show when compared with vitamin D_3. When the metabolism of radioactive vitamin D_3 and vitamin D_2 was compared, it seemed clear that chicks rapidly metabolize and excrete the radioactive vitamin D_2. Although the enzymes that carry out the subsequent activation of the vitamin D molecule are active on the vitamin D_2 compounds in the bird, all the metabolites are one-tenth as active as their vitamin D_3 counterparts.[68] It therefore appears that 24 substitution in some way signals rapid metabolism and excretion of the vitamin D_2 molecule, thereby removing it from biological function and resulting in low biological activity. So far, however, the site of the discrimination has not been exactly described, and the elimination products have not been identified.

TRANSPORT OF VITAMIN D_3 AND ITS METABOLITES IN BLOOD

Both vitamin D and its major metabolites do not circulate in the free form in the plasma. Much work has been expended by a variety of laboratories in studying the proteins of blood which bind vitamin D and its metabolites. It now appears that the major vitamin D transport protein is a 4S material that migrates on disc-gel electrophoresis in the α-globulin region.[69–71] This protein has been isolated in pure form from rats[72] and from humans,[73] showing a molecular weight of approximately 51,000–52,000. It binds 1 mol of 25-OH-D_3 per mole of protein and it appears to bind with much less affinity vitamin D_3 and 1,25-$(OH)_2D_3$. Vitamin D_3 is also bound to β-lipoprotein, and occasionally some binding is found with serum albumin. Thus far, no disease state has been described in which there is a deficiency of the vitamin D transport protein, nor has there been any demonstration that this transport protein is regulated or disturbed by drug administration or various disease states.

OVERALL MECHANISM OF ACTION OF VITAMIN D

In order to consider the functional role of vitamin D and its metabolites, it is essential to have in hand a systematic overall view of the function of vitamin D. A deficiency of vitamin D results in a variety of physiological and pathological disturbances. Under conditions of calcium deprivation and vitamin D deficiency, low-calcium tetany is the major symptomatic condition. However, under conditions of phosphate depletion, low-calcium tetany is not of concern, but instead hypophosphatemia and severe osteomalacia and rickets are the result. Certainly one defect in vitamin D deficiency is a failure of bone mineralization, as revealed by osteomalacia or rickets. This failure of mineralization of newly deposited organic matrix has led investigators to seek a role of vitamin D in the mineralization process. Although it is an intellectually satisfying concept, supporting evidence is lacking. Since it has not been disproved, the possibility must be left open for continued investigation. The major reason for failure of mineralization is an inadequate supply of calcium and phosphorus to the newly forming bone centers. Blood is normally supersaturated with regard to calcium and phosphorus, and it is well known that in rickets and extreme cases of osteomalacia there is a decreased level of these two mineral components in the blood. At least a major function of the vitamin, therefore, is to elevate serum calcium and phosphorus to levels required for normal mineralization or to levels required to prevent low-calcium tetany.[74] The role of vitamin D in the maintenance of serum calcium and phosphorus levels was recognized in the early 1920s and perhaps interpreted in an oversimplified manner, which led to a disregard of this concept in subsequent years.

The elevation of serum calcium in response to vitamin D results from a variety of mechanisms. The best known is that vitamin D stimulates intestinal calcium absorption. This is an active transport process in which calcium is transported against an electrical and chemical gradient with phosphate as the normal accompanying anion.[74] In addition to this process, vitamin D activates a phosphate transport reaction that is independent of the calcium transport reaction, providing another supply of the phosphate anion.[41,75–77] Vitamin D also activates the mobilization of calcium from previously formed bone to the extracellular fluid compartment.[78] This process requires both vitamin D and the parathyroid hormone and represents perhaps one of the most important reactions that is utilized in maintaining serum calcium concentrations at the normal range. It is not known to what extent vitamin D influences renal reabsorption of calcium and phosphorus, although some effect clearly seems likely.

In addition to these well-known effects, it is also suspected that vitamin D has a role in muscle function and metabolism. So far, however, this has not been approached in a systematic way, and the current results available are not convincing. However, clinicians treating patients with vitamin D are often greatly surprised by the marked stimulation of muscle strength and tone by vitamin D preparations. It is likely that the muscle will come under close scrutiny in the next few years and will probably reveal a basic biochemical function for vitamin D in this tissue.

In all these functions of vitamin D, it is now apparent that the vitamin at physiologic doses must be metabolized to $1,25$-$(OH)_2D_3$ or further to an unknown metabolite before these functions can be exercised. Therefore, in considering the mechanism of action of vitamin D in the subsequent discussion, attention will be focused on $1,25$-$(OH)_2D_3$ rather than the parent vitamin or its 25-hydroxy derivative.

MECHANISM OF ACTION OF $1,25$-$(OH)_2D_3$ IN INTESTINE (FIG. 51-5)

In 1923, Orr et al. suggested that vitamin D improves the absorption of calcium based on a study showing a decrease in fecal calcium upon vitamin D administration.[79] Although this important basic work was criticized for a number of years, in 1937, Nicolaysen[80] was able to demonstrate unequivocally that vitamin D improves intestinal calcium absorption. This basic observation was studied repeatedly for approximately two decades, but it was the work of Schachter and Rosen which showed for the first time that vitamin D stimulates the transfer of calcium against a concentration gradient in the small intestine.[81] Subsequently, it was clearly demonstrated that this transfer process occurred against not only a concentration gradient but also an electrical-potential gradient, thus answering the criterion that calcium is transported by an active process.[82–84] Continued investigation has revealed that vitamin D produces an alteration in the microvillus region of the small intestine which permits calcium to enter the mucosal cells.[84] Although Schachter and colleagues believe that vitamin D also affects the transfer of calcium across the basal-lateral membrane,

convincing evidence is lacking. Thus, there is uniform agreement that a site for vitamin D stimulation of intestinal calcium transport is the brush border or microvillus region and there remains the possibility that vitamin D does stimulate transfer across the basal-lateral membrane as well.

Exactly how $1,25$-$(OH)_2D_3$ stimulates intestinal calcium transport has not been convincingly demonstrated. The most popular hypothesis is that $1,25$-$(OH)_2D_3$ combines with a receptor protein in the intestinal cytosol, which then interacts with the intestinal mucosal nuclei, causing the transcription of messenger that codes for calcium transport proteins.[85] These calcium transport proteins, in an ill-defined manner, then function at the brush border surface to facilitate the transport of calcium. The evidence to support this view is the fact that after administration of radioactive $1,25$-$(OH)_2D_3$ the major intestinal subcellular site of location is the nuclear fraction.[86] However, convincing evidence that it is the nuclei that accumulate the $1,25$-$(OH)_2D_3$ has not yet been put forth. Work has been done which demonstrates that $1,25$-$(OH)_2D_3$ accumulates in the chromatin fraction; however, there is some disagreement as to the nature of the chromatin fraction isolated. When chromatin is isolated by published methods to yield homogeneous chromatin, little $1,25$-$(OH)_2D_3$ is found bound.[86] However, when chromatin is isolated by a modified procedure, essentially all of the nuclear-related $1,25$-$(OH)_2D_3$ is found, but the chromatin fraction is highly impure, revealing a variety of other subcellular constituents.[87] Additional evidence includes the demonstration of the existence of a protein in the cytosol of intestinal mucosa from rachitic chicks which binds $1,25$-$(OH)_2D_3$ in a specific manner[88] (Kream and DeLuca, unpublished results) and which then can be shown to bind in a temperature-dependent process to isolated impure chromatin.[88] While this demonstration is quite clear in the chick, so far no specific binding protein has been found in any mammalian species despite intensive investigation (Kream, DeLuca, and Reynolds, unpublished results). In fact, the only binding protein that can be found in the intestine is a 5–6S protein, which prefers to bind 25-OH-D_3 instead of the $1,25$-$(OH)_2D_3$.[89] This 6S protein is found in a number of tissues, many of them nontarget organs, which raises considerable doubt as to whether it represents a receptor or not. Furthermore, new results from this laboratory have demonstrated that the 6S protein can be washed from whole cells, suggesting that the 6S protein may not be a cytoplasmic protein at all but a protein that is loosely bound to the surface of the cells. In any case, uniform acceptance of the existence of a cytosol receptor for $1,25$-$(OH)_2D_3$ is not yet available.

Other evidence for the nuclear-receptor hypothesis in the chick has come from Lawson and Emtage,[90] who have been able to show that polysomes isolated from chicks given vitamin D produce the calcium-binding protein originally described by Wasserman and Taylor, whereas those from rachitic chicks do not produce this substance. Against the receptor hypothesis is the observation that actinomycin D, which is known to bind to DNA and prevent transcription, will not block $1,25$-$(OH)_2D_3$-induced intestinal calcium transport in rats.[91] In the chick, some evidence to show that actinomycin D will prevent the intestinal response to $1,25$-$(OH)_2D_3$ has been presented; however, convincing evidence is lacking, inasmuch as actinomycin D is extremely toxic, especially in the chick.[92]

The nature of the change at the brush-border surface has also received considerable attention. Wasserman and colleagues have demonstrated the existence of a calcium-binding protein that appears in response to vitamin D in the intestinal mucosa of chicks.[93] These investigators have isolated this protein shown to have a molecular weight of the order of 24,000 and to bind four molecules

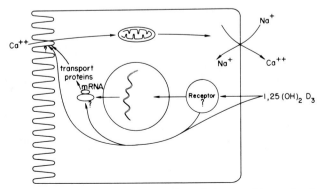

Fig. 51-5. Diagrammatic representation of the possible mechanisms whereby $1,25$-$(OH)_2D_3$ initiates intestinal calcium absorption.

of calcium per mole of protein. With fluorescent antibodies, they have demonstrated that the protein is found in the goblet cells and on the surface of the intestinal epithelial cells but not in the cytoplasm.[94] Other investigators have now disputed this finding and thus the subcellular location of the calcium-binding protein at the present time remains in doubt. The fact that this calcium-binding protein appears in response to vitamin D and that it binds calcium and that other physiologic modifications of calcium transport also modify the level of calcium-binding protein argue strongly for its participation in calcium transport. However, a close quantitative examination of its appearance and disappearance in response to 1,25-$(OH)_2D_3$ does not reveal the same degree of confidence. In the authors' hands the calcium transport response to 1,25-$(OH)_2D_3$ precedes the calcium-binding-protein response.[95] Furthermore, the calcium-binding protein remains high long after the intestinal calcium transport response has subsided to preadministration levels. It therefore appears that if calcium-binding protein is involved in the calcium transport process initiated by 1,25-$(OH)_2D_3$, at least some other modifying factors or some other transport factors must be involved. In a search for these factors, attention has focused on proteins of the brush border which become modified in response to 1,25-$(OH)_2D_3$. A protein of molecular weight of somewhere in the neighborhood of 200,000 has been found which becomes modified under administration of 1,25-$(OH)_2D_3$.[95] This protein, which possesses alkaline phosphatase activity, becomes converted to a protein following 1,25-$(OH)_2D_3$ administration, which migrates on SDS gels with a molecular weight of about 220,000–230,000. This protein has been solubilized from the brush borders, and it appears to possess calcium-binding and alkaline phosphatase activities and appears at the appropriate time in response to 1,25-$(OH)_2D_3$ to play a role in calcium transport. It is, therefore, evident that the actual machinery which is altered by the 1,25-$(OH)_2D_3$ is far from settled; one major candidate is the calcium-binding protein and another is the newly discovered brush-border protein in our laboratory.[95] Still another candidate is the calcium-dependent adenosine triphosphatase activity, which has been much more difficult to pursue.[96] However, the calcium-dependent adenosine triphosphatase activity does not appear to correlate well with intestinal calcium transport, but the insensitivity of the methods of detection may be the cause of the poor correlation. It is therefore evident that the answers to how 1,25-$(OH)_2D_3$ modifies the intestine to permit it to transport calcium are far from satisfied and must remain as a major investigation.

Corradino has devised an embryonic-intestine organ-culture system that responds to vitamin D, 25-OH-D, and 1,25-$(OH)_2D_3$ in an appropriate manner.[97] All these forms of vitamin D at differing concentrations will stimulate the appearance of calcium-binding protein as measured by radioimmunoassay. In this system α-amanitin as well as actinomycin D will block the appearance of the calcium-binding protein in response to the vitamin D substances.[98] Furthermore, 1,25-$(OH)_2D_3$ is the most active substance in this induction, followed by 25-OH-D_3 and finally by vitamin D_3. Corradino has also provided evidence that the calcium-binding protein level is related to the calcium uptake by the embryonic intestine. Although interesting, there is considerable concern that the embryonic intestine and its inductive responses do not represent an adequate model for the calcium transport response to vitamin D in growing animals.

Once the calcium has moved across the brush-border surface, there is considerable doubt as to how the calcium is handled. One view is that mitochondria take up the calcium and serve as a

shuttle.[74] Another view is that the calcium is packaged at the terminal web into vesicles of calcium, which are then extruded past the tight junction of the epithelial cells into the basal-lateral membrane space. In the mitochondrial model the mitochondria are considered to shuttle calcium across the cell and interact with a low calcium environment near the basal-lateral membrane, which is brought about by downhill sodium exchange for calcium reaction. Sodium dependency of the calcium transport system in the intestine has now been well documented in two different laboratories.[99,100] The sodium requirement is for the extrusion of calcium across the basal-lateral membrane.[99] Under conditions of low calcium medium, the mitochondria would give up their calcium, thus completing the transfer mechanism. It is obvious that much remains to be learned about this system but that considerable progress will be made in this understanding by the availability of the active form of vitamin D both in unlabeled and labeled form. The intestinal cytosol-binding protein for 1,25-$(OH)_2D_3$ has been successfully applied to the development of assay systems for the measurement of 1,25-$(OH)_2D_3$ in the plasma, permitting an examination of the effect of various metabolic bone diseases on 1,25-$(OH)_2D_3$ levels[101] (Eisman and DeLuca, submitted for publication).

MECHANISM OF ACTION OF 1,25-$(OH)_2D_3$ ON INTESTINAL PHOSPHATE TRANSPORT

Harrison and Harrison[75] originally discovered that vitamin D stimulates the transfer of phosphate across the distal segments of small intestine. They could not separate the phosphate transport system from the calcium system inasmuch as EDTA treatment prevented phosphate transfer from occurring in the distal small intestine. More recently, evidence has shown that the phosphate transport system is independent of the calcium transport system.[41,76,77] In addition, 1,25-$(OH)_2D_3$ and not 25-OH-D_3 is the active form in this system as well.[41] Little is known concerning the mechanism of phosphate transfer, although it does appear to require sodium for entry of phosphate into the brush border surface;[102] in contrast, the entry of calcium does not require sodium. Beyond this, little is known about this system and much remains to be learned.

THE ROLE OF 1,25-$(OH)_2D_3$ IN BONE

Thus far, no effect of vitamin D or any of its metabolites on the mineralization of bone has been demonstrated. Attempts have been made with tissue culture systems as well as with in vivo measurement. The only suggestive experiments have been at the clinical level in which metabolic bone disease will respond to some form of vitamin D, despite the fact that the serum calcium and phosphorus levels are not changed, suggesting that the treatment of the bone disease involves a local change at the bone site. Beyond that, there is no evidence to support this intellectually appealing idea.

However, vitamin D is known to play an important role in the mobilization of calcium from previously formed bone. This was first demonstrated by Carlsson using radioisotopic techniques and physiologic concentrations of vitamin D.[78] It is certainly well known that large doses of vitamin D will cause a demineralization of bone.[103] However, it can be shown very easily that vitamin-D-deficient animals lacking calcium in the diet develop severe hypocalcemia. In response to a dose of vitamin D, the serum calcium will rise, and the only pool of calcium large enough to support this rise is bone.[104] Thus, there is no question that vitamin D produces a mobilization of calcium from previously formed bone. This process, however, requires the presence of parathyroid hormone[104,105] under physiological conditions. In a recent experiment, it has been shown that the mobilization of calcium from previously formed bone by $1,25\text{-}(OH)_2D_3$ requires the presence of the parathyroid hormone[105] unless extremely high doses of $1,25\text{-}(OH)_2D_3$ are given. In addition to this basic physiologic phenomenon, it has now been clearly demonstrated using cultures of embryonic bone that vitamin D metabolites at very small concentrations will stimulate the movement of calcium from bone to medium. $1,25\text{-}(OH)_2D_3$ at a concentration approaching $10^{-14}M$ will produce very marked bone calcium mobilization.[106,107] Approximately three orders of magnitude greater concentration of either $25\text{-}OH\text{-}D_3$ or the analogue 1α-hydroxyvitamin D_3 ($1\alpha\text{-}OH\text{-}D_3$) is required to produce the same degree of bone calcium mobilization. Vitamin D_3 itself at very high concentrations will produce no response. The organ culture system does not require the parathyroid hormone to be present for $1,25\text{-}(OH)_2D_3$ to exert its effect. Furthermore, with the in vitro model, Reynolds[107] has shown that $1,25\text{-}(OH)_2D_3$ may be the most potent bone-mobilizing agent known, exceeding parathyroid hormone in its biological effectiveness in the embryonic system by a large amount. In any case, it is clear that $1,25\text{-}(OH)_2D_3$ has a profound effect on the utilization of calcium from bone. The mechanism of this effect has not yet been elucidated. However, it is clear from in vivo studies that actinomycin D will completely block $1,25\text{-}(OH)_2D_3$-induced bone calcium mobilization.[108] This contrasts with the failure of actinomycin D in the very same animals to prevent the intestinal calcium transport response.[91] So far, no work has appeared on the possibility of a receptor protein in bone cells for $1,25\text{-}(OH)_2D_3$, and so far, calcium-binding protein has not been found in bone cells known to be responsive to the $1,25\text{-}(OH)_2D_3$. It therefore appears that the mechanism in bone may be somewhat different from that in the intestine, but at present, all evidence suggests that the mechanism in bone involves transcription of DNA to a messenger that must code for calcium-mobilizing proteins.

MECHANISM OF ACTION OF VITAMIN D IN OTHER TISSUES

There have been other suggestions in recent years as to the possible effect of vitamin D metabolites on growth and on muscle function. There seems to be little doubt that vitamin D does stimulate growth in a number of species, and the idea that vitamin D stimulates growth directly is appealing.[109,110] However, any study of this type is always fraught with the criticism that changes in growth response are related to the changes in mineral levels of blood or in mineral levels of tissues and that the basic function of vitamin D is the active transport of calcium and phosphorus, which then secondarily affect growth. Concrete evidence of vitamin D as a growth stimulant, therefore, is lacking. Similarly, studies on the idea that vitamin D functions in muscle are interesting, but, so far, convincing evidence is lacking that vitamin D functions in any way in the metabolism of muscle. However, this system must be examined in view of the well-established clinical observations of improved muscle strength from vitamin D administration to rachitic children.

There has been a report that vitamin D functions in the cross-linking and maturation of collagen.[111] Again this would be an appealing function of the vitamin in view of the failure of mineralization which results from vitamin D deficiency. However, it is known that rachitic matrix will calcify quite well after infusion of calcium and phosphate, which raises considerable question as to whether, in fact, there is a deformity in collagen matrix. In addi-

tion, changes in collagen cross-linking may be merely the result of changes in circulating calcium and phosphorus levels. Again, additional work will have to be done before this can be established on a firm basis.

THE ROLE OF VITAMIN D IN KIDNEY

The possibility that vitamin D is involved in the mineral metabolism of kidney has been under examination since 1941, when Harrison and Harrison suggested that vitamin D might improve renal reabsorption of phosphorus.[112] Although the effects of the early studies were apparently mediated by the parathyroid hormone, the possibility that vitamin D stimulates renal phosphorus reabsorption remains open. There has been much work in this area in recent years, but only recently has the vitamin-D-deficiency experimental model been used. It appears that $1,25\text{-}(OH)_2D_3$ will improve renal reabsorption of phosphorus in animals that are given a constant infusion of parathyroid hormone to produce a constant and stable phosphate excretion pattern.[113] If this result can be confirmed in other laboratories, it will establish very firmly that $1,25\text{-}(OH)_2D_3$ does improve renal reabsorption of phosphorus. In a similarly tenuous position is the possibility that $1,25\text{-}(OH)_2D_3$ improves renal reabsorption of calcium.[114,115] Evidence for this has been presented in dogs and more recently by classic renal physiologic studies in rats. However, the degree of calcium reabsorption is very high in the absence of vitamin D, and the effect of vitamin D is small but consistent. Finally it should be stated that there exists a calcium-binding protein in the kidney of rats and chicks that appears to be sensitive to vitamin D deficiency and repletion.[116] Thus, a role for vitamin D in kidney cells appears to be likely; however, its quantitative importance remains to be assessed, and the nature of its activity in the renal cells also remains unknown.

REGULATION OF VITAMIN D METABOLISM: INTERACTION WITH OTHER HORMONES

REGULATION OF THE RENAL $25\text{-}OH\text{-}D_3\text{-}1$-HYDROXYLASE AND THE RENAL $25\text{-}OH\text{-}D_3\text{-}24$-HYDROXYLASE

Lack of Regulation of the Hydroxylases in Vitamin D Deficiency

The administration of radioactive vitamin D_3 to vitamin-D-deficient animals results in the appearance of sequentially radioactive $25\text{-}OH\text{-}D_3$ and radioactive $1,25\text{-}(OH)_2D_3$ in kidney, blood, and intestine. However, if radioactive vitamin D_3 is given to animals on a high-calcium diet supplemented with a small amount of vitamin D, the sequence is radioactive $25\text{-}OH\text{-}D_3$ and radioactive $24,25\text{-}(OH)_2D_3$, with no $1,25\text{-}(OH)_2D_3$ appearing.[43,117] Similarly, if one examines the renal hydroxylases of chicks maintained on different levels of calcium and phosphorus but in a vitamin-D-deficient state, the only hydroxylase that is evident is the 1-hydroxylase with no evidence of the 24-hydroxylase activity.[118] Thus, it appears that vitamin-D-deficient animals are primed to make $1,25\text{-}(OH)_2D_3$ regardless of their dietary treatment and their serum calcium and phosphorus levels. When vitamin D is given, however, the hydroxylases become subject to regulation.

The first event that is of major importance is that the $25\text{-}OH\text{-}D_3\text{-}24$-hydroxylase appears upon the administration of $1,25\text{-}$

(OH)$_2$D$_3$, as shown in Figure 51-6. Thus, it appears that the 1,25-(OH)$_2$D$_3$ induces the appearance of the 24-hydroxylase, and this induction appears to be important for subsequent regulation by the need for calcium and phosphorus. It is important to realize, as shown in Figure 51-6, that the suppression of 1-hydroxylase activity and the stimulation of 24-hydroxylase activity by 1,25-(OH)$_2$D$_3$ administration requires many hours. It is not a minute-to-minute regulation.

It is only after the administration of 1,25-(OH)$_2$D$_3$ or some form of vitamin D that the 1-hydroxylase can become regulated by calcium and phosphorus needs.[41] Whether or not this is because of the presence of the 25-OH-D$_3$-24-hydroxylase or its messenger remains unknown. In any case, in the vitamin-D-supplemented animal, it is now well established that low-calcium diets stimulate the production of 1,25-(OH)$_2$D$_3$ by stimulating the level of the 25-OH-D$_3$-1-hydroxylase.[118] Animals on normal or high-calcium diets, on the other hand, produce little 1,25-(OH)$_2$D$_3$ and instead produce the 24,25-(OH)$_2$D$_3$. Thus, it seems likely that the adaptation of intestinal calcium absorption to low-calcium diets is mediated by stimulation of 1,25-(OH)$_2$D$_3$ biosynthesis.[120] Nicolaysen and collaborators have demonstrated that animals on a low-calcium diet show increased efficiency of intestinal calcium absorption provided they are given a source of vitamin D. They demonstrated that the adaptation of intestinal calcium absorption was related to the need for calcium and that once the need for calcium was satisfied, the efficiency of intestinal calcium absorption was reduced to normal.[121] They postulated the existence of an endogenous factor elaborated by the skeleton which would inform the intestine of the skeletal needs for calcium. The elaboration or production of this factor apparently required the presence of vitamin D. When it was learned that 1,25-(OH)$_2$D$_3$ or a further metabolite is the active form of the vitamin in intestine, it seemed possible that 1,25-(OH)$_2$D$_3$ might represent the endogenous factor. Consistent with this view is the idea that low-calcium diets stimulate production of 1,25-(OH)$_2$D$_3$. To prove that 1,25-(OH)$_2$D$_3$ was the endogenous factor, it has now been demonstrated that, when 1,25-(OH)$_2$D$_3$ is administered to both rats and chicks, they lose their ability to adapt their intestinal calcium absorption to low-calcium intakes.

The signal for the need for 1,25-(OH)$_2$D$_3$ production is related to serum calcium concentration, as shown in Figure 51-7.[120] It can be shown by either direct measurement in vitro of the 1-hydroxylase enzyme or by the accumulation of 1,25-(OH)$_2$D$_3$ in the blood that serum calcium concentration dictates the biosynthesis of 1,25-

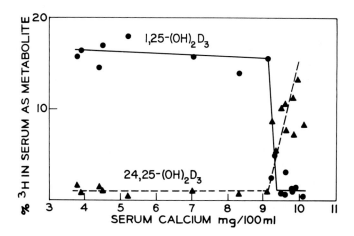

Fig. 51-7. The relationship of serum calcium concentration to the accumulation of 1,25-(OH)$_2$D$_3$ or 24,25-(OH)$_2$D$_3$ in the plasma of rats. Rats were given diets containing a variety of calcium and phosphorus levels. The 1,25-(OH)$_2$D$_3$ and 24,25-(OH)$_2$D$_3$ levels were assessed by chromatographic separation following injection of radioactive 25-OH-D$_3$ 12 hours earlier.

(OH)$_2$D$_3$, either directly or indirectly. Thus, animals having normal serum calcium produce both 24,25-(OH)$_2$D$_3$ and 1,25-(OH)$_2$D$_3$. As they are made hypocalcemic, the animals increase their production of 1,25-(OH)$_2$D$_3$ and suppress the production of 24,25-(OH)$_2$D$_3$. Under conditions ranging from normal to hypercalcemia, 1,25-(OH)$_2$D$_3$ synthesis is shut down and 24,25-(OH)$_2$D$_3$ synthesis is stimulated. Thus the need for calcium dictates biosynthesis of 1,25-(OH)$_2$D$_3$, which clearly establishes this substance as a calcium-mobilizing hormone whose biosynthesis is regulated in some way by serum calcium concentration.

Serum calcium concentration is monitored by the parathyroid glands which, as demonstrated elsewhere in this volume, secrete parathyroid hormone in response to hypocalcemia. It therefore appeared plausible that the parathyroid glands might mediate the control of 1,25-(OH)$_2$D$_3$ synthesis by serum calcium concentration. It could therefore be demonstrated that rats on a low-calcium diet lose their ability to synthesize 1,25-(OH)$_2$D$_3$ in response to hypocalcemia when they are thyroparathyroidectomized and that the biosynthesis of 1,25-(OH)$_2$D$_3$ can be stimulated by the exogenous administration of parathyroid hormone.[122] Thus, parathyroid hormone in some unknown manner stimulates biosynthesis of the 1,25-(OH)$_2$D$_3$ and suppresses the 25-OH-D$_3$-24-hydroxylase.[122] Continued experiments have demonstrated that 1,25-(OH)$_2$D$_3$ exerts its effect on intestine in the complete absence of parathyroid hormone, whereas its effect in stimulating the mobilization of calcium from bone requires the presence of this hormone.[105]

Thus, it is possible to modify the known calcium homeostatic mechanisms, as shown in Figure 51-8. Serum calcium is maintained at 9–10 mg/100 ml, and under conditions of hypocalcemia, parathyroid hormone is secreted by the parathyroid glands. The parathyroid hormone proceeds to the kidney, liver, and bone. In the liver, its function is unknown, but, in the kidney, it is known that the parathyroid hormone activates adenyl cyclase and causes a phosphate diuresis by blocking renal tubular reabsorption of phosphate (this is not shown in the figure). At the same time, it is now known that the parathyroid hormone stimulates production of 1,25-(OH)$_2$D$_3$. The 1,25-(OH)$_2$D$_3$ proceeds to the intestine where, by itself, it activates the intestine to transport calcium. At the bone site the 1,25-(OH)$_2$D$_3$ and the parathyroid hormone must both be present to mobilize calcium from bone. In the kidney, it is likely that both parathyroid hormone and 1,25-(OH)$_2$D$_3$ stimulate renal reabsorption of calcium. These three sources of calcium then drive

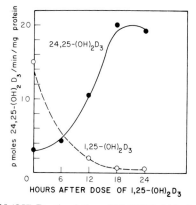

Fig. 51-6. 1,25-(OH)$_2$D$_3$ stimulation of 25-OH-D$_3$-24-hydroxylase activity in chick kidney mitochondria. Rachitic chickens were given a single injection of 325 pmol of 1,25-(OH)$_2$D$_3$ at 0 time, and the hydroxylases were measured in vitro at the times indicated.

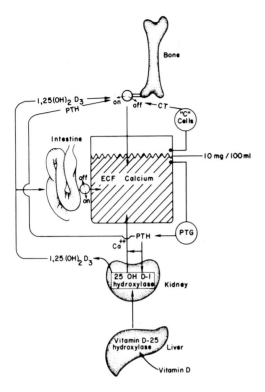

Fig. 51-8. Diagrammatic representation of the calcium homeostatic system as presently conceived. PTG = parathyroid glands; C cells = parafollicular cells of the thyroid.

serum calcium to normal, shutting off parathyroid hormone secretion and completing the low-calcium homeostatic mechanism. From this calcium homeostatic model, it becomes apparent that management of hypoparathyroid and pseudohypoparathyroid patients can best be carried out by the administration of physiologic amounts of 1,25-(OH)₂D₃ plus sufficient amounts of oral calcium. The use of bone calcium to support serum calcium levels under these circumstances is limited because of the lack of the parathyroid hormone. In practice, as will be described elsewhere, 1,25-(OH)₂D₃ or its analogue, 1α-OH-D₃, is very effective as a management agent for these diseases, provided sufficient amounts of oral calcium are provided.[123,124]

THE ROLE OF INORGANIC PHOSPHATE IN THE REGULATION OF 1,25-(OH)₂D₃ SYNTHESIS

As previously pointed out, 1,25-(OH)₂D₃ plays an important role in the elevation of serum inorganic phosphorus concentration. This is especially evident in animals that are made rachitic by both vitamin D and phosphate deprivation, which is the only way rickets can be produced in rats.[125] 1,25-(OH)₂D₃ administration causes a rise in serum inorganic phosphorus in these animals, and the source of phosphorus is from the intestine and probably from bone. The rise in serum phosphorus then provides the basic mechanism for alleviation of the rachitic lesions. In any case, a direct effect of 1,25-(OH)₂D₃ on phosphate metabolism is clearly indicated. Since 1,25-(OH)₂D₃ can be considered a phosphate-mobilizing hormone, it is reasonable to suspect that phosphate might play some role in the regulation of biogenesis of the 1,25-(OH)₂D₃. This can be shown in rats that are thyroparathyroidectomized to remove the calcium-controlling mechanism. If serum inorganic phosphorus is then regulated by dietary deprivation or by other means, a relationship between serum phosphorus concentration and 1,25-

(OH)₂D₃ biosynthesis can be seen (Figure 51-9).[126] Normal serum phosphorus for young growing rats is between 9 and 10 mg/100 ml, and under conditions of thyroparathyroidectomy they synthesize little or no 1,25-(OH)₂D₃ and mostly 24,25-(OH)₂D₃. As they are deprived of phosphate, the production of 1,25-(OH)₂D₃ is stimulated and 24,25-(OH)₂D₃ production is suppressed. Thus the need for phosphorus can stimulate production of 1,25-(OH)₂D₃.

This relationship has recently been questioned by studies with chicks, however.[127] In these experiments the basal diets were calculated to contain approximately 0.35 percent phosphorus. When true phosphate deprivation is carried out in the chick, there is no doubt that the 25-OH-D₃-1-hydroxylase is markedly stimulated.[128]

Inasmuch as there are two mechanisms for switching on 1,25-(OH)₂D₃ production, it has been suggested that the renal-cell level of inorganic phosphate might well be the determining factor.[126] Low renal-cell levels of inorganic phosphorus could be achieved either by parathyroid blocking of phosphate reabsorption in the renal tubules or by phosphate deprivation. Thus, a common denominator for both stimuli might then be renal-cell level of inorganic phorphorus, which could, upon rising to high levels, stimulate 24-hydroxylation or by falling to low levels stimulate 1-hydroxylation.[126] This hypothesis is supported by actual measurements of renal cortical levels of inorganic phosphorus under a variety of physiologic stimuli, but it must still be regarded as an hypothesis.[126]

The mechanism whereby the hydroxylases are regulated remains unknown at present, at least at the cellular and molecular level. Many postulates have appeared, but it is best in a text of this nature to merely state that this is an active area of investigation and that the meaningful physiological mechanism of regulation will involve a mechanism requiring many hours rather than minutes and will likely involve protein and RNA synthesis.

It is well known that phosphate deprivation causes a stimulation of intestinal calcium absorption and bone calcium mobilization. Because phosphate deprivation stimulates 1,25-(OH)₂D₃ production and accumulation in blood and tissues, it would seem

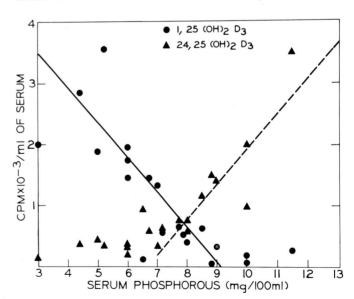

Fig. 51-9. The relationship between serum phosphorus concentration and metabolite accumulation in the serum of thyroparathyroidectomized rats. Serum phosphorus concentration was adjusted by dietary means in the thyroparathyroidectomized rats and the assessment of metabolite accumulation in the serum was determined as described in Figure 51-7. (From Tanaka and DeLuca.[126])

reasonable that at least part of the mechanism of the stimulation might be due to the increased 1,25-$(OH)_2D_3$ production. However, when exogenous 1,25-$(OH)_2D_3$ is administered to animals and the animals then placed on low-phosphate diets, it is evident that they still show a stimulation in intestinal calcium transport independent of 1,25-$(OH)_2D_3$.[129] It, therefore, appears that phosphate deprivation functions in more than one manner to stimulate bone calcium mobilization and intestinal calcium transport. On one hand, it stimulates 1,25-$(OH)_2D_3$ production, and, on the other hand, it directly stimulates the intestine to absorb additional supplies of calcium by some unknown mechanism.

1,25-$(OH)_2D_3$ AS A PHOSPHATE-MOBILIZING HORMONE AND AS A CALCIUM-MOBILIZING HORMONE

It is disturbing to consider that one hormone could have two functions and two signals, namely phosphate mobilization and calcium mobilization, with a signal from low-calcium and low-phosphate levels for production of the same hormone.[130] One can logically explain how one hormone can be a phosphate-mobilizing hormone on one hand and a calcium-mobilizing hormone on the other. The reason for this is that under circumstances of hypocalcemic stimulation of 1,25-$(OH)_2D_3$ biosynthesis, the parathyroid hormone is present, since the parathyroid glands mediate this signal. In the presence of the parathyroid hormone, 1,25-$(OH)_2D_3$, which is made in response to the need for calcium, will stimulate intestinal calcium transport and bone calcium mobilization. In addition, the 1,25-$(OH)_2D_3$ will stimulate the phosphate transport reactions, but the parathyroid hormone, having a marked effect on phosphate diuresis, will essentially cancel the effect of 1,25-$(OH)_2D_3$ on phosphate transport reactions. Under this circumstance, therefore, in response to hypocalcemia, the serum calcium will rise but the serum inorganic phosphorus will remain constant.

Under conditions of hypophosphatemic stimulation of 1,25-$(OH)_2D_3$ synthesis, we know that parathyroid glands are suppressed and that no parathyroid hormone is secreted. As a result, bone calcium mobilization in response to 1,25-$(OH)_2D_3$ is blunted, whereas 1,25-$(OH)_2D_3$ can increase intestinal absorption of both calcium and phosphorus. However, in the absence of parathyroid hormone in the kidney, there is an increase in the fractional excretion of calcium (thus a net loss of calcium in the urine) and a decrease in the fractional excretion of phosphate. Thus under this circumstance, phosphate in the serum will rise, whereas calcium will only rise slightly. It is, therefore, apparent that because of the interaction of 1,25-$(OH)_2D_3$ with the parathyroid hormone, it can function as a phosphate-mobilizing hormone as well as a calcium-mobilizing hormone with a high degree of specificity to correct the original low-calcium or low-phosphate signal.

DISTURBANCES IN THE VITAMIN D ENDOCRINE SYSTEM

With the broadened concept of vitamin D function and regulation, it becomes apparent that various disturbances in the vitamin D endocrine system could result. A mere lack of 1,25-$(OH)_2D_3$ does not necessarily mean that rickets will develop. One must bear in mind the reason for the lack of 1,25-$(OH)_2D_3$. For example, lack of parathyroid hormone means that 1,25-$(OH)_2D_3$ will not be made in response to the need for calcium. However, 1,25-$(OH)_2D_3$ could easily be made in response to the need for phosphorus. In the absence of parathyroid hormone, serum phosphorus remains high, serum calcium remains low, and rickets does not develop. On the other hand, rickets is always associated with hypophosphatemia

with or without hypocalemia. One could logically argue, therefore, that hypocalcemia by itself does not cause rickets but does result in tetany. This discussion merely underscores that a deficiency of production of the active form of vitamin D does not necessarily mean that the same pathological state will ensue, but it implies that the pathological state will be determined by which portion of the vitamin D endocrine system is disturbed.

REGULATION OF PARATHYROID HORMONE SECRETION BY VITAMIN D METABOLITES

There has been much recent interest in the idea that 1,25-$(OH)_2D_3$ or 24,25-$(OH)_2D_3$ or a combination of the two functions to suppress parathyroid hormone secretion. This was first brought about by discovery of the existence of a calcium-binding protein similar to that of Wasserman and Taylor in the parathyroid glands which appears to be vitamin-D-dependent.[131] More recently, Henry and Norman[132] have demonstrated that chick parathyroid glands appear to accumulate 1,25-$(OH)_2D_3$. In addition, a recent report[133] has suggested that in the rat, definite evidence could be obtained for suppression of parathyroid hormone secretion by vitamin D metabolites. However, the results of that study are not convincing, and conflicting reports have appeared from other laboratories. Therefore it is uncertain as to whether or not there is a feedback suppression of parathyroid hormone secretion by any metabolites of vitamin D. Only additional study will allow a clear definition of this interesting idea.

VITAMIN D ANALOGUES OF IMPORTANCE

With the discovery of 1,25-$(OH)_2D_3$ as the probable metabolically active form of the vitamin has come renewed interest in the idea that analogues of 1,25-$(OH)_2D_3$ can be made that would have the specific functions of the vitamin or that would have markedly increased biological activity or, on the other hand, that could serve as an antivitamin. So far the only analogue of great interest is 1α-OH-D_3 (Fig. 51-10), which was synthesized as an exercise in learning the chemical synthesis of 1,25-$(OH)_2D_3$.[134] This analogue is biologically active in anephric animals and can be used clinically as a substitute for 1,25-$(OH)_2D_3$.

It is now clear from the work with [6-^{3}H]1α-OH-D_3 in chicks and rats that this analogue is rapidly metabolized by a hepatic 25-hydroxylase to 1α,25-$(OH)_2D_3$ and that this metabolism precedes the biological response in both the bone and intestine.[135–137] Fur-

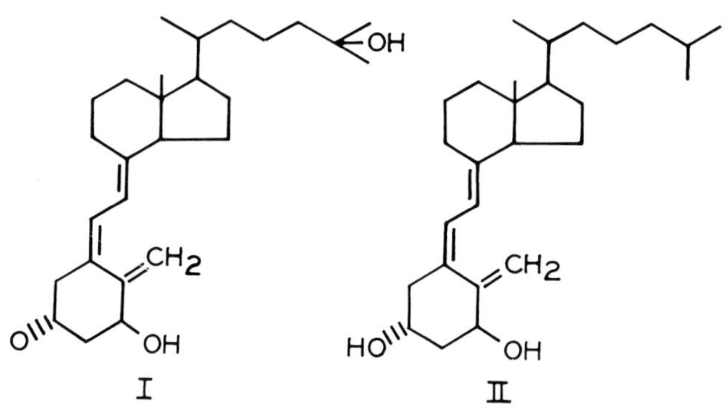

Fig. 51-10. Structures of 1,25-$(OH)_2D_3$ (I) and its synthetic analogue, 1α-OH-D_3 (II).

thermore, when 1α-OH-[6-^{3}H]D$_3$ was given to a patient with renal failure whose serum calcium was maintained with calcium supplementation and 2.5 mg of vitamin D$_2$ daily, it was rapidly metabolized to $1\alpha,25$-(OH)$_2$D$_3$[137a] (Fig. 51-11). Thus the fact that $1\alpha,25$-(OH)$_2$D$_3$ was so easily generated from 1α-OH-D$_3$ in the presence of high exogenous vitamn D$_2$ negates any suggestion that the hepatic 25-hydroxylase would be inactive because of either product inhibition or the presence of excessive amounts of exogenous substrate. This compound has been used effectively in the treatment of renal osteodystrophy, as has $1,25$-(OH)$_2$D$_3$, and in the treatment of hypoparathyroidism and pseudohypoparathyroidism. It is likely that it and its analogue, 1α-OH-D$_2$, may assume considerable importance in clinical circles.[138] In addition to this analogue, 3-deoxy-1α-OH-D$_3$[139,140] has been synthesized, as has been 3-deoxy-$1\alpha,25$-(OH)$_2$D$_3$.[141] These analogues were synthesized with the idea the conformation of the 1-hydroxyl could be fixed in a predominantly axial position and thus potentiate biological activity. Although this interesting idea did not receive support from the studies, the 3-deoxy analogues served to indicate that although the 3-hydroxyl position increases biological activity, it is not essential for the intestine and bone to respond. No antivitamins or superactive analogues have yet been devised, nor have there been any analogues that show extreme preference for activity in one organ over another. Hence, the synthesis of vitamin D analogues will continue to be an interesting area with great potential in the future.

SUMMARY

There is no doubt that vitamin D can now be considered the precursor of at least one hormone whose function it is to mobilize calcium and phosphate from intestine, bone, kidney, and perhaps elsewhere. The possible role of vitamin D in muscle and in the calcification mechanism remains open. In addition, chemical synthesis of new vitamin D analogues can be expected, but even in the absence of that, considerable use of the vitamin D metabolites and their analogues in the treatment of metabolic bone disease can be expected in the near future, not only in renal osteodystrophy and hypoparathyroidism but also in such diverse metabolic bone diseases as osteoporosis and anticonvulsant-induced osteomalacia. Finally, it is clear that the vitamin D system must assume major importance in the calcium homeostatic mechanism.

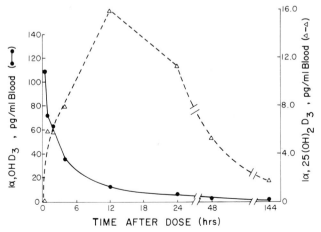

Fig. 51-11. Disappearance of 1α-OH-D$_3$ (—○—) and appearance of $1\alpha,25$-(OH)$_2$D$_3$ (--△--) in the blood of a patient receiving [6-^{3}H]1α-OH-D$_3$ intravenously. (From Holick et al.[137a])

REFERENCES

1. Smerdon, G. T. Daniel Whistler and the English Disease. A Translation and Biographical Note. J. Hist. Med. *5:* 397, 1950.
2. Mellanby, E. An Experimental Investigation on Rickets. Lancet *1:* 407, 1919.
3. McCollum, E. V., Simmonds, N., Becker, J. E., et al. Studies on Experimental Rickets. XXI. An Experimental Demonstration of the Existence of a Vitamin Which Promotes Calcium Deposition. J. Biol. Chem. *53:* 293, 1922.
4. Huldschinsky, K. Heilung von Rachitis durch künstliche Höhensonne. Deutsche Medizinische Wochenschrift *45:* 712, 1919.
5. Steenbock, H., and Black, A. Fat-soluble Vitamins. XVII. The Induction of Growth-promoting and Calcifying Properties in a Ration by Exposure to Ultraviolet Light. J. Biol. Chem. *61:* 405, 1924.
6. Hess, A. F., Weinstock, M., and Helman, F. D. The Antirachitic Value of Irradiated Phytosterol and Cholesterol. J. Biol. Chem. *63:* 305, 1925.
7. Askew, F. A., Bourdillon, R. B., Bruce, H. M., et al. The Distillation of Vitamin D. Proc. Roy. Soc. B*107:* 76, 1931.
8. Windaus, A., Linsert, O., Lüttringhaus, A., et al. Crystalline Vitamin D$_2$. Ann. N. Y. Acad. Sci. *492:* 226, 1932.
9. Schenck, F. Über das kristallisierte vitamin D$_3$. Naturwissenschaften *25:* 159, 1937.
10. DeLuca, H. F., Blunt, K. W., and Rikkers, H. Biogenesis, in *The Vitamins,* edited by W. H. Sebrell, Jr. and R. S. Harris. Academic Press, New York, 1971, vol. 3, p 213-230.
11. Sebrell, W. H., Jr. and Harris, R. S. (eds.). *The Vitamins,* 1st ed., Academic Press, New York, 1954, vol. II, chap. 6, pp. 131–266.
12. Idler, D. R., and Baumann, C. A. Skin sterols. II Isolation of Δ^7-cholesterol. J. Biol. Chem.*195:* 623, 1952.
13. Haddad, J. G., Jr., and Hahn, T. J. Natural and Synthetic Sources of Circulating 25-Hydroxyvitamin D in Man. Nature *244:* 515, 1973.
14. Bills, C. E. Vitamin D Group, in *The Vitamins,* edited by W. H. Sebrell, Jr., and R. S. Harris. Academic Press, New York, 1954, vol. II, pp. 132–223.
14a. Blondin, C. A., Kulkarni, B. D., and Nes, W. R. A Study of the Origin of Vitamin D from 7-Dehydrocholesterol in Fish. Comp. Biochem. Physiol. *20:* 379, 1967.
15. Wasserman, R. H. Active Vitamin D-like Substances in Solanum malacoxylon and other Calcinogenic Plants. Nutr. Rev. *33:* 1, 1975.
15a. Wasserman, R. H. Henion, J. D., et al. Calcinogenic Factor in Solanum malacoxylon: Evidence That It Is 1,25-Dihydroxyvitamin D$_3$-Glycoside. Science *194:* 853, 1976.
16. Greaves, J. D., and Schmidt, C. L. A. The Role Played by Bile in the Absorption of Vitamin D in the Rat. J. Biol. Chem. *102:* 101, 1933.
17. Schachter, D., Finkelstein, J. D. and Kowarski, S. Metabolism of vitamin D. I. Preparation of Radioactive Vitamin D and Its Intestinal Absorption in the Rat. J. Clin. Invest. *43:* 787, 1964.
18. Norman, A. W., and DeLuca, H. F. The Preparation of H^3-Vitamins D$_2$ and D$_3$ and Their Localization in the Rat. Biochemistry *2:* 1160, 1963.
19. Kodicek, E. Metabolic Studies on Vitamin D, in Wolstenholme, G. W. E., O'Connor, C. M. (eds): *Ciba Foundation Symposium on Bone Structure and Metabolism.* edited by G. W. E. Wolstenholme and C. M. O'Connor. Little, Brown, Boston, 1956, pp. 161–174.
20. Avioli, L. V., Lee, S. W., McDonald, J. E., et al. Metabolism of Vitamin D$_3$-^{3}H in Human Subjects: Distribution in Blood, Bile, Feces and Urine. J. Clin. Invest. *46:* 983, 1967.
21. Olson, E. B., Jr., Knutson, J. C., Bhattacharyya, M. H., et al. The Effect of Hepatectomy on the Synthesis of 25-Hydroxyvitamin D$_3$. J. Clin. Invest. *57:* 1213, 1976.
22. Ponchon, G. and DeLuca, H. F. The Role of the Liver in the Metabolism of Vitamin D. J. Clin. Invest. *48:* 1273, 1969.
23. Horsting, M., and DeLuca, H. F. In Vitro Production of 25-Hydroxycholecalciferol. Biochem. Biophys. Res. Commun. *36:* 251, 1969.
24. Bhattacharyya, M., and DeLuca, H. F. Subcellular Location of Rat Liver Calciferol-25-Hydroxylase. Arch. Biochem. Biophys. *160:* 58, 1974.
25. Bhattacharyya, M. H., and DeLuca, H. F. The Regulation of Rat Liver Calciferol-25- Hydroxylase. J. Biol. Chem. *248:* 2969, 1973.
26. Tucker, G. III, Gagnon, R. E., and Haussler, M. R. Vitamin D$_3$-25-Hydroxylase: Tissue Occurrence and Apparent Lack of Regulation. Arch. Biochem. Biophys. *155:* 47, 1973.

27. Blunt, J. W., DeLuca, H. F., and Schnoes, H. K. 25-Hydroxychole-calciferol. A Biologically Active Metabolite of Vitamin D₃. Biochemistry 7: 3317, 1968.

28. Haddad, J. G., and Stamp, T. C. B. Circulating 25-Hydroxyvitamin D in Man. Am. J. Med. 57: 57, 1974.

29. Tanaka' Y., Frank, H., and DeLuca, H. F. Biological Activity of 1,25-Dihydroxyvitamin D₃ in the Rat. Endocrinology 92: 417, 1973.

30. Trummel, C. L., Raisz, L. G., Hallick, R. B., et al. 25-Hydroxydihydrotachysterol₃-Stimulation of Bone Resorption in Tissue Culture. Biochem. Biophys. Res. Commun. 44: 1096, 1971.

31. Boyle, I. T., Miravet, L., Gray, R. W., et al. The Response of Intestinal Calcium Transport to 25-Hydroxy and 1,25-Dihydroxyvitamin D in Nephrectomized Rats. Endocrinology 90: 605, 1972.

32. Holick, M. F., Garabedian, M., and DeLuca, H. F. 1,25-Dihydroxycholecalciferol: Metabolite of Vitamin D₃ Active on Bone in Anephric Rats. Science 176: 1146, 1972.

33. Fraser, D. R. and Kodicek, E. Unique Biosynthesis by Kidney of a Biologically Active Vitamin D Metabolite. Nature 228: 764, 1970.

34. Gray, R., Boyle, I., and DeLuca, H. F. Vitamin D Metabolism: The Role of Kidney Tissue. Science 172: 1232, 1971.

35. Gray, R. W., Omdahl, J. L., Ghazarian, J. G., et al. 25-Hydroxycholecalciferol-1-Hydroxylase: Subcellular Location and Properties. J. Biol. Chem. 247: 7528, 1972.

36. Ghazarian, J. G., and DeLuca, H. F. 25-Hydroxycholecalciferol-1-Hydroxylase: A Specific Requirement for NADPH and a Hemoprotein Component in Chick Kidney Mitochondria. Arch. Biochem. Biophys. 160: 63, 1974.

37. Ghazarian, J. G., Schnoes, H. K., and DeLuca, H. F. Mechanism of 25-Hydroxycholecalciferol 1α-Hydroxylation. Incorporation of Oxygen-18 into the 1α Position of 25-Hydroxycholecalciferol. Biochemistry 12: 2555, 1973.

38. Henry, H. L., and Norman, A. W. Studies on Calciferol Metabolism. IX. Renal 25-Hydroxy-Vitamin D₃-1-Hydroxylase. Involvement of Cytochrome P-450 and Other Properties. J. Biol. Chem. 249: 7529, 1974.

39. Ghazarian, J. G., Jefcoate, C. R., Knutson, J. C., et al. Mitochondrial Cytochrome P₄₅₀: A Component of Chick Kidney 25-Hydroxycholecalciferol-1α-Hydroxylase. J. Biol. Chem. 249: 3026, 1974.

40. Pedersen, J. I., Ghazarin, J. G., Orme-Johnson, N. R., et al. The Isolation of Chick Renal Mitochondrial Ferredoxin Active in the 25-Hydroxyvitamin D₃-1α-Hydroxylase System. J. Biol. Chem. 251: 3933, 1976.

41. Chen, T. C., Castillo, L., Korycka-Dahl, M., et al. Role of Vitamin D Metabolites in Phosphate Transport of Rat Intestine. J. Nutr. 104: 1056, 1974.

42. DeLuca, H. F. The Kidney as an Endocrine Organ for the Production of 1,25-Dihydroxyvitamin D₃, a Calcium-Mobilizing Hormone. New Engl. J. Med. 289: 359, 1973.

43. Boyle, I. T., Gray, R. W., and DeLuca, H. F. Regulation by Calcium of in Vivo Synthesis of 1,25-Dihydroxycholecalciferol and 21,25-Dihydroxycholecalciferol. Proc. Nat. Acad. Sci. USA 68: 2131, 1971.

44. Holick, M. F., Schnoes, H. K., DeLuca, H. F., et al. Isolation and Identification of 24,25-Dihydroxycholecalciferol: A Metabolite of Vitamin D₃ Made in the Kidney. Biochemistry 11: 4251, 1972.

45. Garabedian, M. Pavlovitch, H., Fellot, C., et al. Metabolism of 25-Hydroxyvitamin D₃ in Anephric Rats: A New Active Metabolite. Proc. Nat. Acad. Sci. USA 71: 554, 1974.

46. Knutson, J. C., and DeLuca, H. F. 25-Hydroxyvitamin D₃-24-Hydroxylase: Subcellular Location and Properties. Biochemistry 13: 1543, 1974.

47. Ikeawa, N., Morisaki, N., Koizumi, N., et al. Synthesis and Biological Activity of 24ξ¹- and 24ξ²-Hydroxyvitamin D₃. Biochem. Biophys. Res. Commun. 62: 485, 1975.

48. Seki, M., Koizumi, N., Morisaki, M., et al. Snythesis of Active Forms of Vitamin D. VI. Synthesis of (24R)- and (24S)-24,25-Dihydroxyvitamin D₃. Tetrahedron Letters 1: 15, 1975.

49. Uskoković, M. R., Baggiolini, E., Mahgoub, A., et al. Synthesis of Vitamin D₃ Metabolites, in Vitamin D and Problems Related to Uremic Bone Disease, edited by A. W. Norman, K. Schaefer, H. G. Grigoleit, D. V. Herrath, and E. Ritz. Walter de Gruyter, Berlin, 1975, pp. 279–283.

50. Tanaka, Y., DeLuca, H. F., Ikeawa, N., et al. Determination of Stereochemical Configuration of the 24-Hydroxyl Group of 24,25-Dihydroxyvitamin D₃ and Its Biological Importance. Arch. Biochem. Biophys. 170: 620, 1975.

51. Kleiner-Bossaller, A., and DeLuca, H. F. Formation of 1,24,25-Trihydroxyvitamin D₃ from 1,25-Dihydroxyvitamin D₃. Biochim. Biophys. Acta 338: 489, 1974.

52. Tanaka, Y., Frank, H., DeLuca, H. F., et al. Importance of the Stereochemical Position of the 24-Hydroxyl to Biological Activity of 24-Hydroxyvitamin D₃. Biochemistry 14: 3293, 1975.

53. Boyle, I. T., Omdahl, J. L., Gray, R. W., et al. The Biological Activity and Metabolism of 24,25-Dihydroxyvitamin D₃. J. Biol. Chem. 248: 4174, 1973.

54. Holick, M. F., Baxter, L. A., Schraufrogel, P. K., et al. Metabolism and Biological Activity of 24,25-Dihydroxyvitamin D₃ in the Chick. J. Biol. Chem. 251: 397, 1976.

55. Holick, M. F., Kleiner-Bossaller, A., Schnoes, H. K., et al. 1,24,25-Trihydroxyvitamin D₃: A Metabolite of Vitamin D₃ Effective on Intestine. J. Biol. Chem. 248: 6691, 1973.

56. Frolik, C. A., and DeLuca, H. F. 1,25-Dihydroxycholecalciferol: The Metabolite of Vitamin D Responsible for Increased Intestinal Calcium Transport. Arch. Biochem. Biophys. 147: 143, 1971.

57. Frolik, C. A., and DeLuca, H. F. Metabolism of 1,25-Dihydroxycholecalciferol in the Rat. J. Clin. Invest. 51: 2900, 1972.

58. Tsai, H. C., Wong, R. G., and Norman, A. W. Studies on Calciferol Metabolism. IV. Subcellular Localization of 1,25-Dihydroxyvitamin D₃ in Intestinal Mucosa and Correlation with Increased Calcium Transport. J. Biol. Chem. 247: 5511, 1972.

59. Kumar, R., Harnden, D., and DeLuca, H. F. Metabolism of 1,25-Dihydroxyvitamin D₃: Evidence for Side Chain Oxidation. Biochemistry, 15: 2420, 1976.

60. Harnden, D., Kumar, R., Holick, M. F., et al. Side Chain Metabolism of 25-Hydroxy-[26,27-¹⁴C]vitamin D₃ and 1,25-Dihydroxy-[26,27-¹⁴C]vitamin D₃ in Vivo. Science 193: 493, 1976.

61. Suda, T., DeLuca, H. F., Schnoes, H. K., et al. 25,26-Dihydroxycholecalciferol, A Metabolite of Vitamin D₃ with Intestinal Calcium Transport Activity. Biochemistry 9: 4776, 1970.

62. Higaki, M., Takahashi, M., Suzuki, T., et al. Metabolic activities of Vitamin D in Animals. III. Biogenesis of Vitamin D Sulfate in Animal Tissues. J. Vitaminol. 11: 261, 1965.

63. le Boulch, N., Gulat-Marnay, C., and Raoul, Y. Vitamin D₃ Derivatives of Human and Cow's Milk: Cholecalciferol Sulfate Ester and Hydroxy-25-Cholecalciferol. Internat. J. Vit. Nutr. Res. 44: 167, 1974.

64. Bell, P. A., and Kodicek, E. Investigations on Metabolites of Vitamin D in Rat Bile. Separation and Partial Identification of a Major Metabolite. Biochem. J. 115: 663, 1969.

65. Imrie, M. H., Neville, P. F., Snellgrove, A. W., et al. Metabolism of Vitamin D₂ and Vitamin D₃ in the Rachitic Chick. Arch. Biochem. Biophys. 120: 525, 1967.

66. Jones, G., Schnoes, H. K., and DeLuca, H. F. An in Vitro Study of Vitamin D₃ Hydroxylases in the Chick. J. Biol. Chem. 251: 24, 1976.

67. Jones, G., Schnoes, H. K. and DeLuca, H. F. Isolation and Identification of 1,25-Dihydroxyvitamin D₂. Biochemistry 14: 1250, 1975.

68. Jones, G., Baxter, L. A., DeLuca, H. F., et al. Biological Activity of 1,25-Dihydroxyvitamin D₂ in the Chick. Biochemistry 15: 713, 1976.

69. Rikkers, H., and DeLuca, H. F. An in Vivo Study of the Carrier Proteins of ³H-Vitamins D₃ and D₄ in Rat Serum. Am. J. Physiol. 213: 380, 1967.

70. Belsey, R., Clark, M. B., Bernat, M., et al. The Physiologic Significance of Plasma Transport of Vitamin D and Metabolites. Am. J. Med. 57: 50, 1974.

71. Edelstein, S., Lawson, D. E. M., and Kodicek, E. The Transporting Proteins of Cholecalciferol and 25-Hydroxycholecalciferol in Serum of Chicks and Other Species. Biochem. J. 135: 417, 1973.

72. Botham, K. M., Ghazarin, J. G., Kream, B. E., et al. Isolation of a Potent Inhibitor of 25-Hydroxyvitamin D₃-1-Hydroxylase from Rat Serum. Biochemistry 15: 2130, 1976.

73. Peterson, P. A. Isolation and Partial Characterization of a Human Vitamin D-Binding Plasma Protein. J. Biol. Chem. 246: 7748, 1971.

74. Omdahl, J. L., and DeLuca, H. F. Regulation of Vitamin D Metabolism and Function. Physiol. Rev. 53: 327, 1973.

75. Harrison, H. E., and Harrison, H. C. Intestinal Transport of Phosphate: Action of Vitamin D, Calcium, and Potassium. Am. J. Physiol. 201: 1007, 1961.

76. Kowarski, S., and Schachter, D. Effects of Vitamin D on Phosphate Transport and Incorporation into Mucosal Constituents of Rat Intestinal Mucosa. J. Biol. Chem. 244: 211, 1969.

77. Wasserman, R. H., and Taylor, A. N. Intestinal Absorption of Phosphate in the Chick: Effect of Vitamin D₃ and Other Parameters. J. Nutr. 103: 586, 1973.

78. Carlsson, A. Tracer Experiments on the Effect of Vitamin D on the Skeletal Metabolism of Calcium and Phosphorus. Acta Physiol. Scand. 26: 212, 1952.

79. Orr, W. J., Holt, L. E., Jr., Wilkins, L., et al. The Calcium and Phosphorus Metabolism in Rickets, with Special reference to Ultraviolet Ray Therapy. Am. J. Dis. Child. 26: 362, 1923.

80. Nicolaysen, R. Studies Upon the Mode of Action of Vitamin D. III. The Influence of Vitamin D on the Absorption of Calcium and Phosphorus in the Rat. Biochem. J. 31: 122, 1937.

81. Schachter, D., and Rosen, S. M. Active Transport of Ca^{45} by the Small Intestine and Its Dependence on Vitamin D. Am. J. Physiol. 196: 357, 1959.

82. Schachter, D. Vitamin D and the Active Transport of Calcium by the Small Intestine, in The Transfer of Calcium and Strontium Across Biological Membranes, section IV, edited by R. H. Wasserman. Academic Press, New York, 1963, pp. 197–210.

83. Wasserman, R. H., Kallfelz, F. A., and Comar, C. L. Active Transport of Calcium by Rat Duodenum in Vivo. Science 133: 883, 1961.

84. Martin, D. L., and DeLuca, H. F. Calcium Transport and the Role of Vitamin D. Arch. Biochem. Biophys. 134: 139, 1969.

85. Brumbaugh, P. F., and Haussler, M. R. Specific Binding of 1α,25-Dihydroxycholecalciferol to Nuclear Components of Chick Intestine. J. Biol. Chem. 250: 1588, 1975.

86. Chen, T. C., and DeLuca, H. F. Receptors of 1,25-Dihydroxycholecalciferol in Rat Intestine. J. Biol. Chem. 248: 4890, 1973.

87. Chen, T. C., Weber, J. C., and DeLuca, H. F. On the Subcellular Location of Vitamin D Metabolites in Intestine. J. Biol. Chem. 245: 3776, 1970.

88. Brumbaugh, P. F., and Haussler, M. R. Nuclear and Cytoplasmic Binding Components for Vitamin D Metabolites. Life Sciences 16: 353, 1975.

89. Haddad, J. G., and Birge, S. J. Widespread, Specific Binding of 25-Hydroxycholecalciferol in Rat Tissues. J. Biol. Chem. 250: 299, 1975.

90. Lawson, D. E. M., and Emtage, J. S. 1,25-Dihydroxycholecalciferol: Its Receptor Complexes in the Chick Intestine and Its Control of Calcium-Binding Protein Synthesis, in Calcium-Regulating Hormones, edited by R. V. Talmage, M. Owen, and J. A. Parsons. Excerpta Medica, Amsterdam, 1975, pp. 330–335.

91. Tanaka, Y., DeLuca, H. F., Omdahl, J., et al. Mechanism of Action of 1,25-Dihydroxycholecalciferol on Intestinal Calcium Transport. Proc. Nat. Acad. Sci. USA 68: 1286, 1971.

92. Tsai, H. C., Midgett, R. J., and Norman, A. W. Studies on Calciferol Metabolism. VII. The Effects of Actinomycin D and Cycloheximide on the Metabolism, Tissue and Subcellular Localization, and Action of Vitamin D₃. Arch. Biochem. Biophys. 157: 339, 1973.

93. Wasserman, R. H., Taylor, A. N., and Fulmer, C. S. Vitamin-D-Induced Calcium-Binding Protein and the Intestinal Absorption of Calcium. Biochem. Soc. Spec. Publ. 3: 55, 1974.

94. Taylor, A. N., and Wasserman, R. H. Immunofluorescent Localization of Vitamin D-dependent Calcium-binding Proteins. J. Histochem. Cytochem. 18: 107, 1970.

95. Moriuchi, S., and DeLuca, H. F. The Effect of Vitamin D₃ Metabolites on Membrane Proteins of Chick Duodenal Brush Borders. Arch. Biochem. Biophys. 174: 367, 1976.

96. Melancon, M. J., Jr., and DeLuca, H. F. Vitamin D Stimulation of Calcium-dependent Adenosine Triphosphatase in Chick Intestinal Brush Borders. Biochemistry 9: 1658, 1970.

97. Corradino, R. A. Embryonic Chick Intestine in Organ Culture: Response to Vitamin D₃ and Its Metabolites. Science 179: 402, 1973.

98. Corradino, R. A. 1,25-Dihydroxycholecalciferol: Inhibition of Action in Organ-Cultured Intestine by Actinomycin D and α-Amanitin. Nature 243: 41, 1973.

99. Martin, D. L., and DeLuca, H. F. Influence of Sodium on Calcium Transport by the Rat Small Intestine. Am. J. Physiol. 216: 1351, 1969.

100. Harrison, H. E., and Harrison, H. C. Sodium, Potassium, and Intestinal Transport of Glucose, L-Tyrosine, Phosphate, and Calcium. Am. J. Physiol. 205: 107, 1963.

101. Brumbaugh, P. F., and Haussler, M. R. 1α,25-Dihydroxyvitamin D₃ Receptor: Competitive Binding of Vitamin D Analogs. Life Sciences 13: 1737, 1973.

102. Taylor, A. N. In Vitro Phosphate Transport in Chick Ileum: Effect of Cholecalciferol, Calcium, Sodium and Metabolic Inhibitors. J. Nutr. 104: 489, 1974.

103. Nicolaysen, R., and Eeg-Larsen, N. The Mode of Action of Vitamin D, in Ciba Foundation Symposium on Bone Structure and Metabolism, edited G. W. Wolstenholme and C. M. O'Connor. Little, Brown, Boston, 1956, pp. 175-186.

104. Rasmussen, H., DeLuca, H., Arnaud, C., et al. The Relationship Between Vitamin D and Parathyroid Hormone. J. Clin. Invest. 42: 1940, 1963.

105. Garabedian, M., Tanaka, Y., Holick, M. F., et al. Response of Intestinal Calcium Transport and Bone Calcium Mobilization to 1,25-Dihydroxy-Vitamin D₃ in Thyroparathyroidectomized Rats. Endocrinology 94: 1022, 1974.

106. Stern, P. H., Trummel, C. L., Schnoes, H. K., et al. Bone-resorbing Activity of Vitamin D Metabolites and Congeners in Vitro: Influence of Hydroxyl Substituents in the A Ring. Endocrinology 97: 1552, 1975.

107. Reynolds, J. J., Holick, M. F., and DeLuca, H. F. The Role of Vitamin D Metabolites in Bone Resorption. Calc. Tiss. Res. 12: 295, 1973.

108. Tanaka, Y., and DeLuca, H. F. Bone Mineral Mobilization Activity of 1,25-Dihydroxycholecalciferol, a Metabolite of Vitamin D. Arch. Biochem. Biophys. 146: 574, 1971.

109. Steenbock, H., and Herting, D. C. Vitamin D and Growth. J. Nutr. 57: 449, 1955.

110. Birge, S. J., and Haddad, J. G. 25-Hydroxycholecalciferol Stimulation of Muscle Metabolism. J. Clin. Invest. 56: 1100, 1975.

111. Barnes, M. J., Constable, B. J., Morton, L. F., et al. Bone Collagen Metabolism in Vitamin D Deficiency. Biochem. J. 132: 113, 1973.

112. Harrison, H. E., and Harrison, H. C. The Renal Excretion of Inorganic Phosphate in Relation to the Action of Vitamin D and Parathyroid Hormone. J. Clin. Invest. 20: 47, 1941.

113. Puschett, J. B., Beck, W. S., Jr., and Jelonek, A. Parathyroid hormone and 25-Hydroxy Vitamin D₃: Synergistic and Antagonistic Effects on Renal Phosphate Transport. Science 190: 473, 1975.

114. Gran, F. C. The Retention of Parenterally Injected Calcium in Rachitic Dogs. Acta Physiol. Scand. 50: 132, 1960.

115. Steele, T. H., Engle, J. E., Tanaka, Y., et al. Phosphatemic Action of 1,25-Dihydroxyvitamin D₃. Am. J. Physiol. 229: 489, 1975.

116. Taylor, A. N., and Wasserman, R. H. Vitamin D-Induced Calcium-Binding Protein: Comparative Aspects in Kidney and Intestine. Am. J. Physiol. 223: 110, 1972.

117. Tanaka, Y., and DeLuca, H. F. Stimulation of 24,25-Dihydroxyvitamin D₃ Production by 1,25-Dihydroxyvitamin D₃. Science 183: 1198, 1974.

118. Omdahl, J. L., Gray, R. W., Boyle, I. T., et al. Regulation of Metabolism of 25-Hydroxycholecalciferol by Kidney Tissue in Vitro by Dietary Calcium. Nature New Biol. 237: 63, 1972.

119. Tanaka, Y., Lorenc, R. S., and DeLuca, H. F. The Role of 1,25-Dihydroxyvitamin D₃ and Parathyroid Hormone in the Regulation of Chick Renal 25-Hydroxyvitamin D₃-24-Hydroxylase. Arch. Biochem. Biophys. 171: 521, 1975.

120. Boyle, I. T., Gray, R. W., Omdahl, J. L., et al. Calcium Control of the in Vivo Biosynthesis of 1,25-Dihydroxyvitamin D₃: Nicolaysen's Endogenous Factor, in Taylor S (ed): Endocrinology 1971, Proceedings of the Third International Symposium, edited by S. Taylor. Wm. Heinemann, London, 1972, pp. 468-476.

121. Nicolaysen, R., Eeg-Larsen, N., and Malm, O. J. Physiology of Calcium Metabolism. Physiol. Rev. 33: 424, 1953.

122. Garabedian, M., Holick, M. F., DeLuca, H. F., et al. Control of 25-Hydroxycholecalciferol Metabolism by the Parathyroid Glands. Proc. Nat. Acad. Sci. USA 69: 1673, 1972.

123. Neer, R. M., Holick, M. F., DeLuca, H. F., et al. Effects of 1α-Hydroxyvitamin D₃ and 1,25-Dihydroxyvitamin D₃ on Calcium and Phosphorus Metabolism in Hypoparathyroidism. Metabolism 24: 1403, 1975.

124. Kooh, S. W., Fraser, D., DeLuca, H. F., et al. Treatment of Hypoparathyroidism and Pseudohypoparathyroidism with Metabolites of Vitamin D: Evidence for Impaired Conversion of 25-Hydroxyvitamin D to 1α,25-Dihydroxyvitamin D. New Engl. J. Med. 293: 840, 1975.

125. Tanaka, Y., and DeLuca, H. F. Role of 1,25-Dihydroxyvitamin D₃ in Maintaining Serum Phosphorus and Curing Rickets. Proc. Nat. Acad. Sci. USA 71: 1040, 1974.

126. Tanaka, Y., and DeLuca, H. F. The Control of 25-Hydroxyvitamin D Metabolism by Inorganic Phosphorus. Arch. Biochem. Biophys. 154: 566, 1973.

127. Henry, H. L., Midgett, R. J., and Norman, A. W. Regulation of 25-Hydroxyvitamin D_3-1-Hydroxylase in Vivo. J. Biol. Chem. *249:* 7584, 1974.

128. Baxter, L. A., and DeLuca, H. F. Stimulation of 25-Hydroxyvitamin D_3-1α-Hydroxylase by Phosphate Depletion. J. Biol. Chem. *251:* 3158, 1976.

129. Ribovich, M. L., and DeLuca, H. F. The Influence of Dietary Calcium and Phosphorus on Intestinal Calcium Transport in Rats Given Vitamin D Metabolites. Arch. Biochem. Biophys. *170:* 529, 1975.

130. DeLuca, H. F. Vitamin D: The Vitamin and the Hormone. Fed. Proc. *33:* 22ll, 1974.

131. Oldham, S. B., Fischer, J. A., Shen, L. H., et al. Isolation and Properties of a Calcium-Binding Protein from Porcine Parathyroid Glands. Biochemistry *13:* 4790, 1974.

132. Henry, H. L., and Norman, A. W. Studies on the Mechanism of Action of Calciferol. VII. Localization of 1,25-Dihydroxy-Vitamin D_3 in Chick Parathyroid Glands. Biochem. Biophys. Res. Commun. *62:* 781, 1975.

133. Chertow, B. S., Baylink, D. J., Wergedal, J. E., et al. Decrease in Serum Immunoreactive Parathyroid Hormone in Rats and in Parathyroid Hormone Secretion in Vitro by 1,25-Dihydroxycholecalciferol. J. Clin. Invest. *56:* 668, 1975.

134. Holick, M. F., Semmler, E. J., Schnoes, H. K., et al. 1α-Hydroxy Derivative of Vitamin D_3: A Highly Potent Analog of 1α,25-Dihydroxyvitamin D_3. Science *180:* 190, 1973.

135. Holick, M. F., Holick, S. A., Tavela, T., et al. Synthesis of [6-^{3}H]-1α-Hydroxyvitamin D_3 and Its Metabolism in Vivo to [^{3}H]-1α,25-Dihydroxy-Vitamin D_3. Science *190:* 576, 1975.

136. Holick, M. F., Holick, S. A., Schnoes, H. K., et al. Synthesis of 1α-Hydroxy-[6-^{3}H]Vitamin D_3 and Its Metabolism to 1α,25-Dihydroxy-[6-^{3}H] Vitamin D_3 in the Rat. J. Biol. Chem. *251:* 1020, 1976.

137. Holick, S. A., Holick, M. F., Tavela, T. E., et al. Metabolism of 1α-Hydroxyvitamin D_3 in the Chick. J. Biol. Chem. *251:* 1025, 1976.

137a. Holick, M. F., de Blanco, M. C., Clark, M. B., et al. The Metabolism of [6-^{3}H]1α,Hydroxycholecalciferol in a patient with renal insufficiency. J. Clin. Endocrinol. Metab. *44:* 595, 1977.

138. Lam, H.-Y., Schnoes, H. K., and DeLuca, H. F. 1α-Hydroxyvitamin D_2: A Potent Synthetic Analog of Vitamin D_2. Science *186:* 1038, 1974.

139. Lam, H.-Y., Onisko, B. L., Schnoes, H. K., et al. Synthesis and Biological Activity of 3-Deoxy-1α-Hydroxyvitamin D_3. Biochem. Biophys. Res. Commun. *59:* 845, 1974.

140. Okamura, W. H., Mitra, M. N., Wing, R. M., et al. Chemical Synthesis and Biological Activity of 3-deoxy-1α-Hydroxyvitamin D_3, an Analog of 1α,25-Dihydroxyvitamin D_3, the Active Form of Vitamin D_3. Biochem. Biophys. Res. Commun. *60:* 179, 1974.

141. Okamura, W. H., Mitra, M. N., Procsal, D. A., et al. Studies on Vitamin D and its Analogs. VIII. 3-Deoxy-1α,25-Dihydroxyvitamin D_3, a Potent New Analog of 1α,25-$(OH)_2D_3$. Biochem. Biophys. Res. Commun. *65:* 24, 1975.

52

Calcium and Inorganic-Phosphate Homeostasis

Robert M. Neer

HOMEOSTATIC SYSTEMS

In analyzing homeostatic systems it is useful to subdivide them into controlling and controlled subsystems. For the present discussion, the controlling system consists of parathyroid hormone, 1,25-dihydroxyvitamin D, and (in lower mammals and perhaps humans) calcitonin, plus the kidneys, intestines, and skeleton. The controlled system is the ionized-calcium concentration in serum and the phosphate concentration within cells or serum. The biochemical details of the homeostatic system are outlined in Chapters 40, 43, 47, and 51; here we concentrate on the quantitative and temporal interrelationships of the systems. This is equivalent to treating the parathyroid glands, thyroid, kidneys, intestines, and skeleton as "black boxes" that receive input of calcium and phosphorus from the circulating blood and respond by altering calcium and phosphorus retention by the body or by altering the calcium and phosphorus equilibrium between blood and tissue. Figure 52-1 illustrates these relationships schematically and defines the useful terms: disturbing and controlling signals, and controlled signals.

Under normal circumstances controlling and controlled systems are so tightly integrated that it is difficult to analyze the control process. The integration is due to "cascade effects" and feedback loops. For example, parathyroid hormone increases the blood concentration of ionized calcium and 1,25-dihydroxyvitamin D and decreases the blood concentration of inorganic phosphate. These changes then produce secondary effects on gut, kidney, and bone ("cascade effects"). An analysis of the homeostatic system must attempt to separate the primary effects of parathyroid hormone from the cascade effects produced secondarily and must determine the relative importance of each to calcium and phosphorus homeostasis. An example of the complexity introduced by feedback loops is the following: administration of 1,25-dihydroxyvitamin D increases intestinal calcium absorption and alters skeletal calcium dynamics so as to increase the serum calcium concentration. This produced reciprocal decreases in blood parathyroid hormone concentration (negative feedback loop). The ultimate changes in renal, intestinal, and skeletal handling of phosphorus and calcium will thus reflect the initial increases in 1,25-dihydroxyvitamin D in blood, plus the compensatory decreases in parathyroid hormone concentration in blood. Analysis of homeostatic systems is facilitated if the cascade effects and feedback loops can be totally or partly eliminated, thereby simplifying the responses observed. Such "interrupted chain" and "open loop" studies are essential if one is to untangle the homeostatic process and define the quantitative importance of its various elements.

As a result of new hormone assays, an increasing ability to quantitate controlling signals, and recent experiments designed to eliminate or minimize secondary hormonal effects ("cascades") and negative feedback loops, a general picture of the homeostatic system for calcium and inorganic phosphate is beginning to emerge. This has strikingly changed current ideas about the mechanisms by which inorganic phosphate and calcium concentrations of the serum are normally regulated. Quantitative analysis of calcium and phosphorus homeostasis has also provided an explanation for the pathogenesis of some illnesses. For example, it is now recognized that renal osteodystrophy is in large part an undesirable side effect of serum calcium homeostasis. Finally, analyses of the homeostatic system rationalize observations that at first sight seem paradoxical, such as the lack of correlation between serum concentrations of calcium and parathyroid hormone in patients with secondary hyperparathyroidism. This chapter outlines the major features of the controlling systems, as they are now understood, describes the controlling signals in operational terms, and analyzes the integrated responses of the entire system to variations in calcium or phosphate losses and calcium or phosphate loads of the type commonly seen in clinical practice.

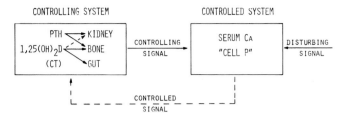

Fig. 52-1. Elementary model of the calcium and inorganic-phosphate homeostatic system. Boxes represent the controlling and controlled subsystems; arrows outside the boxes represent variations in calcium or phosphate input to and output from blood (controlling and disturbing signals) or variations in serum calcium or cellular phosphate concentrations (controlled signals). The controlling system acts to minimize variation of the controlled signal and so overcomes disturbing signals introduced from outside the system.

HOMEOSTATIC REGULATION OF PARATHYROID HORMONE BLOOD LEVELS

Minute-to-minute variations in the blood concentration of parathyroid hormone depend upon its secretion rate, its metabolism or excretion by liver and kidneys, and its volume of distribution within the body. Parathyroid hormone secretion has been examined directly in the venous blood draining the parathyroid glands of calves whose serum calcium concentration was modified by intravenous calcium and/or EDTA infusions (Chapter 44). The complicating effects of parathyroid hormone metabolism and tissue distribution and feedback effects on its own secretion were all eliminated, since the secreted hormone was directly collected, and the serum calcium was exogenously controlled (open-loop experiment). The hormone radioimmunoassays used for this experiment were insensitive to biologically inert carboxy-terminal parathyroid hormone fragments in the calves' blood. These critical experiments define the range of serum calcium concentration over which parathyroid hormone can subserve calcium homeostasis as well as the limits of parathyroid gland adaptation to acute changes in the serum calcium concentration. Normal secretion was 1 ng PTH/kg

of body weight per minute. When the serum calcium concentration in the calf was reduced by a steady EDTA infusion (disturbing signal), parathyroid hormone secretion began to increase, and reached a maximum of 4–5 ng/kg of body weight per minute when the serum calcium in the calf was less than or equal to 7.0 mg/dl (Fig. 52-2A). Conversely, when calcium was infused into the calf to elevate the serum calcium concentration, parathyroid hormone secretion declined and reached a minimum of 0.3 ng/kg of body weight per minute when the serum calcium concentration was greater than 10.5 mg/dl. Parathyroid hormone secretion never stopped completely, even when severe hypercalcemia (serum calcium greater than 14 mg/dl) was induced and maintained for periods of up to 35 hours. Thus the parathyroid secretory response was symmetrical to falling or rising serum calcium concentrations, increased approximately linearly as the serum calcium concentration decreased over the range 10.5–7.0 mg/dl (proportional control), and had finite maximum and minimum secretion rates.[1,2] Qualitatively similar secretory responses occur in organ cultures of human or bovine parathyroid tissue.[3,4] The cumulative data, although still incomplete, suggest that above a serum calcium of 10.5 or below a serum calcium of 7.0 mg/dl, the normal parathyroid gland no longer functions (at least acutely) in an adaptive manner; the maximum and minimum parathyroid hormone secretory rates revealed by these experiments are the normal acute control limits for this portion of the controlling system.

These limits of parathyroid secretory response can be extended, however, if the disturbing signal is chronic. For example, pregnant or lactating cows, whose parathyroid glands have been chronically stressed by calcium losses to the offspring, have an exaggerated parathyroid hormone response to hypocalcemia (Fig. 52-2B). This increased response of the controlling system reflects anatomic hyperplasia of the parathyroid glands.[5] Analogous observations have been made in humans with parathyroid hyperplasia, such as that generated by the disturbing signals of chronic renal failure.[6,7] The time required and the chemical signals involved (such as calcium level) for this functional and anatomic hyperplasia to develop have not been precisely defined. The exact nature of the

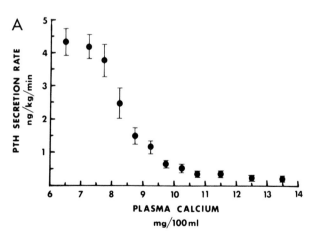

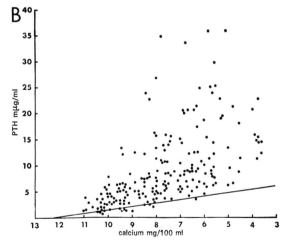

Fig. 52-2A (left). Parathyroid hormone secretory rate as a function of serum calcium concentration in the bovine. Serum calcium concentrations were altered by intravenous calcium infusions over a period of hours, while the venous blood from the parathyroid glands was collected at 15-minute intervals and later assayed for parathyroid hormone. Note the presence of both maximum and minimum secretion rates and the narrow range of calcium concentration separating these two limits. (Reprinted from Mayer, G. P., in Talmage, R. V. et al (eds): Calcium-Regulating Hormones, Proceedings of the Fifth Parathyroid Conference, Amsterdam, Excerpta Medica, 1975, with permission.) **Fig. 52-2B (right).** Serum calcium and parathyroid hormone concentrations in the peripheral blood of cows during parturient hypocalcemia. The solid line is the regression line for PTH levels in normal cows during acute intravenous EDTA infusions. The exaggerated response of the parturient animals reflects the homeostatic hyperplasia of their parathyroid glands in response to a chronic disturbing signal. (Reprinted from Buckle, R. M. et al, in Protein and Polypeptide Hormones, Excerpta Medica, Amsterdam, 1969 (I.C.S. #161), with permission.)

secretory response of the hyperplastic parathyroids is still under analysis (Chapters 43 and 44), but clearly much larger rates of hormone production per unit decrement in calcium are possible after parathyroid hyperplasia.

Parathyroid hyperplasia is not entirely satisfactory as a homeostatic response, however. Although it improves the defense against hypocalcemia, it worsens the defense against hypercalcemia. Some basal hormone secretion is an inherent property of normal parathyroid tissue (Fig. 52-2A). When the parathyroid cell mass is increased, the nonsuppressible parathyroid hormone secretion also increases, either from the additional number of cells and/or from other defects in the control of secretion (Chapters 43 and 44). Thus, when Gittes et al.[8] transplanted multiple normal parathyroid glands into a single recipient animal using genetically inbred animals to ensure acceptance of the transplants, the recipients regularly became hypercalcemic, despite the fact that each of the transplanted glands was normal. A similar phenomenon occurs in patients with secondary hyperparathyroidism if their initiating renal disease or intestinal malabsorption is corrected rapidly (Chapters 59 and 61). Their increased parathyroid cell mass continues to secrete large amounts of parathyroid hormone, although such secretion is rendered unnecessary by cure of the initiating illness (disturbing signal), and hypercalcemia results. The increased amount of nonsuppressible parathyroid hormone secretion will sustain the hypercalcemia until the parathyroid cell mass returns to normal. Thus parathyroid hyperplasia can be initially homeostatic and subsequently antihomeostatic in the same patient as a result of changing circumstances. A truly homeostatic parathyroid hyperplasia would develop in response to a disturbing signal and involute with its disappearance. The involution of parathyroid hyperplasia has been incompletely studied, but in some circumstances hyperplasia in animals and humans appears to be irreversible[9] and therefore antihomeostatic. Thus parathyroid hyperplasia is an important part of the controlling system but can produce disease when the original disturbing signal is reversed by therapy.

Inorganic phosphate also has a major influence on parathyroid function. Although it has no direct effect on parathyroid hormone secretion, changes in the serum inorganic-phosphate concentration alter skeletal calcium uptake and release, thereby altering the serum calcium concentration and indirectly affecting parathyroid hormone secretion.[10-12] Hypophosphatemia decreases skeletal calcium uptake and increases skeletal calcium release, thus tending to raise serum calcium levels.[13-15] Correcting the phosphate depletion reverses these effects.[13-15] Hyperphosphatemia, on the other hand, increases skeletal calcium uptake and tends to lower serum calcium levels without major effects on skeletal calcium release.[15-18] These changes are direct ionic effects, not mediated by changes in circulating parathyroid hormone or vitamin D metabolites, and occur in vivo in both humans and animals and also in vitro[13-18] (see Chapter 40). The net result of these changes is that the serum inorganic-phosphate and calcium concentrations are inversely related if the homeostatic system is uncoupled by parathyroidectomy in animals or humans.[19] Via this indirect route, inorganic phosphate has clinically significant effects on parathyroid hormone secretion. For example, inorganic-phosphate depletion brought on by overdosage with aluminum-hydroxide-containing antacids leads to a suppression of parathyroid hormone secretion.[20,21] At the other extreme, the inorganic-phosphate retention of renal glomerular failure contributes substantially to the reactive hyperparathyroidism of that condition (Chapter 59).

In addition to the serum calcium and phosphate concentrations, serum magnesium and catecholamine concentrations have significant effects on parathyroid hormone secretion. These are ignored here, since they are not directly linked to calcium and phosphorus homeostasis; they are discussed in Chapter 44.

Recently, it has been suggested that 1,25-dihydroxyvitamin D or 24,25-dihydroxyvitamin D or both influence parathyroid hormone secretion and/or parathyroid gland mass, independently of their effects on the serum calcium concentration.[22-27] Parathyroid cells contain a high-affinity protein receptor for 1,25-dihydroxyvitamin D, which has not been found in other tissues except those that are established targets for $1,25(OH)_2D_3$.[20] Several groups have reported that blood parathyroid hormone concentration decreases significantly before the total serum calcium concentration increases when vitamin D deficiency is corrected with vitamin D in humans, or animals.[23-25] Their experiments are very difficult to interpret, since vitamin D and its metabolites rapidly alter skeletal calcium release and intestinal calcium absorption, introducing disturbing calcium-flux signals that could decrease parathyroid hormone secretion before substantial changes in serum ionized calcium could be experimentally detected (see p. 678). Investigators have tried to bypass this difficulty in several ways: (1) by introducing a standard disturbing signal to provoke hypocalcemia or hypercalcemia and so overcome any changes in calcium flux or serum calcium concentration; (2) by perfusing $1,25(OH)_2D_3$ directly through the isolated parathyroid glands in situ and looking for immediate responses (before systemic calcium fluxes or concentrations could possibly change); and (3) by studying the effects of vitamin D metabolites on parathyroid hormone secretion in organ culture in vitro. The first approach has been most successful and suggests that $1,25(OH)_2D_3$ may indeed have a negative feedback effect on parathyroid hormone secretion. Chertow et al. gave vitamin D-deficient rats 130 picomoles of $1,25(OH)_2D_3$, which is probably two to five times the physiological replacement dose. Serum PTH fell 43 percent, and the blood parathyroid hormone response to a subsequent hypocalcemic challenge (phosphate injection) was greatly inhibited.[25] This experiment should be repeated with EDTA challenge and a physiological dose of $1,25(OH)_2D_3$. The in situ perfusion experiments of Care and the thyroid-artery injections of Canterbury et al. used pharmacological doses of $1,25(OH)_2D_3$; they got inconsistent results with lower doses.[26,27] The organ-culture studies of Chertow et al.[25] used very small doses of $1,25(OH)_2D_3$, but their results could not be confirmed by others. This intriguing hypothesis is therefore still under study.

Canterbury et al. injected $24,25(OH)_2D_3$ into the thyroid artery or the peripheral circulation of dogs and rapidly suppressed PTH secretion and peripheral blood PTH levels, even in dogs that were severely hypocalcemic.[27] These experiments employed doses of $24,25(OH)_2D_3$, however, which may have been pharmacological. Since $24,25(OH)_2D_3$ is made primarily in the absence of parathyroid hormone, the further inhibition of PTH secretion by this steroid would represent a positive feedback loop. PTH stimulation by $1,25(OH)_2D_3$, seen in some of the experiments described above, would also represent a positive feedback loop. Positive feedback loops are unstable. They are only compatible with homeostasis if they are integrated with and counterbalanced by a much stronger negative feedback loop. Thus even if further experiments confirm the existence of such positive feedback loops, it seems unlikely that they are a dominant regulatory mechanism under normal circumstances, for such dominance would be incompatible with the known stability of serum calcium concentrations.

The plasma concentrations of parathyroid hormone presented to the body tissues depend not only on the parathyroid hormone secretion rate but also on the parathyroid hormone disappearance rate from plasma. In intact animals or in human patients, parathyroid hormone secreted into the blood is rapidly distributed throughout the extracellular fluid, metabolized by the liver and kidneys, and excreted in the urine (Chapter 45). By using specific radioimmunoassays and/or preliminary chromatography of plasma samples, it is possible to define the kinetics of intact parathyroid hormone metabolites (the lack of such specific analytical methods invalidates many of the earlier studies of parathyroid hormone turnover). The following equations describe *intact* parathyroid hormone disappearance from plasma, where y is the fraction of the injected dose per milliliter of plasma, normalized per kilogram of body weight, and t is time in minutes:

Eq. 1a (calf)[28]: $y = 0.017e^{-1.2t} + 0.0051e^{-0.12t}$
Eq. 1b (dog)[29]: $y = xe^{-0.1t}$
Eq. 1c (rat)[30]: $y = 0.28e^{-0.39t} + 0.098e^{-0.065t} + 0.016e^{-0.0087t}$

The first term in Eqs. 1a and 1c represents rapid hormone mixing and organ uptake, while the second and third terms reflect slower processes. These equations indicate that the pool of intact parathyroid hormone in plasma and extracellular fluid has a mean turnover time of 6 to 11 minutes (calf and dog) or 60 minutes (rat). The longer estimate in the rat may only reflect more complete definition of the slowest components of hormone turnover in that species. Thus parathyroid hormone could theoretically regulate calcium and inorganic-phosphate metabolism on a minute-to-minute basis if its effects on target organs had equally rapid on–off rates.

Two groups have examined the relationship of parathyroid hormone turnover rates to parathyroid hormone blood levels in the calf by infusing intact bovine parathyroid hormone at different rates and measuring the concentration of intact hormone in plasma at intervals until equilibrium was attained.[28,31,32] They found no evidence for nonlinear clearance processes; the rate constants for parathyroid hormone turnover were the same at all the infusion rates, even though the final equilibrium values for intact plasma parathyroid hormone ranged from two to six times normal. Thus there is no suggestion that the rate of parathyroid hormone clearance from plasma is saturable and no suggestion of any threshold for clearance of intact hormone, at least within the normal and supranormal ranges of hormone concentration. Until such evidence is forthcoming, it seems reasonable to assume that variations in parathyroid secretory rates produce parallel variations in blood parathyroid hormone concentration within 6 to 11 minutes (one mean turnover time), with equilibrium concentrations attained soon after.

If one assumes such a linear response, it is meaningful to calculate a constant blood clearance rate for intact parathyroid hormone (metabolic clearance rate):

$$\frac{\text{MCR}}{\text{kilogram of body weight}} = \frac{1}{\int_0^\infty y\,dt} \qquad \text{(Eq. 2)}$$

where y is defined by equations 1a, b, and c, and MCR is the milliliters of plasma cleared of intact parathyroid hormone each minute. MCR per kilogram of body weight calculated in this way averages 13 ml/min/kg in calves infused with bovine parathyroid hormone.[28] Derivation of the metabolic clearance rate permits a useful calculation. At equilibrium, hormone input to and output from plasma must be equal:

hormone secretion = MCR/kg × plasma concentration
(ng/min/kg)   (ml/min/kg)   (ng/ml)

Measurement of the first two terms in calves[1,2,28] allows calculation of the third term. The resultant theoretical value for the normal

bovine plasma concentration of intact parathyroid hormone is < 75 pg/ml, which is well below the detection limit of most assays. This calculation agrees fairly well with two independent estimates of the normal circulating intact parathyroid hormone concentration, based on assays of chromatographed plasma from hyperparathyroid patients[33] and bioassays of intravenously infused bovine parathyroid hormone in dogs.[34] The general agreement helps validate the approximate accuracy of the kinetic analysis.

If one defines the kinetics of intact parathyroid hormone disappearance from peripheral blood and assumes a constant metabolic clearance rate, one can calculate by deconvolution analysis the parathyroid hormone secretory rates necessary to produce the intact parathyroid hormone concentration observed in peripheral blood during an EDTA or calcium infusion.[35] If such calculated values for parathyroid hormone secretory rate in the calf are plotted as a function of the serum calcium concentration, the results agree reasonably with the experimental values determined directly in the calf as described in Figure 52-2A. This helps confirm the validity of the observations made in the animals with isolated parathyroid venous drainage and shows that surgery in the latter animals did not substantially affect the results. Similar calculations might be used to establish parathyroid hormone secretory responses in humans, where direct measurements are impossible.

HOMEOSTATIC REGULATION OF 1,25-DIHYDROXYVITAMIN D BLOOD LEVELS

The circulating blood levels of $1,25(OH)_2D$ are 15–50 pg/ml in healthy adults[36,37] and depend upon the rate of $1,25(OH)_2D$ synthesis and degradation and its tissue distribution within the body. The latter two variables have recently been defined in normal humans,[38] allowing calculation of the metabolic clearance rate and blood production rate of $1,25(OH)_2D_3$. After intravenous injection, tritium-labeled $1,25(OH)_2D$ disappears from plasma much more slowly than does parathyroid hormone and is described by

$$y = 0.58e^{-0.078t} + 0.22e^{-0.0056t} + 0.20e^{-0.00032t} \qquad \text{(Eq. 3)}$$

where y is the fraction of the injected dose per milliliter of plasma, and t is in minutes. The last term accounts for 90 percent of the hormone disappearance curve and has a half-time of 1.5 days. This corresponds to a mean turnover time of 2 days for the $1,25(OH)_2D_3$ in equilibrium with plasma, which means that it takes 2 days for the total pool of $1,25(OH)_2D_3$ to be replaced, on the average.

The kinetics of tritiated $1,25(OH)_2D_3$ disappearance in this study were unaffected by 10-fold variations in the absolute amount of $1,25(OH)_2D_3$ injected (which would have increased the serum $1,25(OH)_2D_3$ concentration by 1.5–15 pg/ml). Thus, within the normal and supranormal ranges of hormone concentration, the kinetics of $1,25(OH)_2D_3$ disappearance are linear, and a constant metabolic clearance rate seems likely. Using Eqs. 2 and 3, the MCR for normal adults is 12.5 ml/min (without correction for body weight). This implies that the total blood $1,25(OH)_2D_3$ turnover rate in a normal adult is about 350 pg/min (MCR in milliters per minute × plasma concentration in picograms per milliliter), or 500 ng/day. This amount of $1,25(OH)_2D_3$ could be provided by 10 μg (400 IU) of absorbed dietary vitamin D or endogenously synthesized vitamin D, if 5 percent of the vitamin D were converted to $1,25(OH)_2D$. This calculation does not include any $1,25(OH)_2D_3$ synthesized and degraded in the kidney without gaining access to the general circulation.

The secretion of $1,25(OH)_2D$ into the blood in vivo can be quantitated using such $1,25(OH)_2D$ tracer studies. Most of the data now available on 1,25(OH)$_2$D secretion rates are nonquantitative, since they are inferred from experiments using only radioactively labeled precursors of 1,25(OH)$_2$D, or measurements of blood 1,-25(OH)$_2$D concentrations. Such techniques measure neither the rate of hormone degradation nor changes in that rate and so do not quantitate hormone turnover. They may thus misinterpret variations in the rate of 1,25(OH)$_2$D degradation as variations in the rate of its secretion. To date, the changes in secretion rates inferred from such experiments have generally been consistent with 1,-25(OH)$_2$D repletion experiments in animals and humans (Chapter 51), but these limitations must be kept in mind in developing a quantitative description of the controlling system.

Serum calcium concentrations in the vitamin D-deficient rat are dependent on the dietary calcium; dietary calcium restriction progressively lowers the serum calcium concentration. When it falls below 9.5 mg/dl, 25-OHD$_3$ conversion to 1,25(OH)$_2$D$_3$ apparently increases, reaching a maximum when the serum calcium concentration is 9.0 mg/dl (Fig. 52-3A). The inferred changes in 1,25(OH)$_2$D production occur over an extremely narrow range of serum calcium concentration, and the maximal conversion rate is 8 to 12 times the minimum.[39] Measurements of serum 1,25(OH)$_2$D$_3$ in normal rats led to the same conclusions (Table 52-1, top). As the serum calcium concentration fell as a result of severe dietary calcium restriction, the mean serum 1,25(OH)$_2$D$_3$ concentration increased from 17 to 90 pg/ml.[40] The parallels between Fig. 52-2A and Fig. 52-3A are obvious, and in fact the serum calcium concentration influences 1,25(OH)$_2$D$_3$ production primarily via induced changes in parathyroid hormone secretion. For instance, when the parathyroid glands are removed, 1,25(OH)$_2$D$_3$ production from 25-OHD$_3$ drops dramatically, and remains low despite severe hypocalcemia.[39–41] Serum 1,25(OH)$_2$D$_3$ concentrations are also low (Table 52-1, lines 4, 5). When parathyroid extract is given to the thyroparathyroidectomized animals, 1,25(OH)$_2$D$_3$ production returns to normal (Fig. 52-4). Thus, 1,25(OH)$_2$D production and secretion by the kidney are under the hormonal control of the parathyroid glands and respond to variations in serum calcium concentrations because of this. This hormonal cascade is homeostatic, since 1,25(OH)$_2$D$_3$ increases the serum calcium concentration and may also directly suppress parathyroid hormone secretion (see above).

The limited data available indicate that a similar control sys-

Table 52-1. Effects of Serum Calcium and Inorganic-Phosphate Concentrations on Serum 1,25(OH)$_2$D$_3$ Concentrations in Intact vs. Chronically Thyroparathyroidectomized Rats

	Calcium (mg/dl)	Inorganic Phosphate (mg/dl)	1,25(OH)$_2$D$_3$ (pg/ml)
Intact animals	11.4	10.0	17
Low-Ca diet	10.1	9.9	90
Low-P diet	13.0	4.8	82
TPTX animals	11.1	10.1	6
Low-Ca diet	8.0	15.7	12
Low-P diet	13.4	5.4	91

Retabulated from ref. (40). All animals were given the same, normal, amount of dietary vitamin D.

tem operates in humans, although the details are still obscure. Mawer et al. have estimated 1,25(OH)$_2$D$_3$ production in patients by injecting radioactively labeled vitamin D or 25-OH-vitamin D, and subsequently measuring radioactively labeled 1,25(OH)$_2$D$_3$ in blood.[42–44] By assaying the specific activity of the injected precursors in the patient's blood, they could correct for differences in tracer dilution by endogenous hormone (a problem avoided in animal studies by the use of D-deficient animals). Some of their studies used vitamin D labeled with ^{3}H at carbon 1 and with ^{14}C elsewhere in the molecule. The 1-hydroxylation of such a tracer causes a loss of ^{3}H and a decrease in the ^{3}H/^{14}C ratio. Their studies suggest that 1,25(OH)$_2$D$_3$ production is increased in patients with primary hyperparathyroidism and decreased in patients with hypoparathyroidism.[43,44] Total serum 1,25(OH)$_2$D$_3$ concentrations are also elevated in patients with primary hyperparathyroidism and may be depressed in untreated patients with hypoparathyroidism (Table 52-2). The doses of vitamin D required to normalize intestinal calcium absorption and serum calcium concentration in hypoparathyroid patients are 1250–2500 μg/day, which is 500 to 1000 times the minimum vitamin D requirement of normal subjects, whereas the doses of 1,25(OH)$_2$D required are only 0.5–4.0 μg/day, little different from the estimated normal daily 1,25(OH)$_2$D turnover.[45–47] This also suggests that 1,25(OH)$_2$D$_3$ production from its precursors is deficient in hypoparathyroid humans. The quantitative relationships between serum calcium concentration and 1,-

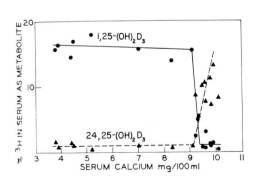

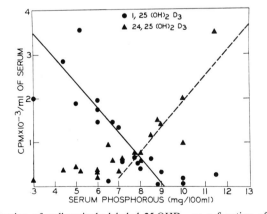

Fig. 52-3. Radioactive 1,25-(OH)$_2$D$_3$ found in plasma 12 hours after injection of radioactively labeled 25-OHD$_3$, as a function of serum calcium concentration in intact rats (A, left) and as a function of serum inorganic phosphate concentration in chronically thyroparathyroidectomized rats (B, right). The effects of calcium are largely abolished by parathyroidectomy, and the effects of inorganic phosphate are masked by those of calcium in intact animals. Note that the effects of inorganic phosphate occur over a broad range of serum concentrations, in contrast to the parathyroid-hormone-mediated effects of calcium. All animals were initially vitamin D-deficient. Serum calcium and inorganic phosphate concentrations were manipulated by varying the dietary calcium and phosphorus. (Reprinted with permission from Boyle, I. T. et al, in Taylor, S. (ed): Endocrinology 1971, Proceedings of the Third International Symposium, London, William Heinemann Medical Books, 1972; and from Tanaka, Y., DeLuca, H. F., *Arch Biochem Biophys 154:* 566–574, 1973.)

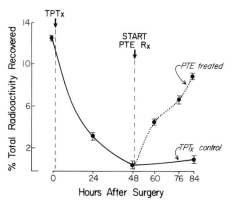

Fig. 52-4. Radioactive 1,25(OH)$_2$D$_3$ in plasma 12 hours after injections of radioactively labeled precursor in vitamin D-deficient rats. Note gradual decrease in apparent 1,25(OH)$_2$D$_3$ production after thyroparathyroidectomy and gradual restoration by treatment with parathyroid extract, 10 units every 6 hours. (Redrawn from Garabedian, M. et al, *Proc Natl Acad Sci USA 69:* 1673–1676, 1972.)

25(OH)$_2$D$_3$ production or serum concentration have not yet been defined in humans.

In intact vitamin D-deficient or vitamin D-sufficient animals, manipulations of the dietary phosphorus induce changes in the serum calcium concentration and secondary changes in parathyroid hormone secretion (see above) and 1,25(OH)$_2$D$_3$ production. Thus phosphate loading increases and *mild* phosphate depletion decreases 1,25(OH)$_2$D$_3$ production.[39,48,48a] Because the effects are mediated via parathyroid hormone, 1,25(OH)$_2$D production correlates with the serum calcium concentration and bears no simple relation to the serum inorganic-phosphate concentration.[39] With *severe* phosphate depletion, however, an alternate control system for 1,25(OH)$_2$D$_3$ production is unmasked. Severe hypophosphatemia, since it suppresses parathyroid hormone secretion (see above), would be expected to decrease renal 1,25(OH)$_2$D$_3$ production. On the contrary, 1,25(OH)$_2$D$_3$ production increases in severely hypophosphatemic animals.[40,49] If the parathyroid glands are removed to uncouple the controlling system, the dramatic effects of phosphate depletion are revealed (Fig. 52-3B).[50] Between serum inorganic-phosphate concentrations of 9 and 5 mg/dl, 1,-25(OH)$_2$D$_3$ apparent production increases 10–15-fold (the normal serum inorganic-phosphate concentration in these animals is approximately 9 mg/dl). The magnitude of the effect is equal to that of parathyroid hormone (Fig. 52-3A), although 10–15-fold may somewhat overestimate the effects of phosphate depletion on 1,-25(OH)$_2$D$_3$ production, since phosphate depletion also retards 1,-25(OH)$_2$D$_3$ degradation rates.[51] Measurements of serum 1,25(OH)$_2$D$_3$ concentrations in vitamin D-sufficient animals confirm these experiments and also suggest that parathyroid hormone and phosphate depletion are equally potent stimuli to 1,25(OH)$_2$D$_3$ production (Table 52-1, lines 2 and 6).

Table 52-2. Serum 1,25(OH)$_2$D Concentrations in Normal, Hyperparathyroid, and Hypoparathyroid Humans

	No. of Pts.	1,25(OH)$_2$D (pg/ml)
Normal adults	29	33 (21–45)
Hyperparathyroidism	20	58 (22–117)
Hypoparathyroidism	10	20 (5–30)

Tabulated from ref. 36. Values are mean ± 2 standard deviations for normals: mean and range for hyperparathyroid and hypoparathyroid patients.

Since 1,25(OH)$_2$D$_3$ increases serum and cellular phosphate by increasing intestinal phosphate absorption and skeletal phosphate release, this subsystem is also homeostatic. When parathyroid hormone is present, 1,25(OH)$_2$D$_3$ production subserves calcium homeostasis, increasing and decreasing in response to changes in the serum calcium concentration and resultant changes in serum parathyroid hormone levels. When parathyroid hormone is suppressed, as with severe phosphate depletion, 1,25(OH)$_2$D$_3$ production subserves phosphate homeostasis, increasing and decreasing in response to the serum inorganic-phosphate concentration or (more probably) changes in intracellular phosphate. DeLuca et al. have suggested that this dual control mechanism may operate via some final common pathway, as outlined in Fig. 52-5, since parathyroid hormone decreases the total phosphorus content of the renal cortex.[50] The biochemical factors regulating renal 25-hydroxyvitamin-D-1α-hydroxylase are extensively discussed in Chapter 51.

Although a similar relationship between 1,25(OH)$_2$D$_3$ production and serum or cellular phosphate concentration exists in humans, its limits have not yet been so fully defined. It has recently been shown, however, that phosphate depletion increases 25-OHD turnover and 1,25(OH)$_2$D blood levels in normal humans, despite simultaneous decreases in their serum parathyroid hormone levels.[20,52] The temporal features of the parathyroid hormone and inorganic phosphate effects on 1,25(OH)$_2$D$_3$ production are undefined in humans. In animals, the "on" and "off" rates for parathyroid hormone's effects on 1,25(OH)$_2$D$_3$ production are symmetrical, detectable within at least 25 hours of parathyroidectomy or parathyroid hormone injection, and complete within 48 hours (Fig. 52-4). The effects of phosphate depletion on serum 1,25(OH)$_2$D$_3$ levels in animals are apparent within 24 hours of initiating a phosphate-deficient diet, well before any decrease in serum inorganic-phosphate concentration.[48a]* The time course for the effects of phosphate repletion in animals is undefined.

Tracer experiments with labeled 25-OHD$_3$ have suggested that magnesium and acidosis influence 1,25(OH)$_2$D$_3$ production in animals, but these experiments have not yet been confirmed with independent techniques and have not been extended to humans at all. Furthermore it is unclear whether the suggested effects in animals are direct, or are mediated via changes in parathyroid hormone secretion, or both.

HOMEOSTATIC CONTROL OF BLOOD PTH AND 1,25(OH)$_2$D LEVELS—A SUMMARY

The above relationships may be summarized as follows: Changes in the serum calcium within the range 7.0–10.5 mg/dl produce reciprocal changes in the parathyroid hormone secretory rate within minutes. Because of the fast turnover time of this hormone, equally rapid changes in the circulating blood parathyroid hormone concentration result. The altered levels of blood parathyroid hormone change the renal production of 1,25(OH)$_2$D$_3$, by altering the activity of the renal 25-hydroxyvitamin-D-1-hydroxylase, but this occurs relatively slowly (Fig. 52-4). Because of the relative slowness of this effect and because the turnover time of 1,25(OH)$_2$D$_3$ is also relatively slow, one can predict that changes in the serum calcium concentration will produce changes in the

---

*Observations such as this are difficult to reconcile with Fig. 52-3B unless one assumes that the controlled signal is actually intracellular "phosphate," which only approximately parallels the serum inorganic phosphate-concentration.

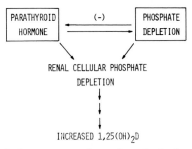

Fig. 52-5. The final common pathway hypothesis for control of 1,-25(OH)$_2$D$_3$ production and/or secretion (also indicated is the fact that phosphate depletion leads to a decrease in parathyroid hormone secretion).

serum 1,25(OH)$_2$D$_3$ only slowly, and 1,25(OH)$_2$D$_3$ can therefore only participate in the control system for serum calcium concentration over time intervals of hours or days, not minutes.

Changes in the serum and/or intracellular inorganic-phosphate concentration will affect the controlling system either directly or indirectly. Under normal circumstances, phosphate affects the controlling system only indirectly by reciprocally altering the serum calcium concentration: Δ inorganic phosphate $\xrightarrow{(-)} \Delta$ serum calcium $\xrightarrow{(-)} \Delta$ PTH $\xrightarrow{(+)} \Delta$ 1,25(OH)$_2$D$_3$, where the minus signs above the arrows indicate a reciprocal effect and the plus signs indicate a positive effect. In this sequence a decrease in serum inorganic-phosphate concentration will decrease 1,25(OH)$_2$D$_3$. The time course and magnitude of these indirect effects will depend on the phosphate-induced changes in the serum calcium concentration.

At the lower extremes of serum inorganic-phosphate concentrations, parathyroid hormone secretion is suppressed, and a partial hypoparathyroid state is induced. The production of 1,-25(OH)$_2$D$_3$ is thereby uncoupled from the serum calcium concentration, and the indirect sequence is no longer operative. In this situation, and in the disease hypoparathyroidism, the direct sequence is dominant: Δ inorganic phosphate $\xrightarrow{(-)} \Delta$ 1,25(OH)$_2$D$_3$.

Note that the controlling system thus reverses its direction in the absence of parathyroid hormone, since a further decrease in serum inorganic phosphate now increases 1,25(OH)$_2$D$_3$. The critical levels of parathyroid hormone and inorganic phosphate needed to make one or the other pathway dominant have not been precisely defined. The indirect pathway subserves calcium homeostasis, while the direct pathway subserves inorganic-phosphate homeostasis. Conflicts between these two goals may thus occur and can lead to disease, as discussed in the final section of this chapter.

REGULATION OF THE CONTROLLING SIGNALS FOR SERUM CALCIUM AND INORGANIC-PHOSPHATE HOMEOSTASIS

From the viewpoint of serum calcium and inorganic-phosphate homeostasis, the proximate controlling signals are the input to the circulating blood of calcium and inorganic phosphate from the intestinal lumen, renal tubules, and skeleton, plus the simultaneous output of these ions from blood to urine and feces and back into the skeleton. These inputs and outputs are determined by the load of calcium and inorganic phosphate in the diet and glomerular filtrate, by the absorptive capacities of the intestinal mucosa and renal tubules, and by the rates of skeletal and extraskeletal uptake and release of calcium and inorganic phosphate (Fig. 52-6). The

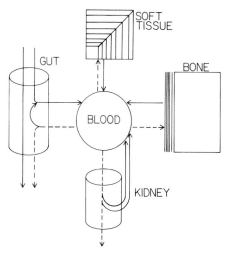

Fig. 52-6. Schematic outline of serum calcium and inorganic phosphate input (solid arrows) and output (interrupted arrows). Arrows on the left represent input from and output to the intestines. Arrows on the right represent input from and output to the skeleton. The vertical lines on the right indicate that substantial portions of the skeletal calcium and inorganic phosphate are unavailable for rapid exchange with the blood mineral. The arrow inferiorly represents output to the glomerular filtrate, while the hooked arrows represent input to the blood from the proximal and distal renal tubules. The square superiorly represents soft tissues, exchange with which is an important aspect of serum phosphate homeostasis but relatively unimportant for serum calcium homeostasis.

absorptive capacities of the intestinal mucosa and renal tubules and the bone cell turnover of mineral are the control points of the homeostatic system, where blood parathyroid hormone and 1,-25(OH)$_2$-vitamin D concentrations are transduced into fluxes of calcium and inorganic phosphate. The chemistry of these transductions is discussed in Chapters 46, 47, and 51. Chapter 40 also discusses the numerous nonhomeostatic factors that influence the fluxes of calcium and inorganic phosphate into and out of the blood.

CALCIUM

The input of calcium from the renal tubules is increased by parathyroid hormone within minutes. The effect disappears rapidly if parathyroid hormone is withdrawn, occurs in the presence or absence of vitamin D, and is directly caused by parathyroid hormone (Chapter 46). The effects of vitamin D metabolites on renal calcium clearance are unimpressive.[53,54] There is no information relating renal calcium clearance to plasma concentrations of biologically active parathyroid hormone, but calcium input from the renal tubule in hypoparathyroid humans decreases as much as 1.5 mg/min, and increases a comparable amount in hyperparathyroid humans, at comparable filtered loads.[117] Serum total calcium concentrations can thus vary 3–6 mg/dl, despite comparable urinary calcium excretion at these two extremes of parathyroid function (Fig. 52-7).

Calcium input from the intestinal lumen is also increased by parathyroid hormone, but human and animal studies strongly suggest that the effect is wholly or primarily indirect via effects on renal 1,25(OH)$_2$D secretion (Chapter 51). The stimulation of intestinal calcium absorption takes hours to develop, which is consistent with the known time lag for parathyroid hormone's stimulation of the renal 25-hydroxyvitamin-D-1-hydroxylase (Fig. 52-4) and the time required for 1,25(OH)$_2$D's effect on the intestine.[55] Parathyroid hormone fails to increase intestinal calcium absorption

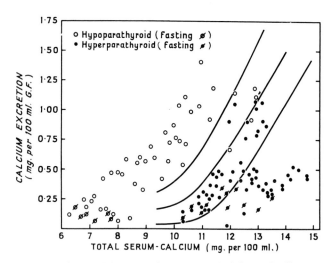

Fig. 52-7. Urinary calcium excretion per 100 ml of glomerular filtrate as a function of the simultaneous total serum calcium concentration in hypoparathyroid and hyperparathyroid humans. The solid lines represent the mean and 95 percent confidence limits for healthy males and females. The serum calcium in the patients and normal volunteers was varied by oral and/or intravenous calcium loading. (Reprinted from Peacock, M. et al, *Lancet 1:* 384–386, 1969, with permission.)

in vitamin D-deficient or anephric animals and humans.[56–60] The magnitude of its effects on intestinal calcium absorption will therefore depend upon the functional capacity of the kidneys and the adequacy of circulating blood levels of 25-OH vitamin D, as well as on the overall efficiency of intestinal digestion and intestinal absorption. If these factors are all normal, parathyroid hormone can increase intestinal calcium absorption in humans from 10 to 20 percent (hypoparathyroidism) to > 70 percent (hyperparathyroidism).[56,78] The threshold dose of parathyroid hormone necessary for a minimal effect and the relationship of the effect to the circulating blood level of biologically active parathyroid hormone are unknown. It is also unclear whether the intestinal calcium absorptive response occurs at the same blood levels of parathyroid hormone as do the renal and skeletal calcium reabsorptive responses. Any change in intestinal calcium absorptive efficiency will also affect the rate of calcium output into the feces, since some of the calcium lost from the blood into the intestinal lumen is reabsorbed.[61] This plays a very limited role in calcium homeostasis, however, since calcium losses from blood to feces vary only slightly, even at the extremes of homeostasis. For example, representative values for such "endogenous fecal calcium" are 110–170 mg/day in hypoparathyroid humans and 40–280 mg/day in hyperparathyroid humans.[62,78]

Calcium input from the skeleton is increased by both parathyroid hormone and 1,25(OH)₂D, and their effects are synergistic. In the absence of vitamin D, parathyroid hormone is relatively ineffective in stimulating skeletal calcium release,[63] and severe hypocalcemia will result despite secondary hyperparathyroidism. This is partly caused by calcium deficiency. Vitamin D deficiency produces a secondary calcium deficiency which, if severe, interferes with the effects of parathyroid hormone on skeletal calcium release.[64] However, calcium repletion of vitamin D-deficient animals only partly restores their skeletal responsiveness to parathyroid hormone.[65] Vitamin D repletion is necessary to restore skeletal responsiveness entirely.[65] The synergism is also illustrated by the fact that 1,25(OH)₂ vitamin D increases skeletal calcium release dramatically in animals with functioning parathyroid glands but has a much smaller effect on skeletal calcium release in parathyroidectomized animals.[66] Thus both parathyroid hormone and 1,-

25(OH)₂D are needed to ensure a normal input of calcium from the skeleton to the blood.

The mechanisms by which parathyroid hormone increases skeletal calcium release are discussed in detail in Chapters 40, 46, and 47. It is only necessary here to note that the dose-response curve is biphasic,[67] and the time course of parathyroid hormone-stimulated skeletal calcium release is also biphasic. An early skeletal calcium release is apparent within minutes, and a second slower skeletal calcium release takes hours or days to develop.[67–69] The interrelationships of these different processes are somewhat vague.[70] At least part of this complexity is due to the fact that parathyroid hormone stimulates 1,25(OH)₂D₃ production, and 1,-25(OH)₂D₃ itself has direct skeletal effects.

Considerable effort has proved that parathyroid hormone mobilizes calcium recently deposited in the skeleton (and presumably on or near crystal surfaces) as well as calcium that has been deposited in the skeleton (and presumably buried deep within crystals) for a long time.[71,72] These two types of bone may be mobilized by different cells (Chapter 46). The quantitative importance of each is unknown, but, for the present analysis, this interesting question is irrelevant; the central question is the magnitude and speed of the net skeletal response, not the detailed features of the response. It is apparent from Table 52-3 that parathyroid hormone can increase blood–bone calcium exchange about 7 mg/min/1.73m², if one compares patients with hypoparathyroidism and primary hyperparathyroidism.[62] This response range is similar to the range of blood–renal tubule calcium exchanges at these same extremes.

The data summarized in Table 52-3 illustrate the fact that parathyroid hormone not only increases the input of calcium from the skeleton but also stimulates calcium output to the skeleton.[62] In the rat, the balance between the two skeletal effects is dose-dependent (Chapter 46). At low doses of parathyroid hormone, skeletal calcium uptake predominates and bone mass increases. At high doses of hormone, the reverse is true. Whether a similar dose-dependent reversal of the net skeletal effect occurs in humans is unknown, an important gap in present knowledge. Based on clinical inference, it is generally assumed that bone catabolism is the dominant effect of parathyroid hormone in humans. Certainly this is true at high hormone doses. However, a synthetic human parathyroid hormone fragment, given to humans in low doses, increases skeletal calcium turnover two to three times without causing net bone catabolism.[73]

Animal experiments suggest that 1,25(OH)₂D or some other vitamin D metabolite also increases skeletal calcium uptake, since vitamin D stimulates bone growth and increases bone mass independently of its effects on serum calcium and inorganic-phosphate concentrations.[74] It is not clear what determines the net balance between calcium input from and calcium output to the skeleton

Table 52-3. Blood/Bone Calcium Exchanges in Hypoparathyroid, Normal, and Primary Hyperparathyroid Humans

Component	Effective Equilibration Time*	Magnitude†		
		Hypo	Normal	Hyper
Fast	1.1 hours	(11.2)	16.6	17.3
Slow	18 hours	(2.0)	3.7	3.1
Slower	8 days	(0.40)	0.66	0.90
Slowest	40+ days	(0.19)	0.24	(0.55)

*Four half-lives.

†Mean value for grams of calcium/day/square meter body surface, from Massin et al.[62] Parentheses embrace values significantly different from normal.

under 1,25(OH)$_2$D stimulation either, but hormone dosage is one important consideration, since large doses of 1,25(OH)$_2$D or its 1-OH analogue cause skeletal calcium release in excess of skeletal calcium uptake.[75,76]

Parathyroid hormone and 1,25(OH)$_2$D also alter the serum inorganic-phosphate concentration (see below). Increases in the serum inorganic-phosphate concentration accelerate calcium output to the skeleton (see p. 671), while decreases in the serum inorganic-phosphate concentration retard calcium output to the skeleton. The balance between calcium output to and input from the skeleton during parathyroid hormone or 1,25(OH)$_2$D stimulation will therefore depend in part upon the hormone's simultaneous effects on phosphate homeostasis. This interaction illustrates the necessity of considering both ions together in any analysis of calcium homeostasis.

Since parathyroid hormone increases the serum calcium concentration, it increases the glomerular filtration of calcium (output) at the same time as it increases renal tubular reabsorption of calcium (input). If parathyroid hormone only affected serum calcium homeostasis via the kidney, it would only increase the serum calcium concentration until these two effects were equal, and the steady-state urinary calcium excretion would be unaffected. However, parathyroid hormone also affects serum calcium homeostasis via the intestines and skeleton. Consequently, it may increase the serum calcium and the load of calcium filtered at the glomerulus more than it stimulates renal tubular reabsorption of calcium. If this happens, hypercalciuria will result. Thus the effects of parathyroid hormone on urinary calcium excretion are variable and depend upon the balance between renal tubular reabsorption of calcium and the net calcium input to blood from bone and gut.

The effects of 1,25(OH)$_2$D (and indirectly of parathyroid hormone) on net calcium input from the intestine are also dependent on the balance between epithelial transport of calcium and the imposed load of calcium. The calcium content of the diet for normal adults in the United States varies from 200 to 1800 mg/day.[77] As the dietary calcium increases within this range, the calcium concentration of the intestinal contents increases substantially, causing increased intestinal calcium absorption (Fig. 52-8). Prior calcium deprivation or sufficiency will alter the magnitude of this effect in young adults (Fig. 52-8) by producing compensatory changes in parathyroid hormone and 1,25 (OH)$_2$D production (page 680). Thus calcium input to the circulation depends upon the balance between PTH or 1,25(OH)$_2$D$_3$ levels and the dietary calcium intake, a fact that has profound homeostatic implications.

It is therefore clear that the effects of 1,25(OH)$_2$D on calcium homeostasis will depend upon the dietary calcium intake and the presence or absence of parathyroid hormone. Similarly, the effects of parathyroid hormone on calcium homeostasis will depend upon the dietary calcium intake, the presence or absence of 25-OH vitamin D, and the ability of the kidneys to synthesize 1,25(OH)$_2$ vitamin D. Finally, the effect of each hormone on skeletal calcium turnover may be qualitatively as well as quantitatively dependent on hormone dosage.

INORGANIC PHOSPHATE

Intestinal absorption of dietary phosphate is enhanced in patients with primary hyperparathyroidism and normal or reduced in patients with hypoparathyroidism.[14,59,80] Small doses of 1,25(OH)$_2$D also increase intestinal phosphate absorption in humans,[81] and the effects of parathyroid hormone on intestinal phosphate absorption in humans are probably indirectly mediated via 1,25(OH)$_2$D. In the rat, this is clearly established.[82] An indirect effect, mediated via 1,25(OH)$_2$D, would explain why acute administration of parathyroid hormone to normal volunteers has no effect on their intestinal phosphate absorption,[83] since it takes several hours for parathyroid hormone to increase blood 1,25(OH)$_2$D levels and several more hours for 1,25(OH)$_2$D to stimulate intestinal phosphate transport.[84] An indirect effect would also explain why intestinal phosphate absorption is slightly reduced in patients with advanced renal failure[56,57] or simple vitamin D deficiency,[59] despite their elevated parathyroid hormone levels. Quantitative data, relating parathyroid hormone blood levels or 1,25(OH)$_2$D blood levels to intestinal phosphate absorption, are not yet available for humans.

The effects of parathyroid hormone and 1,25(OH)$_2$D on renal phosphate handling are complex because the renal excretion of inorganic phosphate is partly dependent on the serum calcium concentration. If calcium is infused intravenously into untreated hypoparathyroid patients, increasing their serum calcium concentration to normal for 2 to 3 consecutive days, the input of inorganic phosphate from the renal tubules is dramatically inhibited, falling to two-thirds of its initial value. Simultaneously, the serum inorganic-phosphate concentration falls to normal.[85] Similar effects can be produced with large doses of oral calcium salts[47] or with small doses of oral 1,25(OH)$_2$D$_3$.[45-47] Animal studies suggest that 1,25(OH)$_2$D$_3$ decreases renal tubular phosphate absorption directly, in addition to its indirect effects via changes in the serum calcium concentration.[86] This is not clear in humans[47] and is under active investigation. These interrelationships are extensively discussed in Chapter 40.

Parathyroid hormone also inhibits inorganic-phosphate input from the renal tubules. The urinary phosphate excretion per 100 ml GFR is increased approximately threefold in hyperparathyroid patients as compared to hypoparathyroid patients with similar serum inorganic-phosphate levels[88,142] (Fig. 52-9). This effect of parathyroid hormone occurs in hypocalcemic and vitamin D-deficient humans and animals.[59,63,89] It is therefore independent of parathyroid hormone's effects on the serum concentration of calcium or 1,25(OH)$_2$D. Furthermore, it occurs in minutes and wears off equally rapidly (Chapter 46).

In addition to the effects of serum calcium, 1,25(OH)$_2$D$_3$, and parathyroid hormone, renal phosphate handling in humans is also

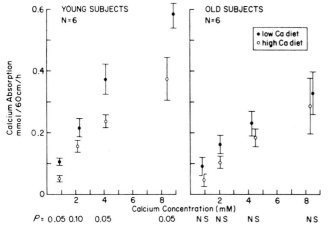

Fig. 52-8. Intestinal calcium absorption as a function of luminal calcium concentration in healthy young and old adults, studied after their adaptation to low or high dietary calcium intakes. The illustrated measurements were made in the jejunum using a triple-lumen intestinal intubation technique. The postprandial luminal calcium concentrations on low-calcium diets normally range from 0.3 to 2.0 mM/liter, and from 3.0 to 8.5 mM/liter on very high dietary calcium intakes.[182] (Reprinted with permission from Ireland, P., Fordtran, J. S., *J Clin Invest 52*: 2672–2681, 1973.)

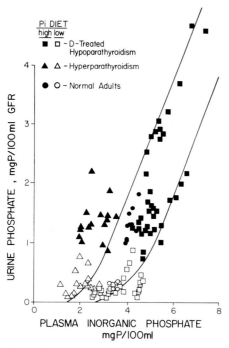

Fig. 52-9. Urinary inorganic phosphate excretion per 100 ml of glomerular filtrate as a function of the serum inorganic phosphate concentration in normal subjects (circles) and in patients with primary hyperparathyroidism (triangles) or vitamin D-treated hypoparathyroidism (squares). Open symbols represent measurements after 3 or more days, equilibration to a low-phosphate diet (<450 mg P/day), while closed symbols represent measurements obtained after similar equilibration to a high-phosphate diet (1900–3400 mg P/day). The solid lines indicate the range of measurements in normal subjects given intravenous infusions of inorganic phosphate to raise the serum concentration acutely. (Plotted from data in references 87, 88, 142, and 143.)

strongly dependent upon the plasma cortisol concentration, and the normal diurnal variation in serum inorganic-phosphate and in renal phosphate clearance is greatly diminished in hypoadrenal patients given evenly spaced doses of replacement glucocorticoid.[90] Gonadal steroids also have a major influence on renal phosphate handling. The hyperphosphatemia and avid renal conservation of phosphate in normal children disappear with puberty,[91] but are restored by surgical castration[92] and partly restored by the natural menopause.[93] Whether these steroidal effects are mediated directly in humans or via changes in vitamin D metabolism[94,95] is presently unclear. Consequently it is still impossible to decide whether these steroidal effects are part of the controlling system for inorganic-phosphate homeostasis or are disturbing signals that challenge it.

The effects of parathyroid hormone and 1,25(OH)$_2$D on the skeletal input and output of inorganic phosphate parallel their effects on skeletal calcium input and output described above. This is true even though skeletal calcium and inorganic phosphate exchange with blood at different rates (see above). Isotope exchange of ^{47}Ca or ^{32}P into preformed skeletal mineral involves only a substitution process, with no net skeletal uptake or release of calcium or phosphate. A net transfer of either ion requires dissolution or precipitation of bone mineral, and this necessarily involves calcium and phosphate in parallel. It is true that as bone crystals mature, their calcium/phosphorus ratio changes,[96] and some dissociation of the two ion fluxes, to or from the skeleton, must accompany this maturation. However, the magnitude of this effect is negligible compared to the other determinants of blood/bone calcium and inorganic-phosphate exchange.

In summary, parathyroid hormone and 1,25(OH)$_2$D together increase inorganic phosphate input to the blood from the intestines and skeleton. Simultaneously, both hormones decrease the input of inorganic phosphate from the renal tubules, both directly and via their effect on the serum calcium concentration. The balance of these effects is such that the urinary phosphate excretion increases dramatically. The effect on the serum inorganic phosphate concentration depends upon the amount of dietary phosphate available to the intestinal mucosa. For example, in thyroparathyroidectomized rats, small doses of 1,25(OH)$_2$D$_3$ increase the serum inorganic-phosphate concentration if the animals receive a low-phosphorus diet but decrease it if the dietary phosphorus is high.[86] This disparity is poorly understood and is discussed further in a later section (see p. 684). Data relating blood levels of biologically active parathyroid hormone or 1,25(OH)$_2$D to serum inorganic-phosphate input and output in humans are not available, and it is not clear whether the renal, intestinal, and skeletal phosphate fluxes all respond to similar blood levels of each hormone.

QUANTITATIVE MEASUREMENTS OF CONTROLLING AND DISTURBING SIGNALS*

CALCIUM

The turnover of serum calcium must be measured with isotopic tracers if one wishes to quantitate the disturbing signals that threaten calcium homeostasis or the controlling signals that preserve it. The importance of doing this is illustrated by an important animal experiment of Ramberg et al.[97] They showed that the level of circulating parathyroid hormone in cows varies with the rate at which calcium is leaving the plasma (V_t in their terminology) and correlates only weakly with the steady-state serum calcium concentration (Fig. 52-10). This apparent paradox is the defining characteristic of a homeostatic system. In the intact animal, increases in the disturbing signal (V_t) transiently decrease the serum calcium concentration, but compensatory increases in parathyroid hormone secretion rapidly and almost completely correct the abnormality in serum calcium concentration. In the new steady state, the serum calcium is therefore practically unchanged, while the serum parathyroid hormone concentration is drastically elevated. Although the interrelationships of the system can be dissected by opening the feedback loop (Fig. 52-2A), an integrated analysis of the serum calcium control system ultimately requires simultaneous measurements of the disturbing signals (V_t), controlling signals (calcium entry from gut and bone), serum parathyroid hormone and serum 1,25(OH)$_2$D$_3$, and controlled signal (serum calcium). The disparity between Fig. 52-2A and Fig. 52-10B dramatically reveals the difference between an open-loop and a closed-loop analysis of the calcium homeostatic system and the necessity for measuring calcium turnover in the latter. Since V_t can be experimentally divided into renal, intestinal, and skeletal components by measuring ^{47}Ca kinetics and excretion, the relative importance of each to the total disturbing signal can be quantitated as well.[98] An important current experimental limitation in humans is the inability to quantitate disturbing and controlling signals that are not labeled with isotopic calcium (i.e., calcium input from diet or bone), except in the steady state.[99] Studies with stable calcium isotopic tracers may soon circumvent that difficulty.[100]

---

*For clarity, we will employ the term "clearance" throughout this discussion to refer to the first-order or pseudo-first-order rate constant for calcium removal from plasma, with units of volume/time. We will use input, output, uptake, release, absorption, or excretion to refer to the actual calcium movements, in milligrams/time.

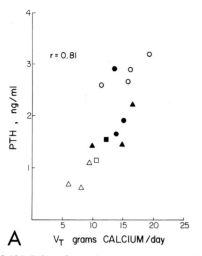

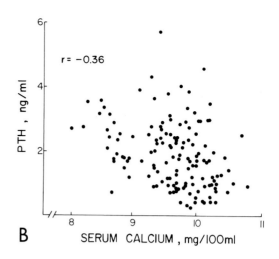

Fig. 52-10A (left). Serum immunoreactive parathyroid hormone as a function of total plasma calcium turnover in the bovine. Each symbol represents a different turnover study; duplicate symbols represent duplicate measurements in the same animal after varying total calcium turnover by means of variations in dietary calcium intake. **Fig. 52-10B (right).** Serum immunoreactive parathyroid hormone vs. the simultaneous serum calcium concentration in the same animals. Values of r are the correlation coefficients for each set of data. Linear regressions are PTH $= 0.19 \, V_t - 0.62$ and PTH $= 3.8 \, (10.3 -$ Ca), when PTH is in nanograms per milliliter, V_t in grams per day, and Ca in milligrams per deciliter. (Modified from Ramberg, C. F., Jr. et al, *J Nutr 106:* 671–679, 1976.)

To quantitate serum calcium turnover, one injects ^{47}Ca or some other calcium isotope intravenously and determines its rate of disappearance from plasma and its rate of excretion in urine and feces. The total ^{47}Ca disappearance, minus the ^{47}Ca excretion, represents the extravascular (largely skeletal) ^{47}Ca uptake. The results with the ^{47}Ca tracer are then extrapolated to total calcium, based on the mean specific activity (^{47}Ca/total Ca) of the plasma.

On closer inspection, the process of vascular/extravascular calcium exchange is rather complex. Immediately after intravenous ^{47}Ca injection, the isotope is rapidly taken up into extravascular tissues, disappearing at a rate of 30–40 g/day. However, after about 1 hour, the rate of ^{47}Ca disappearance gradually slows. Apparently, equilibration is developing between ^{47}Ca in plasma and ^{47}Ca in some extravascular (largely skeletal) calcium mass; i.e., this extravascular mass returns ^{47}Ca to plasma as fast as it takes it up, so this rapid component of blood/bone calcium exchange is no longer revealed by the ^{47}Ca curve. Slower blood/bone exchange processes then become evident, whose presence had been initially screened by the fast exchange. This process continues indefinitely, so that ^{47}Ca exchange between blood and bone can be viewed as a summation of a variety of different exchange rates, varying in speed of equilibration and magnitude of turnover, as shown in Table 52-3.

These different exchange rates reflect the spatial, physical, and biological heterogeneity of skeletal mineral. Physical differences between amorphous calcium phosphate and hydroxyapatite and between partially and fully mineralized bone cause different calcium exchange rates, while spatial differences in the anatomic relation of blood supply to bone crystals cause different times for diffusion of tracer ^{47}Ca. Biological differences in the metabolic activity of different bones and different areas of the same bone are also well known: quantitative autoradiography of bone after ^{45}Ca injection shows that the tracer calcium is taken up both diffusely and in "hot spots." With time, diffuse uptake decreases and tracer in the "hot spots" decreases less; i.e., the skeleton is microscopically heterogeneous with regard to its rate of exchange.[101] To date, it has not been possible to relate the different rates of ^{47}Ca exchange in humans with specific anatomic or biochemical processes in bone.

Some investigators have tried to analyze the rapid and slower phases of human blood/bone calcium exchange separately by di-

viding the total exchange rate into three or four component rates (the total number of components chosen as needed to satisfy the data).[99] Other investigators have viewed such exchanges as a continuum, to be characterized by a mean exchange time.[102] From the viewpoint of serum calcium homeostasis, these analyses are equivalent, since the total mass of calcium entering and leaving the plasma per unit time is calculated to be the same with all methods of analysis.[102] It is also evident (Table 52-3) that parathyroid hormone influences all phases of skeletal calcium turnover in a parallel manner, and this has been carefully established in experimental animals,[71] so that the homeostatic analysis is little affected by the decision to subdivide or aggregate the different exchange rates.

It is difficult to express blood/bone calcium exchanges in terms of pools or compartments because the serum calcium is not a functional pool for calcium. The "extracellular" fluid, an abstraction useful in discussing some ion turnovers, is also a functionally meaningless concept for discussing calcium distribution.[99] Blood calcium and skeletal calcium exchange so rapidly that the serum calcium is functionally one unit with at least some part of the skeletal calcium. For example, 50 percent of a ^{47}Ca dose is in the skeleton only 10 minutes after intravenous injection into a young rat.[103] Furthermore, the injected isotopic calcium tracers never reach equilibrium with the skeletal calcium, so that the apparent calcium "pool" size increases continually with increasing time after isotopic calcium injection. At 1 hour the apparent pool size is 2.5 g of calcium in healthy young adults, increasing to 3–5 g at 6 hours and 5–10 g at 2 days, while the "instantaneous" pool size is 1.2 g.[99] We have arbitrarily selected these times because it is often clinically useful to anticipate the immediate, 1-, 6-, or 48-hour distribution spaces of infused or ingested calcium.

As noted above, the daily turnover of plasma calcium is 30–40 g in healthy young adults.[99] This is about 30 times the instantaneous calcium "pool," so one complete turnover of the plasma calcium takes only about 50 minutes. Nearly all of this turnover represents internal exchanges between blood and bone. (Soft-tissue calcium is less than 1 percent of the total body calcium and exchanges relatively rapidly,[104] while absorption of dietary calcium and fecal and urinary excretion of calcium total only 0.3–0.6 g/day.[99] A moment's consideration of these figures provides some insight into calcium homeostasis. For example, normal urinary and fecal calcium excretion is so slow relative to internal calcium redistribution that changes in renal calcium clearance alter the serum calcium concentration only sluggishly. It is easy to calculate that even if urinary calcium excretion stopped entirely, the serum calcium concentration would hardly change in 1 hour, would increase only 0.2 mg/100 ml in 6 hours, and only 0.8 mg/100 ml in 48 hours (these calculations assume that all other variables remain unaffected and are only intended to illustrate the quantitative and temporal interrelationships of normal adult calcium homeostasis). Doubling renal calcium clearance in a normal adult would lower the serum calcium concentration at the same slow rate (Fig. 52-11). Although in the final steady state, changes in renal calcium clearance can have major effects on the serum calcium concentration, they provide an approach to this ultimate steady state that is too slow for short-term serum calcium homeostasis. The magnitude of net intestinal calcium absorption in adults is normally about the same as renal calcium excretion (another way of stating that adults normally have a net calcium balance of zero). Therefore, major changes in intestinal calcium absorption have similarly slow effects on the serum calcium level (Fig. 52-11). From these considerations, it is necessary to conclude that renal and intestinal calcium clearance can affect serum calcium homeostasis in a major fashion only over long time intervals (weeks), and short-term calcium homeostasis must be accomplished via some combination of renal, intestinal, and skeletal effects.

INORGANIC PHOSPHATE

The fate of inorganic-phosphate molecules entering the plasma is instructive. About 50 percent is excreted in the urine and 5 percent in the feces during the first few days after intravenous administration of isotopically labeled orthophosphate, 30 percent is taken up by the skeleton, and the remainder taken up by the soft tissues, some of which then reappears in blood as phospholipids and other organic-phosphate compounds.[105] Some of the isotopic phosphate also circulates in erythrocytes and granulocytes, in an approximate equilibrium with plasma.[106] These observations emphasize the primacy of the kidney as a route for plasma phosphate disposal.

The total ^{32}P disappearance rate after intravenous injection of ^{32}P-orthophosphate is approximately described by

$$y = 0.75e^{-1.4t} + 0.20e^{-0.35t} + 0.05e^{-0.036t} \qquad \text{(Eq. 4)}$$

where y is the ^{32}P content of whole blood (corrected for isotopic decay), and t is in days.[105] This corresponds to a mean total turnover time of 2.5 days (this is probably an underestimate as a result of incomplete data in the early portions of the disappearance curve). Since plasma inorganic-phosphate exchanges are substantial with many tissues in addition to the skeleton, the determinants of such a curve are considerably more complex than the corresponding plasma calcium disappearance curve. The last term of Eq. 4 represents primarily excretion and skeletal ^{32}P uptake.[107,108] This single exponential describes ^{32}P disappearance from whole blood in adult humans accurately over the interval of 48 hours to 6 weeks after ^{32}P injection.[106] It has a half-life of 19 days, corresponding to a mean blood phosphate turnover time of 27 days as a result of excretion and slow skeletal uptake alone.

Such data can provide an operational definition of the controlling and disturbing signals for inorganic-phosphate homeostasis. If they are combined with measurements of urinary and fecal ^{32}P excretion, the extravascular ^{32}P uptake can be calculated as well. Such measurements are very scanty in humans, and Eq. 4 is based on data from several sources. The general validity of the approach has been demonstrated in animals[107] and in a few human studies.[108]

Pool sizes or "spaces" for inorganic phosphate have been calculated only occasionally[109] in studies of inorganic-phosphate homeostasis. Since the distribution of phosphate is so heterogeneous and is different in the fasting and fed state (Chapter 40), such calculations are only useful analytical devices, not physical entities. In this respect, the phosphate "pool" resembles the calcium "pool." Because human data on phosphate kinetics are so scanty, it is not clear whether plasma phosphate turnover in humans is dominated by skeletal phosphate exchange, extraskeletal phosphate exchange, or glomerular filtrate–renal tubule exchange, and calculations such as those in Fig. 52-11 are unwarranted for phosphate.

HOMEOSTATIC ADAPTATION TO DISTURBING SIGNALS: CLINICAL EXAMPLES

CALCIUM

The response of healthy adult humans to dietary calcium loading or depletion has been studied at calcium intakes of 200–2000 mg/day, which is the normal range of dietary calcium with modern American diets.[77] Figures 52-12 through 52-15, and Table 52-4 summarize the results. As dietary calcium increases, the efficiency of intestinal calcium absorption decreases, falling from ≈ 70 percent efficiency at an intake of 220 mg of calcium per day to ≈ 20 percent efficiency at an intake of 2000 mg of calcium per day. This inverse relationship between dietary calcium load and intestinal calcium absorptive efficiency is exponential, not linear (Fig. 52-12A). This is not the result of saturation of intestinal calcium transport capacity, for intestinal intubation studies in healthy adults[110] show that absorptive efficiency changes in response to dietary calcium, and capacity is not saturated at luminal calcium concentrations that are achieved on such diets (Fig. 52-8, legend). The changes in intestinal calcium absorptive efficiency are more likely the result of changes in $1,25(OH)_2D$ production. In experimental animals, a high-calcium diet decreases $1,25(OH)_2D_3$ production, and this in turn causes a reduction in intestinal calcium absorption. A low-calcium diet, on the other hand, stimulates

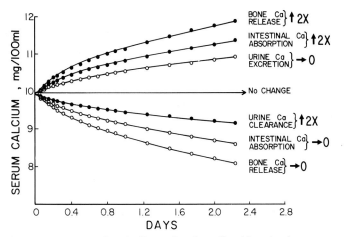

Fig. 52-11. The predicted effects of various disturbing signals on serum calcium concentration in normal adult humans if no homeostatic adaptations occurred. Increments and decrements in serum calcium concentration are plotted as a function of elapsed time in days. Illustrated are the effects of total interruption in renal calcium excretion, intestinal calcium absorption, or the slowest component of skeletal calcium release (○). Also illustrated are the effects of a twofold increase in intestinal calcium absorption, renal calcium clearance, or the slowest component of skeletal calcium release (●). (Calculated from data in reference (99).)

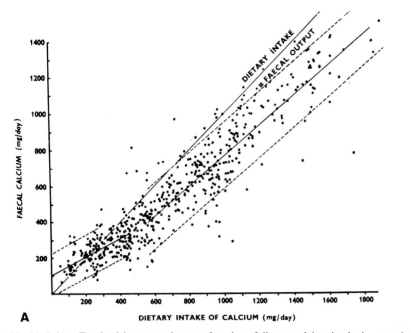

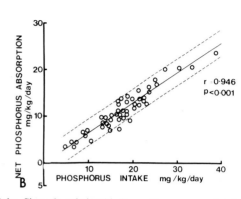

Fig. 52-12A (left). Fecal calcium excretion as a function of dietary calcium intake in normal adults. Since the relationship is curvilinear, regression lines and 95 percent confidence limits have been fitted to the two sections of data independently as indicated. The diagonal line with slope = 1 represents 100 percent absorption. (Reprinted with permission from Stanbury, S. W., in Berlyne, G. M. (ed): Nutrition in Renal Failure, Baltimore, Williams & Wilkins, 1968, p. 118.) **Fig. 52-12B (right).** Intestinal phosphorus absorption vs. dietary intake in normal adults. Note the linearity observed. (Reprinted with permission from Wilkinson, R., in Nordin, B. E. C. (ed): Calcium, Phosphate, and Magnesium Metabolism, New York, Churchill-Livingstone, 1976, p. 36.)

1,25(OH)$_2$D$_3$ production.[111] Vitamin D deficiency eliminates the intestinal adaptation, as does a constant dosage of exogenous 1,25(OH)$_2$D$_3$.[111] Parathyroid hormone deficiency also eliminates the effect,[112] and it seems clear that in these animals, the operative sequence is

$$\Delta \text{ diet Ca} \rightarrow \Delta \text{ Ca absorption} \rightarrow \text{serum Ca}^{(-)} \rightarrow \Delta \text{ PTH} \rightarrow$$
$$\uparrow \underset{\Delta}{\overset{(-)}{\rule{0pt}{0pt}}} \text{Ca absorptive efficiency} \leftarrow \Delta \text{ 1,25(OH)}_2\text{D}$$

Data in humans are less extensive, but it has recently been reported that 1,25(OH)$_2$D$_3$ blood levels in healthy adults are inversely related to the dietary calcium intake.[113] This adaptive mechanism is quite efficient. Had it failed to operate, intestinal calcium absorption in the study summarized in Table 52-4 would have increased from 340 mg/day to 840 mg/day as the diet calcium rose from 850 to 2100 mg/day. Instead, intestinal calcium absorp-

tion rose to only 490 mg/day with the high-calcium diet (Table 52-4). Nonetheless, this additional calcium must be disposed of to preserve homeostasis. Similarly, calcium absorption on the 220-mg intake would have fallen to 88 mg/day without intestinal adaptation. Instead, it only fell to 150 mg/day. The homeostatic stress to the remainder of the body was thus diminished substantially by the intestine.

Because of this intestinal adaptation, changes in dietary calcium have variable and nonlinear effects on urinary calcium excretion.[114] The important renal contribution to calcium homeostasis can be seen clearly only by comparing *absorbed* calcium and urinary calcium (Fig. 52-13). At least two factors cause the linear relationship apparent in that figure. Increased intestinal calcium absorption slightly and transiently increases the serum calcium concentration.[115] This transiently increases the calcium load filtered across the renal glomerulus and simultaneously suppresses the secretion of parathyroid hormone. The increase in filtered load

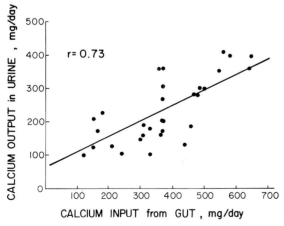

Fig. 52-13. Urinary calcium excretion as a function of calcium input from the intestine in normal adults studied on various dietary calcium intakes. (Plotted from data in references 98 and 99.)

Table 52-4. Normal Adult Response to Varying Dietary Calcium Intake

	220	850	2100
Diet calcium (mg/day)	(low)	(normal)	(high)
Absorbed calcium (mg/day)*	150	340	490
Efficiency (%)†	68%	40%	23%
Renal Ca excretion (mg/day)	150	210	260
Efficiency (arbitrary units)‡	.75	1.0	1.1
Total Ca balance (mg/day)	−110	0	+70
Skeletal Ca uptake (mg/day)**	420	420	420
Efficiency (arbitrary units)‡	1.9	1.9	1.9
Skeletal Ca release (mg/day)**	530	420	350

*Diet minus fecal calcium corrected for endogenous fecal calcium.
†Absorbed calcium/diet calcium.
‡Rate constants for ^{47}Ca removal from plasma into urine or nonexchanging bone.
**Values given were calculated with a compartmental model. Other methods of calculation give results that are identical or are linearly related.[98,102]

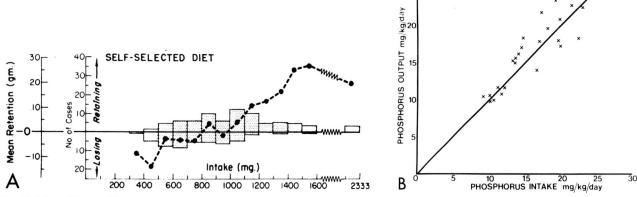

Fig. 52-14A (left). Mean calcium retention or loss (interrupted line) as a function of dietary calcium intake in healthy young adult women studied on a metabolic ward and consuming their customary diets. The shaded bars above and below the zero line show the number of subjects with net calcium retention or loss, respectively, at each calcium intake. Note losses at intakes <500 mg/day, retentions at intakes >1100 mg/day, and apparent homeostatic adaptation between these limits. (Reprinted with permission from Ohlson, M. A., Stearns, G., *Fed Proc 18:* 1077–1085, 1959.) **Fig. 52-14B (right).** Phosphate retention as a function of dietary phosphate intake in healthy adults similarly studied. Note homeostatic adaptation at all intakes. (Reprinted with permission from Nordin, B. E. C. (ed): Calcium, Phosphate, and Magnesium Metabolism, New York, Churchill-Livingstone, 1976, p. 25.)

and the decrease in parathyroid hormone secretion together enhance calcium disposal through the kidneys. Decreases in intestinal calcium absorption have the opposite effect. The relative importance of postprandial changes in load (prerenal factor) and changes in clearance (renal factor) has not been fully investigated, partly because the increments in serum calcium concentration are too small to measure with ease. It is known that shortly after dietary calcium intake is increased or decreased, changes in the serum calcium concentration can be observed in humans (prerenal effect).[115] Later, adaptive changes in renal calcium clearance account for most of the change in renal calcium excretion.[98] For example, after 4 to 6 weeks, equilibration on the 220–850–2100-mg calcium diets in Table 52-4, renal calcium excretion varied in the ratio 0.71 : 1 : 1.24, while renal ^{47}Ca clearance varied in the ratio 0.75 : 1 : 1.10.[98]

Changes in intestinal calcium absorption and renal calcium excretion do not hold calcium balance perfectly constant in healthy

young adults during such dietary variations as shown in Table 52-4, although such variations are within the range of normal dietary calcium. Figure 52-14A summarizes a large number of calcium balance studies in healthy young women and shows that departures from perfect calcium balance are particularly likely to occur on low-normal and high-normal calcium intakes. Negative calcium balances must provoke hypocalcemia, and positive balances must provoke hypercalcemia, unless some additional adaptive mechanism exists to redistribute calcium between the blood and the skeleton. In young adult humans, this is accomplished by varying skeletal calcium release (Table 52-4). Skeletal calcium uptake, interestingly enough, does not change in humans as dietary calcium is altered within the normal range, at least uptake as measured in the fasting steady state.[98]

The contribution of the various organs to homeostasis can be compared by quantitating the fraction of the total dietary perturbation buffered by each. Taking an 850-mg calcium intake as a normal reference point, one obtains the following data:[98]

	Dietary Calcium Perturbation	Percentage of Perturbation Buffered by:		
		Intestine*	Kidney Excretion	Skeletal Ca Release†
Low-calcium diet	−630 mg/day	74%	9%	17%
High-calcium diet	+1250 mg/day	90%	1%	9%

*Diet minus fecal calcium.
†Calculated as in Table 52-4.

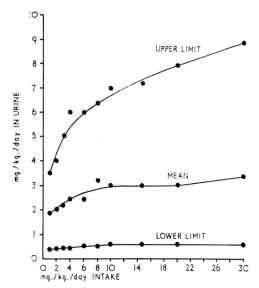

Fig. 52-15. Urinary calcium excretion as a function of dietary calcium intake in healthy subjects. Note the asymmetry of the normal range about its mean. (Reprinted with permission from Peacock, M. et al, *Br Med J 3:* 469–471, 1967.)

Although the intestine is the principal buffer against normal variations in dietary calcium intake, the additional 10 to 25 percent contribution of the kidney and skeleton is obviously essential to prevent hypercalcemia or hypocalcemia. Furthermore, the efficiency of intestinal adaptation is deficient in a significant portion of the normal population. In these individuals, the kidneys play a more important role in the adaptive response to high-calcium diets. This skewed feature of the normal population is evident from Fig. 52-15, which summarizes the data on renal calcium excretion in a large number of normal adults studied on controlled calcium intakes.[114] Skewing of calcium homeostatic mechanisms in normal adults remains unexplained, is associated with the genesis of renal calculi in some people,[116] and will perhaps be clarified by studies of $1,25(OH)_2D_3$ production in normal humans.

The question sometimes arises whether the gut, the kidney, or the skeleton is principally responsible for serum calcium homeostasis in humans. These experimental results demonstrate the inappropriateness of such a question. All three organs are normally responsible. Their responses are presumably integrated by parathyroid hormone, since the changes in $1,25(OH)_2D_3$ production, intestinal and renal calcium conservation, and skeletal calcium release on a low-calcium diet are those produced by increases in circulating parathyroid hormone concentration. Conversely, the changes seen on a high-calcium diet are those expected from parathyroid suppression. Serum parathyroid hormone levels have rarely been compared in humans on low- and high-calcium diets. This probably reflects current difficulties with parathyroid hormone assays (Chapter 45). Formal studies of calcium homeostasis in hypoparathyroid humans subjected to varying calcium intakes are also very limited. It is well known to clinicians, however, that the serum calcium concentration of such individuals is unusually sensitive to variations in dietary calcium intake.

Massive oral calcium loads or intravenous infusions of calcium will surpass or bypass the intestine's adaptive capacity and permit a greater challenge to the homeostatic capacities of the kidney and skeleton. Such experiments provide important insights into calcium homeostasis in hypercalcemic diseases, but the artificiality of extreme calcium loading makes them less relevant to normal calcium homeostasis. Extreme oral calcium loads (such as $CaCo_3$ used as an antacid), intestinal calcium hyperabsorption (such as sarcoidosis), intravenous calcium infusions, or osteolytic bone diseases will increase renal calcium excretion markedly if they increase serum calcium concentrations above normal.[117] At total serum calcium concentrations above 11 mg/100 ml, total serum calcium concentration and renal calcium excretion are experimentally found to be linearly related with a slope of about 0.3 in normal humans (Fig. 52-7). At these serum calcium levels, nearly 50 percent of the calcium filtered by the renal glomeruli is excreted, and the kidneys play a major role in calcium homeostasis.[118] This is clinically evident in many hypercalcemic diseases, which are invariably made rapidly worse by any decrease in renal calcium excretion, such as occurs, for example, in extracellular fluid volume depletion.

In these experimental or pathological situations, the remainder of the infused or absorbed calcium is retained in the skeleton (the induced transient hypercalcemia may also cause pathological calcium deposition in extraskeletal tissues).[119] At total serum calcium concentrations above 11 mg/100 ml, skeletal calcium uptake is also linearly related to total serum calcium concentration with a slope of 0.3 in normal humans (i.e., the skeletal clearance rate for calcium is equal to the renal clearance rate).[120,122] Intestinal excretion of infused calcium is relatively unimportant in the homeostatic defense against such extreme calcium loads.[123]

These linear relationships imply that renal calcium clearance and skeletal calcium clearance from plasma remain constant in normal humans as the total serum calcium concentration is experimentally increased above 11 mg/100 ml by calcium infusions. Since these rate constants are strongly and rapidly influenced by parathyroid hormone, their constancy in turn implies that PTH does not homeostatically regulate serum calcium levels above 11 mg/100 ml in normal humans. This is entirely consistent with the animal data in Fig. 52-2A, which show that PTH secretion is suppressed to a constant basal level at serum total calcium concentrations above 10.5 mg/100 ml. This also explains plots of urine calcium per 100 ml GFR versus serum calcium concentration in hypoparathyroid,

hyperparathyroid, and normal individuals. Such plots (Fig. 52-7) differ primarily with regard to the serum calcium concentration at which significant amounts of calcium begin to appear in the urine, reflecting the different degrees of hypercalcemia necessary to suppress serum PTH concentrations to basal levels in hypoparathyroid, normal, and hyperparathyroid subjects.[124] Above this suppressive level of serum calcium, further increases in calcium concentration affect renal calcium excretion identically in all three groups, as evidenced by similar slopes of the curves in Fig. 52-7. If parathyroid hormone secretion actually became zero in normal individuals during experimentally induced hypercalcemia, one would expect their urinary calcium excretion to increase to that of hypoparathyroid subjects with equivalent serum calcium concentrations. That this does not happen is evidence of the continued secretion of basal nonsuppressible PTH in normal humans at supranormal serum calcium concentrations.

Challenge studies with intravenous calcium infusions have further confirmed the ineffectiveness of normal parathyroid glands in regulating serum calcium concentrations above 11 mg/dl. When calcium is infused intravenously at a constant rate, the resultant Δ serum concentration at equilibrium per Δ disturbing signal (milligrams of calcium infused per kilogram of body weight per hour) indicates the effectiveness of serum calcium homeostasis. If such experiments are done in normal dogs, the effectiveness of serum calcium homeostasis is only two times better than that in thyroparathyroidectomized dogs regardless of the magnitude of the disturbing signal and the severity of the ultimate hypercalcemia.[125,126] Nordin et al. have done such experiments in humans and found only a twofold to fourfold difference in homeostatic effectiveness between hypoparathyroid and hyperparathyroid subjects at serum calcium concentrations above normal. The difference between hypoparathyroid and normal humans is even less, although the data are still not numerous.[122] A twofold difference between normal and hypoparathyroid animals and humans implies that the parathyroid glands play a relatively limited role in calcium homeostasis when the serum calcium concentrations are elevated to 11–18 mg/dl, as they were in these experiments. This is again compatible with the data in Fig. 52-2A. Presumably the homeostatic effectiveness of the parathyroid glands is much greater in the 7.0–10.5 mg/dl range of serum calcium concentrations, since the serum ionized-calcium concentration is normally extremely stable,[127,128] but this has not been formally confirmed.

Calcium deprivation of extreme degree, such as that produced by total starvation, also surpasses or bypasses the adaptive capacity of the intestine, leaving the kidney and skeleton to satisfy homeostatic requirements. Even under these stressful circumstances, the obligate minimum intestinal calcium excretion is 75–100 mg/day, as assessed by balance studies (Fig. 52-12A) or ^{47}Ca kinetic studies.[123] Starvation in addition increases renal calcium clearance, partly as a result of the mild metabolic acidosis of starvation ketosis and partly as a result of obscure mechanisms.[129,130] Thus renal losses of 100–150 mg of calcium per day continue even with total starvation. Under these circumstances, only a short-term sacrifice of skeletal mineral will maintain normocalcemia. Part of this sacrifice occurs in the course of skeletal buffering of the mild starvation ketoacidosis.[131] Buffering the acidosis with exogenous alkali does not prevent maintenance of normocalcemia but does slightly reduce the negative calcium balance. The remainder of the skeletal calcium release is parathyroid-hormone-dependent, and serum PTH levels are mildly elevated during prolonged fasting. The elevated PTH also enhances renal phosphate clearance. This helps dispose of the inorganic phosphate liberated from the skeleton with calcium and prevents phosphate-accelerated skeletal redeposition of the liberated calcium. Thus serum calcium concentrations remain normal, even during prolonged starvation.

During vitamin D deficiency, intestinal calcium absorption is similar to that seen in total starvation. However, severe vitamin D deficiency also interferes with skeletal calcium release in response to parathyroid hormone (see p. 676 and Chapter 51), so that hypocalcemia may result from intestinal calcium malabsorption if vitamin D deficiency is also present.[59,63] During and after infusions of EDTA or citrated blood in large quantities, short-term sacrifices of skeletal mineral are again necessary to restore extracellular fluid calcium rapidly.[132] The reduction is skeletal blood flow that occurs in oligemic patients may delay this homeostatic skeletal response to the challenge of transfused citrate load and prevent maintenance of normocalcemia.[132]

The importance of the parathyroid glands in the defense against such severe disturbing signals has been evaluated with EDTA infusions in animals (and to some extent in patients) who are thyroparathyroidectomized (open loop). In the TPTX dog, EDTA-provoked hypocalcemia fails to evoke any increase in skeletal calcium release, even after hours of moderately severe hypocalcemia.[125,126] Local hypocalcemia in the isolated perfused dog limb stimulates only a limited skeletal calcium release, presumably because parathyroid hormone levels remain normal.[133] Studies of hypoparathyroid patients given EDTA are so limited that it is difficult to deduce whether the same is true in humans, but their recovery from such induced hypocalcemia is clearly delayed.[134] EDTA-induced hypocalcemia will stimulate skeletal calcium release in the thyroparathyroidectomized rat, however,[135] and will also stimulate calcium release from rat bone in organ culture (if PTH is present at a constant amount).[15] It is not clear whether these species differences are quantitative or qualitative,[136] but the clear result in TPTX dogs is that the defense against hypocalcemia is only half as good as normal (i.e., symmetric with the defense against hypercalcemia).[125,126]

It is thus apparent that the relative homeostatic importance of the intestines, kidneys, and skeleton varies with the degree, direction, and source (oral or intravenous) of the challenge to serum calcium homeostasis. The difficulty of ascribing a critical role to one specific organ is perhaps most clearly demonstrated by the fact that oral calcium loads are buffered primarily by the intestine if given in one dose, but if the identical total daily calcium load is subdivided and given orally in daily divided doses, total intestinal calcium absorption is increased, intestinal buffering of the calcium load is partly bypassed, and marked increases in renal calcium excretion occur, together with simultaneous decreases in skeletal calcium release.[137] The essence of any controlling system is the interdependence of its parts. Consideration of one organ in isolation distorts this reality and obscures comprehension of calcium homeostasis, however useful it may be for analysis of other aspects of calcium metabolism. Some clinically significant examples of disturbing signals that threaten serum calcium homeostasis are outlined in Table 52-5; Table 52-6 summarizes the responses of the system to such disturbances.

INORGANIC PHOSPHATE

The capacity of the normal human intestine to absorb phosphate begins to become saturated only at luminal phosphate concentrations far above those encountered on normal diets.[138] Consequently, the intestine plays a relatively limited role in inorganic-phosphate homeostasis, in contrast to its major role in calcium homeostasis. With intakes of 500–2200 mg of phosphorus per day,

the range of dietary phosphate with modern American diets,[139] intestinal phosphate absorption remains a constant fraction (about two-thirds) of the intake (Fig. 52-12B). Although blood 1,25(OH)$_2$D levels (and indirectly parathyroid hormone levels) affect the efficiency of intestinal phosphate transport, the resultant changes in intestinal phosphate absorption appear to be smaller than those caused by normal variations in the diet phosphate. This is clearly established in the rat[82] and is strongly implied in humans. For example, patients deficient in vitamin D or unable to form 1,25(OH)$_2$D because of severe renal failure still absorb substantial amounts of dietary phosphate, although the efficiency of their intestinal phosphate absorption may be somewhat reduced.[56,57,59]

The efficient and unregulated absorption of phosphate by the intestines means that the kidneys must normally excrete a substantial phosphate load and must act alone to maintain phosphate balance on varying phosphate intakes. Figure 52-14B illustrates the efficiency with which this is normally accomplished in healthy adults: net phosphate balance remains constant near zero, despite wide variations in dietary intake (and parallel variations in intestinal phosphate absorption). This variation in renal phosphate excretion is partly the result of variations in the amount of phosphate filtered through the glomerulus, i.e., it is accomplished at the expense of variations in the serum inorganic-phosphate concentration (Fig. 52-16). The remainder of the adaptation is due to homeostatic changes in phosphate input from the renal tubules. Homeostatic renal tubular adjustments are detectable within 24 hours after changes in the dietary phosphate and continue for several days, thereby limiting the variations in serum inorganic-phosphate concentration that would otherwise occur (Fig. 52-16). It is not clear what produces these important adjustments in renal tubular phosphate absorption. Parathyroidectomy does not abolish them in laboratory animals, nor does hypoparathyroidism in patients (Fig. 52-9), and they occur despite constant doses of exogenous 1,25(OH)$_2$D in animals.[86] It is currently unclear whether this renal

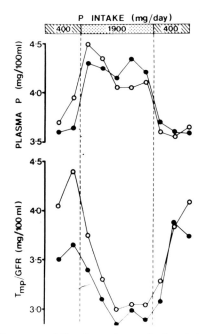

Fig. 52-16. Response of the plasma inorganic-phosphate concentration, and the maximum inorganic-phosphate input from the renal tubules, to variations in the diet phosphorus in two normal adults. (Reprinted with permission from Bijvoet, O. L. M., Morgan, D. B., in Hioco, D. J. (ed): Phosphate et Métabolisme Phosphocalcique, Paris, L'Expansion Scientifique Français, 1971, p. 153.)

Table 52-5. Examples of Clinically Significant Disturbing Signals

Calcium Disturbances	Positive Disturbances That Threaten to ↑ Serum Ca	Negative Disturbances That Threaten to ↓ Serum Ca
Disturbances in serum calcium input		
Input from gut	↑ (e.g., CaCO$_3$ treatment)	↓ (e.g., malabsorption)
Input from bone	↑ (e.g., osteolytic bone disease)	↓ (e.g., osteopetrosis)
Disturbances in serum calcium output		
Output to feces	—————	↑ (e.g., malabsorption)
Output to urine	↓ (e.g., low-sodium diet)	↑ (e.g., furosemide Rx or renal hypercalciuria)
Output to bone or soft tissue	↓ (e.g., hypophosphatemia)	↑ (e.g., hyperphosphatemia)

Inorganic-Phosphate Disturbances	Positive Disturbances That Threaten to ↑ Serum P$_i$	Negative Disturbances That Threaten to ↓ Serum P$_i$
Disturbances in serum inorganic-phosphate input		
Input from gut	↑ (e.g., high-protein diet)	↓ (e.g., AlOH$_3$ Rx or vegetarian diet)
Input from bone	↑ (e.g., osteolytic bone disease)	↓ (e.g., osteopetrosis)
Input from soft tissue	↑ (e.g., fasting)	—————
Disturbances in serum inorganic-phosphate output		
Output to feces		
Output to urine	↓ (e.g., azotemia)	↑ (e.g., osmotic diuresis)
Output to bone	↓ (e.g., growth arrest)	↑ (e.g., healing rickets)
Output to soft tissue	—————	↑ (e.g., postprandial)

tubular adaptation requires any humoral factor; changes in the amounts of phosphate in the renal tubular cells themselves may be the controlling signal (i.e., autoregulation of the controlled signal).[140,141] The importance of this tubular adaptation may be judged from the data in Fig. 52-9, comparing urinary phosphate excretion per 100 ml GFR on low- and high-phosphate diets at comparable serum inorganic-phosphate levels in normal, hypoparathyroid, and hyperparathyroid patients.[87,88,142,143]

More extreme increases in phosphate input involve the controlling system completely. For example, if dietary phosphate is supplemented with large doses of phosphate salts (e.g. 2–3 g of phosphorus daily), efficient intestinal absorption of the ingested phosphate will transiently elevate the serum inorganic-phosphate concentration enough to increase skeletal calcium uptake and provoke reactive transient increases in serum parathyroid hormone levels.[12,144] This will rapidly reduce phosphate input from the renal tubules, supplementing the tubular adaptation described above, although at the expense of an increase in skeletal turnover stimulated by the parathyroid hormone.[145-151] If dietary phosphate supplements of this magnitude are given chronically, the homeostatic system maintains a normal fasting serum inorganic-phosphate concentration,[144,146] but deposits of calcium phosphate are found in the heart and kidneys of experimental animals so treated.[146] Furthermore, the secretion of parathyroid hormone may be increased enough to cause not only increased skeletal turnover but also net bone breakdown and severe osteopenia.[145-150] These complications demonstrate the inadequacy of phosphate homeostasis in the face of massive dietary phosphate loads and illustrate as well the pathological consequences of the normal, unrestrained, intestinal phosphate absorption.

Intravenous infusions of inorganic phosphate trigger a similar series of responses[152] and are the experimental or therapeutic analogue of the massive endogenous phosphate loads released into the vascular space by acute cell death, such as that caused by cancer chemotherapy, severe hemolytic reactions, and massive trauma.[153,154] In these situations, the rate of phosphate input greatly exceeds phosphate output, and severe hyperphosphatemia develops. Phosphate output through the renal glomerulus increases in direct proportion to the serum inorganic-phosphate

concentration, but the input of phosphate from the renal tubules rapidly reaches a maximum, since the tubules normally operate near their maximum reabsorptive capacity.[87] Renal phosphate excretion is therefore determined largely by the glomerular filtration rate when serum inorganic-phosphate levels are significantly elevated above normal (Fig. 52-9). Rapid homeostatic renal tubular adaptations depend primarily on increased secretion of parathyroid hormone, because the other tubular adaptation, which accompanies variations in dietary phosphate, occurs only slowly (Fig. 52-16). Parathyroid hormone secretion is stimulated in hyperphosphatemic patients because large amounts of phosphate and calcium are precipitated or taken up in the skeleton and extraskeletal tissues (Chapter 57). The increased secretion of parathyroid hormone restrains phosphate input from the renal tubule (Fig. 52-9) in a homeostatic manner. Parathyroid hormone also stimulates phosphate input, however, since it causes net skeletal catabolism. This antihomeostatic effect is quantitatively less important than the renal effect in normal humans, but the balance between the two effects depends upon the glomerular filtration rate (see p. 687).

The extreme importance of glomerular filtration to phosphate homeostasis is perhaps best illustrated by the effects of a normal meal on the serum inorganic-phosphate concentration in uremic patients versus normal patients.[155] Normally the serum inorganic phosphate concentration stays the same or goes down after a meal, depending upon the balance between intestinal phosphate absorption, renal phosphate excretion, and postprandial uptake of phosphate into cells along with glucose (Chapter 40). In the uremic patient, however, there is a marked postprandial increase in the serum inorganic-phosphate concentration, since phosphate excretion is impaired. There is a consequent postprandial surge in parathyroid hormone secretion, which does not occur in normal adults.[156] These transient postprandial waves of parathyroid hormone secretion are probably important in the genesis of uremic osteodystrophy. They also emphasize the rapidity with which the controlling system responds to a disturbing signal, and the necessity of considering the transient as well as the steady-state responses of the system in any homeostatic analysis.

Extreme decreases in phosphate input also involve the entire controlling system. Poor dietary intake of phosphate (e.g., a low-

Table 52-6. Summary of Controlling System Responses to Disturbing Signals

Calcium Homeostasis	Responses to Disturbing Signals That Threaten to ↑ Serum Ca	Responses to Disturbing Signals That Threaten to ↓ Serum Ca
Direct responses	↑ Ca output to renal tubules and bones	↓ Ca output to renal tubules and bones
		± ↑ input from bones
	↓ PTH secretion	↑ PTH secretion
	↓ 1,25-(OH)$_2$D secretion*	↑ 1,25-(OH)$_2$D secretion*
Indirect responses (due to changes in blood PTH or 1,25-(OH)$_2$D)	↓ Ca input from gut and bone	↑ Ca input from bone
	↑ Ca output to urine (as GFR permits)	↑ Ca input from gut (as diet Ca permits)
		↑ Ca input from renal tubules
Incidental effects on phosphate homeostasis**	Direct ↑ serum P$_i$ (transient)	± Direct ↑ P$_i$ input from bone
	Direct ↓ P$_i$ input from renal tubules	Direct ↑ P$_i$ input from renal tubules
	Indirect ↓ P$_i$ input from bone (and ± from gut)	Indirect ↑ P$_i$ input from bone (and ± from gut)
	Indirect ↑ P$_i$ input from renal tubules	Indirect ↓ P$_i$ input from renal tubules

Inorganic-Phosphate Homeostasis	Responses to Disturbing Signals That Threaten to ↑ Serum P$_i$	Responses to Disturbing Signals That Threaten to ↓ Serum P$_i$
Direct responses	↓ P$_i$ input from renal tubules	↑ P$_i$ input from renal tubules
	↑ P$_i$ output to bones and soft tissues	↓ P$_i$ output to bones
		↑ P$_i$ input from soft tissue and from bones
	↑ PTH secretion†	↓ PTH secreton†
	↑ 1,25-(OH)$_2$D secretion*	↓ 1,25-(OH)$_2$D secretion*
		↓ 1,25-(OH)$_2$D catabolism‡
		↑ 1,25-(OH)$_2$D secretion‡
Indirect responses (due to changes in blood PTH or 1,25-(OH)$_2$D)	↓ P$_i$ input from renal tubules (as GFR permits)	↑ P$_i$ input from renal tubules (as GFR permits)
	↑ P$_i$ input from bone (and ± from gut)	↑ or ↓ P$_i$ input from bone (and ± from gut)
Incidental effects on calcium homeostasis**	Direct ↑ Ca output to bone	Direct ↓ Ca output to bone
	Indirect ↑ Ca input from bone	Direct ↑ Ca input from bone
	Indirect ↑ Ca input from gut (as diet Ca permits)	Indirect ↑ Ca input from gut (as diet Ca permits)
	Indirect ↑ Ca input from renal tubules	Indirect ↓ Ca input from renal tubules

*Changes in 1,25-(OH)$_2$D secretion result from changes in serum PTH levels.

†Changes in PTH secretion are indirectly produced via effects of inorganic phosphate on calcium input and output, and subserve calcium homeostasis.

‡Changes are produced directly by severe P$_i$ depletion, independently of PTH.

**Note the conflicting directions of the incidental effects, which often make it difficult to predict intuitively the magnitude or direction of the changes in inorganic-phosphate metabolism that accompany primary disturbances in calcium homeostasis, and vice versa.

protein intake), coupled with mild degrees of malabsorption, can produce severe phosphate depletion, as commonly seen in alcoholic patients (Chapter 40). Overdosage with antacids containing aluminum hydroxide, which bind phosphate in the intestine and prevent its absorption, can also produce severe phosphate depletion. Starvation usually does not cause phosphate depletion, since cell catabolism releases enough endogenous phosphate to compensate for the lack of intestinal phosphate absorption.[157] Figure 52-17 illustrates the homeostatic responses to phosphate depletion in a normal adult given large doses of aluminum hydroxide experimentally.[14] The initial response is a total disappearance of inorganic phosphate from the urine as a result of both the renal tubular adaptive response described above and a decrease in parathyroid hormone secretion.[20,21] The decreased parathyroid secretion is caused by the decreased skeletal calcium uptake that accompanies phosphate depletion.[13] After this initial renal adaptation, the efficiency of intestinal phosphate absorption increases and can approach 80 to 90 percent.[14] Despite these changes, cellular phosphate stores are reduced, as revealed by the negative phosphate balance. Finally, as the serum inorganic-phosphate concentration

falls below normal (after weeks of negative phosphorus balance), skeletal breakdown and release of phosphate occur (revealed by the more negative calcium balance near the end of the experiment in Figure 52-17). Similar changes occur in hypoparathyroid humans who have been given large doses of aluminum hydroxide.[14]

This experiment illustrates the fact that hypophosphatemia is a late manifestation of phosphate depletion and that urinary phosphate excretion normally ceases rapidly in a phosphate-depleted human. Continued urinary phosphate excretion in a phosphate-depleted patient is therefore abnormal. The increased efficiency of intestinal phosphate absorption is presumably due to increased secretion of 1,25(OH)$_2$D, stimulated by the phosphate depletion despite the decrease in circulating parathyroid hormone (Fig. 52-3B and Fig. 52-5). This is one of the few instances in which intestinal phosphate absorption increases significantly above 65 to 70 percent of dietary phosphate in normal adults. Increased 1,25(OH)$_2$D secretion is also the presumed reason for the increased intestinal absorption of calcium, which accompanies the increased absorptive efficiency for phosphate. The ultimate breakdown and release of skeletal mineral is also presumably due in part to in-

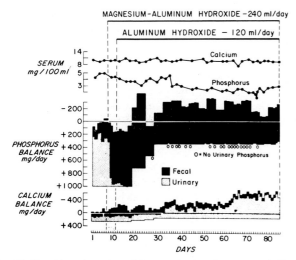

Fig. 52-17. Alterations in calcium and phosphorus metabolism in a healthy adult experimentally depleted of inorganic-phosphate with oral aluminum hydroxide. Serum calcium and inorganic-phosphate concentrations are indicated by the connected dots. Phosphorus and calcium balance data are plotted, with the intake going down from the zero line and the output plotted up from the intake. Positive balance is indicated by a clear space between the zero line and the combined urinary and fecal excretion. Negative calcium or phosphate balance is indicated by extension of the excretory measurements above the zero line. (Reprinted with permission from Lotz, M. et al, *N Engl J Med 278:* 409–415, 1968.)

creased 1,25(OH)$_2$D secretion, although phosphate depletion alone increases skeletal mineral release and decreases skeletal mineral uptake.[13] The hypercalciuria near the end of the experiment is caused by the net skeletal breakdown, combined with the increased intestinal calcium absorption and the absence of parathyroid hormone. Parathyroid hormone plays little part in the defense against phosphate depletion in contrast to its major role in the defense against calcium depletion.

An unexplained facet of inorganic-phosphate homeostasis is the acute effect of calcium infusions on the serum inorganic-phosphate concentration. In thyroparathyroidectomized animals or humans (uncoupled system), calcium infusions transiently increase the serum inorganic-phosphate concentration.[159,160] The effect is too rapid to be due to changes in phosphate balance and must reflect internal redistributions of inorganic phosphate. It is eliminated by endogenous or exogenous calcitonin in animals,[159] but it occurs in adult humans even when the thyroid is present.[160] Subsequently the serum inorganic-phosphate concentration falls as a result of changes in skeletal or renal phosphate handling.[85,161]

Some disturbing signals that threaten inorganic-phosphate homeostasis are outlined in Table 52-5; the compensatory responses of the controlling system are summarized in Table 52-6.

HOMEOSTATIC CONFLICTS AS A PATHOGENETIC FACTOR

VITAMIN D DEFICIENCY

Without vitamin D, the input of calcium from the intestines and skeleton is reduced, leading to a compensatory increase in parathyroid hormone secretion. This enhances renal calcium conservation and also increases the efficiency with which any residual 25-OHD is converted to 1,25(OH)$_2$D. As long as some 1,25(OH)$_2$D remains and severe osteomalacia is avoided, the increased blood

parathyroid hormone levels will also produce a net release of calcium from the skeleton, compensating for the decreased calcium input from the intestine and preserving serum calcium homeostasis.

However, this is accomplished at the expense of phosphate homeostasis. The vitamin D deficiency reduces the input of inorganic phosphate from the intestines, although not so markedly as the input of calcium.[59,82] The secondary hyperparathyroidism, necessary for calcium homeostasis, aggravates this phosphate depletion by decreasing phosphate input from the renal tubules. Severe phosphate depletion therefore becomes increasingly likely, unless skeletal release of phosphate can be increased enough to compensate for both the decreased intestinal input and the decreased renal tubular input of phosphate. The increased blood parathyroid hormone level does enhance skeletal release of phosphate as well as calcium. Furthermore, phosphate depletion itself enhances skeletal release of both ions and simultaneously retards skeletal phosphate and calcium uptake. Although transiently satisfactory, these mechanisms maintain serum homeostasis at the expense of the skeleton. Not only is skeletal mass reduced, but the retardation of skeletal mineralization also leads to osteomalacia. Thus the phosphate depletion, which was in part an unfortunate consequence of calcium homeostasis, ultimately aggravates the skeletal complications of vitamin D deficiency.

UREMIA

As glomerular failure develops, the phosphate filtered across the glomerulus declines. To compensate for this decreased output, phosphate input from the renal tubules, intestines, or skeleton must be diminished correspondingly. Secondary hyperparathyroidism, stimulated by the effects of the retained phosphate on calcium output to the skeleton, plays a major role in this adaptation by diminishing the renal tubular input of phosphate (Chapter 59). An undesirable consequence of secondary hyperparathyroidism, however, is an increased input of phosphate from the intestines and skeleton, which aggravates the phosphate overload. Under normal circumstances these increases are quantitatively less important than the decrease in phosphate input from the renal tubules.[162] Furthermore, in uremia, parathyroid hormone's effects on intestinal and skeletal phosphate input are somewhat limited by the failing kidney's inability to make increased quantities of 1,-25(OH)$_2$D. Therefore, phosphate homeostasis is successful even though it is indirectly mediated via the serum calcium concentration.

As glomerular failure progresses, however, the danger of such an indirect homeostatic loop becomes manifest. Parathyroid hormone can protect against phosphate overload only as long as glomerular output of phosphate is at least equal to the phosphate input from the diet and skeleton. On a 750 mg/day phosphate intake, with 66 percent absorption, the intestinal input is 500 mg P daily. If there is at least 100 mg/day net skeletal calcium release, which is necessary to cover intestinal and urinary calcium losses in the absence of intestinal calcium absorption,[56,123] there will be an accompanying 50 mg/day net skeletal input of P. The combined 550 mg P/day can be filtered at a serum inorganic-phosphate concentration of 4.5 mg/dl and a glomerular filtration rate of 8.5 ml/min, and phosphate homeostasis can be preserved if none of this filtered phosphate is reabsorbed. If any reabsorption occurs, of if the GFR is less than 8.5 ml/min, or if the intestinal phosphate input is unevenly distributed in time (an almost certain eventuality), hyperphosphatemia will develop. This will, however, cause more skeletal calcium uptake and more hyperparathyroidism, and consequently more skeletal phosphate release. A positive feedback loop has thus developed because parathyroid hormone's effects on renal phosphate input are limited by glomerular phosphate output. In this circumstance, secondary hyperparathyroidism aggravates the serum phosphate overload instead of protecting against it. That explains why parathyroidectomy in patients with advanced uremia causes a fall in both serum inorganic-phosphate and calcium concentrations,[163,164] whereas the same operation causes an increase in serum inorganic phosphate and a fall in serum calcium in normal individuals or those with mild renal failure (Chapters 46 and 59). The positive feedback loop would presumably be even worse were the skeletal and intestinal responses to parathyroid hormone not limited by the $1,25(OH)_2D$ deficiency of uremia. Positive feedback develops in this situation because of the indirect sequence of the control loop: $\Delta P_i \xrightarrow{(-)} \Delta Ca \xrightarrow{(-)} \Delta PTH$

HYPOPHOSPHATEMIA

As described above, severe phosphate depletion stimulates renal $1,25(OH)_2D$ production and delays its catabolism, and the $1,25(OH)_2D$ increases the input of phosphate from the intestine and skeleton. Hypophosphatemia itself also increases the input of phosphate from the skeleton and decreases the output of phosphate to the skeleton independently (Chapter 40). Although these measures preserve phosphate homeostasis, they produce undesirable effects on calcium homeostasis. The increased $1,25(OH)_2D$ production increases intestinal calcium absorption and skeletal calcium release. The direct effects of hypophosphatemia on the skeleton also increase skeletal calcium release and decrease skeletal calcium uptake, paralleling changes in skeletal phosphate balance. These changes suppress parathyroid hormone secretion (see p. 671), thereby increasing renal calcium clearance at a time when calcium input to the blood is high. Because of the renal cellular phosphate depletion, $1,25(OH)_2D$ production continues at a high rate despite the decline in circulating parathyroid hormone. Marked hypercalciuria results as an undesirable side effect of inorganic-phosphate homeostasis. This is the disadvantage of having one hormonal system, $1,25(OH)_2D_3$, with major effects on two different ions and with two separate control systems.

This is the presumed genesis of renal calculi in those patients whose idiopathic hypophosphatemia, hypercalciuria, and elevated serum $1,25(OH)_2D$ blood levels can all be corrected by dietary phosphate supplements.[165,166] The basic defect in this subset of hypercalciuric stone-formers is presumably their hypophosphatemia. The hypercalciuria and the renal calculi are unfortunate side effects of the body's attempts to maintain inorganic-phosphate homeostasis.

OSTEOPENIA OF THE ELDERLY

Healthy elderly people absorb calcium from the diet less efficiently than do young adults,[110] particularly when the elderly are on low-calcium diets (Fig. 52-8), for reasons that are a subject of active investigation.[167] The foregoing analysis predicts, and experiment confirms, that the mean and range of normal urinary calcium excretion are therefore lower in elderly (age >60) than in young adults.[168]

How often intestinal calcium malabsorption causes osteopenia in the elderly, by stimulating a homeostatic increase in skeletal calcium release, remains controversial. Riggs et al recently reported that plasma $1,25(OH)_2D$ levels and intestinal calcium absorptive efficiency were decreased in parallel in a group of elderly osteopenic subjects.[167] But it is unclear whether the decrease in

$1,25(OH)_2D$ levels was an etiologically significant primary abnormality in these patients or merely their homeostatically appropriate secondary response to a negative skeletal calcium balance. Two recent studies have independently shown that oral calcium supplements preserve bone mass in elderly women,[169,170] as one would predict if their declining bone mass were caused by homeostatic stress.[171] This "homeostatic theory" for the genesis of senile osteopenia is further discussed in Chapter 71.

GENERAL CONSIDERATIONS

Although the present discussion has focused on serum calcium and inorganic-phosphate homeostasis as influenced by parathyroid hormone and $1,25(OH)_2D$, in the body this control system undoubtedly interacts with others. For example, calcitonin plays an important role in calcium and inorganic-phosphate homeostasis in lower mammals; its importance in humans is not yet clear (Chapters 48 to 50). In experimental animals, diurnal rhythms substantially affect serum calcium and inorganic-phosphate concentrations by modifying the blood levels of calcitonin and/or parathyroid hormone, probably independently of variations in the disturbing signals of serum calcium and phosphate turnover.[172,173] In humans, there are diurnal variations in renal calcium and inorganic-phosphate excretion that are independent of those imposed by food.[174,175] In humans and animals, calcium and inorganic phosphate homeostasis are strongly influenced by the balance between skeletal uptake and release of mineral, which, although sensitive to the blood parathyroid hormone and $1,25(OH)_2D$ concentrations, is also influenced by the mechanical stress, electrical charge, and chemical structure of the organic bone matrix.[176] Skeletal formation and destruction are further linked by a poorly understood local mechanical or cellular control system, so that bone formation and destruction in an area of the skeleton increase and decrease together in normal and pathological conditions.[177] Glucocorticoids and gonadal steroids also have major effects on calcium and inorganic-phosphate turnover, as discussed above and elsewhere in this book, and sodium intake and extracellular fluid volume markedly alter renal calcium and inorganic-phosphate excretion, as reviewed in Chapter 40.

Conflicts between these control systems and the calcium and phosphate homeostatic system may also have pathogenetic significance. To define such conflicts, we must first understand how these other control systems interact with, depend upon, or even dominate the homeostatic system described above. Dissecting such hierarchies of control will require a quantitative description of calcium and inorganic-phosphate homeostasis, correlating measured blood levels of parathyroid hormone and $1,25(OH)_2D$ with the simultaneously measured serum calcium and inorganic-phosphate concentrations, inputs, and outputs. Most of the data currently available are incomplete, omitting several of these quantities. A quantitative description will also be necessary for the temporal aspects of homeostasis, i.e., the initial transient changes in the controlled and controlling signals that precede their final steady-state values. The available data on the transient responses of the controlling system in humans are primarily serial measurements of the blood concentration and urinary excretion of calcium and inorganic phosphate after the acute administration of parathyroid hormone or $1,25(OH)_2D$ and serial measurements of blood parathyroid hormone concentrations after acute calcium or phosphate loads. The other controlling signals have not been measured as a result of technical limitations. More complete data will not only make our description of calcium and inorganic-phosphate homeostasis more quantitative and reveal its dynamic aspects but they may also explain such puzzling observations as the continued secretion of parathyroid hormone in immobilized patients and animals,[178,179] despite a massive input of skeletal calcium[180] and despite the fact that an absence of parathyroid hormone would minimize their skeletal atrophy.[181] Such data may also help us sort out, understand, and ultimately modify the skeletal changes that accompany aging, diabetes mellitus, glucocorticoid excess, and a variety of other conditions that affect multiple controlling signals in the homeostatic system and simultaneously affect bone matrix metabolism.

REFERENCES

1. Mayer, G. P., Habener, J. F., Potts, J. T.: Parathyroid hormone secretion in vivo. Demonstration of a calcium-independent non-suppressible component of secretion. *J Clin Invest 57:* 678–683, 1976.

2. Mayer, G. P.: Effect of calcium and magnesium on parathyroid hormone secretory rate in calves, in Talmage, R. V., Owen, M., Parsons, J. A. (eds): Calcium-Regulating Hormones, Proceedings of the Fifth Parathyroid Conference. Amsterdam, Excerpta Medica, 1975.

3. Sherwood, L. M., Herrman, I., Bassett, C. A.: Parathyroid hormone secretion in vitro: Regulation by calcium and magnesium ions. *Nature 225:* 1056–1058, 1970.

4. Habener, J. F., Kemper, B., Potts, J. T.: Calcium-dependent intracellular degradation of parathyroid hormone: A possible mechanism for the regulation of hormone stores. *Endocrinology 97:* 431–441, 1975.

5. Buckle, R. M., Aurbach, G. D., Potts, J. T.: Adaptive increases in parathyroid glandular activity, in Protein and Polypeptide Hormones. Excerpta Medica International Congress Series #161. Amsterdam, Excerpta Medica, 1969, pp. 389–395.

6. Burckhardt, P., Ruedi, B., Felber, J. P.: The clinical usefulness of the EDTA infusion as a stimulation test for parathyroid function, in Talmage, R. V., Owen, M., Parsons, J. A. (eds): Calcium-Regulating Hormones, Proceedings of the Fifth Parathyroid Conference. Amsterdam, Excerpta Medica, 1975, pp. 75–77.

7. Potts, J. T., Reitz, R. E., Deftos, L. J., et al: Secondary hyperparathyroidism in chronic renal disease. *Arch Intern Med 124:* 408–412, 1969.

8. Gittes, R. F., Radde, I. C.: Experimental model for hyperparathyroidism: Effect of excessive numbers of transplanted isologous parathyroid glands. *J Urology 95:* 595–603, 1966.

9. Bigos, S. T., Neer, R. M., St. Goar, W. T.: Hypercalcemia of seven years' duration after kidney transplantation. *Am J Surg 132:* 83–89, 1976.

10. Sherwood, L. M., Mayer, G. P., Ramberg, C. F., Jr., et al: Regulation of parathyroid hormone secretion: Proportional control by calcium, lack of effect of phosphate. *Endocrinology 83:* 1043–1051, 1968.

11. Fischer, J. A., Binswanger, U., Blum, J. W.: The acute parathyroid hormone response to changes in ionized calcium during phosphate infusions in the cow. *Eur J Clin Invest 3:* 151–155, 1973.

12. Reiss, E., Canterbury, J., Bercovitz, M. A., et al: The role of phosphate in the secretion of parathyroid hormone in man. *J Clin Invest 49:* 2146–2149, 1970.

13. Baylink, D., Wergedal, J., Stauffer, M.: Formation, mineralization and resorption of bone in hypophosphatemic rats. *J Clin Invest 50:* 2519–2530, 1971.

14. Lotz, M., Zisman, E. and Bartter, F. C.: Evidence for a phosphorus-depletion syndrome in man. *N Engl J Med 278:* 409–415, 1968.

15. Raisz, L. G., Neimann, I.: Effect of phosphate, calcium and magnesium on bone resorption and hormonal responses in tissue culture. *Endocrinology 85:* 446–452, 1969.

16. Eisenberg, E.: Effect of intravenous phosphate on serum strontium and calcium. *N Engl J Med 282:* 889–892, 1970.

17. Feinblatt, J., Belanger, L. F., Rasmussen, H.: Effect of phosphate infusion on bone metabolism and parathyroid hormone action. *Am J Physiol 218:* 1624–1631, 1970.

18. Milhaud, G., Perault-Staub, A., Moukhtar, M. S.: Étude de méchanisme de l'effect hypocalcémiant du phosphate mineral et de l'interaction eventuelle avec la thyrocalcitonine. *Compt Rend 266:* 1169–1172, 1968.

19. Parfitt, A. M.: In Kleeman, C. R., Massry, S. G., Coburn, J. W., et al (eds): The clinical physiology of calcium homeostasis, parathyroid hormone, and calcitonin. *Calif Med 114(3):* 16–43, 1971; *114(4):* 19–30, 1971.

20. Dominguez, J. H., Gray, R. W., Lemann, J.: Dietary phosphate deprivation in women and men: Effects on mineral and acid balances, parathyroid hormone, and the metabolism of 25-OH-vitamin D. *J Clin Endocrinol Metab 43:* 1056–1068, 1976.

21. Coburn, J. W., Massry, S. G.: Changes in serum and urinary calcium during phosphate depletion: Studies on mechanisms. *J Clin Invest 49:* 1073–1087, 1970.

22. Brumbaugh, P. F., Hughes, M. R., Haussler, M. R.: Cytoplasmic and nuclear binding components for 1α,25-dihydroxyvitamin D_3 in chick parathyroid glands. *Proc Natl Acad Sci USA 72:* 4871–4875, 1975.

23. Brickman, A. S., Sherrard, D. J., Jowsey, J., et al: 1,25-Dihydroxycholecalciferol: Effect on skeletal lesions and plasma parathyroid hormone levels in uremic osteodystrophy. *Arch Intern Med 134:* 883–888, 1974.

24. Oldham, S. B., Smith, R., Hartenbower, D. L., et al: Effects of 1α,25-dihydroxyvitamin D_3 on serum calcium, immunoreactive parathyroid hormone, and intestinal and parathyroid calcium-binding proteins. *Fed Proc 35:* 534, 1976.

25. Chertow, B. S., Baylink, D. J., Wergedal, J. E., et al: Decrease in serum immunoreactive parathyroid hormone in rats and in parathyroid hormone secretion in vitro by 1,25-dihydroxycholecalciferol. *J Clin Invest 56:* 668–678, 1975.

26. Care, A. D. et al: The effects of vitamin D metabolites and their analogues on the secretion of parathyroid hormone. *Calcif Tissue Res 21 (Suppl):* 142–146, 1976.

27. Canterbury, J. M., Lerman, S., Claflin, A. J., et al: Suppressive effects of 24,25-$(OH)_2D_3$ on parathyroid hormone secretion in dogs. *J Clin Invest 61:* 1375–1383, 1978.

28. Hunziker, W. H., Blum, J. W., Fischer, J. A.: Plasma kinetics of exogenous bovine parathyroid hormone in calves. *Eur J Physiol 371:* 185–192, 1977.

29. Segre, G. V., Niall, H. D., Habener, J. F., et al: Metabolism of parathyroid hormone: Physiological and clinical significance. *Am J Med 56:* 774–784, 1974.

30. Neuman, W. F., Neuman, M. W., Sammon, P. J., et al: The metabolism of labelled parathyroid hormone. III. Studies in rats. *Calcif Tissue Res 18:* 251–261, 1975.

31. Mayer, G. P., Staley, J. A. S., Keaton, J. A., et al: Relation between intravenous infusion rate of PTH and its plasma concentration. 57th Annual Meeting of the Endocrine Society, New York, 1975, p 73.

32. Habener, J. F., Mayer, G. P., Dee, P. C., et al: Metabolism of amino- and carboxy-sequence immunoreactive parathyroid hormone in the bovine: Evidence for peripheral cleavage of hormone. *Metabolism 25:* 385–395, 1976.

33. Habener, J. F., Segre, G. V., Powell, D., et al: Immunoreactive parathyroid hormone in circulation of man. *Nature (New Biol) 238:* 152–154, 1972.

34. Parsons, J. A.: Pharmacology of parathyroid hormone and some of its fragments and analogues, in Talmage, R. V., Owen, M., Parsons, J. A. (eds): Calcium-Regulating Hormones, Proceedings of the Fifth Parathyroid Conference. Amsterdam, Excerpta Medica, 1975, pp. 33–39.

35. Jung, A., Mayer, G. P. and Neer, R. M.: Unpublished observations.

36. Haussler, M. R., Baylink, D. J., Hughes, M. R., et al: The assay of 1α,25-dihydroxyvitamin D: Physiologic and pathologic modulation of circulating hormone levels. *Clin Endocrinol 5:* 151s–165s, 1976.

37. Eisman, J. A., Hamstra, A. J., Kream, B. E., et al: 1,25-Dihydroxyvitamin D in biological fluids: A simplified and sensitive assay. *Science 193:* 1021–1023, 1976.

38. Gray, R. W., Wilz, D. R., Caldas, A. E., et al: Disappearance from plasma of injected ^{3}H-1,25-$(OH)_2$-D_3 in healthy humans, in Norman, A. W., Schaefer, K., Coburn, J. W., et al (eds): Vitamin D. Biochemical, Chemical and Clinical Aspects Related to Calcium Metabolism, Proceedings of the Third Workshop on Vitamin D. New York, Walter de Gruyter, 1977.

39. Boyle, I. T., Gray, R. W., Omdahl, J. L., et al: Calcium control of the in vivo biosynthesis of 1,25-dihydroxyvitamin D_3: Nicolaysen's endogenous factor, in Taylor, S. (ed): Endocrinology 1971, Proceed-

ings of the Third International Symposium. London, William Heinemann Medical Books, 1972.

40. Hughes, M. R., Brumbaugh, P. F., Haussler, M. R., et al: Regulation of serum 1α,25-dihydroxyvitamin D_3 by calcium and phosphate in the rat. *Science 190:* 578–579, 1975.

41. Garabedian, M., Holick, M., DeLuca, F., et al: Control of 25-hydroxycholecalciferol metabolism by the parathyroid glands. *Proc Natl Acad Sci USA 69:* 1673–1676, 1972.

42. Mawer E. B., Backhouse, J., Taylor, C. M., et al: Failure of formation of 1,25-dihydroxycholecalciferol in chronic renal insufficiency. *Lancet 1:* 626–628, 1973.

43. Mawer, E. B., Backhouse, J., Hill, L. F., et al: Vitamin D metabolism and parathyroid function in man. *Clin Sci Mol Med 48:* 349–365, 1975.

44. Mawer, E. B., Backhouse, J., Davies, M., et al: Metabolic fate of administered 1,25-dihydroxycholecalciferol in controls and in patients with hypoparathyroidism. *Lancet 1:* 1203–1206, 1976.

45. Neer, R. M., Holick, M. F., DeLuca, H. F., et al: Effects of 1α-hydroxyvitamin D_3 and 1,25-dihydroxyvitamin D_3 on calcium and phosphorus metabolism in hypoparathyroidism. *Metabolism 24:* 1403–1413, 1975.

46. Kooh, S. W., Fraser, D., DeLuca, H. F., et al: Treatment of hypoparathyroidism and pseudohypoparathyroidism with metabolites of vitamin D: Evidence for impaired conversion of 25-hydroxyvitamin D to 1α, 25-dihydroxyvitamin D. *N Engl J Med 293:* 840–844, 1975.

47. Davies, M., Taylor, C. M., Hill, L. F., et al: 1,25-dihydroxycholecalciferol in hypoparathyroidism. *Lancet 2:* 55–59, 1977.

48. Henry, H. L., Midgett, R. J., Norman, A. W.: Regulation of 25-hydroxyvitamin D_3-1-hydroxylase in vivo. *J Biol Chem 249:* 7584–7592, 1974.

48a. Haussler, M. F., Hughes, M., Baylink, D., et al: Influence of phosphate depletion on the biosynthesis and circulating level of 1,25-dihydroxyvitamin D, in Massry, S. G., Ritz, E. (eds): Phosphate Metabolism. New York, Plenum, 1976, pp. 233–250.

49. Tanaka, Y., Frank, H., DeLuca, H. F.: Intestinal calcium transport stimulation by low phosphorus diets. *Science 181:* 564–566, 1973.

50. Tanaka, Y., DeLuca, H. F.: The control of 25-hydroxyvitamin D metabolism by inorganic phosphorus. *Arch Biochem Biophys 154:* 566–574, 1973.

51. Ribovich, M. L., DeLuca, H. F.: 1,25-Dihydroxyvitamin D_3 metabolism. The effect of dietary calcium and phosphorus. *Arch Biochem Biophys 188:* 164–171, 1978.

52. Gray, R. W., Wilz, D. R., Caldas, A. E., et al: The importance of phosphate in regulating plasma 1,25-$(OH)_2$-vitamin D levels in humans: Studies in healthy subjects, in calcium-stone formers, and in patients with primary hyperparathyroidism. *J Clin Endocrinol Metab 45:* 299–306, 1977.

53. DeLuca, H. F.: Vitamin D endocrine system. *Adv Clin Chem 19:* 125–174, 1977.

54. Ney, R. L., Kelly, G., Bartter, F. C.: Actions of vitamin D independent of the parathyroid glands. *Endocrinology 82:* 760–766, 1968.

55. Spencer, R., Charman, M., Wilson, P., et al: Vitamin D-stimulated intestinal calcium absorption may not involve calcium-binding protein directly. *Nature 263:* 161–163, 1976.

56. Stanbury, S. W.: The intestinal absorption of calcium in normal adults, primary hyperparathyroidism, and renal failure, in Berlyne, G. M. (ed): Nutrition in Renal Failure. Baltimore, Williams & Wilkins, 1968, p 118.

57. Dent, C. E., Harper, C. M., Philpot, G. R.: The treatment of renal-glomerular osteodystrophy. *Q J Med 30:* 1–31, 1961.

58. Baerg, R. D., Kimberg, D. V., Gershon, E.: Effect of renal insufficiency on the active transport of calcium by the small intestine. *J Clin Invest 49:* 1288–1300, 1970.

59. Albright, F., Reifenstein, E. C., Jr.: The Parathyroid Glands and Metabolic Bone Disease. Baltimore, Williams & Wilkins, 1948.

60. Garabedian, M., Tanaka, Y., Holick, M. F., et al: Response of intestinal calcium transport and bone calcium mobilization to 1,25-dihydroxyvitamin D_3 in thyroparathyroidectomized rats. *Endocrinology 94:* 1022–1027, 1974.

61. Milhaud, G., Aubert, J. P., Bourichon, J.: Étude du métabolisme du calcium chez l'homme à l'aide de calcium 45. I. L'absorption du calcium au cours de la digestion. *Pathol Biol 9:* 1761–1768, 1961.

62. Massin, J. P., Vallee, G., Savoie, J. C.: Compartmental analysis of calcium kinetics in man: Application of a four-compartment model. *Metabolism 23:* 399–415, 1974.

63. Rasmussen, H., DeLuca, H., Arnaud, C., et al: The relationship between vitamin D and parathyroid hormone. *J Clin Invest 42:* 1940–1946, 1963.

64. Jowsey, J.: Calcium release from the skeletons of rachitic puppies. *J Clin Invest 51:* 9–15, 1972.

65. Au, W. Y. W., Raisz, L. G.: Restoration of parathyroid responsiveness in vitamin D-deficient rats by parenteral calcium or dietary lactose. *J Clin Invest 46:* 1572–1578, 1967.

66. Garabedian, M., Tanaka, Y., Holick, M. F., et al: Response of intestinal calcium transport and bone calcium mobilization to 1,25-dihydroxyvitamin D_3 in thyroparathyroidectomized rats. *Endocrinology 94:* 1022–1027, 1974.

67. Talmage, R. A., and Talmage, R. V.: Effects of parathyroid hormone on bone calcium without concurrent effects on phosphate, in Talmage, R. V., and Munson, P. L. (eds): Calcium, Parathyroid Hormone, and the Calcitonins, Proceedings of the Fourth Parathyroid Conference. Amsterdam, Excerpta Medica, 1972, pp. 416–421.

68. Parsons, J. A., Robinson, C. J.: A rapid indirect hypercalcemic action of parathyroid hormone demonstrated in isolated blood-perfused bone, in Talmage, R. V., Bélanger, L. F. (eds): Parathyroid Hormone and Thyrocalcitonin (Calcitonin), Proceedings of the Third Parathyroid Conference. Amsterdam, Excerpta Medica, 1968.

69. Rasmussen, H., Arnaud, C. D., Hawker, C.: Actinomycin D and the response to parathyroid hormone. *Science 144:* 1019–1021, 1964.

70. Talmage, R. V., Cooper, C. W., Park, H. Z.: Regulation of calcium transport in bone by parathyroid hormone. *Vitam Horm 28:* 103–140, 1970.

71. Talmage, R. V.: Effect of fasting and parathyroid hormone injection on plasma 45 Ca concentration in rats. *Calcif Tissue Res 17:* 103–112, 1975.

72. Talmage, R. V., Elliott, J. R.: Removal of calcium from bone as influenced by the parathyroids. *Endocrinology 62:* 717–722, 1958.

73. Reeve, J., Hesp, R., Wootton, R., et al: Clinical trial of hPTH(1-34) in "idiopathic" osteoporosis: in Talmage, R. V.: an interim report, and Copp, D. H. (eds): Endocrinology of Calcium Metabolism, Proceedings of the Sixth Parathyroid Conference. Amsterdam, Excerpta Medica, 1978, pp. 71–74.

74. Steenbock, H., Herting, D. C.: Vitamin D and growth. *J Nutr 57:* 449–468, 1955.

75. Raisz, L. G., Trummel, C. L., Holick, M. F.: 1,25-dihydroxycholecalciferol: A potent stimulator of bone resorption in tissue culture. *Science 175:* 768–769, 1972.

76. Peacock, M., Gallagher, J. C., Nordin, B. E. C.: Action of 1α-hydroxyvitamin D on calcium absorption and bone resorption in man. *Lancet 1:* 385–389, 1974.

77. Report of FAO/WHO Expert Group. WHO Technical Report Series #452 FAO/WHO, Geneva, 1970.

78. Milhaud, G., and Bourichon, J.: Étude du métabolisme du calcium chez l'homme à l'aide de calcium 45: l'hyperparathyroidie et l'hypoparathyroidie. *CR Acad Sci Paris 258:* 3398–3401, 1964.

79. Nordin, B. E. C.: Metabolic Bone and Stone Disease. Edinburgh, Churchill-Livingstone, 1973.

80. Stanbury, S. W.: The phosphate ion in chronic renal failure, in Hioco, D. J. (ed): Phosphate et Métabolisme Phosphocalcique. Paris, L'Expansion Scientifique Français, 1971, p 187.

81. Brickman, A. S., Hartenbower, D. L., Norman, A. W., et al: Actions of 1α-hydroxyvitamin D_3 and 1,25-dihydroxyvitamin D_3 on mineral metabolism in man. I. Effects on net absorption of phosphorus. *Am J Clin Nutr 30:* 1064–1069, 1977.

82. Rizzoli, R., Fleisch, H., Bonjour, J. P.: Role of 1,25-dihydroxyvitamin D_3 on intestinal phosphate absorption in rats with a normal vitamin D supply. *J Clin Invest 60:* 639–647, 1977.

83. Walton, J., Williams, M. E., Shea, T., et al: Effects of parathyroid extract on jejunal absorption of phosphate and calcium. *Clin Res 24:* 30a, 1976.

84. Walling, M. W., Kimberg, D. V.: Effects of 1α,25-dihydroxyvitamin D_3 and Solanum glaucophyllum on intestinal calcium and phosphate transport and on plasma Ca, Mg and P levels in the rat. *Endocrinology 97:* 1567–1576, 1975.

85. Eisenberg, E.: Effects of serum calcium level and parathyroid extracts on phosphate and calcium excretion in hypoparathyroid patients. *J Clin Invest 44:* 942–946, 1965.

86. Bonjour, J. P., Preston, C., Fleisch, H.: Effect of 1,25-dihydroxyvitamin D_3 on the renal handling of Pi in thyroparathyroidectomized rats. *J Clin Invest 60:* 1419–1428, 1977.

87. Bijvoet, O. L. M.: Relation of plasma phosphate concentration to renal tubular reabsorption of phosphate. *Clin Sci 37:* 23–36, 1969.

88. Parfitt, A. M.: Phosphate loading and depletion in vitamin D-treated hypoparathyroidism. Phosphate Metabolism: Kidney and Bone (Proceedings of the First International Workshop on Phosphate, June 6–7, 1975), Paris, Nouvelle Imprimerie Fournie, 1976.

89. Steele, T. H., Underwood, J. L., Stromberg, B. A., et al: Renal resistance to parathyroid hormone during phosphorus deprivation. *J Clin Invest 58:* 1461–1464, 1976.

90. Goldsmith, R. S., Siemsen, A. W., Mason, A. D., et al: Primary role of plasma hydrocortisone concentration in the regulation of the normal forenoon pattern of urinary phosphate excretion. *J Clin Endocrinol 25:* 1649–1659, 1965.

91. Greenberg, B. G., Winters, R. W., Graham, J. B.: The normal range of serum inorganic phosphorus and its utility as a discriminant in the diagnosis of congenital hypophosphatemia. *J Clin Endocrinol 20:* 364–379, 1960.

92. Hamilton, J. B., Bunch, L. D., Mestler, G. E., et al: Effect of orchiectomy upon chemical constituents of blood in young mature males, with special reference to sustained increase in the level of serum inorganic phosphorus. *J Clin Endocrinol Metab 16:* 301–321, 1956.

93. Young, M. M., Nordin, B. E. C.: Effects of natural and artificial menopause on plasma and urinary calcium and phosphorus. *Lancet 2:* 118–120, 1967.

94. Carré, M., Ayigbedé, O., Miravet, L., et al: The effect of prednisolone upon the metabolism and action of 25-hydroxy and 1,25-dihydroxyvitamin D₃. *Proc Natl Acad Sci USA 71:* 2996–3000, 1974.

95. Tanaka, Y., Castillo, L., DeLuca, H. F.: Control of renal vitamin D hydroxylases in birds by sex hormones. *Proc Natl Acad Sci USA 73:* 2701–2705, 1976.

96. Richelle, L. J., Onkelinx, C.: Recent advances in the physical biology of bone and other hard tissues, in Bronner, F., Comar, C. (eds): Mineral Metabolism, vol. III. New York, Academic Press, 1969, p 123.

97. Ramberg, C. F., Jr., Mayer, G. P., Kronfeld, D. S., et al: Dietary calcium, calcium kinetics and plasma parathyroid hormone concentration in cows. *J Nutr 106:* 671–679, 1976.

98. Phang, J. M., Berman, M., Finerman, G. A., et al: Dietary perturbation of calcium metabolism in normal man: Compartmental analysis. *J Clin Invest 48:* 67–77, 1969.

99. Neer, R., Berman, M., Fisher, L., et al: Multicompartmental analysis of calcium kinetics in normal adult males. *J Clin Invest 46:* 1364–1379, 1967.

100. Hansen, J. W., Gordan, G. S., Prussin, S. G.: Direct measurement of osteolysis in man. *J Clin Invest 52:* 304–315, 1973.

101. Neuman, W. F., Neuman, M. W.: The Chemical Dynamics of Bone Mineral. Chicago, University of Chicago Press, 1958.

102. Jung, A., Bartholdi, P., Mermillod, B., et al: A critical analysis of methods for analyzing human calcium kinetics. *J Theoret Biol* (in press).

103. Parsons, J. A., Robinson, C. J.: Calcium shift into bone causing transient hypocalcemia after injection of parathyroid hormone. *Nature 230:* 581–583, 1971.

104. Heaney, R. P.: Evaluation and interpretation of calcium kinetic data in man. *Clin Orthop 31:* 153–183, 1963.

105. Jackson, S., Dolphin, G. W.: The estimation of internal radiation dose from metabolic and urinary excretion data for a number of important radionuclides. *Health Phys 12:* 481–500, 1966.

106. Tivey, H., Osgood, E. E., et al: The biological half life of radioactive phosphorus in the blood of patients with leukemia. *Cancer 3:* 992–1017, 1950.

107. Bauer, G. C. H., Carlsson, A., Lindquist, B.: Metabolism and homeostatic function of bone, in Comar, C. L., Bronner, F. (eds): Mineral Metabolism, vol. I. New York, Academic Press, 1961, p 609.

108. Bauer, G. C. H., Carlsson, A., Lindquist, B.: Bone salt metabolism in human rickets studied with radioactive phosphorus. *Metabolism 5:* 573–581, 1956.

109. Walton, R. J., Russell, R. G. G., Smith, R.: Changes in the renal and extrarenal handling of phosphate induced by disodium etidronate (EHDP) in man. *Clin Sci Mol Med 49:* 45–56, 1975.

110. Ireland, P., Fordtran, J. S.: Effect of dietary calcium and age on jejunal calcium absorption in humans studied by intestinal perfusion. *J Clin Invest 52:* 2672–2681, 1973.

111. Boyle, I. T., Gray, R. W., DeLuca, H. F.: Regulation by calcium of in vivo synthesis of 1,25-dihydroxycholecalciferol and 21,25-dihydroxycholecalciferol. *Proc Natl Acad Sci USA 68:* 2131–2134, 1971.

112. Garabedian, M., Holick, M. F., DeLuca, H. F., et al: Control of 25-hydroxycholecalciferol metabolism by the parathyroid glands. *Proc Natl Acad Sci USA 69:* 1673–1676, 1972.

113. Gray, R. W., Caldas, A. E., Adams, N. D., et al: Calcium and plasma 1,25-(OH)₂D-vitamin D in health. *Clin Res 25:* 621A, 1977.

114. Peacock, M., Hodgkinson, A., Nordin, B. E. C.: Importance of dietary calcium in the definition of hypercalciuria. *Br Med J 3:* 469–471, 1967.

115. MacFadyen, I. J., Nordin, B. E. C., Smith, D. A., et al: Effect of variation in dietary calcium on plasma concentration and urinary excretion of calcium. *Br Med J 1:* 161–164, 1965.

116. Epstein, F. H.: Calcium and the kidney. *Am J Med 45:* 700–714, 1968.

117. Peacock, M., Robertson, W. G., Nordin, B. E. C.: Relation between serum and urinary calcium with particular reference to parathyroid activity. *Lancet 1:* 384–386, 1969.

118. Nordin, B. E. C., Peacock, M.: Role of kidney in regulation of plasma calcium. *Lancet 2:* 1280–1283, 1969.

119. Kaltreider, H. B., Baum, G. L., Bogaty, G., et al: So-called "metastatic calcification" of the lung. *Am J Med 46:* 188–196, 1969.

120. Copp, D. H.: Parathyroids and homeostasis of blood calcium, in Rodahl K, Nicholson, J. T., Brown, F. M. (eds): Bone as a Tissue. New York, McGraw-Hill, 1960, p 289.

121. Hausmann, E., Riggs, D. S.: The effectiveness of negative feedback in regulating plasma calcium in the dog. *J Theoret Biol 12:* 350–363, 1966.

122. Marshall, D. H.: Calcium and phosphate kinetics, in Nordin, B. E. C. (ed): Calcium, Phosphate, and Magnesium Metabolism. New York, Churchill-Livingstone, 1976, p 287.

123. Heaney, R. P., Skillman, T. G.: Secretion and excretion of calcium by human gastrointestinal tract. *J Lab Clin Med 64:* 29–41, 1964.

124. Murray, T. M., Peacock, M., Powell, D., et al: Non-autonomy of hormone secretion in primary hyperparathyroidism. *Clin Endocrinol 1:* 235–246, 1972.

125. Riggs, D. S.: The Mathematical Approach to Physiological Problems. Baltimore, Williams & Wilkins, 1963.

126. Riggs, D. S.: A quantitative hypothesis concerning the action of the parathyroid hormone. *J Theoret Biol 12:* 364–372, 1966.

127. Pedersen, K. O.: On the cause and degree of intra-individual serum calcium variability. *Scand J Clin Lab Invest 29–30:* 191–199, 1972.

128. Ladenson, J. H., Bowers, G. N.: Free calcium in serum. II. Rigor of homeostatic control, correlations with total serum calcium, and review of data on patients with disturbed calcium metabolism. *Clin Chem 19:* 575–582, 1973.

129. Lemann, J., Litzow, J. R., Lennon, E. J.: Studies of the mechanism by which chronic metabolic acidosis augments urinary calcium excretion in man. *J Clin Invest 46:* 1318–1328, 1967.

130. Bell, N. H.: Observations concerning the effects of fasting on collagen metabolism in man. *J Clin Endocrinol Metab 29:* 338–345, 1969.

131. Lemann, J., Litzow, J. R., Lennon, E. J.: The effects of chronic acid loads in normal man: Further evidence for the participation of bone mineral in the defense against chronic metabolic acidosis. *J Clin Invest 45:* 1608–1614, 1966.

132. Hinkle, J. E., Cooperman, L. H.: Serum ionized calcium changes following citrated blood transfusion in anaesthetized man. *Br J Anaesth 43:* 1108–1112, 1971.

133. Rodan, G., Liberman, U. A., Paran, M., et al: Lack of physiochemical equilibrium between blood and bone calcium in the isolated perfused dog limb. *Israel J Med Sci 3:* 702–713, 1967.

134. Parfitt, A. M.: Study of parathyroid function in man by EDTA infusion. *J Clin Endocrinol Metab 29:* 569–580, 1969.

135. Rasmussen, H., Anast, C., Arnaud, C.: Thyrocalcitonin, EGTA and urinary electrolyte excretion. *J Clin Invest 46:* 746–752, 1967.

136. Parfitt, A. M.: The actions of parathyroid hormone on bone: Relation to bone remodelling and turnover, calcium homeostasis, and metabolic bone disease. I-IV. *J Clin Endocrinol Metab 25:* 809–844, 909–955, 1033–1069, 1157–1188, 1977.

137. Kales, A. N., Phang, J. M.: Effect of divided calcium intake on calcium metabolism. *J Clin Endocrinol Metab 32:* 83–87, 1971.

138. Jaun, D., Liptak, P., Gray, T. K.: Absorption of inorganic phosphate in the human jejunum and its inhibition by salmon calcitonin. *J Clin Endocrinol Metab 43:* 517–522, 1976.

139. Gillis, J., Neer, R. M.: Unpublished observations.

140. Bijvoet, O. L. M., Morgan, D. B.: The tubular reabsorption of

phosphate in man, in Hioco, D. J. (ed): Phosphate et Métabolisme Phosphocalcique. Paris, L'Expansion Scientifique Français, 1971, p 153.

141. Foulks, J. G., Perry, F. A.: Renal excretion of phosphate following parathyroidectomy in the dog. *Am J Physiol 196:* 554–560, 1959.

142. Eisenberg, E.: Effects of varying phosphate intake in primary hyperparathyroidism. *J Clin Endocrinol 28:* 651–660, 1968.

143. Goldman, R., Bassett, S. H.: Renal regulation of phosphorus excretion. *J Clin Endocrinol Metab 18:* 981–990, 1958.

144. Goldsmith, R. S., Jowsey, J., Dubé, W. J., et al: Effects of phosphorus supplementation on serum parathyroid hormone and bone morphology in osteoporosis. *J Clin Endocrinol Metab 43:* 523–532, 1976.

145. Dietary phosphorus, PTH and bone resorption. *Nutr Rev 31:* 124–126, 1973.

146. Laflamme, G. H., Jowsey, J.: Bone and soft tissue changes with oral phosphate supplements. *J Clin Invest 51:* 2834–2846, 1972.

147. Anderson, G. H., Draper, H. H.: Effect of dietary phosphorus on calcium metabolism in intact and parathyroidectomized adult rats. *J Nutr 102:* 1123–1156, 1972.

148. Krook, L.: On the etiology of primary parathyroid hyperplasia. *Rev Can Biol 24:* 63–69, 1965.

149. Krook, L., Barrett, R. B., Usui, K., et al: Nutritional secondary hyperparathyroidism in the cat. *Cornell Vet 53:* 224–240, 1963.

150. Brown, W. R., Krook, L., Pond, W. G.: Atrophic rhinitis in swine. Etiology, pathogenesis and prophylaxis. *Cornell Vet 56:* Suppl 1, 1966.

151. Harris, W. H., Heaney, R. P., Davis, L. A., et al: Stimulation of bone formation in vivo by phosphate supplementation. *Calcif Tissue Res 22:* 85–98, 1976.

152. Hebert, L. A., Lemann, J., Petersen, J. R., et al: Studies of the mechanism by which phosphate infusion lowers serum calcium concentration. *J Clin Invest 45:* 1886–1894, 1966.

153. Zusman, J., Brown, D. M., Nesbit, M. E.: Hyperphosphatemia, hyperphosphaturia, and hypocalcemia in acute lymphoblastic leukemia. *N Engl J Med 289:* 1335–1340, 1973.

154. Meroney, W. H.: The phosphorus to nonprotein nitrogen ratio in plasma as an index of muscle devitalization during oliguria. *Surg Gynecol Obstet 100:* 309–314, 1955.

155. Canterbury, J. M., Reiss, E., Mahaffey, J. E., et al: Personal communications.

156. Jubiz, W., Canterbury, J. M., Reiss, E., et al: Circadian rhythm in serum parathyroid hormone concentration in human subjects: Correlation with serum calcium, phosphate, albumin, and growth hormone levels. *J Clin Invest 51:* 2040–2046, 1972.

157. Spencer, H., Lewin, I., Samachson, J., et al: Changes in metabolism in obese persons during starvation. *Am J Med 40:* 27–37, 1966.

158. Crawford, J. D., Cribetz, D., Talbot, N. B.: Mechanism of renal tubular phosphate reabsorption and the influence thereon of vitamin D in completely parathyroidectomized rats. *Am J Physiol 180:* 156–162, 1955.

159. Anderson, J. J. B., Talmage, R. V.: The effect of calcium infusion and calcitonin on plasma phosphate in sham-operated and thyroparathyroidectomized dogs. *Endocrinology 93:* 1222–1226, 1973.

160. Hiatt, H. H., Thompson, D. D.: Some effects of intravenously administered calcium on inorganic phosphate metabolism. *J Clin Invest 36:* 573–580, 1957.

161. Rasmussen, H., Tenenhouse, A.: Thyrocalcitonin, osteoporosis and osteolysis. *Am J Med 43:* 721, 1967.

162. Slatopolsky, E., Robson, A. M., Elkan, I., et al: Control of phosphate excretion in uremic man. *J Clin Invest 47:* 1865–1874, 1968.

163. Massry, S. G., Popovtzer, M. M., Coburn, J. W., et al: Intractable pruritois as a manifestation of secondary hyperparathyroidism in uremia. *N Engl J Med 279:* 697–700, 1968.

164. Gill, G., Pallotta, J., Kashgarian, M., et al: Physiologic studies in renal osteodystrophy treated by subtotal parathyroidectomy. *Am J Med 46:* 930–940, 1969.

165. Shen, F. H., Baylink, D. J., Nielsen, R. J., et al: Increased serum 1,25-dihydroxyvitamin D in idiopathic hypercalciuria. *J Lab Clin Med 90:* 955–962, 1977.

166. Shen, F. H., Baylink, D. J., Sherrard, D. J., et al: Idiopathic hypercalciuria: The "phosphate leak" hypothesis and the effects of oral phosphate supplement. *Clin Res 25:* 129A, 1977.

167. Gallagher, J. C., Riggs, B. L., Eisman, J., et al: Impaired production of 1,25-dihydroxyvitamin D in post-menopausal osteoporosis. *Clin Res 24:* 580A, 1976.

168. Davis, R. H., Morgan, D. B., Rivlin, R. S.: The excretion of calcium in the urine and its relation to calcium intake, sex and age. *Clin Sci 39:* 1–12, 1970.

169. Horsman, A., Gallagher, J. C., Simpson, M., et al: Prospective trial of oestrogen and calcium in postmenopausal women. *Br Med J 2:* 789–792, 1977.

170. Recker, R. R., Saville, P. D., Heaney, R. P.: Effect of estrogens and calcium carbonate on bone loss in postmenopausal women. *Ann Intern Med 87:* 649–655, 1977.

171. Bauer, W., Aub, J. C., Albright, F.: Studies of calcium and phosphorus metabolism. V. A study of the bone trabeculae as a readily available reserve supply of calcium. *J Exp Med 49:* 145–166, 1929.

172. Perault-Staub, A. M., Staub, J. F., Milhaud, G.: A new concept for plasma calcium homeostasis in rat. *Endocrinology 95:* 480–484, 1974.

173. Talmage, R. V., Roycroft, J. H., Anderson, J. J. B.: Daily fluctuations in plasma calcium, phosphate, and their radionuclide concentrations in the rat. *Calcif Tissue Res 17:* 91–102, 1975.

174. Min, H. K., Jones, J. E., Flink, E. B.: Circadian variations in renal excretion of magnesium, calcium, phosphorus, sodium, and potassium during frequent feeding and fasting. *Fed Proc 252:* 917–921, 1966.

175. Loutit, J. F., Papworth, D. G.: Diurnal variation in urinary excretion of calcium and strontium. *Proc R Soc Lond (Biol) 162:* 458–472, 1965.

176. Bourne, G. H. (ed): The Biochemistry and Physiology of Bone, vols. 1–4. New York, Academic Press, 1971–1976.

177. Harris, W. H., Heaney, R. P.: Skeletal renewal and metabolic bone disease. *N Engl J Med 280:* 193–202, 253–259, 303–311, 1969.

178. Arnstein, A. R., McCann, D. S., Blumenthal, F. S., et al: Serum immunoreactive parathyroid hormone in patients with paralysis due to spinal cord trauma, in Frame, B., Parfitt, A. M., Duncan, H. (eds): Clinical Aspects of Metabolic Bone Disease. Amsterdam, Excerpta Medica, 1973 p 253.

179. Lerman, S., Canterbury, J. M., Reiss, E.: Parathyroid hormone and the hypercalcemia of immobilization. *J Clin Endocrinol Metab 45:* 425–428, 1977.

180. Heaney, R. P.: Radiocalcium metabolism in disuse osteoporosis in man. *Am J Med 33:* 188–200, 1962.

181. Lindgren, J. V.: Studies of the calcium accretion rate of bone during immobilization in intact and thyroparathyroidectomized adult rats. *Calcif Tissue Res 22:* 41–47, 1976.

182. Fordtran, J. S., Locklear, T. W.: Ionic constituents and osmolality of gastric and small-intestinal fluids after eating. *Am J Dig Dis 11:* 503–521, 1966.

183. Wilkinson, R.: Absorption of calcium phosphorus and magnesium, in Nordin, B. E. C. (ed): Calcium, Phosphate, and Magnesium Metabolism. New York, Churchill-Livingstone, 1976, p 36.

184. Ohlson, M. A., Stearns, G.: Calcium intake of children and adults. *Fed Proc 18:* 1077–1085, 1959.

185. Nordin, B. E. C.: Nutritional considerations, in Nordin, B. E. C. (ed): Calcium, Phosphate, and Magnesium Metabolism. New York, Churchill-Livingstone, 1976, p 25.

53

Clinical Features
of Primary Hyperparathyroidism

Joel F. Habener
John T. Potts, Jr.

SIGNS AND SYMPTOMS

Primary hyperparathyroidism is recognized most commonly between the third and fifth decades, but the disease is seen occasionally in young children[1] and the elderly.[2,3] The incidence of the disease is two to three times higher in women than in men.[2,4] The true incidence of the various symptoms and complications of hyperparathyroidism, however, is difficult to estimate inasmuch as many patients are now being discovered and their hyperparathyroidism is being treated at a time when they are asymptomatic without complications. In addition, some important symptomatic manifestations of primary hyperparathyroidism, particularly articular, neuromuscular, and certain gastrointestinal manifestations, were not appreciated in the earlier studies and hence were not reported.

RENAL MANIFESTATIONS

Before the last decade, kidney involvement, particularly recurrent nephrolithiasis, was reported in 60–70 percent of patients.[5,6] Kidney involvement is less frequent today, but it still remains as one of the most frequent manifestations of primary hyperparathyroidism.

The pathophysiologic effects of excessive parathyroid hormone on the kidney in patients with primary hyperparathyroidism can be considered in two broad categories: anatomic and functional. Under the category of anatomic defects is the occurrence of nephrolithiasis or nephrocalcinosis; under functional defects are included a spectrum of tubular and glomerular disorders that result from the deleterious effects of sustained hypercalcemia and/or excessive concentrations of parathyroid hormone.

Although nephrolithiasis is not seen as frequently as in former years, the overall incidence of this complication remains quite high. In a recent report it was found that in patients with presumptive hyperparathyroidism but without symptoms at the time the diagnosis was established, the incidence of nephrolithiasis detecta-

ble radiographically was still 32 percent.[7] This relatively high incidence of nephrolithiasis might be expected to fall still further as more and more asymptomatic patients with hyperparathyroidism are detected through the application of routine serum calcium measurements in an unselected ambulatory population.

A variety of renal functional abnormalities occur in hyperparathyroidism, even in the absence of detectable nephrocalcinosis and/or nephrolithiasis.[2,8,9] These include elevation of blood urea nitrogen and serum creatinine, reflecting modest to marked reduction in glomerular filtration rate, and numerous renal tubular defects, particularly impairment of proximal tubular function. There is a reduction in net acid secretion, i.e., proximal renal tubular acidosis (proximal, or type II, RTA)[8] as well as aminoaciduria, glycosuria, and decrease in urinary concentrating capacity. These overall defects occur in a continuous spectrum of severity and are influenced by anatomic changes in the kidney, such as diffuse calcium deposition (nephrocalcinosis) and the inflammation due to bacterial infection. Tubular defects involving compromise of proximal tubular function and urinary concentrating ability may be found in the absence of roentgenographically demonstrable renal calcification or evidence of infection.[2,8,10] A difficulty in attempting to assess the incidence and significance of more-subtle tubular disorders is the lack of detailed evaluation of proximal and distal tubular function in most reported series of patients with hyperparathyroidism. With careful evaluation of renal function it is found that inability to excrete acid at normal rates (proximal RTA) is a rather common finding in primary hyperparathyroidism. This situation frequently results in mild hyperchloremic acidosis and reduction in serum bicarbonate. On the other hand,[10,11] hypercalcemia per se, produced experimentally[12] or in disease states associated with hypercalcemia not due to hyperparathyroidism (such as carcinoma and acute vitamin D intoxication), is usually associated with mild alkalosis rather than acidosis.[13,14]

Parathyroid hormone appears to have direct effects on renal tubular function. Certain reports have noted, therefore,[15,16] that hyperchloremia and/or mild reduction in serum bicarbonate serves to distinguish hyperparathyroidism from other causes of hypercalcemia. The distinctions, however, are often subtle; in one study of 13 patients with hyperparathyroidism, no significant departure was found from normal in either serum chloride or serum bicarbonate levels.[17] Palmer et al.[16] noted that some patients did not have elevated plasma chloride. They made the interesting suggestion however, that, in hyperparathyroid patients with hyperchloremia and hypophosphatemia, a discriminant value could be inferred by noting the ratio of chloride to phosphate. Palmer and associates[16] found that the chloride-to-phosphate ratio ranged from 32 to 80 in hyperparathyroidism, with 96 percent of patients having a ratio of higher than 33, whereas the ratio of chloride to phosphate ranged from 17 to 32 in those with hypercalcemia from other causes, with 92 percent having a ratio of less than 30.

Morris and associates[8,18-21] noted close similarities in the abnormalities in renal function in patients with primary hyperparathyroidism and in patients with hereditary fructose intolerance; each disorder is characterized by a proximal-type RTA. Gold et al.[22] have suggested a possible relationship between phosphate depletion and renal bicarbonate wasting. In studies in phosphate-depleted dogs, proximal renal tubular defects similar to those seen in hyperparathyroidism were noted, despite normal circulating levels of parathyroid hormone. Thus phosphate repletion per se might account in part for the restoration of normal proximal tubular bicarbonate and acid handling after successful parathyroid surgery.

Partial or complete reversibility of some or all the defects in glomerular function and tubular function, including acidification mechanisms and renal concentrating ability, has been documented after surgical correction of hyperparathyroidism.[2,7,10,22,23,24] In one brief report, however, a more pessimistic view was presented with regard to the reversibility of renal functional abnormalities after surgical correction of hyperparathyroidism.[25] More detailed study of this problem of reversibility of renal defects associated with hyperparathyroidism seems needed.

SKELETAL MANIFESTATIONS

It is difficult to assess the etiology, frequency, clinical significance, and prognosis of skeletal disease in hyperparathyroidism. These difficulties arise because of the apparently changing pattern of skeletal disease in hyperparathyroidism and because of the technical difficulties involved in the methods required to define pathophysiologic changes in the skeleton in milder forms of disease. Present information suggests that the pathognomonic form of skeletal disease in hyperparathyroidism, osteitis fibrosa cystica, is declining in relative frequency and that a subtle, yet nonetheless clinically significant, form of skeletal disease, simple diffuse osteopenia resembling osteoporosis, is being seen more often.

In an analysis of 138 cases of primary hyperparathyroidism it was noted[2] that in the two decades, 1930–1949, 53 percent of patients had symptomatic, generalized osteitis fibrosa cystica confirmed by radiologic examination, whereas during 1949–1960 only 21 percent were so afflicted. The relative incidence of radiologically demonstrable osteitis fibrosa cystica in the decade 1961–1970 is even lower. For example, in a recent review[26] only 9 percent of 57 patients seen between 1965 and 1973 had skeletal pain or evidence of osteitis fibrosa cystica.

In the present era, patients with primary hyperparathyroidism who have pain referable to the skeleton are most likely to present with findings of diffuse spinal rarefaction indistinguishable from that of senile or postmenopausal osteoporosis rather than the findings of osteitis fibrosa. The degree of osteopenia may be severe. Of 319 patients with surgically proved primary hyperparathyroidism seen at the Mayo Clinic over a recent 3-year period, 14 (4.4 percent) had diffuse osteopenia of the spine with evidence of vertebral crush fractures.[27] Nine of the 14 patients presented with a chief complaint of back pain. In none of the 319 patients, however, was there unequivocal roentgenographic evidence of osteitis fibrosa cystica. The patients with primary hyperparathyroidism demonstrated a statistically higher incidence of diffuse osteopenia of the spine and of vertebral crush fractures compared with a group of age- and sex-matched control patients with degenerative lumbar disc disease. In another recent report of 87 patients with primary

hyperparathyroidism,[28] roentgenographic manifestations of osteopenia were found in the spine in 21 percent of the patients and in the hands in 36 percent. Evidence of osteitis fibrosa (subperiosteal resorption of the phalanges) was noted in only 8 percent of the same patients.[28]

Quantitative analyses by microradiography have shown an average fivefold increase in the rate of bone turnover in all patients with hyperparathyroidism when compared with age-matched control subjects.[29] In addition to the microscopic evidence of increased bone turnover in many patients with primary hyperparathyroidism, evidence of decreased bone density has been found by various sensitive bone densitometric techniques: ^{125}I bone densitometry,[30] x-ray spectrophotometry,[31] and photon absorptiometric analyses.[32]

Using precise and quantitative morphometric techniques on biopsy specimens of iliac bones, Meunier and colleagues[33] evaluated periosteocytic-lacunae size and osteoclastic resorptive surfaces in 40 patients with primary hyperparathyroidism and 62 control subjects. The percentages of total surfaces of trabecular bone involved by osteoclastic resorption and mean surface areas of osteocytic lacunae were significantly higher in hyperparathyroid than in normal subjects.[33]

The reason for the changing pattern of skeletal involvement remains unclear. It may be speculated that the increased bone turnover and consequent osteoporosis is characteristic of patients with milder forms of hyperparathyroidism who lack evidence of extensive bone remodeling, or osteitis fibrosa cystica, seen in severe hyperparathyroidism. These findings may reflect the predominance of the action of low concentrations of parathyroid hormone to promote diffuse osteocytic osteolysis rather than more-localized osteoclast proliferation. The present evidence of multiple effects of parathyroid hormone on the skeleton, including experimental data and clinical evidence (see Chapter 46) of an anabolic effect, makes predictions difficult on a theoretical basis. Even the recognition of multiple actions of the hormone on the skeleton with the possibility that one action, if predominant, will result in a distinctive clinical pattern of bone disease, does not explain why one type of bone lesion rather than another may predominate in patients with apparent similarities in duration and severity of their disease. Other than one report,[34] there are few data concerning correlations between absolute parathyroid hormone levels in blood and the presence or type of bone disease. It is possible that compensatory mechanisms or modifying influences in some way determine whether osteitis fibrosa cystica, osteoporosis, or a normal skeleton will be found in a given patient with hyperparathyroidism. These modifying influences may include: production of calcitonin in response to hypercalcemia; some factor relating to calcium absorption—either dietary content,[35] as originally thought but then doubted,[36] or, more likely, efficiency of intestinal calcium absorption;[37] the levels of active metabolites of vitamin D; or phosphate balance or extracellular fluid concentrations of phosphate. Basically, the pathophysiologic etiology of skeletal changes in this disease remains unclarified.

Clinically, however, a number of features of the bone disease, whether osteitis fibrosa cystica or simple osteopenia, are of importance in providing diagnostic clues to the presence of the disease or in helping to assess the need for surgical treatment as well as the response of the patient after surgical correction. When severe osteitis fibrosa cystica develops, radiologic examinations or bone biopsy can directly establish the diagnosis. The most important roentgenograms for the diagnosis of generalized osteitis fibrosa cystica are those of the hands in the posteroanterior view.[38] In the majority of patients with roentgenographically demonstrable bone lesions, subperiosteal erosion of the radial aspect of the middle phalanges is seen (Fig. 53-1). The skull is the next most frequently involved area.[38] In advanced stages of the disease there is evidence of erosion of the outer cortical surfaces of bone throughout the skeleton, generalized demineralization of bones, and localized destructive lesions, often cystic (Fig. 53-2).

Histologic examination of bone specimens from patients with severe osteitis fibrosa cystica reveals a number of changes that collectively define the presence of parathyroid overactivity. There are a reduction in the number of trabeculae, an increase in multinucleated osteoclasts seen in scalloped areas on the surface of the bone (Howship's lacunae), and a marked replacement of normal cellular and marrow elements by fibrovascular tissue (Fig. 53-3).

The major unsettled issue regarding skeletal manifestations is the frequency, specific relation to hyperparathyroidism, and reversibility, after parathyroidectomy, of the diffuse osteopenia attributed to many patients with the disease. A definite causal relation between hyperparathyroidism and diffuse osteopenia seems likely but requires further study. It will be important to document in prospective studies whether there is indeed a pattern of progressive decrease in bone mineral density detectable by quantitative techniques and whether there is improvement after parathyroidectomy. Such an analysis to establish a causal relation seems particularly necessary, inasmuch as osteoporosis, unrelated to hyperparathyroidism, is so frequenty seen in older patients.

In patients with a documented progressive decline in bone mineral density, application of quantitative morphometric techniques may help to establish the parathyroid etiology of the osteopenia by definite histologic changes. If the osteopenia in such patients is not reversed after parathyroidectomy but its progres-

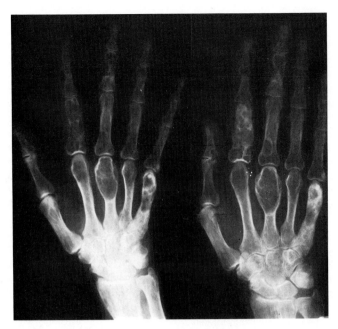

Fig. 53-2. Hand radiographs of patient with hyperparathyroidism and severe osteitis fibrosa cystica before (A) and after (B) removal of parathyroid adenoma. Cystic destruction of bone, subperiosteal resorption, and a pathologic fracture of the second proximal phalanx are evident. Some mineralization has occurred since the parathyroidectomy. (Courtesy of the Department of Radiology, Massachusetts General Hospital.)

sion is simply halted or slowed, it will become even more important to attempt early detection of progressive osteopenia in patients with hyperparathyroidism to prevent further skeletal weakening to the point of pathologic fractures.

NEUROMUSCULAR AND NEUROPSYCHIATRIC MANIFESTATIONS

Profound muscle weakness and atrophy were recognized in several of the earliest described cases of severe hyperparathyroidism.[39-41] Recently pathophysiologic features of neuromuscular involvement in hyperparathyroidism have been studied in greater detail.[26,42] Symptoms include extreme weakness and fatigability, particularly involving proximal musculature (the lower more fre-

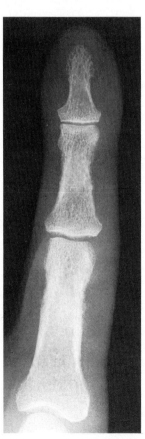

Fig. 53-1. Magnification of radiograph of a finger from a patient with primary hyperparathyroidism, to emphasize typical features. Decreased demineralization in the phalangeal tuft (middle) and subperiosteal bone resorption (middle and right) can be seen. (Adapted from Potts and Deftos, 1974.[34a])

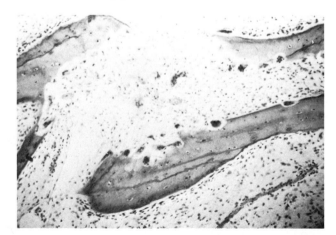

Fig. 53-3. Microscopical appearance of osteitis fibrosa cystica in bone from an iliac crest biopsy. Extensive replacement of marrow with fibrovascular tissue can be seen; osseous trabeculae show evidence of both osteoclastic resorption and areas of osteoblastic bone formation. The classic appearance of dissecting osteitis within lamellar bone of trabeculae is evident. (Courtesy of the Department of Pathology, Massachusetts General Hospital.)

quently than the upper extremities). The muscle weakness may be so profound that an initial diagnosis of amyotrophic lateral sclerosis, muscular dystrophy, or other serious neuromuscular disorders that are irreversible, are entertained, yet there is striking reversal of muscle weakness and atrophy noted in all patients after successful correction of the hyperparathyroidism. Upon examination, gross atrophy may be detectable in involved muscle groups. Electromyographic examinations reveal both short-duration, low-amplitude motor-unit potentials, and abnormally-high-amplitude, long-duration polyphasic potentials, but motor-nerve conduction velocities are normal. Sensory abnormalities are absent. Patten et al.[42] emphasized that the overall findings, including microscopic examination of affected tissue, are consistent with a neuropathic rather than a myopathic origin of the neuromuscular disease.

The overall incidence of this neuromyopathic syndrome in primary hyperparathyroidism is still unknown; however, in the recent prospective study of Patten and associates,[42] 14 of 16 patients showed manifestations of neuromyopathic involvement, at least in mild form. Hence, more-detailed neurologic examination may reveal a much higher incidence of this complication than previously suspected, at least in patients with more severe, symptomatic hyperparathyroidism.

In addition to the neuromyopathic manifestations of hyperparathyroidism, mental disturbances and impairment of higher-central-nervous-system functions are frequently seen.[43,44] Depression, personality changes, psychomotor retardation, memory impairment, and, occasionally, overt psychosis may occur.[44-46] In severe hyperparathyroidism, mental obtundation and coma may be observed.[47] These neuropsychiatric disturbances are thought to be due to the hypercalcemia per se rather than to any direct effects of parathyroid hormone;[44] characteristic electroencephalographic abnormalities have been described in hypercalcemia of many causes.[48,49]

On some occasions after parathyroidectomy there is a striking improvement in a patient's sense of well-being, including relief of fatigue and depression that may not have been noticeable prior to surgery. It should be emphasized, however, that mild depression and vague constitutional complaints cannot alone serve as an indication for surgery because these symptoms are so common in the absence of hyperparathyroidism.

GASTROINTESTINAL MANIFESTATIONS

Peptic ulcer disease in patients with symptomatic primary hyperparathyroidism is seen with such high frequency that most investigators believe that the ulcer disease is causally related to the hyperparathyroidism. Some authors, on the other hand, have questioned whether the frequency of ulcer disease in symptomatic primary hyperparathyroidism is actually higher than it is in the general population.[50] However, in a review of peptic ulcer disease in patients with primary hyperparathyroidism in 10 reported series, evidence of radiologically demonstrable ulcer disease was found in 131 of 928 cases, an overall incidence of 14.2 percent (range 7.7–30.5 percent).[51] It was further concluded that before 1970 the incidence of peptic ulcer disease, based on presumptive or clinical evidence, was probably close to 30 percent. Inasmuch as the prevalence of peptic ulcer disease in the general adult population without hyperparathyroidism is reported to be much lower in the United States—estimates have ranged from a low of 2–3 percent (USPHS National Health Survey, 1960) to as high as 5–10 percent[50]—or in Great Britain (maximum estimate 7.8 percent[52]), it would appear that peptic ulcer disease is a true manifestation of primary hyperparathyroidism.

Some patients with peptic ulcer disease, particularly those with severe symptoms and multiple ulcers, turn out to have Zollinger/Ellison syndrome[53] or the multiple-endocrine-neoplasia syndrome, type I, with gastrin-producing tumors or diffuse hyperplasia of the pancreatic islet cells. These patients, however, constitute a small minority of patients with hyperparathyroidism and peptic ulcers; most patients have no recognized abnormalities of the endocrine pancreas.

The etiologic basis for the increased incidence of ulcer disease in hyperparathyroidism may be increased gastrin secretion with resultant increased gastric acid production induced by the hypercalcemia.[54] Levels of gastrin although elevated are considerably lower than in Zollinger/Ellison syndrome. In hyperparathyroidism both basal acid secretion[55-57] and serum immunoreactive gastrin[55] are increased. Following parathyroidectomy, the excessive acid production, hypergastrinemia, and peptic ulcer symptoms usually return to normal.[54,55,58,59] The weight of the evidence indicates that increased gastrin secretion and hyperacidity in hyperparathyroidism are due to the hypercalcemia and not to direct effects of the parathyroid hormone on gastrin production or on acid production per se. Even in the Zollinger/Ellison syndrome, the hyperacidity, elevated gastrin levels, and peptic ulcer symptoms may be reversed acutely by parathyroidectomy.[55] However, long-term follow-up of some of these patients has revealed ultimate recurrence of the Zollinger/Ellison syndrome despite the persistence of normal parathyroid function.

Although still speculative, the finding of transient improvement in patients with pancreatic tumors and Zollinger/Ellison syndrome suggests that coexistent hyperparathyroidism may lead to an earlier and more severe emergence of peptic symptoms and complications. Despite transient improvement, the underlying and progressive pancreatic tumor leads eventually to a reappearance of the symptoms and signs of the Zollinger/Ellison syndrome.

Pancreatitis, the other major gastrointestinal manifestation of hyperparathyroidism, occurs with a relatively high frequency in patients with primary hyperparathyroidism.[60] Pancreatitis has been the primary diagnostic clue to the presence of otherwise unrecognized hyperparathyroidism in 3 percent of 431 surgically proved cases.[61] Five types of pancreatitis associated with hyperparathyroidism have been described: (1) acute, (2) acute postoperative (after any operation in patients who have unsuspected hyperparathyroidism), (3) recurrent, (4) chronic with pain, and (5) chronic without pain.[62] The most common type is chronic with pain.

Although the association of pancreatitis and hyperparathyroidism is well documented, the basis for it is unknown.[38a,62-65] Whatever the mechanism, the long-standing hypercalcemia per se associated with the hyperparathyroidism seems to predispose to the development of pancreatitis.[62,64] One group has suggested that the hyperparathyroidism develops in response to pancreatitis.[63]

Regardless of the nature of the pathogenic interrelationships between pancreatitis and hyperparathyroidism, awareness of this association has several practical consequences. The diagnosis of hyperparathyroidism should be considered in patients with pancreatitis, particularly those in whom there is no factor present known to be associated with pancreatitis, such as alcoholism or hyperlipidemia, type II.[65] Conversely, one should be aware of the possible development of pancreatitis as a complication of hyperparathyroidism, particularly in parathyroid crisis. It is well documented that both acute and chronic pancreatitis (the latter due to malabsorption) may cause a decrease in serum calcium concentration to deceptively normal or even low levels in hyperparathyroidism. Thus, the findings of even a normal level of serum calcium in the face of pancreatitis may be a clue to the concomitant existence of primary hyperparathyroidism.[62]

ARTICULAR MANIFESTATIONS

A number of articular and periarticular disorders have been recognized in association with primary hyperparathyroidism; chondrocalcinosis with or without acute attacks of pseudogout; juxtaarticular erosions; subchondral fractures; traumatic synovitis; calcific periarthritis; and urate gout.[66-69]

Chondrocalcinosis is characterized by the disposition of calcium pyrophosphate dihydrate (CPPD) crystals in the articular cartilages and menisci (chondrocalcinosis),[70] and occasionally by the occurrence of acute attacks of arthritis (pseudogout) associated with CPPD in the synovial space, usually within polymorphonuclear leukocytes. The incidence of chondrocalcinosis in primary hyperparathyroidism is reported to be 7.5–18 percent.[71,72] The diagnosis of chondrocalcinosis is suggested by radiologic findings of characteristic calcium deposits in articular cartilages (Fig. 53-4); definite diagnosis is established by the finding of CPPD crystals in aspirates of joint fluid.[69] Hyperuricemia is seen frequently in primary hyperparathyroidism[73] and can be attributed to a decreased renal clearance of urates. Approximately 20 percent of patients with pseudogout and hyperparathyroidism have hyperuricemia, a factor that may further confuse the diagnosis of the articular disorder.[69,74]

It is clear that multiple manifestations of articular disease are seen with hyperparathyroidism; certain disorders, such as pseudogout, are so frequently associated with parathyroid disorders that the presence of the former should indeed raise diagnostic suspicion of the latter.

OTHER CLINICAL MANIFESTATIONS

There have been reports that hypertension occurs more frequently in hyperparathyroidism, particularly with elderly patients, than in the general population.[75-77] In some cases, hypertension develops after parathyroidectomy. Britton et al.,[25] however, observed that of 19 patients with hyperparathyroidism and hypertension, in only 1 did the blood pressure return to normal after operation. An additional 17 patients became hypertensive after surgery.

In addition, owing to the high frequency of essential hypertension (at least in the United States—20 percent of the adult population[78]) and the increasing frequency of detection of asymptomatic hyperparathyroidism, it must be concluded that random association of the two diseases might be expected. The presence of hypertension per se (in the absence of multiple endocrine neoplasia, type II) should not serve as an indication for surgery in the expectation of reversal of hypertension.

Skin necrosis, which may be found in patients with hypercalcemia of any cause, has also been found in hyperparathyroidism.[79] Calcification of the cornea (band keratopathy) is occasionally a manifestation of hypercalcemia of whatever cause;[80] however, it is not commonly found in primary hyperparathyroidism when serum phosphorus levels are low and renal glomerular function is maintained.

Certain distinctive clinical features are noted when hyperparathyroidism occurs in children. By 1966 there were reports of 30 proven cases of childhood primary hyperparathyroidism.[1,81-85] The serum calcium levels of the children with primary hyperparathyroidism were unusually high, with the average 14–16 mg/100 ml, and a high incidence of skeletal disease has been noted. It is likely that with the increasing use of screening procedures more instances will be found of hyperparathyroidism in children. The serum levels of calcium and phosphorus, however, will have to be interpreted with respect to the ranges of normal for that age. Data for normal children have been collected and used for this purpose.[86]

ETIOLOGY AND PATHOLOGY

Enlargement of only a single gland is sufficient to cause excessive hormone secretion. In the opinion of the authors and their colleagues, single-gland disease is the most common cause of primary hyperparathyroidism (Table 53-1). The enlarged gland is usually classified as a benign adenoma; only rarely is it a malignant carcinoma. Enlargement and diffuse hyperplasia of all four glands may also be seen (Table 53-1). Hyperplasia involving clear cells as a cause of primary hyperparathyroidism was described many years ago.[87] Later, appropriate emphasis was directed to the frequency of chief-cell hyperplasia as a cause.[88] Although an adenoma of a single gland was regarded, and still is by some, as the most common cause of primary hyperparathyroidism,[89,90] other pathologists and surgeons subscribe to the view that hyperplasia in multiple glands is the most frequent cause of primary hyperparathyroidism.[91] Paloyan and associates[91] reported that in approximately 50 percent of the patients with primary hyperparathyroidism, abnormalities may be found in most of the parathyroid glands if each of the glands is identified surgically, biopsied, and carefully examined by histologic techniques. The changes involve either diffuse hyperplasia and/or a nodular hyperplasia. They stressed that most of all four parathyroid glands should be removed to effect true cure of hyperparathyroidism.

In contrast, Wang et al.[92] have continued to maintain that, in over 80 percent of patients with primary hyperparathyroidism, a single abnormal gland or adenoma is the only abnormality (Table 53-1), and that effective cure can be obtained by the surgical removal of the single abnormal gland. They[92] reported that in only 15 percent of the cases is multiple-gland disease present—an incidence that has remained relatively constant in the period between 1930 and 1976 (Table 53-1).

We still favor the latter view—that an abnormality limited to a single gland is the more common occurrence. Of the 525 new cases operated on at the Massachusetts General Hospital between 1932 and 1973, in 424 only a single gland (adenoma) was excised.[92] In only 3 patients was the assessment incorrect, using as a criterion the requirement of a second operation because of persistent hypercalcemia.

One reason for the continuing uncertainty about the patho-

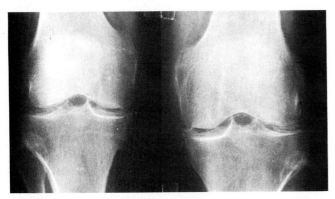

Fig. 53-4. Radiographic appearance of chondrocalcinosis in articular cartilages of the knee. (Courtesy of Dr. S. M. Krane.)

Table 53-1. Hyperparathyroidism at the Massachusetts General Hospital*

	1930–1951	1952–1961	1962–1971	1972–1976	1930–1976
Adenoma	107 (83)†	88 (77)	185 (81)	219 (86)	599 (83)
Single	104 (81)	86 (75)	181 (81)	219 (86)	593 (82)
Double‡	4 (2)	2 (2)	1 (0.4)	0 (0)	6 (1)
Hyperplasia	17 (13)	21 (18)	32 (14)	35 (13.7)	105 (15)
Clear cell	11 (9)	4 (4)	1 (0.4)	3 (1.2)	19 (3)
Chief cell	6 (5)	17 (15)	31 (13.6)	32 (12.5)	86 (12)
Carcinoma	5 (4)	5 (4)	10 (4.4)	2 (0.8)	22 (3)
Total	129	114	227	256	726

*Courtesy of Drs. C. A. Wang, O. Cope, B. Castleman, and S. I. Roth. Cases from Massachusetts General Hospital, including postmortem findings.
†Values in parentheses indicate percentages.
‡Provisional diagnosis only; primary hyperplasia has not been excluded.

logic etiology is that it is often difficult by either gross or histologic examination to distinguish between adenoma and hyperplasia or to decide by objective criteria whether abnormalities are present in only one or all four parathyroid glands. The older criterion used to distinguish between adenoma and hyperplasia, namely, a rim of normal tissue around the tumor nodule in an adenoma ("encapsulation;" Fig. 53-5), may not always be found.[90] Moreover, compression of tissue around an area of hyperplasia may give also the appearance of a capsule ("pseudoencapsulation").[90]

Accordingly, it is difficult to use histologic criteria to reconcile the opposing viewpoints and to determine the frequency of multiple-gland disease. However, inasmuch as these different views of the pathology of hyperparathyroidism have led to different approaches in surgical management of patients, i.e., extensive surgical ablation versus limited extirpation, careful follow-up evaluation of patients seems essential and may help to resolve the controversy. It will be essential to measure both blood calcium and parathyroid hormone levels at intervals in patients who have had a single gland removed to detect, if any, occult recurrence of hyperparathyroidism, which, of course, may lead to symptoms in the future. On the other hand, studies seem necessary in those patients with extensive resection to detect borderline or definite hypoparathyroidism, the principal clinical concern with extensive resection.

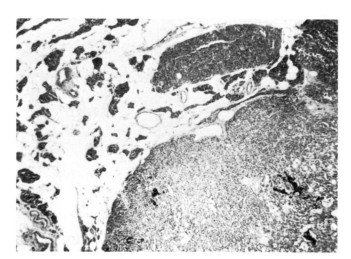

Fig. 53-5. Microscopical appearance of a chief-cell adenoma of the parathyroid gland. Adenoma is in lower right half of the field. Normal parathyroid tissue with characteristic fatty stroma and islands of chief cells and oxyphil cells is seen in the upper left. (Courtesy of the Department of Pathology, Massachusetts General Hospital.)

Parathyroid carcinoma is estimated to be found in approximately 3 percent of patients (Table 53-1).[91,93] Carcinoma of the parathyroid is characterized by the adherence of glandular tissue to surrounding structures. Histologic criteria of malignancy[94] include the presence of nuclear mitotic figures (normally none are seen in an entire section), fibrosis, and capsular or blood-vessel invasion. Analysis of the data of Schantz and Castleman[94] and Wang et al.[92] indicates that many carcinomas of the parathyroid grow slowly and are relatively benign. If the involved parathyroid gland is removed without capsular rupture, long-term follow-up has generally shown no evidence of recurrence,[92] although there are reports of metastases before initial operation.[95]

When the parathyroid carcinoma does become metastatic, spread is usually to the lymphatics on the side of the neck where the original tumor developed.[92] As soon as it becomes hematogenous, parathyroid carcinoma localizes in the lung most frequently and in liver and bone.[95] In 50 cases reviewed by Holmes et al.,[95] 46 of the carcinomas were hyperfunctioning and 4 carcinomas were not associated with excessive parathyroid hormone secretion. A feature often noted with these cases is the marked severity of hypercalcemia (greater than 14 mg/100 ml in 75 percent of cases).

In the past several decades there has been increasing awareness of the hereditary aspects of hyperparathyroidism and the association of familial hyperparathyroidism with other well-defined, associated heritable endocrine disorders. Estimates of incidence in the United States suggest several thousand kindreds in which there is a genetic transmission of hyperparathyroidism and/or other endocrine tumors.

There are two syndromes of multiple hereditary endocrinopathy recognized that are genetically distinct from one another.[95a] The first, now termed multiple endocrine neoplasia, type I (MEN-I), consists primarily of tumors of the parathyroid, pituitary, and pancreas. The second hereditary syndrome, termed multiple endocrine neoplasia, type II (MEN-II), consists of medullary carcinoma of the thyroid, adrenal tumors (pheochromocytoma), and, again, tumors of the parathyroids. (See Chapter 64 for extensive discussion of the latter syndrome.)

Wermer[96] was the first to define the genetic aspects of the earliest recognized multiple-endocrine-neoplasia, or MEN, syndrome, describing a pattern that featured pituitary, pancreatic, and parathyroid tumors (now termed MEN-I). Wermer correctly deduced that the high frequency with which one or more of these tumors was seen in family members from affected kindreds was compatible with an autosomal dominant inheritance.

The other MEN syndrome, MEN-II, was first reported as a suspected separate clinical entity by Sipple.[97] Schimke and Hartmann,[98] Schimke et al.,[99] and Steiner et al.[100] all noted the linkage between pheochromocytoma and medullary carcinoma of the thyroid as originally described by Sipple, plus the additional features of parathyroid tumors and mucosal neuromas. Steiner et al.[100] deduced an autosomal dominant pattern of inheritance in a total of 29 families who exhibited pheochromocytoma, medullary carcinoma of the thyroid, and hyperparathyroidism; they first suggested the term MEN-II for the disorder involving the thyroid and adrenal medulla inasmuch as tumors of the pituitary and pancreas, common in the other type of endocrinopathy (which was then renamed MEN-I), were absent from the kindreds with thyroid and adrenal tumors.

Recent studies suggest that the Zollinger/Ellison syndrome,[101,102] familial medullary carcinoma of the thyroid,[103,104] familial pheochromocytoma,[100] and familial hyperparathyroidism[105] may occur as well-established hereditary syndromes in certain families without any evidence (despite careful screening) of any other endocrine disorder.[105] These findings of familial medullary carcinoma and pheochromocytoma as distinct from MEN-II are discussed in Chapter 64. The genetics of these hereditary endocrine syndromes are not yet fully clarified (Fig. 53-6).

Several explanations, none completely satisfactory, have been offered to explain the etiology of these multiple-endocrine-neoplasia syndromes. There have been speculations, based on the observations of Pearse,[106] that the etiology underlying MEN syndromes involves a primary dysplasia of neuroectoderm.[107] Pearse[106] has discussed the hypothesis that cells originally of neural crest origin ultimately become the cells of origin of secretion of many of the hormones involved in the hereditary endocrine neoplasia (Chapter 64). These cells migrate widely during embryogenesis; the cells can be recognized by their histochemical characteristics (*a*mine *p*recursor *u*ptake plus *d*ecarboxylation—hence the name APUD cells). Such a theory, however, does not account for the clustering of pituitary and pancreatic neoplasia only in kindreds with the MEN-I syndrome and a similar, apparent segregation of parafollicular-cell and adrenal medullary tumors in the MEN-II syndrome; if a common cell type with ultimate dysplasia were the explanation, all endocrine tumors seen in the hereditary syndromes might be expected to appear in an affected kindred.

Another explanation offered for the syndrome is the occurrence of an initial over-production of one hormone leading to a compensatory response of another endocrine organ resulting in hyperplasia and, eventually, neoplasia. Vance et al.[108] offered the hypothesis that nesidioblastosis or hypertrophy of pancreatic islet cells leads to overproduction of insulin and glucagon, which, in turn, stimulates excessive calcitonin release and, ultimately, parathyroid hyperplasia. Similar speculations have involved a stimulus–response associated with medullary carcinoma and parathyroid hyperplasia in MEN-II.

Against this view are the studies of Melvin et al.[109] They established, by serial testing of asymptomatic members of a large kindred with MEN-II syndrome, that elevated blood levels of parathyroid hormone (indicating hyperplasia) with normal blood levels of calcitonin were seen in some patients, whereas in others elevated calcitonin levels (medullary carcinoma) were associated with normal parathyroid hormone levels. These results are consistent with an independent appearance of the discrete forms of endocrine neoplasia. Thus, although a genetic pattern consistent with autosomal dominant inheritance of these syndromes has been demonstrated, a single basic developmental defect explaining the peculiar linkage of some endocrine-gland tumors in the multiple-endocrine-neoplasia syndromes has so far eluded detection.

SUMMARY

Many clinical features of hyperparathyroidism remain unresolved despite the widespread attention it has received recently. The increasing frequency of detection of the disease, particularly in mild form, has led to uncertainty about the natural history of the disease, especially in regard to the indications for surgical treatment versus simple nonoperative medical surveillance (Chapter 57). The true frequency of signs and symptoms is difficult to assess, as discussed above, in view of the different rates of detection of the disease in surveys published prior to the recent decade versus frequency of detection in the present era. The recognition of the frequent hereditary aspects of the disease and the occurrence of associated endocrine disorders in hereditary hyperparathyroidism have added additional requirements to programs of optimal medical management, as discussed in Chapter 57. Despite these continuing uncertainties about treatment or management issues, as reviewed in Chapters 55 and 57, diagnostic criteria, using present clinical data and specialized laboratory techniques such as the radioimmunoassay for parathyroid hormone, are rather precisely established.

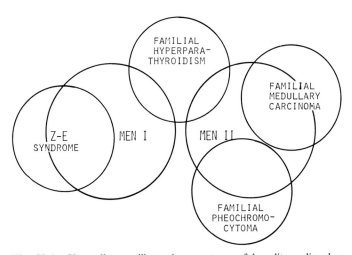

Fig. 53-6. Venn diagram illustrating spectrum of hereditary disorders involving primary hyperparathyroidism. The two multiple-endocrine-neoplasia syndromes (MEN-I and MEN-II) are genetically distinct, inasmuch as certain elements of one syndrome never occur in the other. Familial hyperparathyroidism is common to both. This syndrome, and the other disorders indicated, occur not only as part of the multiple-neoplasia syndromes, but also as separate familial disorders.

REFERENCES

1. Chaves-Carballo, E., Hayles, A. B.: Parathyroid adenoma in children: report of three cases, with unusual articular manifestations in one case. *Am J Dis Child 112:* 553, 1966.
2. Hellström, J., Ivemark, B. I.: Primary hyperparathyroidism: clinical and structural findings in 138 cases. *Acta Chir Scand,* Suppl 294: 12, 1962.
3. Riddick, F. A. Jr.: Primary hyperparathyroidism. *Med Clin North Am 81:* 871, 1967.
4. Watson, L.: Primary hyperparathyroidism. *Clinics Endocrinol Metab 3:* 215, 1974.
5. Krementz, E. T., Race, J. L., Sternberg, W. H., et al: Parathyroid adenoma: problems in diagnosis and management. *Ann Surg 165:* 681, 1967.
6. Yendt. E. R., Gagne, R. J. A.: Detection of primary hyperparathyroidism, with special reference to its occurrence in hypercalciuric

females with "normal" or borderline serum calcium. *Can Med Assoc J 98:* 331, 1968.

7. Purnell, D. C., Smith, L. H., Scholz, D. A., et al: Primary hyperparathyroidism: a prospective clinical study. *Am J Med 50:* 670, 1971.

8. Morris, R. C. Jr., Sebastian, A., McSherry, E.: Renal acidosis. *Kidney Int 1:* 322, 1972.

9. Thorén, L., Werner, I.: Hyperparathyroidism: clinical observations in a series of 85 patients. *Acta Chir Scand 135:* 395, 1969.

10. Epstein, F. H.: Calcium and the kidney. *Am J Med 45:* 700, 1968.

11. Epstein, F. H.: Bone and mineral metabolism in hyperthyroidism. *Ann Intern Med 68:* 490, 1968.

12. Richet, G., Ardaillou, R., Amiel, C., et al: Acidification de l'urine par injection intraveineuse de sels de calcium. *J Urol Nephrol 69:* 373, 1963.

13. Heinemann, H. O.: Metabolic alkalosis in patients with hypercalcemia. *Metabolism 14:* 1137, 1965.

14. Verbanck, M.: Le fonctionnement du rein dans les états d'hypercalcémie: Étude clinique et expérimentale. *Acta Clin Belg* Suppl 1: 1, 1965.

15. Wills, M. R., McGowan, G. K.: Plasma-chloride levels in hyperparathyroidism and other hypercalcaemic states. *Br Med J 1:* 1153, 1964.

16. Palmer, F. J., Nelson, J. C., Bacchus, H.: The chloride–phosphate ratio in hypercalcemia. *Ann Intern Med 80:* 200, 1974.

17. Coe, F. L.: Magnitude of metabolic acidosis in primary hyperparathyroidism. *Arch Intern Med 134:* 262, 1974.

18. Morris, R. C. Jr.: An experimental renal acidification defect in patients with hereditary fructose intolerance. I. Its resemblance to renal tubular acidosis. *J Clin Invest 47:* 1389, 1968.

19. Morris, R. C. Jr.: An experimental acidification defect in patients with hereditary fructose intolerance. II. Its distinction from classic renal tubular acidosis; its resemblance to the renal acidification defect associated with the Fanconi syndrome of children with cystinosis. *J Clin Invest 47:* 1648, 1968.

20. Morris, R. C. Jr.: Renal tubular acidosis: mechanisms, classification and implications. *N Engl J Med 281:* 1405, 1969.

21. Morris, R. C. Jr., McSherry, E., Sebastian, A.: Modulation of experimental renal dysfunction of hereditary fructose intolerance by circulating parathyroid hormone. *Proc Natl Acad Sci USA 68:* 132, 1971.

22. Gold, L. W., Massry, S. G., Arieff, A. I., et al: Renal bicarbonate wasting during phosphate depletion: a possible cause of altered acid-base homeostasis in hyperparathyroidism. *J Clin Invest 52:* 2556, 1973.

23. Edvall, C. A.: Renal function in hyperparathyroidism. A clinical study of 30 cases with special reference to selective renal clearance and renal vein catheterization. *Acta Chir Scand,* Suppl 229, 1958.

24. Purnell, D. C., Scholz, D. A., Smith, L. H., et al: Treatment of primary hyperparathyroidism. *Am J Med 56:* 800, 1974.

25. Britton, D. C., Thompson, M. H., Johnston, I. D. A., et al: Renal function following parathyroid surgery in primary hyperparathyroidism. *Lancet 2:* 74, 1971.

26. Aurbach, G. D., Mallette, L. E., Patten, B. M., et al: Hyperparathyroidism: recent studies. *Ann Intern Med 79:* 566, 1973.

27. Dauphine, R. T., Riggs, B. L., Scholz, D. A.: Back pain and vertebral crush fractures: an unemphasized mode of presentation for primary hyperparathyroidism. *Ann Intern Med 83:* 365, 1975.

28. Genant, H. K., Baron, J. M., Straus, F. H. II, et al: Osteosclerosis in primary hyperparathyroidism. *Am J Med 59:* 104, 1975.

29. Jowsey, J.: Quantitative microradiography: a new approach in the evaluation of metabolic bone disease. *Am J Med 40:* 485, 1966 (editorial).

30. Forland, M., Strandjord, N. M., Paloyan, E., et al: Bone density studies in primary hyperparathyroidism. *Arch Intern Med 122:* 236, 1968.

31. Dalén, N., Hjern, B.: Bone mineral content in patients with primary hyperparathyroidism without radiological evidence of skeletal changes. *Acta Endocrinol 75:* 297, 1974.

32. Pak, C. Y. C., Stewart, A., Kaplan, R., et al: Photon absorptiometric analysis of bone density in primary hyperparathyroidism. *Lancet 2:* 7, 1975.

33. Meunier, P., Vignon, G., Bernard, J., et al: Quantitative bone histology as applied to the diagnosis of hyperparathyroid states. In Frame, B., Parfitt, A. M., Duncan, H. (eds): Clinical Aspects of Metabolic Bone Disease. Amsterdam, Excerpta Medica, 1973, p 215.

34. Bordier, P. J., Arnaud, C.[D.], Hawker, C., et al: Relationship between serum immunoreactive parathyroid hormone, osteoclastic and osteocytic bone resorptions and serum calcium in primary hyperparathyroidism and osteomalacia. In Frame B., Parfitt A. M., Duncan H. (eds): Clinical Aspects of Metabolic Bone Disease. Amsterdam, Excerpta Medica, 1973, p 222.

34a. Potts, J. T., Jr., and Deftos, L. J.: Parathyroid hormone, calcitonin, vitamin D, bone and bone mineral metabolism. In Bondy, P. K., Rosenberg, L. E. (eds): Duncan's Disease of Metabolism. 7th ed. Philadelphia, Saunders, 1974, p. 1225.

35. Albright, F., Reifenstein, E. C. Jr.: The Parathyroid Glands and Metabolic Bone Disease: Selected Studies. Baltimore, Williams & Wilkins, 1948.

36. Dent. C. E.: Some problems of hyperparathyroidism. *Brit Med J 2:* 1419, 1962.

37. Peacock, M.: Renal stone disease and bone disease in primary hyperparathyroidism and their relationship to the action of parathyroid hormone on calcium absorption. In Talmage, R. V., Owen, M., Parsons, J. A. (eds): Calcium-Regulating Hormones, Proceedings of the Fifth Parathyroid Conference. Amsterdam, Excerpta Medica New York, American Elsevier, 1975, p 78.

38. Steinbach, H. L., Gordan, G. S., Eisenberg, E., et al: Primary hyperparathyroidism: a correlation of rotentgen, clinical, and pathologic features. *Am J Roentgenol Radium Ther Nucl Med 6:* 329, 1961.

38a. Potts, J. T. Jr., Deftos, L. J.: Parathyroid hormone, calcitonin, vitamin D, bone and bone mineral metabolism. In Bondy, P. K., Rosenberg, L. E. (eds): Duncan's Diseases of Metabolism. Philadelphia, Saunders, 1974, p 1225.

39. Recklinghausen, F. von: Die fibröse oder deformirende Ostitis, die Osteomalacie und die osteoplastiche Carcinose in ihren gegenseitigen Bieziehungen: In: Festschrift Rudolf Virchow zu seinem 71 Geburtstage. Berlin, Reimer, 1891, p 1.

40. Hirschberg, K.: Zur Kenntniss der Osteomalacie und Ostitis malacissans. *Beitr Pathol Anat 6:* 513, 1889.

41. Mandl, F.: Klinisches und Experimentelles zur Frage der lokalisierten und generalisierten Ostitis fibrosa. (Unter besonderer Berücksichtigung der Therapie der letzteren). *Arch Klin Chir 143:* 1, 245, 1926.

42. Patten, B. M., Bilezikian, J. P., Mallette, L. E., et al: Neuromuscular disease in primary hyperparathyroidism. *Ann Intern Med 80:* 182, 1974.

43. Henson, R. A.: The neurological aspects of hypercalcaemia: with special reference to primary hyperparathyroidism. *J R Coll Physicians Lond 1:* 41, 1966.

44. Petersen, P.: Psychiatric disorders in primary hyperparathyroidism. *J Clin Endocrinol 28:* 1491, 1968.

45. Lehrer. G. M., Levitt, M. F.: Neuropsychiatric presentation of hypercalcemia. *J Mt Sinai Hosp 27:* 10, 1960.

46. Hockaday, T. D. R., Keynes, W. M., McKenzie, J. K.: Catatonic stupor in elderly women with hyperparathyroidism. *Br Med J 1:* 85, 1966.

47. Wilson, R. E., Bernhard, W. F., Polet, H., et al: Hyperparathyroidism: the problem of acute parathyroid intoxication. *Ann Surg 159:* 79, 1964.

48. Moure, J. M. B.: The electroencephalogram in hypercalcemia. *Arch Neurol 17:* 34, 1967.

49. Allen, E. M., Singer, F. R., Melomed, D.: Electroencephalographic abnormalities in hypercalcemia. *Neurology 20:* 15, 1970.

50. Ostrow, J. D., Blanshard, G., Gray, S. J.: Peptic ulcer in primary hyperparathyroidism. *Am J Med 29:* 769, 1960.

51. Barreras, R. F.: Calcium and gastric secretion. *Gastroenterology 64:* 1168, 1973.

52. Doll, R., Jones, F. A., Buckatzsch, M. M.: Occupational factors in the aetiology of gastric and duodenal ulcers. Medical Research Council Special Report Ser No 276. London, Her Majesty's Stationery Office, 1950.

53. Zollinger, R. M., Ellison, E. H.: Primary peptic ulcerations of the jejunum associated with islet cell tumors of the pancreas. *Ann Surg 142:* 709, 1955.

54. Barreras. R. F., Donaldson, R. M. Jr.: Role of calcium in gastric hypersecretion, parathyroid adenoma and peptic ulcer. *N Engl J Med 276:* 1122, 1967.

55. Dent, R. I., James, J. H., Wang, C-A., et al: Hyperparathyroidism: gastric acid secretion and gastrin. *Ann Surg 176:* 360, 1972.

56. Patterson, M., Wolma, F., Drake, A., et al: Gastric secretion and chronic hyperparathyroidism. *Arch Surg 99:* 9, 1969.

57. Ward, J. T., Adesola, A. O., Welbourn, R. B.: The parathyroids, calcium and gastric secretion in man and the dog. *Gut 5:* 173, 1964.

58. McGuigan, J. E., Colwell, J. A., Franklin, J.: Effect of parathyroid-

ectomy on hypercalcemic hypersecretory peptic ulcer disease. *Gastroenterology 66:* 269, 1974.

59. Wilder. W. T., Frame. B., Haubrich. W. S.: Peptic ulcer in primary hyperparathyroidism: an analysis of fifty-two cases. *Ann Intern Med 55:* 885, 1961.

60. Cope, O., Culver. P. J., Mixter. C. G. Jr., et al: Pancreatitis, a diagnostic clue to hyperparathyroidism. *Ann Surg 145:* 857, 1957.

61. Wang, C-A.: Surgery of the parathyroid glands. *Adv Surg 5:* 109, 1971.

62. Mixter, C. G. Jr., Keynes, W. M., Cope, O.: Further experience with pancreatitis as a diagnostic clue to hyperparathyroidism. *N Engl J Med 266:* 265, 1962.

63. Paloyan, E., Lawrence, A. M., Straus, F. H. II, et al: Alpha cell hyperplasia in calcific pancreatitis associated with hyperparathyroidism. *JAMA 200:* 757, 1967.

64. Edmondson, H. A., Berne, C. J., Homann, R. E. Jr., et al: Calcium, potassium, magnesium and amylase disturbances in acute pancreatitis. *Am J Med 12:* 34, 1952.

65. Snodgrass, P. J.: Diseases of the pancreas. In Wintrobe, M. M., Thorn, G. W., Isselbacher, K. J., et al (eds): Harrison's Principles of Internal Medicine, 7th ed. New York, McGraw-Hill, 1974, pp 1568–1579.

66. Bywaters, E. G. L., Dixon, A. St. J., Scott, J. T.: Joint lesions of hyperparathyroidism. *Ann Rheum Dis 22:* 171, 1963.

67. Wang, C-A., Miller, L. M., Weber, A. L., et al: Pseudogout: a diagnostic clue to hyperparathyroidism. *Am J Surg 117:* 558, 1969.

68. Grahame, R., Sutor, D. J., Mitchener, M. B.: Crystal deposition in hyperparathyroidism. *Ann Rheum Dis 30:* 597, 1971.

69. McCarty, D. J. [Jr.]: Diagnostic mimicry in arthritis—patterns of joint involvement associated with calcium pyrophosphate dihydrate crystal deposits. *Bull Rheum Dis 25:* 804, 1975.

70. McCarty, D. J. Jr., Haskin, M. E.: The roentgenographic aspects of pseudogout (articular chondrocalcinosis): an analysis of 20 cases. *Am J Roentgenol 90:* 1248, 1963.

71. McCarty, D. J. Jr.: Crystal deposition disease—calcium pyrophosphate. *Mod Trends Rheumatol 1:* 287, 1966.

72. Dodds, W. J., Steinbach, H. L.: Primary hyperparathyroidism and articular cartilage calcification. *Am J Roentgenol 104:* 884, 1968.

73. Mintz, D. H., Canary, J. J., Carreon, G., et al: Hyperuricemia in hyperparathyroidism. *N Engl J Med 265:* 112, 1961.

74. Scott, J. T., Dixon, A. St. J., Bywaters, E. G. L.: Association of hyperuricaemia and gout with hyperparathyroidism. *Br Med J 1:* 1070, 1964.

75. Hellström, J.: Clinical experiences of twenty-one cases of hyperparathyroidism with special reference to the prognosis following parathyroidectomy. *Acta Chir Scand 100:* 391, 1950.

76. Hellström, J.: Primary hyperparathyroidism: observations in a series of 50 cases. *Acta Endocrinol 16:* 30, 1954.

77. Hellström, J., Birke, G., Edvall, C. A.: Hypertension in hyperparathyroidism. *Br J Urol 30:* 13, 1958.

78. United States National Center for Health Statistics: Vital and Health Statistics: Heart disease in adults: United States 1960–62. USPHS Publ No 1000, Series 11, No 6. Washington, DC, 1964.

79. Anderson, D. C., Steward, W. K., Piercy, D. M.: Calcifying panniculitis with fat and skin necrosis in a case of uraemia with autonomous hyperparathyroidism. *Lancet 2:* 323, 1968.

80. Cogan, D. G., Albright, F., Bartter, F. C.: Hypercalcemia and band keratopathy: report of nineteen cases. *Arch Ophthalmol 40:* 624, 1948.

81. Nolan, R. B., Hayles, A. B., Woolner, L. B.: Adenoma of the parathyroid gland in children: report of case and brief review of the literature. *Am J Dis Child 99:* 622, 1960.

82. Reinfrank, R. F., Edwards, T. L. Jr.: Parathyroid crisis in a child. *JAMA 178:* 468, 1961.

83. Rajasuriy, A. K., Peiris, O. A., Ratnaike, V. T., et al: Parathyroid adenomas in childhood: a case report and a review of the current literature. *Am J Dis Child 107:* 442, 1964.

84. Lloyd, H. M., Aitken, R. E., Ferrier, T. M.: Primary hyperparathyroidism resembling rickets of late onset. *Br Med J 2:* 853, 1965.

85. Steendijk, R.: Metabolic bone disease in children. *Clin Orthop 77:* 247, 1971.

86. Goldsmith, R. S., Furszyfer, J., Johnson, W. J., et al: Etiology of hyperparathyroidism and bone disease during chronic hemodialysis. III. Evaluation of parathyroid suppressibility *J Clin Invest 52:* 173, 1973.

87. Albright, F., Aub, J. C., Bauer, W.: Hyperparathyroidism: a common and polymorphic condition as illustrated by seventeen proved cases from one clinic. *JAMA 102:* 1276, 1934.

88. Cope, O., Barnes, B. A., Castleman, B., et al: Vicissitudes of parathyroid surgery: trials of diagnosis and management in 51 patients with a variety of disorders. *Ann Surg 154:* 491, 1961.

89. Roth, S. I.: Pathology of the parathyroids in hyperparathyroidism: discussion of recent advances in the anatomy and pathology of the parathyroid glands. *Arch Pathol 73:* 495, 1962.

90. Roth, S. I.: Recent advances in parathyroid gland pathology. *Am J Med 50:* 612, 1971.

91. Paloyan, E., Paloyan, D., Pickleman, J. R.: Hyperparathyroidism today. *Surg Clin North Am 53:* 211, 1973.

92. Wang, C. A., Potts, J. T. Jr., Neer, R. M.: Controversy of parathyroid surgery. In Talmage R. V., Owen M., Parsons J. A. (eds): Calcium-Regulating Hormones, Proceedings of the Fifth Parathyroid Conference. Amsterdam, Excerpta Medica, 1975, pp 82–85.

93. Wang, C. A., Cope, O.: Reoperation for hyperparathyroidism. In Hardy J. D. (ed): Rhoad's Textbook of Surgery: Principles and Practice. Philadelphia, Lippincott, 1977.

94. Schantz, A., Castleman, B.: Parathyroid carcinoma: a study of 70 cases. *Cancer 31:* 600, 1973.

95. Holmes, E. C., Morton, D. L., Ketcham, A. S.: Parathyroid carcinoma: a collective review. *Ann Surg 169:* 631, 1969.

95a. Habener, J. F., Potts, J. T. Jr.: Parathyroid physiology and primary hyperparathyroidism. In Avioli L. V., Krane S. M. (eds): Metabolic Bone Disease. Vol. II. New York, Academic (in press).

96. Wermer, P.: Genetic aspects of adenomatosis of endocrine glands. *Am J Med 16:* 363, 1954.

97. Sipple, J. H.: The association of pheochromocytoma with carcinoma of the thyroid gland. *Am J Med 31:* 163, 1961.

98. Schimke, R. N., Hartmann, W. H.: Familial amyloid-producing medullary thyroid carcinoma and pheochromocytoma: a distinct genetic entity. *Ann Intern Med 63:* 1027, 1965.

99. Schimke, R. N., Hartmann, W. H., Prout, T. E., et al: Syndrome of bilateral pheochromocytoma, medullary thyroid carcinoma and multiple neuromas: a possible regulatory defect in the differentiation of chromaffin tissue. *N Engl J Med 279:* 1, 1968.

100. Steiner, A. L., Goodman, A. D., Powers, S. R.: Study of a kindred with pheochromocytoma, medullary thyroid carcinoma, hyperparathyroidism and Cushing's disease: multiple endocrine neoplasia, Type 2. *Medicine 47:* 371, 1968.

101. Ellison, E. H., Wilson, S. D.: The Zollinger-Ellison syndrome: reappraisal and evaluation of 260 registered cases. *Ann Surg 160:* 512, 1964.

102. Fox, P. S., Hofmann, J. W., Decosse, J. J., et al: The influence of total gastrectomy on survival in malignant Zollinger-Ellison tumors. *Ann Surg 180:* 558, 1974.

103. Williams, E. D.: Histogenesis of medullary carcinoma of the thyroid. *J Clin Pathol 19:* 114, 1966.

104. Block, M. A., Horn, R. C. Jr., Miller, J. M., et al: Familial medullary carcinoma of the thyroid. *Trans Am Surg Assoc 85:* 101, 1967.

105. Marx, S. J., Powell, D., Shimkin, P. M., et al: Familial hyperparathyroidism: mild hypercalcemia in at least nine members of a kindred. *Ann Intern Med 78:* 371, 1973.

106. Pearse, A. G. E.: Evolutionary and developmental relationships among the cells producing peptide hormones. In Parsons J. A. (ed): Peptide Hormones. London, Macmillan, 1976, pp 33–46.

107. Weichert, R. F., III: The neural ectodermal origin of the peptide-secreting glands: a unifying concept for the etiology of multiple endocrine adenomatosis and the inappropriate secretion of peptide hormones by nonendocrine tumors. *Am J Med 49:* 232, 1970.

108. Vance, J. E., Stoll, R. W., Kitabchi, A. E., et al: Nesidioblastosis in familial endocrine adenomatosis. *JAMA 207:* 1679, 1969.

109. Melvin, K. E. W., Miller, H. H., Tashjian, A. H. Jr.: Early diagnosis of medullary carcinoma of the thyroid gland by means of calcitonin assay. *N Engl J Med 285:* 1115, 1971.

54

Diagnosis and Differential Diagnosis of Primary Hyperparathyroidism

Joel F. Habener
John T. Potts, Jr.

GENERAL CONSIDERATIONS

Primary hyperparathyroidism is most often searched for in patients with otherwise unexplained hypercalcemia, recurrent kidney stones, peptic ulcer disease, pancreatitis, chondrocalcinosis, diffuse osteoporosis, or, in rarer instances, with symptoms and/or signs of osteitis fibrosa. Blood calcium measurements may lead to detection of hypercalcemia in patients with vague constitutional complaints, lethargy and weakness, gastrointestinal symptoms, atypical arthritis, and myopathy. Also, in recent years, multiphasic routine blood testing in asymptomatic subjects has uncovered hypercalcemia.

Hypercalcemia is an invariant manifestation of hyperparathyroidism. Without definite hypercalcemia, there is almost never a justification for surgical exploration. Repeated measurements of plasma calcium should be made in patients with suspected hypercalcemia. The normal range for serum calcium in most laboratories is 8.6 to 10.4 mg/100 ml. The upper limit of the normal range of serum calcium in females is usually 0.1 to 0.2 mg/100 ml below that of males of the same age, and the values for elderly males may be as much as 0.3 mg/100 ml below those seen in younger males.[1]

Most laboratories determine total calcium, which includes both free or ionized calcium and protein-bound calcium. The serum calcium value must be interpreted in relation to serum protein concentrations because only an abnormality in non-protein-bound calcium reflects an abnormality in calcium metabolism. A rough guide that may be used is the adjustment of the total serum calcium upward or downward by 0.8 mg/100 ml for each gram per 100 ml of serum protein below or above normal, respectively, before any decision is made that a given level of total calcium is truly abnormal. It is important to eliminate errors due to venous stasis during collection of blood; prolonged venous stasis results in an increase in total serum calcium due both to hemoconcentration and to an increase in the fraction of calcium bound to serum proteins.[2] One may detect either a sustained hypercalcemia or a pattern of high-normal blood calciums alternating with occasional slightly elevated values.

It is the latter pattern of blood calcium values that should be emphasized; the hypercalcemia of mild hyperparathyroidism may occasionally present in a subtle or intermittent pattern and thus may confuse the interpretation. Careful scrutiny of reports of "normocalcemic hyperparathyroidism"[3-5] reveals that many of the patients were, in fact, frankly hypercalcemic, although mildly, at some time in the course of their disease (Fig. 54-1). Such patients could more correctly be described, therefore, as having "intermittent hypercalcemia." Some workers, however, have presented data on patients whom they believe represent true "normocalcemic hyperparathyroidism," meaning consistently midnormal values of blood calcium. In one report, several of these patients, who were "recurrent stone-formers" were found at operation to have parathyroid glands that were normal when examined grossly and by light microscopy. Electron microscopy, however, revealed abnormalities in gland histology; after parathyroidectomy, the frequency of stones was reduced.[5a] The variable clinical course of recurrent nephrolithiasis, however, makes it difficult to invoke the presence of mild hyperparathyroidism as the cause even when there is transient improvement after parathyroidectomy. A decreased renal tubular reabsorption of phosphate and resulting phosphaturia are seen in patients with idiopathic hypercalciuria,[6] most of whom do not appear to have hyperparathyroidism; hence, occasional hypophosphatemia in stone-formers cannot be used in support of the concept of normocalcemic hyperparathyroidism. One must be reluctant to consider patients as having primary hyperparathyroidism in the absence of hypercalcemia unless, as emphasized by Reiss and Canterbury,[7] there is known malabsorption or renal failure to modify the calcium-elevating effects of excessive PTH secretion. There eventually may prove to be a substantial number of patients in the catagory of "normocalcemic hyperparathyroidism," but, until a much wider experience is accumulated, the authors stress caution in accepting the concept. Such patients should not be referred to, for purposes of semantic distinc-

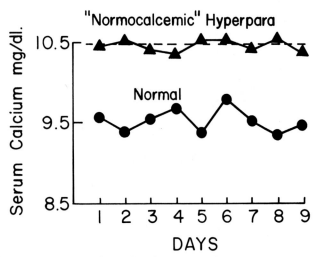

Fig. 54-1. Day-to-day fluctuations in serum calcium that might typically occur in normal individuals and in patients with mild hyperparathyroidism.

tion, as examples of "normocalcemic hyperparathyroidism," but rather as examples of "masked hyperparathyroidism."

The serum inorganic-phosphorus level in primary hyperparathyroidism is usually low but may be normal, especially in patients with abnormal renal function; serum phosphate levels may rise when glomerular filtration rates (GFR) fall to very low levels. The presence of persistent, fasting hypophosphatemia can be useful in pointing to the diagnosis of primary hyperparathyroidism but is less specific than is hypercalcemia, particularly in view of the fact that severe hypercalcemia of any cause may lower serum phosphorus by altering renal tubular handling of phosphate.[8,9] Blood samples should be obtained in the morning, under fasting conditions, inasmuch as there may be a sharp fall in postprandial blood phosphorus levels (Chapter 40). Hypercalciuria also is seen commonly in hyperparathyroidism with hypercalcemia. However, because parathyroid hormone reduces calcium clearance, the urinary excretion of calcium is lower in patients with hyperparathyroidism than in patients with equivalent degrees of hypercalcemia not related to the parathyroids.[10]

Blood alkaline phosphatase[11] and urinary hydroxyproline excretion[12] are usually elevated only when there is substantial bone involvement. Renal involvement can be reflected by a decreased concentrating ability, by specific tubular defects such as tubular acidosis, and, finally, by frank renal failure with the chemical findings of azotemia.[13] Other electrolyte abnormalities such as a mild hyperchloremic acidosis, as described earlier, may also be of diagnostic value.

SPECIAL TESTS

Over the years a number of special tests have been proposed to aid in establishing the diagnosis of hyperparathyroidism. The most useful of all special tests have been the radioimmunoassay for the determination of serum or plasma immunoreactive parathyroid hormone and procedures for the assessment of nephrogenous cyclic AMP excretion. A complete description of the usefulness and pitfalls of the radioimmunoassay for parathyroid hormone is given in Chapter 55.

Some problems have arisen in the interpretation of radioimmunoassay results in patients with hypercalcemia; these problems have resulted from the heterogeneous nature of the circulating hormone (Chapter 45). Most immunoreactive hormone in the

blood of patients with primary hyperparathyroidism consists of biologically inactive COOH-terminal fragments. Cross-reactivity of intact hormone and hormonal fragments may vary with different antisera used in the radioimmunoassays and as a result give quite different values for the concentration of hormone in the blood samples. In most laboratories, however, these problems have been minimized by the use of pooled serum or plasma from hyperparathyroid patients as the assay standard. Even with the use of this assay standard, it has been the general experience that a substantial number of patients (5 to 25 percent in different assays), subsequently found at surgery to have primary hyperparathyroidism, have serum levels of immunoreactive hormone that are consistently within the range of those found in normal individuals (Chapter 55). However, when hormone values are analyzed as a function of the serum calcium, in comparison with the corresponding values in normal individuals, or in individuals with hypercalcemia not due to hyperparathyroidism, the hormone values in hyperparathyroid patients are seen to be abnormal for the given level of serum calcium. In most assays, clearly detectable measurements of immunoreactive parathyroid hormone in the presence of hypercalcemia of any degree strongly indicate the existence of hyperparathyroidism (Chapter 55).

Another problem that arises in the interpretation of immunoassay measurements is encountered in patients with hypercalcemia and malignant tumors of nonparathyroid origin. Some assays quite consistently give undetectable measurements of immunoreactive parathyroid hormone in these patients with hypercalcemia-producing tumors, whereas other assays give detectable, albeit low, measurements of hormone (Chapter 55). The reasons for this disagreement in assay results are at present unknown.

A second, highly useful test for parathyroid gland activity, in addition to the radioimmunoassay, is the assessment of urinary cyclic AMP. As discussed in Chapters 46 and 63, renal excretion of cyclic AMP produced in kidney tubules rises sharply in response to changes in circulating levels of parathyroid hormone. Although vasopressin also has direct effects on renal adenylate cyclase at physiologic concentrations, it contributes little to total urinary cyclic AMP excretion. It has been shown that measurements of the basal level of urinary cyclic AMP excretion could provide a useful test for parathyroid hormone activity. Early attempts to correlate total urinary cyclic AMP with parathyroid gland function were only partly successful, owing to a high degree of overlap in values in patients with known hyperparathyroidism with those values found in normal individuals. Recently, it has been recognized that the variations in GFR and in the amount contributed by extrarenal plasma cyclic AMP are major factors in widening the range of values and thus account for the overlap in values found in persons with and without hyperparathyroidism. Broadus et al.[14] emphasized that the specificity of measurements can be improved greatly by expressing total urinary cyclic AMP as a function of GFR or by determination of the specific nephrogenous component of the urinary cyclic nucleotide. The former determination requires only that the GFR (by creatinine clearance) be measured in addition to total urinary cyclic AMP. Estimation of the nephrogenous component of cyclic AMP requires that the total urinary cyclic AMP be corrected for the contribution made by plasma cyclic AMP. Broadus et al.[14] found diagnostically elevated levels of cyclic AMP excretion expressed as a function of GFR in 89 percent of 51 patients and of nephrogenous cyclic AMP in 91 percent of 52 patients with primary hyperparathyroidism (Fig. 54-2). This group of patients included a subgroup of 26 patients with mild hyperparathyroidism manifested by episodic hypercalcemia (serum calcium less than 10.7 mg/100 ml), a group that is clinically difficult to

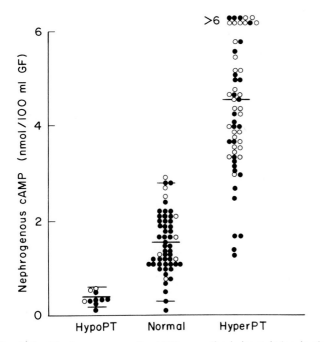

Fig. 54-2. Nephrogenous cyclic AMP as a discriminant index in the differential diagnosis of hyperparathyroidism. Nephrogenous cyclic AMP is expressed as a function of GFR in the control subjects and patients with primary hyperparathyroidism. The open circles depict the subjects and patients with renal impairment (mean creatinine clearance $\leq$ 80 ml/min). The horizontal bars represent the mean values, and the control group is shown as mean ±2 SD (see text). (After Broadus *et al.*: J. Clin. Invest. *60:* 771, 1977.)

differentiate from patients with idiopathic hypercalciuria. Radioimmunoassay for parathyroid hormone, whether singly or in combination with determinations of nephrogenous cyclic AMP, provides the most definitive information for the specific diagnosis of hyperparathyroidism in patients with hypercalcemia.

With regard to other tests, efforts have been made to quantitate the effect of parathyroid hormone on reduction in tubular phosphate reabsorption and increase in urinary phosphate clearance, but these tests have not proved to be uniformly successful.[15] Many factors such as intrinsic renal disease, dietary phosphate intake, and the physiologic diurnal variation in phosphate excretion interfere with the interpretation of phosphate clearance. Calcium infusion to suppress parathyroid secretion and thereby test autonomy of phosphate clearance[16] was utilized before it was realized that the parathyroid glands are responsive to changes in blood calcium levels even in primary hyperparathyroidism.[17]

Therefore, if special tests of renal phosphorus handling are to be used, appropriate caution must be observed in their interpretation. Several convenient indices of phosphate excretion by the kidneys may be determined.[18] Because of the diurnal variation in renal phosphate handling and the fluctuations in plasma phosphate after meals, 24-h urine specimens cannot be used for determinations of phosphate clearance; specimens collected at short intervals in the morning during fasting are needed to give meaningful results.

Phosphate clearance is determined by standard techniques involving simultaneous measurements of urinary and blood phosphate and creatinine concentrations; usually urine samples are collected over a period of 1 to 4 h. Normal subjects have a phosphate clearance of 10.8 + 2.7 ml/min. The tubular resorption of phosphate can be calculated from the phosphate clearance and the glomerular filtration rate, the latter usually determined by

creatinine clearance; in normal subjects, the tubular resorption of phosphate exceeds 85 percent. In some patients with hyperparathyroidism, and unfortunately in other subjects as well, clearance of phosphate is increased or, conversely, resorption of phosphate by the renal tubules is reduced. It is essential to control phosphate intake in such studies because renal tubular phosphate transport, with or without excessive parathyroid effect, will vary with extremes of oral phosphate intake (Chapter 40). Low phosphate intake leads to increased tubular resorption. It is critical that measurements of phosphate clearance be considered quantitatively with respect to phosphate intake (Chapter 40).

Thiazide diuretics in the usual doses of 1 to 2 g daily of chlorothiazide or its equivalent can produce sustained hypercalcemia in patients with hyperparathyroidism and borderline calcium values. Such a response is not usually seen in normal subjects. Although thiazide diuretics may produce transient elevations of blood calcium in normal subjects, normocalcemia returns in a few days despite continued administration. Thiazide administration has, therefore, been suggested as a provocative test for the presence of hyperparathyroidism.[19]

Glucocorticoid administration has been useful in distinguishing the hypercalcemia of hyperparathyroidism from that associated with sarcoidosis, multiple myeloma, vitamin D intoxication, and some malignant diseases with osseous metastases.[20,21] In the last-mentioned diseases, doses of hydrocortisone of 100 mg/day for 10 days usually result in a lowering of the serum calcium to normal levels, whereas calcium levels typically do not fall in primary hyperparathyroidism.

DIFFERENTIAL DIAGNOSIS

GENERAL

Hypercalcemia presents one of the more common diagnostic problems in medicine.[22,23] Although malignant neoplasms with or without skeletal metastases and primary hyperparathyroidism are probably the leading causes of hypercalcemia in adults, other causes must be considered in the differential diagnosis (Table 54-1). The correct diagnosis can be made in many patients after a careful history and physical examination and several routine radiologic procedures and laboratory tests. In many instances there may be obvious manifestations of the responsible disease state, such as widespread malignant disease, thyrotoxicosis, or a history of ex-

Table 54-1. Differential Diagnosis of Hypercalcemia

Malignancy
    Solid Tumors with Osseous Metastases
    Hematologic Tumors Involving Bone: Multiple Myeloma. Lymphoma, and Leukemia
    Pseudohyperparathyroidism
        Ectopic Hyperparathyroidism
        Other Humoral Factors
Primary Hyperparathyroidism
    Primary
    Multiple Endocrine Neoplasia
Sarcoidosis, Tuberculosis, Berylliosis, and Other Granulomatous Diseases
Thyrotoxicosis
Acute Adrenal Insufficiency
Vitamin D Intoxication
Vitamin A Intoxication
Thiazide Diuretics
Immobilization
Milk/Alkali Syndrome
Idiopathic Hypercalcemia of Infancy

cessive ingestion of vitamin D, whereas at other times the underlying cause for the hypercalcemia is not obvious and one must embark on a detailed evaluation of the patient. It is essential, of course, to ensure that true hypercalcemia exists, and repeated determinations of the serum calcium level over a period of a few days are necessary. Patients with hyperparathyroidism, for example, may have levels of calcium that fluctuate in the range from high normal to slightly elevated, and it takes several determinations to establish a truly convincing pattern of hypercalcemia.

It is important to emphasize that hyperparathyroidism is characteristically a chronic disorder; historical information or clinical evidence of the chronicity of a disorder in calcium metabolism such as recurrent renal calculi, chronic peptic-ulcer disease, documented hypercalcemia many months earlier, or even radiographic evidence of renal stone in the absence of symptoms usually favors the diagnosis of hyperparathyroidism rather than malignancy, as has been pointed out by Lafferty.[24] On the other hand, if hypercalcemia was detected only recently without other historical features of chronicity, the search for other causes of hypercalcemia must be particularly thorough.

The serum alkaline phosphatase may be elevated in several conditions that produce hypercalcemic states. A substantially elevated total alkaline phosphatase in the absence of radiologically evident bone disease is an unusual occurrence in primary hyperparathyroidism. Hyperphosphatasia under these circumstances is more consistent with metastatic malignancy or sarcoidosis with hepatic involvement than with hyperparathyroidism. Serum chloride and bicarbonate values may be helpful; a mild hyperchloremic acidosis favors the diagnosis of primary hyperparathyroidism, whereas metabolic alkalosis suggests malignant sarcoidosis, vitamin D intoxication, or milk/alkali syndrome. This situation arises from the bicarbonate-wasting action of parathyroid hormone on the renal tubule. The chloride/phosphate ratio (Chapter 55), especially if above 35, is suggestive of hyperparathyroidism. Persistent azotemia in a well-hydrated patient may point to renal damage secondary to long-standing hypercalcemia and suggests the chronicity of the hypercalcemia. Additional tests might include a sedimentation rate and serum protein electrophoresis or immunoelectrophoresis; the latter may point to multiple myeloma or other non-parathyroid-related disorders, normal in uncomplicated primary hyperparathyroidism. Fraser et al.[25] claimed high usefulness for an all-inclusive analysis of serum phosphorus, alkaline phosphatase, bicarbonate, and urea for the differential diagnosis of hypercalcemia. The diagnosis by this simple analysis in their hands coincided in 197 of 218 cases of hypercalcemia with the diagnosis reached after a long period of detailed clinical investigation.

The necessary roentgenologic procedures in patients with hypercalcemia should include plain films of the lungs, hands, skull, and abdomen (with intravenous pyelogram) to search for, respectively, pulmonary sarcoidosis or malignancy, subperiosteal resorption, enlargement of the sella turcica, and renal calculi or tumor. If occult malignancy is suspected, a complete gastrointestinal series and a bone scan and/or skeletal survey should be performed, in addition to the intravenous pyelogram.

MALIGNANCY

Hypercalcemia is a frequent complication of malignant disease. The elimination of malignancy as the underlying cause of hypercalcemia can be one of the most difficult problems in differential diagnosis, especially because of the association of malignant tumors and the ectopic production of parathyroid hormone. The patient's medical history may therefore be just as important as the physical and laboratory findings in the differentiation.

Hypercalcemia complicating malignancy usually results from one of two basic processes (Table 54-1): (1) osteolytic metastases, more commonly seen in solid tumors such as carcinoma of the breast, kidney, lung, or thyroid, or hematologic malignant conditions with skeletal infiltration such as multiple myeloma;[26] or (2) pseudohyperparathyroidism, defined by Lafferty[24] as a syndrome in which osteolytic metastases are absent, but a humoral agent that causes hypercalcemia is elaborated by tumors of nonparathyroid tissue. Lafferty[24] emphasized that pseudohyperparathyroidism is usually manifested by a rapid, fulminant course with severe symptoms and relatively severe hypercalcemia, often greater than 14 mg/100 ml, that may be distinguished from hypercalcemia resulting from primary hyperparathyroidism or other causes (Table 54-2). In some patients pseudohyperparathyroidism seems due to ectopic production of parathyroid hormone or, perhaps in the majority, to excessive production of humoral substances chemically distinct from parathyroid hormone. Evidence has pointed to prostaglandins as potential mediating agents in some cases of pseudohyperparathyroidism.[27]

Careful skeletal survey including bone scan may be especially helpful in detecting evidence of osteolytic metastases. The entity of pseudohyperparathyroidism remains especially confusing diagnostically in view of conflicting reports concerning the frequency of elevation of parathyroid hormone, prostaglandins, and/or other humoral agents in the syndrome (Chapter 55, Chapter 139). It is hoped that further investigations will clarify the frequency of participation of different humoral agents in the pathophysiology of pseudohyperparathyroidism and improve the specificity of assay techniques for detection of the humoral agents responsible. At present, it is clear that clinical criteria (especially signs of the primary nonparathyroid tumor and the acuteness versus chronicity of the hypercalcemia) rather than specific laboratory tests must be emphasized in the diagnosis (Table 54-2). Alternatively, the particular experience of individual laboratory groups with their assays must be taken into account in interpretation. For example, Arnaud and colleagues (Chapter 55) find a clue to the diagnosis of pseudohyperparathyroidism in their observation that parathyroid hormone values for a given severity of hypercalcemia are lower in patients with cancer than in patients with true primary hyperparathyroidism. In our laboratories, by contrast, virtually all patients with pseudohyperparathyroidism have not had detectable levels of parathyroid hormone, and we find this helpful in the differential diagnosis.

SARCOIDOSIS, TUBERCULOSIS, BERYLLIOSIS, AND OTHER GRANULOMATOUS DISEASES

Abnormalities in calcium metabolism including hypercalcemia, hypophosphatemia, hyperphosphatasia, and hypercalciuria are relatively frequent accompaniments of sarcoidosis[28] and may

Table 54-2. Clinical and Laboratory Criteria Useful in Differential Diagnosis of Primary Hyperparathyroidism versus Pseudohyperparathyroidism

	Pseudohyperparathyroidism	Primary Hyperparathyroidism
Clinical course	Rapid	Gradual
Symptoms	Often severe	Usually mild
Serum calcium	Typically > 14 mg/100 ml	Typically < 14 mg/100 ml
Serum chloride	Typically < 102 mEq/l	Typically > 102 mEq/l
Anemia	Often	Infrequent

mimic those of primary hyperparathyroidism. Goldstein et al.[29] surveyed the reported incidence of hypercalcemia in sarcoidosis. The frequency of hypercalcemia varied quite widely, with estimates ranging from 0.7 to 63 percent, with most series between 10 and 20 percent. The frequency of hypercalcemia was highest in those studies that included many patients examined before corticosteroid therapy was widely used. It seems probable, therefore, that frequent use of corticosteroids, known to lower serum calcium in sarcoidosis,[30] has greatly lowered the incidence of hypercalcemia. Difficulty in establishing a diagnosis in sarcoidosis may result when other manifestations of sarcoidosis such as hepatomegaly, lymphadenopathy, skin lesions, hyperglobulinemia, and respiratory symptoms are minimal or absent. There are several reports of patients with ultimately proved sarcoidosis who underwent neck explorations because of erroneously suspected primary hyperparathyroidism.[20,21,31,32] The situation is further complicated by the occasional occurrence of both sarcoidosis and primary hyperparathyroidism in the same patient.[20,21,33] It was also emphasized that, in analogy with sarcoidosis, other types of chronic granulomatous diseases such as tuberculosis[34] or berylliosis[35] can cause hypercalcemia. Most of the clinical and laboratory data useful in the differential diagnosis of the hypercalcemia of granulomatous disease is based on experience with sarcoidosis rather than with the rarely reported berylliosis or tuberculosis; it is assumed that pathogenesis and general clinical features are similar, however, in all the granulomatous diseases associated with hypercalcemia.

Usually hypercalcemia in sarcoidosis is mild, but levels may occasionally be as high as 18 to 20 mg/100 ml.[36,37] The levels of serum inorganic phosphorus in patients with sarcoidosis, although typically normal, may occasionally be low. In fact, one report suggested that hypophosphatemia may be more common than hypercalcemia in sarcoidosis.[38] Serum alkaline phosphatase levels are frequently elevated, the result of hepatic rather than bone involvement by sarcoid granulomata. The excretion of urinary calcium is more often elevated; hypercalciuria has been reported in from 29 to 36 percent of patients with sarcoidosis.[39,40] Prolonged hypercalcemia and hypercalciuria in sarcoidosis can lead to urolithiasis, nephrocalcinosis, and occasionally to renal failure.

The abnormal calcium metabolism in sarcoidosis is generally regarded as due to an enhanced sensitivity to vitamin D.[41] Patients with sarcoidosis are unusually sensitive to vitamin D either administered exogenously in small doses,[42,43] or formed endogenously by exposure to ultraviolet light.[44] Several lines of evidence indicate that the increased sensitivity to vitamin D in sarcoidosis results in excessive bone resorption as well as increased intestinal absorption of calcium. Metabolic balance studies carried out in patients with sarcoidosis have indicated that hypercalcemia and hypercalciuria can persist in the absence of increased intestinal calcium absorption;[45] hypercalciuria was observed in patients with normal serum and fecal calcium values.[46] Henneman et al.[47] found that the levels of urinary calcium occasionally exceeded calcium intake during carefully performed balance studies.

Thus, it appears that the hypercalcemia and/or hypercalciuria of sarcoidosis is a result of an unusual sensitivity of both bone and intestine to the actions of vitamin D. The metabolic basis of the enhanced sensitivity to vitamin D is unknown. One might speculate, however, that one or more defects may exist in the metabolism of vitamin D to its active hydroxylated metabolites (increased conversion of vitamin D to 1,25-dihydroxycholecalciferol or decreased destruction of 1,25-dihydroxycholecalciferol) or, alternatively, that receptor sites in bone and intestine are unusually responsive to the dihydroxy vitamin.

In those patients in whom the clinical signs and symptoms are not sufficient to distinguish between the diagnosis of primary hyperparathyroidism and sarcoidosis, one or more of several laboratory tests will help to establish the correct diagnosis. An elevated or even a detectable level of serum immunoreactive parathyroid hormone strongly suggests the diagnosis of hyperparathyroidism. In one study of 26 patients with sarcoidosis, serum immunoreactive parathyroid hormone was undetectable or low in 19 and normal in 7 (5 of the latter had been treated with corticosteroids, presumably correcting the vitamin D hypersensitivity at the time of the study).[50] These data include that most patients with sarcoidosis have functional hypoparathyroidism even in the absence of frank hypercalcemia; the increased intestinal absorption of calcium presumably leads to a suppression of parathyroid hormone secretion.

As discussed previously, the cortisone-suppression test is useful in distinguishing between hypercalcemia of sarcoidosis and of hyperparathyroidism.[30] The hypercalcemia of hyperparathyroidism is usually unaffected, whereas that due to sarcoidosis (as well as that due to vitamin D excess) is corrected. Only rarely will the hypercalcemia of hyperparathyroidism respond to corticosteroids. Although some workers have felt that the ameliorative effects of corticosteroids are due to a direct action on sarcoid granulomas in bone,[48] most have interpreted the hypocalcemic effects of glucocorticoids in sarcoidosis as due to an antagonism of vitamin D action. No correlation has been found between hypercalcemia and granulomatous involvement of the skeleton; many patients with demonstrable bone disease do not have hypercalcemia.[49]

A careful examination of the chest roentgenograms may help to establish the diagnosis of hypercalcemic sarcoidosis. Although hilar adenopathy is the classic finding,[51] it has become evident that a diffuse fibroreticular infiltrate in the peripheral lung fields may be present in the absence of detectable hilar adenopathy.[51] Evaluation of pulmonary function also may prove helpful when the roentgenographic changes are equivocal; a low carbon monoxide diffusion and hypoxemia on exercise may be found.

In addition to the special tests of parathyroid hormone assay and cortisone suppression test, other laboratory determinations may be useful in differentiating these two diseases. Although hypophosphatemia may occur, an elevated or normal fasting serum phosphorus level is more consistent with sarcoidosis than with hyperparathyroidism. The finding of a mild hyperchloremia (plasma chloride above 102 mEq/liter) is more consistent with hyperparathyroidism than with sarcoidosis. An elevated sedimentation rate and/or hypergammaglobulinemia is not found in uncomplicated hyperparathyroidism. A definitive procedure, whenever possible, is the establishment of a histologic diagnosis by biopsy of liver or lymph node; a positive Kveim test is also of value.[51]

THYROTOXICOSIS

Severe and symptomatic hypercalcemia is a rare complication of thyrotoxicosis. However, minimal elevations of serum calcium have been reported in as many as 23 percent of patients with hyperthyroidism.[52,53] The cause of hypercalcemia in hyperthyroidism appears to be secondary to increased bone resorption, probably due to direct effects of thyroxine and triiodothyronine on the skeleton.[54-59]

The turnover of calcium by the skeleton is increased by thyroid hormone.[56] Adams and Jowsey[58] found that the serum calcium in 10 hyperthyroid patients averaged 0.5 mg/100 ml higher than it did in a group of matched normal control subjects. The serum protein concentrations in these patients tended to be lower than normal, indicating that the serum ionized calcium was significantly elevated. Serum inorganic-phosphorus levels were high, and urinary clearance decreased, suggesting that parathyroid hormone secretion was suppressed. Castro et al.[60] reported finding low serum parathyroid hormone levels in patients with hyperthyroidism and marked hypercalcemia. Suppression of parathyroid hormone secretion in these patients decreases tubular reabsorption of calcium and leads to hypercalciuria, a finding not infrequently seen in patients with thyrotoxicosis.

Patients with thyrotoxicosis are more sensitive than normal persons to the hypercalcemic effects of parathyroid hormone.[61,62] Epstein[64] emphasized that patients with thyrotoxicosis who develop severe hypercalcemia may have concomitant hyperparathyroidism, inasmuch as the hypercalcemia of uncomplicated thyrotoxicosis is usually mild. The thyrotoxic patient reported by Epstein et al.,[63] with a serum calcium of 15 mg/100 ml, later proved to have a parathyroid adenoma.[65] Breuer and McPherson[66] described 17 patients with thyrotoxicosis and concomitant parathyroid adenomas.

The diagnosis of hyperthyroidism usually offers no difficulties because, in most cases, it is the thyrotoxicosis rather than the hypercalcemia that brings the patient to the physician. However, particularly in the elderly, the signs of thyrotoxicosis may be minimal. During the treatment of a patient with thyrotoxicosis and hypercalcemia, repeated determinations of serum calcium should be made. If the serum calcium does not return toward normal as the thyrotoxicosis is brought under control, another cause for the hypercalcemia, such as hyperparathyroidism, should be suspected.

ADRENAL INSUFFICIENCY

Hypercalcemia can occasionally occur in adrenal insufficiency, most often in acute adrenal failure.[67-69] At least part of the hypercalcemia can be attributed to hemoconcentration and resultant hyperproteinemia. Walser et al.[69] produced adrenal insufficiency in dogs and found that the plasma ionized calcium was normal. They concluded that three alterations combined to produce hypercalcemia: (1) the elevated plasma protein concentration associated with hemoconcentration, (2) an increase in filtrable calcium complexes, especially calcium citrate, and (3) an increase in the affinity of plasma protein for calcium, explained as a consequence of hyponatremia and low ionic strength of plasma. Excessive amounts of a nonfiltrable complex of calcium and phosphate, formed either in vivo or in vitro were also found. The increased calcium concentration of the plasma is not dependent upon increased intestinal absorption of calcium, inasmuch as it occurs on a calcium-free diet.

Hypercalcemia in association with adrenal insufficiency is usually not severe, and blood calcium levels return to normal with adrenal-hormone replacement therapy.

VITAMIN D INTOXICATION

The chronic ingestion of large doses of vitamin D produces hypercalcemia by promoting both increased bone resorption and excessive gastrointestinal absorption of calcium.[70] Usually, ingestion of the large doses of vitamin D_2 and D_3 (in excess of 100,000 U) for several months is necessary for this complication to occur.

The vitamin D intoxication may occur as a complication of the treatment of patients with hypoparathyroidism and with intestinal malabsorption. It may also occur after the inadvertent or intentional ingestion of excessive amounts of the vitamin—a situation that usually can be determined by the history. In the absence of excessive intake, the suspected hypervitaminosis may be investi-

gated by specific competitive-binding assays that will reveal whether there are excessive amounts of vitamin D and its metabolites in the circulation.[71,72]

VITAMIN A INTOXICATION

Excessive ingestion of vitamin A should also be considered in the differential diagnosis of hypercalcemia, although the disorder is infrequently seen. Elevations in the serum calcium to 12 to 14 mg/100 ml with associated symptoms of fatigue and anorexia have been reported in patients who chronically have taken 10 to 20 times the recommended minimum daily requirement (5000 IU) in the mistaken belief that it will be of benefit to them.[73,74] In addition to symptoms attributable to the hypercalcemia, these patients frequently manifest myalgias and diffuse bone pain. Skeletal roentgenograms may be normal, but occasionally they may show multiple sites of distinct, smooth periosteal calcifications along the shafts of the phalanges and metacarpals;[75] it is this unusual roentgenographic appearance that is strongly suggestive of the diagnosis of hypervitaminosis A. The diagnosis may be confirmed by the finding of increased levels of vitamin A in the serum (often twice the upper limit of normal), as well as elicitation of a history of excessive ingestion of the vitamin.

Cessation of ingestion of the vitamin usually leads to prompt amelioration of the symptoms and to healing of the skeletal lesions. Occasionally, if hypercalcemia and other symptoms persist, administration of corticosteroids may prove helpful (doses equivalent to 100 to 200 mg of cortisone daily).

ADMINISTRATION OF THIAZIDE DIURETICS

Administration of diuretics of the benzothiadiazide class[76] to patients with high rates of bone turnover, including those with hyperparathyroidism,[19,77] juvenile osteoporosis,[77] or hypoparathyroidism treated with high doses of vitamin D,[78] results in the appearance de novo of hypercalcemia or aggravation of existing hypercalcemia. This effect appears to be unique to the benzothiadiazide (thiazide) diuretics such as chlorothiazide, hydrochlorothiazide, and chlorthalidone, and is not usually seen with other classes of diuretics such as furosemide, ethacrynic acid, or mercurial diuretics. Although thiazides have been reported to increase serum calcium concentration significantly in normal individuals, the degree of calcium elevation is small and transient.[79,80] Sustained hypercalcemia induced by thiazides implies that an underlying disorder of calcium metabolism exists. The controlled administration of thiazide diuretics has even been proposed as a provocative test for the diagnosis of subclinical primary hyperparathyroidism.[81]

Although a part of the hypercalcemic effects of thiazides can be accounted for by contraction of the extracellular fluid volume and hemoconcentration, sustained hypercalcemia probably arises from actions of the drug on both kidney and bone.[82,82a] The acute administration of thiazides increases urinary calcium excretion,[82] but chronic therapy results in a decrease in calcium in the urine.[78,79,83,84] The latter effect is the basis for the use of these diuretics to lower calcium excretion in idiopathic hypercalciuria.[85,86] The acute hypercalciuric and chronic hypocalciuric actions of thiazides on the kidney may be secondary to the effects of the diuretics on sodium excretion inasmuch as renal tubular resorption of the two cations appears to be coupled; hypercalciuria accompanies the acute natriuretic response, and the chronic effect of lowering of the urinary calcium excretion may reflect the enhancement of proximal tubular resorption of both sodium and calcium in response to sodium depletion.[13]

Two lines of evidence suggest a skeletal action of the drug. The first is that anephric patients maintained on hemodialysis also show a hypercalcemic response to hydrochlorthiazide administration in dosages of 200 mg/day for 2 to 4 weeks.[87] The second is that the hypercalcemic response (both ionized and total calcium) to short-term chlorothiazide infusion was observed in normal subjects and patients with hyperparathyroidism when urinary excretion of calcium (and sodium) was markedly increased.[82] The increased skeletal turnover and consequent hypercalcemia due to thiazides is complex in that it seems to require a synergism with endogenous parathyroid hormone or high doses of vitamin D. The serum calcium levels of hypoparathyroid patients did not rise during chlorothiazide infusion alone, but did when parathyroid extract was infused along with the chlorothiazide. On the other hand, a hypercalcemic response to thiazides administered chronically to patients with postoperative hypoparathyroidism is seen in patients treated with high dosages of vitamin D.[78]

A special point of diagnostic clinical importance should be emphasized. Given the frequency of use of thiazides in hypertensive subjects and the need to establish a correct diagnosis in such patients, if they are hypercalcemic, one can conclude that if patients taking thiazides have been hypercalcemic for at least several weeks since the thiazide therapy was started, they are not normal subjects with a drug reaction, but rather have primary hyperparathyroidism or some other underlying skeletal disorder. Treatment with thiazides should be stopped in these patients because it exaggerates the apparent degree of hypercalcemia, and it is the degree of hypercalcemia that is a factor in judging whether surgery is mandatory.

PROLONGED IMMOBILIZATION

Generalized immobilization of a patient may occasionally lead to hypercalcemia, particularly in patients with high rates of bone turnover, such as those with Paget's disease. Immobilization may also cause hypercalcemia in young patients at a stage of rapid growth and higher bone-turnover rates.[88] The hypercalcemia and associated hypercalciuria resolve when the patient becomes ambulatory.

CHRONIC RENAL FAILURE AND SECONDARY HYPERPARATHYROIDISM

Hypercalcemia may occur in renal disease as a complication of secondary hyperparathyroidism, particularly in subjects undergoing chronic hemodialysis or renal transplantation.[89,90] The pathophysiology and management of this disorder are discussed in Chapters 59, 60, and 61. It should also be kept in mind, however, that primary hyperparathyroidism and hypercalcemia may lead to chronic renal disease and that the hypercalcemia may persist even after renal function has been compromised.

MILK/ALKALI SYNDROME (BURNETT'S SYNDROME)

In this syndrome, hypercalcemia and renal failure occur as a complication of ingestion of large amounts of calcium in some form, usually milk or absorbable antacids.[91] The disorder is less prevalent now than formerly since, in the treatment of peptic ulcers, the nonabsorbable antacids have replaced soluble alkali such as sodium carbonate or bicarbonate or calcium carbonate.[92] The hypercalcemia commonly results in structural damage to the kidney and progressive impairment of renal function; hence, hypercalciuria may not be observed at the time of diagnosis.[93] Renal failure is often, but not invariably, present; it has been established that hypercalcemia precedes the onset of renal damage. The latter can result after only a short course of therapy with soluble alkali and calcium.[94] Calcium carbonate can elevate serum calcium within days in normal individuals, if taken in sufficient quantities. Although the diagnosis is suggested when hypercalcemia coexists with a history of ingestion of excessive absorbable calcium, it should be kept in mind, in view of the high incidence of ulcer disease in hyperparathyroidism,[95] that a "milk/alkali syndrome" may coexist with hyperparathyroidism.

IDIOPATHIC HYPERCALCEMIA OF INFANCY

This is a rare syndrome characterized by hypercalcemia, often in association with multiple congenital facial and cardiovascular lesions.[96-98] The cause of the hypercalcemia is unknown; hypersensitivity to vitamin D has been postulated.[98] The distinctive clinical features and age distribution of the syndrome make it an unlikely problem, however, in the differential diagnosis of most cases of hypercalcemia.

REFERENCES

1. Keating, F. R. Jr., Jones, J. D., Elveback, L. R., et al: The relation of age and sex to distribution of values in healthy adults of serum calcium, inorganic phosphorus, magnesium, alkaline phosphatase, total proteins, albumin, and blood urea. J Lab Clin Med 73: 825, 1969.
2. Krull, G. H., Muller, H., Leijnse, B., et al: Venous-compression test in hyperparathyroidism. Lancet 2: 174, 1969.
3. Yendt, E. R., Gagné, R. J. A.: Detection of primary hyperparathyroidism, with special reference to its occurence in hypercalciuric females with "normal" or borderline serum calcium. Can Med Assoc J 98: 331, 1968.
4. Wills, M. R., Pak, C. Y. C., Hammond, W. G., et al: Normocalcemic primary hyperparathyroidism. Am J Med 47: 384, 1969.
5. Wills, M. R.: Normocalcaemic primary hyperparathyroidism. Lancet 1: 849, 1971.
5a. Shieber, W., Birge, S. J., Avioli, L. V., et al: Normocalcemic hyperparathyroidism with "normal" parathyroid glands. Arch Surg 103: 299, 1971.
6. Hennemann, P. H., Benedict, P. H., Forbes, A. P., et al: Idiopathic hypercalcuria. N Engl J Med 259: 802–807, 1958.
7. Reiss, E., Canterbury, J. M.: The effects of phosphate on parathyroid hormone secretion. In Talmage R. V., Owen M., Parsons J. A. (eds): Calcium-Regulating Hormones, Proceedings of the Fifth Parathyroid Conference. Amsterdam, Excerpta Medica, 1975, p 66.
8. Eisenberg, E.: Effect of serum calcium level and parathyroid extracts on phosphate and calcium excretion in hypoparathyroid patients. J Clin Invest 44: 942, 1965.
9. Schussler, G. C., Verso, M. A., Nemoto, T.: Phosphaturia in hypercalcemic breast cancer patients. J Clin Endocrinol Metab 35: 497, 1972.
10. Nordin, B. E. C., Peacock, M.: Role of kidney in regulation of plasma-calcium. Lancet 2: 1280, 1969.
11. Dent, C. E., Harper, C. M.: Plasma-alkaline-phosphatase in normal adults and in patients with primary hyperparathyroidism. Lancet 1: 559, 1962.
12. Kivirikko, K. I.: Urinary excretion of hydroxyproline in health and disease. Int Rev Connect Tissue Res 5: 93, 1970.
13. Epstein, F. H.: Calcium and the kidney. Am J Med 45: 700, 1968.
14. Broadus, A. E., Mahaffey, J. E., Neer, R. M., et al: Nephrogenous cyclic AMP as a parathyroid function test. J Clin Invest 60: 771, 1977.
15. Strott C. A., Nugent, C. A.: Laboratory tests in the diagnosis of hyperparathyroidism in hypercalcemic patients. Ann Intern Med 68: 188, 1968.
16. Kyle, L. H., Canary, J. J., Mintz, D. H., et al: Inhibitory effects of induced hypercalcemia on secretion of parathyroid hormone. J Clin Endocrinol Metab 22: 52, 1962.

17. Murray, T. M., Peacock, M., Powell, D., *et al:* Non-autonomy of hormone secretion in primary hyperparathyroidism. *Clin Endocrinol 1:* 235, 1972.

18. Goldsmith, R. S.: Hyperparathyroidism. *N Engl J Med 281:* 367, 1969.

19. Duarte, C. G., Winnacker, J. L., Becker, K. L., *et al:* Thiazide-induced hypercalcemia. *N Engl J Med 284:* 828, 1971.

20. Dent, C. E.: Some problems of hyperparathyroidism. *Br Med J 2:* 1419, 1495, 1962.

21. Dent, C. E., Watson, L.: Hyperparathyroidism and sarcoidosis. *Br Med J 1:* 646, 1966.

22. Goldsmith, R. S.: Differential diagnosis of hypercalcemia. *N Engl J Med 274:* 674, 1966.

23. Boonstra, C. E., Jackson, C. E.: Hyperparathyroidism detected by routine serum calcium analysis: Prevalence in a clinic population. *Ann Intern Med 63:* 468, 1965.

24. Lafferty, F. W.: Pseudohyperparathyroidism. *Medicine 45:* 247, 1966.

25. Fraser, P., Healy, M., Rose, N., *et al:* Discriminant functions in differential diagnosis of hypercalcaemia. *Lancet 1:* 1314, 1971.

26. Omenn, G. S., Roth, S. I., Baker, W. H. Jr.: Hyperparathyroidism associated with malignant tumors of nonparathyroid origin. *Cancer 24:* 1004, 1969.

27. Seyberth, H. W., Segre, G. V., Hamet, P., *et al:* Characterization of the group of patients with hypercalcemia of cancer who respond to treatment with prostaglandin synthesis inhibitors. *Trans Assoc Am Physicians 89:* 92, 1976.

28. Winnacker, J. L., Becker, K. L., Katz, S.: Endocrine aspects of sarcoidosis. *N Engl J Med 278:* 427, 483, 1968.

29. Goldstein, R. A., Israel, H. L., Becker, K. L., *et al:* The infrequency of hypercalcemia in sarcoidosis. *Am J Med 51:* 21, 1971.

30. Dent, C. E.: Cortisone test for hyperparathyroidism. *Br Med J 1:* 230, 1956.

31. Klatskin, G., Gordon, M.: Renal complications of sarcoidosis and their relationship to hypercalcemia: With a report of two cases simulating hyperparathyroidism. *Am J Med 15:* 484, 1953.

32. Solomon, R. B., Channick, B. J.: Boeck's sarcoidosis simulating hyperparathyroidism. *Ann Intern Med 53:* 1232, 1960.

33. Burr, J. M., Farrell, J. J., Hills, A. G.: Sarcoidosis and hyperparathyroidism with hypercalcemia: Special usefulness of cortisone test. *N Engl J Med 261:* 1271, 1959.

34. Shai, F., Baker, R. K., Addrizzo, J. R., *et al:* Hypercalcemia in mycobacterial infection. *J Clin Endocrinol Metab 34:* 251, 1972.

35. Tepper, L. B., Hardy, H. L., Chamberlain, R. I.: Toxicity of Beryllium Compounds. Browning E. (ed). Amsterdam, Elsevier, 1961, p 63.

36. Citron, K. M.: Sarcoidosis, hypercalcemia, calcinosis and renal impairment. *Proc R Soc Med 47:* 507, 1954.

37. Ellis, M., Wilson, S.: Sarcoidosis and hypercalcemia: Case report and discussion. *J Tenn Med Assoc 51:* 283, 1958.

38. Putkonen, T., Hannuksela, M., Halme, H.: Calcium and phosphorus metabolism in sarcoidosis. *Acta Med Scand 177:* 327, 1965.

39. Basset, G.: Les désordres humoraux dans la sarcoïdose. *Bull Mem Soc Med Hôp Paris 115:* 583, 1964.

40. James, D. G.: The diagnosis and treatment of ocular sarcoidosis. *Acta Med Scand (176)* Suppl *425:* 203, 1964.

41. Bell, N. H., Gill, J. R. Jr., Bartter, F. C.: On the abnormal calcium absorption in sarcoidosis: Evidence for increased sensitivity to vitamin D. *Am J Med 36:* 500, 1964.

42. Nelson, C. T.: Calciferol in the treatment of sarcoidosis. *J Invest Dermatol 13:* 81, 1949.

43. Larsson, L. G., Liljestrand, A., Wahlund, H.: Treatment of sarcoidosis with calciferol. *Acta Med Scand 143:* 280, 1952.

44. Taylor, R. L., Lynch, H. J. Jr., Wysor, W. G. Jr.: Seasonal influence of sunlight on the hypercalcemia of sarcoidosis. *Am J Med 34:* 221, 1963.

45. Hunt, B. J., Yendt, E. R.: The response of hypercalcemia in sarcoidosis to chloroquine. *Ann Intern Med 59:* 554, 1963.

46. Hendrix, J. Z.: Abnormal skeletal mineral metabolism in sarcoidosis. *Ann Intern Med 64:* 797, 1966.

47. Henneman, P. H., Dempsey, E. F., Carroll, E. L., *et al:* The cause of hypercalcuria in sarcoid and its treatment with cortisone and sodium phytate. *J Clin Invest 35:* 1229, 1956.

48. Anderson, J., Dent, C. E., Harper, C., *et al.* Effect of cortisone on calcium metabolism in sarcoidosis with hypercalcemia: Possibly antagonistic actions of cortisone and vitamin D. *Lancet 2:* 720, 1954.

49. Mather, G.: Calcium metabolism and bone changes in sarcoidosis. *Br Med J 1:* 248, 1957.

50. Cushard, W. G. Jr., Simon, A. B., Canterbury, J. M., *et al:* Parathyroid function in sarcoidosis. *N Engl J Med 286:* 395, 1972.

51. Siltzbach, L. E., James, D. G., Neville, E., *et al:* Course and prognosis of sarcoidosis around the world. *Am J Med 57:* 847, 1974.

52. Rose, E., Boles, R. S. Jr.: Hypercalcemia in thyrotoxicosis. *Med Clin North Am 37:* 1715, 1953.

53. Bryant, L. R., Wulsin, J. H., Altemeier, W. A.: Hyperparathyroidism and hyperthyroidism. *Ann Surg 159:* 411, 1964.

54. Aub, J. C., Bauer, W., Heath, C., et al: Studies of calcium and phosphorus metabolism. III. Effects of thyroid hormone and thyroid disease. *J Clin Invest 7:* 97, 1929.

55. Laake, H.: Osteoporosis in association with thyrotoxicosis. *Acta Med Scand 151:* 229, 1955.

56. Krane, S. M., Brownell, G. L., Stanbury, J. B., *et al:* The effect of thyroid disease on calcium metabolism in man. *J Clin Invest 35:* 874, 1956.

57. Adams, P. H., Jowsey, J., Kelly, P. J., *et al:* Effects of hyperthyroidism on bone and mineral metabolism in man. *Q J Med 36:* 1, 1967.

58. Adams, P. [H.], Jowsey, J.: Bone and mineral metabolism in hyperthyroidism: An experimental study. *Endocrinology 81:* 735, 1967.

59. Krane, S. M., Goldring, S. R.: Hyperthyroidism: skeletal system; hypothyroidism: skeletal system. In Werner S. C., Ingbar S. H. (eds): The Thyroid. New York, Harper & Row, 1976.

60. Castro, J. H., Genuth, S. M., Klein, L.: Comparative response to parathyroid hormone in hyperthyroidism and hypothyroidism. *Metabolism 24:* 839, 1975.

61. Harrison, M. T., Harden, R. McG., Alexander, W. D.: Some effects of parathyroid hormone in thyrotoxicosis. *J Clin Endocrinol 24:* 214, 1964.

62. Bouillon, R., DeMoor, P.: Parathyroid function in patients with hyper- or hypothyroidism. *J Clin Endocrinol Metab 38:* 999, 1974.

63. Epstein, F. H., Freedman, L. R., Levitin, H.: Hypercalcemia, nephrocalcinosis and reversible renal insufficiency associated with hyperthyroidism. *N Engl J Med 258:* 782, 1958.

64. Epstein, F. H.: Bone and mineral metabolism in hyperthyroidism. *Ann Intern Med 68:* 490, 1968.

65. Baxter, J. D., Bondy, P. K.: Hypercalcemia of thyrotoxicosis. *Ann Intern Med 65:* 429, 1966.

66. Breuer, R. I., McPherson, H. T.: Hypercalcemia in concurrent hyperthyroidism and hyperparathyroidism. *Arch Intern Med 118:* 310, 1966.

67. Loeb, R. F.: Chemical changes in the blood in Addison's disease. *Science 76:* 420, 1932.

68. Leeksma, C. H. W., DeGraeff, J., DeCock, J.: Hypercalcemia in adrenal insufficiency. *Acta Med Scand 156:* 455, 1957.

69. Walser, M., Robinson, B. H. B., Duckett, J. W. Jr.: The hypercalcemia of adrenal insufficiency. *J Clin Invest 42:* 456, 1963.

70. Kodicek E.: The absorption of calcium from the intestine. *Proc Nutr Soc 26:* 67, 1967.

71. Belsey, R., DeLuca, H. F., Potts, J. T. Jr.: Competitive binding assay for vitamin D and 25-OH vitamin D. *J Clin Endocrinol Metab 33:* 554, 1971.

72. Haddad, J. G., Chyu, K. J.: Competitive protein-binding radioassay for 25-hydroxycholecalciferol. *J Clin Endocrinol Metab 33:* 992, 1971.

73. Katz, C. M., Tzagouronis, M.: Chronic adult hypervitaminosis A with hypercalcemia. *Metabolism 21:* 1171, 1972.

74. Frame, B., Jackson, C. E., Reynolds, W. A., *et al:* Hypercalcemia and skeletal effects in chronic hypervitaminosis A. *Ann Intern Med 80:* 44, 1974.

75. Caffey, J.: Chronic poisoning due to excess of vitamin A: Description of clinical and roentgen manifestations in 7 infants and young children. *Am J Roentgenol Radium Ther Nucl Med 65:* 12, 1951.

76. Goodman, L. S., Gilman, A.: The Pharmacological Basis of Therapeutics (ed 4). New York, Macmillan, 1970.

77. Parfitt, A. M.: Chlorothiazide-induced hypercalcemia in juvenile osteoporosis and hyperparathyroidism. *N Engl J Med 281:* 55, 1969.

78. Parfitt, A. M.: The interactions of thiazide diuretics with parathyroid hormone and vitamin D: Studies in patients with hypoparathyroidism. *J Clin Invest 51:* 1879, 1972.

79. Seitz, H., Jaworski, Z. F.: Effect of hydrochlorothiazide on serum and urinary calcium and urinary citrate. *Can Med Assoc J 90:* 414, 1964.

80. Stote, R. M., Smith, L. H., Wilson, D. M., et al: Hydrochlorothiazide effects on serum calcium and immunoreactive parathyroid hormone concentrations: Studies in normal subjects. *Ann Intern Med 77:* 587, 1972.

81. van der Sluys, V. J., Birkenhäger, J. C., Smeenk, D.: De invloed van oraal toegediende diuretica op de calcium- en fosfaatstofwisseling. *Ned Tijdschr Geneeskd 109:* 1795, 1965.

82. Popovtzer, M. M., Subryan, V. L., Alfrey, A. C., *et al:* The acute effect of chlorothiazide on serum-ionized calcium: Evidence for a parathyroid hormone-dependent mechanism. *J Clin Invest 55:* 1295, 1975.

82a. Brickman, A. S., Massry, S. G., Coburn, J. W.: Changes in serum and urinary calcium during treatment with hydrochlorothiazide: Studies on mechanisms. *J Clin Invest 51:* 945, 1972.

83. Lamberg, B-A., Kuhlback, B.: Effect of chlorothiazide and hydrochlorothiazide on the excretion of calcium in the urine. *Scand J Clin Lab Invest 11:* 351, 1959.

84. Duarte, C. G., Bland, J. H.: Changes in metabolism of calcium, phosphorus and uric acid after oral administration of chlorothiazide. *Metabolism 14:* 899, 1965.

85. Nassim, J. R., Higgins, B. A.: Control of idiopathic hypercalciuria. *Br Med J 1:* 675, 1965.

86. Yendt, E. R., Gagné, R. J. A., Cohanim, M.: The effects of thiazides in idiopathic hypercalciuria. *Am J Med Sci 251:* 449, 1966.

87. Koppel, M. H., Massry, S. G., Shinaberger, J. H., et al: Thiazide-induced rise in serum calcium and magnesium in patients on maintenance hemodialysis. *Ann Intern Med 72:* 895, 1970.

88. Winters, J. L., Kleinschmidt, A. G. Jr., Frensilli, J. J., *et al:* Hypercalcemia complicating immobilization in the treatment of fractures: A case report. *J Bone Joint Surg 48-A:* 1182, 1966.

89. Freeman, R. M., Lawton, R. L., Chamberlain, M. A.: Hard-water syndrome. *N Engl J Med 276:* 1113, 1967.

90. Segal, A. J., Miller, M., Moses, A. M.: Hypercalcemia during the diuretic phase of acute renal failure. *Ann Intern Med 68:* 1066, 1968.

91. Burnett, C. H., Commons, R. R., Albright, F., *et al:* Hypercalcemia without hypercalcuria or hypophosphatemia, calcinosis and renal insufficiency: A syndrome following prolonged intake of milk and alkali. *N Engl J Med 240:* 787, 1949.

92. Lotz, M., Ney, R., Bartter, F. C.: Osteomalacia and debility resulting from phosphorus depletion. *Trans Assoc Am Physicians 77:* 281, 1964.

93. McMillan, D. E., Freeman, R. B.: The milk alkali syndrome: A study of the acute disorder with comments on the development of chronic condition. *Medicine 44:* 485, 1965.

94. Ivanovich, P., Fellows, H., Rich, C.: The absorption of calcium carbonate. *Ann Intern Med 66:* 917, 1967.

95. Kyle, L. H.: Differentiation of hyperparathyroidism and milk-alkali (Burnett) syndrome. *N Engl J Med 251:* 1035, 1954.

96. Garcia, R. E., Friedman, W. F., Kaback, M. M., *et al:* Idiopathic hypercalcemia and supravalvular aortic stenosis: Documentation of a new syndrome. New Engl J Med 271: 117, 1964.

97. Coleman, E. N.: Infantile hypercalcemia and cardiovascular lesions: Evidence, hypothesis, and speculation. *Arch Dis Child 40:* 535, 1965.

98. Wiltse, H. E., Goldbloom, R. B., Antia, A. U., *et al:* Infantile hypercalcemia syndrome in twins. *N Engl J Med 275:* 1157, 1966.

55

Parathyroid Hormone Assay: General Features

Claude D. Arnaud
Francis P. Di Bella

The first radioimmunoassay of parathyroid hormone (PTH) was described by Berson and co-workers in 1963.[1] Although this paper and several others[2-4] showed that the procedure could be applied to the measurement of PTH in peripheral human serum, it is only recently that it has received widespread attention as a diagnostic tool in the evaluation of the hypercalcemic patients.

The authors' experience using a sensitive radioimmunoassay of serum PTH[4] that is specific for the carboxyl-terminal region of the PTH molecule in the diagnosis of primary hyperparathyroidism is illustrated in Fig. 55-1. Ninety percent of the patients with surgically proved disease had values of serum immunoreactive PTH (iPTH) that exceeded the upper limit of normal, and 10 percent had values that were inappropriately high for the total calcium concentration in the same serum sample. Not shown are serum iPTH values in patients with nonparathyroid hypercalcemia (i.e., sarcoid, vitamin D intoxication). These are low or undetectable except in ectopic hyperparathyroidism due to nonparathyroid cancer (see below).

Results similar to those shown in Fig. 55-1 are not obtained with all radioimmunoassays of PTH (see below). Differences are primarily in the abilities of individual assays to measure low concentrations of serum iPTH and to distinguish between sera from normal subjects and patients with primary hyperparathyroidism.[5]

Although difficult to document, the general availability of radioimmunoassays which give results similar to those shown in Fig. 55-1 has probably caused an evolutionary change in the approach to the laboratory investigation of patients with hypercalcemia. Whereas previously, hypercalcemic patients were first extensively investigated for the presence of nonparathyroid disorders which could cause hypercalcemia,[6] the trend now is to use serum iPTH and calcium measurements to positively assign patients to either a group which is very likely to have a surgically resectable parathyroid lesion(s) or a group which requires further diagnostic evaluation for the cause of hypercalcemia. Caution must be exerted using such an approach, especially in patients with borderline increases in serum iPTH. These patients may have ectopic hyperparathyroidism due to nonparathyroid cancer, and the correct diagnosis may depend on an extensive search for malignancy as well as long-term follow-up with medical treatment of hypercalcemia.

This new laboratory approach to diagnosis should not be construed as a substitute for careful clinical evaluation of patients with hypercalcemia (Chapter 54). Particularly important in this regard are history, physical examination, and laboratory "signposts" which suggest the presence of familial disease or nonparathyroid hypercalcemia (Chapters 53 and 54). These cautionary notes notwithstanding, the practical advantages of using the PTH assay in combination with the serum total calcium as principal and definitive diagnostic probes are clear. Patients can be evaluated on an outpatient basis because only fasting serum is required, thereby frequently eliminating the costs of hospitalization and the multiple indirect testing required for a diagnosis of primary hyperparathyroidism by exclusion.[6]

INFLUENCE OF ASSAY SPECIFICITY ON CLINICAL UTILITY

Ideally, radioimmunoassay of serum PTH would consistently separate all patients with primary hyperparathyroidism from normal subjects. This is more than can be expected from any diagnostic test, and the PTH assay is no exception. In fact, there has been enormous variability of individual assays in producing results which approach this ideal degree of differentiation. Current knowledge suggests that this problem is due to the complexities involved in the reactions of multivalent antisera (used in different radioimmunoassays) with the multiple forms of circulating PTH[7-12] (Chapter 45).

Most antisera used in PTH assays contain multiple populations of antibodies directed at different regions of the PTH molecule. However, because they are used in the greatest possible dilution, the antibody population that is present in highest concentration and has the highest affinity for the PTH molecule is predominantly operative in the resulting assay. Theoretical exceptions to this include antisera that contain antibody populations in equivalent concentrations and have similar affinities for different regions of the PTH molecule, or antibody populations that are present in high concentrations and are directed against a specific conformational property of PTH.[13] Assays developed with such antisera might be expected to react with more than one region of the PTH molecule.

If circulating PTH comprised only the intact molecule, these immunologic considerations might be academic. However, there is good evidence that circulating PTH, at least in hyperparathyroid patients, is a complex mixture of intact hormone and fragments of the hormone (Chapter 45). The quantity of carboxyl-terminal frag-

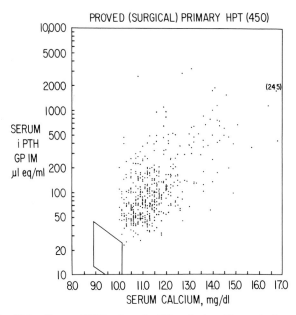

Fig. 55-1. Serum iPTH values in 450 patients with surgically proved primary hyperparathyroidism as a function of serum calcium concentration. Serum iPTH was measured with a radioimmunoassay using GP1M antiserum.[2] The area enclosed by the solid lines represents the normal range ± 2SD for serum iPTH and serum calcium. Note that there is a 10 percent overlap of serum iPTH with the normal range but that greater than 95 percent of normal sera and all hyperparathyroid sera have measurable iPTH. Formal discriminative analysis of serum iPTH and serum calcium separates 100 percent of hyperparathyroid patients from normal subjects. (From Arnaud, et al: Excerpta Medical International Congress Series No. 270, 1973, p. 281)

ments far exceeds intact hormone; amino-terminal fragments, if they exist, represent a small fraction of total serum iPTH.[11–14]

Carboxyl-terminal fragments of PTH cannot be measured with assays using predominantly amino-terminal-specific antisera. The latter assays can be used to detect only intact PTH and any amino-terminal fragments present in blood; there is general agreement[5] that such assays measure only 10–20 percent of the total quantity of iPTH in the serum. In contrast, assays using carboxyl-terminal-specific antisera measure both intact PTH and carboxyl-terminal fragments but cannot detect amino-terminal fragments. The latter assays measure more than 90 percent of the iPTH in serum. Therefore, amino-terminal-specific assays give values for serum iPTH which are 5–10 times lower than carboxyl-terminal-specific assays.[11–14]

We and others[12–15] have found that carboxyl-terminal-specific assays are far superior to amino-terminal-specific assays in distinguishing normal subjects from patients with primary and secondary (renal failure) hyperparathyroidism. This empiric observation seems paradoxical because it would be expected that assays measuring the amino-terminal, biologically active region of the hormone molecule would reflect the state of hyperparathyroidism better than those measuring the carboxyl-terminal, biologically inactive region. At the present time, there is no direct explanation of this paradox, but there are several recently discovered phenomena which may ultimately prove to be important in understanding it. The first relates to the relatively longer survival times of carboxyl-terminal fragments in the circulation (hours) than the intact hormone (minutes)[10,12,16] (Chapter 45). It is possible that measurements of peripheral serum carboxyl-terminal fragments of iPTH may better reflect the integrated secretory rate of PTH over a period of hours than do measurements of the rapidly metabolized

intact molecule. The second explanation relates to the recent reports[12,17] that carboxyl-terminal fragments of PTH are released into the circulation in relatively large quantities; we find that parathyroid tumor venous effluent contains 70 percent intact PTH and 30 percent carboxyl-terminal and amino-terminal fragments of PTH. Similar measurements in the venous effluent of normal parathyroid glands have not been made. However, if normal glands released smaller quantities of carboxyl-terminal fragments relative to intact hormone than did parathyroid tumors, carboxyl-terminal fragments in the peripheral circulation might represent a form of "tumor marker" which could only be detected by carboxyl-terminal-specific PTH assays.

PRACTICAL APPLICATION OF A CARBOXYL-TERMINAL-"SPECIFIC" RADIOIMMUNOASSAY OF PTH IN DIFFERENTIAL DIAGNOSIS OF PRIMARY HYPERPARATHYROIDISM

Almost all of the radioimmunoassays of PTH in human serum use (1) antisera directed against bovine or porcine PTH; (2) bovine PTH as a radiolabeled ligand (^{131}I or ^{125}I); and (3) human hyperparathyroid serum as a standard. Although desirable,[13] few laboratories have used human PTH as an immunogen for the production of species-specific antisera because of the unavailability of sufficient quantities of human PTH. Hyperparathyroid serum is used as standard in assays because it provides the most nearly uniform mixture of circulating species of PTH available and, in most instances, produces immunodilution curves which are similar to those produced by sera from patients with all forms of hyperparathyroidism.[4] Clear exceptions to this exist[18] (unpublished observations).

Unfortunately, fragments of the human PTH molecule are necessary to definitively characterize individual antisera with regard to their amino-terminal or carboxyl-terminal specificity (Chapter 45). These are not currently available. In practice, an assay which fails to recognize synthetic bovine PTH 1–34* and easily quantitates subnanogram quantities of intact human PTH (standard calibrated against highly purified human PTH) is worth empiric evaluation by studying its use in the measurement of iPTH in human serum.

The features of an assay which may provide near-ideal clinical utility in measuring steady-state concentrations of serum iPTH include:

1. Consistently low or undetectable values in all patients with surgical or idiopathic hypoparathyroidism.
2. The ability to measure iPTH in greater than 95 percent of normal sera and to demonstrate a negative relationship between serum iPTH and total serum calcium over the normal range for the total serum calcium.
3. Low or undetectable values in all patients with hypercalcemia associated with nonparathyroid disorders except cancer (see below).
4. The ability to measure values greater than the upper limit of normal in 90 percent of patients with surgically proved hyperparathyroidism.

From a technical point of view, scrupulous attention should be paid to quality control of assays when they are employed in

*Synthetic bovine PTH 1–34 based on the sequence proposed by Niall and co-workers (residue No. 22 being glutamic acid) originally synthesized by that group (see Chapter 42 for details) has been made commercially available by Beckman Bioproducts (Palo Alto, Calif.).

patient evaluations. Aside from usual careful statistical observations of intra- and interassay variations of standards (low and high serum controls), the authors' laboratory requires the following control measures to be performed in all assays:[4]

1. Values of "antibody-bound" radiolabeled PTH are corrected for "nonspecific binding" ("damaged hormone") generated by each unknown serum.
2. "Nonspecific" inhibition of the reaction between antibody and radiolabeled PTH by hypoparathyroid serum added to incubation mixtures in varying dilutions is determined. Hormone "values" in unknown sera are not considered valid unless the inhibition of the immune reaction is significantly greater than that produced by equivalent dilutions of hypoparathyroid serum.
3. Unknown sera are routinely studied in multiple dilutions. To be valid, at least two of the values for percent bound of B/F must fall on the standard curve, and the iPTH concentrations thus generated must agree within 15 percent.

Approximately 10 percent of sera in the assay that the authors' laboratory routinely uses gives "invalid" results when criterion 3 is applied. The most common aberration observed is a progressive increase in iPTH values as an individual serum is studied in increasing dilution. Although assay artifacts can produce such a result, it is most frequently observed in patients with ectopic hyperparathyroidism or renal lithiasis (Chapter 54).

It is likely, at least in the case of ectopic hyperparathyroidism (pseudohyperparathyroidism), that these "nonparallel" immunodilution curves are caused by different molecular forms or a different ratio of molecular forms of PTH in sera from patients with hyperparathyroidism due to nonparathyroid cancer as compared with those from patients with hyperparathyroidism of parathyroid origin.[18] The authors' laboratory has obtained evidence in support of this thesis.[19] In fractionation experiments, sera from patients with ectopic hyperparathyroidism were found to contain quantities of intact or a large-molecular-weight form(s) of iPTH approximately equal to the quantity of intact iPTH in the sera of patients with primary hyperparathyroidism with similar degrees of hypercalcemia, but the relative quantities of circulating carboxyl-terminal fragments were considerably less.

These observations have practical importance because they tend to explain the interesting and useful paradox illustrated in Fig. 55-2.[20] Values of serum iPTH, measured with a carboxyl-terminal-specific assay, were much lower for a given serum calcium in ectopic hyperparathyroidism than in primary hyperparathyroidism. It would appear, then, that the lower values are likely to be due to the relatively low concentrations of circulating carboxyl-terminal fragments of PTH in ectopic hyperparathyroidism, and that this difference is made more evident when carboxyl-terminal-specific assays are used to measure serum iPTH. One alternative to this explanation is that the relatively low serum iPTH values in ectopic hyperparathyroidism are due to an obligate uncontrolled low level of PTH secretion by the parathyroid glands in these hypercalcemic patients. The author believes that this is unlikely in the majority of cases because serum iPTH is either well below the normal range or undetectable in patients with hypercalcemia of nonparathyroid origin (sarcoid, vitamin D intoxication). Another is based on a recent report suggesting that excessive secretion of prostaglandins by nonparathyroid cancer may be responsible for the syndrome of pseudohyperparathyroidism in some patients[21] (Chapter 54). It should also be recognized that malignant tissue has the potential of producing more than one humoral agent in abnormal quantities, and it is possible that the severe hypercalcemia

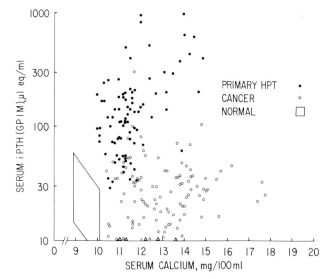

Fig. 55-2. Relationship between serum iPTH and serum calcium in primary hyperparathyroid patients (●) and hypercalcemic patients with cancer (○). Note that for a given serum calcium value, serum iPTH is lower in patients with cancer. Of 105 patients with cancer, 5 had undetectable serum iPTH (△). Area enclosed with solid lines indicates normal range ± 2 SD for serum iPTH and serum calcium. (From Benson et al: *Am J Med 56:* 821,1974.[20])

frequently observed in patients with cancer may be due to the combined effects of several ectopically secreted hypercalcemic substances.

Irrespective of the pathophysiology involved, the relationships shown in Fig. 55-2 have helped greatly in determining the course of action to be followed in some hypercalcemic patients who are suspected of having cancer (e.g., high erythrocyte sedimentation rate, weight loss) but in whom proof is lacking. If serum calcium values are greater than 12.5 mg/dl, and serum iPTH is within the normal range or only slightly increased, more intensive efforts are made to identify a neoplastic lesion, and the patient is followed-up with temporizing medical treatment. If the situation is not clarified after 6–12 months, the patient is reevaluated for parathyroid surgery.

FUTURE DEVELOPMENTS

At the present time, it is extremely difficult to prospectively produce carboxyl-terminal-specific antisera which produce radioimmunoassays of PTH with the sensitivity required to produce results similar to those shown in Figs. 55-1 and 55-2. As far as the authors know, assays of this requisite sensitivity exist in only a few laboratories in the world. Furthermore, the antisera employed in these laboratories are scarce and unavailable for distribution.

The major problem in producing ideal antisera appears to be the lack of sufficiently large quantities of suitable human antigen. Too-little human PTH has been available to use for this purpose because most of it is being diverted to completion of the amino acid sequence analysis of the hormone. This is proper because once the correct, complete amino acid sequence of human PTH is known, regions of the carboxyl-terminal part of the molecule can be synthesized in large quantities and used as immunogens. However, the time required for this to be accomplished is not known. Recent observations in the authors' laboratory may provide a substitute approach which will help greatly in providing an earlier solution to this difficult problem. In the course of isolating human PTH for sequence analysis from parathyroid tumors, a fraction was identified that contained large quantities of immunoreactive carboxyl-terminal fragments of the hormone without significant contamination with intact or amino-terminal fragments of PTH.[22] This fraction has been successfully used in a pilot study to produce antisera to the carboxyl-terminal region of human PTH.

Other approaches are being continually evaluated as work proceeds in several laboratories to better understand the complex nature of the heterogeneity of circulating PTH and to better define the specific region(s) of the PTH molecule with which assays must react to obtain diagnostic discrimination between primary disorders of parathyroid function and those due to metabolic disorders which mimic hyperparathyroidism (Chapters 45 and 54). However, it is clear that with proper selection, performance, and interpretation, the present generation of PTH assays are of great value in the differential diagnosis of primary hyperparathyroidism.

REFERENCES

1. Berson, S. A., Yalow, R. S., Aurbach, G. D., Potts, J. T. Jr.: Immunoassay of bovine and human parathyroid hormone. *Proc Natl Acad Sci USA 49:* 613, 1963.
2. Berson, S. A., Yalow, R. S.: Parathyroid hormone in plasma in adenomatous hyperparathyroidism, uremia and bronchogenic carcinoma. *Science 154:* 907, 1966.
3. Reiss, E., Canterbury, J. M.: A radioimmunoassay for parathyroid hormone in man. *Proc Soc Exp Biol Med 128:* 501, 1968.
4. Arnaud, C., Tsao, H. S., Littledike, E. T.: Radioimmunoassay of human parathyroid hormone in serum. *J Clin Invest 50:* 21, 1971.
5. Arnaud, C.: Parathyroid hormone: coming of age in clinical medicine. *Am J Med 55:* 577, 1973.
6. Goldsmith, R. S.: Hyperparathyroidism. *N Engl J Med 281:* 367, 1969.
7. Berson, S. A., Yalow, R. S.: Immunochemical heterogeneity of parathyroid hormone in plasma. *J Clin Endocrinol Metab 28:* 1037, 1968.
8. Arnaud, C. D., Tsao, H., Oldham, S. B.: Native human parathyroid hormone: an immunochemical investigation. *Proc Natl Acad Sci USA 67:* 415, 1970.
9. Arnaud, C. D., Sizemore, G. W., Oldham, S. B., et al: Human parathyroid hormone: glandular and secreted molecular species. *Am J Med 50:* 630, 1971.
10. Canterbury. J. M., Reiss, E.: Multiple immunoreactive molecular forms of parathyroid hormone in human serum. *Proc Soc Exp Biol Med 140:* 1393, 1972.
11. Segre, G. V., Habener, J. F., Powell, D, et al: Parathyroid hormone in human plasma: immunochemical characterization and biological implications. *J Clin Invest 51:* 3163, 1972.
12. Silverman, R., Yalow, R. S.: Heterogeneity of parathyroid hormone: clinical and physiologic implications. *J Clin Invest 52:* 1958, 1973.
13. Fischer, J. A., Binswanger, U., Dietrich, F. M.: Human parathyroid hormone: immunological characterization of antibodies against a glandular extract and the synthetic amino-terminal fragments 1–12 and 1–34 and their use in the determination of immunoreactive hormone in human sera. *J Clin Invest 54:* 1382, 1974.
14. Arnaud, C. D., Goldsmith, R. S., Bordier, P. J., et al: Influence of immunoheterogeneity of circulating parathyroid hormone on results of radioimmunoassays of serum in man. *Am J Med 56:* 785, 1974.
15. Arnaud, C. D., Goldsmith, R. S., Sizemore, G. W., et al: Studies on characterization of human parathyroid hormone in hyperparathyroid serum: practical considerations. Excerpta Medica International Congress Series No. 270, 1973, pp 281–290.
16. Reiss, E., Canterbury, J. M.: Spectrum of hyperparathyroidism. *Am J Med 56:* 794, 1974.
17. Flueck, J. A., Di Bella, F. P., Edis, A. J., et al: Immunoheterogeneity of parathyroid hormone in venous effluent serum from hyperfunctioning parathyroid glands. *J Clin Invest 60:* 1367, 1977.
18. Riggs, B. L., Arnaud, C. D., Reynolds, J. C., et al: Immunologic differentiation of primary hyperparathyroidism from hyperparathyroidism due to nonparathyroid cancer. *J Clin Invest 50:* 2079, 1971.
19. Benson, R. C., Jr, Riggs, B. L., Pickard, E. M., et al: Immunoreactive forms of circulating parathyroid hormone in primary and ectopic hyperparathyroidism. *J Clin Invest* 54:175, 1974
20. Benson, R. C. Jr., Riggs, B. L., Pickard, B. M., et al: Radioimmunoassay of parathyroid hormone in hypercalcemic patients with malignant disease. *Am J Med 56:* 821, 1974.
21. Seyberth, H. W., Segre, G. V., Morgan, B. S., et al: Prostaglandins as mediators of hypercalcemia associated with certain types of cancer. *N Engl J Med 293:* 1278, 1975.
22. Di Bella, F. P., Gilkinson, J. B., Flueck, J. [A.], et al: Carboxyl-terminal fragments of human parathyroid tumors unique new source of immunogens for the production of antisera potentially useful in the radioimmunoassay of parathyroid hormone in human serum. *J Clin Endo Metab 46:* 604, 1978.

56

Special Localizing Techniques for Parathyroid Disease

Harvey Eisenberg
Johanna A. Pallotta

GENERAL CONSIDERATIONS

The diagnosis of hyperparathyroidism is generally made from chemical determinations. Surgical exploration usually proceeds without further diagnostic studies and is successful in 80 to 95 percent of patients (Chapters 53 and 58). This success rate is clearly dependent upon the expertise of the surgeon. The need for special localization techniques arises primarily in patients who have undergone unsuccessful explorations and in patients who have had prior neck surgery which makes subsequent neck exploration more difficult and hazardous. Preoperative localization studies may also prove beneficial in some or all patients who have not had prior surgery.

Unsuccessful parathyroid explorations usually result from an unusual neck location, from a mediastinal location, or from difficulty in distinguishing single- from multiple-gland disease by surgical inspection or frozen-section biopsy.[1] At the initial exploration, the surgeon has usually identified the histology of at least one parathyroid gland, and the subsequent problem is most often one of localizing a solitary lesion when the glands previously identified were of normal histology. Occasionally, a single hyperplastic gland has been left behind in a multiple-gland resection. Not infrequently, the surgeon has failed to recognize the presence of hyperplasia or has encountered asymmetric hyperplasia and mistakenly taken out only the largest glands and labeled them multiple adenomas.[2] In these circumstances, and in cases in which the histological findings are unclear or in which glands have not been identified histologically at the initial exploration, the problem of determining single- versus multiple-gland disease is present, as is the need for specific localization. In our experience, it is not valid to accept visual identification of a parathyroid gland, even when this is given by an experienced neck surgeon. Histological confirmation is essential to determine which glands have been found at previous explorations and what the nature of the disease process is. When a gland has been missed on prior neck exploration, the tendency is to direct a subsequent exploration to the mediastinum. This is partic-ularly true when repeat surgery is to be performed by the same surgeon. In the great majority of cases of prior unsuccessful neck explorations, however, the abnormal gland is still in the neck or reachable from a neck approach (Chapter 58). This is true even when initial explorations have been performed by experienced neck surgeons. In general, lesions in the neck are missed as a result of: (1) lack of descent of the abnormal parathyroid gland into the usual region of a neck exploration, (2) an intrathyroidal location, or (3) a relatively medial and posterior location, such as the tracheo-esophageal groove. Because of the difficulty in dissection in the previously explored neck and the increased risk of nerve damage, it is important to try to limit repeat exploration to the appropriate side of the neck, as well as to eliminate unnecessary mediastinal exploration. In the case of mediastinal lesions, it is important to determine whether the lesion is in the anterior, middle, or posterior mediastinum and whether it projects into the base of the neck or is as far as the caudad pericardium.[3,4] Precise localization in the mediastinum may allow a neck approach if the lesion hangs down from a vascular pedicle off the inferior thyroid artery into the thymus gland or upper mediastinum. If the gland is lateral in the upper anterior mediastinum, a simple rib-splitting approach may be used rather than submitting the patient to a full sternal split. Occasionally, the lesion may be within the pericardium, which requires a cardiac approach.[3]

Preoperative localization techniques need to be highly accurate if they are to benefit these patients significantly. They must be able to localize the parathyroid abnormality specifically and to differentiate solitary- from multiple-gland disease. An incorrect preoperative localization, whether false negative or false positive, is potentially harmful to the patient and may often result in unnecessary extensive exploration in areas such as a scarred neck or mediastinum. The techniques that have been proposed for localization for parathyroid disease include both noninvasive and invasive modalities.

NONINVASIVE MODALITIES

The noninvasive techniques are barium swallow,[5] selenomethionine scanning,[6] thermography,[7] a squeeze test with peripheral parathyroid hormone sampling,[8] and, most recently, computerized axial tomography.[9]

The invasive techniques include arteriography[3,10,11] and venous catheterization[11,12] for selective sampling and parathyroid hormone level determination.[3,12]

The most commonly used noninvasive technique is the barium

swallow.[14] This study may prove helpful for large posterior neck lesions or for lesions hiding in the tracheoesophageal groove. However, displacements of the esophagus are far more likely to be caused by thyroid enlargements or by previous surgery than by parathyroid lesions.

Radioisotope scanning has the potential advantage of providing an agent selectively metabolized by the parathyroids for demonstration by scanning techniques. Unfortunately, selenomethionine has proved to be a relatively ineffective agent for this purpose.[15] It is taken up not only by the parathyroid glands but also by the thyroid and salivary glands, scar tissue, and lymph nodes. This agent has had some usefulness for relatively superficial lesions but is not well suited for lesions deeper in the neck or in the chest.

Thermography has in one series been suggested as a very accurate technique for the detection of parathyroid lesions.[16] This technique depends upon the increase in temperature related to decreased blood flow through these metabolically active lesions. Although parathyroid tumors are hypervascular, the abnormally rich plexus of these lesions transports blood less rapidly than does normal tissue. This also accounts for the persistent staining seen on arteriography. Thermography has the disadvantage of being positive for anything that would increase metabolic activity or decrease blood flow, and thus positive thermograms include thyroid lesions as well as inflammatory nodes or inflammations from scar tissue of previous surgery. Nevertheless, the potential value of this technique exists and awaits confirmation from other laboratories.

Most recently, computerized axial tomography (CAT) has made a significant impact as a valid radiologic technique for tumor localizations throughout the body.[9] This device uses x-ray beams and computer processing to achieve extremely high-contrast sensi-

tivity in an x-ray examination, achieving 98 percent contrast transfer as compared to less than 50 percent in conventional examinations. CAT scanning with its contrast enhancement allows one to image and differentiate the soft tissues of the body, albeit with relatively poor resolution for soft-tissue masses. Masses in the range of 2–3 cm can be visualized. Our preliminary impression is that there may be some benefit to this technique in localizing anterior mediastinal tumors, with which surrounding fatty tissues silhouette denser parathyroid lesions. The technique may also be useful in detecting larger tumors greater than 2–3 cm in both the neck and mediastinum. The problem still remains that most parathyroid lesions are below the resolution limits of this technique and that the x-ray coefficient of absorption of thyroid nodules and lymph nodes is indistinguishable from parathyroid tissue.

Although the noninvasive techniques mentioned above have the great advantage of safety to the patient, their high incidence of false-positive as well as false-negative interpretations has seriously limited their value for both tumor localization and for differentiating single- from multiple-gland disease.

INVASIVE MODALITIES

ARTERIOGRAPHY

Selective arteriography and selective venous sampling for parathyroid hormone levels are currently the most accurate techniques for the localization of abnormal functioning parathyroid tissue and for the differentiation of single- from multiple-gland disease. As with surgery itself, considerable technical expertise is necessary for optimal results and safety.

Arteriography (Fig. 56-1) requires selective injections into the

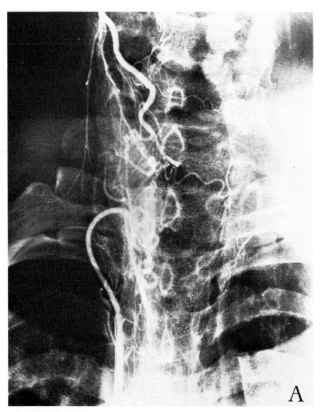
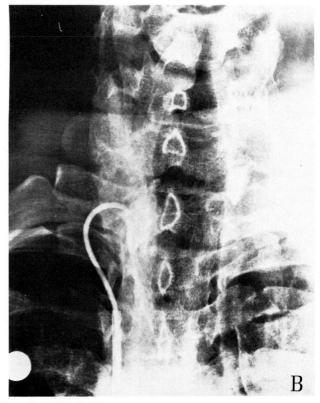

Fig. 56-1. Arteriography (right-lower-pole adenoma). (*a*) Arterial phase of injection of deep right inferior thyroid artery with reflux through normal collaterals into superior thyroid artery. (*b*) Parenchymal phase showing hypervascular adenoma silhouetted against normal thyroid blush.

inferior or superior thyroid or internal mammary arteries.[3,4] Such injections will produce a vascular-tumor blush in over 95 percent of cases, including adenoma, hyperplasia, or carcinoma. Less selective injections into the aorta or subclavian or carotid arteries will usually only demonstrate very large lesions. Fortunately, lymph nodes and scar tissue do not visualize on selective angiography, as these are avascular structures. Thyroid nodules are richly vascularized, however, and are indistinguishable angiographically from enlarged parathyroid glands. The distinction from a parathyroid lesion is generally made by showing a circumscribed tumor blush to be separate from the thyroid gland. This requires a preliminary thyroid scan that will indicate the position and mass of the intact or remnant thyroid gland. Also, the scan will usually show thyroid nodules. Multiple radiographic projections and high-resolution filming techniques (magnification) are frequently necessary. In approximately 10 to 15 percent of cases, it is not possible to differentiate thyroid from parathyroid tissue angiographically, which results primarily in false-positive interpretations.[3,4,17,18] In our experience, however, failure to show a tumor blush in the area of a tumor is distinctly unusual (2 percent). Selective angiography involves a significant morbidity, which is related primarily to transient pain occurring with intra-arterial subselective injections. Also, central-nervous-system complications, both intracerebral and of the spinal cord, may occur in 1 to 5 percent of cases.[19] This should limit the use of these procedures to patients with prior unsuccessful explorations, as well as to experienced angiographers, in whose hands the complication rate is less than 1 percent.[3,4,18] Arteriography will usually show the specific position of abnormal glands in either unusual neck or mediastinal locations and has proved valuable in predicting a proper surgical approach.

VENOUS CATHETERIZATION AND HORMONE ASSAY

All the localization techniques discussed so far have provided demonstration of the morphology of an enlarged parathyroid gland. These studies do not provide any information about the functional activity of the parathyroid glands. At the present time, in fact, the exact relationship between the gross pathology and histology of parathyroid glands and their functional activity is not clear. This is of paramount importance, since parathyroid disease, like most other endocrine disorders, is primarily a functional disturbance (Chapter 53). It has been shown in patients with MEA syndrome that parathyroid glands can be normal by conventional histological techniques, despite the presence of marked functional hyperactivity.[20,21] These findings in patients with MEA disease comprise a large percentage of the series by Black in which he showed electron-microscopic abnormalities in supposedly normal glands.[2,22] Some surgical groups routinely resect three and one-half glands at any parathyroid exploration because of the difficulty in distinguishing adenoma from hyperplasia on gross inspection or frozen sections.[23,24]

The technique of selective venous sampling offers the opportunity to selectively determine the functional activity of the parathyroid glands (Fig. 56-2). As with the arteriography, the technical aspects of these procedures are essential to their success. Nonselective sampling from large veins of the neck provides relatively poor accuracy (40 percent), and it is of little help in differentiating single- from multiple-gland disease.[25,26] Although it is impossible to catheterize the parathyroid veins themselves, as these are tiny branches draining into the thyroid plexus, extensive selective small-vein sampling of the thyroid plexus and thymic veins has proved to be highly accurate in determining regional hyperactivity.

Although these studies are long and tedious, they have an insignificant complication rate and a relatively low morbidity. In the previously explored patient, a technical problem is encountered with these studies in that the surgeons usually ligate veins during a neck dissection. Fortunately, these ligations occur at the surface of the thyroid gland, and the origins of the thyroid plexus remain open, receiving the drainage from the parathyroid glands. The origins of the superior thyroid veins can always be found, and the inferior thyroid veins are patent in about 85 percent of cases. When these veins are not patent, alternate pathways are predictable into the vertebral, thyrocervical, or thymic veins.

Clear differences are seen in the venous drainage patterns of patients with adenoma as compared to those with hyperplasia. In adenomas present in the neck, hormone elevations are only seen unilaterally, whereas, in hyperplasia, hormonal elevations are seen throughout the thyroid venous plexus bilaterally. Striking local elevations have been seen in patients with adenomas as small as 4 mm (Fig. 10). Very often, marked neck-vein elevations have been seen in either adenoma or hyperplasia, when peripheral levels have been undetectable. Occasionally, a very large adenoma may demonstrate some crossover at the level of the inferior thyroid veins. This has not been observed at the level of the superior veins. Thus, in the circumstance in which elevations are obtained in the superior and inferior thyroid veins on one side and there is a lesser but significant elevation of the inferior thyroid veins in the contralateral side, interpretation is for either a very large adenoma or hyperplasia. This differential diagnosis is then easily made by surgical inspection. Elevations of parathyroid hormone in the superior thyroid veins are highly accurate for predicting a neck location and for predicting the appropriate side. These elevations are usually specific for an upper-pole lesion; occasionally, however, a large lower-pole lesion will extend cephalad to involve upper parathyroid veins. When interpreting elevations in the inferior thyroid veins, one must be aware that the upper-pole parathyroid glands drain through the inferior thyroid vein as well as the superior thyroid veins. One must also be careful to look for thymic branches draining up from the chest into the thyroid plexus and to attempt to catheterize these selectively when they are noted. One must also be careful to observe flow patterns in thyroid veins following surgical intervention, as this may occasionally cause deviations in flow to the contralateral side of the neck.

An integral part of interpretation of hormone values from the neck-vein catheterization is the consideration of what to expect from normal glands. The catheter position may also be important, as gradients of hormone may occur. It is still uncertain how often or whether or not gradients from the parathyroid glands are detectable. This issue is obviously pertinent to the question of false-positive localizations from normal gland activity. For obvious reasons, there has not been extensive experience of catheterization studies in normocalcemic human subjects. In the experience of Shimkin,[27] significant gradients were demonstrated in normocalcemic patients with normal glands identified at surgery. Experiments in cows confirm that gradients are detectable readily from the venous effluent of normal glands.[28] However, the cumulative data from our own experiences and that of others[3,4,18] indicate that the gradients are not seen from the opposite side of the neck in patients with parathyroid adenoma, suggesting that these glands are either totally or nearly totally suppressed. We have studied several normocalcemic patients with extensive neck-vein sampling in which no gradients were observed from the thyroid veins. In addition, venous catheterization has been used in our hands to diagnose and localize a parathyroid adenoma in normocalcemic, renal-stone-forming patients. In this group, the extensive sampling

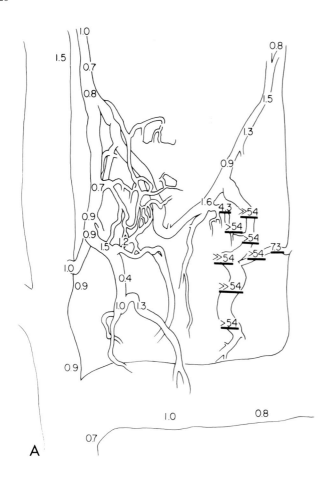

A

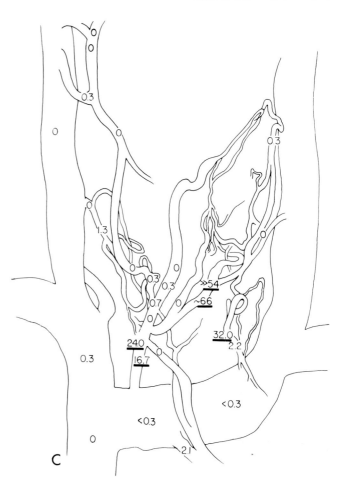

C

Fig. 56-2. Venous catheterization and parathyroid hormone assay. Typical patterns of: (*a*) adenoma (left lower pole), (*b*) diffuse hyperplasia, and (*c*) small localized adenoma (4 mm).

throughout the thyroid plexus demonstrated a somewhat broad area of regional hyperactivity and minimized the false-positive effect of a very local gradient from a specific catheter position. In patients with known hyperparathyroidism, a thorough neck sampling with no elevations has been used to interpret a mediastinal location. In patients with hypercalcemia in whom the diagnosis of hyperparathyroidism was uncertain, extensive neck sampling was used to rule out the presence of the disease with high probability. In patients with parathyroid carcinoma and recurrent hypercalcemia following a removal of neck tumor, venous catheterization has been used to establish or rule out the presence of recurrent neck disease, as well as to assess the hepatic circulation for evidence of peripheral metastases. One unsettled issue concerns the possible confusion that might arise in distinguishing the pattern seen in a patient with chief-cell hyperplasia from that seen in a normal patient.

In the previously explored patient, it is generally important to specifically visualize the parathyroid lesions by arteriography after localizing them regionally by venous sampling and distinguishing single- from multiple-gland hyperactivity. The venous-catheterization study can then be used to limit the arteriographic study, which carries a higher morbidity and potential complications. The venous catheterizations are also used to confirm that an abnormal blush seen on arteriogram is parathyroid tissue rather than thyroid, thereby minimizing false-positive interpretations. An alternative approach is to use arteriography as the initial procedure, which may potentially eliminate the need for venous study when arteriographic findings are definitive (75 percent). This approach also

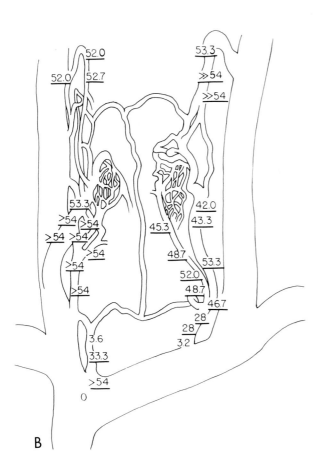

B

determines venous anatomy and flow pathways prior to venous catheterization. We have individualized the initial choice of studies based on the previous surgical and histological data. When a single gland is missing, arteriography has been the initial study. In all other circumstances, venous catheterization has preceded arteriography. Only on occasion has the venous study alone been considered sufficient for precise localization. The use of these techniques in combination is illustrated in the following cases.

ILLUSTRATED CASE STUDIES

CASE I

H. H. is a 52-year-old male with a 20-year history of renal colic and a right nephrolithotomy confirming the presence of calcium stones.

In 1971, after evaluations at another hospital for persistent hypercalcemia (calcium 11.6–13.3, phosphate 1.9, normal creatinine), a neck exploration was performed. At surgery, no parathyroid glands could be identified. A total thyroidectomy was performed. No parathyroid tissue was evident on pathological examination. Postoperatively, the patient continued to have calcium and phosphate abnormalities. Selenomethionine scan suggested a mediastinal localization. In April 1972, a venous catheterization showed a step-up in the left superior thyroid vein.

In June 1972, surgery was repeated and both neck and mediastinal explorations were negative.

In January 1974, the patient was readmitted with calcium 13 and phosphorus 2.7. Venous catheterization again showed an increased parathyroid hormone level in the left superior and left middle thyroid veins. A left superior thyroid arteriogram showed an adenoma of the left upper pole at the carotid bifurcation, well above the area of a usual neck exploration (Fig. 56-3).

At surgery, a 3×2-cm adenoma was excised. The calcium level dropped to 7.0 postoperatively.

Representative parathyroid hormone levels from the venous catheterization:

Left superior	13.5 ng/ml
Left middle	40 ng/ml
Deeper left middle	7.75
Left superior	.80
Low left middle	40
Left costovertebral	3.50
Left thyrocervical	.65
Right middle	0.4
Deeper right middle	0.45
Right superior	0.75
Right costovertebral	1.5
SVC	1.50
RA	2
IVC	.65

Discussion

This case illustrates several points. This patient was one of several in whom venous catheterization was correct but insufficient for surgical localization when used alone. The arteriographic localization showed the need for a modified approach for neck exploration, since the usual low transverse neck incision does not permit access to the undescended gland. This is an often forgotten location and one that was seen in 8 patients in our experience. It is important to note that even though the middle-thyroid-vein elevations were the highest levels seen, the presence of significant

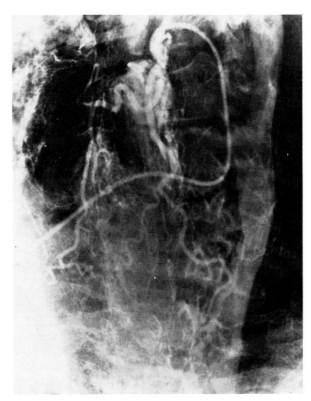

Fig. 56-3. Arteriography of undescended left-superior-pole adenoma at carotid bifurcation.

elevations in the superior thyroid veins usually indicates an upper-pole localization.

CASE II

D. C. is a 62-year-old female admitted with persistent hyperparathyroidism despite prior surgery.

Her hypercalcemia became symptomatic 3 years prior to admission. Fifteen years earlier, she had undergone a subtotal thyroidectomy with removal of a thyroid adenoma of the left lobe. She was maintained on thyroid suppression. One year prior to admission, she developed coma from hypercalcemia and was managed medically. Bone scan, barium swallow, IVP, hand films, and chest x-ray were negative. A parathyroid hormone level was 363 pg/ml at a time when the serum calcium was 12.8 mg/100 ml (nl 255 pg/ml + 561 SD).

At exploratory neck surgery, both right and left inferior glands were removed. The left superior gland was not identified. Pathological reports showed that the patient had two adenomas, a 1.5× 0.7-cm clear-cell adenoma removed from the right neck and a 2.0× 1.7-cm chief-cell adenoma removed from the left side of the neck.

Postoperatively, the patient still complained of nausea and lethargy and her serum calcium was in the range of 12 mg/100 ml. Selective venous catheterization for parathyroid hormone levels was performed in the authors' laboratory. The results of these studies revealed bilateral step-ups in venous parathyroid hormone levels obtained from the right inferior thyroid vein and left superior thyroid vein. Subsequent arteriography revealed possible lesions of the right lower pole and at the left superior pole high in the neck.

In December 1975, she underwent exploration of the neck at Beth Israel Hospital with removal of an enlarged left superior parathyroid (1.5×2 cm) located posterior to the recurrent laryngeal nerve just as it entered the larynx; this was found with difficulty and required unusually high dissection. The patient also had a subtotal resection of a normal-appearing right inferior parathyroid gland. Pathology showed hyperplasia in both glands. Postoperatively, she did well, with normocalcemia confirming cure of the hyperparathyroidism without hypoparathyroidism.

The case illustrates the value of venous catheterization in a patient in whom there was difficulty intraoperatively and pathologically in differentiating single- from multiple-gland disease. Arteriography was essential in directing the surgery on the left after an extensive, difficult neck dissection and thyroid resection failed to reveal parathyroid tissue.

INDICATIONS FOR LOCALIZATION TECHNIQUES

It is generally accepted by those cooperating groups of surgeons, pathologists, internists, and radiologists that the major use of the procedure is in patients with confirmed disease requiring surgical correction who have been previously explored unsuccessfully. Because of the high accuracy of selective sampling and because of the safety of the procedure, the authors have also considered the use of these techniques in patients without prior exploration, both in special circumstances and for routine cases. A specific circumstance in which these studies may be helpful is in elderly patients who are relatively poor surgical candidates. It is clear in these patients that the amount of surgical exploration and anesthesia time is considerably reduced by preoperative venous catheterization. These studies, although long and tedious, produced no significant morbidity. In addition, these studies were performed in patients with severe hypercalcemia, where the importance of a successful exploration on the first attempt was stressed. If the lesion is missed, these patients can be very difficult

to manage during the 4 to 6 weeks necessary between original and subsequent exploration. Another use for venous catheterizations in previously unexplored patients may be to establish a diagnosis of hyperparathyroidism in patients with hypercalcemia from other coexistent or suspected diseases, such as myeloma, sarcoidosis, and metastatic malignancy, or in patients with normocalcemic hyperparathyroidism. In addition to these special circumstances, there is good reason to consider venous sampling in routine cases. This is particularly pertinent, since they may play a role in the serious controversy that exists as to the optimal surgical approach to parathyroid disease. As noted previously, some surgical groups routinely resect three and one-half glands at initial exploration because of the difficulty in distinguishing adenoma from hyperplasia on gross inspection or frozen section. Although a rough correlation has been established between gland size and calcium level, it has also been noted that histologically normal glands may hypersecrete and that large glands may be functionally inactive.[21]

Another surgical approach, and one that we endorse, is for a limited parathyroid exploration whenever possible. Here, if rapid intraoperative identification of an adenoma is achieved, additional exploration is limited to the biopsy of a normal gland. This approach is based upon statistics indicating that multiple adenomas are rare and that the finding is usually single-gland disease (adenoma, 85 percent) or hyperplasia (15 percent) (Chapter 58). In follow-up statistics of 3 to 15 years, this limited surgical approach was successful in 96 percent of 340 cases, with marked improvement in complications and morbidity in comparison to a 4-gland exploration.[29,30] The high accuracy of selective venous sampling in differentiating single- from multiple-gland abnormality in the unexplored patient (Table 56-1) would make this a logical precursor to a routine limited parathyroid exploration, allowing a limited exploration in all patients with adenoma. At the very least, these studies

Table 56-1.

Data		
Solitary Lesions		
Adenomas	95	101
Residual hyperplastic gland	6	
Multiple Lesions		
Hyperplasia	18	
Residual hyperplastic gland	4	30
Carcinoma	8	
Previous Exploration		70
Unexplored		71
diagnostic problems	10	

Patients with Prior Exploration (70)

	prospective accuracy	retrospective	false +	false −
Selective Thyroid Arteriography 66	59/66	60/66	7 thyroid nodules	none
Selective Thyroid Venous Sampling 59	55/59	—	cross drainage 2	single vs. multiple 2
Artery + Vein	64/70 (91%)	65/70 (92%)		

Patients without Prior Exploration

		prospective accuracy
Selective Venous Sampling:	Hyperplasia	16/17 (94%)
	Adenoma	52/54 (97%)

would minimize the chances of an unsuccessful exploration. Furthermore, these studies have proved to be of considerable help in the operating room to the surgeon and pathologist in making a difficult decision between the diagnosis of hyperplasia and adenoma.

Hyperplasia can often be grossly asymmetric, both morphologically and functionally. In fact, another important controversy in parathyroid surgery is whether or not three-and-one-half gland resection is always necessary for hyperplasia, especially in cases of gross asymmetry. In 23 cases of hyperplasia, with only 2 glands removed, 50 percent of the patients remained normocalcemic for up to 5 to 10 years. With the use of selective venous sampling, the functional assessment of the individual glands may allow one to tailor the parathyroid resections to the functional abnormality in asymmetric hyperplasia. These venous-sampling studies have at times shown marked hypersecretion in patients with histologically normal glands. The potential of venous studies in understanding the relation between morphology and function in parathyroid disease, or, more appropriately, in recognizing the dynamic spectrum of parathyroid disease, is yet to be realized. The single biggest drawback is technical complexity.

SUMMARY

Preoperative localization techniques for parathyroid disease need to be highly accurate if they are to significantly benefit both patients who have had previous unsuccessful surgery and those without prior exploration. The techniques must be able to predict the surgical approach accurately and to differentiate solitary- from multiple-gland involvement. The noninvasive modalities, with few exceptions, have not proved capable of these objectives because of their high incidence of false-positive as well as false-negative findings. Still, techniques such as computed axial tomography, thermography, and radioisotope scanning should be pursued in the interests of safety and comfort to the patient. Inasmuch as these are noninvasive procedures, they may be utilized in routine cases, but they should be interpreted with great caution. It should be emphasized that incorrect direction to a surgical exploration may ultimately do more harm than good to the patient.

At the present time, morphological demonstration of abnormal parathyroid glands is best accomplished by selective arteriography (Fig. 56-4). This technique carries significant morbidity but can be performed safely in experienced laboratories. Because of its potential CNS complications, the technique should be limited to the previously explored patient. Selective venous catheterization, when properly performed, provides functional assessment of the parathyroid glands. Ultimately, understanding the functional aspects of parathyroid disease may well be a better guide to therapy than any morphological assessment, whether by radiology, surgery, or even histopathology. The venous studies, although safe, are limited by their technical complexity and await the development of less-expensive and quicker assays as well as simplification in catheterization techniques. In the final analysis, one uses those techniques that are available, with continuing review of cost-effectiveness, and interprets them in the light of their limitations.

REFERENCES

1. Black, B. M., Problems in the treatment of hyperparathyroidism. *Surg. Clin. North Am. 41:* 1061, 1961.
2. Black, B. M., Haff, R. C., Surgical pathology of parathyroid chief cell hyperplasia. *Am J Clin Pathol 53:* 565–579, 1970.
3. Eisenberg, H., Pallotta, J. A., Sherwood, L., Selective arteriography,

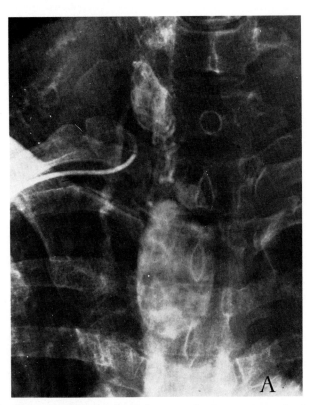
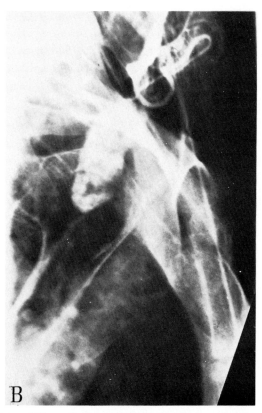

Fig. 56-4. Arteriography. (*a*) Left-upper-pole adenoma descending behind thyroid into middle mediastinum. (*b*) Lateral view shows lesion extending above sternum, allowing neck approach.

venography and venous hormone assay in diagnosis and localization of parathyroid lesions. *Am J Med 56:* 810–820, 1974.

4. Doppman, J. L., Wells, S. A., Shimkin, P. M., et al, Parathyroid localization by angiographic techniques in patients with previous neck surgery. *Br J Radiol 46:* 403–418, 1973.

5. Stevens, A. C., Jackson, C. E.: Localization of parathyroid adenomas by esophageal cine-roentgenography. *Am J Roentgenol 99:* 233, 1967.

6. DiGiulio, W., Morales, J.: An evaluation of parathyroid scanning using Se⁷⁵-methionine. *J Nucl Med 7:* 380, 1966.

7. Samuels, B. I., Dowdy, A. H., Leeky, J. W.: Parathyroid thermography. *Radiology 104:* 575–578, 1972.

8. Reiss, E., Canterbury, J. M.: Primary hyperparathyroidism: application of radioimmunoassay to differentiation of adenomas and hyperplasia and to preoperative localization of hyperfunctioning parathyroid glands. *N Engl J Med 280:* 1381, 1969.

9. Carter, B.: Personal communication.

10. Doppman, J. L., Hammond, W. G., Melson, G. L., et al: Staining of parathyroid adenomas by selective arteriography. *Radiology 92:* 527, 1969.

11. Doppman, J. L., Hammond, W. G.: Localization of parathyroid adenoma. *N Engl J Med 281:* 1248, 1969.

12. Shimkin, P., Powell, D., Doppman, J. L., et al: Parathyroid venous sampling. *Radiology 104:* 571, 1972.

13. Doppman, J. L., Hammond, W. G.: The anatomic basis of parathyroid venous sampling. *Radiology 95:* 603, 1970.

14. Ackerman, N., Winer, N.: Evaluation of methods for localizing parathyroid tumors. *Ann Surg 122:* 699, 1971.

15. DiGiulio, W., Morales, J. O.: The value of selenomethionine (Se⁷⁵) scan in preoperative localization of parathyroid adenomas. *JAMA 209:* 1873, 1969.

16. Samuels, B. I., Dowdy, J., et al: Parathyroid thermography. *Radiology 104:* 575–578, 1972.

17. Doppman, J. L., Hammond, W. G., Melson, G. L., et al: Staining of parathyroid adenomas by selective arteriography. *Radiology 92:* 527, 1969.

18. Doppman, J. L., Parathyroid localization arteriography and venous sampling. *Radiol Clin North Am 14(2):* 163–187, 1976.

19. Personal communications to authors.

20. Haff, R. C., Black, W. C., Ballinger, W. F.: Primary hyperparathyroidism: changing clinical, surgical and pathological aspects. *Ann Surg 171:* 85, 1970.

21. Castleman, B.: Case records of Massachusetts General Hospital. *N Engl J Med. 294(1):* 37, 1976.

22. Black, B. M.: The parathyroids. Proceedings of Symposium on Advances in Parathyroid Research. Springfield Ill. Thomas, 1961, p 427.

23. Haff, R. C., Arusky, R.: Trends in current management of primary hyperparathyroidism. *Surgery 75:* 715, 1974.

24. Paloyan, E., Paloyan, D., Pickleman, J. R.: Hyperparathyroidism today. *Surg Clin North Am 53:* 211, 1973.

25. Dunnegan, L. J., Watson, C., Kaufman, S., Pallotta, J., et al: Primary hyperparathyroidism: preoperative evaluation and correlation with surgical findings. *Am J Surg 128:* 471–477, 1974.

26. O'Riordan, J. L. H., Kendall, B. E., Woodhead, J. S.: Preoperative localization of parathyroid tumors. *Lancet 2:* 1172, 1971.

27. Shimkin, P., Powell, D.: Parathyroid hormone level in thyroid vein blood of patients without abnormalities of calcium metabolism. *Ann Intern Med 78:* 714–716, 1973.

28. Mayer, G. P., Habener, J. F., Potts, J. T., Jr.: Parathyroid hormone secretion in vivo: Demonstration of a calcium-independent, nonsuppressible component of secretion. *J Clin Invest 57:* 678–683, 1976.

29. Wang, C. A.: Personal communication.

30. Wang, C. A.: The anatomic basis of parathyroid surgery. *Ann Surg 183:* 271–275, 1976.

57

Medical Management of Hypercalcemia and Hyperparathyroidism

Robert M. Neer
John T. Potts, Jr.

MEDICAL TREATMENT OF HYPERCALCEMIA

The acute treatment of hypercalcemia is usually successful. With modern management, the serum calcium concentration can be decreased 3–9 mg/dl (0.75–2.25 mM/liter) in 24 to 48 hours in most patients. This is enough to relieve acute symptoms, prevent death from hypercalcemic crisis, and permit diagnostic evaluation. However, the chronic management of hypercalcemia is still very unsatisfactory unless the underlying cause can be corrected, because the available therapies are inconvenient or toxic or have intolerable side effects.

Hypercalcemia develops because skeletal calcium release is excessive, intestinal calcium absorption is excessive, or renal calcium excretion is inadequate. In patients with primary hyperparathyroidism, all three abnormalities are present, and a multifaceted therapeutic approach is reasonable. In other hypercalcemic conditions the abnormalities are more localized, and understanding the particular pathogenesis helps guide therapy. For example, hypercalcemia in patients with osteolytic mestastases or acute immobilization is primarily due to excessive skeletal calcium release and is therefore hardly affected by a severe restriction of the patients' dietary calcium. On the other hand, patients with vitamin D hypersensitivity or vitamin D intoxication have excessive intestinal calcium absorption; severe restriction of their dietary calcium is extremely beneficial (although it may not totally cure their hypercalcemia, since overdoses of vitamin D metabolites cause excessive skeletal calcium release as well). Decreased renal function or extracellular fluid depletion will decrease urinary calcium excretion in anyone. If other abnormalities, such as increased bone breakdown, prevent a compensatory decline in calcium entry into the circulation, hypercalcemia will develop. This may happen, for example, when patients with resorptive bone disease become dehydrated. In such situations, increasing the urinary calcium excretion may cure the hypercalcemia even if the other abnormalities of calcium turnover remain.

HYDRATION AND MILD DIURESIS

The first principle of treatment is to increase urinary calcium excretion by maximizing glomerular filtration, maximizing urinary sodium excretion, and administering furosemide or ethacrynic acid. Many hypercalcemic patients are dehydrated because of vomiting, inanition, or hypercalcemia-induced defects in urinary concentrating ability. The resultant drop in glomerular filtration is accompanied by an additional drop in renal tubular sodium and calcium clearance. Restoring a normal extracellular fluid volume will correct these abnormalities and increase urine calcium excretion by 100–300 mg/day (2.5–7.5 millimoles/day). Increasing urinary sodium excretion to 400–500 mEq/day will increase urinary calcium excretion even further than simple rehydration. In the normal kidney, sodium clearance and calcium clearance are very closely linked during water or osmotic diuresis, independent of any changes in urine ionic strength or acidity (see Chapter 40).[1] Finally, administering conventional doses of furosemide or ethacrynic acid twice daily will depress the tubular reabsorptive mechanism for calcium and potentiate the above maneuvers (unless the diuretic is allowed to provoke dehydration).[2] The combined use of these three maneuvers will increase urinary calcium excretion to 400–800 mg/day (10–20 mM/day) in a hypercalcemic patient. Since this is a substantial percentage of the exchangeable calcium pool, the serum calcium concentration usually falls 1–3 mg/dl (0.25–0.75 mM/liter) within 24 hours. The combination of fluids, sodium, and furosemide or ethacrynic acid is also adaptable to chronic outpatient treatment, if necessary, using sodium chloride tablets. The usual precautions regarding potassium and magnesium depletion during chronic therapy are necessary; calcium-containing renal calculi are a potential but unlikely complication.

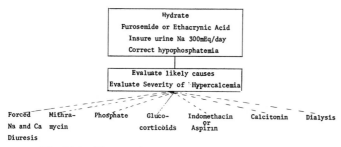

Fig. 57-1. Therapeutic strategy in treating hypercalcemia.

FORCED DIURESIS

Under life-threatening circumstances, the above therapy can be pursued much more aggressively,[3] giving 6 liters of isotonic saline (900 mEq sodium) daily plus furosemide in doses up to 100 mg every 1 to 2 hours or ethacrynic acid in doses up to 40 mg every 1 to 2 hours. Urinary calcium excretions exceeding 1000 mg/day (25 mM/day) are possible, and the serum calcium may decrease by 2–4 mg/dl (0.5–1.0 mM) within 24 hours. Severe potassium and magnesium depletion are inevitable unless replacements are given; pulmonary edema can obviously be precipitated. The potential complications can be averted by intensive monitoring of central venous pressure and plasma or urine electrolytes, but the demands on the patient and medical staff are significant. A bladder catheter is usually necessary after the first 24 hours to allow the patient to sleep.

PHOSPHATE

Patients with primary hyperparathyroidism are frequently hypophosphatemic, and hypercalcemia of other causes may also be complicated by hypophosphatemia. Hypophosphatemia decreases the rate of calcium uptake into bone,[4–8] increases intestinal calcium absorption,[9,10] and both directly and indirectly stimulates bone breakdown.[4,10,11] All these effects aggravate hypercalcemia, and correcting the hypophosphatemia will lower the serum calcium concentration. The usual treatment is 1–3 g of phosphate phosphorus per day for several days, given in four divided doses to prevent hyperphosphatemia. This can be continued indefinitely if necessary to maintain the serum inorganic phosphate concentration above 3.1 mg/dl (1.0 mM/liter). It is not clear that any toxicity will occur if the phosphate therapy only restores serum inorganic phosphate concentrations to normal, but this question has not been adequately studied. It is important to realize that the effects of oral phosphate supplements on the serum inorganic phosphate concentration may be transient; fasting serum levels should be monitored at least daily at first.

Raising the serum inorganic phosphate concentration above normal will further decrease serum calcium levels. This has long been known,[12] but the deliberate induction of hyperphosphatemia has only recently been considered an acceptable therapy for hypercalcemia. Goldsmith and Ingbar[13,14] reintroduced the use of oral phosphate, beginning with a dose of 2000 mg phosphate phosphorus daily, or intravenous phosphate, beginning with a dose of 1500 mg phosphate phosphorus over 6 to 8 hours. Serum calcium levels fell 1.8 to 10.6 mg/dl (mean fall 5.6 mg/dl) in 15 patients with malignancy and initially normal serum inorganic phosphate concentrations. Hypercalcemia due to other causes also responds to this therapy: hyperparathyroidism,[12,13,15–17] sarcoidosis,[13,18] vitamin D intoxication,[13] and multiple myeloma.[19] Oral or intravenous phosphate is one of the most dramatically effective treatments available for severe hypercalcemia. In fact, fatal hypocalcemia can be produced by excessive dosage;[14,19–21] frequent serum calcium determinations are necessary if intravenous phosphate is being administered.[14]

Unlike sodium chloride, sodium phosphate does not remove calcium from the body. In fact, urine calcium generally declines after oral or intravenous phosphate administration,[12,13,15,16] and fecal calcium declines or remains the same.[12,16,18] The decline in serum calcium therefore reflects a redistribution of calcium within the body. Studies of strontium and calcium kinetics during intravenous phosphate therapy[22,23] indicate a rapid efflux of calcium from the circulation, with no change in calcium entry to the circulation. Similar results are obtained in rats[23–25] if parathyroid stimulation (by induced hypocalcemia) is avoided. These results suggest acute precipitation of some calcium phosphate salt, as does the fact that the serum calcium concentration begins to fall within minutes of the beginning of a phosphate infusion.[16] Precipitation of calcium salts along the vein receiving the infusion has in fact been seen on radiographs.[26] The decrease in serum calcium levels during intravenous phosphate therapy is directly and linearly proportional to the mean ion product of calcium × phosphate achieved during the infusion.[16] This also suggests a precipitation phenomenon. The calculated in vivo "solubility product," 2.5×10^{-6} mol/liter, obtained from this linear relationship agrees surprisingly closely with the solubility product for $CaHPO_4$ determined in vitro at physiological temperature, pH, and ionic strength.[16] (This molar product for ultrafiltrable calcium and phosphate corresponds to a Ca × P product of about 58, using total calcium and total inorganic phosphorus in milligrams per deciliter.)

It seems unlikely that the calcium precipitates only in bone. Metastatic calcification has been reported in patients receiving oral or intravenous phosphate therapy for hypercalcemia,[13,17,20,21,26] but such observations are difficult to interpret, since hypercalcemia itself can cause metastatic calcification. Laboratory experiments, however, clearly indicate that inorganic phosphate treatment of hypercalcemia produces calcium deposits in the heart, kidney, and other tissues.[27,28] Furthermore, hyperphosphatemia causes similar deposits in normocalcemic animals.[29–31] In normocalcemic patients, a high blood phosphate can cause marked periarticular calcium deposits,[32] and the soft-tissue calcifications of uremia, which are due in part to the hyperphosphatemia, may resolve when the serum phosphate is reduced.[33] It has long been known that hyperphosphatemia may lead to the intravascular formation[34] and precipitation[35] of colloidal calcium phosphate, which is subsequently phagocytosed by the reticuloendothelial system and later slowly released into the circulation. Although it seems likely that correction of hypercalcemia with phosphate does produce some soft-tissue calcification, it is not clear that this is permanent[35,22] if therapy is brief. Furthermore, the few available studies fail to demonstrate any functional toxicity of acute phosphate therapy.[13,36] In view of this and the severity of hypercalcemic symptoms in some patients, administration of oral or intravenous phosphate to the point of hyperphosphatemia remains a justifiably popular emergency treatment.

Use of phosphate for the chronic treatment of hypercalcemia is more controversial but will remain necessary in the absence of less-toxic alternatives (see Summary). If chronic phosphate therapy is necessary, it should be given in the lowest possible dose, and the serum inorganic phosphate (checked 1 or 2 hours after an oral dose) should be kept below 5.5 mg/dl if possible, in hopes of minimizing soft-tissue calcification.

It is unclear whether precipitation of calcium salts accounts entirely for the hypocalcemic effect of supplemental phosphate. Small effects on bone calcium release would have been missed by the kinetic studies cited above. Sensitive morphologic techniques do reveal an effect of hyperphosphatemia on skeletal resorption, opposite to that of hypophosphatemia,[4] if parathyroid stimulation is avoided, and high phosphate levels depress skeletal calcium release in organ culture.[37] Finally, although serum inorganic-phosphate levels return to baseline values within 18 hours after intravenous phosphate therapy, serum calcium levels are not restored for 2 to 4 days.[16] Dual effects on calcium exchange may thus be responsible for the redistribution of body calcium.

Inorganic phosphate is commercially available in liquid, powder, and capsule form for oral use and as a liquid for intravenous use. Preparations differ in their content of phosphorus and associated cations and pH, as shown in Table 57-1.

MITHRAMYCIN

For the acute management of hypercalcemia, mithramycin is a therapeutic agent of major importance. It is a cytotoxic substance derived from an actinomycete of the genus *Streptomyces* and is successfully used in the treatment of certain testicular tumors. It has only limited effects on other malignancies, but it strikingly and consistently inhibits bone resorption. It consequently lowers serum and urine calcium and urine hydroxyproline excretion even in patients without apparent skeletal disease,[38] and studies in mice show that it localizes in areas of active bone resorption.[39] These observations suggest a direct skeletal effect, which is further confirmed by the drug's effect on Paget's disease of bone: urinary hydroxyproline and blood alkaline phosphatase fall markedly, and the excessive skeletal turnover falls to or toward normal.[40]

Mithramycin must be given intravenously, either as a freshly prepared injection or as a 4- to 24-hour infusion. The usual dose for the treatment of hypercalcemia is 25 μg/kg body weight; 10 μg/kg can be effective for chronic therapy in some patients. One or two doses per week is usually sufficient; treatment should not be repeated until hypercalcemia recurs because the toxicity is strikingly dependent on the frequency of treatment and the total dosage.[41,42]

Perlia et al.[43] treated 32 patients with hypercalcemia unresponsive to adequate hydration and a low-calcium diet. One patient had a parathyroid adenoma; the others had various malignancies. Serum calcium, which ranged from 11.8–18.4 mg/dl before mithramycin treatment, fell to normal in every patient! In 30 of 41 hypercalcemic episodes, one dose was sufficient to lower serum calcium levels to normal within 48 hours. Occasionally, the serum calcium concentration fell more slowly after a single dose, reaching normal levels only after 3 to 4 days. If no response occurred during the first 24 to 48 hours, the 25 μg/kg dose was repeated daily until the serum calcium began to fall. Smaller doses were generally ineffective. The duration of action was variable—usually several days.

Elias et al.[44,45] reported similar results in 11 patients with hypercalcemia due to malignant disease and in 1 patient with a parathyroid adenoma. Serum and urine calcium and phosphorus declined strikingly and 10 of 12 patients achieved a normal serum calcium. The mean decrement in serum calcium concentration was 5.3 mg/dl; responses ranged from a decrease of 1.6 mg/dl to a decrease of 11.0 mg/dl. Prior hydration had failed to control the serum calcium, which was 12.8–19.5 mg/dl before mithramycin therapy. The drug was effective in patients with and without skeletal metastases and with a variety of malignancies. The serum inorganic phosphate was normal in 10 of 12 patients before therapy but fell below 3.0 mg/dl in 8 of 12 after mithramycin, presumably as a result of the decrease in bone resorption. Preventing the hypophosphatemia would presumably have made the effects on the serum calcium concentration even more striking. Singer et al.[46] obtained a therapeutic response to mithramycin in a patient with a functioning parathyroid carcinoma after vigorous hydration, oral sodium phosphate, and calcitonin in combination had failed to control the serum calcium. Serum calcium and phosphorus and urinary hydroxyproline fell from elevated values to normal, while serum immunoreactive parathyroid hormone increased 1.5-fold. This further increase in parathyroid hormone indicates that the response was due to mithramycin's effects on the target organs rather than effects on the functioning parathyroid carcinoma.

Mithramycin has serious toxic effects that require careful monitoring if repeated doses are used. The major side effects are thrombocytopenia (with normal bone-marrow megakaryocytes), hepatocellular necrosis with increased LDH and SGOT levels and decreased clotting factors, and resultant epistaxis, bruising, hemorrhage, and bleeding gums. Azotemia and proteinuria occur; renal function should be carefully followed, since the hypercalcemia itself may have caused significant renal tubular or glomerular damage. Hypocalcemia can occur.[38] Hypophosphatemia and hypokalemia may also develop, and nausea, vomiting, stomatitis, and facial swelling can occur.[41,42] Toxicity is rare when only one or two doses are used and can be minimized by repeating single doses only when hypercalcemia recurs.[44] Toxic effects can usually be reversed by stopping the drug; hemorrhage may be an exception.[39–45,47]

GLUCOCORTICOIDS

Glucocorticoids increase urinary calcium excretion and decrease intestinal calcium absorption in humans when given in pharmacological doses (e.g., 40–100 mg prednisone daily in divided doses),[48–50] but they also cause a negative skeletal calcium balance.[51,52] In normal subjects and in patients with primary hyperparathyroidism, glucocorticoids neither increase nor decrease the serum calcium concentration.[53] In patients with hypercalcemia due to certain osteolytic malignancies, however, glucocorticoids are strikingly effective as a result of their antitumor effect. The malignancies causing glucocorticoid-responsive hypercalcemia are, classically, hematologic malignancies such as multiple myeloma, leukemias, Hodgkin's disease, and other lymphomas; carcinoma of the breast also responds frequently, at least early in the course of the disease. Other malignancies occasionally produce a glucocorticoid-responsive hypercalcemia, but this is unpredictable, and more reliable remedies are available for the hypercalcemia in such

Table 57-1

	1000 mg P	mEq Na	mEq K
Oral phosphate preparations			
Neutraphos® (1250 mg capsule)	4 caps	28.5	28.5
Neutraphos-K® (1450 mg capsule)	4 caps	—	57
Phos-Tabs® (860 mg tablet)	6 tabs	—	51
Fleets Phospho-Soda® (liquid)	6.7 ml	40	—
Intravenous phosphate preparations			
In-Phos®	40 ml	65	8
Hyper-Phos-K®	15 ml	—	50

Doses of phosphate are usually described in milligrams of phosphate phosphorus (as above), since clinical laboratories use such units to report serum and urine concentrations of inorganic phosphate. 1000 mg phosphate phosphorus = 33 mM. Milliequivalents are inappropriate units, since the valence is variable.

situations.[54] Glucocorticoids are very effective in treating hypercalcemia resulting from vitamin D poisoning or from the vitamin D hypersensitivity of sarcoidosis and tuberculosis.[53,55,56] The mechanism of action in the latter circumstances is unclear. In all the above situations the hypocalcemic effect develops over several days, and the usual glucocorticoid dosage is 40–100 mg prednisone (or its equivalent) daily in four divided doses. The side effects of chronic glucocorticoid therapy are well known but may be acceptable in some circumstances.

INDOMETHACIN/ASPIRIN

Malignancies often cause excessive bone breakdown and hypercalcemia without actually metastasizing to bone. The hormonal mediator of this hypercalcemia is parathyroid hormone or a related peptide in some patients, a prostaglandin of the E series in other patients, and is still undefined in the remainder (see Chapters 54 and 55).[57] Since prostaglandin synthesis can be blocked by indomethacin or aspirin, these drugs sometimes cure the hypercalcemia in such patients.[57,58] The analytical methods necessary to define prostaglandin excess are not widely available, and a therapeutic trial is the accepted diagnostic maneuver. Indomethacin, 25 mg every 6 hours, or aspirin in sufficient doses to produce a serum salicylate level of 20–30 mg/dl will generally lower the serum calcium concentrations to or toward normal over several days if prostaglandin excess is the initiating factor.[57,58] Hypercalcemia due to parathyroid hormone excess, or other causes, is not affected by this treatment.[58] Although this treatment is less predictable than some of the other available remedies for hypercalcemia caused by extraosseous malignancies, its low toxicity and specific action on the etiologic humoral agent make it particularly attractive if chronic therapy is necessary in such patients. Its effectiveness can be most safely evaluated by first controlling the hypercalcemia with other agents and then attempting to maintain normocalcemia with the inhibitors of prostaglandin synthesis. Apparent success can be confirmed by temporarily withdrawing the therapy and following the response of the serum calcium concentration over the ensuing week. Present experience suggests that therapeutic responses to aspirin or indomethacin are unlikely in patients with osteolytic metastases, even if prostaglandin excess is also present.[58]

DIALYSIS

Hypercalcemia complicated by severe renal failure is difficult to manage; if treatment is necessary, dialysis is often the first choice. Peritoneal dialysis will remove 500–2000 mg (12.5–50 mM) of calcium in 24 to 48 hours and lower the serum calcium concentration by 3–12 mg/dl (0.75–3.0 mM/liter), if calcium-free dialysis fluid is used.[59] Standard commercial peritoneal dialysis fluids generally contain 5–8 mg Ca/dl (1.25–2.0 mM/liter), which is higher than the normal serum ionized-calcium concentration. Dialysis with these standard fluids cannot be expected to relieve hypercalcemia. With calcium-free fluids and 30-minute exchanges of 2 liters each, ultrafiltrable calcium clearances exceed the urea clearances.[59] Equilibration of plasma and peritoneal fluid calcium concentrations takes 90–120 min.[60,61] Peritoneal calcium clearance can be increased approximately 30 percent by using 7 percent rather than 1.5 percent dextrose in the dialysis fluid.[60,61] The addition of albumin to the dialysis solution could theoretically increase calcium removal, but calculations suggest that the benefit is trivial compared to the expense.

Hemodialysis is equally effective.[62] The membranes currently used in artificial kidneys are quite permeable to calcium, and its dialysance is only limited by the flow rates of blood and dialysate. The dialysance of ultrafiltrable calcium approaches that of urea.[63,64] Large calcium transfers can thus occur over relatively short intervals if the dialysate is calcium-free. In addition to special salt mixtures, this may also require the use of distilled or deionized water if the local tap water contains much calcium. Hemodialysis solutions prepared with hard water may contain 15 mg Ca/dl (3.25 mM/liter).[65]

Since commercial dialysis solutions contain little or no inorganic phosphate, phosphate clearances are high during peritoneal dialysis[60] and phosphate dialysances are high during hemodialysis.[64] Large quantities of phosphate are therefore lost during conventional dialyses, and serum inorganic phosphate concentrations usually fall. If phosphate depletion develops, the hypercalcemia will be aggravated. Therefore the serum inorganic-phosphate concentration should be measured after dialysis, and phosphate supplements added to the diet or to subsequent dialysis fluids if necessary.

CALCITONIN

Calcitonin decreases the skeletal release of calcium, phosphorus, and hydroxyproline within minutes of its intravenous injection.[66,67] The subsequent changes in serum calcium and phosphorus depend upon the initial magnitude of skeletal resorption: subjects with the most rapid bone turnover show the greatest reduction in serum calcium concentration.[68] In the doses used clinically, calcitonin also increases the renal clearance of calcium and phosphorus (and sodium).[69,70] Increased skeletal uptake of phosphorus is also an initial effect of the drug in animals.[71] Further details of the hormone's effects are provided in Chapter 50.

Calcitonin is only moderately effective in lowering the serum calcium concentration in hypercalcemic patients (a 1–4 mg/dl or 0.25–1.0 mM/liter fall can be expected). The most impressive results have been seen in patients with hypercalcemia due to immobilization,[72] thyrotoxicosis,[73] or vitamin D intoxication.[74,75] These situations are all characterized by a high rate of bone turnover. Surprisingly, calcitonin has been less effective than phosphate or mithramycin in patients with hypercalcemia due to malignancy[76,77] or hyperparathyroidism,[72,75] conditions in which bone turnover is also high.

After several hours or days, escape from the hypocalcemic effects of calcitonin occurs in patients and in animals.[78–80] An analogous phenomenon is seen in tissue culture, where it can be blocked by glucocorticoids.[80] The effectiveness of calcitonin in animals is related to the serum inorganic-phosphate level. Phosphate loading enhances[81] and phosphate depletion inhibits[82] the hypocalcemic effect of the hormone. Since hypophosphatemia is a primary effect of calcitonin, a self-negating effect exists. Limited studies suggest that this does not account for the escape from the hormone's action.[78] However, synergism of calcitonin and inorganic phosphate in patients with hypercalcemia warrants further study.

Calcitonin is effective by intravenous, intramuscular, or subcutaneous injection, but it is inert when taken by mouth or sublingually. Porcine calcitonin must be given every 3 to 6 hours for maximum effect; salmon calcitonin is more potent and can be given in doses of 25–50 U every 6 to 8 hours.[83] In dilute solutions, calcitonin adheres to glass, and heat-inactivated human albumin (1 mg/ml) or some other protein must be added to the solution if it is given by continuous infusion.

Calcitonin is expensive. Its most appealing characteristic is its freedom from toxic effects. Used in combination with other drugs, it might allow a reduction in dose of the more potent, but more toxic, alternatives.

SUMMARY

The various therapies are listed in Table 57-2, with their particular indications and principal toxicities. The choice of therapy depends upon the basic disease, the severity of the hypercalcemia, the serum inorganic-phosphate level, and the patient's renal, hepatic, and bone-marrow function. Mild hypercalcemia (< 12 mg/dl or 3 mM/liter) can usually be managed by good hydration, sodium chloride, and small doses of furosemide or ethacrynic acid. Severe hypercalcemia (> 15 mg/dl or 3.75 mM/liter) requires certain and speedy correction. Aggressive sodium/calcium diuresis with large doses of furosemide and ethacrynic acid works rapidly but should only be attempted if appropriate monitoring is available and cardiac function is adequate. Mithramycin may well be the drug of choice, since it has the advantage of great effectiveness and simplicity of use; the principal contraindication is the question of toxicity. Renal, hepatic, or bone-marrow disease may preclude its use. If hypophosphatemia is present, it should be corrected with oral or, rarely, intravenous phosphate repletion. Intermediate degrees of hypercalcemia can be treated with some combination of these remedies and/or glucocorticoids, with the choice dependent upon the underlying disease. Phosphate supplements should be avoided if hyperphosphatemia is already present. Severe dietary calcium restriction should only be employed if intestinal hyperabsorption is present. Glucocorticoids and prostaglandin-synthesis inhibitors work slowly over several days and should not be relied upon as the sole treatment for life-threatening hypercalcemia. Dialysis should be reserved for hypercalcemia complicating acute or chronic renal failure.

The only really satisfactory treatments for chronic outpatient therapy are dietary calcium restriction, sodium chloride, furosemide and ethacrynic acid, and indomethacin. The more effective remedies (mithramycin, phosphate, glucocorticoids) all have significant toxicity or side effects, so that chronic treatment is more appropriately directed at the underlying disease.

An important point to stress is that the treatment of hypercalcemia must be approached in the context of overall patient care. If the underlying disease is unknown or has a reasonable chance of successful definitive therapy, then treatment of the hypercalcemia should be aggressive. If it can be ascertained that the patient suffers from a disease process, such as malignancy, for which all

Table 57-2. Summary of Useful Treatments for Hypercalcemia

Therapy	Dose	Particular Indications	Complications	Precautions
Hydration	p.r.n.	Universal	—	—
High urine Na	300 mEq/day excreted Na	Universal	—	—
Furosemide or ethacrynic acid	40–160 mg/day 50–200 mg/day	Universal	K and Mg	Measure serum K and Mg
Prednisone or equivalent	5–15 mg/6 hours	Breast cancer Lymphomas Leukemias Multiple myeloma D poisoning Sarcoid Tuberculosis	Cushing's syndrome if chronic Rx	Alternate-day Rx for chronic use
Indomethacin	25 mg/6 hours by mouth	"Humor tumor"	Na retention GI bleeding Headache	Monitor
Mithramycin	10–25 µg/Kg i.v., repeat p.r.n.	Universal	Liver toxicity Kidney toxicity Marrow toxicity	Rx p.r.n. Monitor platelets, CBC, BUN, SGOT
Phosphate	250–750 mg P/6 hours by mouth	Serum P < 3 mg/dl or 1 mM/liter	Ectopic calcification	Keep serum P below 5–6 mg/dl
Forced diuresis	4–6 liters fluid i.v./day containing: 600–900 mEq Na plus furosemide/2–4 hours plus at least 60 mEq K/day plus at least 60 mEq Mg/day	Universal	Pulmonary edema K and Mg	Intensive monitoring, including venous pressure and serum Mg and K
Calcitonin	2 units/Kg/4 hours subcutaneously	Paralysis Immobilization D poisoning	—	—
Dialysis	Low-Ca bath	Acute renal failure	Multiple	Monitor serum P after dialysis

definitive or effective ameliorative measures have been exhausted, then aggressive therapy of the hypercalcemia may not be indicated. The sedative effects of severe hypercalcemia can sometimes be a blessing.

MEDICAL TREATMENT OF HYPERPARATHYROIDISM

MANAGEMENT OF ASYMPTOMATIC HYPERPARATHYROIDISM

The widespread use of the clinical chemistry laboratory as a medical screening device and wider studies of hyperparathyroid patients' families are bringing to medical attention considerable numbers of asymptomatic hypercalcemic patients. Radioimmunoassays for parathyroid hormone and other modern methods usually permit a diagnosis in such patients without a neck exploration. As a result, the indications for parathyroid surgery in a hypercalcemic patient are now almost exclusively therapeutic. If the hypercalcemia is discovered accidentally, and the patient is asymptomatic, the need for such surgery is often not clear. The appropriate treatment of such patients is endlessly debated, as the prospect of neck surgery for asymptomatic disease is unsettling to patients and doctors alike. Since few surgeons are really experienced at parathyroid exploration, the final results of surgery can be unsettling as well. Surgery can be particularly difficult in these patients with mild hyperparathyroidism because the mildly abnormal parathyroid gland is often only slightly enlarged. However, without surgical cure, renal function may deteriorate, renal calculi and infection may occur, hypercalcemic crisis may ensue, or osteoporosis, bone cysts, and fractures may become disabling. Balancing the risks and benefits of prophylactic surgery is often done intuitively or by emotional and social criteria, beyond the usual assessment of "operability."

Very useful information on the natural history of this disease is provided by a report from the Mayo Clinic of 147 surgically untreated or incompletely treated patients with primary hyperparathyroidism, 134 of whom had mild asymptomatic disease.[84] Over a 5-year period 20 percent of these patients required surgery (which was unsuccessful in 5 of 29 patients), 58 percent were without deterioration, and 4 percent died of unrelated causes. The remaining 18 percent were lost to follow-up. There is a need for parallel follow-up studies in a group of surgically treated patients, since renal deterioration has been reported in some patients despite successful surgery,[85] possibly related to renal infection, prior nephrocalcinosis, or renal calculi.

When faced with such a patient, it is first important to confirm the diagnosis and the lack of symptoms (see Chapter 53 concerning the variable symptoms of primary hyperparathyroidism), measure the creatinine clearance and renal tubular function, and search for urinary-tract calculi or infection. If renal function is impaired, or if infection or calculi are present, the patient's lack of symptoms is illusory, and surgery is warranted if possible. It is important to recall that hypercalcemia causes a functional defect in urinary concentrating capacity that is reversible and so is not an indication for surgery. The skeletal mass should be evaluated simultaneously, including quantitative measurements of metacarpal cortical width[86] or phalangeal mass[87] if possible. Gamma-ray absorptiometry of the hand or forearm is particularly sensitive and useful for detecting early bone loss in such patients[88,89] but is not yet widely available.

If bone mass is already low (for whatever reason), parathyroid surgery is advisable to prevent further bone loss from the hyperparathyroidism. Lastly, if the hypercalcemia is severe (above 13 mg/dl or 3.25 mM/liter), the risks of more-severe life-threatening hypercalcemia are great enough to warrant surgery. Other considerations are the age and general health of the patient and the skill of the available parathyroid surgeons. The difficulties of lifelong follow-up for an asymptomatic illness are notorious. Many young patients will therefore warrant surgery simply because of their unwillingness or inability to maintain a regular follow-up. The final consideration should be the patient's anxieties, either about surgery and anesthesia or about having an uncorrected abnormality. These anxieties may influence therapy significantly if consideration of the preceding factors produces only equivocal arguments for or against parathyroid surgery.

Such a review dictates surgery for many of these patients, but a significant residue of truly asymptomatic patients without complications will remain. In these patients, serial quantitative measurement of renal glomerular and tubular function and bone mass at 6-month and later at 12-month intervals is extremely helpful. Patients with developing complications will be detected early, before significant permanent damage occurs, and will accept surgery more readily when apprised of the reasons. The majority of patients, who will show no deterioration or symptoms, can be reassured and reevaluated yearly. Until it is possible to predict which patients will deteriorate and which will not, this empirical approach is the only alternative to universal prophylactic surgery. At the present time, it is probably wise to resist any temptation to treat such patients with inorganic phosphate or other remedies. If treatment is necessary, the patient is no longer asymptomatic, and the primary therapeutic approach should still be surgery. The indications for medical treatment of hyperparathyroidism (other than observation) are relatively limited (see below).

MEDICAL TREATMENT OF SYMPTOMATIC PRIMARY HYPERPARATHYROIDISM

Occasionally, patients with symptomatic primary hyperparathyroidism must be treated medically because repeated surgery is unsuccessful, or coincidental illness makes surgery inadvisable, or the patient refuses surgery. This difficult situation is aggravated by the fact that hyperfunctioning parathyroid glands generally remain responsive to changes in the serum calcium concentration.[90] Therefore, remedies that decrease the serum calcium concentration will increase the serum parathyroid hormone concentration, aggravating the tendency to bone dissolution. It is therefore advisable to lower the serum calcium concentration only enough to eliminate symptoms, minimize the dangers of hypercalcemic crisis, and keep the urinary calcium excretion below 300 mg/day (7.5 mM/day). Maintaining a serum calcium below 11–12 mg/dl (2.75–3.0 mM/liter) will usually accomplish this. Although it is generally assumed that the risk of ectopic calcification in the kidneys, blood vessels, joint cartilage, heart, and elsewhere is directly proportional to the serum calcium concentration, there are no controlled clinical observations to support this, and animal experiments suggest the contrary.[91] In fact, many patients with mild asymptomatic hyperparathyroidism (serum calcium 10.3–11.5 mg/dl or 2.6–2.9 mM/liter) never develop significant ectopic calcification despite many years of follow-up (see above). Since total correction of the hypercalcemia may aggravate the bone disease and inconvenience the patient without necessarily producing any corresponding benefit, moderate correction seems reasonable until more clinical information is available.

Many patients with primary hyperparathyroidism are significantly phosphate depleted because of the increased renal phosphate clearance induced by the parathyroid hormone excess. In these patients, it is possible to decrease the serum calcium concentration, without harming the skeleton, by correcting the phosphate deficiency. As outlined above, and as described in greater detail in Chapter 52, the correction of severe phosphate depletion can produce a positive skeletal calcium and phosphorus balance and an improvement in bone mass despite a secondary increase in the serum parathyroid hormone concentration. Albright et al. demonstrated such a sequence in 2 of 4 patients with primary hyperparathyroidism treated with supplemental oral phosphate to correct severe phosphate depletion.[92] Whether the skeletal benefits of phosphate repletion and the general benefits of the resultant decrease in the serum calcium concentration outweigh the risks of the increased parathyroid hormone secretion in all patients with surgically untreatable primary hyperparathyroidism is unclear.[93] At present, it seems reasonable to give dietary phosphate supplements only if necessary to maintain the fasting serum inorganic phosphate concentrations within the normal range, following the general principles for phosphate therapy of hypercalcemia outlined above.

Patients with primary hyperparathyroidism are sometimes vitamin-D-deficient, as revealed by low serum concentrations of 25-hydroxyvitamin D.[94,95] This will aggravate the skeletal disease by superimposing vitamin-D-deficiency osteomalacia upon the already-present hyperparathyroid bone disease. On the other hand, vitamin D deficiency will limit intestinal calcium absorption and skeletal calcium release, thus moderating the hypercalcemia (see Chapter 52). Correcting any vitamin D deficiency in such patients will therefore aggravate the hypercalcemia, even though it may improve the bone disease. The balance between these two effects is impossible to predict at present, and the results of such therapy can only be established by a cautious therapeutic trial. In some patients the benefits clearly outweigh the risks,[94] and the need and risks of such therapy should be carefully evaluated before parathyroid surgery in any hyperparathyroid patient with severe bone disease.

POSTOPERATIVE MANAGEMENT

Medical issues that may arise in the days and weeks after parathyroid surgery include the adequacy of the surgery, the functional adequacy of the residual parathyroid tissue left behind, and the appropriate oral or parenteral intake of calcium, inorganic phosphate, or magnesium. The adequacy of surgery, as well as the function of the residual parathyroid tissue, is best evaluated by serial postoperative determinations of serum calcium, inorganic phosphate, and parathyroid hormone. If surgery was adequate, the serum calcium usually falls by several milligrams per deciliter within the first 24 hours, and the nadir is reached in 4 or 5 days at values of 8.0–8.4 mg/dl (2.0–2.1 mM/liter).[96] However, there is a great individual variation in this pattern of response, and the nadir in the serum calcium concentration may not be reached for as long as several weeks after operation.[96] If hypercalcemia persists longer than this, the surgery was inadequate or a second cause of hypercalcemia is coincidentally present. For a discussion of the differential diagnosis of hypercalcemia, see Chapter 54. Techniques to localize residual parathyroid tissue, as well as general surgical considerations, are discussed in Chapters 56 and 58.

In some patients, hypocalcemia is a significant and even dangerous postoperative problem. Its frequency varies greatly, depending on the presence or absence of associated medical complications and the surgical approach used. There are several possible causes. First, hypocalcemia may be due to inadequate residual parathyroid tissue, that is, true hypoparathyroidism, either temporary or permanent. Temporary hypoparathyroidism is due to operative trauma or ischemia, severe postoperative hypomagnesemia (serum magnesium less than 1.0 mEq/liter), or simply delayed recovery of secretory function by the residual normal glands, which presumably had been suppressed by the hypercalcemia. Transient hypoparathyroidism on this basis is a diagnosis of exclusion. Second, hypocalcemia may be caused by the excessive calcium uptake of a healing osteomalacic skeleton or, rarely, rapid intra-abdominal precipitation of calcium due to intraoperative pancreatitis. Albright and Reifenstein reported that a marked drop in calcium was particularly likely in patients with very high serum alkaline-phosphatase levels and other evidence of osteitis fibrosa preoperatively. Their serum calcium concentration often fell below 7 mg/dl (1.75 mM/liter) postoperatively. Accelerated skeletal uptake of calcium is probably the major factor responsible for the severe hypocalcemia in these patients. The abrupt reduction in circulating levels of parathyroid hormone in patients who are successfully operated upon arrests the excessive bone resorption but not the excessive new bone formation. Hypocalcemia results. Hypophosphatemia and hypomagnesemia may occur simultaneously as a result of unbalanced skeletal uptake of these elements as well. Serial bone biopsies taken after parathyroidectomy in such patients have shown a marked postoperative osteoblastic response manifested by the deposition of large amounts of osteoid in areas previously involved by osteoclastic resorption.[97]

Third, hypocalcemia may be due to partial skeletal or intestinal resistance to the action of parathyroid hormone, which limits the severity of the hypercalcemia preoperatively and limits the adequacy of serum calcium homeostasis postoperatively. This occurs in patients whose primary hyperparathyroidism is complicated by renal failure, vitamin D deficiency or intestinal malabsorption, or severe magnesium depletion. In the experience of the authors over the last 10 years, patients with severe renal failure have difficulty maintaining a normal serum calcium concentration after parathyroid surgery. This difficulty arises even though the residual parathyroid tissue continues to provide concentrations of circulating hormone well above the upper limit of normal. The management of such patients is similar to the approach used in hypocalcemic renal failure of any cause (Chapter 62). Dihydrotachysterol may be helpful as well as 1,25-dihydroxycholecalciferol (Chapter 62). Significant magnesium depletion and severe hypomagnesemia occasionally appear in patients with primary hyperparathyroidism preoperatively and more often postoperatively.[98–102] Hypomagnesemia per se may be responsible for persistent and refractory hypocalcemia, and, unless magnesium levels are restored to normal, it may be difficult or impossible to correct postoperative hypocalcemia in such patients. The hypocalcemia associated with magnesium depletion arises from an impairment of the secretion of parathyroid hormone from the residual parathyroid gland[103–105] and from a magnesium-sensitive blockade of the peripheral tissues' responsiveness to parathyroid hormone.[106] Repletion of magnesium leads to a prompt restoration of the normal secretory activity of the parathyroids and target-organ responsiveness to the action of the hormone.

The origin of the hypomagnesemia in hyperparathyroidism is not entirely understood. Although in normal subjects, parathyroid hormone acts at the level of the kidney to promote magnesium reabsorption, as well as calcium reabsorption,[107] in patients with hyperparathyroidism, excessive filtered loads of magnesium resulting from skeletal breakdown predominate over renal conservation effects (analogous to findings with calcium excretion).

Severe magnesium deficiency in a hypocalcemic patient should therefore be promptly corrected whenever detected (e.g., serum Mg^{++} levels below 1.0 mEq/liter). $MgCl_2$ is sufficiently soluble to be effective by mouth, but preparations of this compound are not widely available, and oral repletion with other magnesium salts is likely to cause diarrhea. Therefore, repletion should usually be parenteral. The extent of total-body magnesium deficiency is usually at least 150–200 mEq if hypomagnesemia is present.[108] Inasmuch as the depressant effect of magnesium on central and peripheral neural function is not seen below 4 mEq/liter (normal range: 1.5–2.0 mEq/liter), intravenous magnesium replacement can be accomplished safely. An intravenous dose of 80–120 mEq can be given over 8 to 12 hours to the average-size adult if severe hypomagnesemia is detected, provided renal function is not impaired.[108] The magnesium is given either as an intravenous infusion over 8 to 12 hours or in divided doses intramuscularly ($MgSO_4$ USP is the preparation normally used, available as a 50% solution, 4 mEq/ml, or as a less-concentrated 20% solution). If hypocalcemia is due to hypomagnesemia, blood calcium usually returns to normal within 24 to 48 hours, together with normal rates of parathyroid hormone secretion and/or peripheral response to the hormone.[103,105,106] Since magnesium is primarily an intracellular cation, serum magnesium levels are a poor guide to the adequacy of magnesium repletion. If in doubt, another guide is the restoration of normal rates of excretion of magnesium. Urinary excretion of 70 to 90 percent of the administered dose[108] of magnesium will occur when the intracellular deficit is corrected.

Serum parathyroid hormone levels are indispensable for the final differential diagnosis of postparathyroidectomy hypocalcemia, but serum inorganic-phosphate levels may provide an early clue to the diagnosis. If the hypocalcemia is due to hypoparathyroidism, hyperphosphatemia will also develop as a consequence of the loss of parathyroid hormone action on renal phosphate clearance, an effect that predominates over changes in skeletal release and intestinal uptake of phosphate. All the other causes of postoperative hypocalcemia are accompanied by hypophosphatemia as a result of rapid repair of bone mineral deficits or persistent (but now reactive and appropriate) hyperparathyroidism in the residual glands. Renal insufficiency, if present, will limit the applicability of this test.

Oral calcium supplementation may suffice as treatment for mild symptomatic hypocalcemia in the postoperative period. Assuming that hypomagnesemia has been eliminated, the therapeutic objective is to support the blood calcium level while awaiting restoration of balance between skeletal uptake and normal parathyroid function. Because intestinal absorption of calcium remains elevated for at least several days after parathyroidectomy,[96] addition to the diet of several grams of elemental calcium per 24 hours (given as any of several preparations, plus liberal use of milk as tolerated) will often lessen symptoms of increased neuromuscular irritability. If hypocalcemia is severe and/or continues, intravenous calcium is necessary to avoid serious consequences of tetany, laryngospasm, and convulsions. The rate and duration of intravenous calcium therapy are determined by the severity of symptoms, and the response to therapy is assessed by monitoring both blood calcium levels and signs of neuromuscular irritability. An infusion of 0.5–2 mg Ca/kg body weight per hour usually relieves symptoms. In most instances, parenteral therapy will be required for only a few days. If the requirement for parenteral calcium continues for more than 4 or 5 days, replacement therapy with vitamin D (or its analogues) and/or high-dose oral calcium should be initiated, since the persistent hypocalcemia suggests that hypoparathyroidism may be present or that there may be a large bone mineral deficit.

Ten days or longer may be required for the calcium-raising action of large doses of vitamin D plus oral calcium to become manifest.[96] This can be shortened, in the authors' experience, if daily loading doses of 300,000–400,000 IU of vitamin D are used until the serum calcium just begins to rise, and then immediately switched to maintenance doses of 50,000–100,000 IU/day (adult dose). The recent finding that 1-hydroxycholecalciferol or 1,25-dihydroxycholecalciferol can raise serum calcium to normal within 24 to 48 hours after initiation of treatment indicates that in the future these rapidly acting derivatives of vitamin D may be preferred, regardless of whether the hypocalcemia is permanent or transient[109,110] (Chapter 62).

MANAGEMENT ISSUES IN HEREDITARY HYPERPARATHYROIDISM

The incidence of hereditary endocrinopathies is strikingly high in patients with primary hyperparathyroidism. In one recent series of 100 consecutive families, 11 percent had such a syndrome.[111] Numerous practical issues in the overall medical management of patients with familial hyperparathyroidism and/or multiple-endocrine-neoplasia syndromes have become evident. It is becoming clear that appropriate screening procedures can be developed to permit early detection of hyperplasia and/or neoplasia of endocrine tissue other than the parathyroids in an affected member of an involved kindred. The pituitary tumors of the MEN-1 syndrome can be arrested by noninvasive treatment such as proton-beam therapy if detected early.[112] If they are undetected until late in the evolution of gland enlargement, however, irreversible consequences such as impairment of vision and other complications secondary to the space-occupying lesion may occur, and surgery is then the only available therapy. Skull radiographs and immunoassays for growth hormone and especially prolactin are helpful in the presymptomatic diagnosis of such tumors. Many pituitary tumors, even when small, are associated with excessive prolactin secretion with or without amenorrhea and galactorrhea,[113] so that serum prolactin assays are a particularly valuable screening test. Acromegaly was found in 27 percent of 55 cases involving abnormality of the pituitary in one review published in 1964.[114] Overproduction of ACTH, TSH, or gonadotropins by pituitary tumors is less common.

Recent reviews have stressed the great value of the immunoassay for gastrin as an important adjunct to studies of gastric physiology in the diagnosis of Zollinger/Ellison syndrome. Recognition of the presence of Zollinger/Ellison syndrome in the MEN-1 syndrome leads to special management decisions; total rather than subtotal gastrectomy leads to improved long-term survival, despite the occurrence of metastases arising from the pancreatic, gastrin-producing tumors.[115,116]

Similar detailed medical management issues have been clarified in the diagnosis and treatment of affected members of kindreds afflicted with various components of the MEN-II syndrome (see Chapter 64). Careful attention to these issues in the hereditary endocrine syndromes promises to lead to significant improvement in the morbidity and mortality of these patients and represents an important adjunct to the medical management of heritable hyperparathyroidism.

REFERENCES

1. Walser, M.: Calcium clearance as a function of sodium clearance in the dog. *Am J Physiol 200:* 1099, 1961.
2. Walser, M.: Treatment of hypercalcemias. *Mod Treatment 7:* 662, 1970.
3. Suki, W. N., et al: Acute treatment of hypercalcemia with furosemide. *N Engl J Med 283:* 836, 1970.
4. Baylink, D., et al: Formation, mineralization, and resorption of bone in hypophosphatemic rats. *J Clin Invest 50:* 2519, 1971.
5. Lotz, M., et al: Osteomalacia and debility resulting from phosphorus depletion. *Trans Assoc Am Physicians 77:* 281, 1964.
6. Bloom, W. L., Flinchum D.: Osteomalacia with pseudofractures caused by the ingestion of aluminum hydroxide. *JAMA 174:* 1327, 1960.
7. Freeman, S., McLean F.: Experimental rickets: Blood and tissue changes in puppies receiving diet very low in phosphorus with and without vitamin D. *Arch Pathol 32:* 387, 1941.
8. Nagant, C., Krane, S.: The treatment of adult phosphate diabetes and Fanconi syndrome with neutral sodium phosphate. *Am J Med 43:* 508, 1967.
9. Lotz, M., et al: Evidence for a phosphorus-depletion syndrome in man. *N Engl J Med 278:* 409–415, 1968.
10. Tanaka, Y., Deluca, H.: The control of 25 hydroxyvitamin D metabolism by inorganic phosphorus. *Acta Biochem Biophys 154:* 566, 1973.
11. Day, H. G., McCollum, E. V.: Mineral metabolism, growth, and symptomatology of rats on diet extremely deficient in phosphorus. *J Biol Chem 130:* 269, 1939.
12. Albright, F., et al: Studies in parathyroid physiology; Effect of phosphate ingestion in clinical hyperparathyroidism. *J Clin Invest 11:* 411, 1932.
13. Goldsmith, R. S., Ingbar, S. H.: Inorganic phosphate treatment of hypercalcemia of diverse etiologies. *N Engl J Med 274:* 1, 1966.
14. Goldsmith, R. S., Ingbar, S. H.: Phosphate, sulfate, and hypercalcemia. *Ann Intern Med 67:* 463, 1967.
15. Eisenberg, E.: Effects of varying phosphate intake in primary hyperparathyroidism. *J Clin Endocrinol Metab 28:* 651, 1968.
16. Hebert, L. A., et al: Studies of the mechanism by which phosphate infusion lowers serum calcium concentration. *J Clin Invest 45:* 1886, 1966.
17. Dent, C. E.: Some problems of hyperparathyroidism. *Br Med J 2:* 1495, 1962.
18. Pak, C. Y., et al: Control of hypercalcemia with cellulose phosphate. *J Clin Endocrinol Metab 28:* 1828, 1968.
19. Goldsmith, R. S., et al: Phosphate supplementation as an adjunct in the therapy of multiple myeloma. *Arch Intern Med 122:* 128, 1968.
20. Shackney, S., Hasson, J.: Precipitous fall in serum calcium, hypotension, and acute renal failure after intravenous phosphate therapy for hypercalcemia. Report of two cases. *Ann Intern Med 66:* 906, 1967.
21. Breuer, P. I., LeBauer, J.: Caution in the use of phosphates in the treatment of severe hypercalcemia. *J Clin Endocrinol Metab 27:* 695, 1967.
22. Eisenberg, E.: Effect of intravenous phosphate on serum strontium and calcium. *N Engl J Med 282:* 889, 1970.
23. Milhaud, C. R., et al: Étude du mécanisme de l'effet hypocalcémiant du phosphate minéral et de l'interaction èventuelle avec la thyrocalcitone. *C R Acad Sci (Paris) 266:* 1169, 1968.
24. Pechet, M. M., et al: Regulation of bone resorption and formation. Influences of thyrocalcitonin, parathyroid hormone, neutral phosphate, and vitamin D_3. *Am J Med 43:* 696, 1967.
25. Feinblatt, J., et al: Effect of phosphate infusion on bone metabolism and parathyroid hormone action. *Am J Physiol 218:* 1624, 1970.

26. Carey, R. W., et al: Massive extraskeletal calcification during phosphate treatment of hypercalcemia. *Arch Intern Med 122:* 150, 1968.
27. Schneeberger, E. E., Morrison, A. B.: Increased susceptibility of magnesium-deficient rats to a phosphate-induced nephropathy. *Am J Pathol 50:* 549, 1967.
28. Spaulding, S. W., Walser, M.: Treatment of experimental hypercalcemia with oral phosphate. *J Clin Endocrinol Metab 31:* 531, 1970.
29. Hamuro, Y., et al: Acute induction of soft tissue calcification with transient hyperphosphatemia in the KK mouse by modification of dietary contents of calcium, phosphorus and magnesium. *J Nutr 100:* 404, 1970.
30. Jowsey, J., Balasubramanian, P.: Effect of phosphate supplements on soft-tissue calcification and bone turnover. *Clin Sci 42:* 289, 1972.
31. Craig, J. M.: Observations on the kidney after phosphate loading in the rat. *Arch Pathol 68:* 306, 1959.
32. Wilber, J. F., Slatopolsky, E.: Hyperphosphatemia and tumoral calcinosis. *Ann Intern Med 68:* 1043, 1968.
33. Parfitt, A. M.: Soft tissue calcification in uremia. *Arch Intern Med 124:* 544, 1969.
34. Grollman, A.: Condition of inorganic phosphorus of blood with special reference to calcium concentration. *J Biol Chem 72:* 565, 1927.
35. Gersh, I.: Improved histochemical methods for chloride, phosphate-carbonate and potassium applied to skeletal muscle. *Anat Rec 70:* 331, 1938.
36. Stamp, T. C. B.: The hypocalcaemic effect of intravenous phosphate administration. *Clin Sci 40:* 55, 1971.
37. Raisz, C., Nilmann, I.: Effect of phosphate, calcium and magnesium on bone resorption and hormonal responses in tissue culture. *Endocrinology 85:* 446, 1969.
38. Parsons, V., et al: Effects of mithramycin on calcium and hydroxyproline metabolism in patients with malignant disease. *Br Med J 1:* 474, 1967.
39. Kennedy, B. J., et al: Studies with tritiated mithramycin in C_3H mice. *Cancer Res 27:* 1534, 1967.
40. Ryan, W. G., et al: Effects of mithramycin on Paget's disease. *Ann Intern Med 70:* 549, 1969.
41. Brown, J. H., Kennedy, B. J.: Mithramycin in the treatment of disseminated testicular neoplasms. *N Engl J Med 272:* 111–118, 1965.
42. Ream, N. W., et al: Mithramycin therapy in disseminated germinal, testicular cancer. *JAMA 204:* 1030, 1968.
43. Perlia, C. P., et al: Mithramycin treatment of hypercalcemia. *Cancer 25:* 389, 1970.
44. Elias, E., et al: Control of hypercalcemia with mithramycin. *Ann Surg 175:* 431, 1972.
45. Elias, E., et al: Hypercalcemia crisis in neoplastic diseases: Management with mithramycin. *Surgery 71:* 631, 1972.
46. Singer, F., et al: Mithramycin treatment of intractable hypercalcemia due to parathyroid carcinoma. *N Engl J Med 283:* 634, 1970.
47. Kofman, S., et al: Mithramycin in the treatment of embryonal cancer. *Cancer 17:* 938, 1964.
48. Pechet, M. M., et al: Metabolic studies with a new series of 1,4-diene steroids. II. Effects in normal subjects of prednisone, prednisolone, and 9-α-fluoroprednisolone. *J Clin Invest 38:* 691, 1959.
49. Laake, H.: The action of corticosteroids on the renal reabsorption of calcium. *Acta Endocrinol (Kbh) 34:* 60, 1960.
50. Caniggra, A., Gennari, C.: In *Clinical Aspects of Metabolic Bone Disease,* ed B. Frame, A. Parfitt, H. Duncan. Excerpta Medica, Amsterdam, 1973, p. 333.
51. Jowsey, J.: Quantitative microradiography. A new approach in the evaluation of metabolic bone disease. *Am J Med 40:* 485, 1966.
52. Storey, E.: Cortisone-induced bone resorption in the rabbit. *Endocrinology 68:* 533, 1961.
53. Dent, C. E., Watson, L.: The hydrocortisone test in primary and tertiary hyperparathyroidism. *Lancet 2:* 662, 1968.
54. Fulmer, D. H., et al: Treatment of hypercalcemia. Comparison of intravenously administered phosphate, sulfate and hydrocortisone. *Arch Intern Med 129:* 923, 1972.
55. Verner, J. V., Jr., et al: Vitamin D intoxication: Report of two cases treated with cortisone. *Ann Intern Med 48:* 765, 1958.
56. Henneman, P. H., et al: Cause of hypercalciuria in sarcoid and its treatment with cortisone and sodium phytate. *J Clin Invest 35:* 1229, 1956.
57. Seyberth, H. W., et al: Prostaglandins as mediators of hypercal-

cemia associated with certain types of cancer. *N Engl J Med 293:* 1278, 1975.

58. Seyberth, H. W., et al: Characterization of the groups of patients with the hypercalcemia of cancer who respond to treatment with prostaglandin synthesis inhibitors. *Trans Assoc Am Physicians 89:* 92, 1976.

59. Nolph, K. D., Stoltz, M., Maher, J. F.: Calcium free peritoneal dialysis. Treatment of vitamin D intoxication. *Arch Intern Med 128:* 809, 1971.

60. Stoltz, M. L., et al: Factors affecting calcium removal with calcium-free peritoneal dialysis. *J Lab Clin Med 78:* 389, 1971.

61. Garrett, J. J., Cuddihee, R. E.: Calcium absorption during peritoneal dialysis. *Trans Am Soc Artif Intern Organs 14:* 372, 1968.

62. Eisenberg, E., Gottch, F. A.: Normocalcemic hyperparathyroidism culminating in hypercalcemic crisis. Treatment with hemodialysis. *Arch Intern Med 122:* 238, 1968.

63. Schreiner, G.: Dialysis of poisons and drugs—annual review. *Trans Am Soc Artif Intern Organs 18:* 563, 1972.

64. Wolf, A. V., et al: Artificial kidney function: Kinetics of hemodialysis. *J Clin Invest 30:* 1062, 1951.

65. Free, R. M., et al: Hard-water syndrome. *N Engl J Med 276:* 1113, 1967.

66. Milhaud, G., et al: Étude du mecanisme de l'action hypocalcémiante de la thyrocalcitonine. *C R Acad Sci (Paris) 261:* 813, 1965.

67. Krane, S. M., et al: Acute effects of calcitonin on bone formation in man. *Metabolism 22:* 51, 1973.

68. Milhaud, G., et al: In *Parathyroid Hormone and Thyrocalcitonin (Calcitonin),* ed. R. V. Talmage, L. F. Belanger. Excerpta Medica, Amsterdam, 1968. p. 86ff.

69. Haas, H. G., et al: Renal effects of calcitonin and parathyroid extract in man. Studies in hypoparathyroidism. *J Clin Invest 50:* 2689, 1971.

70. Bijvoet, O., et al: Natriuretic effect of calcitonin in man. *N Engl J Med 284:* 681, 1971.

71. Talmage, R. V., et al: The influence of calcitonins on the disappearance of radiocalcium and radiophosphorus from plasma. *Endocrinology 90:* 1185, 1972.

72. Neer, R. M., et al: Pharmacology of calcitonin: Human studies, In *Calcitonin 1969,* ed. S. Taylor, G. Foster. London, Heinemann, 1970, pp 547–554.

73. Bijvoet, O., et al: Effects of calcitonin on patients with Paget's disease, thyrotoxicosis, or hypercalcemia. *Lancet 1:* 876, 1968.

74. Buckle, R., et al: Vitamin D intoxication treated with porcine calcitonin. *Br Med J 3:* 205, 1972.

75. West, T. E. T., et al: Treatment of hypercalcemia with calcitonin. *Lancet 1:* 675, 1971.

76. Kammerman, S., Canfield, R.: Effect of porcine calcitonin on hypercalcemia in man. *J Clin Endocrinol Metab 31:* 70, 1970.

77. Foster, G. W., et al: Effect of thyrocalcitonin in man. *Lancet 1:* 107, 1966.

78. Neer, R. M., et al: Escape from calcitonin (CT) during therapy of hypercalcemia. *Clin Res 18:* 676, 1970.

79. Sorensen, O. H., Hindberg, I.: Calcitonin and bone. *Lancet 1:* 1061, 1970.

80. Raisz, L., et al: Induction, inhibition and escape as phenomena of bone resorption. In *Calcium, Parathyroid Hormone, and Calcitonin,* ed. R. V. Talmage, P. C. Munson. Amsterdam, Excerpta Medica, 1972, p. 446.

81. Hirsch, P. F., Cooper, C. W.: In *Parathyroid Hormone and Thyrocalcitonin (Calcitonin),* ed. R. V. Talmage, L. Belanger. Amsterdam, Excerpta Medica, 1968, p. 381 ff.

82. Kennedy, J. W., Talmage, R. V.: In *Parathyroid Hormone and Thyrocalcitonin (Calcitonin),* ed. R. V. Talmage, L. Belanger. Amsterdam, Excerpta Medica, 1968, p. 407ff.

83. Habener, J. F., et al: Explanation for unusual potency of salmon calcitonin. *Nature New Biol 232:* 91, 1971.

84. Purnell, D. C., et al: Treatment of primary hyperparathyroidism. *Am J Med 56:* 800, 1974.

85. Britton, D. C., et al: Renal function following parathyroid surgery in primary hyperparathyroidism. *Lancet 2:* 74, 1971.

86. Hassain, M., Smith, D. A., Nordin, B. E. C.: Parathyroid activity and postmenopausal osteoporosis. *Lancet 1:* 809, 1970.

87. Colbert, C., Mazess, R. B., Schmidt, P. B.: Bone mineral determination in vitro by radiographic photodensitometry and direct photon absorptiometry. *Invest Radiol 5:* 336, 1970.

88. Forland, M., et al: Bone density studies in primary hyperparathyroidism. *Arch Intern Med 122:* 236, 1968.

89. Pak, C. Y. C., et al: The hypercalciurias. Causes, parathyroid function, and diagnostic criteria. *J Clin Invest 54:* 387, 1974.

90. Murray, T. M., et al. Non-autonomy of hormone secretion in primary hyperparathyroidism. *Clin Endocrinol.* 1(3): 235, July 1972.

91. Jowsey, J., et al: Effect of phosphate supplements on soft tissue calcification and bone turnover. *Clin Sci 42:* 289, 1972.

92. Albright, F., et al: Studies in parathyroid physiology: Effect of phosphate ingestion in clinical hyperparathyroidism. *J Clin Invest 11:* 411, 1932.

93. Dudley, F. J., Blackburn, C. R. B.: Extraskeletal calcification complicating oral neutral-phosphate therapy. *Lancet 2:* 628, 1970.

94. Woodhouse, N. J. Y., Dagle, F. H., Joplin, G. H.: Vitamin D deficiency and primary hyperparathyroidism. *Lancet 2:* 283, 1971.

95. Lumb, G. A., and Stanbury, S. W.: Parathyroid function in human vitamin D deficiency, and vitamin D deficiency in primary hyperparathyroidism. *Am J Med 56:* 833, 1974.

96. Albright, F., Reifenstein, E. C., Jr.: *The Parathyroid Glands and Metabolic Bone Disease: Selected Studies.* Baltimore, Williams and Wilkins, 1948.

97. Habener, J., Potts, J. T., Jr: Parathyroid physiology in primary hyperparathyroidism. In *Metabolic Bone Disease,* ed. L. V. Avioli, S. M. Krane. New York, Academic Press, vol. 2, 1978.

98. Harmon, M.: Parathyroid adenoma in a child: Report of a case presenting as central nervous system disease and complicated by magnesium deficiency. *Am J Dis Child 91:* 313, 1956.

99. Barnes, B. A., Krane, S. M., and Cope, O.: Magnesium studies in relation to hyperparathyroidism. *J Clin Endocrinol Metab 17:* 1407, 1957.

100. Agna, J. W., and Goldsmith, R. E.: Primary hyperparathyroidism associated with hypomagnesemia. *N Engl J Med 258:* 222, 1958.

101. Potts, J. T., Jr. and Roberts, B.: Clinical significance of magnesium deficiency and its relation to parathyroid disease. *Am J Med Sci 235:* 206, 1958.

102. Sutton, R. A. L.: Plasma magnesium concentration in primary hyperparathyroidism. *Br Med J 1:* 529, 1970.

103. Anast, C. S., Winnacker, J. L., Forte, L. R. and Burns, T. R.: Evidence for impaired release of parathyroid hormone in magnesium deficiency. In *Program and Abstracts,* 57th Annual Meeting, Endocrine Society, 1975, abstract 47, p. 74.

104. Singer, F. R., Segre, G. V., Habener, J. F., and Potts, J. T., Jr.: Peripheral metabolism of bovine parathyroid hormone in the dog. *Metabolism 24:* 139, 1975.

105. Rude, R. K., Oldham, S. B., Sharp, C. F., Singer, F. R.: Parathyroid hormone secretion in magnesium deficiency. In *Program and Abstracts,* 59th Annual Meeting, Endocrine Society 1977, abstract 357.

106. Estep, H. L., Martinez, G. R., Jones, D.: Parathyroid hormone unresponsiveness and 3′,5′-AMP excretion. In *Program and Abstracts,* 51st Annual Meeting, Endocrine Society, 1969, abstract 145.

107. MacIntyre, I., Boss, S., Troughton, V. A.: Parathyroid hormone and magnesium homeostasis. *Nature 198:* 1058, 1963.

108. Shils, M. E.: Experimental human magnesium depletion. *Medicine 48:* 61, 1969.

109. Neer, R. M., Holick, M. F., DeLuca, H. F., Potts, J. T., Jr.: Effects of 1α-hydroxy-vitamin D$_3$ and 1,25-dihydroxy-vitamin D$_3$ on calcium and phosphorus metabolism in hypoparathyroidism. *Metabolism 24:* 1403, 1975.

110. Kooh, S. W., Fraser, D., DeLuca, H. F., et al: Treatment of hypoparathyroidism and pseudohypoparathyroidism with metabolites of vitamin D: Evidence for impaired conversion of 25-hydroxyvitamin D to 1,25-dihydroxyvitamin D. *N Engl J Med 293:* 840, 1975.

111. Jackson, C. E., Frame, B., Block, M. A.: The spectrum of hereditary hyperparathyroidism. 6th Parathyroid Conference (in press).

112. Kjellberg, R. N., and Kliman, B.: Bragg peak proton treatment for pituitary-related conditions. *Proc Roy Soc Med 67:* 32, 1974.

113. Daughaday, W. H.: The adenohypophysis. In *Textbook of Endocrinology,* 5th edition, ed. R. H. Williams. Philadelphia. W. B. Saunders, 1974, p. 31.

114. Ballard, H. S., Frame, B., Hartsock, R. J.: Familial multiple endocrine adenoma–peptic ulcer complex. *Medicine 43:* 481, 1964.

115. Fox, P. S., Hofmann, J. W., Wilson, S. D., DeCosse, J. J.: Surgical management of the Zollinger-Ellison syndrome. *Surg Clin North Am 54:* 395, 1974.

116. Friesen, S. R.: Effect of total gastrectomy on the Zollinger-Ellison tumor: Observations by second-look procedures. *Surgery 62:* 609, 1967.

58

Surgical Management of Primary Hyperparathyroidism

Chiu-an Wang

Foremost for the surgeon in the management of primary hyperparathyroidism is to find and resect the diseased parathyroid glands. It is essential, therefore, for the surgeon to be familiar with the anatomic distribution of the parathyroid glands and to be able to differentiate a normal from an abnormal gland.

LOCATION OF NORMAL PARATHYROID GLANDS

Despite its widespread distribution, the pattern of location of the normal parathyroid gland is fairly predictable.[1] The parathyroid has a close embryologic relationship with the thyroid and the thymus glands. Originating from the fourth branchial pouch, the upper, or superior, gland is invariably associated with the lateral thyroid lobe and accordingly is commonly found at the cricothyroid junction (77 percent) or in the dorsum of the upper pole of the thyroid (22 percent) (Fig. 58-1A,B). Rarely, it may be found in an ectopic location such as the midretropharyngeal or retroesophageal space (Fig. 58-1C) Because of this unique relationship with the thyroid, the upper gland is generally found easily at surgery.

The lower, or inferior, gland, on the other hand, has a much wider distribution than the upper. With the thymus, it originates from the third branchial pouch. As the thymus descends caudally, the lower gland invariably migrates with it until it reaches the level of the lower pole of the thyroid, where it is dissociated from the thymus. Of the lower glands, nearly half are normally found on the surface of the lower pole of the thyroid (42 percent) (Fig. 58-2A) or near the lower pole (15 percent) (Fig. 58-2C). The remaining glands are located within the thymic tongue (39 percent); rarely, one descends deep into the mediastinum (2 percent) (Fig. 58-2B). A small number are left high in the neck or alongside the carotid sheath as a result of an anomalous development (2 percent) (Fig. 58-2D).

PATHOLOGIC DISPLACEMENT OF DISEASED PARATHYROID GLANDS

Theoretically, because the normal parathyroid gland falls in a rather constant pattern of distribution, it can easily be found; in practice, however, difficulties in finding the abnormal gland are frequently encountered. While a gland that is confined beneath the surgical capsule of the thyroid almost never moves far, even when enlarged and diseased, a parathyroid which lies outside the capsule is often displaced into the superior posterior or superior anterior mediastinum. This unique anatomy of the parathyroid gland explains why some diseased glands are more elusive than others.

INTRAOPERATIVE PATHOLOGIC DIAGNOSIS

Broadly speaking, there are two pathologic entities of hyperparathyroidism—neoplasia and hyperplasia.[2] (See discussion in Chapter 53.) In the experience of the Massachusetts General Hospital, of the patients with neoplasia, 81 percent have an adenoma and 3 percent a carcinoma; 15 percent of the patients have diffuse hyperplasia. The so-called "double adenomas," if they ever exist, are extremely rare (Table 58-1). Neoplasia is a localized process, involving only one gland; the remaining three glands are generally free of the disease, and, in fact, in the presence of hypercalcemia, the uninvolved glands are invariably suppressed and atrophic. Under such circumstances, the uninvolved glands are small in size, yellowish tan in color,* and soft in consistency. These glands often have a sharp edge. These macroscopic features aid greatly in distinguishing a suppressed normal from a diseased gland.

In contrast, primary hyperplasia, whether of the chief- or the clear-cell type, is a diffuse disease process involving all four glands and even a supernumerary fifth or sixth gland. While hyperplastic glands may differ in size—some are large, others small—they are invariably uniformly beefy red and bulbous. Thus, diagnosis of primary hyperplasia as opposed to neoplasia can often be made based on the macroscopic features of at least one other gland. If the second gland is normal, the enlarged gland is an adenoma (or, rarely, carcinoma). If the second gland is also diseased, one can safely conclude that the patient has primary hyperplasia.[3,4]

Histologically, stromal fat cells are abundant in a normal gland but few or none occur in a diseased gland. On the basis of the quantity of stromal fat cells, an experienced pathologist can usually determine whether a parathyroid of normal size is diseased or not by frozen-section Sudan fat stain, and thus differentiate neoplasia from hyperplasia.

SURGICAL APPROACH

That the extent of surgery depends on the pathologic diagnosis is obvious. For an adenoma, simple excision of the diseased gland is all that is needed. A biopsy of an uninvolved second gland

---

*Because the number of stromal fat cells is relatively fewer in the gland of a young person, the normal gland of a child and an adolescent generally appears yellowish brown.

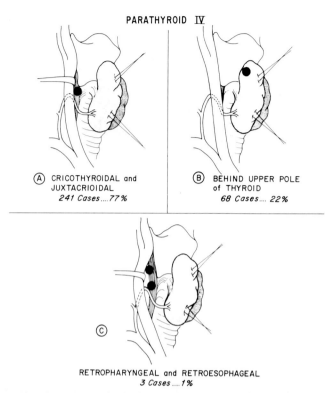

PARATHYROID IV

(A) CRICOTHYROIDAL and JUXTACRIOIDAL
241 Cases....77%

(B) BEHIND UPPER POLE of THYROID
68 Cases.... 22%

(C) RETROPHARYNGEAL and RETROESOPHAGEAL
3 Cases....1%

Fig. 58-1. Anatomic distribution of 312 upper parathyroid glands

must be taken for confirmation. For primary hyperplasia, removal of one or even two is inadequate for cure. Most of the hyperfunctioning tissue must be excised, leaving generally about 75 mg of hyperplastic tissue in situ with an intact blood supply. Hyperparathyroidism would invariably continue if the surgery had been

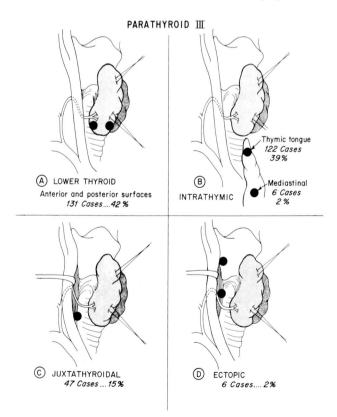

PARATHYROID III

(A) LOWER THYROID
Anterior and posterior surfaces
131 Cases....42%

(B) INTRATHYMIC
Thymic tongue
122 Cases
39%

Mediastinal
6 Cases
2%

(C) JUXTATHYROIDAL
47 Cases....15%

(D) ECTOPIC
6 Cases....2%

Fig. 58-2. Anatomic distribution of 312 lower parathyroid glands.

Table 58-1. Primary Hyperparathyroidism: 702 Cases Successfully Treated at the Massachusetts General Hospital (1930–1975)

Pathologic Entity	No. of Cases	Percent
Neoplasia	598	85
Single adenoma	571	81
Double adenoma*	6	1
Carcinoma	21	3
Hyperplasia	104	15
Chief cell	84	12
Clear cell	20	3

*Tentative diagnosis.

inadequate.[5] Conversely, excessive excision or inadvertent injury to the blood supply of residual tissue leads to hypoparathyroidism.

In the case of a carcinoma, the neoplasm must be excised with a margin of normal tissue. Rupture of the tumor capsule must be carefully avoided, or local implants invariably develop, and recurrence is prone to ensue. Conventional radical neck dissection with removal of lymph glands as a prophylactic procedure is seldom indicated, as the disease is rarely spread by the lymphatics.[6]

Surgery of the parathyroid is demanding, and its success depends in a large measure on the skill and experience of the surgeon. He must understand where to find the glands and recognize the normal as well as the diseased. A meticulous technique and bloodless field are essential. Since the first operation often affords the best and possibly the last chance to cure the disease, cursory exploration should be discouraged.

POSTOPERATIVE CARE

In a majority of the patients, the postoperative course is uneventful. Complications are few. After successful surgery, the serum calcium is reversed to a normal range, usually from the first postoperative day on. In patients with little or no skeletal involvement, a drop of serum calcium of 2–3 mg/100 ml from the preoperative level signifies surgical success. In patients with underlying severe bone disease, the fall in calcium is even more dramatic, and the serum calcium may plummet to a level of 7 mg/100 ml or lower, at which level tetany invariably ensues. Tingling in the fingers, toes, and lips accompanied by circumoral pallor is a commonplace occurrence. In most cases, symptoms are self-limiting and rarely require calcium therapy. If a strongly positive Chvostek or Trousseau sign is present, accompanied by listlessness and a feeling of impending doom, vigorous calcium therapy is needed.

UNUSUAL POSTOPERATIVE COMPLICATIONS

Of the unusual postoperative complications, renal colic is the commonest. It is triggered by the return of smooth-muscle tone of the ureter with the reversal of hypercalcemia. The peristaltic contraction of the ureter forces the stone to move downward. If it is small, the stone may pass uneventfully, but, if large, it may require surgical removal. It is of historical interest that the first patient diagnosed as having hyperparathyroidism in this country, Captain Charles Martell, was successfully treated but unfortunately died from an obstructive ureteric stone 6 weeks after a mediastinal exploration.[7]

Next in frequency, intraoperative acute pancreatitis may occur in patients with severe hyperparathyroidism. Though its pathogenesis remains obscure, it is highly possible that surgical manipulation of a large parathyroid mass causes a sudden outpouring of parathyroid hormone that may, in turn, by some mechanism as yet unknown, precipitate and trigger acute pancreatitis.[8] We encountered 3 patients with this serious complication, all of whom had severe hyperparathyroidism and large tumors; fortunately, all recovered after conservative medical therapy. Experience has taught us to handle a large parathyroid tumor mass with utmost gentleness at the time of its removal.

Occasionally, a patient may develop acute psychosis, or even severe mental derangement immediately after surgery. Whether or not this is the result of the operation is difficult to ascertain. In contrast, some patients who previously suffered from mental confusion and amnesia have noticeably improved after successful surgery. Whatever the relationship between mental derangement and hyperparathyroidism, a psychiatric evaluation by a competent, medically oriented psychiatrist prior to surgery is important in any patient who shows signs of mental instability.

Hemorrhage, infection, or injury to the recurrent laryngeal nerve are rare complications, but they may occur.[9] However, these complications can generally be avoided if the surgeon is familiar with the anatomy of the neck, if he is meticulous in his technique, and if he understands the anatomic distribution of the parathyroid glands.

MEDIASTINAL EXPLORATION

Of the 702 patients with primary hyperparathyroidism successfully surgically treated at the Massachusetts General Hospital between 1930 and 1975, 23 (3 percent) required a mediastinal exploration. The initial exploration of the neck was unrewarding either because the diseased parathyroid had been ectopic in location or because it had been displaced into the mediastinum. As a rule, before mediastinal exploration is undertaken, the missing gland must be excluded from the neck or within the thyroid. Experience has shown that over 80 percent of the missing glands were located in the neck or were retrievable from a neck incision.[10] If the hypercalcemia is mild and the disease is not severe, it is better to postpone further exploration rather than attempt mediastinal exploration immediately. Localization of the missing diseased gland is often desirable prior to reexploration and can be carefully carried out by venous catheterization and radioimmunoassay for parathyroid hormone, either alone (see Chapter 56) or in conjunction with arteriography. In experienced hands, these studies are useful in approximately 80 percent of the patients.[11,12]

Of paramount importance is the decision about how best to manage the diseased gland when it is found. In many patients who have had one or more negative parathyroid explorations, one or two normal glands have frequently been excised by intent or damaged by accident, particularly by the use of Bovie cautery. In this instance, removal of the entire diseased gland often results in permanent hypoparathyroidism, which in itself may be worse than the disease. Careful judgment must be exercised as to how much functioning tissue (unless it is cancerous) should be left behind with a viable blood supply so that the patient has neither persistent hyperparathyroidism nor permanent hypoparathyroidism from the surgery. We prefer to leave in situ about a 75-mg remnant of the tissue in an easily accessible place in the neck marked with a 2-cm-long black silk for identification in the event that further resection of the remnant is needed. If the diseased gland is in the mediastinum of a patient in whom all the normal parathyroid tissues have either been excised or destroyed, a sliver of the hyperfunctioning benign tissue is minced and implanted in the subcutaneous or the platysma-muscle layer. We have not found it necessary or advisable to transplant the tissue to a new locale, as advocated by others.[13,14]

SUMMARY

Between 1930 and 1975, 712 patients with primary hyperparathyroidism were cared for by the physicians and surgeons at the Massachusetts General Hospital. Of these, 702 were successfully operated upon and the hyperparathyroidism was corrected. Ten were considered failures; in these patients the diseased gland was not found and hyperparathyroidism continued. These were patients who had had multiple unsuccessful explorations prior to reoperation, with 6 patients previously operated on elsewhere.

Our experience has shown that the successful management of patients with hyperparathyroidism demands an interdisciplinary collaboration of the internist, pathologist, radiologist, and surgeon. Each plays an important role independent of the other; nevertheless, all should be actively involved in the care of these patients. As for the surgeon, he alone must possess the experience in recognizing a parathyroid gland when he sees one, and in differentiating a normal from a diseased gland. His knowledge of the pathologic anatomy of the disease and the skill involved in knowing how to ferret out the diseased gland are indispensable, and they come only from painstaking learning of the distribution of the normal gland, the displacement of the diseased gland, and the anatomy of the neck in general.

REFERENCES

1. Wang, C. A.: The anatomic basis of parathyroid surgery. *Ann Surg 188:* 271, 1976.
2. Castleman, B., Mallory, T. B.: The pathology of the parathyroid gland in hyperparathyroidism. *Am J Pathol 11:* 1, 1935.
3. Wang, C. A.: Surgery of the parathyroid glands. *Adv Surg 5:* 109, 1971.
4. Cope, O.: The story of hyperparathyroidism at the Massachusetts General Hospital. *N Engl J Med 274:* 1174, 1966.
5. Cope, O., Keynes, W. M., Roth, S. I., Castleman, B.: Primary chief-cell hyperplasia of the parathyroid glands: a new entity in the surgery of hyperparathyroidism. *Ann Surg 148:* 375, 1958.
6. Wang, C. A., Cope, O.: Carcinoma of the parathyroid glands, in Nealon, T. F., Jr. (ed): Management of the Patient with Cancer. Philadelphia, Saunders, 1965, pp 425–434.
7. Bauer, W., Federman, D. D.: Hyperparathyroidism epitomized: the case of Captain Charles E. Martell. *Metabolism 11:* 21, 1962.
8. Haverback, B. J., Dyce, B., Bundy, H., Edmondson, H. A.: Trypsin, trypsinogen and trypsin inhibitor in human pancreatic juice. *Am J Med 29:* 424, 1960.
9. Wang, C. A.: The use of the inferior cornu of the thyroid cartilage in identifying the recurrent laryngeal nerve. *Surg Gynecol Obstet 140:* 91, 1975.
10. Wang, C. A.: Parathyroid reexploration: a clinical and pathological study of 112 patients. *Ann Surg 186:* 140, 1977.
11. Bilezikian, J. P., Doppman, J. L., Shimkin, P. M., Powell, D., Wells, S. A., Heath, D. A., Ketcham, A. S., Monchik, J., Mallette, L. E., Potts, J. T., Aurbach, G. D.: Preoperative localization of abnormal parathyroid tissue: cumulative experience with venous sampling and arteriography. *Am J Med 55:* 505,514 1973.
12. Seldinger, S. I.: Localization of parathyroid adenomata by arteriography. *Acta Radiol 42:* 353, 1954.
13. Wells, S. A., Ellis, G. J., Gunnells, J. C., Schneider, A. B., Sherwood, L. M.: Parathyroid autotransplantation in primary parathyroid hyperplasia. *N Engl J Med 295:* 57, 1976.
14. Cope, O.: Hyperparathyroidism—too little, too much surgery? *N Engl J Med 295:* 100, 1976.

59

Secondary Hyperparathyroidism: Pathophysiology and Etiology

Jane E. Mahaffey
John T. Potts, Jr.

The Nature of the Adaptation—Functional Autonomy versus Growth
    Autonomy
Clinical Disorders Associated with Secondary Hyperparathyroidism

Secondary hyperparathyroidism can be defined as *hypertrophy* of the parathyroids and consequent *excessive secretion* of parathyroid hormone found in diverse situations in which there is resistance to the biological actions of PTH at the bone, kidney, and intestine. Most evidence suggests that it is the hypocalcemia resulting from resistance to hormone action that triggers the hypertrophy of the glands. Whether hypocalcemia is indeed the stimulus to growth of the parathyroids and, if so, whether the mediation of the calcium effect is direct or indirect is unknown. Increased secretion of hormone per se (over hours to days in response to hypocalcemia without an increase in parathyroid tissue mass) should be distinguished from secondary hyperparathyroidism in which hyperplasia of the glands and much greater secretory capacity as well as increased secretion of hormone are involved.[1] The importance of recognizing the glandular hyperplasia present in states of secondary hyperparathyroidism is underlined by the recent appreciation that glands which have become hyperplastic, especially in chronic renal failure, may not always return to normal size or function when the cause of original resistance is removed. Compensatory adaptation of the parathyroids (secondary hyperparathyroidism) seems to be called into play when resistance to hormone action is severe or prolonged. In addition to a deficiency in hormone action per se, there are often additional factors that contribute to hypocalcemia, such as serum phosphate elevation or uremia. The complex issues involved in the pathology of secondary hyperparathyroidism have recently been critically reviewed.[1a]

Certain special features of the normal physiology of parathyroid function may explain the invariable development of glandular hyperplasia as part of the adaptive response in secondary hyperparathyroidism. Important in the genesis of secondary hyperparathyroidism is the fact that the total amount of preformed hormone stored in the gland is small in relation to the normal hormone secretion rate. (The biosynthetic pathways of parathyroid hormone production and the physiology of secretion are discussed in Chapters 43 and 44.) The fractional turnover of hormone in the gland is high even with basal rates of secretion; this situation contrasts greatly with the storage capacity in many other endocrine organs in which polypeptide hormones are stored in large quantities in relation to their basal secretory rates.[2,3] The maximal secretion rate of the parathyroids is only approximately five times

the basal secretion rate.[4–6] It is not surprising, therefore, that to overcome hypocalcemia in the presence of prolonged resistance to PTH action, greater rates of secretion may be necessary than can be obtained via maximal stimulation of normal parathyroid glands. Under such circumstances, an increase in the mass of functioning parathyroid tissue develops, presumably in some way mediated by chronic hypocalcemia.

Hyperplastic parathyroid glands undergo an increase in both the relative and absolute numbers of chief cells and show an absence or marked decrease in fat cells.[7] Studies at the ultrastructural level reveal a marked increase in the number of chief cells in the active phase of the secretory cycle rather than a resting stage whenever there is chronic stimulation of the parathyroids. Active cells have an increased Golgi apparatus, decreased amount of glycogen, and an increase in electron-dense secretory granules (Chapter 41). However, even the active-phase cell can become relatively depleted of secretory granules after continuous stimulation. It is therefore postulated that chronic stimulation increases the gland weight and volume by increasing the number of cells in the active phase as well as by increasing cell division so that the ultimate mass of parathyroid tissue increases as much as 100-fold.[8–13]

THE NATURE OF THE ADAPTATION— FUNCTIONAL AUTONOMY VERSUS GROWTH AUTONOMY

Several central questions are posed concerning the adaptation of the parathyroids in secondary hyperparathyroidism. The first issue concerns the nature of the cellular or secretory response in secondary hyperparathyroidism to changes in serum calcium level. Are the hyperplastic parathyroids *functionally autonomous*? The second issue involves the *reversibility* of the *abnormal growth* of the parathyroids, the cellular hypertrophy, and/or the increased number of cells characteristic of secondary hyperparathyroidism. Are the hyperplastic parathyroids resistant to involution?

In regard to the first issue, the nature of feedback control of hormone production by blood calcium in normal and abnormal parathyroid glands, several aspects of known physiological and pathophysiological mechanisms must be considered. Hormone secretion is always partially responsive to changes in blood calcium levels, even in adenomas. But conversely, an elevated blood calcium may never completely suppress hormone production, even in normal glands.* Hence, it seems established that *total autonomy of function* is not characteristic even of parathyroid adenomas; autonomy of function in various disorders of the parathyroids, such as secondary hyperparathyroidism, if present, must be more subtle than simply a fixed output of hormone independent of blood calcium.

The precise nature of the abnormal cellular control of hormone secretion in secondary hyperparathyroidism (as well as the cellular defect in primary hyperparathyroidism) has not yet been defined. The example of secondary hyperparathyroidism most extensively studied has been that of the parturient cow. The amount of PTH secretion for any given calcium level is always excessive in animals with hyperplastic parathyroids but varies from one animal to the next (Fig. 59-1). This increased slope of response clearly implies either increased secretion per cell for the same stimulus (as compared to normal cells) or merely an increase in the number of cells actively secreting hormone but in a manner quantitatively identical to that of a normal cell.†

Similar to these results in cows with secondary hyperparathyroidism, findings in patients with hyperparathyroidism, both primary and secondary, also show an increased slope of the response function relating PTH secretion rate and blood calcium. Again, as in studies in animals, it is unclear whether exaggerated hormone secretion reflects simply the increased mass of functioning cells or increased function per cell.

The principal unsettled issue in primary and secondary hyperparathyroidism is whether there are defects in the cellular response to calcium alteration, i.e., partially autonomous or defective control of hormone production. It is difficult to analyze the situation in man because of the heterogeneity of circulating hormone. However, with regard to defective control of secretion, useful data about secretory control in normal glands have been provided by Mayer,[5] who circumvented difficulties due to the heterogeneity of circulating hormone by direct analysis of effluent blood in vivo in cows. His results (Chapter 44) demonstrate that in normal cows, a decrease in secretion occurs when the calcium is raised from 9 mg/100 ml to 11 mg/100 ml; however, no further suppression occurs as calcium is raised above that point despite many hours of hypercalcemia in the 12–16 mg/100 ml range (Fig. 59-2). This low but persistent level of calcium-independent secretion of PTH in normal glands could be expected to become a problem in patients with secondary hyperparathyroidism; i.e., there would be an increased mass of parathyroid tissue and therefore a higher level of calcium-independent secretion.

A model of more extreme defective control is shown in Figure 59-3. In this concept, there is a set-point error whereby the point of suppression, maximal stimulation, and half-maximal stimulation of PTH production, i.e., the response function, is shifted away from normal toward a higher calcium concentration (as well as being steeper). Such a set-point defect would clearly account for hyper-

---

*Initial studies of parathyroid gland sensitivity to calcium suppression in patients with primary hyperparathyroidism showed divergent results between those with adenomas and those with primary hyperplasia; patients with adenomas showed no suppression.[14] Later studies documented suppression and stimulation in both instances.[15] It now appears that much of the discrepancy in the previous studies can be accounted for by the considerable heterogeneity of circulating forms of parathyroid hormone and variations in its recognition by various antisera (Chapter 45).

†These studies in cows performed prior to 1968 when the heterogeneity of circulating hormone was first identified by Berson and Yalow[16] did not provide direct measures of secretion of active hormone and therefore did not permit precise analysis of pathophysiological mechanisms of secretion.

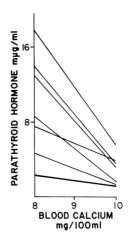

Fig. 59-1. Peripheral PTH levels in relation to plasma calcium in parturient cows with secondary hyperparathyroidism. The heavy line (—) illustrates the response of normal cows for comparison.

calcemia in primary hyperparathyroidism (excessive hormone production that is not shut off despite hypercalcemia due to the set-point defect) but could be present also in secondary hyperparathyroidism even though patients are not hypercalcemic as a result of the associated resistance to hormone action. The importance of considering this possible pathophysiological defect in secondary hyperparathyroidism is the explanation it provides for the appearance of hypercalcemia when the resistance to hormone action is reversed. An underlying set-point defect in control of hormone production, for example, could account for the hypercalcemia sometimes seen in secondary hyperparathyroidism (such as after renal transplantation); once the block to hormone action has been removed by successful renal transplantation, secondary hyperparathyroidism then becomes analogous to primary hyperparathyroidism. In this model, the set-point defect permits excessive hormone production (Fig. 59-3), despite hypercalcemia after renal function is restored.

Such cellular defects may exist in secondary hyperparathyroidism in man, particularly in renal failure, but do not seem to be evident in cows with secondary hyperparathyroidism. In these animals, artificially induced hypercalcemia leads to a rapid suppression of hormone production at a level of calcium similar to

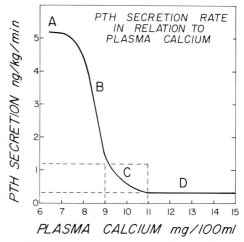

Fig. 59-2. PTH secretion rate in relation to plasma calcium as determined by analysis of parathyroid effluent blood in vivo in normal cows (see text, G. P. Mayer, Chapter 44).

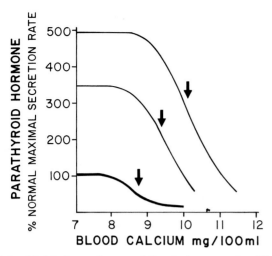

Fig. 59-3. Model of set-point-error defect for hyperparathyroidism. The heavy line (—) represents the normal (a replot of A, B, C of Fig. 59-2), with the thin lines (—) representing moderate and severe examples of hyperparathyroidism. All data are illustrated for comparison as percent of normal maximal secretion rate of PTH in response to changing calcium concentration. The arrows denote the different points of half-maximal stimulation in each case.

that causing suppression in normal animals; a set-point defect is not seen (Fig. 59-4).

An alternate pattern of defective control, favored by the authors as probably being present in secondary hyperparathyroidism, is illustrated in Figure 59-5. In this model, as in the set-point

model, the increased mass of tissue is responsible for the increased slope of response; in contrast to the set-point defect, however, a high level of hormone secretion above 11 mg/100 ml calcium is caused merely by the nonsuppressible secretion seen even in normal glands but exaggerated in hyperplasia due to tissue mass. In such a pathophysiological mechanism, in contrast to the mechanism illustrated in Figure 59-3, there is no defect in control of hormone production by any individual cell. Rather, each cell functions normally without a set-point defect, but the increased number of parathyroid cells is responsible for excessive hormone production in the zone of nonsuppressible secretion above 11 mg/100 ml of calcium. The latter phenomenon could then account for reported cases of posttransplant hypercalcemia if the glands do not involute; a set-point defect need not be postulated.

These issues, in turn, focus attention on the second question, autonomy of tissue growth. In primary hyperparathyroidism, whether resulting from adenoma or primary chief-cell hyperplasia, there seems by definition to be autonomy in growth. There was originally no resistance to hormone action to trigger an adaptive response, and little if any evidence of spontaneous involution is found. Most have believed that in secondary hyperparathyroidism, on the other hand, spontaneous involution does occur when resistance to hormone action is removed. In chronic renal failure, for example, therapy with vitamin D metabolites, high calcium intake, and agents to reduce phosphate absorption often lead to increases in basal blood calcium, a reduced stimulation of the parathyroids, and, then, it has generally been believed, involution of the increased parathyroid tissue mass. However, it is by no means certain that involution occurs in all individuals with secondary hyperparathyroidism.[17] In fact, as outlined in Figure 59-6, it is difficult to detect involution of the hyperplastic glands in secondary hyperparathyroidism merely by measurements of basal hormone concentration during therapy. Figure 59-6 illustrates the difficulty incurred when trying to use changes in basal levels of parathyroid hormone as an indicator of involution of tissue mass and associated defects in secretion. In the case of secondary hyperparathyroidism, a change in the degree of stimulation (i.e., rise in serum calcium level as a result of treatment) per se would be expected to produce a fall in the secretion of PTH along the abnormal slope of response without necessarily implying an invo-

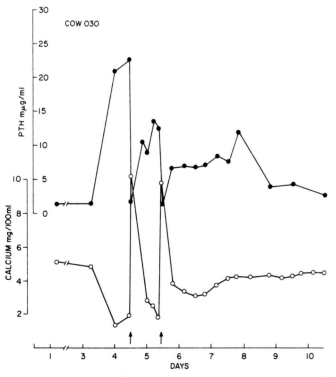

Fig. 59-4. Suppression of PTH by calcium infusion in a hypocalcemic parturient cow with secondary hyperparathyroidism. Note that PTH measurements are on peripheral blood samples, not effluent blood as in Fig. 59-2; hormone concentrations approached 1–2 ng/ml. Completeness of suppression of hormone output was not seen, but the marked fall with a calcium level no higher than 10 mg/100 ml did not indicate a "set-point" defect.

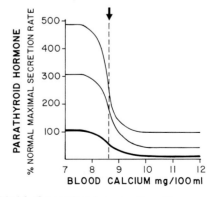

Fig. 59-5. Model of secondary hyperparathyroidism associated with an increased mass of tissue. The heavy line (—) represents the normal (Fig. 59-1), and the thin (—) lines represent moderate and severe examples of hyperparathyroidism. All data are illustrated as percent normal maximal secretion rate of PTH (as in Fig. 59-3). The arrow denotes the identical point of half-maximal stimulation common to both normal and hyperparathyroid subjects. Note should be made of the increasing level of nonsuppressible secretion secondary to the increased mass of normally responsive tissue.

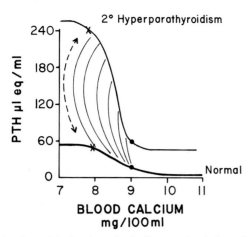

Fig. 59-6. A model showing criteria for true involution of excessive secretion of PTH in secondary hyperparathyroidism. The heavy (—) line represents the PTH response to a changing blood calcium in normals; the thin line (—) represents that in secondary hyperparathyroidism. As noted, a rise in serum calcium from low levels (X) to normal levels (●) results in a fall in PTH in both cases. Involution of secondary hyperparathyroidism can only be known to have occurred if the PTH response to change in blood calcium changes from the abnormal response curve (— line) to the normal response curve (—), as illustrated by the arrow (→).

lution of the hyperplasia. Rather than assessing involution by the absolute level of PTH, it seems clear that the information needed to prove whether involution occurs is whether the parathyroid response function (hormone production as a function of calcium) returns to a normal pattern. Such information could be achieved by a deliberate lowering of blood calcium with any of several measures such as EDTA infusion. A return to a normal curve would offer the best criterion of true involution (Fig. 59-6). A failure to see a normal secretory response curve would suggest that in such individuals, the hyperplastic parathyroids have failed to involute. In such a situation, the autonomy of growth results in a persistence of an inappropriately large tissue mass and hence a high secretion of hormone despite normal or even elevated blood calcium levels *without* the implication of an autonomy in function of individual cells.

Some patients with chronic renal failure, for example, develop severe parathyroid hyperplasia as evidenced by basal PTH levels 20- to 30-fold elevated and clinically significant osteitis fibrosa cystica. Their medical histories usually reveal a long duration of disease complicated by chronic uncompensated stimuli to PTH secretion (↑ phosphorus, ↓ calcium). Some observers now find that, at least in some patients of this type, once the disease has progressed to this degree of severity, despite apparently successful reversal of factors responsible for hormone resistance (giving vitamin D, restricting phosphate intake) there is little effect on the parathyroid hyperfunction over periods of as long as several years. Although formal studies of gland function such as those described above were not made, the persistence of osteitis fibrosa, other symptoms such as pruritus, and chemical abnormalities such as high calcium, phosphate, and parathyroid hormone levels[18-20] suggest the failure of involution of the parathyroids. Even more dramatically in some patients, sudden reversal of the previous resistance to the biologic effect of PTH as accomplished by renal transplantation can actually lead to severe post-renal-transplant hypercalcemia.[17]

Development of hypercalcemia with or without renal transplant or progressive osteitis fibrosa cystica has been described in the past by the term "tertiary hyperparathyroidism" because of a presumption in such cases that an adenoma develops in one or more of the previous hyperplastic glands, thus explaining nonsuppressibility of parathyroid function. However, as discussed above, autonomy is not characteristic even of adenomas, and abnormalities in control of secretion occur with hyperplastic glands (Figs. 59-3 and 59-5). The development of adenomas is clearly not responsible for hypercalcemia in patients with renal failure, since parathyroid hyperplasia, not adenoma, is found in most such cases at operation. Therefore, these patients would seem to establish that there can be a failure of involution of hyperplastic parathyroids despite removal of the original stimulus, resistance to hormone action. The defective control of hormone secretion associated with the hyperplasia and secondary hyperparathyroidism, whether it be of the set-point-error type (Fig. 59-3) or simply exaggerated nonsuppressible secretion from normally functioning cells present in excess (Fig. 59-5), accounts for excessive PTH production.

The more common example of the clinical problem in reversal of secondary hyperparathyroidism is that of the patient who, after initiation of dialysis or early transplantation, reverts to a state of normal calcium levels but continues to have parathyroid hormone hypersecretion, albeit mild. Whether such patients will eventually revert to a truly euparathyroid status is not clear from current experience or literature reports. More detailed studies of the process of involution (Fig. 59-6) may eventually resolve the issue. To a lesser extent, similar problems are occasionally encountered in patients with long-standing vitamin D deficiency[21,22] or steatorrhea and malabsorption.[23]

The above considerations of the pathophysiological characteristics and the ultimate resolution of the abnormality in function or growth in severe secondary hyperparathyroidism are, in most instances, not associated with serious clinical issues in the many forms of hyperparathyroidism that are mild or short-lived. For example, the typical patient with dietary vitamin D deficiency or anticonvulsant use has a mild elevation (1.5- to 3-fold) in parathyroid hormone secretion consistent with the degree of compensation necessary to maintain a normal calcium. In addition, such patients clinically show no evidence of osteitis fibrosa cystica. Experimentally, severe vitamin D deficiency will produce hyperplastic parathyroid glands in animals[24] (similar to the hyperplastic tissue found at surgery in some of the first-described cases of pseudohypoparathyroidism).[25] However, administration of vitamin D with reversal of the cause for resistance to PTH action is followed by a prompt return of basal PTH levels to normal, suggesting that with mild hyperparathyroidism there is no growth autonomy in such D-deficient rats. Vitamin D therapy in high dose with associated improvement of bone, intestinal, and renal transport of calcium and phosphate in patients with pseudohypoparathyroidism is usually accompanied by signs of abatement of the hyperparathyroidism.

In the future, a clearer understanding of the frequency and completeness of involution of secondary hyperparathyroidism should become possible by the application and interpretation of serial provocative tests of patterns of secretion in individual patients (Fig. 59-6). Such an approach should allow a more appropriate assessment of the effectiveness of various therapeutic modalities and indications for surgical therapy.

CLINICAL DISORDERS ASSOCIATED WITH SECONDARY HYPERPARATHYROIDISM

Since the initial description by Fuller Albright of the compensatory nature of hyperparathyroidism as manifested by osteitis fibrosa cystica in renal failure, an ever-increasing spectrum of disease processes has been found to be accompanied by secondary

Table 59-1. Disorders Associated with Secondary Hyperparathyroidism

A. Vitamin D-deficiency rickets
  1. Dietary vitamin D deficiency
  2. Malabsorption of vitamin D and calcium
    a. Primary small-bowel disease
    b. Short-bowel syndrome
    c. Postgastrectomy syndrome
  3. Drug-induced osteomalacia
    a. Anticonvulsants (Dilantin, phenobarbital)
    b. Cholestyramine
    c. Laxative abuse
B. Vitamin D-dependent rickets
C. Vitamin D-resistant rickets
  (X-linked hypophosphatemia) *after* treatment with phosphate
D. Pseudohypoparathyroidism
E. Hypomagnesemia
F. Chronic renal failure
  1. Early stages with phosphate retention inducing hypocalcemia
  2. Late, severe phase with
    a. Deficiency of renal 1-hydroxylase activity
    b. Deficient intestinal absorption secondary to uremia

hyperparathyroidism, as noted in Table 59-1. With the advent of the immunoassay for PTH, secondary hyperparathyroidism has been documented to play a role in physiological adaptation to a number of disease states.[1a] The common denominator of all these disorders is an increased stimulation of parathyroid secretion, presumably by a chronic tendency to hypocalcemia. At any given point in the course of the patient's disease, however, hypocalcemia may be difficult to document because the compensatory hypersecretion of PTH has resulted in a partial correction of the hypocalcemia.

The mechanism responsible for the tendency to hypocalcemia can be grouped into disorders associated with (1) a deficiency of active $1,25(OH)_2D_3$ (vitamin D deficiency, malabsorption syndrome, vitamin D-dependent rickets, and anephric states); (2) a depression of serum calcium by progressive or persistent hyperphosphatemia (phosphate retention in chronic renal failure, and phosphate-treated vitamin D-resistant rickets); and (3) a resistance of renal and bone target organs to biologically active parathyroid hormone (hypomagnesemia, pseudohypoparathyroidism).

In view of the variety of etiologies, it is not surprising to find a wide range in the presenting clinical and biochemical parameters.

Points of importance in establishing the cause of the hyperparathyroidism include several clinical issues. In the *medical history,* a dietary profile, drug-ingestion history (anticonvulsants, diuretics, laxatives, cholestyramine), bowel symptoms or history of bowel surgery, symptoms of renal failure, and symptoms of hypocalcemia are important. In reviewing a *family history,* one must take note of relatives with short stature, with or without deformity, skeletal abnormalities such as shortened metacarpals or metatarsals, convulsive disorders, tetany, mental retardation, or familial renal disease. On *physical examination,* attention should be paid to any evidence of skeletal deformities of long bones or metacarpals and metatarsals, bone tenderness, positive Trousseau or Chvostek signs, muscle weakness, or subcutaneous calcification. Appropriate *laboratory data* will include serum calcium, magnesium, and PTH values; fasting serum phosphorus; serum 25-OH-D_3 levels ($1,25(OH)_2D_3$ levels when they become available routinely); alkaline phosphatase, albumin, and total protein measurement; and parameters of renal function including estimates of glomerular filtration rate. Appropriate *x-rays* may include chest, spine, pelvis, and long-bone films to look for osteomalacia, hand films for subperiosteal resorption, and skull films to look for basal-ganglia calcification.

Interpretation of these data should allow one to reach a tentative diagnosis as to the cause of the problem as shown in Table 59-2. Detailed descriptions of the syndromes clinically analyzed under the topics of osteomalacia (Chapter 70), inherited defects in vitamin D metabolism (Chapter 66), acquired disorders in vitamin D metabolism (Chapter 67), pseudohypoparathyroidism (Chapter 63), and renal osteodystrophy (Chapters 60 and 61) are presented by other authors. Table 59-2 gives a brief review of features pertinent to the manifestations of secondary hyperparathyroidism in each of the several disease categories with emphasis on differential diagnostic features.

REFERENCES

1. Burckhardt, P., Ruedi, B., Felber, J. P.: The clinical usefulness of the EDTA infusion as a stimulation test for parathyroid function, in Talmage, R. V., Owen, M., and Parsons, J. A., (eds): Calcium-Regulating Hormones, Proceedings of the Fifth Parathyroid Conference, Oxford, United Kingdom, 1974. Amsterdam, Excerpta Medica, 1975.
1a. Prien, E. L., Jr., Pyle, E. B., Krane, S. M.: Secondary hyperparathy-

Table 59-2.

	PTH	Ca	Mg	P	GFR	25OHD	Alk'ptase	Response to PTH Renal/Bone	
Vitamin D deficiency, dietary	sl ↑	N, ↓	N	↓,N	N	↓	↑	N,sl ↓ *	↓
Anticonvulsant osteomalacia	sl ↑	N, ↓	N	↓	N	N, ↓	sl ↑	—	—
Malabsorption	↑	↓	sl ↓,↓↓	↓	N	↓	↑	N	↓
Mg⁺⁺ deficiency	↑,N,↓	↓	↓↓	↓,N	N	—	N	↓	↓
Phosphate-treated X-linked hypophosphatemia	↑	↓	N	↓	N	N	↑,N	↓ **	—
Autosomal recessive vit. D-dependent rickets	↑	↓	N	↓	N	N	↑	—	—
Chronic renal failure	N, ↑,↑↑	N,↓	↓,N,↑	N,↑	↓	N,↓	N,↑	↓	↓
Pseudohypoparathyroidism	↑	↓	N	↑	N	N	N	↓	↓

*TRCa response decreased while TRP response intact.
**TRP maximally "inhibited," may return to normal response to PTH briefly when given iv $1,25(OH)_2D_3$.

roidism, in Greep, R. O., and Astwood, F. B., (eds): Handbook of Physiology, Section 7, Endocrinology, Washington, DC, American Physiological Society, 1976, vol. 7, pp. 383–410.

2. Finkelstein, J. W., Roffwarg, H. P., Boyer, R. M., et al: Age-related change in twenty-four-hour spontaneous secretion of growth hormone. *J Clin Endocrinol Metab 35:* 665–670, 1972.

3. Humbel, R. E., Bosshard, H. R., Zahn, H.: Chemistry of insulin, in Greep, R. O., and Astwood, F. B., (eds): Handbook of Physiology, Section 7, Endocrinology. Washington, DC, American Physiological Society, 1972, vol. 1, chap 6, p 111.

4. Sherwood, L. M., Potts, J. T., Jr., Care, A. D., et al: Evaluation by radioimmunoassay of factors controlling the secretion of parathyroid hormone. *Nature 209:* 52–57, 1966.

5. Mayer, G. P., Habener, J. F., Potts, J. T., Jr.: Parathyroid hormone secretion in vivo: demonstration of a calcium-independent, nonsuppressible component of secretion. *J Clin Invest 57:* 678–683, 1976.

6. Habener, J. F., Potts, J. T., Jr.: Chemistry, biosynthesis, secretion, and metabolism of parathyroid hormone, in Astwood, E. B., and Greep, R. O., (eds): Handbook of Physiology, Section 7, Endocrinology. Washington DC, American Physiological Society, 1976, chap 13, p 313.

7. Roth, S. I.: Recent advances in parathyroid gland pathology. *Am J Med 50:* 612–622, 1971.

8. Albright, F., Drake, T. G., Sulkowitch, H. W.: Renal osteitis fibrosa cystica: report of a case with discussion of metabolic aspects. *Bull Johns Hopkins Hosp 60:* 377–399, 1937.

9. Dreskin, E. A., Fox, T. A.: Adult renal osteitis fibrosa with metastatic calcification and hyperplasia of one parathyroid gland: Report of a case. *Arch Intern Med 86:* 533–557, 1950.

10. Gilmour, J. R.: The Parathyroid Glands and Skeleton in Renal Disease. New York & London, Oxford Medical Publications, 1947, p 157.

11. Herbert, F. K., Miller, H. G., Richardson, G. O.: Chronic renal disease, secondary parathyroid hyperplasia, decalcification of bone and metastatic calcification. *J Pathol Bacteriol (London) 53:* 161–182, 1941.

12. Pollak, V. E., Schneider, A. F., Freund, G., et al: Chronic renal disease with secondary hyperparathyroidism. *Arch Intern Med 103:* 200–218, 1959.

13. Stanbury, S. W., Lumb, G. A.: Parathyroid function in chronic renal failure. A statistical survey of the plasma and biochemistry in azotaemic renal osteodystrophy. *Q J Med 35:* 1–25, 1966.

14. Reiss, E., Canterbury, J. M.: Primary hyperparathyroidism: Application of radioimmunoassay to differentiation between adenoma and hyperplasia and to pre-operative localization of hyperfunctioning parathyroid glands. *N Engl J Med 280:* 1381–1385, 1969.

15. Murray, T. M., Peacock, M., Powell, D., et al: Non-autonomy of hormone secretion in primary hyperparathyroidism. *Clin Endocrinol 1:* 235–246, 1972.

16. Berson, S. A., Yalow, R. S.: Immunochemical heterogeneity of parathyroid hormone in plasma. *J Clin Endocrinol 28:* 1037–1047, 1968.

17. Bigos, S. T., Neer, R. M., St. Goar, W. T.: Hypercalcemia of seven years' duration after kidney transplantation. *Am J Surg 132:* 83–89, 1976.

18. Katz, A. D., Kaplan, L.: Parathyroidectomy for hyperplasia in renal disease. *Arch Surg 107:* 51–55, 1973.

19. Pletka, P., Strom, T., Bernstein, D. S., et al: Secondary hyperparathyroidism in human kidney transplant recipients. Program of Proceedings of the Fifth International Congress of Nephrology, Mexico City, 1972, p 156.

20. Wilson, R. E., Roth, S. I.: Case records of the Massachusetts General Hospital: Case 13, 1974. *N Engl J Med 290:* 793–799, 1974.

21. Richards, A. J.: Vitamin D deficiency and hyperparathyroidism. *Proc R Soc Med 65:* 1018, 1972.

22. Lumb, G. A., Stanbury, S. W.: Parathyroid function in human vitamin D deficiency and vitamin D deficiency in primary hyperparathyroidism. *Am J Med 56:* 833, 1974.

23. Connor, T., Toskes, P., Mahaffey, J., et al: Parathyroid function during chronic magnesium deficiency. *Johns Hopkins Med J 131:* 100–117, 1972.

24. Roth, S. I., Au, W. Y. W., Kunin, A. S., et al: Effect of dietary deficiency in vitamin D, calcium, and phosphorus on the ultrastructure of the rat parathyroid gland. *Am J Pathol 53:* 631, 1968.

25. Elrick, H., Albright, F., Bartter, F. C., et al: Further studies on pseudohypoparathyroidism: report of four new cases. *Acta Endocrinol 5:* 199, 1950.

60

Secondary (Adaptive) Hyperparathyroidism

Eric Reiss
Eduardo Slatopolsky

INTRODUCTION

The term *secondary hyperparathyroidism* implies that a pathophysiologic abnormality external to the parathyroid glands initiates the secretion of increased amounts of parathyroid hormone (PTH) by the parathyroid glands. The extraparathyroidal abnormality leads to a reduction in the serum ionized-calcium concentration. This stimulates increased PTH secretion, which in turn raises calcium concentrations toward normal. Secondary hyperparathyroidism thus is believed to represent an adaptive response that serves to protect calcium homeostasis[1] (see Chapter 59).

In the secondary form of hyperparathyroidism, the stimulus to PTH secretion is known; the adaptation, if successful, will restore serum calcium from low toward normal concentrations. However, elevated levels of PTH typically do not result in hypercalcemia. Secondary hyperparathyroidism thus would stand in contrast to primary hyperparathyroidism, in which the increased PTH secretion is presumed to arise from an abnormality intrinsic to the parathyroid glands. Moreover, in the primary form, hypercalcemia is the rule, and it is presumed that the excessive levels of PTH are pathologic and of a nonadaptive nature.

Despite the fact that the term *secondary hyperparathyroidism* is deeply ingrained in medical literature and in medical teaching, the differential features cited above are neither unambiguous nor fundamental. Indeed, there is growing evidence that a sharp distinction between primary and secondary hyperparathyroidism may be specious.[2] For example, it is not possible at the present stage of knowledge to conclude that the same stimulus believed to be responsible for secondary hyperparathyroidism, a decrease in ionized calcium, may not also antedate at least some forms of primary hyperparathyroidism.[3] Moreover, some patients with the primary form are normocalcemic and some with the secondary form may become hypercalcemic.[4,5]

The present discussion is concerned with the pathogenesis and characteristics of the most common form of secondary hyperparathyroidism, namely, that seen in chronic progressive renal disease. The pathophysiology of this entity, which will be termed *renal hyperparathyroidism,* has been studied in greater detail than any other form of hyperparathyroidism, and it not only lends itself well to an examination of pathogenetic concepts, but highlights the ambiguities noted above. It seems likely that renal hyperparathyroidism, which is seen in spontaneous renal disease in man and can be induced in animals with experimentally induced renal disease, may represent a model which will direct future investigations into other forms of hyperparathyroidism.

CHRONIC RENAL FAILURE: ETIOLOGIC CONSIDERATIONS

Systematic investigations into the pathogenesis of renal hyperparathyroidism were not initiated until approximately 15 years ago. This relates to the fact that before the introduction of chronic hemodialysis and renal transplantation as life-supporting measures for patients with terminal renal disease, hyperparathyroidism was more of a pathologic curiosity than a clinical abnormality of major importance; patients typically died before the skeletal manifestations of hyperparathyroidism became clinically significant. However, once it became possible to maintain patients alive long beyond the natural history of their disease, renal hyperparathyroidism emerged as an entity that could seriously limit the degree of rehabilitation and restoration of well-being of a chronically uremic patient.[6] The increasing recognition of the potentially grave consequences of renal hyperparathyroidism served to spark a widespread search for clues to the pathogenesis of the abnormality. This search was greatly facilitated by the introduction of a radioimmunoassay of PTH.[7] The latter provided the missing and essential tool required for a critical examination of various pathogenetic mechanisms.

A THEORY

The theoretical model to be described evolved from the studies of Bricker and his associates concerning the adaptations that occur in the course of progressive loss of nephrons in chronic renal disease.[8] The central tenet of the theory is that early renal hyperparathyroidism comes into being as a result of the requirements of phosphate homeostasis in the face of declining renal function.

When functioning nephrons are destroyed by disease, the glomerular filtration rate (GFR) falls, and the amount of phosphate filtered through the glomeruli of the residual functioning nephrons falls pari passu. Assuming that the dietary intake of inorganic phosphorus remains unchanged and that no alterations occur in

THEORY: PATHOGENESIS OF EARLY RENAL HYPERPARATHYROIDISM

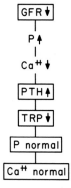

Fig. 60-1. Items enclosed within rectangles represent established observations in human chronic renal disease and in an experimental model studied in the dog. The intermediate steps of a tendency toward hyperphosphatemia and hypocalcemia are conjectural. (From Reiss and Canterbury: Am. J. Med 50:679, 1971.)

either intestinal absorption of phosphate or in bone metabolism, the serum phosphate concentration must rise with each fall in GFR until the amount of phosphate excreted per residual nephron increases sufficiently to reestablish phosphate balance. An elevation of serum phosphate characteristically is associated with a reciprocal decrease in the ionized-calcium concentration of the serum. The latter leads to an increase in PTH secretion, which in turn reduces the tubular reabsorption of phosphate (TRP) and increases the rate of phosphate excretion per residual nephron. As a result of these changes, the serum phosphate concentration is restored to normal, as is the ionized calcium. This schema is depicted in Fig. 60-1.

SUPPORTING EVIDENCE

For this theory to be tenable, it must be demonstrated that (1) the basic features of the model are fulfilled in naturally occurring progressive renal disease as well as in experimental renal disease, (2) PTH secretion is influenced by the requirements for phosphate homeostasis, and (3) renal hyperparathyroidism is preventable and/or reversible by altering the requirements for phosphate homeostasis.

All of the features depicted in rectangles in Fig. 60-1 are known to be characteristic of early renal insufficiency. Some of the essential data were provided in 1954 by Goldman and Bassett, who demonstrated that a decrease in TRP occurred in patients with advancing renal disease and that the latter was associated with the continued maintenance of normophosphatemia until GFR fell to levels as low as 25 ml/min.[9] The progressive fall in TRP constitutes a remarkable adaptation that permits a decreasing number of nephrons faced with a decreasing total filtered load of phosphate to excrete the same amount of phosphate in the urine per day as is excreted by a normal complement of nephrons. How this adaptation occurs has been elucidated only recently.

Convincing evidence has been presented that increasing levels of circulating PTH account in large part for the fall in TRP.[10,11] The serum or plasma PTH levels increase early in the course of advancing chronic renal disease.[11] Moreover, the PTH levels tend to rise progressively as GFR falls if phosphorus intake remains constant. Finally, there is a reasonable correspondence between rising levels of PTH and the falling values for TRP.

While the foregoing evidence interrelating renal hyperparathy-

roidism with increasing phosphaturia per nephron is generally accepted, not all of the recorded observations are consonant with the thesis. However, most of the discrepant observations can be readily explained by recent information about the metabolism of PTH and by the varying affinity characteristic of different antisera employed in radioimmunoassay in the reported studies[12-14]

Thus, current evidence shows that the kidney serves as a principal organ of metabolism of PTH and that metabolism accounts in large measure for the presence of PTH fragments in the blood.[15] Additionally, the kidney may represent an important route of hormone catabolism. All of this suggests the need for caution in extrapolating from serum or plasma PTH levels to the long-term rates of PTH secretion in the presence of renal disease (Chapters 45 and 59). Nevertheless, there is little doubt that PTH secretion increases early in the course of renal insufficiency and increases progressively as renal function declines (Fig. 60-2). There is some question as to whether the serum calcium concentration is in fact maintained at a normal level throughout the course of early renal disease, and, in some studies, a small but definite reduction in ionized-calcium concentrations has been observed. This issue remains unresolved, but resolution should emerge readily with the development of simpler methods for the precise and accurate determination of ionized-calcium concentrations in biologic fluids.

Disagreement also existed for many years as to whether altering serum phosphate concentration influenced PTH secretion. The

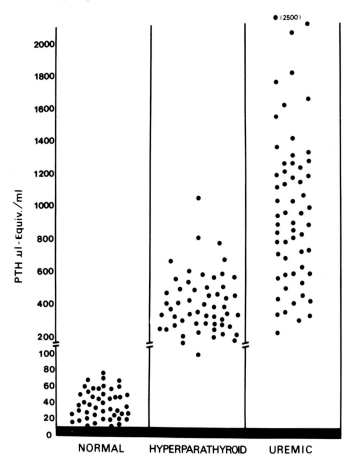

Fig. 60-2. Immunoassay results in normal subjects, patients with hypercalcemic (primary) hyperparathyroidism, and uremic patients. The data were obtained with a polyvalent antiserum that has high affinity for the carboxy-terminal fragment of PTH.[13] Note the generally higher assay results in uremia than in hypercalcemic hyperparathyroidism. This has been a consistent observation in many laboratories, including the original report by Berson and Yalow.[10]

introduction of the radioimmunoassay of PTH, however, provided a definite answer to this question both in animal and human studies. Elevation of serum phosphate concentrations either from intravenous infusions or oral administration of phosphate does indeed result in increased levels of circulating PTH.[16,17] However, this is now known not to be a direct effect of phosphate per se. Rather, as already suggested, hyperphosphatemia leads to a decrease in ionized calcium, and the latter in turn triggers PTH secretion (Fig. 60-3). When phosphate and calcium are given concomitantly in amounts that will raise the serum phosphorus concentration substantially but maintain the serum calcium concentration at a normal level, circulating levels of PTH do not change.[16] From a biologic point of view, however, the fact that the hypocalcemia, rather than hyperphosphatemia, accounts for increased PTH secretion does not militate against the thesis that in renal failure, hyperparathyroidism results from a primary failure to maintain phosphate homeostasis.

The long-term effects of altering the dietary phosphate intake on PTH secretion have been thoroughly studied. Clark and Rivera-Cordero have recently reviewed this problem and have contributed important new data.[18] In many species, increasing the dietary intake of phosphate results in loss of bone mass. Decreasing the calcium/phosphate ratio of the diet results in a striking increase in volume and weight of parathyroid glands. In an extensive series of studies, Laflamme and Jowsey[19] and Jowsey et al.[20] have been able to demonstrate increasing serum PTH levels with increasing phosphate intake. Associated with rising levels of serum PTH was clear-cut evidence of loss of bone mass. In contrast to the acute phosphate-loading experiments previously quoted, their careful experiments provided no clue to the trigger for increased PTH secretion. Total serum calcium concentration in dogs adapted to high phosphate intakes remained unchanged from control values, while the serum phosphorus concentration actually tended to decrease. Presumably, periods of hypocalcemia stimulated PTH secretion in these long-term experiments, as they did in the acute experiments, but examination of the steady-state levels of serum

calcium and phosphorus provided no clue concerning the genesis of this experimentally induced hyperparathyroidism.

We have provided evidence supporting the theory that the requirements for phosphate homeostasis play an important role in the genesis of renal hyperparathyroidism.[21,22] Studies were performed in healthy adult dogs in which a stepwise reduction of renal mass was produced so that observations could be made in the transition from normal renal function to advanced renal insufficiency. One group of dogs was maintained on a phosphorus intake of 1200 mg/day; a second group was maintained on a low phosphate intake of 100 mg/day. As the GFR declined in the dogs on the 1200-mg diet, serum PTH levels increased dramatically. By contrast, no increase of serum PTH was observed in the dogs maintained on the 100-mg phosphate diet despite the development of severe renal insufficiency. Thus, a low-phosphorus diet prevented the development of renal hyperparathyroidism. Further studies showed that severe restriction of phosphate intake was not required to prevent renal hyperparathyroidism in this model. When the phosphate intake was reduced in exact proportion to the reduction of GFR, the increase in serum PTH was likewise prevented. More recently, these studies have been extended in chronic experiments that more nearly simulate naturally occurring chronic renal failure. Reduction of the phosphate intake in proportion to the reduction in GFR prevented renal hyperparathyroidism in dogs with experimental renal disease for as long as 1 year.

CRITIQUE

The most serious criticism of the theory arises from the failure to document the signals for increased PTH secretion, that is, episodes of hyperphosphatemia and hypocalcemia. This criticism is dampened somewhat by the fact that in an effectively functioning adaptive system the signals initiating the need for adaptation are obscured. That raising the serum phosphorus concentration decreases the ionized calcium concentration is well established on the basis of many observations, but the mechanism by which the calcium decreases is poorly understood. As indicated earlier, one may question whether serum levels of PTH under the condition of renal insufficiency appropriately reflect long-term PTH secretory rates. This does not appear to be a strong objection since it seems highly unlikely that abnormalities in renal metabolism and/or excretion of PTH play an important role with only minimal decreases of the GFR. On the other hand, such abnormalities could well contribute to the very high levels of serum PTH characteristic of advanced renal failure.[10]

LATE RENAL HYPERPARATHYROIDISM

In contrast to the evidence that phosphate plays a decisive role in the pathogenesis of the hyperparathyroidism in the early stages of chronic renal failure, other factors also assume importance as renal failure becomes more advanced. Of these, abnormalities in the metabolism of vitamin D may well be of the greatest importance (Chapters 51 and 67). In animals with normal renal function, the metabolism of vitamin D and that of phosphate are closely interrelated,[23] and this is likely to be true in uremia. However, evidence concerning this point is fragmentary.

Intestinal malabsorption of calcium has long been known to be characteristic of the uremic state.[24] Recent studies have demonstrated that the decrease in net calcium absorption is due to impairment of active transport of calcium with no apparent effect on the portion of calcium absorption that is passively mediated.[25]

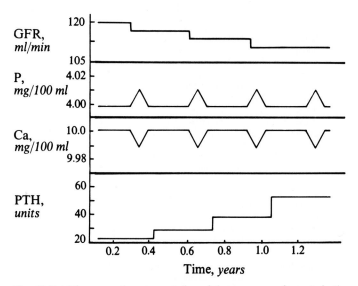

Fig. 60-3. Diagrammatic representation of the sequence of events in the genesis of renal hyperparathyroidism. As the GFR falls, there is a tendency toward phosphate retention. This triggers hypocalcemia and increased PTH secretion. As the result of the phosphaturic effect of PTH, serum phosphorus and serum calcium return to normal. This sequence is repeated with each fall of the GFR. The overall result is maintenance of the normal serum calcium and phosphorus concentrations at the expense of increasing serum PTH levels.

Intestinal absorption of cholecalciferol and of 25-hydroxycholecalciferol (25-OH-D$_3$) is normal in uremia, as are circulating concentrations of 25-OH-D$_3$.[26] However, circulating levels of 1,25-dihydroxycholecalciferol (1,25-(OH)$_2$D$_3$) have been found to be low in uremic patients.[27] In view of these data and the evidence that kidney represents the only tissue capable of 1-α-hydroxylation of 25-OH-D$_3$, it has been suggested that defective functioning of the 1-α-hydroxylase in diseased kidneys represents a key factor in the development of impaired calcium homeostasis in uremia. Indeed, small doses of 1,25-(OH)$_2$D$_3$ administered to uremic patients promptly restore calcium absorption to normal.[28]

The problem in disordered homeostasis in uremia is more complex than has been suggested in the preceding paragraphs. For example, there is some evidence that the malabsorption of calcium in uremia can be accounted for, at least in part, by defective synthesis of a calcium-binding protein in the intestine.[29] This defect appears to be independent of the action of vitamin D or its metabolites and is probably related to the overall decrease in protein synthesis that is characteristic of the uremic state. Furthermore, it has been recently demonstrated that the administration of 25-OH-D$_3$ in doses of 100–500 μg/day can correct intestinal malabsorption of calcium even in anephric patients.[30]

RESISTANCE TO PTH

Despite very high levels of circulating PTH, hypocalcemia of some degree is characteristic of advanced renal failure. The failure of PTH to maintain or to restore the calcium to normal requires explanation. In a careful series of experiments, Massry et al. have demonstrated that the calcemic response to injected PTH is markedly blunted in patients with renal insufficiency.[31] This phenomenon has been documented not only in advanced renal insufficiency but also in moderate renal failure (creatinine clearance 52 ml/min) and in acute renal failure. It is not reversed by hemodialysis and is not related to the severity of the hyperparathyroidism present. Of the factors known to influence skeletal responsiveness to PTH, an abnormality of vitamin D metabolism again appears to be most likely. It has long been known that skeletal responsiveness to PTH is severely blunted in rachitic animals.[32] This problem has been reexamined in recent years, and while the correct explanation remains in doubt, the basic observation has been confirmed repeatedly. Until the abnormalities of vitamin D metabolism in uremia are better understood, a thorough understanding of the skeletal resistance to PTH will not be possible.

Phosphate retention is also an important factor in the genesis of hypocalcemia. When the serum phosphorus concentration is carefully controlled in uremic patients, the serum calcium concentration rises. While the mechanism by which phosphate exerts this effect is unknown, it seems likely that it involves some action on the metabolism of vitamin D.

HYPERCALCEMIA

When bones of uremic patients are studied by biopsy, a startling array of metabolic lesions is encountered.[33] Some patients show predominantly the lesions of osteitis fibrosis; others, those of osteomalacia; and the majority, a combination of these and other abnormalities. In some patients the adaptive hyperparathyroidism overshoots the mark of compensation, and hypercalcemia supervenes. How frequently this occurs is not clear from the literature, but it is probably a rare event. One must assume that these patients

have severe hyperparathyroidism, limited abnormalities of vitamin D metabolism, and some defect that permits an adaptive response to become maladaptive. Evidence has been presented that a very large secretory mass of parathyroid tissue may account for the development of hypercalcemia.[11,34,35] PTH secretion cannot be suppressed to zero by any known means.[36,37] Hence a very large mass of functioning parathyroid tissue may yield enough unsuppressible secretion to cause hypercalcemia in susceptible individuals (Chapter 59).

It is apparent that much has been learned about the genesis of hyperparathyroidism and that much remains to be learned. A theoretical framework exists on which further studies can be based. The theory concerning the role of phosphate in the genesis of early renal hyperparathyroidism has strong support, but it undoubtedly represents an oversimplification. Similarly, possible abnormalities of vitamin D metabolism in late renal hyperparathyroidism represent an interesting basis for speculation, but the current formulations are clearly incomplete. There is much evidence that the actions and metabolism of vitamin D and PTH are intimately interrelated. This interrelationship is the subject of intensive current investigation, and it appears highly likely that the results of basic and physiologic studies will soon have direct applicability to further understanding of the genesis of renal hyperparathyroidism.

REFERENCES

1. Albright, F., Reifenstein, E. C. Jr.: The parathyroid glands and metabolic bone disease. Baltimore, Williams & Wilkins, 1948.
2. Reiss, E., Canterbury, J. M.: Spectrum of hyperparathyroidism. Am J Med 56: 794, 1974.
3. Coe, F. L., Canterbury, J. M., Firpo, J. J., Reiss, E.: Evidence for secondary hyperparathyroidism in idiopathic hypercalciuria. J Clin Invest 52: 134, 1973.
4. Wills, M. R., Pak, C. Y. C., Hammond, W. G., Bartter, F. C.: Normocalcemic primary hyperparathyroidism. Am J Med 47: 384, 1969.
5. Davies, D. R., Dent, C. E., Willcox, A. Hyperparathyroidism and steatorrhea. Br Med J 2: 1133, 1956.
6. Bricker, N. S., Slatopolsky, E., Reiss, E., Avioli, L. V.: Calcium, phosphorus, and bone in renal disease and transplantation. Arch Intern Med 123: 543, 1969.
7. Berson, S. A., Yalow, R. S., Aurbach, G. D., Potts, J. T., Jr: Immunoassay of bovine and human parathyroid hormone. Proc Natl Acad Sci USA 49: 613, 1963.
8. Bricker, N. S.: On the pathogenesis of the uremic state: an exposition of the "trade-off" hypothesis. N Engl J Med 286: 1093, 1972.
9. Goldman, R., Bassett, S. H.: Phosphorus excretion in renal failure. J Clin Invest 33: 1623, 1954.
10. Berson, S. A., Yalow, R. S.: Parathyroid hormone in plasma in adenomatous hyperparathyroidism, uremia, and bronchogenic carcinoma. Science 154: 907, 1966.
11. Reiss, E., Canterbury, J. M., Kanter, A. Circulating parathyroid hormone concentration in chronic renal insufficiency. Arch Intern Med 124: 417, 1969.
12. Habener, J. F., Powell, D., Murray, T. M., Mayer, G. P., Potts, J. T., Jr.: Parathyroid hormone: secretion and metabolism in vivo. Proc Natl Acad Sci USA 68: 2986, 1971.
13. Canterbury, J. M., Reiss, E.: Multiple immunoreactive molecular forms of parathyroid hormone in human serum. Proc Soc Exp Biol Med 140: 1393, 1972.
14. Arnaud, C. D., Goldsmith, R. S., Bordier, P. J., Sizemore, G. W.: Influence of immunoheterogeneity of circulating parathyroid hormone on results of radioimmunoassays of serum in man. Am J Med 56: 785, 1974.
15. Hruska, K. A., Kopelman, R., Rutherford, W. E., Klahr, S., Slatopolsky, E.: Metabolism of immunoreactive parathyroid hormone in the dog: the role of the kidney and the effects of chronic renal disease. J Clin Invest 56: 39, 1975.

16. Sherwood, L. M., Mayer, G. P., Ramberg, C. F., Jr., Kronfeld, D. S., Aurbach, G. D., Potts J. T., Jr.: Regulation of parathyroid hormone secretion: proportional control by calcium, lack of effect of phosphate. *Endocrinology 83:* 1043, 1968.

17. Reiss, E., Canterbury, J. M., Bercovitz, M. A., Kaplan, E. L. The role of phosphate in the secretion of parathyroid hormone in man. *J Clin Invest 49:* 2146, 1970.

18. Clark, I., Rivera-Cordero, F.: Effects of endogenous parathyroid hormone on calcium, magnesium and phosphate metabolism in rats. II. Alterations in dietary phosphate. *Endocrinology 96:* 360, 1974.

19. Laflamme, G. H., Jowsey, J.: Bone and soft tissue changes with oral phosphate supplements. *J Clin Invest 51:* 2834, 1972.

20. Jowsey, J., Reiss, E., Canterbury, J. M.: Long-term effects of high phosphate intake on parathyroid hormone levels and bone metabolism. *Acta Orthop Scand 45:* 801, 1974.

21. Slatopolsky, E., Caglar, S., Pennell, J. P., Taggart, D. D., Canterbury, J. M., Reiss, E., Bricker, N. S.: On the pathogenesis of hyperparathyroidism in chronic experimental renal insufficiency in the dog. *J Clin Invest 50:* 492, 1971.

22. Slatopolsky, E., Caglar, S., Gradowska, L., Canterbury, J., Reiss, E., Bricker, N. S.: On the prevention of secondary hyperparathyroidism in experimental chronic renal disease using "proportional reduction" of dietary phosphorus intake. *Kidney Int 2:* 147, 1972.

23. Tanaka, Y., DeLuca, H. F. The control of 25-hydroxyvitamin D metabolism by inorganic phosphorus. *Arch Biochem Biophys 154:* 566, 1973.

24. Liu, S. H., Chu, H. I.: Studies of calcium and phosphorus metabolism with special reference to pathogenesis and effects of dihydrotachysterol (A.T. 10) and iron. *Medicine* (Baltimore) *22:* 103, 1943.

25. Parker. T. F., Vergne-Marini. P., Hull. A. R., Pak. C. Y. C., Fordtran, J. S.: Jejunal absorption and secretion of calcium in patients with chronic renal disease on hemodialysis. *J Clin Invest 54:* 358, 1974.

26. Aviolo L. V., Birge, S. J., Slatopolsky, E.: The nature of vitamin D resistance of patients with chronic renal disease. *Arch Intern Med 124:* 451, 1969.

27. Brumbaugh, P. F., Haussler, D. H., Bressler, R., Haussler, M. R.: Radioreceptor assay for 1α, 25-dihydroxyvitamin D_3. *Science 183:* 1089, 1974.

28. Brickman, A. S., Coburn, J. W., Norman, A. W. Action of 1,25-dihydroxycholecalciferol, a potent kidney-produced metabolite of vitamin D_3, in uremic man. *N Engl J Med 287:* 891, 1972.

29. Avioli, L. V.: Intestinal absorption of calcium. *Arch Intern Med 129:* 345, 1972.

30. Rutherford, E., Blondin, J., Hruska, K., Kopelman, R., Klahr, S., Slatopolsky, E.: The effect of 25-hydroxycholecalciferol (25-OH-D_3) on calcium absorption in uremia. Proceedings of the American Society of Nephrology. Washington DC, 1974 (abstract).

31. Massry, S. G., Coburn, J. W., Lee, D. B. N., Jowsey, J., Kleeman, C. R.: Skeletal resistance to parathyroid hormone in renal failure. *Ann Intern Med 78:* 357, 1973.

32. Harrison, H. C., Harrison, H. E., Park, E. A.: Vitamin D and citrate metabolism: effect of vitamin D in rats fed diets adequate in both calcium and phosphorus. *Am J Physiol 192:* 432, 1958.

33. Rasmussen, H., Bordier, P.: The Physiological and Cellular Basis of Metabolic Bone Disease. Baltimore, Williams & Wilkins, 1974.

34. Stanbury, S. W.: Bone disease in uremia. *Am J Med 44:* 714, 1968.

35. Gittes, R. F., Radde, I.: Experimental hyperparathyroidism from multiple isologous parathyroid transplants. *Endocrinology 78:* 1015, 1966.

36. Targovnik, J. H., Rodman, J. S., Sherwood, L. M. Regulation of parathyroid hormone secretion in vitro: quantitative aspects of calcium and magnesium ion control. *Endocrinology 88:* 1477, 1971.

37. Mayer, G. P., Habener, J. F., Potts, J. T., Jr.: Parathyroid hormone secretion in vivo. *J Clin Invest 57:* 678, 1976.

61

Management of Secondary Hyperparathyroidism

Claude D. Arnaud, Jr.
Philippe J. Bordier

INTRODUCTION

The successful management of disorders of mineral and bone metabolism associated with chronic renal failure depends upon a detailed understanding of their pathogenesis and natural history. Many authors have considered the current concepts of the pathogenesis and have concluded that it is complex and involves many interrelated factors. It is clear, however, that the failure of the diseased kidney to excrete phosphorus normally is central among these. Not only does the resulting hyperphosphatemia cause hypocalcemia and secondary hyperparathyroidism, but it may be responsible for inhibiting the enzymatic conversion of 25-hydroxyvitamin D (25-OH-D) to the physiologically important metabolite of vitamin D, 1,25-dihydroxyvitamin D, or 1,25-$(OH)_2$D, by the renal tubular enzyme, 1α-25-(OH)-D_2 hydroxylase. The classic biochemical and physiologic abnormalities of mineral and bone metabolism observed in patients with chronic renal failure include, therefore, hypocalcemia, hyperphosphatemia, decreased intestinal calcium absorption and negative calcium balance, marked increases of circulating parathyroid hormone (PTH), and a bizarre osseous disease in which both osteitis fibrosa and osteomalacia are prominent features.

The natural history of the disorders of mineral and bone metabolism associated with chronic renal failure is less well understood. The reason for this is that prior to the advent of hemodialysis, renal osteodystrophy and soft-tissue mineralization were little more than medical oddities and not worth serious study because the life expectancy of patients with chronic renal failure was so dismal.

NATURAL HISTORY AND MANAGEMENT DURING EARLY CHRONIC RENAL FAILURE

Recently, we[3] studied a group of untreated patients with chronic renal failure of varying severity and duration not undergoing hemodialysis in an attempt to learn something about the natural history of the mineral sequelae. In spite of the obvious limitations imposed on the interpretations of the results by the cross-sectional design of the study, it was possible to roughly stage their development as functions of time and severity. This staging scheme is illustrated in Fig. 61-1. The first detectable abnormality of those shown appears to be an increase in serum immunoreactive parathyroid hormone (iPTH). This occurs before glomerular filtration rates decrease[1] below 40 ml/min and before there are detectable changes in the serum phosphorus or serum calcium. This is not unexpected if, as has been suggested, increased PTH secretion represents the major mechanism by which the organism adapts to renal phosphate retention. The important question is whether this adaptive mechanism, which appears to be so successful in maintaining extracellular calcium and phosphorus homeostasis, is in the best interest of the patient or whether an externally applied therapeutic measure designed to accomplish the same thing might serve him better in the long run.

It is clear from our studies that all of the pateints with mild to moderate degrees of chronic renal failure (serum creatinine, 3.0mg/dl or less) had histomorphometric evidence of excess circulating PTH in bone biopsies as well as subperiosteal bone resorption on hand radiographs. These observations strongly suggest that the maintenance of normal levels of serum calcium and phosphorus in patients with chronic renal failure by adaptive increases in PTH secretion occurs as a result of an important trade-off—loss of osseous integrity. In fact, it is quite likely that sometime during the progressive loss of nephrons, hyperparathyroidism becomes self-perpetuating. That is, phosphorus as well as calcium is released from bone during the process of PTH-induced bone resorption, and the initial perturbation causing hyperparathyroidism—hyperphosphatemia—is augmented by the very adaptive process originally called upon to control it. Thus, there is every reason to believe that the negative feedback system which exists between bone and the parathyroid glands when a normal kidney is present is transformed into a biologically unstable "positive feedback" system when a kidney is present which cannot excrete phosphorus. The chronology of this transformation is unknown, but it must be extremely complex depending on many variables, including, at the very least, dietary calcium, phosphorus, and vitamin D and the rapidity with which the patient loses nephrons.

Presently, there is little effort made by physicians to interrupt the adaptive cycle described and prevent the development of the pathologic "positive feedback" relationship between bone and the parathyroid glands early in the course of renal failure. This is probably due to the fact that patients are generally asymptomatic and reluctant to take medicines. In addition, no long-term prospec-

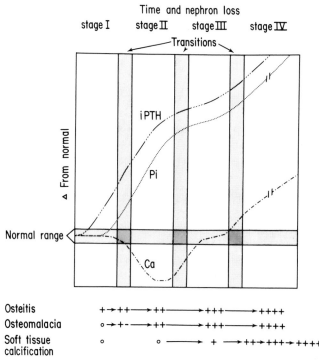

Fig. 61-1. Staging of biochemical and osseous abnormalities in renal osteodystrophy as a function of time and nephron loss. (From Bordier et al.: *Kidney Int 7:* Suppl 2 p S102, 1975)

tive studies have been reported showing that appropriate therapy instituted early and directed at preventing the development of positive phosphorus balance, negative calcium balance, and hyperparathyroidism will significantly decrease the incidence or the severity of the mineral and bone complications in the late stages of renal failure or during the hemodialysis and postkidney-transplant periods. However, extensive investigations by the Mayo Clinic group[4–6] showed that restoration of serum calcium and phosphorus levels toward normal by the use of oral phosphate binding gels and dialysate calcium concentrations of 6–7 mg/dl in hemodialyzed patients decreased serum levels of iPTH (Fig. 61-2) and caused improvement in established renal osteodystrophy (Fig. 61-3). It is therefore likely that the part of the syndrome of renal osteodystrophy due to hyperparathyroidism could be prevented if active steps were taken early in the course of chronic renal failure to avoid the need by the organism to bring into play adaptive increases in PTH secretion. Since the stimulus to PTH secretion is hypocalcemia induced by hyperphosphatemia, it is logical to assume that combined dietary restriction of phosphate either by feeding of a low-phosphate diet or the administration of phosphate-binding gels and relatively large doses of absorbable calcium might be successful in restoring extracellular calcium and phosphorus homeostasis to normal.

There is one serious difficulty in this approach. Early in the development of chronic renal failure, serum calcium and phosphorus concentrations are usually within the range of normal. Thus, it is not possible under such circumstances to know if a therapeutic effort is successful unless serum iPTH is measured serially. This can be difficult because of the interpretive problems caused by the immunoheterogeneity of circulating PTH and the varying specificities of commercially available PTH radioimmunoassays. In practice, we have found carboxyl-terminal-specific assays (Chapter 55) to be most useful for this purpose. Although an increased serum

level may reflect diminished clearance of carboxyl-terminal PTH fragments by diseased kidneys, it is our experience that the institution of the therapy noted above results in a progressive decline of serum iPTH values into the normal range. This result would imply either a decrease in PTH secretion or improved clearance of carboxyl-terminal fragments by the kidney. The possibility that the treatment given (phosphate restriction and calcium supplementation) would result in the latter alternative is remote, and it is our belief that the decreases in serum iPTH we have observed actually reflect our success in directly interrupting the development of adaptive hyperparathyroidism.

Thus it appears that the single most important indication for considering a patient with chronic renal failure for treatment with dietary restriction of phosphate and calcium supplementation is a serum iPTH value which is clearly in the abnormally high range. Although treatment with dietary restriction of phosphate may be sufficient, reduction in serum iPTH might require the addition of phosphate-binding antacids to the therapeutic regimen. There are many aluminum-containing phosphate-binding antacids on the market. Alu-Caps, the high-potency liquid Basaljel, and aluminum hydroxide-containing cookies (either commercially prepared or baked by the patient) appear to be the most effective and the best tolerated because of the almost complete absence of the taste of the aluminum compound. Most recently, Slatopolski (personal communication) has found that bread sticks containing an aluminum-based gel are very effective and exceptionally well tolerated. The patient should be offered a variety of preparations and dosage forms, and generally he will choose a combination which suits him. Dosage needs to be adjusted for each patient, and prolonged

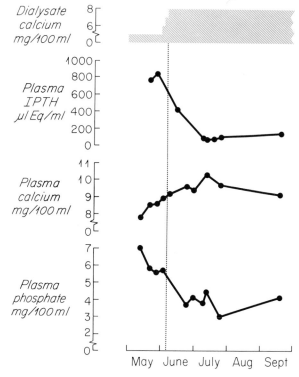

Fig. 61-2. Serial values of plasma iPTH, calcium, and phosphorus during the treatment of a patient with end-stage renal failure (stage-2 renal osteodystrophy; see Fig. 61-1) by reduction of plasma phosphorus by oral administration of aluminum-hydroxide gel and subsequent gradual increase in dialysate calcium concentration to 8 mg/dl. (From Goldsmith et al.: *Am. J. Med. 50:* 692, 1971)

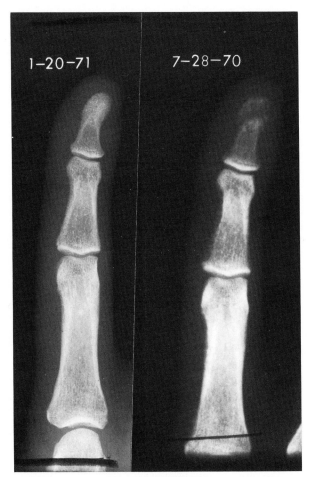

Fig. 61-3. Roentgenographic appearance of index finger of a patient with stage-3–4 renal osteodystrophy before and after 6 months of treatment similar to that described in Fig. 61-2. (From Vosik et al.: Mayo Clin. Proc. *47:* 110, 1972)

NATURAL HISTORY AND MANAGEMENT DURING LATE STAGES OF CHRONIC RENAL FAILURE AND DURING HEMODIALYSIS

Most patients with end-stage renal failure present with the mineral and osseous abnormalities found in the second stage (Fig. 61-1). Varying degrees of hypocalcemia and hyperphosphatemia and increases in serum iPTH (carboxyl-terminal assay using GP1M antiserum) in the range of 10–20-times normal are found. Patients may have complaints of bone pain but more often than not they are relatively asymptomatic. Soft tissue calcification is generally not a prominent feature of this stage unless patients have been inadvertently treated with high-phosphate diets (i.e., milk) and intoxicating doses of vitamin D, in which case they really occupy stages 3 and 4.

The hypocalcemia of stage 2 is probably reflective of the development of severe vitamin D deficiency as a result of the progressive destruction of the $1\alpha,25\text{-}(OH)_2D$ hydroxylase system along with the kidneys. Patients in this stage of the development of renal osteodystrophy can produce only minimal quantities of 1,25-$(OH)_2D$ and, as a result, osteomalacia is superimposed on the osteitis fibrosa which developed during stage 1. It is probably the degree and duration of the hypocalcemia of stage 2 which determines whether or not patients enter stages 3 and 4. Since these stages tend to be much less reversible by medical means (see below) than stage 1 or 2, we think it is extremely important to assume a rather aggressive stance when confronted with a patient whose disease has been determined to approximate stage 2.

In treating patients with stage-2 disease, it is important to recognize that the hypocalcemia probably reflects a fortuitous protective adaptation of the organism to severe hyperparathyroidism; that is, the permissive influence of vitamin D on the bone-resorbing action of PTH[7–9] has been largely removed by the final destruction of the kidneys, and, in essence, the devastating effects of the enormously high concentrations of circulating PTH have been naturally averted. Thus, it is probably important to delay the introduction of vitamin D or one of its biologically active metabolites or analogues until such time when hyperparathyroidism has been at least partly brought under control. This can be done in almost all nondialyzed patients by vigorously restoring serum calcium and phosphorus to normal using the simple manipulations described in the previous section. The initiation of the regimen can be most easily accomplished in the hospital and should not require more than 1 week. After a trend downward in serum iPTH has been established, it would seem logical to introduce some form of vitamin D therapy. At this writing, the most effective metabolite(s) or analogue(s) has not been determined yet, and it is quite possible that combination therapy may be necessary to restore both intestinal calcium absorption and bone formation processes to normal.

It is likely that patients treated prophylactically as described in the previous section will reach end-stage renal failure and the time when it is necessary to enter them into a hemodialysis program with only minor hyperparathyroidism and renal osteodystrophy. These patients should present few problems in continuing prophylaxis. Since PTH-induced release of phosphate from bone into the circulation is probably not much greater than normal, dietary phosphate need not be restricted vigorously, and the dose of phosphate-binding agent needed to maintain serum phosphorus in the normal range should not be beyond the tolerance of the average patient. Although it is possible that these patients may require only supplemental vitamin D_2 or D_3 to avoid the development of osteomalacia, ideal therapeutic regimens will probably include vitamin D metabolites or analogues.

hypophosphatemia should be avoided at all costs. Initial doses should range between 0.25 and 0.5 g/day with further adjustments upward if hypophosphatemia does not ensue or serum iPTH does not decrease. The antacids should always be taken with meals.

It should be recognized that low-phosphate diets are also low in calcium. Therefore, if it is elected to control enteral absorption of phosphate by feeding a diet low in phosphorus, it will be absolutely necessary to supplement the patient with some form of calcium-containing drug. We use calcium carbonate preferentially because it is cheap and well tolerated and it combats renal acidosis at the same time it supplies calcium. Calcium should be given to the patient who is on a normal diet as well because of the generally decreased enteral absorption of calcium in chronic renal failure. Doses of elemental calcium should be monitored because rarely some patients develop hypercalcemia. However, doses as high as 5.0 g/day may be tolerated well.

We have maintained patients with early renal failure on relatively small doses of vitamin D_2 (1000–2000 U/day) with the idea of providing no more than 10 times the daily requirement. It is quite possible that treatment with a biologically active vitamin D metabolite will be found advantageous in the future, but it is our current opinion that if it is found to be important to treat the abnormalities of mineral and bone metabolism of early chronic renal failure, it will always be necessary to carefully regulate calcium and phosphate intake.

Patients who have not received prophylactic treatment and enter hemodialysis in stages 2, 3, or 4 should be considered as having sustained negative calcium balance for a long period of time and as suffering from a form of hyperparathyroidism which is self-perpetuating (see above). Successful medical treatment requires intensive efforts (1) to interrupt the positive feedback relationship between bone and the parathyroid glands, (2) to produce positive calcium balance, and (3) to treat vitamin D deficiency if it exists.

Patients with stage-2 renal osteodystrophy should respond to the treatment regimen outlined for patients in stage 2 not on hemodialysis. The important consideration in patients on hemodialysis is not to aggravate negative calcium balance by using dialysate calcium concentrations below 5.7 mg/dl.[4,6,10,11] Under these conditions, patients almost uniformly lose calcium into the dialysate during hemodialysis.[4] In fact, it is possible and probably desirable to use hemodialysis as a means of producing positive calcium balance by employing dialysate calcium concentrations of 6.5–8.0 mg/dl.[4] However, this should not be attempted until serum phosphorus concentrations are decreased below 5.0 mg/dl because of the danger of inducing extraosseous mineralization with calcium-×-phosphorus products in the serum of 70 or greater. This approach is demonstrated in Fig. 61-2, where the combined reduction of plasma phosphate to 3.0 mg/dl and the gradual introduction of dialysate calcium concentration of 8.0 mg/dl resulted in an increase in the plasma calcium from 8.0 to 10.0 mg/dl and a concomitant and permanent decrease in plasma iPTH from values up to 20 times normal to values just above the upper limits of normal within a period of 2.5 months. This patient fulfilled all of the criteria for stage-2 renal osteodystrophy.

The question of whether patients with stages-3 and -4 renal osteodystrophy (serum calcium normal or increased above normal, serum phosphorus increased above 8.0 mg/dl, and serum iPTH greater than 50–100-times normal) can or should be treated with the regimen illustrated in Fig. 61-2 is controversial. It is clear it can be successfully applied to these patients if heroic efforts are expended. We have described such a patient and her course after institution of the described regimen.[5] The resolution of this patient's subperiosteal bone resorption within 6 months of the institution of intensive treatment is illustrated by the radiographs shown in Fig. 61-3.

However, in practice, it is probable that patients with stage 3 or 4 renal osteodystrophy should be treated initially with subtotal parathyroidectomy in order to decrease the size of the parathyroid gland mass followed by the institution of the regimen described for patients with stage-2 renal osteodystrophy. The reason that this rather radical approach is probably justified is that we have found that the mineral complications and persistence of hyperparathyroidism in patients after renal transplantation are less in patients whose hyperparathyroidism and osteodystrophy were well controlled prior to transplantation. It generally takes much longer to bring stage-3 and -4 patients under control, and success is less frequent than in patients with stage-2 disease. Therefore, considering the unpredictable availability of donor kidneys for transplantation and the probable desirability of having hyperparathyroidism and renal osteodystrophy under control prior to transplantation, it is important to decide as soon as possible whether or not patients have stage-3 or -4 renal osteodystrophy. When in doubt, an intensive regimen of medical treatment should be instituted, and if

marked improvement in hyperparathyroidism and osteodystrophy is not observed (3–4 months), serious consideration should be given to subtotal parathyroidectomy.

FUTURE PROSPECTS

It is clear that there is great need for the ultimate in prophylaxis—the prevention of kidney disease. However, until this happens, it will be important to concentrate on developing convenient means of preventing the development of the syndrome of renal osteodystrophy in patients with established kidney disease that is expected to progress to end-stage renal failure. At the present time, we do not know if such an approach will be successful in the long-term management of patients, and there are several crucial elements of the prophylaxis regimen described in this chapter which are lacking or not entirely satisfactory. The most important of these from a therapeutic point of view is a preparation of oral phosphate-binding agent which will be enthusiastically accepted by all patients. A reliable, inexpensive PTH radioimmunoassay for patient follow-up is another. It is difficult to predict when these will become available.

REFERENCES

1. Arnaud, C.: Hyperparathyroidism and renal failure. *Kidney Int 4:* 89, 1973.
2. Goldsmith, R. S., Johnson, W. J., Arnaud, C. D.: The hyperparathyroidism of renal failure: pathophysiology and treatment. *Clin Endocrinol Metab 3:* 305, 1974.
3. Bordier, P. J., Marie, P. J., Arnaud, C. D.: Evolution of renal osteodystrophy: correlation of bone histomorphometry and serum mineral and immunoreactive parathyroid hormone values before and after treatment with calcium carbonate or 25-hydroxycholecalciferol. *Kidney Int 7:* [Suppl] 2 p S102, 1975.
4. Goldsmith, R. S., Furszyfer, J., Johnson, W. J., Fournier, A. E., Arnaud, C. D.: Control of secondary hyperparathyroidism during long-term hemodialysis. *Am J Med 50:* 692, 1971.
5. Vosik, W. M., Anderson, C. F., Steffee, W. P., Johnson W. J., Arnaud, C. D., Goldsmith, R. S.: Successful medical management of osteitis fibrosa due to "tertiary" hyperparathyroidism. *Mayo Clin Proc 47:* 110, 1972.
6. Fournier, A. E., Arnaud. C. D., Johnson. W. J., Taylor. W. F., Goldsmith, R. S.: Etiology of hyperparathyroidism and bone disease during hemodialysis. II. Factors affecting serum immunoreactive parathyroid hormone. *J Clin Invest 50:* 599, 1971.
7. Harrison, H. C., Harrison, H. E., Park, E. A.: Vitamin D and citrate metabolism: effect of vitamin D in rats fed diets adequate in both calcium and phosphorus. *Am J Physiol 192:* 432, 1958.
8. Rasmussen, H., DeLuca, H., Arnaud, C. D., Hawker, C., von Stedingk, M.: The relationship between vitamin D and parathyroid hormone. *J Clin Invest 42:* 1940, 1963.
9. Arnaud, C, Rasmussen, H., Anast, C.: Further studies on the interrelationship between parathyroid hormone and vitamin D. *J Clin Invest 45:* 1955, 1966.
10. Fournier, A. E., Johnson, W. J., Taves, D. R., Beabout, J. W., Arnaud, C. D., Goldsmith, R. S.: Etiology of hyperparathyroidism and bone disease during chronic hemodialysis. I. Association of bone disease with potentially etiologic factors. *J Clin Invest 50:* 592, 1971.
11. Johnson, W. J., Goldsmith, R. S., Beabout, J. W., Jowsey, J., Kelly, P. J., Arnaud, C. D.: Prevention and reversal of progressive secondary hyperparathyroidism in patients maintained by hemodialysis. *Am J Med 56:* 827, 1974.

62

Surgical, Idiopathic, and Other Varieties of Parathyroid Hormone-Deficient Hypoparathyroidism

A. Michael Parfitt

Impairment of parathyroid function is traditionally divided into three categories: surgical hypoparathyroidism (SHP), idiopathic hypoparathyroidism (IHP), and pseudohypoparathyroidism (PHP), listed in order of their formulation as clinical entities. Today, a more complex system of classification is necessary, but a logical primary subdivision is into those disorders associated with parathyroid hormone (PTH) deficiency, which will be described here, and those associated with PTH excess, which will be discussed in the next chapter.

A classic technique of experimental endocrinology is to study the effects of complete extirpation of a gland, but one of several curious features of the development of knowledge about the parathyroid glands is that the results of their accidental removal were observed before their existence was generally recognized. This interesting story will not be related here, but several excellent accounts are available.[1,2]

BIOCHEMICAL EFFECTS OF PTH DEFICIENCY AND THEIR PATHOGENESIS

HYPOCALCEMIA AND HYPOCALCIURIA

The hypocalcemia in hypoparathyroidism (HP) results from a fall in the level of the blood–bone calcium equilibrium, and a reduction in both renal tubular reabsorption and in gastrointestinal absorption of calcium.[3] Renal 1-hydroxylation of 25-hydroxycholecalciferol (25-OH-D_3) is thought to be defective in HP, since 1-hydroxylated compounds are effective in doses which are modestly greater than the physiologic requirement.[4] Lack of PTH produces hypocalcemia both directly and via deficiency of 1,25-dihydroxycholecalciferol ($1,25\text{-}(OH)_2D_3$).

Depending on the degree of PTH deficiency, the plasma calcium in HP can vary from about 5.0 mg/100 ml to low normal levels.[5] The lowest values, which occur with complete absence of PTH, reflect the level of equilibration corresponding to the solubility of bone mineral in body fluids. At all levels of severity the plasma calcium in HP is less stable than normal. It varies more with changes in calcium intake and shows much greater reciprocal fluctuation with plasma phosphate than in normal subjects.[3] Consequently, when PTH is only moderately deficient, hypocalcemia may only occur when the intake of calcium is deficient or the intake of phosphate is excessive.[5]

As well as determining the steady-state level of plasma calcium, PTH also participates in the correction of deviations from the steady-state level. Optimal recovery from induced hypocalcemia is dependent on a rapid increase in PTH secretion. By analogy with the early stages of Addison's disease, as parathyroid cell mass is reduced, a point may be reached where maximally stimulated cells are able to maintain a nearly normal basal level of hormone secretion, but are unable to further augment secretion in response to increased physiologic demand. The recovery from induced hypocalcemia will then be retarded and incomplete. Based on these considerations, five grades of severity of HP have been defined. Grades 1 and 2 refer to diminished reserve in response to an EDTA challenge but with no or with inconstant spontaneous hypocalcemia, respectively, and grades 3, 4, and 5 refer to hypocalcemia below 8.5, 7.5, and 6.5 mg/100 ml, respectively.

The urinary excretion of calcium is low (Table 62-1), but, for the same degree of hypocalcemia, urinary calcium is higher in HP than in normals or patients with osteomalacia because of impaired tubular reabsorption of calcium due to lack of PTH action.

HYPERPHOSPHATEMIA

The other major consequence of PTH deficiency is elevation of plasma phosphate. PTH is the most important (but not the only) factor controlling the renal tubular reabsorption of phosphate and the phosphate threshold (Transfer Maximum for Phosphate/Glo-

Table 62-1. Metabolic Data in HP Classified According to Severity

Quantity	Grade				
	1	2	3	4	5
No. of cases	10	10	9	8	5
Plasma Ca (mg/100 ml)	9.54 ± 0.13	9.21 ± 0.15	8.14 ± 0.09	6.86 ± 0.07	5.80 ± 0.14
Urine Ca (mg/24 h)	127 ± 22	122 ± 23	64 ± 11	47 ± 9	46 ± 10
Urine Ca (μg/100 ml C_{Cr})	99 ± 9	87 ± 12	50 ± 8	36 ± 7	36 ± 8
Plasma P (mg/100 ml)	3.79 ± 0.13	4.13 ± 0.34	4.16 ± 0.21	5.06 ± 0.22	5.64 ± 0.32
TmP/GFR (mg/100 ml)	3.30 ± 0.18	3.25 ± 0.32	4.31 ± 0.27	5.59 ± 0.38	6.23 ± 0.49
Urine P (mg/24 h)	674 ± 80	654 ± 38	455 ± 60	469 ± 68	518 ± 111
Urine P (μg/100 ml C_{Cr})	480 ± 41	566 ± 57	401 ± 56	359 ± 55	397 ± 90

	1 + 2	3 + 4 + 5	Difference	P
No. of cases	20	22		
Urine P (mg/24 h)	664 ± 42	485 ± 41	179 ± 59	< 0.005
Urine P (μg/100 ml C_{Cr})	523 ± 42	385 ± 35	138 ± 54	< 0.02

Upper panel shows means + SE in each grade. Lower panel compares phosphate excretion in grades 1,and 2 (normocalcemic) and grades 3–5 (hypocalcemic). C_{cr} = creatinine clearance.

merular Filtration Rate, or TmP/GFR). In conjunction with the load of phosphate requiring excretion, this threshold regulates the plasma phosphate level. In HP, TmP/GFR is usually increased,[6] but the phosphate load may be decreased, partly because of reduced gastrointestinal absorption of phosphate and partly because of reduced bone turnover. Moreover, less PTH is needed to inhibit phosphate reabsorption than to raise the plasma calcium.[5] Consequently, hyperphosphatemia is a much less constant finding than hypocalcemia, and with moderate hypocalcemia (grade 3) the plasma phosphate is usually normal (Table 62-1).

OTHER EFFECTS

PTH regulates bone turnover by its action on osteoprogenitor cell proliferation into osteoclasts, and in HP bone turnover is reduced, whether measured by kinetic or morphologic techniques.[3] This is unrelated to the hypocalcemia, but is manifested by decreased surface remodeling of bone and decreased urinary excretion of total hydroxyproline (THP). The alkaline phosphatase level is not consistently altered.

PTH reduces the renal tubular reabsorption of bicarbonate as well as phosphate, and in HP both the renal threshold and plasma level of bicarbonate are frequently raised. Although the cerebrospinal fluid calcium does not fall as much as the plasma calcium, the sensitivity of the respiratory center to CO_2 is increased.[7] Consequently, respiratory compensation for the raised plasma bicarbonate is incomplete, and the plasma pH may be elevated in HP.[8]

CLINICAL EFFECTS OF PTH DEFICIENCY AND THEIR PATHOGENESIS

Hypocalcemia is not only the chief consequence of PTH deficiency but is the main cause of its various clinical manifestations. Many of these result from increased irritability of the nervous system, both peripheral and central.

TETANY

In the strict sense, tetany is a purely motor phenomenon of spontaneous tonic muscular contractions, but it is convenient to use the term in a wider sense to denote the entire symptom complex due to increased neural excitability.

Overt Tetany

A typical attack[9] begins with sensations of tingling in the tips of the fingers, around the mouth, and less commonly in the feet. These gradually increase in severity and spread proximally along the limbs and over the face, and may be followed by numbness. The muscles of the extremities and the face then begin to feel tense and later go into spasm, progressing in the same pattern as the preceding sensory symptoms. The spasm is frequently described as carpopedal, although the hand and forearm are more commonly involved than the feet and legs. The first change is adduction of the thumb, followed in order by flexion of the metacarpophalangeal joints, extension of the interphalangeal joints without separation of the fingers, and flexion of the wrist and elbow joints to produce the classic main d'accoucheur posture. Pain depends on the degree of tension developed in the muscle, and may be very severe. Less commonly, similar changes occur in the lower limbs with plantar flexion of the toes, arching of the foot, and contraction of the calf muscles. Rarely, in a severe and prolonged attack the muscles of the face are involved, with wrinkled forehead, staring gaze, pursed lips, depression of the angles of the mouth, and accentuation of the nasolabial grooves.[1] Spasm of the cranial muscles may produce headache. Tetany is rarely dangerous but it is frequently alarming, and the patient may be hyperventilating, both as a result of anxiety and as a reflex component of the syndrome.[2] Both hypocapnia[7] and increased adrenalin secretion[10] worsen the tetany and produce their own effects, such as peripheral and circumoral pallor, sweating, and tachycardia.

Experimentally, a nerve exposed to a low concentration of calcium exhibits a reduced threshold of excitation, repetitive responses to a single stimulus, impairment of accommodation, and, finally, continuous activity.[11,12] The manifestations of tetany are due to spontaneous discharges of both sensory and motor fibers in peripheral nerves.[9] These discharges originate in the proximal part of the nerve even though the symptoms are felt earliest in the extremities.[13] During an attack of tetany the EMG shows repetitive motor-unit action potentials, usually grouped as doublets, occasionally as single or triple spikes, corresponding to individual motor units excited by single or multiple discharges from a single focus.[12,14] Other causes of muscle spasm such as tetanus, myokymia, or stiff-man syndrome have different EMG characteristics.

Latent Tetany

Lesser degrees of neural excitability may be recognized by various signs for latent tetany. The neurologic examination may otherwise be negative. The deep tendon reflexes may be increased, decreased, or unchanged. Chvostek's sign[15] is elicited by tapping the facial nerve about 2 cm anterior to the earlobe just below the zygomatic process (Chvostek I) or between the zygomatic arch and the corner of the mouth (Chvostek II). Chvostek I results from direct mechanical stimulation of the facial nerve, and Chvostek II mainly from reflex stimulation. The responses consist of twitching of muscles supplied by the facial nerve and can be ranked in a semiquantitative manner:[16] grade 1, twitching of the lip at the angle of the mouth only; grade 2, twitching of the alae nasi in addition; grade 3, contraction of the orbicularis oculi in addition; and grade 4, contraction of all the muscles innervated on that side. The sign may be noticed by the patient during shaving. A grade-1 response as an isolated observation is of no clinical significance since it is observed in 25 percent of normal adults and in an even higher proportion of children.

Trousseau's sign is elicited by inflating a sphygmomanometer cuff on the upper arm to above the systolic blood pressure. The sensory and motor manifestations of tetany occur in sequence within 2 minutes, culminating in a typical attack of carpal spasm. The responses can be ranked semiquantitatively:[16] grade 1, a spasm which can be overcome by the patient: grade 2, a spasm which can be overcome by the examiner, but not by the patient: grade 3, a spasm which cannot be overcome by the examiner, occurring after 1 min: grade 4, the same occurring in less than 1 min. The response depends on the induction of ischemia of the ulnar nerve immediately subjacent to the cuff.[9,13] When the cuff is released, the muscles take about 5–10 s to relax; spasm which disappears immediately is unlikely to be genuine. A grade-3 or -4 Trousseau sign is always pathologic, but a grade-1 or -2 response may occur in about 4 percent of normal subjects. In one case of the author, a negative response occurred in one arm and a grade-4 response in the other; no explanation could be found.

Erb's sign[1,2] is a diminished threshold of response to galvanic stimulation, now of historical interest only. Of the neural effects of hypocalcemia, impaired accommodation is more precisely and reproducibly measured. Accommodation is an increase in the threshold of excitation in response to an increase in the intensity of the stimulus, and changes can be detected very quickly in response to alterations in treatment.[17]

Variations in Clinical Expression

If a typical attack is witnessed or well described, the diagnosis of tetany will be obvious, but many variations are possible. The patient may describe the muscle spasm as a cramp or as stiffness or clumsiness. In chronic stable HP the patient may be more-or-less continuously liable to mild paresthesiae and cramps rather than to clearly defined attacks of tetany, or may develop carpal spasm only during prolonged use of the hand and forearm, for example, during writing or knitting. Tetany is frequently precipitated by hyperventilation, whether due to emotional distress or to exercise. Only sensory symptoms may occur, and carpal-tunnel decompression may be performed before the correct diagnosis is made. If the spasm is more severe in the legs than in the arms, the patient may complain of limping or difficulty in walking and may be subject to

falls. Occasionally, only one side of the body is affected.[18] Spasm of the muscles of the larynx (laryngismus stridulus) fixes the vocal cords in the midline, leading to stridor, crowing respiration, and cyanosis. This used to be a frequent manifestation of infantile vitamin D deficiency, but, in adults with HP, laryngeal stridor is usually a result of vocal-cord paralysis.[19] Nevertheless, reversible laryngeal spasm may occasionally be the presenting feature,[20] and minor difficulties with vocalization are not uncommon. One patient of the author's could no longer sing in church, a loss which she attributed to age until her voice recovered with treatment.

The irritability of autonomic ganglia is also increased by hypocalcemia[21] and an amazing variety of symptoms has been attributed to spasm of smooth muscle.[1] This has been reasonably well documented in the esophagus, leading to dysphagia;[4] in the small intestine, leading to abdominal pain and pseudoobstruction;[22] in the sphincter of Oddi, leading to biliary colic;[23] and in the bronchi, leading to wheezing and shortness of breath.[24]

The clinical expression of hypocalcemia is modified by many other factors.[2] In infants, carpopedal spasm is rare, but tremors, twitches, and convulsive seizures are more common than in adults; this may be due to the frequently associated hypomagnesemia. Carpopedal spasm occurs in older children but is less common than in adults.[25] The effects of a rapidly falling calcium level are more marked than those of a stable calcium at a lower level, and both overt and latent tetany may rarely be absent in longstanding hypocalcemia. Tetany may be masked without a change in plasma calcium by hypokalemia,[26] hypermagnesemia, metabolic acidosis, uremia,[27] or a fall in plasma phosphate induced by probenecid.[28] Tetany may be worsened by withdrawal of thyroid medication in patients who also have hypothyroidism, and may be precipitated by infection or by diuretic administration. Finally, symptoms may be worse just before menstruation[2] and during pregnancy,[29] even though the plasma calcium level is unchanged; this is probably because of sodium and water retention.[30] There is no evidence of any relationship of symptoms to the onset of the menopause[31] despite many statements to this effect.

Other Causes of Tetany

Although tetany is most typically associated with hypocalcemia, there are several other causes, such as metabolic alkalosis, hyperkalemia, hypokalemia, and hypomagnesemia.[2,23] The most important is hyperventilation. This lowers the ionized calcium, partly because alkalosis increases the calcium-binding capacity of proteins and partly because of the accumulation of organic acids which complex calcium.[27] More important, alkalosis has an independent effect of increasing neural excitability which is synergistic with that of hypocalcemia.[7] Hypocapnia produces many other effects, including peripheral vasoconstriction with a pale and moist skin, dizziness, tinnitus, blurring of vision, lightheadedness, and eventually syncope due to cerebral vasoconstriction and tissue hypoxia.[32] With voluntary hyperventilation, symptoms of tetany may not occur for 10 min and overt carpopedal spasm not for 20 min.[33] Consequently, when hyperventilation reflects an underlying psychoneurosis, overt tetany is present only in a minority of cases.[32] Some individuals are unusually susceptible to the effects of respiratory alkalosis, and a much shorter period of overbreathing induces tetany as the earliest symptom.[33] The chemical changes in the blood may easily escape detection,[27,33] leading to a diagnosis of idiopathic or constitutional tetany.[28,27] Hyperventilation is a common feature of hypocalcemic tetany, and patients with unrecognized HP who are anxious and overbreathing are not uncommonly dismissed from emergency rooms as hysterical.

CONVULSIVE SEIZURES

Hypocalcemia increases neuronal irritability in the central as well as in the peripheral system, and fits resembling those of epilepsy are an important manifestation of HP. In children, convulsions are a common nonspecific manifestation of a variety of illnesses, but they are particularly liable to occur in hypocalcemia. There are two distinct types of seizure, although intermediate cases undoubtedly occur, and some patients may get both kinds. First, hypocalcemia lowers the excitation threshold for preexisting subclinical epilepsy.[34] The attacks are indistinguishable from those occurring in the absence of hypocalcemia and may be of any form—focal, Jacksonian, petit mal, or grand mal.[35] The EEG shows the same range of findings as in epilepsy with normocalcemia, and remains abnormal with successful treatment of the HP even though the number of seizures is reduced.[34] The other type of seizure is more aptly referred to as cerebral tetany rather than epilepsy. The attacks consist essentially of generalized tetany followed by prolonged tonic spasms. There may be either an aura of the sensory symptoms of tetany or no aura at all, and tongue-biting, loss of consciousness, incontinence, and postictal confusion may not occur.[36,37] They may sometimes be precipitated by hypoxia in patients with laryngeal obstruction or stridor.

Hypocalcemia frequently produces distinct changes in the EEG.[38,39] These may be seen with either clinical type of seizure or occur in patients who have no seizures at all. There is irregularity and fragmentation of the postcentral background activity, a shift in frequency from delta (< 4 Hz) to theta ($4-8$ Hz), and increased low-voltage fast activity. Most characteristic are paroxysmal bursts of high-voltage slow waves at $2-5$ Hz, which occur with increasing frequency and duration at lower calcium levels. These bursts are a nonspecific response to a variety of metabolic derangements, which include hyper- as well as hypocalcemia. If the plasma calcium falls below 6.5 mg/100 ml, irregular sharp spike and wave patterns may appear. The abnormality shows a general resemblance to the pattern found with hyperventilation.[32] The spike and waves and paroxysmal slow bursts may disappear within a few days of raising the plasma calcium, but the abnormal background may not improve for several weeks, and the response to photic stimulation may not become normal for several months.[42]

Successful treatment of the HP will usually prevent both types of seizure and reduce or abolish the need for anticonvulsants; in fact, standard anticonvulsants are not only ineffective but may, by anti-vitamin D effects, aggravate the seizure disorder.[41]

OTHER MANIFESTATIONS OF HP

Tetany is related to the severity of hypocalcemia and not to its duration, but many of the other complications require a certain period of time to develop. In chronic hypocalcemia, many kinds of organ dysfunction may occur, but those which produce clinical effects are not always those which would be predicted from current knowledge of the multiple effects of calcium on cell functions at the molecular level.[42,43] For example, the participation of ionic calcium in blood coagulation is known in considerable detail, but spontaneous bleeding is never caused by HP.

To qualify as a genuine manifestation of the disease, a clinical phenomenon must either be reversed by the correction of hypocalcemia or be shown to occur more commonly than in a properly matched control group. Some clinical phenomena are commoner in SHP than in normal subjects, but are not more common than in thyroidectomized subjects of the same age and sex.[34] Another

factor to be considered in SHP is the presence or absence of hypothyroidism.

Basal-Ganglion Calcification and Extrapyramidal Syndromes[35,44–46]

In longstanding HP, small irregular discrete areas of calcification may be seen about $3-5$ cm above the sella in the lateral view of the skull and about $2-4$ cm from the midline in the frontal view.[35,44] Localization is best accomplished by tomography.[45] The lesions consist of deposits of calcium salts and iron in a basophilic material rich in glycosaminoglycans which accumulates in and around the walls of small blood vessels in the basal ganglia. Such lesions also occur in the dentate nucleus of the cerebellum. In SHP, the average interval between operation (presumed to mark the onset of the hypoparathyroid state) and radiographic detection of basal-ganglia calcification is 17 years.[46] The lesions occur in all varieties of HP which remain untreated for a sufficiently long time. Basal-ganglion calcification may occur in a variety of other conditions;[35] of particular interest is a familial form which has certain points of resemblance to PHP.

There may either be no neurologic disability or a variety of extrapyramidal syndromes, including classic Parkinsonism, choreoathetosis (either spontaneous or kinesiogenic), and dystonic spasms (either spontaneous or precipitated by phenothiazine drugs).[35] The neurologic disability usually improves with successful treatment of the HP but occasionally gets worse.

Papilledema and Raised Intracranial Pressure[35,40,47,48]

Swelling of the optic disc is an occasional finding. It is usually of moderate degree (not more than 3 diopters) and unaccompanied by hemorrhages. Most instances have been in long-standing untreated disease, but papilledema has developed acutely within 2 weeks of thyroid surgery. There are no symptoms, and vision is not impaired; its importance is in the frequent mistaken diagnoses of cerebral tumor, especially since the patient usually also has seizures. It occurs in all types of HP, but is less frequent in PHP than in IHP or SHP. The swelling begins to subside within a few days of treatment and has usually disappeared within 4 weeks, although some cases take much longer, and some residual pallor of the disc may persist indefinitely. The cause is unclear.

Psychiatric Disorders[35,49]

In longstanding HP, many kinds of psychoneurosis, psychosis, and organic brain syndrome have been described, but in a defined population serious psychopathology is uncommon. Subnormal intelligence occurs in about one-fifth of children with IHP; it correlates with prolonged untreated hypocalcemia irrespective of its cause. Intelligence may increase with treatment or remain unchanged despite improvement in personality. The wide variety of other syndromes suggests that, as with seizures, hypocalcemia has triggered a disorder to which the patient was already predisposed.

Changes in the Skin and Related Structures[50–52]

The acute hypocalcemia of SHP may rarely be followed by a temporary arrest of growth of the hair and fingernails. The affected hair loses its luster, and with resumption of growth (which may occur spontaneously even in the absence of treatment) it falls out extensively. The fingernails also may be shed or may show transverse ridging when growth is resumed.[50]

In chronic HP, the skin may be dry and scaling, the nails brittle and fissured longitudinally, and the hair coarse, dry, fractured, and easily shed. These changes must be distinguished from those due to infection with Candida,[37] and from alopecia occurring as an independent component of the multiple-endocrine-deficiency, autoimmune–candidiasis (MEDAC) syndrome (see below).

A variety of much-more-severe skin lesions has occurred in isolated cases of chronic HP, including atopic eczema, exfoliative dermatitis, and impetigo herpetiformis.[51,52] Psoriasis may be exacerbated or may occur for the first time within a few weeks of the onset of SHP. These diverse lesions all improve considerably or disappear after normocalcemia is restored. Occasionally hypocalcemia from any cause may lead to secondary Candida infection of the skin; this improves with a rise in plasma calcium and is another instance of the nonspecific effect of hypocalcemia on skin health.

Changes in the Teeth[53,54]

Hypocalcemia affects a tooth only when it begins during the development of that tooth; teeth already formed are not affected. Hypoplasia of the enamel, with pitting, staining, superficial fractures, and increased liability to caries is the most characteristic finding. The corresponding dentin is irregular and may be completely dysplastic. There may also be delayed eruption and blunting of the roots with gaps between the teeth because some are missing altogether.

Lenticular Cataract[55,56]

This is the commonest complication of chronic hypocalcemia. Cataracts begin as discrete punctate or lamellar opacities in the cortex of the lens but separated from the capsule by a clear zone. They may occur in several distinct layers and are more evident in the posterior pole than in the anterior, but radially they are of even distribution. Eventually they may become confluent and produce total opacity of the lens. Such cataracts are not specific for HP and occur in several other metabolic disorders, but they are distinct from senile cataracts, which are frequently confined to one segment of the lens. Small opacities may be no commoner than in control subjects. It usually takes at least 5–10 years for cataracts to reach a size which interferes with vision. With treatment, further progression is arrested, and rarely the opacities may even become smaller.[57,58]

Concerning pathogenesis, cataracts occur in vitamin D deficiency with low phosphorus and high PTH and in chronic renal failure with high phosphorus and high PTH. Consequently, the hypocalcemia which occurs in all three conditions is the most likely immediate cause. The high calcium content of the affected lens is due to dystrophic calcification; it is common to cataracts of all types and does not result from lack of a PTH effect on a calcium transport system.[56]

Intestinal Malabsorption[59,60]

Long-standing HP may rarely be complicated by intestinal malabsorption and steatorrhea, which disappear with correction of the hypocalcemia. A vicious circle may be established, the malabsorption further worsening the hypocalcemia. Jejunal biopsy may show partial villous atrophy which does not respond to a gluten-free diet but is reversible with vitamin D. There is a suggestion that bile salt deficiency may be involved.[61] Radiologic examination of the bowel may show puddling and flocculation resembling sprue even in the absence of steatorrhea. Gastric and intestinal contractability improve when the plasma calcium rises. Achlorhydria may

occur, and megaloblastic anemia due to selective impairment of vitamin B_{12} absorption without steatorrhea has been described in two cases.[62] Malabsorption secondary to hypocalcemia must be distinguished from primary intestinal malabsorption with acquired resistance to PTH leading to hypocalcemia and elevated plasma phosphate.[63]

Cardiovascular Manifestations[64–66]

Hypocalcemia delays ventricular repolarization and increases the QT_c and ST intervals on ECG. These quantities vary inversely with plasma calcium over the range 16–4 mg/100 ml, but a prediction of plasma calcium from QT_c is very inaccurate because of the wide scatter.[64] With prolongation of electrical systole, the ventricles may fail to respond to the next atrial impulse, producing 2:1 heart block.

Calcium ion has a positive inotropic effect on the myocardium and is essential for coupling of excitation and contraction, but clinically detectable effects of hypocalcemia on heart muscle function are rare in current experience. Nevertheless, there are several well-documented instances in both children[65] and adults[31] of chronic HP leading to congestive cardiac failure requiring digitalization and diuretic therapy, the need for which was abolished after restoration of normocalcemia for a few weeks or months. In HP, calcium infusion may increase both cardiac output and blood pressure,[66] suggesting that cardiac function may have been suboptimal even without clinical manifestations. In earlier periods[1] cardiac tetany was often reported in hypocalcemic infants with advanced, untreated rickets who developed dyspnea, tachycardia, and sudden death due to cardiac arrest in diastole.[1]

Osseous and Locomotor Manifestations[67–71]

There are many reports of increased cortical thickness and trabecular bone density in IHP.[37] Most of these are unsupported by objective evidence, but abnormal width of the lamina dura is evident in a few instances.[67] It has been claimed that the rate of progression of involutional osteoporosis is reduced in HP. This could be predicted as a consequence of reduced bone turnover, but an attempt to confirm the finding in a much larger series of patients with SHP was unsuccessful.[68] Calcific periarthritis of the shoulder has been reported,[69] but may be a result of treatment with vitamin D.

Fatigue and weakness which improve with treatment are common symptoms, but objective confirmation of muscle disease is usually lacking. However, one case of severe myopathy has been reported[70] accompanied by striking elevation of serum creatine phosphokinase and lactic dehydrogenase which returned to normal with treatment. Elevation of these enzymes in the absence of muscle weakness may be quite common in hypocalcemia.[71] In another case there was a marked increase in the severity and duration of the muscle paralysis induced by curarization in preparation for surgery.[35]

Complete Absence of Symptoms and Signs

The adaptation which occurs to long-standing hypocalcemia has already been mentioned; occasionally this is so successful that all manifestations of HP may be absent. Unexpected hypocalcemia is commonly found as a result of multichannel biochemical screening, but is usually due to some cause other than HP, such as hypoproteinemia. No case of previously unrecognized HP was discovered at Henry Ford Hospital in the first 2 years of availability of multichannel screening. In striking contrast is the increased recognition of primary hyperparathyroidism, which suggests that completely asymptomatic HP is exceedingly uncommon.

CAUSES OF PTH DEFICIENCY[72]

These are classified in Table 62-2 as idiopathic, acquired, and reversible.

IDIOPATHIC

As originally defined, the term IHP referred to all cases not due to surgical damage or some other equally well-defined cause. Within this group a number of distinct syndromes can now be recognized and the term IHP should perhaps be restricted to those cases remaining after these syndromes have been removed, but, as a matter of convenience, if not of logic, the traditional definition of IHP will be retained.

Isolated Persistent Neonatal HP[73]

HP manifest at or soon after birth is most likely due to congenital absence of the parathyroid glands; parathyroid antibodies are not found. Most cases are sporadic, but both X-linked recessive and autosomal recessive inheritance occur.

Branchial Dysembryogenesis[74-76] (III–IV-Pharyngeal-Pouch Syndrome; DiGeorge Syndrome)

Congenital absence of the parathyroid glands may also be associated with congenital absence of the thymus. In addition to neonatal tetany, affected infants suffer from repeated severe infections because of profoundly depressed cell-mediated immunity. They frequently have maldevelopment of the first and fifth branchial clefts as well. The former produces a characteristic set of facial abnormalities—hypertelorism, antimongoloid slant of the eyes, asymmetrical ears which are low set and notched, abnormally short philtrum of the lip, and micrognathia. The latter produces a wide variety of congenital aortic-arch or conotruncal anomalies, such as right-sided arch or Fallot's tetralogy. Most of the patients die in infancy or early childhood from infection or from heart failure, but, if the cardiovascular lesion is mild or surgically remediable and the defective immunity partial rather

Table 62-2. Causes of PTH-Deficient Hypoparathyroidism

Idiopathic
  Isolated persistent neonatal HP
  Branchial dysembryogenesis
  MEDAC syndrome (*m*ultiple *e*ndocrine *d*eficiency, *a*utoimmune–*c*andidiasis.)
  Isolated late onset HP
Acquired
  Postsurgical (thyroid, parathyroid, or radical neck)
  Post-^{131}I therapy (any reason)
  Hemosiderosis (any cause)
  Secondary neoplasia
  Miscellaneous possible causes (amyloid, TB, trauma, sarcoidosis, asparaginase)
Reversible
  Neonatal hypocalcemia, physiologic and pathologic
  Transient congenital dysplasia
  Maternal hyperparathyroidism
  Suppression by hypercalcemia
  Hypomagnesemia

than complete, survival into adolescence or adult life is possible. Consequently, the syndrome should be considered in IHP occurring at any age. In one personal case previously reported[74] parathyroid function improved to nearly normal after 8 years of treatment.

Multiple-Endocrine-Deficiency, Autoimmune,–Candidiasis (MEDAC) Syndrome: Juvenile Familial Endocrinopathy—Hypoparathyroidism, Addison's Disease, and Candidiasis (HAM Syndrome)

This is a genetic disorder transmitted as an autosomal recessive comprising hypofunction of several endocrine glands, often associated with organ-specific autoantibodies, variable involvement of other organs, and recurrent Candida infections.[77-79] The major independent components are HP, Addison's disease, and chronic mucocutaneous candidiasis, at least two of which are present in most patients with the syndrome. The sexes are equally affected.

Candidiasis usually appears first in early childhood and affects the skin, finger- and toenails, oropharynx, and vagina.[80] The lesions may be of trivial extent or may cover almost the whole body. The affected nails are pitted and friable, and the changes are sometimes confused with those due to hypocalcemia.[37] Most patients with chronic mucocutaneous candidiasis are not destined to develop endocrine deficiency, but they are clinically indistinguishable from those who are. In many patients there is subtle evidence of impaired cell-mediated immunity and reduction or absence of delayed cutaneous hypersensitivity to Candida. There may also be deficiency of a candidicidal substance normally present in the blood.[80a] Despite this, systemic candidiasis is rare in the MEDAC syndrome and occurs only if there are other predisposing factors such as diabetes mellitus.[80b] The candidiasis is refractory to both local antifungal therapy and to treatment of the HP, but may respond to diiodohydroxyquin or to systemic amphotericin alone or combined with transfer factor.[81] Occasionally, a related immunologic defect leads to infection with other fungi, such as *Trichophyton rubrum*.[82] Recurrent staphylococcal infections of the skin are also common in these patients.

Symptoms of HP develop on the average about 4 years after the onset of candidiasis (mean age, 9 years), the interval ranging from 0 to 20 years, and of Addison's disease on the average after a further 5 years (mean age, 14 years). The HP does not differ clinically from IHP occurring in isolation; lymphocytic infiltration has been noted in a few cases.[83] In addition to the early age of onset, the Addison's disease is associated with an unusually high mortality.

There are additional components of the syndrome. Keratoconjunctivitis may be noted in as many as 50 percent of patients.[84] In mild cases, slight redness of the eye, photophobia, and blepharospasm may occur, and, in severe cases, ulceration, scarring, and vascularization may lead to corneal opacity and impairment of vision. Keratoconjunctivitis may be a hypersensitivity response to Candida infection rather than an independent component of the syndrome, but has occurred in the absence of candidiasis. Alopecia may occur in 30 percent of the cases and may be partial or total with loss of eyebrows and eyelashes as well.[85] Enamel hypoplasia and other varieties of dental dysplasia may precede hypocalcemia[86] or occur in its absence.[80] Pernicious anemia, despite its early onset, is of the adult type (gastric atrophy with loss of all secretory components, and presence of antibodies to parietal cells and intrinsic factor) rather than of the juvenile type (selective deficiency of intrinsic factor without antibodies). It usually occurs 5–10 years after the onset of HP. Hepatitis progressing to cirrhosis of the liver has been reported.[80] Premature ovarian failure may give rise to primary or secondary amenorrhea, and the ovarian pathology may resemble gonadal dysgenesis.[82] Autoimmune thyroiditis resembles that seen in isolation.

The immunologic aspects of the syndrome are confusing.[83,87] There is poor correlation between the presence or absence of antibodies and the presence or absence of clinical manifestations in different members of a kindred.[87] The presence of antibodies, however, may provide clues to endocrine deficiency before clinical manifestations occur. The significance of antibodies found in apparently normal family members is unclear. Finally, there is not yet any evidence that antibodies are directly involved in the destruction of parathyroid tissue.

Isolated Late-Onset HP

The three categories considered above comprise distinct clinical entities, but the remaining cases of idiopathic hypoparathyroidism are much less clearly defined. Fragmentary information available concerning genetics, age of onset, presence or absence of parathyroid antibodies, and pathology has suggested subdivision into autoimmune and nonautoimmune categories, each of which may be hereditary or sporadic.

In the commonest group, the onset is usually between the ages of 2 and 10 years, and females are affected twice as often as males. About 3 cases of 4 are sporadic, with a high incidence of parathyroid antibodies in the patients but not in other family members. In about one-quarter of the cases there is evidence of autosomal recessive inheritance, and antibodies may be found in relatives as well as in the patient. Some of these cases will be formes frustes of the MEDAC syndrome, but isolated HP is a genetically distinct disorder.[87]

In a much smaller number, successive generations are affected, suggesting autosomal dominant inheritance, and parathyroid antibodies are absent. The age of onset covers a wider range (1 month to 20 years), and is often much earlier in the child than in the parent.[73]

When IHP first produces symptoms in adult life, it is almost invariably sporadic, and without antiparathyroid antibodies. The onset may be at any age up to the eighth decade. The duration of symptoms before diagnosis and institution of treatment is longest in this group. In the few cases examined pathologically, fatty replacement[88] or atrophy with fatty infiltration and fibrosis[89] has been found. In the very elderly, ischemia is a plausible cause but has never been proven.

ACQUIRED

Surgical Hypoparathyroidism

This is by far the most common variety. With the increasing use of ^{131}I for the treatment of hyperthyroidism, the incidence of thyroid operations has diminished in major medical centers, but the frequency in the total population remains high. With decreasing surgical experience, the incidence of parathyroid injury may increase so that the number of new cases of tetany may remain the same or even rise.[90]

It is important to distinguish between hypocalcemia and tetany because the therapeutic and prognostic implications are quite different. Mild asymptomatic hypocalcemia may reflect a nonspecific response to surgery or anesthesia,[91] or sudden reversal of negative bone and calcium balance if hyperthyroidism had been incompletely controlled before operation. Release of calcitonin during manipulation of the thyroid[92] has been suggested but is difficult to interpret due to lack of hypocalcemia following calcitonin administration to normal subjects even in large doses (Chapter 50). This reversal has been suggested as the mechanism for most cases of early hypocalcemia after thyroidectomy for hyperthyroidism because, when parathyroidectomy complicates radical neck surgery, tetany rarely occurs before 3 days and is often delayed for 1 week.[93] The "hungry bone" phenomenon may well determine the time of onset of the hypocalcemia, but the mechanism of hypocalcemia and the prognosis of tetany are different problems. In 49 of the author's cases of postthyroidectomy tetany, this event occurred during the first 24 hours in 11 and during the second 24 hours in 18. Earlier onset and lesser severity of tetany increased the chance of eventual recovery. However, whatever the time of onset, more than half the cases were eventually found to need vitamin D permanently and many of the rest showed impaired parathyroid function even though they needed no treatment; the findings of others have been similar.[94] By contrast, in patients who do not develop symptoms, impaired calcium homeostasis revealed by EDTA eventually reverts completely to normal, usually within 1 year.[95]

The mechanism of the parathyroid injury is unclear. The incidence of postoperative tetany diminishes progressively with age,[90] is much higher in women than in men, and is higher after operations for hyperthyroidism than for nontoxic goiter. The incidence decreases with the extent of resection and is highest with radical neck surgery for thyroid cancer,[96] but it diminishes with increasing surgical experience and skill, and with the use of special techniques of dissection.[96] Injury to the recurrent laryngeal nerve is more common in patients with parathyroid injury than in those without.[19] However, short of removing all four glands, which almost never occurs except in operations for cancer, there is no relationship between the occurrence of tetany and the presence or absence of parathyroid tissue in the excised specimen.[97] The incidence increases with the number of ligatures close to the parathyroid gland.[95] This suggests that parathyroid injury is a result of ischemia and reflects the extent of dissection and hemostasis necessary to achieve a dry operative field.

About half the patients who develop postoperative tetany will eventually recover sufficiently for treatment to be withdrawn. Such patients may regain persistent normocalcemia without symptoms (grade 1) or they may be liable to intermittent hypocalcemia, for example, during episodes of gastroenteritis (grade 2). Recovery frequently takes place within a few weeks to 6 months (occasionally as long as 36 months), but these patients have permanent latent hypoparathyroidism. Prolonged hypocalcemia and apparent resistance to treatment may also reflect continuation of the hungry-bone phenomenon[98] and the long time required for bone turnover to return to normal.[99] Apparent clinical recovery, but with persistent impairment of response to EDTA infusion,[100] may occasionally be followed by the delayed recurrence of clinically overt HP and persistent hypocalcemia. In two personally documented cases this relapse occurred 6 and 13 years after surgery, but much longer delays might be possible.

In the remaining cases of postoperative tetany, hypocalcemia persists because of permanent chronic HP. This requires treatment indefinitely, usually with vitamin D in some form, occasionally with calcium supplements alone. Many patients with chronic SHP probably retain a small remnant of functioning tissue; its failure to regenerate is presumably due to fibrosis or ischemia.

A less frequent course is the subsequent discovery of chronic

HP in the absence of tetany in the early postoperative period.[31] It is usually assumed that such patients have had asymptomatic hypocalcemia ever since the operation, but chronic HP may occur after a period of normocalcemia[101] as long as 23 years after operation. The explanation for this late onset is unknown. One possibility is continuing fibrosis in and around the thyroid leading to parathyroid strangulation. Whatever the explanation, the practical lesson is clear—HP should be suspected in every patient with a scar in the neck, however long ago the operation and whether or not the plasma calcium has previously been normal.

Any differences noted in clinical features between IHP and SHP reflect differences in the severity of PTH deficiency and in the length of delay before diagnosis. When the effects of age are discounted, patients with the same degree of hypocalcemia have the same level of plasma phosphate in both SHP and IHP.[51] Similarly, in SHP which is not diagnosed for 10 years or more, the incidence of long-term complications such as cataracts and basal-ganglion calcification is the same as in IHP.[31]

Irradiation Damage

[131]I administration for the treatment of hyperthyroidism or thyroid cancer or for the deliberate induction of hypothyroidism has very occasionally been followed by HP, usually transient but occasionally permanent with cataracts and persistent need for vitamin D.[102,103] The parathyroids are unusually resistant to irradiation, and the incidence is unrelated to the dose; possibly intrathyroidal location of the parathyroid glands increases the risk. Diminished functional reserve determined by a number of techniques has been found to be surprisingly common in ^{131}I-treated patients, but this may be related to associated hypothyroidism.[104]

Iron Overload

Hemochromatosis may cause siderosis and clinical failure of the pancreatic islets, and, occasionally, of the pituitary; the parathyroid glands are uniformly infiltrated with iron at autopsy.[105] Clinical HP has been described in a variety of diseases characterized by increased iron storage, and in one such case due to thalassemia siderosis, fibrosis and atrophy of the parathyroid glands were found at autopsy.[106]

Neoplastic Infiltration

As in the adrenal gland, microscopic evidence of metastatic disease is fairly common, occurring in 6 percent of one large series.[107,124] However, clinical HP is rare; it was found in only 2 of 41 cases of metastases, in both of which more than 75 percent of the parathyroid parenchyma was replaced by tumor. Exclusion of osteoblastic metastases and of the effects of antimitotic therapy on the gland would be necessary to make an antemortem diagnosis.

Miscellaneous Pathologic Processes[1]

Pathologic involvement of the parathyroid can occur in syphilis, miliary tuberculosis, amyloidosis (both primary and secondary), hemorrhage due to external trauma, and sarcoidosis, but there is no well-documented case of clinical HP due to any of these causes. In rabbits, parathyroid necrosis can be produced by asparaginase;[108] the use of this substance in the treatment of leukemia has been associated with hypocalcemia, but the mechanism has not been established.

REVERSIBLE

This can be due to delayed maturation of parathyroid function, suppression of normal glands by hypercalcemia or impaired hormone synthesis because of magnesium depletion.

Neonatal Hypocalcemia and Tetany[109–112]

After birth the plasma calcium usually falls from the high levels found in cord blood to a value 1–2 mg/100 ml below the normal level of infancy, the lowest point occurring within 24–48 hours and then recovering spontaneously. Early neonatal tetany represents an exaggeration of this normal phenomenon, which occurs especially in association with maternal diabetes, prematurity, low birth weight, or respiratory distress. Compared to infants without tetany, the PTH level is lower and slower to rise to normal.[109–114] Late neonatal tetany occurring after about 1 week usually follows cow's milk feeding and is associated with hyperphosphatemia and more severe symptoms.[110,112]

Transient Congenital Parathyroid Dysplasia[113,114]

This condition is characterized by severe persistent hypocalcemia, which is occasionally delayed for several weeks after birth, elevated plasma phosphate, and a need for vitamin D therapy to restore normocalcemia. At this stage, the condition is indistinguishable from persistent isolated neonatal HP, but, after 3–6 months, parathyroid function returns to normal, and treatment can be withdrawn. Some cases may represent a severe and protracted form of late neonatal tetany.[112]

Maternal Primary Hyperparathyroidism[72,115]

Infants born to mothers with primary hyperparathyroidism not uncommonly develop severe hypocalcemia. Symptoms usually begin within the first 2 weeks, and complete recovery usually occurs after about 3 months, although one case of permanent HP has occurred.[116] The mother's disease may otherwise be asymptomatic, so that neonatal tetany may be the first clue to the diagnosis. The cause is presumed to be depression of fetal parathyroid function because of transmission of maternal hypercalcemia via the placenta, but in 1 case the level of PTH in the infant was raised, and the hypocalcemia was attributed to hypomagnesemia and target-cell resistance to PTH.[117]

Suppression by Hypercalcemia

A normal parathyroid gland secretes less hormone in the face of hypercalcemia. When the hypercalcemia is corrected, recovery of normal function depends on quiescent cells reentering a secretory phase of the cell cycle and not on regeneration of new tissue. Such temporary suppression of parathyroid function may contribute to symptomatic hypocalcemia after removal of a parathyroid adenoma, although reversal of hyperparathyroid bone disease and deliberate or accidental trauma to the other glands are usually more important factors. A rare but interesting variant is the occurrence of hypocalcemic tetany as the presenting manifestation of primary hyperparathyroidism with bone disease, due to spontaneous infarction of an adenoma.[118]

Hypomagnesemia

A frequent manifestation of magnesium depletion is hypocalcemia. The causes are multiple and include abnormalities in the crystal structure of bone and consequent disturbances of the blood–bone equilibrium, impaired target-cell response to PTH, and impaired synthesis of PTH, presumably because of deficiency of a magnesium-dependent enzyme.[119] Primary congenital hypomagnesemia[110,120] is a disorder characterized by selective gastrointestinal malabsorption of magnesium, hypocalcemia, and convulsive seizures occurring between 1 and 4 months of age. The hypocalcemia is refractory to the administration of calcium but responds quickly to magnesium replacement. PTH levels, when measured, have been low or absent in the untreated state and have returned to normal with magnesium replacement, the need for which seems to be permanent.

Hypocalcemia due to magnesium depletion also occurs in adults. The plasma phosphate is usually reduced but is occasionally raised to produce a clinical and biochemical resemblance to primary hypoparathyroidism.[121] Normal or raised PTH levels have been recorded in adults with hypomagnesemia, so that the other factors mentioned may be relatively more important than in infants.

DIAGNOSIS OF HP

In the fullest sense, diagnosis in HP comprises (1) the recognition that the patient's symptoms are manifestations of tetany, (2) the differentiation of hypocalcemic from other forms of tetany, (3) the differentiation of HP from other causes of hypocalcemia, and (4) categorization of the type of HP. Only the third of these steps remains to be discussed.[45]

In most cases the diagnosis is obvious once it is considered, but as in hypofunction of other endocrine glands, the ultimate criterion is the demonstration of a subnormal hormone level in the blood. Despite unresolved problems in the methodology of parathyroid radioimmunoassay, measurements of immunoassayable PTH have confirmed that the PTH level in HP is undetectable or clearly below that expected for the level of plasma calcium,[122] and that different degrees of parathyroid deficiency can occur.

Although inconstant, hyperphosphatemia or other evidence of impaired phosphate reabsorption is present in the majority of patients. However, the combination of low calcium and high phosphate can occur in several other conditions (Table 62-3). Some index of renal function should always be obtained; a low PTH level may identify HP in patients who also have renal failure. The plasma magnesium should be measured routinely in all hypocalcemic patients. The precipitation of hypocalcemic tetany by massive oral or i.v. phosphate loads, or by cell breakdown during cytotoxic therapy, is of great interest but should not pose any diagnostic problem. The differentiation of IHP from PHP is described in the next chapter; the type of HP cannot be predicted with certainty from the patient's physical habitus.[123] There are many other causes of hypocalcemia, most of which should not be difficult to distinguish from HP (Table 62-3).

The recognition of latent HP would be accomplished most reliably by demonstrating a subnormal increment in plasma PTH in response to a hypocalcemic challenge. A diagnostic test based on this principle has not yet been standardized, but delayed recovery from hypocalcemia induced by EDTA can be used to assess parathyroid function provided the patient is euthyroid.[106,122] The occurrence of hypocalcemia in response to cellulose phosphate and a low-calcium diet has a similar significance.[124]

TREATMENT OF HP

Unless or until an oral preparation of pure human PTH can be supplied, the treatment of HP will consist primarily of the use of some form of vitamin D with or without supplemental calcium. Most patients will therefore require life-long administration of pharmacologic amounts of a potentially toxic medication which is an imperfect replacement for what they are lacking. Despite these considerable theoretical disadvantages, with appropriate attention

Table 62-3. Causes of Hypocalcemia Other Than Hypoparathyroidism

Vitamin D deficiency
Vitamin D dependency
Chronic renal failure*
Hypomagnesemia (may have low, normal, or high P)*
Intestinal malabsorption (of vitamin D, Ca, Mg)*
Induced by calcium depletion
   Normocalcemic hypoparathyroidism
   Medullary carcinoma of the thyroid
   Osteopetrosis
Dietary or absorptive phosphorus excess (usually impaired PTH action on bone is also needed)*
   Neonatal, delayed maturation
   Renal failure, resistance
   Hypoparathyroidism, especially pseudo-
Osteoblastic metastases in bone
Healing of osteitis fibrosa after surgery for hyperparathyroidism
Healing of high-turnover osteoporosis after surgery for hyperthyroidism
Drug induced
   Rapid infusion of phosphate
   Calcitonin
   Mithramycin, actinomycin
   Glucagon
   Viomycin
   Exchange resin in noncalcium phase
   Colchicine
   Imidazole
   Ethanol
Transient
   Acute renal failure*
   Magnesium infusion
   Muscle necrosis with dystrophic calcification
   Malignant hyperthermia*
   White-phosphorus burns*
   Sudden hyperphosphatemia due to cytotoxic therapy*
   Acute pancreatitis
   Chelating agents
      Citrate in massive transfusions
      EDTA (total Ca may be normal)
   Hemodialysis with Ca-free dialysate
   Hypertonic dehydration in children
   Calcitonin release during thyroid surgery
   Following major surgery of any kind
   Onset of healing in rickets or osteomalacia
   Hyperkalemic periodic paralysis
Fall in protein-bound calcium
   Hemodilution
   Hypoalbuminemia from any cause

*Also accompanied by hyperphosphatemia.

to detail, results comparable to those of replacement therapy for other endocrine deficiencies can be achieved.[125]

VITAMIN D AND ANALOGUES

Ergocalciferol (vitamin D_2), which for historical reasons is used instead of the naturally occurring cholecalciferol (vitamin D_3), and the synthetic analogue dihydrotachysterol (DHT) are the principal agents available. The physiologic metabolites 25-OH-D_3 and $1\alpha,25$-(OH)$_2$-D_3 and the synthetic analogue 1α-OH-D_3 are under active clinical investigation but have not yet been released for general use.

Of those effects of vitamin D which have been demonstrated to occur in patients with HP, increased gastrointestinal absorption of both calcium and phosphate are the most consistent.[126] The external balances do not usually change since the urinary excretion

Table 62-4. Clinical Comparison of Substances with Vitamin D Action

Characteristic	D_2 or D_3	DHT	25-OH-D_3	1α-OH-D_3 $1\alpha,25$-$(OH)_2$-D_3
Daily dose to prevent rickets (μg)	2–10	100–200	1–5	0.2–1
Relative potency	1	1/50*	2	10
Daily dose in hypoparathyroidism (μg)	750–3000	250–1000	50–200	0.5–2
Relative potency	1	3*	15	1500
Time to restore normocalcemia (weeks)*	4–8	1–2	2–4	3–6 days
Time to reach maximum effect (weeks)†	4–12	2–4	4–20	3–6 days
Persistence after cessation (weeks)	6–18‡	1–3	4–12	3–6 days

*Note that DHT is less potent than vitamin D in the treatment of rickets but more potent in the treatment of hypoparathyroidism.
†For constant daily dose; shorter if a loading dose is given.
‡Up to 18 months after severe intoxication.

increases by the same amount as net absorption, as with a pharmacologic dose of vitamin D in a normal individual.[127]

The extent to which increased absorption raises the plasma level depends on the GFR and the prevailing characteristics of tubular reabsorption. The acute effect of vitamin D and its metabolites on the kidney are unclear (Chapter 51). In most patients with HP, the decreased calcium reabsorption characteristic of PTH deficiency persists, so that urinary calcium tends to be high during treatment. In other patients, calcium reabsorption may either increase[128] or decrease.[129] The increased TmP/GFR invariably falls with treatment,[126] an effect most likely secondary to the rise in plasma calcium.[130] The change in plasma phosphate depends on the balance between the fall in TmP/GFR and the increase in phosphate absorption; occasionally there is a temporary rise in serum phosphate, but in most cases phosphate eventually falls to a high normal level.

Vitamin D also raises the level of the blood–bone equilibrium,[3] even though urinary hydroxyproline excretion does not change.[131] The calcium fluxes between blood and bone increase before any change in calcium absorption or plasma calcium is detectable,[132] and, in most patients with treated HP, recovery from EDTA-induced hypocalcemia is almost normal.[133]

Although there are no systematic differences in the effects of different forms of vitamin D, there are crucial differences in the doses needed and in the times of onset and offset of these effects (Table 62-4). The information for 25-OH-D_3 is less complete[125] than it is for D_2 and DHT,[134] and, for the 1-hydroxylated derivatives, only short-term data are available.[4,135] The slow onset of action of D_2 and D_3 probably reflects the need for 25-hydroxylation, whereas persistence of action after cessation is a function of storage in body tissues.[134]

CALCIUM SALTS

Supplemental calcium increases the flux of calcium through the body by about 5–10 percent of the amount given, depending on the prevailing efficiency of absorption. When given without vitamin D, the average increase in plasma calcium is about 0.5 mg/100 ml/g elemental calcium, with quite wide variation. Frequent small doses are better absorbed than fewer larger ones. The commonest mistake in the use of calcium preparations is thinking in terms of weight of salt, rather than quantity of elemental calcium; when prescribed in equimolar amounts there is not much difference between one salt and another. Intravenous calcium is usually given as the gluconate, available in ampules of 10 percent solution, 10 ml containing 90 mg of calcium. The effect of a single injection is short lived, but continuous i.v. infusion will raise the plasma level by

about 0.5 mg/100 ml/100 mg calcium load/24 h, again depending on GFR and the characteristics of tubular reabsorption.

PRACTICAL ASPECTS OF TREATMENT

In acute HP with tetany (most common soon after neck surgery) the objectives of treatment are to relieve symptoms and forestall laryngeal obstruction or seizures; these are unlikely if the vocal cords are mobile and the plasma calcium is kept above 7.0 mg/100 ml—the level is otherwise unimportant. In adults, depending on the severity, 10–20 ml of 10 percent calcium gluconate is given by slow i.v. push, allowing not less than 1 min/10 ml. In patients who are digitalized, particular caution is needed, and EKG control is advisable. If the patient can swallow, oral calcium should be begun immediately, starting with 200 mg calcium every 2 hours of wakefulness, increasing each dose progressively to 500 mg if required. If i.v. calcium is needed again within 6 hours, continuous i.v. administration is advisable, beginning with 10 ml of 10 percent solution added to 500 ml of i.v. fluid every 6 hours.

If symptomatic hypocalcemia is prolonged or difficult to control, DHT should be given. A well-tried regimen is 4 mg/day for 2 days, then 2 mg/day for 2 days, then 1 mg/day until further dose adjustments are indicated. This will increase the plasma calcium to normal within 1 week or less (Fig. 62-1). Oral calcium can be continued until the plasma calcium rises above normal; even if some overshoot occurs, normocalcemia is quickly restored when

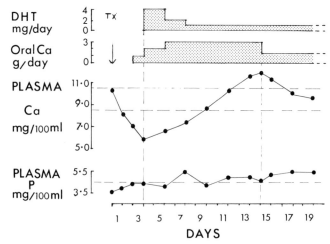

Fig. 62-1. Rapid response to DHT in a patient with medullary carcinoma of the thyroid subjected to total resection of thyroid and parathyroid glands and consequent postoperative tetany.

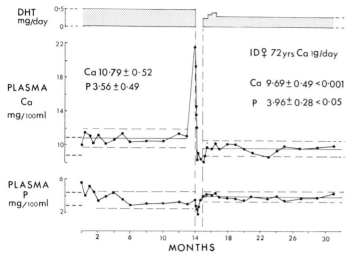

Fig. 62-2. Abrupt onset of severe hypercalcemia in a patient with SHP taking DHT. The dose had been too high for many months before, with slight but nonprogressive hypercalcemia. After recovery, the patient was restabilized on a smaller dose.

the oral calcium is withdrawn. Apart from its rapidity of onset, another major advantage of DHT is that it is noncumulative, so that the effect abates quickly when it is withdrawn[136,137] (Fig. 62-2). The rapid offset of DHT also enables recovery to be easily tested. If treatment is withdrawn, hypocalcemia will recur within 2 weeks if parathyroid function has failed to improve. Both $1\alpha(OH)D_3$ and $1\alpha,25(OH)_2D_3$, but not $25\text{-}OH\text{-}D_3$, act even more quickly than DHT (Table 62-4), and one or other of these may become the drug of choice when a rapid effect is needed.[4,135]

In contrast to acute HP, in which control of symptoms is paramount, in chronic HP the object of treatment is to keep the plasma calcium in the lower half of the normal range. This is usually high enough to control symptoms and prevent complications such as cataracts, while limiting the degree of hypercalciuria. Symptoms may improve or even disappear despite persistence of hypocalcemia, and so cannot be used as a guide to treatment. Vitamin D_3 is much cheaper than DHT, but fine regulation of dose is more difficult. Treatment should begin with a low dose, cautiously increased by small increments, allowing time for the maximum response to be observed (Table 62-4). This policy minimizes the risk of hypercalcemia and enables drug equilibrium to be achieved, and thus the plasma level and body stores of parent substance and metabolites remain stable because the amount metabolized or excreted each day balances exactly the amount given.[134] If the dose is increased too quickly or by too-large increments, it will be impossible to tell if the final dose selected is higher than is needed to attain this equilibrium. When this happens, the plasma calcium may remain normal for a long time, but it is inevitable that vitamin D poisoning will eventually occur (Fig. 62-2).

The dietary calcium should be made up to about 1.0 g daily from all sources. Calcium supplements are not otherwise necessary, except in patients in the grade-3 category who may attain normocalcemia without vitamin D. Although untreated patients may get tetany with extra phosphate, variation in phosphate intake has little effect on plasma calcium in patients on vitamin D.[138] In patients with persistent hyperphosphatemia, dietary phosphate restriction may reduce the risk of soft-tissue calcification.[139] Vitamin D may lead to renal wasting of magnesium and an occasional

patient becomes severely magnesium, depleted and refractory to treatment.[140]

Most patients treated according to these principles are restored to good health.[125] The doses required for maintenance usually fall within the ranges of 1.0–3.0 mg/day for D_2 and 0.3–1.0 mg/day for DHT. Episodes of hypo- or hypercalcemia are rare, and their causes, such as dispensing error, change in calcium intake, or thiazide diuretic,[141] are easily identified.[125] Poor results[142,143] are largely due to serious defects in most commercially available vitamin D preparations.[125] The main problem with long-term treatment is impairment of both glomerular and tubular function and an increased risk of nephrolithiasis and nephrocalcinosis. These complications may occur without hypercalcemia and may be due to hypercalciuria or to a direct nephrotoxic effect of vitamin D.[139]

REFERENCES

1. Shelling, D. H.: The Parathyroids in Health and Disease. St. Louis, Mosby, 1935.
2. Fourman, P., Royer, P.: Calcium Metabolism and the Bone (ed 2). Oxford, Blackwell, 1968.
3. Parfitt, A. M.: The actions of parathyroid hormone on bone: relation to bone remodelling and turnover, calcium homeostasis and metabolic bone disease. Part 2, PTH and bone cells: bone turnover and plasma calcium regulation. Metabolism. *25:* 909, 1976.
4. Kooh, S. W., Fraser, D., DeLuca, H. F., et al: Treatment of hypoparathyroidism and pseudohypoparathyroidism with metabolites of vitamin D: evidence for impaired conversion of 25-hydroxy vitamin D to 1,25 dihydroxy vitamin D. *N Engl J Med 293:* 840, 1975.
5. Parfitt, A. M.: The spectrum of hypoparathyroidism. *J Clin Endocrinol Metab 34:* 152, 1972.
6. Aperia, A., Broberger, O., Bergstrand, O. G., et al: Renal response to intravenous phosphate load in idiopathic hypoparathyroidism and pseudohypoparathyroidism. *Acta Paediatr Scand 56:* 357, 1967.
7. Edmondson, J. W., Brashear, R. F., Li, T. K.: Tetany: quantitative interrelationship between calcium and alkalosis. *Am J Physiol 228:* 1082, 1975.
8. Barzel, U. S.: Systemic alkalosis in hypoparathyroidism. *J Clin Endocrinol Metab 29:* 917, 1969.
9. Kugelberg, E.: Neurologic mechanism for certain phenomena in tetany. *Arch Neurol Psychiatry 52:* 507, 1946.
10. Harvey, A. M., Lilienthal J. L.: Observations on the nature of tetany. The effect of adrenaline. *Bull Johns Hopkins Hosp 71:* 163, 1948.
11. Brink, F.: The role of calcium in neural processes. *Pharmacol Res 6:* 243, 1954.
12. Katzmann, R., Pappius, H. M.: Brain Electrolytes and Fluid Metabolism. Baltimore, Williams & Wilkins, 1973.
13. Lewis, T.: Trousseau's phenomenon in tetany. *Clin Sci 4:* 361, 1942 (Dec.).
14. Layzer, R. B., Rowland, L. P.: Cramps. *N Engl J Med 285:* 31, 1971.
15. Hoffman, E.: The Chvostek sign. A clinical study. *Am J Surg 96:* 33, 1958.
16. Schaaf, M., Payne, C. A.: Effect of diphenyl hydantoin and phenobarbital in overt and latent tetany. *N Engl J Med 274:* 1228, 1966.
17. Wigton, R. S., Brink, F.: Studies of accommodation of nerve in parathyroid deficiency. *J Clin Invest 23:* 898, 1941.
18. Simpson, J. A.: The neurological manifestations of hypoparathyroidism. *Brain 75:* 76, 1952.
19. Shearman, B. T., Clubb, J. S., Neale, F. C., et al: Vocal-cord paralysis and voice changes in patients with surgical hypoparathyroidism. *Br Med J 3:* 619, 1965.
20. Williams, G. T., Brown, M.: Laryngospasm in hypoparathyroidism *J Laryngol 88:* 369, 1970.
21. Levy, H. A.: Unusual clinical manifestations of chronic hypoparathyroidism. *Med Clin North Am 21:* 243, 1947.
22. Taybi, H., Keele, D.: Hypoparathyroidism: a review of the literature and report of two cases in sisters, one with steatorrhoea and intestinal pseudo-obstruction. *Am J Roentgenol 88:* 432, 1962.

23. Woodhouse, N. J. Y.: Hypocalcemia and hypoparathyroidism. *Clin Endocrinol Metab 3:* 323, 1974.
24. Sussman, R. M., Edinburgh, A.: Chronic idiopathic hypoparathyroidism simulating cardiac asthma. *N Engl J Med 256:* 734, 1957.
25. Soper, R. J., Mason, E. E., Buckwalter, J. A.: Hypoparathyroidism in children and adolescents. *Pediatrics 20:* 1097, 1950.
26. Engel, F. L., Martin, S. P., Taylor, H.: On the relation of potassium to the neurological manifestations of hypocalcemic tetany. *Bull Johns Hopkins Hosp 84:* 285, 1949.
27. Fanconi, A., Rose, G. A.: The ionized, complexed and protein-bound fractions of calcium in plasma. *Q J Med 27:* 463, 1958.
28. Pascale, I. R., Dubin, A., Hoffman, W. S.: Influence of Benecid on urinary excretion of phosphate in hypoparatharodism. *Metabolism 3:* 462, 1954.
29. Meyer, B.: Tetany and pregnancy. A clinical study. *Acta Endocrinol Suppl 43:* 1–146, 1959.
30. McQuarrie, I., Hansen, A. E., Ziegler, M. R.: Studies on the convulsive mechanism in idiopathic hypoparathyroidism. *J Clin Endocrinol 1:*789, 1941.
31. Parfitt, A. M.: Delayed recognition of post-surgical hypoparathyroidism. *Med J Aust 1:* 702, 1967.
32. Ames, F.: The hyperventilation syndrome. *J Ment Sci 101:* 466, 1955.
33. McCance, R. A.: Spontaneous overbreathing tetany. *Q J Med 1:* 247, 1932.
34. Basser, L. S., Neale, F. C., Ireland, A. W., et al: Epilepsy and electroencephalographic abnormalities in chronic surgical hypoparathyroidism. *Ann Intern Med 71:* 507, 1969.
35. Frame, B.: Neuromuscular manifestations of parathyroid disease. In: Vinken P. B., Bruyn G. W. (eds.): Handbook of Clinical Neurology, vol 27. Amsterdam, North Holland, 1976.
36. Bartter, F. C.: The parathyroid gland and its relationship to diseases of the nervous system. *Proc Assoc Res Nerv Ment Dis 32:* 1, 1953.
37. Bronsky, D., Kushner, D. S., Dubin, A., et al: Idiopathic hypoparathyroidism and pseudohypoparathyroidism; case report and review of the literature. *Medicine 37:* 317, 1958.
38. Roth B., Newsimal O.: EEG study of tetany and spasmophilia. *Electroencephalogr Clin Neurophysiol 17:* 36, 1969
39. Swash, M., Rowan, A. J.: Electroencephalographic criteria for hypocalcemia and hypercalcemia. *Arch Neurol 26:* 218, 1972.
40. Kerr, D.: Papilloedema and fits in hypoparathyroidism. *Q J Med 22:* 243, 1953.
41. Stamp, T. C. B.: Effects of long-term anticonvulsant therapy on calcium and vitamin D metabolism. *Proc R Soc Med 67:* 64, 1974.
42. Manery, J. F.: Effects of calcium ions on membranes. *Fed Proc 25:* 1804, 1966.
43. Rasmussen, H., Bordier, P. M.: The Physiological and Cellular Basis of Metabolic Bone Disease. Baltimore, Williams & Wilkins, 1974.
44. Bennett, J. C., Maffly, R. H., Steinbach, H. L.: The significance of bilateral basal ganglion calcification. *Radiology 72:* 368, 1959.
45. Schneider, A. B., Sherwood, L. M.: Pathogenesis and management of hypoparathyroidism and other hypocalcemic disorders. *Metabolism 24:* 871, 1975.
46. Smith, K. D., Geraci, A., Luparello, F. J.: Basal ganglion calcification in postoperative hypoparathyroidism. *N Y State J Med 73:* 1807, 1973.
47. Walsh, F. B., Murray, R. C.: Ocular manifestations of disturbances in calcium metabolism. *Am J Ophthalmol 36:* 1657, 1953.
48. Palmer, R. F., Searles, H. H., Boldrey, E. B.: Papilledema and hypoparathyroidism simulating brain tumor. *J Neurosurg 16:* 378, 1959.
49. Denko, J. D., Kaelbling, J. R.: The psychiatric aspects of hypoparathyroidism. *Acta Psychiatr Scand 38 Suppl 164:* 1, 1962.
50. Simpson, J. A.: Dermatological changes in hypocalcemia. *Br J Dermatol 66:* 1, 1954.
51. Dent,, C. E., Garretts, M.: Skin changes in hypocalcaemia. *Lancet 1:* 142, 1960.
52. Risum, G.: Psoriasis exacerbated by hypoparathyroidism with hypocalcaemia. *Br J Dermatol 89:* 309, 1973.
53. Hinrichs, E. M.: Dental changes in idiopathic juvenile hypoparathyroidism. *Oral Surg 9:* 1102, 1956.
54. Gorlin, R. J., Goldman, H. M.: Thoma's Oral Pathology (ed 5). St. Louis, Mosby, 1970.
55. Bellows, J. G.: Cataract and Anomalies of the Lens. St. Louis, Mosby, 1944.
56. Ireland, A. W., Hornbrook, J. N., Neale, F. C., et al: The crystalline lens in chronic surgical hypoparathyroidism. *Arch Intern Med 122:* 408, 1968.
57. Jordan, A., Kelsall, A. R.: Observations on a case of idiopathic hypoparathyroidism. *Arch Intern Med 87:* 242, 1951.
58. Drury, M. I., Loughlin, S. O., Sweeney, E. C., et al: Idiopathic hypoparathyroidism: a report of four cases. *Irish J Med Sci 140:* 513, 1971.
59. Clarkson, B., Kowlessar, O. D., Horwith, I. M., et al: Clinical and metabolic study of a patient with malabsorption and hypoparathyroidism. *Metabolism 9:* 1093, 1960.
60. Russell, R.: Hypoparathyroidism and malabsorption. *Br Med J 3:* 781, 1967.
61. Lorenzy, R., Burr, I. M.: Idiopathic hypoparathyroidism and steatorrhoea; a new aid in management. *J Pediatr 85:* 522, 1974.
62. Gay, J. D. L., Grimes, J. D.: Idiopathic hypoparathyroidism with impaired vitamin B_{12} absorption and neuropathy. *Can Med Assoc J 107:* 54, 1972.
63. Muldowney, F. P., Donohue, J., Ryan, C.: Bone disease in intestinal malabsorption. *Mod Treat 7:* 686, 1970.
64. Yu, P. N. G.: The electrocardiographic changes associated with hypercalcemia and hypocalcemia. *Am J Med Sci 224:* 413, 1952.
65. Aryanpur, I., Farhoudi, A., Zangeneh, F.: Congestive heart failure secondary to idiopathic hypoparathyroidism. *Am J Dis Child 122:* 738, 1973.
66. Boen, S. T., Leijnse, B., Gerbrandy, J.: Influence of serum calcium concentration on QT interval and circulation. *Clin Chim Acta 7:* 432, 1962.
67. Forbes, G. B.: Clinical features of idiopathic hypoparathyroidism in children. *Ann N Y Acad Sci 64:* 432, 1956.
68. Parfitt, A. M.: Metacarpal cortical dimensions in hypoparathyroidism, primary hyperparathyroidism and chronic renal failure. Proceedings of the XII European Symposium on Calcified Tissues. *Calcif Tissues Res 22 Suppl:* 329–331, 1977.
69. Dimich, A., Bedrossian, P. B., Wallach, S.: Hypoparathyroidism. Clinical observations in 34 patients. *Arch Intern Med 120:* 444, 1967.
70. Wolf, S. M., Lusk, W., Weisberg, L.: Hypocalcemic myopathy. *Bull Los Angeles Neurol Soc 37:* 167, 1972.
71. Stoner, R. E., Williams, J. B., Connor, T. B., et al: Inverse correlation between serum calcium concentration and lactic dehydrogenase activity. *Metabolism 20:* 464, 1972.
72. Nusynowitz, M. L., Frame, B., Kolb, F. O.: The spectrum of the hypoparathyroid states. *Medicine 55:* 105, 1976.
73. Barr, D. G. D., Prader, A., Esper, U., et al: Chronic hypoparathyroidism in two generations. *Helv Paediatr Acta, 26:* 507, 1971.
74. Miller, M. J., Frame, B., Posnanski, A. K., et al: Branchial anomalies in idiopathic hypoparathyroidism. Branchial dysembryogenesis. *Henry Ford Hosp Med Bull 20:* 3, 1972.
75. Taitz, L. S., Zarate-Salvador, C., Schwartz, E.: Congenital absence of the parathyroid and thymus glands in an infant (III and IV pharyngeal-pouch syndrome). *Pediatrics 38:* 412, 1966.
76. Freedom, R. M., Rosen, F. S., Nadas, A. S.: Congenital cardiovascular disease and anomalies of the third and fourth pharyngeal pouch. *Circulation 46:* 165, 1972.
77. Wuepper, K. D., Fudenberg, H. H.: Moniliasis, "autoimmune" poly endocrinopathy, and immunologic family study. *Clin Exp Immunol 2:* 71, 1967.
78. Hermann, P. E., Ulrich, J. A., Markowitz, H.: Chronic mucocutaneous candidiasis as a surface expression of deep-seated abnormalities. *Am J Med 47:* 503, 1969.
79. Rimoin, D. L., Schimke, R. W.: Genetic Disorders of the Endocrine Glands. St. Louis, Mosby, 1971.
80. Kirkpatrick, C. H., Rich, E. R., Bennett, J. E.: Chronic mucocutaneous candidiasis. Model building in cellular immunity. *Ann Intern Med 74:* 955, 1971.
80a. Louria, D. B., Shannon, D., Johnson, G., Caroline, L., Okas, A., Taschdjian, C.: The susceptibility to moniliasis in children with endocrine hypofunction. *Trans Assoc Am Physicians 80:* 236, 1967.
80b. Podolsky, S., Ferguson, B. D.: Fatal systemic candidiasis following treatment of Addisonian crisis in a juvenile diabetic. *Diabetes 19:* 438, 1970.
81. Kirkpatrick, C. H., Smith, T. K.: Chronic mucocutaneous candidiasis: immunologic and antibiotic therapy. *Ann Intern Med 80:* 310, 1974.
82. Kleerekoper, M., Basten, A., Penny R., et al: Idiopathic hypoparathyroidism with primary ovarian failure. *Arch Intern Med 134:* 944, 1974.

83. Irvine, W. J., Barnes, E. W.: Adrenocortical insufficiency. *Clin Endocrinol Metab 1:* 549, 1972.

84. Gass, J. D. M.: The syndrome of keratoconjunctivitis, superficial moniliasis, idiopathic hypoparathyroidism and Addison's disease. *Am J Ophthalmol 54:* 660, 1962.

85. Stankler, L., Bewsher, P. D.: Chronic mucocutaneous candidiasis, endocrine deficiency and alopecia areata. *Br J Dermatol 86:* 238, 1972.

86. Greenberg, M. S., Brightman, V. J., Lynch, M. A., et al: Idiopathic hypoparathyroidism, chronic candidiasis and dental hypoplasia. *Oral Surg 28:* 42, 1969.

87. Spinner, M. W., Blizzard, R. M., Gibbs, J., et al: Familial distribution of organ-specific antibodies in the blood of patients with Addison's disease and hypoparathyroidism and their relatives. *Clin Exp Immunol 5:* 461, 1969.

88. Drake, T. G., Albright, F., Bauer, W., et al: Chronic idiopathic hypoparathyroidism. Report of 6 cases with autopsy findings in one. *Ann Intern Med 12:* 1751, 1934.

89. Treusch, J. V.: Idiopathic hypoparathyroidism. Follow-up study including autopsy findings of a case previously reported. *Ann Intern Med 56:* 484, 1962.

90. Parfitt, A. M.: The incidence of hypoparathyroid tetany after thyroid operations. Relationship to age, extent of resection and surgical experience. *Med J Aust 1:* 1103, 1971.

91. Clowes, G. H., Simeone, F. A.: Acute hypocalcemia in surgical patients. *Ann Surg 146:* 530, 1957.

92. Kaplan, E. L., Starostik, R., Peskin, G. W., et al: Calcitonin-like responses in man during thyroid surgery. *J Clin Endocrinol Metab 28:* 740, 1968.

93. Michie, W., Stowers, J. M., Duncan, T., et al: Mechanism of hypocalcemia ater thyroidectomy for thyrotoxicosis. *Lancet 1:* 508, 1971.

94. Wade, J. S. H., Fourman, P., Deane, L.: Recovery of parathyroid function in patients with transient hypoparathyroidism after thyroidectomy. *Br J Surg 52:* 493, 1965.

95. Wade, J. S. H., Goodall, P., Deane, L., et al: The course of partial parathyroid insufficiency after thyroidectomy. *Br J Surg 52:* 497, 1965.

96. Attie, J. M., Kharif, R. A.: Preservation of parathyroid glands during total thyroidectomy. Improved techniques utilizing microsurgery. *Am J Surg 130:* 399, 1975.

97. Girling, J. A., Murley, R. S.: Parathyroid insufficiency after thyroidectomy. *Br Med J 1:* 1323, 1967.

98. Dent, C. E., Harper, C. M.: Hypoparathyroid tetany (following thyroidectomy) apparently resistant to vitamin D. *Proc R Soc Med 51:* 489, 1958.

99. Krane, S.: Selected features of the clinical course of hypoparathyroidism. *JAMA 178:* 472, 1961.

100. Parfitt, A. M.: Study of parathyroid function in man by EDTA infusion. *J Clin Endocrinol Metab 29:* 569, 1969.

101. Thompson, N. W., Harness, J. K.: Complications of total thyroidectomy for carcinoma. *Surg Gynecol Obstet 131:* 861, 1970.

102. Orme, M. C. L'E, Connoley, M.: Hypoparathyroidism after iodine-131 treatment of thyrotoxicosis. *Ann Inter Med 75:* 136, 1971.

103. Helous, A., Tyan, E., Zara, M.: Nouveau cas de tétanie après traitment d'une thyrotoxicose per l'iode radioactif. *Ann Endocrinol 25:* 238, 1964.

104. Goldsmith, R. E., King, L. R., Zalme, E., et al: Serum calcium homeostasis in radioiodine-treated thyrotoxic subjects as measured by ethylene diamine tetra-acetate infusion. *Acta Endocrinol 58:* 565, 1968.

105. Macdonald, R. A., Mallory, G. K.: Hemochromatosis and hemosiderosis. Study of 211 autopsied cases. *Arch Intern Med 105:* 686, 1960.

106. Oberklaid, F., Seshadri, R.: Hypoparathyroidism and other endocrine dysfunction complicating thalassemia major. *Med J Aust 1:* 304, 1975.

107. Horwitz, C. A., Myers, W. P. L., Foote, F. W.: Secondary malignant tumors of the parathyroid glands. Report of two cases with associated hypoparathyroidism. *Am J Med 52:* 797, 1972.

108. Young, D. M., Olson, H. M., Prieur, D., et al: Clinicopathologic and ultrastructural studies of L-asparaginase-induced hypocalcemia in rabbits. An experimental animal model of acute hypoparathyroidism. *Lab Invest 29:* 374, 1973.

109. David, D., Anast, C. S.: Calcium metabolism in newborn infants. The interrelationship of parathyroid function and calcium, magnesium and phosphorus metabolism in normal, "sick" and hypocalcemic newborns. *J Clin Invest 54:* 287, 1974.

110. Rosli, A., Fanconi, A.: Neonatal hypocalcemia. "Early type" in low-birth-weight infants. *Helv Paediatr Acta 28:* 443, 1973.

111. Fairney, A.: The role of parathyroid hormone in the aetiology of neonatal hypocalcemia. *Postgrad Med J 51 Suppl 3:* 18, 1975.

112. Barltrop, D.: Neonatal hypocalcemia. *Postgrad Med J 51 Suppl 3:* 7, 1975:

113. Fanconi, A., Prader, A.: Transient congenital idiopathic hypoparathyroidism. *Helv Paediatr Acta 22:* 342, 1967.

114. Rosenbloom, A. L.: Transient congenital idiopathic hypoparathyroidism. *South Med J 66:* 666, 1973.

115. Better, O. S., Levi, J., Greif, E., et al: Prolonged neonatal parathyroid suppression. A sequel to asymptomatic maternal hyperparathyroidism. *Arch Surg 106:* 722, 1973.

116. Bruce, J., Strong, J. A.: Maternal hyperparathyroidism and parathyroid deficiency in the child. *Q J Med, 24:* 307, 1950.

117. Monteleone, J. A., Lee, J. B., Tashjian, A. H., et al: Transient neonatal hypocalcemia, hypomagnesemia and high serum parathyroid hormone with maternal hyperparathyroidism. *Ann Intern Med 82:* 670, 1975.

118. Northcutt, R. C., Levinson, J. P., Earnest, J. B.: Hypocalcemia resulting from infarction of a parathyroid adenoma. *Ann Intern Med 70:* 353, 1969.

119. Anast, C. S., Mohs, J. M., Kaplan, S. L., et al: Evidence for parathyroid failure in magnesium deficiency. *Science 177:* 606, 1972.

120. Suh, S. M., Tashjian, A. H., Matsuo, N., et al: Pathogenesis of hypocalcemia in primary hypomagnesemia: normal end-organ responsiveness to parathyroid hormone, impaired parathyroid gland function. *J Clin Invest 52:* 153, 1973.

121. Medalle, R., Waterhouse, C.: A magnesium-deficient patient presenting with hypocalcemia and hyperphosphatemia. *Ann Intern Med 79:* 76, 1972.

122. Parfitt, A. M.: Investigation of disorders of the parathyroid gland. *Clin Endocrinol Metab 3:* 451, 1974.

123. Moses, A. M., Rao, K. T., Coulson, R., et al: Parathyroid hormone deficiency with Albright's hereditary osteodystrophy. *J Clin Endocrinol 39:* 496, 1974.

124. Parfitt, A. M.: Effect of cellulose phosphate on calcium and magnesium homeostasis. Studies in normal subjects and patients with latent hypoparathyroidism. *Clin Sci Mol Med 49:* 83, 1975.

125. Parfitt, A. M.: Adult hypoparathyroidism: Treatment with 25-hydroxy cholecalciferol. *Arch Intern Med* (in press).

126. Hunt, G., Morgan, D. B.: The early effects of dihydrotachysterol on calcium and phosphorus metabolism in patients with hypoparathyroidism. *Clin Sci 38:* 713, 1970.

127. Dent, C. E., Harper, C. M., Morgan, M. E., et al: Insensitivity to vitamin D developing during the treatment of postoperative tetany. Its specificity as regards the form of vitamin D taken. *Lancet 2:* 687, 1955.

128. Nordin, B. E. C.: Metabolic Bone and Stone Disease. London, Churchill Livingston, 1973.

129. Liberman, V. A., Chaichenko, J., Samuel, R.: A possible mechanism for the increased urinary calcium excretion induced by 1α-hydroxycholecalciferol treatment to hypoparathyroid patients. vitamin D: Biochemical, chemical and clinical aspects related to calcium metabolism. A. W. Norman et al. (eds). Berlin. De Gruyter. 1977 pp. 797–799.

130. Eisenberg, E.: Effects of serum calcium level and parathyroid extracts on phosphate and calcium excretion in hypoparathyroid patients. *J Clin Invest 44:* 942, 1965.

131. Mautalen, C. A.: Total urinary hydroxyproline excretion after administration of vitamin D to patients with hypoparathyroidism. *J Clin Endocrinol Metab 31:* 595, 1970.

132. Bell, N. H., Bartter, F. C., Smith, H.: The effect of vitamin D on ^{47}Ca metabolism in man. *Trans Assoc Am Physicians 126:* 165, 1963.

133. Parfitt, A. M.: Dual mechanism of recovery from acute hypocalcemia. *Clin Res 17:* 146, 1969.

134. Parfitt, A. M. Frame, B.: Drug treatment of rickets and osteomalacia. *Semin Drug Treat 2,* 83–115, 1972.

135. Neer, R. M., Holick, M. F., DeLuca, H. F., et al: Effect of 1α hydroxy-vitamin D_3 and 1,25-dihydroxy-vitamin D_3 on calcium and phosphorus metabolism in hypoparathyroidism. *Metabolism 24:* 1403, 1975.

136. Harrison, H. E., Lifshitz, F., Blizzard, R. M.: Comparison between

crystalline dihydrotachysterol and calciferol in patients requiring pharmacologic vitamin D therapy. *N Engl J Med 276:* 894, 1967.

137. Dymling, J. F., Ryd, H.: Crystalline dihydrotachysterol (Digratyl) in the treatment of hypoparathyroidism. *Acta Med Scand 184:* 333, 1968.

138. Parfitt, A. M., Frame, B.: Phosphate loading and depletion in vitamin-D-treated hypoparathyroidism. Implications for different physiologic models of phosphate reabsorption. Phosphate Metabolism: Kidney and Bone. L. V. Avioli et al. (eds.) Paris, Armour Montague, 1976.

139. Parfitt, A. M.: Renal function and phosphate metabolism in vitamin D treated hypoparathyroidism. Phosphate Metabolism. S. G. Massry, E. Ritz (eds.). New York, Plenum Press, 1977.

140. Rosler, A., Rabinowitz, D.: Magnesium-induced reversal of vitamin-D resistance in hypoparathyroidism. *Lancet 1:* 803, 1973.

141. Parfitt, A. M.: Thiazide-induced hypercalcemia in vitamin-D-treated hypoparathyroidism. *Ann Intern Med 77:* 557, 1972.

142. Ireland, A. W., Clubb, J. S., Neale, F. C., et al: The calciferol requirements of patients with surgical hypoparathyroidism. *Ann Intern Med 69:* 81, 1968.

143. Avioli, L. V.: The therapeutic approach to hypoparathyroidism. *Am J Med 57:* 34, 1974.

63

Pseudohypoparathyroidism

John T. Potts, Jr.

INTRODUCTION

Pseudohypoparathyroidism is a rare hereditary disorder characterized by symptoms and signs of hypoparathyroidism in association with distinctive skeletal and developmental defects. The cause of the disease differs from that of true hypoparathyroidism; in the latter there is deficient parathyroid hormone (PTH) production. Pseudohypoparathyroidism is due to deficient end-organ response to endogenous hormone. In fact, pseudohypoparathyroidism is characterized by excessive secretion of PTH and hyperplasia of the parathyroids, a response to the resistance to hormone action at the target tissues—the kidney and the bone.

The term *pseudopseudohypoparathyroidism* has been applied to the syndrome in which there are distinctive developmental anomalies in family members who lack evidence of hypoparathyroidism.

Studies over the past decade indicate that defective response of target-cell receptors and/or adenylyl cyclase to PTH is the biochemical defect in the disease (Fig. 63-1). The defective production of target-cell cAMP then leads to a failure of intracellular actions necessary to maintain normal calcium and phosphate transcellular transport. The resultant hypocalcemia in turn leads to a loss of negative feedback on the parathyroids, with resultant parathyroid hyperplasia and hypersecretion (Fig. 63-1).

Although this basic formulation of the pathophysiology remains valid, more recent findings have indicated qualifications or exceptions to this proposed sequence of pathophysiologic events in certain patients thought to represent examples of the syndrome.

Many aspects of pseudohypoparathyroidism remain unclarified, including the relation between the skeletal and developmental defects and the hypoparathyroidism.

The genetics of this disorder, proposed by some to be sex-linked dominant, are still under review, particularly the suggestion that a defective sex chromosome may be responsible for both the hypoparathyroidism and the growth and developmental defects.

PATHOPHYSIOLOGY

In pseudohypoparathyroidism there is an inadequate flow of calcium into extracellular fluid because of the reduced effectiveness of PTH in some or all of the target cells.

PTH-driven bone resorption is defective, reducing the normal rate of entry of calcium into blood and extracellular fluid. The loss of normal hormone action to reduce urinary calcium clearance results in calcium losses from extracellular fluid and a further drain on normal calcium homeostasis. Intestinal calcium absorption is defective. Since most, if not all, of the effects of the hormone on intestinal calcium absorption are thought to reflect the stimulation of production of 1,25-$(OH)_2$-D (1,25-dihydroxyvitamin D) in renal tissue, it must be assumed that this target tissue response of PTH, i.e., stimulation of the renal 25-hydroxyvitamin-D-1-hydroxylase (25-OH-D-1-hydroxylase), is also defective. This deficient action of the hormone overall on calcium transport systems in bone, kidney, and intestine leads to a serious reduction in extracellular-fluid calcium concentration. In addition, owing to the failure of the normal action of PTH to promote phosphate excretion in the kidney, hyperphosphatemia develops. Hypocalcemia per se also reduces the effectiveness of renal phosphate clearance so that PTH ineffectiveness, both directly and via its hypocalcemic effect, seriously impairs normal renal phosphate clearance mechanisms. There are several important physiologic consequences of the hyperphosphatemia.[1] It is well known that a high blood phosphate concentration tends to lower blood calcium in many experimental situations or in disease states; the mechanism of the phosphate effect is still unclear. Present data indicate that an elevated blood phosphate concentration leads to an increased rate of deposition of calcium from extracellular fluid into bone and also into extraosseous tissues. In addition, there is evidence that a high blood phosphate concentration inhibits bone resorption.

The metabolic effects of hyperphosphatemia appear to act synergistically with deficient calcium transport to produce severe hypocalcemia. In response to the persistent hypocalcemia in untreated subjects with pseudohypoparathyroidism, secondary hyperparathyroidism develops. All patients who have been examined have markedly increased peripheral concentrations of hormone.[1-4] As is consistent with secondary hyperparathyroidism (Chapter 59), calcium infusion lowers hormone concentrations toward undetectable values. Hormone production is still under the control of blood calcium concentration, but is excessive at every level of calcium concentration. The excessive hormone production seems to be a compensatory mechanism that is only partly, if at all, effective.

Because all patients with the complete syndrome by definition are hypocalcemic and hyperphosphatemic, it has generally been accepted that both bone and kidney are unresponsive. From the time of earliest clinical investigations of the syndrome, however, there was evidence contradictory to the thesis of complete end-organ unresponsiveness. It was observed in the early studies of patients with the syndrome that some patients showed an essentially normal phosphaturia following the injection of PTH.[5] There have also been reports that repeated intramuscular injections of parathyroid extract caused a slight rise in blood calcium. Four of

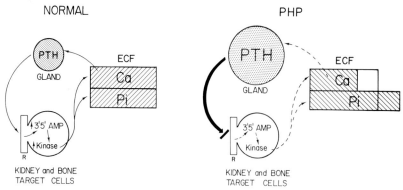

Fig. 63-1. Normal effects of PTH on cAMP production in target tissues followed by stimulation of calcium (Ca) and phosphate (Pi) transport systems essential to maintaining a normal extracellular fluid (ECF) level of each mineral ion. In pseudohypoparathyroidism, the indicated block at the receptor prevents normal cAMP accumulation, hence there is defective ion transport, resulting in hypocalcemia and hyperphosphatemia in ECF. With hypocalcemia, the negative feedback on the parathyroids, operating in normals, is reduced, and thus parathyroid hyperplasia and hypersecretion develop. (From Potts, in Stanbury et al. (eds): The Metabolic Basis of Inherited Disease (ed 4), 1978. Courtesy of McGraw-Hill)

the original 13 patients studied by Chase et al.[3] showed a detectable, even though subnormal, increase in 3′,5′-AMP after injections of parathyroid extract. One patient had a completely normal rise in cAMP after the administration of the hormone to kidney tissues obtained post mortem and studied in vitro.

During the study of 1 patient with pseudohypoparathyroidism previously treated with vitamin D, Nagant and Krane[6] found that the removal of all four parathyroid glands was accompanied by a striking fall in serum calcium requiring a massive increase in vitamin D to restore serum calcium toward normal. These findings suggest that, at least in some patients, especially when on chronic vitamin D treatment, there is a significant contribution to extracellular-fluid calcium from PTH-driven bone resorption when sufficient parathyroid hypersecretion has developed, despite relative bone resistance to parathyroid action.

Other evidence in favor of at least partial responsiveness of target organs to PTH is the report[7] that the degree of hypercalciuria in patients with pseudohypoparathyroidism is less marked than in patients with true hypoparathyroidism when the patients are compared after restoration of normal blood calcium in each group by high-dose vitamin D and oral calcium supplements. This result, in the light of more recent knowledge of physiologic mechanisms, can reasonably be interpreted to mean that there is a partial response of renal calcium conservation in pseudohypoparathyroidism by the high endogenous PTH produced in these patients, in contrast to the total lack of this effect in true hypoparathyroidism.

Recently, considerable confusion concerning the pathophysiology of this disorder has arisen from a series of articles documenting certain features noted in pseudohypoparathyroid patients and analyzing pathophysiologic mechanisms. One line of reasoning has been that bone and renal defects may vary independently in such a way that one organ tissue, e.g., bone, may be completely normal. Other observations lead to the designation of subgroups or distinct categories of patients because of apparent uncoupling between urinary cAMP responses on the one hand and blood and urine calcium and phosphate responses on the other.

It is the author's present contention that most of the apparently distinctive patterns of tissue response are not as distinctive as they may seem, but can be explained as quantitative differences in manifestations of a single underlying defect—clearly defective but still partly responsive receptors in both kidney and bone.

Reports have accumulated concerning more than a dozen patients with hypocalcemia and hyperphosphatemia in whom evidence of osteitis fibrosa has been found by both x-ray films and biopsy.[8-14] This has led to the speculation that the renal end-organ

defect may be the most severe, if not the sole, abnormality in some patients. Some authors have attributed the hypocalcemia solely to the hyperphosphatemia and have speculated that the skeleton is fully responsive; accordingly, it is argued that osteitis develops because of secondary hyperparathyroidism with a responsive skeleton.[8-14]

On the one hand, the clinical features in some of these patients suggest that many may not be typical, either genetically or with regard to physical findings, of patients with true pseudohypoparathyroidism. On the other hand, however, it is also possible that these patients do have the same genetic and biochemical defects as the majority of patients with pseudohypoparathyroidism. The appearance of osteitis fibrosa cystica in some patients may be simply another reflection of the complex picture that occurs in calcium, phosphate, and skeletal homeostasis when there is the combination of partial unresponsiveness to a homeostatic mechanism, PTH, and a compensatory excessive production of the hormone. For example, there is a similar paradox in chronic renal failure, in which the sequence of hormone resistance, hypocalcemia, and hyperphosphatemia, and compensatory overproduction of hormone culminates, in some patients, with frank osteitis fibrosa cystica, a manifestation of excessive hormone action.

This problem and the analogy between some patients with chronic renal failure and pseudohypoparathyroidism was recently carefully reviewed.[15] The compensatory mechanism, PTH overproduction, may eventually overshoot; such a phenomenon must explain this paradox in PTH-resistant states such as renal failure or pseudohypoparathyroidism. In pseudohypoparathyroidism in particular, differing degrees of bone and renal responsiveness on the one hand and of parathyroid hyperplasia on the other could explain the occurrence of osteitis in certain patients. This would not imply a fundamental difference in pathophysiology between patients with pseudohypoparathyroidism who develop bone disease and those who do not.

Recently, even greater complexity with regard to pathophysiologic mechanisms in pseudohypoparathyroidism has been introduced. First, several reports note discordant responses between urinary cAMP production versus phosphaturia and calcium elevation in either untreated patients or treated patients who had elevation of blood calcium after high-dose vitamin D therapy and/or calcium infusion. Second, the term *pseudohypoparathyroidism type II* has been introduced into classification schemes to explain the responses, seen in several patients, differing from classic responses in pseudohypoparathyroidism, in that cAMP response is normal despite other features of pseudohypoparathyroidism.

With regard to quantitatively unusual responses, the initial observation,[16] subsequently confirmed and extended,[17] was that in certain patients the failure of exogenously administered PTH to cause phosphaturia or elicit hypercalcemia was reversed by restoration of blood calcium to normal by chronic high-dose vitamin D therapy; that is, the phosphaturic and hypercalcemic responses to exogenous hormone were fully evident after treatment with vitamin D. In the patient of Suh et al.,[16] there was no test of urinary cAMP response to exogenous PTH before or after vitamin D therapy, but, in the patient reported by Stögmann and Fischer,[17] the urinary cAMP response to administered hormone remained absent to severely blunted below normal, even after vitamin D therapy had restored a normal phosphaturic and hypercalcemic response to hormone.

The persistently blunted cAMP responses with normal phosphaturic and hypercalcemic responses to PTH in certain patients treated with high-dose vitamin D therapy need not imply, as has been at least suggested,[17] a dissociation between cAMP production and phosphaturia in patients with pseudohypoparathyroidism.

Several issues must be considered in the interpretation of these findings. Some reports have clearly indicated a persistence of blunted phosphaturic and hypercalcemic responses to exogenous PTH in a number of patients with pseudohypoparathyroidism, despite high-dose vitamin D therapy;[18,19] in fact, the majority of the patients with blunted responses in calcium and phosphate transport studied originally by Chase et al.[3,20,21] were already on high-dose vitamin D replacement at the time of testing with hormone. On the other hand, the improvement in hypercalcemic response in certain patients, given the cumulative evidence that resistance is only partial in many patients with pseudohypoparathyroidism, is predictable. With more effective levels of biologically active vitamin D, the bone responsiveness to administered PTH would be greater because of the synergism of vitamin D and PTH actions on bone mineral release. In addition, stimulation of intestinal calcium absorption may occur if much greater tissue and blood levels of vitamin D and 25-OH-D are provided, allowing the partially effective, high endogenous levels of PTH to permit more formation of $1,25\text{-(OH)}_2\text{-D}$. These considerations seem plausible in explaining why, in some patients, high-dose vitamin D therapy increased hypercalcemic effectiveness of PTH without requiring a fundamental difference in pathophysiologic mechanisms. The improved phosphaturic action of the hormone, although not explainable by vitamin D administration, is expected merely because of the correction of the severe hypocalcemia per se.[1,22,23]

With regard to a related issue, the apparent dissociation between urinary cAMP and phosphaturic response per se, too little is known at present about basic aspects of hormone action to relate quantitatively the degree of cAMP response and the degree of renal tubular ion transport response.[24] The cAMP measured reflects an overflow of excess intracellular cAMP into urine.[24] With deficient intracellular production of cAMP, an absent or nearly absent urinary cAMP excretion need not imply totally defective intracellular response of adenylyl cyclase to PTH. The unitary pathophysiologic explanation is that the intracellular response to minimal cAMP production is greatly augmented by high-dose vitamin D therapy.

Two recent reports[26,27] describing cases labeled as examples of pseudohypoparathyroidism type II, however, represent a more serious challenge to any unitary concept of pathophysiologic mechanisms in that urinary cAMP responses are normal, but mineral-ion transport is still defective. Each of the two patients had hypocalcemia (only moderate in one)[26] and elevated basal PTH levels (measured only once in the more severely hypocalcemic subject).[27] These findings suggested pseudohypoparathyroidism

rather than hypoparathyroidism. Urinary cAMP responses to administered PTH, however, were found to be brisk at levels typical of normal or hypoparathyroid subjects rather than of pseudohypoparathyroid patients. On the other hand, neither subject showed a phosphaturic response to PTH when initially studied or a hypercalcemic response to administered PTH (4 days). The patient studied by Rodriguez et al.[26] showed a normal phosphaturic response to PTH after acute or subacute elevation of calcium to normal.

It is difficult to relate findings in these interesting reports to pathophysiologic mechanisms in true pseudohypoparathyroidism. It may be that these patients represent a disease state superficially related to but pathophysiologically distinct from pseudohypoparathyroidism. The supposition is that neither patient responds in renal or bone tissue to normally produced cAMP; that is, although they are examples of PTH resistance, the locus of defect is beyond the step of cAMP production rather than at the level of the hormone receptor–cyclase complex as in classic pseudohypoparathyroidism.

Additional information and tests on other patients resembling the subjects of the two recent reports will clearly be required to define the pathophysiologic mechanisms and to clearly establish whether there is indeed a variant of pseudohypoparathyroidism with a locus of metabolic defect different from that in the majority of patients. A more detailed discussion of these issues concerning the pathophysiology of pseudohypoparathyroidism appears in a recent review.[23]

An alternative suggestion has been made recently with regard to pathophysiology in pseudohypoparathyroidism. It has been proposed that the entire defect in pseudohypoparathyroidism is a deficiency of circulating $1,25\text{-(OH)}_2\text{-D}$ before treatment.[25] This conclusion seems unwarranted in view of the clearly deficient responses to administered PTH, both renal and bone, that persist in pseudohypoparathyroidism despite high-dose vitamin D therapy.[18,19]

Improvement in intestinal calcium absorption, restoration of serum calcium to normal, and reduction in circulating PTH levels are all predictable with high-dose vitamin D therapy without implying that such therapy restores physiologic mechanisms completely to normal—that is, the $1,25\text{-(OH)}_2\text{-D}$ deficiency is the single defect in pseudohypoparathyroidism.[25]

Thus, despite unresolved questions about variation or changes in end-organ sensitivity in some patients with pseudohypoparathyroidism, the overall evidence suggests that the disturbances in calcium and phosphorus metabolism in most patients with pseudohypoparathyroidism result from at least partial unresponsiveness of the receptors in both bone and kidney, and, indirectly, in intestine. The latter effect, as well as part of the reduced responsiveness of bone, involves deficient production of $1,25\text{-(OH)}_2\text{-D}$; PTH-specific responses in kidney and bone are blunted owing to a defect at the level of the cyclase–receptor–hormone interaction site.

Little can be said at the present time about the pathophysiology of the multiple skeletal and developmental defects in these patients. The genetics of the disorder are compatible with an abnormality in the X chromosome. Since identical features of short stature, abnormal metacarpals and metatarsals, and other physical signs of the disease are found without hypocalcemia or hyperphosphatemia in patients with pseudopseudohypoparathyroidism (who have an apparently normal renal-cell adenylyl cyclase system), it seems likely that the skeletal and developmental defects are an independently inherited aspect of the illness, reflecting abnormal X-chromosome function, rather than a consequence of hypoparathyroidism per se.

CLINICAL FEATURES

Most of the symptoms of pseudohypoparathyroidism reflect increased neuromuscular irritability resulting from the abnormally low concentration of calcium in the blood and extracellular fluid. The average age at onset of symptoms is about 8 years.[28,29] Symptoms include tetany, convulsions, muscle cramps, and seizures. Episodes of laryngeal spasm are reported. Poor vision may occur as a result of cataracts. (See Chapter 62 for a detailed analysis of symptom complexes associated with hypoparathyroidism.)

Signs of the disease detected on physical and laboratory examination are referable either to the hypoparathyroidism or to the associated skeletal and developmental defects. Hypocalcemia and hyperphosphatemia are present in untreated pseudohypoparathyroidism as in hypoparathyroidism of any cause. Alkaline phosphatase is usually normal, except for the small number of patients discussed above in whom there is evidence of osteitis fibrosa. A complication, particularly of the hyperphosphatemia, is the frequent occurrence of soft-tissue calcifications. In pseudohypoparathyroidism the mineral deposits in ectopic sites may include the development of true bone. True bone formation in ectopic sites is never seen in idiopathic hypoparathyroidism.[5,30,31] Amorphous deposits of calcium and phosphate are also found in subcutaneous tissue and particularly in the basal ganglia. Calcification of the basal ganglia is noted in as many as 50 percent of the patients. Most patients with the asymptomatic variant, pseudopseudohypoparathyroidism, do not have ectopic calcium deposits, although the original patient reported with pseudopseudohypoparathyroidism had extensive ectopic calcification despite normal blood calcium and phosphate concentrations.[31]

The multiple skeletal and developmental abnormalities that are found in both pseudohypoparathyroidism and pseudopseudohypoparathyroidism include short stature, round face, short neck, thick, stocky body build, and multiple discrete abnormalities in individual bones of the skeleton (Fig. 63-2).[28–30,32] The latter abnor-malities include shortness of the metacarpal and metatarsal bones and sometimes the phalanges. These defects seem to be due to premature closure of the epiphyses (Fig. 63-3). The most classic finding is an abnormally short fourth and fifth metacarpal or metatarsal. This defect may be unilateral. When only one digit is involved, it is invariably the fourth; the least-frequently involved is the second. When the hand is closed, the knuckles on the affected fingers are replaced by dimples (Fig. 63-3). Exostoses are frequently reported. Usually there are only one or two detected, but occasionally multiple exostoses are found. Radius curvus may be present in some patients. There may be only a mild curvature or there may be extreme bowing with displacement of the epiphysis.[32]

Although, as discussed above, a few patients with the syndrome have shown evidence of osteitis fibrosa, the usual picture on x-ray examination in pseudohypoparathyroidism is a normal or even increased density, particularly in the skull.[28,29] The calvarium may be thickened. In addition, multiple abnormalities are detected in tooth formation. Although the nails may be fragile, the moniliasis commonly found in true hypoparathyroidism is not found in pseudohypoparathyroidism.[28,29] Mental deficiency is rather common in patients with pseudohypoparathyroidism. It seems most probable that this is part of the inherited syndrome rather than a consequence of hypocalcemia. In any event, there is little improvement in mental status even with adequate therapy with calcium and vitamin D. The frequency of these signs and symptoms is indicated in Table 63-1.[28,29]

Two other features have been described that appear to be part of the abnormal genetic inheritance. Distinctive impairments in olfaction and taste have been reported in the majority of patients examined.[33] In addition, unusual dermatoglyphic abnormalities have been detected, including features such as frequent hypothenar patterns and distally located triradii.[34]

The incidence of either frank diabetes or an abnormal glucose tolerance curve is greatly increased. Signs of hypothyroidism have been noted with a frequency considerably greater than expected

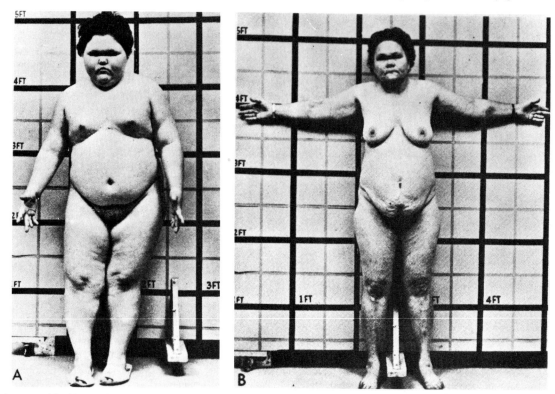

Fig. 63-2. A. A young girl with pseudohypoparathyroidism. B. Her mother with pseudopseudohypoparathyroidism. Both exhibit short stature, obesity, rounded faces, and shortened metacarpals. Only the girl had the chemical abnormalities of hypoparathyroidism. (From Potts, in Stanbury et al. (eds): The Metabolic Basis of Inherited Disease (ed 4), 1978. Courtesy of McGraw-Hill)

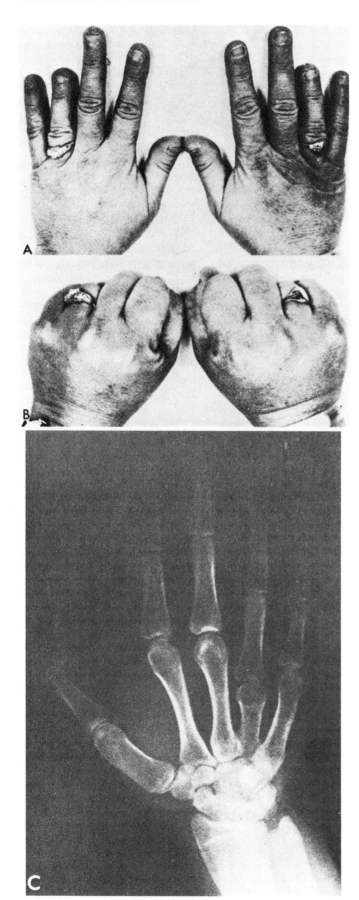

Fig. 63-3. Hands of a patient with pseudohypoparathyroidism. A. Note the shortened fourth finger. B. Note the "absent" fourth knuckle. C. Film shows the shortened fourth metacarpal. (From Potts, in Stanbury et al. (eds): The Metabolic Basis of Inherited Disease (ed 4), 1978. Courtesy of McGraw-Hill)

Table 63-1. Incidence of Signs and Symptoms in Pseudohypoparathyroidism*

	Percent
Signs	
Hypocalcemia	100
Soft-tissue calcifications	
Subcutaneous tissue	60
Cataracts	35
Basal ganglia	50
Skeletal Abnormalities	
Increased density	15
Decreased density	15
Thickened calvaria	20
Developmental abnormalities	
Round face, short neck	75
Thick-set, stocky body build	50
Brachydactyly	
Metacarpals	70
Metatarsals	40
Symptoms	
Tetany	65
Convulsions	65
Muscle cramps	40
Laryngeal spasm	10
Paresthesias	10
Mental and personality changes	10
Parkinsonism	10

*The reported incidence of complications and symptoms listed here reflects earlier observations[28,29] with emphasis on findings prior to treatment, and does not reflect recent case reports involving patients with unusual manifestations.[23]

for random occurrence. Certain studies have indicated that hypothyroidism is due to isolated thyrotropin deficiency.[35-37]

However, an extensive study of 8 of 10 patients with pseudohypoparathyroidism revealed early primary hypothyroidism with minimal symptoms, elevated basal thyrotropin levels, and an exaggerated thyrotropin response to infused thyroid-releasing hormone.[38] Hence, although the mechanism of this defect in the hypothalamic–pituitary–thyroid axis remains unclear, it is evident that a careful clinical and full thyroid-function assessment should be performed in all patients because of the surprisingly high incidence of thyroid dysfunction.

GENETICS

The hereditary aspects of pseudohypoparathyroidism have been well established.[4,5,30,39] Pseudohypoparathyroidism is usually found within kindreds in which some other family members also have pseudohypoparathyroidism or the metabolically normal variant of the disorder, pseudopseudohypoparathyroidism. The variable expression of metabolic abnormalities in affected individuals is not understood.

In a detailed review, Mann et al.[39] analyzed the incidence of the disorder in a total of 22 families. It was concluded that the two disorders, pseudohypoparathyroidism and pseudopseudohypoparathyroidism, were genetically linked and were transmitted as a sex-linked dominant disorder. In support of this contention, it was found that the sex incidence of affected females to males was 2:1. At present, this view that pseudohypoparathyroidism is inherited as a sex-linked dominant seems plausible, but cannot be unequivocally accepted. The disease is extremely rare, so that the total number of patients or involved siblings is small for statistical analysis. Furthermore, acceptance of cases as authentic examples of the syndrome on the basis of literature reports is difficult, particularly with respect to the metabolically normal individuals, i.e., those with pseudopseudohypoparathyroidism. Certain developmental defects, such as short stature, short metacarpal or metatarsal bones, or even basal-ganglia calcification are found in Turner's syndrome, Gardner's syndrome, basal-cell-nevus syndrome, or other hereditary disorders.[40] These disorders are believed to be genetically distinct from pseudohypoparathyroidism, since some of them are associated with chromosomal defects, appear to be autosomal dominant traits, and/or have apparently normal renal adenylyl cyclase responses.[40] Hence, the finding of skeletal or developmental defects per se cannot be used as an absolute indication of pseudopseudohypoparathyroidism. These difficulties in interpreting published case reports help to explain the uncertainty about proposed genetic mechanisms. For example, four cases of apparent male-to-male transmission are recorded.[39] This mode of inheritance does not fit in with sex-linked dominance.

The possibility has not been excluded that the X chromosome is structurally deficient. In addition, even if the concept of simple sex-linked dominant inheritance is accepted, it is difficult to explain the occurrence of developmental defects in pseudopseudohypoparathyroidism without coexistent abnormality in renal adenylyl cyclase responses or calcium or phosphate metabolism if the genetic defect is identical in pseudohypoparathyroidism and pseudopseudohypoparathyroidism.

Aurbach[41] has proposed that this discrepancy might be explained, at least in females, by the Lyon hypothesis, i.e., one or other of the X chromosomes might be inactivated to a relatively greater extent. Thus, if the abnormal X chromosome is inactivated, the adenylyl cyclase enzyme system would be competent, and pseudopseudohypoparathyroidism would be the result in the affected individual. The assumption is made that the developmental (pseudopseudohypoparathyroidism) only as distinct from biochemical abnormalities (pseudohypoparathyroidism) results from the presence of the abnormal X chromosome during fetal development despite later inactivation of the defective X chromosome. If, on the other hand, the normal X chromosome is inactivated, then the adenylyl cyclase system would be deficient, and pseudohypoparathyroidism would be the clinical result. This explanation could not account for the occurrence of pseudopseudohypoparathyroidism in the male, nor is it consistent with the concept of random inactivation of the X chromosome. Clearly, further analysis of these issues concerning inheritance patterns and cytogenetic defects is required.

DIAGNOSIS

Typically, the diagnosis of pseudohypoparathyroidism is first considered in a patient who has symptoms of hypocalcemia and is found to have both hypocalcemia and hyperphosphatemia in the presence of normal renal function. Clinically, pseudohypoparathyroidism is more likely than true hypoparathyroidism if the unusual skeletal and developmental defects are detected or if there is a family history of other siblings with short stature and skeletal anomalies. A definitive diagnosis of pseudohypoparathyroidism must be established through application of specific laboratory tests. Two principal tests should be employed, namely, the PTH radioimmunoassay, and measurement of urinary cAMP excretion following the administration of PTH.

Patients with symptomatic hypocalcemia, particularly if the history and physical examination suggest chronicity of the hypocalcemia (such as gradual onset of symptoms and evidence of ectopic calcification), would be expected to have secondary hyperparathyroidism if the parathyroid glands are functional. If no, or

only low, levels of PTH are detected by radioimmunoassay, notwithstanding the stimulus of marked hypocalcemia, then true hypoparathyroidism is the most likely diagnosis; if elevated concentrations of PTH are found, then hypoparathyroidism based on end-organ resistance is more likely.[1,35] If high circulating concentrations of hormone are found, the renal end-organ resistance to the PTH can be demonstrated by measuring the urinary excretion of cAMP in response to the injection of a standard dose of PTH. Typical responses in normal subjects, patients with idiopathic or postsurgical hypoparathyroidism, pseudohypoparathyroidism, and pseudopseudohypoparathyroidism are shown in Figure 63-4. Chase et al. found that there was a 10- to 20-fold increase in urinary cAMP excretion in all groups, except those with pseudohypoparathyroidism, in whom a clearly blunted response was noted.[3]

Another approach to a demonstration of PTH unresponsiveness has been the administration of several hundred units of parathyroid extract daily for 1 week or more. As discussed above, only a few patients with pseudohypoparathyroidism have been tested in this manner and there is not much experience with the response to such a test procedure in normal subjects. Even so, the lack of any rise in serum calcium despite the administration of PTH for 7 to 10 days has occasionally been useful as a further indication of PTH unresponsiveness.

The differential diagnosis of pseudohypoparathyroidism involves two principal categories of illness: (1) other causes of hypocalcemia, and (2) other unusual syndromes featuring skeletal and developmental anomalies that may simulate many of the constitutional features of pseudohypoparathyroidism.

With regard to the latter issue, patients with a variety of unusual skeletal and developmental defects—including the basal-cell-nevus syndrome,[42–44] familial calcification of the cerebral basal ganglia,[45,46] Gardner's syndrome,[47,48] and Turner's syndrome—share certain features observed in pseudohypoparathyroidism. There have also been occasional reports that these patients are unresponsive to PTH.[47] These findings have led some to suspect that these diseases are related to pseudohypoparathyroidism. Most of these patients, however, have not been reported to have any abnormalities in calcium and phosphorus metabolism; reported tests showing parathyroid responsiveness in these circumstances were indirect. Studies by Aurbach and associates[40] have established that such phenotypically similar patients have a normal excretion of cAMP following the administration of PTH. It was also observed that patients with Gardner's syndrome, vitamin D-resistant rickets, and the basal-ganglia-calcification syndrome had higher baseline rates of excretion of cAMP than normal subjects.[40] This has also been observed in primary hyperparathyroidism and in biochemically normal subjects with pseudopseudohypoparathyroidism.[40] Although further study of these unusual syndromes will undoubtedly be required in order to understand fully many features of these diseases, it does not appear that they are genetically or biochemically related to true pseudohypoparathyroidism.

A detailed analysis of the differential diagnosis of hypocalcemic states per se is provided in the chapter on hypoparathyroidism (Chapter 62). In distinguishing true hypoparathyroidism (any of several variants) from pseudohypoparathyroidism, in addition to obvious clinical features such as a history of previous thyroid surgery, hypoparathyroidism is indicated rather than pseudohypoparathyroidism by three criteria: (1) the lack of any findings of skeletal and developmental defects; (2) a lack of detectable or appropriately elevated PTH despite hypocalcemia; and, (3) if necessary, a demonstration of a brisk rise in urinary cAMP excretion after administration of PTH.

The issues related to differential diagnosis become quite com-

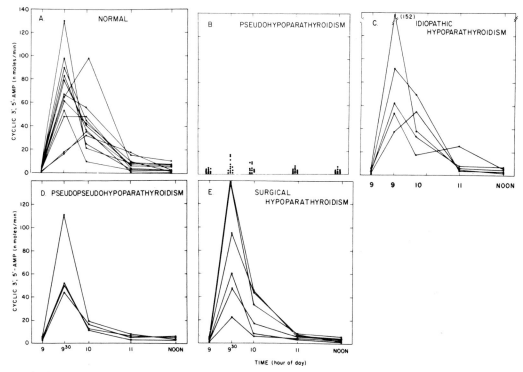

Fig. 63-4. cAMP excretion in urine in response to the injection of PTH (300 USP units of PTH given at 9 A.M.). (From Potts, in Stanbury et al. (eds): The Metabolic Basis of Inherited Disease (ed 4), 1978. Courtesy of McGraw-Hill)

plex if the unusual syndromes or atypical cases discussed above, such as pseudohypoparathyroidism type II, are included; the three criteria used to distinguish hypoparathyroidism from pseudohypoparathyroidism do not hold according to those published case reports.

The author prefers to reserve the category *pseudohypoparathyroidism* for those patients with definite developmental defects of classic type (best if there is also a positive family history), elevated PTH, and severely blunted urinary cAMP responses. The category *hypoparathyroidism* then applies to those who meet the three criteria listed above: lack of developmental defects, absent PTH, and normal urinary cAMP. It is possible that distinctive variants of deficient parathyroid function will eventually emerge from further study of unusual patients, e.g., a disease category due to elaboration of immunologically competent but biologically inert hormone or a category reflecting a failure to respond to normally generated second messenger, cAMP, in target tissues (the defect suspected in the patients reported as having pseudohypoparathyroidism type II). In the author's opinion, more careful demonstration of such defects will be required, however, before accepting the view that discrete syndromes or categories other than simple hypoparathyroidism or classic pseudohypoparathyroidism exist.

TREATMENT

The basic principles outlined under treatment of hypoparathyroidism in Chapter 62 apply to pseudohypoparathyroidism as well, and hence are not repeated in detail. The proper dose of vitamin D or the equivalent, more potent analogue is used to overcome the block in renal 1-hydroxylase[49–51] to restore efficiency of intestinal calcium absorption toward normal, plus sufficient supplemental oral calcium (1–2 g of elemental calcium) to maintain a satisfactory blood calcium. The general approach used in any form of hypoparathyroidism is to achieve a symptom-free low to midnormal blood calcium level by proper adjustment of vitamin D and oral

calcium; 24-hour urine calcium excretion should then be determined. In hypoparathyroidism, careful observation must be made to ensure that 24-hour urine calcium values do not exceed the 400–500 mg/24-hour range, thereby running the risk of kidney stones. Although the problem of hypocalcemic or normocalcemic hypercalciuria is less frequent in pseudohypoparathyroidism,[7] each patient should be checked during establishment of optimum treatment schedules.

Although there have been no recent reports of careful quantitative comparisons between replacement-therapy requirements (vitamin D or its active metabolite) and oral calcium supplements in pseudohypoparathyroidism versus hypoparathyroidism, it seems quite plausible that the partial responsiveness to endogenous hormone in the former will lead, in many patients with pseudohypoparathyroidism, to lower therapeutic requirements, especially calcium supplements, than are needed in patients with true hypoparathyroidism.

REFERENCES

1. Deftos, L. J., Potts, J. T. Jr.: Parathyroid hormone, calcitonin, vitamin D, bone and bone mineral metabolism. In Bondy, P. K., Rosenberg, L. E. (eds): Duncan's Diseases of Metabolism (ed 7). Philadelphia, Saunders, 1974, p 1225.
2. Tashjian, A. H. Jr., Frantz, A. G., Lee, J. B.: Pseudohypoparathyroidism: assays of parathyroid hormone and thyrocalcitonin. *Proc Natl Acad Sci USA 56:* 1138, 1966.
3. Chase, L. R., Melson, G. L., Aurbach, G. D.: Pseudohypoparathyroidism: defective excretion of 3′,5′-AMP in response to parathyroid hormone. *J Clin Invest 48:* 1832, 1969.
4. Lee, J. B., Tashjian, A. H., Streeto, J. M., et al: Familial pseudohypoparathyroidism. *N Engl J Med 279:* 1179, 1968.
5. Elrick, H., Albright, F., Bartter, F. C., et al: Further studies on pseudohypoparathyroidism: report of four new cases. *Acta Endocrinol 5:* 199, 1950.
6. Nagant de Deuxchaisnes, C., Krane, S. M.: unpublished,
7. Litvak, J., Moldawer, M. P., Forbes, A. P., et al: Hypocalcemic

hypercalciuria during vitamin D and dihydrotachysterol therapy of hypoparathyroidism. *J Clin Endocrinol Metab 18:* 246, 1958.

8. Bell, N. H., Gerard, E. S., Bartter, F. C.: Pseudohypoparathyroidism with osteitis fibrosa cystica and impaired absorption of calcium. *J Clin Endocrinol Metab 23:* 759, 1963.

9. Kolb, F. O., Steinbach, H. L.: Pseudohypoparathyroidism with secondary hyperparathyroidism and osteitis fibrosa. *J Clin Endocrinol Metab 22:* 59, 1962.

10. Zampa, G. A., Zucchelli, P. C.: Pseudohypoparathyroidism and bone demineralization: case report and metabolic studies. *J Clin Endocrinol Metab 25:* 1616, 1965.

11. Allen, E. H., Millard, F. J. C., Nassim, J. R.: Hypo-hyperparathyroidism. *Arch Dis Child 43:* 295, 1968.

12. Singleton, E. B., Teng, C. T.: Pseudohypoparathyroidism with bone changes simulating hyperparathyroidism (report of a case). *Radiology 78:* 388, 1962.

13. Costello, J. M., Dent, C. E.: Hypo-hyperparathyroidism. *Arch Dis Child 38:* 397, 1963.

14. Cohen, R. D., Vince, F. P.: Pseudohypoparathyroidism with raised plasma alkaline phosphatase. *Arch Dis Child 44:* 96, 1969.

15. Prien, E. L. Jr., Pyle, E. B., Krane S. M.: Secondary hyperparathyroidism. In Greep, R. O., Astwood, E. B. (sec eds), Aurbach, G. D. (vol ed), Geiger, S. R. (bk ed): Handbook of Physiology, sec 7: Endocrinology, vol 7: Parathyroid Gland. Washington D.C., American Physiological Society, 1976, p 383.

16. Suh, S. M., Fraser, C., Kooh, S. W.: Pseudohypoparathyroidism: responsiveness to parathyroid extract induced by vitamin D_2 therapy. *J Clin Endocrinol Metab 30:* 609, 1970.

17. Stögmann, W., Fischer, J. A.: Pseudohypoparathyroidism: disappearance of the resistance to parathyroid extract during treatment with vitamin D. *Am J Med 59:* 140, 1975.

18. McDonald, K. M.: Responsiveness of bone to parathyroid extract in siblings with pseudohypoparathyroidism. *Metabolism 21:* 521, 1972.

19. Moses, A. M., Breslau, N., Coulson, R.: Renal responses to PTH in patients with hormone-resistant (pseudo) hypoparathyroidism. *Am J Med 61:* 184, 1976.

20. Aurbach, G. D., Houston, B. A.: Determination of 3′,5′-adenosine monophosphate with a method based on a radioactive phosphate exchange reaction. *J Biol Chem 243:* 5935, 1968.

21. Chase, L. R., Aurbach, G. D.: Cyclic AMP and the mechanism of action of parathyroid hormone. Proceedings of the Third Parathyroid Conference, Parathyroid Hormone and Thyrocalcitonin (Calcitonin). Amsterdam, Excerpta Medica, 1968, p 247.

22. Potts, J. T. Jr.: Disorders of parathyroid glands. In Wintrobe, M. M., Thorn, G. W., Adams, R. D., et al (eds): Harrison's Principles of Internal Medicine (ed 7). New York, McGraw-Hill, 1974, p 1951.

23. Potts, J. T. Jr.: Pseudohypoparathyroidism. In Stanbury, J. B., Wyngaarden, J. B., Fredrickson, D. S. (eds): The Metabolic Basis of Inherited Disease (ed 4). New York, McGraw-Hill 1978, p 1350.

24. Aurbach, G. D.: Cyclic nucleotides and biochemical actions of parathyroid hormone and calcitonin. In Greep, R. O., Astwood, E. B. (sec eds), Aurbach, G. D. (vol ed), Geiger, S. R. (bk ed): Handbook of Physiology, sec 7: Endocrinology, vol 7: Parathyroid Gland. Washington DC, American Physiological Society, 1976, p 353.

25. Sinha, T. K., DeLuca, H. F., Bell, N. H.: Evidence for a defect in the formation of a 1α,25-dihydroxyvitamin D in pseudohypoparathyroidism. *Clin Res 23:* 538A, 1975.

26. Rodriguez, H. J., Villarreal, H., Klahr, S., et al: Pseudohypoparathyroidism type II: restoration of normal renal responsiveness to parathyroid hormone by calcium administration. *J Clin Endocrinol Metab 39:* 693, 1974.

27. Drezner, M., Neelon, F. A., Lebavitz, H. E.: Pseudohypoparathyroidism type II: a possible defect in the reception of the cyclic AMP signal. *N Engl J Med 289:* 1056, 1973.

28. Bronsky, D., Kushner, D. S., Dubin, A., et al: Idiopathic hypoparathyroidism and pseudohypoparathyroidism: case reports and review of the literature. *Medicine* (Baltimore) *37:* 317, 1958.

29. Aurbach, G. D., Potts, J. T. Jr.: The parathyroids. In Levine R., Luft R. (eds): Advances in Metabolic Disorders, vol 1. New York, Academic, 1964, p 45.

30. Albright, F., Burnett, C. H., Smith, P. H., et al: Pseudohypoparathyroidism—an example of the "Seabright-Bantam syndrome." *Endocrinology 30:* 922, 1942.

31. Albright, F., Forbes, A. P., Henneman, P. H.: Pseudopseudohypoparathyroidism. *Trans Assoc Am Physicians 65:* 337, 1952.

32. Bartter, F. C.: Pseudohypoparathyroidism and pseudopseudohypoparathyroidism. In Stanbury, J. B., Wyngaarden, J. B., Fredrickson, D. S. (eds): The Metabolic Basis of Inherited Disease. New York, McGraw-Hill, 1966, p 1024.

33. Henkin, R. I.: Impairment of olfaction and of the tastes of sour and bitter in pseudohypoparathyroidism. *J Clin Endocrinol Metab 28:* 624, 1968.

34. Forbes, A. P.: Fingerprints and palm prints (dermatoglyphics) and palmar-flexion creases in gonadal dysgenesis, pseudohypoparathyroidism and Klinefelter's syndrome. *N Engl J Med 270:* 1268, 1964.

35. Aurbach, G. D.: Genetic disorders involving parathyroid hormone and calcitonin. *Birth Defects 7:* 48, 1971.

36. Winnacker, J. L., Becker, K. L., Moore, C. F.: Pseudohypoparathyroidism and selective deficiency of thyrotropin: an interesting association. *Metabolism 16:* 644, 1967.

37. Zisman, E., Latz, M., Jenkins, M. E., et al: Studies in pseudohypoparathyroidism. *Am J Med 46:* 464, 1969.

38. Werder, E. A., Illig, R., Bernasconi, S., et al: Excessive thyrotropin response to thyrotropin-releasing hormones in pseudohypoparathyroidism. *Pediatr Res 9:* 12, 1975.

39. Mann, J. B., Alterman, S., Hills, A. G.: Albright's hereditary osteodystrophy comprising pseudohypoparathyroidism and pseudopseudohypoparathyroidism: with a report of two cases representing the complete syndrome occurring in successive generations. *Ann Intern Med 56:* 315, 1962.

40. Aurbach, G. D., Marcus, R., Winickoff, R. N., et al: Urinary excretion of 3′,5′-AMP in syndromes considered refractory to parathyroid hormone. *Metabolism 19:* 799, 1970.

41. Aurbach, G. D.: Parathyroids. In Beeson, P. B., McDermott, W. (eds): Cecil and Loeb Textbook of Medicine (ed 14). Philadelphia, Saunders, 1975, p 1808.

42. Block, J. B., Clendenning, W. E.: Parathyroid hormone responsiveness in patients with basal-cell nevi and bone defects. *N Engl J Med 268:* 1157, 1963.

43. Gorlin, R. J., Goltz, R. W.: Multiple nevoid basal-cell epithelioma, jaw cysts and bifid rib: a syndrome. *N Engl J Med 262:* 908, 1960.

44. Clendenning, W. E., Block, J. B., Radde, I. G.: Basal-cell nevus syndrome. *Arch Dermatol, (Chicago) 90:* 38, 1964.

45. Roberts, P. D.: Familial calcification of the cerebral basal ganglia and its relation to hypoparathyroidism. *Brain 82:* 599, 1959.

46. Matthews, W. B.: Familial calcification of the basal ganglia with response to parathormone. *J Neurol Neurosurg Psychiatry 20:* 172, 1957.

47. Trygstad, C. W., Zisman, E., Witkop, C. J. Jr., et al: Resistance to parathyroid extract in Gardner's syndrome. *J Clin Endocrinol Metab 28:* 1153, 1968.

48. Gardner, E. J.: Follow-up study of a family group exhibiting dominant inheritance for a syndrome including intestinal polyps, osteomas, fibromas and epidermal cysts. *Am J Hum Genet 14:* 376, 1962.

49. Kooh, S. W., Fraser, D., DeLuca, H. F., et al: Treatment of hypoparathyroidism and pseudohypoparathyroidism with metabolites of vitamin D to 1α,25-dihydroxyvitamin D. *N Engl J Med 293:* 840, 1975.

50. Neer, R. M., Holick, M. F., DeLuca, H. F., et al: Effects of 1α-hydroxy-vitamin D_3 and 1,25-dihydroxy-vitamin D_3 on calcium and phosphorus metabolism in hypoparathyroidism. *Metabolism 24:* 1403, 1975.

51. Sinha, T. K., Bell, N. H.: 1,25-dihydroxyvitamin D, and pseudohypoparathyroidism. *N Engl J Med 294:* 612, 1976.

Medullary Carcinoma and Other Disorders Involving Calcitonin

64

Medullary Carcinoma of the Thyroid

E. D. Williams

The recognition that medullary carcinoma of the human thyroid gland is a separate entity from other thyroid tumors,[1] and that it is a tumor derived from the parafollicular, or C cells,[2] has led to a considerable volume of work on this tumor. The clinical syndromes it is associated with, the hormones it produces, chief among them calcitonin, and the link between these cells and the cells of the diffuse endocrine system of the gastrointestinal tract have been investigated. These observations, however, can best be seen in the historical perspective of growth in three separate strands of knowledge, which must be woven together to enable us to understand the pathophysiology of medullary carcinoma, its diagnosis, and its treatment. These three strands are the study by anatomists and histologists of the cytology of the thyroid, the study by pathologists of the different types of tumors of the thyroid, and the study by biochemists and physiologists of the hormones controlling calcium metabolism.

The first observations that established the existence of a second type of epithelial cell in the thyroid were those of Baber in 1876.[3] His work in the dog was confirmed and extended to other species by numerous observers. The study of the morphology of these cells was helped by the discovery that they could be distinguished from the follicular cells by silver impregnation techniques[4] and more recently by the presence of masked metachromasia.[5] We currently recognize that there are two morphologically quite separate types of epithelial cells in the mammalian thyroid, the follicular cell, and the C, or parafollicular, cell. The C cell usually lies between the follicular cell and the basement membrane (Fig. 64-1), or forms small solid nests of cells in an apparent interfollicular position. Electron microscopy shows that it lacks the distended cisternae of the follicular cell and contains electron-dense secretory granules of the type seen in the polypeptide-hormone-producing endocrine cells. Getzowa suggested that the embryologic origin of these cells was different from that of the thyroid follicular cell as long ago as 1907.[6] Her suggestion that these cells were derived from the ultimobranchial body was supported in 1937 by Godwin.[7] Pearse and Carvalheira[8] demonstrated by cytochemical techniques that these cells were carried to the thyroid by the ultimobranchial body, but the quail chick transplant work of Le Douarin and Le Lievre[9] showed that the precursor cells reached the ultimobranchial body from the neural crest. The mammalian thyroid is thus clearly established as a dual endocrine gland. The major component is the follicular cells, which are derived from the thyroglossal duct, and can be regarded as modified intestinal cells, secreting into and absorbing from a lumen. The minor component is the C cells, which are derived from the neural crest, and are true endocrine cells.

The separate identification of two types of tumors derived from these two cell types was hindered by the controversy between those anatomists who were convinced that there were two cell types, and those who regarded the parafollicular cells as degenerate follicular cells. In man, however, medullary carcinoma was separated as a tumor before C cells were recognized in the human thyroid. The early history of this separation is briefly reviewed elsewhere.[10] The tumor was clearly established as an entity by the work of Hazard et al.,[1] who recognized that it did not show follicular or papillary differentiation, but separated it from the anaplastic carcinomas, with which it had previously been classified. The regular occurrence of stromal amyloid in medullary carcinoma was an important diagnostic feature. Comparative studies in human and rat tumors led to the suggestion that medullary carcinoma was of parafollicular-cell origin.[2]

The recognition of the existence of calcitonin as a second hormone concerned with calcium regulation proceeded quite separately from the identification of parafollicular cells and their tumors. Copp and his group[11,12] presented evidence for the existence of a hypocalcemic factor in the dog, and suggested that it originated in the parathyroids. Hirsch et al[13] showed that in the rat, a hypocalcemic factor was found in the thyroid. Foster et al.[14] repeated Copp's experiment in the goat, an animal in which the parathyroid and thyroid are anatomically separate, and found that this factor, named *calcitonin* by Copp, was derived from the

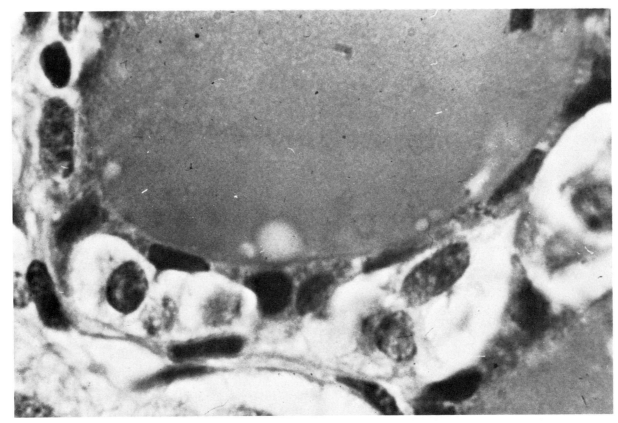

Fig. 64-1. C cells in the rat thyroid. The cells show a pale cytoplasm, and lie between the follicular cells and the basement membrane. They are unusually numerous in this photomicrograph. PAS. ×900.

thyroid. The parafollicular-cell origin of calcitonin within the thyroid was demonstrated by immunolocalization techniques (Fig. 64-2), and the name C cell was suggested.[15]

The cell, the hormone, and the tumor were firmly linked together when it was demonstrated that medullary carcinoma of the thyroid contained and secreted large amounts of calcitonin.[16,17] The decade that has elapsed since medullary carcinoma was firmly established as a calcitonin-secreting tumor of thyroid C cells has seen many advances in our knowledge of this tumor.

SPORADIC AND GENETIC MEDULLARY CARCINOMA

Medullary carcinoma may be inherited in a number of distinct syndromes which will be discussed in detail later. In one of these syndromes there is a relatively high frequency of occurrence of spontaneous mutations. The use of the terms *familial* or *inherited* medullary carcinoma is therefore not satisfactory, and the term *genetic* medullary carcinoma is applied when there is evidence of the presence of a syndrome known to be heritable or direct evidence of inheritance. The term *sporadic* medullary carcinoma is used for cases with no evidence of a genetic factor.

INCIDENCE

Medullary carcinoma has been reported to comprise between 3.5 and 10 percent of all thyroid carcinomas,[1,18] with a mean figure of 6.8 percent.[19] Several factors may influence this variation in reported incidence. First, the incidence of thyroid carcinomas derived from the follicular cell is known to show geographic variation. Second, the diagnostic criteria or the accuracy of their application for both C-cell and follicular-cell tumors may well vary in different areas. Third, the existence of a large family with many affected members in one area will lead to a considerable increase in frequency of occurrence of this tumor in the hospital serving that population.

Despite the importance of these factors, it seems likely that there is a geographic variation in the incidence of sporadic medullary carcinoma. A study of the incidence of medullary carcinoma in two well-defined populations, Iceland and northeast Scotland, has shown that it accounted for 5 percent of all thyroid cancers in Iceland, an area with an unusually high incidence of papillary carcinomas, but that no cases occurred in a 20-year period in a population of 500,000 people in northeast Scotland.[20] Although the numbers in this study were small, the Icelandic incidence is similar to the 3.5 percent incidence reported in a large recent study in Norway,[21] and the incidence in northeast Scotland confirmed previous personal communications that this tumor is rare in Scotland. Possible reasons for this variation in incidence will be discussed later.

In contrast to the other types of thyroid cancer, and to most thyroid disease, the incidence in males and females is almost equal. In sporadic cases the female-to-male ratio is 1.3:1, in genetic cases it is 1:1. The age at presentation varies widely, from infancy to old age, with the majority of sporadic cases presenting in the fourth, fifth, and sixth decades.

PATHOLOGY

The histopathologic features of this tumor have been described in detail elsewhere.[10,18] The tumor is a solid, often hard mass, well circumscribed but not encapsulated. At a light-microscope level it is composed of sheets of cells with abundant granular

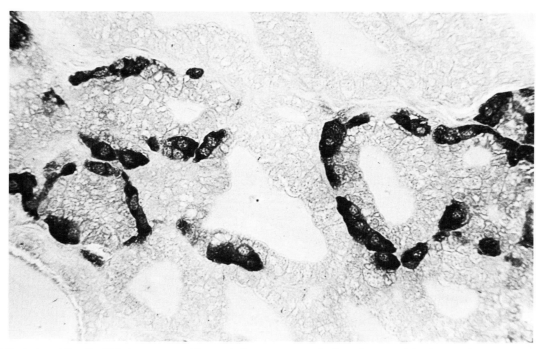

Fig. 64-2. Calcitonin in rat C cells. This immunoperoxidase technique uses an antibody to human calcitonin. The C cells are darkly staining with relatively unstained nuclei. The follicular cells can just be distinguished. Peroxidase. ×350.

cytoplasm. Typically it contains irregular masses of amyloid and often much collagen, and it lacks papillary or follicular differentiation (Fig. 64-3) On electron microscopy, characteristic small electron-dense membrane-limited secretory granules can be seen (Fig. 64-4). The tumor may be composed of fusiform cells forming a whorling pattern, and rarely the more-rapidly growing forms may show a pattern reminiscent of an oat-cell carcinoma. While the tumors may rarely show formation of ductular structures, good evidence of true follicular formation is lacking. In the primary tumor, nonneoplastic follicles are often included in the tumor, and rarely more than one type of tumor may occur in the same gland.

A small number of tumors in which no amyloid can be detected by conventional methods can be accepted as medullary carcinomas.

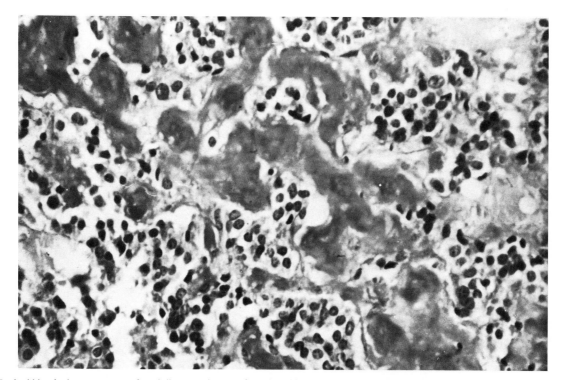

Fig. 64-3. Typical histologic appearance of medullary carcinoma of the thyroid. The amorphous amyloid lies between solid groups of regular tumor cells. H&E. ×200.

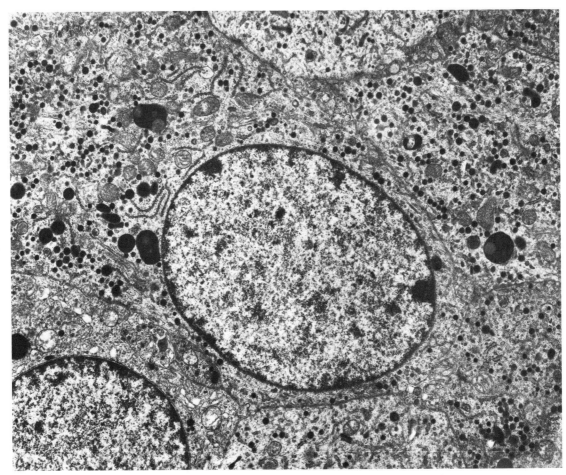

Fig. 64-4.   Electron micrograph of medullary carcinoma showing a light cell with numerous small electron-dense secretory granules. ×14,000.

CLINICAL PRESENTATION AND SPREAD

The majority of patients present with a thyroid mass, often with palpable cervical lymph nodes. At operation, involved cervical lymph nodes are found in two-thirds of the patients.[18] The other common site for early extrathyroid tumor spread is the upper mediastinum, where massive secondary tumor deposits may be found (Fig. 64-5). Spread beyond the neck and mediastinum usually occurs late in the natural history of the disease, with the lungs, liver, adrenal, and bones being the most common sites. Metastases to bone are sometimes osteoblastic, although lytic metastasis to the spine with paralysis due to cord compression is not infrequent in disseminated medullary carcinoma.

Of the various hormonally mediated syndromes associated with medullary carcinoma, diarrhea is the most prominent clinically. It is present in about one-quarter of all patients, and may be the presenting complaint.

CALCITONIN

Calcitonin is consistently produced by medullary carcinoma of the thyroid (Fig. 64-6). The tumor, like the normal C cell, contains electron-dense membrane-limited secretory granules, which are thought to be the site of calcitonin storage. The concentration of calcitonin in the tumor may be as much as 5000 times the concentration of calcitonin in normal human thyroid.[17] It seems unlikely from electron microscopic studies that the individual cell contains more calcitonin than the individual normal cell, and it is probable that this ratio gives some idea of the relative frequency of

C cells in the human thyroid. The chemistry and action of calcitonin are discussed elsewhere.

The measurement of serum calcitonin is of value in establishing the diagnosis of medullary carcinoma, in establishing the presence of metastases, and in following the effects of treatment.[22] It is of particular value in family studies on the genetic group, especially if stimulation tests such as calcium infusion, pentagastrin infusion, or alcohol are used.

The finding of a high serum calcitonin in a patient is not by itself proof of the presence of medullary carcinoma. Excess calcitonin may be found in association with other tumors, particularly oat-cell carcinoma of the lung, carcinoids, and carcinoma of the breast,[23,24] and in patients with the Zollinger/Ellison syndrome.[25] The obvious interpretation of these findings is that the calcitonin is being secreted as an ectopic hormone by these tumors. However, evidence on this point is conflicting. It seems likely that in some tumors this is indeed correct. However, no calcitonin was found by immunoperoxidase staining in a number of G-cell tumors of the pancreas, while in one such case C cells were apparently more numerous than normal in the thyroid.[26] In one case of adenocarcinoma of the lung with hypercalcitoninemia, the calcitonin level fluctuated with radiotherapy of the tumor, but its origin was shown by catheterization studies to be from thyroid, not tumor.[27] It therefore seems likely that in some cases high levels of calcitonin are due to production of a calcitonin-releasing factor, either directly by the tumor, or as a result of tumor-induced changes in some other tissue—for example, bone. A raised plasma calcitonin has also been recorded in pyknodysostosis[28] (Chapter 65).

PROSTAGLANDINS

Evidence that some medullary carcinomas contain and secrete prostaglandin E_2 and F_2 was presented by Williams et al.[29] Grimley et al.[30] found evidence of prostaglandin production by medullary carcinoma in tissue culture. A number of other authors have reported cases with elevated levels of circulating prostaglandins.[31–34] However, its absence has also been the subject of a number of reports, most recently by Ménagé et al.,[35] and it is clearly not consistently produced in large amounts.

AMYLOID

The occurrence of a material with the staining properties of amyloid was one of the features that led to the pathologic separation of medullary carcinoma from other thyroid tumors. While a few tumors of similar morphology may contain no demonstrable amyloid, it remains a characteristic of the great majority of this group of tumors, and it may be present in large amounts. The amyloid is produced by the tumor cells themselves, as has been shown by morphologic and tissue culture studies.

The first indication that the amyloid from medullary carcinoma of the thyroid differs from the amyloid associated with chronic infections came from a study by Benditt and Eriksen,[36] who found that the amino acid composition of amyloid from several patients with chronic infections was consistent, and was different from that found in a case of medullary carcinoma. Pearse et al.,[37] using histochemical techniques, found that the amyloid associated with endocrine tumors differed from that associated with chronic infections in its negative reaction to tyrosine and tryptophan—although Benditt and Eriksen had found little difference in tyrosine content.

Tashjian et al.[38] found that antibodies to calcitonin reacted with the amyloid in sections of medullary carcinoma, although the interpretation of this observation is made more difficult by the finding that the amyloid may contain cellular fragments, including secretory granules.[39] However, Sletten et al.[40] have prepared and partially characterized amyloid fibril proteins from medullary carcinoma. The main fibril component was found to differ from other

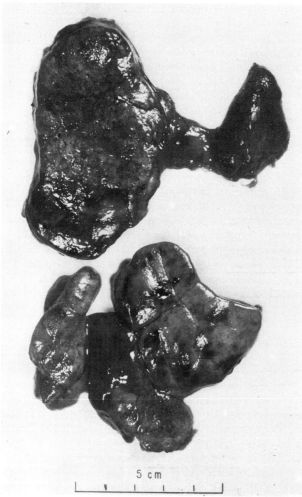

Fig. 64-5. Macroscopic appearance of medullary carcinoma of the thyroid. The greater part of the right lobe of the thyroid is replaced by a solid tumor. The lower mass of tumor was removed from the upper anterior mediastinum.

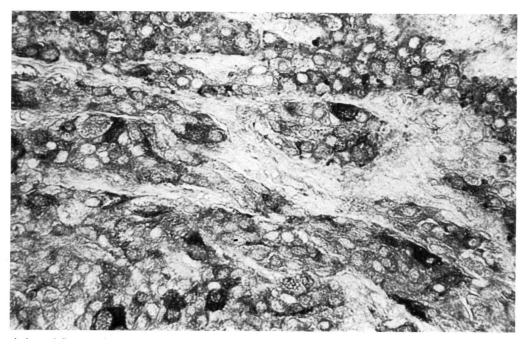

Fig. 64-6. Calcitonin in medullary carcinoma. The cords of tumor cells show a variable content of calcitonin, demonstrated with an immunoperoxidase technique. ×400.

known amyloid proteins, and the AA and light-chain variable fragments found in other amyloids were not present in medullary carcinoma amyloid. The amino acid composition of the amyloid protein from medullary carcinoma differed considerably from calcitonin, but it contained an amino acid sequence identical to residues 9–19 in human calcitonin. Sletten et al. suggest that the main protein component of amyloid in medullary carcinoma may represent a prohormone of calcitonin. While further work is needed on this point, it seems likely that the amyloid is related either to calcitonin prohormone or a hormonal breakdown product, perhaps in association with another component.

BIOGENIC AMINES

It has been known for many years that the thyroid in some species has a high content of 5-hydroxytryptamine (5-HT).[41] Falck et al.[42] showed that in the sheep thyroid, the amine was confined to the parafollicular (C) cells. It has also been shown that C cells contain dopa decarboxylase, and are able to take up dopa and 5-hydroxytryptophan, and decarboxylate them, respectively, to dopamine and 5-HT.[43,44]

It is therefore not surprising that some patients with medullary carcinoma show a raised urinary excretion of 5-hydroxyindolacetic acid, although the majority do not show elevated levels.[45,46] High levels of 5-HT have been recorded in the tumor itself,[45,47] which has also been shown to have a high dopa decarboxylase content.[45,47,48] It is rather more surprising that high levels of histaminase have been found in both tumor and serum in patients with medullary carcinoma.[49,50] Elevated serum histaminase levels were detected in somewhat over half the patients tested and in many of the tumors examined.[48,50] The flare response after intradermal histamine injection may be absent in patients with medullary carcinoma of the thyroid.[51,52] While there has been speculation that this may be related to the raised levels of histaminase, the patients reported with absent flare have also had multiple mucosal neuromas. It seems likely that the abnormal response to histamine is due to a neural abnormality leading to an abnormal axon reflex.

ACTH AND CORTICOTROPIN-RELEASING HORMONE

Cushing's syndrome has been recorded on a number of occasions with carcinoma of the thyroid, and an analysis of the reports up to 1968 showed that the association was specifically with medullary carcinoma of the thyroid.[53] This has been amply confirmed since that time, and when adequate investigation has been carried out it has in most cases been found that ectopic production of ACTH was the cause of the Cushing's syndrome. Production of both calcitonin and ACTH by the same tumor has been demonstrated, and removal of the thyroid carcinoma has led to regression of the Cushing's syndrome.[54,55] Recently a case of medullary carcinoma of the thyroid with Cushing's syndrome, in which the tumor produced both ACTH and a substance with corticotropin-releasing hormone (CRH) activity has been reported.[56] In addition, the tumor produced large amounts of calcitonin, and also a substance which stimulated prolactin production. The preoperative investigation had shown partial dexamethasone suppression and lysine vasopressin and metyrapone stimulation, and a 30-fold gradient of CRH activity was demonstrated between thyroid artery and vein. As well as secreting immunoreactive, biologically active ACTH, a larger form, possibly "big ACTH," was present in the tumor. The genetic implication of the production of both CRH and

ACTH by the same tumor are considerable. However, the identity of CRH was not proven, and further work is needed on this subject. One point of interest is whether these multiple polypeptide-hormone-secreting tumors contain individual cells that secrete more than one polypeptide hormone. The evidence so far suggests that each cell generally produces only one polypeptide hormone,[57,58] although somatostatin and calcitonin have both been found in a subpopulation of C cells in rat thyroid.[58a]

OTHER HUMORAL FACTORS

High levels of carcinoembryonic antigen have been found in all 13 cases of medullary carcinoma tested, and in only 3 of 65 cases of other types of thyroid disease.[59] As mentioned above, a substance with prolactin-stimulating activity has been found in one patient, associated with galactorrhea;[56] gynecomastia was recorded in one other case.[60] An osteoblast-stimulating factor has been described in the parafollicular cells of grey-lethal mice,[61] and it is of interest that osteopetrosis has been described in the children of a patient with medullary carcinoma of the thyroid.[62] Finally, high levels of nerve-growth factor have been found in the plasma of a patient with medullary carcinoma of the thyroid.[63]

HUMORALLY MEDIATED SYNDROMES

The range of substances secreted by medullary carcinoma of the thyroid is considerable, and it is not surprising that a variety of clinical syndromes due to humoral factors may be found in association with this tumor, whether sporadic or genetic. The most common of these is diarrhea. Attention was drawn to this by Williams,[45] who found that severe diarrhea was relatively common in patients with medullary carcinoma, and that it was very frequent in patients with widespread tumors. These findings have been confirmed on a number of occasions, and the combined results of the two largest series show that diarrhea was present in about 20 percent of all patients with medullary carcinoma and in about half of the patients with disseminated carcinoma.[10,46] It is surprising that although the diarrhea has been known to be associated with the tumor for over 10 years, the humoral factor concerned is not yet identified with certainty. There is no doubt that the diarrhea is humorally mediated, as resection of tumor may lead to great improvement in the diarrhea.[45,64–66] One reason that the humoral factor has not yet been identified may be because several of the factors which medullary carcinoma may produce are likely to increase gut motility. Certainly, prostaglandins may lead to hypermotility, and calcitonin itself may lead to borborygmi and increased jejunal secretion of water and electrolytes.[67,68] It has also been shown to stimulate intestinal alkaline phosphatase activity.[69] 5-HT also leads to intestinal hypermotility, although in the carcinoid syndrome, kinins may also be involved.

The diarrhea is characterized by intestinal hypermotility, which may be extreme, with undigested food in the very frequent watery stools. Bernier et al.[65] found that steatorrhea was mild or absent, and that there was excessive loss of water and electrolytes in the stools. Jejunal absorption is normal, but, in the ileum, Na^+, Cl^-, and water were secreted into the lumen, while bicarbonate was absorbed—the reverse of normal.[31] These findings, and the abnormalities in intestinal transit, have been reported after administration of prostaglandin $F_2\alpha$. Nutmeg, which contains a prostaglandin-synthetase inhibitor, given orally leads to improvement in the diarrhea.[34,70] While prostaglandins seem most consistently implicated, they have not always been demonstrable in patients with diarrhea[35] and a multifactorial cause still seems likely.

This conclusion is supported by the variable occurrence of the other symptoms which may be associated with diarrhea. Flushing is the most common of these, occurring in one-third of the patients with diarrhea; in some cases there is pronounced episodic flushing, which, as in the carcinoid syndrome, may be induced by alcohol ingestion.[45,46]

Cushing's syndrome is another important humorally mediated complication of medullary carcinoma; it is found in approximately 5 percent of cases.[82] Treatment, as for other tumors that produce ectopic ACTH, is resection of tumor where possible, otherwise adrenalectomy.

The frequency of occurrence of diarrhea and Cushing's syndrome appears to be similar in both genetic and sporadic medullary carcinoma.

GENETICALLY MEDIATED SYNDROMES

One of the most interesting features of medullary carcinoma is the part it plays in a variety of genetically determined syndromes. Williams[71] and Schimke and Hartmann[72] pointed out that the link, reviewed by Sipple[73], between pheochromocytoma and thyroid carcinoma was specifically with medullary carcinoma of the thyroid, and Schimke and Hartmann recognized that this condition was inherited as an autosomal dominant. It is now evident that medullary carcinoma may be inherited without pheochromocytoma, that it may be inherited together with pheochromocytoma, or that it may be inherited with multiple mucosal neuromas, pheochromocytomas, ganglioneuromatosis of the gastrointestinal tract, and a number of associated abnormalities. Each of these three syndromes is separately inherited, and together they comprise about 20 percent of all cases of medullary carcinoma.[74–77]

Only a small number of families with inherited medullary carcinoma without pheochromocytomas or neuromas have been described; the largest reported is that of Block et al.[78] In the majority of cases where adequate investigation has been carried out, the medullary carcinoma has been found to be bilateral. Of 7 reported families, 3 showed parathyroid disease, which will be discussed later. The average age at presentation was 28 years.

Well over 20 families with inherited medullary carcinoma and pheochromocytoma have been reported. The average age of presentation is about 36 years. Whereas in autopsy studies in the adult, bilateral medullary carcinoma and bilateral pheochromocytoma are the usual findings, either tumor may lead to the initial clinical presentation. Some of these patients have had parathyroid disease, and 1 family also showed cutaneous fibromas. In general, however, these patients do not show any cutaneous abnormalities.

The third inherited form is the association of medullary carcinoma with pheochromocytomas, multiple mucosal neuromas, intestinal ganglioneuromatosis, marfanoid habitus, muscular weakness, high arched palate, pes cavus, and a number of other abnormalities. This syndrome was first defined by Williams and Pollock,[79] who reported 2 cases, one of which was known to be familial, and reviewed the literature up to that time. Since then there have been a considerable number of individual case reports, and six other reports of families affected by this syndrome. The average age of presentation with the medullary carcinoma of the thyroid in cases with neuromas is 19. The thyroid tumor presents earlier than do other inherited types of medullary carcinoma, and the prognosis is worse. The reported patients have been followed

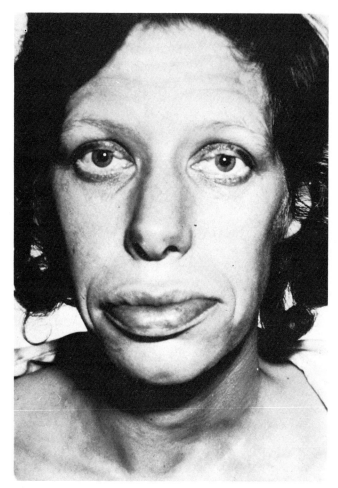

Fig. 64-7. Facial appearance of the fully developed syndrome of multiple mucosal neuromas. Note the eyelid neuromas and the thickened "bumpy" lips. (Case 2, from Williams and Pollock: 1959)

for various periods of time, but half were dead at the time they were reported, all of whom died before the age of 37, with a mean age of 27 years. No chromosomal abnormalities can be detected.[80]

These patients have very characteristic faces (Fig. 64-7) with thick, nodular, rather everted lips, thickened eyelids with small polypoid greyish tumors on the contact margins, usually near the inner canthus (Fig. 64-8), and similar small polypoid lesions in the anterior third of the tongue, particularly near the tip and lateral

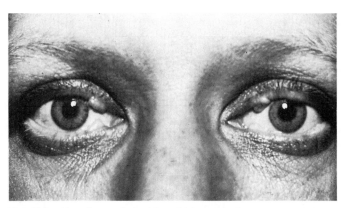

Fig. 64-8. Eyes in a patient with multiple mucosal neuromas (same case as in Fig. 64-7). (Case 2, from Williams and Pollock: 1959)

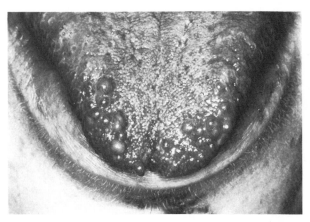

Fig. 64-9. Tongue in a patient with multiple mucosal neuromas.

border (Fig. 64-9). These lesions are usually present at birth, although in a minority of cases they appear to arise in adult life. Ganglioneuromatosis of the intestine probably occurs in the majority of the patients, and may be associated with the presence of diverticulosis in childhood or with areas of megacolon.[81]

MEDULLARY CARCINOMA IN GENETICALLY MEDIATED SYNDROMES

The medullary carcinomas found in these inherited syndromes are commonly bilateral and are found in the midportions of the lateral lobes of the gland[82] (Fig. 64-10). While they are usually symmetrical, occasionally they may be grossly asymmetrical.[83] In the very young patients belonging to families with inherited medullary carcinoma, C-cell hyperplasia has been described in the absence of carcinoma.[84] Histologically, these tumors are not separable from sporadic medullary carcinomas.

PHEOCHROMOCYTOMAS IN GENETICALLY MEDIATED SYNDROMES

The pheochromocytomas found in these inherited syndromes with medullary carcinoma are usually bilateral, may be multiple, and are occasionally extraadrenal. When the pheochromocytoma is unilateral, the opposite adrenal commonly shows diffuse or

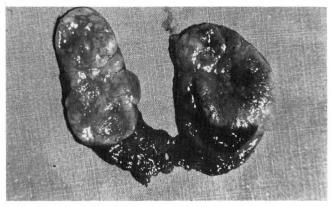

Fig. 64-10. Bilateral primary medullary carcinomas in a patient with genetically determined disease.

nodular hyperplasia; rarely both adrenals may show hyperplasia or no abnormality.[85,86] The pheochromocytomas are not histologically distinguishable from sporadic pheochromocytomas, although occasionally metastatic medullary carcinoma may be found in the adrenal medullary tumors. Malignant pheochromocytomas have been described by several authors.

The incidence of malignancy in sporadic pheochromocytomas varies widely in different series; using strict criteria, its incidence is only 2.5 percent.[87] In 15 patients with medullary carcinoma and pheochromocytoma, a total of 25 pheochromocytomas was found, of which 4 were associated with metastasis, and another 3 showed invasion without metastasis.[85] The incidence of malignancy in pheochromocytomas associated with medullary carcinoma may therefore well be higher than it is in patients with sporadic pheochromocytomas.

One particular point of interest in the pheochromocytomas in these syndromes is the high proportion of adrenalin that they produce. This has been noted on several occasions.[88–91] In a study of 21 pheochromocytomas from patients without medullary carcinoma, whether familial or not, the amount of adrenalin was always less than that of noradrenalin. By contrast, in 13 tumors from patients with medullary carcinoma, the amount of adrenalin was always greater than the amount of noradrenalin, usually forming more than 70 percent of the total catecholamine content.[90] In one extraadrenal tumor (without evidence of associated adrenal cortex) adrenalin comprised 46 percent of the total—more than in any of the intraadrenal cases not associated with medullary carcinoma. These observations, together with the finding that pheochromocytomas associated with medullary carcinoma may contain 5-HT[47] and calcitonin,[92] show that these pheochromocytomas differ biochemically from sporadic pheochromocytomas and from inherited pheochromocytomas not associated with medullary carcinoma. These observations also provide support for the suggestion that in man, the enzyme noradrenalin N-methyltransferase may exist in two forms or may have two controlling mechanisms. One may be steroid-inducible, as found in most pheochromocytomas, and one may be unaffected or little affected by steroids, and present in pheochromocytomas associated with medullary carcinoma.

NEUROMAS IN INHERITED MEDULLARY-CARCINOMA SYNDROMES

The mucosal lesions found in the inherited syndrome are neuromas—that is, they consist of bundles or sheets of nerve fibers, usually poorly separated from the surrounding tissue (Fig. 64-11). In the eyelid, lip, and tongue, they usually lack ganglion cells, which presumably implies that there is an increased number of ganglion cells elsewhere, perhaps in the trigeminal ganglion. Prominent medullated nerves may be seen in the cornea.[93] In the gastrointestinal tract, the major histologic lesion is an enlargement of Auerbach's plexus, with rounded masses of both ganglion cells and nerve fibers producing a very striking picture (Fig. 64-12). This is often prominent in the esophagus, and may extend throughout the gastrointesinal tract to the anus. Similar changes may also be found in other viscera (for example, the pancreas), and peripheral-nerve hypertrophy has been described.[81,94]

Despite the fact that the neuromas in this condition are sometimes mistakenly referred to as neurofibromas, the multiple-mucosal-neuroma syndrome is quite distinct from Recklinghausen's disease. It must be stressed that multiple mucosal neuromas are not seen in occasional patients in a family with inherited medullary carcinoma and pheochromocytomas—either all affected members

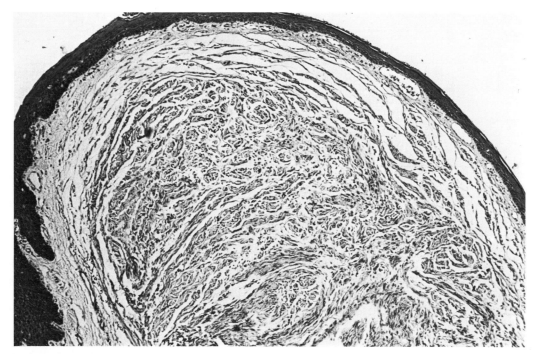

Fig. 64-11. Histology of one of the mucosal neuromas from the patient shown in Fig. 64-9. The lesion is composed of nerve fibers. H&E ×75.

in a family show this condition, or none of them do. The degree of involvement in a family may, however, vary. Occasional examples of multiple mucosal neuromas are not found in families with true Recklinghausen's neurofibromatosis. There is, however, a single case report of medullary carcinoma in one patient belonging to a family with cutaneous neurofibromatosis and pheochromocytomas.[95] While neurofibromatosis may affect the eyelids, tongue, and gut, it is usually diffuse in the eyelid, and does not form the characteristic polypoid lesion at the mucocutaneous junctions of multiple mucosal neuromas. In the tongue, it usually causes a single tumor, and, in the gut, in contrast to multiple mucosal neuromas, it may give multiple tumors or occasionally affect a localized segment. Calcitonin and amyloid have been reported as occurring in mucosal neuromas in this syndrome.[92,96]

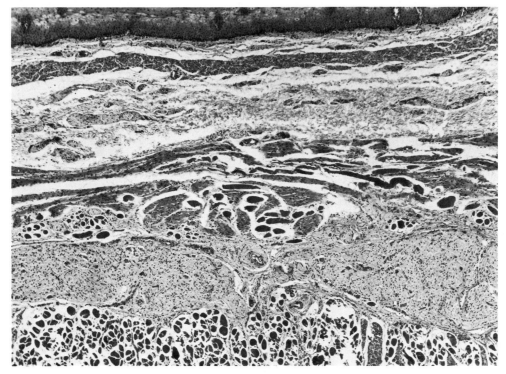

Fig. 64-12. Ganglioneuromatosis of the esophagus in a patient with multiple mucosal neuromas. A greatly enlarged Auerbach plexus is shown. H&E. ×33.

PARATHYROIDS IN INHERITED MEDULLARY-CARCINOMA SYNDROMES

Parathyroid involvement is not uncommon in familial medullary carcinoma, and it has been described in all three patterns of inherited disease. Symptomatic hyperparathyroidism has been described on a number of occasions; more recently, attention has been focused on biochemical and structural abnormalities in the absence of clinical disease. The clinical features of hyperparathyroidism do not differ from those seen in association with a single parathyroid adenoma, except that renal stones appear rather frequently. In the earlier case reports, the pathology usually described was that of an adenoma, but when all glands have been examined it is apparent that it is common for more than one gland to be involved. However, when careful parathyroid studies have been carried out, it has been shown that in a number of cases the parathyroid pathology has been chief-cell hyperplasia.[97] Hyperplasia may be found at thyroidectomy in a considerable number of patients, and raised parathyroid hormone (PTH) levels are common in some families. The incidence of hypercalcemia differs widely in different families. It was not present in any of the 13 cases studied directly by Melvin et al.,[82] even though 4 had renal stones and 1 of these and another 3 showed consistently elevated PTH levels. In contrast, 9 of 25 members of the family studied by Keiser et al.[97] showed hypercalcemia. Both these families showed inherited medullary carcinoma and pheochromocytoma without mucosal neuromas. In families with medullary carcinoma without pheochromocytoma or neuromas, hyperparathyroidism also occurs. A parathyroid adenoma was found in 1 of 9 patients with thyroid carcinoma from a family with inherited medullary carcinoma,[78] and a second member of the family had renal stones. In another family, 2 of 4 siblings with medullary carcinoma of the thyroid showed hypercalcemia due to a parathyroid adenoma.[98]

Parathyroid disease, however, seems relatively rare in families with multiple mucosal neuromas. The only well-documented case is the one reported by Bartlett et al.,[99] although Ljungberg[100] reported an apparently nonfamilial case who showed renal stones. Serum calcium and PTH were normal in 12 patients with multiple mucosal neuromas studied by Chong et al.[74] Ljungberg[100] also recorded a case of hyperparathyroidism in a sporadic case of medullary carcinoma; the parathyroid tumor weighed 130 g and was, not surprisingly, regarded as an adenoma.

PTH studies have been carried out in many patients with familial medullary carcinoma; in some there has been a surprising lack of correlation between the hormone levels, the calcium, and the histologic evidence of parathyroid hyperplasia.[82] A paradoxical increase in PTH secretion during calcium infusion in patients with medullary carcinoma has been recorded.[101]

OTHER TUMORS AND CONGENITAL ABNORMALITIES IN INHERITED MEDULLARY-CARCINOMA SYNDROMES

A variety of other tumors have been recorded in association with medullary carcinoma. Some are certainly coincidental. It is worth noting, however, that bilateral adrenal ganglioneuromas together with pheochromocytomas have been documented.[102] A rectal carcinoid in a patient with multiple mucosal neuromas has been recorded.[75] Bilateral Wilms tumors and congenital heart disease were found in a child whose mother had medullary carcinoma and pheochromocytoma.[103] Congenital heart disease has also been recorded in a sibling of a patient with multiple mucosal neuromas.[75]

GENERAL COMMENTS ON THE INHERITED SYNDROMES ASSOCIATED WITH MEDULLARY CARCINOMA

It can be seen from the previous section that medullary carcinoma plays a major role in a complex set of inherited endocrine tumors. Analysis of the inheritance of the tumor shows that in all three of the major variants of inherited medullary carcinoma, the tumor is inherited as a dominant of almost complete penetrance.[10] Nomenclature of these syndromes poses a problem. Various authors refer to them by different terms: some use *Sipple's syndrome* for all forms indiscriminately, others use *multiple-endocrine-neoplasia (MEN) IIa and IIb,* yet others *MEN II and MEN III.* They should however, be viewed in the whole spectrum of inherited endocrine neoplasia, ranging from an inherited liability to tumors of one gland, to an inherited liability to tumors of four different endocrines. For the purposes of this discussion, and for the purposes of patient care, it is important to define the inherited complex accurately. Indeed, it is of particular importance to delineate the disease processes present in the family and not assume that that family will resemble others in the pattern of disease displayed. The best usage of the terms is to apply *MEN II* to the whole complex of syndromes associated with genetically mediated medullary carcinoma. Further subdivision is best achieved by qualification of the term—e.g., MEN II with neuromas, or MEN II without pheochromocytomas—rather than a formal subdivision which may need revision.

One of the most significant observations is that both the inherited medullary carcinomas and the inherited pheochromocytomas may be accompanied, and are probably preceded, by hyperplasia. This would suggest that either the C cells and the adrenal medullary cells have a genetic abnormality that predisposes to continued growth and eventual tumor formation, or that they are being subjected to a continued abnormal stimulus to growth with the same result. It is well known from animal studies that a long-continued stimulus to growth of an endocrine gland leads to tumor formation. This has been shown, for example, in rat thyroid and pituitary. The same situation leads to tumor formation in man, as in the development of thyroid follicular tumors in dyshormonogenesis, and parathyroid tumors in the hyperplastic glands of chronic renal failure. The tumors that arise in these situations of chronic stimulation are commonly multiple.

The suggestion that these tumors arise as a result of continued nonneoplastic growth receives support from the observation that in a patient with glucose-6-phosphate dehydrogenase mosaicism, both medullary carcinoma and pheochromocytoma contained only one form of the enzyme. This suggests that the tumors each originated from a single clone of cells, and make it unlikely that all the patient's C cells and all her adrenal medullary cells took part in the neoplastic process.[104]

In the author's opinion, the most likely explanation is the production in excess of a substance or substances that stimulates C-cell and adrenal medullary growth. Alternatively, the cells may have a genetic defect that renders them sensitive to the growth-promoting effect of an inappropriate hormone. Either of these mechanisms could be the result of a single gene defect, and both could result in tumors on a background of hyperplasia. It was pointed out in 1969 that the intestinal changes in patients with multiple mucosal neuromas resembled those produced in experimental animals by the administration of nerve-growth factor, and it was suggested that an excess of this substance might mediate all or part of this syndrome.[105] Recently Bigazzi[63] has found high levels of nerve-growth factor in the serum of a patient with familial medullary carcinoma.

It is therefore a tenable hypothesis to suggest that the syndrome of multiple mucosal neuromas is due to high plasma levels of a substance with nerve-growth-factor properties, which stimulates growth of C cells, adrenal medullary cells, and some parasympathetic ganglia. This requires the assumption of a second, perhaps related, growth factor which stimulates C and adrenal medullary cells, and yet a third which stimulates C cells only. It is clear that many problems remain unanswered, not least the variability of parathyroid involvement.

The variability in the behavior of medullary carcinoma between those families with multiple mucosal neuromas and those without is not only important when discussing the pathogenesis, but also in relation to treatment and prognosis. In addition, it is relevant to the frequency of occurrence of isolated cases. One striking finding on reviewing the literature is the high proportion of reports of individual cases of multiple mucosal neuromas with medullary carcinoma and pheochromocytoma without a family history, and the high proportion of reports of cases of medullary carcinoma and pheochromocytoma with a family history. Obviously, severe facial disfigurement, present in some cases with mucosal neuromas, may militate against the likelihood of having children. However, when to this is added the earlier age of presentation of medullary carcinoma and the frequency of death before the end of the reproductive period in those cases with multiple mucosal neuromas, it is obvious that fertility in patients with this syndrome is likely to be considerably reduced. Under these circumstances the maintenance of a constant gene pool in the population requires a relatively high proportion of cases due to spontaneous mutation as compared to inheritance.

TREATMENT OF MEDULLARY CARCINOMA

It is clear from the foregoing that it is essential to establish whether a patient with medullary carcinoma belongs to the sporadic or genetic groups. Obviously, if a patient shows the multiple-mucosal-neuromas syndrome, then the medullary carcinoma is genetically determined, whether or not a family history is present—and as discussed above, in many cases it will not be present. In the absence of mucosal neuromas a patient is more likely to belong to the genetic group if the medullary carcinoma is bilateral, if he belongs to a young age group, or if there are symptoms suggestive of pheochromocytoma or hyperparathyroidism, or if there is a family history of medullary carcinoma, pheochromocytoma, or hyperparathyroidism. However, irrespective of these findings it is advisable to screen for pheochromocytoma before any operations are undertaken on a patient with medullary carcinoma. Obviously, pheochromocytoma, if present, should be dealt with first. Because of the high proportion of adrenalin produced by these tumors, it has been suggested that beta-adrenergic blockade should be used, as well as alpha-adrenergic blockade, during surgery.[106]

SURGICAL TREATMENT

The extent of surgical treatment which should be undertaken depends in part on the spread of the disease, in part on the associated hormonal complications, and in part on whether the tumor belongs to the genetic or sporadic group. In the presence of distant spread it may still be worth resecting a large mass of tumor to control severe diarrhea or Cushing's syndrome.

In the absence of metastatic disease outside the neck, the accepted treatment is surgery. However, the extent of surgical treatment advised varies in different centers. There is general agreement that in symptomatic familial cases, a total thyroidectomy should be carried out, with either a modified or a radical neck dissection.[74,107] In the children of patients with familial medullary carcinoma, several studies have shown that serum calcitonin measurements, with or without alcohol, calcium infusion, pentagastrin infusion, or other stimulation tests, can be used to identify children with tumors or with C-cell hyperplasia before tumors have developed.[97,106,107] In a 5-year follow-up of 12 patients submitted to thyroidectomy solely on the basis of abnormal calcitonin values, 7 were disease free by all criteria, 2 were known to have metastatic disease present immediately after surgery, and 1 has converted from a normal calcitonin response postoperatively to an abnormal calcitonin response despite total thyroidectomy.[106] While it is possible to demonstrate medullary carcinoma or C-cell hyperplasia in childhood, before any clinical symptoms appear, it does not necessarily follow that it is best to submit these children to radical surgery.

If the cases reported by Ljungberg[100] and Melvin et al.[82] are analyzed together—as they belong to the same family—7 patients died from medullary carcinoma, at an average age of 60 years, with a range of 50–76 years. Ten patients ranging in age from 50 to 64 were alive; medullary carcinoma was found at operation for thyroid enlargement in 8 and diagnosed by calcitonin screening tests in 2. It is therefore clear that in this family the inheritance of medullary carcinoma is compatible with a long life. Six cases in this family were known to have died from medullary carcinoma; the mean survival from presentation to death was 13 years. In contrast, the survival in 8 sporadic cases reported by Ljungberg[100] was 4½ years. The decision as to whether to carry out thyroidectomy in children with proven occult medullary carcinoma must take into account these observations as well as the possibility of chronic illness from metastatic medullary carcinoma. On balance it seems likely that in members of families with inherited medullary carcinoma without mucosal neuromas, thyroidectomy should be undertaken only with firm evidence of the presence of tumor. As criteria for diagnosis, two positive responses to provocative tests have been recommended.[106] However, a rigorous search for evidence of medullary carcinoma should be undertaken in families with mucosal neuromas, followed by radical surgery when this is positive. Several authors have stressed the importance of recognizing the presence of pheochromocytomas, and in some families these have proved far more life-threatening at an early age than have the medullary carcinomas.[77,108]

The operative treatment of sporadic medullary carcinoma varies considerably from center to center, and no series yet provides an adequate number of cases separated into sporadic and the various genetic groups, treated by differing techniques and followed for a sufficiently long time to enable any firm judgements to be made on the ideal treatment. The Mayo Clinic group[74] recommended an aggressive approach, even though there was no difference in recurrence rates between subtotal and total thyroidectomy. Because of the known distribution of C cells in the thyroid, it has been proposed that the operation of choice for nonfamilial medullary carcinoma is a bilateral 90 percent upper-pole thyroidectomy, leaving remnants at both lower poles, together with both lower parathyroids.[109]

It is clearly not possible to make an authoritative statement on the surgical treatment of any form of medullary carcinoma, heritable or sporadic, which will cover all eventualities. Where there is no evidence suggesting that the tumor belongs to the genetic group, it would seem logical to carry out a lobectomy on the side with the main tumor mass, and a subtotal lobectomy on the opposite side. This approach covers not only those cases where there is spread across the midline, but also the possibility that the tumor will be bilateral, despite the lack of any other evidence of inheritance.

NONSURGICAL THERAPY

Although medullary carcinoma was initially thought to be radioresistant, it has been found to respond to high-voltage therapy.[110] In one patient triiodothyronine therapy induced regression of both the primary tumor and metastases.[111] This observation has not been confirmed; indeed, Goltzman et al.[22] found that neither T_3 suppression of thyroid-stimulating hormone nor its stimulation by thyroid-releasing hormone influenced the secretion of calcitonin by medullary carcinoma. Furthermore, suppression therapy with thyroxine for over 1 year had no effect on tumor growth as assessed clinically and by calcitonin production (J. T. Potts, Jr., personal communication, 1977). The diarrhea in this condition may be helped by codeine treatment. More recently, large doses of nutmeg have been claimed to control the diarrhea.[34,70] Treatment of the Cushing syndrome, which may be associated—as may the other hormonally mediated syndromes—with either the sporadic or the genetic forms of medullary carcinoma, is by resection of the medullary carcinoma when this is feasible, and adrenalectomy when this is not. It should be remembered that pheochromocytoma is also one of the tumor types associated with ectopic ACTH production,[112] so that in heritable medullary-carcinoma syndromes this is an alternative possible cause of Cushing's syndrome.

IMMUNE RESPONSE IN PATIENTS WITH MEDULLARY CARCINOMA

Some patients with medullary carcinoma have been shown to have a cell-mediated immune response to tumor antigens. Most of the patients studied have belonged to families with inherited medullary carcinoma because of the opportunity that a tumor with such well-defined inheritance allows for the study of the development of tumor immunity during the early stages of tumor growth. The methods used have included leukocyte-adherence inhibition,[113] lymphocyte-proliferation responses, and migration-inhibition studies.[114,115] The results showed that there was evidence of a cell-mediated immune response to tumor extracts in somewhat over

half the patients studied, and Maluish et al.[113] showed that blocking factors were present in the serum of patients with progressive medullary carcinoma. Family members at risk of developing the disease have also been studied, with contradictory results: one group has found no immune response to tumor antigen,[114] and another has found a significant response in half of those at risk.[115] The value of these in vitro tests in terms of tumor diagnosis is probably small. However, immune responses may play a role in determining the variation in age of presentation of familial cases and in controlling the rate of tumor progression.

MEDULLARY-CARCINOMA EQUIVALENTS IN ANIMALS

The similarities between the naturally occurring rat thyroid tumor (Fig. 64-13) and human medullary carcinoma were pointed out in 1966.[2] It has now been shown by electron microscopy that these tumors show the same ultrastructural characteristics as C cells,[116] and that they contain and secrete calcitonin (Fig. 64-14).[117–119] Radioimmunoassay and immunolocalization techniques have utilized antibodies raised against human calcitonin, which shows a marked cross reaction with rat calcitonin. Calcitonin has now been extracted both from rat thyroid and rat C-cell tumors, and its amino acid composition has been determined.[120,121] This naturally occurring thyroid carcinoma in the rat is therefore a potentially useful model of medullary carcinoma in man.

It is known that hypercalcemia stimulates calcitonin synthesis and release in C cells.[122] However, mild hypercalcemia induced by excess dietary calcium does not increase the incidence of C-cell tumors in rats.[123] Vitamin D administration is known to increase calcitonin secretion and to lead to hyperplasia of C cells.[124,125] While it has generally been assumed that the effect of vitamin D is mediated through hypercalcemia, it is possible that D or one of its metabolites also has a direct effect on the C cell. These studies in animals suggest that both variation in dietary calcium and in dietary vitamin D may be relevant to the geographic variation in incidence of medullary carcinoma in man.

Thyroid radiation to the newborn rat led to an increase in incidence in C-cell tumors in the adult rat.[123] This sequence has been recorded in man,[75] but not enough studies have been carried

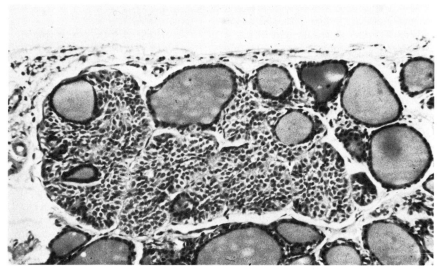

Fig. 64-13. Spontaneous C-cell tumor in a rat. Note the lobular arrangement of the tumor, caused by proliferation of the C cells between the follicular cells and the follicular basement membranes. H&E. ×210.

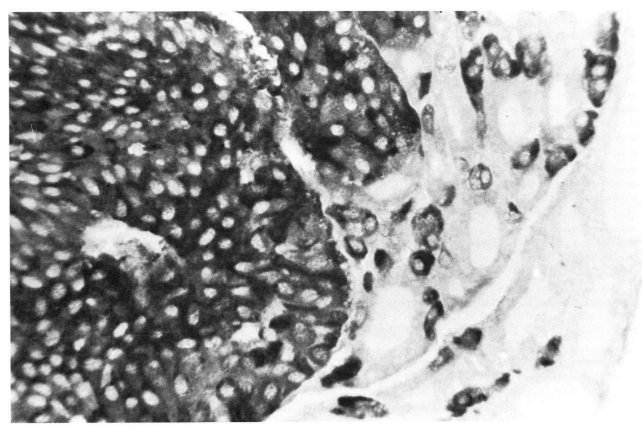

Fig. 64-14. Calcitonin in rat C-cell tumor. The tumor cells contain variable amounts of immunoreactive calcitonin, demonstrated with an antibody to human calcitonin and an immunoperoxidase method. ×800.

out to know if radiation is a significant factor in the genesis of medullary carcinoma in man. C-cell tumors are also described in other animals, and are of particular interest in cattle. As early as 1959, Jubb and McEntee[126] drew attention to the occurrence of tumors at the vasculostromal hilus in old bulls and suggested that these tumors were of ultimobranchial origin. This observation was confirmed[127] and it was suggested that an excessive intake of dietary calcium in the bull led to C-cell tumors and an associated osteopetrosis.[128] These tumors have also been shown to contain calcitonin.[129] A particularly interesting finding was that two of the three bulls with ultimobranchial tumors subjected to complete necropsy also had bilateral pheochromocytomas. It is difficult to reconcile the findings in man that bilateral pheochromocytomas and bilateral medullary carcinoma form a genetically determined heritable syndrome with the suggestion that the bilateral ultimobranchial tumors in bulls, often associated with bilateral pheochromocytomas, are due to a high dietary calcium. If environmental factors are the cause of these tumors in bulls, then the possibility must be considered that the adrenal medullary hyperplasia and neoplasia are secondary to hyperplasia and neoplasia of C cells.

Another species in which a C-cell tumor has been reported is the sheep. Calcinosis was found in a 5-year-old sheep which died suddenly with bilateral C-cell tumors of the thyroid and bilateral adrenal medullary hyperplasia.[130] Calcinosis has been attributed in South American studies to the ingestion of *Solanum malacoxylon,* and this has been found to cause C-cell hyperplasia in sheep, guinea pigs, and rats.[131] As the active constituent of *Solanum malacoxylon* is now known to be the glucuronide of 1,25-dihydroxycholecalciferol, this raises again the possibility that vitamin D, either directly or through D-induced hypercalcemia, or

through a combination of these two or as yet unknown mechanisms, is a potent stimulus to C-cell hyperplasia and neoplasia.

Few human tumors have such a well-documented counterpart occurring in a variety of animals. The mechanisms that link C-cell tumors with tumors of other endocrines are likely to be similar in man and those other mammalian species, and are therefore available for experimental elucidation. The next decade may see as great an advance in this area as the last decade has seen in our understanding of the pathophysiology of the C cell and its tumors.

REFERENCES

1. Hazard, J. B., Hawk, W. A. and Crile, G. Jr. Medullary (solid) carcinoma of the thyroid—A clinicopathologic entity. *J. Clin. Endocrinol. 19:* 152, 1959.
2. Williams, E. D. Histogenesis of medullary carcinoma of the thyroid. *J. Clin. Pathol. 19:* 114, 1966.
3. Baber, E. D. Contributions to the minute anatomy of the thyroid gland of the dog. *Philos. Trans. R. Soc. Lond. Biol. 166:* 557, 1876.
4. Nonidez, J. F. Further observations on parafollicular cells of mammalian thyroid. *Anat. Rec. 53:* 339, 1932.
5. Solcia, E., Vassallo, G., and Capella, C. Selective staining of endocrine cells by basic dyes after acid hydrolysis. *Stain. Technol. 43:* 257, 1968.
6. Getzowa, S. Über die Glandula parathyroidea, intrathyroideale Zellhaufen derselben und Reste des postbranchialen Korpers. *Virchows Arch. Path. Anat. 188:* 181, 1907.
7. Godwin, M. C. Complex IV in the dog with special emphasis on the relation of the ultimobranchial body to interfollicular cells in the postnatal thyroid gland. *Am. J. Anat. 60:* 299, 1937.
8. Pearse, A. G. E. and Carvalheira, A. F. Cytochemical evidence for an ultimobranchial origin of rodent thyroid C cells. *Nature 214:* 929, 1967.

9. Le Douarin, N., and Le Lièvre, Ch. Démonstration de l'origine neurale des cellules à calcitonine du corps ultimobranchial chez l'embryon de poulet. *C. R. Acad. Sci.* D *270:* 2857, 1970.

10. Williams. E. D. Medullary carcinoma of the thyroid. In: Recent Advances in Pathology, 9th ed. Edited by C. V. Harrison and K. Weinbren. Edinburgh, Churchill Livingstone, 1975, pp. 156–182.

11. Copp, D. H., and Cameron, E. C. Demonstration of a hypocalcemic factor (calcitonin) in commercial parathyroid extract. *Science 134:* 2038, 1961.

12. Copp, D. H., Cameron, E. C., Cheney, B. A., Davidson, A. G. F., and Henze, K. G. Evidence for calcitonin—a new hormone from the parathyroid that lowers blood calcium. *Endocrinology 70:* 638, 1962.

13. Hirsch, P. F., Gauthier, G. F., and Munson, P. L. Thyroid hypocalcemic principle and recurrent laryngeal nerve injury as factors affecting the response to parathyroidectomy. *Endocrinology 73:* 244, 1963.

14. Foster, G. V., MacIntyre, I., and Pearse, A. G. E. Calcitonin production and the mitochondrion-rich cells of the dog thyroid. *Nature 203:* 1029, 1964.

15. Bussolati, G., and Pearse, A. G. E. Immunofluorescent localization of calcitonin in the "C" cells of the pig and dog thyroid. *J. Endocrinol. 37:* 205, 1967.

16. Milhaud, G., Tubiana, M., Parmentier, C., and Coutris, G. Epithelioma de la thyroïde sécrétant de la thyrocalcitonine. *C. R. Acad. Sci.* D (Paris) *266:* 608, 1968.

17. Cunliffe, W. J., Black, M. M., Hall, R., Johnston, I. D. A., Hudgson, P., Shuster, S., Gudmundsson, T. V., Joplin, G. F., Williams, E. D., Woodhouse, N. J. Y., Galante, L., and MacIntyre, I. A calcitonin-secreting thyroid carcinoma. *Lancet 2:* 63, 1968.

18. Williams, E. D., Brown, C. L., and Doniach, I. Pathological and clinical findings in a series of 67 cases of medullary carcinoma of the thyroid. *J. Clin. Pathol. 19:* 103, 1966.

19. Fletcher, J. R. Medullary (solid) carcinoma of the thyroid gland. *Arch. Surg. 100:* 257, 1970.

20. Williams, E. D., Doniach, I., Bjarnason, O., and Michie, W. Thyroid cancer in an iodide rich area—a histopathological study. *Cancer 39:* 215, 1977.

21. Normann, T., Johannessen, J. V., Gautvik, K. M., Olsen, B. R., and Brennhovd, I. O. Medullary carcinoma of the thyroid—diagnostic problems. *Cancer 38:* 366, 1976.

22. Goltzman, D., Potts, J. T. Jr., Ridgway, E. C., and Maloof, F. Calcitonin as a tumor marker. *N. Engl. J. Med. 290:* 1035, 1974.

23. Milhaud, G., Calmette, C., Taboulet, J. Julienne, A., and Mouktar, M. S. Hypersecretion of calcitonin in neoplastic conditions. *Lancet 1:* 462, 1974.

24. Coombes, R. D., Hillyard, C., Greenberg, P. B., and MacIntyre, I. Plasma-immunoreactive-calcitonin in patients with non-thyroid tumours. *Lancet 1:* 1080, 1974.

25. Sizemore, G. W., Go, V. L. W., Kaplan, E. L., Sanzenbacher, L. J., Holtermuller, K. H., and Arnaud, C. D. Relations of calcitonin and gastrin in the Zollinger–Ellison syndrome and medullary carcinoma of the thyroid. *N. Engl. J. Med. 288:* 641, 1973.

26. LiVolsi, V. A., Feind, C. R., LoGerfo, P., and Tashjian, A. H. Jr. Whence the calcitonin. *N. Engl. J. Med. 289:* 1314, 1973.

27. Silva, O. L., Becker, K. L., Primack, A., Doppman, J. L., and Snider, R. H. Hypercalcitonemia in bronchogenic cancer. *J.A.M.A. 234:* 183 1975.

28. Baker, R. K., Wallach, S., and Tashjian, A. H. Jr. Plasma calcitonin in pycnodysostosis: intermittently high basal levels and exaggerated responses to calcium and glucagon infusions. *J. Clin. Endocrinol. Metab. 37:* 46, 1973.

29. Williams, E. D., Karim, S. M. M., and Sandler, M. Prostaglandin secretion by medullary carcinoma of the thyroid. *Lancet 1:* 22, 1968.

30. Grimley, P. M., Deftos, L. J., Weeks, J. R., and Rabson, A. S. Growth in vitro and ultrastructure of cells from a medullary carcinoma of the human thyroid gland: transformation by simian virus 40 and evidence of thyrocalcitonin and prostaglandins. *J. Natl. Cancer Inst. 42:* 663, 1969.

31. Isaacs, P., Whittaker, S., and Turnberg, L. A. The mechanisms for the diarrhoea associated with medullary thyroid carcinoma. *Eur. J. Clin. Invest. 3:* 240, 1973.

32. Levin, D. L., Perlia, C., Tashjian, A. H. Jr. Medullary carcinoma of the thyroid gland: the complete syndrome in a child. *Pediatrics 52:* 192, 1973.

33. Schaison, G., Nathan, C., and Gilbert-Dreyfus. Exploration biologique dans trois cas de cancers médullaires de la thyroïde. *Ann. Endocrinol.* (Paris) *35:* 291, 1974.

34. Barrowman, J. A., Bennett, A., Hillenbrand, P., Rolles, K., Pollock, D. J., and Wright, J. T. Diarrhoea in thyroid medullary carcinoma: role of prostaglandins and therapeutic effect of nutmeg. *Br. Med. J. 3:* 11, 1975.

35. Ménagé, J. J., Besnard, J. C., Guilmot, J. L., Vandooren, M., and Neel, J. N. Preuves de l'absence de sécrétion de prostaglandines par un carcinome médullaire de la thyroïde avec diarrhée motrice. *Nouv. Presse Med. 4:* 2862, 1975.

36. Benditt, E. P., and Eriksen, N. Chemical classes of amyloid substance. *Am. J. Pathol. 65:* 231, 1971.

37. Pearse, A. G. E., Ewen, S. W. B., and Polak, J. M. The genesis of apudamyloid in endocrine polypeptide tumours: histochemical distinction from immunamyloid. *Virchows Arch. Zellpathol. 10:* 93, 1972.

38. Tashjian, A. J. Jr., Wolfe, H. J., and Voelkel, E. F. Human calcitonin. Immunologic assay, cytologic localization and studies on medullary thyroid carcinoma. *Am. J. Med. 56:* 840, 1974.

39. Newman, G. R., Williams, E. D. Electron microscopic findings in medullary carcinoma of the thyroid. (in preparation)

40. Sletten, K., Westermark, P., and Natvig, J. B. Characterization of amyloid fibril proteins from medullary carcinoma of the thyroid. *J. Exp. Med. 143:* 993, 1976.

41. Paasonen, M. K. 5-Hydroxytryptamine in mammalian thyroid gland. *Experientia 14:* 95, 1958.

42. Falck, B., Larson, B., von Mecklenburg, C., Rosengren, E., and Svenaeus, K. On the presence of a second specific cell system in mammalian thyroid gland. *Acta Physiol. Scand. 62:* 491, 1964.

43. Håkanson, R., Owman, Ch., and Sundler, F. Aromatic L-amino acid decarboxylase in calcitonin-producing cells. *Biochem. Pharmacol. 20:* 2187, 1971.

44. Pearse, A. G. E. 5-hydroxytryptophan uptake by dog thyroid 'C' cells, and its possible significance in polypeptide hormone production. *Nature 211:* 598, 1966.

45. Williams, E. D. Diarrhoea and thyroid carcinoma. *Proc. R. Soc. Med. 59:* 602, 1966.

46. Steinfeld, C. M., Moertel, C. G., and Woolner, L. B. Diarrhea and medullary carcinoma of the thyroid. *Cancer 31:* 1237, 1973.

47. Falck, B., Ljungberg, O., and Rosengren, E. On the occurrence of monoamines and related substances in familial medullary thyroid carcinoma with phaeochromocytoma. *Acta Pathol. Microbiol. Scand. 74:* 1, 1968.

48. Atkins, F. L., Beaven, M. A., and Keisner, H. R. Dopa decarboxylase in medullary carcinoma of the thyroid. *N. Engl. J. Med. 289:* 545, 1973.

49. Baylin, S. B., Beaven, M. A., Engelman, K., and Sjoersdma, A. Elevated histaminase activity in medullary carcinoma of the thyroid gland. *N. Engl. J. Med. 283:* 1239, 1970.

50. Baylin, S. B., Beaven, M. A., Keiser, H. R., Tashjian, A. H. Jr., and Melvin, K. E. W. Serum histaminase and calcitonin levels in medullary carcinoma of the thyroid. *Lancet 1:* 455, 1972.

51. Baum, J. L. Abnormal intradermal histamine reaction in the syndrome of phaeochromocytoma, medullary carcinoma of the thyroid gland and multiple mucosal neuromas. *N. Engl. J. Med. 284:* 963, 1971.

52. Gorlin, R. J. Skin test for medullary thyroid carcinoma. *N. Engl. J. Med. 284:* 983, 1971.

53. Williams, E. D., Morales, A. M., and Horn, R. D. Thyroid carcinoma and Cushing's syndrome. *J. Clin. Pathol. 21:* 129, 1968.

54. Donahower, G. F., Schumacher, O. P., and Hazard, J. B. Medullary carcinoma of the thyroid—a cause of Cushing's syndrome. Report of two cases. *J. Clin. Endocrinol. 28:* 1199, 1968.

55. Melvin, K. E. W., Tashjian, A. H., Jr., Cassidy, C. E., and Givens, J. R. Cushing's syndrome caused by ACTH- and calcitonin-secreting medullary carcinoma of the thyroid. *Metabolism 19:* 831, 1970.

56. Birkenhager, J. C., Upton, G. V. Seldenrath, J. H., Kreiger, D. T., and Tashjian, A. H. Jr. Medullary thyroid carcinoma: ectopic production of peptides with ACTH-like, corticotrophin releasing factor-like and prolactin production-stimulating activities. *Acta Endocrinol. 83:* 280, 1976.

57. Bordi, C., Anversa, P., Vitali-Mazza, L. Ultrastructural study of a calcitonin-secreting tumor. *Virchows Arch. Pathol. Anat. 357:* 145, 1972.

58. Bussolati, G., van Noorden, S., and Bordi, C. Calcitonin and ACTH-producing cells in a case of medullary carcinoma of the thyroid. *Virchows Arch. Pathol. Anat. 360:* 123, 1973.

58a. van Noorden, S., Polak, J. M., and Pearse, A. G. E. Single cellular origin of somatostatin and calcitonin in the rat thyroid gland. *Histochemistry 53:* 243, 1977.

59. Ishikawa, N., and Hamada, S. Association of medullary carcinoma of the thyroid with carcinoembryonic antigen. *Br. J. Cancer 34:* 111, 1976.

60. Baum, J. L., and Adler, M. E. Phaeochromocytoma, medullary thyroid carcinoma, multiple mucosal neuroma. *Arch. Ophthalmol. 87:* 574, 1972.

61. Marks, S. C. The parafollicular cell of the thyroid gland as the source of an osteoblast-stimulating factor. *J. Bone Joint Surg. 51-A:* 875, 1969.

62. Verdy, M., Beaulieu, R., Demers, L., Sturtridge, W. C., Thomas, P., and Kumar, M. A. Plasma calcitonin activity in a patient with thyroid medullary carcinoma and her children with osteopetrosis. *J. Clin. Endocrinol. Metab. 32:* 216, 1971.

63. Bigazzi, M., Revoltella, R., Casciano, S., and Vigneti, E. High level of a nerve growth factor in the serum of a patient with medullary carcinoma of the thyroid gland. *Clin. Endocrinol. 6:* 105, 1977.

64. Bernier, J. J., Bouvry, M., Cattan, D., and Prost, A. Diarrhée motrice par cancer médullaire thyroïdien. *Presse Med. 75:* 593, 1967.

65. Bernier, J. J., Rambaud, J. C., Cattan, D., and Prost, A. Diarrhoea associated with medullary carcinoma of the thyroid. *Gut 10:* 980, 1969.

66. Debray, Ch., Leymarios, J., Tourneur, R., and Chariot, J. Les cancers thyroïdiens médullaires diarrhéogènes. *Ann. Med. Intern. 120:* 73, 1969.

67. Edwards, I. R., and Smith, A. H. The mechanism of the diuretic response to porcine calcitonin in normal subjects. *Clin. Sci. 42:* 5P, 1972.

68. Gray, T. K., Bieberdorf, F. A., and Fortran, J. S. Thyrocalcitonin and the jejunal absorption of calcium, water, and electrolytes in normal subjects. *J. Clin. Invest. 52:* 3084, 1973.

69. Lechi, C., De Bastiani, G., and Zatti, M. In vitro stimulation of apparent intestinal alkaline phosphatase activity by thyrocalcitonin. *Clin. Chim. Acta 57:* 171, 1974.

70. Fawell, W. N., and Thompson, G. Nutmeg for diarrhea of medullary carcinoma of thyroid. *N. Engl. J. Med. 289:* 108, 1973.

71. Williams, E. D. A review of 17 cases of carcinoma of the thyroid and phaeochromocytoma. *J. Clin. Pathol. 18:* 288, 1965.

72. Schimke, R. N., and Hartmann, W. H. Familial amyloid-producing medullary thyroid carcinoma and phaeochromocytoma. *Ann. Intern. Med. 63:* 1027, 1965.

73. Sipple, J. H. The association of pheochromocytoma with carcinoma of the thyroid gland. *Am. J. Med. 31:* 163, 1961.

74. Chong, G. C., Beahrs, O. H., Sizemore, G. W., Woolner, L. H. Medullary carcinoma of the thyroid gland. *Cancer 35:* 695, 1975.

75. Dunn, E. L., Nishiyama, R. H., Thompson, N. W. Medullary carcinoma of the thyroid gland. *Surgery 73:* 848, 1973.

76. Gordon, P. R., Huvos, A. G., and Strong, E. W. Medullary carcinoma of the thyroid gland—a clinicopathologic study of 40 cases. *Cancer 31:* 915, 1973.

77. Beaugie, J. M., Brown, C. L., Doniach, I., and Richardson, J. E. Primary malignant tumours of the thyroid: the relationship between histological classification and clinical behaviour. *Br. J. Surg. 63:* 173, 1976.

78. Block, M. A., Horn, R. C. Jr., Miller, J. M., Barrett, J. L., and Brush, B. E. Familial medullary carcinoma of the thyroid. *Ann. Surg. 166:* 403, 1967.

79. Williams, E. D., and Pollock, D. J. Multiple mucosal neuromata with endocrine tumours: a syndrome allied to von Recklinghausen's disease. *J. Pathol. Bacteriol. 91:* 71, 1966.

80. Nankin, H., Hydovitz, J., and Sapira, J. Normal chromosomes in mucosal neuroma variant of medullary thyroid carcinoma syndrome, *J. Med. Genet. 7:* 374, 1970.

81. Carney, J. A., Go, V. L. W., Sizemore, G. W., and Hayles, A. B. Alimentary-tract ganglioneuromatosis. *N. Engl. J. Med. 295:* 1287, 1976.

82. Melvin, K. E. W., Tashjian, A. H. Jr., and Miller, H. H. Studies in familial (medullary) thyroid carcinoma. *Recent Prog. Horm. Res. 28:* 399, 1972.

83. Cope, C. L., and Williams, E. D. A case of diarrhoea and goitre. *Br. Med. J. 3:* 293, 1967.

84. Wolfe, H. J., Melvin, K. E. W., Cervi-Skinner, S. J., Al Saadi, A. A., Juliar, J. F., Jackson, C. E., Tashjian, A. H. Jr. C-cell hyperplasia preceding medullary thyroid carcinoma. *N. Engl. J. Med. 289:* 437, 1973.

85. Carney, J. A., Sizemore, G. W., and Sheps, S. G. Adrenal medullary disease in multiple endocrine neoplasia, type 2. *Am. J. Clin. Pathol. 66:* 279, 1976.

86. DeLellis, R. A., Wolfe, H. J., Gagel, R. F., Feldman, Z. T., Miller, H. H., Gang, D. L., and Reichlin, S. Adrenal medullary hyperplasia, *Am. J. Pathol. 83:* 177, 1976.

87. Neville, A. M. The adrenal medulla. In: Functional Pathology of the Human Adrenal Gland. Edited by T. Symington. London, Livingstone, 1969, pp. 219–324.

88. von Studnitz, W., and Ljungberg, O. Familiär auftretendes Adrenalin produzierendes Phäochromocytom in Kombination mit medullärem Thyreoidea-Carcinom. *Klin. Wochenschr. 48:* 144, 1970.

89. Ljungberg, O., Cederquist, E., and von Studnitz, W. Medullary thyroid carcinoma and phaeochromocytoma: a familial chromaffinomatosis. *Br. Med. J. 1:* 279, 1967.

90. Sato, T., Kobayashi, K., Miura, Y., Sakuma, H., Yoshinaga, K., and Nakamura, K. High epinephrine content in the adrenal tumors from Sipple's syndrome. *Tohoku J. Exp. Med. 115:* 15, 1975.

91. Marks, A. D., and Channick, B. J. Extra-adrenal phaeochromocytoma and medullary thyroid carcinoma with phaeochromocytoma. *Arch. Intern. Med. 134:* 1106, 1974.

92. Voelkel, E. F., Tashjian, A. H. Jr., Davidoff, F. F., Cohen, R. B., Perlia, C. P., and Wurtman, R. J. Concentrations of calcitonin and catecholamines in pheochromocytomas, a mucosal neuroma and medullary thyroid carcinoma. *J. Clin. Endocrinol. Metab. 37:* 297, 1973.

93. Robertson, D. M., Sizemore, G. W., and Gordon, H. Thickened corneal nerves as a manifestation of multiple endocrine neoplasia. *Trans. Am. Acad. Ophthalmol. Otolaryngol. 79:* 772, 1975.

94. Joosten, E., Gabreëls-Festen, A., Horstink, M., Gabreëls, F., Jaspar, H., Korten, J., and Vingerhoets, H. Hypertrophy of peripheral nerves in the syndrome of multiple mucosal neuromas, endocrine tumours and Marfanoid habitus. Autonomic disturbances and sural nerve findings. *Acta Neuropathol.* (Berl.) *30:* 251, 1974.

95. Pages, A., Marty, C. H., Baldet, P., and Peraldi, R. Le syndrome neurofibromatose-carcinome médullaire thyroïdien-phéochromocytome. *Arch. Anat. Pathol.* (Paris) *18:* 137, 1970.

96. Thliveris, J. A., Dubé, W. J., and Banerjee, R. Comparative ultrastructure of thyroid, tongue, and eyelid lesions in the neuroma phenotype of medullary carcinoma of the thyroid. *Virchows Arch. Pathol. Anat. 369:* 249, 1976.

97. Keiser, H. R., Beaven, M. A., Doppman, J., Wells, S. Jr., and Buja, L. M. Sipple's syndrome: medullary thyroid carcinoma, pheochromocytoma, and parathyroid disease. *Ann. Intern. Med. 78:* 561, 1973.

98. Markey, W. S., Ryan, W. G., Economou, S. G., Sizemore, G. W., Arnaud, C. D. Familial medullary carcinoma and parathyroid adenoma without pheochromocytoma. Report of two cases. *Ann. Intern. Med. 78:* 898, 1973.

99. Bartlett, R. C., Myall, R. W. T., Bean, L. R., and Mandelstam, P. A neuropolyendocrine syndrome: mucosal neuromas, pheochromocytoma and medullary carcinoma. *Oral Surg. 31:* 206, 1971.

100. Ljungberg, O. On medullary carcinoma of the thyroid. *Acta Pathol. Microbiol. Scand.* **A,** Suppl. No. 231, 1972.

101. Deftos, L. J., and Parthemore, J. G. Secretion of parathyroid hormone in patients with medullary thyroid carcinoma. *J. Clin. Invest. 54:* 416, 1974.

102. Delorme, F., and Giroux, L. Épithéliome médullaire à stroma amyloïde associé à des phéochromocytomes et à des ganglioneuromes dans les deux surrénales. *Union Med. Can. 104:* 601, 1975.

103. Lynch, H. T., and Green, G. S. Wilms' tumor and congenital heart disease. Report of a case and family. *Am. J. Dis. Chil. 115:* 723, 1968.

104. Baylin, S. B., Gann, D. S., and Hsu, S. H. Clonal origin of inherited medullary thyroid carcinoma and pheochromocytoma. *Science 193:* 321, 1976.

105. Williams, E. D. Medullary carcinoma of the thyroid. In: Calcitonin 1969: Proceedings of the 2nd International Symposium. London, Heinemann, 1970, pp. 483–486.

106. Gagel, R. F., Melvin, K. E. W., Tashjian, A. H. Jr., Miller, H. H., Feldman, Z. T., Wolfe, H. J., DeLellis, R. A., Cervi-Skinner, S., Reichlin, S. Natural history of the familial medullary thyroid carcinoma–pheochromocytoma syndrome and the identification of preneoplastic stages by screening studies: a five-year report. *Trans. Assoc. Am. Physicians 88:* 177, 1975.

107. Miller, H. H., Melvin, K. E. W., Gibson, J. M., Tashjian, A. H. Jr. Surgical approach to early familial medullary carcinoma of the thyroid gland. *Am. J. Surg. 123:* 438, 1972.

108. Smits, M., and Huizinga, J. Familial occurrence of phaeochromocytoma. *Acta Genet. 11:* 137, 1961.

109. Roediger, W. E. W. Thyroidectomy for non-familial medullary carcinoma. *Br. J. Surg. 63:* 343, 1976.

110. Tubiana, M., Milhaud, G., Coutris, G., Lacour, J., Parmentier, C., and Bok, B. Medullary carcinoma and thyrocalcitonin. *Br. Med. J. 4:* 87, 1968.

111. Wahner, H. W., Cuello, C., and Aljure, F. Hormone-induced regression of medullary (solid) thyroid carcinoma. *Am. J. Med. 45:* 789, 1968.

112. Azzopardi, J. G., and Williams, E. D. Pathology of 'non-endocrine' tumours associated with Cushing's syndrome. *Cancer 22:* 274, 1968.

113. Maluish, A. E., Halliday, W. J., Bartley, P. C., and Lloyd, H. M. Immunological reactions in medullary carcinoma of the thyroid. *Clin. Immunol. Immunopathol. 5:* 303, 1976.

114. George, J. M., Williams, M. A., Almoney, R., and Sizemore, G. W. Medullary carcinoma of the thyroid. *Cancer 36:* 1658, 1975.

115. Rocklin, R. E., Gagel, R., Feldman, Z., and Tashjian, A. H. Jr. Cellular immune responses in familial medullary thyroid carcinoma. *N. Engl. J. Med. 296:* 835, 1977.

116. Boorman, G. A., van Noord, M. J., and Hollander, C. F. Naturally occurring medullary thyroid carcinoma in the rat. *Arch. Pathol. 94:* 35, 1972.

117. Boorman, G. A., Heersche, J. N. M. & Hollander, C. F. Transplantable calcitonin-secreting medullary carcinomas of the thyroid in the WAG/Rij rat. *J. Natl. Cancer Inst. 53:* 1011, 1974.

118. Bollman, R., and Pearse, A. G. E. Calcitionin secretion and APUD characteristics of naturally occurring medullary thyroid carcinomas in rats. *Virchows Arch. Zellpathol. 15:* 95, 1974.

119. Triggs, S. M., Hesch, R. D., Woodhead, J. S., and Williams, E. D. Calcitonin production by rat thyroid tumours. *J. Endocrinol. 66:* 37, 1975.

120. Burford, H. J., Ontjes, D. A., Cooper, C. W., Parlow, A. F., and Hirsch, P. F. Purification, characterization and radioimmunoassay of thyrocalcitonin from rat thyroid glands. *Endocrinology 96:* 340, 1975.

121. Byfield, P. G. H., Matthews, E. W., Heersche, J. N. M., Boorman, G. A., Girgis, S. I., and MacIntyre, I. Isolation of calcitonin from rat thyroid medullary carcinoma. *FEBS Lett. 65:* 238, 1976.

122. Care, A. D., Cooper, C. W., Duncan, T., and Orimo, H. A study of thyrocalcitonin secretion by direct measurement of in vivo secretion rates in pigs. *Endocrinology 83:* 161, 1968.

123. Triggs, S. M., and Williams, E. D. Experimental carcinogenesis in the rat thyroid follicular and C cells. *Acta Endocrinol. 85:* 84, 1977.

124. Young, D. M., and Capen, C. C. Thyrocalcitonin: response to experimental hypercalcaemia induced by vitamin D in cows. In: Calcitonin 1969: Proceedings of the 2nd International Symposium. London, Heinemann, 1970, pp. 141–153.

125. Triggs, S. M., and Bailey-Wood, R. Excessive vitamin D content of a standard iron-deficient diet for rats. *Br. J. Nutr. 35:* 277, 1976.

126. Jubb, K. V., and McEntee, K. The relationship of ultimobranchial remnants and derivatives to tumors of the thyroid gland in cattle. *Cornell Vet 49:* 41, 1959.

127. Williams, E. D. 5-Hydroxindoles and the thyroid. In: Advances in Pharmacology, vol. 6, part B. Edited by S. Garahini and P. A. Shore. New York, Academic, 1968, pp. 151–155.

128. Krook, L., Lutwak, L., and McEntee, K. Dietary calcium, ultimobranchial tumors and osteopetrosis in the bull. *Am. J. Clin. Nutr. 22:* 115, 1969.

129. Black, H. E., Capen, C. C., and Young, D. M. Ultimobranchial thyroid neoplasms in bulls. *Cancer 32:* 865, 1973.

130. Neumann, F., and Klopfer, U. Calcinosis in sheep associated with C-cell adenoma of the thyroid. *Vet. Med. Small Anim. Clin. 70:* 1209, 1975.

131. Carrillo, B. J. Efecto de la intoxicación de Solanum malacoxylon en la morfología de las células parafoliculares de la tiroides. *Rev. Invest. Agropec.,* **Ser. 4,** *Patol. Anim. 10:* 41, 1973.

65

Clinical Uses of the Calcitonin Assay

Leonard J. Deftos

INTRODUCTION

As discussed in Chapter 64, it is now well established that medullary thyroid carcinoma (MTC) is a tumor of the calcitonin-producing cells (C cells) of the thyroid gland. In the neoplastic state, these cells secrete an abnormal amount of calcitonin into peripheral plasma. Since these circulating levels of plasma calcitonin can be most conveniently measured by radioimmunoassay, the radioimmunoassay for human calcitonin has become an important clinical tool in the diagnosis and management of patients with MTC.[1,2]

DIAGNOSIS

The majority of patients with established MTC have basal calcitonin levels which are clearly distinguishable from normal. In these patients, the relatively simple procedure of measurement of plasma calcitonin by radioimmunoassay can be diagnostic of the presence of the tumor. However, basal calcitonin measurement may not be diagnostic in a small but significant percentage of the patients whose basal plasma calcitonin levels are indistinguishable from normal in many radioimmunoassay systems[1–3]. In addition, plasma calcitonin can fluctuate in patients with the tumor from abnormal levels to levels indistinguishable from normal.[3]

Most of the patients with plasma calcitonin that is borderline or indistinguishable from normal have very early stages of the tumor. In such patients the disease is represented by only hyperplasia of the C cells or by foci of tumor confined to the thyroid gland.[2,4] With the increasing appreciation of the familial distribution of the tumor, patients with early disease are being discovered with increasing frequency. These patients are candidates for effective surgical management of the tumor and even surgical cure.[5] In order to identify patients who have definite but early disease, several approaches have been utilized to improve the discriminatory value of the assay.

One approach has been to improve the sensitivity of the calcitonin assay. In early procedures, the upper limit of "normal" was 300–1000 pg/ml.[6,7] With improved assay sensitivity, the upper limit of normal has been reduced to under 100–200 pg/ml in most but not all assay procedures.[8–11] This sensitivity has permitted the diagnosis of MTC to be made in patients in whom basal calcitonin levels would have been considered indistinguishable from normal by earlier, less sensitive assays. Improvement in sensitivity of the calcitonin assay has been paralleled by more-sensitive histologic and immunohistologic criteria for the identification of neoplastic C cells in the thyroid, including C-cell hyperplasia, an intermediate or early stage in the development of medullary carcinoma.[4,12]

In addition to improved assay sensitivity, provocative testing of calcitonin secretion is used for early and more-definitive diagnosis (Fig. 65-1). Three agents have been evaluated as calcitonin secretagogues. Glucagon was one of the first provocative agents used, but it has been largely abandoned as a clinical test because of its unreliability and potential side effects.[13] Calcium and pentagastrin are now commonly used.[8,9,14] Both agents are reliable calcitonin secretagogues. Their administration can produce abnormal increases in plasma calcitonin in patients with a consistent clinical history of MTC who either have borderline or normal basal levels of the hormone. Pentagastrin (Peptavalon, Ayerst) is usually given intravenously at a dose of 0.5 μg/kg by i.v. push. Plasma samples are collected frequently for calcitonin measurement since the stimulation of hormone secretion is brisk (Fig. 65-1). This procedure has been clinically useful in evaluating patients with known or suspected MTC.[14] The early calcitonin response makes the procedure relatively brief and the sampling convenient. Rapid sampling is important to detect the peak calcitonin response. One disadvantage of the procedure is that it regularly causes an unpleasant feeling, including epigastric distress. This is usually transient and seldom needs therapy, but it does make the patient less willing to undergo repeated testing. Another disadvantage is that, at the time of this writing, pentagastrin is not approved by the FDA for this use. Hence, its administration requires an approved experimental protocol.

Several procedures have been reported for calcium administration. Calcium is given intravenously as either the chloride salt, which is 36 percent calcium by weight, or the gluconate salt, which is 8.9 percent calcium by weight. The early procedures described were 2–4-h infusions of calcium at a dose of 3–5 mg/kg/h.[6,15] Plasma samples were collected at hourly intervals, and the increase in plasma calcitonin was proportional to the rise in calcium. A disadvantage of this procedure is its duration, which made its use as an ambulatory screening procedure cumbersome. Morbidity is also a problem, at least in some patients. Nausea and vomiting are seen toward the end of this infusion. Therefore, we introduced a shorter calcium infusion in which calcium was given at a dose of 3 mg/kg over 10 min.[16] In our hands, this has been a reliable provocative test for calcitonin secretion; it has a short duration and

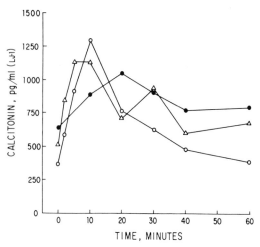

Fig. 65-1. Provocative tests for calcitonin secretion in a patient with medullary thyroid carcinoma. Pentagastrin infusion at a dose of 0.5 μg/kg by i.v. push (○) produced a brisk increase in plasma calcitonin in this patient. Calcium (gluconate) infusion at a dose of 2 mg/kg by i.v. push (△) produced a similar pattern of calcitonin secretion, whereas calcium (chloride) given over 10 min at a dose of 3 mg/kg (●) produced a more gradual increase in plasma calcitonin. Pentagastrin given during a 10-min infusion (data not shown) produced a secretory response indistinguishable from that of the 10-min calcium infusion. Therefore, the secretory response produced by calcium and pentagastrin is a function of their route of administration.

a convenient sampling schedule and is relatively free of side effects. The success with this procedure suggested that the rate of administration was as important as the agent used for provocative testing. This has led to the administration of calcium by i.v. push, similar to pentagastrin, at a dose of 2 mg/kg (Fig. 65-1).[17] This procedure results in a pattern of calcitonin secretion similar to that produced by gastrin, but, like rapid gastrin administration, it is accompanied by patient distress and needs further evaluation and, perhaps, modification.

There is no convincing evidence at this time that either pentagastrin or calcium is inherently superior as a calcitonin secretagogue in clinical testing for patients with MTC. In the majority of patients with the tumor, both agents are reliable calcitonin secretagogues. However, there is evidence to suggest that for any given patient, one agent, calcium or pentagastrin, may be superior to the other as a secretagogue. False negative tests have been reported for both agents[9] and we have observed that for a few patients with very early MTC, calcium results in a diagnostic increase in plasma calcitonin, whereas pentagastrin does not, and vive versa. Therefore, if the clinical situation strongly suggests MTC, but a given provocative test is not diagnostic, the alternative procedure should probably be used.

LOCALIZATION AND CLINICAL MANAGEMENT

In addition to being useful in the diagnosis of MTC, the immunoassay for human calcitonin can also be used in conjunction with selective venous catheterization to document the location and extent of tumor.[18] By assaying plasma samples collected at catheterization from potential tumor sites it is possible to demonstrate gradients of hormone concentration which correlate with tumor location. Such information can be useful in planning therapy. Selective venous catheterization may even have a potential role in primary diagnosis. It is possible that the ultimate in early diagnosis of the tumor could be accomplished by calcitonin measurement in

samples collected at thyroid venous catheterization during optimal provocative testing. However, the practical difficulties of such a procedure probably preclude its clinical application except in special circumstances. Another diagnostic use of the assay is to distinguish between abnormal ectopic and eutopic calcitonin secretion. As discussed later, some nonthyroidal tumors can also secrete excessive amounts of calcitonin (ectopic calcitonin production). Assay of selective venous samples can be used to distinguish such patients from those with MTC. Another indication for localization studies is evidence of recurrent disease. Venous catheterization can be used to determine whether recurrence is due to metastatic tumor or tumor localized in the neck, where surgery is feasible.[18]

Serial measurements of plasma calcitonin can be used to monitor the effectiveness of therapy in patients with MTC and other calcitonin-producing tumors (ectopic calcitonin production, see below). Measurements made during and after surgical and/or chemotherapeutic treatment can be used, along with other clinical parameters, to evaluate the effectiveness of therapy and to screen for recurrent disease.[9]

DIFFERENTIAL DIAGNOSIS OF HYPERCALCITONINEMIA

Until recently, an elevated plasma calcitonin was considered diagnostic of MTC. However, further studies with radioimmunoassays of improved sensitivity and varying specificity have developed a more complicated picture. Patients with hypercalcemic states may have elevated plasma calcitonin.[10,19] In addition, nonthyroidal tumors can also be associated with calcitonin excess. Although reported for a variety of tumors, the most notable examples are oat-cell carcinoma of the lung and carcinoma of the breast.[20–22] In most instances the tumor is secreting calcitonin ectopically. Some of the tumors responsible for this phenomenon seem to be embryologically related in their neural-crest origin to the C cells of the thyroid gland. However, with some tumors, the thyroid seems to be the source of excess calcitonin.[23] It has been speculated that the tumor is directly or indirectly responsible for stimulating the secretion of thyroidal calcitonin through one of several mechanisms.[24] In such cases, selective venous catheterization can be used to determine the thyroidal origin of the calcitonin.[23]

It also seems possible that advantage can be taken of the immunochemical heterogeneity of plasma calcitonin (Chapter 49) to identify the origin of hypercalcitoninemia (Fig. 65-2). There is some evidence to suggest that different tissues may produce immunochemically distinguishable forms of calcitonin.[25,26] The evidence is more convincing, however, that the plasma calcitonin in another hypercalcitoninemic state, renal disease, is immunochemically distinguishable from MTC calcitonin.[27] It may be that normal human thyroidal calcitonin has an immunochemically distinct pattern. In either of these circumstances, calcitonin assays of differing immunochemical specificity may be of clinical value.

SUMMARY

Plasma calcitonin is diagnostically elevated in the majority of patients with MTC. In those few patients in whom basal levels of the hormone are not abnormal, provocative testing with calcium or pentagastrin can establish the presence of neoplasia by producing a diagnostic increase in calcitonin. Assay of samples collected at

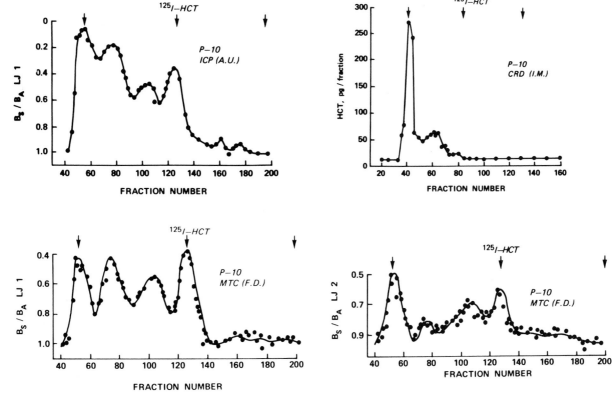

Fig. 65-2. Immunochemical heterogeneity of calcitonin in vivo. Chromatography (Bio Gel P-10) fractions of plasma were assayed from a patient with the following: *A.*, A calcitonin-producing islet-cell carcinoma of the pancreas. *B.*, Chronic renal disease. *C, D,* Medullary thyroid carcinoma. Antiserum LJ-1 was used for all samples except *D*; the pattern produced by LJ-1 (*C*) was compared to that produced by antiserum LJ-2 (*D*). Arrows represent void and salt volumes of the columns and the elution position of ^{125}I-HCT.

selective venous catheterization can be used to establish the extent and location of tumor. Such procedures can also help to identify ectopic calcitonin production by nonthyroidal tumors. Serial calcitonin measurements can be used to evaluate the treatment of calcitonin-producing tumors. Plasma calcitonin exists in multiple immunochemical forms, and distinct immunochemical patterns of plasma calcitonin may prove to be characteristic of certain disease states, but this issue is still under evaluation. The clinical setting in conjunction with the appropriate use of calcitonin assay (including catheterization) is usually sufficient to establish the cause of excessive calcitonin secretion from among the hypercalcitoninemic states that have been identified.[28]

REFERENCES

1. Deftos, L. J. An Immunoassay for Human Calcitonin I: The Method. *Metabolism 20:* 1122, 1971.
2. Melvin, K. E. W., Miller, H. H., and Tashjian, A. H., Jr. Early Diagnosis of Medullary Thyroid Carcinoma of the Thyroid Gland by Means of Calcitonin Assay. *N. Engl. J. Med. 285:* 1115, 1971.
3. Deftos, L. J. Radioimmunoassay for Calcitonin in Medullary Thyroid Carcinoma. *J.A.M.A. 227:* 403, 1974.
4. Wolfe, H. J., Melvin, K. E. W., Cervi-Skinner, S. J., al Saadi, A. A., Juliar, J. F., Jackson, C. E., and Tashjian, A. H., Jr. Cell Hyperplasia Preceding Medullary Thyroid Carcinoma. *N. Engl. J. Med. 289:* 437, 1973.
5. Hill, C. S., Jr., Ibanez, M. L., Samaan, N. A., Ahearn, M. J., and Clark, R. L. Medullary (Solid) Carcinoma of the Thyroid Gland: An Analysis of the M. D. Anderson Hospital Experience with Patients with the Tumor, Its Special Features, and Its Histogenesis. *Medicine 52:* 141, 1973.
6. Tashjian, A. H., Jr., Howland, B. D., Kenneth, B. A., Melvin, K. E. W., and Hill, C. S., Jr. Immunoassay of Human Calcitonin: Clinical Measurement, Relation to Serum Calcium and Studies in Patients with Medullary Carcinoma. *N. Engl. J. Med. 283:* 890, 1970.
7. Samaan, N. A., Hill, C. S., Jr., Beceiro, J. R., and Schultz, P. N. Immunoreactive Calcitonin in Medullary Carcinoma of the Thyroid and in Maternal and Cord Serum. *J. Lab. Clin. Med. 81:* 671, 1973.
8. Parthemore, J. G., and Deftos, L. J. Calcitonin Secretion in Normal Human Subjects, *J. Clin. Endocr. Metab. 47:* 184, 1978.
9. Gagel, R. F., Melvin, K. E. W., Tashjian, A. H., Jr., Miller, H. H., Feldman, Z. T., Wolfe, H. J., Delellis, R. A., Cervi-Skinner, S., and Reichlin, S. Natural History of the Familial Medullary Thyroid Carcinoma–Pheochromocytoma Syndrome and the Identification of Preneoplastic Stages by Screening Studies: Five-Year Report. *Tr. Assoc. Am. Physicians 88:* 177, 1975.
10. Silva, O. L., Snider, R. H., and Becker, K. L. Radioimmunoassay of Calcitonin in Human Plasma. *Clin. Chem. 20:* 337, 1974.
11. Sizemore, G. W., and Heath, H. H., III. Immunochemical Heterogeneity of Calcitonin in Plasma of Patients with Medullary Thyroid Carcinoma. *J. Clin. Invest. 55:* 111, 1975.
12. McMillan, P. J., Hooker, W. M., and Deftos, L. J. Distribution of Calcitonin-Containing Cells in Human Thyroid. *Am. J. Anat. 140:* 73, 1974.
13. Deftos, L. J., Goodman, A. D., Engelman, K., and Potts, J. T., Jr. Suppression and Stimulation of Calcitonin Secretion in Medullary Thyroid Carcinoma. *Metabolism 20:* 428, 1971.
14. Hennessy, J. F., Wells, S. A., Jr., Ontjes, D. A., and Cooper, C. W. A Comparison of Pentagastrin Injection and Calcium Infusion as Provocative Agents for the Detection of Medullary Carcinoma of the Thyroid. *J. Clin. Endocrinol. Metab. 39:* 487, 1974.
15. Deftos, L. J., Bury, A. E., Habener, J. F., Singer, F. R., and Potts, J. T., Jr. Immunoassay for Human Calcitonin II: Clinical Studies. *Metabolism 20:* 1129, 1971.
16. Parthemore, J. G., Bronzert, D., Roberts, G., and Deftos, L. J. A Short Calcium Infusion in the Diagnosis of Medullary Thyroid Carcinoma. *J. Clin. Endocrinol. Metab. 39:* 108, 1974.

17. Rude, R. K., and Singer, F. R. Y. Comparison of a 1-Minute Calcium Injection with Pentagastrin Injection in the Diagnosis of Medullary Thyroid Carcinoma. *Clin. Res. 25:* A162, 1977.

18. Goltzman, D., Potts, J. T., Jr., Ridgway, E. C., and Maloof, F. Calcitonin as a Tumor Marker. Use of the Radioimmunoassay for Calcitonin in the Postoperative Evaluation of Patients with Medullary Thyroid Carcinoma. *N. Engl. J. Med. 290:* 1035, 1974.

19. Parthemore, J. G. Compensatory Hypercalcitoninism in Primary Hyperparathyroidism. Proceedings of the 59th Annual Meeting of the Endocrine Society, 1977, p. 235.

20. Milhaud, G., Calmette, C., Jullienne, A., et al. Calcitonin Disorders and Therapeutic Use. In: Calcium, Parathyroid Hormone and the Calcitonins. Talmage, R. V., and Munson, P. L., eds. Amsterdam, Excerpta Medica, 1972, pp. 66–70.

21. Silva, O. L., Becker, K. L., Primack, A., Doppman, J., and Snider, R. H. Ectopic Secretion of Calcitonin by Oat-Cell Carcinoma. *N. Engl. J. Med. 290:* 1122, 1974.

22. Hillyard, C. J., Coombes, R. G., Greenberg, P. B., Galante, L. S., and MacIntyre, I. Calcitonin in Breast and Lung Cancer. *Clin. Endocrinol. 5:* 1, 1976.

23. Silva, O. L., Becker, K. L., Doppman, J. L., Snider, R. H., and Moore, C. F. Calcitonin Levels in Thyroid-Vein Blood of Man. *Am. J. Med. Sci. 269:* 37, 1975.

24. Deftos, L. J., Roos, B. A., and Parthemore, J. G. Calcium and Skeletal Metabolism. *West. J. Med. 123:* 447, 1975.

25. Deftos, L. J., Roos, B. A., Bronzert, D., and Parthemore, J. G. Immunochemical Heterogeneity of Calcitonin in Plasma. *J. Clin. Endocrinol. Metab. 40:* 407, 1975.

26. Roos, B. A., Parthemore, J. G., Lee, J., and Deftos, L. J. Calcitonin Heterogeneity: In Vivo and In Vitro Studies. *Calcif. Tissues Res. 22S:* 298–302, 1977.

27. Lee, J. Parthemore, J. G., and Deftos, L. J. Calcitonin Secretion in Renal Disease. *Calcif. Tissues Res. 22S:* 154–157, 1977.

28. Fujimoto, Y., Oka, A., Fukumitsu, M., Obara, T., and Akisada, M.: Physical and Radiological Findings Specific for Medullary Carcinoma of the Thyroid Gland. *Endocrinologica Japan 22:* 225-232, 1975.

66

Disorders Associated with Hereditary or Acquired Abnormalities in Vitamin D Function: Hereditary Disorders Associated with Vitamin D Resistance or Defective Phosphate Metabolism

Donald Fraser

Charles R. Scriver

Calciopenic Rickets
Phosphopenic Rickets
Hereditary Vitamin-D Dependency
X-Linked Hypophosphatemia

With the discovery and subsequent therapeutic application of vitamin D in the 1920s, it soon became evident that not all rickets and osteomalacia could be attributed to simple deficiency of vitamin D. The first detailed study of a "nonnutritional" condition, which thereafter became known as "vitamin-D-resistant osteomalacia," was published by Albright and colleagues in 1937.[1] Five years later, attention was drawn to a form of osteomalacia accompanied by "phosphate diabetes," the term used by Robertson et al.[2] to distinguish a condition they believed to be different from that reported by Albright. In the wake of these classical reports, many other syndromes were subsequently described. An early review by Fraser and Salter[3] listed 10 discrete conditions in the category of "refractory" rickets and came to some accord with the mechanisms underlying the lesions; the list is now even longer.[4,5]

In the interval since Albright's original report, many efforts have been made to explain why some patients fail to respond to normal exposure to sunlight and an adequate dietary intake as dual sources of vitamin D. However, to say that such patients are completely refractory to vitamin D is rarely correct; in most instances, they are refractory only to the usual requirement of normal individuals* but are reponsive, at least to a degree, to pharmacological doses of the vitamin.

Recently, the terms "calciopenia" and "phosphopenia" have been proposed as a simple expedient to focus attention on the

aberrant processes, i.e., disturbances primarily involving calcium availability or phosphorus availability.[7,8]

CALCIOPENIC RICKETS

Rickets or osteomalacia can occur when the availability of calcium to the skeleton is impaired. Simple dietary restriction of calcium can cause rickets. However, to induce rickets in the experimental animal, the degree of restriction must be extreme, and, in the human, such extremes of dietary restriction have almost never been observed. The iatrogenic cases of Maltz et al.[9] and Kooh et al.[10] are rare examples of diet-induced calciopenia resulting in rickets.

The more usual cause of calciopenia in the human is impairment of calcium absorption by the intestine. Intestinal calcium absorption depends to a great extent upon vitamin D, and it follows that calciopenia would result from vitamin D deficiency. Further, it has been shown in the past decade that to exert physiological action at the target cells, vitamin D_2 (ergocalciferol) and vitamin D_3 (cholecalciferol) must be hydroxylated, first in the liver at the carbon-25 position in the side chain and then in kidney at the 1 position in the A ring. The resultant 1,25-dihydroxyvitamin D possesses hormonelike activity with respect to calcium transport. (The mechanisms and regulation of vitamin D-hormone biosynthesis are discussed elsewhere in this chapter.) It follows, therefore, that calciopenia could result from deficient intake of vitamin D, defective metabolism of vitamin D to 1,25 dihydroxyvitamin D, excessive destruction or excretion of vitamin D metabolites, or impaired responsiveness of target organs to the vitamin D hormone. In the context of this chapter, we believe that autosomal recessive vitamin D dependency is a model disease in the calciopenic group.

Primary abnormalities of the absorbing epithelium of the intes-

---

*In North America, the recommended daily intake of vitamin D to prevent rickets during growth is 400 IU (10 μg) of crystalline vitamin D_2 or vitamin D_3.[6]

tine (viz. celiac disease) can occasionally lead to rickets of the calciopenic type by interfering with absorption of calcium and probably also vitamin D.

PHOSPHOPENIC RICKETS

This term connotes that a defect in the availability of phosphate anion is the primary event in the pathogenesis of rickets. Relatively little is known about the mechanisms involved in membrane transport of phosphate beyond the fact that an anion carrier appears to be involved. The best-studied anion carrier is in the erythrocyte,[11,12] and this carrier is probably not identical to that in renal epithelium. Inorganic phosphate (P_i) is present in the blood in freely ultrafiltrable form, and large amounts appear in the glomerular filtrate. Thus the availability of P_i for bone mineralization depends in part upon efficient mechanisms for phosphate reclamation by the renal tubules. Renal tubular reabsorption of phosphate observes a maximum rate (Tm P_i),[13] suggesting that there may be a limitation in the capacity of a membrane carrier or in the intracellular events that contribute to transepithelial transport of the ion.[14] Although there is evidence that vitamin D plays a direct role in intestinal phosphate reabsorption,[15–17] there is little to indicate that the vitamin D hormone holds the same primacy for intestinal phosphate transport that it does for calcium absorption, and there is no evidence that it plays a role in renal phosphate reabsorption. If carrier mediation is of quantitative importance in phosphate transport, it follows that mutation could cause phosphopenia as a primary event. We believe that X-linked hypophosphatemia is a model disease in this respect. In the same vein, but with different mechanisms involved, we believe that the various forms of the Fanconi syndrome[18] can produce phosphopenic rickets by virtue of the defect in the tubular reclamation of phosphate ion that characterizes the various diseases included in the syndrome. Examples of the Fanconi syndrome are cystinosis, hereditary tyrosinemia, and oculocerebrorenal syndrome; and the hypophosphatemic tubulopathies secondary to Wilson's disease, lead, and other toxic agents.

While recognizing the two primary mechanisms—calciopenia and phosphopenia—that can result in rickets, we should recall that calciopenia can, in turn, produce hypophosphatemia (phosphopenia) by a linked event, namely secondary hyperparathyroidism. The phenomenon is well illustrated in the later stages of vitamin D deficiency in man[19] and experimental animals.[20] C-terminal-immunoreactive-parathyroid-hormone (iPTH) levels in serum are elevated in stages II and III of vitamin D deficiency,[21,22] and there is increased fractional excretion of phosphate, connoting an impairment in tubular reabsorption.[19] The generalized tubulopathy of vitamin D deficiency (phosphaturia, generalized aminoaciduria, tubular acidosis) is thus related, in a complex manner, to the depletion of vitamin D hormone and calcium ion in tissues[7] and to the excess of PTH, which itself will further deplete cellular stores of calcium.[23] Decrease of the cytoplasmic calcium concentration will decrease plasma membrane permeability;[24] it also increases "tight-junction" permeability.[25] The result of these combined events is likely to be impairment of net transtubular absorption of solute. Hypophosphatemia will result because of the important role normal tubular reclamation plays in the maintenance of phosphate homeostasis. It follows that determination of serum iPTH (measured with C-terminal antiserum) can serve as a useful test by which calciopenic rickets accompanied by secondary hyperparathyroidism and hypophosphatemia can be distinguished from the primary forms of phosphopenic rickets. This distinction will be further illustrated in the discussions to follow.

The distinguishing features of hereditary vitamin D dependency, X-linked hypophosphatemia, and the Fanconi syndrome are indicated in Table 66-1. In our experience, X-linked hypophosphatemic rickets is about three times more prevalent than vitamin D dependency, which in turn is somewhat more prevalent than the Fanconi syndrome.

HEREDITARY VITAMIN D DEPENDENCY

CLINICAL DESCRIPTION

Hereditary vitamin D-dependency rickets, which has also been named "pseudo-vitamin-D-deficiency rickets" has only recently become familiar as a distinct condition. This form of rickets has all the clinical features of the advanced stage of vitamin D deficiency, but it occurs in spite of vitamin D intakes that would ordinarily be prophylactic.[3,26–28] Prominent signs are usually evident before 6 months of age. Features include hypocalcemia, often with tetany or convulsions; hypophosphatemia; marked elevation of the alkaline phosphatase activity; and skeletal deformities (Fig. 66-1a). Generalized hyperaminoaciduria is a constant feature, and the plasma iPTH concentration is increased. Radiographically, the growth plates are acutely and severely rachitic, and the bones show general undermineralization, sometimes with pathological fractures (Fig. 66-2a). The permanent teeth show marked hypoplasia of the enamel.[28] Treatment is with very high doses of vitamin D. Important features that distinguish this disease from X-linked hypophosphatemia and the Fanconi syndrome are the dramatic and complete healing of the biochemical and skeletal lesions (Figs. 66-1b and 66-2b) and the resumption of the normal rate of growth that result from high-dosage vitamin D therapy. The condition is inherited as an autosomal recessive trait.

PATHOGENESIS

Several postulates were advanced to explain the syndrome. It was first suggested that bone and epiphyseal cartilage lacked the ability to mineralize in a normal manner. This early idea was discarded when slices of costochondral junction, removed from untreated patients, were found to mineralize in vitro when incubated in the patient's own serum to which had been added calcium and inorganic phosphate in amounts sufficient to raise the concentration of these ions to the physiological range.[29] Slices that were incubated in the patient's unaltered serum as a control failed to mineralize. The fact that the plasma Ca × P ion product of patients was far below normal offered a simple explanation for the defective mineralization.

Attention was then directed to the mechanisms for calcium and phosphate homeostasis.[30] Intestinal absorption of ^{47}Ca in the untreated proband was considerably below that of controls. No other component of intestinal absorption was abnormal. These findings, in conjunction with external calcium balance data, suggested that defective intestinal absorption of calcium was a critical abnormality in vitamin D dependency.

It is evident that vitamin D dependency has many features in common with severe vitamin D-deficiency rickets, hence the name "pseudodeficiency rickets."[26,31] Furthermore, all the biochemical and radiological signs of active rickets heal completely when patients are given large (pharmacological) doses of vitamin D. The term that we prefer, "hereditary vitamin D dependency," empha-

Table 66-1. Features of the Common Types of Vitamin D-Refractory Rickets

	X-Linked Hypophosphatemia	Vitamin D Dependency	Fanconi Syndrome
Genetics	X-linked dominant or sporadic (a rare autosomal dominant condition has been reported)	Autosomal recessive	Autosomal recessive (unless due to a toxic agent).
Onset of physical signs	12 to 18 mo. (hypophosphatemia present shortly after birth)	3 to 12 mo. (biochemical signs present shortly after birth)	Infancy, childhood, adulthood.
Mode of presentation	Onset of bowlegs when starting to walk, short stature, slight to severe deformities.	Irritability, tetany, convulsions, delayed walking, severe rickets, failure to thrive, bulging fontanel (in some cases).	Infancy: irritability, anorexia, failure to thrive, polydipsia, polyuria, dehydration. Childhood: bowlegs or knock-knees, short stature, rickets, polyuria, polydipsia.
Additional physical signs	Healthy, short and stocky, strong. Females usually less severely affected than males, and may have no deformities or dwarfism. Saggital craniosynostosis common. No enamel hypoplasia in permanent teeth, but pulp spaces enlarged. No urinary symptoms.	Severe rapidly increasing deformities, short stature, physically weak, enamel hypoplasia in permanent teeth. No urinary symptoms.	Cystinosis: cystine deposits in cornea, conjunctiva, leukocytes, rectal mucosa, bone marrow, cultured fibroblasts; photophobia; hair usually grey-blonde.
Radiographs	Mild to severe "chronic" rickets; shafts usually wide, cortices thick, coarse trabecular pattern, total skeletal calcium increased.[41] Some hypophosphatemic females have no physical or radiographic abnormalities.	Severe rachitic changes in growth plates and shafts; bones have thin cortices and tend toward osteoporosis.	Mild to severe rickets; osteoporosis in most cases.
Plasma			
Ca	Normal	Moderate to marked decrease	Normal to moderately decreased
Pi	Marked decrease	Decreased when syndrome well established	*Early:* marked decrease *Late:* normal or increased
Alk.p'tase	Slight to moderate increase	Increased, usually markedly	Moderate increase
Electrolytes	Normal	Normal	Serum K decreased
Acid/base	Normal		Mild acidosis
BUN, creatinine	Normal	Normal	*Early:* normal *Late:* increased
Amino acids	Normal	Normal	Normal (except in hereditary tyrosinemia)
iPTH	Normal	Increased	
Urine			
Protein	0	0	+ to + + +
Glucose	0	0 (occasionally +)	+ to + + +
pH	Normal range	Normal (in some cases, mild proximal RTA)	Acid
Concentration	Normal range	Normal range	Dilute
Amino acids	Normal	Generalized aminoaciduria	Generalized aminoaciduria
Prognosis	Probably require lifelong therapy in most cases; normal life expectancy; remain hypophosphatemic; males and most females remain stunted and deformed.	Require lifelong therapy; Normal life expectancy; with vitamin D therapy, condition is compatible with normal mineral balance, bone mineralization, and growth.	Cystinosis: Infant (Type I): severe uremia by end of 1st decade Adolescent (Type III): good life-expectancy. Other forms of Fanconi: variable
Therapy	Phosphate supplements Vitamin D	Vitamin D ~ 40–50 μg/kg/day	Phosphate supplements Potassium supplements Sodium bicarbonate Vitamin D Calcium

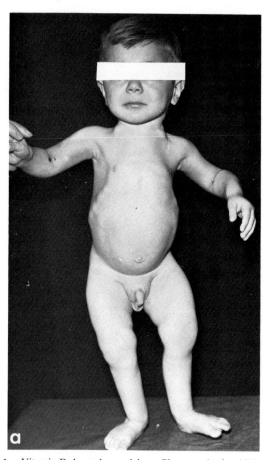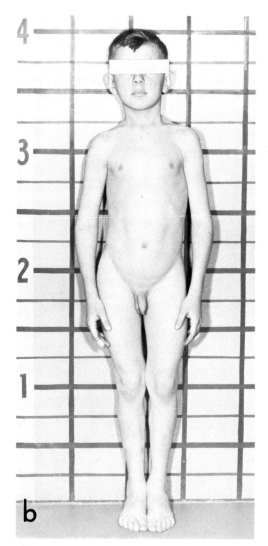

Fig. 66-1. Vitamin D-dependency rickets. Photograph of a child (*a*) before treatment, aged 3 years. Note severe deformities of long bones, "beading" of the costochondral junctions, and prominent Harrison sulci. The child could not walk without support. (*b*) The same child, aged 11 years, after treatment with vitamin D_2, 50,000–75,000 IU/day. The child was growing normally and the deformities had improved greatly.

sizes the genetic nature of the condition and the dependence on vitamin D at pharmacological levels to achieve a normal clinical and biochemical status.

Three mechanisms have been suggested to explain vitamin D dependency: (1) vitamin D is poorly absorbed, (2) vitamin D is inadequately converted to 1,25-dihydroxyvitamin D (1,25-$(OH)_2D$), and (3) the target tissues—bone, intestine, and kidney— are unable to respond satisfactorily to physiological concentrations of the active metabolite. Specific malabsorption of vitamin D is ruled out because normal levels of the vitamin are demonstrable in serum of untreated patients by the rat tibia-line test.[30] Moreover, assays of vitamin D and 25-hydroxyvitamin D reveal extremely high concentrations in patients who are given large doses of the vitamin during therapy.[30,32,33] Of the two remaining possibilities, recent evidence favors the likelihood that the condition results from a block in vitamin D metabolism.[34] It does not appear that the target organs are refractory to the active metabolite of vitamin D.

Evidence of a block in vitamin D metabolism has been obtained indirectly by observing the response of patients given vitamin D and its 25-hydroxy and 1α,-25-dihydroxy analogues.[34] Massive doses of vitamin D_2 and D_3, in the order of 1000–3000 μg/day (100 to 300 times the normal requirement) are required to maintain

biochemical and radiographic healing in vitamin D dependency. The maintenance requirement of 25-hydroxyvitamin D_3 (25-OHD_3), the first product of vitamin D metabolism, is also very high (200–900 μg/day) in the same patients.[34,35] By contrast, a very much smaller dose of 1α,25-$(OH)_2D_3$ (1 μg/day or less) is required to correct hypocalcemia, augment intestinal calcium absorption, establish positive calcium balance, and initiate radiographic healing in hereditary vitamin D dependency. A similar response is achieved with very small doses of the synthetic analogue 1α-OH-vitamin D_3.[33] Estimates based on such data indicate that the ratios of the dose requirements of vitamin D/25-$(OH)D_3$/1α,25-$(OH)_2D_3$ are on the average 1700:700:1.[34]

If one assumes that vitamin D and 25-OHD function in the normal individual through production of 1,25-$(OH)_2D$ (and all the physiological evidence favors this assumption), then the ratios of the requirements of vitamin D/25-OHD_3/1α,25-$(OH)_2D_3$ can be taken as an indirect measure of the efficiency of vitamin D metabolism. Conversion of vitamin D to 25-OHD appears normal in hereditary vitamin-D-dependency rickets, the 3:1 ratio for dose requirements of vitamin D/25-OHD_3 being similar to that in the rachitic rat.[36] However, to interpret the significance of the large difference in requirement of 25-OHD_3 and 1α,25-$(OH)_2D_3$ in vita-

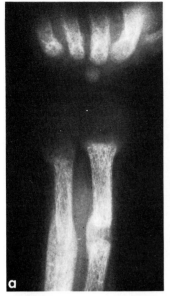
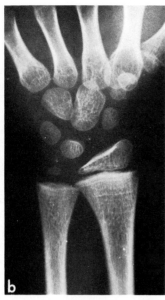

Fig. 66-2. Vitamin D-dependency rickets. Radiograph of the child's forearm (*a*) before treatment, aged 2 years. Note changes of severe rickets. No bone mineral can be detected in the epiphyses and at the zones of provisional calcification. The cortices are very poorly mineralized, the trabecular pattern is coarse, and there are healed pathological fractures in the midshafts of the radius and ulna. (*b*) Radiograph of forearm, aged 8 years, after treatment with vitamin D_2, 50,000–75,000 IU/day. The radiographic appearance is normal.

min D dependency requires a knowledge of the relative efficacies of these two metabolites under circumstances where optimal metabolism of vitamin D would be expected. Vitamin D deficiency is such a model. Kooh et al.[37] have shown, in two infants with vitamin D deficiency, that the dose of 25-OHD$_3$ required to initiate biochemical healing was only three times that of $1\alpha,25$-(OH)$_2$D$_3$. The ratio is virtually the same as that observed in rachitic rats and chicks.[36,38]

The most appealing interpretation of the data assigns the cause of vitamin D-dependency to an inborn error in conversion of 25-hydroxyvitamin D to 1,25-dihydroxyvitamin D, due to a recessively inherited deficiency of 25-hydroxyvitamin D-1-hydroxylase in the kidney (Fig. 66-3). The minute, possibly physiological doses of $1\alpha,25$-(OH)$_2$D$_3$ are thought to cure the rachitic lesions by bypassing the inherited enzyme deficiency. Confirmation of the hypothesis awaits direct evidence of a deficiency of 1-hydroxylase activity in the kidney. No evidence has yet been obtained that the target organs are refractory to the active metabolite of vitamin D.

One explanation for the response of patients to pharmacological doses of vitamin D is that the enzymatic mutation does not ablate hydroxylase activity completely but allows the production of sufficient amounts of 1,25-(OH)$_2$D, albeit inefficiently, to achieve normal mineral metabolism. Alternatively, because of the high concentration of 25-hydroxyvitamin D in the plasma, this metabolite may become bound to nuclear chromatin in sufficient amounts to exert direct physiological action in the absence of the final active metabolite.[34]

Hereditary vitamin D-dependency rickets is the first of what may prove to be a long list of inborn errors of vitamin D-hormone biosynthesis. Indeed, investigation of probands in different pedigrees may reveal different mechanisms for their dependence on pharmacological doses of vitamin D. Obviously, a block in conversion of vitamin D to 25-hydroxyvitamin D would cause the same

phenotypic abnormalities, and evidence of this block in metabolism should be sought in future pedigrees of the disease.

TREATMENT

As has already been emphasized, one of the important features of hereditary vitamin-D-dependency rickets is the complete healing of the biochemical and radiographic abnormalities that occurs with large doses of vitamin D. The dose required is very large—as much as 100 to 300 times the normal daily requirement. The response of patients to these large doses of vitamin D corresponds exactly to the response of vitamin D-deficient individuals to physiological intakes of the vitamin.

The method of establishing the optimal therapeutic dose of vitamin D in vitamin D-dependency rickets illustrates a therapeutic principle that is also applicable to a number of other vitamin D-refractory syndromes, including X-linked hypophosphatemia, Fanconi's syndrome, renal osteodystrophy, and hypoparathyroidism. Using a high-potency vitamin D_2 or D_3 preparation and starting with a less than adequate dose, the intake is slowly increased by small increments, with repeated assessment of response, until healing has occurred. In our experience, 25 μg (1000 IU) of vitamin D_2 or D_3 per kilogram of body weight per day is an appropriate starting dose in hereditary vitamin D-dependency rickets. Initially, response is evaluated at intervals of 6 to 8 weeks, because the full effect of a given dose is achieved only after such a period, presumably because the vitamin is dispersed to many storage depots. If, after that time, no biochemical or radiographic improvement has occurred, the dose of vitamin D should be increased by 25 percent; if signs of healing are evident, the increment should be only 15 percent. Similar increases in dosage should be made at 6-week to 3-month intervals until the appropriate maintenance dose has been achieved. At each assessment, plasma calcium, inorganic phosphate, and alkaline phosphatase are determined; A-P radiographs of the knees and wrists are obtained at longer intervals.

Once the suitable dose has been established, the patient needs less frequent assessment. However, plasma calcium and phosphate concentrations should be accurately monitored at intervals not longer than 3 or 4 months on a lifelong basis. There is an

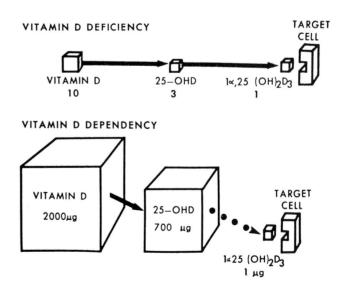

Fig. 66-3. Schematic diagram illustrating comparative therapeutic efficacies of vitamin D, 25-OHD$_3$ and 1,25-(OH)$_2$D$_3$ in (*a*) vitamin D deficiency and (*b*) hereditary vitamin D dependency. The diagram illustrates the hypothesis that hereditary vitamin D dependency is due to a defect in the 1-hydroxylation step of vitamin D metabolism.

advantage in conducting these assessments in the same medical center. For patients who live far from the hospital, provision of return-addressed mailing tubes by which serum samples can be conveniently shipped for analysis has been useful. The physical status of the patient, radiographs of the knees and wrists, and the renal function and urinary amino acid excretion should be evaluated at least annually to confirm that these parameters remain normal. The maintenance requirement of vitamin D_2 or D_3 is usually about 40–50 μg/kg body weight per day, the requirement increasing more or less in proportion to body weight. However, the maintenance requirement varies somewhat from patient to patient, and the optimum dose must be worked out for each individual by careful trial. Furthermore, small variations in requirement are likely to occur from time to time, and the dose of vitamin D should be increased or decreased by 15 percent of the previous dose, as indicated by the biochemical and radiographic responses. The necessity for high-dosage vitamin D treatment is lifelong.

In our opinion, the single most important indicator of vitamin D overdosage is hypercalcemia as determined by accurate measurement of the plasma calcium on frequent occasions. Additional signs are polyuria, nocturia, hypercalciuria, polydipsia, anorexia, and weight loss. Since the effective therapeutic dose is little less than the minimum toxic dose, mild hypervitaminosis D is likely to occur from time to time during treatment. On the other hand, if parent and physician are alert, and if vitamin D is discontinued at the earliest evidence of vitamin D intoxication, the hypercalcemia disappears within a few days, and no detectable residual damage occurs. If, after 2 weeks without medication, all clinical and biochemical evidence of vitamin D intoxication has disappeared, maintenance vitamin D therapy is resumed, with a dose 15 percent less than that which produced the hypercalcemia. The Sulkowich test is not a suitable means of regulating vitamin D dosage.

The objective of treatment is to employ the minimum dosage of vitamin D that maintains the plasma calcium and inorganic phosphate concentrations and the alkaline phosphatase activity within the normal range and establishes a radiographically normal appearance at the epiphyseal plates of the knees and wrists. With this therapy, catch-up growth is to be expected during the early months of treatment, and thereafter growth of the skeleton should occur at a normal rate. The newly formed metaphyseal bone should be radiographically normal when the appropriate dosage is being given, and eventually the entire skeleton should become normal in appearance.

Several high-potency vitamin D preparations are available. All those in North America contain vitamin D_2. Products with the vitamin in liquid form (see Appendix I) have a major advantage over capsules because the liquid preparations permit the physician to prescribe any dose of vitamin D required, in contrast to the inflexibility of treatment with capsules. The most dependable and practical way for the parents or patient to measure the dose is by use of a tuberculin syringe from which the appropriate volume of medication is given directly into the patient's mouth.

We and others have treated several patients with 25-OHD$_3$ on a long-term basis. In our patients, the dose required to maintain normal plasma calcium and phosphorus levels and normal bone architecture has been in the range of 200–900 μg/day.[34] Rosen et al.[39] have maintained patients on much smaller intakes than this, but the possibility that their probands had a different form of the disease cannot be excluded. In our experience, 25-OHD$_3$ is a satisfactory agent for treating vitamin D-dependency rickets. However, 25-OHD$_3$ is no less likely to cause hypercalcemia than is

vitamin D, nor is disappearance of hypercalcemia appreciably faster when the agent is withheld. Despite the smaller dose needed to control the rachitic disease, the drug offers no substantial advantages over vitamin D.

With the demonstration that biochemical and radiographic healing could be initiated with minute doses of 1α,25-(OH)$_2$D$_3$, and the demonstration that very small doses of 1α-OHD$_3$ can be substituted for 1α,25-(OH)$_2$D$_3$, the feasibility of using these active agents in therapy has become a practical question.[33,34] The more rapid onset of 1α,25-(OH)$_2$D$_3$ and 1α-OHD$_3$ and the shorter duration of effect[33,34,37] could theoretically be of advantage over vitamin D. However, until 1α,25-(OH)$_2$D$_3$ and 1α-OHD$_3$ become more readily available for clinical trial, and until there has been more experience with dosage, vitamin D remains the agent of choice.

Patients with hereditary vitamin D-dependency rickets respond satisfactorily to treatment with dihydrotachysterol (DHT), but the dose required is large. The theoretical possibility that the configuration of the rotated A ring of the DHT molecule would provide an antirachitic agent of much superior potency, approaching that of 1α,25-(OH)$_2$D$_3$, has not been borne out in practice. Daily doses in the 500–1000 μg range appear to be needed.[31] We do not believe the agent has any special advantages over vitamin D, and it is more expensive.

INHERITANCE AND RECURRENCE RISK

The inheritance of vitamin D dependency is almost certainly autosomal recessive. Heterozygotes show no biochemical or clinical manifestations by any of the available tests.[28] One expects that, when eventually practicable, assay of 25-hydroxyvitamin-D-1-hydroxylase activity in the kidney will reveal a partial deficiency of this enzyme in carriers of the mutation. It will be of interest to know whether the 1,25(OH)$_2$D levels in plasma are lower than normal in heterozygotes.

The recurrence risk for the trait is 1 in 4 at the birth of each sib of a homozygous proband. Biochemical diagnosis can be made within weeks after birth. Treatment can be started at that time, and, accordingly, the phenotypic manifestations can be prevented.

X-LINKED HYPOPHOSPHATEMIA

X-linked hypophosphatemia is a dominantly inherited disease of variable phenotypic expression.[40] A low plasma inorganic phosphate concentration is the constant feature and is present from early infancy in all individuals. In males, the hemizygous mutant allele always causes rickets and short stature, while in heterozygous females, the genetic defect is variably expressed, some individuals showing no physical or radiographic abnormalities and others showing various degrees of rickets and stunted growth (Fig. 66-4).

Characteristically, the plasma P$_i$ concentration is very low— but to establish hypophosphatemia, one must take into account the patient's sex and age, factors that influence the normal plasma P$_i$ concentration (Fig. 66-5). The plasma calcium is normal, urinary amino acid excretion is normal, and the plasma iPTH level is within the normal range.

Rickets, when present, develops later than in hereditary vitamin D dependency. Genu varum first becomes evident about the time the child commences to walk, and the plasma alkaline phosphatase activity is then moderately increased. Dwarfism often becomes a conspicuous feature. Radiographically (Fig. 66-6a), the

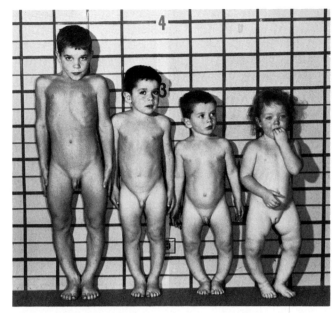

Fig. 66-4. X-linked hypophosphatemia in three male sibs and a female first cousin. Note genu varum, femoral and tibial torsion, and short stature. Palpation revealed enlargement of the costochondral junctions.

growth plates show varying degrees of long-standing rachitic activity. The long bones, particularly the femora, show bowing, the cortices are thickened, and the trabeculae are prominent and coarse. In individuals who have rickets and dwarfism, the skeleton contains more calcium than normal by the end of puberty.[41]

In contrast to the enamel hypoplasia seen in vitamin D dependency, the permanent teeth have a normal appearance. High doses of vitamin D have a beneficial effect on the skeletal lesions, but, in contrast to the situation in vitamin D dependency, the rachitic lesions do not heal completely (see below).

PATHOGENESIS

Impaired Tubular Phosphate Reclamation

X-linked hypophosphatemia (XLH) emerges as a selective disorder of transepithelial transport of orthophosphate (P_i).[7,42-44] Net tubular reabsorption, or reclamation, of P_i is impaired, even at the low concentrations of serum phosphate in affected patients, and maximal tubular reabsorption of phosphate (TmP_i) during phosphate loading is far below normal.[43,45] Indeed, secretion (or "negative reabsorption") of phosphate by the renal tubule occurs in hemizygous male patients under certain circumstances.[43] On the other hand, there is ordinarily a net, albeit decreased, reabsorption of phosphate by the kidney of the XLH patient; this residual reabsorptive function is insensitive to further inhibition by parathyroid hormone infusion but is enhanced by calcium infusion.[43-46]

There is some evidence that a defect also exists in phosphate transport by the intestine. If this is confirmed, XLH could be assigned to the class of inborn errors of membrane transport that affect epithelial transport tissues in general. Impaired intestinal phosphate absorption is suggested by oral-phosphate-loading studies[47] and by in vitro measurements of phosphate uptake by intestinal mucosa obtained by biopsy.[48] On the other hand, other investigators have not found abnormal intestinal transport of P_i in XLH patients.[49,50] It is not clear at present whether the discrepancies between the various reports reflect genetic heterogeneity among patients or are attributable to differences in methodology.

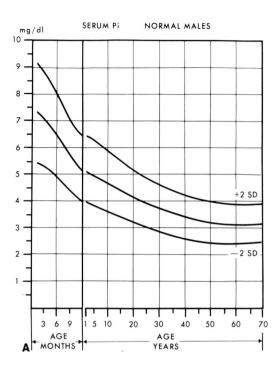

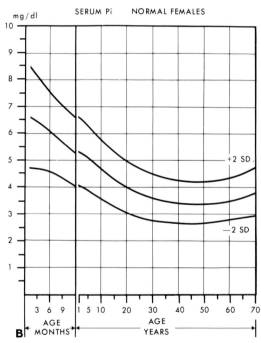

Fig. 66-5. Age-related variation in normal serum inorganic phosphate concentrations in males and females. The curves depict the mean and 95% confidence limits. Data for infants aged 0–6 months are from Owen, G. M., Garry, P., and Fomon, S. J., *Pediatrics 31:* 495, 1963. Data for subjects 1 year of age and older are from Greenberg, B. G., Winters, R. W., and Graham, J. B., *J. Clin. Endocrinol. Metab. 20:* 364, 1960.

The "Hyperresponsive-Tubule" Hypothesis

As an explanation of the impaired reclamation of P_i by the kidney, some investigators have proposed that the renal tubules are hyperresponsive to circulating PTH in XLH[51,52] and other forms of vitamin-D-refractory rickets. This hypothesis has arisen from the finding that plasma levels of iPTH are essentially normal in untreated patients[42,53,54] and the observation that no further

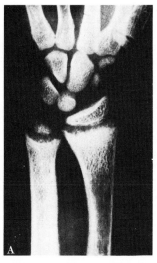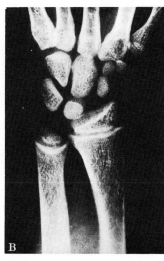

Fig. 66-6. X-linked hypophosphatemia: radiographs of the wrist of an affected boy (*a*) before treatment, aged 12 years. Note increased thickness at the epiphyseal plates, fraying of the metaphyses, and prominent coarseness of the trabecular pattern—evidence of long-standing rachitic activity of moderate intensity. The cortices are thickened and appear laminated. (*b*) After 1 year's treatment with vitamin D_2, 100,000 IU/day. Mineral has been deposited at the zones of provisional calcification, the epiphyseal plates are of normal thickness, and there is no evidence of rachitic activity. However, the trabecular pattern remains coarse—evidence of persistent osteomalacia.

impairment of renal P_i reclamation occurs when PTH is administered.[42]

So far, the weight of evidence is against hyperresponsiveness of the renal tubule to PTH. In the XLH phenotype, altered tubule function is limited strictly to phosphate-ion transport; there is no impairment in amino acid reabsorption and no increase in the basal level or urinary 3'5'-adenosine monophosphate (cyclic AMP), as would be expected were parathyroid hormone hyperresponsiveness the basis of the tubular transport defect.[44] Indeed, in keeping with our present concepts concerning the interrelations of PTH, calcium ion, and the transport functions of the normal renal tubule, urinary cyclic AMP and, usually, urinary amino acid excretion increase when exogenous PTH is given in XLH, and the urinary calcium excretion decreases appropriately.[7,55]

Three reports of subtotal parathyroidectomy in the XLH phenotype provide important additional evidence against the "hyperresponsive-tubule" hypothesis.[56-58] The removal of sufficient parathyroid tissue to cause hypocalcemia of several weeks' duration caused no significant improvement in tubular reabsorption of phosphate and did not correct the hypophosphatemia.

Comment

It is noted elsewhere that under certain circumstances, the amount of P_i secreted in the urine can exceed the amount filtered by the glomeruli.[43,59] This phenomenon, which we have referred to as "negative phosphate reabsorption" or "phosphate secretion," implies a net flux of P_i from the peritubular blood through the epithelial cell of the tubule into the urine. One possible explanation could be a defect in the luminal membrane of the tubule cell secondary to an altered transmembrane equilibrium of P_i such that back-flux of P_i takes place from the cytosol of the tubule cell into the urine. In this instance, uptake of P_i from the blood at the basal (peritubular) membrane of the tubule cell need not be abnormal. Indeed, if it were normal, it might serve to sustain the mitochon-

drial content of P_i within the tubule cell because phosphate, like calcium, can equilibrate with a mitochondrial compartment during movement through the cell.[60] Second, this might sustain the apical (luminal) cytoplasmic pool of P_i and presumably could thus provide for the back-flux of P_i into the urine at the luminal membrane of the cell.

Studies in Erythrocytes of XLH Patients

In investigating the extent of the impairment of transmembrane transport of P_i in XLH, the entry of P_i into the XLH erythrocyte was examined under a wide range of conditions.[11] No abnormality was found. A perturbation of phosphate-dependent metabolism does take place in the XLH erythrocyte; however, this abnormality can be attributed quite simply to the diminished concentration of plasma P_i characteristic of the disease.

TREATMENT

Response to Vitamin D

Vitamin D alone has a beneficial effect on the rachitic lesions in XLH if the vitamin is given in sufficiently large doses. The optimum dose is arrived at by the procedure described for treatment of vitamin-D-dependency rickets, and to have any beneficial effect on the skeleton, it must be close to the toxic range without causing hypercalcemia. Plasma P_i then increases slightly, although not to the physiological range, serum alkaline phosphatase activity decreases but rarely reaches the normal value, skeletal deformities such as genu varum tend to improve, and the rachitic lesions in the growth plates heal radiographically.[3,61] However, the characteristic coarse trabecular pattern rarely disappears, wide osteoid seams persist on microscopic examination, and the bones probably never heal completely[44] (Fig. 66-6*b*).* Vitamin D therapy alone rarely corrects dwarfism completely[62] and, even if started in early infancy, may fail to prevent its development.[63,64] In a number of cases, increasing deformities and dwarfism remain problems despite optimal treatment with vitamin D. As with the treatment of vitamin D dependency with large doses of vitamin D, care must be taken to avoid vitamin D intoxication. The plasma calcium level should be accurately measured at least every 3 months. High-dosage vitamin D treatment has sometimes caused permanent renal damage;[65] however, such changes can be avoided by regular monitoring of the clinical, biochemical, and radiographic status.[66]

Response to Vitamin D Hormone

The response to $1\alpha,25\text{-}(OH)_2D_3$ in XLH has been examined.[67] Perhaps through its effect on calcium concentrations within cells, rapid intravenous infusion of $1\alpha,25\text{-}(OH)_2D_3$ at the 1-μg dose level promoted a transient improvement of phosphate reclamation by the renal tubule; the phosphaturic response to bovine PTH was also restored transiently. However, long-term treatment with $1\alpha,25\text{-}(OH)_2D_3$ does not cure the condition at these dose levels, whether administered intravenously or by mouth: serum P_i does not return to normal, and, in our experience, the rachitic process does not heal completely. We conclude that $1\alpha,25\text{-}(OH)_2D_3$ by itself and at low dosage levels is inadequate as a therapeutic agent in XLH. The finding is not surprising if XLH is indeed a primary abnormality of transepithelial transport of phosphate. Whether

---

*It should be noted that a normal alkaline phosphatase value in XLH does not necessarily indicate that the bone lesions are healed; not uncommonly, particularly in adult patients, radiographic and histological evidence of osteomalacia may be present without elevation of plasma alkaline phosphatase activity.

$1\alpha,25\text{-}(OH)_2D_3$ or the $1\alpha\text{-}OH$ analogue has any practical advantage over vitamin D as an adjunct to phosphate supplementation has not yet been clearly shown.

Response to Oral Phosphate Supplementation

The evidence for a phosphopenic mechanism as the cause of XLH rickets suggests that phosphate replacement would be the appropriate way to neutralize the effect of the mutant allele.[68] It has long been known that dietary phosphate will heal rachitic bone lesions in animals. Lilly et al.[69] described this phenomenon in rats and reviewed the relevant literature as far back as 1872. Subsequently, several investigators[29,63,70,71] observed that intravenous infusion of phosphate promoted rapid healing of rickets in human hypophosphatemic states without the aid of high doses of vitamin D. Fraser et al.,[72] Wilson et al.,[59] and Gerbeaux-Balsan[49] observed radiographic improvement of the rachitic lesions and found positive external balances for phosphorus and calcium in XLH after oral supplementation with phosphate salts. However, the healing effect was evident only during the first 1 to 2 months of treatment, after which rachitic lesions again appeared in spite of the phosphate supplementation.[72] Reports of "failed phosphate treatment" have also appeared in the literature,[64,73] but the latter reports seem to reflect more a failure on the part of the patient to comply with the prescribed oral phosphate therapy than a failure on the part of patient's bones to respond to phosphate.

The facilitative diffusional mode of phosphate transport, evident for example in the erythrocyte membrane, permits phosphate to pass from the intestinal lumen into the bloodstream and to enter cells even if other mechanisms of phosphate transport are impaired by the mutant allele. The objective in children is to attain serum P_i levels of about 4 mg/dl. The response of the serum inorganic-phosphate level to pulsed phosphate loading is short-lived—the plasma concentration reaches a peak in about $1\frac{1}{2}$ hours and has usually returned to baseline within 4 hours. For this reason, phosphate supplements must be given every 4 hours, and the child should receive a dose five times daily.[68,74] Any of the four phosphate formulations mentioned in Appendix II may be employed, depending upon the child's preference. Initially, phosphate supplementation may cause diarrhea, but with persistence the patient normally develops a tolerance to the regimen, usually within 1 or 2 weeks. To begin treatment in a 1-year-old child, we administer 0.125 g t.i.d. on the first day, 0.25 g t.i.d. on the second day, 0.25 g q.i.d. on the third day, and 0.25 g q. 4 h. five times a day on the fourth and succeeding days. The latter dose provides 1.25 g supplemental phosphorus daily. Older children tolerate considerably larger doses. The supplement is given with meals when possible. Depending on the child's body weight and the response of his plasma P_i level and skeleton, treatment should be adjusted to provide 1–5 g elemental phosphorus per day. Phosphate supplementation involves the intake of appreciable loads of sodium and, for some preparations, potassium, but we have not observed hypertension in our series of XLH patients.

Phosphate loading decreases the level of ionized calcium and thus causes the concentration of plasma iPTH to increase.[68,75] Characteristic bone changes and hyperaminoaciduria with aminopeptiduria will appear if sustained secondary hyperparathyroidism occurs. In addition, the elevated levels of parathyroid hormone, through action on the residual parathyroid hormone-sensitive component of tubular phosphate reabsorption, will cause an even greater impairment in renal phosphate reclamation. This phenomenon probably explains why, after Fraser et al. obtained good initial healing of rachitic lesions with oral phosphate supplements,[63] the rachitic lesions gradually returned in spite of persistent treatment.[72]

Vitamin D must be used as an adjunct to phosphate therapy to avoid these complications. The dosage of vitamin D ranges from 0.1 to 1.25 mg (4000–50,000 IU) per day, depending on the amount of phosphate taken by the patient. Should secondary hyperparathyroidism appear (aminoaciduria, elevated iPTH, subperiosteal bone resorption), phosphate treatment should be withheld temporarily to allow calcium homeostasis to be regained,[68] or in some cases the dose of vitamin D may need to be increased.

Regular treatment with orthophosphate supplements by mouth in doses ranging from 1 to 5 g of elemental phosphorus per day will heal the rickets of XLH. The average radiographic density of bone monitored by photodensitometry of a standard x-ray image of a middle phalanx has revealed satisfactory bone density when compared with age-matched control subjects. Of greater clinical importance, a striking increase in the linear growth velocity occurs after initiation of treatment with supplemental phosphate. Glorieux et al.[68] observed that the average linear growth velocity in children with untreated XLH was only 63 percent of normal; when treated with vitamin D alone in the traditional manner, the growth rate was not greatly improved. However, in patients receiving phosphate treatment and vitamin D, the average growth rate was approximately twice the pretreatment rate. The lower segment, which is the fastest-growing portion of the body in childhood, is included in this acceleration of growth. Others have also shown that phosphate therapy permits true catch-up growth in XLH, and this reduces the hazard of dwarfism.[15,76]

A regimen that requires the preschool or school child to take phosphate supplements five times a day over a prolonged period is not easily accommodated by the patient or his family. The schedule of dosing is inconvenient. The night dose of phosphate is particularly difficult to organize, but is nonetheless very important. The taste of the various phosphate mixtures is rather unpleasant. Despite these problems, the benefits of oral phosphate supplementation far outweigh the drawbacks. Therefore, if maximum long-term benefits are to be achieved, it is essential to provide continuous support and reinforcement to the patient and his family. This is best accomplished through regular home visits by a member of the treatment team.[74] The role of this individual is to provide encouragement regarding the benefits of treatment through information about the response of the patient's serum P_i levels and demonstrations of evidence that catch-up growth and radiographic healing are taking place. We recommend, in addition, that the consumption rate of the phosphate supplement be monitored, thus giving some indication that the prescribed dose is being administered regularly.

REFERENCES

1. Albright, F., Butler, A. H. and Bloomberg, E. Rickets resistant to vitamin D therapy. *Am. J. Dis. Child.* 59: 529, 1937.
2. Robertson, B. R., Harris, R. C. and McCune, D. J. Refractory rickets: Mechanism of therapeutic action of calciferol. *Am. J. Dis. Child,* 64: 948, 1942.
3. Fraser, D. and Salter, R. B. The diagnosis and management of the various types of rickets. *Pediatr. Clin. North Am.* 5: 417, 1958.
4. Smith, R. The pathophysiology and management of rickets. *Orthop. Clin. North Am.* 3: 601, 1972.
5. Arnaud, S. B. and Stickler, G. B. Rickets, in, Conn, H. F. and Conn, R. B., Jr. (Eds.), Current Diagnosis, 4th ed. W. B. Saunders Co., Philadelphia, 1974, p. 655.
6. Recommended Dietary Allowances, 8th rev. ed. National Academy of Sciences, Washington, D.C., 1974, pp. 54–56.

7. Scriver, C. R. Rickets and the pathogenesis of impaired tubular transport of phosphate and other solutes. *Am. J. Med. 57:* 43, 1974.

8. Fraser, D. and Scriver, C. R. Familial forms of vitamin D-resistant rickets revisited. X-linked hypophosphatemia and autosomal recessive vitamin D dependency. *Am. J. Clin. Nutr. 29:* 1315, 1976.

9. Maltz, H. E., Fish, M. B. and Holliday, M. A. Calcium-deficiency rickets and the renal response to calcium infusion. *Pediatrics 46:* 865, 1970.

10. Kooh, S. W., Fraser, D., Reilly, B. J., Hamilton, J. R., Gall, D. G., and Bell, L. Rickets due to calcium deficiency. *N. Engl. J. Med. 297:* 1264, 1977.

11. Tenenhouse, H. S. and Scriver, C. R. Orthophosphate transport in the erythrocyte of normal subjects and of patients with X-linked hypophosphatemia. *J. Clin. Invest. 55:* 644, 1975.

12. Cabantchik, Z. I. and Rothstein, A. Membrane proteins related to anion permeability of human red blood cells. I. Localization of disulfenic stibbene binding sites in proteins involved in permeation. *J. Membr. Biol. 15:* 207, 1974.

13. Bijvoet, O. L. M. Relation of plasma phosphate concentration to renal tubular reabsorption of phosphate. *Clin. Sci. 37:* 23, 1969.

14. Scriver, C. R., Chesney, R. W. and McInnes, R. R. Genetic aspects of renal tubular transport. Diversity and topology of carriers. *Kidney Int. 9:* 149, 1976.

15. Harrison, H. E., Harrison, H. C., Lifshitz, F. and Johnson, A. D. Growth disturbance in hereditary hypophosphatemia. *Am. J. Dis. Child. 112:* 290, 1966.

16. Chen, T. C., Castillo, L., Koricka-Dahl, M. and DeLuca, H. F. Role of vitamin D metabolites in phosphate transport of rat intestine. *J. Nutr. 104:* 1056, 1974.

17. DeLuca, H. F., Tanaka, Y. and Castillo, L. Interrelations between vitamin D and phosphate metabolism, in Talmage, R. V., Owen, M., Parsons, J. A. (Eds.), Calcium-Regulating Hormones. Proceedings of the Fifth Parathyroid Conference, Oxford, 1974. Excerpta Medica, ICS 346, Amsterdam, 1975, pp. 305–317.

18. Leaf, A. The syndrome of osteomalacia, renal glucosuria, aminoaciduria, and increased phosphorus clearance (the Fanconi syndrome), in Stanbury, J. B., Wyngaarden, J. B. and Fredrickson, D. S. (Eds.), The Metabolic Basis of Inherited Disease, 2nd ed. McGraw-Hill, New York, 1966, p. 1205.

19. Fraser, D., Kooh, S. W. and Scriver, C. R. Hyperparathyroidism as the cause of hyperaminoaciduria and phosphaturia in human vitamin D deficiency. *Pediatr. Res. 1:* 425, 1967.

20. Grose, J. and Scriver, C. R. Parathyroid-dependent phosphaturia and aminoaciduria in the vitamin D-deficient rat. *Am. J. Physiol 214:* 370, 1968.

21. Arnaud, C., Glorieux, F. and Scriver, C. R. Serum parathyroid hormone levels in acquired vitamin D deficiency of infancy. *Pediatrics 49:* 837, 1972.

22. Fischer, J. A., Binswanger, U., Fanconi, A., Illig, R., Baerlocher, K. and Prader, A. Serum parathyroid hormone concentrations in vitamin D-deficiency rickets of infancy: Effects of intravenous calcium and vitamin D. *Horm. Metab. Res. 5:* 381, 1973.

23. Borle, A. B. Regulation of the mitochondrial control of cellular calcium homeostasis and calcium transport of phosphate, parathyroid hormone, calcitonin, vitamin D and cyclic AMP, in Talmage, R. V., Owen, M., Parsons, J. A. (Eds.), Calcium-Regulating Hormones. Proceedings of the Fifth Parathyroid Conference, Oxford, 1974. Excerpta Medica, ICS 346, Amsterdam, 1975, p. 217.

24. Baker, P. F. Transport and metabolism of calcium ions in nerve. *Progr. Biophys. Mol. Biol. 24:* 177, 1972.

25. Rose, B. and Loewenstein, W. R. Permeability of cell junction depends on local cytoplasmic calcium activity. *Nature 254:* 250, 1975.

26. Prader, A., Illig, R. and Heierli, E. Ein besondere Form der primaren vitamin-D-resistenten Rachitis mit Hypocalcämie und autosomal-dominantem Erbgang: die hereditäre Pseudo-Mangelrachitis. *Helv. Paediatr. Acta 16:* 452, 1961.

27. Scriver, C. R. Vitamin D dependency. *Pediatrics 45:* 361, 1970.

28. Arnaud, C., Maijer, R., Reade, T., Scriver, C. R. and Whelan, D. T. Vitamin D dependency: An inherited postnatal syndrome with secondary hyperparathyroidism. *Pediatrics 46:* 871, 1970.

29. Fraser, D., Jaco, N. T., Yendt, E. R., Munn, J. D. and Liu, E. The induction of in vitro and in vivo calcification in bones of children suffering from vitamin D-resistant rickets without recourse to large doses of vitamin D. *Am. J. Dis. Child. 93:* 84, 1957 (abstract).

30. Hamilton, J. R., Harrison, J., Fraser, D., Radde, I., Morecki, R. and Paunier, L. The small intestine in vitamin D-dependent rickets. *Pediatrics 45:* 364, 1970.

31. Fanconi, A. and Prader, A. Die hereditäre Pseudo-Mangelrachitis *Helv. Paediatr. Acta 24:* 423, 1969.

32. Fanconi, A., Prader, A. Pseudo-vitamin-D-deficiency rickets, in Bartrop, D. and Burland, W. L. (Eds.), Metabolism in Paediatrics. Oxford, Blackwell Scientific Publications, 1969, pp. 19–26.

33. Reade, T. M., Scriver, C. R., Glorieux, F. H., Nogrady, B., Delvin, E., Poirier, R., et al. Response to crystalline 1α-hydroxyvitamin D_3 in vitamin D dependency. *Pediatr. Res. 9:* 593, 1975.

34. Fraser, D., Kooh, S. W., Kind, H. P., Holick, M. F., Tanaka, Y. and DeLuca, H. F. Pathogenesis of hereditary vitamin-D-dependent rickets. An inborn error of vitamin-D metabolism involving defective conversion of 25-hydroxyvitamin D to 1α,25-dihydroxyvitamin D. *N. Engl. J. Med. 289:* 817, 1973.

35. Balsan, S. and Garabedian, M. 25-Hydroxycholecalciferol. A comparative study in deficiency rickets and different types of resistant rickets. *J. Clin. Invest. 51:* 749, 1972.

36. Tanaka, Y., Frank, H. and DeLuca, H. F. Biological activity of 1,25-dihydroxyvitamin D_3 in the rat. *Endocrinology 92:* 417, 1973.

37. Kooh, S. W., Fraser, D., DeLuca, H. F., Holick, M. F., Belsey, R. E., Clark, M. B., Murray, T. M. Treatment of hypoparathyroidism and pseudohypoparathyroidism with metabolites of vitamin D: Evidence for impaired conversion of 25-hydroxyvitamin D to 1α,25-dihydroxyvitamin D. *N. Engl. J. Med. 293:* 840, 1975.

38. Norman, A. W. and Wong, R. G. Biological activity of the vitamin D metabolite 1,25-dihydroxycholecalciferol in chickens and rats. *J. Nutr. 102:* 1709, 1972.

39. Rosen, J. F. and Finberg, L. Vitamin D-dependent rickets: Actions of parathyroid hormone and 25-hydroxycholecalciferol. *Pediatr. Res. 6:* 552, 1972.

40. Williams, T. F. and Winters, R. W. Familial (hereditary) vitamin D-resistant rickets with hypophosphatemia, in Stanbury, J. B., Wyngaarden, J. B. and Fredrickson, D. S. (Eds.), The Metabolic Basis of Inherited Disease, 3rd ed. McGraw-Hill, New York, 1972, chap 60, pp. 1465–1485.

41. Harrison, J. E., Cumming, W. E., Fornasier, V., Fraser, D. Kooh, S. W. and McNeill, K. G. Increased bone mineral content in young adults with familial hypophosphatemic vitamin D-refractory rickets. *Metabolism 25:* 33, 1976.

42. Arnaud, C., Glorieux, F. and Scriver, C. R. Serum parathyroid hormone in X-linked hypophosphatemia. *Science 173:* 845, 1971.

43. Glorieux, F. and Scriver, C. R. X-linked hypophosphatemia: Loss of a PTH-sensitive component of phosphate transport. *Science 175:* 997, 1972.

44. Glorieux, F. H. and Scriver, C. R. Transport, metabolism and clinical use of inorganic phosphate in X-linked hypophosphatemia, in Frame, B., Parfitt, A. M. and Duncan, H. (Eds.), The Clinical Aspects of Metabolic Bone Disease. Excerpta Medica, ICS 270, Amsterdam, 1973, p. 421.

45. Fraser, D., Leeming, J. M., Cerwenka, E. A., Kenyeres, K. Studies of the pathogenesis of the high renal clearance of phosphate in hypophosphatemic vitamin D-refractory rickets of the simple type. *Am. J. Dis. Child. 98:* 586, 1959 (abstract).

46. Fraser, D., Leeming, J. M. and Cerwenka, E. A. Über die Handhabung von Phosphat durch die Nieren bei hypophosphatämischer vitamin-D-resistenter Rachitis der einfachen Art und bei Cystinspeicherkrankheit. Reaktion auf verlängerte Calciuminfusion. *Helv. Paediatr. Acta 14:* 497, 1959.

47. Condon, J. R., Nassim, J. R. and Rutter, A. Pathogenesis of rickets and osteomalacia in familial hypophosphatemia. *Arch. Dis. Child. 46:* 269, 1971.

48. Short, E. M., Binder, H. J. and Rosenberg, L. E. Familial hypophosphatemic rickets: defective transport of inorganic phosphate by intestinal mucosa. *Science 179:* 700, 1973.

49. Gerbeaux-Balsan, S. L'absorption intestinale du phosphore dans le rachitisme vitamino-résistant hypophosphatémique héréditaire. Effets de fortes surcharges de phosphore et des régimes très pauvres en calcium. *Rev. Fr. Etudes Clin. Biol. 10:* 65, 1965.

50. Glorieux, F. H., Morin, C. L., Travers, R., Delvin, E. E. and Poirier, R. Intestinal phosphate transport in familial hypophosphatemic rickets. *Pediatr. Res. 10:* 691, 1976.

51. Arnstein, A. R. and Hanson, C. A. Nature of renal phosphate leak. *N. Engl. J. Med. 281:* 1427, 1969.

52. Short, E. M., Morris, R. C., Sebastian, A. and Spencer, M. Exaggerated phosphaturic response to circulating parathyroid hormone in patients with familial X-linked hypophosphatemic rickets. *J. Clin. Invest. 58:* 152, 1976.

53. Lewy, J. E., Cabana, E. C., Repetto, . A., Canterbury, J. M. and

Reiss, E. Serum parathyroid hormone in hypophosphatemic vitamin D-resistant rickets. *J. Pediatr. 81:* 294, 1972.

54. Fanconi, A., Fischer, J. A. and Prader, A. Serum parathyroid hormone concentrations in hypophosphatemic vitamin D-resistant rickets. *Helv. Paediatr. Acta 29:* 187, 1974.

55. Scriver, C. R., McInnes, R., Tenenhouse, H., Reade, T. and Glorieux, F. H. The further delineation of acquired vitamin D deficiency, autosomal recessive vitamin D dependency and X-linked hypophosphatemia, in Talmage, R. V., Owen, M. and Parsons, J. A. (Eds.), Calcium-Regulating Hormones. Proceedings of the Fifth Parathyroid Conference. Excerpta Medica, ICS 346, Amsterdam, 1975, p. 421.

56. Talwalkar, Y. B., Musgrave, J. E., Buist, N. R. M., Campbell, R. A. and Campbell, J. R. Vitamin D-resistant rickets and parathyroid adenomas. *Am. J. Dis. Child 128:* 704, 1974.

57. Scriver, C. R., Glorieux, F. H., Reade, T. M. and Tenenhouse, H. S. X-linked hypophosphatemia and autosomal recessive vitamin D dependency. Models for the resolution of vitamin-D-refractory rickets. Edited by J. Stern. Soc. Study Inborn Errors Metab. Sympos. No. 12. Churchill-Livingstone, Edinburgh, 1975.

58. Wilson, D. R. Personal communication, 1975.

59. Wilson, D. R., York, S. E., Jaworski, Z. F. and Yendt, E. R. Studies in hypophosphatemic vitamin D-refractory osteomalacia in adults. Oral phosphate supplements as an adjunct to therapy. *Medicine (Balt.) 44:* 99, 1965.

60. Borle, A. B. Calcium metabolism at the cellular level. *Fed. Proc. 32:* 1944, 1973.

61. Fraser, D. Treatment of rickets, in Conn, H. F. (Ed.), Current Therapy. W. B. Saunders Co., Philadelphia, 1972, p. 407.

62. Parfitt, A. M. Hypophosphatemic vitamin D-refractory rickets and osteomalacia. *Orthop. Clin. North Am. 3:* 653, 1972.

63. Fraser, D., Geiger, D. W., Munn, J. D., Slater, P. E., Jahn, R., and Liu, E. Calcification studies in clinical vitamin D deficiency and in hypophosphatemic vitamin D-refractory rickets: The induction of calcium deposition in rachitic cartilage without the administration of vitamin D. *Am. J. Dis. Child. 96:* 460, 1958 (abstract).

64. Stickler, G. B., Hayles, A. B. and Rosevear, J. W. Familial hypophosphatemic vitamin D-resistant rickets. *Am. J. Dis. Child. 110:* 664, 1965.

65. Nigrin, G., Cochrane, W. A., Janigan, D. and Ernst, A. Results of calcium infusion and renal biopsy studies in refractory rickets. *Am. J. Dis. Child 104:* 478, 1962 (abstract).

66. Paunier, L., Kooh, S. W., Conen, P. E., Gibson, A. A. M. and Fraser, D. Renal function and histology after long-term vitamin D therapy of vitamin D refractory rickets. *J. Pediatr. 73:* 833, 1968.

67. Glorieux, F. H., Scriver, C. R., Holick, M. F. and DeLuca, H. F. X-linked hypophosphatemic rickets. Inadequate therapeutic response to 1,25-dihydroxycholecalciferol. *Lancet 2:* 287, 1973.

68. Glorieux, F. H., Scriver, C. R., Reade, T. M., Goldman, H. and Roseborough, A. Use of phosphate and vitamin D to prevent dwarfism and rickets in X-linked hypophosphatemia. *N. Engl. J. Med. 287:* 481, 1972.

69. Lilly, C. A., Peirce, C. B. and Grant, R. L. The effects of phosphates on the bones of rachitic rats. *J. Nutr. 9:* 25, 1935.

70. Steendijk, R. The effect of a continuous intravenous infusion of inorganic phosphate on the rachitic lesions in cystinosis. *Arch. Dis. Child 36:* 321, 1961.

71. Scriver, C. R., Goldbloom, R. B. and Roy C. C. Hypophosphatemic rickets with renal hyperglycinuria, renal glucosuria and glycylprolinuria. A syndrome with evidence for renal tubular secretion of phosphorus. *Pediatrics 34:* 357, 1964.

72. Fraser, D. and Kooh, S. W. (unreported data).

73. Frame, B., Smith, R. W., Jr., Fleming, J. L. and Manson, G. Oral phosphates in vitamin D-refractory rickets and osteomalacia. *Am. J. Dis. Child. 106:* 147, 1963.

74. Clow, C., Reade, T. and Scriver, C. R. Management of hereditary metabolic disease. The role of allied health personnel. *N. Engl. J. Med. 284:* 1292, 1971

75. Reiss, E. and Canterbury, J. M. The effects of phosphate on parathyroid hormone secretion, in Talmage, R. V., Owen, M. and Parsons, J.

A. (Eds.), Calcium-Regulating Hormones. Proceeds of the Fifth Parathyroid Conference, Excerpta Medica, ICS 346, Amsterdam, 1975, p. 66.

76. West, C. D., Blanton, J. C., Silverman, F. N. and Holland, N. H. Use of phosphate salts as an adjunct to vitamin D in the treatment of hypophosphatemic vitamin D refractory rickets. *J. Pediatr. 64:* 469, 1964.

APPENDIX I: SOME HIGH-POTENCY VITAMIN-D_2 PREPARATIONS IN LIQUID FORM

Radiostol Liquid (Allen & Hanbury), 100,000 IU vit D_2 per milliliter.

Drisdol (Winthrop), 10,000 IU vit D_2 per milliliter.

Calciferol (Kremers-Urban), 500,000 IU vit D_2 per milliliter (should be diluted to 100,000 IU/ml before dispensing).

APPENDIX II: PHOSPHATE SUPPLEMENTS FOR ORAL ADMINISTRATION IN X-LINKED HYPOPHOSPHATEMIA

ACIDIC PHOSPHATE (JOULIE'S SOLUTION)

Ingredients:

Dibasic sodium phosphate (Na_2HPO_4 $7H_2O$, reagent grade)	102.0 g
Phosphoric acid (NF 85 percent)	58.80 g
Distilled water to	1000 ml

Dissolve the phosphate salt in approx. 750 ml warm water, to which has been added the phosphoric acid. Make the solution up to 1 liter with distilled water. Store at room temperature.

The concentration of phosphorus in this solution is 2.76 g/100 ml; the pH is 4.3. The solution is often better accepted than neutral phosphate solution. It can be flavored to the child's preference. When taken between meals and at bedtime, it should be followed immediately by a drink of the patient's choice (100–200 ml).

NEUTRAL PHOSPHATE SOLUTION

Ingredients:

$NaH_2PO_4 \cdot H_2O$ reagent grade	18.2 g
$Na_2HPO_4 \cdot 7H_2O$ reagent grade	145.0 g
Distilled water to	1000 ml

Mix the phosphate salts and dispense in dry form as packets. The parent should dissolve the packet of salts in distilled water by gentle warming. Store at 4°C in refrigerator. Shake well if precipitate forms. Each batch lasts several days.

The concentration of phosphorus in this solution is 2.08 g/100 ml: the pH is neutral.

PROPRIETARY FORMULATIONS

Phosphate-Sandoz (Sandoz). Each effervescent tablet provides 0.50 g phosphorus as the Na and K salts.

Neutra-Phos (Willen). When the powder or capsule is dissolved as instructed, the concentration of phosphorus (as the Na and K salts) is 0.33 g/100 ml.

67

Acquired (Noninherited) Disorders of Vitamin D Function

Theodore J. Hahn
Louis V. Avioli

ANTICONVULSANT-DRUG-INDUCED OSTEOMALACIA

Recently, it has become apparent that chronic administration of a variety of drugs can produce significant disorders in vitamin D, mineral, and bone metabolism. The one factor common to all of these agents is that they are potent inducers of hepatic microsomal mixed-oxidase activity. The clinical abnormalities most commonly seen include hypocalcemia, elevated serum bone alkaline phosphatase, reduced serum levels of biologically active vitamin D metabolites, and radiographic changes of rickets and/or osteomalacia. Histologic examination in such cases reveals osteomalacia and varying degrees of increased osteoclastic activity. Although the anticonvulsant drugs have been most commonly implicated in this disorder, various agents appear to have the potential to produce osteomalacia.

The earliest reports of anticonvulsant osteomalacia appeared in the European literature. In retrospect, this may have been partly a function of the generally lower levels of vitamin D intake and sunlight exposure in certain European populations. In 1968, Kruse reported hypocalcemic and radiologic evidence of rickets in 15 percent of a German pediatric outpatient population.[1] Subsequently, English investigators reported hypocalcemia in 23–30 percent of institutionalized adult and pediatric epileptic patients receiving long-term anticonvulsant drug therapy.[2,3] More recently, this disorder has been reported in epileptic populations throughout the world, with the incidence of hypocalcemia, clinical evidence of osteomalacia, or deficient bone mineral content varying from 4 to 75 percent depending on the population studied and the level of sensitivity of the diagnostic techniques employed.[4–9] The clinical severity of drug-induced osteomalacia varies considerably, ranging from subclinical decreases in bone mass, detectable only by the most sensitive techniques, to marked hypocalcemia and severe osteopenia with multiple, recurrent bone fractures.

PATHOPHYSIOLOGY

For a number of years it has been known that many drugs, including virtually all of the common anticonvulsants and many of the major and minor tranquilizers, are capable of inducing hepatic microsomal mixed oxidase enzyme activity.[10] Since steroids share the hepatic microsomal degradation pathways with foreign substances, induction of these enzyme systems leads to an increased catabolism of a variety of steroid hormones, which results in accelerated production of polar, hydroxylated biologically inactive products that are eliminated in the bile and urine. This has been particularly well demonstrated in the case of estrogens, progesterone, and corticosteroids.[9]

In the presence of an intact hypothalamic–pituitary axis, normal feedback control mechanisms increase the endogenous production of steroid hormones so that normal levels of biologically active hormones are maintained. This feedback control system almost certainly explains why clinical evidence of drug-induced deficiencies of adrenal and gonadal steroids have not been reported. On the other hand, chronic administration of hepatic microsomal-inducing agents, particularly phenobarbital and diphenylhydantoin, significantly reduces the biologic effects of *exogenously* administered steroid hormones.[11,12] Since vitamin D and its biologically active metabolites bear a structural similarity to the steroid hormones, it has become apparent that the vitamin D sterols are at risk of sharing a similar fate.

Vitamin D activity in man is derived from two sources: (1) vitamin D_2 (ergocalciferol), produced synthetically from the irradiation of 7-dehydroergocalciferol, and (2) vitamin D_3 (cholecalciferol), the naturally occurring form, derived from solar ultraviolet irradiation of 7-dehydrocholesterol in the skin and from ingestion of vitamin D_3-containing animal and fish oils. Vitamin D_2 is the form generally contained in multivitamin preparations and vitamin-supplemented foods, and in the United States accounts for the major portion of vitamin D intake. Both forms appear to have equal biologic activity in man. Although vitamin D metabolite production is subject to some degree of product feedback control at the level of the hepatic vitamin-D-25-hydroxylase system and a greater degree of control at the level of renal 1-hydroxylation, under conditions of deficient vitamin D intake, diminished cutaneous production, or increased metabolite utilization, this renal feedback regulation is often inadequate to maintain normal levels of biologically active vitamin D metabolites, and a clinical state of vitamin D deficiency occurs.

Anticonvulsant drugs do not appear to interfere with the intestinal absorption of vitamin D.[13] However, in man and animals, chronic anticonvulsant drug therapy is associated with a marked decrease in the plasma half-life of vitamin D and an increased appearance of polar metabolites other than the known biologically active products.[14,15] Additionally, in animals, chronic administration of phenobarbital increases in vivo liver microsomal uptake and metabolism of vitamin D,[16] enhances biliary excretion of vitamin D metabolites, and accelerates in vitro liver microsomal catabolism of vitamin D, 25-hydroxycholecalciferol ($25\text{-}OH\text{-}D_3$), and 1,25-dihydroxycholecalciferol ($1,25\text{-}(OH)_2D_3$) to polar inactive products.[14,15] In view of these observations it would appear likely that chronic anticonvulsant-drug therapy should lead to decreased body levels of vitamin D metabolites through increased liver microsomal catabolism. Not surprisingly, significant reductions in serum levels of 25-OH-D have been repeatedly demonstrated in patients receiving chronic anticonvulsant-drug therapy.[4,5,17,18] Serum calcium levels in these patients show a direct correlation with serum 25-OH-D levels.[4,5] Moreover, concomitant with the decrease in serum calcium, there is an appropriate secondary increase in serum parathyroid hormone (PTH) levels.[18] Thus, drug-induced increased catabolism of vitamin D and its metabolites most certainly plays a major role in the production of anticonvulsant osteomalacia.

However, recent evidence suggests that the anticonvulsant drugs may also have direct effects on mineral and bone metabolism independent of their effects on vitamin D. This is particularly true in the case of diphenylhydantoin, which has been demonstrated to alter ion transport across cell membranes by virtue of its effect on membrane-bound ATPase transport systems. For example, when diphenylhydantoin is administered to rats in doses that do not appear to alter vitamin D metabolism, there is significant inhibition of intestinal calcium absorption, while comparable doses of phenobarbital do not produce this effect.[19] Additionally, both diphenylhydantoin and phenobarbital have been shown to have direct effects on bone calcium mobilization and bone response to PTH, calcitonin, and $1,25\text{-}(OH)_2D_3$.[20,21]

Based on current knowledge, it appears that anticonvulsant drugs produce their deleterious effects on mineral and bone metabolism through at least two mechanisms: (1) a dose-related stimulation of hepatic mixed oxidase microsomal enzyme systems, resulting in increased catabolism and excretion of vitamin D and its biologically active products, a consequent decrease in intestinal calcium absorption, and, as a result, decreased serum calcium levels, secondary hyperparathyroidism, and decreased availability of mineral to calcify bone; and (2) direct inhibitory effects on intestinal calcium transport and bone metabolism.

CLINICAL FEATURES

It might be considered surprising that although the anticonvulsant drugs have been widely employed for many years it is only recently that their adverse effect on mineral metabolism became apparent. Certainly, increased awareness of the existence of the disorder partly accounts for the recent burgeoning of reported cases. However, the primary factor in the delayed awareness of anticonvulsant osteomalacia probably reflects the broad spectrum of clinical presentation.

An occasional patient will present the full-blown clinical picture: a history of repeated bone fractures, physical findings of rickets with bone deformities (in children), hypocalcemia, hypophosphatemia, and radiographic signs of rickets (in children) or severe osteopenia with pseudofractures (in adults). Even more rarely, a patient may experience a significant *increase* in seizure frequency with the institution of higher doses of anticonvulsant drugs, presumably due to increased neuromuscular instability resulting from progressive hypocalcemia.[22] Occasionally, proximal myopathy similar to that seen in other forms of severe vitamin D deficiency may occur.[23,24] The basis for the myopathy is unclear, but it may be related to the fact that vitamin D metabolites appear to play an important role in the maintenance of intracellular phosphate concentrations required to maintain normal ATP levels in muscle.[25]

On the other hand, the usual patient has a much more subtle presentation: bone symptoms may be minimal or absent; serum calcium, phosphate, and alkaline phosphatase levels in a random blood specimen may be within the normal range; and routine radiographs may fail to detect any bone abnormalities. In most large series, the *mean* reduction in serum calcium in groups of anticonvulsant-treated patients as compared to control subjects averages 0.3–0.8 mg/dl, with the incidence of frank hypocalcemia varying from 4 to 30 percent and the incidence of elevated serum alkaline phosphatase levels ranging between 24 and 40 percent.[1-9,17] Serum phosphate levels are occasionally reduced but often lie within the normal range.

However, with the recent development of more sensitive means of detecting abnormalities in vitamin D and bone metabolism, significant derangements in mineral metabolism have been found in the group of patients who do *not* manifest obvious biochemical abnormalities. Serum 25-OH-D levels in randomly selected anticonvulsant-treated patients are routinely reduced by 40–70 percent when compared to matched controls.[4,5,17] The use of photon-absorption bone-mass measurements has also led to increased detection of osteopenia in these populations. Whereas routine radiographic techniques cannot detect a reduction in bone mass less than 30–50 percent, the photon-absorption technique has an accuracy of 4 percent in the estimation of bone loss.[26] Using photon-absorption measurements, mean bone mass in various epileptic populations routinely shows a 10–30 percent reduction from age-normal values.[5,27,28]

RISK FACTORS

The above figures represent mean values from large population surveys. However, within any group of anticonvulsant-treated patients there are wide variations in the severity of the disorder. It has become apparent that there are a number of risk factors predisposing to increased severity of drug-induced mineral disorders. The more important factors are discussed below.

Drug Dose and Duration of Therapy

Multiple-drug regimens have been demonstrated to produce more severe reductions in serum calcium, serum 25-OH-D, and bone mass than do single-drug regimens. Moreover, the larger the total daily dose of drug, the more severe the derangements in mineral metabolism.[3-5] Additionally, the incidence of abnormalities increases with duration of therapy, with significant changes in mineral parameters being observed after as little as 6 months of treatment.[7,8] Early reports suggested that there was a definite relationship between drug type and the severity of induced abnormalities, with Pheneturide, primidone, diphenylhydantoin, and phenobarbital ranked in decreasing order of potency.[3] These initial observations are yet to be specifically confirmed. However, considering the varying potency of drugs in inducing hepatic microsomal oxidases and the additional factor of potential direct effects on membrane transport of ions and amino acids, it is likely that various agents *do* differ in their ability to derange mineral metabolism. At present all that can be said with certainty is that all of the commonly used anticonvulsant drugs have been implicated in the production of anticonvulsant osteomalacia and that their effect increases with increasing dosage.

Vitamin D Intake

It has been shown that serum 25-OH-D levels correlate positively with vitamin D intake in normal subjects and patients on anticonvulsant drugs.[4,5] However, at any given level of vitamin D intake, serum 25-OH-D levels are lower in patients receiving anticonvulsant drugs, with the degree of reduction depending on dose of drugs[4,5] received (Fig. 67-1). Conversely, at any given drug dose level, the lower the mean daily intake of vitamin D, the more likely is the development of clinical manifestations of vitamin D deficiency. Comparisons of serum 25-OH-D levels in anticonvulsant-treated and control subjects suggest that multiple-drug regimens increase the intake of vitamin D required to maintain normal 25-OH-D levels by 400–1000 IU/day.[4,5] The changes in levels of other vitamin D metabolites are currently unknown but presumably follow a similar pattern.

Sunlight Exposure

The major source of vitamin D activity in man is sunlight exposure with conversion of cutaneous 7-dehydrocholesterol to vitamin D_3. In situations in which exposure to solar irradiation is limited, the risk of significant vitamin D deficiency is increased. Thus, biochemical and radiographic evidence of drug-induced osteomalacia is more common in institutionalized patients confined indoors than in patients with adequate sunlight exposure.[3,9] Even among outpatients, in whom the incidence of detectable abnormalities is usually lower, individuals with limited sunlight exposure have significantly lower serum calcium and 25-OH-D levels than do those who habitually spend much of their time outdoors (Fig. 67-2).[4] Additionally, serum 25-OH-D levels may be slightly lower in blacks than in whites with similar sunlight exposure, presumably because of decreased penetration of solar ultraviolet irradiation to the stratum granulosum layer of the skin where 7-dehydrocholesterol is converted to vitamin D_3.[4]

An additional consideration in persons living in the temperate zone is the seasonal change in vitamin D levels. Serum 25-OH-D levels are highest in the summer months, when sunlight exposure is maximum, and fall to lowest levels in the late winter.[29] This correlates well with the observation that the highest incidence of nutritional rickets occurs in the winter months.[30] Therefore, it is logical to assume that in susceptible patients receiving anticonvulsant therapy, the time of greatest risk for deranged mineral metabolism is during the winter.

Physical Activity

The most potent known stimulator of bone formation in adults is physical stress, which appears to act through induction of piezoelectric forces in bone, resulting in increased osteoblastic activity. Enforced immobilization markedly decreases bone-forming activity with a resultant negative calcium balance and loss of bone mass. Even lesser degrees of immobilization, such as the limitation of activity occurring with advanced rheumatoid arthritis, produce significant generalized decreases in bone mass readily detectable by photon-absorption densitometry.[31] Thus, it is not

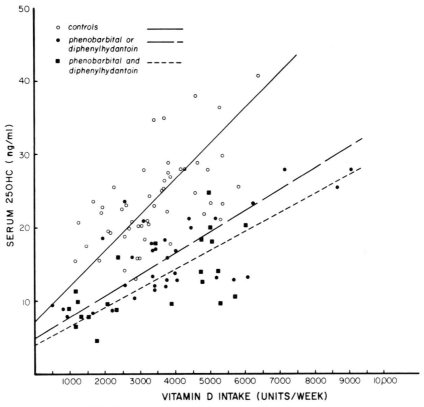

Fig. 67-1. Serum 25-hydroxycholecalciferol (25OHD) concentration vs. vitamin D intake in normals and patients receiving single or combined anticonvulsant-drug therapy. (From Hahn, T. J., Hendin, B. A., Scharp, C. R., et al. Serum 25-hydroxycalciferol levels and bone mass in children on chronic anticonvulsant therapy. *New Eng. J. Med 292:* 550–554, 1975.

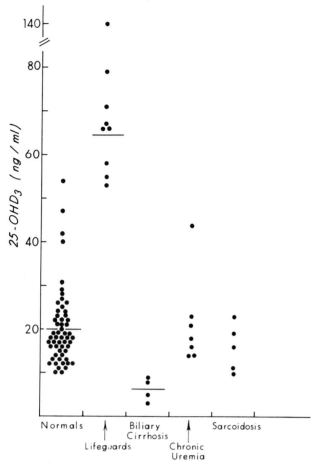

Fig. 67-2. Plasma 25OHD levels in patients with disorders of hepatic and renal function. Note the effect of sunlight exposure also (i.e. lifeguards).

surprising that radiographic evidence of bone disorders is most severe in nonambulatory patients.[9] Indeed, a significant portion of the osteopenia seen in many patients with seizure disorders may be the result of decreased physical activity due to the sedative effect of anticonvulsant drugs and/or associated neurologic disorders.

Coexisting Diseases

Disorders that interfere with the normal absorption, biologic activation, or end-organ localization of the vitamin D sterols predispose to disordered mineral metabolism. Thus, patients with fat malabsorption, liver disease (see below), or decreased functional renal mass (see below) are more prone to develop vitamin-D-deficiency syndromes, and the concurrence of such disorders with anticonvulsant-drug therapy would increase the likelihood of clinically significant bone disease. Additionally, it has been reported that severe recurrent infections may alter the response to vitamin D and thereby produce increased risk of severe mineral disorders in drug-treated patients.[9]

Individual Susceptibility

Certain individuals receiving anticonvulsant drugs appear to have disproportionately severe disorders of mineral metabolism, even when the above factors are taken into consideration. It has been suggested that increased susceptibility to drug induction of liver microsomal enzymes or differing basal drug-degradation rates may be operative in these individuals. Although there is ample precedent for individual variations in rates of hepatic drug metabo-

lism and enzyme induction, the role of this factor in anticonvulsant osteomalacia remains speculative.

DIAGNOSIS AND MANAGEMENT

The most important aid in the diagnosis of anticonvulsant osteomalacia is a high index of suspicion. As a preliminary step the physician determines if there are high-risk factors present (multiple-drug regimens, poor vitamin D intake, limited sunlight exposure, etc.), and the patient should be questioned about bone pain, fractures, and worsening seizure control associated with increased drug dose.

The most sensitive means of rapidly establishing the diagnosis of drug-induced osteomalacia are measurements of serum 25-OH-D and determination of bone mass by photon-absorption densitometry. Where these techniques are not available, one has to rely on more conventional diagnostic techniques. Serum calcium, phosphorus, and alkaline phosphatase should be determined on multiple occasions. When the mean serum calcium and phosphorus values are at or below the lower limits of normal, a significant derangement of mineral metabolism is likely. An elevated serum alkaline phosphatase per se does not unequivocally indicate osteomalacia, since *liver* alkaline phosphatase levels can rise rapidly after initiation of anticonvulsant therapy at a time when bone alkaline phosphatase is normal.[4] However, at the very least, an elevated alkaline phosphatase indicates hepatic enzyme induction and should be an indication for more intensive investigation of the patient's mineral and skeletal status. A carefully collected 24-hour-urine calcium can be a sensitive diagnostic aid, since urinary calcium excretion is in essence an integral of the serum ionized-calcium level and additionally reflects the effects of PTH on calcium resorption at the renal tubule. Urinary calcium excretion of less than 80 mg/24 hours in an adult on a normal (600–800 mg) calcium intake is good presumptive evidence of decreased intestinal calcium absorption. In children, values must be related to normal levels for age.

When there is reason to suspect a drug-induced disorder of mineral metabolism, the patient should be carefully examined for radiographic evidence of bone disease. In children, one should search for evidence of demineralization and the epiphyseal changes of rickets; in adults the suggestive findings include demineralization, multiple old fractures (often poorly healed), and pseudofractures. A very useful confirmatory aid is a needle bone biopsy under local anesthesia with the patient prelabeled with tetracycline, 250 mg four times per day for 2 days prior to biopsy.[32] Undecalcified bone sections are then examined for the presence of increased osteoid tissue and increased osteoclastic activity.[3] However, in many cases of severe disease the diagnosis can be established by the other techniques described above.

TREATMENT

Overt Disease

In patients with clinically obvious bone disease a variety of regimens have been employed. Christiansen and co-workers have reported that vitamin D in doses of 2000–4000 U/day in combination with 400 mg calcium/day for 3 months produces a 3–5 percent increase in bone mass as measured by photon-absorption densitometry in various groups of pediatric and adult patients with drug-induced osteomalacia.[27,33] Additionally, it has been suggested that vitamin D in a dose of 4000 U/day can significantly reduce seizure incidence in patients with drug-induced mineral disorders presumably by normalizing serum ionized-calcium levels.[34] Although it has been suggested that vitamins D_2 and D_3 may differ in their therapeutic efficacy in this disorder, this remains to be confirmed.[33] On the other hand, other investigators have reported that vitamin D$_2$ in doses of 2000–6000 U/day for as long as 7 months may be ineffective in healing bone lesions, while 15,000 U/day for 10 weeks may produce significant healing.[35]

Several authors have suggested that 25-OH-D in relatively smaller doses (100–2000 U/day) may be more rapidly effective than vitamin D. This suggestion has some theoretical basis since serum 25-OH-D levels are much more rapidly increased by 25-OH-D than by vitamin D administration[36] and 25-OH-D administration bypasses the requirement for hepatic accumulation and metabolism of vitamin D.

However, in the current state of the art, vitamin D and calcium supplementation are the mainstays of therapy. In adults with clinically or radiologically apparent bone disease and/or definite hypocalcemia, an initial dose of 50,000–75,000 U of vitamin D (50,000 U/m^2 surface body area) per *week* in divided doses plus 500 mg of supplemental calcium per day should be maintained for a period of 4–6 months. In children, doses are reduced according to body area. After normalization of biochemical and radiographic parameters (serum 25-OH-D, bone mass, serum and urine calcium) patients can then be maintained on approximately 10,000 U of vitamin D per week. When this regimen is employed it is essential to follow serum and urine calcium levels carefully so that vitamin D and calcium supplementation can be adjusted to individual requirements and inadvertent vitamin D overdosage can be avoided.

Prophylactic Treatment

There is a considerable controversy as to whether vitamin D supplementation should be given to all patients receiving anticonvulsant-drug therapy, even when gross parameters of mineral metabolism are normal. The potential objections to this approach include the economic burden of chronic vitamin D supplementation and the ever-present possibility of inadvertent overdosage. On the other hand, in many institutions the single most costly medical problem in seizure patients is the treatment of pathologic bone fractures due to demineralization of bone. Additionally, since bone mass progressively decreases with age after the third decade,[37] the combined effects of drug-induced demineralization and the aging process lead to an increase in clinically significant osteopenia in older patients who have been maintained on anticonvulsant drugs throughout life.

If one accepts the premise that prophylactic vitamin D supplementation is of value, the question arises as to when therapy should be initiated. It has been reported that a decrease in bone mass can be demonstrated in patients who have received anticonvulsant therapy for 1 year or less,[27] and Liakakos et al.[6] have reported that administration of vitamin D 4000 U/day concomitant with the initiation of anticonvulsant therapy prevents the pathologic rise in serum alkaline phosphatase and urinary hydroxyproline seen in patients not supplemented with vitamin D. It has been the general experience that significant reductions in serum 25-OH-D and elevations in bone alkaline phosphatase generally occur only after 6 months or more of therapy. Additionally, preliminary animal data suggest that a brief paradoxical rise in serum 25-OH-D occurs after initiation of drug therapy, presumably due to a temporary competitive block of catabolic pathways.[38] Therefore, the most reasonable current approach is to recommend prophylactic vitamin D supplementation (10,000 U/week) only in patients who have been on therapy for 6 months or longer. Additionally, the dose of supplemental vitamin D must always be individually adjusted on the basis of individual requirements and response.

STEROID-INDUCED OSTEOPENIA

Since the original description of Cushing's syndrome, it has been recognized that chronically maintained supraphysiologic levels of corticosteroids can produce severe bone loss.[39,40] Radiographic and histologic studies of patients with Cushing's syndrome have shown that the great majority have severe loss of bone mass.[40,41] Furthermore, the bone changes have a characteristic distribution; the osteopenia is more severe in those regions of the skeleton having a high content of trabecular bone (vertebrae, ribs) and is less striking in the long bones, which are predominantly cortical.[39–41] Consequently, rib fractures and compression deformities of vertebrae are common occurrences in patients with steroid-induced osteopenia.

It is not surprising, therefore, that the administration of supraphysiologic doses of exogenous corticosteroids or corticotropin often produces clinically significant bone loss. This problem has been noted by many investigators, most of whom have emphasized the high incidence of vertebral compression fractures in children and adults treated with corticosteroids.[42–44] The incidence of *symptomatic* steroid-induced osteopenia seems to be highest in children and in women over 50.[43,44] In the former group a high initial bone turnover rate seems to be the predisposing factor; in the latter group, the relatively low initial bone mass can rapidly be reduced to levels of clinically significant osteopenia. Numerous recent studies have clarified the physiologic basis of steroid-induced osteopenia, and these advances have in turn suggested new means of decreasing the severity of the disorder.

Histologic studies of bone after prolonged corticosteroid administration have demonstrated both decreased bone formation and increased resorption, the latter manifested by increased osteoclast number, activity, and resorption sites.[45,46] The decrease in formation rate has generally been attributed to direct corticosteroid inhibition of osteoblast function. This view is supported by the demonstration that moderate doses of steroids decrease both the synthesis of bone collagen by preexisting osteoblasts and the conversion of precursor cells to functioning osteoblasts.[45–49] This is apparently a direct steroid effect since addition of cortisone to bone cells in culture markedly reduces protein synthesis.[49]

Increased bone resorption rates following moderate-dose steroid administration have been variously attributed to either direct stimulation of osteoclast activity or an indirect effect mediated by increased parathyroid secretion. However, it has been shown that corticosteroids do not directly stimulate bone resorption in vitro.[50] Furthermore, parathyroidectomy totally abolishes the osteoclastic response to corticosteroids in animals.[51] Finally, it has recently been demonstrated that chronic corticosteroid administration in man is associated with elevated serum PTH levels.[31,52] This appears to be due, at least in part, to the decreased intestinal calcium absorption produced by corticosteroid administration.[53,54]

The basis of the steroid-induced reduction in intestinal calcium absorption remains controversial. Initial studies of this phenomenon suggested that corticosteroid therapy might impair the conversion of vitamin D to 25-OH-D in man.[55] However, subsequent studies in animals demonstrated that cortisone administration does not alter either the conversion of vitamin D to 25-OH-D or the conversion of 25-OH-D to 1,25(OH)$_2$D.[56,57] Moreover, we have recently demostrated that serum 25-OH-D concentrations in patients with steroid-induced osteopenia are identical to those in matched non-steroid-treated subjects.[58] Thus, if steroids do indeed impair vitamin D metabolism, the alterations must occur at a point subsequent to the formation of 25-OH-D.

Recent animal studies have suggested that massive doses of

delta-1-prednisone in the rat may decrease 1,25-$(OH)_2$D formation.[59] However, the relevance of this observation to vitamin D states in patients receiving moderate doses of corticosteroids is uncertain. Moreover, recent studies have suggested that patients receiving corticosteroid therapy may have elevated 1,25-$(OH)_2$D levels,[60] which would be an appropriate response to their state of secondary hyperparathyroidism.[31,52]

Therefore, based on currently available data, the most probable explanation for the steroid-induced decrease in intestinal calcium absorption is that corticosteroids directly inhibit intestinal calcium transport processes, possibly through decreased synthesis of a carrier protein. Thus, current evidence strongly suggests that the mechanism of corticosteroid-induced osteopenia is (1) direct inhibition of bone formation and (2) indirect stimulation of bone resorption through inhibition of intestinal calcium absorption with a consequent increase in PTH secretion.

Based upon the higher hormone responsiveness of trabecular relative to cortical bone, it would be predicted that skeletal areas with a high trabecular bone content would be the first to exhibit radiographic changes in patients with corticosteroid excess. Indeed, in patients with Cushing's syndrome, trabecular thinning and loss in the vertebral bodies, followed by compression fracture, is one of the earliest radiographic findings. Precise quantitation of the relationship between cortical and trabecular bone is not possible by routine radiographic techniques. However, with the increased precision afforded by photon-absorption bone-mass measurements,[37] such comparisons have recently become feasible.

The relationship between cortical and trabecular bone mass has been examined in a variety of demineralizing disorders using photon-absorption measurement of bone mass in the radius at a midshaft point composed primarily of cortical bone and at a distal point 3 cm from the radial head, which contains a relatively high proportion of trabecular bone.[37] The midshaft and distal measurements (MM and DM, respectively) are expressed as g/cm^2.

In patients with senile osteoporosis and rheumatoid arthritis not treated with steroids, bone mass in the diaphyseal and metaphyseal sites is decreased to a similar degree (Fig. 67-1). However, steroid treatment in patients with rheumatoid arthritis and nonrheumatic disorders produced a strikingly greater loss at the metaphyseal (trabecular) site. This pattern of increased metaphyseal loss mimics that seen in patients with primary hyperparathyroidism or secondary hyperparathyroidism due to intestinal malabsorption syndromes.[37] It should be noted that despite similar steroid doses, patients with rheumatoid arthritis had a greater degree of bone loss at both the diaphyseal and metaphyseal sites. This presumably reflects the additive effects of relative immobilization osteoporosis. There is not a greater bone loss in females, when adjusted for age–sex norms in steroid-treated females, indicating the *absence* of a sex predilection per se for steroid-induced bone loss. Thus the increased incidence of symptomatic steroid-induced osteopenia in women very probably reflects their lower initial bone mass.[61] A definite relationship can be demonstrated between duration of corticosteroid therapy and the degree of reduction in bone mass.[37] Despite similar daily steroid doses, patients who have been treated for more than 3 years show a greater DM and MM loss, and a greater disproportion between DM and MM than do patients treated for 1–3 years.

Having defined some of the basic physiologic changes in steroid osteopenia, the question of prevention and reversibility arises. Improved radiographic bone density and histologic evidence of increased bone formation have been observed in patients with Cushing's syndrome following adrenalectomy.[40,62] Moreover, we have observed histologic evidence of a striking "rebound"

increase in osteoblastic function and new bone formation in several patients following cessation of steroid therapy.[63] Presumably, this reflects a normal response of the osteoblast to increased stress stimulation in weakened bone after release from steroid inhibition.

Translating these observations into practical patient management terms is difficult. Obviously, discontinuation of steroid therapy would be beneficial to the skeletal system but is often impossible. Maintaining the steroid dose at the lowest possible level should theoretically be helpful. Recent animal data suggest that alternate-day steroid regimens may produce less severe bone loss than do daily regimens.[64] However, this remains to be conclusively demonstrated in man. Aside from these measures one would like to have a more direct way of stimulating bone formation and/or decreasing bone resorption; however, increasing an individual's level of physical activity is currently the only practical way of stimulating bone formation and there are obvious limits to this modality. On the other hand, since the increased bone resorptive activity in steroid osteopenia appears to be the result of a secondary hyperparathyroidism resulting from steroid inhibition of intestinal cacium absorption, it should be theoretically possible to suppress bone resorption by stimulating intestinal calcium absorption and thereby normalizing PTH activity.

There are recent data to suggest that this approach is feasible. A regimen of vitamin D 50,000 U three times weekly plus calcium 500 mg/day has been shown to suppress serum immunoreactive PTH (iPTH) concentrations to normal levels and produce a significant increase in trabecular bone mass over a 1-year period in a group of steroid-treated patients as compared to a matched group of nonsupplemented controls.[31] Similarly, 25-OH-D at a dose of 40–60 μg/day has been shown to rapidly increase intestinal calcium absorption to near-normal levels, normalize serum iPTH, reverse bone histologic evidence of increased osteoclastic activity, and produce significant increases in trabecular and cortical bone mass.[31]

These results strongly indicate that stimulation of intestinal calcium resorption can suppress PTH secretion, decrease bone resorption, and produce a net increase in bone mass. Several questions remain, however. First, will the effects of such treatment produce lasting, clinically significant effects? Since bone formation and resorption are often "coupled," a reduction in resorption rate might ultimately result in a parallel reduction in formation. On the other hand, steroid osteopenia is itself an "uncoupled" state with resorption rates greater than formation rates. Suppression of resorption would thus restore a more normal equilibrium. The question of clinical effects remains to be answered by large-scale controlled clinical trials. However, the well-established relationship between measured bone mass and fracture risk[65] suggests that improving bone mass is very likely to reduce the risk of pathologic fracture.

Second, should high-risk patients be started on supplementation at the time steroid therapy is begun? Although the current data strongly suggest that the *average* risk of fracture, as measured by loss of bone mass, increases with duration of therapy,[37] the response of an individual patients is much less predictable. Although we are inclined to favor prophylactic supplementation (e.g., in premenopausal white females with subnormal basal bone mass and a family history of clinical osteopenia), its effectiveness remains to be proven. Moreover, it should be remembered that supplementation with vitamin D or its metabolites carries the risk of intoxication and potentially serious renal and vascular damage. Although adverse side effects have not been observed in patients treated with vitamin D or 25-OH-D as outlined above, frequent careful monitoring of serum and urine calcium levels must be maintained.

Accumulated data would suggest that high-risk patients in whom steroid-induced osteopenia is documented may benefit from regimens designed to stimulate intestinal calcium absorption. Currently, vitamin D 50,000 IU 2–3 times weekly plus supplemental calcium (500 mg/day) appears to be a reasonable regimen. When 25(OH)D becomes commercially available it would appear to be the agent of choice. Whichever regimen is used, monitoring of serum and urine calcium at 1–2-month intervals is essential to avoid inadvertent intoxication.

VITAMIN D DEFICIENCY AND BONE DISEASE ASSOCIATED WITH CHRONIC RENAL FAILURE

It has been demonstrated with biologic assay techniques that vitamin D activity (i.e., antirachitic activity) in the serum of untreated patients with chronic uremia is lower than that observed in either a well-fed, healthy population or in malnourished individuals with terminal cachexia.[66,67] In addition, patients with acute rapidly progressive[68] or terminal uremia[66] require a greater intake of vitamin D and higher levels of assayable antirachitic activity for biologic effectiveness than do normal individuals. This well-recognized phenomenon of vitamin D resistance in renal failure has been variably attributed to uremic toxins interfering with the normal production of biologically active vitamin D metabolites, or to the response of the end organs (i.e., bone and intestine) to these metabolites. Studies with radioactive isotopic forms of vitamin D[69,70] and 25-OH-D[70–72] in subjects with renal failure, anephric animals,[73,74] and animals with experimentally induced chronic renal failure[75] have stressed the loss of renal parenchyma rather than the loss of renal excretory function as the primary cause for the malabsorption of calcium. It appears logical to assume that a reduction in functioning renal mass would result in decreased 1,25-$(OH)_2D$ synthesis and a subsequent reduction in the intestinal mucosal concentration of 1,25-$(OH)_2D$. Results demonstrating that small doses of 1,25-$(OH)_2D$ augment calcium absorption and raise the serum calcium of uremic man[76,77] are consistent with this hypothesis, as is the failure of intermittent hemodialysis[78–80] to reverse the calcium malabsorption and intestinal resistance to vitamin D. The observation that reductions in intestinal calcium absorption become apparent only when glomerular filtration rates reach levels of 25–30 ml/min[81,82] are also consistent with the hypothesis that calcium malabsorption attending the progressive evolution of renal failure in man is due primarily to decreased generation of biologically active vitamin D metabolites.

In addition, alterations in the metabolism of vitamin D or its hydroxylated metabolites may result in the accumulation of structurally related abnormal metabolites[69–72] which compete with 1,25-$(OH)_2D$ for receptor sites in the cytosol or nucleus of specific target organs. Moreover, tissue 1,25-$(OH)_2D$ receptor sites may exhibit a relative rather than an absolute specificity for diol and triol vitamin D-related sterols, and as such are readily available to 25-OH-D and vitamin D as well.[83,84] Demonstrated in vitro effectiveness of vitamin D[85] and 25-OH-D[86] on calcium transport and in vivo intestinal responses to dihydrotachysterol,[87,88] a compound structurally similar to 1,25-$(OH)_2D$, supports this contention. It may be premature to assume that negative feedback hormonal and ionic control mechanisms for 25-OH-D and 1,25-$(OH)_2D$ generation by the liver and kidney, respectively, are intact in the uremic subject. Although, in theory, the attendant hypocalcemia and resultant secondary hyperparathyroidism observed in patients with chronic renal insufficiency should compensate for the decrease in 1,25-$(OH)_2D$ production anticipated by the loss of renal mass, this obviously is not the case since circulating 1,25-$(OH)_2D$ levels are decreased in uremic patients.[89]

When quantitated in uremic patients, plasma 25-OH-D levels are normal, low, or increased,[90–93] and a significant direct correlation obtains between calcium and 25-OH-D plasma concentrations.[90] Since large doses of 25-OH-D are effective in raising serum calcium in the anephric state,[94,95] it appears likely that the renal conversion of 25-OH-D to 1,25-$(OH)_2D$ is not an obligatory step for its biological effect on bone or intestine. In fact, the progressive osteomalacia observed in untreated uremic patients with osteodystrophy may result, at least in part, from the decreased biologic availability of 25-OH-D.[90] Although the cause for decreased circulating 25-OH-D in patients with advanced renal failure has been attributed primarily to poor nutrition and inadequate exposure to sunlight, it should be emphasized that the circulating antirachitic activity of serum obtained from uremic patients is still lower than that of malnourished sedentary patients with terminal cachexia.[67] The intestinal absorption of vitamin D is normal in uremic patients,[69] and circulating 25-OH-D levels ultimately increase following vitamin D feeding. These observations are reminiscent of documented alterations of vitamin D metabolism in patients receiving anticonvulsants whose levels of circulating 25-OH-D are low[14,16]—an effect attributed to a malfunctioning hepatic microsomal cytochrome P-450 enzyme system.[12,16] This may also be the case in patients with chronic renal failure on normal or marginally low vitamin D intakes since, as noted previously for Dilantin and phenobarbital, microsomal cytochrome P-450 metabolic pathways are also impaired by uremia.[96] Finally, one must acknowledge reports that vitamin D metabolites other than 25-OH-D generated at extrarenal sites are biologically activated by the kidney[97] and that trace metals which may, in fact, accumulate in either nontreated or dialyzed patients with renal insufficiency[98] may impair the renal hydroxylation of 25-OH-D to 1,25-$(OH)_2D$.[99]

THERAPEUTIC RESPONSE TO VITAMIN D METABOLITES IN UREMIA

Reports of vitamin D intoxication in the anephric uremic state,[100] and others citing a direct effect of 25-OH-D on bone metabolism in vitro[101,102] and in vivo in the anephric state[103] collectively suggest that this hydroxylated metabolite may prove useful in reversing renal osteodystrophy in man. Preliminary studies by Bordier et al. reveal that the osteomalacic component of the osteodystrophy of uremic adults is less resistant to 25-OH-D_3 (i.e., 30–500 μg/day) than to vitamins D_2 and D_3.[104] 25-OH-D_3, in doses of 100 μg/day for 3–9-month periods, effectively reverses the skeletal abnormalities of uremic adults undergoing intermittent hemodialysis with concomitant increments in intestinal calcium absorption and a decrease in circulating alkaline phosphatase and PTH (Fig. 67-3).[104] Recently, Witmer et al. also reported that 25-OH-D_3, in doses of 25–200 μg/day, effectively reversed the skeletal lesions toward normal in uremic children resistant to vitamin D in doses of 345–386 μg/day.[105] Although 100–200-μg daily doses of 25-OH-D_3 are still considerably higher than those required to heal dietary rickets or the rickets attending malabsorption syndromes, they are much lower than those of vitamin D_2 or D_3 used unsuccessfully in azotemic osteodystrophy by others. 1,25-$(OH)_2D_3$ has also been used successfully in vitamin D-resistant uremic patients with osteodystrophy;[107–110] improvements in bone mass and calcium absorption and a decrease in circulating PTH have been documented on doses of 0.68–2.7 μg/day. Limited long-term therapeutic trials with this agent are promising.[106,110] In one instance, in

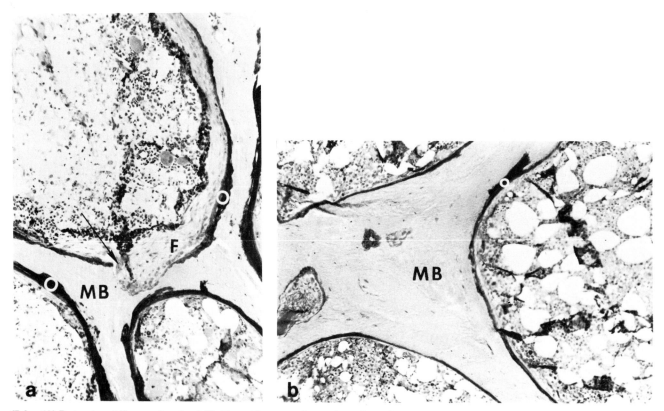

Fig. 67-3. (A) Pretreatment iliac-crest undecalcified-bone biopsy specimen of a patient with chronic renal disease and secondary hyperparathyroidism. Numerous osteoclasts (arrows), marrow fibrosis (F), and wide osteoid seams (O) are present. MB represents mineralized bone (Goldner × 250). (B) Post-treatment biopsy specimen of the same patient noted in Figure 3A. Patient was treated with 25OHD$_3$ (100 μg/day) for 3 months. Therapy was attended by a 3-fold increment in calcium absorption and a 50% decrease in circulating immunoreactive PTH. Osteoclast number was decreased and marrow fibrosis virtually eliminated. Osteoid (O) was also decreased, and marrow fibrosis markedly decreased. MB represents mineralized bone (Goldner × 100).

a 14-year-old child given 0.68 μg daily for over 3 months, there was radiographic demonstration of progressive healing of the skeletal lesions radiographically (detectable after 4 weeks of therapy) with a fall in alkaline phosphatase. This response was attended by a complete reversal of the secondary hyperparathyroidism and osteomalacic bone lesions noted on iliac-crest specimens biopsied prior to the intervention of 1,25-(OH)$_2$D$_3$ therapy.[106] Of additional interest is the observation that during the 1,25-(OH)$_2$D$_3$ treatment period, muscular weakness also improved when judged clinically and by electromyographic testing.

The most recent synthetic vitamin D$_3$ analogue used for the treatment of vitamin D-resistant renal osteodystrophy is 1α-hydroxycholecalciferol (1α-OH-D$_3$).[111-113] This analogue has biologic activity comparable on weight basis to 1,25-(OH)$_2$D$_3$ in the stimulation of intestinal calcium transport and bone calcium mobilization in the normal and anephric state.[114] Unlike 1,25-(OH)$_2$D$_3$, which is more effective when administered intravenously rather than orally,[110] the response to 1α-OH-D$_3$ is rapid, with daily doses of 2.5 μg effectively reversing the skeletal defects of patients with nutritional osteomalacia by 8–10 days.[115] Doses as small as 10 μg/day for 2–3 days in uremic patients have been associated with a 2–3-fold increase in calcium absorption, an elevation in serum calcium, and a fall in circulating alkaline phosphatase.[112] More-prolonged treatment (i.e., 9–10 weeks) with daily doses of 1.0–2.0 μg reveal progressive increments in both calcium absorption and skeletal mineral.[112] 1α-OH-D$_3$ is biologically effective in the anephric state,[115] although it appears to be rapidly metabolized in the liver to 1α,25-(OH)$_2$D$_3$, the latter considered to be the ultimate metabolically active form.[115a]

VITAMIN D DEFICIENCY AND BONE DISEASE ASSOCIATED WITH HEPATIC AND GASTROINTESTINAL DISEASE

One of the major advances in the elucidation of the mechanism of action of vitamin D has been the delineation of the role of the liver in the metabolism of vitamin D, particularly with regard to the regulation of 25-OH-D formation. Although recent exciting discoveries of the role of the kidney in precise regulation of the formation of 1,25-(OH)$_2$D have temporarily overshadowed the physiologic role of 25-OH-D, several recent observations have served to refocus attention on the important role of 25-OH-D in mineral metabolism. First, it has been observed that the 100-fold-higher circulating levels of 25-OH-D relative to 1,25-(OH)$_2$D approximately inversely parallels the difference in in vitro potency of the two metabolites.[116-119] Secondly, elevation of serum 25-OH-D concentration to supraphysiologic levels has been shown to stimulate calcium absorption in anephric man.[100] Third, in cases of vitamin D intoxication serum, 25-OH-D levels are 20–30-fold elevated, whereas 1,25-(OH)$_2$D levels have been reported to be normal.[120] Finally, 25-OH-D but not 1,25-(OH)$_2$D has been shown to directly stimulate muscle accumulation of phosphate in vitro.[25]

Among the earliest studies of the role of the liver in vitamin D metabolism in man were those of Avioli and co-workers. These investigators observed that after an intravenous dose of 4000 IU of tritiated vitamin D$_3$ (^{3}H-D$_3$), approximately 5 percent of the radioactivity was excreted in the bile within 48 hours.[121] Of this amount approximately 9 percent was unaltered vitamin D$_3$ and 40 percent was glucuronides of vitamin D and more-polar metabolites. Moreover, in patients with cirrhosis, the plasma ^{3}H-D$_3$ half-life was increased by 25–50 percent and the urinary vitamin D-glucuronide excretion was decreased by 36 percent; this suggests impaired vitamin D metabolism in the presence of hepatocellular dysfunction.[121]

Perhaps most important, these investigators were the first to demonstrate a biphasic plasma radioactivity disappearance curve after intravenous injection of ^{3}H-D$_3$ in humans, with an initial rapid fall for 3 hours, a subsequent rise for the next 5 hours, and then a constant exponential decrease.[121] Subsequently, Ponchon and DeLuca demonstrated a similar biphasic disappearance curve for the total plasma radioactivity in rachitic rats following injection of 10 IU of ^{3}H-D$_3$. Approximately 90 min after injection, a striking rebound in plasma radioactivity occurred.[122] Concurrently, hepatic radioactivity dropped sharply from 43.9 percent of the injected dose at 90 min to 1.4 percent at 120 min.[122] Silicic acid column chromatography demonstrated that the rebound in plasma radioactivity was accounted for by the appearance of the recently discovered 25-OH-D metabolite.[123] On this basis it was postulated that the liver is the major site of transformation of vitamin D to 25-OH-D$_3$. In support of this hypothesis, it was subsequently demonstrated that portacaval shunting diminished, and mean total vascular isolation of the liver almost completely eliminated, the conversion of ^{3}H-vitamin D$_3$ to ^{3}H-25-OH-D$_3$ and more-polar metabolites.[123] Shortly thereafter, it was demonstrated that vitamin D$_3$ could be converted to 25-OH-D$_3$ in isolated perfused rat liver and liver homogenates.[124] Subsequently, it was shown that vitamin D$_2$ and dihydrotachysterol also undergo 25-hydroxylation in the liver prior to expression of their biologic activity.[125–127]

More recently, the uniqueness of the liver's role in the 25-hydroxylation of vitamin D has been challenged by Tucker et al., who demonstrated that significant conversion of vitamin D$_3$ to 25-OH-D$_3$ can occur in homogenates from chick intestine and kidney as well as liver.[128] Later studies by Olson et al. in rats who had been completely hepatectomized by a two-stage procedure demonstrated that at 6 hours after a 10-IU dose of ^{3}H-D$_3$, 0.4 percent of the injected dose appeared in a plasma peak that comigrated with 25-OH-D$_3$ by Sephadex LH-20 chromatography as opposed to 1.2 percent in sham-operated controls.[129] However, only half of the apparent ^{3}H-25-OH-D$_3$ from hepatectomized rats comigrated with authentic 25-OH-D$_3$ on hydroxyallylsoxypropyl Sephadex columns. Moreover, apparent extrahepatic production of 25-OH-D$_3$ occurred in the presence of plasma ^{3}H-D$_3$ levels which were four times that of the control animals, the higher plasma levels attributed to absence of hepatic processing of ^{3}H-D$_3$. These data, combined with the observation that the liver takes up the majority of an injected dose of ^{3}H-D$_3$,[122,130,131] indicate that the liver plays the predominant role in the 25-hydroxylation of vitamin D.

Hepatic vitamin-D-25-hydroxylase activity apparently appears early in fetal development but does not reach maximal activity until some weeks after birth. Moriuchi and DeLuca have demonstrated that conversion of vitamin D$_3$ to 25-OH-D$_3$ occurs in the chick embryo as early as 9 days of age.[132] However, the 25-hydroxylase activity in liver homogenates from 18-day chick embryos is one-half that of 3-week-old chicks raised on a vitamin D-deficient diet.[132] In addition, Hillman and Haddad have demonstrated that serum 25-OH-D levels decline significantly from immediate postnatal values and do not increase in response to usual vitamin D supplements in premature infants born prior to 38 weeks of gestation.[133] The fact that plasma clearance of 25-OH-D$_3$ is not different in early- and late-weanling animals[134] suggests immaturity of the hepatic 25-hydroxylase in premature infants.

The high incidence and severity of bone disease in patients with severe liver disease and the higher requirements for vitamin D usually observed in chronic hepatic insufficiency[135,136] indicate the importance of normal hepatic functioning to normal vitamin D metabolism. Although an intact liver is required for normal 25-hydroxylation of vitamin D, the absorption of vitamin D depends upon normal functioning of the biliary system and intact fat absorption across the intestine and into the lacteals. Thus, the question of the relative roles of hepatocellular dysfunction, intestinal viability, and deficient fat absorption in the vitamin D deficiency of chronic liver disease is still unanswered.

It has been demonstrated that there is a definite decrease in plasma disappearance of vitamin ^{3}H-D$_3$ and decreased urinary vitamin-D$_3$-glucuronide excretion in cirrhotic patients.[121] Decreased serum 25-OH-D concentrations have been documented in patients with portal[137,138] and biliary[138,139] cirrhosis (Fig. 67-2). Recently Imawari and Goodman have shown that low 25-OH-D levels in cirrhotic patients also are attended by marked decreases in the serum-binding protein (DBP) which binds both vitamin D and its biologically active metabolites.[140] Studies of patients with biliary cirrhosis with osteomalacia have demonstrated marked malabsorption of vitamin D.[141] Subnormal increases in serum 25-OH-D are also observed following 25-OH-D administration in patients with fat malabsorption.[142,143] Thus the recently recognized enterohepatic recirculation of 25-OH-D,[144] as well as biliary excretion of unaltered vitamin D, suggests that depletion of body stores may occur in addition to malabsorption of ingested sterol.

In a recent large series, Long and colleagues demonstrated decreased serum 25-OH-D levels in patients with chronic alcoholic hepatitis, cirrhosis, chronic active hepatitis, symptomatic biliary cirrhosis, and acute and chronic biliary disease.[138] However, serum 25-OH-D values were normal in a group of patients with presymptomatic biliary cirrhosis. Additionally, serum 25-OH-D levels in patients with hepatic disease with a recent history of prolonged exposure to sunshine tended to be normal, suggesting that decreased precursor availability may be the more important factor in decreased serum 25-OH-D in patients with liver disease. However, the interplay of mechanisms producing low serum 25-OH-D levels in patients with liver disease is at best undefined and requires considerable investigation to determine their relative contributions to the development of hepatic osteodystrophy.

It appears rather premature to assign the pivotal defect in skeletal and mineral metabolism of cirrhotic patients to simple vitamin D deficiency or its abnormal bioactivation to 25-OH-D or 1,25-(OH)$_2$D. There appears little doubt that patients with parenchymal liver disorders have significant osteopenia. Although osteomalacia has been well documented in patients with primary biliary cirrhosis, osteoporosis appears to be a more common cause for the progressive bone disease of cirrhotic patients. In addition to potential alterations in vitamin D metabolism, documented elevations in circulating free cortisol, reduced somatomedin levels, magnesium deficiency, metabolic acidosis due to elevations in blood lactic or pyruvic acids, secondary hyperparathyroidism, and direct cytotoxic effects of ethanol on intestine and bone probably all contribute to the osteopenia.

Osteopenia (osteomalacia and osteoporosis) is also relatively common after gastric surgery. Estimates of the incidence of bone disease vary between 14 and 26 percent, depending on the diagnostic criteria used.[45–151] The pathogenesis of the bone disease following gastrectomy is still virtually unknown, with inadequate intake of calcium and protein, steatorrhea, and a malabsorption of calcium and vitamin D often considered the most likely etiologic factors. Despite a variety of assertions to the contrary, no quantitative relationship exists between the amount of fecal fat and the proportion of ingested calcium excreted in the feces. In addition, it has been demonstrated that vitamin D absorption may be normal or only slightly abnormal in gastrectomized patients with osteomalacia, and that steatorrhea alone is not the major cause of the impaired vitamin absorption, since vitamin D absorption can be normal in patients with steatorrhea.[152] Moreover, the intestinal absorption of calcium in gastrectomized individuals may be, in fact, increased and not responsive to vitamin D.

The potpourri of conflicting evidence regarding the relationship between gastrointestinal and hepatic dysfunction and osteopenia may also result from an inadequate appraisal of intestinal cell functions. The intestinal response to vitamin D depends on the integrity of the mucosal cell: it has been established that vitamin D via its active metabolites promotes DNA synthesis and intestinal cell growth, both of which precede the stimulated cellular transport of calcium. The "resistance" to vitamin D observed in certain patients with coeliac disease when gluten-free diets are discontinued,[153] as in others with tropical sprue and folic acid deficiency,[154] exemplifies the permissive requirement of cellular integrity for the maximal expression of vitamin D metabolites on intestinal calcium absorption.

REFERENCES

1. Kruse, R. Osteopathien dei antiepileptischer langzeit-therapie (vorlaufige mitteilung). *Monatsschr. Kinderheilkd. 116:* 378, 1968.
2. Williams, R. Altered calcium metabolism in epileptic children on anticonvulsants. *Br. Med. J. 2:* 202, 1971.
3. Richens, A., and Rowe, D. J. F. Disturbance of calcium metabolism by anticonvulsant drugs. *Br. Med. J. 3:* 73, 1970.
4. Hahn, T. J., Hendin, B. A., Scharp, C. R., and Haddad, J. G., Jr. Effect of chronic anticonvulsant therapy on serum 25-hydroxycalciferol levels in adults. *N. Engl. J. Med. 287:* 900, 1972.
5. Hahn, T. J., Hendin, B. A., Scharp, C. R., Boisseau, V. C., and Haddad, J. G., Jr. Serum 25-hydroxycalciferol levels and bone mass in children on anticonvulsant therapy. *N. Engl. J. Med. 292:* 550, 1975.
6. Liakakos, D., Papadopoulos, Z., Vlachos, P., Boviatsi, E., and Varonos, D. D. Serum alkaline phosphatase and urinary hydroxyproline values in children receiving phenobarbital with and without vitamin D. *J. Pediatr. 87:* 291, 1975.
7. Rodbro, P., Christiansen, C., and Lund, M. Development of anticonvulsant osteomalacia in epileptic patients on phenytoin treatment. *Acta Neurol. Scand. 50:* 527, 1974.
8. Tolman, K. G., Jubiz, W., Sannella, J. J., Madsen, J. A. et al. Osteomalacia associated with anticonvulsant drug therapy in mentally retarded children. *Pediatrics 56:* 45, 1975.
9. Lifshitz, F., and Maclaren, N. K. Vitamin D-dependent rickets in institutionalized mentally retarded children receiving long-term anticonvulsant therapy: I. A survey of 288 patients. *J. Pediatr. 83:* 612, 1973.
10. Conney, A. H. L. Pharmacologic implications of microsomal enzyme induction. *Pharmcol. Rev. 19:* 317, 1967.
11. Jubiz, W., Meikle, A. W., and Levinson, R. A. Effect of diphenylhydantoin on the metabolism of dexamethasone: mechanism of the abnormal dexamethasone suppression in humans. *N. Engl. J. Med. 283:* 11, 1970.
12. Levin, W., Welch, R. M., and Conney, A. H. Effect of chronic phenobarbital treatment on the liver microsomal metabolism and uterotrophic action of 17B-estradiol. *Endocrinology 80:* 135, 1967.
13. Schaefer, K., Kraft, D., and von Herrath, D. Intestinal absorption of vitamin D_3 in epileptic patients and phenobarbital-treated rats. *Epilepsia 13:* 509, 1972.
14. Hahn, T. J., Birge, S. J., Scharp, C. R., and Avioli, L. V. Phenobarbital-induced alterations in vitamin D metabolism. *J. Clin. Invest. 51:* 741, 1972.

15. Silver, J. Neale, G., and Thompson, G. R. Effect of phenobarbitone treatment on vitamin D metabolism in mammals. *Clin. Sci. Mol. Med. 46:* 433, 1974.
16. Hahn, T. J., Scharp, C. R., and Avioli, L. V. Effect of phenobarbital administration on the subcellular distribution of vitamin D_3-^{3}H in rat liver. *Endocrinology 94:* 1489, 1974.
17. Stamp, T. C. B., Round, M. M., Rowe, D. J. F., and Haddad, J. G. Plasma levels and therapeutic effect of 25-hydroxycholecalciferol in epileptic patients taking anticonvulsant drugs. *Br. Med. J. 4:* 9, 1972.
18. Bouillon, R., Reynaert, J., Cloes, J. H., Lissens, W., and DeMoor, P. The effect of anticonvulsant therapy on serum levels of 25-hydroxy-vitamin D, calcium and parathyroid hormone. *J. Clin. Endocrinol. Metab. 41:* 1130, 1975.
19. Koch, H. V., Kraft, D., von Herrath, D., et al. Influence of diphenylhydantoin and phenobarbital on intestinal calcium transport in the rat. *Epilepsia 13:* 829, 1972.
20. Jenkins, M. V., Harris, M., and Wills, M. R. The effect of phenytoin on parathyroid extract and 25-hydroxycholecalciferol-induced bone resorption: adenosine 3'5' cyclic monophosphate production. *Calcif. Tissues Res. 16:* 163, 1974.
21. Hahn, T. J., Halstead, L. R., Scharp, C. R., et al. Enhanced biotransformation and biologic efficacy of vitamin D following phenobarbital administration in the rat. *Clin. Res. 23:* 111A, 1975.
22. Glynne, A., Hunter, I. P., and Thomson, J. A. Pseudohypoparathyroidism with paradoxical increase in hypocalcemic seizures due to long-term anticonvulsant therapy. *Postgrad. Med. J. 48:* 632, 1972.
23. Dent, C. E., Richens, A., Rowe, D. J. F., and Stamp, T. C. B. Osteomalacia with long-term anticonvulsant therapy in epilepsy. *Br. Med. J. 4:* 69, 1970.
24. Marsden, C. D., Reynolds, E. H., Parsons, V., Harris, R., and Duchan, L. Myopathy associated with anticonvulsant osteomalacia. *Br. Med. J. 4:* 526, 1973.
25. Birge, S. J., and Haddad, J. G. 25-Hydroxycholeciferal stimulation of muscle metabolism. *J. Clin. Invest. 56:* 1100, 1975.
26. Lachman, C. Osteoporosis: the potentialities and limitations of its roentgenologic diagnosis. *Am. J. Roentgenol. Radium Ther. Nucl. Med. 74:* 712, 1955.
27. Christiansen, C., Rodbro, P., and Lund, P. Incidence of anticonvulsant osteomalacia and effect of vitamin D: controlled therapeutic trial. *Br. Med. J. 4:* 695, 1973.
28. Linde, J., Molholm-Hansen, J., Siersbaek-Nielsen, K., and Fugland-Fredriksen, V. Bone density in patients receiving long-term anticonvulsant therapy. *Acta Neurol. Scand. 47:* 650, 1971.
29. Haddad, J. G., Jr., and Hahn, T. J. Natural and synthetic sources of circulating 25-hydroxyvitamin D in man. *Nature 244:* 515, 1973.
30. Loomis, W. F. Seasonal variations in the incidence of osteomalacia. *Science 157:* 501, 1967.
31. Hahn, T. J., and Hahn, B. H. Osteopenia in patients with rheumatic diseases: principles of diagnosis and therapy. *Semin. Arthritis Rheum. 6:* 165, 1976.
32. Frost, H. M. Tetracycline-based histological analysis of bone remodeling. *Calcif. Tissue Res. 3:* 211, 1969.
33. Christiansen, C., Rodbro, P., and Nielsen, C. T. Iatrogenic osteomalacia in epileptic children. A controlled therapeutic trial. *Acta Pediatr. Scand. 64:* 219 1975.
34. Christiansen, C., Rodbro, P., and Ole, S. Anticonvulsant action of vitamin D in epileptic patients: A controlled pilot study. *Br. Med. J. 2:* 258, 1974.
35. Maclaren, N. K., annd Lifshitz, F. Vitamin-D-dependency rickets in institutionalized, mentally retarded children on long-term anticonvulsant therapy: II. The response to 25-hydroxycholecalciferol and vitamin D. *Pediatr. Res. 7:* 914, 1973.
36. Haddad, J. G., Jr. and Rojanasathit, S. Acute administration of 25-hydroxycholecalciferol in man. *J. Clin. Endocrinol. Metab. 284:* 290, 1976.
37. Hahn, T. J., Boisseau, V. C., and Avioli, L. V. Effect of chronic corticosteroid administration on diaphyseal and metaphyseal bone mass. *J. Clin. Endocrinol. Metab. 39:* 274, 1974.
38. Hahn, T. J., Halstead, L. R., Scharp, C. R., and Haddad, J. G. Enhanced biotransformation and biologic efficacy of vitamin D following phenobarbital administration in the rat. *Clin. Res. 23:* 111A, 1975.
39. Sussman, M. L., and Coplman, B. The roentgenologic appearance of the bones in Cushing's syndrome. *Radiology 39:* 288, 1942.
40. Howland, W. J., Pugh, D. G., and Sprague, R. G. Roentgenologic

changes of the skeletal system in Cushing's syndrome. *Radiology 71:* 69, 1958.

41. Soffer, L. J., Iannaccone, A., and Gabrilove, J. L. Cushing's syndrome: a study of fifty patients. *Am. J. Med. 30:* 129, 1961.

42. Curtiss, P. H., Clark, W. S., and Herndon, C. H. Vertebral fractures resulting from prolonged cortisone and corticotropin therapy. *J.A.M.A. 156:* 467, 1954.

43. Bradley, B. W. D., and Ansell, B. M. Fractures in Still's disease. *Ann. Rheum. Dis. 19:* 135, 1960.

44. Saville, P. D., and Kharmosh, O. Osteoporosis of rheumatoid arthritis. Influence of age, sex and corticosteroids. *Arthritis Rheum. 10:* 423, 1967.

45. Frost, H. M., and Villaneuva, A. R. Human osteoblastic activity III. The effect of cortisone on lamellar osteoblastic activity. *Henry Ford Hosp. Med. Bull. 9:* 97, 1961.

46. Jowsey, J., and Riggs, B. L. Bone formation in hypercortisolism. *Acta Endocrinol. 63:* 21, 1970.

47. Thompson, J. S., Palmieri, G. M. A., and Crawford, R. L. The effect of porcine calcitonin on osteoporosis induced by adrenal cortical steroids. *J. Bone Joint Surg. 54A:* 1490, 1972.

48. Stoerk, H. C., Peterson, A. C., and Jelinck, V. C. The blood calcium lowering effect of hydrocortisone in parathyroidectomized rats. *Proc. Soc. Exp. Biol. Med. 114:* 690, 1963.

49. Peck, W. A., Brand, J., et al. Hydrocortisone-induced inhibition of protein synthesis and uridine incorporation in isolated bone cells in vitro. *Proc. Natl. Acad. Sci. U.S.A. 57:* 1599, 1967.

50. Stern, P. H. Inhibition by steroids of parathyroid hormone-induced ^{45}Ca release from embryonic rat bone in vitro. *J. Pharmacol. Exp. Ther. 168:* 211, 1969.

51. Jee, W. S. S., Park, H. Z., Roberts, W. E., et al. Corticosteroids and and bone. *Am. J. Anat. 129:* 477, 1970.

52. Fucik, R. F., Kukreja, S. C., Hargis, G. K., et al. Effect of glucocorticoids on function of the parathyroid gland in man. *J. Clin. Endocrinol. Metab. 40:* 152, 1975.

53. Wajchenberg, B. L., Periera, V. A., Kieffer, J., et al. Effect of dexamethasone on calcium metabolism and ^{47}Ca kinetics in normal subjects. *Acta Endocrinol. 61:* 173, 1969.

54. Collins, E. J., Garrett, E. R., and Johnston, R. L. Effect of adrenal steroids on radio-calcium metabolism in dogs. *Metabolism 11:* 716, 1962.

55. Avioli, L. V., Birge, S. J., and Lee, S. W. Effects of prednisone on vitamin D metabolism in man. *J. Clin. Endocrinol. Metab. 28:* 1341, 1968.

56. Kimberg, D. V., Baerg, R. D., Gershon, E., et al. Effect of cortisone treatment on the active transport of calcium by the small intestine. *J. Clin. Invest. 50:* 1309, 1971.

57. Favus, M. J., Kimberg, D. V., Millar, G. N., et al. Effects of cortisone administration on the metabolism and localization of 25-hydroxycholecalciferol in the rat. *J. Clin. Invest. 52:* 1328, 1973.

58. Hahn, T. J., Halstead, L. R., and Haddad, J. G. Serum 25-hydroxyvitamin D concentrations in patients receiving chronic corticosteroid therapy. *J. Lab. Clin. Med. 90:* 399, 1977.

59. Carre, M., Ayegbede, O., Miravet, L., et al. The effect of prednisolone upon the metabolism and action of 25-hydroxy and 1,25-dihydroxyvitamin D_3. *Proc. Natl. Acad. Sci. U.S.A. 71:* 2996, 1974.

60. Hahn, T. J., unpublished observations.

61. Avioli, L. V. Senile and postmenopausal osteoporosis. In Stollerman G. H. (ed): Advances in Internal Medicine, vol. 21. Chicago, Yearbook, 1976, p. 391.

62. Riggs, B. L., Jowsey, J., and Kelly, P. J. Quantitative microradiographic study of bone remodeling in Cushing's syndrome. *Metabolism 15:* 773, 1966.

63. Teitelbaum, S. L., and Hahn, T. J. Unpublished observations.

64. Sheagren, J. N., Jowzey, J., Bird, D. C., at el. Effect on bone growth of daily versus alternate-day corticosteroid administration: an experimental study. *J. Lab. Clin. Med. 89:* 120, 1977.

65. Wilson, C. R. The use of in vivo bone mineral determination to predict the strength of bone. Norland-Cameron Bone Mineral Analyzer Applications, Note No. 3. Norland-Cameron Instruments, Ft. Atkinson, Wisc., 1972.

66. Lumb, G. A., Mawer, E. B., and Stanbury, S. W. The apparent vitamin D resistance of chronic renal failure. *Am. J. Med. 50:* 421, 1971.

67. Ritz, E., and Jantzen, R. Vitamin D Aktivitat im Serum uramischer Patienten. *Klin. Wochenschr. 47:* 1112, 1969.

68. Bell, N. H., and Bartter, F. C. Transient reversal of hyperabsorption of calcium and of abnormal sensitivity to vitamin D in a patient with sarcoidosis during episodes of nephritis. *Ann. Intern. Med. 61:* 702, 1964.

69. Avioli, L. V., Birge, S., Lee, S. W., and Slatopolsky, E. The metabolic fate of vitamin D_3-^{3}H in chronic renal failure. *J. Clin. Invest. 47:* 2239, 1969.

70. Gray, R. W., Weber, H. P., Dominguez, J. H., and Lemann, J., Jr. The metabolism of vitamin D_3 and 25-hydroxyvitamin D_3 in normal and anephric humans. *J. Clin. Endocrinol. Metab. 39:* 1045, 1974.

71. Piel, C. F., Roof, B. S., and Avioli, L. V. Metabolism of tritiated 25-hydroxycholecalciferol in chronically uremic children before and after successful renal homotransplantation. *J. Clin. Endocrinol. Metab. 37:* 944, 1973.

72. Mawer, E. B., Taylor, C. M., Blackhouse, J., et al. Failure of formation of 1,25-dihydroxycholecalciferol in chronic renal insufficiency. *Lancet 1:* 626, 1973.

73. Gray, R., Boyle, I., and DeLuca, H. F. Vitamin D metabolism: the role of kidney tissue. *Science 172:* 1232, 1971.

74. Hill, L. F., van den Berg, C. J., and Mawer, E. B. Vitamin D metabolism in experimental uraemia: effects on intestinal transport of ^{45}Ca and on formation of 1,25-dihydroxycholecalciferol in rat. *Nature 232:* 189, 1971.

75. Avioli, L. V., Birge, S. J., and Slatopolsky, E. The nature of vitamin D resistance of patients with chronic renal disease. *Arch. Intern. Med. 124:* 451, 1969.

76. Henderson, R. G., Ledingham, J. G., Oliver, D. O., et al. Effects of 1,25-dihydroxycholecalciferol on calcium absorption, muscle weakness, and bone disease in chronic renal failure. *Lancet 1:* 379, 1974.

77. Brickman, A. S., Coburn, J. W., Massry, S. G., et al. 1,25-Dihydroxyvitamin D_3 in normal man and patients with renal failure. *Ann. Intern. Med. 80:* 161, 1974.

78. Genuth, S. M., Vertes, V., and Leonards, J. R. Oral calcium absorption in patients with renal failure treated by chronic hemodialysis. *Metabolism 18:* 124, 1969.

79. Brickman, A. S., Coburn, J. W., Rowe, P. H., et al. Impaired calcium absorption in uremic man: evidence for defective absorption in the proximal small intestine. *J. Lab. Clin. Med. 84:* 791, 1974.

80. Messener, R. P., Smith, H. T., Shapiro, F. L., et al. The effect of hemodialysis, vitamin D, and renal homotransplantation on the calcium malabsorption of chronic renal failure. *J. Lab. Clin. Med. 74:* 472, 1969.

81. Coburn, J. W., Hartenbower, D. L., and Massry, S. G. Intestinal absorption of calcium and the effect of renal insufficiency. *Kidney Int. 4:* 96, 1973.

82. Schaefer, K., Schaefer, P., Poeppe, P., et al. Uraemic osteopathy. The relationship between disturbances in intestinal calcium absorption and renal function. *Germ. Med. Mon. 13:* 575, 1968.

83. Brumbaugh, P. F., and Haussler, M. R. 1 α,25-Dihydroxycholecalciferol receptors in intestine. *J. Biol. Chem. 249:* 1251, 1974.

84. Brumbaugh, P. F., and Haussler, M. R. Nuclear and cytoplasmic receptors for 1,25-dihydroxycholecalciferol in intestinal mucosa. *Biochem. Biophys. Res. Commun. 54:* 74, 1973.

85. Corradino, R. A. Embryonic chick intestine in organ culture: interaction of adenylate cyclase system and vitamin D_3-mediated calcium absorptive mechanism. *Endocrinology 94:* 1607, 1974.

86. Olson, E. B., and DeLuca, H. F. 25-Hydroxycholecalciferol: direct effect on calcium transport. *Science 165:* 405, 1969.

87. Kaye, M., and Sagar, S. Effect of dihydrotachysterol on calcium absorption in uremia. *Metabolism 21:* 815, 1972.

88. Kaye, M., Chatterjee, G., Cohen, G. H., et al. Arrest of hyperparathyroid bone disease with dihydrotachysterol in patients undergoing chronic hemodialysis. *Ann. Intern. Med. 73:* 225, 1970.

89. Brumbaugh, P. F., Haussler, D. H., Bressler, R., et al. Radioreceptor assay for 1 α,25-dihydroxyvitamin D_3. *Science 183:* 1089, 1974.

90. Bayard, F., Bec, Ph., Ton That, H., et al. Plasma 25-hydroxycholecalciferol in chronic renal failure. *Eur. J. Clin. Invest. 3:* 447, 1973.

91. Eastwood, J. B., Stamp, T. C. B., Harris, E., et al. Vitamin D-deficiency in the osteomalacia of chronic renal failure. *Lancet 2:* 1209, 1976.

92. Lund, B., Sorenson, H. O., Nielsen, P., et al. 25-Hydroxycholecalciferol in chronic renal failure. *Lancet 2:* 372, 1975.

93. Shen, F. H., Baylink, D. J., Sherrard, D. J., et al. Serum immunoreactive parathyroid hormone and 25-hydroxyvitamin D in patients

with uremic bone disease. *J. Clin. Endocrinol. Metab. 40:* 1009, 1975.

94. Pavlovitch, H., Garabedian, M., and Balsan, S. Calcium-mobilizing effect of large doses of 25-hydroxycholecalciferol in anephric rats. *J. Clin. Invest. 52:* 2656, 1973.

95. Counts, S. J., Baylink, D. J., Shen, F. H., et al. Vitamin D intoxication in an anephric child. *Ann. Intern. Med. 82:* 196, 1975.

96. Leber, H. W., and Schutterle, G. Oxidative drug metabolism in liver microsomes from uremic rats. *Kidney Int. 2:* 152, 1972.

97. Garabedian, M., Pavlovitch, H., Fellot, C., et al. Metabolism of 25-hydroxyvitamin D_3 in anephric rats: a new active metabolite. *Proc. Natl. Acad. Sci. U.S.A. 71:* 554, 1974.

98. Alfrey, A. C., and Smythe, W. R. Trace element abnormalities in chronic uremia. Artificial Kidney-Chronic Uremia Program. National Institute of Arthritis, Metabolism, and Digestive Diseases, January 13–15, 1975, p. 29.

99. Feldman, S. L., and Cousins, R. J. Influence of cadmium on the metabolism of 25-hydroxycholecalciferol in chicks. *Nutr. Rep. Int. 8:* 4, 1973.

100. Counts, S. J., Baylink, D. J., Shen, F. H., et al. Vitamin D intoxication in an anephric child. *Ann. Intern. Med. 82:* 196, 1975.

101. Raisz, L., Trummel, C. L., and Simmons, H. Induction of bone resorption in tissue culture: prolonged response after brief exposure to parathyroid hormone on 25-hydroxycholecalciferol. *Endocrinology 90:* 744, 1972.

102. Reynolds, J. J., Holick, M. F., and DeLuca, H. F. The effects of vitamin D analogues on bone resorption. *Calcif. Tissue Res. 15:* 333, 1974.

103. Pavlovitch, H., Garabedian, M., and Balsan, S. Calcium-mobilizing effect of large doses of 25-hydroxycholecalciferol in anephric rats. *J. Clin. Invest. 52:* 2656, 1973.

104. Bordier, P. J., Maries, P. J., and Arnaud, C. D. Evolution of renal osteodystrophy: correlation of bone histomorphometry and serum mineral and immunoreactive parathyroid hormone values before and after treatment with calcium carbonate or 25-hydroxycholecalciferol. *Kidney Int. 7:* S102, 1975.

105. Witmer, G., Margolis, A., Fontaine, O., et al. Effects of 25-hydroxycholecalciferol on bone lesions of children with terminal renal failure. *Kidney Int. 10:* 395, 1976.

106. Henderson, R. G., Ledingham, J. G., Oliver, D. P., et al. Effects of 1,25-dihydroxycholecalciferol on calcium absorption, muscle weakness, and bone disease in chronic renal failure. *Lancet I:* 379, 1974.

107. Brickman, A. S., Coburn, J. W., and Massry, S. G. 1,25-Dihydroxy-vitamin D_3 in normal man and patients with renal failure. *Ann. Intern. Med. 80:* 161, 1974.

108. Brickman, A. S., Coburn, J. W., and Norman, A. W. Action of 1,25-dihydroxycholecalciferol, a potent, kidney-produced metabolite of vitamin D_3 in uremic man. *N. Engl. J. Med. 287:* 891, 1972.

109. Brickman, A. S., Sherrard, D. J., Jowsey, J., et al. 1,25-Dihydroxy-cholecalciferol. *Arch. Intern. Med. 134:* 883, 1974.

110. Ahmed, K. Y., Wills, M. R., Varghese, Z., et al. Long-term effects of small doses of 1,25-dihydroxycholecalciferol in renal osteodystrophy. *Lancet 1:* 629, 1978.

111. Catto, G. R. D., MacLeod, M., Pelc, B., et al. 1α-Hydroxychole-calciferol: a treatment for renal bone disease. *Br. Med. J. 1:* 12,1975.

112. Chalmers, T. M., Hunter, J. O., Davie, M. W., et al. 1-Alpha-hydroxycholecalciferol as a substitute for the kidney hormone; 1,25-dihydroxycholecalciferol in chronic renal failure. *Lancet 2:* 696, 1973.

113. Peacock, M., Gallagher, J. C., and Nordin, B. E. C. Action of 1α-hydroxyvitamin D_3 on calcium absorption and bone resorption in man. *Lancet 1:* 385, 1974.

114. Holick, M. F., Semnler, E. J., Schnoes, H. K., et al. 1α-Hydroxy derivative of vitamin D_3: a highly potent analog of 1α,25-dihydroxy-vitamin D_3. *Science 180:* 190, 1973.

115. Pechet, M. M., and Hesse, R. H. Metabolic and clinical effects of pure crystalline 1α-hydroxyvitamin D_3 and 1α-dihydroxyvitamin D_3. *Am. J. Med. 57:* 13, 1974.

115a. Holick, M. F., de Blanco, M. C., Clark, M. B., et al. The metabolism of [6-^{3}H]1α,hydroxycholecalciferol to [6-^{3}H]1α,25-dihydroxy-cholecalciferol in a patient with renal insufficiency. *J. Clin. Endocrinol. Metab. 44:* 595, 1977.

116. Raisz, L. G., Trummel, C. L., Holick, M. F., et al. 1,25-Dihydrox-ycholecalciferol: a potent stimulator of bone resorption in tissue culture. *Science 175:* 768, 1972.

117. Corradino, R. A. Embryonic chick intestine in organ culture: response to vitamin D_3 and its metabolites. *Science 179:* 402, 1973.

118. Haddad, J. G., Jr., and Hahn, T. J. Natural and synthetic sources of circulating 25-hydroxyvitamin D in man. *Nature 244:* 515, 1973.

119. Haussler, M. R., Baylink, D. J., Hughes, M. R., et al. The assay of 1α,25-dihydroxyvitamin D_3: physiologic and pathologic modulation of circulating hormone levels. *Clin. Endocrinol. 5:* 151s, 1976.

120. Hughes, M. R., Baylink, D. J., Jones, P. C., et al. Radioligand receptor assay for 25-hydroxyvitamin D_2/D_3 and 1 α-25-dihydroxy-vitamin D_2/D_3. Application to hypervitaminosis D. *J. Clin. Invest. 58:* 61, 1976.

121. Avioli, L. V., Lee, S. W., McDonald, J. E., et al. Metabolism of vitamin D_3-^{3}H in human subjects: distribution in blood, bile, feces and urine. *J. Clin. Invest. 46:* 983, 1967.

122. Ponchon, G., and DeLuca, H. F. The role of the liver in the metabolism of vitamin D. *J. Clin. Invest. 48:* 1273, 1969.

123. Ponchon, G., Kennan, A. L., and DeLuca, H. F. "Activation" of vitamin D by the liver. *J. Clin. Invest. 48:* 2032, 1969.

124. Horsting, M., and DeLuca, H. F. In vitro production of 25-hydrox-ycholecalciferol. *Biochem. Biophys. Res. Commun. 36:* 251, 1969.

125. Suda, T., DeLuca, H. F., Schnoes, H., et al. 25-Hydroxyergocalciferol: a biologically active metabolite of vitamin D_2. *Biochem. Biophys. Res. Commun. 35:* 182, 1969.

126. Holick, R. B., and DeLuca, H. F. 25-Hydroxy-dihydrotachysterol$_3$ of biosynthesis in vivo and in vitro. *J. Biol. Chem. 246:* 5733, 1971.

127. Suda, T., Holick, R. B., DeLuca, H. F., et al. 25-Hydroxydihydro-tachysterol. Synthesis and biological activity. *Biochemistry 9:* 1651, 1970.

128. Tucker, G., III, Gagnon, R. E., Haussler, M. R. Vitamin D_3-25-hydroxylase: tissue occurrence and apparent lack of regulation. *Arch. Biochem. Biophys. 155:* 47, 1973.

129. Olson, E. B., Jr., Knutson, J. C., Bhattacharyya, M. H., et al. The effect of hepatectomy on the synthesis of 25-hydroxyvitamin D_3. *J. Clin. Invest. 57:* 1213, 1976.

130. Norman, A. W., and DeLuca, H. F. The preparation of ^{3}H-vita-mins D_2 and D_3 and their localization in the rat. *Biochemistry 2:* 1160, 1963.

131. Rojanasathit, S., and Haddad, J. G. Hepatic accumulation of vita-min D_3 and 25-hydroxyvitamin D_3. *Biochim. Biophys. Acta 42:* 12, 1976.

132. Moriuchi, S., and DeLuca, H. F. Metabolism of vitamin D_3 in the chick embryo. *Arch. Biochem. Biophys. 164:* 165, 1974.

133. Hillman, L. S., and Haddad, J. G. Perinatal vitamin D metabolism III: serial blood 25-hydroxyvitamin D concentrations in term and premature infants after birth. *J. Pediatr. 86:* 928, 1975.

134. Mendelsohn, M., and Haddad, J. G. Post-natal fall and rise in blood 25-hydroxycholecalciferol in the rat. *J. Lab. Clin. Med. 86:* 32, 1975.

135. Osk-Upmark, E. Osteomalacia hepatica. *Acta Med. Scand. 99:* 204, 1939.

136. Atkinson, M., Nordin, B. E. C., and Sherlock, S. Malabsorption and bone disease in prolonged obstructive jaundice. *Q. J. Med. 25:* 299, 1956.

137. Garcia-Pascual, B., Peytremann, A., Courvosier, B., et al. A simplified competitive protein assay for 25-hydroxycalciferol. *Clin. Chem. Acta 68:* 99, 1976.

138. Long, R. G., Wills, M. R., Skinner, R. K., et al. Serum 25-hydroxyvitamin D in untreated parenchymal and cholestatic liver disease. *Lancet 2:* 650, 1976.

139. Haddad, H. G., and Chyu, K. J. Competitive protein-binding radioassay for 25-hydrocholecalciferol. *J. Clin. Endocrinol. Metab. 33:* 992, 1971.

140. Imawari, M., and Goodman, D. W. S. Immunological and immunoassay studies of the binding protein for vitamin D and its metabolites in human serum. *J. Clin. Invest. 59:* 432, 1977.

141. Thompson, G. R., Lewis, B., and Booth, C. C. Absorption of vitamin D_3-^{3}H in control subjects and patients with intestinal malabsorption. *J. Clin. Invest. 45:* 94, 1966.

142. Stamp, T. C. B. Intestinal absorption of 25-hydroxycholecalciferol. *Lancet 2:* 121, 1974.

143. Teitelbaum, S., Halverson, J., and Haddad, J. G. Abnormalities of circulating 25-hydroxyvitamin D following jejunal–ileal bypass for obesity: evidence of an adaptive response. *Ann. Intern. Med. 86:* 289, 1977.

144. Arnaud, S. B., Goldsmith, R. S., Lambert, P. W., et al. 25-Hydroxy-vitamin D_3: Evidence of an enterohepatic circulation in man. *Proc. Soc. Exp. Biol. Med. 149:* 570, 1975.

145. Deller, D. J., Edwards, R. G., and Addison, M. Calcium metabolism and the bones after partial gastrectomy. *Ann. Med. 12:* 295, 1963.

146. Pulvertaft, C. N. Gastric resection and metabolic bone disease. *Postgrad. Med. J. 44:* 618, 1968.

147. Worstman, J., Pack, C. Y. C., Bartter, F. C., et al. Pathogenesis of osteomalacia in secondary hyperparathyroidism after gastrectomy. *Am. J. Med. 52:* 556, 1972.

148. Pryor, J. P., O'Shea, M. J., Brooks, P. L., et al. The long-term metabolic consequences of partial gastrectomy. *Am. J. Med. 51:* 5, 1971.

149. Eddy, R. L. Metabolic bone disease after gastrectomy. *Am. J. Med. 50:* 442, 1971.

150. Morgan, D. B., Hunt, G., and Paterson, C. R. The osteomalacia syndrome after stomach operations. *Q. J. Med. 39:* 395, 1970.

151. Garrick, R., Ireland, A. W., and Posen, S. Bone abnormalities after gastric surgery. *Ann. Intern. Med. 75:* 221, 1971.

152. Thompson, G. R., Neale, G., Watts, J. M., et al. Detection of vitamin D deficiency after partial gastrectomy. *Lancet 1:* 457, 1966.

153. Nassim, J. R., Savile, P. D., Cook, P. B., et al. The effects of vitamin D and gluten-free diet in idiopathic steatorrhea. *Q. J. Med. 28:* 141, 1958.

154. Haddock, L., and Vasquez, M. Antirachitic activity of sera of patients with tropical sprue. *J. Clin. Endocrinol. Metab. 25:* 859, 1966.

68

Disorders Associated with Renal Calcium-Stone Disease

Munro Peacock
William G. Robertson
Robert W. Marshall

INTRODUCTION

The presence of renal stones is usually obvious clinically; the patient is often only too aware that there is a foreign body in the urinary tract causing pain, abnormal micturition, and damage which are relieved only by the stone's passage or by its surgical removal. Occasionally the first episode is misinterpreted, but sooner or later the diagnosis is firmly established since the condition tends to be recurrent. Investigation of the urinary tract by x-ray techniques usually confirms that a stone is present since most stones in man are composed largely of radiopaque salts. Although renal stone disease has been recognized for many centuries and is relatively easy to diagnose clinically, it remains a difficult problem to manage in terms of pathogenesis, treatment, and prevention.

The stone most commonly formed in patients from Europe and North America is composed mainly of calcium oxalate and/or phosphate, with minor geographic variations in composition[1–4] (Table 68-1). This is in contrast to countries where endemic bladder stone disease is still common and the stones, in addition, contain large amounts of urates.[5] Stones composed of magnesium ammonium phosphate, produced in patients with recurrent urinary tract infection, are common throughout the world, whereas uric acid and cystine stones are relatively uncommon.[1–4]

Patients with calcium-containing stones can sometimes be

shown to suffer from a well-defined disease such as primary hyperparathyroidism or congenital hyperoxaluria. In the majority, however, this is not the case, and these patients are diagnosed as having idiopathic calcium-stone disease. The elucidation of the "causes" of calcium-stone disease involves the questions of why stone-forming salts precipitate and aggregate in urine during its passage through the renal tract, why stone formation is episodic,[6,7] and why its incidence is increasing.[8] It is clear from several studies that the mean recurrence rate of calcium-stone formation is approximately 5–10 years.[7,8] The mean rate, however, does not reflect the great variation between patients; some patients pass stones every month while others may only have a single episode. The variation is partly due to what is defined as a stone episode. In our studies it has been useful to define a stone episode as the passage of a stone or its surgical removal. A stone episode rate can thus be estimated and related to the etiologic factors considered to be important in stone formation and its treatment.

Some stone-forming patients, however, have no definable episode rate, either because the stones remain within the kidney or they are too small to collect. In the latter case, there is usually a history of renal colic or passage of gravel, and there is little doubt from our own observations on crystalluria that small aggregates or "stones," 300 μm in diameter, cause renal colic. This raises the question of the definition of a renal stone. If the material passed can be seen by the naked eye, i.e., if it has a diameter of approximately 500–1000 μm, it can safely be called a stone; when several of these small stones are passed during a bout of renal colic, only one episode is recorded. As defined by these criteria, the stone episode rate is useful for assessing the activity of the disease and its response to treatment, but it underestimates the real situation in many patients and excludes those with x-ray evidence of kidney stones who have never passed a stone nor required surgery. It is obvious that more definitive criteria are needed to distinguish stone-forming patients from normal subjects and to monitor the effect of treatment on stone formation. As discussed in the following sections, it may be that the amount and type of crystalluria present will prove to be a more accurate guide.

URINARY FACTORS INVOLVED IN RENAL CALCIUM-STONE FORMATION

It is clear from Table 68-2 that stone formation is a disorder associated with the precipitation of sparingly soluble salts and acids. If so, the process should be subject to the chemical laws of

Table 68-1. Frequency (%) of Urinary Tract Stones from Four Countries, Classified According to Composition

Stone Type	Country			
	USA*	Scandinavia†	Germany‡	Britain§
Calcium oxalate	32.7	13.1	38.7	13.3
Calcium oxalate/ calcium phosphate	34.3	37.4	17.7	45.0
Magnesium ammonium phosphate	19.0	30.9	24.1	28.4
Calcium phosphate	5.3	7.9		7.6
Uric acid	5.8	8.8	15.3	2.7
Cystine	2.9	1.2	1.5	3.0
Other	—	0.7	2.6	—
Total number of stones	1000	600	1190	264

*Data from Prien.[1]
†Data from Lagergren.[2]
‡Data from Richter and Sucker.[3]
§Data from Nordin and Hodgkinson.[4]

crystal nucleation, growth, and aggregation. Of the many theories advanced to explain the mechanism of stone formation, the simplest proposes that it takes place in four stages. First, there is a nucleation phase during which crystal embryos are formed from urine excessively oversaturated with one or more of the stone-forming salts. Second, there is a period during which the primary crystallites grow and perhaps aggregate to produce larger secondary particles. Third, one of these secondary particles must become large enough within the transit time of urine through the urinary tract to become trapped at some narrow section. Finally, this trapped particle acts as a nidus, or growth point, for the formation of a stone.

In support of this hypothesis it has been shown that periods of crystalluria may trigger off stone formation in animals[9] and in man.[10-12] Thus patients with recurrent calcium oxalate stones pass more calcium oxalate crystals in their urine than normal subjects, and these are generally larger and more aggregated than those of normal subjects.[11] Moreover, these abnormal crystals (which may be up to 300 μm in diameter) exist in calyceal urine and are therefore likely to have at least started forming in the collecting ducts (maximum diameter 200 μm at the ducts of Bellini). It is possible that the largest of such particles may become trapped in the papillary region or become lodged in one of the lower calyces of the kidney and act as a nidus for the formation of a stone. In this connection it has been noted that the passage of large aggregates in the urine is often accompanied by attacks of renal colic,[11] and that the severity of the disorder (as defined by the stone episode rate) is related to the percentage of large crystals and aggregates in the urine (Fig. 68-1).

Table 68-2. Solubilities of Some Stone-Forming and Non-Stone-Forming Salts and Acids in Water at 37°C

	Compound	Solubility (g/l)
Urine salts and acids forming stones	Calcium oxalate	0.0071
	Calcium phosphate	0.08
	Uric acid	0.08
	Cystine	0.17
	Magnesium ammonium phosphate	0.36
Urine salts not forming stones	Calcium sulphate	2.1
	Calcium citrate	2.2
	Magnesium sulphate	293
	Magnesium chloride	361
	Ammonium chloride	420
	Calcium chloride	560

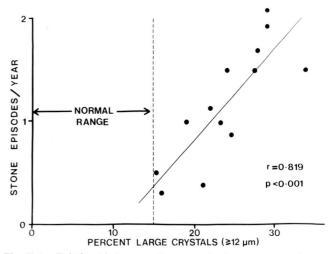

Fig. 68-1. Relationship between the stone episode rate over a period of 10 years and the percentage of large calcium oxalate crystals in the urine of 13 recurrent calcium-stone formers. (From Robertson, in Fleisch et al (eds): Urolithiasis Research, 1976. Courtesy of Plenum).

FACTORS CONTROLLING THE PRODUCTION OF LARGE CRYSTALS AND AGGREGATES

The two main factors controlling the growth and aggregation of calcium salts in urine are the degree of saturation of urine and the level of activity of various inhibitors of crystallization.

Saturation of Urine

If renal stone formation is an extracellular phenomenon occurring in the urinary tract, then the level of saturation with each of the stone-forming salts will determine, first, whether crystals can form at all and, second, whether they are likely to aggregate and grow into a stone. It was recognized by the early crystallographers that new crystals do not develop readily in just-saturated solutions. Indeed, often a very high level of supersaturation is required before spontaneous precipitation takes place. It has been suggested that there is a zone of "metastable" supersaturation, which, in the case of a salt, lies between its solubility product (the point at which the salt is in equilibrium with its bathing medium) and its formation product (the point at which the salt precipitates spontaneously by homogeneous nucleation) (Fig. 68-2). Within the metastable zone a solution may exist for long periods without precipitation taking place. If, however, a nucleating material is added to such a solution, heterogeneous nucleation followed by crystal growth may take place at saturation levels below the formation

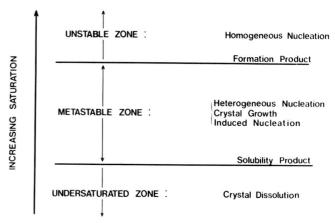

Fig. 68-2. Possible regions of saturation of a solution of a sparingly soluble salt or acid in relation to its solubility and formation products.

product.[13,14] Solutions below the solubility product are undersaturated and will dissolve added crystals of the salt concerned.

The measurement of the saturation of urine with the various stone-forming salts is a complex procedure requiring the measurement of the activity products of each salt. These cannot be measured directly and must be calculated from the ionic activities of each ion involved. Computer programs have been written to calculate the saturation of urine with calcium oxalate, calcium phosphate, magnesium ammonium phosphate,[15] cystine, uric acid, sodium urate, and ammonium urate (Robertson, unpublished results). Essentially this involves measuring the *total* concentrations of all the main ionizable species in urine and calculating their *free ionized* concentrations from a knowledge of the extent to which they complex with one another.

These calculations show that the levels of uric acid and cystine in the urine of uric-acid-stone formers, cystine-stone formers, and infected stone formers frequently exceed the levels of spontaneous precipitation of uric acid, cystine, and calcium phosphate and/or magnesium ammonium phosphate, respectively. Thus crystalluria is common in these patients. Calcium-stone formers, especially those who have active, recurrent disease, also pass urine generally oversaturated with calcium phosphate and/or calcium oxalate and are therefore at frequent risk of crystalluria.[16] In contrast, the patients who have had only one stone episode have lower saturation levels, intermediate between those of patients with recurrences and those of normal subjects and are at less risk of crystalluria than are patients with recurrences.[17] These differences in the saturation of urine with calcium salts can be related to differences in urinary calcium, oxalate, and pH.

Of the various chemical factors influencing the saturation of urine with calcium salts, the concentration of oxalate and an alkaline pH are potentially the most critical. Thus, increasing either urinary pH or the concentration of oxalate to the upper limit of their normal ranges is sufficient to produce calcium phosphate and calcium oxalate crystalluria, respectively, in virtually the entire population. On the other hand, increasing the concentration of calcium within and even beyond the normal range of urinary calcium does not lead to spontaneous crystalluria of either calcium oxalate or phosphate in most normal subjects. However, persistent hypercalciuria does increase the risk of calcium crystalluria by raising urine saturation to a plateau value near the saturation level of both calcium salts so that a relatively small increase in either urinary oxalate or pH will cause crystalluria. It is significant that, with recurrent calcium-stone formation, there are both hypercalciuria and an increased excretion of oxalate, and, in some patients, a more-alkaline urine than normal.

The persistent passage of excessively supersaturated urine by patients with recurrent calcium stones is paralleled by an increase in calcium oxalate and calcium phosphate crystalluria (Fig. 68-3). Only a few normals, however, pass urines sufficiently supersaturated to form crystals spontaneously. This is the first important difference between patients with recurrent stones and controls.

Urinary Inhibition of Crystallization

The second important difference lies in the size and habit of the crystals excreted by the two groups. The crystals of the stone formers are larger and more aggregated than those of normal subjects, and the initiation of stone formation seems to be related to the propensity to form these abnormally large particles.

Why then do normal subjects pass only small crystals, whereas the patient with recurrent calcium stones pass much larger crystals in their urine? One of the factors likely to promote crystal growth and aggregation in the urines of the stone formers is their continuously high level of supersaturation. Indeed, there is a

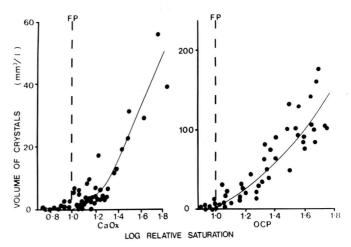

Fig. 68-3. Volume of crystals of calcium oxalate (CaOx) and octocalcium phosphate (OCP) in fresh urine in relation to their corresponding saturation levels. Saturation is expressed on a log-relative saturation scale in which 0 corresponds to the solubility product and 1 to the formation product (FP) of the salt concerned. (From Robertson et al.: N. Engl. J. Med. *294:* 249, 1976).

broad relationship between these variables in their urines. However, there is no corresponding relationship in normal urine. At any given level of supersaturation, normal subjects always pass smaller crystals than do the stone formers, suggesting that normal urine contains some protective element which prevents the formation of large crystals and aggregates and allows any calcium oxalate which precipitates to be passed harmlessly as small particles. Patients with recurrent calcium stones appear to have less protection against growth and aggregation and are at risk of the primary crystals growing freely under the existing supersaturated conditions.

In vitro evidence for the existence of an inhibitor of calcium oxalate crystallization in normal urine has been established by several groups of workers.[18-22] It is believed by some that most of the inhibitory activity lies in the acid mucopolysaccharide (AMPS) fraction of urine,[23,24] and that only a small proportion is normally attributable to the concentration of pyrophosphate.[21,23] Patients with recurrent calcium stones have significantly less inhibitory activity in their urine than normal subjects have (Fig. 68-4). This

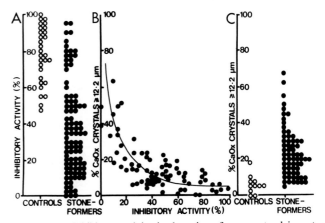

Fig. 68-4. A. Inhibitory activity in the urine of recurrent-calcium-stone formers and controls. B. Relationship between the percentage of large calcium oxalate (CaOx) crystals excreted in fresh urine and the level of inhibitory activity at a given supersaturation. C. Percentage of large CaOx crystals in fresh urine from recurrent-calcium-stone formers and controls. (From Robertson, in Fleisch et al. (eds): Urolithiasis Research, 1976. Courtesy of Plenum).

may not always result from a reduced excretion of AMPS, since in the stone formers who have a tendency to hyperuricosuria, a reduced inhibitory activity may be caused by an effective reduction in the concentration of the AMPS by its adsorption onto colloidal particles of sodium urate or uric acid.

At a constant level of supersaturation, the percentage of large crystals excreted in urine is inversely related to the inhibitory activity. Calcium-stone formers have lower inhibitory activities and higher supersaturation levels than normal subjects have, and thus have more risk of forming large crystals and aggregates of calcium salts (Fig. 68-4). This observation has led to the concept that stone formation is caused by an imbalance in the relationship between urine saturation and inhibitory activity.[25]

ROLE OF SATURATION–INHIBITION IMBALANCE IN STONE FORMATION

Figure 68-5 shows the relationship between inhibitory activity and urine saturation in normal subjects and in patients with recurrent stones. Clearly the best separation between the groups is defined, not by either variable alone, but by a line relating these factors. Discriminant analysis positions the line of best separation as shown in Figure 68-5. When the distance of each individual urine from the line is measured and replotted, the overlap between normal subjects and formers of recurrent calcium stones is reduced to about 4 percent (Fig. 68-6). This measurement has been termed the *saturation–inhibition index of stone formation* since it appears to act as a quantitative indicator of the risk of forming calcium oxalate stones.[25] Thus both the passage of large crystals and the severity of the disorder (as defined by the stone episode rate of the patient) correlate with the saturation–inhibition index of the individual stone former.

FACTORS INFLUENCING THE RISK OF STONE FORMATION

The foregoing evidence from studies in patients in whom recurrent calcium-stone formation is active supports the model of stone formation outlined previously. However, a large proportion of calcium-stone formers form stones much less frequently than this subgroup does. It is more difficult to account for the initiation of stones in this group from their urinary biochemistry, although they do tend to have higher urinary calcium and oxalate excretions than normal. The risk of crystalluria is less in these patients than in the group with the most recurrence,[26] and it has to be postulated that these patients only occasionally exceed the formation product

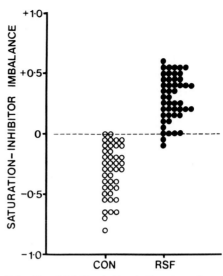

Fig. 68-6. Saturation–inhibition indices in the urines of recurrent-calcium-stone formers (RSF) and controls (CON). (From Robertson, in Fleisch et al. (eds): Urolithiasis Research, 1976. Courtesy of Plenum).

of one of the calcium salts. To prove this point would require collecting every urine sample from a large number of such calcium-stone formers over a long time, a task which is quite impracticable. Nevertheless, it is possible to show that there are various underlying fluctuations in urinary biochemistry which might account for the occasional transient period of oversaturation and crystalluria and that, by studying only random urines, the critical period of high risk may be missed.

The first factor which alters the precipitability of urine is the diurnal variation in the excretion of stone-forming salts and of water. These changes mainly reflect the diurnal pattern of eating and drinking. In addition, there is a diurnal variation in the excretion of the AMPS inhibitor of crystallization; very low levels of protection occur during the night.

The second factor which may cause intermittent changes in urine saturation are dietary and/or absorptive fluctuations. Thus increases in the dietary intake of calcium, phosphate, and oxalate may alter the urinary excretion of these ions.

Variations in diet may also alter the excretion of inhibitors; for example, phosphate intake[27] influences the excretion of pyrophosphate, one of the inhibitors of the crystallization of calcium salts.

The third factor causing fluctuations in the precipitability of urine is the seasonal variation in the urinary excretion of stone-forming salts[28] and, in hot climates, the excretion of water. In Britain, the main variables appear to be the urinary excretion of calcium and oxalate. Both reach a peak in the summer and lead to a marked increase in the number of calcium-stone formers at risk of crystalluria, as shown by an increase in the stone episode rate during the summer months.[28]

MODEL OF STONE FORMATION

Figure 68-7 summarizes the hypothesis that stone formation takes place in four stages: a nucleation phase, which results in crystalluria; a growth and aggregation phase, producing large crystals and aggregates; a trapping phase, during which a critical particle is retained at some point in the urinary tract; and, finally, a growth phase, during which the trapped particle grows into a stone.

There are two main chemical factors which control this process. First, excessive supersaturation of urine with one of the stone-forming salts is required to trigger off spontaneous nuclea-

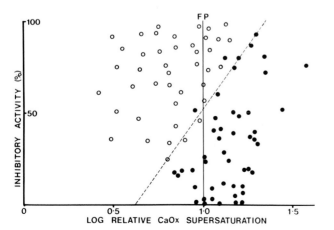

Fig. 68-5. Inhibitory activity plotted in relation to urine saturation with calcium oxalate (CaOx) in recurrent-calcium-stone formers (0) and controls (0). (From Robertson et al. N. Engl. J. Med. *294:* 249, 1976).

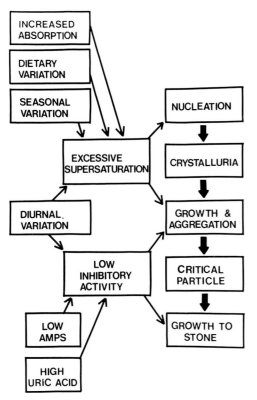

Fig. 68-7. Model of calcium-stone formation. (From Robertson, in Fleisch et al. (eds): Urolithiasis Research, 1976. Courtesy of Plenum).

tion and to support the subsequent growth of primary crystals. Second, a low level of protective inhibitory activity is necessary to permit further growth and aggregation of the primary particles. Finally, there are a number of factors which influence the levels of supersaturation and inhibitory activity in urine. These include variations in dietary intake and intestinal absorption, diurnal and seasonal fluctuations in the urinary excretion of stone-forming salts, and variations in the effective concentration of the AMPS inhibitor of crystalluria.

It is clear from the previous discussion that we consider that all stone formation is multifactorial. The more abnormal factors there are, the greater is the risk of forming stones. The diagnosis, prevention, and treatment of stone disease therefore largely depend on establishing the abnormalities in the stone-forming factors. Certain diseases, such as primary hyperparathyroidism, give

Table 68-3. Classification and Sex Distribution of 502 Unselected Patients with Upper Urinary Tract Stone Disease.

Type of Stone Disease	Number	%	Male (%)	Female (%)
Calcium				
Idiopathic	319	63.5	85.3	14.7
Hyperparathyroid	39	7.8	35.9	64.1
Infected	128	25.5	33.6	66.4
Metabolic*	16	3.2	62.5	37.5

*Includes patients with cystinuria and uric acid stones.

rise to specific abnormalities which increase the risk of calcium-stone disease. But even in patients with these diseases, individual variation in stone formation and recurrence occur, depending on the degree to which the factors involved in stone formation are affected. It is important, therefore, not only to diagnose any primary disease "causing" stone formation but also to establish to what extent the stone-forming factors are affected. The treatment and the prevention of stone disease can thus be designed to treat not only the primary disease but also the associated problem of renal stone disease.

CLASSIFICATION OF RENAL CALCIUM-STONE FORMERS

In dealing clinically with a large number of patients presenting with stone disease, the first step is the classification of the patients into the broad diagnostic groups of calcium-stone disease, infected stone disease, and metabolic stone disease, which includes uric-acid-stone disease and cystine-stone disease (Table 68-3). Patients with infected stone disease pass stones of magnesium ammonium phosphate with or without calcium phosphate, have a history of recurrent urinary tract infection, and pass infected urines (usually with urea-splitting bacteria). Patients with uric-acid-stone disease pass uric-acid stones and have abnormalities in plasma and urine uric acid and/or urine pH. Patients with cystine-stone disease pass cystine stones and have cystinuria. Having diagnosed and excluded these forms of renal stone disease, the second step is the further classification of patients with calcium-stone disease into several diagnostic subgroups. This is best done by using multiple, rather than single, diagnostic criteria and by directing the investigations toward elucidating the factors involved in stone formation (Table 68-4).

Table 68-4. Summary of the Main Biochemical Abnormalities in Idiopathic (ISF), Hyperparathyroid (HSF), Renal Tubular Acidotic (RTA), and Hyperoxaluric (HOx) Stone Formers, and Effect of Renal Failure (RF) on the Biochemical Parameters

	Stone Analysis Ox>PO₄	24-hr Urine Ca	PO₄	Ox	pH	Crystalluria CaOX	CaPO₄	Urinary Inhibitory Activity	Calcium Absorption	Plasma Ca	PO₄	PTH	1,25(OH)₂D₃	HCO₃
ISF														
Pure	↑↑	↑	=	↑	=	↑	↑	↓	↑	=	↓	↓	↑	=
Mixed	↑	↑	=	↑	↑	↑	↑	↓	↑	=	↓	↓		=
HSF														
Mild	↓	↑↑	↑	↑	↑↑	↑	↑↑	↓	↑↑	↑	↓↓	↑	↑	↓
Severe	↓	↑↑	↑	↑	↑↑	↑	↑↑	↓	↑↑	↑↑	↓↓	↑↑		↓
RTA	↓↓	↑	=	=	↑↑	?	?	?	=	=	↑	=	=	↓↓
HOx	↑↑	=	=	↑↑	=	↑↑	=	?	=	=	=	=	=	=
RF	—	↓↓	=	=	↓	↓	↓	?	↓↓	=	↑↑	↑↑	↓↓	↓↓

Key: ↑↑, grossly increased; ↑, increased; =, normal; ↓, decreased; ↓↓, grossly decreased; ?, not yet determined.

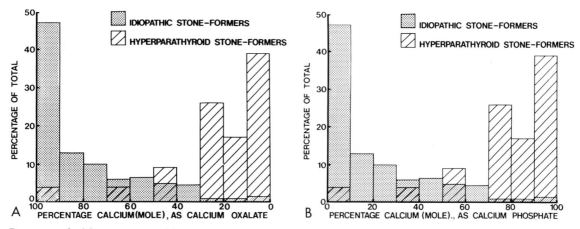

Fig. 68-8. Percentage of calcium present as calcium oxalate (A) and as calcium phosphate (B) in 200 unselected upper urinary tract stones from idiopathic calcium stone formers (▨) and 23 unselected upper urinary tract stones from hyperparathyroid stone formers (▧).

IDIOPATHIC STONE FORMERS

Idiopathic is rather an unfortunate term to use in classifying these patients; it wrongly implies that little is known about the factors involved in their stone formation and that they form a homogeneous group. We have retained it however, since although its diagnostic criteria have never been firmly established, it is universally used.

Patients with idiopathic stone formation make up the largest subgroup of patients with calcium-stone disease (Table 68-3). Idiopathic stone formation is uncommon in children, reaches its peak incidence between the ages of 30 and 50, and is much more common in males than females[4,7,8] (Table 68-3).

Stone Analysis

Quantitative stone analysis shows that idiopathic stone formers pass stones of almost pure calcium oxalate (Fig. 68-8A). Approximately 40 percent of idiopathic stone formers, however, pass stones containing a significant amount of phosphate (i.e., >20 percent by weight as calcium phosphate) and can be classified as "mixed"-stone formers[29,30] (Fig. 68-8B). Analysis of the urine of these two groups shows that both have raised urinary activity products for calcium oxalate and calcium phosphate, but that the mixed-stone formers have a higher urinary calcium phosphate activity product mainly because of a higher urinary pH. There is little doubt that stone formation in these two groups reflects the composition of the prevailing urine in which it is formed.

Urine Biochemistry

Calcium. Hypercalciuria is a striking feature of patients with idiopathic stone formation.[31] The hypercalciuria is mainly of the absorptive type[32,33] (Fig. 68-9), although in some studies a significant number of patients with tubular hypercalciuria have been described.[34,35] It is confusing and serves no useful purpose to continue to call the hypercalciuria of this condition *idiopathic*, and it should be avoided. The hypercalciuria should be defined in terms of the organ mainly involved in its cause, namely, absorptive from the gut, resorptive from bone, and tubular from the kidney.[33]

Oxalate. The urine oxalate is raised in idiopathic stone formers.[11,29,36] The cause of this increase is still unknown. In most studies there is a direct relationship between urine calcium and oxalate,[36] which is present even on a fixed dietary intake of calcium and oxalate.[30] Since in fact an increase in dietary calcium decreases urine oxalate, and a decrease in dietary calcium increases urine oxalate,[37] the relationship cannot be due simply to

dietary and digestive factors. It could be that there is either hyperabsorption of both calcium and oxalate or that hyperabsorption of calcium results in less complexed oxalate being present in the bowel, thus promoting oxalate absorption.

pH. Urine pH is normal in idiopathic stone formers. However, if the patients with "mixed" calcium oxalate/phosphate stones are examined as a group, their urinary pH is significantly raised.[29,30] It

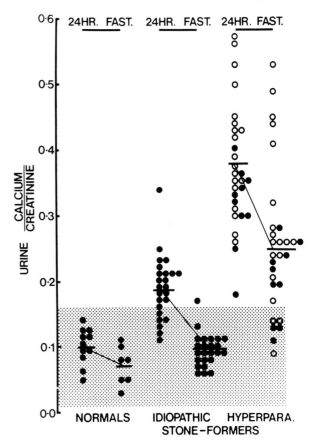

Fig. 68-9. Urine calcium/creatinine ratio in 24-hour nonfasting urine (24 hr) and fasting urine (Fast) in normal subjects and idiopathic and hyperparathyroid stone formers (males ●, females ○) on a fixed dietary intake of 800 mg/day. Decrease in the urine calcium/creatinine ratio in each group due to fasting is indicated by a line joining the mean values. Normal range for fasting urine calcium/creatinine ratio is indicated by the shaded area. (From Peacock et al., in Avioli et al. (eds): Phosphate Metabolism: Kidney and Bone, 1976. Courtesy Armour-Montagu).

is unclear at present whether the high urinary pH of "mixed"-stone formers is a manifestation of an underlying abnormality or whether it represents the upper end of the normal urine pH distribution.

Crystalluria and Inhibitors of Crystal Growth and Aggregation. As previously discussed, patients with idiopathic stone disease are significantly different from normals in the amount and type of crystals in the urine. It is probable that these differences may prove to be useful in differentiating this type of stone disease from others; also, the urines of idiopathic stone formers are deficient in inhibitors of crystal growth and aggregation. The urinary pyrophosphate inhibitors are normal, and the difference in inhibitory activity is due to a deficiency, or possibly an inactivation, of the mucopolysaccharide inhibitors.

Plasma Biochemistry

Calcium. The plasma calcium in idiopathic stone formers is normal when it is measured after an overnight fast[38] (Fig. 68-10). However, it may be raised if the patient is not fasting and calcium is still being cleared from absorption. Tubular reabsorption of calcium is also generally normal in the fasting state and during calcium infusion.[32] However, if tubular reabsorption is measured from clearance studies performed over short time intervals (1–2 hours) it is important to have the patient completely fasted (>12 hours) to avoid a decrease in tubular reabsorption secondary to calcium absorption, which may be mistaken for a "tubular leak."

Phosphate. In contrast to plasma calcium, the plasma phosphate is lower in idiopathic stone formers than in normal subjects when assessed in the fasting state. The hypophosphatemia is due to a decreased tubular reabsorption of phosphate[30,39] (Fig. 68-11). It is unlikely to be due either to phosphate depletion or an increase in glomerular filtration rate, since the 24-hour urine phosphate and creatinine are normal in idiopathic stone formers.[15]

Parathyroid Hormone (PTH). The plasma PTH is in the lower half of the normal range in idiopathic stone formers[30,35] (Fig. 68-10). This is compatible with the hypothesis that hyperabsorption of calcium suppresses PTH secretion in idiopathic stone formation and is not the result of increased PTH secretion. Some workers, however, have described a significant number of idiopathic stone formers with raised levels of PTH and a tubular leak of calcium and have argued that hyperabsorption of calcium results from secondary hyperparathyroidism induced by the calcium "leak."[34]

Vitamin D. Plasma 25-OH-D_3 (25-hydroxyvitamin D_3) is normal in idiopathic stone formers (Peacock, unpublished results), and,

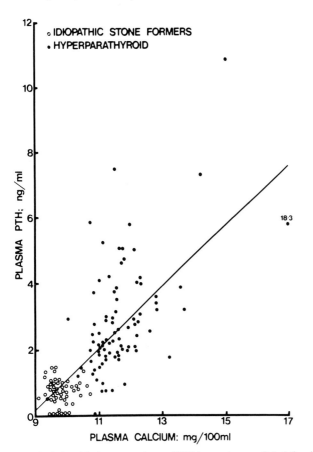

Fig. 68-10. Relationship between plasma PTH (normal range 0.5–1.5 ng/ml) and plasma calcium (normal range 9–10.6 mg/100 ml) in idiopathic stone formers (○) and hyperparathyroid patients with and without renal stone disease (●). (From Peacock et al., in Avioli et al. (eds): Phosphate Metabolism: Kidney and Bone, 1976. Courtesy Armour-Montagu).

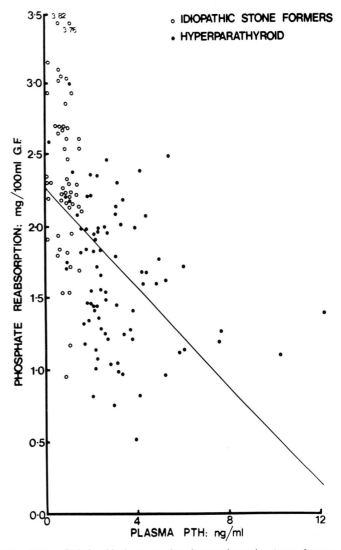

Fig. 68-11. Relationship between phosphate reabsorption (normal range 2–3.5 mg/100 ml glomerular filtrate) and plasma PTH (normal range 0.5–1.5 ng/ml) in idiopathic stone formers (○) and hyperparathyroid patients with and without renal stone disease (●). (From Peacock et al., in Avioli et al. (eds): Phosphate Metabolism: Kidney and Bone, 1976. Courtesy Armour-Montagu).

although the seasonal rise in urinary calcium coincides with the seasonal rise in plasma 25-OH-D₃, it is still not clear whether these two parameters are related. It has been reported however, that the plasma, 1,25-(OH)₂-D₃ (1,25-dihydroxyvitamin D₃) is raised in patients with idiopathic stone disease.[40] If this observation is confirmed, then it is clear that hyperabsorption of calcium is secondary to an increased production of 1,25-(OH)₂-D₃ despite a suppression of PTH. Since hypophosphatemia is known to stimulate 1,25-(OH)₂-D₃ production, it has therefore been postulated that the hypophosphatemia of idiopathic stone formers may be the primary abnormality responsible for hyperabsorption.[40]

Absorption

Calcium. The hyperabsorption of calcium in patients with idiopathic stone disease is well established[33,35,39,41] (Fig. 68-12). Various hypotheses have been put forward to explain it: (1) it may be caused by increased sensitivity of the gut to vitamin D;[42] (2) it may be due to increased PTH secretion secondary to a tubular leak of calcium;[34] (3) it may be caused by an increased 1,25-(OH)₂-D₃ production stimulated by low plasma phosphate;[40] or (4) it may represent the upper end of the normal range for calcium absorption.[43] In our experience, secondary hyperparathyroidism from a ''tubular leak'' of calcium is rare. Although the role of 1,25-(OH)₂-D₃ in hyperabsorption represents an exciting new concept, more

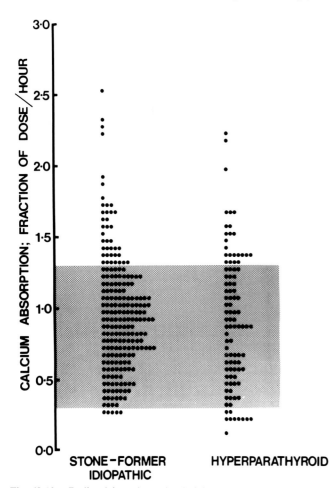

Fig. 68-12. Radiocalcium absorption in idiopathic stone formers and hyperparathyroid patients with and without stone disease. Normal range is indicated by the shaded area. (From Peacock et al., in Avioli et al. (eds): Phosphate Metabolism: Kidney and Bone, 1976. Courtesy Armsur Montagu).

studies are required—especially in relation to hypophosphatemia, which is neither a constant nor a universal feature of hyperabsorption—before passing judgement. It may be that all these mechanisms, to a lesser or greater extent, are involved since hyperabsorption of calcium leading to hypercalciuria is only another of the risk factors in calcium-stone disease.

Phosphate. There is no indication that there is a net increase in phosphate absorption since the 24-hour urine phosphate both on a free or on a fixed diet is not increased as compared to normal subjects.[15,30]

Oxalate. The 24-hour urine oxalate is increased in idiopathic stone formers.[11,29,36] This may be due to an increase in oxalate absorption. Measurements of oxalate absorption, however, have shown no difference between idiopathic stone formers and normal subjects (Wilkinson and Hodgkinson, personal communication). It may be that hyperabsorption of calcium, however, by increasing the amount of free oxalate in the bowel, allows more oxalate to be absorbed.

Bone Metabolism

It is generally true that idiopathic stone disease and clinical bone disease are mutually exclusive. It is very rare in our experience for patients with either osteoporosis or osteomalacia to have a history of idiopathic calcium-stone disease. In idiopathic stone formers the urinary hydroxyproline excretion (Fig. 68-13) and the alkaline phosphatase are normal.[39]

Apart from the passage of a stone and possibly the passage of large calcium oxalate crystals in the urine, there is no single abnormality which distinguishes idiopathic stone formers from normal subjects. Various biochemical disorders can be defined but they occur together in only a small percentage of the patients. Hypophosphatemia, for example, occurs in only about 10 percent of patients, and the plasma phosphate of idiopathic stone formers does not correlate with calcium absorption (Peacock, unpublished data). It seems unlikely, therefore, that idiopathic stone formation as defined by the passage of a calcium oxalate and/or phosphate stone represents a homogeneous condition and that only one disorder accounts for the biochemical disorders which have so far been described. Since, however, stone formation is multifactorial it is easy to understand how these biochemical abnormalities increase the risk of oversaturation with calcium oxalate and calcium phosphate of urine that is defective in inhibitors.

HYPERPARATHYROID STONE FORMERS

Hyperparathyroid stone formers make up about 8 percent of patients with calcium-stone disease (Table 68-3). All patients with primary hyperparathyroidism, however, do not develop calcium-stone disease; only about 60 percent of patients do so.[44–46] As will be subsequently discussed, this apparent anomaly is due to some primary hyperparathyroid patients being at greater risk of stone formation than others. Primary hyperparathyroidism occurs most commonly in postmenopausal women, and hyperparathyroid stone formers are usually female (Table 68-3). The stone disease is recurrent but, unlike idiopathic calcium-stone disease, there is occasionally an associated nephrocalcinosis, which may also occur in the absence of renal stone disease. Although both these conditions are associated with primary hyperparathyroidism and involve deposition of calcium salts, they need not involve the same biochemical mechanisms.

Stone Analysis

The stones from hyperparathyroid stone formers are mainly composed of calcium phosphate with a variable amount of oxalate[30,47] (Fig. 68-8A,B). The urine activity products for calcium oxalate and especially phosphate are increased, and the composition reflects to a large extent the urine in which the stone forms. The increased activity products are due mainly to increased concentrations of urine calcium and oxalate and to a higher urinary pH.[30]

Urine Biochemistry

Calcium. Hypercalciuria, which is both absorptive and resorptive in origin, is present in most hyperparathyroid stone formers[33,39] (Fig. 68-9). It is due to the action of PTH on calcium absorption and on bone resorption. After successful parathyroidectomy the urine calcium returns to normal.[30]

Oxalate. Urine oxalate shows the same relationship to urine calcium in hyperparathyroid stone formers as in idiopathic stone formers and it is likely that the same mechanisms are involved.[30]

pH. Urine pH in primary hyperparathyroid patients is raised.[30] The most acceptable explanation is that PTH acts on the renal tubule to decrease the tubular reabsorption of bicarbonate.[48]

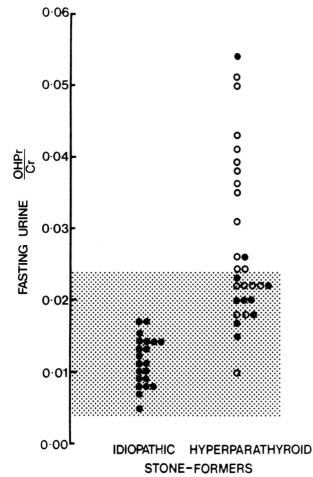

Fig. 68-13. Fasting urine hydroxyproline/creatinine ratio in idiopathic and hyperparathyroid stone formers (males ●, females ○). Normal range is indicated by the shaded area. (From Peacock et al., in Avioli et al. (eds): Phosphate Metabolism: Kidney and Bone, 1976. Courtesy Armour-Montagu).

Phosphate. There is a slight but significant increase in the urine phosphate,[30] probably reflecting the action of PTH on phosphate absorption.

Crystalluria and Inhibitors of Crystal Growth and Aggregation. From the limited studies which have been done on hyperparathyroid stone formers, it seems that the same pattern exists as is seen in idiopathic stone formers: the inhibitors are lower in the hyperparathyroid patients with stone disease as compared to those without (Peacock and Robertson, unpublished data).

Plasma Biochemistry

Calcium. The majority of patients with primary hyperparathyroidism have a raised plasma calcium,[45,46] which in the absence of renal failure or vitamin D deficiency is directly related to the plasma PTH concentration[39] (Fig. 68-10). The raised plasma calcium in the fasting state is due to a combination of increased tubular reabsorption of calcium and increased bone resorption. In hyperparathyroid stone formers the bone is rarely severely affected, and the rise in fasting plasma calcium largely results from the action of PTH on the renal tubule. In primary hyperparathyroidism with renal failure or vitamin D deficiency, the plasma calcium is low relative to the plasma PTH. Indeed, in some patients it may be so low that the plasma calcium lies in the normal range. This may account for some of the patients who have been classified as having "normocalcemic" hyperparathyroidism.[46] It is probable, however, that many of the so-called normocalcemic hyperparathyroid patients have mild primary hyperparathyroidism and the plasma calcium and PTH are both at the upper end of the normal range. Certainly, accurate and repeated measurements of plasma calcium (and ionized calcium if it can be done more accurately) and PTH are required to separate this group of patients from normal subjects and from idiopathic stone formers.

Phosphate. The action of PTH to decrease tubular reabsorption of phosphate results in most hyperparathyroid stone formers having a low plasma phosphate.[45] The relationship, however, between plasma phosphate or phosphate reabsorption and plasma PTH is poor, which suggests that although PTH is important, other factors are involved (Fig. 68-11).

PTH. Although plasma PTH is raised in most patients with hyperparathyroid stone disease, it cannot be taken as an absolute criterion for establishing the diagnosis (Fig. 68-10). Although radioimmunoassay can measure plasma levels of PTH, it is not very reproducible, and the immunochemical heterogeneity of plasma PTH makes the assay rather nonspecific.[49] Furthermore, milder forms of primary hyperparathyroidism may have plasma PTH in the upper end of the normal range since the glands are not completely autonomous.[50]

Vitamin D_3. Patients with primary hyperparathyroidism may have osteomalacia and low plasma 25-OH-D_3 concentrations. This, however, is extremely rare in those patients who are actively forming stones. The levels of 1,25-$(OH)_2$-D_3 are high from the action of PTH on the renal 1α-hydroxylase to increase 1,25-$(OH)_2$-D_3 production.[40]

Bicarbonate. Some authors have stressed the importance of low bicarbonate and high chloride levels in hyperparathyroid patients due to the action of PTH on the tubular reabsorption of bicarbonate.[48] In hyperparathyroid stone formers these changes are not remarkable and are rarely of use in diagnosis.

Absorption

Calcium. Calcium absorption is increased in hyperparathyroid stone formers by the action of PTH on the gut, indirectly through its action on 1,25-(OH)$_2$-D$_3$ production (Fig. 68-12). Following parathyroidectomy the hyperabsorption returns to normal. Hyperparathyroid patients with stone disease have a higher absorption of calcium than those without stone disease, some of whom may even have malabsorption of calcium.[44] The relative malabsorption of calcium probably accounts for their lower urinary calcium and is one of the factors which protects them from developing stones. It is likely that vitamin D deficiency and renal failure are the main causes of this relative malabsorption. Certainly, the high urine calcium from hyperabsorption is an important risk factor in the stone formation of hyperparathyroidism.

Phosphate. Phosphate absorption tends to be increased in patients with hyperparathyroidism due either to a direct action of PTH on phosphate transport or to a secondary action from its effect on calcium absorption.[51]

Oxalate. Little is known about the absorption of oxalate in primary hyperparathyroidism. As previously discussed, however, there may be an increase in oxalate absorption as a result of the hyperabsorption of calcium.

Bone Metabolism

There is usually biochemical evidence of increased bone turnover in patients with primary hyperparathyroidism. The hydroxyproline excretion is raised (Fig. 68-13) and there may be a rise in alkaline phosphatase. However, hyperparathyroid stone formers are usually only mildly affected, and many have hydroxyproline excretions at the upper end of the normal range.[39] Bone biopsy of the iliac crest, however, shows that even in the patients who are only mildly affected there tends to be an increase in resorbing and forming surfaces (Peacock, unpublished data).

The action of PTH in man results in several abnormalities which result in an increased risk of forming calcium phosphate and oxalate stones in the urinary tract. The most important factors are probably the increase in urine calcium and pH. However, in the individual patient, high urinary oxalate and phosphate, low urinary volume, and low urinary inhibitors also play a role. Some patients with primary hyperparathyroidism never form stones since they pass urine with a normal calcium and oxalate concentration and high inhibitory power. Unlike idiopathic stone formers, patients with hyperparathyroid stone disease form a more uniform diagnostic group, and consequently are easier to treat.

DIFFERENTIATION BETWEEN IDIOPATHIC STONE FORMERS AND MILD HYPERPARATHYROID STONE FORMERS

It is obvious from the previous discussion that these two conditions can have several abnormalities in common apart from the passage of a calcium-containing stone: the increased calcium absorption and urine calcium, the decreased tubular reabsorption of phosphate, and possibly the raised plasma 1,25-(OH)$_2$-D$_3$ level. In addition, the idiopathic mixed-stone formers have urine pH and stone analysis very similar to that of the hyperparathyroid stone formers. The diagnostic problem at present seems to center around

the accurate measurement of plasma calcium, either total or ionized, and plasma PTH. The estimations must be done from blood taken at a fixed time after a meal, probably at least 12 hours, to avoid the changes caused by calcium absorption, which is equally high in both conditions; there is little argument that repeated estimations increase the separation between the two groups. Even with these precautions, however, an overlap occurs. Rather than force a patient into one or the other of the diagnostic groups, it is probably more advisable to leave these patients in a separate category for at least 6 months while repeated tests are carried out. This avoids unnecessary parathyroid operations in idiopathic stone formers and unsuccessful parathyroid operations in hyperparathyroid stone formers, since the glands are often only slightly enlarged at this "stage" of the disease. The patients, however, must be prepared to be followed regularly at the clinic and have the stone disease treated in its own right as previously outlined.[30] Stimulation and suppression tests of parathyroid function have been advocated as methods of diagnosing mild hyperparathyroidism,[34,35,50] but they have not been found generally useful, probably because of the problems in measuring small changes in parathyroid secretion.

STONE FORMERS WITH RENAL TUBULAR ACIDOSIS

Only a very small percentage of calcium-stone formers are found to have renal tubular acidosis. These patients usually have a very high stone episode rate, and radiography of the kidneys shows multiple small stones often closely associated with the renal pyramids, which may be mistakenly diagnosed as medullary sponge kidneys. There may be an associated nephrocalcinosis. The stone disease can present in late childhood or early adulthood and there is sometimes a family history of stone disease. The striking biochemical abnormality is the passage of persistently alkaline urine which does not acidify normally after an oral acid load. Acidemia may be severe but it can be mild. The urine activity product for calcium phosphate is persistently high and the stone composition is almost always pure calcium phosphate. These patients may have other metabolic abnormalities, such as glycosuria, which are unrelated to the production of renal stones, but hypercalciuria, if it is present, is an important risk factor.[52]

HYPEROXALURIC-STONE FORMERS

Mild hyperoxaluria, as previously mentioned, is a feature of both idiopathic stone formers and hyperparathyroid stone formers. Large increases in urine oxalate, however, are seen in two uncommon groups of patients with renal stone disease. In the first group the patients have congenital hyperoxaluria in which there are defects in oxalate metabolism and the stone disease usually presents in childhood. These unfortunate patients have very high urine calcium oxalate activity products, pass almost pure calcium oxalate stones, and invariably die in renal failure with the kidneys destroyed by deposits of calcium oxalate.[53] The second group consists of patients who have hyperoxaluria induced by extensive surgery to the small bowel, usually because of Crohn's disease. The stone disease is milder than in congenital hyperoxaluria and it is less common to see tissue destruction from calcium oxalate deposits—probably because their plasma oxalate is never as high as that of those patients with the congenital form of the disease. The mechanisms involved in this hyperoxaluria are still unknown, although increased absorption of dietary oxalate is an important factor.[54]

DISEASES ASSOCIATED WIH RENAL CALCIUM-STONE FORMATION

Vitamin D intoxication, the milk/alkali syndrome, adrenocortical hyperfunction, acromegaly, and sarcoidosis are all diseases which may be associated with renal stone disease. Few detailed studies have been done to establish the abnormalities giving rise to stone formation in these conditions or even to determine which type of stone is produced. However, it is clear that certain risk factors for stone formation are present, such as hypercalciuria and alkaline urine, and it is likely that the stone formation in these diseases can be explained in the same terms as in the commoner forms of stone disease.

COMPLICATIONS OF URINARY TRACT INFECTION AND RENAL FAILURE IN THE DIAGNOSIS OF RENAL CALCIUM-STONE DISEASE

Obstruction in the urinary tract, especially if it becomes chronic, invariably leads to urinary tract infection. It is not uncommon therefore, for patients with a long history of calcium-stone disease to present eventually with urinary tract infection and stones largely composed of magnesium ammonium phosphate. The risk factors which gave rise to calcium-stone disease have been superseded by those factors which give rise to infected stone disease.[45] In general, the treatment of these patients is directed toward clearing the obstruction and making the urine sterile with appropriate antibiotics.

Similarly, calcium-stone disease may also lead to impairment of renal function. When this occurs the diagnosis of the type of calcium-stone disease becomes much more difficult. Even mild renal failure can give rise to a fall in calcium absorption and a decrease in urine calcium, a rise in plasma phosphate and a decrease in phosphate reabsorption, and a fall in plasma calcium and an elevation of plasma PTH (Table 68-4). These are all changes which make the biochemical classification of calcium-stone formers more difficult and call for great experience in the interpretation of the investigations. If the renal failure progresses, most of the risk factors for calcium-stone formation disappear and the patient passes mainly undersaturated urine. Although the stones in the kidney may not dissolve, especially if they are of the calcium oxalate type, the activity of the disease is greatly reduced.

TREATMENT

IDIOPATHIC STONE FORMERS

Although surgical treatment of calcium-stone disease is indicated if there is ureteral or intrarenal obstruction, it is clear that surgery has no place in the prevention of recurrence of renal stone.[55,56] The prevention of calcium-stone disease and its recurrence, therefore, lies in the medical management of the patient.

It has been shown above that calcium-stone formation is caused by an imbalance in the relationship between the saturation of urine with calcium salts and the level of protective inhibitory activity. Treatment, therefore, may be directed at either reducing urine saturation or increasing inhibitory activity, or reducing saturation and increasing inhibitory activity simultaneously. Not only must treatment be effective in these respects, but it must also be continuous, and the patient should be made to realize that to avoid further stones, treatment probably has to be lifelong. Idiopathic calcium-stone disease can be treated in several ways.

1. The saturation of urine with calcium salts may be reduced by giving a low-calcium, low-oxalate, high-fluid regimen to reduce the concentrations of calcium and oxalate in the urine. This lowers urine saturation[37] and significantly reduces the stone recurrence rate to about 40 percent of the pretreatment rate[57] (Fig. 68-14A). The main problems with dietary therapy are that the diet is unattractive and, for many patients, difficult to adhere to at all times.

2. Urine saturation may be reduced by administration of cellulose phosphate,[58,59] which complexes calcium in the intestine and thereby reduces the intestinal absorption and urinary excretion of calcium.[60,61] Preliminary reports suggest that cellulose phosphate may effectively reduce the rate of recurrence of calcium stones.[59,61] Long-term studies are necessary to evaluate this form of therapy (Fig. 68-14B), since it may lead to stimulation of the parathyroids and bone disease in some patients[62] and to reduced serum levels of magnesium, iron, copper, and zinc.[63] Cellulose phosphate may therefore have only limited application.

3. Administration of thiazide diuretics lowers the urinary excretion of calcium,[64] possibly through the effect of extracellular volume contraction on stimulating the tubular reabsorption of calcium. Urine saturation is reduced[58,65] (Fig. 68-14C) and there is a reduction in stone recurrence.[64,66] Potassium supplements have to be administered in conjunction with these drugs.

4. Since no simple method is known to increase the urinary excretion of the naturally occurring AMPS inhibitor of calcium oxalate crystallization in urine, attempts have been made to increase the protection against crystal growth and aggregation by the feeding of synthetic inhibitors of crystallization. Ethane-1-hydroxy-1,1-diphosphonate (EHDP) is an effective inhibitor of calcium oxalate crystallization in vitro and in animals in vivo.[67] Studies in man show that, although there is an apparent reduction in the short-term stone recurrence rate,[68] there is often an increase in calcium oxalate crystalluria as a result of a dramatic rise in urinary oxalate.[69] It is also known that EHDP, in the high doses required to increase urinary inhibitory activity, may produce significant changes in bone.[70] It seems unlikely, therefore, that this form of therapy will ever become acceptable unless the side effects can be overcome.

5. Some forms of treatment have been designed to reduce urine saturation *and* increase inhibitory activity simultaneously. The first of these involves the oral administration of magnesium supplements (usually given as magnesium oxide). It was thought that magnesium, by complexing with phosphate and oxalate ions, would reduce urine saturation with calcium salts[71,72] and also increase the inhibitory activity, since it appeared from some studies,[73] but not others,[74,75] to block the crystallization of calcium salts. There is only fragmentary evidence that magnesium supplements reduce the stone formation rate in man.[72]

6. A more promising alternative is to administer supplements of orthophosphate (1–1.5 g P/day). This form of therapy reduces urine saturation[76,77] by decreasing urine calcium,[60] and increases inhibitory activity[76] by increasing urinary pyrophosphate.[27,76] The net result is to produce a great improvement in the saturation–inhibition index and in the frequency of passage of large crystals and aggregates in the urine[76] (Fig. 68-15). Successful reduction of the stone recurrence rate has been reported from a number of centers.[27,76,78–80] Addition of phosphate supplements to the low-calcium, low-oxalate diet reduces the stone episode rate in those patients who have only partially responded to the diet alone (Fig. 68-14A). Few side effects, apart from occasional diarrhea, have been reported with this therapy and long-term studies have failed to find any evidence of parathyroid stimulation.[78]

7. Finally, there are reports that many patients with calcium

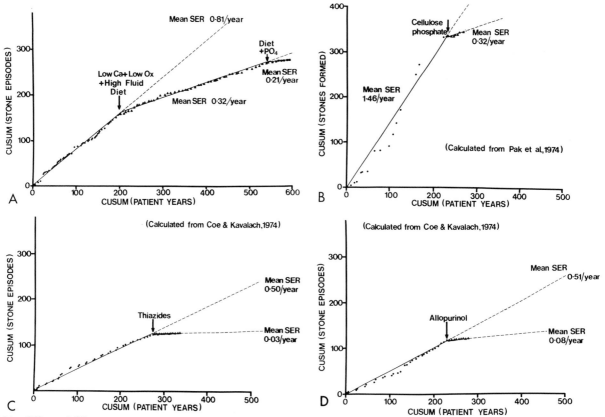

Fig. 68-14. Effects of different treatments on the mean stone episode rate (SER) of recurrent-calcium-stone formers. A. Low-calcium, low-oxalate diet ± orthophosphate supplements. B. Cellulose phosphate.[59] C. Thiazides.[66] D. Allopurinol.[66] The data are presented in the form of cusum plots, i.e., the cumulative sum of the stone episodes of all the patients plotted in relation to the cumulative patient years. The values for each patient are plotted before and during therapy. The slope of the regression line through each pretreatment and treatment period is the average stone episode rate of the group as a whole.

oxalate stones also have hyperuricosuria.[66,81] These patients may be treated with the xanthine oxidase inhibitor, allopurinol, which reduces the urinary excretion of uric acid.[66] Preliminary studies indicate a beneficial effect of reducing urinary uric acid on the rate of calcium oxalate stone formation (Fig. 68-14D). The mechanism by which this is achieved is not yet clear. One school of thought believes that hyperuricosuria leads to spontaneous precipitation of

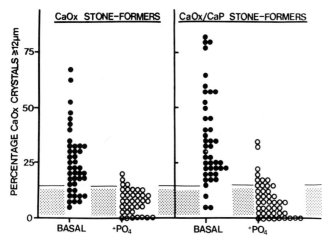

Fig. 68-15. Percentage of large calcium oxalate (CaOx) crystals in the urines of patients with "pure" CaOx stones and "mixed" CaOx/calcium phosphate (CaP) stones before and during treatment with orthophosphate supplements (1 g P/day extra in the diet). Shaded area represents the normal range of large crystals.

crystals of sodium urate which, in turn, act as nucleators of calcium oxalate crystallization.[82,83] However, crystals of sodium urate are not observed in the urines of hyperuricosuric patients, so that this mechanism seems unlikely. An alternative explanation proposes that hyperuricosuria leads to the formation of *colloidal* sodium urate.[24,84] This, in turn, is thought to be stabilized by adsorption of the AMPS inhibitor of crystallization, thereby reducing the effective concentration of AMPS available to inhibit the crystallization of calcium oxalate.[24] Reduction of urinary uric acid would decrease the amount of sodium urate colloid formed and release AMPS to inhibit the formation of large crystals of calcium oxalate.

HYPERPARATHYROID STONE FORMERS

The principles of treatment of hyperparathyroid stone formers are the same as those outlined above for idiopathic stone formers. Since, however, all the urinary abnormalities are caused by the action of excessive PTH secretion, the treatment of choice is parathyroidectomy.[45] If successful, not only does the urine saturation decrease, largely because of the fall in urine calcium and pH, but the urine saturation remains normal after parathyroidectomy and the stone recurrence rate is reduced permanently (Fig. 68-16).

In some patients, however, parathyroidectomy may fail to remove all the abnormal parathyroid tissue, and, in others parathyroidectomy may not be feasible because of infirmity or age. In these patients the high urine saturation can be reduced by medical treatment. Probably the safest procedure is a very high fluid

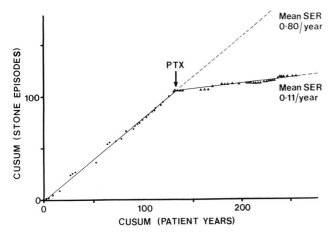

Fig. 68-16. Effect of parathyroidectomy (PTX) on the mean stone episode rate (SER) of a group of hyperparathyroid stone formers. Data are presented in the form of a cusum plot as described in Fig. 68-14.

intake, which should be maintained throughout the 24 hours (Fig. 68-17). A high fluid intake is also useful after successful parathyroidectomy in those patients who have stones in the kidney. A very substantial reduction in urine saturation occurs and probably helps to partially dissolve the stones and allow them to be passed (Fig. 68-17). In those patients whose urine calcium is mainly absorptive, a reduction in dietary calcium may be helpful. Oral orthophosphate can also be given with benefit in a dose of 1 g/day. Both these treatments, however, carry the risk of stimulating the parathyroid glands and increasing bone resorption. If they are used, regular plasma PTH and urinary hydroxyproline estimation must be done to monitor any increase in bone resorption. Reduc-

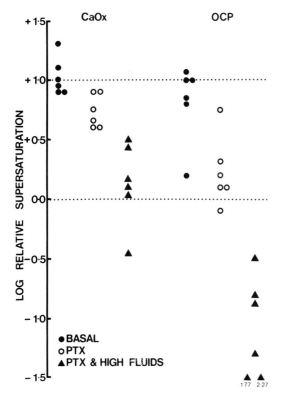

Fig. 68-17. Saturation of urine with calcium oxalate (CaOx) and octocalcium phosphate (OCP) in hyperparathyroid stone formers before and after parathyroidectomy (PTX) ± a high fluid intake. (From Peacock et al., in Finlayson et al. (eds.): Colloquium on Renal Lithiosis, 1976. Courtesy The University Presses of Florida.)

tion of urine pH can be achieved by a small daily dose of acid in the form of ammonium sulphate 2–4 g/day. The long-term effect of this treatment on bone, however, has never been properly assessed. In some female patients a large fraction of the urine calcium may be resorptive from bone, as indicated by a high urinary hydroxyproline excretion. Estrogens in the form of ethinyl estradiol 25–50 μg/day can be used in these patients to reduce the urine calcium.[85] It is clear, therefore, that medical management of the hyperparathyroid stone former is possible although each patient must be assessed individually.

RENAL-STONE FORMERS WITH RENAL TUBULAR ACIDOSIS

Although these patients form a small percentage of the calcium stone formers they are a difficult clinical problem because they have very recurrent stone disease which is difficult to manage. The basic defect is a failure to acidify the urine normally. The condition may be associated with severe acidemia, hypokalemia, decreased phosphate and glucose tubular reabsorption, and osteomalacia.[52] In the patients with recurrent stone disease, however, the condition is usually uncomplicated and the defect in acidification may only be identified following an acid-load test. The aim of the treatment in these patients is to reduce the urine pH to below 6.2 and thus prevent the precipitation of calcium phosphate. If the patient is not acidemic this can often by achieved by an oral dose of acid. An acceptable preparation is ammonium sulphate in gelatin capsules, usually 2–6 g/day. Since the urine pH has a marked circadian rhythm, the capsules should be taken every 6 hours throughout the 24 hours. In the acidemic patients, however, the problem is more difficult since these patients are usually already under maximum acid stress and may require *alkali* to prevent severe acidemia.

In some patients other risk factors may be present, such as hypercalciuria. This may be absorptive and can be reduced by a low-calcium diet. More commonly, it is tubular in origin. Alkali has been used to increase the tubular reabsorption of calcium and so decrease the urine calcium. However, it would seem illogical in the patients with the milder form of the disease to decrease the urine calcium at the expense of increasing urine pH. Bendrofluazide 5–10 mg/day with potassium salts decreases urine calcium without the adverse effect on urine pH.

HYPEROXALURIC-STONE FORMERS

In the congenital form of this disease the prognosis is very poor and, indeed, the patient is often in severe renal failure at the time he presents clinically. Various forms of "specific" treatment have been advocated to block the endogenous production of oxalate.[86] Only the use of high doses of pyridoxine 100–300 mg/day seem to have a consistent effect on urinary oxalate excretion, and even on this dose the urine oxalate remains well above the normal range.[87] The general approach, therefore, must be to increase fluid intake, reduce dietary oxalate as much as possible, and give pyridoxine. There is also some evidence that oral orthophosphate may be of some help in reducing calcium oxalate crystalluria and it can be added to the regimen.[88]

In the hyperoxaluria associated with small-bowel disease, a very striking reduction in the raised urine oxalate occurs on restriction of dietary oxalate.[54] These patients also tend to have a low urine volume because of the loss of fluid through the bowel. If the urine oxalate concentration can be maintained in the normal range by dietary oxalate restriction and high fluids, the prognosis is good.

REFERENCES

1. Prien, E. Studies in urolithiasis II. Relationships between pathogenesis, structure and composition of calculi. *J Urol 61:* 821, 1949.
2. Lagergren, C. Biophysical investigations of urinary calculi. *Acta Radiol* (Stockh) [Suppl] *133:* 1, 1956.
3. Richter, E., Sucker, I. Uber die Zusammensetzung von Harnsteinen. *Urol Int 22:* 178, 1967.
4. Nordin, B. E. C., Hodgkinson, A. Urolithiasis. In Dock, W., Snapper, I. (eds): Advances in Internal Medicine, vol 13. Chicago, Year Book, 1967, p. 155.
5. Lonsdale, K. Human stones. Science *159:* 1199, 1968.
6. Williams, R. E. The natural history of renal lithiasis. In Hodgkinson, A., Nordin, B. E. C. (eds): Renal Stone Research Symposium. London, Churchill, 1969, p. 65.
7. Blacklock, N. J. The pattern of urolithiasis in the Royal Navy. In Hodgkinson, A., Nordin, B. E. C. (eds): Renal Stone Research Symposium. London, Churchill, 1969, p. 33.
8. Andersen, D. A. Historical and geographical differences in the pattern of incidence of urinary stones considered in relation to possible aetiological factors. In Hodgkinson, A., Nordin, B. E. C. (eds): Renal Stone Research Symposium. London, Churchill, 1969, p. 7.
9. Vermeulen, C. W., Ellis, J. E., Hsu, T. C. Experimental observations on the pathogenesis of urinary calculi. *J Urol 95:* 681, 1966.
10. Sengbusch, R. von, Timmermann, A. Das kristalline Calciumoxalat im menschlichen Harn und seine Beziehung zur Oxalatstein-Bildung. *Urol Int 4:* 76, 1957.
11. Robertson, W. G., Peacock, M., Nordin, B. E. C. Calcium crystalluria in recurrent renal stone-formers. *Lancet 2:* 21, 1969.
12. Valyasevi, A., Dhanamitta, S. Studies of bladder stone disease in Thailand. XVII. Effects of exogenous source of oxalate on crystalluria. *Am J Clin Nutr 27:* 877, 1974.
13. Robertson, W. G. Factors affecting the precipitation of calcium phosphate in vitro. *Calcif Tissue Res 11:* 211, 1973.
14. Meyer, J. L., Smith, L. H. Growth of calcium oxalate crystals. I. A model for urinary stone growth. *Invest Urol 13:* 31, 1975.
15. Robertson, W. G., Peacock, M., Nordin, B. E. C. Activity products in stone-forming and non-stone-forming urine. *Clin Sci 34:* 579, 1968.
16. Robertson, W. G., Peacock, M., Nordin, B. E. C. Calcium oxalate crystalluria and urine saturation in recurrent renal stone-formers. *Clin Sci 40:* 365, 1971.
17. Robertson, W. G. Physical chemical aspects of calcium stone-formation in the urinary tract. In Fleisch, H., Robertson, W. G., Smith, L. H., Vahlensieck, W. (eds): Urolithiasis Research. New York, Plenum, 1976, p. 25.
18. Fleisch, H., Bisaz, S. The inhibitory effect of pyrophosphate on calcium oxalate precipitation and its relation to urolithiasis. *Experientia 20:* 276, 1964.
19. Dent, C. E., Sutor, D. J. Presence or absence of inhibitor of calcium oxalate crystal growth in urine of normals and of stone-formers. *Lancet 2:* 775, 1971.
20. Robertson, W. G., Peacock, M. Calcium oxalate crystalluria and inhibitors of crystallisation in recurrent renal stone-formers. *Clin Sci 43:* 499, 1972.
21. Meyer, J. L., Smith, L. H. Growth of calcium oxalate crystals. II. Inhibition by natural urinary crystal growth inhibitors. *Invest Urol 13:* 36, 1975.
22. Rose, M. B. Renal stone formation. The inhibitory effect of urine on calcium oxalate precipitation. *Invest Urol 12:* 428, 1975.
23. Robertson, W. G., Peacock, M., Knowles, C. F. Calcium oxalate crystalluria and inhibitors of crystallisation in recurrent renal stone-formers. In Delatte, L. C., Rapado, A., Hodgkinson, A. (eds): Urinary Calculi. Basel, Karger, 1973, p. 302.
24. Robertson, W. G., Knowles, C. F., Peacock, M. Urinary acid mucopolysaccharide inhibitors of calcium oxalate crystallisation. In Fleisch, H., Robertson, W. G., Smith, L. H., Vahlensieck, W. (eds): Urolithiasis Research. New York, Plenum, 1976, p. 331.
25. Robertson, W. G., Peacock, M., Marshall, R. W., et al. Saturation-inhibition index as a measure of the risk of calcium oxalate stones formation in the urinary tract. *N Engl J Med 294:* 249, 1976.
26. Dyer, R., Nordin, B. E. C. Urinary crystals and their relation to stone formation. *Nature 215:* 751, 1967.
27. Edwards, N. A., Russell, R. G. G., Hodgkinson, A. The effect of oral phosphate in patients with recurrent renal calculus. *Br J Urol 37:* 390, 1965.

28. Robertson, W. G., Peacock, M., Marshall, R. W., et al. Seasonal variations in the composition of urine in relation to calcium stone-formation. *Clin Sci Mol Med 49:* 597, 1975.
29. Marshall, R. W., Cochran, M., Robertson, W. G., et al. The relation between the concentration of calcium salts in the urine and renal stone composition in patients with calcium-containing renal stones. *Clin Sci 43:* 433, 1972.
30. Peacock, M., Marshall, R. W., Robertson, W. G., et al. Renal stone disease in primary hyperparathyroidism and idiopathic stone-formers: diagnosis, etiology and treatment. In Finlayson, B., Thomas, W. C. (eds.). Colloquium on Renal Lithiasis. Gainesville, University Presses of Florida, 1976, p. 338.
31. Flocks, R. H. Calcium and phosphorus excretion in the urine of patients with renal or ureteral calculi. *JAMA 113:* 1466, 1939.
32. Peacock, M., Nordin, B. E. C. The hypercalciuria of renal stone disease. In Hodgkinson, A., Nordin, B. E. C. (eds): Renal Stone Research Symposium. London, Churchill, 1968, p. 253.
33. Nordin, B. E. C., Peacock, M., Wilkinson, R. Hypercalciuria and calcium stone disease. *Clin Endocrinol Metab 1:* 169, 1972.
34. Coe, F. L., Canterbury, J. M., Firpo, J. J., et al. Evidence for secondary hyperparathyroidism in idiopathic hypercalciuria. *J Clin Invest 52:* 134, 1973.
35. Pak, C. Y. C., Ohata, M., Lawrence, E. C., et al. The hypercalciurias. *Clin Invest 54:* 387, 1974.
36. Hodgkinson, A. Relations between oxalic acid, calcium, magnesium and creatinine excretion in normal men and male patients with calcium oxalate kidney stones. *Clin Sci Mol Med 46:* 357, 1974.
37. Marshall, R. W., Cochran, M., Hodgkinson, A. Relationships between calcium and oxalic acid intake in the diet and their excretion in the urine of normal and renal-stone-forming subjects. *Clin Sci 43:* 91, 1972.
38. Peacock, M., Knowles, F., Nordin, B. E. C. Effect of calcium administration and deprivation on serum and urine calcium in stone-forming and control subjects. *Br Med J 2:* 729, 1968.
39. Peacock, M., Marshall, R. W., Robertson, W. G., et al. Hypercalciuria and recurrent renal calcium stone disease: effect of oral phosphate. In Avioli, L., Bordier, Ph., Fleisch, H., Massry, S., Slatopolsky, E. (eds.): Phosphate Metabolism: Kidney and Bone. Paris, Armour-Montagu, 1976, p. 63.
40. Haussler, M. R., Baylink, D. J., Hughes, M. R., et al. The assay of $1\alpha,25$-dihydroxy vitamin D_3: physiologic and pathologic modulation of circulating hormone levels. *Clin Endocrinol 5:* 151S, 1976.
41. Henneman, P. H., Benedict, P. H., Forbes, A. P., et al. Idiopathic hypercalciuria. *N Engl J Med 259:* 802, 1958.
42. Flocks, R. H. Calcium urolithiasis: the role of calcium metabolism in the pathogenesis and treatment of calcium urolithiasis. *J Urol (Baltimore) 43:* 214, 1940.
43. Nordin, B. E. C., Peacock, M., Marshall, D. H. Calcium excretion and hypercalciuria. In Fleisch, H., Robertson, W. G., Smith, L. H., Vahlensieck, W. (eds): Urolithiasis Research. New York, Plenum, 1976, p. 101.
44. Peacock, M. Stone and bone disease in primary hyperparathyroidism and their relationship to the action of parathyroid hormone on calcium absorption. In Talmage, R. W., Owen, M. (eds): Calcium-Regulating Hormones. Amsterdam, Excerpta Medica, 1975, p.78.
45. Albright, F., Reifenstein, E. C. The Parathyroid Glands and Metabolic Bone Disease. London, Bailliere, Tindall and Cox, 1948, p. 62.
46. Purnell, D. C., Smith, L. H., Scholz, D. A., et al. Primary hyperparathyroidism: a prospective clinical study. *Am J Med 50:* 670, 1971.
47. Hodgkinson, A., Marshall, R. W. Changes in the composition of urinary tract stones. *Invest Urol 13:* 131, 1975.
48. Froeling, P. G. A., M., Bijvoet, O. L. M. Kidney-mediated effects of parathyroid hormone on extracellular homeostasis of calcium, phosphate and acid–base balance in man. *Neth J Med 17:* 174, 1974.
49. Potts, J. T., Murray, T. M., Peacock, M., et al. Parathyroid hormone: sequence, synthesis, immunoassay studies. *Am J Med 50:* 639, 1971.
50. Murray, T. M., Peacock, M., Powell, D., et al. Non-autonomy of hormone secretion in primary hyperparathyroidism. *Clin Endocrinol 1:* 235, 1972.
51. Peacock, M. Parathyroid hormone. In B. E. C. Nordin (ed): Calcium, Phosphate and Magnesium Metabolism. London, Churchill Livingstone, 1976, p. 425.
52. Seldin, D. W., Wilson, J. D. Renal tubular acidosis. In Stanbury, J. B., Wyngaarden, J. B., Fredrickson, D. S. (eds): The Metabolic Basis of Inherited Disease (ed 4). New York, McGraw-Hill, 1972, p. 1548.

53. Williams, H. E., Smith, L. H. Disorders of oxalate metabolism. *Am J Med 45:* 715, 1968.

54. Chadwick, K. S., Modha, K., Dowling, R. H. Mechanism for hyperoxaluria in patients with ileal dysfunction. *N Engl J Med 289:* 172, 1973.

55. Sutherland, J. W. Recurrence following operations for upper urinary tract stones. *Br J Urol 26:* 22, 1954.

56. Williams, R. E. The results of conservative surgery for stone. *Br J Urol 44:* 292, 1972.

57. Nordin, B. E. C., Robertson, W. G., Barry, H., et al. Dietary treatment of recurrent calcium stone disease. In Hioco, D. (ed): Rein et Calcium. Paris, Sandoz, 1972, p. 345.

58. Marshall, R. W., Barry, H. Urine saturation and the formation of calcium-containing renal calculi: the effects of various forms of therapy. In Delatte, L. C., Rapado, A., Hodgkinson, H. (eds): Urinary Calculi. Basel, Karger, 1973, p. 164.

59. Pak, C. Y. C., Delea, C. S., Bartter, F. C. Successful treatment of recurrent nephrolithiasis (calcium stones) with cellulose phosphate. *N Engl J Med 290:* 175, 1974.

60. Parfitt, A. M., Higgins, B. A., Nassim, J. R., et al. Metabolic studies in patients with hypercalciuria. *Clin Sci 27:* 463, 1964.

61. Blacklock, N. J., MacLeod, M. A. The effect of cellulose phosphate on intestinal absorption and urinary excretion of calcium. *Br J Urol 46:* 385, 1974.

62. Pak, C. Y. C. Idiopathic renal lithiasis: new developments in evaluation and treatment. In Fleisch, H., Robertson, W. G., Smith, L. H., Vahlensieck, W. (eds): Urolithiasis Research. New York, Plenum, 1976, p. 213.

63. Pietrek, J., Kokot, F. Treatment of patients with calcium-containing renal stones with cellulose phosphate. *Br J Urol 45:* 136, 1973.

64. Yendt, E. R., Guay, G. F., Garcia, D. A. The use of thiazides in the prevention of renal calculi. *Can Med Assoc J 102:* 614, 1970.

65. Woelfel, A., Kaplan, R. A., Pak, C. Y. C. Effect of hydrochlorothiazide therapy on the crystallization of calcium oxalate in urine. *Metabolism 26:* 201, 1977.

66. Coe, F. L., Kavalach, A. G. Hypercalciuria and hyperuricosuria in patients with calcium nephrolithiasis. *N Engl J Med 291:* 1344, 1974.

67. Fraser, D., Russell, R. G. G., Pohler, O., et al. The influence of disodium-ethane-1-hydroxy-1,1-diphosphonate (EHDP) on the development of experimentally induced urinary stones in rats. *Clin Sci 42:* 197, 1972.

68. Baumann, J. M., Ganz, U., Bisaz, S., et al. Verebreichung eines Diphosphonats zur Steinprophylaxe. *Helv Chir Acta 41:* 421, 1974.

69. Robertson, W. G., Peacock, M., Marshall, R. W. The effect of ethane-1-hydroxy-1,1-diphosphonate (EHDP) on calcium oxalate crystalluria in recurrent renal stone-formers. *Clin Sci 47:* 13, 1974.

70. Jowsey, J., Riggs, B. L., Kelly, P. J., et al. The treatment of osteoporosis with disodium ethane-1-hydroxy-1,1-diphosphonate. *J Lab Clin Med 78:* 574, 1971.

71. Gershoff, S. N., Prien, E. L. Effect of daily MgO and vitamin B_6 administration to patients with recurring calcium oxalate kidney stones. *Am J Clin Nutr 20:* 393, 1967.

72. Moore, C. A., Bunce, G. E. Reduction in frequency of renal calculus formation by oral magnesium administration. *Invest Urol 2:* 7, 1967.

73. Mukai, T., Howard, J. E. Some observations on the calcification of rachitic rat cartilage by urine. *Bull Johns Hopkins Hosp 112:* 279, 1963.

74. Robertson, W. G., Peacock, M., Nordin, B. E. C. Inhibitors of the growth and aggregation of calcium oxalate crystals in vitro. *Clin Chim Acta 43:* 31, 1973.

75. Hodgkinson, A., Marshall, R. W. Stone composition, urine saturation and treatment of patients with calcium-containing renal stones. In Hioco, D. (ed): Rein et Calcium. Paris, Sandoz, 1972, p. 319.

76. Robertson, W. G., Peacock, M., Marshall, R. W., et al. Effect of oral orthophosphate on calcium crystalluria in stone-formers. In Fleisch, H., Robertson, W. G., Smith, L. H., Vahlensieck, W. (eds): Urolithiasis Research. New York, Plenum, 1976, p. 339.

77. Burdette, D. C., Thomas, W. C., Finlayson, B. Urinary supersaturation with calcium oxalate before and during orthophosphate therapy. *J Urol 115:* 418, 1976.

78. Smith, L. H., Thomas, W. C., Arnaud, C. D. Orthophosphate therapy in calcium renal lithiasis. In Delatte, L. C., Rapado, A., Hodgkinson, A. (eds): Urinary Calculi. Basel, Karger, 1973, p. 188.

79. Horn, H-D. Der Einfluss einer oralen Phosphat-Applikation auf den Verlauf der Urolithiasis bei Kranken mit calciumhaltigen Steinen. *Urologe 6:* 223, 1967.

80. Oliver, I., Weinberger, A., Bar-Meir, S., et al. Orthophosphate treatment of calcium lithiasis associated with idiopathic hypercalciuria. *Urol Int 29:* 414, 1974.

81. Smith, M. J. V., Hunt, L. D., King, J. S., et al. Uricemia and urolithiasis. *J Urol 101:* 637, 1969.

82. Coe, F. L., Lawton, R. L., Goldstein, R. B., et al. Sodium urate accelerates precipitation of calcium oxalate in vitro. *Proc Soc Exp Biol Med 149:* 926, 1975.

83. Pak, C. Y. C., Arnold, L. H. Heterogeneous nucleation of calcium oxalate by seeds of monosodium urate. *Proc Soc Exp Biol Med 149:* 930, 1975.

84. Porter, P. Colloidal properties of urates in relation to calculus formation. *Res Vet Sci 7:* 128, 1966.

85. Gallagher, J. C., Wilkinson, R. The effect of ethinyloestradiol on calcium and phosphorus metabolism of post-menopausal women with primary hyperparathyroidism. *Clin Sci Mol Med 45:* 785, 1973.

86. Williams, H. E., Smith, L. H. Primary hyperoxaluria. In Stanbury, J. B., Wyngaarden, J. B., Fredrickson, D. S. (eds): The Metabolic Basis of Inherited Disease (4th ed). New York, McGraw-Hill, 1972, p. 196.

87. Gibbs, D. A., Watts, R. W. E. Action of pyridoxine in primary hyperoxaluria. *Clin Sci 38:* 277, 1970.

88. Van den Berg, C. J., Cahill, T. M., Smith, L. H. Crystalluria. In Fleisch, H., Robertson, W. G., Smith, L. H., Vahlensieck, W. (eds): Urolithiasis Research. Plenum, New York, 1976, p. 365.

69

Metabolic Bone Disease: Introduction and Classification

Stephen M. Krane
Alan L. Schiller

NORMAL BONE: STRUCTURE, ORGANIZATION, AND GROWTH

Bone is a dynamic tissue and its formation and resorption are continuous processes throughout the life of the organism. The skeleton is vascular and receives about 10 percent of the cardiac output. Its structure is designed to carry out the mechanical functions of providing a protective covering for neural structures, giving rigid support to the extremities and the joints, and serving as levers and points of attachment for the muscles required for locomotion and prehension. Bone also provides a reservoir of calcium, phosphorus, magnesium, sodium, and other ions essential for a variety of homeostatic functions.

The properties of bone depend upon its chemical structure and biologic organization. Mechanical demands require a tissue that is rigid but resists forces that would break brittle materials, and yet is light enough to be responsive to muscle pull. The combination of dense compact bone and cancellous bone, reinforced at points of stress, results in an organ ideally suited to its functions.[1,2] For example, although bone is three times lighter than cast iron, it has the tensile strength of cast iron, is very much more flexible, and has a high modulus of elasticity.[3] These properties of bone, in turn, result from the unique organization of the extracellular portion. This consists of an inorganic mineral phase, which makes up about two-thirds of the weight of bone, small amounts of water, and an organic portion which is mainly ($\sim$90–95 percent) collagen.[1,2] Other minor components include proteoglycans, a number of noncollagenous proteins,[4,5] lipid, and newly described acidic proteins which contain γ-carboxyglutamic acid.[6–8] The mineral phase consists of mixtures of poorly crystallized hydroxyapatite and another calcium-phosphate solid. The latter lacks a coherent x-ray diffraction pattern, has a lower Ca:P ratio than pure hydroxyapatite, and has been termed *amorphous* calcium phosphate.[1,2,9,10] Younger bone tissue has a larger proportion of amorphous calcium phosphate than does older bone tissue.

Bone tissue contains several types of cells (Fig. 69-1).[11,12] The *osteoblast* (Fig. 69-2) is an active synthetic cell concerned with production and modulation of matrix components and probably translocation of the mineral ions from the extracellular fluid to the inorganic mineral phase. The osteoblasts become encased in bone matrix, which eventually is mineralized almost to the cell membrane. These trapped cells, now called *osteocytes,* gradually lose their synthetic activities (Fig. 69-3). Bone-resorbing cells, which are classically multinucleated, are termed *osteoclasts* (Figs. 69-4 and 69-5). The osteoblasts and osteoclasts are thought to be derived from a population of dividing cells near bone surfaces, termed *osteoprogenitor cells.*[13] The latter probably arise from more-primitive mesenchymal stem-cell precursors, always present in bone as small cells in bone connective tissue (Figs. 69-6 and 69-7). Although the osteoclast is a syncitium of a number of cells which fuse into a single cell (Figs. 69-8 and 69-9), there is no direct evidence for conversion of osteoblasts or osteocytes directly into osteoclasts, or osteoclasts into osteoblasts.

Bone has been classified microscopically into two types of tissue: woven bone (Fig. 69-10), which is normal in the embryo or as part of reaction to injury in the adult; and lamellar bone (Fig. 69-11), the type characteristic of the normal adult skeleton.[2,14] Woven bone can be deposited rapidly but it is a rather weak structure replaced in the adult skeleton by lamellar bone. Lamellar bone is structurally sound and is normally laid down more slowly. Postnatal bone is almost all lamellar but of varying degree of perfection.[2] It is primarily the organization of the collagen fibers that defines these two types of bone tissue and produces the lamellar or woven structure with their characteristic birefringent pattern seen by polarized light microscopy. Therefore, the definition of woven bone includes the following three features: a nonparallel array of collagen fibers in an irregular, haphazard pattern; many osteocytes per unit area of matrix; and variation in the osteocyte size and shape. Lamellar bone, on the other hand, has virtually the opposite properties: a parallel orderly arrangement of collagen fibers; few osteocytes per unit area of matrix; and uniform osteocytes which tend to have lacunae parallel to the collagen-fiber long axis. Lamellar bone may be further subdivided into bone of the cortex (circumferential lamellar bone, concentric lamellar bone, or osteones, that surround the vascular canals and comprise the haversian systems, and interstitial lamellar bone) and bone making up the cancellous bone in the medulla.

In lamellar bone most of the mineral phase is within the collagen fibrils located predominantly in the pore (hole) areas (Fig. 69-12) created by the specific packing arrangement of the component collagen molecules.[1,2,15,16] However, in woven bone, mineral is found elsewhere, e.g., in membrane-bound vesicles (Fig. 69-13) and lying free between the fibrils, at times causing woven bone to be more radiodense than lamellar bone. Such vesicles, which were first observed in calcifying cartilage, are rich in lipid, average about 1000 Å, are enclosed by a trilamellar membrane, and are rich in

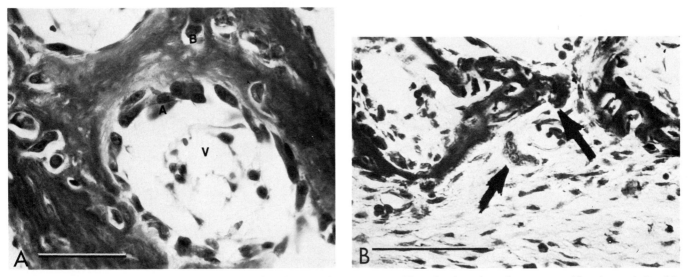

Fig. 69-1. A. Woven bone showing prominent osteoblastic activity (A), large osteocytes (B), and an irregular collagen pattern. Note the proximity of the bone to a small vessel (V). All bone tissue, woven or lamellar, needs a good vascular supply. H&E. Calibration marker: 50 μm. B. Another example of woven bone, illustrating osteoblastic activity and osteoclasts (arrows) surrounded by a loose connective-tissue stroma. Again note the small capillaries adjacent to the bone. This picture also illustrates the exquisite control of bone remodeling: on one surface resorption is prominent and on the opposite surface bone deposition is found. H&E. Calibration marker: 100 μm.

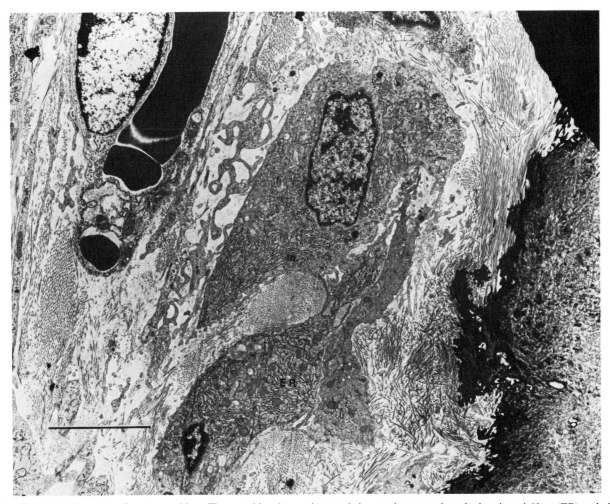

Fig. 69-2. Electron micrograph of a rat osteoblast. The osteoblast has a characteristic prominent rough endoplasmic reticulum (ER) and abundant mitochondria (M). Many collagen fibrils, which are secreted by the osteoblast, lie adjacent to the cell. The region of collagen fibrils between the cell and the dark-black tissue is unmineralized bone tissue (osteoid). The black region represents mineralized bone. There is always a thin rim of osteoid present in newly deposited bone; often, however, it is only apparent in electron micrographs. Note the proximity of the osteoblast to a capillary. Calibration marker: 6 μm. (Courtesy of Dr. M. Holtrop)

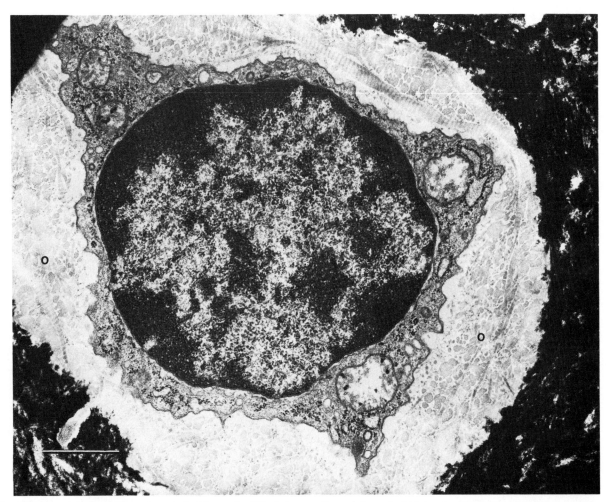

Fig. 69-3. Electron micrograph of an osteocyte (rat) trapped within its lacuna, the periphery of which is osteoid (O). Note that the secretory machinery, particularly the rough endoplasmic reticulum, which is prominent in the osteoblast, is much reduced in this new osteocyte. In old osteocytes there is virtually no endoplasmic reticulum apparent. The dark tissue is mineralized bone. Calibration marker: 1 μm. (Courtesy of Dr. M. Holtrop)

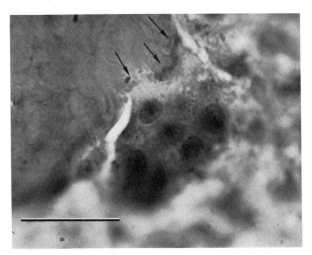

Fig. 69-4. Osteoclast with multiple nuclei, illustrating the region of the ruffled border (arrows), where active bone resorption is taking place. Part of the cell is out of focus because its large size precludes the whole cell from lying in the same plane of focus. H&E. Calibration marker: 40 μm.

phosphatases such as ATPase, pyrophosphatase, and alkaline phosphatase.[17-20] There has been considerable interest in the possible roles of these vesicles in the initiation of mineralization in cartilage and in bone. However, in lamellar bone, which is the adult bone structure, the mineral phase must be largely within the collagen fibrils.[2] Unfortunately, the mechanisms whereby mineral is so deposited remains to be elucidated. One hypothesis that is favored states that a change in phase occurs from ions (particularly calcium and P_i) in solution, through ion clusters, to the solid, which is somehow nucleated by specific organic macromolecules inside or outside the cell.[1,2] The nucleation agent in bone may well be collagen, but other components could also serve that role.

In the embryo and in the growing child, bone develops in two ways.[23] The first, *endochondral bone formation* (Fig. 69-14), occurs by replacing previously calcified cartilage (which contains type II collagen) with new bone matrix (which now contains type I collagen, a different gene product) using the calcified cartilage as a scaffold.[21,22] In all bones, but particularly those of the calvarium, bone is also laid down directly from pluripotential connective tissue without the calcified-cartilage model in a process termed *intramembranous bone formation* (Fig. 69-15).

It is possible that there are degrees of "perfection" of lamellation in lamellar bone[2] which may depend upon the rate at which it is deposited (Figs. 69-16 and 69-17). In all bones, lamellar bone is found in both the trabeculae (or cancellous bone) and in the cortex,

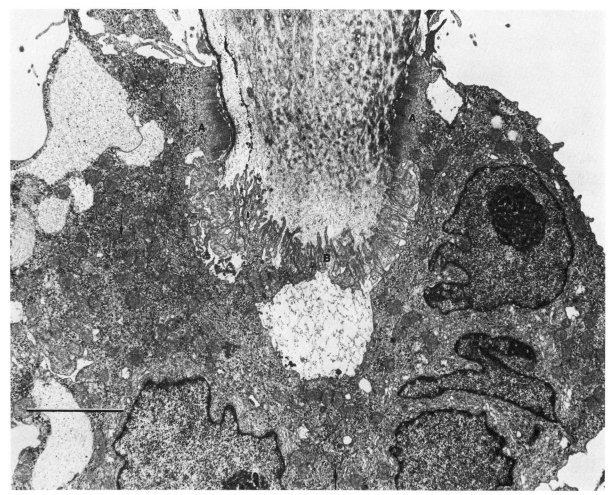

Fig. 69-5. Electron micrograph of a decalcified section of bone (rat) showing an osteoclast resorbing bone. A spicule of bone is surrounded by the "clear zone" (A) of the osteoclast, a relatively organelle-free portion of the cell which may act to fasten the cell to the bone and isolate the bone from the extracellular milieu. The ruffled border (B), with its many interdigitating projections of cell membrane, is the actively resorbing part of the cell. The remaining cytoplasm contains abundant mitochondria and an endoplasmic reticulum with a rosette type of pattern of ribosomes (arrow) represented as clusters of black dots. The multiple nuclei are also seen in various planes of cutting. Calibration marker: 5 μm. (Courtesy of Dr. M. Holtrop)

deposited in highly ordered arrangement around blood vessels along their longitudinal course, forming the haversian systems, or osteones. Growth in length of bones is dependent upon proliferation of cartilage cells in the growth plate followed by maturation of these cells and endochondral ossification. Growth in width and thickness is accomplished by formation of bone at the periosteal surface, and resorption at the endosteal surface; the rates are unequal, formation exceeding resorption. In adults after epiphyseal-plate closure, growth in length ceases, but endochondral bone formation can be reactivated in certain conditions only in limited regions beneath the articular surface.

Frost has used the term *modeling* to include those processes which establish the ultimate architecture of the skeleton at the macroscopic level.[24] Modeling therefore subsides at age 18–20 as most of the endochondral sequence also subsides and bone growth ceases. *Remodeling* of bone, in contrast, is a continuous process from the earliest embryonic bone until death. Remodeling involves all of the bone surfaces: periosteal, haversian, and cortical–endosteal, and seems essential to preservation of the mechanical strength of bone. It is the deviation of this remodeling activity that forms the basis for the development of metabolic bone disease, particularly that seen in adults, where there is interference with

this normally orderly process of resorption and formation. The presence of activity at bone surfaces can be demonstrated using a number of techniques which include quantitative assessment of cellular activity using mineralized thin sections,[12,25] microradiography of thick mineralized sections,[26] and fluorescence of marker tetracyclines which bind at regions of newly mineralized bone (Fig. 69-18).[27]

Overall, there is a tight coupling of formation and resorption of bone.[23,24,28] From the time longitudinal growth has ceased, bone mass has reached its adult proportions and remains at this level for 2 to 3 decades. Since there is no net gain or loss of skeletal mass, and remodeling is continuous, formation and resorption must be essentially equal. This probably results not from coordinated activity of randomly distributed osteoblasts and osteoclasts, but rather from the coupling of activity of "packets" of interacting cells (Fig. 69-19), which Frost has termed *basic multicellular units*, which are involved in the turnover of a relatively small volume of bone.[24] Remodeling is not uniform. Most surfaces at any one time are not involved either in resorption or formation (Fig. 69-20).[11,12,25,26] Active resorption surfaces are covered by active osteoclasts and are usually irregular in configuration. Inactive resorption surfaces are irregular scalloped surfaces without osteoclasts. Bone forma-

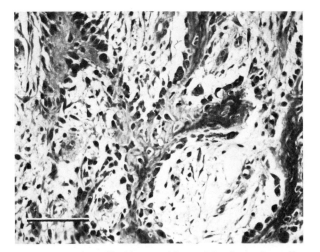

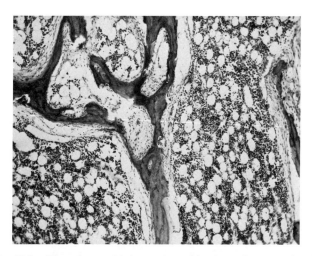

Fig. 69-6. Woven bone lined by osteoblasts arising from a loose fibrovascular stroma, characteristic of intramembranous bone formation. H&E. Calibration marker: 100 μm.

Fig. 69-7. Dissecting osteitis in a patient with primary hyperparathyroidism, illustrating the pluripotentiality of the bone marrow, which normally should be hematopoietic in this case. However, a loose fibrous stroma closely applied to the bone may be the source of the osteoclastic cells upon stimulation by parathyroid hormone. Most of the marrow remains normal—only those areas closest to the bone have been transformed into the appropriate tissue by the hormonal stimulation.

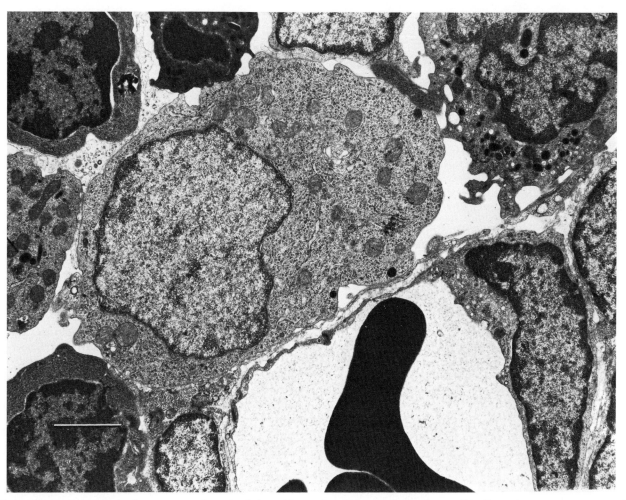

Fig. 69-8. Electron micrograph of rat marrow after stimulation with parathyroid hormone. The large cell in the center may represent a primitive osteoclast since the rosette pattern of ribosomes and mitochondria is apparent. The single nucleus in this plane of section may be one of many such structures in the cell. The other cells are marrow elements; there also is a capillary with a red blood cell in the lumen. Calibration marker: 2 μm. (Courtesy of Dr. M. Holtrop)

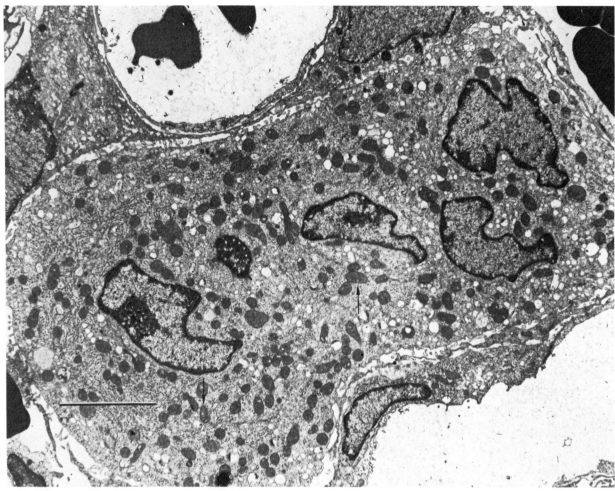

Fig. 69-9. Electron micrograph of rat marrow showing an early osteoclast, but at a stage later than in Fig. 69-8, with more classic features i.e., multiple nuclei and abundant mitochondria (arrow). A prominent endoplasmic reticulum with ribosomes arranged in rosettes is not seen. This large cell is very close to and wedged between two capillaries but it is not applied to bone, making the specific identity of this cell uncertain. Calibration marker: $5\,\mu$m. (Courtesy of Dr. M. Holtrop)

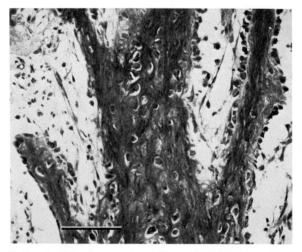

Fig. 69-10. Section of woven bone illustrating haphazard collagen arrangement, hypercellularity, and osteocyte pleomorphism, all of which characterize woven-bone tissue. The osteoblastic rimming and loose fibrovascular stroma can be seen with either woven or lamellar bone and do not define the bone tissue. H&E. Calibration marker: $100\,\mu$m.

tion surfaces are characterized by the presence of osteoid (unmineralized bone). Active bone formation surfaces are covered by plump osteoblasts, and inactive surfaces are smooth and naked, lacking osteoblasts. Temporally, resorption precedes formation and is more intense. Frost estimates that resorption lasts about 1 month in a normal 30-year-old adult, and formation about 3 months.[24] The total duration of activity of the typical bone unit (termed *sigma* by Frost), which increases with increasing age, lasts about 5 months at age 65. Quantitative morphometric data have now been obtained and indicate that in transiliac biopsies from normal adults, the osteoid surface averages 10 percent of the total surface, and thickness of the osteoid seam is $9–10\,\mu$m, with normal seams usually not in excess of $12–13\,\mu$m. The resorption surface is usually 2–4 percent of the total bone surface.[29–31]

Kinetic studies using isotopes such as ^{47}Ca and breakdown products of collagen provide different estimates of the extent of bone formation and resorption. It is currently impossible to prove the assumptions essential for the calculations. However, estimates are that the size of the calcium "pool" is ~5000 mg. This consists of the extracellular-fluid calcium, soft-tissue calcium, and a portion of the exchangeable pool of bone. Movement from this pool into and out of bone is ~500 mg/day in normal adults.[32,33] If this

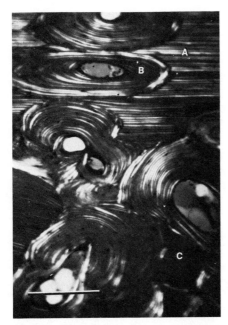

Fig. 69-11. Partially polarized section of human cortex showing lamellar bone. The adult human cortex consists of circumferential lamellar bone (A) and haversian systems made up of concentric lamellar bone (B), or osteones. The bone between haversian bone is the interstitial lamellar bone (C). All types of lamellar bone have a parallel arrangement of collagen fibers, more matrix than cells, and uniform osteocytes. H&E. Calibration marker: 200 μm.

MECHANISMS OF BONE MINERALIZATION AND RESORPTION

Bone mineralization is an orderly process in which the inorganic mineral is deposited in relation to an organic matrix (Figs. 69-12 and 69-21). Since the mineral is composed of calcium and phosphorus, the concentration of these ions in the plasma and extracellular fluid influences the rate at which the mineral phase is formed. In vitro, mineralization can proceed, and crystals of hydroxyapatite grow at concentrations of calcium and phosphorus similar to those in an ultrafiltrate of plasma. The concentration of these ions at the sites of mineralization is not known, however, and it is possible that the cells involved (osteoblasts, osteocytes) somehow regulate the local concentration of calcium, phosphorus, and other ions, or other aspects of the mineralizing environment such as pH. Collagens from a variety of sources can catalyze the nucleation of a mineral phase of calcium and phosphorus from solutions of these ions, and the mineral in the initial phase is deposited in a specific location in the holes produced by the particular packing arrangement of the collagen molecules.[1,2] It is likely that the organization of collagen influences the amount and type of mineral phase that is formed. The collagen of bone is similar in its primary structure to that of skin (contains two α1(I) chains and one α2 chain) but differs by virtue of modification of that structure in hydroxylation, glycosylation, and the type, number, and distribution of intermolecular cross-links.[21,22,47,48] Other posttranslational modifications of collagen structure such as phosphorylation may also be necessary for mineralization.[1,2] In addition, there is evidence that the "holes" in the packing structure of

calcium is in newly formed bone, and the total skeletal calcium is ~1100 g, then ~1/6 of the skeleton could be deposited and resorbed annually. This figure is probably high, but, unfortunately, there are no established independent means to verify it.[28]

In the process of bone resorption, matrix, which is mostly collagen, is also resorbed. Peptides containing amino acids that are unique to collagen[21,22] (hydroxyproline and hydroxylysine) are present in plasma and are excreted in the urine.[28,34] Since hydroxyproline[35] and hydroxylysine[36] are not reutilized for collagen biosynthesis, quantitation of their excretion should provide an index of bone collagen resorption. Unfortunately, measurement of urinary hydroxyproline excretion is not a quantitative marker for collagen degradation since free hydroxyproline liberated from peptides is metabolized to other products not included in the hydroxyproline determination.[37,38] Quantitation of urinary hydroxylysine and its glycosides gives a better estimate of collagen breakdown[39] since the hydroxylysine glycosides are not metabolized to the same extent as hydroxyproline, and the ratio of the different glycosides indicates the predominant source of the degradation products, whether from bone or elsewhere.[39-42] Normal adults on low-gelatin (collagen) diets excrete less than 40 mg hydroxyproline per 24 h, most of which is derived from bone. Almost all of this is in the form of small peptides.[34,43] A small portion (~5–10 percent) of the total urinary hydroxyproline is in the form of higher-molecular-weight material (~5000 daltons) which has a typical collagen structure.[44-46] Excretion of this material reflects collagen synthesis more than degradation. Estimates of bone resorption based on collagen degradation are lower than those based on [47]Ca kinetics by a factor of ~3 because of the irregular biodegradation of free hydroxyproline, but still indicate considerable turnover.

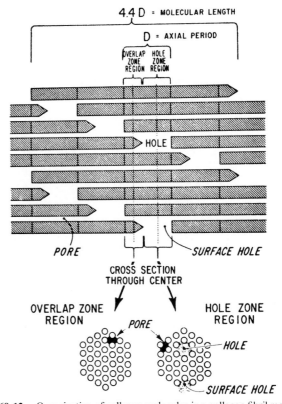

Fig. 69-12. Organization of collagen molecules in a collagen fibril modified by Glimcher[2] and Katz and Li[15,16] from the model proposed by Hodge and Petruska[63]. (From Glimcher, in Aurbach (ed): Handbook of Physiology, sect 7, vol 7, 1976. Courtesy of the American Physiological Society)

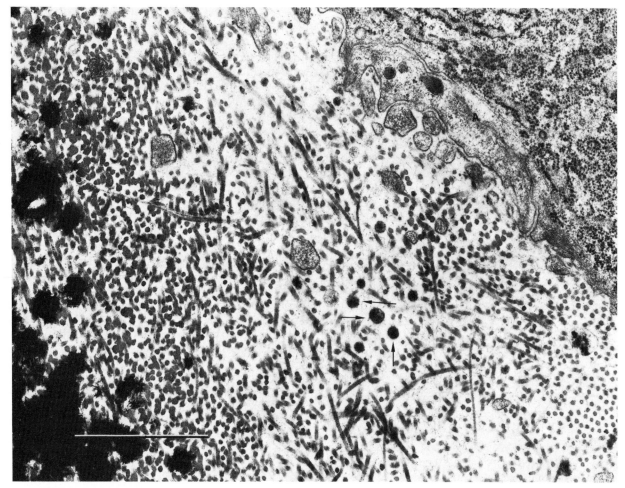

Fig. 69-13. Electron micrograph of rat woven bone showing the interface between an osteoblast (A) and newly laid-down osteoid. Small membrane-bound vesicles containing mineral (arrows) are seen among the collagen fibrils. The black area at the periphery represents fully mineralized woven bone. At least two similar vesicles are also seen within the osteoblast in support of the concept of cellular secretion of such vesicles which then lie between collagen fibrils of woven bone. Calibration marker: 0.5 μm. (Courtesy of Dr. M. Holtrop)

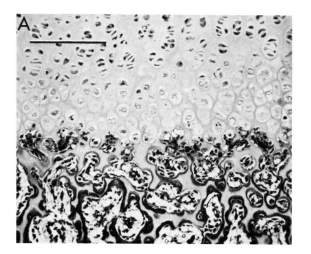

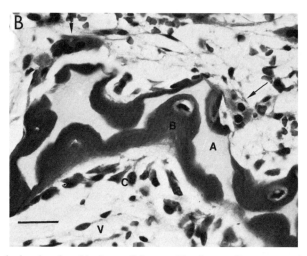

Fig. 69-14. A. Endochondral ossification is a process by which cartilage is resorbed and replaced by bone. Columns of hyaline cartilage are seen being resorbed from below by osteoclasts (now termed *chondroclasts*) and loose fibrovascular stroma, leaving thin sheets of cartilage. These sheets of cartilage are then coated with bone, usually woven, by osteoblastic differentiation of the mesenchymal marrow. Such a cartilage–bone composite is called a *primary trabeculum.* H&E. Calibration marker: 200 μm. B. Higher-power view of endochondral ossification showing a cartilage core (A) surrounded by woven bone (B). Again, note the osteoclastic activity (arrow) on one surface and osteoblasts on the opposite side (C). The net effect of such cellular control is to destroy this primary trabeculum and replace it with bone. The presence of vessels (V) closely associated with the bone is striking here. H&E. Calibration marker: 20 μm.

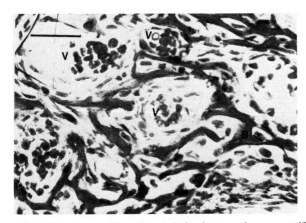

Fig. 69-15. Woven bone (B) produced during intramembranous ossification. The bone tissue appears to be arising directly from bone cells, which in turn are derived from the loose connective tissue. There is no cartilage precursor or model in this process. Lamellar and woven bone can be produced by this process. Again, note the vascularity (V) of the periosseous tissue. H&E. Calibration marker: 50 μm.

the collagen (Fig. 69-12) are larger in normally mineralized collagen of bone and dentin than the holes in normally unmineralized collagen such as tendon.[2,15,16] Other noncollagenous organic components, such as glycoproteins, may also play a role in the formation and localization of the mineral phase of bone. The recently described acidic proteins containing γ-carboxyglutamic acid may be involved in binding of calcium ions and somehow regulate calcification locally.[6,7]

In order to explain how collagens from tissues normally not mineralized can catalyze nucleation of an inorganic phase from solutions of calcium and P_i at a concentration similar to that of normal extracellular fluid, regulation of mineralization by inhibitory substances has been suggested.[1,2] Inorganic pyrophosphate is a potent inhibitor of mineralization at concentrations several orders of magnitude below those necessary to bind calcium ions.[49] Since alkaline phosphatase, present in osteoblasts and other cells, can catalyze the hydrolysis of inorganic pyrophosphate at neutral pH, this enzyme could play a role in the regulation of mineralization by controlling the concentrations of pyrophosphate. In addi-

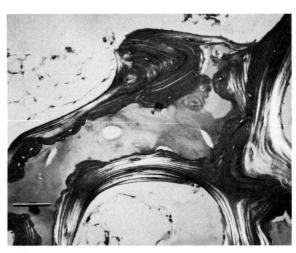

Fig. 69-17. Lamellar bone, viewed under polarized light, which surrounds a core of hyaline cartilage. Contrast with Fig. 69-14B, where woven bone is present because of rapid remodeling of endochondral ossification. Here the cartilage is slowly growing and being resorbed, allowing time for lamellar bone to be laid down. This finding is commonly seen below the cartilaginous cap of an osteochondroma, a slowly growing lesion of bone. Note also the relatively inactive marrow, which is largely fat with little if any mesenchymal differentiation. H&E. Calibration marker: 100 μm.

tion, macromolecular inhibitors such as the proteoglycans may also influence the rate and extent of mineralization.[50] Since in cartilage and bone undergoing calcification, membrane-bound vesicles containing mineral have been identified outside the cells, it has been suggested that this is the initial mineral phase, at least in early mineralization in the embryo.[17–20] In later stages of ossification, however, the mineral is probably on or within the collagen fibrils.

It was pointed out earlier that in bone the initial mineral phase

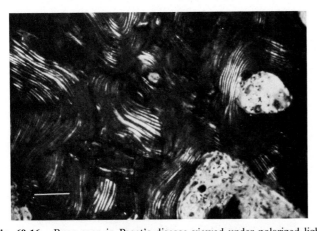

Fig. 69-16. Bone seen in Paget's disease viewed under polarized light, illustrating various units of lamellar bone haphazardly cemented together with other units of lamellar bone. The interfaces between these units produce the mosaic pattern diagnostic of Paget's disease. This is a good example of lamellar bone rapidly laid down, but in a disorganized fashion. H&E. Calibration marker: 100 μm.

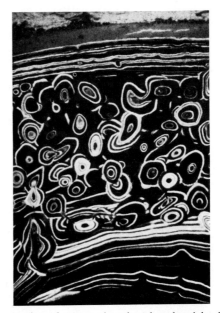

Fig. 69-18. Section of cortex viewed under ultraviolet light showing autofluoresence of tetracycline-labeled bone. This antibiotic binds to newly mineralized bone and autofluoresces under ultraviolet light. Such a technique is useful in determining bone dynamics. In this case, newly mineralized haversian systems in various stages of development are seen sandwiched between the endosteal and periosteal circumferential lamellar bone (see also Fig. 69-11). (Courtesy of Dr. E. Uehlinger)

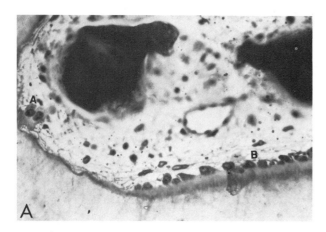
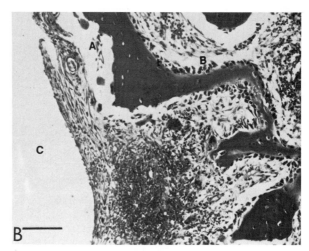

Fig. 69-19. A. "Cutting cone" in the cortex with its typical cell population of a leading front of osteoclasts (A) followed by osteoblasts (B) to illustrate the bone remodeling unit of initial resorption and subsequent bone formation. This is a thick (100-μm) mineralized section of cortex, hence the poor focus of the central vessels. Note the presence of loose connective-tissue stroma surrounding the vessels which give rise to the active bone cells. (Courtesy of Dr. J. Jowsey) B. Photomicrograph illustrating balance and control between formation and resorption of bone. The lining of an expanding bone cyst (C) is walled off by a woven-bone shell. However, on the cyst side, osteoclasts (A) are active, allowing for expansion of the cyst, whereas osteoblasts (B) are prominent on the opposite surface of the bone shell, allowing for continuous bone deposition in order to keep pace with the cyst expansion. H&E. Calibration marker: 100 μm.

probably represents the "amorphous" solid with a relatively low calcium/phosphorus molar ratio. With maturation, part of the amorphous solid is converted to a poorly crystalline hydroxyapatite.[9,10] Even mature bone from old animals still contains considerable amounts of the amorphous calcium phosphate. Fluoride ions, when incorporated into the mineral phase, tend to decrease the proportion of amorphous calcium phosphate and increase crystallinity,[51] an effect which may explain in part the apparent therapeutic usefulness of fluoride administration in osteoporosis.[52]

The concentrations of calcium and phosphorus ions in the extracellular fluid affect the dissolution and formation of the mineral phase of bone. A "solubility product" for bone mineral is difficult to calculate, however, since the mineral itself is of variable composition, and the true nature of species in solution governing this solubility product is not known.[1] Nevertheless, when the concentrations of calcium and phosphorus, particularly the latter, in extracellular fluid are excessive, a mineral phase may be formed in areas that are not normally mineralized. Conversely, when the

concentration of mineral ions is deficient, formation of bone mineral is impaired.

When bone is resorbed, calcium and phosphorus ions from the solid phase are released into solution in the extracellular fluid, and subsequently the organic matrix is also resorbed. It is not entirely clear how these processes occur. A decrease in pH, the presence of a chelating substance, and the operation of a cellular pump mechanism to shift the equilibrium between solid and solution are possible explanations for mineral release. Resorption occurs at specific sites either adjacent to osteoclasts or surrounding osteocytes and requires normal metabolism of these cells. The matrix is resorbed presumably through the action of collagenases[53] released from the resorbing cells; these enzymes attack collagen in a specific manner but are incapable of degrading the protein before the mineral phase is removed. The rate at which resorption occurs is influenced by several hormones, particularly parathyroid hormone, calcitonin, and vitamin D, and is accelerated by the action of other substances, such as heparin, prostaglandins of the E

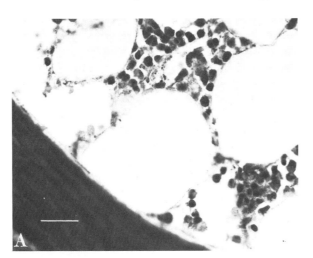
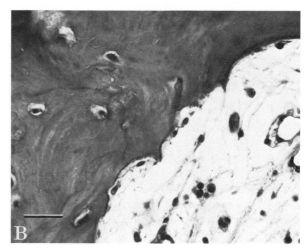

Fig. 69-20. A. Inactive formation surface with a smooth demarcation of lamellar bone from the unreactive fatty and hematopoietic marrow. H&E. Calibration marker: 20 μm. B. Inactive resorption surface with scalloped bone surface lacking osteoclasts. This is a focus in Paget's disease, showing units of lamellar bone and a loose connective-tissue stroma. H&E. Calibration marker: 20 μm.

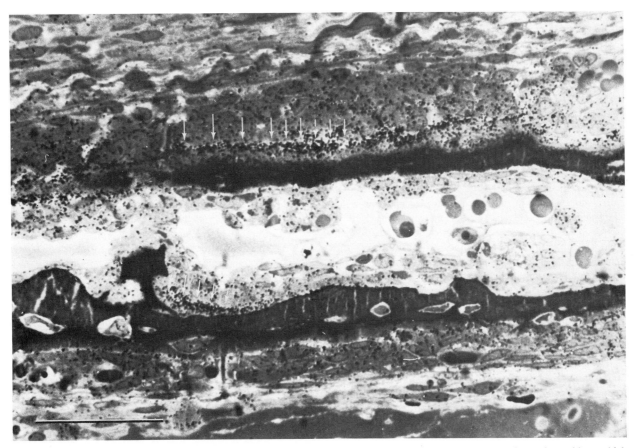

Fig. 69-21. Autoradiograph of a rat calvarium labeled with tritiated proline. The line of black dots (arrows) indicates a front of osteoblasts which actively synthesize collagen fibrils and hence incorporate the labeled proline. The black linear tissue is mineralized bone of the inner and outer tables of the skull. Calibration marker: 40 μm. (Courtesy of Dr. M. Holtrop)

series, and a factor from mononuclear cells termed *osteoclast-activating factor.*[54]

CONCEPT OF METABOLIC BONE DISEASE

Metabolic bone disease is a term introduced by Albright and Reifenstein[55] to include disorders of the skeleton that are generalized (involving *all* of the skeleton *to some degree*) and are therefore subject to humoral influences. Albright and Reifenstein assumed that *all* bones in metabolic bone disease might be involved, although not necessarily to the *same extent.* This definition therefore excludes a disorder such as Paget's disease of bone, in which "normal" bone is always found. Therefore, although Paget's disease may be *widespread,* it is never *generalized.* However, the situation in Paget's disease is so distinctive insofar as the intensity of the abnormality in remodeling is concerned, that it is often considered, as in this volume (Chapter 72), with the metabolic bone diseases.

We have emphasized that continuous remodeling of the skeleton occurs normally. Any alteration of the coupling of formation and resorption would result not only in alteration of the total bone mass but also in the form and distribution of bone. It was also stated that remodeling is not a generalized random phenomenon but involves packets, or units, of bone cells. Signals must be received and interpreted by osteoprogenitor cells to proliferate and function as bone-resorbing cells coupled to the activity of bone-forming cells. One must remember that in all bones the marrow has the ability to modulate into a loose connective tissue which gives

rise on demand to osteoblasts and osteoclasts. The nature of the factors influencing these local cellular modulations remains to be determined.

Hormones, especially parathyroid hormone, calcitonin, and vitamin D, have profound and complex effects, not only on resorption, as discussed above, but also on remodeling, modeling, and growth. In attempting to interpret these effects it is not easy to decide whether a given phenomenon in states of hormone deprivation is explained by the specific lack of one hormone, even if replacement therapy reverses the abnormality, or is the result of a combined effect of many hormones. It should also be emphasized that the ultimate skeletal dimensions are dependent not only on alterations in *rate* of growth but also on *duration* of growth as determined by the duration of the endochondral sequence. Although a detailed review of hormonal effects on growth will not be attempted here, several points may be made.

Decreased thyroid function not only delays growth but also retards maturation of the skeleton as evidenced by delayed endochondral ossification and closure of the epiphyseal plate. The effect on maturation is manifested by delay in appearance of secondary centers of ossification.[56,57] When ossification centers do appear in the untreated hypothyroid child, they have an abnormal fragmented or stippled radiographic appearance (epiphyseal dysgenesis).[58] The hypothyroid dwarf retains infantile skeletal proportions, in contrast to the hypopituitary dwarf, who usually has proportions consistent with his skeletal age. Growth and maturation are then accelerated when thyroid hormones are administered. Direct skeletal actions of T_4 and T_3 have been shown,[59,60] although some of the effects of thyroid hormones may result from interactions with growth hormone (through somatomedin). The effects of thyroid hormones are also modulated by the predetermined growth potential of the specific bone at the time of exposure and may appear paradoxical. For example, in vitro T_3 reduces growth of an already rapidly growing bone, whereas it accelerates growth of a slower-growing bone.

Lack of pituitary growth hormone causes decreased bone growth (pituitary dwarf), while an excess (in children) yields gigantism. Growth hormone can stimulate cartilage growth and endochondral ossification. In adults, this reactivation can take place only in the thin rim of epiphyseal cartilage, which lies just below the true articular cartilage, because the cartilage of the growth plate has been replaced by bone and also because the true articular cartilage does not participate in endochondral ossification. The increase in size of the bones of the acromegalic hand is thus accounted for by two processes: (1) stimulation of periosteal growth, and (2) activation of endochondral ossification at the articular cartilage, which occupies a proportionally larger percentage of total skeletal volume in small bones than in the large long bones. In contrast with thyroid hormones, which act directly in vitro on bone and cartilage preparations, growth hormone requires the formation of somatomedins before it can act in vitro.[61]

In the absence of sex hormones, both growth and maturation are retarded.[62] The total duration of growth is prolonged, since epiphyses do not close at the appropriate age, resulting in variable skeletal dimensions in hypogonadal individuals. Administration of sex hormones to deficient subjects during an expected period of growth then accelerates growth. Since maturation is also increased, however, cartilage proliferation is only of short duration, resulting in short stature.

CLASSIFICATION OF METABOLIC BONE DISEASE

Metabolic bone diseases result from disorders in remodeling, irrespective of whether disease occurs in the growing or nongrowing skeleton. In the following suggested classification of generalized metabolic bone diseases, effects on the endochondral sequence would have to be considered when applying it to children. The classification is based upon the relationship of the mineral phase to the matrix in the bone that is formed and the relative rates of formation and resorption of bone. Possible examples are provided, but other conditions could also be included. Paget's disease and related disorders (e.g., hyperphosphatasia) are not considered in this classification even though they are characterized by abnormal remodeling, since normal bone is always present, and the remodeling abnormality is still focal rather than generalized.

I. Ratio of inorganic/organic phase (mineral/matrix): low. Resorption may range from low to high depending upon the disorder.
    A. *Osteomalacia* (*rickets* in growing subjects)—due to failure to mineralize newly formed matrix (Chapters 67 and 70). Histologically, this state is characterized by increased surface of bone covered by osteoid as well as by increased thickness of the osteoid seam.
II. Ratio of inorganic/organic phase (mineral/matrix): normal. Rate of bone resorption exceeds that of bone formation.
    A. *Osteitis fibrosa*—excessive destruction of bone (e.g., in hyperparathyroidism) out of proportion to rate of bone formation. Bone formation, however, is also high in attempt at repair. Osteoclasts are abundant, and replace-

ment of fatty and hematopoietic marrow with fibrous stroma is characteristic (Chapter 53).
    B. *Osteoporosis*—resorption higher than formation. Formation rate usually normal or decreased depending upon etiology (Chapter 71). Osteoclasts are usually not abundant, and fibrous conversion of marrow is not seen.
III. Ratio of inorganic/organic phase: normal. Rate of bone formation exceeds that of bone resorption.
    A. *In hypoparathyroidism*—histologically, however, the changes in kinetics are not accompanied by changes in morphology that enable sufficient distinction from normal bone.
IV. Ratio of inorganic/organic phase: low. Rate of bone formation exceeds that of bone resorption.
    A. *Osteopetrosis*—rate of resorption low, but bone formed may be poorly mineralized. Thus, even though bone mass is increased, bone that is formed is osteomalacic. Histologically, the characteristic finding in the medulla is calcified cartilage surrounded by poorly mineralized woven and/or lamellar bone. This occurs because the primary spongiosa of endochondral ossification is not resorbed properly and persists into adult life. Osteoclasts can be seen but apparently are nonfunctional.
    B. *Osteitis fibrosa in healing phase*—Bone resorption ceases, and formation continues at same or increased rate after removal of parathyroid adenoma or other hyperfunctioning parathyroid tissue. Therefore, the histology of healing osteitis fibrosa is primarily that of maximal osteoblastic activity with minimal osteoclasts. There may be a prominent osteoid seam as the trabeculae and osteones fill in with new bone, often lamellar bone.

In Chapters 70–72 osteoporosis, osteomalacia, and Paget's disease are considered in detail in view of the prevalence of the disorders and their relation to hormonal function either in pathogenesis or treatment. The clinical features of other forms of metabolic bone disease are discussed in several recent reviews.[11,12,64–66]

REFERENCES

1. Glimcher, M. J., Krane, S. M.: The organization and structure of bone and the mechanism of calcification. In Ramachandran, G. N., Gould, B. S. (eds): A Treatise on Collagen. Biology of Collagen, vol 2B. New York, Academic, 1968, p 68.
2. Glimcher, M. J.: Composition, structure, and organization of bone and other mineralized tissues and the mechanism of calcification. In Aurbach, G. D. (ed): Handbook of Physiology. Endocrinology. Parathyroid Gland, sect 7, vol 7. Washington, DC, American Physiological Society, 1976, p 25.
3. Ascenzi, A., Bell, G. H.: Bone as a mechanical engineering problem. In Bourne, G. H. (ed): The Biochemistry and Physiology of Bone, vol 1. New York, Academic, 1972, p 311.
4. Herring, G. M.: The organic matrix of bone. In Bourne, G. H. (ed): The Biochemistry and Physiology of Bone, vol 1. New York, Academic, 1972, p 127.
5. Dickson, I.: The composition and antigenicity of sheep cortical bone matrix proteins. *Calcif Tissue Res 16:* 321, 1974.
6. Hauschka, P. V., Lian, J. B., Gallop, P. M.: Direct identification of the calcium-binding amino acid, γ-carboxyglutamate, in mineralized tissue. *Proc Natl Acad Sci USA 72:* 3925, 1975.
7. Price, P. A., Otsuka, A. S., Poser, J., et al: Characterization of a γ-carboxyglutamic acid-containing protein from bone. *Proc Natl Acad Sci USA 73:* 1447, 1976.
8. Stenflo, J.: Vitamin K, prothrombin and γ-carboxyglutamic acid. *N Engl J Med 296:* 624, 1977.

9. Posner, A. S.: Crystal chemistry of bone mineral. *Physiol Rev 49:* 760, 1969.
10. Termine, J. D.: Mineral chemistry and skeletal biology. *Clin Orthopaed 85:* 207, 1972.
11. Rasmussen, H., Bordier, P.: The Physiological and Cellular Basis of Metabolic Bone Disease. Baltimore, Williams & Wilkins, 1974, p 1.
12. Schenk, R. K., Olah, A. J., Merz, W. A.: Bone cell counts. In Frame, B., Parfitt, A. M., Duncan, H. (eds): Clinical Aspects of Metabolic Bone Disease. Amsterdam, Excerpta Medica, 1973, p 103.
13. Owen, M.: Cellular dynamics of bone mineral. In Bourne, G. H. (ed): The Biochemistry and Physiology of Bone, vol 3. New York, Academic, 1971, p 271.
14. Jaffe, H. J.: Metabolic, Degenerative, and Inflammatory Diseases of Bones and Joints. Philadelphia, Lea & Febiger, 1972, p 44.
15. Katz, E. P., Li, S.-T.: The intermolecular space of reconstituted collagen fibrils. *J Mol Biol 73:* 351, 1973.
16. Katz, E. P., Li, S.-T.: Structure and function of bone collagen fibrils. *J Mol Biol 80:* 1, 1973.
17. Anderson, H. C.: Vesicles associated with calcification in the matrix of epiphyseal cartilage. *J Cell Biol 41:* 59, 1969.
18. Bonucci, E.: Fine structure and histochemistry of "calcifying globules" in epiphyseal cartilage. *Z Zellforsch Mikrosk Anat 103:* 192, 1970.
19. Anderson, H. C., Reynolds, J. J.: Pyrophosphate stimulation of calcium uptake into cultured embryonic bones. Fine structure of matrix vesicles and their role in calcification. *Dev Biol 34:* 211, 1973.
20. Anderson, H. C.: Calcium-accumulating vesicles in the intercellular matrix of bone. In: Hard-Tissue Growth, Repair and Remineralization. Amsterdam, Elsevier, 1973, p 213.
21. Miller, E. J.: A review of biochemical studies on the genetically distinct collagens of the skeletal system. *Clin Orthopaed 92:* 260, 1973.
22. Miller, E. J.: Biochemical characteristics and biological significance of the genetically-distinct collagens. *Mol Cell Biochem 13:* 165, 1976.
23. Johnson, C.: The kinetics of skeletal remodeling. A further consideration of the theoretical biology of bone. *Birth Defects 2:* 66, 1966.
24. Frost, H. M.: The origin and nature of transients in human bone remodeling dynamics. In Frame B., Parfitt, A. M., Duncan, H. (eds): Clinical Aspects of Metabolic Bone Disease. Amsterdam, Excerpta Medica, 1973, p 124.
25. Teitelbaum, S. L., Rosenberg, E. M., Richardson, C. A., et al: Histological studies of bone from normocalcemic post-menopausal osteoporotic patients with increased circulating parathyroid hormone. *J Clin Endocrinol Metab 42:* 537, 1976.
26. Jowsey, J.: Microradiography. A morphological approach to quantitating bone turnover. In Frame, B., Parfitt, A. M., Duncan H. (eds): Clinical Aspects of Metabolic Bone Disease. Amsterdam, Excerpta Medica, 1973, p 114.
27. Jowsey, J., Kelly, P. J., Riggs, B. L., et al: Quantitative microradiographic studies of normal and osteoporotic bone. *J Bone Joint Surg 47A:* 785, 1965.
28. Krane, S. M.: Skeletal remodeling and metabolic bone disease. In Talmage, R. V., Owen, M., Parsons, J. A. (eds): Calcium-Regulating Hormones. Amsterdam, Excerpta Medica, 1975, p 57.
29. Meunier, P., Vignon, G., Bernard, J., et al: La lecture quantitative de la biopsie osseuse, moyen de diagnostic et d'étude de 106 hyperparathyroidies primitives, secondaires et paranéoplastiques. *Rev Rhum 39:* 635, 1972.
30. Courpron, P., Meunier, P., Eduard, C., et al: Données histologiques quantitative sur le vieillissement osseux humain. *Rev Rhum 40:* 469, 1973.
31. Merz, W. A., Schenk, R. K.: A quantitative histological study on bone formation in human cancellous bone. *Acta Anat (Basel) 76:* 1, 1970.
32. Aubert, J. P., Milhaud,, G.: Méthode de mésure des principales voies du métabolisme calcique chez l'homme. *Biochim Biophys Acta 39:* 122, 1960.
33. Nagant de Deuxchaisnes, C., Krane, S. M.: The treatment of adult phosphate diabetes and Fanconi syndrome with neutral sodium phosphate. *Am J Med 43:* 508, 1967.
34. Kivirikko, K. I.: Urinary excretion of hydroxyproline in health and disease. *Int Rev Connect Tissue Res 5:* 93, 1970.
35. Stetten, M. R.: Some aspects of metabolism of hydroxyproline studied with aid of isotopic nitrogen. *J Biol Chem 181:* 31, 1949.
36. Sinex, F. M., Van Slyke, D. D., Christman, D. R.: The source and

state of the hydroxylysine of collagen. II. Failure of free hydroxylysine to serve as a source of the hydroxylysine or lysine of collagen. *J Biol Chem 234:* 918, 1958.
37. Weiss, P. H., Klein, L.: The quantitative relationship of urinary peptide hydroxyproline excretion to collagen degradation. *J Clin Invest 48:* 1, 1969.
38. Efron, M. L., Bixby, E. M., Pryles, C. V.: Hydroxyprolinemia. II. A rare metabolic disease due to deficiency of the enzyme "hydroxyproline oxidase." *N Engl J Med 272:* 1299, 1965.
39. Cunningham, L. W., Ford, J. D., Segrest, J. P.: The isolation of identical hydroxylysyl glycosides from hydrolysates of soluble collagen and from human urine. *J Biol Chem 242:* 2570, 1967.
40. Pinnell, S. R., Fox, R., Krane, S. M.: Human collagens: differences in glycosylated hydroxylysines in skin and bone. *Biochim Biophys Acta 229:* 119, 1971.
41. Askenasi, R.: Urinary hydroxylysine and hydroxylysyl glycoside excretions in normal and pathological states. *J Lab Clin Med 83:* 673, 1974.
42. Krane, S. M., Kantrowitz, F. G., Byrne, M., et al: Urinary excretion of hydroxylysine and its glycosides as an index of collagen degradation. *J Clin Invest 59:* 819, 1977.
43. Meilman, E., Urivetzky, M. M., Rapoport, C. M.: Urinary hydroxyproline peptides. *J Clin Invest 42:* 40, 1963.
44. Krane, S. M., Munoz, A. J., Harris, E. D., Jr.: Collagen-like fragments: excretion in urine of patients with Paget's disease of bone. *Science 157:* 713, 1967.
45. Krane, S. M., Munoz, A. J., Harris, E. D. Jr.: Urinary polypeptides related to collagen synthesis. *J Clin Invest 49:* 716, 1970.
46. Haddad, J. G. Jr., Couranz, S., Avioli, L. V.: Nondialyzable urinary hydroxyproline as an index of bone collagen formation. *J Clin Endocrinol Metab 30:* 282, 1970.
47. Tanzer, M. L.: Cross-linking of collagen. Science *180:* 561, 1973
48. Bailey, A. J., Robins, S. P., Balian, G.: Biological significance of the intermolecular cross-links of collagen. *Nature 251:* 105, 1974.
49. Russell, R. G. G.: Metabolism of inorganic pyrophosphate. *Arthritis Rheum 19:* 465, 1976.
50. Howell, D. S., Pita, J. C., Marquez, J. F., et al: Demonstration of macromolecular inhibitor(s) of calcification and nucleational factor(s) in fluid from calcifying sites in cartilage. *J Clin Invest 48:* 630, 1969.
51. Posner, A. S., Eanes, E. D., Zipkin, I.: X-ray diffraction analysis of the effect of fluoride on bone. In Richelle, L. J., Dallemagne, M. J. (eds): Proceedings of the Second European Symposium on Calcified Tissues. Liége, Université de Liége, 1965, p 79.
52. Riggs, B. L., Jowsey, J.: Treatment of osteoporosis with fluoride. *Semin Drug Treat 2:* 27, 1972.
53. Harris, E. D. Jr., Krane, S. M.: Collagenases. *N Engl J Med 291:* 557, 605, 652, 1974.
54. Raisz, L. G.: Mechanisms of bone resorption. In Aurbach G. D. (ed): Handbook of Physiology. Endocrinology. Parathyroid Gland. sect 7, vol 7. Washington, DC, American Physiological Society, 1976, p 117.
55. Albright, F., Reifenstein, E. C. Jr.: The Parathyroid Glands and Metabolic Bone Disease. Baltimore, Williams & Wilkins, 1948.
56. Krane, S. M., Goldring, S. R.: Skeletal system. In Werner S. C., Ingbar S. H. (eds): The Thyroid. New York, Harper and Row, 1978, p. 727.
57. Greenberg, A. H., Najjar, S., Blizzard, R. M.: Effects of thyroid hormone on growth, differentiation, and development. In Greer, M. A., Solomon, D. H. (eds): Handbook of Physiology. Endocrinology. Thyroid. sect 7, vol 3. Washington, DC, American Physiological Society, 1974, p 377.
58. Wilkins, L. W.: Hormonal influences on skeletal growth. *Ann NY Acad Sci 60:* 763, 1955.
59. Fell, H. B., Mellanby, E.: The effect of L-triiodothyronine on the growth and development of embryonic chick limb-bones in tissue culture. *J Physiol 133:* 89, 1956.
60. Mundy, G. R., Shapiro, J. L., Bandelin, J. G., et al: Direct stimulation of bone resorption by thyroid hormones. *J Clin Invest 58:* 529, 1976.
61. Cheek, D. B., Hill, D. E.: Effect of growth hormone on cell and somatic growth. In Knobil E., Sawyer W. H. (eds): Handbook of Physiology. Endocrinology. The Pituitary Gland and Its Neuroendocrine Control. sect 7, vol 4. Washington, DC, American Physiological Society, 1974, p 159.
62. Gardner, W. U., Pfeiffer, C. A.: Influence of estrogens and androgens on the skeletal system. *Physiol Rev 23:* 139, 1943.

63. Hodge, A. J., Petruska, J. A.: Recent studies with the electron microscope on ordered aggregates of the tropocollagen macromolecule. In Ramachandran, G. N. (ed): Aspects of Protein Structure. New York, Academic, 1963, p 289.

64: Krane, S. M.: Metabolic bone disease, section 13: Disorders of bone and bone mineral metabolism. In Thorn, G. W., Adams, R. D., Braunwald, E., Isselbacher, K. J., Petersdorf, R. G. (eds): Harrison's Principles of Internal Medicine (ed 8). New York, McGraw-Hill, 1977, ch 355, p 2028.

65. Avioli, L., Krane, S. M. (eds): Metabolic Bone Disease, vol. I. New York, Academic, 1977; vol. II, l978.

66. Jowsey, J.: Metabolic Diseases of Bone. Philadelphia, Saunders, 1977.

70

Disorders of Calcification: Osteomalacia and Rickets

Steven R. Goldring

Stephen M. Krane

Osteomalacia and rickets are disorders of calcification. In osteomalacia there is a failure to mineralize the newly formed organic matrix (osteoid) of bone in a normal manner. In rickets, a disease of children, the growth plate at the epiphysis is also involved in a process characterized by defective calcification of cartilage, delayed maturation of the cellular sequence, and disorganization of the arrangement of the cartilage cells, resulting in thickening of the epiphyseal plate. A number of different disorders are associated with osteomalacia in adults and rickets in children.[1-3] The pathogenesis of the mineralization defect, the biochemical alterations, the clinical manifestations, and the therapeutic approaches differ in these conditions, and a systematic approach to osteomalacia is therefore essential.

MINERALIZATION DEFECT

Mineralization of bone is a complex process in which the calcium-phosphate inorganic mineral phase is deposited in relation to the organic matrix in a highly ordered fashion. Optimal mineralization can take place at bone-forming surfaces only if (1) cellular activity of bone-forming cells is adequate, (2) matrix is normal in composition and is synthesized at a normal rate, (3) the supply of mineral ions (calcium and inorganic phosphate) from the extracellular fluid is sufficient, (4) the pH at sites of mineralization is appropriate (~ 7.6), and (5) the concentration of inhibitors of calcification is controlled. These regulatory mechanisms have already been considered in Chapter 69. It is possible that clinical disorders of mineralization can be attributed to defects at several of these control steps, examples of which are shown in Table 70-1.

Since the mechanism of defective mineralization is not the same in all of the above disorders, biochemical indices such as serum levels of calcium and phosphate will also differ. Moreover, the relative imbalance in matrix synthesis and its mineralization will vary, depending upon the underlying disease mechanism. Thus, although it is clinically useful to consider changes in a "calcium-phosphate product" in certain forms of rickets and osteomalacia, it should be emphasized that there are other conditions in which defective mineralization occurs in the face of normal or even elevated "calcium-phosphate products." Even when a low "product" is raised, for example, by increasing the serum phosphate concentration in phosphate-depleted animals, the rise in the product itself may not be the only biological event to explain the change in mineralization, since profound alterations in metabolic behavior and modifications of the matrix accompany phosphate depletion and repletion.[4]

Rickets and osteomalacia are disorders of skeletal turnover. The defects can all be ascribed to insufficient mineralization of newly forming matrix (cartilage and bone), not to the removal of mineral from mature bone. The pathogenesis of the alterations in the rachitic growth plate has recently been reviewed, and mechanical explanations for the deformities provided.[1] The characteristic changes occur in the maturation zone, whereas the resting and proliferative zones show normal histological features (Fig. 70-1). In the maturation zone the height of the cell columns is increased, and the cells are closely packed and irregularly aligned. The hypertrophic cells are sparse in number and irregularly distributed. The increase in thickness of the plate is also accompanied by an increase in the transverse diameter, which may extend beyond the ends of the bone, resulting in characteristic cupping or flaring. In experimental rickets the water content of the plate is increased,[5] and a number of metabolic abnormalities have been observed, including decreased glycogen content and altered pattern of glycolysis.[4]

Estimates from tetracycline labeling indicate that the appositional growth rate in normal bone is about 1 μm per day.[6] It has also been suggested that complete mineralization of the osteoid in normal bone requires approximately 10 to 21 days.[7] Thus the thickness of the osteoid seam normally does not exceed 20 μm and is usually not greater than 13 μm. The surface of bone covered by osteoid is normally less than 20 percent, and the active surface covered by osteoid is considerably less. (See reviews by Rasmussen and Bordier,[8] Bordier and Tun Chot,[9] and Byers.[10]) The major histological criteria for establishment of osteomalacia are the increased osteoid surface and the increased thickness of the osteoid

Table 70-1. Examples of Disorders in Which Mechanisms Responsible for Mineralization Control Differ

Disorder	Possible Mechanism
1. Postoperative hyperparathyroidism	1. Rate of matrix synthesis exceeds rate of mineralization
2. Fibrogenesis imperfecta ossium	2. Defective collagenous matrix
3. Adult phosphate diabetes	3. Phosphate concentration deficient at mineralization sites
4. Nutritional (vitamin D-deficient osteomalacia)	4. Calcium and phosphate concentrations deficient (? role of deficient vitamin D itself)
5. Systemic acidosis	5. pH inadequate for mineralization
6. Hypophosphatasia	6. Concentration of inhibitor (? inorganic pyrophosphate) excessive

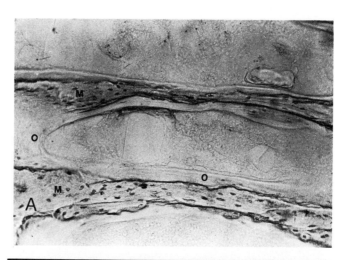

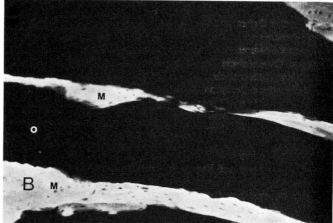

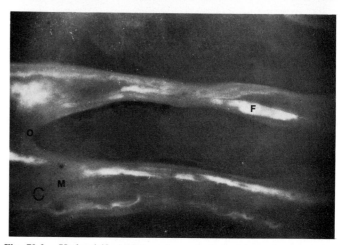

seam (Fig. 70-2).[1,3,8–10] The "calcification front" at the junction of mineralized bone and osteoid is also abnormal in osteomalacia, and some consider this alteration critical in diagnosis.[9] The architecture of the bone cells and matrix in osteomalacic bone is usually normal, although some cellular abnormalities have been described, such as osteocyte perilacunar defects.[11,12] These defects are probably nonspecific.[13] The collagen of the osteoid is largely lamellar, although foci of woven bone are occasionally seen (Fig. 70-3).[10]

When bone is examined histologically, it is essential that undemineralized sections are used. In usual practice, however, with classic clinical, radiological, and biochemical findings, bone biopsy is not necessary to arrive at the diagnosis of osteomalacia. Techniques for biopsy have been standardized in several laboratories and have been facilitated by the design of special trocars for this purpose.[10] The most commonly biopsied site is the iliac crest; sample size ranges from 5 to 10 mm in diameter and should include both inner and outer cortices. Growth plates from long bones in children are usually not biopsied, although an open wedge biopsy of growth cartilage of the iliac apophysis may occasionally be obtained without the possible hazard of altering subsequent skele-

Fig. 70-2. Undecalcified thick sections of a bone biopsy from a patient with adult-onset hypophosphatemic osteomalacia (renal-tubular-phosphate leak) (case 1, ref. 22). Sections were examined under different conditions. (A) Unstained. (B) Microradiograph. (C) Ultraviolet photomicrograph demonstrating fluorescence (F) of tetracycline administered 14 hours prior to biopsy. Note mineralized bone (M) and osteoid (O).

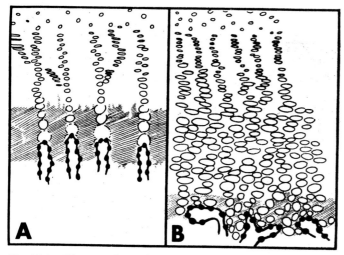

Fig. 70-1. Diagram of postulated mechanism involved in causing increased length of cartilage columns in the growth plate in rickets. In the normal plate (A), the calcified zone (shaded area) provides tunnels for the ingrowth of vascular buds which are involved presumably in destruction of the cells of the hypertrophic zone most distal from the growth plate, thereby limiting growth in length of the column. In the rachitic plate (B), the calcium-deficient zone does not provide tunnels, and the normal vascular mechanism limiting growth in length of the columns is lost. (From H. J. Mankin, *Journal of Bone and Joint Surgery,* 56A: 101–129, 352–386, 1974.)

tal proportions. Mineralized specimens of bone are most satisfactorily embedded in plastic media, which provide preservation of tissue architecture not usually attained with paraffin-embedding techniques, since the tinctorial distinction between mineralized and unmineralized bone is markedly decreased by decalcification of the specimen. Undecalcified sections should therefore be obtained to adequately differentiate osteoid from mineralized bone,

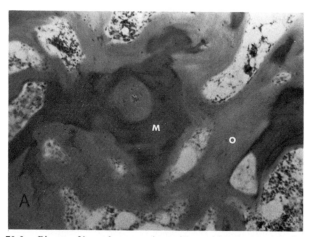
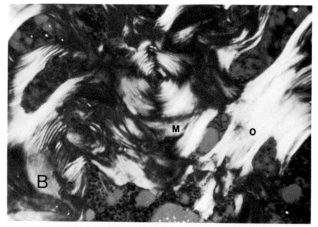

Fig 70-3. Biopsy of bone from a patient with nutritional osteomalacia (partially decalcified sections stained with hematoxylin and eosin. (*A*) Viewed with transmitted nonpolarized light. (*B*) Viewed under polarized light with analyzer. Note that most of bone is lamellar whether mineralized (M) or osteoid (O).

although in severely affected individuals, undecalcified paraffin sections may show the osteoid satisfactorily if the samples can be properly cut. Plastic-embedded specimens can be prepared using grinding procedures or sectioning with a heavy-duty sledge microtome. A number of different staining techniques can then be used to demonstrate the osteoid and apply quantitative morphometric analysis (Fig. 70-4).[14]

In normal bone, a "calcification front" is seen at the junction of the osteoid seam and newly mineralized bone.[8,9] This region can be demonstrated by an intense fluorescence of tetracycline, which is deposited in this zone if the antibiotic is administered prior to obtaining the biopsy (Fig. 70-5). In normal individuals, the osteoid seam/bone junctions fluoresce intensely, whereas in osteomalacia

the fluorescence is less well defined (more diffuse) or even absent (Fig. 70-2*C*). The calcification front may also be demonstrated by staining the sections with toluidine blue or the dye Solochrome-cyanine R. There is not universal agreement, however, concerning the requirement for abnormality in the calcification front in the diagnosis of osteomalacia.[3]

It is apparent that if a wide osteoid seam is demonstrated in osteomalacia, the rate at which matrix is formed must be greater than that at which it is mineralized. In most forms of human osteomalacia, matrix biosynthesis is probably not occurring at a normal rate, even though the total osteoid surface is increased. In rats, in which the process can be adequately quantitated, the osteomalacia of vitamin D deficiency is associated with a de-

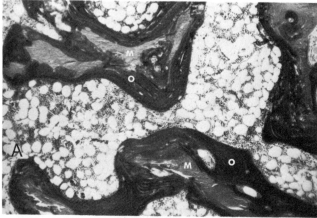
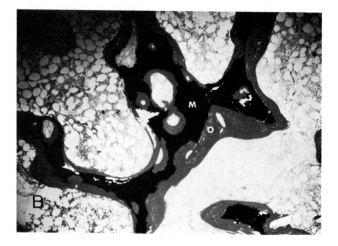
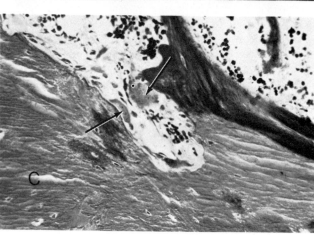

Fig. 70-4. Thin sections of iliac-bone biopsy from a patient with renal osteodystrophy on chronic hemodialysis. (*A*) Goldner stain. (*B*) Von Kossa stain. (*C*) High power of an area from (*A*) showing osteoclasts (arrow) resorbing mineralized bone. Mineralized bone (M) is readily distinguished from osteoid (O).

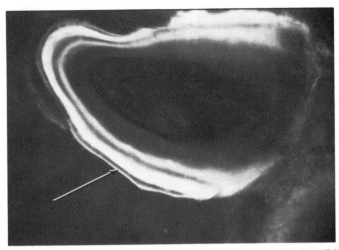

Fig. 70-5. Thick section of undemineralized bone from a man with mild phosphate diabetes (case 4, ref. 22). This patient received tetracycline on several occasions months before the biopsy was taken. The fluorescence of the region corresponding to the earliest dose of tetracycline (arrow) is sharp and characteristic of a normal calcification front. Compare with Fig. 70-2C where the tetracycline deposition is irregular and diffuse.

creased rate of matrix formation.[15] Despite these observations in rats, the level of serum alkaline phosphatase is elevated in many but not all forms of human rickets and osteomalacia. Although the level of alkaline phosphatase in serum probably reflects osteoblastic "activity" in bone, the rate of matrix biosynthesis cannot be adequately estimated from the levels of this enzyme alone. Since the lag time in mineralization is also prolonged, and the rate of mineralization slowed, the net result is an increase in the thickness of the osteoid seam. Not only is the *rate* of matrix synthesis altered in such situations but the matrix itself may be modified. Indeed, the hydroxylation of certain lysyl residues of bone collagen is increased in vitamin D deficiency as well as in other experimental hypocalcemic states.[16–18]

CLINICAL FEATURES OF RICKETS AND OSTEOMALACIA

The clinical manifestations of rickets, although they vary to some extent depending upon the underlying disorder, are mainly related to skeletal pain and deformity, fracture of the abnormal bones, slippage of epiphyses, and disturbances in growth.[1–3] Hypocalcemia when it occurs may be symptomatic. In some children, especially those with vitamin D deficiency, muscular weakness and hypotonia may be prominent. Dent and Stamp[2] have indicated nine factors that underlie the clinical manifestations of rickets, and they are modified here as follows:

1. Failure of the calcification mechanism affects predominantly those parts of the skeleton whose growth is most rapid.
2. Rickets affects endochondral bone more than intramembranous bone, poosibly because of the more-rapid growth of the former. Only when rickets is severe is bone such as that in the midshaft involved clinically.
3. Proximal and distal ends of bones do not grow at the same rate, and rickets affects the most rapidly growing area.
4. Different bones grow at different rates at different stages of development. At the time when rickets is active, these factors determine the clinical expression. For example,

the skull is growing rapidly at birth, and craniotabes is therefore a manifestation of congenital rickets. During the first year the upper limbs and rib cage grow rapidly, and therefore abnormalities at these sites are prominent, e.g., rachitic rosary. Signs of rickets at the wrist are usually seen at the ulnar side, since the growth rate of the distal ulnar epiphysis is relatively greater than that of the distal radial epiphysis.
5. Deformities in mild chronic rickets are most often due to disordered growth at the epiphyseal plate rather than to bending at the shafts.
6. In some forms of rickets the radiological changes include those of secondary hyperparathyroidism (subperiosteal resorption, most commonly at the metaphyses).
7. Deformities that occur before the age of 4 years correct themselves if the rickets is cured, whereas if rickets is persistent to a later age, the deformities are permanent (dwarfism, bowleg, and knock-knee).
8. "Late" rickets, which occurs at the time of the pubescent growth spurt, produces dramatic disturbances, and results in knock-knee.
9. Adult manifestations of osteomalacia, such as Looser's zones and increased biconcavity of vertebral bodies, are seen in young children only when the rickets is very severe.

In infants and young children, especially in severe, classic rickets, listlessness and irritability are common. In infants, myopathy is characteristic and is manifested by floppiness and hypotonia. In older children the weakness may present as a proximal myopathy similar to that observed in the adult. Other findings in infants include parietal flattening or frontal bossing, softening of the calvarium (craniotabes), and widening of the sutures. The thickened growth plates may be evident clinically as the rachitic rosary at the rib ends or may even simulate juvenile rheumatoid arthritis when areas such as the wrists are involved. Indentation of the lower ribs at the site of attachment of the diaphragm is known as Harrison's groove, or sulcus. Pelvic deformities also occur, and the skeleton is more prone to fractures. Pain may not be prominent, and, when present, it is greater at the knees and on weight-bearing points. Dental eruption may be delayed, and enamel defects are common.

In contrast, osteomalacia in adults may be difficult to detect on clinical grounds alone. Diffuse skeletal pain and muscular weakness may be present in the absence of a specific pattern. Pain is often prominent about the hips and may produce an antalgic gait. Fractures may occur about the rib cage and vertebral bodies, as well as in long bones, and lead to progressive deformities. Muscular weakness is particularly prominent.[19] In one series of 45 patients with osteomalacia, it was present in almost half.[20] The weakness is primarily proximal in distribution (which contributes to the waddling gait) and is often associated with wasting, discomfort on movement, and hypotonia with preservation of brisk reflexes.[21] The same myopathy is seen in patients with all types of osteomalacia, with the exception of those with X-linked hypophosphatemic osteomalacia. In adults with acquired renal tubular phosphate leak, in contrast to children with the X-linked form, proximal muscle weakness may also be profound and is correctable by phosphate repletion.[22] Although electromyograms occasionally show myopathic changes and muscle biopsies rarely show denervation,[19] in one series of 6 patients with osteomalacia of different etiologies, muscle biopsies revealed nonspecific changes including neurogenic atrophy or type II fiber atrophy of uncertain cause.[23] These patients had electromyographic changes of neurogenic muscle disease consistent with the histological changes. None of these patients had severe hypophosphatemia (lowest recorded phosphatemia was 2.7 mg/dl). Thus the neuromuscular disease of osteomalacia has multiple causes, and it usually responds to specific therapy of the underlying disorder, such as vitamin D in nutritional osteomalacia, alkalinization in acidosis, and phosphate repletion in the adult form of hypophosphatemic osteomalacia. There may be a role for the secondary hyperparathyroidism (when it occurs) in the production of the neuromuscular disease, since changes similar to those described in osteomalacia have also been found in primary hyperparathyroidism.[24] The role of hypophosphatemia per se in muscular weakness is discussed in Chapter 40.

RADIOLOGICAL FEATURES

Radiological changes in the skeleton in rickets and osteomalacia reflect the histopathological changes.[1,2] In rickets the alterations are most evident at the epiphyseal growth plate, which is increased in thickness, cupped, and reveals a haziness at the diaphyseal border due to decreased calcification of the hypertrophic zone and inadequate mineralization of the primary spongiosa (Fig. 70-6). Variation in the pattern of the rachitic changes is influenced by differences in rates of growth of bones or portions of bones as discussed earlier. The trabecular pattern of the metaphyses is abnormal, the cortices of the diaphyses may be thinned, and bowing of the shafts may be present.

In osteomalacia there is usually some decrease in bone density associated with loss of trabeculae, blurring of trabecular margins, and variable degrees of thinning of the cortices.[2,4] In some patients the radiological changes are indistinguishable from those seen in osteoporosis. The finding that suggests osteomalacia more specifically is the presence of radiolucent bands ranging from a few millimeters to several centimeters in length, usually oriented perpendicularly to the surface of the bone (Fig. 70-7). They tend to occur symmetrically and are particularly common at the inner aspects of the femur, especially near the femoral neck, in the pelvis, in the outer edge of the scapula, in the upper fibula, and in the metatarsals. These translucent bands are referred to as pseudofractures, Looser's zones, or umbauzonen. They are often multiple, occasionally occurring at 10 to 15 sites in a single individual.[22,25] Such multiple symmetrical pseudofractures occurring in individuals with osteomalacia of a variety of etiologies have been referred to as Milkman's syndrome.[26,27] The abnormalities in Milkman's original cases[28,29] were also considered by Albright and Reifenstein[27] as manifestations of osteomalacia. The pseudofractures most often occur at sites where major arteries cross the bones and have been thought to be secondary to the mechanical stress of the pulsating vessel. Arteriography in some cases,[22,30,31] but not all,[32] has indicated that the origins of the pseudofractures correspond to the location of major arteries (Fig. 70-8). Trauma of some sort, whether related to arterial pulsation or other factors, must be responsible for the symmetry of the lesions and predilection for the described sites. The histopathology of Looser's zones, according to Ball and Garner,[33] is that of premalacic lamellar bone, some of which is surrounded by lamellar osteoid at the edge of the defect. In addition, there are foci of woven bone, some of which is mineralized and some not. This accounts for the lower radiological mineral density of the pseudofracture compared to the surrounding bone. Subperiosteal erosions along the diaphyseal cortices extending to the metaphyses may be seen when secondary hyperparathyroidism is present. Widening (or pseudowidening) of the sacroiliac joints with hazy margins has also been observed, sometimes sug-

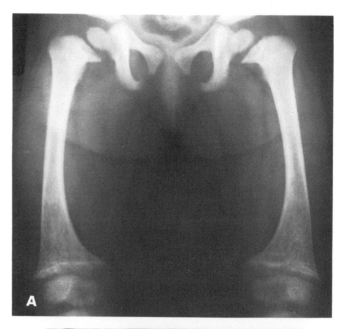

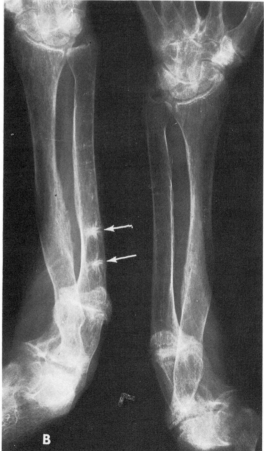

Fig. 70-6(A) Rickets in a child with Fanconi syndrome showing typical cupping of distal femoral epiphyses. (B) Osteomalacia in an 80-year-old woman who had a history compatible with hypophosphatemic rickets dating to early childhood. Note multiple pseudofractures (arrows).

gesting ankylosing spondylitis (which osteomalacia may mimic clinically).[22]

In some patients with osteomalacia, increased rather than decreased radiological density of bones may be observed.[25] This is

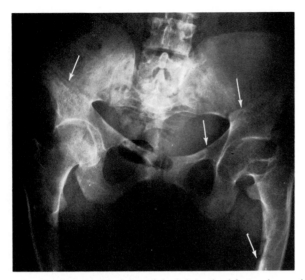

Fig. 70-7. Roentgenogram of the pelvis and proximal femurs in a patient with adult phosphate diabetes (case 2, ref. 22). Note pseudofractures or Looser's zones (arrows).

seen particularly in patients with renal tubular phosphate leaks, as opposed to vitamin D deficiency (Fig. 70-9). In such patients there may be a striking degree of thickening of the cortices and trabeculae of the spongy bone, at times associated with exostotic spurs. This hyperostosis has been noted in untreated patients. It is not usually observed in individuals with generalized defects in proximal renal tubular reabsorption. Despite the increase in mass of bone per unit volume, microscopically the trabeculae are covered with abnormally thickened osteoid seams typical of osteomalacia. Similar findings may be noted in patients with chronic renal failure. The reason for the hyperostosis is unknown; the bone is still architecturally abnormal and subject to fracture with relatively minimal trauma.

A comprehensive classification of rickets and osteomalacia is shown in Table 70-2. A detailed discussion of all these conditions will not be included here, since selected areas are covered in other chapters. Fraser and Scriver have discussed vitamin D dependency and X-linked hypophosphatemic rickets in Chapter 66, and Hahn and Avioli, in Chapter 67, have discussed anticonvulsant and drug-induced osteomalacia, intestinal and hepatic etiologies, effects of glucocorticoids, and renal osteodystrophy. The ensuing discussion therefore includes major types of rickets and osteomalacia that have not been previously discussed.

NUTRITIONAL OSTEOMALACIA

Writings of the 17th century in Scotland and England vividly documented the association between poverty, undernutrition, and the occurrence of infantile rickets. Reports from Glasgow in the late 1800s and 1900s drew further attention to the widespread prevalence of infantile rickets in the industrialized regions of Britain. In 1923, the work of the Vienna Council finally established the link between rickets, dietary deficiency of vitamin D, and correction of vitamin D deficiency by irradiation with sunlight. Following the discovery that rickets was a vitamin-deficiency disease, fortification of certain foods with vitamin D reduced the incidence of nutritional rickets in Europe and the United States to negligible levels, and by the 1940s, deficiency of vitamin D was no longer regarded as an important cause of osteomalacia and rickets.[27]

The studies of Dunnigan et al.[34] and of Arneil and Crosbie[35] in Glasgow and Benson et al.[36] in London have documented the reappearance of nutritional osteomalacia and rickets as a public-health problem in Britain. The new population at risk exists primarily among the large number of immigrants arriving in Britain since the 1950s from India, Pakistan, and other Commonwealth countries. Unique dietary and social customs have played a significant role in the emergence of osteomalacia and rickets in this population. Another large group of individuals in whom nutritional osteomalacia is being recognized with increasing frequency include housebound and other elderly subjects.[37–40] Additional cases are also being recognized among food faddists, especially those on vegetarian or fat-free diets.[37]

In normal individuals, vitamin D is provided from two sources: (1) dietary supplementation with ergocalciferol (D_2), which is an irradiation product obtained from plants, and (2) the natural vitamin, cholecalciferol (D_3), produced in human skin by the action of ultraviolet light on the physiological precursor, 7-dehydrocholesterol. Since most foods (with the exception of fatty fish) contain only small amounts of D_3, individuals must rely upon either adequate sunlight exposure or dietary supplements of ergocalciferol for maintenance of adequate vitamin D supply.

With the availability of a reliable assay for 25-hydroxyvitamin D,[40] it has become possible to study vitamin D status in individuals who have no evidence of obvious clinical disease. Several groups of investigators have documented marked seasonal variations in plasma 25-hydroxyvitamin D both in Britain[41–44] and in the United States,[45] independent of age and sex. These variations parallel changes in sun exposure, with higher levels occurring in late-summer months and fall. These observations point out the critical

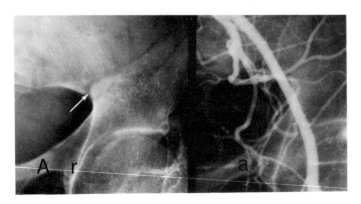

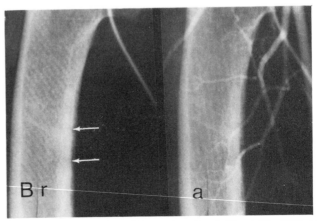

Fig. 70-8. Roentgenograms (r) and corresponding arteriograms (a) in a patient with adult-onset phosphate diabetes (case 2, ref. 22, see Fig. 70-7). (*A*) Pelvis. (*B*) Femur. Note that origin of Looser's zones (arrows) corresponds with crossing of major vessels.

in children with severe vitamin D-deficient rickets, in order to avoid the development of tetany.

Other investigators have reported successful treatment of nutritional rickets and osteomalacia with either 1,25-dihydroxyvitamin D, or 1α-hydroxyvitamin D.[66,67] Similar beneficial effects have not been achieved with dihydrotachysterol,[49] and therefore in light of the multiple other preparations, this compound should not be used for treatment of these disorders at this time. Phosphate supplements are not indicated in deficiency rickets or osteomalacia because of the potential hazard of severe hypocalcemia and tetany.

In summary, rickets and osteomalacia are being recognized with increasing frequency in selected populations. The availability of assays of serum 25-hydroxyvitamin D has permitted detection of these disorders prior to the development of overt clinical disease.

ACIDOSIS AND OSTEOMALACIA

Acidosis resulting from a number of different causes has been associated with osteomalacia. The mechanisms of bone loss and the mineralization defects are complex, and the problem is by no means settled. Albright and his colleagues[27] suggested that acidosis produces slow dissolution of the mineral phase of bone in an attempt to buffer retained hydrogen ion. This process is associated with hypercalciuria. Support for this concept has been obtained by studies in patients with renal tubular acidosis in whom retention of hydrogen ion is greater than that theoretically required to produce the observed decrease in plasma bicarbonate.[68] In further studies in normal individuals, it has also been observed that in induced metabolic acidosis, the excess of retained hydrogen ion is balanced by the increase in urinary calcium excretion.[69,70] This has been ascribed to increased bone dissolution. The effects of acidosis on increasing bone resorption may be cellularly mediated.[71,72] For example, in vitro, comparable small decreases in pH produce greater calcium release from living than from dead bones.

However, hypercalciuria and increased bone resorption that accompany most acidotic states do not themselves produce osteomalacia, and other mechanisms must be invoked to explain the occurrence of clinically significant skeletal mineralization defects. Some of these factors include the following.

Maintenance of a critical-level pH range is essential for mineralization to proceed normally. In rats, where it is possible to obtain micropuncture samples at calcification sites in the growth plate, the pH is ~7.6.[73,74] An independent decrease in systemic pH alone could thus inhibit mineralization by lowering pH at calcification sites. Acidosis can also affect phosphate metabolism[75] by altering renal tubular handling of the anion and changing the species of phosphate in solution (Chapter 40). In patients with chronic acidosis (e.g., with ureterosigmoidostomy), treatment with alkali alone can restore a low serum phosphate level to normal when the acidosis is treated. This is accompanied by increased phosphate reabsorption, presumably secondary to increased phosphate T_m. Secondary hyperparathyroidism may be an important factor in the altered phosphate handling.[75] Harrison and colleagues[76] have emphasized that acidosis may also alter the response to exogenous vitamin D. They showed that doses of vitamin D that were ineffective in producing rises in intestinal calcium absorption and serum calcium levels in the presence of acidosis were effective when the acidosis was corrected. More-recent studies have indicated that in rats made acidotic with ammonium chloride feeding, conversion of cholecalciferol to 1,25-dihydroxycholecalciferol measured in the intestine was diminished[77] despite the presence of hypocalcemia and hypophosphatemia, both of which usually stimulate formation of this metabolite.

Rickets and osteomalacia secondary to acidosis are most often a complication of distal renal tubular acidosis.[1,2,78-80] In most of the reported cases,[2,81] healing of the bone disease can result from correction of the acidosis with sodium bicarbonate alone (5–10 g/day). Healing is slow, and the response may be hastened by the addition of vitamin D (up to 15 mg/day have been required). Occasionally, vitamin D toxicity may develop unexpectedly, and these patients must therefore be carefully monitored. Vitamin D is usually not necessary once the osteomalacia is cured. Continued use of vitamin D may be necessary, however, for complete healing in those individuals in whom the glomerular filtration rate is low.[2,81,82]

In several of the syndromes associated with more widespread renal tubular reabsorptive defects, systemic acidosis may contribute to the pathogenesis of osteomalacia. Some of these are inherited, such as various forms of the Fanconi syndrome, with and without cystinosis, and Lowe's syndrome (oculocerebrorenal syndrome). Some patients with renal tubular phosphate leaks may also have mild acidosis, especially in those associated with excessive urinary excretion of glycine.[83-86] The clinical picture is variable in these cases, and the specificity of the hyperglycinuria has not been established. Detailed considerations of the general features of these syndromes have been published,[1,78-80,87] and other aspects are considered elsewhere in this chapter.

Osteomalacia may also be a complication of the acidosis produced by ureterosigmoidostomy, a procedure formerly used in the treatment of patients with carcinoma of the bladder.[75] Reabsorption of chloride and hydrogen ions from urine in the colon is responsible for the acidosis. An example of Looser's zones seen in such individuals is shown in Fig. 70-10. Keeping the rectosigmoid empty by frequent drainage may prevent or correct the acidosis and thus prevent the development of the osteomalacia. Although it is rarely used at present as a diuretic, we have encountered typical osteomalacia (Fig. 70-11) in a patient with acidosis presumably resulting from chronic acetazolamide therapy. This individual was receiving phenobarbital and phenytoin, as well, for severe seizure disorders, but when the acetazolamide alone was discontinued and plasma bicarbonate increased, the osteomalacia showed evidence of healing both radiologically and clinically. Acetazolamide does

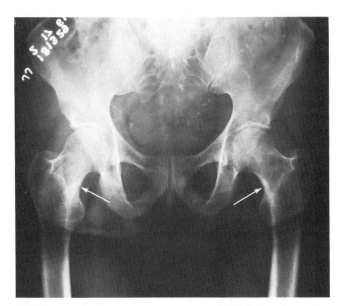

Fig. 70-10. Roentgenogram of pelvis and femora of a 60-year-old man with ureterosigmoidostomy. Note Looser's zones (arrows).

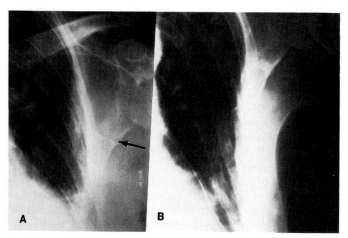

Fig. 70-11. Roentgenogram of left scapula from a 42-year-old woman with acidosis due in part to chronic acetazolamide therapy. (*A*) Before and (*B*) 6 months after discontinuing acetazolamide. Note Looser's zone (arrow) in pretreatment roentgenogram.

have direct inhibitory effects on bone resorption in animals independent of pH,[88] and therefore exact interpretation of the course in this patient is not possible at this time. The contributory role of acidosis in the osteodystrophy of chronic renal failure is considered elsewhere.

DIETARY PHOSPHATE DEPLETION

In man, phosphate depletion and resultant hypophosphatemia may lead to the development of rickets or osteomalacia by mechanisms discussed earlier. A state of phosphate depletion can be produced either by inadequate dietary supply of this element or by excessive losses through urine or stool (Chapter 40). It is difficult to produce selective deficiency of phosphorus by dietary means alone, since most foods contain this element in concentrations sufficient to prevent hypophosphatemia and bone disease (Chapter 40). Several authors have reported the occurrence of severe phosphate depletion and hypophosphatemia associated with osteomalacia in patients ingesting large quantities of nonabsorbable antacids, usually as a form of self-medication for dyspepsia.[89–92] Studies in these patients as well as in normal volunteers have revealed that ingestion of nonabsorbable antacids in large doses is associated with a rapid decline in urinary phosphorus to undetectable levels.[90,91] This is accompanied by a marked increase in fecal phosphorus presumably related to binding of dietary phosphate with the antacid, resulting in a complex that is poorly absorbed from the gastrointestinal tract. With continued ingestion of the antacid, serum phosphorus levels gradually decrease, eventually leading to signs and symptoms of hypophosphatemia. The early decline in urinary phosphorus cannot be accounted for by a decrease in filtered load, since serum phosphorus concentrations and renal function are initially unchanged; the mechanism of the early hypophosphaturia is uncertain. In addition to the changes in phosphorus handling, these individuals also develop hypercalciuria. Since serum calcium levels have remained unchanged despite marked hypophosphatemia, the hypercalciuria also cannot be attributed to changes in filtered loads of calcium. Urinary calcium excretion occasionally has exceeded dietary calcium intake, and, therefore, a portion of the urinary calcium excreted is presumably of skeletal origin. However, these individuals lack overt evidence of increased bone resorption, and it is more likely that the rise in urinary calcium excretion is related to impaired bone mineraliza-

tion, a concept that is supported by the association of this syndrome with osteomalacia. In general, clinically significant bone disease is quite rare, despite the wide use of nonabsorbable antacids for treatment of peptic-ulcer disease. This suggests that although the medication interferes with intestinal phosphate absorption, this defect is compensated for by ample supply of dietary phosphorus in milk and dairy products. A similar syndrome of phosphate depletion has been described in patients with renal failure receiving large quantities of aluminum hydroxide gel.[93]

Hypophosphatemia has also been observed in both chronic and acute alcoholism[94,95] (Chapter 40). Bone densitometric studies and tetracycline-labeled bone biopsies obtained from chronic alcoholics have revealed an increased frequency of bone disease compared to sex- and race-matched controls.[96] The bone abnormalities include changes consistent with mixtures of osteoporosis, osteomalacia, and osteitis fibrosa. The precise role and mechanism of phosphate depletion and hypophosphatemia in the development of bone disease in these individuals are uncertain.

IMPAIRED RENAL TUBULAR PHOSPHATE REABSORPTION

In 1937 Albright and co-workers[97] reported their studies of a 16-year-old boy with long-standing rickets in whom standard doses of vitamin D failed to produce clinical improvement. Healing of the bone disease eventually occurred, but only after administration of extremely high doses of vitamin D. The results of their studies led to the introduction of the concept of "vitamin D resistance" in certain types of rickets. Since this initial report, so-called vitamin D-resistant rickets has been classified into several clinical and biochemical subtypes, the most common of which is the X-linked, dominantly inherited form discussed in detail in Chapter 66. Affected individuals usually present with clinical and roentgenographic evidence of rickets within the second or third year of life. Another X-linked form has been identified in which the bone disease first becomes manifest in the fourth or fifth decade without evidence of earlier rachitic abnormalities.[98] In other patients, the disease occurs sporadically in the absence of an associated family history of bone disease and/or hypophosphatemia. As in the X-linked form of the disease, the cardinal biochemical disturbance is the abnormally low serum phosphorus level, presumably secondary to a primary renal tubular phosphorus leak. Plasma calcium levels are always normal, and serum alkaline phosphatase activity is usually raised, although, in some individuals, the elevations are minimal.[97,99] The results of measurements of calcium balance in untreated patients are variable, but balance tends to be slightly negative or zero, accompanied by normal urinary excretion of hydroxyproline peptides.[22,99,100] The diagnosis of the latter disorder is dependent upon the demonstration of impaired renal tubular phosphorus absorption and the presence of osteomalacia, i.e., widened osteoid seams and increased osteoid surface on bone biopsy. As in the X-linked disease, other causes of osteomalacia, such as those listed in Table 70-2, must be excluded, particularly primary vitamin D deficiency, malabsorption, renal insufficiency, generalized renal tubular disorders, neurofibromatosis, and certain mesenchymal tumors. Evaluation of patients with possible adult-onset hypophosphatemic osteomalacia should thus include general tests of renal function (creatinine clearance, acidification, and concentrating ability, and analysis of urinary amino acid excretion), tests of intestinal absorptive capacity (fecal fat, D-xylose absorption), and careful search for the presence of occult tumors.

The mode of presentation of patients with adult hypophosphatemic osteomalacia or phosphate diabetes, as it has occasionally been termed, is characteristic. In contrast to individuals with the X-linked form, patients with the sporadic disease often develop prominent myopathy similar to that seen in other forms of rickets or osteomalacia. Deformities of the limbs are frequently absent (possibly indicating normophosphatemia during the growth period), but these patients may experience severe bone pain related to vertebral-body collapse or femoral-neck fractures. As in other forms of osteomalacia, roentgenograms often reveal extensive pseudofractures. Some subjects may also have isolated renal hyperglycinuria and occasionally renal glycosuria in addition to the hypophosphatemia. Generalized aminoaciduria or acidification defects are not usually seen in these individuals.

The pathogenesis of the hypophosphatemia in these patients remains controversial. In the X-linked form of the disease, which has been more extensively studied, there is evidence for a primary defect in the membrane transport of inorganic phosphate.[101–103] In addition, there may also be an associated defect in intestinal phosphate transport.[104–106] The possible role of parathyroid hormone and altered vitamin D metabolism in the pathogenesis of the X-linked form of hypophosphatemia is considered in Chapter 66.

Although abnormal metabolism of vitamin D or altered renal and intestinal response to this vitamin may exist in patients with adult, sporadic hypophosphatemia, complete healing of the bone disease (as shown by biopsy) can be effected with oral phosphate supplements alone (Fig. 70-12).[22] The first changes associated with the institution of oral phosphate therapy have been a rise in serum phosphorus level often accompanied by a fall in serum calcium level and a decrease in urinary calcium excretion. Initially, fecal calcium excretion has remained high, but with prolonged phosphate supplements, fecal calcium excretion has decreased and positive calcium balance developed.

Although usually normal prior to treatment, serum immunoreactive parathyroid hormone levels have been elevated during the initial stages of therapy with phosphate, suggesting that phosphate supplementation results in stimulation of some degree of increased secretion of parathyroid hormone by inducing hypocalcemia. The

mechanism of the hypocalcemia may be related to a phosphate-induced increased rate of mineralization and increased net movement of calcium into bone. There is also an increase in urinary hydroxyproline excretion accompanying initiation of therapy, presumably reflecting increased bone (matrix) resorption related either to a primary effect of phosphate supplementation or secondary to increased parathyroid hormone secretion. Cessation of phosphate supplementation has resulted in a rapid fall in urinary hydroxyproline excretion and return of the immunoreactive parathyroid hormone levels to normal. These findings suggest that parathyroid hormone is playing a secondary rather than a primary role in the genesis of the renal tubular phosphate leak.

A variety of neutral phosphate salts are available for oral supplementation, including sodium and potassium salts or mixtures of the two. The rise in serum phosphorus level after an oral dose of phosphate is transient,[22,104,107] and therefore patients receiving this medication require administration of frequent doses. The precise amount of phosphate must be individualized in each patient, and, in those individuals with severe leaks, as high as 1000 mg of elemental phosphorus are required every 4 to 6 hours to effect a sustained elevation in serum phosphorus level. The efficacy of therapy cannot be assessed with a single fasting determination of phosphatemia, and multiple measurements of serum levels at various times after each dose are required. Opening of the capsules and dissolution of the salt in water or liquid may improve intestinal absorption and enhance serum phosphorus levels. Most patients initially experience some degree of gastrointestinal distress, including cramps and diarrhea, with initiation of therapy, and therefore the initial doses should be low, with gradual titration to higher levels as tolerated. Glorieux et al.[108] have shown that simultaneous use of phosphate and vitamin D has resulted in accelerated healing in a group of patients with the X-linked form of hypophosphatemic osteomalacia. Vitamin D itself or various analogs have a "phosphate-sparing" effect, allowing use of lower doses of oral phosphate supplements. Whether the improved serum phosphorus levels seen with vitamin D are related to increased intestinal absorption of phosphate or decreased renal loss

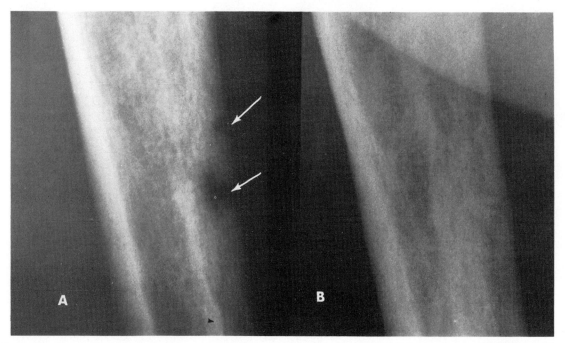

Fig. 70-12. Roentgenogram of right femur of a patient with phosphate diabetes (case 2, ref. 22). (*A*) Before therapy. (*B*) Eleven weeks after starting phosphate therapy. Arrows indicate Looser's zones.

(due to decreased secondary hyperparathyroidism) is a question that needs to be clarified. We have observed improved phosphate tolerance in our patients on oral phosphate with vitamin D, 1α-hydroxyvitamin D, and dihydrotachysterol. The dosages have been adjusted to obtain maximal serum phosphorus levels without raising urinary calcium excretion. In our hands, calcium supplements are not required during early phases of treatment, as has been suggested by others.[99] With healing of the osteomalacia, serum phosphorus levels can be maintained with lower doses of supplemental phosphorus, at least in some patients. Lowering of phosphate requirements has not been related to decreased glomerular filtration rate, since general renal function has been well maintained.

TUMOR-ASSOCIATED RICKETS AND OSTEOMALACIA

In 1959, Prader el al.[109] described the case of an 11-year-old girl who, over the course of a year, developed severe symptomatic rickets accompanied by hypophosphatemia, increased renal phosphate clearance, and mild hypocalcemia. The child was found to have a huge tumor in the left chest that on biopsy was interpreted as a reparative giant-cell granuloma of a rib. Following excision of the tumor, the rickets healed without any specific therapy. It was postulated that the giant-cell reparative granuloma may have produced a "rachitogenic substance." A case reported earlier by McCance[110] was subsequently considered to be an example of this situation,[111] as was the patient reported by Hauge.[112]

Since that time there have been several reports of patients in whom osteomalacia has been associated with various types of tumor.[113-119] In a recent review of the literature, 11 cases were described, the authors adding 2 additional cases of their own.[120] Other examples not mentioned in this review have also been reported.[3] In addition to the reparative giant-cell granuloma described by Prader el al.,[109] this syndrome has been associated with cavernous or sclerosing hemangioma, angiosarcoma, hemangiopericytoma, nonossifying fibroma, and a number of mesenchymal tumors difficult to classify on histological grounds. Some of the tumors have involved soft tissues and not bone.[120] In most of the reported cases, the removal of the tumor resulted in clinical cure of the osteomalacia or rickets, although, in some, early recurrence of the tumor or inadequate removal of the malignancy presumably prevented good clinical response.[3] In the patient reported from our service (Fig. 70-13),[114] the tumor was a malignant giant-cell sarcoma that was first detected clinically after the osteomalacia was

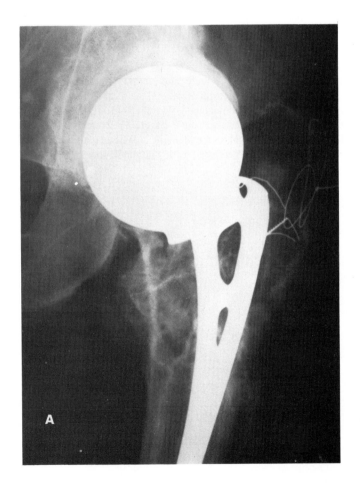

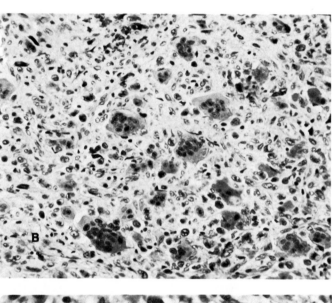

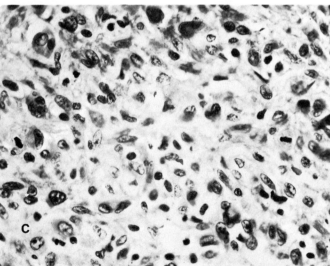

Fig. 70-13 (*A*)   Roentgenogram of left femur of a 56-year-old man showing irregularity of cortex at site of giant-cell sarcoma.[114] (*B*) Sections of the tumor showing giant cells surrounded by atypical stromal cells. The latter are seen at higher power in (*C*).

successfully treated with phosphate supplements and vitamin D. When the tumor, which involved the upper femur, was resected by hind-quarter amputation, the hypophosphatemia improved, despite cessation of phosphate and vitamin D therapy. Four years later, hypophosphatemia recurred, associated with the reappearance of pulmonary metastases. The patient died 2 years thereafter of a massive pulmonary embolus, at which time the lungs were filled with metastatic tumor.

All these patients have demonstrated hypophosphatemia, high phosphate clearance, and normal or near-normal serum calcium level. In a few, renal glycosuria has been present. When measured, serum immunoreactive parathyroid hormone levels have usually been normal,[115,118,120] although high values have also been reported.[117] The size of the tumors has ranged from very large, in the original case of Prader et al.,[109] to one as small as 1×1 cm. In several instances the tumor was not detected until years after development of clinical osteomalacia.[3,120] On the other hand, clinical response has occurred on an average of 16 weeks (range 24 hours to 17 months) after removal of the tumor.[120]

The cause of the syndrome is still unknown. A preliminary report has appeared suggesting that there may be inhibition of formation of 1,25-dihydroxyvitamin D by some factor in the giant cell tumor.[121] Before surgery, serum levels of the metabolite were low. After resection of the tumor, 1,25-$(OH)_2$-D concentration increased, associated with a rise in serum phosphate level and a decrease in renal phosphate clearance. These observations await confirmation.

Hypophosphatemic osteomalacia may also occur in association with neurofibromatosis, although the nature of the association is unclear.[1,3,122–124] Dent and Gertner[125] have also described 3 patients with fibrous dysplasia who had concomitant hypophosphatemic osteomalacia or rickets. Two of the patients were adults with polyostotic fibrous dysplasia, and the third was an 8-year-old child with fibrous dysplasia of the facial bones and rickets. In the child, resection of most of the dysplastic bone was accompanied by improvement in the metabolic bone disease. The authors were aware of 5 previously reported cases in which fibrous dysplasia in children was associated with hypophosphatemia and rickets. The immunoreactive parathyroid hormone levels in the cases of Dent and Gertner[125] were not elevated. These authors suggested that the occurrence of hypophosphatemia and bone disease in patients with fibrous dysplasia is analogous to other forms of "tumor" osteomalacia.

GENERAL RENAL TUBULAR DISORDERS

In addition to the individuals previously described with so-called vitamin D-resistant rickets and osteomalacia attributable solely to a primary renal phosphate leak, a further subset of patients with rickets or osteomalacia of renal origin can be identified. The disorder in these individuals is characterized by a generalized dysfunction of the proximal renal tubules leading to excessive loss of amino acids, glucose, phosphate, uric acid, and bicarbonate in the absence of a primary disturbance in glomerular function. The metabolic consequences of these disturbances are systemic acidosis, hypophosphatemia, and dehydration, which in turn lead to growth disturbance and development of rickets or osteomalacia. These disorders have been classified under the general heading of de Toni/Debré/Fanconi syndrome or renal Fanconi syndrome. They may be further classified into primary renal types, in which the underlying defect is located within the tubular cells, and the prerenal types, in which toxic metabolic substances outside the kidney lead to derangements in tubular function (see Table 70-2). These disorders occur in adults as well as in children.

Dent and Harris were the first to describe a patient with presumed familial adult-onset idiopathic Fanconi syndrome[126] with an autosomal recessive pattern of inheritance. These patients usually present at the age of 40 with signs and symptoms of hypokalemia and osteomalacia. They do not have cystinosis, and no other systemic disease has been identified. Healing of the bone disease has occurred with the use of vitamin D, alkali, and potassium. Brodehl[127] described another patient with presumed idiopathic Fanconi syndrome of the sporadic type who presented at the age of 7 with muscle weakness and bone pain attributable to osteomalacia. Renal biopsy showed no crystalline material, and electron-microscopic studies revealed the presence of abnormal giant mitochondria. This grouping of patients with idiopathic renal Fanconi syndrome is somewhat artificial, and in time the specific biochemical derangements responsible for the tubular dysfunction may be identified.

In cystinosis (Lignac/de Toni/Fanconi syndrome),[128] glycogenosis,[127] and Lowe's syndrome,[129] the renal disease is associated with a more generalized systemic metabolic disorder. The precise metabolic defect in each of these diseases is unknown. In cystinosis, there is an accumulation of cystine in many tissues, including the kidneys, resulting in tubular dysfunction and later in renal glomerular failure. Recent experience with renal transplantation in patients with cystinosis has shown reaccumulation of cystine in the transplanted kidney without the reappearance of the Fanconi syndrome, suggesting that a primary renal-tubular-cell defect may exist in these patients.[130] Whether a similar pathogenetic mechanism occurs in glycogenosis and in Lowe's syndrome is not known, since the underlying metabolic defect in these syndromes remains obscure.

In Wilson's disease, tyrosinemia,[131] and the other inborn errors of metabolism outlined in Table 70-2, Fanconi syndrome may be an accompaniment of the generalized systemic disease and lead to the development of bone disease. In Wilson's disease the clinical and pathologic manifestations are presumably related to the toxic effects of excessive accumulation of copper in liver, kidney, brain, and cornea. Most patients present with signs and symptoms secondary to liver disease, hemolytic anemia, or neurologic disease. However, occasionally, renal dysfunction and associated osteomalacia may predominate. Mayan et al.[132] were the first to describe a patient with Wilson's disease in whom Fanconi syndrome and rickets were the initial presenting features. Although the bone disease responded promptly to oral vitamin D supplementation, the tubular dysfunction persisted. Renal biopsy from this patient did not reveal evidence of "swan neck" deformity. The renal tubular abnormalities in these individuals include aminoaciduria, glucosuria, uricosuria, hypercalciuria, and renal tubular acidosis. Studies by Wilson and Goldstein[133] have suggested that the defect in acidification is presumably related to a distal rather than a proximal tubular defect. The presence of hypercalciuria and the frequent occurrence of renal lithiasis are consistent with a distal tubular abnormality. Several investigators have shown that treatment of Wilson's disease with D-penicillamine significantly improves the renal tubular acidification defect.[133,134] As was mentioned earlier, in patients with coexistent rickets or osteomalacia, healing of the bone disease can be accomplished with oral vitamin D supplements alone.

The development of Fanconi syndrome in plasma-cell myeloma has been attributed to the toxic effects of Bence Jones protein on the proximal renal tubules.[135] Although extremely rare, osteomalacia may develop as a consequence of the renal phosphate wasting and resultant hypophosphatemia.

Fanconi syndrome and osteomalacia have been observed in patients with heavy metal poisoning, particularly cadmium.[136,137] The bone disease is presumably secondary to hypophosphatemia and systemic acidosis produced by impaired tubular function. A similar syndrome has been described in lead intoxication[138] and in patients exposed to outdated tetracycline.[139]

In the various types of so-called prerenal Fanconi syndrome, the specific treatment of the underlying disorder often results in disappearance or improvement in the renal tubular dysfunction, thus allowing healing of the associated bone disease. In several of the above disorders, improvement in the bone disease can also be achieved by correcting the acidosis and hypophosphatemia, i.e., supplementation with alkali, oral phosphate, and vitamin D.

HYPOPHOSPHATASIA

Hypophosphatasia is a heritable disorder characterized by deficiency in alkaline phosphatase, increased urinary excretion of phosphorylethanolamine, and skeletal disease that includes osteomalacia and rickets.[140-143] The disease may present in infancy, where it is associated with hypercalcemia, renal failure, and increased intracranial pressure. These infants may show enlarged sutures of the skull, craniostenosis, delayed dentition, enlarged epiphyses, and prominent costochondral junctions. Genu valgum or varum may develop subsequently. The histological picture is indistinguishable from other forms of rickets. In older children, it is manifested in a less severe form and may present as rickets alone. In this group, serum calcium and phosphorus levels are usually normal. In adults, even though osteopenia may be seen, the disorder tends to be mild, and osteomalacia may not be the primary pathological process.[143-145]

The alkaline phosphatase levels in recorded cases have been lower than those for age-matched controls. The plasma levels and urinary excretion of phosphorylethanolamine are markedly elevated in affected individuals and higher than controls in the putative heterozygotes.[145-150] Although it has been suggested that phosphorylethanolamine is the "true substrate" for alkaline phosphatase in bone, there is no positive evidence for this except that this phosphate ester (like others) is hydrolyzed by alkaline phosphatase.

Alkaline phosphatase from bone, cartilage, and other tissues is a pyrophosphatase at neutral pH,[151,152] although one chromatographic form of alkaline phosphatase from cartilage[153] does not hydrolyze inorganic pyrophosphate (PP_i). Since the concentrations of PP_i in plasma[154] and urine[155] are invariably increased in patients with hypophosphatasia, and PP_i has been shown to be an inhibitor of calcification[156] in several systems, it has been proposed that the mineralization defect in hypophosphatasia is due to insufficient alkaline phosphatase to permit normal hydrolysis of PP_i.[157]

Therapy is a problem. Vitamin D has been ineffective, and phosphate supplements are probably not indicated. Glucocorticoids are probably also ineffective.[143] When osteotomies are performed, healing has been slow.[97]

CALCIFICATION INHIBITORS

The skeletal abnormalities that result from ingestion of excessive amounts of fluoride ion include increases in total osteoid surface.[159] These occur despite adequate vitamin D intake. When fluoride ion in doses of 13–41 mg/day has been administered to patients with osteoporosis, the new bone formed is poorly mineralized and has other histological features of osteomalacia.[160] These findings also occur in normal individuals consuming excessive amounts of fluoride. There is evidence that the mineralization defect can be overcome by increasing dietary intake of calcium and vitamin D (50,000 U twice weekly).

The diphosphonate, disodium etidronate (EHDP), has been used in the treatment of a large number of patients with Paget's disease of bone.[161-167] In patients who have received 10–20 mg/kg/day for several months or longer, bone biopsies in a number of individuals have revealed increased osteoid surface as well as increased thickness of the osteoid seams.[163-166] In individuals who received the drug for periods of 3 to 17 months, especially at the higher dose range, there has been an increased incidence of fractures associated with spotty increased radiolucency of involved bones.[166] An example of changes in bone histology produced after 18 months of therapy with EHDP at 10–20 mg/kg/day is shown in Fig. 70-14. Here the mineralized pagetic bone is encased by lamellar osteoid, which in some instances exceeds 150 μm. The thick osteoid is located almost entirely around the pagetic bone, not around normal bone.[165] In patients with osteoporosis who have been treated with EHDP, broad osteoid seams have also been observed surrounding osteoporotic bone within 3 months of starting the drug.[168] Others have noted decreased tetracycline uptake at the calcification fronts.[165] The data suggest that EHDP primarily acts by inhibiting osteoclastic resorption, although at first bone formation continues at a high rate.[164,166] The new bone is poorly mineralized as a result of an additional direct effect of EHDP on mineralization and/or an imbalance of bone resorption and formation. At some time in the course of therapy, osteoblastic activity decreases, the rate of matrix synthesis slows, and the osteoid seams decrease. The gross radiological abnormalities are reversed within months after the EHDP is discontinued.[166] It is also possible that the mineralization defect is due in part to altered metabolism of vitamin D and inadequate formation of 1,25-dihydroxycholecalciferol, as has been shown in animals receiving large doses of EHDP.[3,169]

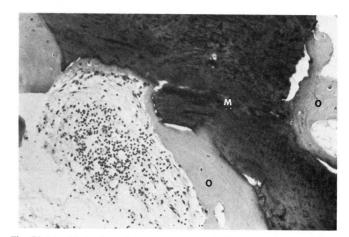

Fig. 70-14. Undemineralized section stained with hematoxylin and eosin of femoral head from a patient with Paget's disease of bone who had been treated with the diphosphonate, disodium etidronate, initially for 12 months with 1 mg/kg/day followed by an additional 12 months with 10 mg/kg/day. He had no therapy for 3 months prior to total hip replacement when this specimen was obtained. Note mineralized pagetic bone (M) surrounded by lamellar nonpagetic osteoid (O).

HYPERPARATHYROIDISM AND HYPOPARATHYROIDISM

In individuals with hyperparathyroidism who have excessive bone resorption and high rates of bone formation, thick osteoid seams may be seen. The mineralization defects are especially prominent in the early period following operative therapy of the hyperparathyroidism when chemical osteomalacia (low levels of serum calcium and phosphorus) is associated with histological changes in bone as discussed by Albright and Reifenstein.[27] An example of this finding is shown in Fig. 70-15. However, in some patients with hyperparathyroidism, frank osteomalacia has coexisted with untreated hyperparathyroidism.[3] Radiological findings have included typical Looser's zones and vertebral hyperostosis. Some of the cases have been associated with intestinal malabsorption or "privational" vitamin D deficiency. Serum calcium levels have tended to be relatively or absolutely low. Stanbury, who has reviewed the problem in detail,[3] proposed that the syndrome is the bony expression of primary hyperparathyroidism modified by vitamin D deficiency.

It should also be noted that hypercalcemia and autonomous hyperparathyroidism may be associated with hypophosphatemic rickets and osteomalacia.[86,170] In a recent review, it was suggested that primary hyperparathyroidism was a chance occurrence in these individuals rather than a manifestation of the hypophosphatemic rickets or a complication of therapy.[171]

Hypoparathyroidism has also been associated with osteomalacia on rare occasions.[172] The mechanism may be related to a decrease in formation of 1,25-dihydroxyvitamin D owing to lack of parathyroid hormone per se as well as hyperphosphatemia.[173]

OSTEOPETROSIS

The association of radiologically dense bones and increased bone mass with rickets and osteomalacia has been discussed previously. Rickets also may occur in the severe (recessive) form of osteopetrosis. Affected children may have low levels of serum phosphorus and calcium and increased activity of alkaline phosphatase.[174,175] Dent described an osteopetrotic child with gross

aminoaciduria and increased urinary hydroxyproline excretion[175] whose rickets failed to respond to high doses of vitamin D (15 mg/day).

The morphological changes in cartilage and bone include in addition to rickets, decreased osteoclastic and chondroclastic resorption, and abnormal-appearing osteoclasts.[176] It is not clear why abnormal matrix mineralization should occur in this disorder. One possible explanation is a decreased local supply of mineral ions secondary to decreased resorption in the face of relatively high rates of bone formation.

FIBROGENESIS IMPERFECTA OSSIUM

Fibrogenesis imperfecta ossium[177-181] is a rare disorder characterized by progressively disabling skeletal pain and tenderness, forced immobilization, muscular weakness and atrophy, and contractures. It has been described in men over the age of 50. Levels of calcium and phosphorus in the serum are normal, but alkaline phosphatase activity is increased. The radiological abnormalities are generalized and consist of thickened and amorphous-appearing trabeculae with spotty increase in density, reduced cortical thicknesses, and occasionally pseudofractures. Histologically, there is an increase in thickness of "osteoid" which occurs diffusely on bone surfaces. Its appearance is distinctive and is best seen using polarized light microscopy. The "osteoid" lacks the lamellar structure and typical birefringence that is characteristic of the other osteomalacic states. Electron-microscopic studies[181] of the "osteoid" region have shown small-diameter collagen fibers that are immature and arranged in loops and dense areas that have been termed whorls. A single study of bone from a patient with fibrogenesis imperfecta ossium has revealed that the collagen was more soluble in neutral salt and dilute acetic acid. This was interpreted as indicative of defective cross-linking.[182] However, direct evidence for defective cross-linking or the chemical nature of the putative defect has not been obtained.

Several of these patients have been treated with dihydrotachysterol or ergocalciferol in doses that produced hypercalcemia. This has resulted in decreased skeletal pain, although the radiological abnormalities have persisted. The etiology and pathogenesis of this interesting disorder have not been defined.

AXIAL OSTEOMALACIA

Axial osteomalacia is a term introduced by Frame et al.[183] in 1961 to describe a disorder occurring in three individuals, all males. The characteristic roentgenological findings have included a coarsened and spongelike trabecular pattern in the bones of the cervical spine and, to a lesser degree, in the ribs, lumbar spine, and pelvis. The skull and appendicular skeleton have been uninvolved. Bone biopsies have revealed wide osteoid seams compatible with osteomalacia. The authors interpreted the serum chemical findings as inconsistent with other forms of osteomalacia. However, the serum phosphorus level in one of the original cases was 2.6 mg/dl and in the other two, 3.1 mg/dl. Three other cases have been reported,[11,184] also in males. In one,[184] the serum phosphorus level was 3.0 mg/dl and in the other two,[11] the range was 1.2 to 3.4 and 1.4 to 3.8 mg/dl. It has been suggested[179] that axial osteomalacia and fibrogenesis imperfecta ossium are the same conditions, although others[180] have disputed this idea. The presence of definite or borderline hypophosphatemia in the reported cases raises questions as to whether axial osteomalacia is a distinct entity or belongs

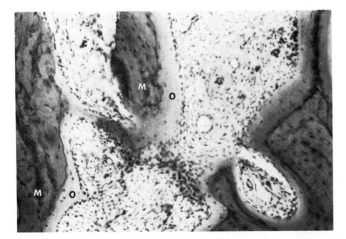

Fig. 70-15. Section of bone from patient with hyperparathyroidism and osteitis fibrosa cystica taken 8 days following removal of a parathyroid adenoma.[27] Even in this demineralized section stained with hematoxylin and eosin, mineralized bone (M) can be distinguished from the thickened osteoid seam (O).

in one of the several categories of hypophosphatemic osteomalacia discussed earlier.

REFERENCES

1. Mankin, H. J.: Rickets, osteomalacia and renal osteodystrophy. *J Bone Joint Surg 56-A:* 101–128, 352–386, 1974.
2. Dent, C. E., Stamp, T. C. B: Vitamin D, rickets and osteomalacia, in Avioli, L. V. and Krane, S. M. (eds): Metabolic Bone Disease. New York, Academic Press, 1977, p 237.
3. Stanbury, S. W.: Osteomalacia. *Clin Endocrinol Metab 1:* 239–266, 1972.
4. Krane, S. M., Parsons, V., Kunin, A. S.: Studies of the metabolism of epiphyseal cartilage, in Basset, C. A. L. (ed): Cartilage Degradation and Repair. Washington, National Research Council, 1967, p 43.
5. Howell, D. S.: Histologic observations and biochemical composition of rachitic cartilage with special reference to mucopolysaccharides. *Arthritis Rheum 8:* 337–354, 1965.
6. Lee, W. R.: Bone formation in Paget's disease. A quantitative microscopic study using tetracycline markers. *J Bone Joint Surg 49-B:* 146–153, 1967.
7. Frost, H, M,: Tetracycline-based histological analysis of bone remodeling. *Calcif Tissue Res 3:* 211–237, 1969.
8. Rasmussen, H., Bordier, P.: The Physiological and Cellular Basis of Metabolic Bone Disease. Baltimore, Williams and Wilkins, 1974, p 1.
9. Bordier, P. J., Tun Chot, S.: Quantitative histology of metabolic bone disease. *Clin Endocrinol Metab 1:* 197–215, 1972.
10. Byers, P. D.: The diagnostic value of bone biopsies, in Avioli, L. V., Krane, S. M. (eds): Metabolic Bone Disease. New York, Academic Press, 1977, p 184.
11. Arnstein, A. R., Frame, B., Frost, H.: Recent progress in osteomalacia and rickets. *Ann Intern Med 67:* 1296–1330, 1967.
12. Engfeldt, B., Zetterström, R., Winberg, J.: Primary vitamin-D resistant rickets. III Biophysical studies of skeletal tissue. *J Bone Joint Surg 38-A:* 1323–1334, 1956.
13. Bohr, H. H.: Microradiographic studies in osteomalacia, in Hioco, D. J. (ed): L'osteomalacie. Paris, Masson, 1967, p 117.
14. Jaworski, Z. F. G., Kloswvych, S., Cameron, E. (eds): Proceedings of the First Workshop on Bone Morphometry. Ottawa, University of Ottawa Press, 1973 p 1.
15. Baylink, D., Stauffer, M., Wergedal, J., Rich, C.: Formation mineralization and resorption of bone in vitamin-D deficient rats. *J Clin Invest 49:* 1122–1134, 1970.
16. Toole, B. P., Kang, A. H., Trelstad, R. L., Gross, J.: Collagen heterogeneity within different growth regions of long bones of rachitic and non-rachitic chicks. *Biochem J 127:* 715–720, 1972.
17. Barnes, M. J., Constable, B. J., Morton, L. F., Kodicek, E.: Bone collagen metabolism in vitamin-D deficiency. *Biochem J 132:* 113–115, 1973.
18. Barnes, M. J., Constable, B. J., Morton, L. F., Kodicek, E.: The influence of dietary calcium deficiency and parathyroidectomy on bone structure. *Biochem Biophys Acta 328:* 373–382, 1973.
19. Prineas, J. W., Stuart Mason, A., Henson, R. A.: Myopathy in metabolic bone disease. *Br Med J 1:* 1034–1036, 1965.
20. Smith, R., Stern, G.: Myopathy osteomalacia and hyperparathyroidism. *Brain 90:* 593–602, 1967.
21. Schott, G. D., Wills, M. R.: Muscle weakness in osteomalacia. *Lancet 1:* 626–629, 1976.
22. Nagant de Deuxchaisnes, C., Krane, S. M.: The treatment of adult phosphate diabetes and Fanconi syndrome with neutral sodium phosphate. *Am J Med 43:* 508–543, 1967.
23. Mallett, L. E., Patten, B. M., King Engel, W.: Neuromuscular disease in secondary hyperparathyroidism. *Ann Intern Med 82:* 474–483, 1975.
24. Aurbach, G. D., Mallette, L. E., Patten, B. M., Heath, D. A., Doppman, J. L., Bilezikian, J. P.: Hyperparathyroidism: Recent studies. *Ann Intern Med 79:* 566–581, 1973.
25. Steinbach, H. L., Noetzli, M.: Roentgen appearance of the skeleton in osteomalacia and rickets. *Am J Roentgenol Radiother 91:* 955–972, 1964.
26. de Sèze, S., Lichtwitz, A., Ryckewaert, A., Bordier, P., Hioco, D., Mazabraud, A.: Le syndrome de Looser-Milkman. Étude de 60 cas. *Sem Hôp 34:* 2005–2025, 1962.
27. Albright, F., Reifenstein, E. C., Jr.: The Parathyroid Glands and Metabolic Bone Disease. Baltimore, Williams and Wilkins, 1948, p 1.
28. Milkman, L. A.: Pseudofractures (hunger osteopathy, late rickets, osteomalacia): Report of a case. *Am J Roentgenol 24:* 29–37, 1930.
29. Milkman, L. A.: Multiple spontaneous idiopathic symmetrical fractures. *Am J Roentgenol 32:* 622–634, 1934.
30. Steinbach, H. L., Kolb, F. O., Gilfillan, R.: A mechanism of the production of pseudofractures in osteomalacia (Milkman's syndrome). *Radiology 62:* 388–394, 1954.
31. LeMay, M., Blunt, J. W. Jr.: Factor determining the location of pseudofractures in osteomalacia. *J Clin Invest 28:* 521–525, 1949.
32. Jackson, W. P. U., Dowdle, E., Linder, G. C.: Vitamin-D resistant osteomalacia. *Br Med J 1:* 1269–1274, 1958.
33. Ball, J., Garner, A.: Mineralization of woven bone in osteomalacia. *J Pathol Bacteriol 91:* 563–568, 1966.
34. Dunningan, M. G., Paton, J. O. J., Haase, S., McNicol, G. W., Gardner, M. D., Smith, C. M.: Late rickets and osteomalacia in the Pakistani community in Glasgow. *Scott Med J 7:* 159–167, 1962.
35. Arneil, G. C., Crosbie, J. C.: Infantile rickets returns to Glasgow. *Lancet 2:* 423–425, 1963.
36. Benson, P. F., Stroud, C. E., Mitchell, N. J., Nicolaides, A.: Rickets in immigrant children in London. *Br Med J 5337:* 1054–1056, 1963.
37. Dent, C. E., Smith, R.: Nutritional osteomalacia. *Q J Med 38:* 195–209, 1969.
38. Chalmers, J., Conacher, W. D. H., Gardner, D. L., Scott, P. J.: Osteomalacia—a common disease in elderly women. *J Bone Joint Surg 49B:* 403–423, 1967.
39. Gough, K. R., Lloyd, O. C., Wills, M. R.: Nutritional osteomalacia. *Lancet 2:* 1261–1264, 1964.
40. Haddad, J. G., Chyu, K. J.: Competitive protein-binding radioassay for 25-hydroxycholecalciferol. *J Clin Endocrinol Metab 33:* 992–996, 1971.
41. Corless, D., Boucher, B. J., Beer, M., Gupta, S. P., Cohen, R. D.: Vitamin D status in long-stay geriatric patients. *Lancet 1:* 1404–1406, 1975.
42. Hodkinson, H. M., Round, P., Stanton, B. R., Morgan, C.: Sunlight, vitamin D and osteomalacia in the elderly. *Lancet 1:* 910–912, 1973.
43. Stamp, T. C. B., Round, J. M.: Seasonal changes in human plasma levels of 25-hydroxyvitamin D. *Nature 247:* 563–565, 1974.
44. Lester, E., Skinner, R. K., Wills, M. R.: Seasonal variation in serum 25-hydroxyvitamin D in the elderly in Britain. *Lancet 1:* 979–988, 1977.
45. Haddad, J. G., Stamp, T. C. B.: Circulating 25-hydroxyvitamin D in man. *Am J Med 57:* 57–62, 1974.
46. Tech Rep Ser Wld Hlth Org *452:* 34, 1970.
47. Exton-Smith, A. N., Hodkinson, H. M., Stanton, B. R.: Nutrition and metabolic bone disease in old age. *Lancet 2:* 999–1001, 1966.
48. McLennan, W. J., Caird, F. I., MacLeod, C. C.: Diet and bone rarefaction in old age. *Age Ageing 1:* 131–140, 1972.
49. Stamp, T. C. B.: Factors in human vitamin D nutrition and in the production and cure of classical rickets. *Proc Nutr Soc 34:* 119–130, 1975.
50. Arneil, G. C.: Symposium on osteomalacia and rickets. Nutritional rickets in children in Glasgow. *Proc Nutr Soc 34:* 101–109, 1975.
51. Stanbury, S. W., Torkington, P., Lumb, G. A., Adams, P. H., Preenie de Silva, Taylor, C. M.: Asian rickets and osteomalacia: Patterns of parathyroid response in vitamin D deficiency. *Proc Nutr Soc 34:* 111–117, 1975.
52. Goel, K. M., Logan, R. W., Arneil, G. C., Sweet, E. M., Warren, J. M., Shanks, R. A.: Florid and subclinical rickets among immigrant children in Glasgow. *Lancet 1:* 1141–1145, 1976.
53. Freece, M. A., McIntosh, W. B., Tomlinson, S., Ford, J. A., Dunnigan, M. G., O'Riordan, J. L. H.: Vitamin D deficiency among Asian immigrants to Britain. *Lancet 1:* 907–910, 1973.
54. Loomis, W. F.: Skin-pigment regulation of vitamin D biosynthesis in man. *Science 157:* 501–506, 1967.
55. Ford, J. A., Calhoun, E. M., McIntosh, W. B., Dunnigan, M. G.: Rickets and osteomalacia in the Glasgow Pakistani community: 1961–71. *Br Med J 2:* 677–680, 1967.
56. Doxiadia, S., Angelis, C., Karatzas, P., Vrettas, C., Lapatsanis, P.: Genetic aspects of nutritional rickets. *Arch Dis Child 51:* 83–90, 1976.
57. Wills, M. R., Day, R. C., Phillips, J. B., Bateman, E. C.: Phytic acid and nutritional rickets in immigrants. *Lancet 1:* 771–773, 1972.

58. Dent, C. E., Rowe, D. J. F., Round, J. M., Stamp, T. C. B.: Effect of chapattis and ultraviolet irradiation on nutritional rickets in an Indian immigrant. *Lancet 1:* 1282–1284, 1973.

59. Bordier, P. L., Hioco, D., Hepner, G. W., Thompson, G. R.: Effect of intravenous vitamin D on bone and phosphate metabolism in osteomalacia. *Calcif Tissue Res 4:* 78–83, 1969.

60. Teitelbaum, S. L., Rosenberg, E. M., Bates, M., Avioli, L. V.: The effects of phosphate and vitamin D therapy in osteopenic, hypophosphatemic osteomalacia of childhood. *Clin Orthop 116:* 38–47, 1976.

61. Scriver, C. R.: Rickets and the pathogenesis of impaired tubular transport of phosphate and other solutes. *Am J Med 57:* 43–49, 1974.

62. Arnaud, C. D., Glorieux, F., Scriver, C. R.: Serum parathyroid hormone levels in acquired vitamin D deficiency of infancy. *Pediatrics 49:* 837–840, 1972.

63. Muldowney, F. P., Freaney, R., McGeeney, D.: Renal tubular acidosis and aminoaciduria in osteomalacia of dietary or intestinal origin: *Q J Med 148:* 517–548, 1968.

64. Whittle, H., Neale, G., McLaughlin, M., et al.: Intravenous vitamin D in the detection of vitamin D deficiency. *Lancet 1:* 747–750, 1969.

65. Naylor, R., Mandy, R., Paul, J.: Detecting the early stages of osteomalacia with the intravenous vitamin D test. *Geriatrics,* 1977, p 52–56.

66. Balsan, S., Garabedian, M., Sorgniard, R., Holick, M. F., DeLuca, H. F.: 1,25-dihydroxyvitamin D₃ and 1α-hydroxyvitamin D₃ in children: Biologic and therapeutic effects in nutritional rickets and different types of vitamin D resistance. *Pediatr Res 9:* 586–593, 1975.

67. Bordier, P. H., Pechet, M. M., Hesse, R., Marie, P., Rasmussen, H.: Response of adult patients with osteomalacia to treatment with crystalline 1α-hydroxyvitamin D₃. *N Engl J Med 291:* 866–871, 1974.

68. Goodman, A. D., Lemann, J., Jr., Lennon, E. J., Relman, A. S.: Production, excretion and net balance of fixed acid in patients with renal acidosis. *J Clin Invest 44:* 495–506, 1965.

69. Lemann, J., Jr., Lennon, E. J., Goodman, A. D., Litzow, J. R., Relman, A. S.: The net balance of acid in subjects given large loads of acid or alkali. *J Clin Invest 44:* 507–517, 1965.

70. Lemann, J., Jr., Litzow, J. R., Lennon, E. J.: The effects of chronic acid loads in normal man: Further evidence for the participation of bone minerals in the defense against chronic metabolic acidosis. *J Clin Invest 45:* 1608–1614, 1966.

71. Raisz, L. G.: Physiologic and pharmacologic regulation of bone resorption. *N Engl J Med 282:* 909–916, 1970.

72. Raisz, L. G.: Mechanisms of bone resorption, in Aurbach, G. D. (ed): Handbook of Physiology, Endocrinology, Parathyroid Gland, Section 7. Washington DC, American Physiological Society, 1976, vol. VII, p 117.

73. Howell, D. S., Pita, J. C., Marquez, J. F., Madruga, J. E.: Partition of calcium, phosphate, and protein in the fluid phase aspirated at calcifying sites in epiphyseal cartilage. *J Clin Invest 47:* 1121–1132, 1968.

74. Howell, D. S.: Review article, Current concepts of calcification. *J Bone Joint Surg 53A:* 250–258, 1971.

75. Donohoe, J. F., Freaney, R., Muldowney, F. P.: Osteomalacia in uretero-sigmoidostomy. *Irish J Med Sci 2:* 523–530, 1969.

76. Harrison, H. E., Harrison, H. C.: Physiology of vitamin D, in Rodahl, K., Nicholson, J. T., Brown, E. M., Jr., (eds): Bone as a Tissue. New York, McGraw-Hill, 1960, p 300.

77. Lee, S. W., Russell, J., Avioli, L. V.: 25-hydroxycholecalciferol to 1,25-dihydroxycholecalciferol: Conversion impaired by systemic metabolic acidosis. *Science 195:* 994–996, 1977.

78. Morris, R. C., Jr.: Renal tubular acidosis. Mechanisms, classification and implications. *N Engl J Med 281:* 1405–1413, 1969.

79. Morris, R. C., Jr., Sebastian, A., McSherry, E.: Renal acidosis. *Kidney Int 1:* 322–340, 1972.

80. Seldin, D. W., Wilson, J. D.: Renal tubular acidosis, in Stanbury, J. B., Wyngaarden, J. B., Fredrickson, D. S. (eds): The Metabolic Basis of Inherited Disease. New York, McGraw-Hill, 1972, p 1548.

81. Richards, P., Chamberlain, M. J., Wrong, O. M.: Treatment of osteomalacia of renal tubular acidosis by sodium bicarbonate alone. *Lancet 2:* 994–997, 1972.

82. York, S. E., Yendt, E. R.: Osteomalacia associated with renal bicarbonate loss. *Can Med Assoc J 94:* 1329–1342, 1966.

83. Dent, C. E., Harris, H.: Hereditary forms of rickets and osteomalacia. *J Bone Joint Surg 38-B:* 204–226, 1956.

84. Kallmeyer, J., Dunea, G., Schwartz, F. D.: Hypophosphatemic osteomalacia with hyperglycosuria. *Ann Intern Med 66:* 136–141, 1967.

85. Scriver, C. R., Goldbloom, R. B., Roy, C. C.: Hypophosphatemic rickets with renal hyperglycosuria, renal glycosuria and glycyl-prolinuria. A syndrome with evidence for renal tubular secretion of phosphorus. *Pediatrics 34:* 357–371, 1964.

86. Henneman, P. H., Dempsey, E. F., Carroll, E. L., Henneman, D. H.: Acquired vitamin D-resistant osteomalacia: A new variety characterized by hypercalcemia, low sodium bicarbonate and hyperglycinuria. *Metabolism 11:* 103–116, 1962.

87. Schneider, J. A., Seegmiller, J. E.: Cystinosis and the Fanconi syndrome, in Stanbury, J. B., Wyngaarden, J. B., Fredrickson, D. (eds): The Metabolic Basis of Inherited Disease. New York, McGraw-Hill, 1972, p 158.

88. Waite, L. C., Volkert, W. A., Kenny, A. D.: Inhibition of bone resorption by acetazolamide in the rat. *Endocrinology 87:* 1129–1139, 1970.

89. Bloom, W. L., Flinchum, D.: Osteomalacia with pseudofractures caused by ingestion of aluminum hydroxide. *JAMA 174:* 1327–1330, 1960.

90. Lotz, M., Zisman, E., Bartter, F. C.: Evidence for a phosphorus-depletion syndrome in man. *N Engl J Med 278:* 409–415, 1968.

91. Lotz, M., Ney, R., Bartter, F. C.: Osteomalacia and debility resulting from phosphorus depletion. *Trans Assoc Am Physicians 77:* 281–295, 1964.

92. Dent, C. E., Winter, C. E.: Osteomalacia due to phosphate depletion from excessive aluminium hydroxide ingestion. *Br Med J 1:* 551–552, 1974.

93. Baker, L. R. I., Ackrill, P., Cattell, W. R., Stamp, T. C. B., Watson, L.: Iatrogenic osteomalacia and myopathy due to phosphate depletion. *Br Med J 3:* 150–152, 1974.

94. Territo, M. C., Tanaka, K. R.: Hypophosphatemia in chronic alcoholism. *Arch Intern Med 134:* 445–447, 1974.

95. Stein, J. H., Smith, W. O., Ginn, H. E.: Hypophosphatemia in acute alcoholism. *Am J Med Sci 252:* 78–83, 1966.

96. Biosseau, V. C., Teitelbaum, S. J., Avioli, L. V.: Bone loss in chronic alcoholism. *Clin Res 22:* 567A, 1974.

97. Albright, F., Butler, A. M., Bloomberg, E.: Rickets resistant to vitamin D therapy. *J Clin Dis Child 54:* 529–547, 1937.

98. Frymoyer, J. W., Hodgkin, W.: Adult-onset vitamin-D-resistant hypophosphatemic osteomalacia. *J Bone Joint Surg 59A:* 101–106, 1977.

99. Dent, C. E., Stamp, T. C. B: Hypophosphatemic osteomalacia presenting in adults. *Q J Med 158:* 303–329, 1971.

100. Ray, R. D., Mueller, K. H., SanKaran, B., Menson, E. D., Schwartz, T. B: Metabolic diseases of bone. Kinetic studies. *Med Clin North Am 49:* 241–258, 1965.

101. Glorieux, F., Scriver, C. R.: Loss of a parathyroid-sensitive component of phosphate transport in X-linked hypophosphatemia. *Science 175:* 997–1000, 1972.

102. Robertson, B. R., Harris, R. C., McCune, D. J.: Refractory rickets. Mechanism of therapeutic action of calciferol. *Am J Dis Child 64:* 948–952, 1942.

103. Dent, C. E.: Rickets and osteomalacia from renal tubular defects. *J Bone Joint Surg 34B:* 266–274, 1952.

104. Condon, J. R., Nassim, J. R., Rutter, A.: Pathogenesis of rickets and osteomalacia in familial hypophosphatemia. *Arch Dis Child 46:* 269–272, 1971.

105. Short, E. M., Binder, H. J., Rosenberg, L. E.: Familial hypophosphatemic rickets: defective transport of inorganic phosphate by intestinal mucosa. *Science 179:* 700–702, 1973.

106. Glorieux, F. H., Morin, C. L., Travere, R., Delvin, E. E., Pointer, R.: Intestinal phosphate transport in familial hypophosphatemic rickets. *Pediatr Res 10:* 691, 1976.

107. Frame, F., Manson, G.: Refractory rickets and osteomalacia. *Henry Ford Hosp Med Bull 8:* 293–298, 1960.

108. Glorieux, F. M., Scriver, C. R., Reade, T. M., Goldman, H., Roseborough, A.: Use of phosphate and vitamin D to prevent dwarfism and rickets in X-linked hypophosphatemia. *N Engl J Med 87:* 481–487, 1972.

109. Prader, A., Illig, R., Uehlinger, E., Stalder, G.: Rachitis infolge Knochentumors. *Helv Paediatr Acta 14:* 554–565, 1959.

110. McCance, R. A.: Osteomalacia with Looser's nodes (Milkman's syndrome) due to raised resistance to vitamin-D acquired about the age of 15 years. *Q J Med 16:* 33–50, 1947.

111. Dent, C. E., Friedman, M.: Hypophosphatemic osteomalacia with complete recovery. *Br Med J 1:* 1676–1679, 1964.
112. Hauge, B. N.: Vitamin-D resistant osteomalacia. *Acta Med Scand 153:* 271–282, 1956.
113. Yoshkiawa, S., Kawabata, M., Hatsuyama, Y., Hosokawa, O., Fujita, T.: Atypical vitamin-D resistant osteomalacia. Report of a case. *J Bone Joint Surg 46-A:* 998–1007, 1964.
114. Case Records of the Massachusetts General Hospital (Case 38-1965) *N Engl J Med 273:* 494–504, 1965.
115. Salassa, R. M., Jowsey, J., Arnaud, C. D.: Hypophosphatemic osteomalacia associated with "nonendocrine" tumors. *N Engl J Med 283:* 65–70, 1970.
116. Evans, S. J., Azzopardi, J. G.: Distinctive tumors of bone and soft tissue causing acquired vitamin-D resistant osteomalacia. *Lancet 1:* 353–354, 1972.
117. Olefsky, J., Kempson, R., Jones, H., Reavan, G.: "Tertiary" hyperparathyroidism and apparent "cure" of vitamin-D resistant rickets after removal of an ossifying mesenchymal tumor of the pharynx. *N Engl J Med 286:* 740–745, 1972.
118. Pollack, J. A., Schiller, A. L., Crawford, J. D.: Rickets and myopathy cured by removal of a nonossifying fibroma of bone. *Paediatrics 52:* 364–371, 1973.
119. Moser, C. R., Fessel, W. J.: Rheumatic manifestations of hypophosphatemia. *Arch Intern Med 134:* 674–678, 1974.
120. Linovitz, R. J., Resnick, D., Keissling, P., Kondon, J. J., Sehler, B., Nejdl, R. J., et al: Tumor-induced osteomalacia and rickets: A surgically curable syndrome. *J Bone Joint Surg 58-A:* 419–423, 1976.
121. Drezner, M. K., Feinglos, M. N.: Tumor-induced inhibition of 25-hydroxycholecalciferol (25(OH)D₃) 1α-hydroxylase activity. *Clin Res 25:* 390, 1977.
122. Hernberg, C. A., Edgren, W.: Looser-Milkman's syndrome with neurofibromatosis Recklinghausen and general decalcification of the skeleton. *Acta Med Scand 136:* 26–33, 1949.
123. Swann, G. F.: Pathogenesis of bone lesions in neurofibromatosis. *Br J Radiol 27:* 623–629, 1954.
124. Saville, P. D., Nassim, J. R., Stevenson, F. H., Muelligan, L., Carey, M.: Osteomalacia in von Recklinghausen's neurofibromatosis. Metabolic study of a case. *Br Med J 1:* 1311–1313, 1955.
125. Dent, C. E., Gertner, J. M.: Hypophosphatemic osteomalacia in fibrous dysplasia *Q J Med 45:* 411–420, 1976.
126. Dent, C. E., Harris, M.: Hereditary forms of rickets and osteomalacia. *J Bone Joint Surg 38B:* 204–226, 1956.
127. Brodehl, J.: Tubular Fanconi syndromes with bone involvement, in Bickel, H., Stern, J. (eds): Inborn Errors of Calcium and Bone Metabolism. Baltimore, University Park Press, 1976, pp 191–213.
128. Schneider, J. A., Seegmiller, J. E.: Cystinosis and the Fanconi syndrome, in Stanbury, J. B., Wyngaarden, J. B., Fredrickson, D. (eds): The Metabolic Basis of Inherited Disease. New York, McGraw-Hill, 1972, p 1581.
129. Lowe, C. U., Ferrey, M., MacLachlin, E. A.: Organic aciduria, decreased renal ammonia production, hydrophthalmos and mental retardation. *Am J Dis Child 83:* 164, 1952.
130. Briggs, W. A., Kominami, N., Merrill, J. P., Wilson, R. E.: Kidney transplantation in Fanconi syndrome. *N Engl J Med 286:* 25, 1972.
131. Rosenberg, L. E., Scriver, C. R.: Disorders of amino acid metabolism, in Bondy, P. K. (ed): Duncan's Diseases of Metabolism. Philadelphia, Saunders, 1969, pp 366–515.
132. Morgan, H. G., Stewart, W. K., Lowe, K. G., Stowers, J. M., Johnstone, J. M.: Wilson's disease and the Fanconi syndrome. *Q J Med 31:* 361–383, 1962.
133. Wilson, D. M., Goldstein, N. P.: Bicarbonate excretion in Wilson's disease (hepatolenticular degeneration). *Mayo Clin Proc 49:* 394–400, 1974.
134. Walshe, J. M.: Effect of penicillamine on failure of renal acidification in Wilson's disease. *Lancet 1:* 775–778, 1968.
135. Snapper, I., Kahn, A.: Determination of Bence Jones protein in urine and serum, in Myelomatosis, Fundamentals and Clinical Features. Baltimore, University Park Press, 1971, pp 203–204.
136. Adams, R. G., Harrison, J. F., Scott, P.: The development of cadmium-induced proteinuria, impaired renal function, and osteomalacia in alkaline-battery workers. *Q J Med 38:* 425–443, 1969.
137. Emerson, B. T.: "Ouch-Ouch" disease: the osteomalacia of cadmium nephropathy. *Ann Intern Med 73:* 854–855, 1970.
138. Chisolm, J. J., Jr., Leahy, N. B.: Aminoaciduria as a manifestation of renal tubular lead injury in lead intoxication and a comparison with patterns of aminoaciduria seen in other diseases. *J Pediatr 160:* 1–17, 1962.
139. Gross, J. M.: Fanconi syndrome (adult type) developing secondary to the ingestion of outdated tetracycline. *Ann Intern Med 48:* 523–528, 1963.
140. Rathbun, J.R.: Hypophosphatasia. *Am J Dis Child 75:* 822–831, 1948.
141. Sobel, E. H., Clark, L. C., Fox, R. P., Robinow, M.: Rickets, deficiency of "alkaline" phosphatase activity and premature loss of teeth in childhood. *Pediatrics 11:* 309–321, 1953.
142. Fraser, D.: Hypophosphatasia. *Am J Med 22:* 730–746, 1957.
143. Bartter, F. C.: Hypophosphatasia, in Stanbury, J. B., Wyngaarden, J. B., Frederickson, D. S. (eds): The Metabolic Basis of Inherited Disease. New York, McGraw-Hill, 1972, p 1295.
144. Bethune, J. E., Dent, C. E.: Hypophosphatasia in the adult. *Am J Med 28:* 615–622, 1960.
145. Birtwell, V. M. Jr., Riggs, B. L., Peterson, L. F. A., Jones, J. D.: Hypophosphatasia in an adult. *Arch Intern Med 120:* 90–93, 1967.
146. Fraser, D., Yendt, E. R., Christie, F. H. E.: Metabolic abnormalities in hypophosphatasia. *Lancet 1:* 286, 1955.
147. McCance, R. A.: The excretion of phosphorylethanolamine and hypophosphatasia. *Lancet 1:* 131, 1955.
148. McCance, R. A., Fairweather, D. V. I., Barrett, A. M., Morrison, A. B.: Genetic, clinical, biochemical and pathological features of hypophosphatasia. *Q J Med 25:* 523–538, 1956.
149. Goyer, R. A.: Ethanolamine phosphate excretion in a family with hypophosphatasia. *Arch Dis Child 38:* 205–207, 1963.
150. Rasmussen, K.: Phosphorylethanolamine and hypophosphatasia. *Dan Med Bull 15:* (Suppl 2): 1–112, 1968.
151. Fernley, H. N., Walker, P. G.: Studies on alkaline phosphatase: Inhibition by phosphate derivatives and the substrate specificity. *Biochem J 104:* 1011–1018, 1967.
152. Moss, D. W., Eaton, R. H., Smith, J. K., Whitby, L. G.: Association of inorganic pyrophosphatase activity with human alkaline phosphatase preparations. *Biochem J 102:* 53–57, 1967.
153. Arsenis, C., Rudolph, J., Hackett, M. H.: Resolution, purification and characterization of the orthophosphate releasing activities from fracture callus calcifying cartilage. *Biochim Biophys Acta 391:* 301–315, 1975.
154. Russell, R. G. G., Bisaz, S., Donath, A., Morgan, D. B., Fleisch, H.: Inorganic pyrophosphate in plasma in normal persons and in patients with hypophosphatasia, osteogenesis imperfecta and other disorders of bone. *J Clin Invest 50:* 961–969, 1971.
155. Russell, R. G. G.: Excretion of inorganic pyrophosphate in hypophosphatasia. *Lancet 2:* 899–902, 1970.
156. Fleisch, H., Neuman, W. F.: Mechanisms of calcification: Role of collagen, polyphosphates and phosphatase. *Am J Physiol 200:* 1291–1300, 1961.
157. Russell, R. G. G.: Metabolism of inorganic pyrophosphate (PPi). *Arthritis Rheum 19:* 465–478, 1976.
158. Jacobson, D. P., McClain, E. J.: Hypophosphatasia in monozygotic twins. A case report. *J Bone Joint Surg 49A:* 377–380, 1967.
159. Teotia, S. P. S., Teotia, M.: Endemic skeletal fluorosis in children: Evidence of secondary hyperparathyroidism, in Frame, B., Parfitt, A. M., Duncan, H., (eds): Clinical Aspects of Metabolic Bone Disease. Amsterdam, Excerpta Medica, 1973, p 232.
160. Riggs, B. L., Jowsey, J.: Treatment of osteoporosis with fluoride. *Semin Drug Treat 2:* 27–33, 1972.
161. Smith, R., Russell, R. G. G., Bishop, M.: Diphosphonates and Paget's disease of bone. *Lancet 1:* 945–947, 1971.
162. Smith, R., Russell, R. G. G., Bishop, M. C., Wood, C. G., Bishop, M.: Paget's disease of bone. Experience with a diphosphonate (disodium etidronate) in treatment. *Q J Med 42:* 235–256, 1973.
163. Khairi, M. R. A., Johnston, C. C., Jr., Altman, R. D., Wellman, H. N., Serafini, A. N., Sankey, R. R.: Treatment of Paget's disease of bone (osteitis deformans) *JAMA 230:* 562–567, 1974.
164. deVries, H. R., Bijvoet, O. L. M.: Results of prolonged treatment of Paget's disease of bone with disodium ethane-1-hydroxy-1,1-diphosphonate (EHDP) *Neth J Med 171:* 281–298, 1974.
165. Guncaga, J., Lauffenburger, T., Lentnen, C., Dambacker, M. A., Haas, H. G., Fleisch, H., Olah, A. J.: Diphosphonate treatment of Paget's disease of bone. A correlated metabolic, calcium kinetic and morphometric study. *Horm Metab Res 6:* 62–69, 1974.
166. Kantrowitz, F. G., Byrne, M. H., Schiller, A. L., Krane, S. M.: Clinical and biochemical effects of diphosphonate in Paget's disease of bone. *Arthritis Rheum 18:* 407, 1975.

Osteoporosis

R. G. G. Russell

Osteoporosis literally means "porosity of the bone." Alternative terms are "osteopenia" or "thin bones." Osteoporosis is often defined simply as a state in which the mass of calcified bone is reduced, but for clinical purposes it is perhaps preferable to restrict the term to a state in which fractures have occurred after bone mass has been reduced to a level at which the structural integrity of the skeleton is impaired.

The condition can arise in a variety of ways. It is customarily divided into two main groups: primary, or idiopathic, when the cause is unknown, and secondary when osteoporosis is associated with other clinical conditions (see Table 71-1). Since loss of bone is a feature of normal aging, osteoporosis should not be viewed exclusively as a disease process. This is particularly true of the so-called idiopathic osteoporosis that occurs in postmenopausal or elderly women. This type of osteoporosis increases in incidence with age and is the most common metabolic bone disease; it is therefore of great social and economic importance and a major cause of disability and morbidity. It probably affects more than 10 million people in the United States alone and is responsible for the majority of the 1 million fractures occurring in the elderly each year.[1]

With few exceptions, osteoporosis is a generalized disorder of the skeleton, and in view of the importance of hormones in calcium homeostasis, it is appropriate to discuss it in this section. Recent accounts of osteoporosis include those of Avioli,[2] Morgan,[3,4] Nordin,[5] Paterson,[6] Barzel,[7] Thomson and Frame,[8] and Fourman and Royer.[9]

CLINICAL FEATURES

Patients with reduced bone mass often have no symptoms, but when present the cardinal sympton is bone pain due to fracture, whether radiologically visible or not. The most common fractures occur at the wrist or femoral neck, usually associated with trauma, or in the vertebrae. Vertebral crush fractures are associated with sudden onset of severe localized back pain, often precipitated by muscular effort or trauma. Pain may radiate anteriorly and is often exacerbated by movement and relieved by rest. This pain tends to improve over 3 to 8 weeks, but further episodes of crush fracture cause recurrence of symptoms. Chronic low-grade back pain may ensue, and osteoporosis is probably one of the most common causes of this in the community. Bone tenderness is sometimes present, but neurological complications are surprisingly infrequent.

The signs of generalized osteoporosis are usually those of the spinal lesion. There may be a marked dorsal kyphosis (dowager's or widow's hump) and, rarely, a scoliosis, usually with a measurable loss in height due to collapse of the vertebral bodies. In normal adults, total height is approximately equal to the span but is less following loss of height in osteoporosis. Crown to pubis distance is normally nearly equal to the pubis to heel distance but becomes relatively shortened (upper segment shortening) in osteoporosis, and this process may lead to a transverse skin crease across the abdomen. The lower ribs may eventually come into contact with the iliac crest and cause pain.

Patients with primary osteoporosis are often otherwise well. Symptoms and signs of the other associated conditions may be present in secondary osteoporosis.

PROGNOSIS

Osteoporosis itself is only rarely a fatal disease and then usually because of continued collapse of the thoracic cage leading to respiratory complications. This is particularly true of the young adult form but may occur in myeloma.

In the vast majority of patients, attacks of pain are followed by periods of remission, regardless of treatment. Radiological severity does not necessarily indicate a poor outcome. In the elderly,

Table 71-1. Causes of Osteoporosis

Primary ("idiopathic")
  Juvenile
  Young adults
  Postmenopausal
  Old age
Secondary
  Endocrine
    Cushing's syndrome
    Hyperthyroidism
    Hyperparathyroidism
    Hypogonadism, including postoophorectomy
    Diabetes mellitus
  Pregnancy and lactation
  Nutritional
    Protein malnutrition
    Ascorbic acid deficiency
    Low calcium intake
    Alcoholism
    Vitamin D deficiency
  Gastrointestinal
    Malabsorption
    Stomach operations
  Congenital; inherited
    Osteogenesis imperfecta
    Chromosome abnormalities
  Liver disease
  Renal disease
    Chronic renal failure
    Hemodialysis
  Drugs
    Corticosteroids
    Anticonvulsants
    Methotrexate
    Heparin
  Immobilization; disuse
    Generalized
      Bed rest
      Paraplegia
      Spina bifida
      Neurological
      Space flight
    Localized
      Postfracture
      Sudeck's atrophy
  Rheumatoid arthritis
  Neoplasms
    Myeloma
    Secondary deposits and diffuse neoplasia
    Monocytic leukemias
    Mast-cell disease
  Other causes
    Smoking
    Disappearing bones
    Transient or migratory osteoporosis

however, hip fractures in particular usually require enforced confinement to bed, and significant mortality occurs from secondary complications in this group.

BIOCHEMICAL FEATURES

There are no biochemical changes that are characteristic of osteoporosis. Plasma calcium, phosphate, alkaline phosphatase, and acid phosphatase levels are normal, but the alkaline phosphatase level may be raised during fracture healing. The urinary calcium level is usually normal, although in certain types of osteoporosis, e.g., juvenile, or after immobilization or in thyroid disease, it may be increased. Biochemical changes of associated disorders may, of course, be present.

RADIOLOGICAL FEATURES

Reduced bone mass leads to loss of radiographic intensity. In the vertebrae, this accompanies a loss of normal trabecular pattern, so that the end plates of the vertebral bodies, and even the intervertebral discs, may become relatively more prominent (Fig. 71-1). Vertebrae change shape as they undergo mechanical failure and become wedge-shaped (Figs. 71-2 and 71-3). Herniation of the intervertebral discs occurs, so that protrusion of the disc into the body takes place, either to produce a generalized pattern of "cod fish" vertebrae or a localized protrusion of the nucleosus pulposus into the vertebral body to produce a "Schmorl node."

In long bones, osteoporosis is visible as thinning of the cortex, which can be measured quantitatively in the metacarpals or femurs.

Localized osteoporosis can lead to striking x-ray changes, e.g., loss of trabecular bone at the ends of the metacarpals and phalanges in rheumatoid arthritis.

PATHOGENIC MECHANISMS—GENERAL CONSIDERATIONS

The amount of bone represents the balance between the rates of bone formation and bone destruction. A diminution in bone mass can arise in a number of ways. During growth, a sustained reduction in the rate of bone formation will eventually result in a reduced bone mass at maturity. After the growth phase, a decrease in bone mass requires an increase in the net rate of bone destruction relative to formation. There are at least four ways in which this can happen.

1. Increased rates of resorption with normal rates of formation,
2. Diminished rates of formation with normal rates of resorption,
3. Rates of both formation and resorption decreased, but formation increased more than resorption,

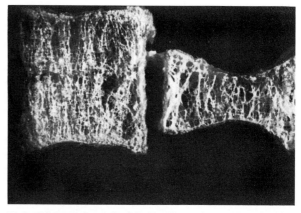

Fig. 71-1. Macerated vertebral bodies illustrating compression fracture. The vertebral body on the left is basically normal. The vertebral body on the right is severely misshapen, rectangular, and shows the convexities produced by the expanding intervertebral disc into an osteoporotic bone.

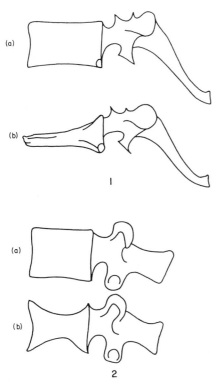

Fig. 71-2. Tracing of x-rays of (1) thoracic and (2) lumbar vertebrae. (a) normal; (b) osteoporotic. (From Fourman and Royer.[9])

4. Both formation and resorption increased, but resorption increased more than formation.

Changes in bone formation and resorption rates are often considered equivalent to corresponding changes in calcium metabolism. Although it is true that there are close relationships between the formation and destruction of all skeletal components (mineral and organic), it can be misleading to consider the changes only in terms of altered calcium metabolism, since this may obscure primary changes in the turnover of matrix components, e.g., in osteogenesis imperfecta. When viewed in terms of calcium homeostasis, however, a diminution in bone mass must represent a net increase in removal of calcium from the skeleton compared with deposition. The disturbances in calcium metabolism that can, in theory, lead to this state of affairs are

1. Inadequate dietary intake,
2. Impaired intestinal absorption of calcium or excessive intestinal losses of calcium in secretions,
3. Increased urinary losses of calcium.

Each of these changes in calcium metabolism has been proposed to be of etiological importance in the development of senile and other types of osteoporosis.

When individual causes of osteoporosis are considered, it is helpful to bear in mind the theoretical ways in which bone mass can be reduced so that possible etiological factors can be appreciated.

METHODS OF ASSESSMENT OF BONE MASS

Accurate methods of measuring bone mass are required for the purposes of diagnosis and for following changes in populations or individuals and the response to treatment. It is estimated that at least 20 percent of spinal mineral needs to be lost before even a skilled radiologist can be confident about the loss. Subjective evaluation can be improved somewhat by comparing x-ray densities with standards such as a step wedge, which consists of pieces of aluminium of various thickness. Use of fine-grain industrial film,[10] particularly for hand bones, makes it possible to detect subtle changes in bone turnover and texture.

Another technique of some value using straightforward x-rays is that of grading bone loss at the upper end of femur on a seven-point scale that depends on changes in the trabecular pattern[11] (Fig. 71-4).

Quantitative and accurate measurements of the *cortical thickness* of long bones is possible using precision calipers to measure periosteal (D) and endosteal (d) diameters. This is the least expen-

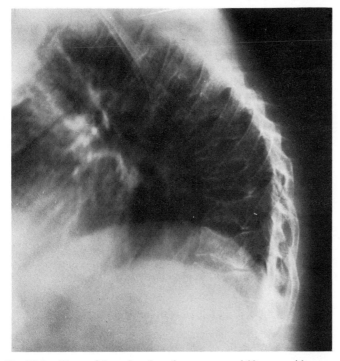

Fig. 71-3. X-ray of thoracic spine of a women aged 33 years with severe osteoporosis and vertebral compression fractures presenting in early adult life.

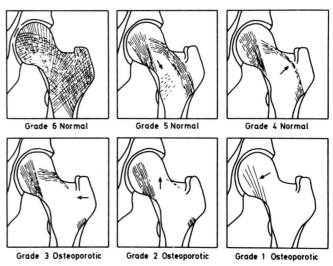

Grade 6 Normal   Grade 5 Normal   Grade 4 Normal

Grade 3 Osteoporotic   Grade 2 Osteoporotic   Grade 1 Osteoporotic

Fig. 71-4. Bone trabecular patterns of upper end of femur with increasing severity of osteoporosis. Arrows show progressive radiological disappearance of trabecular groups. (Adapted from Singh et al.[11])

sive noninvasive technique, with a precision in the order of ± 2 percent. The metacarpal bones, especially the right second metacarpal, are most commonly used, but other bones that have been utilized include the second to fourth metacarpal of both hands or the femur, radius, or humerus.[12] The best measurement is probably the simplest, that of cortical thickness of a bone expressed as $D - d$, i.e., external diameter (D) minus internal diameter (d). Attempts to produce other indices, such as $(D - d)/D$ or $D^2 - d^2$, do not increase precision, because dividing by D itself, although thought to be correct for body size, introduces a systematic error.[3,4] Age-dependent changes in metacarpal cortical thickness can be readily seen not only in populations but also in individuals, so that the response of treatment can be followed in particular patients.

The other now widely used[13] quantitative technique capable of precision in the order of 2 percent is that based on the *photon-beam-absorptiometry* method introduced by Cameron and Sorenson[14] in which the degree of attenuation by bone of gamma-ray emission from isotopic sources (e.g., ^{125}I or ^{247}Am) is measured. Instruments for this purpose are now commercially available. The techniques are best suited to limb bones such as those distal or midshaft of the radius and ulna to give estimates of predominantly trabecular or cortical bone, respectively. Photon densitometry has the advantage over cortical-thickness measurements because it measures both cortical porosity and trabecular bone in addition to narrowing of the cortex due to endosteal resorption. This may be important, since in men the earliest bone loss involves increased intracortical porosity, whereas in women endosteal bone loss is the major event.[15]

Ultrasound pulse echo has also been used as a method of assessing bone mass but has not so far offered significant advantages over other densitometric techniques.

Bone histology, e.g., of iliac bone, is another method that can be used to measure bone mass. The amount of bone present in a given cross-sectional area is measured. This approach is complicated by considerable sampling errors,[16] and the precision is not very high, but the data obtained correlate broadly with other methods.

An ideal approach to avoid the problems inherent in sampling only selected sites within the skeleton is to measure *total-body calcium.* This can be done by *neutron activation,* a technique still used in only a few centers,[17] but theoretically capable of precision in the order of ± 2 percent. The ^{49}Ca produced by irradiation of stable ^{48}Ca with neutrons is measured in a total-body counter. Adaptations of this technique have been applied to measuring calcium in the spine and the hand[18] and have been successful in following the changes produced by treatment.

Although x-ray *appearances* may be helpful in a qualitative manner in assessing the degree of skeletal damage and the presence or absence of fractures, they are too insensitive to provide precise quantitative data. In the future, it is likely that computer-based *total body x-ray scanners,* which are currently under development, will offer a valuable alternative method. It might be anticipated that these will be particularly suitable for difficult sites, such as the spine.

PRIMARY OSTEOPOROSIS

There are four types of primary osteoporosis, which are classified according to the age of onset: juvenile, adult, postmenopausal, and senile. The last two are by far the most important in terms of numbers of people affected.

JUVENILE OSTEOPOROSIS

This rare condition[19,20] occurs in childhood or adolescence (ages 8 to 15 approximately). Bone pain and fractures are the presenting features, together with loss of height. The condition appears to be self-limiting over a 4- to 5-year period, but deformities may persist. Malabsorption of calcium, together with increased urinary loss, has been demonstrated, as has some degree of radiological reversal. There is no known treatment. The etiology is unknown, and although it is possibly a variant of osteogenesis imperfecta, it differs from the classic form in that there is no family history, the onset is later, and the histology of bone is normal apart from reduction in quantity. Moreover, it affects the vertebrae rather than the peripheral skeleton, and some of the other changes of osteogenesis imperfecta, such as ligamentous laxity, blue sclerae, and dental abnormalities, are missing.

ADULT OSTEOPOROSIS

This type of osteoporosis occurs in adults aged 20 to 40, excluding that associated with secondary diseases or with pregnancy or lactation. The clinical features resemble those in older patients except for the age of onset. This condition is uncommon but can be relentlessly progressive and can even result in death from respiratory complications due to collapse of the thoracic cage.

POSTMENOPAUSAL AND SENILE OSTEOPOROSIS

Osteoporosis, presenting with fractures, particularly of the wrist, increases steeply in incidence among females between the ages of 40 and 60. There is an obvious relation to the menopause and lack of estrogen.

Most patients with osteoporosis, however, present past the age of 60 years with vertebral crush fractures or fractured neck of the femur. There is still a preponderance of women over men, and although this group is often considered to be distinct from the "postmenopausal" group and to have "senile" osteoporosis, it seems more likely that this is an extension of the process that starts at the menopause. Indeed, some authors reserve the term "senile osteoporosis" for men and consider all women with osteoporosis to be part of the single postmenopausal variety. It is clear, however, that both varieties cannot be considered without taking into account the skeletal changes that occur in everyone with aging, and, for this reason, it is convenient to discuss them together while looking for additional factors that account for the increased incidence in women. With regard to the effects of aging, a key question is whether patients who present with fracture represent one end of the spectrum of normal bone loss with aging or whether other factors predispose to clinically significant osteoporosis.

Bone Loss with Age

A slow loss of bone in both sexes and in all races appears to be part of normal aging. The debate continues as to whether clinically recognizable osteoporosis represents part of this aging process or whether it is due to more rapid bone loss in particular individuals as a result of other factors.

In the past 20 years, many studies have demonstrated that in normal persons the amount of bone diminishes with age (for reviews, see Morgan[3,4] and others[21-25]), with a mean difference between young persons (20 to 30 years) and the elderly (70 to 80 years) of about 30 percent. The majority of these studies have been cross-sectional population surveys, but longitudinal surveys demonstrating losses of comparable magnitude in individuals have begun to appear.[13,13a,25,26]

The loss of both cortical and trabecular bone begins between the ages of 40 and 50 in women and between 50 and 60 in men. The annual rate of loss is about 1 percent per year in women and is probably somewhat lower in men, and it appears to be linear with time, although, beyond the age of 80 years, there are few data and the rate of loss may level off. Newton-John and Morgan[27,28] have pointed out that the distribution of values for metacarpal cortical thickness is normal and that the variance does not increase with age, suggesting that the entire population loses bone at a uniform rate, rather than there being subpopulations in which bone loss is excessive. This has been confirmed for forearm bone mineral content measured by photon absorptiometry.[13] The implication, therefore, is that persons with the least bone at maturity are those with least bone in later life; others, however, have demonstrated unequal rates of bone loss in individuals.[10,21,25,26] The apparent discrepancies can only be resolved with further work but may indicate that rates of bone loss are either not constant with time or are directly related to bone mass at maturity.[13,23,29]

In normal persons the rate of loss may be greater in the axial than in the peripheral skeleton, but the normal variation in these rates is unknown, and this relationship requires further study because it may influence whether fractures occur mainly in the peripheral or axial skeleton.

The amount of bone at any given age seems higher in Negroes[30] than in Caucasians, who in turn have higher values than Chinese[25] or Eskimos.[31] Among Caucasians, Anglo-Saxon women have lower values. Once loss begins, the amount of bone may be related to the amount present at maturity and also to overall body size. The racial differences may be genetic or dietary in origin, in the latter case perhaps related to calcium or protein intake or to muscle mass, which correlates with skeletal mass.[32-34]

Changes in Bone Composition with Age

Albright's definition of osteoporosis was "too little bone but what bone there is is normal." There is no reason to modify this, since by currently available techniques, osteoporotic bone is normal in chemical composition. The amount of bone, i.e., mass of bone per unit volume of bone tissue, is reduced, but its mineral content per unit mass is normal. This distinguishes it from the bone in osteomalacia in which the mineral content per unit mass is decreased as a result of the presence of unmineralized matrix (osteoid). This classic distinction between the bone in osteoporosis and osteomalacia still holds, although it must be realized that the two conditions may coexist.

Histological and microradiographic techniques clearly demonstrate the increased porosity of cortical bone with age (Fig. 71-5). There are associated histological changes in that closure of osteons, and filling in of lacunal has suggested to some that death of bone cells occurs with age.

With the exception of inherited disorders such as osteogenesis imperfecta, there is scant evidence that the matrix components are altered either in kind or in amount in osteoporosis. This is true of collagen, the major structural protein of bone, and also of the proteins and glycosoaminoglycans of the bone. As the total amount of bone is diminished, however, these components are reduced in proportion. There is evidence that the amount of collagen may be reduced both in bone and skin in the osteoporosis of the elderly,[35-37] suggesting that there is generalized age-dependent change in connective tissue.[38,39] The amount of cross-linked collagen that is nonextractable may increase relative to other fractions

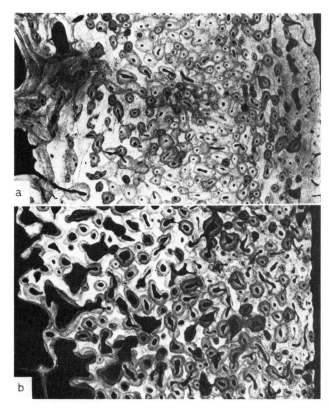

Fig. 71-5. Microradiographs of the femoral cortex of a 17-year-old male (a) and a 77-year-old female (b) (X 20) to show increased porosity (osteoporosis) in the older bone. (From Jowsey, reproduced in Fourman & Royer.[9])

with age. There is also an increase in the proportion of chondroitin sulfate relative to hyaluronic acid and keratosulfate with advancing age. Methods available for measuring amounts and structure of connective-tissue components are still probably not sufficiently sophisticated to detect minor abnormalities, e.g., in the structure of glycosoaminoglycans or of collagen. The diminution of mechanical strength of whole bone with age appears to be accounted for entirely by diminution in the amount of bone rather than in its quality.

Changes in Bone Turnover and Remodeling with Age

As bone mass diminishes with age, the destruction rate must be greater than the bone formation rate. Techniques available for studying these rates are far from satisfactory but include the use of radioisotopes of calcium (^{45}Ca, ^{47}Ca), with or without metabolic balances, and various histological techniques, including microradiography,[40] assessment of bone cell populations, and use of multiple tetracycline markers.[41]

Calcium kinetic techniques[42] demonstrate that bone mineralization and resorption rates fall with age. However, this technique cannot determine whether the fall is due simply to reduction in bone mass, with the rate of events at individual bone surfaces remaining relatively constant. Unfortunately, the histological data do not clearly resolve this point.

Frost[43] and Schenk and Merz[44] concluded on the basis of tetracycline labeling that bone formation diminishes with age, whereas bone resorption remains constant. Quantitative assessment of cell counts also suggests that resorption surfaces are unchanged.[45] In contrast, microradiographic data[40] indicate that iliac bone surfaces engaged in resorption increase with age, whereas those engaged in formation remain constant. Interpretation of microradiographic data requires caution, however, because measurement of linear surfaces that show past or present resorptive or formative activity cannot give absolute values for the current rates (i.e., per unit time) of these events. Despite these unresolved differences, alleged changes in cortical or trabecular bone turnover may be overshadowed by increased resorption concentrated on the endosteal surfaces of long bones, leading to thinning of the cortex with age. This process, which is not measured by the usual histological technique, is obviously important in producing the characteristic radiological appearances of osteoporosis.

There is little evidence at present that the performance of individual osteoblasts or osteoclasts changes with aging.

Calcium and Phosphate Metabolism

With aging, several changes are observed.[5] There is an increase in plasma phosphate levels in females after the age of 40, probably as a result of enhanced renal tubular reabsorption of phosphate, a rise in plasma alkaline phosphatase levels, and a fall in intestinal calcium absorption and urinary calcium excretion, which is more noticeable in women than in men; but there is no detectable change in urinary peptide-bound hydroxyproline.

The Fracture Syndromes: Wrist, Vertebrae, and Proximal Femur

Although osteoporosis may be said to be present if the mass of bone falls below some arbitrary limit with respect to age and sex, the condition becomes of clinical significance only when structural failure and fracture ensue.

The three major types of fracture are forearm (distal radius and ulna—Colles' fracture), femoral-neck fracture, and the vertebral crush fracture. There is some evidence that the changes leading to each of these presentations may be slightly different. Forearm fractures occur in postmenopausal women, whereas proximal-femur fractures occur in elderly women and men. Vertebral crush fractures also occur in this older age group.

Several workers (e.g., Nordin[5]) have proposed that the amount of bone that needs to be lost in order to risk sustaining a forearm fracture is less than that needed to increase the risk of femoral-neck fracture. This would explain the earlier onset and the relatively minor reduction in bone-mass measurements in this population compared with age-matched controls. It is questionable whether patients who sustain vertebral crush fractures have an accentuated loss from the spine compared with the peripheral skeleton. As a population, a generalized reduction of bone mass can be demonstrated, so that, for example, metacarpal cortical thickness is diminished in patients with vertebral crush fractures. There is, however, a considerable overlap with normal, so that in any individual the value may be within the normal range, and, conversely, there are many individuals with a reduction in bone mass who remain free of fractures. Patients with femoral-neck fractures usually have clearly visible radiological diminution of bone at the affected site, so that the ''Singh score'' is grade 3 or less, but these patients also have a diminution in metacarpal cortical thickness as a group, although again there is an overlap with normal.

The group of patients with proximal-femur fractures differ from the others not only in being older but also in that osteomalacia, as defined by an increased amount of osteoid tissue covering trabecular surfaces in bone biopsies, occurs in approximately 30 percent of the patients.[46,47] This suggests that some degree of vitamin D deficiency may contribute to this particular mode of

presentation, and there is some evidence for this in that 25-hydroxycholecalciferol has been found to be low in this group,[47] although not in all series;[48] 1,25-hydroxycholecalciferol levels have also been claimed to be reduced,[49] although only by a small margin.

PATHOGENESIS OF AGE-DEPENDENT CHANGES IN BONE AND OF POSTMENOPAUSAL AND SENILE OSTEOPOROSIS

In theory, many factors could predispose to osteoporosis during aging. Those that are under serious consideration currently include dietary factors, genetic predisposition, hormonal disturbances, or local changes in bone cells or marrow. It is likely that osteoporosis will turn out to be multifactorial in origin and that the relative importance of the several causative factors will vary in different patients. Once again, in view of the universal changes in bone mass that occur with aging, it is important to know in terms of pathogenesis whether patients who sustain fractures as a result of osteopenia differ in any qualitative rather than quantitative way from normal. Opinion is divided. Although most authors continue to view osteoporosis as a disease process superimposed on the aging phenomenon, others argue that patients with clinically important osteoporosis represent those persons who lie at the lower end of the normal distribution of bone mass, by analogy with the distribution of hypertension in the population (Figs. 71-6 and 71-7). These apparently opposing views may be reconciled to some extent if it is proposed that the factors leading to reduced bone mass in later years are also not uniformly distributed in the population. Thus, for example, intestinal ability to absorb calcium on a given dietary intake of calcium and vitamin D may also be lower in patients with clinically evident osteoporosis. Another way of viewing this is to propose that environmental factors resulting in reduced bone mass have an exaggerated effect in a susceptible subpopulation.

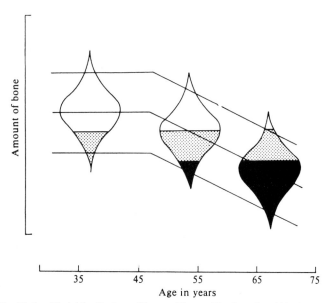

Fig. 71-6. Model for the loss of bone with age. The dotted and black areas represent the proportion of the population at each age who have an amount of bone less than arbitrary figures corresponding to mean − 1 standard deviation and mean − 2.5 standard deviation, respectively, for women aged between 30 and 40. Note the nonlinear increase in proportion of patients with thin bones. (From Morgan.[4])

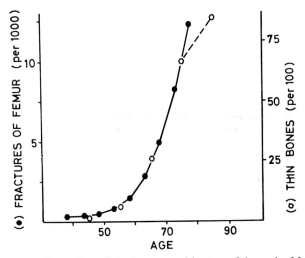

Fig. 71.7. Comparison of the frequency of fracture of the neck of femur (per 1000 per 10 years) and the frequency of thin bones (less than mean − 2.5 standard deviation in persons aged 20 to 40 years) in women according to age. Note the similar changes with age. Compare with Fig. 71-6. (From Morgan.[4])

Calcium Deficiency Due to Inadequate Calcium Intake or Malabsorption of Calcium or Vitamin D Deficiency

Calcium deficiency due to a low dietary intake or malabsorption of calcium is an attractive explanation for osteoporosis, but the evidence that it occurs is still controversial. In experimental animals skeletal calcium can be shown to be directly related to dietary intake, and calcium deficiency produces a reversible osteopenia,[50] which is particularly evident during growth. In man, some studies[24,51] report no relationship between dietary intake and bone density, but others claim a significant correlation between the two.[52] There are also studies which suggest that patients with osteoporosis consume less calcium than do controls.[53-56] Avoidance of a major dietary source of calcium in the form of milk, because of lactase deficiency,[57] is a potentially important cause of calcium deficiency.[58] However, simple calcium deficiency resulting from low dietary intake does not correlate with the incidence of osteoporosis on a worldwide scale.[59]

Calcium deficiency can arise even in the face of adequate dietary intake if malabsorption of calcium occurs. It is significant, therefore, that calcium absorption diminishes with age in both men and women[60-63] and that the adaptation to low dietary intakes is also impaired with aging.[62] The reason for this change is not established. It may reflect mild dietary deficiency of vitamin D or age-dependent, vitamin D-independent decline in efficiency of intestinal absorption. Alternatively, it may indicate diminished intestinal responsiveness to 1,25-dihydroxyvitamin D or progressive failure by the kidney to sustain its production of 1,25-dihydroxyvitamin D. Indeed, renal impairment is claimed by some to be an important factor in the development of osteopenia.[64] In true malabsorption syndromes, impairment of calcium absorption is associated with osteopenia, presumably as a result of malabsorption of both calcium and vitamin D, accentuated in some conditions, such as gluten-sensitive enteropathy, by a defective intestinal response to 1,25-(OH)₂-D due to villous atrophy.

Deficiency of vitamin D or disturbances in its metabolism might therefore be expected to be particularly prevalent in osteoporosis in the elderly. There are reports, as mentioned above, that 25-OH-D levels are low in patients with proximal-femur fractures, but others claim the levels to be normal.[48] There is a relationship between osteopenia and exposure to sunlight.[32] In the United Kingdom, osteomalacia, as defined by excessive coverage of trabecular surfaces in bone with osteoid, is present in about 30 percent of patients with proximal-femur fractures,[46] suggesting that vitamin D deficiency might be common. This is not surprising in view of the low intakes of vitamin D in the United Kingdom where few foods are fortified and the northern latitude results in low exposure to sunlight, particularly in the elderly housebound population. The importance in the United States of marginal states of vitamin D deficiency, which may lead to osteopenia rather than frank osteomalacia, is still unclear. There are, however, seasonal variations in plasma 25-OH-D, suggesting the importance of sunlight exposure, and even recent claims that 1,25dihydroxyvitamin D levels are lower, although only slightly so, in patients with vertebral crush fractures than in age-matched controls.[49]

Other Dietary Components

Suggestions that osteoporosis may be due to other dietary deficiencies, e.g. vitamin C, are only speculative. However, the high-protein diets characteristically ingested by Western civilizations and also notably by Eskimos[65] have been invoked as causative agents, since they are acid producing, and acidosis is a recognized predisposing factor to osteopenia in man and experimental animals. Increased acid loads also arise from the increased consumption of soft drinks, and this burden of acid is partly buffered at the expense of bone, leading to increased urinary losses of calcium.[66]

Reduced Bone Mass at Maturity

If bone loss with age is universal and uniform, then skeletal mass will reach a particular critical limit sooner in those who have less bone to begin with. Therefore, any cause of reduced bone mass at maturity may predispose to osteoporosis later, and the best protection would be to have a large skeletal mass at maturity. Apart from the reduced calcium availability discussed above, another factor that could be important is physical activity, since muscle mass is known to be related to bone mass.[34] This may be related to the prevalence of osteoporosis among individuals of small body size,[33] i.e., "little, thin old ladies."

Endocrine Factors—Mechanism of Changes with Age

The loss of ovarian function at the menopause is the currently most attractive explanation for the loss of bone that begins in females around this age. There are small but detectable rises after the menopause in fasting urine calcium levels and also in hydroxyproline values, both presumably derived from the skeleton. This is also seen in women who undergo oophorectomy, which thereby brings about an early menopause.[5]

The other changes with age are not currently readily explained, apart from suggestions that they are part of the senescence process, which merely begs the question. One recent, but unproven, suggestion referred to above is that the gradual reduction in intestinal absorption of calcium is due to impaired production of 1,25-dihydroxycholecalciferol by the aging kidney.

The precise mechanisms of estrogen action on bone are not known. Even though only high concentrations of estrogens will block resorption induced by parathyroid hormone (PTH) in tissue culture, it seems likely that the administration of estrogen in therapeutic doses to patients achieves a similar effect (Fig. 71-8).

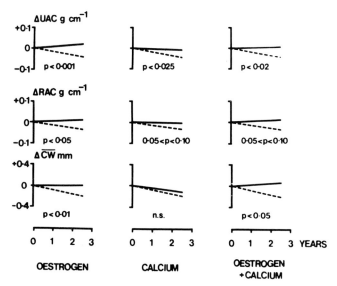

Fig. 71-8. A comparison of the loss of bone from the ulna (ΔUAC), radius (ΔRAC), and metacarpal (ΔCW) in controls (dotted) and in groups of postmenopausal women treated with estrogen (as ethinyl estradiol, 25–50 μg daily for 3 weeks out of 4) alone, or calcium (as 2 Sandocal tablets/day, 800 mg Ca/day) alone, or with a combination of both. Ulnar and radial density were measured by photon absorption, and metacarpal cortical width on radiographs. Note significant reduction of bone loss during treatment with estrogen. (From A. Horsman, et al., *Calcif. Tissues Res. 22* (Suppl.): 217-224, 1977.)

Thus, estrogens probably delay loss of bone in postmenopausal women.[67–76] Heaney[77] and Jasani et al.[78] have proposed that bone is more readily resorbed by parathyroid hormone when estrogen activity is reduced. The involvement of the parathyroid in postmenopausal bone loss is implied by the greater loss seen in hyperparathyroid postmenopausal women than in hypoparathyroid[79] or normal women.[80] Even though parathyroid hormone levels have not been shown to be raised in women with postmenopausal osteoporosis,[81] it has been proposed that there may be a steady stimulus to parathyroid hormone secretion by reduced plasma calcium during the night after intestinal calcium absorption is complete and calcium is still being excreted in the urine. When there is no estrogen to restrict the action of parathyroid hormone on bone, a greater amount of bone is resorbed,[5] and this results in the raised fasting urinary calcium levels seen in these patients. The renal conserving effect of PTH on calcium is lost because PTH is maintained at normal or subnormal levels[81] by calcium derived mainly from the diet by day and from bone at night. An additional feature is that the renal conserving mechanism is also unable to achieve urinary calcium levels below about 1 mmole per 24 hours in the face of a normal plasma calcium,[82] so that there is an obligatory minimum daily loss of calcium of this amount. If dietary absorption of calcium cannot keep up with this, a negative calcium balance inevitably ensues. Few direct data are available, however, to support this intriguing concept of parathyroid hormone/estrogen homeostatic balance as causative in osteoporosis.

There are other measurable changes in endocrine status with aging that might contribute to loss of bone. Declining androgen function, relative to glucocorticoid secretion, is one such change.[83] Furthermore, growth hormone, which has marked effects on bone, is secreted less well in response to hypoglycemia in postmenopausal women, perhaps because of estrogen deficiency.[84]

Endocrine Abnormalities in Osteoporosis

There is little convincing evidence that patients with "idiopathic" postmenopausal or senile osteoporosis systematically differ from normal in pituitary, thyroid, parathyroid, pancreatic, or adrenal function. In other words, although there may be age-related changes in these systems contributing to loss of bone, it remains to be shown that these changes are exaggerated in patients with clinically significant osteoporosis. Overt abnormalities in any of these systems are, of course, well-recognized causes of secondary osteoporosis.

With regard to sex hormones, although an attractive hypothesis, there is not much evidence to suggest that estrogen levels are lower in osteoporotic patients that in age-matched controls. Thus, Riggs et al.[85] found no difference in plasma estrogen levels, although Nordin et al.[85a] have reported lower levels. There is also evidence for estrogen deficiency in that vaginal-smear maturation index is reduced in such patients[5] and there are raised gonadotrophic levels and sparse pubic and axillary hair.[83] Recent studies have also proposed altered estrogen-receptor activity in osteoporosis.[86] Clearly, further work is needed in this area.

In the case of androgens, although plasma testosterone levels do not appear to differ in osteoporotic patients compared with normals of the same age,[85] there is evidence that the rise in adrenal androgens in response to ACTH is impaired.[83]

Another unconfirmed suggestion is that osteoporotic patients are relatively deficient in calcitonin[87] and therefore have an impaired ability to prevent bone resorption.

Physical Activity

Since immobilization leads to rapid loss of bone, it is possible that reduced physical activity in the elderly may aggravate bone loss, although it is hard to prove that this is an important etiological factor.

Fluoride

There are several reports suggesting that osteoporosis may be more common in regions where the water is low in fluoride.[88,89] In contrast, high intakes of fluoride lead to skeletal fluorosis.

Hereditary

There is some evidence that idiopathic osteoporosis is more common among relatives, but it is uncertain whether this indicates inherited or environmental causes. This is also true of racial differences, such as the relative resistance to osteoporosis among Negroes. It seems likely that inherited minor disturbances in bone matrix production, e.g., collagen biosynthesis and structure, may turn out to be more common than normal in osteoporosis. Skin is thinner,[36] and its collagen content is reduced in patients with clinically significant osteoporosis.

Local Factors in the Pathogenesis of Osteoporosis

Skeletal remodeling is a complex process that involves coordination of events occurring at periosteal, intracortical, and endosteal sites as well as within trabecular bone. Remodeling responds to mechanical stress and to hormone activity, but there must also be elegant control mechanisms of which we are not yet aware. Osteoporosis could arise from a localized disorder of this remodeling. Thus, endosteal resorption may be exaggerated to give rise to progressive loss of cortical thickness. Bone marrow may itself be involved in these processes, and one suggestion is that mast cells containing heparin contribute to bone resorption.[90]

SECONDARY OSTEOPOROSIS

CONGENITAL OR INHERITED FORMS

Osteogenesis Imperfecta

Osteogenesis imperfecta is a well-recognized, rather common inherited abnormality of bone in which bone formation is defective and produces skeletal deformities and fracture. The condition shows a remarkable range of severity and clinical presentation, and it is likely that more than one abnormality is involved.[91] The most probable explanation is that it is due to a defect in collagen biosynthesis or structure, and in view of the great complexity of the collagen molecule, it is not surprising that more than one abnormality could occur. These patients have thin bones that fracture with minimal trauma but heal readily, often with exuberant callus formation.

Chromosomal and Inherited Disorders

These topics have been reviewed elsewhere.[2,91] Osteopenia is a feature of children with XO (Turner's syndrome) gonadal dysgenesis, Klinefelter's (XXY) syndrome,[92] and other chromosomal disorders, including XXXY and XXXXY individuals and Down's syndrome (trisomy 21). Factors that result in diminished bone mass during growth and prior to gonadal maturity are likely to differ from those responsible for loss of bone during adult life. It is therefore interesting that in Down's syndrome the osteopenia appears to reverse at puberty.[92]

NUTRITIONAL DISTURBANCES

Protein Malnutrition

There is evidence in experimental animals as well as in man that prolonged intake of diets poor in protein may result in less-calcified bone.

Vitamin C Deficiency and Iron-Storage Disease

Osteopenia is a feature of juvenile scurvy and is also sometimes seen in scorbutic adults, although presumably it requires a prolonged deficiency of vitamin C to produce significant changes. The osteoporosis found in Bantu males in South Africa[93,94] has been claimed to be due to siderosis resulting from consumption of alcoholic drinks stored in iron containers.

The accumulation of iron is thought to lead to vitamin C depletion by promoting its oxidation, a situation that can be reproduced experimentally in guinea pigs. Hemochromatosis can also result in a variable osteopenia, perhaps produced by a similar mechanism, although hypogonadism due to iron deposition in the testes is also a possibility.[95]

Vitamin C is involved in the hydroxylation of proline and lysine in collagen, so osteopenia due to vitamin C deficiency may reflect acquired abnormalities in collagen biosynthesis and maturation.

Low Calcium Intake

Low intakes of dietary calcium have already been invoked as a possible contributing factor in so-called idiopathic osteoporosis. There have been claims, mostly as sporadic case reports, that osteoporosis develops secondary to prolonged low calcium intakes.

Alcoholism

Saville[96] found thin bones in young alcoholics at autopsy. Excessive alcohol intake has been shown to result in diminished bone mass during life[97] and in increased femoral-neck fractures in man.[98]

The mechanism is unclear[2] but could be due to generalized poor nutrition, resulting particularly in low intakes of calcium, vitamin C, and protein. Alternatively, it might be due to liver disease, perhaps leading to disturbances in vitamin D metabolism. Since ethanol increases urinary excretion of magnesium, magnesium depletion may occur in alcoholics, and this in turn may lead to alterations in parathyroid status.

PREGNANCY AND LACTATION

Rapidly progressive osteoporosis, particularly of the spine leading to crush fracture, can occur during pregnancy or lactation. There are already extra demands on calcium metabolism at these times to meet the needs of the growing fetus and to provide milk for the newborn infant. The losses of calcium from the mother can be in the order of 200 mg per day, but this is usually compensated for by increased intestinal absorption, which may in turn be mediated by increased synthesis of 1,25-dihydroxyvitamin D. Indeed, 1,25-dihydroxyvitamin D levels are reported to be high in the later stages of pregnancy and during lactation.[99] Studies on small numbers of patients have shown that negative calcium balances may exist during lactation,[100] but there is no evidence that multiparity or repeated periods of lactation are significantly related to fracture incidence later in life.[101] The patients who present with rapidly progressive osteoporosis during pregnancy or lactation thus differ markedly from normal. They usually have no sign of vitamin D deficiency, and evidence for altered metabolism of vitamin D has not been sought. It is possible that many of them have some inherent defect of the skeleton that is revealed during this time, and we have seen patients with a family history of the early adult form of osteoporosis presenting after childbirth.

ENDOCRINE DISEASE

Disordered secretion of any of the hormones (PTH, growth hormone, glucocorticoids, and thyroid hormones or gonadal steroids) that have actions on bone may result in osteopenia.

Adrenal Glands

Glucocorticoid excess may be caused by a tumor of the adrenal glands or by adrenal hyperplasia secondary to excessive ACTH from the anterior pituitary or from nonendocrine tumors such as carcinoma of the bronchus. Therapy with corticosteroids or with ACTH or it synthetic analogues may produce the same results.

Osteoporosis is a well-recognized feature of long-standing glucocorticoid excess (for review, see Avioli[2]). It was present in Cushing's original cases. Radiological osteoporosis is often present and said to be more marked in the axial skeleton and skull than in the periphery. Radiological rarefaction of the spine occurs in about half the patients,[102] and Doyle[29] demonstrated reduced ulnar mineral content in about one-third of patients with Cushing's syndrome. Patients may present with backache or fracture, which is often painless. In children, e.g., asthmatics on treatment with steroids, the bone changes may be severe and complicated by growth retardation. The bone loss that accompanies glucocorticoid excess seems to be irreversible in adults but partly reversible in children.

The mechanism is still debated. Part of the confusion arises because of the multitude of experimental data that might be relevant. The effect of glucocorticoid administration to animals is complicated by variable effects at different doses, by significant species differences, and by the differences between growing and skeletally mature animals.

Glucocorticoids appear to impair calcium absorption in man,[103] and there may be an increase in urinary calcium leading occasionally to renal stones. It is not clear whether the renal handling is itself altered or whether the excessive urinary calcium is derived from bone. Impaired absorption and increased urinary losses both tend to give rise to a negative balance. These various effects seem to occur at doses above 15 mg per day of prednisolone or its equivalent.

In bone itself, histological findings suggest that bone formation may be diminished and bone resorption increased.[43,104] In culture, steroids depress bone resorption and also depress collagen biosynthesis. In growing children, this latter effect may predominate to produce the skeletal changes and growth retardation.

Thyroid Disease

Hyperthyroidism is frequently accompanied by well-recognized changes in mineral metabolism (for review, see Goldring and Krane[105]). Plasma calcium may be raised transiently or continuously. This is usually associated with hypercalciuria, even though intestinal absorption of calcium seems to be decreased, so that a negative calcium balance occurs. Plasma phosphate is often raised as a result of an elevation in the renal threshhold for phosphate, best expressed at TmP/GFR.

In bone[106] there is an increase in rates of bone formation and destruction; these changes in turnover can be demonstrated by increased resorption by osteoclasts, increased osteoblastic activity, and, often, widened osteoid seams caused, not by impaired mineralization, but by accelerated matrix deposition. There may also be marrow fibrosis (osteitis fibrosa). The increased bone turnover accounts for the increased urinary excretion of hydroxyproline and hydroxylysine in peptides derived from collagen, findings that may be of value in diagnosis.[107] Levels of plasma alkaline phosphatase derived from bone are also often raised.

Although both formation and destruction of bone are increased, there is a progressive loss of bone in hyperthyroidism leading to skeletal rarefaction indistinguishable from that seen in other forms of osteoporosis. The mechanism underlying the changes in skeletal metabolism that occur in hyperthyroidism are not fully understood but are probably due in part to the direct effects of thyroid hormones (T_4 or T_3) on the bone. Recently, T_4 has been shown to stimulate bone resorption directly in tissue culture but only after the several days' delay so characteristic of the other metabolic effects of thyroid hormone.[108] The osteoporosis can be visualized as a progressive diminution in bone mass due to resorption exceeding formation, coupled with intestinal malabsorption of calcium and increased urinary losses. There is some evidence that changes in mineral metabolism and skeletal turnover occur in all patients with hyperthyroidism, although the changes only rarely attain clinical significance. The bone loss may be reversible in young patients but not in older ones.[109] The tendency to hypercalcemia may suppress parathyroid secretion,

and this may account for the increase in TmP/GFR, but this suggestion requires further documentation. Patients with thyrotoxicosis are also said to exhibit increased skeletal sensitivity to parathyroid hormone,[110] but the biochemical basis of this requires cautious interpretation because the mass of the target organ (i.e., the bone cell population) capable of responding to PTH must be considerably increased, and it is difficult to distinguish between this and increased responsiveness of individual cells, i.e., altered receptor activity.

Although the skeletal changes in hyperthyroidism only infrequently result in bone pain and fracture, the possibility of thyroid disease should be borne in mind as a possible cause of these symptoms in any elderly patient with osteoporosis. Similarly, hypercalcemia in a thyrotoxic patient should alert one to the coexistence of hyperparathyroidism, the incidence of which appears increased in this group.[111]

Acromegaly

There are characteristic skeletal changes in active acromegaly in which there is an excess of growth hormone. These changes include generalized overgrowth of bone leading to cortical thickening and coarsening of structure. The skull vault is thickened, phalangeal tufts enlarge, and vertebrae enlarge owing to new bone deposition around the bodies. The characteristic facial appearances are produced by thickening of the orbital ridges and maxillary bones and the enlargement of the mandible by growth at the condyles to produce prognathism.

The changes in long bones have given rise to the belief that acromegaly causes osteoporosis but the x-ray appearances of apparent cortical thinning are due to subperiosteal deposition of bone and enlargement of the marrow cavity. Thus, although there are sporadic case reports of osteoporosis in acromegaly, a survey of over 50 cases by Doyle[29] showed that ulnar densitometry was usually normal. Furthermore, fractures are uncommon.[112,113] The most obvious disturbance in calcium and phosphate metabolism is the increased tubular reabsorption of phosphate leading to raised plasma phosphate levels. This is probably a direct effect of growth hormone on the renal tubule[114] but is also possibly due to suppression of parathyroid hormone secretion. The increased plasma phosphate could be an etiological factor in promoting periosteal apposition of bone, since similar appearances are occasionally seen in generalized bone dysplasias and in some patients with tumoral calcinosis.

Plasma calcium levels are usually normal, but hypercalcemia can occur, and an increase in urinary calcium is common. Intestinal calcium absorption is normal or raised. With the exception of the change in intestinal absorption, the changes in calcium metabolism resemble those of hyperthyroidism and could be explained by increased bone turnover, as can be demonstrated by calcium kinetic studies,[115] with a tendency to parathyroid suppression.

Hyperparathyroidism

Hyperparathyroidism as a cause of bone loss and fracture has been discussed earlier in the section dealing with clinical disorders of the parathyroid glands.

Hypogonadism and Hypopituitarism

Apart from the bone loss that occurs after natural or surgically induced menopause, estrogen deficiency may also account for the osteoporosis in other situations, e.g., in Turner's syndrome and perhaps in juvenile osteoporosis, but further evaluation is required. In males, hypogonadism may also lead to reduced bone mass, which may account for their osteopenia in adult life.[83]

Diabetes Mellitus

For many years, a statistically significant association between osteoporosis and diabetes mellitus has been suggested,[116-118] and hip fractures are said to be more common.[118] Forearm-bone mineral content is reduced[119,120] in juvenile and maturity-onset diabetics, suggesting that a decrease in bone formation could be intrinsic to the disorder. Skeletal abnormalities exist in the fetuses of diabetic mothers.[121] The rate of osteoid formation is decreased,[43,122] but the pathogenic mechanisms need further study. Insulin stimulates amino acid uptake by bone cells and also stimulates collagen synthesis. An impairment of these processes in diabetes could be responsible for diminished bone formation. There is some evidence that insulin may protect against osteopenia, whereas oral antidiabetic drugs may exacerbate it.[120]

GASTROINTESTINAL DISEASE

Malabsorption Syndromes

Malabsorption syndromes are perhaps better recognized as causes of osteomalacia, but bone loss can occur in malabsorption, even in the absence of osteomalacia.[123] The mechanism is probably that malabsorption of both vitamin D and calcium occurs in many of these patients, but those who receive adequate vitamin D from other sources, e.g., by the action of sunlight on skin, are protected from osteomalacia but may develop osteoporosis. In patients with gluten-sensitive enteropathy, the lack of intestinal villi means that there is no target organ for vitamin D to act on in the gut, and malabsorption of calcium inevitably occurs, so that fecal losses can even exceed dietary intake.

Another interesting example is the osteopenia of lactose intolerance in which malabsorption of calcium can be demonstrated.[124,125] The possibility that lactase deficiency contributes to senile osteoporosis was mentioned earlier.[57]

Stomach Operations

After gastrectomy, a small number of patients may develop osteomalacia, but a larger number show accelerated loss of bone after the age of 50 in women and 60 in men.[126,127]

LIVER DISEASE

Chronic liver disease both in children and in adults can lead to reduced bone mass. Although osteomalacia is a well-recognized complication of obstructive liver disease, bone loss and fracture can occur in the absence of osteomalacia. The mechanism is unclear and unlikely to be simple. There is evidence both for malabsorption of vitamin D as well as for defective conversion to 25-hydroxyvitamin D in obstructive liver disease, and plasma 25-hydroxyvitamin D levels are often subnormal.[128] This may account for intestinal malabsorption of calcium, which has also been recorded in parenchymatous liver disease.[129] The osteoporosis associated with chronic alcohol ingestion may bring in other causative factors, e.g., suboptimal nutrition. It is possible that the low albumin levels so characteristic of liver disease bear some relationship to diminution in bone mass, because albumin is preferentially taken up from the plasma during bone matrix synthesis.[130] Similarly, other proteins synthesized in the liver may be important for proper bone matrix synthesis. Thus the plasma concentrations of the glycoprotein designated $\alpha2HS$ can be shown to be inversely correlated with rates of bone matrix deposition.[131]

KIDNEY DISEASE

Chronic renal disease produces a variety of disturbances in calcium metabolism, and osteopenia may be one of these. Malabsorption of calcium is an early event in the development of renal failure, and a negative calcium balance may often be demonstrated. This malabsorption is probably due to an impaired renal production of 1,25-dihydroxyvitamin D combined with a reduced ability of the intestine to respond to this hormone.[132] This diminished production of 1,25-$(OH)_2$-D [133] may be due to renal tissue damage per se or to the hyperphosphatemia that accompanies renal impairment. The rise in plasma phosphate levels, coupled with malabsorption of calcium, tends to lower plasma calcium levels and thereby to stimulate secretion of parathyroid hormone. The changes of secondary hyperparathyroidism, both radiological and histological, are the most common to be seen in chronic renal failure. Osteomalacia is less common and cannot be explained solely by lack of active metabolites of vitamin D, since it is no more common in patients who have had a total nephrectomy, which removes all sources of 1,25-$(OH)_2$-D.[134]

The secondary hyperparathyroidism that accompanies renal failure may in itself be responsible for some diminution in bone mass, but it seems that the most severe osteoporosis occurs in patients on long-term hemodialysis.[135] Possible causative factors are reduced dietary intake and poor absorption of calcium, calcium losses in dialysis fluid, and the immobilization that accompanies prolonged hospitalization.

After renal transplantation, although secondary hyperparathyroidism tends to resolve, often over a prolonged period, the administration of steroids and antimetabolite drugs, together with a phosphate-losing nephropathy, is a continuing possible cause of diminishing bone mass.

RHEUMATOID ARTHRITIS

Patients with untreated rheumatoid arthritis often show severe generalized osteoporosis with fractures,[136,137,137a] and in addition there is accentuated loss of trabecular bone around the joints, possibly due to local factors arising from the diseased joints, such as prostaglandins, which can stimulate bone resorption. The etiology of the generalized osteoporosis is complex and is usually considered to be partly due to prolonged immobilization as a result of pain and disability, which is exacerbated in those patients on steroids.[36] Recently, it has been proposed that there is an increased incidence of hyperparathyroidism in patients with rheumatoid arthritis on the basis of elevated plasma calcium and plasma alkaline phosphatase.[138a] Bone resorbing factors other than prostaglandins are probably also produced by the abnormal synovial tissue and may also be responsible for bone loss.

IMMOBILIZATION

Generalized

Immobilization such as that incurred by prolonged periods of bed rest leads to bone loss that comes on very rapidly, as indicated by abrupt rises in urinary calcium and urinary total hydroxyproline levels. The loss can be confirmed by densitometric techniques and is particularly marked in weight-bearing bones. In the initial stages, 0.5 percent of the body stores of calcium can be lost per month.[139] These findings led to concern about the effects of bone loss during prolonged immobilization in *space flight*.[140] The potential losses are now considered to be less severe than first thought.[141]

Neurological Disease

Immobilization due to neurological disease, e.g., paraplegia and tetraplegia, is also a potent cause of bone loss and is associated with increased urinary calcium and hydroxyproline and sometimes with intestinal malabsorption of calcium. Loss of weightbearing may be important, but altered blood flow is another potential causative factor. The losses may be greater from the peripheral than from the central skeleton. There is often associated ectopic calcification, particularly around the hips in paraplegic patients. Stone formation is a frequent complication, partly as a result of the increased urinary calcium but often complicated by urinary tract infection.[5]

In *spina bifida*, children whose lower limbs are paralyzed often have severe osteoporosis, and fractures of the leg bones occur in as many as half the patients. These fractures heal readily, often with extensive callus formation.

Local

Local immobilization, e.g., after fractures or as a result of painful joints, can lead to rapid loss of bone, a situation that can be easily mimicked in experimental animals. This type of loss is largely reversible, and it is misleading to use these experimental models to elucidate pathogenic mechanisms in other types of osteoporosis. The mechanisms may include loss of mechanical forces and changes in blood flow.

Sudeck's Atrophy

This term is used to describe a clinically recognizable form of localized osteoporosis occurring in painful limbs after trauma or fracture.

DRUGS

Corticosteroids

The effect of corticosteroids have already been discussed. Osteopenia accompanying corticosteroid therapy has been described in patients with asthma, with various skin disorders (e.g., psoriasis), with rheumatoid arthritis, or with ulcerative colitis. Although steroids undoubtedly affect calcium metabolism in some of these conditions, the underlying medical disorder may also be a contributing factor.

Anticonvulsants

Drugs in this group, such as barbiturates and phenytoin, are now well recognized as causes of rickets or osteomalacia.[142] Osteopenia, even in the absence of the Looser zones or epiphyseal changes of rickets or osteomalacia, may be a striking radiological feature.

The mechanism of the osteomalacia is said to be a drug-induced stimulation of microsomal enzymes in the liver that causes ineffective metabolism of 25-OH-D to inactive products, thereby inducing an acquired deficiency of vitamin D. However, these drugs may have direct effects on intestinal calcium absorption and on bone (see Chapter 67), and further work needs to be done before the action on calcium and skeletal metabolism is properly understood.

Antimetabolites

Osteopenia has been reported in patients on treatment with anticancer drugs, especially methotrexate.[143] Although bone loss might be due to the primary disease being treated, e.g., leukemia[144] or psoriasis,[2] methotrexate does cause intestinal malabsorption of calcium and increased urinary excretion of calcium;[145,146] both of the latter effects would tend to diminish bone mass if methotrexate were given for long periods.

Heparin

Severe osteoporosis and spontaneous fractures can occur in patients on long-term heparin therapy.[147,148] It has been difficult to reproduce this condition experimentally, and the cause is unknown. Several theoretical explanations exist, including effects on bone cells and matrix synthesis.[148] In addition, heparin is a potent inhibitor of crystal aggregation and is also an activator of bone collagenase.[149] It is tempting to compare the effects of heparin therapy with the skeletal demineralization that occurs in systemic mastocytosis,[2,147] since mast cells contain heparin. Thus, heparin could play a role in urticaria pigmentosa and in the bone loss in renal-disease patients on long-term dialysis who require heparin before each dialysis. Moreover, mast cells may be increased in the bone of patients with postmenopausal or senile osteoporosis.[90,149a,150]

NEOPLASTIC BONE DISEASE

Myelomatosis and diffuse bone neoplasia can produce clinical and radiological features of osteoporosis leading to pathological fractures, particularly of the vertebrae but also of long bones. These fractures obviously indicate an impairment of the mechanical stability of the bone. There is evidence that tumors produce bone-resorbing substances that might be responsible for these effects. Prostaglandins, particularly of the E series, are one group of such bone-resorbing substances, and some patients with hypercalcemia due to malignancy respond to treatment with inhibitors of prostaglandin synthesis, such as indomethacin.[151] Other resorbing substances include the so-called osteoclast-activating factors (OAF), which may be peptides and which have been described from myeloma cells and other sources.[152]

MONOCYTIC LEUKEMIA

These patients deserve mention because they may exhibit a triad of changes that may be related, i.e., osteoporosis, increased excretion of lysozyme, and hypokalemia. The problem has been little studied, and, although direct involvement by neoplasm is a possible cause of the osteoporosis, it is interesting to recall that lysozyme, the product of the malignant monocytes, is thought to play some role in calcification,[153] possibly as an inhibitor of proteolytic enzyme activity. Furthermore, since bone extracellular fluid has been claimed to have a high concentration of potassium,[154] it is possible that hypokalemia interferes with bone metabolism by lowering bone extracellular-fluid potassium.

OTHER CAUSES

Smoking

There is some evidence that women who smoke have less bone and a higher incidence of vertebral crush fractures than age-matched nonsmoking controls.[155,156] Nutritional or constitutional factors could play a role; thus, smoking is associated with a premature menopause, low ascorbic acid levels, and a mild acidosis in those patients with impaired pulmonary function. Obesity seems to protect against osteoporosis in smokers, and it is possible that this is related to the enhanced estrogen production, perhaps by adipose tissue itself,[157,158] associated with obesity.[159]

Disappearing Bones

Rarely, part of the skeleton may disappear completely and be replaced by fibrous tissue.[160] This remarkable condition usually affects one or more limb bones, and there may be a history of fracture or injury. It may be an extreme form of Sudeck's atrophy, and synonyms are "phantom bones" or massive osteolysis. The cause is unknown.

Transitory or Regional Migratory Osteoporosis

This is another uncommon, poorly understood condition in which a painful and localized loss of bone occurs, usually in the upper femurs but also in other sites. Reversal usually occurs. There may be more than one form, and there is evidence of an association with type IV hyperlipoproteinemia.[161,162]

Mast-Cell Disease

In urticaria pigmentosa, bone loss sometimes occurs, and there are increased numbers of mast cells.[163] Mast cells are said to be increased in some patients with postmenopausal osteoporosis[90] and also in chronic renal failure. Since mast cells contain heparin, it is possible that the mechanism of any bone loss is analogous to that caused by heparin therapy, as described earlier.

MANAGEMENT

The treatment objectives are to relieve symptoms and to prevent recurrence of fractures. Neither of these desired benefits is easy to attribute to any given treatment so far tried. Furthermore, the evaluation of therapeutic measures aimed at an increase in bone mineral mass is also not straightforward.

GENERAL MEASURES

The patient who presents with fractures or pain should be investigated in sufficient depth to exclude remediable associated disease.

Treatment of fractures is beyond the scope of this discussion. As far as possible, bed rest and immobilization should be kept to a minimum, not only because they exacerbate bone loss but also because, in the elderly, they lead to a bedbound state. Orthopedic braces and corsets sometimes offer relief, analgesics are helpful, and physical therapy can hasten rehabilitation.

General dietary advice is important in order to ensure adequate intakes of vitamins C and D and calcium. In view of the high incidence of borderline vitamin D deficiency, at least in the United Kingdom, it is reasonable to advocate supplements of vitamin D (1000 U per day), together with a pint of milk a day.

SPECIFIC MEASURES

A large number of different therapeutic regimens have been proposed for the treatment of osteoporosis, a sure indication of their unsatisfactory nature. The purpose of treatment is to prevent continuing bone loss and, if possible, to restore bone mass, thereby reducing the risk of further fracture.

Theoretical Aspects

Among the problems in finding an effective drug treatment, four are particularly important. First, an effective agent must be capable of increasing the rate of bone formation relative to that of bone destruction so that bone loss is slowed down or reversed. However, as described previously, there exists a poorly understood but extremely effective mechanism for linking rates of bone formation to rates of resorption,[164] so that there are no proven ways in which these rates can be dissociated and turned to therapeutic advantage. Thus the short-term improvements in calcium balance claimed for each new drug have usually failed to be maintained over the long run. The second problem is related in that there is much evidence to suggest that bone loss is usually irreversible. The notable exception is the acute loss due to immobilization (e.g., after fractures), which does reverse. The reason for the irreversibility is not clear, although it has been proposed that once individual spicules of trabecular bone have disappeared completely, there is no structure left on which new bone can be deposited.

The third problem is concerned with assessment of therapeutic benefit. The methods of measuring bone mass need to be very precise in order to measure the very small changes that would represent a beneficial result, and individual patients need to be studied for prolonged periods in order to assess the results. One year is a minimum and 5 to 15 years the ideal. Even if improvements in the quantity of bone can be demonstrated, it would still require a long-term trial involving hundreds, if not thousands, of patients in order to show a convincing reduction in symptoms or in fracture rate. Most studies have not been properly controlled, and very rarely have they been conducted on a double-blind basis, so that the symptomatic benefits claimed are generally due to the underlying natural history of the disorder plus a possible placebo effect rather than to the drug used. Fourth, the currently used animal models for osteoporosis on which drugs might be evaluated leave much to be desired. Most have serious flaws in terms of mimicking human disease. At best, they may help in understanding the pharmacology of the drugs; at worst, they can be frankly misleading.

Drugs

The most popular current regimens are estrogen to reduce bone loss or a combination of fluoride, calcium, and vitamin D to restore bone mass. Others that have been used are calcium supplements (oral and parenteral), phosphate, vitamin D and its metabolites, diphosphonates, calcitonin, androgens and anabolic steroids, and combinations thereof. There is no evidence that any of these regimens relieve symptoms and reduce the incidence of further fractures.

Estrogens. One of the current rationales for giving estrogens to postmenopausal women is that they should prevent bone loss associated with declining ovarian function. There is now reasonable evidence that this occurs. Early but uncontrolled studies[165] and recent long-term follow-ups[73] have suggested that vertebral fracture rate and loss of height might be reduced. Several other studies have now shown that estrogens reduce bone loss and may even increase bone mass whether started soon after the menopause[68,138] or several years later.[70,71,166]

Oral contraceptives also seem to increase bone mass,[167] and there is evidence that multiparity may protect against subsequent bone loss.[83,167]

Estrogens are thought to act mainly by reducing bone resorption, and they do reverse the rise in fasting urine calcium levels associated with the menopause.[5] They increase calcium retention in the short term, but there is a subsequent compensatory diminution in bone formation, so that a negative calcium balance may return.[76] In one study,[168] the estrogens appeared most effective in those patients showing the least change in plasma cortisol.

Although there are other medical grounds for advocating temporary or permanent estrogen replacement after the menopause, particularly if this occurs early (e.g., after surgical oophorectomy), the hazards have yet to be fully assessed. Those of greatest concern are the occurrence of thromboembolism and of genital or mammary neoplasia, but the risks, if any, in the postmenopausal population are still uncertain.[169-174]

Various treatment regimens have been advocated, but cyclic administration of ethinyl estradiol (50 μg per day), given for 3 of every 4 weeks, is becoming a common mode of therapy.

Fluoride, Calcium, and Vitamin D. Fluoride increases bone formation and in high doses can lead to skeletal fluorosis. At doses of 50–150 mg per day, new bone is laid down but does not mineralize well unless calcium and vitamin D supplements are given as well.

Striking increases in radiological density of the spine can be demonstrated in patients with osteoporosis on a regimen such as sodium fluoride (50 mg daily), oral calcium (1 g per day), and vitamin D (50,000 IU twice per week),[175,176] but it is not certain whether this new bone is as mechanically sound as normal bone. Moreover, numerous side effects occur, particularly in joints, so that this approach, although promising, should still be considered experimental.

Vitamin D and Its Metabolites. Since the discovery of biologically active metabolites of vitamin D, namely 1,25-dihydroxyvitamin D and its analogue, 1α-hydroxycholecalciferol, there has been interest in using them to treat osteoporosis. There is little evidence in man that osteoporosis itself is due to deficiency of vitamin D metabolites, although it is not unreasonable to propose that with aging, defective production of 1,25-$(OH)_2$-D_3 or defective target-organ responses in the intestine could account for the fall in calcium absorption with age, which in turn might be responsible for the gradual loss of bone with age. Several reports have shown that small doses of these 1α-hydroxylated derivatives of vitamin D (1–2 μg per day) increase calcium absorption in the elderly.[177]

There is little reason to believe or evidence to show, however, that this increase in calcium absorption would lead to an increase in bone mass, although if given early enough, it might prevent bone loss. Some of the claims for increases in bone mass may include responses in patients who have significant osteomalacia.[177] The idea of using these metabolites in conjunction with other therapy, e.g., fluoride, to increase bone matrix production and perhaps the use of calcitonin to reduce bone resorption offers some theoretical advantages, although the treatment regimens would then become rather complex. There have been encouraging preliminary results combining 1α-hydroxycholecalciferol with estrogens in reducing metacarpal bone loss in osteoporotic women.[178]

Calcium Supplements. Given orally or intravenously, calcium supplements have been advocated on the grounds that they not only provide a source of calcium but also reduce bone resorption by suppressing parathyroid secretion. There seems little to lose by offering all patients an adequate calcium intake of at least 1 g per day by adding supplements if necessary. Moreover, there is some evidence that oral supplements can reduce bone loss in postmenopausal females (Fig. 71-8).[166,179]

There has also been considerable interest in the effects of parenteral administration of calcium in the form of prolonged infusions over many days. This regimen has been reported to give positive calcium balances that may continue for many months after the infusions stop and is associated with relief of symptoms.[180,181] Many doubts about these effects have arisen as a result of subsequent experiments, and the beneficial effects are now being questioned.[182] There are reports, however, that calcium infusions relieve bone pain in other situations, e.g., in Paget's disease.

Phosphate Supplements. Phosphate therapy has been given on the grounds that it may stimulate bone formation and enhance collagen synthesis as well as reduce bone resorption. High doses of phosphate can be associated with secondary hyperparathyroidism, however, and there is little evidence for a beneficial effect in postmenopausal osteoporosis.[183] Phosphate was ineffective at preventing bone loss due to acute immobilization in healthy adults.[139]

Androgens. Androgens have been advocated in elderly males in much the same way as estrogens have in females. Pharmacologic doses do lead to positive nitrogen balance and short-term positive calcium balances, but they have virilizing side effects, and their long-term value in increasing bone mass and reducing fracture rate remains uncertain.[73]

Anabolic Steroids. Anabolic steroids (e.g., norethandrolone) are similar in action to androgens but are less virilizing. They are also of unproven long-term value and have lost most of their former popularity.

Calcitonin. Calcitonin offers an attractive treatment since it reduces bone resorption, but there is no evidence in osteoporotic patients that it increases bone mass in the long term, presumably because bone formation is reduced to a corresponding extent.[184,185]

Parathyroid Hormone. Recently, low doses of parathyroid hormone have been shown to produce positive calcium balances over a period of 6 months or more in osteoporotic patients.[186] There is an increase in intestinal calcium absorption, presumably accompanied by an increased deposition of calcium in bone. If these observations are borne out by further work, this approach alone or in combination with other therapy may represent a significant advance.

Growth Hormone. Growth hormone has been shown to increase bone formation in experimental animals[187] but has not been subjected to clinical trials.

Diphosphonates. Diphosphonates reduce bone resorption, but again, evidence suggests that bone formation is also diminished.[188] Saville and Heaney[189] have demonstrated a reduction in both bone formation and bone resorption rate in osteoporotic patients given diphosphonates. With the compound currently in use (sodium etidronate), it therefore seems unlikely that bone mass can be increased or fracture rate reduced, but it is possible that other compounds or combinations with other agents might achieve this.

PREVENTION OF OSTEOPOROSIS

In view of the scale of the problem and its importance in social and economic terms, the question of preventing osteoporosis is a pertinent one. With increased medical screening programs, it is likely that increased numbers of patients at risk will be recognized. What should be done? At present, there is insufficient evidence to indicate that any one treatment is satisfactory for asymptomatic patients with osteoporosis. Simple measures such as ensuring adequate intakes of calcium and vitamin D and encouraging physical activity, together with, in some instances, the cautious use of estrogens, can be advocated.

A wider question is whether one should seek out patients potentially at risk and offer them prophylactic therapy. This seems not only impracticable but also unwise at the present time, because no therapy has been satisfactorily proven to be effective. However, potentially useful therapies are going to have to be studied on large numbers of patients over long periods of time if any progress is to be made, and centers with an interest in osteoporosis have a responsibility to attempt to answer some of these questions.

REFERENCES

1. Iskrant, A. P., Smith, R. W., Jr.: Osteoporosis in women 45 years and over related to subsequent fractures. *Public Health Rep. 84:* 33–38, 1969.
2. Avioli, L. V., Osteoporosis: Pathogenesis and Therapy. In Avioli, L. V., Krane, S. M. (eds) *Metabolic Bone Disease*, *Vol. I.* New York, Academic Press, 1977, pp. 307–385.
3. Morgan, D. B.: Ageing and osteoporosis, in particular spinal osteoporosis. *Clin. Endocrinol. Metab. 2:* 187-201, 1973.
4. Morgan, D. B.: Osteomalacia, Renal Osteodystrophy, and Osteoporosis. Springfield, Charles C Thomas, 1973, pp. 248-257.
5. Nordin, B. E. C.: Metabolic Bone and Stone Disease. Baltimore, Williams and Wilkins Company, 1973.
6. Paterson, C. R.: Metabolic Disorders of Bone. Oxford, Blackwell Scientific Publications, 1974.
7. Barzel, U. S.: Osteoporosis, New York, Grune & Stratton, 1970.
8. Thomson, D. L., Frame B.: Involutional osteopenia. Current concepts. *Ann. Intern. Med. 85:* 789-803, 1976.
9. Fourman, P., Royer, P.: Calcium metabolism and the bone, ed. 2. Oxford and Edinburgh, Blackwell Scientific Publication, 1968.
10. Meema, H. E., Meema, S.: Microradioscopic bone structure of the hand in thyrotoxicosis, renal osteodystrophy and acromegaly. In Frame, B., Parfitt, A. M., Duncan, H. (eds.): Clinical Aspects of Metabolic Bone Disease. Amsterdam, Excerpta Medica, 1973, pp. 10-19.
11. Singh, M., Riggs, B. L., Beabout, J. W. et al.: Femoral trabecular pattern index for evaluation of spinal osteoporosis. *Ann. Intern. Med. 77:* 63-67, 1972.
12. Horsman, A.: Bone mass. In Nordin, B. E. C. (ed.): Calcium Phosphate and Magnesium Metabolism. London, Churchill Livingstone, 1976, chap. 10, pp. 357-404.
13. Smith, D. M., Khairi, M. R. A., Johnston, C. C., Jr.: The loss of bone mineral with ageing and its relationship to risk of fracture. *J. Clin. Invest. 56:* 311-318, 1975.
13a. Smith, R. W., Goeller, E. G., Knutson, L.: Skeletal involution of ageing. Relationships of vertebral, metacarpal and femoral changes. *J. Lab. Clin. Med, 64:* 1004, 1964.
14. Cameron, J. R., Sorenson, J.: Measurement of bone mineral in vivo: An improved method. *Science 142:* 230-232, 1963.
15. Meema, H. E., Meema, S.: Cortical bone mineral density versus cortical thickness in diagnosis of osteoporosis: A roentgenologic densitometric study. *J. Am. Geriatr. Soc. 17:* 120-141, 1969.
16. Ellis, H. A., Peart, K. M.: Quantitative observations on mineralized and non-mineralized bone in the iliac crest. *J. Clin. Pathol. 25:* 277-286, 1972.
17. Cohn, S. H., Ellis, K. J., Wallach, S.: In vivo neutron activation analysis. *Am. J. Med. 57:* 683-686, 1974.
18. Catto, G. R. D., MacLeod, M., Pelc, B., Kodicek, E. 1αHydroxycholecalciferol: A treatment for renal bone disease. *Br. Med. J. 1:* 12-14, 1975.
19. Dent, C. E., Friedman, M.: Idiopathic juvenile osteoporosis. *Q. J. Med. 34:* 177, 1965.
20. Jowsey, J., Johnson, K. A.: Juvenile osteoporosis: Bone findings in seven patients. *J. Pediatr. 81:* 511–517, 1972.
21. Dequeker, J.: Bone Loss in Normal and Pathological Conditions. Leuven, Leuven University Press, 1972.
22. Dequeker, J.: Bone and ageing. *Ann. Rheum. Dis. 34:* 100-115, 1975.
23. Doyle, F.: Involutional osteoporosis. *Clin. Endocrinol. Metab. 2:* 187-201, 1973.
24. Garn, S. M.: The Earlier Gain and the Later Loss of Cortical Bone. Springfield, Charles C Thomas, 1970.
25. Garn, S. M., Rohmann, C. G., Wagner, B.: Bone loss as a general phenomenon in man. *Fed. Proc. 26:* 1729-1736, 1967.
26. Adams, P., Davies, G. T., Sweetnam, P.: Osteoporosis and the effects of ageing on bone mass in elderly men and women. *Q. J. Med. 39:* 601-615, 1970.
27. Newton-John, H. F., Morgan, D. B.: Osteoporosis: Disease or senescence? *Lancet 1:* 232-233, 1968.
28. Newton-John, H. F., Morgan, D. B.: The loss of bone with age, osteoporosis and fractures. *Clin. Orthop. 71:* 229-252, 1970.
29. Doyle, F. H.: Radiologic assessment of endocrine effects on bone. *Radiol. Clin. North Am. 5:* 289-302, 1967.
30. Trotter, M., Broman, G. E., Peterson, R. R.: Densities of bones of white and negro skeletons. *J. Bone Joint Surg. 42A:* 50–58, 1960.
31. Mazess, R. B., Jones, R.: Weight and density of Sadlermint Eskimo long bones. *Hum. Biol. 44:* 537-548, 1972.
32. Smith, R. W., Jr., Rizek, J.: Epidemiologic studies of osteoporosis in women of Puerto Rico and southwestern Michigan with special reference to age, race, national origin and to other related or associated findings. *Clin. Orthop. 45:* 31-48, 1966.
33. Saville, P. D.: The syndrome of spinal osteoporosis. *Clin. Endocrinol. Metabol. 2:* 177-185, 1973.
34. Doyle, F., Brown, J., Lachance, C.: Relationship between bone mass and muscle weight. *Lancet 1:* 391-393, 1970.
35. McConkey, B., Fraser, G. M., Bligh, A. S.: Transparent skin and osteoporosis. *Lancet 1:* 693-695, 1963.
36. McConkey, B., Walton, K. W., Carney, S. A., Lawrence, J. C., Ricketts, C. R.: Significance of the occurrence of transparent skin. *Ann. Rheum. Dis. 26:* 291, 1967.
37. Meema, H. E., Reid, D. B. W.: The relationship between skin and cortical bone thickness in old age with special reference to osteoporosis and diabetes mellitus: A roentgenographic study. *J. Gerontol. 24:* 28-32, 1969.
38. Kivirikko, K. I.: Urinary excretion of hydroxyproline in health and disease. *Int. Rev. Connect. Tiss. Res. 5:* 93, 1970.
39. Dequeker, J., Merlevede, W.: Collagen content and collagen extractability pattern of adult human trabecular bone according to age, sex and amount of bone mass. *Biochem. Biophys. Acta. 244:* 410-420, 1971.
40. Jowsey, J., Kelly, P. J., Riggs, B. L. et al: Quantitative microradiographic studies of normal and osteoporotic bone. *J. Bone Joint Surg. 47A:* 785-806, 1965.
41. Frost, H. M.: Tetracycline-based histological analysis of bone remodelling. *Calcif. Tissue Res. 3:* 211-237, 1969.
42. Bell, N. H.: Dynamics of bone metabolism. *Ann. Rev. Med. 18:* 299, 1967.
43. Frost, H. M.: Bone Dynamics in Osteoporosis and Osteomalacia. Springfield, Charles C Thomas, 1966.
44. Schenk, R. K., Merz, W. A.: Histologisch-morphometrische Untersuchungen über Altersatrophie und senile Osteoporose in der Spongiosa des Beckenkammes. *Deutsch. Med. Wochenschr. 94:* 206, 1969.
45. Rasmussen, H., Bordier, P.: The Physiological and Cellular Basis of Metabolic Bone Disease. Baltimore, Williams and Wilkins Co., 1974.
46. Aaron, J. E., Gallagher, J. C., Anderson, J. et al.: Frequency of osteomalacia and osteoporosis in fractures of the proximal femur. *Lancet 1:* 229-233, 1974.
47. Faccini, J. M., Exton–Smith, A. N., Boyde, A.: Disorders of bone and fracture of proximal femur. *Lancet 1:* 1089–1092, 1976.
48. Lund, B., Sorensen, O. H., Christensen, A. B.: 25-Hydroxycholecalciferol and fractures of the proximal femur. *Lancet 2:* 300-302, 1975.
49. Gallagher, J. C., Riggs, L., Eisman, J. et al: Impaired intestinal calcium absorption in postmenopausal osteoporosis: Possible role of vitamin D metabolites and PTH. *Clin. Res. 24:* 360A, 1976.
50. Jowsey, J., Gershon-Cohen, J. L.: Clinical and experimental osteoporosis. In Blackwood, H. J. J. (ed.): *Bone and Tooth.* Oxford, Pergamon, 1964, pp. 35-44.
51. Smith, R. W., Frame, B.: Concurrent axial and appendicular osteoporosis. *N. Engl. J. Med. 273:* 73-78, 1965.

52. Hurxthal, L. M., Vose, C. P.: The relation of dietary calcium intake to radiographic bone density in normal and osteoporotic persons. *Calcif. Tissue Res. 4:* 245, 1969.

53. Nordin, B. E. C.: Osteomalacia, osteoporosis and calcium deficiency. *Clin. Orthop. 17:* 235-237, 1960.

54. Lutwak, L.: Osteoporosis—a mineral deficiency disease? *J. Am. Diet. Assoc. 44:* 173-175, 1964.

55. Bassan, J., Frame, B., Frost, H.: Osteoporosis: A review of pathogenesis and treatment. *Ann. Intern. Med. 58:* 539-550, 1970.

56. Riggs, B. L., Kelly, P. J., Kinney, V. R. et al.: Calcium deficiency and osteoporosis. *J. Bone Joint Surg. 49A:* 915-924, 1967.

57. Birge, S. J., Jr., Keutman, H. T., Cuatrecasas, P., Whedon, G. D.: Osteoporosis, intestinal lactase deficiency and low dietary calcium intake. *New Engl. J. Med. 276:* 445-448, 1967.

58. Editorial: Osteoporosis and primary intestinal lactase deficiency. *Nutr. Rev. 25:* 274-276, 1967.

59. Chalmers, J., Ho, K. C.: Geographical variations in senile osteoporosis. *J. Bone Joint Surg. 52B:* 667-675, 1970.

60. Avioli, L. V., McDonald, J. E., Singer, R. A., Henneman, P. H.: A new oral isotopic test of calcium absorption. *J. Clin. Invest. 44:* 128-139, 1965.

61. Bullamore, J. R., Gallagher, J. C., Wilkinson, R., Nordin, B. E. C., Marshall, D. H.: Effect of age on calcium absorption. *Lancet 2:* 535-537, 1970.

62. Ireland, P., Fordtran, J. S.: Effect of dietary calcium and age on jejunal calcium absorption in humans studied by intestinal perfusion. *J. Clin. Invest. 52:* 2672-2681, 1973.

63. Spencer, H., Menczel, J., Lewin, I. et al.: Absorption of calcium in osteoporosis. *Am. J. Med. 37:* 223-234, 1964.

64. Berlyne, C. M., Ben-Ari, J., Kushelevsky, A. et al.: The aetiology of senile osteoporosis: Secondary hyperparathyroidism due to renal failure. *Q. J. Med. 44:* 505-521, 1975.

65. Cahill, G. F.: *J. A. M. A. 227:* 448, 1974.

66. Lemann, J., Litzow, J. R., Lennon, E. J.: Studies on the mechanism by which chronic metabolic acidosis augments urinary calcium excretion in man. *J. Clin. Invest. 46:* 1318, 1967.

67. Aitken, J. M., Hart, D. M., Anderson, J. B., Lindsay, R., Smith, D. A., Speirs, C. F.: Osteoporosis after oophorectomy for nonmalignant disease in premenopausal women. *Br. Med. J. 2:* 325-328, 1973.

68. Aitken, J. M., Hart, D. M., Lindsay, R.: Oestrogen replacement therapy for prevention of osteoporosis after oophorectomy. *Br. Med. J. 3:* 515-518, 1973.

69. Davis, M. E., Stranjord, N. M., Lanzl, L. H.: Estrogens and the ageing process. The detection, prevention and retardation of osteoporosis. *J. A. M. A. 196:* 219, 1966.

70. Meema, H. E., Meema, S.: Prevention of postmenopausal osteoporosis by hormone treatment of the menopause. *Can. Med. Assoc. J. 99:* 248–251, 1968.

71. Meema, S., Bunker, M. L., Meema, H. E.: Preventive effect of estrogen on postmenopausal bone loss. *Arch. Intern. Med. 135:* 1436-1440, 1975.

72. Henneman, P. H.: Treatment of postmenopausal osteoporosis with gonadal steroids. *Semin. Drug Treat.:* 15-19, 1972.

73. Gordan, G. S., Picchi, J., Roof, B. S.: Antifracture efficacy of long-term estrogens for osteoporosis. *Trans. Assoc. Am. Physicians 86:* 326-332, 1973.

74. Young, M. M., Jasani, C., Smith, D. A. et al.: Some effects of ethinyl oestradiol on calcium and phosphorus metabolism in osteoporosis. *Clin. Sci. 34:* 417, 1968.

75. Riggs, B. L., Jowsey, J., Kelley, P. J. et al.: Effects of sex hormones on bone primary osteoporosis. *J. Clin. Invest. 48:* 1065-1072, 1969.

76. Riggs, B. L., Jowsey, J., Goldsmith, R. S. et al.: Short- and long-term effects of estrogen and synthetic anabolic hormones in postmenopausal osteoporosis. *J. Clin. Invest. 51:* 1659-1663, 1972.

77. Heaney, R. P.: A unified concept of osteoporosis. *Am. J. Med. 39:* 877, 1965.

78. Jasani, C., Nordin, B. E. C., Smith, D. A. et al.: Spinal osteoporosis and the menopause. *Proc. R. Soc. Med. 58:* 441-444, 1965.

79. Hossain, M., Smith, D. A., Nordin, B. E. C.: Parathyroid activity and postmenopausal osteoporosis. *Lancet 1:* 809, 1970.

80. Pak, Y. C., Stewart, A., Kaplan, R. et al.: Photon absorptiometric analysis of bone density in primary hyperparathyroidism. *Lancet 2:* 7-8, 1975.

81. Riggs, B. L., Arnaud, C. D., Jowsey, J. et al.: Parathyroid function in primary osteoporosis. *J. Clin. Invest. 52:* 181-184, 1973.

82. Robertson, W. G., Morgan, D. B.: The distribution of urinary calcium excretions in normal persons and stone-formers. *Clin. Chim. Acta 37:* 503-508, 1972.

83. Smith, R. W., Jr.: Dietary and hormonal factors in bone loss. *Fed. Proc. 26:* 1737-1746, 1967.

84. Frantz, A. G., Rabkin, M. T.: Effects of estrogen and sex difference on secretion of human growth hormone. *J. Clin. Endocrinol. Metab. 25:* 1470-1480, 1965.

85. Riggs, B. L., Ryan, R. J., Wahner, H. W. et al.: Serum concentrations of estrogen, testosterone and gonadotropins in osteoporotic and nonosteoporotic post-menopausal women. *J. Clin. Endocrinol. Metab. 36:* 1097-1099, 1973.

85a. Nordin, B. E. C., Horsman, A., Gallagher, J. C.: Effect of various therapies on bone loss in women. In Kuhlencordt, F., Kruse, H. O. (eds.): *Calcium Metabolism, Bone and Metabolic Bone Disease.* Berlin, Springer, 1975, p. 233.

86. Bartizal, F. J., Coulam, C. B., Gaffey, T. A. et al.: Impaired binding of estradiol to target tissue in postmenopausal osteoporosis (PMO): A possible molecular basis for the disease (abstract). *Clin. Res. 23:* 534A, 1975.

87. Heath, H. III, Sizemore, G. W.: Women have lower basal and stimulated plasma calcitonin levels than men. In *Program of the Fifty-Seventh Annual Meeting of Endocrine Society.* 1975, p. 77.

88. Bernstein, D. S., Sadowsky, N., Hegsted, D. M., Guri, C. D., Stare, F. J.: Prevalence of osteoporosis in high and low-fluoride areas in North Dakota. *J. A. M. A. 198:* 499, 1966.

89. Alffram, P. A., Herneborg, J., Nilsson, B. E. R.: The influence of a high fluoride content in the drinking water on the bone mineral mass in man. *Acta Orthop. Scand. 40:* 137, 1969.

90. Frame, B., Nixon, R. K.: Bone marrow factors in osteoporosis. In Barzel, U.S. (ed.): *Osteoporosis.* New York, Grune & Stratton, 1970, pp. 238-250.

91. McKusick, V. A.: *Heritable Disorders of Connective Tissue, ed. 4.* St. Louis, C. V. Mosby, 1972.

92. Garn, S. M., Poznanski, A. K.: Transient and irreversible bone losses. In Barzel, U.S. (ed.): *Osteoporosis.* New York, Grune & Stratton, 1970, p. 114.

93. Lynch, S. R., Seftel, H. C., Wapnick, A. A., Charlton, R. W., Bothwell, T. H.: Some aspects of calcium metabolism in normal and osteoporotic Bantu subjects with special reference to the effects of iron and ascorbic acid depletion. *S. Afr. J. Med. Sci. 35:* 45-56, 1970.

94. Wapnick, A. A., Lynch, S. R., Seftel, H. C., Charlton, R. W., Bothwell, T. H., Jowsey, J.: The effect of siderosis and ascorbic acid depletion on bone metabolism with special reference to osteoporosis in Bantu. *Br. J. Nutr. 25:* 367-376, 1971.

95. Leading Article: Bone and joint changes in haemochromatosis. *Br. Med. J. 3:* 191-192, 1969.

96. Saville, P. D.: Changes in bone mass with age and alcoholism. *J. Bone Joint Surg. 47A:* 492-499, 1965.

97. Nilsson, B. E., Westlin, N. E.: Changes in bone mass in alcoholics. *Clin. Orthop. Rel. Res. 90:* 229-245, 1973.

98. Nilsson, B. E.: Spinal osteoporosis and femoral neck fracture. *Clin. Orthop. 68,* 93-95 1970.

99. Haussler, M. R.: Biochemical, physiological and clinical applications of radiological assay for 1,25-dihydroxyvitamin D. In Norman, A., et al. (eds.): Vitamin D, Berlin, W. de Gruytel, 1977, 473–482.

100. Atkinson, P. J., West, R. R.: Loss of skeletal calcium in lactating women. *J. Obstet. Gynaecol. Br. Commonw. 77:* 555-560, 1970.

101. Walker, A. R. P.: The human requirement of calcium: Should low intakes be supplemented? *Am. J. Clin. Nutr. 25:* 518-530, 1972.

102. Innacone, A., Gabrilone, J. L., Braham, S. A., Soffer, L. J.: Osteoporosis in Cushing's syndrome. *Ann. Intern. Med. 52:* 570, 1960.

103. Gallagher, J. C., Aaron, J., Horsman, A., Wilkinson, R., Nordin, B. E. C.: Corticosteroid osteoporosis. *Clin. Endocrinol. Metab. 2:* 355-368, 1973.

104. Jowsey, J., Gershon-Cohen, J.: Effect of dietary calcium levels on production and reversal of experimental osteoporosis in cats. *Proc. Soc. Exp. Biol. Med. 116:* 437-441, 1964.

105. Goldring, S., Krane, S. M.: Metabolic bone disease. In Stanbury, J. (ed.) *Thyroid Disorders.* (in press).

106. Krane, S. M., Brownwell, G. L., Stanbury, J. B., Corrigan, H.: The effect of thyroid disease on calcium metabolism in man. *J. Clin. Invest. 35:* 874, 1956.

107. Kivirikko, K. I., Laitinen, O., Lamberg, B. A.: Value of urine and

serum hydroxyproline in the diagnosis of thyroid disease. *J. Clin. Endocrinol. 25:* 1347, 1965.

108. Mundy, G. R., Shapiro, J. L., Bardelin, J. G., Canalis, E. M., Raisz, L. G.: Direct stimulation of bone resorption by thyroid hormones. *J. Clin. Invest. 58:* 529-534, 1976.

109. Fraser, S. A., Anderson, J. B., Smith, D. A., Wilson, G. M.: Osteoporosis and fractures following thyrotoxicosis. *Lancet I:* 981-983, 1971.

110. Castro, J. H., Genuth, S. M., Klein, L.: Comparative response to parathyroid hormone in hyperthyroidism and hypothyroidism. *Metabolism 24:* 839-848, 1975.

111. Parfitt, A. M., Dent, C. E.: Hyperthyroidism and hypercalcaemia. *Q. J. Med. N.S. 39:* 171-187, 1970.

112. Riggs, B. L., Randall, R. V., Wahner, H. W., Jowsey, J., Kelly, P. J., Singh, M.: The nature of the metabolic bone disorder in acromegaly. *J. Clin. Endocrinol. Metab. 34,* 911-918, 1972.

113. Aloia, J. F., Roginsky, M. S., Jowsey, J., Dombrowski, C. S., Skukla, K. K., Cohn, S. H.: Skeletal metabolism and body composition of acromegaly, *J. Clin. Endocrinol. Metab. 35:* 543–551, 1972.

114. Corvilain, J., Abramow, M.: Growth hormone and renal control of plasma phosphate. *J. Clin. Endocrinol. 34:* 452-459, 1972.

115. Bell, N. H., Bartter, F. C.: Studies of ^{47}Ca metabolism in acromegaly. *J. Clin. Endocrinol. 27:* 178-184, 1967.

116. Albright, F., Reifenstein, E. C.: The Parathyroid Glands and Metabolic Bone Disease. Baltimore, Williams and Wilkins, 1948.

117. Hernberg, C. A.: Skelettveränderungen bei Diabetes mellitus der Erwachsenen. *Acta Med. Scand. 143:* 1; 1952.

118. Menczel, J., Makin, M., Robin, G., Jaye, I., Naor, E.: Prevalence of diabetes mellitus in Jerusalem. Its association with pre-senile osteoporosis. *Israel J. Med. Sci. 8:* 918, 1972.

119. Jurist, J. M.: In vivo determinations of the elastic response in bone. II: Ulnar resonant frequency in osteoporotic, diabetic and normal subjects. *Phys. Med. Biol. 15:* 427-434, 1972.

120. Levin, M. E., Boisseau, V. C., Avioli, L. V.: Effects of diabetes mellitus on bone mass in juvenile and adult onset diabetes. *New Eng J Med 294:* 241–245, 1976.

121. Pederson, J.: In The Pregnant Diabetic and Her New Born: Problems and Management. Baltimore, Williams and Wilkins, 1967, p. 60.

122. Wu, K., Schubeck, K., Frost, H. M., Villanueva, A.: Haversian bone formation rates determined by a new method in a mastodon and in human diabetes mellitus and osteoporosis. *Calc. Tiss. Res. 6:* 204-219, 1970.

123. Parfitt, A. M., Nassim, J. R., Collins, J., Hilb, A.: Metabolic studies in a case of fibrocystic disease of the pancreas. *Arch. Dis. Child. 37:* 25-33, 1962.

124. Condon, J. R., Nassim, J. R., Millard, F. J. C., Hilbe, A., Stainthorpe, E. M.: Calcium and phosphorus metabolism in relation to lactose tolerance. *Lancet 1:* 1027–1029, 1970.

125. Güller, R., Kayasseh, L., Haas, H. G.: Osteoporose und Laktoseintoleranz. *Schweiz. Med. Wochensch. 103:* 107-109, 1973.

126. Morgan, D. B., Pulvertaft, C. N., Fourman, P.: Effects of age on the loss of bone after gastric surgery. *Lancet 2:* 772–773, 1966.

127. Fujita, T., Okuyama, Y., Handa, N., Orimo, H., Ohata, M., Yoshikawa, M. et al.: Age-dependent bone loss after gastrectomy. *J. Am. Geriatr. Soc. 19:* 840-846, 1971.

128. Skinner, R. K., Long, R. G., Sherlock, S., Wills, M. R.: 25-Hydroxylation of vitamin D in primary biliary cirrhosis. *Lancet 1:* 720-721, 1977.

129. Whelton, M. J., Kehayoglou, A. K., Agnew, J. E., Turnberg, L. A., Sherlock, S.: ^{47}Calcium absorption in parenchymatous and biliary liver disease. *Gut 1:* 987-983, 1971.

130. Owen, M. E., Triffit, J. T., Melick, R. A.: Albumin in bone. In Vaughan, J., Soggnaes, R. (eds.): Hard Tissue Growth Repair and Remineralisation. *Ciba Found. Symp. 11.* (N. S.) 1973.

131. Triffit, J. T., Gebauer, Owen, M. E.: Synthesis by the liver of a glycoprotein which is concentrated in bone matrix. In Nielsen, S. P., Hjorting-Hansen, E. (eds.) Calcified Tissues. Copenhagen, Fadl's Forlag, 1975, pp. 437–442.

132. Coburn, J. W., Brickman, A. S., Kurokawa, K., Massry, S. G., Bethune, J. E., Harrison, H. E., Norman, A. W.: Action of 1,25 (OH)$_2$ cholecalciferol in normal man and patients with hypophosphataemic resistant rickets, pseudohypoparathyroidism and uraemia. In Taylor, S. (ed.): Endocrinology. London, Heinemann, 1974.

133. Mawer, E. B., Backhouse, J., Taylor, C. M., Lumb, G. A., Stanbury, S. W.: Failure of formation of 1,25-dihydroxycholecalciferol in chornic renal insufficiency. *Lancet 1:* 626-628, 1973.

134. Bordier, P. J., Tun Chot, S., Eastwood, J. B., Fournier, A., de Wardener, H. E.: Lack of histological evidence of vitamin D abnormality in the bones of anephric patients. *Clin. Sci. 44:* 33-41, 1973.

135. Parfitt, A. M., Massry, S. G., Winfield, A. C.: Osteopenia and fractures occurring during maintenance hemodialysis. *Clin. Orthop. 87:* 287-302, 1972.

136. Duncan, H.: Bone dynamics of rheumatoid arthritis treated with adrenal corticosteroids. *Arthritis Rheum. 10:* 216, 1967.

137. Bjelle, A. O., Nilsson, B. E.: Osteoporosis in rheumatoid arthritis. *Calcif. Tissue Res. 5:* 327, 1970.

137a. Saville, P. D., Karmosh, O.: Osteoporosis of rheumatoid arthritis: Influence of age, sex and corticosteroids. *Arthritis Rheum. 10:* 423, 1967.

138. Lindsay, R., Hart, D. M., Aitken, J. M. et al.: Long-term prevention of postmenopausal osteoporosis by oestrogen. *Lancet 2:* 1038-1040, 1976.

138a. Lindsay, R., Kennedy, A. C.: Aspects of bone disease in rheumatoid arthritis. In Kanis, J. A. (ed.): Bone Disease and Calcitonin. Eastbourne, Armour, 1977, pp. 171–179.

139. Hulley, S. B., Vogel, J. M., Donaldson, C. L., Bayers, J. H., Friedman, R. J., Rosen, S. N.: The effect of supplemental oral phosphate on the bone mineral changes during prolonged bed rest. *J. Clin. Invest. 50:* 2506–2518, 1971.

140. Mack, P. B., LaChance, P. L.: Effects of recumbency and space flight on bone density. *Am. J. Clin. Nutr. 20:* 1194, 1967.

141. Whedon, G. D., Lutwak, L., Rambaut, P., Whittle, M., Leach, C., Reid, J. and Smith, M.: Effect of weightlessness on mineral metabolism: Metabolic studies on Skylab orbital space flights. In Pors Nielsen, S., and Hjorting-Hansen, E. (eds.): Calcified Tissues. Copenhagen, Fadl's Forlag, 1975, pp. 423-430.

142. Editorial. Anticonvulsant osteomalacia. *Br. Med. J. 2:* 1340-1341, 1976.

143. Nesbit, M., Krivit, W., Heyn, R., Sharp, H.: Acute and chronic effects of methtrexate on hepatic, pulmonary and skeletal systems. *Cancer 37:* 1048-1054, 1976.

144. Ragab, A. H., Frech, R. S., Vietti, T. J.: Osteoporotic fractures secondary to methotrexate therapy of acute leukaemia in remission. *Cancer 25:* 580-585, 1970.

145. Nevinny, H. B., Hall, T. C.: Prevention of hormone-induced hypercalciuria by use of methotrexate. *Cancer Chemother. Rep. 16,* 305, 1962.

146. Nevinny, H. B., Krant, M. J., Moore, E. W.: Metabolic studies of the effects of methotrexate. *Metabolism 14:* 35, 1965.

147. Griffith, G. C., Nichols, G., Asher, J. D., Flanagan, B.: Heparin osteoporosis. *J. A. M. A. 193:* 91-94, 1965.

148. Avioli, L. V.: Heparin-induced osteopenia. In Bradshaw, R. A., Wessler, S. (eds.): Heparin: Structure, Function, and Clinical Implications. New York, Plenum Press, 1975, pp. 375-388.

149. Harris, E. D., Krane, S. M.: Collagenases. *N. Engl. J. Med. 291:* 557-563, 605-609, 652-661, 1974.

149a. Frame, B., Nixon, R. K.: Bone marrow mast cells in osteoporosis of ageing. *N. Engl. J. Med. 279:* 626, 1968.

150. Kruse, H. P., Kuhlencordt, F., Ringe, J. D.: Correlation of clinical, densitometric and histo-morphometric data in osteoporosis. In Nielsen, S. P., Hjorting-Hansen, E. (eds.): Calcified Tissues. Copenhagen, Fadl's Forlag, 1975, 457-461.

151. Seyberth, H. W., Segre, G. V., Morgan, J. L. et al.: Prostaglandins as mediators of hypercalcemia associated with certain types of cancer. *N. Engl. J. Med. 293:* 1278-1283, 1975.

152. Mundy, G. R., Luben, R. A., Raisz, L. G., Oppenheim, J., Buell: Bone resorbing activity in supernatants from lymphoid cell lines. *N. Engl. J. Med. 290,* 867-871, 1974.

153. Kuettner, K. E., Wezeman, F. H., Simmons, D. J. et al.: Lysozyme in preosseus cartilage. *Lab. Invest. 27,* 324-330, 1972.

154. Neuman, W. F.: The milieu interieur of bone: Claude Bernard revisited. *Fed. Proc. 28:* 1846-1850, 1969.

155. Daniell, H. W.: Osteoporosis of the slender smoker. *Arch. Intern. Med. 136:* 298, 1976.

156. Editorial: Smokers' bones. *Br. J. Med. 3:* 201, 1976.

157. Schindler, A. E., Ebert, A., Friedrich, E.: Conversion of androstenedione to estrone by human fat tissue. *J. Clin. Endocrinol. Metab. 35:* 627-630, 1972.

158. Grodin, J. M., Siiteri, P. K., MacDonald, P. C.: Source of oestro-

gen production in postmenopausal women. *J. Clin. Endocrinol. Metab. 36:* 207-214, 1973.

159. De Waard, F., Baanders van Halewijn, E. A.: Further cytological observations concerning oestrogenic activity in post-menopausal women. *Acta Endocrinol. 38:* 515, 1961.

160. Phillips, R. M., Bush, O. B., Hall, H. D.: Massive osteolysis (phantom bone, disappearing bone). *Oral Surg., Oral Med., Oral Pathol. 34:* 886–896, 1972.

161. Hunder, G. G., Kelley, P. J.: Bone scans in transient osteoporosis. *Ann. Intern. Med. 75:* 134, 1971.

162. Pinals, R. S., Jabbs, J. M.: Type IV hyperlipoproteinaemia and transient osteoporosis. *Lancet 2:* 929, 1972.

163. Ives, D. R., Thompson, D. M.: Urticaria pigmentosa with spinal osteoporosis. *Proc. R. Soc. Med. 66:* 175-176, 1973.

164. Harris, W. H., Heaney, R. P.: Skeletal renewal and metabolic bone disease. *N. Engl. J. Med. 280:* 193-202, 253-259, 303-311, 1969.

165. Wallach, S., Henneman, P. H.: Prolonged estrogen therapy in postmenopausal women. *J. A. M. A. 171:* 1637-1642, 1959.

166. Nordin, B. E. C., Gallagher, J. C., Aaron, J. C. et al.: Post-menopausal osteopenia and osteoporosis. *Front. Horm. Res. 3:* 131-149, 1975.

167. Goldsmith, N. F., Johnston, J. O.: Bone mineral: Effects of oral contraceptives, pregnancy, and lactation. *J. Bone Joint Surg. 57A:* 657-668, 1975.

168. Aitken, J. M., Hall, P. E., Rao, L. G. S. et al.: Hypercortisolaemia and lack of skeletal response to oestrogen in postmenopausal women. *Clin. Endocrinol. 3:* 167-174, 1974.

169. Weiss, N. S., Szekely, D. R., Austin, D. F.: Increasing incidence of endometrial cancer in the United States. *N. Engl. J. Med. 294:* 1259-1262, 1976.

170. Smith, D. C., Prentice, R., Thompson, D. J. et al.: Association of exogenous estrogen and endometrial carcinoma. *N. Engl. J. Med. 293:* 1164-1167, 1975.

171. Weiss, N. S.: Risks and benefits of estrogen use (editorial). *N. Engl. J. Med. 293:* 1200-1202, 1975.

172. Ziel, H. K., Finkle, W. D.: Increased risks of endometrial carcinoma among users of conjugated estrogens. *N. Engl. J. Med. 293:* 1167-1170, 1975.

173. Mack, T. M., Pike, M. C., Henderson, B. E. et al.: Estrogens and endometrial cancer in a retirement community. *N. Engl. J. Med. 294:* 1262-1267, 1976.

174. Gordan, G. S., Greenberg, B. G.: Exogenous estrogens and endometrial cancer. *Postgrad. Med. 59(6):* 66-67, 1976.

175. Riggs, B. L., Jowsey, J., Kelly, P. J., Hoffman, D. L., Arnaud, C. D.: Studies on pathogenesis and treatment in post-menopausal and senile osteoporosis. *Clin. Endocrinol. Metab. 2:* 317-332, 1973.

176. Parsons, V., Mitchell, C. J., Reeve, J., Hesp, R.: The use of fluoride, vitamin D and calcium supplements in the treatment of patients with axial osteoporosis. *Calcif. Tissues Res. 22 (Suppl.):*236–240, 1977.

177. Lund, B., Hjarth, L., Kjaer, I. et al.: Treatment of osteoporosis of ageing with 1α-hydroxycholecalciferol. *Lancet 3:* 1168-1171, 1975.

178. Marshall, D. H., Nordin, B. E. C.: The effect of 1α-hydroxyvitamin D_3 with and without oestrogens on calcium balances and bone loss in post-menopausal women. *Clin. Endocrinol. 7:* 159s–168s, 1977.

179. Riggs, B. L., Jowsey, J., Kelly, P. J. et al.: Effect of oral therapy with calcium and vitamin D in primary osteoporosis. *J. Clin. Endocrinol. Metab. 42:* 1139-1144, 1976.

180. Pak, C. Y. C., Zisman, E., Evens, R. et al.: The treatment of osteoporosis with calcium infusions. Clinical studies. *Am. J. Med. 47:* 7-16, 1969.

181. Jowsey, J., Hoye, R. C., Pak, C. Y. C. et al.: The treatment of osteoporosis with calcium infusions. Evaluation of bone biopsies. *Am. J. Med. 47:* 17-22, 1969.

182. Walton, J., Dominguez, M., Bartter, F. C.: Effect of calcium infusions in patients with post-menopausal osteoporosis. *Metabolism 24:* 849-854, 1975.

183. Goldsmith, R. S.: Treatment of osteoporosis with phosphate. *Semin. Drug Treat. 2:* 35-37, 1972.

184. Wallach, S., Aloia, J., Cohn, S.: Treatment of osteoporosis with calcitonin. *Semin. Drug Treat. 2:* 21-25, 1972.

185. Cohn, S. H., Dombrowski, C. S., Hauser, W. et al.: Effect of porcine calcitonin on calcium metabolism in osteoporosis. *J. Clin. Endocrinol. Metab. 33:* 719-728, 1971.

186. Reeve, J., Hesp, R., Williams, D. et al.: Anabolic effect of low doses of a fragment of human parathyroid hormone on the skeleton in post-menopausal osteoporosis. *Lancet 1:* 1035-1038. 1976.

187. Harris, W. H., Heaney, R. P., Jowsey, J. et al.: Growth hormone: The effect on skeletal renewal in the adult dog. *Calcif. Tiss. Res. 10:* 1-13, 1972.

188. Russell, R. G. G., Fleisch, H.: Pyrophosphate and diphosphonates in skeletal metabolism. *Clin. Orthop. Rel. Res. 108:* 241-263, 1975.

189. Saville, P. D., Heaney, R.: Treatment of osteoporosis with diphosphonates. *Semin. Drug Treat. 2:* 47-50, 1972.

72

Paget's Disease

I. MacIntyre,
Imogen M. A. Evans,
N. J. Y. Woodhouse

INTRODUCTION

Paget's disease is a common disorder of bone, often familial and affecting people mainly of Western European stock. It is characterized by the presence of excessive numbers of osteoclasts and osteoblasts, an increased turnover of bone mineral and collagen, and the formation of structurally weakened bone tissue. The most frequently involved sites are the lumbosacral spine, pelvis, femora, skull, and tibiae. Affected bones are expanded and lose their normal architectural pattern; deformity, bone pain, and fractures are common complications, but occur in only a small proportion of affected individuals. Clinical presentation before the age of 40 is unusual. A similar bone disease, known as hereditary bone dysplasia with hyperphosphatasemia, occurs in young children.

PATHOPHYSIOLOGY

The initial stages of Paget's disease are characterized histologically by evidence of increased bone turnover in the absence of deposition of woven bone. With progression of the disease, lamellar bone, both cortical and cancellous, is replaced by woven bone, the haversian systems disappear, and bone architecture becomes highly disorganized. During this process islands of lamellar bone are left surrounded by large areas of the predominant woven bone. The latter is then replaced by disorganized lamellar bone, giving rise to the characteristic mosaic structure. Eventually, newly deposited woven bone, which is not normally present after the age of 14 or 16 years, or disorganized lamellar bone may comprise anywhere from 20 to 80 percent of the bone tissue. Another characteristic feature of Paget's disease is the increased extent of the osteoid

volume with a normal calcification front. This would seem to indicate that the bone remineralization is not delayed, the increase in osteoid reflecting the accelerated new bone formation.

At the level of the bone cells, the increased osteoid volume is associated with an increased number of active bone surface cells, i.e., osteoblasts and osteoclasts. The osteoclasts, apart from being present in increased numbers, also exhibit marked variation in size and may contain anywhere from a few to over 100 nuclei in a section. Such osteoclasts are the cellular hallmark of Paget's disease. The osteoblasts also vary in size, shape, and staining properties; very large cells with irregularly shaped nuclei are often noted. It is these characteristics that have led some workers to consider Paget's disease as a benign bone neoplasm. The osteocytes are also involved in the disease process and extensive osteocytic osteolysis is seen. Even in the initial stages of the disease, before woven bone has been laid down, a marked increase in osteocytic osteolysis occurs in lamellar bone associated with an increased number of osteoclasts on the overlying bone surface. When Paget's disease "burns out" in any one area, the cellular activity returns to normal but the characteristic architectural abnormalities of the bone persist.[1]

A raised cardiac output is a common finding in patients with radiologically extensive bone disease and this is due to an increase in bone blood flow through dilated arterioles, capillaries, and venous sinuses. Anatomic arteriovenous shunts have not been demonstrated; the raised venous oxygen levels are due to the increased flow of blood through the bone.[2] In addition to the presumed increase in blood flow through bone,[49] a recent report emphasized that much of the increased blood flow to involved areas represents increased cutaneous flow.[50] In patients with a reduced myocardial reserve, extensive Paget's disease may sometimes precipitate high-output congestive cardiac failure.

The turnover of bone mineral may be 20 times greater than normal in extensive Paget's disease, but, provided the rates of bone resorption and formation are equal, calcium balance should be maintained. Sometimes, usually in association with long periods of immobilization, the rate of bone resorption exceeds that of bone formation and the resulting increase in extracellular fluid calcium reduces parathyroid hormone secretion. Hypercalciuria then occurs and the patient goes into negative calcium balance. If the capacity of the kidney to excrete this calcium load is exceeded, hypercalcemia will result.[3] In the later stages of Paget's disease some patients have heavily mineralized and dense bones and presumably have been in positive calcium balance during this mineralization phase.

Serum alkaline phosphatase levels are raised, reflecting the increased bone formation. This enzyme is produced by the osteoblasts that are present in increased numbers and it is also likely that the individual cells are more active in enzyme production in Paget's disease.[4] The levels of alkaline phosphatase correlate well with histologic measurements of active bone formation surface, i.e., that part of the osteoid surface which is covered by active osteoblasts.

Serum acid phosphatase levels are also raised in some patients, particularly in those with extensive disease. This enzyme has a wide tissue distribution but in Paget's disease the increased levels probably result from increased osteoclastic activity.

Urinary peptide-hydroxyproline levels are elevated due to the increased rate of bone collagen synthesis and destruction (turnover). More than 95 percent of the hydroxyproline in the urine is excreted as hydroxyproline-containing peptides which exist in several forms (e.g., di- and tri-peptides and larger-molecular-weight species). The smaller peptides reflect bone resorption, while the larger peptides are associated with an increase in bone formation. Measurement of total urinary hydroxyproline, therefore, reflects bone collagen turnover as a whole, and dialysis or gel filtration is necessary if separate information about bone resorption and formation is required.[5]

Calcium kinetic measurements are also useful in assessing disease activity. Using radioactive isotopes of calcium (^{45}Ca or ^{47}Ca) or strontium (^{85}Sr) or stable strontium, it can be shown that uptake by pagetic bone is increased above normal. Although the rapid bone turnover invalidates the calculation of bone formation rate by this means, the measurements can be regarded as indices of total skeletal calcium turnover, and in this light they may be used to monitor disease activity and response to treatment.

In general, the serum alkaline phosphatase and urinary hydroxyproline levels correlate well, patients with localized Paget's disease having much lower values than those with extensive disease. The levels of alkaline phosphate and urinary hydroxyproline may vary independently, at least to some degree, with the extent of disease being influenced by the degree of osteolytic versus osteosclerotic change. Patients may also have localized active and symptomatic or monostotic Paget's disease with "normal" alkaline phosphatase and hydroxyproline values, as the normal range is relatively large; in such patients clinical examination, isotope scanning, or bone biopsy may reveal activity of the disease.

EPIDEMIOLOGY AND PATHOLOGY

Sir James Paget's elegant account is the first detailed description of the clinical features and natural history of the disease.[6] There are, however, earlier mentions of the same disease under different names. Although Paget's disease has been recognized by medical practitioners for only 100 years, it is now well established that it occurred in ancient times and there are several well documented examples (Fig. 72-1A, B).

Necropsy studies in Germany and England suggest that between 3 and 4 percent of the population over 40 have Paget's disease; the incidence increases with age to reach 10 percent in the ninth decade. These postmortem figures are substantiated by one small population survey of normal men and women.[7] From Collins' data and population statistics it has been estimated that 750,000 people in England and Wales have Paget's disease.[8] Necropsy and population data are not yet available from other countries, but Paget's disease is considered common in Western Europe, Australia, and New Zealand, and less common in North

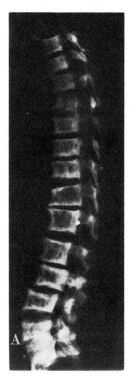
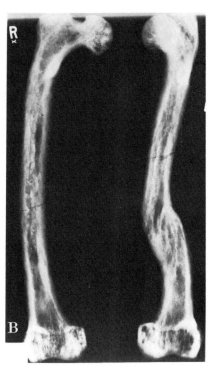

Fig. 72-1. Anglo-Saxon skeleton. Radiographs confirming the presence of extensive Paget's disease in an ancient skeleton found in Jarrow Monastery. A. Classic "window frame" appearance of the diseased vertebrae is readily apparent. B. Paget's disease involves both femurs. A healed pathologic fracture can be seen in the left femur. There are also two postmortem fractures. (From Wells and Woodhouse: Med. Hist. *19:* 396, 1975)

America.[13] It is reputedly rare in Scandinavia, parts of Switzerland, the Near and Far East, and Africa, but cases do occur in these localities and are increasingly reported. Thus, while there is clearly a geographic variation, this may be more apparent than real in some areas.

The majority of individuals with Paget's disease are asymptomatic. Most of them will never know they have the disease and in some it will be diagnosed by chance during medical examination for other reasons, particularly during radiology of the genitourinary tract. Collins has estimated that no more than 5 percent of patients will be symptomatic.[9] However, this figure is based on small numbers and may be inaccurate.

The incidence of familial disease in large series has varied from 1.2 to 7.7 percent.[52] The latter figure conforms with our own experience, but is likely to prove a gross underestimate, as relatives may not be available for examination or, if they are, they have not been followed up for many years. Several examples of Paget's disease in identical twins have been reported.[53]

In the past, Paget's disease has been linked with Hashimoto's thyroiditis, pseudoxanthoma elasticum, and diabetes mellitus. Angioid streaks in the retina have been reported in 8–15 percent of patients with advanced Paget's disease.[51,52] It is possible that these are chance associations, with the recognition that Paget's disease is so common. We are impressed, however, by the occurrence of primary hyperparathyroidism in Paget's disease: 3 cases have occurred in 90 patients seen at the Hammersmith and King's College hospitals, and Paget's disease has been observed in 6 of 66 patients with primary hyperparathyroidism.[10] This would seem to be more than a chance association, but its validity awaits confirmation.

Sir James Paget regarded the disease as one of slow and

relentless progression; this clinical observation is supported by serial observations of the serum alkaline phosphatase level. In some patients, however, the disease may progress rapidly, producing radiologic changes in months, and in others it may remain static for years. In 8 of 20 patients radiographed after 2 years, extension of the disease occurred; no change was observed in the remainder.[11] Spontaneous radiologic healing of the disease has not been reported.

The radiologic spectrum of Paget's disease comprises three phases, reflecting the morbid anatomic changes (Fig. 72-2). Thus progression is seen from the early osteolytic stage to the final phase of predominant sclerosis with an intermediate mixed phase combining both lytic and sclerotic features. The periosteal surface appears to be an exception, as it does not show osteolytic (resorptive) features and the initial change noted is the apposition of new bone in layers. The overall process, viewed radiologically, is usually one of slow progression over the years, but in some cases the radiologic changes remain static for long periods of time and in others the disease can be seen to advance in the space of a few months. In any one patient with multiple affected bones the rate of progression may not be uniform in all areas.

The osteolytic phase is exemplified in the skull by the condition known as *osteoporosis circumscripta,* a well-demarcated area of decalcification seen commonly in the frontal and occipital regions. In the skull this lytic phase may persist longer than it does elsewhere before progressing to sclerosis, perhaps because it is not subjected to the mechanical stresses which affect other bones. The osteolytic phase is also seen in the long bones, where intracortical resorption clefts appear and grow in the long axis of the bone. Sometimes a V-shaped lytic edge, representing a massive resorption front, is seen to advance along the shaft, and this is usually followed by a repair phase with abnormal periosteal and endosteal

bone formation. Incomplete transverse fractures occur quite frequently in this lytic zone; they are often multiple and are especially noted in the femora and tibiae.

As the disease progresses new bone formation occurs, manifested by sclerosis, expansion of bone, and coarse trabeculation. The bony architecture becomes grossly distorted as normal trabeculae are replaced by those which are abnormal both in thickness and in orientation. As a result, the medullary cavity may be obliterated with loss of corticomedullary differentiation. In the skull the changes are first noted in the outer table, where areas of sclerosis appear, which, interspersed with areas of rarefaction, give rise to the so-called "cotton wool" appearance. Subsequently, differentiation between inner and outer tables is lost and the bony overgrowth may result in gross enlargement.

The long bones may also be greatly thickened and, in addition, the effects of weight bearing may be apparent. The new bone which is so vigorously laid down is structurally weak and, as a result, the femora and tibiae are often bowed both anteriorly and laterally. In the pelvis, deformity may also occur as the diseased bone is compressed, with the formation of *protrusio acetabuli.* Mechanical stress, however, is not the sole factor leading to marked distortion, as deformity is often readily seen in non-weight-bearing long bones such as the humeri and phalanges. In the vertebral column the changes range from enlargement and sclerosis of a single vertebral body (which may resemble an osteoblastic metastasis) to widespread involvement, and compression fractures occur quite frequently. Occasionally, marked enlargement of the vertebral bodies in an anterior–posterior direction results in protrusion into the spinal cord.

It must always be remembered that the radiologic picture of Paget's disease indicates past and not necessarily present disease activity. Thus, in a "burnt out" case, extensive radiologic changes will persist despite normal biochemical parameters. To date, radiologic natural regression of the disease has not been documented. When assessing the results of therapy it must be borne in mind that the only firm criterion of regression is a reduction in bone size, improved bone organization being hard to assess and virtually impossible to quantitate.[12]

The radiologic diagnosis of Paget's disease does not usually present many problems, although with extensive skeletal involvement it is often impossible to diagnose a coexistent primary or secondary bone neoplasm. Isolated involvement of a vertebral body may be confused with an osteoblastic metastasis, but when affected by Paget's disease, the vertebra is usually enlarged as well as sclerotic in appearance. The presence of lytic deposits in the ribs would also mitigate against the diagnosis of Paget's disease, which uncommonly affects these bones and, when it does so, tends to cause diffuse enlargement. Osteitis fibrosa cystica, particularly in the skull, may cause some confusion, but x-rays of the hands (and serum biochemistry) usually provide the answer: in hyperparathyroidism phalangeal erosions are present, in contrast to the cortical thickening of Paget's disease.[12]

Recently, radionuclide bone scans have been increasingly used in Paget's disease. ^{85}Sr-, ^{87m}Sr-, ^{18}F-, ^{137m}Ba-, and ^{99m}Tc-labeled diphosphonate have all been shown to be capable of demonstrating Paget's disease (Fig. 72-3). Aside from documenting the extent of the disease, bone scans are of value in revealing early lesions which may not be noted radiologically and they may serve as a better guide to disease activity in patients with widespread skeletal involvement. They may also be very useful in assessing the effects of therapy in cases of localized Paget's disease in which no biochemical abnormalities are apparent and in studying areas that are difficult to evaluate radiologically such as the scapulae and

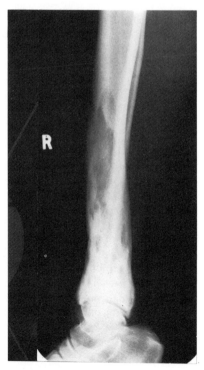

Fig. 72-2. Radiograph of the lower end of a diseased right tibia showing several classic features. A. Expansion and deformity of the bone. B. V-shaped resorption front in the anterior cortex. C. Loss of the normal corticomedullary function, bone sclerosis, and an abnormal trabecular pattern.

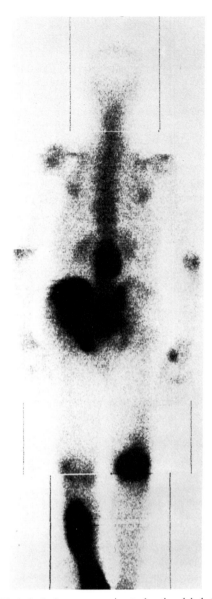

Fig. 72-3. Whole-body bone scan using technetium-labeled diphosphonate in a patient with extensive Paget's disease. The increased skeletal uptake of isotope corresponds to the diseased areas of bone seen on the radiographs and is indicated by the dense black areas seen in the photograph. In some patients increased isotope uptake may be seen in radiologically normal bone. Bone histology is necessary to confirm Paget's disease as similar findings may occur with other bone lesions.

clavicles. Other causes of increased radionuclide uptake such as osteoarthritis have to be distinguished from Paget's disease. It has now been found possible to quantitate the scanning data and it is hoped that such measurements will provide a useful tool when assessing the efficacy of any therapeutic regimen.[14,15]

CLINICAL FEATURES

Deformity is most readily seen in the long bones and skull. The femora and tibiae are bowed anteriorly and laterally while the skull and facial bones are sometimes hugely thickened. The skin temperature overlying the diseased bones may be increased with dilation of the superficial temporal arteries. Bruits may be heard over vascular bone tissue but these are rare. When the spinal cord is diseased there may be loss of height and the development of

kyphosis; the pelvis may soften and become triradiate and there may be protrusio acetabuli. Degenerative joint disease and loss of joint cartilage may be seen in joints surrounded by Paget's disease but are not necessarily a consequence of the disease, as even in severe protrusio the cartilage may be well preserved. Nevertheless, structural abnormalities around joints, particularly the hip and knee, often produce limitation of movement and pain.

Severe bone pain sometimes occurs and is described as aching, throbbing, stabbing, burning, or shooting; its cause is unknown. Affected bones may be tender to pressure, while localized pain or tenderness may be due to fissure fractures or to the development of sarcoma. If the pain is confined to the bone and there is no adjacent joint disease the diagnosis of painful Paget's disease can be made with some certainty. With spinal or pelvic Paget's disease the diagnosis is usually made retrospectively if the disease is brought under control by medical means.

Three types of fracture commonly occur: fissure, complete, and vertebral fractures. Fissure fractures may be painful; they are usually seen on the convex surface of the femora or tibiae and may proceed to form a complete fracture. Complete fractures also occur most often in the lower limbs, sometimes spontaneously but normally after mild trauma. They are usually transverse and heal rapidly, non-union occurring in only 10 percent of cases. Vertebral fractures are usually painless, but they are potentially dangerous.

Deafness is a common complication of Paget's disease in the skull. It may be due to fixation of the stapes footplate or malleolus, blockage of the eustachian tube or external meatus, or involvement of the cochlea. Contrary to popular opinion, deafness is rarely due to compression of the eighth nerve by temporal-bone enlargement. A mixed conductive and neurosensory loss is the usual finding. Other cranial nerves may be involved, particularly when there is considerable bone thickening; with platybasia, cerebellar and long-tract signs may be seen.

Crush fractures of the vertebrae may cause spinal cord compression, and dislocation of cervical vertebrae has been reported. With the exception of deafness, nervous-system involvement by Paget's disease is uncommon. Immobilization after fractures may result in excessive bone resorption and hypercalcemia.

Increased cardiac outputs (2–3 times normal) can occur in patients with extensive and biochemically active disease.[54] This is due to an increase in bone blood flow and reduction in peripheral vascular resistance. Wide pulse pressures and warm extremities are seen.

Osteogenic sarcoma is fortunately a rare complication of Paget's disease, as it carries a virtually hopeless prognosis. It has been estimated that about 0.15 percent of patients with the disease will eventually develop sarcoma[16] and the average survival from the time of diagnosis is 12 months. The risk of developing sarcoma is about 30 times greater in persons over 40 years of age who have Paget's disease than in the rest of the population, and the peak incidence occurs at age 65 years, an age when osteogenic sarcoma is almost unknown in countries where Paget's disease is rare. In 20 percent of cases the tumor is apparently multicentric in origin. Sarcoma usually occurs in patients with polyostotic Paget's disease in whom a predilection for the humerus has been noted.[13]

HEREDITARY BONE DYSPLASIA WITH HYPERPHOSPHATASEMIA

This rare disorder was first described as *fragile bones and macrocranium* in 1956 by Bakwin and Eiger.[17] Subsequently it has been called by many different names, including *juvenile Paget's disease, congenital and hereditary hyperphosphatasia, chronic idiopathic hyperphosphatasia,* and others. It occurs in both sexes and is clinically detected in early childhood due to the marked skeletal deformities and excessive bone fragility leading to fractures. Although the disease is usually generalized, bone pain and tenderness do not always occur. Skull involvement is commonly seen together with mixed conductive and neurosensory deafness. As in adult Paget's disease, the affected bones are expanded, with loss of the normal corticomedullary junction, and biochemically serum alkaline and acid phosphatase and urinary hydroxyproline are greatly increased. Histologic examination reveals immature woven bone in areas normally occupied by mature lamellar bone. The trabeculae lack the cartilaginous core remnant characteristic of normal bone and also demonstrate intense osteocytic osteolysis. Until more is known about the etiology of both this condition and adult Paget's disease any precise relationship between the two conditions must remain in doubt, although there are obvious similarities.[18,19]

ETIOLOGY

The year 1977 marks the centenary of Sir James Paget's original description of the disease of bone which bears his name, and although it is no longer believed that the condition is one of chronic inflammation, the etiology remains elusive. Abnormalities of the nervous system, syphilis, unidentified toxins, altered immunity, and aberrant behavior by several endocrine glands have all been suggested and subsequently dismissed.

Some patients with Paget's disease give a positive family history and it seems likely that there is a genetic element to the condition; the pattern of inheritance, where it can be ascertained, appears to be one of autosomal dominance with incomplete penetrance.[52] The individual or familial association of Paget's disease with pseudoxanthoma elasticum and angioid retinal streaks has led to the consideration of the condition as a hereditary disorder of connective tissue. Biochemical support for this idea was provided recently by the demonstration that polymeric collagen (extracted from the skin) is decreased both in amount and in stability when compared with matched controls.[20] However, the latest ideas concerning the etiology of Paget's disease revive the possibility of an infectious origin in that two groups of workers have noted nuclear inclusions in the osteoclasts that may be specific for the disease and that resemble viral particles.[21,22] Interesting though these ideas may be, the true nature of Paget's disease remains unknown at the present time and none of the therapeutic approaches used to date has shed any light on this problem.

TREATMENT

GENERAL ISSUES

Given our very rudimentary knowledge of the etiology of Paget's disease, the treatment of the condition poses obvious problems which, until quite recently, were further enhanced by a patent lack of suitably objective criteria upon which to base a therapeutic assessment. Although the etiology remains elusive, therapeutic efficacy can now be gauged by biochemistry (alkaline phosphatase and hydroxyproline), bone histology, calcium kinetics, and quantitative bone scanning in addition to radiologic changes, thus lending some degree of objective assessment of response to the subjective assessment of pain relief.

When considering any therapeutic approach it must be borne in mind that Paget's disease is most frequently asymptomatic, and even when symptoms are present they may not be directly referable to the disease process *per se;* e.g., the bone pain may be

osteoarthritic rather than pagetic in origin. It is important, therefore, to judiciously avoid the widespread and indiscriminate use of any therapeutic regimen without first weighing potentially serious side effects, both acute and long term, against the expected benefits of treatment.

In the past treatment has included parathyroidectomy, radiotherapy, corticosteroids, aspirin, iodides, fluoride, and glucagon, all of which have been largely ineffective.[67] In recent years inter in the medical treatment of Paget's disease has been renewed chiefly because of the introduction of three new therapeutic agents—mithramycin, diphosphonates, and the calcitonins—which act to curb the excessive activity of pagetic bone cells. These agents have been studied in the reasonable hope that anything that induces biochemical and histologic improvement may subsequently suppress disease activity, prevent complications, and even effect a "cure."

MITHRAMYCIN

Mithramycin is a cytotoxic antibiotic produced by *Streptomyces plicatus* which inhibits RNA synthesis and has been used in the treatment of a variety of malignancies. After noting that hypocalcemia was a side effect of mithramycin therapy, its use in Paget's disease was entertained and favorable results, with relief of bone pain and reduction in serum alkaline phosphatase and urinary hydroxyproline levels and in skeletal calcium turnover (as measured using ^{85}Sr), were first reported in 1969.[23] Its mode of action is presumably a direct cellular effect on the osteoclasts and osteoblasts wherein it binds to the nuclear DNA, thus preventing RNA and protein synthesis.

Subsequently, several reports have attested to the efficacy of mithramycin in Paget's disease when given either as an intravenous infusion or as a bolus intravenous injection (15–25 μg/kg body weight/day) over various periods of time.[24-26] Gastrointestinal symptoms (nausea and vomiting) were seen as side effects in most patients and evidence of more serious toxicity (hepatic, renal, and hematologic) was also apparent in some. Most recently, mithramycin has been given on an outpatient basis and toxic manifestations were minimized.[27] Despite the latter report, it is rarely justified to use such a toxic agent when other forms of treatment are available that are more efficacious and do not carry the burden of such serious side effects.

DIPHOSPHONATES

Diphosphonates are stable analogues of pyrophosphate possessing a P-C-P rather than a P-O-P grouping, which confers resistance to enzymatic (and chemical) hydrolysis. Introduction of these agents for therapeutic use in Paget's disease was based on knowledge of the actions of pyrophosphate, the anionic end product of cell metabolism which circulates in small amounts in body fluids and is hydrolyzed by cellular pyrophosphatases. Pyrophosphate forms a film (or "chemisorbs") on the surface of bone mineral, markedly delaying accretion and loss of ions, and it also strongly inhibits conversion of amorphous calcium phosphate to the crystalline hydroxyapatite form. Experimentally, pyrophosphate inhibits formation and dissolution of hydroxyapatite crystals *in vitro* and prevents vitamin D–induced ectopic calcification in animals *in vivo*. The diphosphonates, being resistant to enzymatic breakdown, are effective when administered orally and, apart from their pyrophosphatelike actions on the bone surface mineral, they may also exert a direct effect on the bone cells *in vivo*.

One of the diphosphonates, disodium ethane-1-hydroxy-1,1-diphosphonate (disodium etidronate, or EHDP) has been studied in Paget's disease. It was first shown to be effective by Smith et al.

in 1971[28] as assessed by a decrease in serum alkaline phosphatase and total urinary hydroxyproline levels. These preliminary findings, indicating a reduction in bone turnover, have been confirmed and, in addition, quantitative radionuclide (^{18}F or ^{87m}Sr) scans have shown improvement (decreased uptake) over pagetic bone with treatment.[29-31]

EHDP is given orally and gut absorption in man ranges between 1 and 10 percent of the administered dose; it is highest when given in the fasting state. EHDP accumulates to an appreciable extent only in bone and it is not metabolized, being excreted in the urine as unchanged diphosphonate.[30] The doses used clinically have ranged between 1 and 20 mg/kg body weight/day for treatment periods of up to 12 months in duration. The clinical (pain relief) and biochemical (suppression of raised alkaline phosphatase and hydroxyproline) responses are dose related, moderate to marked improvement being noted with the 20 mg/kg dose.[30,31] Recently, however, several cases of increased pain during treatment have been reported.[32-34] A single course of treatment has been shown to maintain biochemical remission for at least 2 years following cessation of therapy.[30]

EHDP has not yet been shown to cause improvement or resolution of the disease as determined radiologically, but bone biopsies have shown apparent histologic suppression of the pagetic process even with doses lower than 10 mg/kg/day. Bone resorption and deposition are reduced as assessed by cellular morphology and, in addition, the pagetic marrow fibrosis is replaced by normal hematopoietic tissue.[30]

EHDP is generally well tolerated by patients, with mild diarrhea being the only symptomatic side effect noted with regularity; this effect can be avoided if the agent is not given on an empty stomach (without affecting absorption significantly).

Plasma phosphate increases in a dose-related fashion. This effect, apparently renal in origin, occurs within a few days of starting treatment, reaches a plateau at about 2 weeks, and takes a similar period of time to revert to normal with cessation of therapy. Studies in animals and human subjects have not shown either interference with parathyroid hormone secretion or renal toxicity.[55,62,63] Calcium absorption and vitamin D metabolism seem normal[30] in man at the doses used, although high doses in animals, greater than the therapeutic dose, caused impaired formation of 1,25-dihydroxycholecalciferol.[35] However, EHDP regularly causes an increase in unmineralized osteoid tissue with doses of 10 mg/kg/day and above.[30] Recently, a reduction in dose of EHDP to 5mg/kg/day has been recommended for therapy beyond six months[55,62] because of an apparently more favorable ratio of desired effects, improvement in clinical status and in biochemical parameters, versus undesired effects such as osteomalacia[30,55] or actual symptomatic deterioration[62] with prolonged therapy at 20mg/kg.[62] Combined therapy with low doses of diphosphonate and calcitonin was reported to have greater effect on the biochemistry than has calcitonin alone.[56] But there is no evidence to date that combined therapy confers any additional clinical advantages over calcitonin, and further long-term studies are necessary before it is possible to draw conclusions on the efficacy of this approach. At present, however, it does not appear safe to advise combined treatment in patients in whom osteolytic lesions are prominent.

CALCITONIN

Calcitonin acts specifically on the bone cells to reduce the abnormally raised turnover rate of bone tissue in Paget's disease. Cellular activity becomes more orderly and healing of the disease may sometimes be seen in serial radiographs. Relief of bone pain has frequently been reported. These features, together with the absence of any serious side effects, make calcitonin, in the opinion of the authors, the treatment of choice for Paget's disease at present.

Three species of calcitonin are available for use in man: natural porcine and synthetic human and salmon.

Biochemical Changes

Calcitonin acts on two major target organs—bone and kidney. Bone is the more important site of action, the major physiologic effect being the inhibition of bone resorption (Chapter 50). An acute injection of calcitonin lowers the plasma calcium and phosphate, and these effects are associated with a marked decrease in the number of active osteoclasts. The most striking and immediate effect of an acute injection of calcitonin is a fall in the level of total urinary hydroxyproline, which occurs within hours of administration of the hormone.[57] Clearly, the magnitude of the hypocalcemic and hypophosphatemic response to calcitonin will depend to a large extent on the bone turnover; the greater the movement of calcium and phosphorus into and out of the bone (turnover), the greater the hypocalcemic and hypophosphatemic effects.[57]

Daily administration of calcitonin continues to produce transient hypocalcemia and hypophosphatemia following the injection, but overall the serum calcium and phosphate levels remain within the normal range. These effects become less obvious as the bone turnover rate decreases with treatment. The urinary total hydroxyproline levels fall rapidly at the onset of calcitonin therapy, while the serum alkaline phosphatase tends to remain elevated for around 1–2 weeks before starting to decrease. After 4 weeks or more the declining alkaline phosphatase levels closely parallel the change in hydroxyproline excretion.

These biochemical changes, reflecting a rapid reduction in bone turnover, occur within the first few months of starting treatment. Subsequently, three general patterns of biochemical response are seen: the serum alkaline phosphatase and urinary hydroxyproline levels either (1) return slowly toward normal, (2) level out above the normal range (plateau), or (3) return toward pretreatment values (relapse). The reason or reasons for these differences are not entirely clear but, in general, patients who relapse are the most severely affected. In some cases in which animal calcitonins are being used, relapse is associated with the presence of high-titer antibodies directed against either the porcine or the salmon hormone; in these cases there will be a response to the human hormone.[46,47]

The plateau response tends to be seen in cases of intermediate severity; in most cases, it probably reflects continuing disease activity, but, in some patients, it may reflect a normal bone turnover in a larger-than-normal bone-tissue mass. It should also be noted that healing of hereditary bone dysplasia with hyperphosphatasemia was observed on roentgenograms during this phase (Figure 72-4A). To date, there is no evidence to suggest that secondary hyperparathyroidism is responsible for the development of either relapse or the plateau response to treatment.[53]

Histology

Interpretation of results obtained by quantitative histologic measurements is potentially unreliable in a patchy disorder of bone. Inaccuracies can be minimized, however, by serial biopsies taken from a small area of uniformly diseased pelvic bone. Under these circumstances histologic studies have shown an immediate reduction in osteoclast numbers preceding a reduction in the active osteoblast surface. Furthermore, progressively more lamellar and less woven bone is seen during treatment. These morphologic changes correlate well with the biochemical response to treatment and emphasize the point that calcitonin therapy produces healing of the Paget's disease process.

Calcium Balance

In the early treatment phase calcium balance becomes positive or more positive as urinary and fecal calcium excretion falls; this improvement in balance may persist for months. There is presumably a relatively greater inhibition of bone resorption than formation and a net gain of skeletal calcium; this deduction is supported by the sequential histologic changes. Measurement of total body calcium by the technique of neutron activation analysis shows that this calcium retention as observed by the initial balance studies is not sustained and a subsequent loss of bone mass occurs, presumably as a result of bone remodeling.[36]

Radiology

Radiologic improvement has been observed after months or years of treatment in adult patients and in 3 patients with hereditary bone dysplasia with hyperphosphatasemia.[12,18,19,65] The changes were most dramatic in the growing children, as might be expected, but the same changes were present to a lesser extent in the adults. The criteria for healing of the disease are a reduction in

bone volume, condensation of the cortex, loss of abnormal trabecular bone, and the reappearance of a normal corticomedullary junction (Fig. 72-4B).

Clinical Effects

In most reported series striking relief of bone pain was claimed by many patients. Although these studies were not controlled by double-blind trials, pain relief coincided with a loss of bone tenderness, reduction in skin temperature, and metabolic, kinetic, or histologic evidence of a reduction in bone turnover.[36-40,57,66] Withdrawal of treatment also resulted in relapse of disease activity and bone pain in some patients.[58] These facts suggest that calcitonin is of real value in the management of bone pain in Paget's disease. Relief of pain usually occurs within the first few weeks but may be delayed 6 months or more. Any patient with severe pain not managed by simpler or cheaper means should be given a trial course of calcitonin even if gross degenerative joint disease is present as well. The clinical response may sometimes be dramatic.[37-40]

Regression of neurologic signs (motor and sensory) in the lower limbs has also been reported in patients with spinal-cord compression and vertebral Paget's disease.[59,60] These changes were associated with good functional improvement which took place over several months. The mechanism of this change is not

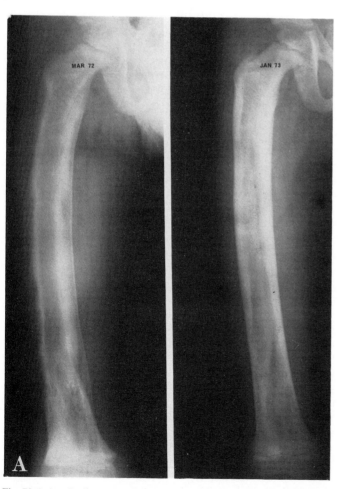
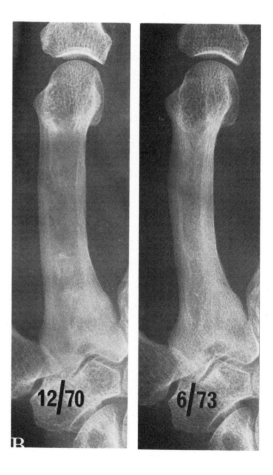

Fig. 72-4. A. Radiographs of the right femur in a patient with juvenile Paget's disease before and after 10 months of treatment with calcitonin. A striking improvement in the appearance of the diseased bone is seen. (From Doyle et al.: Br. J. Radiol. *47:* 9, 1974) B. Radiographs of a diseased metacarpal in an elderly patient with Paget's disease. After 30 months of calcitonin treatment there has been a considerable reduction in bone volume. (From Doyle et al.: Br. J. Radiol. *47:* 1, 1974)

known but may be due to alteration in blood flow or to remodeling of the diseased bone tissue.

Improvement in hearing is unusual in the short term[41,42] and has only been reported in occasional cases. A progressive fall in cardiac output may be seen in some patients with initially elevated values (Fig. 72-5).[61] An immediate fall in serum and urinary calcium levels and improvement in renal function was observed in one patient with immobilization of hypercalcemia. The serum calcium subsequently remained within the normal range during long-term calcitonin treatment in this patient.[61]

Indications for Calcitonin Treatment

On the available evidence it is difficult to decide how best to treat many patients with symptomatic Paget's disease. The following indications and treatment regimens are intended only as guidelines and may be modified in the light of further experience. It is unclear at present whether calcitonin should be given as single or multiple courses or as life-long therapy. Currently there are four situations that warrant at least a trial course of calcitonin: bone pain, immobilization hypercalcemia, spinal-cord compression, and deformity and repeated bone fractures.

In patients with bone pain, treatment should be tried for at least 6 months or until pain relief occurs. Repeat courses of the hormone may then be given when necessary. A short course (1–2 weeks) may be adequate to control hypercalcemia during immobilization, but treatment will be determined by serum and urinary calcium levels. Only a few patients with cord compression have so far been treated, but when surgery has failed or is impossible, it would seem reasonable to give calcitonin for at least 6 months. If improvement occurs, then life-long treatment is probably necessary. The evidence for treatment with regard to deformity and

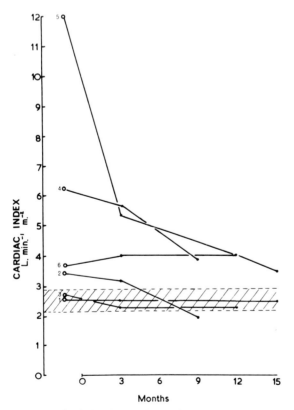

Fig. 72-5. Cardiac index in 6 patients with Paget's disease before and during calcitonin treatment. A substantial reduction in cardiac index is seen in 3 of the 4 patients (Nos. 2, 4, and 5) with initially elevated levels. Data from Woodhouse et al. Brit. Med. J. *4:* 686, 1975.

bone fractures is clear cut in hereditary bone dysplasia with hyperphosphatasemia where cessation of bone fractures and remodeling of the diseased bone occurs. The situation in adult patients is more difficult as radiologic improvement may take years to accomplish. Evidence of bone healing in adult Paget's disease and hereditary bone dysplasia with hyperphosphatasemia suggests a possible prophylactic role for calcitonin in selected patients. In theory it might be possible to achieve complete healing of the disease, but this would probably take as many years to occur as the disease took to develop. Therefore, only young patients can be considered in this category. Of more practical importance, perhaps, is arresting the disease process and preventing further complications. With such a variable natural history, selection of patients with Paget's disease is difficult, and the expected benefits of calcitonin therapy should be carefully weighed against the possible necessity for life-long injections and the considerable cost involved.

Pharmacologic Issues

Calcitonin may be given intravenously, intramuscularly, or subcutaneously. In the initial studies the intramuscular route was used and intramuscular injections continue to be routine in many centers. If the hormonal preparation used is in aqueous solution it seems advisable to use the subcutaneous route as this may minimize any side effects; it is also simpler for the patient to give his own injections subcutaneously and it is our practice to encourage patients to do this whenever practicable.

Comparison of the potencies of the three calcitonins currently in use is at best only approximate.[43] Usually only the calcium-lowering action of the hormone is considered when potency is assessed. The reason for the greater apparent potency of salmon calcitonin is not fully understood but may be partly explained by the apparent resistance of this form of calcitonin to enzymatic degradation.[64] The Medical Research Council (MRC) Unit is a measure of the calcium-lowering ability of intravenously administered calcitonin in the rat, and the standard currently in use (MRC Research Standard B) is a porcine standard.

Bearing these points in mind, on a weight basis 100 MRC units is equivalent to 1 mg of the pure porcine or human preparations and to 0.025 mg of the pure salmon calcitonin. In practice, the therapeutic effect of 50–100 MRC units of any calcitonin is similar in man.[43,44]

Complications of Treatment

Antibodies to porcine and salmon calcitonin develop in 50 percent or more of cases and their presence is dependent on the dose used and the duration of treatment.[45,46] In most instances they are of low titer and do not interfere with treatment—a situation analogous to that seen in insulin-requiring diabetics.[46] In approximately 10 percent of patients, antibody titers are sufficiently raised to produce a clinical and biochemical relapse. Treatment may then be changed successfully to human calcitonin, which is not antigenic.[46,47] No serious side effects have occurred using any calcitonin. In approximately 20–30 percent of patients, flushing and a feeling of warmth in the face and hands may occur within a few minutes of the injection and last about 1 hour; this may also be associated with mild nausea. These side effects can be minimized by using the subcutaneous route of injection, giving the calcitonin on retiring to bed, or giving metoclopramide (10 mg orally) one-half hour prior to the injection. Rare complications include diarrhea and vomiting, pain at the injection site, and the development of a rash (nonhuman calcitonins). Withdrawal of treatment is seldom necessary.

SUMMARY

Paget's disease is very common in some countries, and although symptomatic disease occurs in only a small proportion of cases, many patients would benefit from treatment when the disease is considered on a world-wide basis.

At the present time the most rational form of treatment would seem to be calcitonin, as this hormone can reduce excessive bone turnover and may be of symptomatic benefit without incurring undesirable side effects. The only therapy approved by regulatory agencies in the United Kingdom and North America (at the time of writing) is calcitonin. The ultimate therapeutic usefulness of the other agents such as diphosphonates is still being evaluated. Radiologic healing of the disease as seen in some patients raises the possibility that prophylactic treatment may prevent the development of many severe complications of Paget's disease. Calcitonin is undoubtedly the treatment of choice for the juvenile condition, hereditary bone dysplasia with hyperphosphatasemia.[48]

REFERENCES

1. Rasmussen, H., and Bordier, P. The Physiological and Cellular Basis of Metabolic Bone Disease. Baltimore, Williams & Wilkins, 1974.
2. Rhodes, B. A., Greyson, N. D., Hamilton, C. R., White, R. I., Giargiana, F. A., and Wagner, H. N. Absence of anatomic arteriovenous shunts in Paget's disease of bone. N. Engl. J. Med. 287: 686, 1972.
3. Albright, F., and Reifenstein, E. C. The Parathyroid Glands and Metabolic Bone Disease. London, Bailliere, Tindall and Cox, 1948.
4. Moss, D. W., and Butterworth, P. B. Enzymology and Medicine. London, Pitman Medical, 1974.
5. Krane, S. M., Munoz, A. J., and Harris, E. D. Urinary polypeptides related to collagen synthesis. J. Clin. Invest. 49: 716, 1970.
6. Paget, J. On a form of chronic inflammation of bones (osteitis deformans). Med. Chir. Trans. 60: 37, 1877.
7. Hobson, W., and Pemberton, J. The Health of the Elderly at Home. London, Butterworth, 1955, p. 137.
8. Woodhouse, N. J. Y. Paget's disease and calcitonin therapy. In: Ninth Symposium on Advanced Medicine. London, Pitman Medical, 1973, p. 202.
9. Collins, D. H. Paget's disease of bone. Incidence and subclinical forms. Lancet, 2: 53, 1956.
10. Dent, C. E. Personal communication.
11. Grainger, R. G., and Laws, J. W. Paget's disease—active or quiescent. Br. J. Radiol. 30: 120, 1957.
12. Doyle, F. H. Pennock, J., Greenberg, P. B., Joplin, G. F., and MacIntyre, I. Radiological evidence of a dose-related response to long-term treatment of Paget's disease with human calcitonin. Br. J. Radiol. 47: 1, 1974.
13. Barry, H. C. Paget's Disease of Bone. Edinburgh, Livingstone, 1969, p. 42.
14. Miller, S. W., Castronovo, F. P., Pendergrass, H. P., and Potsaid, M. S. Technetium 99M labeled diphosphonate bone scanning in Paget's disease. Am. J. Roentgenol. 121: 177, 1974.
15. Lavender, P. J., Evans, I. M. A., Arnot, R., Bowrings, S., Joyce, F. H., Joplin, G. F., and MacIntyre, I. A comparison of radiography and radioisotope scanning in the detection of Paget's disease and in the assessment of response to human calcitonin. Brit. J. Radiol. 50: 243, 1977.
16. Price, C. H. G. The incidence of sarcoma in south-west England and its relationship to Paget's disease of bone. J. Bone Joint Surg. 44B: 366, 1962.
17. Bakwin, H., and Eiger, M. S. Fragile bones and macrocranium. J. Pediatr. 49: 558, 1956.
18. Doyle, F. H., Woodhouse, N. J. Y., Glen, A. C. A., Joplin, G. F., and MacIntyre, I. Healing of the bones in juvenile Paget's disease treated by human calcitonin. Br. J. Radiol. 47: 9, 1974.
19. Whalen, J. P., Horwith, M., Krook, L., MacIntyre, I., Mena, E., Viteri, F., Torun, B., and Nunez, E. A. Calcitonin treatment in hereditary bone dysplasia with hyperphosphatasaemia: a radiographic and histologic study of bone. Am. J. Roentgenol. 129: 29, 1977.

20. Francis, M. J. O., and Smith, R. Evidence of a generalised connective tissue defect in Paget's disease of bone. Lancet 1: 841, 1974.
21. Rebel, A., Malkani, K., Basle, B., and Bregeon, C. Particularités ultrastructurales des osteoclastes de la Maladie de Paget. Rev Rhum. 41: 767, 1974.
22. Singer, F. R., Neer, R. M., Goltzman, D., Krane, S. M., and Potts, J. T., Jr. Treatment of Paget's disease of bone and hypercalcemia with salmon calcitonin. In Taylor, S. (ed.): Endocrinology 1973: Proceedings of the Fourth International Symposium. London, William Heinemann Medical Books Limited, 1974, p. 397.
23. Ryan, W. G., Schwartz, T. B., and Perlia, C. P. Effects of mithramycin on Paget's disease of bone. Ann. Intern. Med. 70: 549, 1969.
24. Ryan, W. G., Schwartz, T. B., and Northrop, G. Experiences in the treatment of Paget's disease of bone with mithramycin. J.A.M.A. 213: 1153, 1970.
25. Condon, J. R., Reith, S. B. M., Nassim, J. R., Millard, F. J. C., Hilb, A., and Stainthorpe, E. M. Treatment of Paget's disease of bone with mithramycin. Br. Med. J. 1: 421, 1971.
26. Elias, E. G., and Evans, J. T. Mithramycin in the treatment of Paget's disease of bone. J. Bone Joint Surg. 54-A: 1730, 1972.
27. Lebbin, D., Ryan, W. G., and Schwartz, T. B. Outpatient treatment of Paget's disease of bone with mithramycin. Ann. Intern. Med. 81: 635, 1974.
28. Smith, R., Russell, R. G. G., and Bishop, M. Diphosphonates and Paget's disease of bone. Lancet, 1: 945, 1971.
29. Altman, R. D., Johnston, C. C., Khairi, M. R. A., Wellman, H., Serafini, A. N., and Sankey, R. R. Influence of disodium etidronate on clinical and laboratory manifestations of Paget's disease of bone (osteitis deformans). N. Engl. J. Med. 289: 1379, 1973.
30. Russell, R. G. G., Smith, R., Preston, C., Walton, R. J., and Woods, C. G. Diphosphonates in Paget's disease. Lancet 1: 894, 1974.
31. Khairi, M. R. A., Johnston, C. C., Altman, R. D., Wellman, H. N., Serafini, A. N., and Sankey, R. R. Treatment of Paget's disease of bone (osteitis deformans). Results of a one-year study with sodium etidronate. J.A.M.A. 230: 562, 1974.
32. Fromm, G., Schajowicz, F., and Mautalen, C. A. Disodium ethane-1-hydroxy-1-1-diphosphonate (E.H.D.P.) in Paget's disease. Lancet 2: 666, 1975.
33. Haddad, J. Personal communication.
34. Ibbertson, H. K. Personal communication.
35. Hill, L. F., Lumb, G. A., Mawer, E. B., and Stanbury, S. W. Indirect inhibition of the biosynthesis of 1,25-dihydroxycholecalciferol in rats treated with a diphosphonate. Clin. Sci. 44: 335, 1973.
36. Wallach, S., Avramides, A., Flores, A., Bellavia, J., and Cohn, S. Skeletal turnover and total body elemental composition during extended calcitonin treatment of Paget's disease. Metabolism 24: 745, 1975.
37. Haddad, J. G., Birge, S. J., and Avioli, L. V. Effects of prolonged thyrocalcitonin administration on Paget's disease of bone. N. Engl. J. Med. 283: 549, 1970.
38. Woodhouse, N. J. Y., Reiner, M., Bordier, Ph, Kalu, D. N., Fisher, M., Foster, G. V., Joplin, G. F., and MacIntyre, I. Human calcitonin in the treatment of Paget's bone disease. Lancet 1: 1139, 1971.
39. Greenberg, P. B., Doyle, F. H., Fisher, M. T., Hillyard, C. J., Joplin, G. F., Pennock, J., and MacIntyre, I. Treatment of Paget's disease of bone with synthetic human calcitonin. Am. J. Med. 56: 867, 1974.
40. Woodhouse, N. J. Y. Clinical applications of calcitonin. Br. J. Hosp. Med. 11: 677, 1974.
41. Grimaldi, P. M. G. B., Mohamedally, S. M., and Woodhouse, N. J. Y. Deafness in Paget's disease: effect of salmon calcitonin. Br. Med. J. 2: 726, 1975.
42. Menzies, M. A., Greenberg, P. B., Joplin, G. F. Otological studies in patients with deafness due to Paget's disease before and after treatment with synthetic human calcitonin. Acta Otolaryngol. 79: 378, 1975.
43. Galante, L. S. The effect of bioassay methods on the potencies of porcine, human and salmon calcitonins. Ph.D Thesis, University of London, 1972.
44. Galante, L., Joplin, G. F., MacIntyre, I., and Woodhouse, N. J. Y. The calcium lowering effect of synthetic human, porcine and salmon calcitonin in patients with Paget's disease. Clin. Sci. 44: 605, 1973.
45. Haddad, J. G., and Caldwell, J. G. Calcitonin resistance: clinical and immunological studies in subjects with Paget's disease of bone treated with porcine and salmon calcitonins. J. Clin. Invest. 51: 3133, 1972.
46. Singer, F. R., Aldred, J. P., Neer, R. M., Krane, S. M., Potts, J. T.,

and Bloch, K. J. An evaluation of antibodies and clinical resistance to calcitonin. *J. Clin. Invest. 51:* 2331, 1972.

47. Rojanasathit, S., Rosenberg, E., and Haddad, J. G. Paget's bone disease: response to human calcitonin in patients resistant to salmon calcitonin. *Lancet 2:* 1412, 1974.

48. Horwith, M., Nunez, E. A., Krook, L., Viteri, F., Torun, B., Mena, E. Suh, S. M., Eisenberg, E., MacIntyre, I., and Whalen, J. P. Hereditary bone dysplasia with hyperphosphatasaemia. Response to synthetic human calcitonin. In I. MacIntyre and A. G. E. Pearse (eds.): Endocrinology 1975. Molecular Endocrinology. Supplement to Clinical Endocrinology, vol.5. London, Blackwell, 1975, p. 341s.

49. Demmler, K.: Die Vaskularisation des Paget-Knochens. *Deut Med Wochenschr 99:* 91, 1974.

50. Heistad, D. D., Abboud, F. M., Schmid, P. G., et al.: Regulation of blood flow in Paget's disease of bone. *J. Clin. Invest. 55:* 69, 1975.

51. Paton, D.: The Relation of Angioid Streaks to Systemic Disease. Springfield, Ill., Charles C Thomas, 1972.

52. McKusick, V.: Heritable Disorders of Connective Tissue. St. Louis, C. V. Mosby, 1972.

53. Burckhardt, P. M., Singer, F. R., Potts, J. T., Jr.: Parathyroid function in patients with Paget's disease treated with salmon calcitonin. *Clin. Endocrinol. 2:* 15, 1973.

54. Lequime, J., Denolin, H.: Circulatory dynamics in osteitis deformans. *Circulation 12:* 215, 1955.

55. Khairi, M. R. A., Altman, R. D., DeRosa, G. P., et al.: Sodium etidronate in the treatment of Paget's disease of bone. *Ann. Intern. Med. 87:* 656, 1977.

56. Hosking, D. J., Bijvoet, O. L., Van Aken, J., et al.: Paget's bone disease treated with diphosphonate and calcitonin. *Lancet 1:* 615–617, 1976.

57. Singer, F. R., Keutmann, H. T., Neer, R. M., et al.: Pharmacological effects of salmon calcitonin in man. In Talmage, R. V., Munson, P. L.

(eds.): Calcium, Parathyroid Hormone and the Calcitonins. Excerpta Medica, Amsterdam, 1972, p. 89.

58. Avramides, A., Flores, A., DeRose, J., et al.: Paget's disease of the bone: observations after cessation of long-term synthetic salmon calcitonin treatment. *J. Clin. Endocrinol. Metab. 42 (3):* 459, 1976.

59. Melick, R. A., Ebeling, P., Hjorth, R. J.: Improvement in paraplegia in vertebral Paget's disease treated with calcitonin. *Br. Med. J. 1 (6010):* 627, 1976.

60. Wallach, S.: Paget's disease: new treatment for an old disease. *Am. Fam. Physician 13 (1):* 78, 1976.

61. Woodhouse, N. J., Crosbie, W. A., Mohamedally, S. M.: Cardiac output in Paget's disease: response to long-term salmon calcitonin therapy. *Br. Med. J. 4 (5998):* 686, 1975.

62. Canfield, R., Rosner, W., Skinner, J., et al.: Diphosphonate therapy of Paget's disease of bone. *J. Clin. Endocrinol. Metab. 44:* 96, 1977.

63. Yarrington, J. T., Capen, C. C., Black, H. E., et al.: Experimental parturient hypocalcemia in cows following prepartal chemical inhibition of bone resorption. *Am. J. Path. 83:* 569, 1976.

64. Potts, J. T., Jr. Aurbach, G. D.: Chemistry of the calcitonins. In Geiger, S. R. (ed.); Aurbach, G. D. (vol. ed.); Greep, R. O. Astwood, E. B. (sec. ed.): Handbook of Physiology, Sec. VII. Washington, DC, Parathyroid Gland. American Physiological Society, 1976, p. 423.

65. Nagant de Deuxchaisnes, C., Rombouts-Lindemans, C., Huaux, J. P., et al.: Roentgenologic evaluation of the efficacy of calcitonin in Paget's disease of bone. In MacIntyre and Szelke (eds.): Molecular Endocrinology, Amsterdam, Elsevier, 1977, p. 213.

66. Evans, I. M. A., Doyle, F. H., Banks, L., et al.: Paget's disease: results of long-term treatment with synthetic human calcitonin. In MacIntyre and Szelke (eds.): Molecular Endocrinology, Amsterdam, Elsevier, 1977, p. 235.

67. Singer, F. R., Schiller, A. L., Pyle, E. B., et al.: Paget's disease of bone. In Avioli, L. V., Krane, S. M. (eds.): Metabolic Bone Disease, Vol. 2, New York, Academic Press, 1978, p. 489.

73

Synopsis

John T. Potts, Jr.

The 33 chapters in this section dealing with parathyroid hormone, calcitonin, vitamin D., and bone and bone mineral metabolism, cover the basic and clinical issues pertinent to the disturbances in calcium, phosphate, and bone metabolism now recognized with increasing frequency in our population. The broad range of topics precludes a simple synopsis of diagnosis and treatment. The purpose of this brief summary is to serve as a guide to the material covered in the individual chapters, to explain the organization of the section, and to stress certain concepts important in our present understanding and pertinent to future clinical and basic research goals in calcium and bone metabolism.

The last one-and-a-half decades have been an extraordinarily productive period in understanding basic features of the physiological role and the mode of action of parathyroid hormone, calcitonin, and vitamin D. Calcitonin was not known to exist as a hormone prior to the pioneering studies of Copp, Munson, MacIntyre, and their associates as outlined in Chapters 48, 49, and 50. Their work led to the discovery of calcitonin, a polypeptide hormone now appreciated to be widely represented in the vertebrate species. In man and other mammalian vertebrates, calcitonin in adult life is a hormone of the thyroid gland. As emphasized in Chapter 48, and also in Chapter 64, it has been found, however, that calcitonin arises from a group of cells derived from the neural crest that migrate during embryogenesis first into the ultimobranchial body and then, in mammals, into the thyroid gland. In submammalian vertebrates, calcitonin-producing cells remain outside the thyroid gland in the ultimobranchial body, a discrete endocrine tissue in adult life. Appreciation of the ultimobranchial origin of calcitonin in submammalian vertebrates opened the way for the isolation, chemical characterization, and synthesis of calcitonin from the ultimobranchial body of the Pacific-coast salmon (Chapter 48). Salmon calcitonin is now the form of calcitonin most widely used for therapeutic purposes in the United States. Its physiological action to block bone resorption led to its introduction as a drug in clinical medicine, particularly in the control of Paget's disease of bone (Chapter 72). In addition to its use as a drug in disorders associated with increased bone destruction, the other major medical importance of calcitonin is that it serves as an exquisitely sensitive marker for tumors (medullary carcinoma) arising from the cell of origin of calcitonin in the thyroid in man, the parafollicular cell. Its occurrence as part of hereditary endocrine disorders and the malignant character of the lesion led to use of assays for calcitonin in the early diagnosis and improved treatment of patients with medullary carcinoma (Chapters 64 and 65). These findings, in turn, provided the opportunity to determine the amino acid sequence of calcitonin from man by isolation of calcitonin from medullary-carcinoma tissue (Chapter 72). Synthetic human calcitonin is now also widely used in therapy of Paget's disease as an alternative form of therapy to animal or fish calci-

tonin (Chapter 72). Despite the clear medical importance of calcitonin and the extensive study of its physiology and mode of action, the true biological role, if any, of calcitonin in adult humans is completely unknown. Thus calcitonin remains an enigma. The classic clinical endocrine correlates of defects in hormone production, namely diseases associated with excessive or deficient production of the hormone, do not seem to apply to calcitonin. Patients presumably devoid of calcitonin, such as those with a congenital or acquired absence of the thyroid given only replacement therapy with thyroxine, have no evidence of deficiency in calcium or bone metabolism or other metabolic activity. Medullary carcinoma constitutes a serious challenge to survival (Chapter 64), yet it is tumor growth per se and not metabolic consequences of the vastly excessive calcitonin production associated with the malignant growth of the parafollicular cells that is responsible for the morbidity and mortality in patients with medullary carcinoma of the thyroid. The true biological role of calcitonin may simply be yet undiscovered. Calcitonin may play a more important role in calcium or bone metabolism during embryonic or early childhood, or, in adult humans, may play a still undiscovered metabolic role distinct from its action on blockade of bone resorption and its effects on calcium and phosphorus metabolism.

The physiological role of parathyroid hormone, by contrast, is clearly central in calcium and phosphate metabolism and in bone metabolism. Clinically severe problems associated with excessive parathyroid hormone production, whether primary or secondary, have been recognized with increased frequency in the last decade. Although much less common, absolute or relative deficiency of parathyroid hormone action is associated with severe abnormalities in calcium and phosphate metabolism and requires intensive medical therapy. Many aspects of the chemical basis of biological activity for parathyroid hormone, as well as the biosynthesis, secretion, metabolism, and mode of action of the hormone, are well understood, as outlined in Chapters 42 through 47. Many of the recent basic studies, particularly on the biosynthesis of parathyroid hormone, have involved new insights in the molecular biology of endocrine physiology. Studies on parathyroid hormone have uncovered previously unsuspected complexity in successive stages of intracellular processing of molecular precursors of the secreted form of the hormone, and in turn have served as model systems for parallel investigations with other polypeptide hormones. The ultimate physiological or clinical significance of many of these new studies relating to the complex intracellular control of parathyroid hormone biosynthesis and release are not yet understood in physiological or clinical terms. It seems likely that the basic information gained will shed new insight on cellular defects associated with excessive or deficient production of parathyroid hormone in the disease states associated with abnormal hormone secretion. The heterogeneity of circulating parathyroid hormone

(Chapter 45) has posed serious interpretive problems in the physiological and clinical utility of blood assay methods based on antisera derived by immunization with purified hormone extracted from parathyroid glands in man and the bovine species. Present information concerning the origins of the fragments of the circulating hormone smaller in size than the polypeptide of 84 amino acids extracted from the gland, as well as the problems posed for the present generation of immunoassays for parathyroid hormone when they are applied to detect the concentration of biologically active peptide in blood, are discussed in Chapters 45 and 55. Information concerning initial steps of hormone action at the receptor level (Chapter 47) has proven helpful in understanding the disease entity pseudohypoparathyroidism, in which defective receptor response in renal and bone tissue is believed responsible for the hypoparathyroidism secondary to peripheral resistance to hormone action (Chapter 63).

Perhaps the most intense investigation related to calcium and bone metabolism at the present time is that involving the biosynthesis, metabolism, and mode of action of vitamin D. As outlined by DeLuca and Holick in Chapter 51, vitamin D is actually a hormone in conditions of adequate sunlight, and successive hydroxylations under metabolic control are required to produce the circulating active form of the hormone, 1,25-dihydroxyvitamin D. An almost explosive range of information has developed in the last decade concerning structure/activity relations in vitamin D metabolites, organ specificity of hydroxylations, the role of plasma transport proteins and intracellular receptors for vitamin D metabolites, and ultimate biological expression of active forms of vitamin D. The overall integrated activity of the two hormones, parathyroid hormone and vitamin D, on calcium and phosphate metabolism including absorption, distribution, and excretion of the mineral ions, as well as present understanding of the complex processes of homeostasis of calcium and phosphate, are analyzed in Chapters 40 and 52.

The organization of the chapters dealing with clinical disorders in calcium and bone metabolism represented a dilemma that is a reflection of the integrative approach necessary in analyzing diseases due to disorders in calcium metabolism, bone turnover, or excessive or deficient action of parathyroid hormone and vitamin D. It is for example, impossible to assess present clinical information concerning the bone disease osteomalacia, a disorder associated with defective bone mineralization, without considering the manner in which apparently quite different pathophysiologic defects result in a common tissue response in the skeleton. Yet in order to focus, for purposes of an endocrine textbook, on disorders associated with hereditary or acquired deficiencies in vitamin D action, Chapters 66 and 67 have dealt specifically with disorders in vitamin D function and should be read in conjunction with Chapter 70 dealing with osteomalacia per se. In Chapter 70, the skeletal manifestations of osteomalacia are examined, and etiologies other than those involving clear deficiencies in vitamin D action are considered.

Similarly, organizational difficulties are encountered in discussing clinical indications for and results achieved from therapy employing vitamin D and vitamin D metabolites, especially 1,25-dihydroxyvitamin D. The latter compound has been synthesized, introduced in widespread clinical trials, and, at the time of this writing, is about to be released for general therapeutic use. The organization of the clinical chapters into primary hyperparathyroidism, secondary hyperparathyroidism, hypoparathyroidism, hereditary or acquired abnormalities in vitamin D function, and, finally, endocrine aspects of metabolic bone disease, a useful separation of chapters from one point of view, has necessitated

multiple references to vitamin D therapy; hence Chapters 51, 59, 61, 62, 63, 66, 67, 69, 70, and 71 all touch on some aspects of vitamin D therapy. In addition to the main subsection headings of clinical disorders in calcium and bone metabolism listed above, there is a section on medullary carcinoma and other disorders involving calcitonin. These sections are logically included in the general area of bone and bone mineral metabolism even though medullary carcinoma of the thyroid is not per se involved in disorders of calcium or skeletal metabolism. This is largely because many cases of medullary carcinoma arise in the setting of hereditary endocrine-neoplasia syndromes and are often linked with hyperparathyroidism in affected kindreds. These syndromes of multiple-endocrine-neoplasia type I (MEN I) and type II (MEN II) are described in Chapters 53 and 64.

It was felt essential to devote several chapters to metabolic bone disease and clearly to place it in the section dealing with disorders of calcium and phosphate metabolism. It must be understood, however, that there is little reason to suspect a primary disorder in calcium or phosphate metabolism or in the function of parathyroid hormone, calcitonin, or vitamin D in several of the disorders treated in Chapters 69–72. Similarly, a general chapter (Chapter 68) is devoted to renal calcium-stone disease with an emphasis on metabolic abnormalities in calcium absorption or calcium excretion when they have been identified in the pathogenesis of the disorders. As a survey of Chapters 68–72 reveals, a clear knowledge of the specific pathogenesis is often lacking in many of the disease syndromes associated with nephrolithiasis or bone disease, in sharp contrast to disorders clearly associated with abnormal production or expression of action of parathyroid hormone or vitamin D metabolites. Chapter 69 serves as a general introduction to basic concepts in bone growth and remodeling and systematic classification of the often-confusing entities encountered in metabolic bone disease, thus serving a general role similar to that provided by the basic chapters dealing with parathyroid hormone and vitamin D physiology, metabolism, and mode of action.

With regard to an overall synopsis of diagnosis and therapy, only a few general comments are appropriate in view of the broad scope of organ systems, hereditary defects, and disease entities considered in this section. The principal issues pertinent to clinical expression and diagnosis of primary hyperparathyroidism, including special features involving the use and interpretation of the parathyroid hormone immunoassay and considerations in the surgical and medical management of the disease, are covered in Chapters 53–58. The diagnosis is usually easy to establish, but uncertainties concerning the natural history of hyperparathyroidism leave unsettled how frequently surgical intervention is needed in asymptomatic patients (Chapter 57).

The diagnosis of secondary hyperparathyroidism seen in chronic renal failure is readily made, but optimum management, including the proper attention to dietary control, especially that of phosphate, the use of synthetic active metabolites of vitamin D, and considerations appropriate for evaluating the pathophysiological consequences of parathyroid hyperplasia and its successful involution secondary to therapy, represent particularly perplexing treatment issues with highly variable patterns of disease from one individual to another. It is difficult to make uniform therapeutic recommendations in these disorders, but Chapters 59–61 attempt to summarize present concepts and suggested therapeutic guidelines.

The differential diagnosis between hypoparathyroidism due to peripheral resistance to parathyroid hormone action versus that due to deficient hormone production, as well as optimum guidelines for successful management through oral calcium supplements and vitamin D or vitamin D metabolites, are outlined in Chapters 62 and 63. The diagnosis of medullary carcinoma and the utility of the calcitonin assay in this process are discussed in Chapters 64 and 65. The possibility of early detection of the disease at a completely preclinical stage has led to encouragement that the previously high mortality of this disorder could be greatly lessened. Clear evidence that improved mortality in medullary carcinoma is associated with early recognition and surgery is not yet evident, but seems likely; detailed long-term clinical evaluation of patients with early detection and treatment compared to historical controls will be required to settle this issue.

Although the pathogenesis of hereditary and acquired disorders associated with abnormalities in vitamin D function (Chapters 66 and 67) is not yet by any means clear, clinical experience has made it possible to propose schedules of combined therapy that have proven therapeutic benefit. The pathogenesis of the many apparently diverse syndromes associated with calcium nephrolithiasis is logically analyzed by Drs. Peacock, Robinson, and Marshall in Chapter 68, but it is clear that much further work will be required before many discrete metabolic defects can be identified. Again, however, recent experience with therapy with high phosphate intake, thiazides, and even inhibitors of uric acid production have been reported to be of considerable clinical benefit. Rigorous clinical evaluation of the successful therapy in these patients with recurrent kidney stones is extremely difficult because of the highly variable natural history of stone formation and the secondary complications that often follow initial renal damage secondary to nephrolithiasis.

With regard to metabolic bone disease, specific therapeutic intervention tailored to the pathogenesis of different syndromes associated with osteomalacia can often be followed with reasonable expectation of success (Chapters 66, 67, and 70). Unfortunately, the same cannot be stated for the extremely prevalent problem of osteoporosis (Chapter 71). Recent studies do suggest that both estrogens and an adequate calcium intake might play an important role in reducing the incidence of the disease through prevention of accelerated bone mineral loss. Therapeutic problems are extraordinarily difficult once osteoporosis is far advanced. Much greater success has been accomplished in Paget's disease with judicious use of calcitonin and/or newer agents such as the diphosphonates. In this situation, therapy is not directed at the pathogenesis of the disease, but serves to override the abnormal skeletal response that follows the still-unknown initial lesion in the bone (Chapter 72).

The rapid advances made in the last decade in understanding normal skeletal remodeling, the homeostatic role of parathyroid hormone and vitamin D, and the pathophysiology of certain syndromes associated with abnormal bone and bone mineral metabolism, leave the strong impression that many more insights will be achieved over the next several decades in many of the other disorders discussed in this section, for which, at present, specific pathogenesis is still unknown.

Pancreatic Islets

74

Anatomy and Ultrastructural Organization of Pancreatic Islets

Paul E. Lacy
Marie H. Greider

The islets of Langerhans are scattered throughout the mammalian pancreas, with a greater number in the tail than in the body and head of the pancreas.[1-3] The total mass of endocrine tissue comprises approximately 1–2 percent of the wet weight of the adult human and rat pancreas.[3] By the collagenase technique, the total number of islets in the pancreas of an adult rat has been estimated to be approximately 1000, based upon the insulin content of the isolated islets and the total amount of insulin present within the rat pancreas.[4] The islets in the adult rat pancreas range in size from 50 to 400 μm, with the main part of the islet volume composed of medium-sized islets, approximately 200 μm in diameter.[3] The medium-sized islets correspond to those isolated by the collagenase technique and do not include the small islets with diameters less than 200 μm. The intravital neutral red technique permits identification of all islets, including the small, medium, and large islets. With the neutral red technique, the average number of islets observed was 13,500 per rat pancreas,[5] 26,000 per guinea pig pancreas,[6] and 876,000 per adult human pancreas.[7]

EMBRYOLOGY OF THE ISLETS

Embryologically, the mammalian pancreas develops from two diverticula of the duodenum, one forming part of the head and the other forming the rest of the head, the body, and the tail. Tech-

niques have been developed for the in vitro culture of the developing rat pancreas, thus permitting biochemical, electron microscopic, and hormonal studies on the development and differentiation of islet cells.[8-10] The dorsal lobe first appears midway through the 11th day and the ventral lobe appears approximately 12 hours later.[8] The two lobes soon fuse in the in vivo situation, whereas they develop separately in the in vitro cultures, thus allowing for separate analysis of each lobe. Afer 7 days in culture, the two lobes have a similar degree of morphologic differentiation, the same content of exocrine enzymes, and similar levels of insulin. In contrast, the dorsal lobe has 5–6 times the glucagon content of the ventral pancreas.

In the developing rat pancreas in vivo, insulin is first assayable during the period of the initial formation of the pancreatic diverticulum (11th day of gestation).[9-11] The concentration of insulin increases to a stable level from day 12 to day 14 and then increases dramatically between days 14 and 20. Glucagon is also present on the 11th day, but at levels 100 times higher than insulin, and it remains essentially constant during the remainder of development, with levels comparable to that present in the adult pancreas. Ultrastructural studies indicate that alpha cells with secretory granules are present on day 11 and granulated beta cells appear after the 15th day of development and soon become the dominant cell type.[10] The early appearance of alpha cells and glucagon suggests that this hormone may play a significant role in embryogenesis.[11]

An interaction between mesenchymal tissue and embryonic epithelial tissue in the development of several epithelial organs has been demonstrated. Differentiation of salivary gland epithelia occurs only in the presence of salivary mesenchyme, whereas pancreatic epithelia can develop normally in the presence of a wide variety of mesodermal tissues.[12] A partially purified mesenchymal factor for pancreatic epithelium has been isolated from chick embryos. This factor stimulates DNA, RNA, and protein synthesis in embryonic pancreatic epithelium.[12] Recent studies indicate that the factor may be interacting with the plasma membrane since the factor was active when it was bound to Sepharose beads.[13] The mesenchymal factor also appears to affect the differentiation of embryonic pancreatic epithelia into acinar tissue and beta cells. These fascinating studies are of fundamental importance in attempting to understand the biochemical events controlling cellular differentiation into acinar and endocrine cells of the pancreas and eventually determining whether abnormalities in these control mechanisms play a role in setting the stage for the subsequent development of diabetes mellitus.

It has been generally accepted that the endocrine cells of the pancreas develop from pancreatic ducts which are of endodermal origin. Pearse et al. have suggested that islet cells and enterochromaffin cells of the intestinal tract originate from neuroectodermal cells of the neural crest that have migrated to the foregut and its derivatives.[14,15] The major basis for this postulation is that cytochemically the endocrine cells of the pancreas contain fluorogenic amines and will take up precursors of these amines, such as 3,4-dihydroxyphenylalanine and 5-hydroxytryptophan, similar to cells of the neural crest. In a beautiful series of studies, Le Douarin et al.[16,17] have shown that the C cell of the thyroid is derived from the neural crest. This was accomplished by grafting rhombencephalic primordium from quail embryos into chick embryos in which the rhombencephalon had been removed. The nuclei of the quail cells contain a large mass of heterochromatic DNA, which is absent in cells of chick embryos. Thus a biologic marker exists which permitted the demonstration of the migration of the neural crest cells to the thyroid to form the C cells of the thyroid. Similar studies were accomplished to determine whether enterochromaffin cells were of neurocrestal origin.[18] These investigations revealed that the neural crest cells form the ganglion cells of the intestinal tract, but they do not migrate into the endoderm to form enterochromaffin cells. Recently Phelps[19] removed the neural groove from rat embryos prior to the formation of the neural crest. Pancreatic tissue removed from these embryos and maintained in tissue culture became differentiated and formed beta cells. Thus it would appear that the endocrine cells of the pancreas and the enterochromaffin cells of the intestine are not derived from the neural crest cells as suggested by Pearse et al.

GENERAL ULTRASTRUCTURAL FEATURES

The islet cells are arranged as cords along the capillary channels within the islets and individual cells are surrounded by distinct plasma membranes. The plasma membranes of animal cells in general are now considered to be a fluid mosaic in which particulate components of the membrane may be translocated.[20] Presumably the same concept would apply to the islet cells. With freeze-etch electron microscopy, intramembranous particles have been demonstrated in the plasma membrane of islet cells similar to findings in other types of cells. Initial studies with freeze-etch electron microscopy by Orci et al.[21] have shown that the number of intramembranous particles is decreased in the beta cells of severely diabetic Chinese hamsters in comparison with normal beta cells. The chemical composition of these intramembranous particles and their possible role in hormone secretion is entirely unknown at the present time.

The plasma membranes of adjacent islet cells are attached at specific focal points by desmosomes. It is of interest that these intracellular junctions can be increased in number by incubating the islets with pronase[22] and that within 24 hours after injecting islets into the portal system of the liver, desmosomes can be observed between liver cells and islet cells.[23] In addition to desmosomes, another specialized structure of the plasma membrane, called a *gap junction,* has been demonstrated between alpha and beta cells as well as between individual beta cells.[24] In other cells, it has been shown that gap junctions permit electrical conductivity between cells as well as permitting the passage of low molecular weight substances from one cell to another.[25] It is unknown whether the gap junctions between islet cells affect electrical conductivity or permit the passage of low molecular weight sub-

stances. Since it is now possible to obtain monolayer cultures of islet cells, it should be feasible to determine whether there is a functional interchange of material between islet cells and whether the potential for intercellular communication does exist within the islets of Langerhans.

The secretory granules of islet cells contain the stored hormonal products of the cells and these granules are surrounded by smooth membranous sacs (Fig. 74-1). The mitochondria of islet cells are relatively small in comparison with mitochondria of adjacent acinar cells. Islet cells contain varying amounts of rough endoplasmic reticulum and numerous polysomes scattered throughout the cytoplasm. The Golgi complex is usually located near the nucleus and consists of parallel arrays of smooth membranes and numerous small vesicles. The size of the Golgi complex varies with the functional status of the individual cell.

In the normal islet cell, there are relatively few lysosomes; however, in damaged cells or in those in which hormonal secretion has been suppressed, distinct lysosomes can be observed. Numerous ceroid bodies are present in the islet cells of the normal adult human pancreas. These intracytoplasmic bodies are autofluorescent and contain lipid and lysosomal enzymes. The origin of these structures is unknown.

A microtubule–microfilament system is present in the islet cells. In the normal beta cell, microtubules can be observed adjacent to the plasma membrane as well as scattered throughout the cytoplasm. In the elongated processes of beta cells in monolayer cultures, it is possible to see a more organized arrangement of the microtubules. Under these conditions, the cytoplasmic processes contain long bundles of microtubules which separate linear columns of beta granules (Fig. 74-1).[24] Microfilaments (50–70 Å in diameter) are present as a web just beneath the plasma membrane and probably occur as individual fibers in the interior of the cell (Fig. 74-2).[24] In other types of cells, it has been shown that microfilaments will complex with heavy meromyosin and therefore

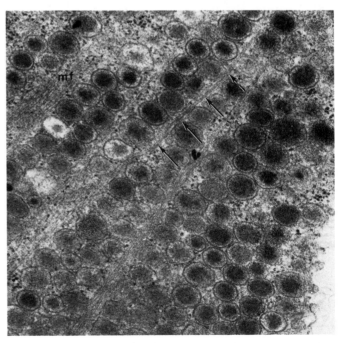

Fig. 74-1.   Electron micrograph of a beta cell in a monolayer cell culture of neonatal (7.5 days) rat pancreas. Rows of microtubules (arrows) separate linear columns of beta granules. Microfilaments (mf) are also present. ×35,000. (From Orci et al.: J. Ultrastruct. Res. *43:* 270, 1973)

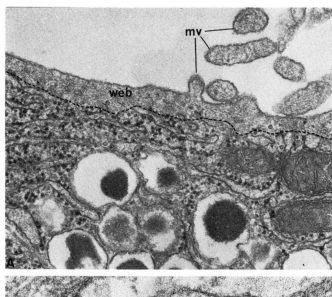

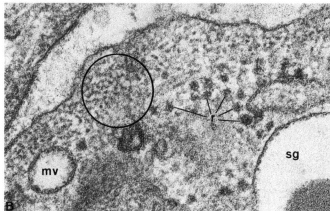

Fig. 74-2. Electron micrograph of normal beta cells of the rat. (A). The cell web of microfilaments is present just beneath the plasma membrane and extends into the microvillous processes (mv). ×40,000. (B). At higher magnification, the network of microfilaments of the cell is demonstrated more clearly. Microvesicles (mv) and ribosomes (r) are present in the cell web. sg, secretory granule. ×125,000. (From Orci et al.: Science *175:* 1128, 1972)

probably contain actin.[26] In monolayer cultures of islet cells, actin has been demonstrated beneath the plasma membrane of these cells by the immunofluorescent technique.[27]

ALPHA CELLS

A variety of light microscopic techniques can be used for the identification of alpha cells, the cells that synthesize and store glucagon. However, none of these staining procedures are truly specific in terms of reacting with a substance unique to alpha cells. Alpha cells were identified by transmission electron microscopy by examining profiles of the cells in a section stained by light microscopic techniques and locating the same cells in an adjacent ultra-thin section.[28] Bussolati et al.[29] have now achieved correlative histochemical and immunocytochemical staining of alpha cells by transmission electron microscopy.

Alpha cells can be differentiated from other types of islet cells on the basis of the ultrastructural appearance of their secretory granules. In man, alpha granules are round with a closely applied membranous sac, and the center of the granule is extremely electron dense with a less dense area surrounding it (Fig. 74-3).

The distribution of alpha cells within the islets varies in differ-

ent species: in the rat and mouse, the alpha cells form a rim at the periphery of the islet; in the horse, they are present in the center of the islet; and in man and the guinea pig, the alpha cells are scattered throughout the islet. In the chicken, pigeon, and duck, large islets in the splenic lobe are composed primarily of alpha cells, with delta cells at the periphery of the islets, whereas small islets composed of beta cells and a peripheral rim of alpha and delta cells are present throughout the rest of the pancreas. Alpha cells comprise approximately 20–25 percent of the islet cell population in adult mammals.

BETA CELLS

Beta cells, which synthesize and store insulin,[30] can be identified with specific staining procedures such as aldehyde fuchsin or aldehyde thionin.[31] Apparently, these reagents react with sulfhydryl groups within insulin. Beta granules have a remarkably different ultrastructural appearance in certain species.[28] In the rat and mouse, beta granules are round and relatively dense, with a distinct space separating the granules from the encasing membranous sacs. In beta cells of man, the dog, and the bat, the granules have rectangular profiles with a crystalline matrix containing lines of repeating periodicity of approximately 50 Å (Fig. 74-3). In the cat,

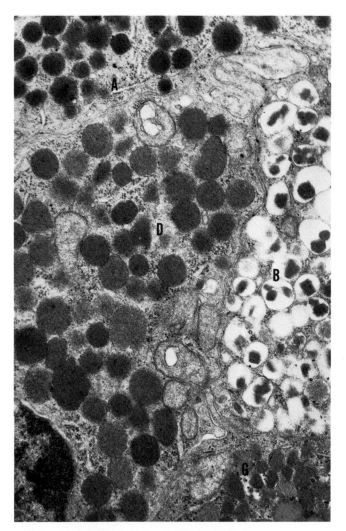

Fig. 74-3. Electron micrograph of portions of an alpha (A), beta (B), and delta (D) cell of a normal human islet. Also present is part of a cell with small secretory granules (G) that may represent a gastrin cell. ×32,000.

beta granules are found with a central dense rhomboid-shaped crystalline structure which is surrounded by pale amorphous material. In the chicken, the granules are composed of sheaves of long, needlelike crystals within the membranous sacs. The reason for this marked species difference in ultrastructural appearance of the granules is unknown. The fluorescent-antibody technique has been used to demonstrate insulin in the beta cells in different species and the immunoperoxidase technique for electron microscopy has demonstrated insulin within individual beta granules.[32] Beta cells comprise approximately 75–80 percent of the islet cell population in the normal adult human islet.

C CELLS

The C cell was first described by Bensley[6] in 1911 as a clear, nonstainable cell in the islets of the guinea pig pancreas. This cell has been identified by electron microscopy.[28,33] It does not contain secretory granules and has only a few mitochondria and a small amount of endoplasmic reticulum.

DELTA CELLS

The delta cell was first identified in human islets by Bloom[34] in 1931 using the Mallory-Heidenhain stain, which imparted a blue color to the cytoplasm of the delta cell. Silver stains have also been used to identify the delta cell.[35] Unfortunately, there is tremendous confusion in the literature as to the terminology that should be applied to this cell and whether a subtype of the delta cell exists.[36] The reason for this confusion is that cytochemical stains do not exist for the specific and uniform identification of the cell, and the secretory product of the cell has not been clearly established. By electron microscopy, a cell is present in human islets and in the islets of other species which contains large, round secretory granules (250–450 nm) with a low electron opacity (Fig. 74-3). The ultrastructural appearance of the secretory granules of these cells is distinctly different from alpha or beta granules and there is general agreement that this represents the delta cell. Another cell, which has been included under the term delta cell, is one which contains small granules (150–250 nm) that are electron opaque and resemble the secretory granules in the gastrin cell (G cell) of the gastric mucosa and the neoplastic islet cells of ulcerogenic tumors (Figs. 74-4 and 74-5).[37] Regrettably, this confusion will remain until the secretory products of these cells are identified and localized by

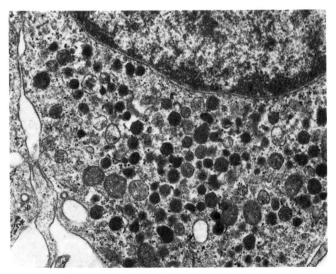

Fig. 74-4. Electron micrograph of a gastrin cell (G cell) in normal human gastric mucosa. ×20,000.

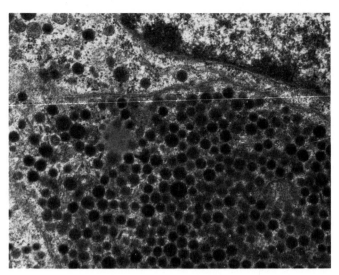

Fig. 74-5. Electron micrograph of a neoplastic islet cell in an ulcerogenic tumor. ×20,000.

electron microscopic immunochemical techniques to the appropriate cell.

E CELLS

Thomas, in 1937, described a new type of cell in the islets of the opossum using light microscopic techniques.[38] In his survey of the islets of 41 species representing 25 families of mammals, the cell type, designated the E cell, was unique to the opossum. The large cytoplasmic granules stained magenta, a color which differentiated the cell from the alpha, beta, and delta cells in tissues stained by Thomas' variation of Mallory's azan stain. By electron microscopy, Munger et al.[39] observed a fourth type of islet cell in the opossum pancreas which was believed to be the E cell. The cells contained relatively large (350–400 nm), irregular-shaped granules of moderate electron density that were distinctly different from the secretory granules of alpha, beta, and delta cells.

F (X) CELLS

By means of tinctorial staining methods, Bencosme and Liepa[40] reported the presence of another type of islet cell in the dog and cat pancreas which they called an X cell (for unknown). In the dog, the X cell was located primarily in the islets of the uncinate process of the pancreas, and alpha cells were not present in these islets. In the cat, the X cell was distributed more uniformly throughout the pancreas and was present not only in the islets but also in the ducts and acini. The ultrastructural features of this cell were described by Munger et al.[39] and the cell was renamed the F cell. The secretory granules of the F cell were moderately electron dense with a marked variability in profile, ranging from kidney-shaped to round granules, and they were distinctly different in ultrastructural appearance from secretory granules of the alpha, beta, delta, and E cells.

STORED HORMONES IN THE ISLETS

Glucagon has been localized to the alpha cell and insulin to the beta cell using electron microscopic immunochemical techniques.[29,32] Other hormones have been localized to the islets; however, the specific cell type producing these hormones has not been established. Gastrin has been demonstrated in cells of human islets using the light microscopic fluorescent-antibody technique.[41] Morphologic studies with electron microscopy indicate that certain cells in human islets contain secretory granules that resemble the secretory granules of the gastrin cell of the gastric mucosa (G cell) and neoplastic cells of ulcerogenic tumors.[37] Electron microscopic immunochemical studies are needed to establish whether this islet cell is the gastrin-containing cell of human islets.

Kimmel et al.[42] have isolated a hormone from the chicken pancreas which is chemically and biologically different from insulin, glucagon, gastrin, and other polypeptide hormones. This hormone has been called *avian pancreatic polypeptide* (APP). Biologically, APP is a powerful gastric secretagogue, stimulating HC1 as well as pepsin secretion, and it accelerates glycogenolysis without altering blood glucose levels.[43] Immunofluorescent studies revealed APP to be present in individual cells scattered throughout the exocrine portion of the chicken pancreas.[44] Ultrastructurally, these cells are endocrine in type and contain secretory granules which are different from alpha, beta, and delta granules.

A peptide which appears to be homologous to APP has been isolated from human, pig, sheep, and beef pancreas. This hormone has been called human pancreatic polypeptide (HPP) and has the same molecular size as APP (36 amino acids) but a different amino acid sequence.[45,46] Immunofluorescent studies have demonstrated HPP in cells located at the periphery of human islets as well as in a few cells interspersed between exocrine cells and between the epithelial cells of small and medium-sized pancreatic ducts.[47]

Somatostatin is a hormone which has been isolated from the hypothalamus; it inhibits glucagon and insulin release from the islets.[48,49] Fluorescent-antibody studies have demonstrated somatostatin in islet cells of the guinea pig, rat, man, sheep, ox, and pig.[50–52] Immunochemical ultrastructural studies indicate that somatostatin is present in delta cells.[53]

It is apparent from the description of the morphology of the islet cells and the hormones localized to the islets that distinct types of islet cells exist that have not been assigned a specific hormone and distinct hormones have been localized to islets that have not been assigned to a specific type of islet cell. Future electron microscopic studies with specific ultrastructural immuno-

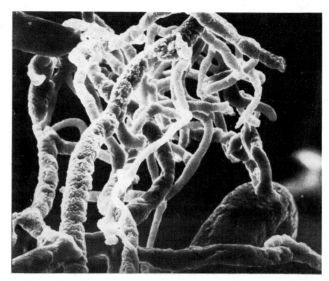

Fig. 74-7. Scanning electron micrograph of the capillary network within an islet. The vascular system of the pancreas was injected with a plastic and the parenchyma was digested away, leaving a cast of the capillaries in an islet attached to larger vessels. ×400. (Courtesy of Dr. Edward W. Dempsey and Dr. Mabel Purkerson)

chemical techniques should resolve these problems and should assist in determining the role of these hormones in maintaining homeostasis and delineating new and as yet unrecognized endocrine dysfunctions based upon either hypersecretion or hyposecretion of these hormones.

VASCULAR STRUCTURE OF THE ISLETS

The blood flow through the pancreas can be visualized in a small, anesthetized animal by light microscopic observations of a transilluminated portion of the pancreas.[54–56] The islets appear as highly vascularized, round to ovoid structures containing small, polygonal cells. Morphologic studies of the islets indicate that the endocrine cells are arranged in short bands or cords of cells separated by a network of capillaries. Each islet cell is close to a capillary (Fig. 74-6), thus allowing for the rapid transport of hormones into the vascular system. Figure 74-7 illustrates the three-dimensional appearance of the capillary network within an islet as visualized by scanning electron microscopy.

The islets are vascularized by 1–3 arterioles and 1–6 venules, depending upon the size of the islet. Upon entering the islet, the arterioles terminate abruptly into capillaries. The rate of blood flow in the islet capillaries is not influenced by the administration of glucagon, hydrocortisone, glucose, or alloxan, whereas epinephrine does cause a temporary interruption of blood flow through the islets.[55] McCuskey and Chapman[56] observed that although total blood flow through the islets is normally constant, flow through individual capillaries may be intermittent. Endothelial cells appear to be responsible for this focal intermittent flow within the islets.

Capillaries of the pancreatic islets are composed of fenestrated endothelial cells (Fig. 74-6),[28] a feature typical of capillaries of other endocrine glands. The fenestrated areas are composed only of the fused plasma membranes or portions of the unit membranes and are considered to be areas that may permit the rapid exchange of material across the endothelium. Marked permeability of islet capillaries has been demonstrated by electron microscopic studies on the transport of horseradish peroxidase (40,000 mol wt)

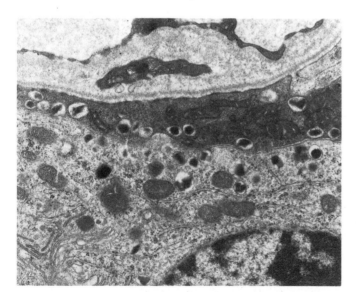

Fig. 74-6. Electron micrograph of a portion of a capillary adjacent to a human beta cell. Fenestrated areas are present in the endothelial cytoplasm. The capillary is separated from the beta cell by two basement membranes with a cross section of a fibroblast between the two basement membranes. ×17,500.

from the blood stream to the pericapillary space of the sand rat.[57] Forty seconds after intravenous injection of the enzyme, peroxidase activity can be detected at the level of the basement membranes and, shortly thereafter, throughout the intercellular spaces. In contrast, the time for transport of horseradish peroxidase across a nonfenestrated capillary, as in the heart, is approximately 5 minutes, or seven times longer.[58]

Hormonal products released into the extracellular fluid surrounding the islet cells must traverse several anatomic structures before entering the blood stream—two basement membranes and the endothelium. The space between the two basement membranes may contain collagen fibers, fibroblasts, and nerve fibers (Fig. 74-6), whereas in some areas the two membranes may be closely apposed. In hyalinized islets of diabetic patients, amyloid deposits have been identified between the two basement membranes.[59] Similar amyloid deposits have been observed in islet cell tumors.[60] Thus in pathologic states another potential anatomic barrier may be present between the endocrine cell and the capillary lumen.

INNERVATION OF THE ISLETS OF LANGERHANS

Nerve fibers enter the pancreas from the celiac ganglion (sympathetic) and the vagus nerves (parasympathetic). These fibers terminate in the pancreas as perivascular, periacinar, and periinsular nerve plexuses.[61,62] Cholinergic nerve fibers have been demonstrated in the islets of the rat, cat, and rabbit using light microscopic techniques for the demonstration of cholinesterase.[63] Fluorescence microscopy has been used to demonstrate adrenergic nerve fibers in the islets of several different species.[64] With this technique, the islets of the golden hamster were observed to contain the highest density of adrenergic fibers, whereas the islets of the dog and cat contained fewer fibers.[65] These light microscopic techniques have clearly demonstrated the presence of adrenergic and cholinergic nerve fibers in the islets; however, the number of these fibers in the islets varies from species to species. With electron microscopy, unmyelinated nerve fibers have been demonstrated in the islets, and the fibers were either surrounded by Schwann cells, were present between the basement membranes of the capillaries, or were closely apposed to the islet cells.[66] Nerve fibers and presumed synapses have been reported in association with alpha, beta, and delta cells.[67-69]

The role of the autonomic nervous system in the control of hormonal release from the islets is not clearly established. Either vagal stimulation or the addition of acetylcholine to pancreatic pieces maintained in vitro will stimulate insulin release.[70] Epinephrine inhibits glucose-induced insulin release.[71] It is possible that the autonomic nervous system has a modulating effect on insulin secretion in the normal subject and may play a role in the pathogenesis of abnormal islet function in the diabetic patient. Orci et al.[72] have reported the absence of autonomic nerve fibers in the islets of the spiny mouse, which has a hereditary form of spontaneous diabetes.

BETA CELL SECRETION

Twenty years ago, information concerning the mechanism of secretion of the beta cell was extremely meager. At that time, special stains had been developed for demonstrating beta granules by light microscopy, and it could be shown that beta cells became degranulated when they were stimulated with glucose. This loss of beta granules could be correlated with a diminished insulin content using the arduous procedure of the mouse convulsion assay for determining the insulin content of the pancreas. During this 20-year interval, remarkable advances have been made in attempting to understand the mechanisms for the formation, storage, and release of insulin from the beta cell. These advances have been due in part to the development of a wealth of techniques and tools such as the following: transmission electron microscopy; procedures for the isolation of mammalian islets; subcellular fractionation of the islets; tissue culture of islet cells; immunoassay for insulin, glucagon, and gastrin; biochemical methods for measuring quantitatively the glucose substrates in the beta cell; and procedures for determining transport of glucose and other agents into the beta cell. By using these biochemical, metabolic, and ultrastructural techniques, it has been possible to gain some insight into the mechanisms by which the beta cell responds to glucose stimulation and subsequently releases insulin into the vascular system. There still remain a tremendous number of unanswered basic questions concerning these processes. In this section, the present state of knowledge concerning the mechanism of beta cell secretion will be reviewed and those areas in which further information is needed will be indicated.

SYNTHESIS OF BETA GRANULES

Stimulation of the beta cell by glucose results in the increased formation of proinsulin in the endoplasmic reticulum. This has been demonstrated by electron microscopic autoradiographic studies as well as by studies on subcellular fractions of the islets.[73,74] The newly formed proinsulin is transported by an energy-requiring mechanism to the Golgi complex.[75] In the Golgi sacs, pale granules can be observed which are presumably immature beta granules. There is evidence that an enzyme or enzyme system exists in the Golgi membranes which apparently is responsible for the splitting of the C peptide from proinsulin and converting it to insulin.[76,77]

The beta granules are packaged in the Golgi complex and released into the cytoplasm, acquiring a membranous sac from the Golgi complex which completely surrounds the individual granules. At some point, zinc is transported into the beta granule. Little or no information is available concerning the control mechanism for the transport of zinc into the granules or the mechanism by which this is accomplished. Apparently the C peptide fragment is also enclosed in this sac with the beta granule. The insulin within the beta granule is transformed into a crystalline state and, by negative staining, it has been shown with electron microscopy that the matrix of the mature beta granule contains lines of periodicity that are approximately 50 Å apart.[78] This distance is consistent with a hexameric form of crystalline zinc insulin. Thus the mature beta granule probably represents a microcrystal of zinc insulin.

RELEASE OF BETA GRANULES

Ultrastructural studies with transmission electron microscopy have demonstrated that, following glucose stimulation, beta granules could be observed adjacent to the plasma membrane; they have also demonstrated evidence for fusion of the membranous sac around the beta granule with the plasma membrane and the resultant liberation of the granule into the extracellular space. This simple process for the release of beta granules was called *emiocytosis*.[79,80] Since the concept of emiocytosis was based entirely on serial morphologic examination of beta cells, additional definitive evidence was needed to determine the validity of this proposed mechanism of secretion. The utilization of in vitro techniques for the study of beta cell secretion provided further evidence in sup-

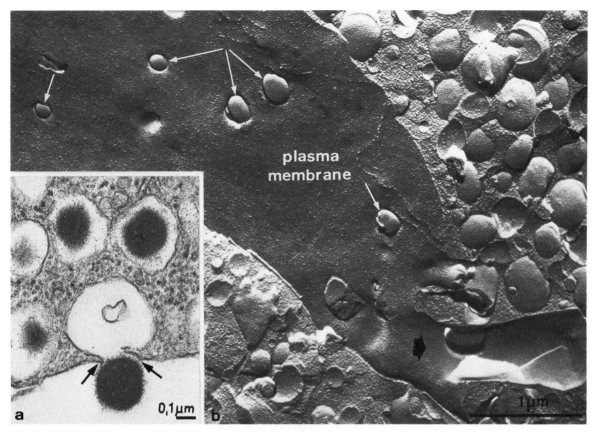

Fig. 74-8. Isolated islets exposed to a high (3.0 mg/ml) glucose concentration. (A.) Thin section of part of a beta cell. A granule–core is being discharged into the extracellular space through the opening resulting from the coalescence of the membrane limiting the granule with the plasma membrane (arrows). ×56,000. Freeze-fracture replica. On the exposed face of the plasma membrane there are several exocytotic (emiocytotic) stomata (thin arrows). The channel extending in the cytoplasm (large arrow) is possible the result of the fusion of the membrane of several granules whose cores could be discharged through a single aperture in the plasma membrane. ×31,000. (Courtesy of Dr. Lelio Orci, Geneva).

port of emiocytosis as the mechanism of beta granule release. Incubation in vitro of isolated beta granules with agents which stimulate insulin secretion did not produce disintegration or solubilization of the beta granules.[81] The final evidence in support of the concept of emiocytosis was obtained in the elegant studies of Orci et al. using freeze-etch electron microscopy.[82] In these studies, they demonstrated a direct continuity of the plasma membrane of the beta cell with the walls of the membranous sac and a portion of a beta granule protruding into the extracellular space surrounding the beta cell (Fig. 74-8). Thus, it is now accepted that the final step in the release of insulin is by the simple process of emiocytosis. In other cell systems, this process has been called *exocytosis*. While the naming of a particular process is of little consequence, the only reason we prefer to use the term *emiocytosis* is that it is based upon the word *emesis* and, as will be indicated subsequently, there are at least superficial similarities between vomiting and the ejection of beta granules.

In emiocytosis, the mechanism of fusion of the membranous sac encasing the granule with the plasma membrane is unknown. In other endocrine glands, such as the adrenal medulla, it has been demonstrated that the membranes surrounding chromaffin granules are markedly different in lipid composition in comparison with the plasma membrane of the chromaffin cell.[83] Chromaffin granules are also released by emiocytosis.[84] Lysolecithin has been demonstrated in chromaffin granule membranes and it is absent or present in very small quantities in the plasma membrane of the medullary cells of the adrenal. Since lysolecithin causes lysis of red blood cells, it has been suggested that it may be responsible for the fusion

of membranes in emiocytosis of chromaffin granules in the adrenal medulla.[85] There is no information available concerning the composition of the membranous sacs surrounding the beta granules. This is an important area that requires intensive study to determine the similarity and dissimilarity of the membranous sacs to the plasma membrane and to attempt to determine the mechanism by which fusion occurs.

The continued release of beta granules by emiocytosis would result in the addition of a large amount of new membranes to the plasma membrane of the cell unless a mechanism existed for either recycling or for degradation of the membranous sacs after they were incorporated into the plasma membrane. In the parotid gland, Amsterdam et al.[86] have demonstrated that zymogen granules of parotid acinar cells are released by emiocytosis and that the membranous sacs encasing the granules fuse with the apical plasma membrane of the acinar cells, resulting in a marked dilatation of the lumen of the acini. After the release of the granules, the plasma membrane is pinched off and returned to the interior of the cell as microvesicles. Using horseradish peroxidase as an extracellular marker, a similar phenomenon of membrane removal has been demonstrated in the beta cell using electron microscopy.[24] Prior to stimulation, the peroxidase was present at the cell surface, whereas following stimulation, microvesicles containing peroxidase could be demonstrated in the cytoplasm as well as the Golgi complex and lysosomes. Since it is probable that the composition of the membranous sacs encasing the granule is different from the plasma membrane, this would imply that the sacs encasing the granule could be recognized and removed specifically for recycling and/or degradation. No information is available as to how this might be accomplished.

ROLE OF THE MICROTUBULE–MICROFILAMENT SYSTEM IN THE INTRACELLULAR TRANSPORT OF BETA GRANULES

The concept of emiocytosis implies that beta granules have been moved to the surface of the beta cell prior to being released. Many had suggested that this was accomplished simply by brownian movement and that the secretory granules came in contact with the plasma membrane by random chance. In order to study the movement of beta granules, phase cinemicroscopy of monolayer cultures of beta cells was accomplished. Quantitative methods were used to assess the movement of the granules, and it was found that glucose and other insulin secretagogues enhanced the movement of beta granules, whereas the absence of calcium in the medium caused a cessation of movement of the granules.[87] The rate of movement of single beta granules was determined and found to be approximately 1.5 μm/s, which compares very well with the rapid component of movement of macromolecules in peripheral nerves. The movement of a single beta granule is shown in Figure 74-9. The granule moved for a distance of 2.4 μm at a rate of 1.2 μm/s, paused for 2.0 s, and moved again at a rate of 1.4 μm/s, paused again for 0.6 s, and moved again at a rate of 1.3 μm/s. The total distance moved by this single granule was approximately

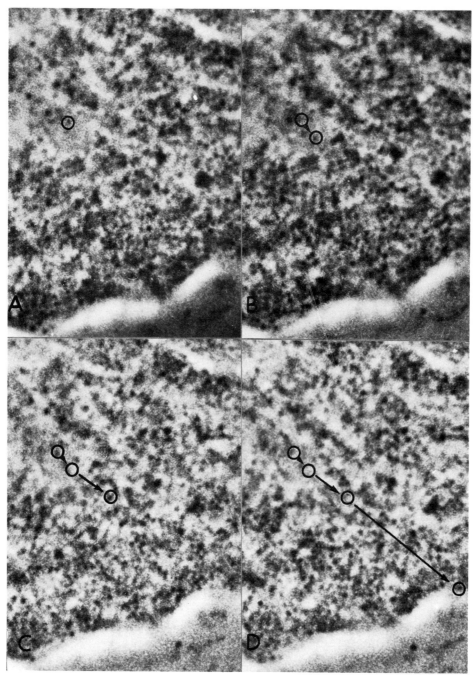

Fig. 74-9. Photomicrographs of four frames of a movie film showing the movement of a beta granule in the cytoplasm of a beta cell. The beta granule encircled in (A) moved a distance of 2.4 μm at a rate of 1.2 μm/s (B); paused for 2 s; moved a distance of 3.8 μm at a rate of 1.4 μm/s, (C); paused 0.6 s; moved a distance of 5.0 μm at a rate of 1.3 μm/s (D). Approximately ×4,200.

11.2 μm. Thus, it is apparent that beta granule movement is not by a brownian movement but is one which is unidirectional in type, which suggests that an internal structural element is present that either guides the granule along a straight line or provides a propelling force for the movement of the granule. It has been proposed that the microtubule–microfilament system is responsible for the intracellular translocation of beta granules to the cell surface.[88]

In the normal beta cell, microtubules can be observed throughout the cytoplasm of the beta cell. In monolayer cultures of beta cells in which elongated processes are present, microtubules have been demonstrated forming columns within these cytoplasmic processes, which are separated by columns of beta granules (Fig. 74-1).[24] Microfilaments are observed predominately as a web beneath the plasma membrane of the beta cell (Fig. 74-2).[89] Presumably, microfilaments are also scattered throughout the cytoplasm of the beta cell, although this point is difficult to establish at the present time. At the plasma membrane, the microtubules blend with the microfilaments.

A variety of agents are available which will either destroy the microtubules or interfere with their function. In a series of studies, it was demonstrated that colchicine, vinblastine, and vincristine (agents which destroy microtubules), as well as deuterium oxide, hexylene glycol, and ethyl alcohol (agents which stabilize microtubules) inhibited the release of insulin following stimulation with either glucose or tolbutamide.[88,90,91] These agents had no effect on calcium uptake by the isolated islets nor did they affect insulin formation by the beta cells. Thus, it was proposed that the microtubules were in some way involved in the translocation of the beta granules to the cell surface.

The microfilamentous system is composed of tiny fibers (50–70 Å in diameter) which apparently contain actin.[26] This system can be altered by using cytochalasins which are extracts of moulds. In the initial studies with cytochalasins, it was suggested that cytochalasin B causes a disruption of the microfilamentous system in many cell types.[92] More recently, Miranda et al.[93] have suggested that the cytochalasins induce a state of hypercontraction of the microfilaments, since the compacted feltlike masses induced by the cytochalasins bind heavy meromyosin, and these masses do not occur when inhibitors of energy metabolism are present in the medium. In addition, it has been shown that cytochalasin B inhibits glucose transport into fibroblasts,[94] and, in studies in our own laboratory, the agent also inhibits glucose transport into the beta cell.[95] Thus the primary site of action of the cytochalasins is not clearly defined. They presumably affect the plasma membrane with respect to hexose transport, but they also affect the microfilamentous system.

Cytochalasin B produces an enhancement of glucose-induced and tolbutamide-induced insulin release.[89] Using perifusion studies, it was demonstrated that this enhancement occurs in both the first and second phase of insulin release.[96] Orci et al. suggested that this enhancing effect of cytochalasin B was due to a partial removal of the microfilamentous web from beneath the plasma membrane, thus exposing an additional membranous surface and removing a barrier to the emiocytosis of the beta granules.[89] An interesting paradox exists since, on the one hand, cytochalasin B enhances glucose-induced insulin release and, on the other, it inhibits the rate of transport of glucose into the beta cell.

From the evidence available, it would appear that the microtubules and microfilaments should be considered as a single functional system. Since the microfilaments contain actin, they would be the logical mediators of a propellant force to move secretory granules in the beta cell. The microtubules could be a dynamic scaffolding for the microfilaments and the two then function as a synergistic unit. If this scaffolding of microtubules were destroyed, then the beta granules could not be directed to the cell surface. If a hypercontraction of the microfilaments was induced, such as with the cytochalasins, then the number of granules reaching the cell surface would be increased per unit time. This synergistic action of the microtubule–microfilament system could explain how columns of beta granules could be moved to the plasma membrane and, as observed with electron microscopy, three to four granules would be released at a single locus on the plasma membrane. It could also explain the biphasic pattern of insulin release, since those granules associated with the system would be released first, and stored granules as well as newly formed granules would then become associated with the system and finally reach a state of equilibrium forming the second phase of secretion. At the present time, this concept is still a working hypothesis, since it requires the establishment, from a biochemical standpoint, of a direct association of the membranous sac surrounding the beta granules with the microtubule–microfilament system. Hopefully, this can be accomplished by subcellular fractionation of the islets under appropriate conditions.

CALCIUM METABOLISM AND INSULIN RELEASE

Extracellular calcium is an absolute requirement for the induction of insulin release from the beta cell.[97] Malaisse-Lagae et al. have shown that the accumulation of ^{45}Ca is increased following glucose stimulation and that the amount of bound calcium accumulating in the islet cell is proportional to the degree of stimulation.[98] In further studies, these investigators have shown that glucose apparently inhibits the efflux of calcium from islet cells, whereas dibutyrl cAMP apparently mobilizes bound calcium in the beta cell.[99] Ultrastructural histochemical studies have shown that the distribution of calcium in the beta cell is changed following stimulation with glucose.[100] In the nonstimulated condition, calcium is present predominantly on the plasma cell membrane and, following glucose stimulation, calcium is found on and within the membranous sacs encasing beta granules. This shift in calcium localization may be related to the change in membrane potential that has been observed in electrophysiologic studies of beta cells following glucose stimulation.[101]

Since the microtubule–microfilament system is involved in the translocation of beta granules following glucose stimulation, it has been suggested that calcium may be the trigger for the induction of contraction or change in physical conformation of this system with the resultant intracellular transport of the beta granules to the cell surface, where they are released by emiocytosis.[80,102] The modulating effect of cAMP on glucose-induced insulin release could be due to the shifting of calcium from a bound form to a free form in which it could interact with the microtubule–microfilament system. Studies on calcium metabolism in beta cells have been limited predominantly to investigations of bound calcium within these cells. Information is needed with respect to the acute effects of glucose on the transport of calcium across the beta cell membrane. Information is also needed to determine the site of storage of calcium in the nonstimulated beta cell, such as in mitochondria or endoplasmic reticulum, and to determine whether calcium is shifted to other organelles such as the microtubule–microfilament system following glucose stimulation. These investigations should be feasible using subcellular fractions of the islets under different experimental conditions. Studies such as these should indicate the interrelationship of acute glucose stimulation with respect to calcium transport and finally whether calcium is the intracellular trigger initiating a contraction or change in conformation of the microtubule–microfilament system.

ROLE OF PLASMA MEMBRANE IN BETA CELL SECRETION

Until recently, it has been assumed that the induction of insulin release from the beta cell was due to the metabolism of glucose. Matschinsky et al. have shown that this concept is incorrect, since no significant changes in substrate and ATP levels could be demonstrated in islets following acute glucose stimulation.[103] They have suggested that glucose may be interacting with specific receptors on the plasma membrane of the beta cell. The problem of establishing the existence of glucoreceptors on the beta cell membrane is more difficult than for other endocrine tissues since the stimulating agent is not a protein and it is transported into the cell.

The diabetogenic action of alloxan in vivo can be prevented by the simultaneous administration of either D-glucose, D-mannose, or 3-0-methyl-D-glucose.[104–106] In our laboratory, we have been using alloxan as a possible in vitro probe for establishing the existence of glucoreceptors on the plasma membrane. In a series of studies, it was demonstrated that exposure of isolated rat islets to alloxan in vitro for a 5-minute period inhibited subsequent glucose-induced insulin release, yet tolbutamide-induced insulin release remained intact.[107] Concomitant exposure of the isolated islets with alloxan and high concentrations of either D-glucose, D-mannose, or 3-0-methyl-D-glucose resulted in protection of the beta cells from alloxan. L-glucose, which is not transported into the beta cell, provided no protection. A stereospecificity for the protection of glucose against the diabetogenic action of alloxan in vivo has been reported.[108] The alpha anomer of D-glucose provided greater protection against alloxan in vivo than the beta anomer.

In recent studies, we have shown that theophylline and caffeine will also protect islet cells from the inhibitory effect of alloxan and that the mechanism of protection by these agents is not through the metabolism of cAMP.[109] Theophylline has been shown in other cell types to inhibit glucose transport.[110] Cytochalasin B also protects the islets against the inhibitory action of alloxan, whereas cytochalasin D does not provide protection.[111] Both of these agents enhance glucose-induced insulin release; however, cytochalasin B inhibits hexose transport,[95] whereas cytochalasin D does not affect the rate of transport of glucose into the islet cells.[111] Alloxan has no effect on the rate of hexose transport in the isolated islets, and alloxan alone induces a short burst of insulin release.[112]

The interpretation of these findings at the present time is that alloxan may be interacting with a glucoreceptor site which is in close proximity to the hexose transport site and that the protective agents are in some way covering the glucoreceptor as they are being transported. Information is needed as to whether alloxan is transported into the islet cells or whether it is bound to the plasma membrane. With this information, it would be possible to study the competitive action of agents which protect the beta cell against alloxan. A digestion filtration technique has been developed which provides a large number of islets from a single rat pancreas.[113] This procedure should make it feasible to attempt to obtain plasma membrane fractions which could be used for studies on binding of labeled alloxan and glucose. Hopefully, these approaches may lead to the establishment and characterization of specific receptors for glucose on the beta cell membrane.

MODEL OF BETA CELL SECRETION

A model is proposed which describes the possible steps linking the specific stimulus by glucose with the resultant secretion of insulin (Fig. 74-10). The model is presumptuous since there are large gaps in our information. However, it is of value for testing various hypotheses with respect to insulin secretion and for com-

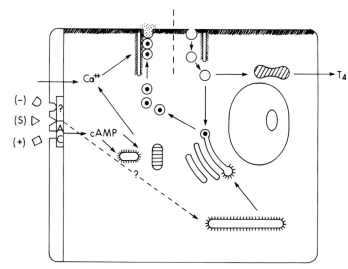

Fig. 74-10. Model of beta cell secretion (see text).

paring the mechanism of secretion in the beta cell with other endocrine glands.

It is proposed that in the beta cell specific glucoreceptors exist on the plasma membrane which recognize D-glucose and preferentially recognize the alpha anomer of D-glucose. As a result of the interaction of D-glucose with the receptor, the adenylate cyclase system is activated and very probably the beta cell membrane becomes more permeable to calcium, resulting initially in an influx of ionic calcium into the cell. This resultant change in ionic flux would be associated with the change in membrane potential which has been described for the beta cell. cAMP would play only a modulating role in insulin secretion by releasing bound calcium from the organelles of the cell. The ionic calcium within the cell in association with other factors would initiate a contraction of the microtubule–microfilament system, with a resultant displacement of columns of beta granules to the cell surface, where they would be released by emiocytosis. This immediate release of insulin would form the first phase of secretion. The second phase of release would be due to stored and newly formed granules becoming associated with the microtubular–microfilamentous system and being released by emiocytosis. The membranous sacs which encased the beta granules fuse with the plasma membrane and are subsequently pinched off by the microtubular–microfilamentous system and appear again as microvesicles in the cytoplasm. The microvesicles either are returned to the Golgi complex or fuse with the lysosomes and become degraded.

In comparing the proposed model for the release of insulin from the beta cell with other endocrine glands, it appears that there are areas of similarity and dissimilarity. For example, in the thyroid the colloid within a thyroid follicle is analogous to a single, huge secretory granule that is surrounded by several cells. Following stimulation of the thyroid with thyroid-stimulating hormone, cellular projections are formed at the apical surface of the follicular cells which engulf portions of the colloid and transfer the material into the cell by endocytosis. The colloid droplets move toward the basal portion of the cell, where they fuse with lysosomes, resulting in the proteolytic digestion of thyroid globulin and the release of thyroxine and triiodothyronine.[114] This entire sequence of events can be mimicked by the addition of dibutyrl cAMP.[115] Antimicrotubular agents inhibit the release of thyroid hormones from thyroid glands incubated in vitro, and cytochalasin B also blocks the release of thyroid hormone,[116] indicating that the microtubule–microfilament system is involved in the endocytotic process in the thyroid cell. The secretion of thyroid hormone in the thyroid gland would be analogous to the recycling of membrane from the beta cell following the release of beta granules. Thus the secretion of hormone by the thyroid gland would employ only one portion of the secretory process of the beta cell.

Glucose not only stimulates the immediate release of stored hormone from the beta cell, it also initiates the new formation of insulin within the cell. Following glucose stimulation, proinsulin formation is stimulated within the endoplasmic reticulum by a mechanism which is as yet unknown. Proinsulin is then transported by an energy-requiring mechanism to the Golgi complex, where the C peptide of proinsulin is apparently removed. The newly formed insulin is then packaged into secretory granules that are surrounded by membranous sacs derived from the Golgi complex; it is then released into the cytoplasm of the beta cell. Zinc enters the secretory granule at some stage in this development, resulting in the formation of microcrystals of zinc insulin, which is the mature form of beta granules.

ALPHA CELL SECRETION

Compared with the information available on the intracellular events associated with beta cell secretion, relatively little information is available with respect to the mechanism of glucagon secretion by the alpha cells. Emiocytosis has been described as the mechanism of release of alpha granules.[117] The possible role of the microtubule–microfilament system in alpha secretion is not clear at the present time. In the normal islet, glucose suppresses glucagon release from the alpha cells, whereas in the diabetic patient, hyperglucagonemia is present and glucagon secretion is not suppressed by glucose.[118] It is unknown whether glucose causes suppression of glucagon secretion by interacting with a specific receptor for glucose on the plasma membrane of the alpha cell or whether suppression occurs as a result of the intracellular metabolism of glucose. The recent demonstration of gap junctions between alpha and beta cells raises the intriguing possibility of a direct interaction between alpha and beta cells through the transport of metabolites from one cell to the other.[24] The resolution of the basic mechanisms responsible for the formation, storage, and release of glucagon from the alpha cell is an exciting challenge for future investigations.

REFERENCES

1. Opie, E. L. On the histology of the islands of Langerhans of the pancreas. *Johns Hopkins Hosp. Bull. 11:* 205, 1900.
2. Hellman, B. The frequency distribution of the number and volume of the islets of Langerhans in man. I. Studies on non-diabetic adults. *Acta Soc. Med. Upsal. 64:* 432, 1959.
3. Hellman, B. Methodological approaches to studies of the pancreatic islets. *Diabetologia 6:* 110, 1970.
4. Steinke, J., and Patel, T. Variable glucose response and extractable insulin content of single pancreatic rat islets. *Diabetes 20:* 327, 1971.
5. Haist, R. E., and Pugh, E. J. Volume measurement of the islets of Langerhans and the effect of age and fasting. *Am. J. Physiol. 152:* 36, 1948.
6. Bensley, R. R. Studies on the pancreas of the guinea pig. *Am. J. Anat. 12:* 297, 1911.
7. Clark, E. The number of islands of Langerhans in the human pancreas. *Anat. Anz. 43:* 81, 1913.
8. Spooner, B. S., Walther, B. T., and Rutter, W. J. Development of the dorsal and ventral mammalian pancreas *in vivo* and *in vitro. J. Cell. Biol. 47:* 235, 1970.
9. Clark, W. R., and Rutter, W. J. Synthesis and accumulation of insulin in the fetal rat pancreas. *Develop. Biol. 29:* 468, 1972.
10. Pictet, R. L., Clark, W. R., Williams, R. H., and Rutter, W. J. An ultrastructural analysis of the developing embryonic pancreas. *Develop. Biol. 29:* 436, 1972.
11. Rall, L. B., Pictet, R. L., Williams, R. H., and Rutter, W. J. Early differentiation of glucagon-producing cells in embryonic pancreas: a possible developmental role for glucagon. *Proc. Natl. Acad. Sci. U.S.A. 70:* 3478, 1973.
12. Ronzio, R. A., and Rutter, W. J. Effects of a partially purified factor from chick embryos on macromolecular synthesis of embryonic pancreatic epithelia. *Develop. Biol. 30:* 307, 1973.
13. Levine, S., Pictet, R., and Rutter, W. Control of cell proliferation and cytodifferentiation by a factor reacting with the cell surface. *Nature [New Biol.] 246:* 49, 1973.
14. Pearse, A. G. E. Common cytochemical and ultrastructural characteristics of cells producing polypeptide hormones (the APUD series) and their relevance to thyroid and ultimobranchial C cells and calcitonin. *Proc. R. Soc. [B] 170:* 71, 1968.
15. Pearse, A. G. E., Polak, J. M., and Heath, C. M. Development, differentiation and derivation of the endocrine polypeptide cells of the mouse pancreas. *Diabetologia 9:* 120, 1973.
16. Le Douarin, N., and Le Lièvre, C. Démonstration de l'origine neurale des cellules à calcitonine du corps ultimobranchial chez l'embryon de Poulet. *C. R. Acad. Sci. Paris 270:* 2857, 1970.
17. Le Douarin, N., Fontaine, J., and Le Lièvre, C. New studies on the neural crest origin of the avian ultimobranchial glandular cells. Interspecific combinations and cytochemical characterization of C cells based on the uptake of biogenic amine precursors. *Histochemistry 38:* 297, 1974.
18. LeDouarin, N., and Teillet, M. A. The migration of neural crest cells to the wall of the digestive tract in avian embryo. *J. Embryol. Exp. Morphol. 30:* 31, 1973.
19. Phelps, P. Evidence that the endocrine pancreatic cells are not derived from the neural crest. *Anat. Rec. 181:* 449, 1975.
20. Berlin, R. D., Oliver, J. M., Ukena, T. E., and Yin, H. H. The cell surface. *Physiol. Med. 292:* 515, 1975.
21. Orci, L., Amherdt, M., Malaisse-Lagae, F., Perrelet, A., Dulin, W. E., Gerritsen, G. C., Malaisse, W. J., and Renold, A. E. Morphological characterization of membrane systems in A and B cells in Chinese hamsters. *Diabetologica 10:* 529, 1974.
22. Unger, R. H., and Renold, A. E. Pronase effect on pancreatic beta cell secretion and morphology. *Science 180:* 647, 1973.
23. Griffith, R. C., Sharp, D. W., Ballinger, W. F., and Lacy, P. E. A morphologic study of intrahepatic portal vein islet isografts. *Diabetes 24:* 449, 1975.
24. Orci, L. A portrait of the pancreatic B cell. The Minkowski Award Lecture, 1973. *Diabetologia 10:* 163, 1974.
25. Payton, B. W., Bennett, M. V. L., and Pappas, G. D. Permeability and structure of functional membranes at an electronic synapse. *Science 166:* 1641, 1969.
26. Ishikawa, H., Bischoff, R., and Holtzer, H. Formation of arrowhead complexes with heavy meromyosin in a variety of cell types. *J. Cell Biol. 43:* 312, 1969.
27. Gabbini, G., Malaisse-Lagae, F., Blondel, B., and Orci, L. Actin in pancreatic islet cells. *Endocrinology 95:* 1630, 1974.
28. Lacy, P. E. Electron microscopic identification of different cell types in the islets of Langerhans of the guinea pig, rat, rabbit and dog. *Anat. Rec. 128:* 255, 1957.
29. Bussolati, G., Capella, C., Vassalo, G., and Solcia, E. Histochemical and ultrastructural studies on pancreatic A cells. Evidence for glucagon and non-glucagon components of the granules. *Diabetologica 7:* 181, 1971.
30. Lacy, P. E. Electron microscopic and fluorescent antibody studies on islets of Langerhans. *Exp. Cell Res. [Suppl.] 7:* 296, 1959.
31. Gomori, G. Aldehyde-fuchsin: a new stain for elastic tissues. *Am. J. Clin. Pathol. 20:* 665, 1950.
32. Misugi, K., Howell, S. L., Greider, M. H., Lacy, P. E., and Sorenson, G. D. The pancreatic beta cell. Demonstration of peroxidase-labeled antibody technique. *Arch. Pathol. 89:* 97, 1970.
33. Caramia, F., Munger, B. L., and Lacy, P. E. The ultrastructural basis for the identification of cell types in the pancreatic islets. I. Guinea pig. *Z. Zellforsch. 67:* 533, 1965.
34. Bloom, W. A new type of granular cell in the islets of Langerhans of man. *Anat. Rec. 49:* 363, 1931.
35. Hellerstrom, C., and Hellman, B. Some aspects of silver impregnation of the islets of Langerhans in the rat. *Acta Endocrinol. 35:* 518, 1960.
36. Greider, M. H., Bencosme, S. A., and Lechago, J. The human

pancreatic islet cells and their tumors. I. The normal pancreatic islets. *Lab. Invest. 22:* 344, 1970.

37. Greider, M. H., Rosai, J., and McGuigan, J. E. The human pancreatic islet cells and their tumors. II. Ulcerogenic and diarrheogenic tumors. *Cancer 33:* 1423, 1974.

38. Thomas, T. B. Cellular components of the mammalian islets of Langerhans. *Am. J. Anat. 62:* 31, 1937.

39. Munger, B. L., Caramia, F., and Lacy, P. E. The ultrastructural basis for the identification of cell types in the pancreatic islets. II. Rabbit, dog and opossum. *Z. Zellforsch. 67:* 776, 1965.

40. Bencosme, S. A., Liepa, E. Regional differences of the pancreatic islets. *Endocrinology 57:* 588, 1955.

41. Greider, M. H., and McGuigan, J. E. Cellular localization of gastrin in the human pancreas. *Diabetes 20:* 389, 1971.

42. Kimmel, J. R., Pollock, H. G., and Hazelwood, R. L. A new polypeptide hormone. *Fed. Proc. 30:* 1318, 1971.

43. Hazelwood, R. L., Turner, S. D., Kimmel, J. R., and Pollock, H. G. Spectrum effects of a new polypeptide (third hormone?) isolated from the chicken pancreas. *Gen. Comp. Endocrinol. 21:* 485, 1973.

44. Larsson, L. I., Sundler, F., Hakanson, R., Pollock, H. G., and Kimmel, J. R. Localization of APP, a postulated new hormone, to a pancreatic endocrine cell type. *Histocemistry 42:* 377, 1974.

45. Lin, T. M., and Chance, R. E. Spectrum gastrointestinal actions of a new bovine pancreas polypeptide (BPP). *Gastroenterology 62:* 852, 1972.

46. Lin, T. M., Evans, D. C., and Chance, R. E. Action of a bovine pancreatic polypeptide (BPP) on pancreatic secretion in dogs. *Gastroenterology 66:* 852, 1974.

47. Larsson, L. I., Sundler, F., and Hakanson, R. Immunochemical localization of human pancreatic polypeptide (HPP) to a population of islet cells. *Cell Tissue Res. 156:* 167, 1975.

48. Brazeau, P., Vale, W., Burgus, R., Ling, N., Butcher, M., Rivier, J., and Guillemin, R. Hypothalamic polypeptide that inhibits the secretion of immunoreactive pituitary growth hormone. *Science 179:* 77, 1973.

49. Koerker, D. J., Ruch, W., Chideckel, E., Palmer, J., Goodner, C. J., Ensinck, J., and Gale, C. C. Somatostatin: Hypothalamic inhibitor of the endocrine pancreas. *Science 184:* 482, 1974.

50. Luft, R., Efendic, S., Hokfelt, T., Johannson, O., and Arimura, A. Immunohistochemical evidence for the localization of somatostatin-like immunoreactivity in a cell population of the pancreatic islets. *Med. Biol. 52:* 428, 1974.

51. Dubois, M. P. Immunoreactive somatostatin is present in discrete cells of the endocrine pancreas. *Proc. Natl. Acad. Sci. 72:* 1340, 1975.

52. Hokfelt, T., Efendic, S., Hellerstrom, C., Johansson, O., Luft, R., and Arimura, A. Cellular localization of somatostatin in endocrine-like cells and neurons of the rat with special references to the A_1-cells of the pancreatic islets and to the hypothalamus. *Acta Endocrinol. 80:* 1, 1975.

53. Pelletier, G., Le Clerc, R., Arimura, A., and Schally, A. V. Immunohistochemical localization of somatostatin in the rat pancreas. *J. Histochem. Cytochem. 23:* 699, 1975.

54. O'Leary, J. L. An experimental study of the islet cells of the pancreas *in vivo. Anat. Rec. 45:* 27, 1930.

55. Bunnag, S. C., Bunnag, S., and Warner, N. E. Microcirculation in the islets of Langerhans of the mouse. *Anat. Rec. 146:* 117, 1963.

56. McCuskey, R. S., and Chapman, T. M. Microscopy of the living pancreas *in situ. Am. J. Anat. 126:* 395, 1969.

57. Like, A. A. The uptake of exogenous peroxidase by the beta cells of the islets of Langerhans. *Am. J. Pathol. 59:* 225, 1970.

58. Karnovsky, M. J. The ultrastructural basis of capillary permeability studied with peroxidase as a tracer. *J. Cell Biol. 35:* 213, 1967.

59. Lacy, P. E. Electron microscopy of the beta cell of the pancreas. *Am. J. Med. 31:* 851, 1961.

60. Porta, E. A., Yerry, R., and Scott, R. E. Amyloidosis of functioning islet cell adenoma of the pancreas. *Am. J. Pathol. 41:* 623, 1962.

61. Gentes, M. Note sur les terminaisous nerveuses des ilots de Langerhans du pancreas. *C. R. Soc. Biol. 54:* 202, 1902.

62. Pensa, A. Osservazioni sulla distribugione du vasi sanguigni e dei nervi nel pancreas. *Intern. Meschr. Anat. Physiol. 22:* 90, 1905.

63. Coupland, R. E. The innervation of pancreas of the rat, cat and rabbit as revealed by the cholinesterase technique. *J. Anat. 92:* 143, 1958.

64. Lever, J. D., Spriggs, T. L. B., and Graham, J. D. P. A formol-fluorescence, fine-structural and autoradiographic study of the adrenergic innervation of the vascular tree in the intact and sympathectomized pancreas of the cat. *J. Anat. 103:* 15, 1968.

65. Cegrell, L. The occurrence of biogenic monoamines in the mammalian endocrine pancreas. *Acta Physiol. Scand. [Suppl.] 314:* 1, 1968.

66. Lacy, P. E. Electron microscopy of the normal islets of Langerhans. Studies in the dog, rabbit, guinea pig and rat. *Diabetes 6:* 498, 1957.

67. Esterhuizen, A. C., Spriggs, T. L. B., and Lever, J. D. Nature of islet-cell innervation in the cat pancreas. *Diabetes 17:* 33, 1968.

68. Legg, P. G. The fine structure and innervation of the beta and delta cell in the islets of Langerhans of the cat. *Z. Zellforsch. 80:* 307, 1967.

69. Kobayashi, S., and Fujita, T. Fine structure of mammalian and avian pancreatic islets with special reference to D cells and nervous elements. *Z. Zellforsch. 100:* 340, 1969.

70. Frohman, L. A., Ezdinli, E. Z., and Javid, R. Effect of vagotomy and vagal stimulation on insulin secretion. *Diabetes 16:* 443, 1967.

71. Malaisse, W., Malaisse-Lagae, F., Wright, P. H., and Ashmore, J. Effects of adrenergic and cholinergic agents upon insulin secretion *in vitro. Endocrinology 80:* 975, 1967.

72. Orci, L., Lambert, A. E., Amherdt, M. L., Cameron, D., Kanazawa, Y., and Stauffacher, W. The autonomous nervous system and the B cell; metabolic and morphological observations made in spiny mice *(Acomys cahirius)* and in cultured foetal rat pancreas. *Acta Diabetol. Lat. 7 [Suppl 1]:* 184, 1970.

73. Bauer, G. E., Lindall, A. W., Dixit, P. K., Lester, G., and Lazarow, A. Studies of insulin biosynthesis. Subcellular distribution of leucine-H^3 radioactivity during incubation of goosefish islet tissue. *J. Cell Biol. 28:* 413, 1966.

74. Howell, S. L., Kostianovsky, M., and Lacy, P. E. Beta granule formation in isolated islets of Langerhans: a study by electron microscopic radioautography. *J. Cell Biol. 42:* 695, 1969.

75. Howell, S. L. Role of ATP in the intracellular translocation of proinsulin and insulin in the rat pancreatic beta cell. *Nature [New Biol.] 235:* 85, 1972.

76. Grant, P. T., and Coombs, T. L. Proinsulin, a biosynthetic precursor of insulin. *Biochemistry 6:* 69, 1970.

77. Kemmler, W., and Steiner, D. F. Conversion of proinsulin to insulin in a subcellular fraction from rat islets. *Biochem. Biophys. Res. Commun. 41:* 1223, 1970.

78. Greider, M. H., Howell, S. L., and Lacy, P. E. Isolation and properties of secretory granules from rat islets of Langerhans. II. Ultrastructure of beta granule. *J. Cell Biol. 41:* 162, 1969.

79. Lacy, P. E. Electron microscopy of the beta cell of the pancreas. *Am. J. Med. 31:* 851, 1961.

80. Lacy, P. E. Beta cell secretion—from the standpoint of a pathobiologist. *Diabetes 19:* 895, 1970.

81. Howell, S. L., Young, D. A., and Lacy, P. E. Isolation and properties of secretory granules from rat islets of Langerhans. III. Studies of the stability of the isolated beta granules. *J. Cell Biol. 41:* 167, 1969.

82. Orci, L., Amherdt, M., Malaisse-Lagae, F., Rouiller, C., and Renold, A. E. Insulin release by emiocytosis: demonstration with freeze-etching technique. *Science 179:* 82, 1973.

83. Blaschko, H., Firemark, H., Smith, A. D., and Winkler, H. Lipids of the adrenal medulla. Lysolecithin, a characteristic constituent of chromaffin granules. *Biochem. J. 104:* 545, 1967.

84. Douglas, W. W., and Poisner, A. M. On the relation between ATP splitting and secretion in the adrenal chromaffin cell: extrusion of ATP (unhydrolyzed) during release of catecholamines. *J. Physiol. 183:* 249, 1966.

85. Howell, J. I., and Lucy, J. A. Cell fusion induced by lysolecithin. *FEBS Lett. 4:* 147, 1969.

86. Amsterdam. A., Ohad, I., and Schramm, M. Dynamic changes in the ultrastructure of the acinar cell of the rat parotid gland during the secretory cycle. *J. Cell Biol. 41:* 753, 1969.

87. Lacy, P. E., Finke, E. H., and Codilla, R. C. Cinemicrographic studies on beta granule movement in monolayer culture of islet cells. *Lab. Invest. 33:* 570, 1975.

88. Lacy, P. E., Howell, S. L., Young, D. A., and Fink, C. J. New hypothesis of insulin secretion. *Nature 219:* 1177, 1968.

89. Orci, L., Gabbay, K. H., and Malaisse, W. J. Pancreatic beta cell web. Its possible role in insulin secretion. *Science 175:* 1128, 1972.

90. Malaisse, W. J., Malaisse-Lagae, F., Walker, M. O., and Lacy, P. E. The stimulus–secretion coupling of glucose-induced insulin release. V. The participation of a microtubular–microfilamentous system. *Diabetes 20:* 257, 1971.

91. Lacy, P. E., Walker, M. O., and Fink, C. J. Perifusion of isolated rat islets *in vitro:* participation of the microtubular system in the biphasic release of insulin. *Diabetes 21:* 987, 1972.

92. Wessells, N. K., Spooner, B. S., Ash, J. F., Bradley, M. O., Luduena, M. A., Taylor, E. L., Wrenn, J. T., and Yamada, K. M. Microfilaments in cellular and developmental processes. *Science 171:* 135, 1971.

93. Miranda, A. F., Godman, G. C., and Tanenbaum, S. W. Action of cytochalasin D on cells of established lines. II. Cortex and microfilaments. *J. Cell Biol. 62:* 406, 1974.

94. Kletzien, R. F., Perdue, J. F., and Springer, A. Cytochalasin A and B: inhibition of sugar uptake in cultured cells. *J. Biol. Chem. 247:* 2964, 1972.

95. McDaniel, M. L., King, S., Anderson, S., Fink, C. J., and Lacy, P. E. Effect of cytochalasin B on hexose transport and glucose metabolism in pancreatic islets. *Diabetologia 10:* 303, 1974.

96. Lacy, P. E., Klein, N. J., and Fink, C. J. Effect of cytochalasin B on the biphasic release of insulin in perifused rat islets. *Endocrinology 92:* 1458, 1973.

97. Grodsky, G. M., and Bennett, L. L. Cation requirements for insulin secretion in the isolated perfused pancreas. *Diabetes 15:* 910, 1966.

98. Malaisse-Lagae, F., and Malaisse, W. J. Stimulus–secretion coupling of glucose-induced insulin release. III. Uptake of ^{45}calcium by isolated islets of Langerhans. *Endocrinology 88:* 72, 1971.

99. Malaisse, W. J. Insulin secretion—multifactional regulation for a single process of release. Minkowski Award Lecture, 1972. *Diabetologia 9:* 167, 1973.

100. Herman, L., Sato, T., and Hales, C. N. The electron microscopic localization of cations to pancreatic islets of Langerhans and their possible role in insulin secretion. *J. Ultrastruct. Res. 42:* 298, 1973.

101. Dean, D. M., and Matthews, E. K. The bioelectrical properties of pancreatic islet cells. Effect of diabetogenic agents. *Diabetologia 8:* 173, 1972.

102. Malaisse, W. J., and Malaisse-Lagae, F. A possible role for calcium in the stimulus–secretion coupling of glucose-induced insulin secretion. *Acta Diabetol. 7:* 264, 1970.

103. Matschinsky, F. M., Ellerman, J. E., Krzanowski, J., Kotler-Brajtburg, J., Landgraf, R., and Fertel, R. The dual function of glucose in islets of Langerhans. *J. Biol. Chem. 246:* 1007, 1971.

104. Bhattacharya, G. Protection against alloxan diabetes by mannose and fructose. *Science 117:* 230, 1953.

105. Carter, W. J., and Younathan, E. S. Studies on protection against the diabetogenic effect of alloxan by glucose. *Proc. Soc. Exp. Med. 109:* 611, 1962.

106. Zawalich, W. S., and Beidler, L. M. Glucose and alloxan interactions in the pancreatic islets. *Am. J. Physiol. 224:* 963, 1973.

107. Tomita, T., Lacy, P. E., Matschinsky, F. M., and McDaniel, M. L. Effect of alloxan on insulin secretion in isolated rat islets perifused *in vitro. Diabetes 23:* 517, 1974.

108. Rossini, A. A., Berger, M., Shadden, J., and Cahill, G. F. Beta cell protection to alloxan necrosis by anomers of D-glucose. *Science 183:* 424, 1974.

109. Lacy, P. E., McDaniel, M. L., Fink, C. J., and Roth, C. Effect of methylxanthines on alloxan inhibition of insulin release. *Diabetologia 11:* 501, 1975.

110. Plagemann, P. G. W., and Sheppard, J. R. Competitive inhibition of the transport of nucleosides, hypoxanthines, choline and deoxyglucose by theophylline, papaverine and prostaglandins. *BBRC 56(4):* 869–875, 1974.

111. McDaniel, M. L.; Roth, C.; Fink, C. J.; Fyfe, G. and Lacy, P. E. Effects of cytochalasins B and D on alloxan inhibition of insulin release. *Biochem. Biophys. Res. Commun. 66:* 1089, 1975.

112. McDaniel, M. L., Anderson, S., Fink, C. J., Roth, C., and Lacy, P. E. Effect of alloxan on permeability and hexose transport in rat pancreatic islets. *Endocrinology 97:* 68, 1975.

113. Shibata, A., Ludvigsen, C. W., Jr., McDaniel, M. L., and Lacy, P. E. Standardization of a digestion–filtration method for isolation of pancreatic islets. *Diabetes 25:* 667, 1976.

114. Nadler, N. J. Anatomical features. In R. O. Greep and E. B. Astwood (eds): Handbook of Physiology, Sec. 7, Endocrinology, vol. 3, Thyroid. Baltimore, Williams & Wilkins, 1974, pp. 39–54.

115. Dumont, J. E., Willems, C., Van Sande, J., and Neve, P. Regulation of the release of thyroid hormones: role of cyclic AMP. *Ann. N. Y. Acad. Sci. 185:* 291, 1971.

116. Wolff, J., and Williams, J. A. The role of microtubules and microfilaments in thyroid secretion. *Rec. Prog. Horm. Res. 29:* 229, 1973.

117. Gomez-Acebo, J., Parrilla, R., and R-Candela, J. L. Fine structure of the A and D cells of the rabbit endocrine pancreas *in vivo* and incubated *in vitro.* I. Mechanism of secretion of the A cells. *J. Cell Biol. 36:* 33, 1968.

118. Unger, R. H., and Orci, L. The essential role of glucagon in the pathogenesis of diabetes mellitus. *Lancet 1:* 14, 1975.

75

Biosynthesis of Insulin and Glucagon

Donald F. Steiner
Howard S. Tager

INTRODUCTION

The classical experiments of Von Mering and Minkowski at the close of the 19th century clearly demonstrated that the pancreas plays an important role in the prevention of diabetes.[1] However, it was not until Banting and Best, in 1921, ligated the exocrine duct in dogs, allowing the destructive acinar tissue to atrophy, that potent preparations of insulin could routinely be prepared. The name *insulin,* which was based on the belief that the hormone was derived from the islets of Langerhans, actually was suggested as early as 1909 by deMayer and later again in 1917 by Sir Edward Sharpey-Schaffer. Preparative methods based on those of Banting and Best were rapidly developed for the commercial preparation of the hormone, and within 1 year insulin was being administered to patients with diabetes.

The chemical nature of insulin was a more elusive problem, although the fact that it was destroyed by proteolytic enzymes suggested that it was indeed a protein. At that time, however, it was not appreciated that proteins might function as hormones as well as enzymes and produce such dramatic biologic effects as the lowering of blood sugar and the enhancement of carbohydrate utilization. When J. J. Abel first succeeded in crystallizing insulin in 1926 there was great controversy as to whether the crystals of protein he had obtained were actually the active biologic principle or merely the vehicle for a smaller active moiety.[2] Such controversies seem remarkable in the light of our detailed present-day knowledge of the structure and biologic properties of insulin, but it is important to remember that many of the modern techniques of protein chemistry were developed through the clinical need for insulin, which made it abundantly available to the biochemist as an object for study.

Despite many recent advances in our understanding of the formation and secretion of insulin, we still lack complete insight into the molecular details of its action. We are similarly deficient in our understanding of why diabetes afflicts many humans as well as many other animal species. This chapter will selectively review our present knowledge of the chemistry and properties of insulin and glucagon and their precursors, and the biosynthetic mechanisms of the alpha and beta cells. The mechanism of biosynthesis of insulin via proinsulin has served as a model for the study of many other hormonal systems. As a result of these and related studies it is now generally recognized that most peptide hormones are heterogeneous in the circulation and that the interconversion and metabolism of these various forms adds additional complexity to the normal physiologic regulation of endocrine secretion. We will try to relate these findings, wherever possible, to pathologic states in man, particularly diabetes and benign or malignant endocrine tumors.

ISOLATION, PROPERTIES, AND STRUCTURE OF INSULIN

ISOLATION AND CHARACTERIZATION

Insulin occurs throughout the vertebrate kingdom and immunologic and biologic evidence indicates its presence in the digestive systems of some invertebrate species.[3] The early recognition that ethanol or acid–ethanol extraction of pancreas inhibited proteolytic destruction of insulin has provided the basis for most modern preparative procedures.[4] Acid–ethanol also extracts proinsulin, C-peptide, and glucagon from islet tissue in most species. The acid–ethanol extracts are partially purified by fractional precipitation and isoelectric precipitation with organic solvents to solubilize fats, and can then be further resolved by gel filtration[5] and ion exchange chromatography.[6,7] Salting-out from acidic solutions is not effective for recovering small amounts of insulin and may lead to significant losses of C-peptide.[8] For most analytical as well as preparative purposes it is preferable to omit salting-out steps and to proceed directly to gel filtration, a convenient and highly reproducible method that separates proinsulin from insulin and thus permits specific immunoassays to be made for insulin, C-peptide, and proinsulin, as well as for glucagon and its precursors. A suitable flow sheet for extraction of the pancreas of most mammals is shown in Figure 75-1.

Yields of insulin vary dependent on the source: for mammalian pancreas, 10–15 μmol/kg wet weight; for fetal calf pancreas,

PREPARATION of INSULIN, PROINSULIN and C-PEPTIDE

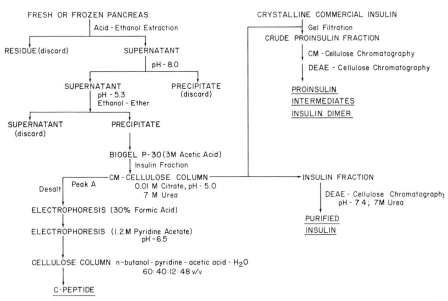

Fig. 75-1. Flow diagram for the isolation of proinsulin, insulin, and C-peptide from fresh pancreas or from commercial insulin preparations. For methodologic details see Steiner et al.[7,38]

60–70 μmol/kg; for fish islets, 300–500 μmol/kg; for isolated rat islets of Langerhans, 2–3 mmol/kg.

With modern methods of purification, the biologic activity of most mammalian insulin preparations ranges from 26 to 30 IU/mg. The bovine insulin standard of the International Union of Pure and Applied Chemistry is stated to have an activity of 25 IU/mg dry weight.[4] Although crystallization with zinc is a powerful method for purification of insulin, it is now generally recognized that even repeated crystallization does not eliminate all impurities from insulin. Most crystalline preparations contain glucagon, desamido insulin, proinsulin and intermediate cleavage forms, ethyl esters of insulin, dimers of insulin, and higher aggregates of insulin and proinsulin with unknown components. Gel filtration of crystalline preparations separates these components into essentially three fractions:[7] *a component*—material of high molecular weight eluting essentially in the void volume, i.e., aggregates; *b component*—proinsulin, intermediate cleavage products of proinsulin, and insulin dimers; *c component*—insulinlike components including desamido forms, arginyl insulins (B_{31} and B_{32} arginine residues), glucagon, and C-peptide. Further purification of the insulin-containing fractions by ion exchange chromatography, using urea-containing buffers or 60 percent ethanol as dispersing agents, yields preparations that are better than 99 percent pure, i.e., the "monocomponent" or "single-component" insulins now being offered commercially. These preparations are apparently less antigenic than crystalline insulin preparations and show promise for therapeutic application.[9]

The assay of insulin, like most other protein hormones, has always presented difficulties with regard to precision and sensitivity. The various in vivo blood sugar–lowering assays that often are used by pharmaceutical houses require too much material to be very useful for most experimental laboratories. When sufficient amounts of hormone are available (i.e., >0.5 mg), polyacrylamide gel electrophoresis with appropriate standards can provide a wealth of useful information regarding the homogeneity and quality of the preparations.[6,7,10] This method also gives indications as to the state of amidation of the insulin or proinsulin, which may reflect the harshness of the acid conditions applied in the extrac-

tion, and this method also can reveal the extent to which autolysis may have occurred in the pancreas prior to extraction. Other routinely used biochemical methods for assessing the purity of proteins are equally applicable, of course, but it must be borne in mind that even though all tests indicate that homogeneity has been achieved, the biologic activity of the preparation must be examined directly to ascertain that no chemical damage to the hormone has occurred.

The recent introduction of hormone-binding assays using isolated plasma membrane preparations promises to provide more sensitive and reliable methods for screening material for biologic potency in vivo since these methods have thus far demonstrated a good correlation between binding and measured biologic potency.[11–13] However, both binding tests and immunoassays can be misleading since neither necessarily measures the true biologic effectiveness of the hormone. Thus the thorough characterization of any insulin preparation should include measurements of biologic potency with isolated fat cells or liver cells, as well as measurements of binding characteristics, and full characterization of the protein in terms of its molecular weight, composition, homogeneity, and, if possible, amino acid composition and sequence. For more detailed information regarding the physicochemical properties of insulin several recent reviews are recommended.[4,14,15]

INSULIN STRUCTURE

The determination of the primary structure of bovine insulin by Ryle and his associates[16] provided the first known protein structure and it also laid to rest the prevalent notions that proteins were not defined chemical entities. This demonstration thus provided an important cornerstone of molecular biology which led to the recognition of the existence of the genetic code. The primary structures of insulins from more than 25 vertebrate species have been determined in the interval since the pioneering studies of Ryle and co-workers.[4,17–19] These results, summarized in Figure 75-2, indicate that amino acid substitutions can occur at many positions within either chain without greatly altering the biologic effectiveness of the hormone as measured in various bioassay systems. On the other hand, certain structural features are conserved throughout vertebrate evolution, including the positions of the three disulfide bonds, the N-terminal and C-terminal regions of the A chain, and the hydrophobic residues in the C-terminal region of the B chain, as well as others. Since chemical modifications in any of these regions tend to markedly reduce or abolish biologic activity, these evidently play important roles in maintaining important secondary and tertiary structural features needed for biologic activity.[4,20] The C-terminal hydrophobic sequence of the B chain (residues 23–27) also plays an important role in the formation of insulin dimers as described below.

As might be anticipated from the extensive amino acid substitutions that occur between mammalian and piscine insulins, it is not surprising that the immunologic cross-reactivity between these proteins is rather weak. Generally, very low cross-reactivity can be detected by means of conventional immunoassays, especially when the heterologous insulin is used as the labeled tracer. For detailed considerations of insulin antigenicity in relation to its structure several recent reviews are recommended.[4,21]

The elucidation by Blundell and co-workers of the three-dimensional structure of porcine insulin, initially at a resolution of 2.8 Å and with recent refinements at 1.9 Å, represents an important breakthrough in the study of peptide hormone structure. The results have proven invaluable in interpreting much of the available chemical data on the properties of insulin.[22] Detailed knowledge of the spatial organization of the molecule also promises to provide further insight into the molecular mechanism of binding and action of insulin. The hexameric unit of crystalline zinc insulin (Fig. 75-3) consists of three dimers arranged around a major threefold axis which passes through two zinc atoms, each of which is coordinated with the imidazole groups of three B_{10} histidine residues and is located just above or below the plane of the hexamer.[23] The insulin dimers are held together in the crystals by hydrogen bonds between the peptide groups of residues 24 and 26 within the C-terminal region of the B chain, forming an antiparallel beta pleated sheet structure. The locations in space of the known invariant amino acids within the insulin monomer are shown in Figure 75-4.

Preliminary x-ray diffraction studies on hagfish insulin crystals suggest a very similar arrangement of the molecular backbone of the insulin in this very primitive cyclostome.[18,24] These results are consistent with the conservation in hagfish insulin of many primary structural features known to be concerned with the formation of the characteristic secondary and tertiary structure of the hormone. Taken altogether, these results suggest that despite

some variations in certain species such as the guinea pig and coypu,[18] the molecular structure of insulin, as well as its tendency to form isologous dimers, has remained remarkably constant throughout vertebrate evolution. The fact is further reflected in the relatively high interspecies crossover of biologic potency among the known insulins; most fish insulins are only slightly less active than mammalian insulins, and even the highly substituted hagfish insulin has been found to have 5–10 percent of the biologic activity of bovine or porcine insulin in various mammalian test systems.[25]

These findings also imply that the receptor(s) for insulin have changed relatively little throughout vertebrate evolution. This conservatism is similar to that seen in many other proteins, including various enzymes and the electron carrier, cytochrome C. Thus cytochrome C molecules from distant species all function similarly in mammalian mitochondrial preparations.[26] On this basis one might speculate that the structure of insulin and its receptor protein(s) does not simply represent arbitrary lock-and-key design to subserve simple recognition purposes, but rather the insulin–receptor complex fulfills some specific chemical function in the plasma membrane either enzymatically as a catalytic unit or possibly as an intramembrane ionophore or translocase.[27] The insulin receptor is discussed in greater detail in Chapter 87.

BIOSYNTHETIC PATHWAY TO INSULIN

Until 1967 it was generally believed that insulin is formed via the combination of separately synthesized A and B chains.[28] The discovery of proinsulin, a precursor form which includes the B and A chains within a single 9000-dalton polypeptide chain, finally disproved this hypothesis.[29] The structure of a representative mammalian proinsulin is shown in Figure 75-5. During the intracellular transport of proinsulin from its site of biosynthesis in the rough endoplasmic reticulum of the beta cell it is slowly cleaved, yielding insulin and a peptide fragment known as the C-peptide; both peptides are then stored in the secretion granules along with small amounts of residual proinsulin and its intermediate cleavage forms.[30] More recently, limited proteolysis also has been found to occur in the formation of a variety of small peptide hormones and other secreted proteins such as serum albumin[31,32] as well as many viral capsule proteins,[33,34] and even connective tissue structural proteins such as collagen.[35] The distinctive feature of insulin biosynthesis which sets it apart from classical zymogen activation is the intracellular proteolytic conversion of the precursor to the

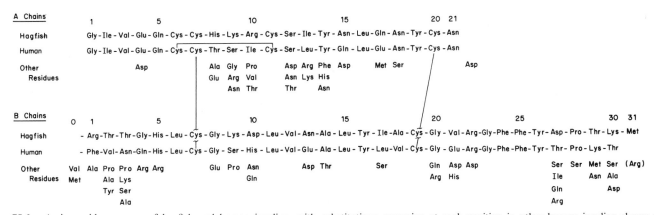

AMINO ACID SEQUENCES OF SOME VERTEBRATE INSULINS

Fig. 75-2. Amino acid sequence of hagfish and human insulins, with substitutions occurring at each position in other known insulins shown for comparison.

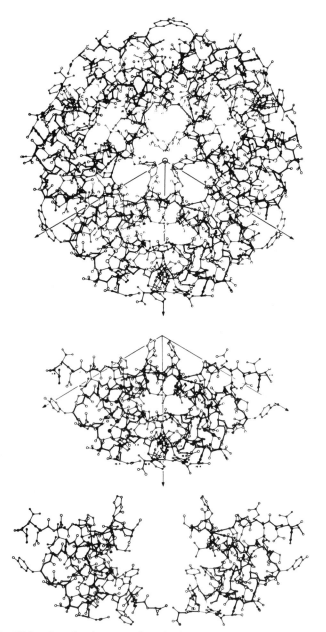

Fig. 75-3. Complete hexamer of porcine insulin showing the development of dimers from monomers and their organization into the hexamer. (From Blundell et al.: Adv. Protein Chem. 26: 279, 1972)

hormone prior to its storage and secretion from the beta cells.[36] The intracellular localization and precise mechanism of this proteolytic process in the beta cell represents an important problem which is discussed in greater detail in the section on the conversion of proinsulin to insulin.

STRUCTURE AND PROPERTIES OF PROINSULIN

Methods for the isolation of proinsulin and related peptides were described in the preceding section. Mammalian proinsulins range in length from 78 (dog) to 86 (human, horse, rat) amino acid residues.[6,37] The variations in length in these proteins occur only in the connecting polypeptide portion which links the carboxyl terminus of insulin B chain to the amino terminus of the insulin A chain (Fig. 75-5). All the known mammalian proinsulins have pairs of basic residues at either end of the connecting peptide that link the connecting polypeptide to the insulin chains. These residues are excised during the conversion of proinsulin to insulin,[38] and the resulting products are native insulin and the C-peptide.

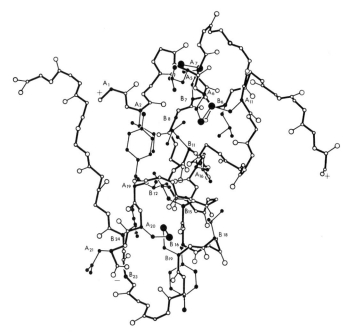

Fig. 75-4. View of a porcine insulin monomer oriented perpendicular to the threefold axis. Only the side chains of known invariant residues are shown. (From Blundell et al.: Adv. Protein Chem. 26: 279, 1972)

Despite its considerably larger molecular size, proinsulin is remarkably similar to insulin in many properties, including solubility, isoelectric point,[30] self-associative properties,[39] and reactivity with insulin antisera.[28,40,41] These observations, and evidence from other studies, strongly suggest that the conformation of the insulin moiety in proinsulin is nearly identical to that of insulin itself.[30] It is of interest that the connecting peptide is much larger than would seem to be required to bridge the short 8-Å gap between the ends of the B and A chains (Fig. 75-4). Although the connecting peptide may be folded over a portion of the surface of the insulin monomer, it does not completely mask the "active site," since intact proinsulin still exhibits 3–5 percent biologic activity in several systems in vitro.[42,43] It is unlikely that any significant cleavage or "activation" of proinsulin occurs in the tissues to account for this level of intrinsic activity.[44] The connecting peptide also does not obscure those surfaces of the monomer which interact to form dimers and hexamers.[45,46] A hypothetical arrangement of the connecting peptide moiety in a proinsulin hexamer is shown in Figure 75-6. As discussed later, this hexameric structure, having the C-

HUMAN PROINSULIN

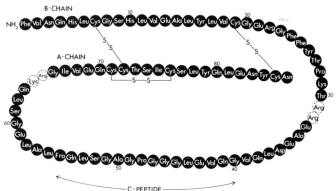

Fig. 75-5. Covalent structure of human proinsulin. Circles in dashes indicate sites of cleavage. (From Oyer, et al.: J. Biol. Chem. 246: 1375, 1971)

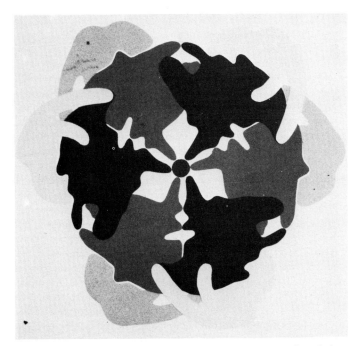

Fig. 75-6. Hypothetical proinsulin hexamer arrangement as viewed along the threefold axis of the hexamer. The connecting peptide portion is shown in lighter gray around the periphery of the darker outline of an insulin hexamer arranged according to the data of Blundell et al.[23] The central density represents the two zinc atoms in coordination linkage to the six (three above and three below hexamer plane) histidine side chains at position 10 in the B chain.

peptide oriented externally, may play a role in the efficient conversion of proinsulin to insulin in the beta cells. The three-dimensional structure of proinsulin has not yet been determined, although crystallization has been accomplished by Low and co-workers.[47–49]

PRECURSOR RELATIONSHIP OF PROINSULIN TO INSULIN

By means of isolated islet preparations[50,51] the precursor–product relationship between proinsulin and insulin have been carefully documented in a variety of biosynthetic experiments.[52–56] The intracellular proteolytic conversion of proinsulin to insulin continues even when protein synthesis is inhibited with cycloheximide, indicating that continuous protein synthesis is not necessary for the transformation of proinsulin to insulin.[52] By carefully char-

acterizing rat islet proteins labeled with various precursor amino acids by means of polyacrylamide gel electrophoresis, Clark and Steiner[57] have shown the existence of two proinsulins, one corresponding to each of the two rat insulins.[58] Both rats and mice[59] have two nonallelic insulin genes, each coding for a proinsulin. The two rat proinsulins and their corresponding C-peptides have been isolated and their structures are known.[60–62] In addition to the intact proinsulins, several intermediate forms have been identified in rat islets.[57,63] These are partly cleaved forms of rat proinsulin which have two chains, as in insulin, but still retain the connecting peptide, or fragments thereof, attached to the A or B chains. During a "chase" incubation of islets labeled with ^{3}H-leucine, radioactivity is transferred from these components, as well as from proinsulin, to insulin.[57]

Comparative studies of insulin biosynthesis in the cod[64] and angler fish,[65] as well as in such primitive vertebrates as cyclostomes,[66] indicate the formation and cleavage of a proinsulin similar in size to the mammalian proteins. A requirement for trypsin-like cleavage has been demonstrated for both of the fish proinsulins, and an interesting intermediate cleavage form, having an N-terminal tripeptide A-chain extension, has been isolated from anglerfish islets by Yamaji et al.[67] A number of reports have appeared of the biosynthesis, isolation, and characterization of intermediate forms of mammalian proinsulins in various species.[57,63,68–72]

PREPROINSULIN, PRECURSOR OF PROINSULIN

With recent improvements in the methods for large-scale islet isolation and the development of systems for the cell-free translation of messenger RNA (mRNA), it has become possible to examine directly the initial polypeptide products encoded in the insulin mRNA extracted from islets or islet cell tumors. Wheat germ ribosomal systems have been shown to be especially suitable for this purpose as they contain very little endogenous mRNA and are also very low in nucleolytic and proteolytic activity. Translation of islet nucleic acid extracts in this system gives rise to a major immunoreactive peptide having a molecular weight of 11,500.[73–76] Our analysis of this material[74] shows that it consists of the rat proinsulins with N-terminal peptide extensions that are 23 residues long and account for its higher molecular weight (Fig. 75-7). We have recently detected a similar precursor in normal islets and in islet cell tumors by incorporation studies using slab gel electrophoresis with fluorography, and have shown that this component turns over very rapidly.[180] The peptide extension, which has a strongly hydrophobic character, is evidently removed very rapidly in vivo, probably before the peptide chain is completed—a situation that is

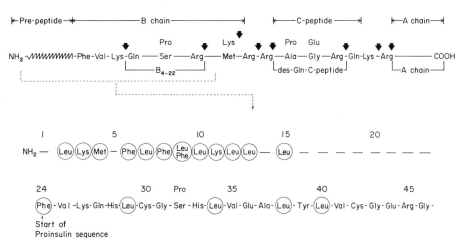

Fig. 75-7. Proposed structure and partial amino acid sequence of the rat preproinsulins. (From Chan et al.: Proc. Natl. Acad. Sci. U.S.A. *73:* 1964, 1976)

analogous to the evanescent incorporation of fMet or Met at the N-terminus of nascent peptides in bacterial and eukaryocitic systems.

We have designated this material as *preproinsulin,* using the prefix *pre,* rather than *pro,* in order to include it in a new class of rapidly cleaved precursor forms of secreted proteins which are just beginning to be widely recognized. Some other presecretory proteins which have been studied include the myeloma L-chain precursors,[77,78] preproparathyroid hormone,[79] prezymogen proteins in the pancreas,[80] honeybee prepromellitin,[81] prepro-(serum) albumin,[181] and many others. It has been suggested that the hydrophobic N-terminal extensions of these precursors promote the association of ribosomes with the membrane of the endoplasmic reticulum, thereby leading to the vectorial discharge of the nascent secretory peptide across the membrane into the cisternal space.[77,82,83] as illustrated in Figure 75-8. This "signal hypothesis," as it has been called, appears to provide a simple and plausible explanation for the initial sequestration of secretory proteins during their biosynthesis, and thus represents an important conceptual addition to the familiar Palade-Jamieson model of secretory cell organization.[84]

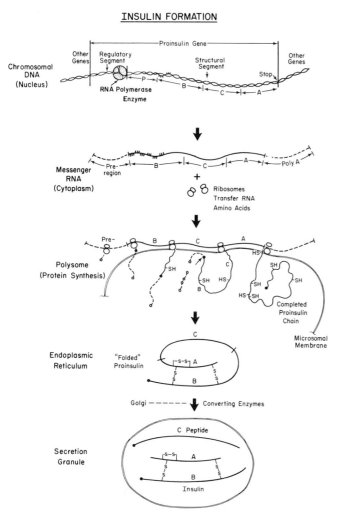

INSULIN FORMATION

Fig. 75-8. Simplified scheme depicting molecular biologic aspects of insulin formation. The proinsulin gene is represented schematically (upper panel). RNA polymerase is necessary for the transcription of preproinsulin messenger RNA (mRNA) from the gene, and this then serves to guide the formation of preproinsulin chains on the polyribosomes. Preproinsulin is vectorially discharged and cleaved to proinsulin (center panel). The proinsulin is then transferred to the Golgi region where conversion to insulin and storage in secretion granules begins (see Fig. 75-9).

We have recently isolated and characterized the mRNA for preproinsulin from rat islet tumor extracts.[85] The mRNA coding for preproinsulin is retained on columns of oligo-dT-cellulose, indicating the presence of a polyadenylate region presumably located at the 3' end, as in the case of many other mRNA molecules from eukaryotic cells. Our preliminary results[182] also strongly suggest that this messenger is capped at the 5'-terminus with a 7-methyl guanosine residue, as is the case with a number of other mRNAs from eukaryotic cells or animal viruses.[73,86] Using electrophoresis on polyacrylamide gels containing formamide, we have estimated that the rat preproinsulin mRNA has a molecular weight of about 210,000, and it sediments on sucrose gradients in salt-containing buffers with an S value of 9.3. Thus, preproinsulin mRNA should contain about 600 nucleotides. Since the preproinsulin sequences alone would require about 330 nucleotides, and since the poly A component could account for up to 100 additional residues, it is unlikely that both of the rat proinsulin molecules derived from the two nonallelic insulin genes in this species are represented in a single polycistronic mRNA transcript. As studies on the isolation of preproinsulin mRNA proceed, it should become possible to utilize the purified material or its complementary DNA transcript as a probe for the identification of the insulin gene and also as starting material for "cloning" this gene in a suitably safe host bacterium.[73,87] Only when the entire polynucleotide sequence of the insulin gene becomes known will it be possible to approach an understanding of the regulation of its expression in normal and diabetic individuals or animals.

BIOSYNTHETIC ORGANIZATION OF THE BETA CELL

The beta cells of the islets of Langerhans share many features with other cells that elaborate secretory proteins (Fig. 75-9). The participation of the Golgi apparatus in the formation of beta granules was suggested as early as 1944 by Hard.[88] Later Munger[89] confirmed by electron microscopy that secretion granule formation occurs within the Golgi apparatus. He identified "progranules" with altered morphology near the Golgi body. Subsequent studies by electron microscopic autoradiography[90,91] have confirmed that newly synthesized peptide material passes via the Golgi apparatus into beta cell secretory granules. The overall process appears to be strikingly similar to that occurring in the pancreatic exocrine cells[84,92,93] and in many other secretory cells.

It is now well established that proinsulin, in common with many other exportable proteins, is synthesized by ribosomes associated with the rough endoplasmic reticulum[94] and it comprises the major biosynthetic product found in the microsomal fraction.[95] Evidence was reviewed in the preceding section indicating that proinsulin is in turn derived from a larger precursor, preproinsulin, which is rapidly cleaved to proinsulin in the microsomes. After the biosynthesis and cleavage of the preproinsulin chain, peptide chain folding and sulfhydryl oxidation occur rapidly in the cisternal spaces. The folded proinsulin is then transported to the Golgi apparatus (Fig. 75-9) in a process requiring about 20 min.[30,90–93] Addition to pancreatic islets of antimycin or other energy poisons after short labeling periods with [3H]-leucine completely blocks the subsequent transformation of the newly formed proinsulin to insulin.[96] However, if the addition of antimycin is delayed until about 30 min after the beginning of the postlabeling period, there is no inhibition of subsequent conversion, indicating that once newly synthesized proinsulin has reached the Golgi apparatus, its transformation no longer requires energy. Howell, using electron microscopic autoradiography has demonstrated that dinitrophenol prevents the transfer of labeled proteins from the rough endoplasmic

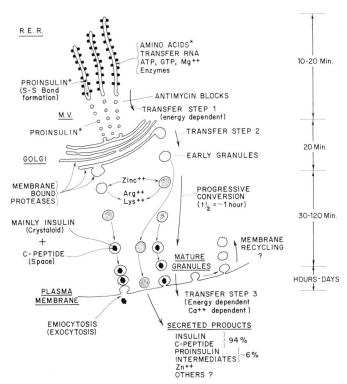

BETA GRANULE FORMATION

Fig. 75-9. Schematic summary of the insulin biosynthetic machinery of the pancreatic beta cells. See text for details regarding this process. RER, rough endoplammic reticulum; MV, microvesicles. (From Steiner and Rubenstein, in: Proceedings of the Eighth Midwest Conference on Endocrinology and Metabolism, 1973)

reticulum to the Golgi apparatus in the beta cells.[97] The chemical basis for this energy requirement in the intracellular translocation of peptides[98] is not known.

The conversion of proinsulin to insulin in intact rat islet cells behaves like a first-order reaction having a half-time of about 1 hour.[36] Peak labeling of proteins in the Golgi apparatus is observed 30–40 min after biosynthetic labeling of islets with tritiated amino acids; relatively little radioactivity remains in this region after 1 hour.[90,91] Thus, it is likely that conversion is initiated in the Golgi apparatus or in newly formed secretion granules, or "progranules," as these leave the Golgi region, and that it continues for many hours within the granules as they collect in the cytosol (Fig. 75-9).

CONVERSION OF PROINSULIN TO INSULIN

The major types of proteolytic cleavage required for the conversion of proinsulin to insulin are summarized in Figure 75-10. This scheme requires the conjoint action of a trypsinlike protease with another having specificity similar to that of carboxypeptidase B. The latter enzyme is necessary to remove the C-terminal basic residues left after tryptic cleavage, giving rise to the important naturally occurring products—the C-peptide and native insulin. We have shown that appropriate mixtures of pancreatic trypsin and carboxypeptidase B can quantitatively convert proinsulin to insulin in vitro.[99] This model system can account for the known major intermediate forms and products that occur naturally in pancreatic extracts.[38,69] Several activities have been reported which produce insulinlike material from proinsulin in extracts of whole pancreas[100] or in homogenates of islets of Langerhans,[101–104]

but the intracellular origin and mechanism of action of these enzymes remain uncertain.

In some species, such as rats and probably also pigs and humans, additional cleavages occur in the C-peptide region of proinsulin which appear to be due to a chymotrypsinlike enzyme.[63,71] The role of this additional C-peptide cleavage in conversion remains unclear, however, and it probably occurs only in species in which the proinsulin C-peptide contains sites of high chymotryptic sensitivity. These findings suggest that the beta granules may contain a mixture of proteases, having specificities similar to those of the exocrine pancreatic proteases. Thus the specific cleavage of precursor forms may be dictated partially by the high sensitivity of certain regions in the substrate molecules to a variety of known proteases, as well as by restricted specificities or special substrate adaptations on the part of the converting proteases. Further discussions of this interesting problem appear elsewhere.[30,105,106]

BETA GRANULE FORMATION

Morphologic studies of newly formed secretory granules in a variety of cells suggest that these particles undergo biochemical maturation after their formation in the Golgi apparatus (Fig. 75-9). Thus, in the beta cells the "progranules," or condensing vacuoles,[93] characteristically are less dense than the mature granule inclusions and have a uniform density throughout.[89] A variety of biochemical changes may take place in these granules as they remain in the cytoplasm of the cell, including of course the proteolysis of proinsulin to insulin. Morphologic studies of mature insulin-secretion granules indicate that the dense central inclusion is crystalline with repeat-unit spacings that are closely similar to those observed in ordinary zinc insulin crystals.[107,108] Thus, as insulin is liberated from proinsulin, it evidently tends to crystallize with zinc. The C-peptide liberated in the conversion process probably remains in the clear space surrounding the dense insulin crystal since there is no evidence for cocrystallization of the C-peptide with insulin.

The role of zinc in secretion granule formation is not understood. The available evidence indicates that most of the islet zinc is present in the granules and is liberated proportionately with insulin during secretion.[109,110] However, the mechanism for accumulation

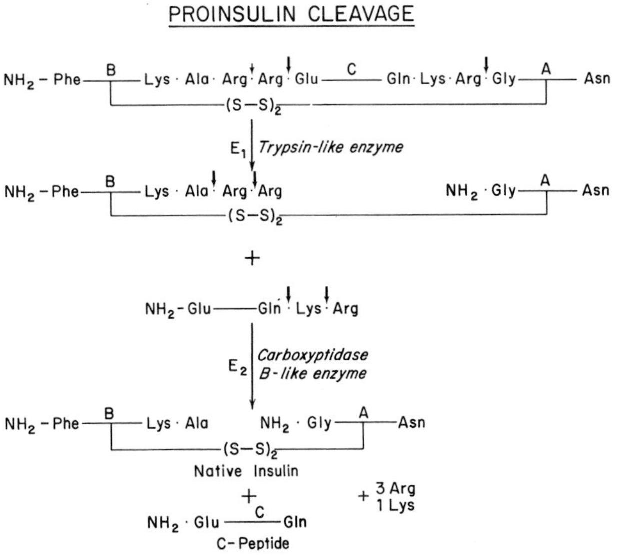

PROINSULIN CLEAVAGE

$NH_2 - Phe$ —B— $Lys \cdot Ala \cdot Arg \cdot Arg \downarrow Glu$ —C— $Gln \cdot Lys \cdot Arg \downarrow Gly$ —A— Asn
$(S-S)_2$

E_1 *Trypsin-like enzyme*

$NH_2 - Phe$ —B— $Lys \cdot Ala \downarrow Arg \cdot Arg$ $NH_2 \cdot Gly$ —A— Asn
$(S-S)_2$

+

$NH_2 - Glu$ —— $Gln \downarrow Lys \downarrow Arg$

E_2 *Carboxyptidase B-like enzyme*

$NH_2 - Phe$ —B— $Lys \cdot Ala$ $NH_2 \cdot Gly$ —A— Asn
$(S-S)_2$
Native Insulin
+   + 3 Arg
$NH_2 \cdot Glu$ ——C—— Gln 1 Lys
C-Peptide

Fig. 75-10. Stages in the cleavage of proinsulin insulin by the combined action of trypsinlike and carboxypeptidase B–like proteases. (See text for details.)

of zinc within the granules is not known. Both proinsulin and insulin have been shown to bind zinc.[45,111] However, the insulins of a few species, including the guinea pig and coypu[58] and the hagfish,[37,112] lack the histidine residue at position 10 of the B chain required for zinc binding during the association of insulin dimers into hexamers.[23] As mentioned earlier, most mammalian proinsulins probably also can exist as hexamers stabilized by two zinc atoms coordinated with the six B-10-histidines, as in the case of insulin, but these also evidently can bind larger amounts of zinc at additional sites without precipitating from solution.[111] This property may allow proinsulin to play a role in zinc accumulation in the islet cells. The metal ions also might regulate the conversion process in some way and subsequently aid in the sequestration of the newly formed insulin in an osmotically inactive and biochemically stable crystalline form (Fig. 9).

The pH of the granule interior is not known, but we may assume that it is near pH 6.0 in the mature granules since the optimal pH for insulin crystallization in vitro also is about 6.0.[68] However, this pH is unfavorable for disulfide exchange reactions, which occur more readily under mildly alkaline conditions. Accordingly, the pH in the cisternal spaces of the rough endoplasmic reticulum, where proinsulin folding and sulfhydryl oxidation occur, may be somewhat above neutrality. As the secretory products move to the Golgi apparatus and proteolysis begins, the cationic arginine and lysine residues liberated during conversion may diffuse out of the granules and be replaced by hydrogen ions, resulting in a decrease in the intragranular pH. This gradual acidification as the granules mature could create appropriate conditions for the formation of the crystalline zinc insulin inclusions.[113] Clearly, the biosynthesis of insulin via the precursors preproinsulin and proinsulin and their intracellular transport, proteolysis, and ultimate storage in secretory granules are closely integrated, both topographically and biochemically, inside the beta cell.

C-PEPTIDE AS A PRODUCT OF PROINSULIN TRANSFORMATION

Due to the localization of the proinsulin conversion process within secretion granules, the C-peptide accumulates along with insulin in equimolar amounts[38] and is secreted along with the hormone by exocytosis of the granule contents.[114] In contrast, our evidence suggests that the prepeptide is rapidly degraded after cleavage.[180] The amino acid sequences of C-peptides from nine mammalian and one avian species have been combined in the composite diagram shown in Figure 75-11.[17,61,62,115–119] These peptides exhibit a much higher rate of mutation acceptance than do the corresponding insulins, a finding consistent with the possibility that this region in the proinsulin molecule does not have any specific hormonal function. Among known proteins, only the fibrinopeptides have a higher rate of mutation acceptance than the proinsulin C-peptides. The much lower rate of mutation acceptance of insulin, on the other hand, is similar to that of many other functional proteins, such as hemoglobin or cytochrome C.[120] Certain regions of the relatively large connecting peptide may serve specific functions, such as facilitating the folding of the proinsulin polypeptide chain and the formation of the correct disulfide bonds,[121] or guiding the enzymatic cleavage of proinsulin to insulin. Several acidic residues are consistently present in the connecting peptides. These tend to offset the cationic charges due to the basic residues at the cleavage sites, so that the isoelectric pH of proinsulin is nearly the same as that of insulin, i.e., pH 5.1–5.5.[30,122,123]

Recent studies have shown that relatively short cross-linking reagents inserted between the amino groups at A_1 and B_{29} lysine (ϵ)

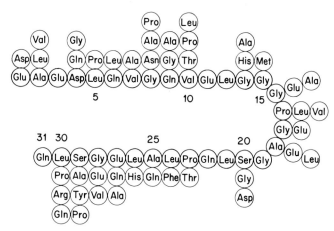

Fig. 75-11. Amino acid sequence of human proinsulin C-peptide combined with the known substitutions occurring in eight other mammalian species; one avian C-peptide is also included. Deletions occur in the dog (residues 4–11), pig (residues 18 and 19), sheep and ox (residues 22–26), and guinea pig (residues 25 and 26). (These sequences do not include the basic residues at either end which link the C-peptide to the insulin chains.)

of insulin can replace the proinsulin C-peptide in promoting the correct reoxidation of the sulfhydrils in high yield.[124,125] Thus it is apparent that the C-peptide region of proinsulin must serve other functions, as indicated above. The recent finding of larger precursors for many other short peptide hormones ranging from 10 to 40 residues in length suggests that length may be an important constraint. The length of peptide chain required to span the large ribosomal subunit and the microsomal membrane is at least 65 residues in extended configuration.[182] Thus the initial sequestration step in the biosynthesis of secretory proteins may require a minimum peptide length greater than this number of residues. This rather simple hypothesis can account for the existence of many of the proproteins. It is also possible that translational constraints such as mRNA sequence, size, or secondary structure may play a role in dictating the primary structure of some regions within proinsulin.

Synthesis of several mammalian C-peptides has been accomplished recently by classical fragment-condensation approaches.[126–131] The synthetic porcine C-peptide, containing all four terminal basic residues, was tested for its ability to promote the recombination of insulin A and B chains in vitro, but failed to influence the yield.[126] Synthetic porcine and bovine C-peptides cross-react well with antibodies directed against the corresponding natural proinsulins or C-peptides, and fragments of these peptides have been successfully utilized to study the antigenic determinants in this region of the proinsulin molecule.[128,129,132]

PROPERTIES AND STRUCTURE OF GLUCAGON

Although the existence of a pancreatic, hyperglycemic factor was postulated in the early 1920s,[133] the peptide hormone glucagon was not isolated until 30 years later.[134] Using a crude fraction obtained during the commercial preparation of insulin, Staub et al. succeeded in both purifying and crystallizing the pancreatic stimulator of hyperglycemia.[134] As well as reporting that the peptide lacked the amino acids cystine, proline, and isoleucine and contained methionine and tryptophan (in contrast to bovine and porcine insulin), they noted the nearly neutral isoelectric pH of the peptide and the tendency of the highly purified material to form fibrils at acidic pH. The availability of the pure hormone thus eliminated any continuing doubt as to the existence of a unique glucagon and made possible a great number of experiments regarding its chemistry and mechanism of action.

In 1957, Bromer et al. reported the amino acid sequence of porcine glucagon as shown in Figure 75-12, and noted the sensitivity of the peptide to digestion by trypsin.[135] Since that time, the glucagons from cattle[136] and man[137] have been isolated and their sequences determined. Remarkably, the arrangements of amino acid residues in the glucagons of these three species are identical. Furthermore, the amino acid compositions of the hormones from the rabbit[138] and the rat[139] are unchanged from the composition of the porcine peptide. More recently, glucagons from three avian species have been isolated and their sequences examined. Two of these, the hormones from the turkey[140] and chicken,[141] appear to be identical, and their amino acid sequences differ from the common sequence of the known mammalian glucagons only by substitution of the penultimate asparagine (residue 28) by serine. The other hormone, from the duck,[142] differs by two residues: asparagine 28 is replaced by serine and serine 16 is replaced by threonine. Neither of these changes, however, appears to be a major one, notwithstanding a poorer reactivity of duck glucagon with antisera directed toward the mammalian hormone.[142] The isolation of anglerfish glucagon has also been reported.[143] Although its NH_2-terminus is histidine and its overall length appears to be the same as that of other glucagons, compositional studies indicated that several amino acid substitutions have occurred. The notably high degree of structural conservatism within the glucagons from these various species undoubtedly reflects evolutionary constraints placed on the mechanism of action of the hormone as well as, perhaps, on the biosynthesis of the hormone itself.

Investigations on the secondary and tertiary structure of glucagon have been given considerable attention during the past 10 years. Early x-ray analysis of crystalline glucagon[144] and optical rotatory dispersion studies of glucagon in concentrated solution[145] indicated that the hormone assumes a largely α-helical conformation. The extent of α-helix formation in solution, however, is dependent on both peptide concentration[145–148] and on the characteristics of added solutes.[149–151] Solutions of glucagon at high dilution possess relatively little easily defined secondary structure.[148,151,152] Nevertheless, measurements of temperature effects on circular dichroism,[153] of rates of tritium exchange,[154] and of solution viscosities[148] may indicate that the conformation of glucagon even in dilute solution is not that of a random coil. It is clear that, coincident with the assumption of helicity in more concentrated solutions, glucagon monomers associate into trimers[145,155] and possibly higher oligomers. This association is accompanied by changes in the optical rotatory dispersion[145] and circular dichroic[146,148] spectra of the solutions and in a shift in the pK_a of a single tyrosine residue in the peptide.[146,156]

A major development in our understanding of glucagon structure is the recent report of Sasaki and his co-workers on the complete x-ray analysis of crystalline glucagon at 3 Å resolution.[157] The crystals used for their studies were grown at pH 9.2 (within the basic range often used for analysis of glucagon structure in solution), but they were soaked at a more neutral pH prior to analysis. Some small changes in the crystal structure which occurred after the pH change emphasize the pH dependency of glucagon structure both in the crystal and in solution. The peptide exists in the crystal as a trimer with a high percentage of helical secondary structure. Residues 10–25 occur in α-helix and residues 5–9 and 26–29 in a less regular, right-handed helical conformation. The NH_2-terminal pentapeptide is apparently more flexible and its conformation is less well defined. The association of glucagon monomers within the trimer is by means of hydrophobic interactions, with the result that hydrophobic residues become buried within the oligomer. Thus, on several grounds, the analyses of the solution structure and the crystal structure of the hormone are both consistent and complementary. The exact structure of monomeric glucagon in very dilute solution remains unsolved, but the possibility of induction of α-helicity by interaction of the peptide with hydrophobic membrane recognition sites has been considered.[156] Continued investigations of glucagon analogues having altered helix-forming capabilities[158–160] should prove both informative and rewarding.

GLUCAGON BIOSYNTHESIS AND PROGLUCAGON

Evidence concerning the biosynthesis of glucagon by way of a higher molecular weight precursor has accumulated from two separate lines of experimentation. The first relates to the detection, in either serum or pancreas extracts, of peptides larger than glucagon which are reactive with antiglucagon sera; the second involves the in vitro biosynthesis of glucagon-related peptides, usually in isolated islets, using radioactively labeled amino acids. In 1970 Rigopoulou et al. first reported that acid–ethanol extracts of pancreas from four mammalian and one avian species contain small amounts of higher molecular weight peptides reactive with antiglucagon serum.[161] Most of these glucagonlike peptides were about 9000 daltons, although two appeared to be considerably larger. Furthermore, the larger component from dog pancreas was converted by trypsin to peptides immunologically indistinguishable from those of trypsin-treated glucagon. Often, as an adjunct to biosynthetic studies, similar higher molecular weight, glucagon-immunoreactive components have been detected by others in islets of the anglerfish,[162,163] pigeon,[164–167] guinea pig,[168,169] rat,[170] and human,[171] and in rat pancreas.[172] Noe and Bauer also showed that limited tryptic digestion of the higher molecular weight glucagon component from anglerfish islets resulted in an initial increase in total immunoreactivity followed by a drop in immunoreactivity after longer incubation periods.[162] This sequence of events presumably represents release of glucagon from the precursor followed by degradation of the released hormone.

Attempts to directly examine the biosynthesis of glucagon have generally been based on incorporation of tritium-labeled tryptophan, which occurs in glucagon but not in insulin, into the proteins of isolated pancreas or islet preparations. Higher molecular weight biosynthetic products having many of the properties expected of proglucagon have been detected in the islet tissues of

```
 1   2   3   4   5   6   7   8   9  10  11  12  13  14
NH2-His-Ser-Gln-Gly-Thr-Phe-Thr-Ser-Asp-Tyr-Ser-Lys-Tyr-Leu-


15  16  17  18  19  20  21  22  23  24  25  26  27  28  29
-Asp-Ser-Arg-Arg-Ala-Gln-Asp-Phe-Val-Gln-Trp-Leu-Met-Asn-Thr-CO2H
     Thr                                             Ser


30  31  32  33  34  35  36  37
-Lys-Arg-Asn-Asn-Lys-Asn-Ile-Ala-CO2H
```

Fig. 75-12. Primary structures of glucagon and a fragment of proglucagon. The identical sequences of human, bovine, and porcine glucagon are shown. The two replacements found in avian glucagon are shown beneath the sequence. The primary structure of the extension found at the C-terminus of a fragment of porcine/bovine proglucagon is shown at the bottom of the figure. (See text for details.)

birds,[164–167] fish,[16,163] and mammals.[168–172] Whether incubation with the radioactive amino acid precursor is continuous, or whether it is brief, followed by incubation with unlabeled amino acid or with inhibitors of protein synthesis, identification of labeled proglucagon usually proceeds from coelution of radioactive and immunoreactive peptides after gel filtration. Most of these larger forms have apparent molecular weights in the range 9000–12,000 daltons.[162,163,171,172] The precursor from pigeons, however, may be significantly larger.[164,166] Hellerström et al. have suggested that guinea pig proglucagon may dimerize under selected conditions.[169]

Conversion of radioactively labeled proglucagon to glucagon in anglerfish,[162,163] rat,[172] and human[171] islet tissues during pulse-chase experiments in vitro seems to require several hours, or, in the case of guinea pig islets, perhaps even days.[169] O'Connor and Lazarus have also reported difficulty in detecting conversion of a 8200-dalton, glucagonlike peptide during 16 hours of incubation of pigeon islets.[167] It has often been noted that the biosynthesis of proglucagon and glucagon is stimulated by lowering the glucose concentration in the incubation medium. Furthermore, limited proteolysis of partially purified proglucagon by trypsin results in a product having the expected physical and chemical properties of glucagon. Thus, although the quantitative study of proglucagon conversion to glucagon within the pancreatic islet remains a difficult task, evidence for the existence of the precursor in a variety of species is unequivocal.

Three proglucagon-related peptides have now been isolated. We reported the isolation and sequence determination of a 37-residue peptide from crystalline glucagon which contained the primary structure of the hormone at its NH$_2$-terminus.[173] The remainder of the sequence as shown in Figure 75-12 is Lys-Arg-Asn-Asn-Lys-Asn-Ile-Ala. The structure of this peptide, which is probably a fragment of bovine or porcine proglucagon, is consistent with the tryptic sensitivity of proglucagon and suggests that, as for proinsulin, both trypsinlike and carboxypeptidase B–like enzymes may be required for the conversion of the precursor in vivo. Interestingly, Moody has demonstrated that the 10,000-dalton glucagonlike immunoreactive peptide from intestine has an amino acid sequence at its COOH-terminus which is nearly identical to that shown above for the extension on pancreatic glucagon (Moody, personal communication). The difference between the two sequences is due to inversion of two residues and it is likely that this apparent discrepancy will be resolved in the near future. The complete sequence analyses of both intestinal glucagonlike immunoreactivity and the precursor of pancreatic glucagon will provide important information on the structural relatedness of the two peptides. Recent studies on the heterogeneity of crude glucagon have indicated the presence of up to 20 or 30 high molecular weight glucagonlike forms. The quantities of each peptide are very low, however, and it seems likely that many of these may be artifacts of tissue processing.

Trakatellis et al. have reported the isolation of anglerfish proglucagon.[143] The peptide contains 78 amino acids and is converted by very small amounts of trypsin to glucagon. Preliminary evidence suggested that the glucagon moiety of the precursor is NH$_2$-terminal and that, interestingly, the peptide may contain an unusually high amount of glutamic acid and leucine. Since the molecular weight of anglerfish proglucagon hs been reported to be about 12,000,[162,163] however, it is not clear if this isolated peptide represents the entire hormone precursor. O'Connor and Lazarus have recently applied the technique of immunoabsorption to the isolation of small amounts of an 8200-dalton, glucagonlike peptide from bovine pancreas.[174] Although the precursor nature of this peptide has been questioned by the same group,[167] the material does stimulate lipolysis in isolated fat cells and adenylate cyclase

in pancreatic islets. It does not, however, stimulate hepatic adenylate cyclase nor does it induce hyperglycemia in the rat.

Recent attention has also been paid to examining the physical properties in circulating immunoreactive glucagon in the serum of humans. Valverde et al.[175] and Weir et al.[176] both showed that the bulk of such material in the fasting state is associated with protein components having molecular weights of approximately 150,000. The glucagon immunoreactive protein, by a variety of criteria, is stable and does not appear to be the result of the improper handling of sera. Although its properties are not altered by treatment with urea or with glucagon itself, at this stage the possibility of its being the result of a nonspecific interaction cannot be ruled out.

A 9000-dalton immunoreactive component has also been detected in human serum.[175,177,178] It is of special interest that this component of circulating immunoreactive glucagon predominates in the plasma of patients with chronic renal failure.[177,178] Kuku et al. have demonstrated that suppression of glucagon secretion by oral glucose and stimulation of secretion by intravenous arginine are manifested in these patients, as in normal individuals, largely by changes in the circulating levels of glucagon rather than by changes in the levels of the larger component.[178] In addition, levels of the 9000-dalton plasma material are increased in the rat by nephrectomy.[178] These findings suggest that the higher molecular weight material, which is likely to be proglucagon or a fragment thereof, is metabolized and is cleared from the circulation largely by the kidney, as is the case for proinsulin.[179] At this time, the detailed chemistry of proglucagon and the exact mechanisms for its conversion and degradation in vivo remain topics for further investigation. Nevertheless, theoretical considerations regarding the biosynthesis of small peptides[73,182] as well as accumulated chemical and biosynthetic evidence leave little doubt that glucagon is synthesized by way of a precursor which must be at least three times the size of the hormone.

REFERENCES

1. Von Mering, J., Minkowski, O.: Diabetes mellitus nach pankreas extirpation. *Arch Exp Pathol Pharmacol Leipzig 26:* 371, 1890.
2. Murnaghan, J. H., Talalay, P.: John Jacob Abel and the crystallization of insulin. *Perspect Biol Med 10:* 334, 1967.
3. Falkmer, S., Emdin, S., Havu, N., et al: Insulin in invertebrates and cyclostomes. *Am Zool 13:* 625, 1973.
4. Humbel, R. E., Bosshard, H. R., Zahn, H.: Chemistry of insulin, in Steiner, DF, Freinkel, N. (eds): Handbook of Physiology. Endocrinology I. Williams & Wilkins, Baltimore, 1972, ch 6, p 111.
5. Davoren, P. R.: The isolation of insulin from a single cat pancreas. *Biochim Biophys Acta 63:* 150, 1962.
6. Chance, R. E., Ellis, R. M., Bromer, W. W.: Porcine proinsulin: characterization and amino acid sequence. *Science 161:* 165, 1968.
7. Steiner, D. F., Hallund, O., Rubenstein, A. H., et al: Isolation and properties of proinsulin, intermediate forms and other minor components from crystalline bovine insulin. *Diabetes 17:* 725, 1968.
8. Tager, H., Rubenstein, A. H., Steiner, D. F.: Methods for the assessment of peptide precursors. Studies on insulin biosynthesis, in O'Malley B. W., Hardman J. G. (eds): Hormones and Cyclic Nucleotides: Methods in Enzymology, vol 37, part B. New York, Academic, 1975, p 326.
9. Bruni, B., O'Alberto, M., Osenda, M., et al: Clinical trial with monocomponent lente insulins. *Diabetologia 9:* 492, 1973.
10. Mirsky, I. A., Kawamura, K.: Heterogeneity of crystalline insulin. *Endocrinology 78:* 1115, 1966.
11. Freychet, P., Roth, J., Neville, D. M.: Insulin receptors in the liver: Specific binding of [^{125}I] insulin to the plasma membrane and its relation to insulin bioactivity. *Proc. Natl. Acad. Sci. USA 68:* 1833, 1971.
12. Freychet, P., Brandenburg, D., Wollmer, A.: Receptor-binding assay of chemically modified insulins. Comparison with in vitro and in vivo bioassays. *Diabetologia 10:* 1, 1974.

13. Glieman, J., Gammeltoft, S.: The biological activity and the binding affinity of modified insulins determined on isolated rat fat cells. *Diabetologia 10:* 105, 1974.

14. Klostermeyer, H., Humbel, R. E.: The chemistry and biochemistry of insulin. *Angew Chem Int Edit 5:* 807, 1966.

15. Tager, H. S., Steiner, D. F.: Peptide hormones. *Ann Rev Biochem 43:* 509, 1974.

16. Ryle, A. P., Sanger, F., Smith, L. F., et al: The disulfide bonds of insulin. *Biochem J 60:* 541, 1955.

17. Dayhoff, M. O. (ed): Atlas of Protein Sequence and Structure, vol 5, suppl 1. Bethesda, Md, Biomedical Research Foundation, 1973.

18. Smith, L. F.: Amino acid sequences of insulins. *Diabetes 21 [Suppl 2]:* 457, 1972.

19. Peterson, J. D., Steiner, D. F., Emdin, S. O., et al: The amino acid sequence of the insulin from a primitive vertebrate, the Atlantic hagfish (Myxine glutinosa). *J Biol Chem 250:* 5183, 1975.

20. Carpenter, F. H.: Relationship of structure to biological activity of insulin as revealed by degradative studies. *Am J Med 40:* 750, 1966.

21. Arquilla, E. R., Miles, P. V., Morris, J. W.: Immunochemistry of insulin, in Steiner D. F., Freinkel N. (eds): Handbook of Physiology. Endocrinology I. Baltimore, Williams & Wilkins, 1972, ch 9, p 159.

22. Blundell, T. L., Dodson, G. G., Hodgkin, D. C., et al: Insulin: the structure in the crystals and its reflection in chemistry and biology. *Adv Protein Chem 26:* 279, 1972.

23. Blundell, T. L., Dodson, G. G., Dodson, E., et al: X-ray analysis and the structure of insulin. *Rec Prog Horm Res 27:* 1, 1971.

24. Cutfield, J. F., Cutfield, S. M., Dodson, E. J., et al: The low resolution crystal structure of hagfish insulin. *J Mol Biol 87:* 23, 1974.

25. Emdin, S. O., Gammeltoft, S., Gliemann, J.: The degradation, binding affinity and potency of insulin from the Atlantic hagfish determined on isolated rat fat cells. *J. Biol. Chem. 252:* 602, 1977.

26. Acher, R.: Recent discoveries in the evolution of proteins. *Angew Chem Int Edit 13:* 186, 1974.

27. Steiner, D. F.: Insulin and the regulation of hepatic biosynthetic activity. *Vitam Horm 24:* 1, 1966.

28. Steiner, D. F., Clark, J. L., Nolan, C., et al: Proinsulin and the biosynthesis of insulin. *Rec Prog Horm Res 25:* 207, 1969.

29. Steiner, D. F., Oyer, P. E.: The biosynthesis of insulin and a probable precursor of insulin by a human islet cell adenoma. *Proc Natl Acad Sci USA 57:* 473, 1967.

30. Steiner, D. F., Kemmler, W., Clark, J. L., et al: The biosynthesis of insulin, in Steiner D. F., Freinkel N (eds): Handbook of Physiology. Endocrinology I. Baltimore, Williams & Wilkins, 1972, ch 10, p 175.

31. Geller, D. M., Judah, J. D., Nicholls, M. R.: Intracellular distribution of serum albumin and its possible precursors in rat liver. *Biochem J 127:* 865, 1972.

32. Judah, J. D., Gamble, M., Steadman, J. H.: Biosynthesis of serum albumin in rat liver. Evidence for the existence of ''proalbumin.'' *Biochem J 134:* 1083, 1973.

33. Jacobson, M. R., Baltimore, D.: Morphogenesis of poliovirus. I. Association of the viral RNA with coat protein. *J Mol Biol 33:* 369, 1968.

34. Kiehn, E. D., Holland, J. J.: Synthesis and cleavage of enterovirus polypeptides in mammalian cells. *J Virol 5:* 358, 1970.

35. Bornstein, P.: The biosynthesis of collagen. *Ann Rev Biol Chem 43:* 567, 1974.

36. Steiner, D. F.: Evidence for a precursor in the biosynthesis of insulin. *Trans NY Acad Sci [II] 30:* 60, 1967.

37. Steiner, D. F., Peterson, J. D., Tager, H. S., et al: Comparative aspects of proinsulin and insulin structure and biosynthesis, in Pirart J, Malaisse W. J. (eds): Proceedings of the 8th Congress of the International Diabetes Federation, Brussels, July 1973. International Congress Ser. 312. Amsterdam, *Excerpta Medica,* 1973, p 119.

38. Steiner, D. F., Cho, S., Oyer, P. E., et al: Isolation and characterization of proinsulin C-peptide from bovine pancreas. *J Biol Chem 246:* 1365, 1971.

39. Frank, B. H., Veros, A. J.: Physical studies on proinsulin: association behavior and conformation in solution. *Biochem Biophys Res Commun 32:* 155, 1968.

40. Rubenstein, A. H., Melani, F., Pilkis, S., et al: Proinsulin: secretion, metabolism, immunological and biological properties. *Postgrad Med J [Suppl] 45:* 476, 1969.

41. Rubenstein, A. H., Mako, M., Welbourne, W. P., et al: Comparative immunology of bovine, porcine, and human proinsulin and C-peptides. *Diabetes 19:* 546, 1970.

42. Narahara, H. T.: Biological activity of proinsulin, in Fritz I. (ed): Insulin Action. New York, Academic, 1972, p 63.

43. Gliemann, J., Sorensen, H. H.: Assay of insulin-like activity by the isolated fat cell method. IV. The biological activity of proinsulin. *Diabetologia 6:* 499, 1970.

44. Lazarus, N. R., Penhos, J. E., Tanese, T., et al: Studies on the biological activity of porcine proinsulin. *J Clin Invest 49:* 487, 1970.

45. Frank, B. H., Veros, A. J.: Interaction of zinc with proinsulin. *Biochem Biophys Res Commun 38:* 284, 1970.

46. Steiner, D. F.: Cocrystallization of proinsulin and insulin. *Nature 243:* 528, 1973.

47. Fullerton, W. W., Potter, R., Low, B. W.: Proinsulin crystallization and preliminary x-ray diffraction studies. *Proc Natl Acad Sci USA 66:* 1213, 1970.

48. Rosen, L. S., Fullerton, W. W., Low, B. W.: Proinsulin: further crystallization and x-ray crystallographic studies of bovine and porcine prohormone. *Arch Biochem Biophys 152:* 569, 1972.

49. Low, B. W., Fullerton, W. W., Rosen, L. S.: Insulin/proinsulin, a new crystalline complex. *Nature 248:* 339, 1974.

50. Moskalewski, S.: Isolation and culture of the islets of Langerhans of the guinea pig. *Gen Comp Endocrinol 5:* 342, 1965.

51. Lacy, P. E., Kostianovsky, M.: Method for the isolation of intact islets of Langerhans. *Diabetes 16:* 35, 1967.

52. Steiner, D. F., Cunningham, D. D., Spigelman, L., et al: Insulin biosynthesis: evidence for a precursor. *Science 157:* 697, 1967.

53. Tung, A. K., Yip, C. C.: The biosynthesis of insulin and ''proinsulin'' in fetal bovine pancreas. *Diabetologia 4:* 68, 1968.

54. Lin, B. J., Haist, R. E.: Insulin biosynthesis: effects of carbohydrates and related compounds. *Can Physiol Pharmacol 47:* 791, 1969.

55. Morris, G. E., Korner, A.: The effect of glucose on insulin biosynthesis by isolated islets of Langerhans in the rat. *Biochim Biophys Acta 208:* 404, 1970.

56. Tanese, T., Lazarus, N. R., Devrim, S., et al: Synthesis and release of proinsulin and insulin by isolated rat islets of Langerhans. *J Clin Invest 49:* 1394, 1970.

57. Clark, J. L., Steiner, D. F.: Insulin biosynthesis in the rat: demonstration of two proinsulins. *Proc Natl Acad Sci USA 62:* 278, 1969.

58. Smith, L. F.: Species variation in the amino acid sequence of insulin. *Am J Med 40:* 662, 1966.

59. Markussen, J.: Mouse insulins—separation and structures. *Int J Protein Res 3:* 149, 1971.

60. Sundby, F., Markussen, J.: Rat proinsulins and C-peptides. Isolation and amino acid compositions. *Eur J Biochem 25:* 147, 1972.

61. Markussen, J., Sundby, F.: Rat proinsulin C-peptides. Amino acid sequences. *Eur J Biochem 25:* 153, 1972.

62. Tager, H. S., Steiner, D. F.: Primary structures of the proinsulin connecting peptides of the rat and the horse. *J Biol Chem 247:* 7936, 1972.

63. Tager, H. S., Emdin, S. O., Clark, J. L., et al: Studies on the conversion of proinsulin to insulin. II. Evidence for a chymotrypsin-like cleavage in the connecting peptide region of insulin precursors in the rat. *J Biol Chem 248:* 3476, 1973.

64. Grant, P. T., Coombs, T. L.: Proinsulin, a biosynthetic precursor of insulin, in Campbell P. N., Greville G. D. (eds): Essays in Biochemistry, vol 6. London, Academic, 1971, p 69.

65. Trakatellis, A. C., Schwartz, G. P.: Biosynthesis of insulin in anglerfish islets. *Nature 225:* 548, 1970.

66. Steiner, D. F., Peterson, J. D., Tager, H., et al.: Comparative aspects of proinsulin and insulin structure and biosynthesis. *Am. Zoologist 13:* 591, 1973.

67. Yamaji, K., Tada, K., Trakatellis, A. C.: On the biosynthesis of insulin in anglerfish islets. *J Biol Chem 247:* 4080, 1972.

68. Kemmler, W., Steiner, D. F., Borg, J.: Studies on the conversion of proinsulin to insulin. III. Studies in vitro with a crude secretion granule fraction isolated from islet of Langerhans. *J Biol Chem 248:* 4544, 1973.

69. Nolan, C., Margoliash, E., Peterson, J. D., et al: The structure of bovine proinsulin. *J Biol Chem 246:* 2780, 1971.

70. Tung, A. K., Yip, C. C.: Biosynthesis of insulin in bovine fetal pancreatic slices: the incorporation of tritiated leucine into a single-chain proinsulin, a double-chain intermediate, and insulin in subcellular fractions. *Proc Natl Acad Sci USA 63:* 442, 1969.

71. Chance, R. E.: Chemical, physical, biological and immunological studies on porcine proinsulin and related polypeptides, in Rodriquez R. R., Vallance-Owen J. J. (eds): Proceedings of the 7th Congress of the International Diabetes Federation. Amsterdam, *Excerpta Medica,* 1971, p 292.

72. Kitabchi, A. E., Stentz, F. B.: Degradation of insulin and proinsulin by various organ homogenates of rat. *Diabetes 21:* 1091, 1972.

73. Lernmark, A., Chan, S. J., Choy, R., et al: Biosynthesis of insulin and glucagon: a view of the current state of the art, in: Polypeptide Hormones: Molecular and Cellular Aspects, CIBA Foundation Symposium 41. Amsterdam, Elsevier/*Excerpta Medica,* North-Holland, 1976, p 7.

74. Chan, S. J., Keim, P., Steiner, D. F.: Cell-free synthesis of rat preproinsulins: characterization and partial amino acid sequence determination. *Proc Natl Acad Sci USA 73:* 1964, 1976.

75. Permutt, M. A., Biesbroeck, J., Chyn, R., et al: Isolation of a biologically active messenger RNA from fish pancreatic islets by oligo (2′-deoxythymidylic acid) affinity chromatography, in: Polypeptide Hormones: Molecular and Cellular Aspects, CIBA Foundation Symposium 41. Amsterdam, *Elsevier/Excerpta Medica,* North-Holland, 1976, p. 97.

76. Lomedico, P. T., Saunders, G. F.: Preparation of pancreatic mRNA: cell-free translation of an insulin-immunoreactive polypeptide. *Nucleic Acids Res 3:* 381, 1976.

77. Milstein, C., Brownlee, G. G., Harrison, T. M., et al: A possible precursor of immunoglobulin light chains. *Nature* [New Biol] *239:* 117, 1972.

78. Schecter, I., Burstein, Y.: Partial sequence of the precursors of immunoglobulin light-chains of different subgroups; evidence that the immunoglobulin variable-region is larger than hitherto known. *Biochem Biophys Res Commun 68:* 489, 1976.

79. Kemper, B., Habener, J. F., Mulligan, R. C., et al: Pre-proparathyroid hormone: a direct translation product of parathyroid messenger RNA. *Proc Natl Acad Sci USA 71:* 3731, 1974.

80. Devillers-Thiery, A., Kindt, T., Scheele, G., et al: Homology in amino-terminal sequence of precursors to pancreatic secretory proteins. *Proc Natl Acad Sci USA 72:* 5016, 1975.

81. Suchanek, G., Kindas-Mugge, I., Kreil, G., et al: Translation of honeybee promelittin messenger-RNA. Formation of a larger product in a mammalian cell-free system. *Eur J Biochem 60:* 309, 1975.

82. Blobel, G., Dobberstein, B.: Transfer of proteins across membranes. I. Presence of proteolytically processed and unprocessed nascent immunoglobulin light chains on membrane bound ribosomes of murine myeloma. *J Cell Biol 67:* 835, 1975.

83. Blobel, G., Dobberstein, B.: Transfer of proteins across membranes. II. Reconstitution of functional rough microsomes from heterologous components. *J Cell Biol 67:* 852, 1975.

84. Palade, G.: Intracellular aspects of the process of protein synthesis. *Science 189:* 347, 1975.

85. Duguid, J. R., Steiner, D. F.: Partial purification and characterization of the mRNA for rat preproinsulin. *Proc Natl Acad Sci USA 73:* 3539, 1976.

86. Muthukrishnan, S., Both, B. W., Furuichi, Y., et al: 5′-Terminal 7-methylguanosine in eukaryotic mRNA is required for translation. *Nature 255:* 33, 1975.

87. Morrow, J. F., Cohen, S. N., Chang, A. C. Y., et al: Replication and transcription of eukaryotic DNA in Escherichia coli. *Proc Natl Acad Sci USA 71:* 1743, 1974.

88. Hard, L.: The origin and differentiation of the alpha and beta cells in the pancreatic islets of the rat. *Am J Anat 75:* 369, 1944.

89. Munger, B. L.: A light and electron microscopic study of cellular differentiation in the pancreatic islets of the mouse. *Am J Anat 103:* 275, 1958.

90. Howell, S. L., Kostianovsky, M., Lacy, P. E.: Beta granule formation in isolated islets of Langerhans: a study by electron microscopic radioautography. *J Cell Biol 42:* 695, 1969.

91. Orci, L., Lambert, A. E., Kanazawa, Y., et al: Morphological and biochemical studies of B cells of fetal rat endocrine pancreas in organ culture. Evidence for proinsulin biosynthesis. *J Cell Biol 50:* 565, 1971.

92. Jamieson, J. D., Palade, G. E.: Intracellular transport of secretory proteins in pancreatic exocrine cell. I. Role of peripheral elements of Golgi complex. *J Cell Biol 34:* 577, 1967.

93. Jamieson, J. D., Palade, G. E.: Intracellular transport of secretory proteins in pancreatic exocrine cell. II. Transport to condensing vacuoles and zymogen granules. *J Cell Biol 34:* 597, 1967.

94. Permutt, M. A., Kipnis, D. M.: Insulin biosynthesis: studies of islet polyribosomes. *Proc Natl Acad Sci USA 69:* 505, 1972.

95. Sorensen, R. L., Steffes, M. W., Lindall, A. W.: Subcellular localization of proinsulin to insulin conversion in isolated rat islets. *Endocrinology 86:* 88, 1970.

96. Steiner, D. F., Clark, J. L., Nolan, C., et al: The biosynthesis of insulin and some speculations regarding the pathogenesis of human diabetes, in: The Pathogenesis of Diabetes Mellitus, Proceedings of

the 13th Nobel Symposium. Stockholm, Almqvist and Wiksell, 1970, p 123.

97. Howell, S. L.: Role of ATP in the intracellular translocation of proinsulin and insulin in the rat pancreatic B cell. *Nature* [New Biol] *235:* 85, 1972.

98. Jamieson, J. D., Palade, G. E.: Intracellular transport of secretory proteins in the pancreatic exocrine cell. IV. Metabolic requirements. *J Cell Biol 39:* 589, 1968.

99. Kemmler, W., Peterson, J. D., Steiner, D. F.: Studies on the conversion of proinsulin to insulin. I. Conversion in vitro with trypsin and carboxypeptidase B. *J Biol Chem 246:* 6786, 1971.

100. Yip, C. C.: A bovine pancreatic enzyme catalyzing the conversion of proinsulin to insulin. *Proc Natl Acad Sci USA 68:* 1312, 1971.

101. Zühlke,, H., Jahr, H., Schmidt, S., et al: Catabolism of proinsulin and insulin. Proteolytic activities in Langerhans islets of rat and mice pancreas in vitro. *Acta Biol Med Germ 33:* 407, 1974.

102. Smith, R. E.: Summary of discussion. *Diabetes 21:* 581, 1972.

103. Smith, R. E., vanFrank, R. M.: Substructural localization of an enzyme in B cells of rat pancreas with the ability to convert proinsulin to insulin. *Endocrinology 94* [*Suppl*]: A190 1974 (abstract).

104. Sorensen, R. L., Shank, R. D., Lindall, A. W.: Effect of pH on conversion of proinsulin to insulin by a subcellular fraction of rat islets. *Proc Soc Exp Biol Med 139:* 652, 1972.

105. Steiner, D. F., Kemmler, W., Tager, H. S., et al: Proteolytic mechanisms in the biosynthesis of polypeptide hormones, in: Proteases and Biological Control. Cold Spring Harbor Laboratory, 1975, p 531.

106. Zühlke, H., Steiner, D. F., Lernmark, A., et al: Carboxypeptidase B-like and trypsin-like activities in isolated rat pancreatic islets, in: Polypeptide Hormones: Molecular and Cellular Aspects, CIBA Foundation Symposium 41. Amsterdam, Elsevier/*Excerpta Medica,* North-Holland, 1976, p 183.

107. Greider, M. H., Howell, S. L., Lacy, P. E.: Isolation and properties of secretory granules from rat islets of Langerhans. II. Ultrastructure of the beta granule. J Cell Biol 41:162, 1969.

108. Lange, R. H., Boseck, S., Ali, S. S.: Cristallographische interpretation der feinstruktur der B-granula in den Langerhansschen inseln der ringelnatter, natrix n. natrix (L.). *Z Zellforsch 131:* 559, 1972.

109. Falkmer, S.: Sulfhydryl compounds and heavy metals in islet morphology and metabolism, in Rodriquez R. R., Vallance-Owen J. J. (eds): Proceedings of the 7th Congress of the International Diabetes Federation. Amsterdam, Excerpta Medica, 1971, p 219.

110. Logothetopoulos, J., Maneko, M., Wrenshall, G. A., et al: Zinc, granulation, and extractable insulin of islet cells following hyperglycemia or prolonged treatment with insulin, in: The Structure and Metabolism of the Pancreatic Islets, Wenver-Gress Center International Symposium Series, vol 3. Oxford, Pergamon, 1964, p 333.

111. Grant, P. T., Coombs, T. L., Frank, B. H.: Differences in the nature of the interaction of insulin and proinsulin with zinc. *Biochem J 126:* 433, 1972.

112. Peterson, J. D., Coulter, C. L., Steiner, D. F., et al: Structural and crystallographic observations on hagfish insulin. *Nature 251:* 239, 1974.

113. Steiner, D. F., Rubenstein, A. H.: Recent studies on the biosynthesis, secretion and metabolism of proinsulin and C-peptide, in: Proceedings of the 8th Midwest Conference on Endocrinology and Metabolism, 1973, p 43.

114. Rubenstein, A. H., Clark, J. L., Melani, F., et al: Secretion of proinsulin C-peptide by pancreatic B cells and its circulation in blood. *Nature 224:* 697, 1969.

115. Ko, A. S. C., Smyth, D. G., Markussen, J., et al: The amino acid sequence of the C-peptide of human proinsulin. *Eur J Biochem 20:* 190, 1971.

116. Smyth, D. G., Markussen, J., Sundby, F.: The amino acid sequence of guinea pig C-peptide, *Nature 248:* 151, 1974.

117. Oyer, P. E., Cho, E., Peterson, J. D., et al: Studies on human proinsulin. Isolation and amino acid sequence of the human pancreatic C-peptide. *J Biol Chem 246:* 1375, 1971.

118. Peterson, J. D., Nehrlich, S., Oyer, P. E., et al: Determination of the amino acid sequence of the monkey, sheep and dog proinsulin C-peptides by a semi-micro Edman degradation procedure. *J Biol Chem 247:* 4866, 1972.

119. Sundby, F., Markussen, J.: Preparation method for the isolation of C-peptides from ox and pork pancreas. *Horm Metab Res 2:* 17, 1970.

120. Dayhoff, M. O. (ed): Atlas of Protein Sequence and Structure, vol 5. Bethesda, Md, Biomedical Research Foundation, 1972.

121. Steiner, D. F., Clark, J. L.: The spontaneous reoxidation of reduced beef and rat proinsulins. *Proc Natl Acad Sci USA 60:* 622, 1968.

122. Kohnert, K. D., Ziegler, M., Zühlke, H., et al: Isoelectric focusing of proinsulin and intermediate in polyacrylamide gel. *FEBS Lett 28:* 177, 1972.

123. Kohnert, K. D., Zühlke, H., Ziegler, M., et al: Isolierung und partielle charakterisierung von kristall-insulin sowie proinsulinhaltiger b-komponente aus human-pankreas. *Acta Biol Med Germ 31:* 515, 1973.

124. Busse, W. D., Hansen, S. R., Carpenter, F. H.: Carbonylbis (L-methionyl) insulin. A proinsulin analog which is convertible to insulin. *J Am Chem Soc 96:* 5949, 19744.

125. Brandenburg, D., Wollmer, A.: The effect of a non-peptide interchain cross-link on the reoxidation of reduced insulin. Hoppe-Seylers *Z Physiol Chem 354:* 613, 1973.

126. Geiger, R., Wissman, H., Weidenmuller, H. L., et al: Rekombination der A- und B-ketten von schweine insulin in anwesenheit von synthetischem C-peptid der schweine-proinsulins. *Z Naturforsch 24b:* 1489, 1969.

127. Yanaihara, N., Hashimoto, T., Yanaihara, C., et al: Studies on the synthesis of proinsulin. I. Synthesis of partially protected tritriaconta-peptide related to the connecting peptide fragment of porcine proinsulin. *Chem Pharm Bull* (Tokyo) *18:* 417, 1970.

128. Yanaihara, N., Hashimoto, T., Yanaihara, C., et al: Synthesis of polypeptides related to porcine proinsulin. *Diabetes 21 [Suppl 2]:* 476, 1972.

129. Yanaihara, N., Sakura, N., Yanaihara, C., et al: Studies on the synthesis of proinsulin. III. Synthesis of polypeptides related to the connecting peptide segment of bovine proinsulin. *J Am Chem Soc 94:* 8243, 1972.

130. Naithani, V. K.: Studies on polypeptides. I. The synthesis of C-peptide of porcine proinsulin. Hoppe-Seylers *Z Physiol Chem 353:* 1806, 1972.

131. Naithani, V. K.: Studies on polypeptides. IV. The synthesis of C-peptide of human proinsulin. Hoppe-Seylers *Z Physiol Chem 354:* 659, 1973.

132. Naithani, V. K.: Immunoassays of the nine synthetic porcine C-peptide sequences. *Horm Metab Res 5:* 53, 1973.

133. Kimball, C. P., Murlin, J. R.: Aqueous extracts of pancreas; some precipitation reactions of insulin. *J Biol Chem 58:* 337, 1923.

134. Staub, A., Sinn, L., Behrens, O. K.: Purification and crystallization of glucagon. *J Biol Chem 214:* 619, 1955.

135. Bromer, W. W., Sinn, L. G., Behrens, O. K.: Amino acid sequence of glucagon. V. Location of amide groups, acid-degradation studies, and summary of sequential evidence. *J Am Chem Soc 79:* 2807, 1957.

136. Bromer, W. W., Boucher, M. E., Koffenberger,, J. E.: Amino acid sequence of bovine glucagon. *J Biol Chem 246:* 2822, 1971.

137. Thomsen, J., Kristiansen, K., Brunfeldt, K., et al: The amino acid sequence of human glucagon. *FEBS Lett 21:* 315, 1972.

138. Sundby, F., Markussen, J.: Rabbit glucagon: Isolation, crystallization and amino acid composition. *Horm Metab Res 4:* 56, 1972.

139. Sundby, F., Markussen, J.: Isolation, crystallization and amino acid composition of rat glucagon. *Horm Metab Res 3:* 184, 1971.

140. Markussen, J., Frandsen, E., Heding, L. G., et al: Turkey glucagon: crystallization, amino acid composition and immunology. *Horm Metab Res 4:* 360, 1972.

141. Pollock, H. G., Kimmel, J. R.: Chicken glucagon, isolation and amino acid sequence studies. *J Biol Chem 250:* 9377, 1975.

142. Sundby, F., Frandsen, E. D., Thomsen, J., et al: Crystallization and amino acid sequence of duck glucagon. *FEBS Lett 26:* 289, 1972.

143. Trakatellis, A. C., Tada, K., Yamaji, K., et al: Isolation and partial characterization of anglerfish proglucagon. *Biochemistry 14:* 1508, 1975.

144. King, M. V.: A low-resolution structural model for cubic glucagon based on packing of cylinders. *J Mol Biol 11:* 549, 1965.

145. Blanchard, M. H., King, M. V.: Evidence of association of glucagon from optical rotary dispersion and concentration-difference spectra. *Biochem Biophys Res Commun 25:* 298, 1966.

146. Gratzer, W. B., Beaven, G. H.: Relation between conformation and association state, a study of the association equilibrium of glucagon. *J Biol Chem 244:* 6675, 1969.

147. Panijpan, B., Gratzer, W. B.: Conformational nature of monomeric glucagon. *Eur J Biochem 45:* 547, 1974.

148. Epand, R. M.: Studies on the conformation of glucagon. *Can J Biochem 49:* 166, 1971.

149. Bornet, H., Edelhoch, H.: Polypeptide hormone interaction. I. Glucagon detergent interaction. *J Biol Chem 246:* 1785, 1971.

150. Schneider, A. B., Edelhoch, H.: Polypeptide hormone interaction. III Glucagon binding to lysolecithin. *J. Biol Chem 27:* 4986, 1972.

151. Gratzer, W. B., Beaven, G. H., Rattle, H. W. E.: A conformational study of glucagon. *Eur J Biochem 3:* 276, 1968.

152. Edelhoch, H., Lippoldt, R. L.: Structural studies on polypeptide hormones. I. Fluorescence. *J Biol Chem 244:* 3876, 1969.

153. Epand, R. M.: Reversible unfolding of glucagon by urea and temperature changes. *Arch Biochem Biophys 148:* 325, 1972.

154. McBride-Warren, P. A., Epand, R. M.: Evidence for the compact conformation of monomeric glucagon. Hydrogen-tritium exchange studies. *Biochemistry 11:* 3571, 1972.

155. Gratzer, W. B., Creeth, J. M., Beaven, G. H.: Presence of trimers in glucagon solution. *Eur J Biochem 31:* 505, 1972.

156. Frank, B. H., Pekar, A. H.: Physical properties of nitroglucagons and aminoglucagons. *J Biol Chem 249:* 4846, 1974.

157. Sasaki, K., Dockerill, S., Adamiak, D. A., et al: X-ray analysis of glucagon and its relationship to receptor binding. *Nature 257:* 751, 1975.

158. Epand, R. M.: Conformational properties of cyanogen bromide–cleaved glucagon. *J Biol Chem 247:* 2132, 1972.

159. Lin, M. C., Wright, D. E., Hruby, V. J., et al: Structure–function relationships in glucagon: properties of highly purified Des-His-monoiodo- and [Des-Asn^{28},Thr^{29}](homoserine lactone^{22})-glucagon. *Biochemistry 14:* 1559, 1975.

160. Epand, R. M., Wheeler, G. E.: The effects of the trinitrophenylation of the amino groups of glucagon on its conformational properties and on its ability to activate rat liver adenylyl cyclase. *Biochim Biophys Acta 393:* 236, 1975.

161. Rigopoulou, D., Valverde, I., Marco, J., et al: Large glucagon immunoreactivity in extracts of pancreas. *J Biol Chem 245:* 496, 1970.

162. Noe, B. D., Bauer, G. E.: Evidence for glucagon biosynthesis involving a protein intermediate in islets of the anglerfish (Lopius americanus). *Endocrinology 89:* 642, 1971.

163. Noe, B. D., Bauer, G. E.: Precursor from anglerfish islet tissue. *Proc Soc Exp Biol Med 142:* 210, 1973.

164. Tung, A. K., Zerega, F.: Biosynthesis of glucagon in isolated pigeon islets. *Biochem Biophys Res Commun 45:* 387, 1971.

165. Tung, A. K.: Biosynthesis of avian glucagon: evidence for a possible high molecular weight biosynthetic intermediate. *Horm Metab Res 5:* 416, 1973.

166. Tung, A. K.: Glucagon biosynthesis in avian pancreatic islets: evidence for medium-sized biosynthetic intermediates. *Can J Biochem 52:* 1081, 1974.

167. O'Connor, K. J., Lazarus, N. R.: Studies on the biosynthesis of pancreatic glucagon in the pigeon (Columa livia). *Biochem J 156:* 279, 1976.

168. Hellerström, C., Howell, S. L., Edwards, J. C., et al: Investigation of glucagon biosynthesis in isolated pancreatic islets of guinea pigs. *FEBS Lett 27:* 97, 1972.

169. Hellerström, C., Howell, S. L., Edwards, J. C., et al: Biosynthesis of glucagon in isolated pancreatic islets of guinea pigs. *Biochem J 140:* 13, 1974.

170. Petersen, K.-G., Heilmeyer, P., Kerp, L.: Synthesis of proinsulin and large glucagon immunoreactivity in isolated Langerhans islets from EMC-virus infected mice. *Diabetologia 11:* 21, 1975.

171. Noe, B. D., Bauer, G. E., Steffes, M. W.: Glucagon biosynthesis in human pancreatic islets: preliminary evidence for a biosynthetic imtermediate. *Horm Metab Res 7:* 314, 1975.

172. O'Connor, K. J., Gay, A., Lazarus, N. R.: The biosynthesis of glucagon in perfused rat pancreas. *Biochem J 134:* 473, 1973.

173. Tager, H. S., Steiner, D. F.: Isolation of a glucagon-containing peptide: primary structure of a possible fragment of proglucagon. *Proc Natl Acad Sci USA 70:* 221, 1973.

174. O'Connor, K. J., Lazarus, N. R.: The purification and biological properties of pancreatic big glucagon. *Biochem J 156:* 265, 1976.

175. Valverde, I., Villanveva, M. L., Lozano, I., et al: Presence of glucagon immunoreactivity in the globulin fraction of human plasma ("bid plasma glucagon"). *J Clin Endocrinol Metab 39:* 1090, 1974.

176. Weir, G. C., Knowlton, S. D., Martin, D. B.: High molecular weight glucagon-like immunoreactivity in plasma. *J Clin Endocrinol Metab 40:* 296, 1975.

177. Kuku, S. F., Zeidler, A., Emmanouel, D. S., et al: Heterogeneity of plasma glucagon: patterns in patients with chronic renal failure and diabetes. *J Clin Endocrinol Metab 42:* 173, 1976.

178. Kuku, S. F., Jaspan, J. B., Emmanouel, D. S., et al: Heterogeneity

of plasma glucagon: circulating components in normal subjects and patients with chronic renal failure. *J Clin Invest 58:* 742, 1976.

179. Katz, A. I., Rubenstein, A. H.: Metabolism of proinsulin, insulin and C-peptide in the rat. *J Clin Invest 52:* 1113, 1973.

180. Patzelt, C., Labrecque, A. D., Duguid, J. R., et al.: Detection and kinetic behavior of preproinsulin in pancreatic islets. *Proc Natl Acad Sci USA* 1978 (in press).

181. Strauss, A. W., Donohue, A. M., Bennett, C. D., et al.: Rat liver preproalbumin: *In vitro* synthesis and partial amino acid sequence. *Proc Natl Acad Sci USA 74:* 1358, 1977.

182. Patzelt, C., Chan, S. J., Duguid, J., et al.: Biosynthesis of Polypeptide Hormones in intact and cell-free systems. FEBS Proceedings 1978 (in press).

76

Metabolism of Pancreatic Islets and Regulation of Insulin and Glucagon Secretion

Franz M. Matschinsky

Anthony A. Pagliara

Walter S. Zawalich

Michael D. Trus

INTRODUCTION

The pancreatic islets serve as fuel homeostats for the organism. Insulin-producing β cells greatly outnumber the other cellular constituents of the typical mammalian pancreatic islet and they play the predominant physiologic role; the consequences of impairment of this function are dramatically manifest in human and experimental diabetes. The distinctive characteristics of the β cell are their ability to function as a fuel receptor cell that monitors minute-to-minute changes in the organism's supply of small calorigenic molecules (i.e., glucose, amino acids, ketone bodies, and fatty acids) and to respond to alterations in fuel supply with an appropriate change in insulin secretion.

Many other cells in the body have similar chemoreceptor capacities and respond to changes in the concentrations of metabolic fuels in the blood with alterations in hormonal secretion or neuronal activity. The glucagon-secreting α cells of the pancreatic islets and of the gastrointestinal mucosa constitute another system of this type. The anatomic association of these two fuel homeostatic systems within the pancreatic islets has led to speculation concerning the significance of anatomic relationships between the α and β cells, and it has been hypothesized that diabetes mellitus may be the result of a primary lesion affecting both of these cell types.[1] Another equally important fuel homeostatic system is comprised of the hypothalamus, the anterior pituitary, and the adrenal cortex.[2] Here the chemoreceptor function is apparently confined to the central nervous system, and the final message is elaborated by the endocrine glands. In still another fuel homeostatic system, neuronal elements of the central nervous system that are still undefined serve as the chemoreceptors and the adrenal medulla or the peripheral autonomic nervous system produce the final message.[2] These fuel homeostatic systems are linked with the β cells through regulatory loops. Consequently, β cell dysfunction can affect these interrelated fuel receptor homeostatic systems; this is dramatically exemplified by the increased glucagon, growth hormone, corticosteroid, and catecholamine secretion that results from the experimental induction of acute severe circulating insulin deficiency.

With this general background in mind, this chapter will consider the function of the pancreatic islet cells with emphasis on the metabolic specialization of the pancreatic endocrine cells related to their function as fuel homeostats.

PHYSIOLOGIC FUEL RECEPTOR FUNCTIONS OF THE PANCREATIC α AND β CELLS

The two predominant cell types of the mammalian pancreatic islets respond to a wide variety of physiologic and unphysiologic calorigenic molecules. First, the physiologically important substances shall be discussed and classified as stimulators, inhibitors, or inert substances (Table 76-1). Beta cells are stimulated by physiologic concentrations of D-glucose, L-amino acids, fatty acids, and ketone bodies to secrete insulin. There are no known β-cell inhibitors among the known fuel molecules of the mammalian organism. Transport metabolites such as lactate, pyruvate, and glycerol do not appear to alter insulin release, a fact of some importance. The insulin-releasing action of amino acids, ketone bodies, and possibly of fatty acids is dependent upon the presence of substimulatory levels of glucose;[3,4] these substances are best termed *glucose-dependent stimulators of insulin secretion*. Thus, glucose plays a predominant role in the regulation of normal β cell

Table 76.1. Fuel Receptor Function of Pancreatic Islet Cells

Stimulators	Inhibitors	Inert Molecules
β Cells		
D-glucose		Lactate
L-Amino acids		Pyruvate
Fatty acids		Glycerol
Ketone bodies		
α_2 Cells		
L-Amino acids	D-glucose	Lactate
Fatty acids		Pyruvate
		Glycerol

function. Pancreatic α cells are stimulated to secrete glucagon by L-amino acids[4,5] and by fatty acids.[6,7] D-Glucose is the physiologic inhibitor of α cells.[1,4] Lactate, pyruvate, and glycerol seem to be inert with regard to modifying α-cell secretion, as they are with regard to β cell secretion. However, in contrast to their effect on β cell secretion, ketone bodies do not appear to stimulate glucagon release by pancreatic α cells.[7]

The actions and interactions of these physiologic fuel molecules on pancreatic islet cells has been demonstrated most clearly by *in vitro* studies of the isolated, perfused mammalian pancreas.[4,8] However, the results obtained from studies carried out in man are generally in agreement with those obtained from these *in vitro* studies,[1,9] and many of the initial observations concerning the modification of β cell and α cell secretion by physiologic fuels were, of course, made in man.

The typical responses of the α and β cells to a square wave of a maximal physiologic stimulus is a biphasic increase in the secretion of their characteristic hormones (Fig. 76-1). Thus, in the isolated perfused pancreas 20 mM glucose elicits a rapid burst of insulin release with a peak that occurs about 1 min after the wave of increased glucose concentration reaches the pancreas; this is followed by a resting period lasting several minutes and then by a slowly rising second phase of insulin secretion. A return to perfusion with glucose-free fluid results in instantaneous cessation of insulin secretion. Similar profiles of insulin secretion are observed with saturating levels of a physiologic amino acid mixture (15 mM)[4] or with D,L-β-hydroxybutyrate (20 mM),[3] provided that a basal glucose concentration greater than 2.5 mM is present in the perfusion medium. However, medium-chain-length fatty acids do not stimulate the typical biphasic response.[7]

The increased secretion of glucagon by the α cells that results from exposure to a square wave pulse of a physiologic mixture of

20 L-amino acids (15 mM) in the absence of glucose is also biphasic in nature (Fig. 76-1). Glucose suppression of amino acid–stimulated glucagon secretion is rapid and is complete within 5 min after the perfused pancreas is exposed to 10 mM glucose (Fig. 76-2). When glucose is removed from the perfusate it takes almost 15 min before the initial rate of amino acid–stimulated glucagon release is resumed.

The dynamics of the alterations in the release of insulin and glucagon induced by physiologic fuels are concentration dependent. Low concentrations of glucose (6–7 mM)[10] or amino acids (1–2 mM)[4] merely elicit a transient burst of secretory activity, and the biphasicity of the secretory response manifests itself as the stimulus level is increased. Many concentration-dependency curves of islet cell responses to physiologic fuel molecules are distinctly sigmoidal (Fig. 76-3).[4,8,10] The β cell threshold for glucose is close to 5 mM, and that for an amino acid mixture 1 mM, provided that a basal glucose concentration is present. The steep portions of the dose–response curves for insulin release correspond to the ranges of glucose and amino acids found in blood postprandially. The concentration-dependency curve of glucose suppression of amino acid–induced glucagon release is also sigmoidal; half maximal suppression occurs at a glucose concentration of approximately 3 mM. Expressed in a different fashion, glucose suppression of α cell function is not greatly relieved unless the glucose level falls below 4 mM. In the absence of glucose the dose–response curve for amino acid–stimulated glucagon release is clearly hyperbolic. However, when 5 mM glucose is present in the perfusate, the concentration of the amino acid mixture must exceed a threshold of 1 mM before the α cells respond; i.e., in the presence of glucagon the dose–response curve for amino acid–stimulated glucose release is sigmoidal.

If one considers the physiologic serum levels of the major fuel molecules discussed, it is evident that the chemostatic properties of the α and β cells are ideal. It is also obvious that minor shifts in the concentration-dependency curves to the left or right might have profound consequences for the fuel homeostasis of the organism. Such alterations of the setting of pancreatic islet chemostat are most likely mediated under physiologic conditions by the autonomic nervous system, the endocrine system, and nutritional factors (see below).

Various hypotheses have been proposed to explain the biphasic secretory response of the α and β cells to physiologic fuel molecules and the sigmoidal shape of the dose–response curves.[10] It has been postulated that the biphasic hormone-release profile is due to compartmentalization of the hormone stores into a readily releasable pool and a slowly releasable pool, and it is assumed that

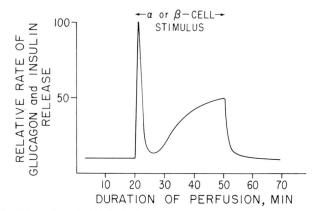

Fig. 76-1. A typical biphasic hormone-releasing profile as seen with the isolated perfused pancreas from different species as a result of α or β cell stimulation.[4,10]

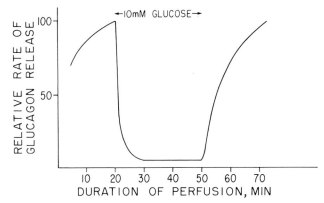

Fig. 76.2 Typical response of the pancreatic α cell to glucose as seen in the isolated perfused pancreas stimulated by a physiologic mixture of amino acids.[4,8]

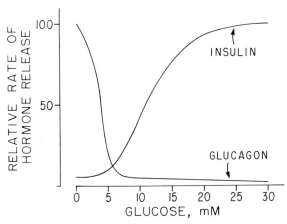

Fig. 76-3. Dose–response curves of glucose suppression of glucagon release stimulated by amino acids and of glucose stimulation of insulin secretion as obtained by in vitro studies with the isolated perfused pancreas of the rat.[4,8]

the transfer of hormone from one pool to the other is a limiting step. Extensive computer modeling has been employed to provide evidence to support this concept. Another hypothesis holds that the multiphasic release profile might be due to feedback inhibition of secretion by the hormone released. There is, indeed, experimental evidence to support such a concept. A recent report provides an example of this evidence. In experiments employing electrophysiologic techniques, it was found that insulin, at levels that occur during stimulated insulin release, results in hyperpolarization of β cells and a decrease in the number of cells that exhibit spike activity on exposure to high glucose.[11] An alternative version of the feedback explanation suggests that the site of feedback inhibition may be located in the metabolic sequence essential for triggering hormone release, e.g., in the glycolytic pathway in the case of glucose-induced insulin release. This is a theoretically appealing hypothesis, but one for which there is, as yet, no experimental support.

The sigmoidal nature of the dose–response curve for glucose-induced insulin secretion has been attributed to a Gaussian distribution of thresholds for stimulation among the β cells.[10] Although this concept received support from electrophysiologic studies, alternative explanations must be considered. For example, the sigmoidal nature of the dose–response curve might well be due to cooperative processes at the level of the putative chemoreceptors. The profusion of hypotheses to explain these characteristics of the α and β cell secretion induced by physiologic fuel molecules illustrates how limited our knowledge is.

STRUCTURE–ACTIVITY RELATIONSHIPS OF PHYSIOLOGIC AND PHARMACOLOGIC ISLET CELL STIMULATORS AND INHIBITORS

The foregoing discussion of the effects of physiologic concentrations of the major metabolic fuel molecules on the release of insulin and glucagon by the pancreatic β cells and α cells was designed to document the well-designed capacity of the pancreatic islet to serve as a chemoreactive fuel homeostat. To explore the basis of the capacities of the pancreatic islet cells to serve this function, however, it is necessary to consider data derived from what in the broadest sense can be considered pharmacologic studies, i.e., studies utilizing unphysiologic concentrations of major fuel molecules, substances that bear a structural relationship to major fuels, and metabolites that are not major fuels.

The effects of a variety of sugars, sugar derivatives, and sugar alcohols on the release of insulin and glucagon have been examined. These substances are best classified as stimulators, potentiators, inhibitors, and inert agents. D-Glucose, D-mannose, D-glyceraldehyde, dihydroxyacetone, and D-glucosamine qualify as stimulators of insulin secretion by the β cells.[3,12] D-Glucose, D-mannose, and D-glyceraldehyde have been shown to inhibit amino acid–stimulated glucagon release by the α cells.[1,7,12] The α anomer of glucose has been shown to be a more potent stimulator of insulin release than the β anomer of glucose, and it is also a more potent inhibitor of amino acid–stimulated glucagon release.[13,14] Various sugar molecules function as potentiators or activators when tested with basal substimulatory levels of glucose alone or with similar levels of glucose plus a phosphodiesterase inhibitor; fructose, N-acetyl-glucosamine, and galactose belong in this category.[15] This is analogous to the glucose dependence of certain physiologic stimulators such as the amino acids and ketone bodies (as discussed above).

Of considerable theoretical interest are data related to the effects of compounds known to be metabolic inhibitors in other tissues—e.g., D-mannoheptulose, which inhibits glucose phosphorylation, and 2-deoxyglucose, which inhibits the utilization of glucose-6-phosphate in the glycolytic sequence, but has been suggested to inhibit glucose utilization at other sites. Mannoheptulose and 2-deoxyglucose greatly potentiate the action of tolbutamide or pyruvate in stimulating insulin secretion by explants of embryonic pancreas.[16] (Studies of insulin secretion by embryonic pancreas explants are carried out in the presence of caffeine since in the absence of caffeine or theophylline fetal or neonatal β cells exhibit a relatively poor response to glucose alone.) 2-Deoxyglucose also enhances the actions of D-glyceraldehyde and α-ketoisocaproate in isolated perifused islets from adult rat.[17] There are three powerful inhibitors of glucose- or mannose-stimulated insulin release: mannoheptulose, 2-deoxyglucose, and glucosamine.[18] Little is known of the possible effects of these agents on α cell function, but they seem to cause hyperglucagonemia in the intact organism.[19] In the dog and in man xylitol and sorbitol have been reported to increase circulating insulin levels and decrease plasma glucagon levels, but it is difficult to classify their actions since in vitro data are lacking. In the dog and in man xylitol has a high potency in vivo, but most investigators have been unsuccessful in efforts to demonstrate effects on insulin secretion in the rat despite the use of a variety of experimental systems. L-Glucose, 3-O-methylglucose, gold thioglucose, and 1,5-anhydroglucitol can be classified as inert with regard to effects on the secretion of insulin.[3,15]

Structure–activity studies have also been carried out with regard to the effects of amino acids on secretion by the islet cells. It is important to note that individual amino acids are inert at levels similar to those found in plasma under physiologic conditions. Most amino acids can serve individually as stimulators of islet cells at appropriate concentrations, but the orders of potencies vary greatly from species to species and depend upon the experimental setting.[4,5,8] Maximal rates are usually obtained at very high levels (greater than 10 mM) and potencies are modified by basal glucose concentrations.

Leucine deserves special attention among the amino acids that stimulate islet cells.[3,7,20] It is widely held that the β cells can be readily stimulated by L-leucine in the absence of a basal glucose concentration. In acute experiments with the isolated perfused rat pancreas carried out at 33–35C, it was found that leucine causes insulin release only when low concentrations of glucose are also present; in these studies it was found that in the presence of a basal glucose concentration L-leucine functions as a mixed agonist and antagonist, i.e., it exhibits stimulatory as well as inhibitory properties. However, if the pancreas was preperfused for a short period at 37–38C (15 min), or for 90 min at 33–35C, with saline lacking glucose or other fuels, leucine (20 mM) caused a prompt biphasic insulin release. An intriguing finding in these studies was that the responsiveness of the β cells to glucose was inversely related to their responsiveness to leucine. The response of the α cells to leucine in the isolated perfused rat pancreas was a transient monophasic secretion that was not significantly altered by preperfusion with medium free of glucose and other fuels.

It is not clear at present whether the response of the β cells to leucine *in vivo* is more accurately reflected by the response observed in the isolated perfused pancreas that has not been preperfused with fuel-free medium, or that observed in tissue preperfused in this manner. The change in the chemosensitivity of the β cells to leucine under these conditions, whatever its nature, may be relevant for our understanding of the leucine hypersensitivity observed in certain clinical hypoglycemic syndromes and following treatment with sulfonylureas.[59] The data suggest that the sensitivity of the β cells to leucine is inversely related to the energy potential of the β cell.

The response of the islet cells to a series of metabolites of amino acids has also been studied.[3,20] Phenylpyruvate, α-ketoisocaproate, α-keto-β-methylvalerate, and α-ketocaproate are powerful stimulators of insulin release, and most are effective in the absence of glucose. The insulin-secretory response to all four of these amino acid metabolites is biphasic. The dose–response curve to α-ketoisocaproate is sigmoidal; detailed data concerning the concentration dependency of the effects of the other metabolites on insulin secretion is not available as yet. The transamination metabolite of alanine, pyruvate, was found to be inert in the isolated perfused rat pancreas with regard to stimulating insulin secretion; this is in contrast to the stimulatory effects of the comparable metabolites of leucine, valine, and their isomers. It is important to note that certain nonmetabolizable amino acid analogues—2-endoaminonorbonane-2-carboxylic acid (BCH), 4-amino-1-guanylpiperidine-4-carboxylic acid (GPA), and α-aminoisobutyric acid—can cause insulin release.[21] With regard to glucagon secretion, α-ketoisocaproate (10 mM) stimulated secretion by the α cells in the isolated perfused pancreas. During the first phase the rate of glucagon release increased 10-fold above the basal level (from 2 to 20 ng/min), but with continued prolonged infusion the rate fell to approximately twice the basal rate, and there was little evidence of a sustained response.

The response of the islet cells to this wide spectrum of physiologic and unphysiologic fuel molecules and their derivatives or analogues was considered at some length to provide an indication of the broad chemoreceptive capacity of these cells, and to serve as an introduction to a discussion of the mechanisms that may underlie stimulation or inhibition of hormone release by these molecules.

SYNCYTIAL, HUMORAL, NEURONAL, AND PHARMACOLOGIC MODULATION OF HORMONE RELEASE AS RELATED TO FUEL STIMULATION OF PANCREATIC ISLET CELL SECRETION

The discussion of the effects of fuel molecules on the regulation of pancreatic islet cell secretion up until this point might lead one to assume that the pancreatic endocrine cells behave as independent autonomous units. There is, however, circumstantial evidence that this may not be the case. Thus, there is a theoretical possibility that islet cells behave like a syncytium and that a fraction of the chemoreceptive cells may function as pacemaker cells within the islet organ.[22] In addition, the islet cell hormones (insulin, glucagon, and somatostatin)[23] are potential modulators of α and β cell functions, and there are a great number of possible interactions between these and other hormones and various fuel molecules that must be considered in efforts to understand the effects of fuel molecules on islet cell secretion.[24] The modulating effects of the adrenergic and cholinergic limbs of the autonomous nervous system on islet cell secretion add to the complexity of the problem;[2] thus, it is conceivable that fuel molecules affect ganglion cells, nerve terminals, or an autonomous nerve plexus within the islet organ. These superimposed potential regulatory systems must be dissected one by one and their possible contributions considered. Each of these systems may respond in a peculiar manner to glucose provision or glucose deprivation. From these comments it should be apparent that interpretations of the effects of fuel molecules on hormone release from the pancreatic islets observed in the isolated perfused pancreas and other systems must be made with reservations.

Because of the vast scope of the topic of neural modulation of islet cell function, this discussion will be restricted to those aspects which promise to contribute to our understanding of the fuel-receptor function of the islet cells. Acetylcholine has a pronounced stimulatory effect only when the β cells are supplied with basal glucose concentrations.[7,25] Under these conditions, 1 μM acetylcholine causes biphasic insulin release that is indistinguishable in its profile and magnitude from that stimulated by 16–20 mM glucose. Many investigators have shown that β-adrenergic agents optimally exert their stimulatory action on the β cells in the presence of glucose.[26] Similarly, glucagon stimulates insulin secretion only when glucose is present.[27] It is not known how specific this permissive action of glucose may be; other fuels, such as fructose, pyruvate, or leucine, may be able to function as permissive agents. The α cells are stimulated by both the adrenergic and cholinergic limbs of the autonomic nervous system.[28] In contrast to the situation in the β cells, this neural stimulation of α cell secretion is largely independent of exogenous fuel molecules. It is not known whether cholinergic and adrenergic agents potentiate the stimulation of α cells by fuel molecules such as amino acids.

One of the most potent drugs affecting islet cell function is tolbutamide, a member of the sulfonylurea family. The action of tolbutamide on insulin secretion by β cells is glucose independent,[29] but potentiation by glucose has been observed.[30] The profile of the insulin secretion stimulated by tolbutamide is clearly biphasic[29,30] (Fig. 76-4). This effect is observed with concentrations as low as 10 μg/ml and the dose–response curve is very steep. Tolbutamide also inhibits amino acid–stimulated glucagon release (Fig. 76-4); dramatic inhibitory effects are observed with tolbutamide concentrations as low as 10 μg/ml. The inhibition of glucagon secretion was instantaneous and a half maximal response was observed within 30 seconds after adding the drug. In the isolated perfused pancreas of rats starved for 3 days, tolbutamide stimulation of β cell secretion is abolished but tolbutamide inhibition of α cell secretion can still be demonstrated.[31] Tolbutamide inhibition of α-cell secretion has not been consistently observed by other workers.[32] In part, this discrepancy may reflect efforts to study tolbutamide inhibition of α cell secretion without providing a stimulus to glucagon secretion such as amino acids. The demonstration that tolbutamide inhibits glucagon release has considerable theoretical pharmacologic significance and may have therapeutic implications. An agent that stimulates insulin release and also suppresses α-cell function would, according to some views, be a highly desirable

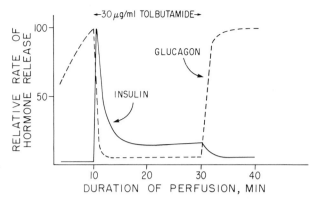

Fig. 76-4. Effect of tolbutamide on α and β cells of the isolated perfused rat pancreas continuously exposed to a physiologic amino acid mixture at 10 mM.[31]

agent in diabetics with a significant β cell reserve and apparent α cell hyperfunction.

Current concepts of the function of the pancreatic islet as a chemoreceptive fuel homeostat rest on the premise that its two major cellular constituents, the α cells and β cells, function as antagonists; their hormonal secretions have opposing effects on specific aspects of fuel homeostasis, and their release is altered in an opposite manner by a variety of natural substances and drugs (e.g., glucose, alloxan, tolbutamide, and epinephrine). We believe that these actions are primary, i.e., that the α cells as well as the β cells have specific receptor mechanisms for these substances. Glucose, alloxan, and tolbutamide stimulate insulin secretion by the β cells but inhibit glucagon secretion by the α cells; epinephrine inhibits β cell secretion but stimulates α cell secretion. A major objective of current research is to elucidate the processes underlying these opposite on–off switches in the two cell types.

An alternative formulation advanced by Samols et al.[33,34] suggests that the opposite effects of these modulators of islet cell secretion are hormonally mediated; in this hypothesis, the inhibition of the α cells by glucose might be an indirect effect resulting from the effect of glucose-stimulated insulin release on the α cells rather than a direct action of glucose on the α cells. Similarly, according to this hypothesis, the stimulation of insulin secretion by amino acids might be the indirect result of amino acid–stimulated glucagon release on the β cells rather than a direct effect on the β cells.[33,34] This hypothesis is incompatible with most of the data now available. First, exogenous insulin does not suppress normal α cells, at least not acutely.[35] Second, β-hydroxybutyrate, which is a powerful stimulant to insulin secretion in the presence of a basal glucose concentration, does not alter α cell secretion in the isolated perfused rat pancreas under these conditions, nor does it alter glucagon secretion in the absence of glucose.[7] Third, glucose and tolbutamide suppression of α cell secretion can be completely dissociated from concomitant insulin release;[31] moreover, optimal insulin release occurs in most instances when glucagon is suppressed, which makes insulin and glucagon unlikely mediators for inhibition or activation, respectively, of the opposite cell type. This does not, however, preclude the possibility that there are chronic influences of insulin on α cell function or of glucagon on β cell function.

The functional complexity of the pancreatic islet must be kept in mind when the biochemistry of the islet cells is considered. In most studies concerned with the biochemistry of the islet cells, the morphologic and functional heterogeneity of the islet tissue is, for technical reasons, neglected. The interpretation of most of the resulting biochemical data on islet tissue is therefore subject to significant restrictions.

BIOCHEMICAL BASIS OF SIGNAL RECOGNITION AND THE PROCESS OF STIMULUS SECRETION COUPLING

A number of theoretically possible biochemical mechanisms can be formulated that might explain the phenomenology presented in the preceding description of the chemoreceptor capabilities of α and β cells of the pancreatic islets. At least three such mechanisms come to mind:[18,36–38]

1. The islet cells might recognize the fuel molecules as such through fuel receptors most likely located in the cell membrane. This concept is most aptly called the *fuel receptor model,* and more specifically the *glucoreceptor or amino acid receptor model of stimulus recognition.* The term *regulator site model* has also been used to express this concept.

2. Recognition of a fuel molecule may be mediated through events connected with the metabolism of fuel molecules. For example, a change of the constellation of glycolytic metabolites or cofactors may constitute the trigger for glucose-induced insulin release or glucose suppression of stimulated glucagon release. In more general terms, stimulus recognition may be a function of energy, phosphate, or redox potentials or of the intracellular pH as altered by metabolic processes. This concept is best called the *fuel metabolism model of stimulus recognition. Substrate site model* is another expression used to describe this concept.

3. A priori, the two mechanisms may function simultaneously. For example, glucose might be recognized unmodified by a glucoreceptor, which leads to altered hormone release, provided that metabolism of the sugar furnishes a cofactor or cofactors essential for release to occur.

Activator or potentiator molecules (e.g., amino acids or ketone bodies) may be recognized similarly through any one of these three processes. Currently, it is not known which of these hypothetical mechanisms operate in the islet cells. It is not surprising that the fuel metabolism model of fuel recognition has been favored by many investigators, because it appeals to common sense and fits most data; more recently the fuel receptor model as formulated under process 2 or 3 has been invoked to explain a number of phenomena not easily explained by the metabolism model alone. This issue is introduced at this point in the discussion since it constitutes the framework that led to most of the biochemical studies of islet cells to be reviewed in the following sections.

NATURE OF HEXOSE METABOLISM IN ISLET CELLS

Because glucose plays such an important role in the regulation of insulin and glucagon secretion, the glucose metabolism of islet cells has been thoroughly studied during the past decade. As a result of this, a fairly accurate picture has emerged. First, islet tissue readily metabolizes glucose, as indicated by countless *in vitro* studies with isolated islets from experimental animals and man.[18,39–42] Maximal rates of glucose utilization are observed at approximately 30 mM glucose, the rates reaching levels as high as

30 μmol/g tissue/h. This rate is comparable to the rate of glucose utilization observed in brain in situ, but the rate of glucose utilization by isolated pancreatic islets may be artificially high due to the loss of lactate into the incubation medium. Mannose is utilized at rates similar to that observed with glucose; however, higher substrate concentrations are required to achieve the maximal rates.[18,43] Fructose, D-glucosamine, and N-acetylglucosamine also serve as substrates for glycolysis.[18,43] The rate of D-glucosamine utilization is low and does not exceed 5 μmol/g tissue/h. D-galactose does not serve as a substrate in isolated pancreatic islets.[18]

Detailed concentration-dependency studies of glucose metabolism have been performed with isolated islets. Most investigators have found that rates of glucose utilization, lactate production, and CO_2 production, plotted as a function of glucose levels, result in a sigmoidal curve with an inflection point at approximately 10 mM, resembling the glucose-dependency curve of insulin release.[18,40,44,45] However, hyperbolic concentration-dependency curves of glucose utilization and lactate formation were observed in one recent study.[41] It remains to be seen which of the two applies to the islets in vivo.

Since this question is of particular importance for the understanding of islet cell metabolism and function, the data which seem to be the most detailed are reproduced here (Figs. 76-5 and 76-6). The capacity to metabolize glucose was nonlinearly related to glucose-stimulated insulin release. The glucose threshold for insulin release was 5.5 mM; at this concentration glucose utilization had reached a rate of 50 pmol/islet/h. At glucose levels which caused maximal insulin release ($\approx$15 mM) glucose consumption had doubled to 100 pmol/islet/h. The data show that coupling between the two processes, if it exists, is nonlinear, implicating a threshold phenomenon triggered by an event connected to glucose metabolism. Glucose metabolism and mannose metabolism are competitively blocked by mannoheptulose or 2-deoxyglucose. The effects of mannoheptulose on glucose metabolism and glucose-induced insulin release by isolated rat islets are illustrated in Figures 76-7 and 76-8. Mannoheptulose, at 5 mM, exhibits half maximal effects on glucose use and insulin release. Relatively small alterations of glucose utilization, from 90.7 $\pm$ 13 to 57.5 $\pm$ 2.8 pmol/islet/h, are accompanied by complete blockage of insulin release. Interestingly, there seems to be a mannoheptulose-resistant component of islet glucose metabolism. However, there is no effect of these two inhibitors on fructose metabolism.[43] Glucose and fructose metabolism seem to occur through independent pathways, as judged from the previous data and from the absence of isotope dilution when appropriate substrate mixtures are employed. Another inhibitor widely used in such studies is iodoacetate. Iodoacetate inhibits glucose metabolism and glucose-induced insulin release, but the action of this agent is complex and results in a shift to the left of the metabolism–response relationship of isolated islets in vitro (Fig. 76-8). The data seem to indicate, however, that glycolysis and glucose-induced insulin release are associated.

Experiments have been performed to determine to what extent the major known pathways of glucose metabolism in mammalian cells are functioning in islet tissue. The issue is unsettled. The majority of investigators state that approximately 50 percent of the glucose used is converted to lactate, and 50 percent to CO_2 and H_2O, to a large extent through the citric acid cycle and to a minor extent through the pentose–phosphate pathway.[18,45–47,50] Most investigators also feel that the pentose–phosphate shunt is not stimulated by high glucose concentrations.[46] Glucose conversion to glycogen or incorporation of glucose metabolites into other macromolecules is quantitatively insignificant.[46] However, there is ample

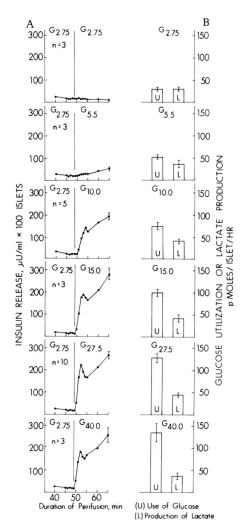

Fig. 76-5. Glucose dependency of insulin release, glucose utilization and, lactate formation studied with isolated pancreatic islets. A. Insulin-releasing profiles at increasing levels of glucose. B. Corresponding rates of glucose utilization (U) and lactate accumulation (L). (From Zawalich and Matschinsky: Endocrinology *100:* 1, 1977.)

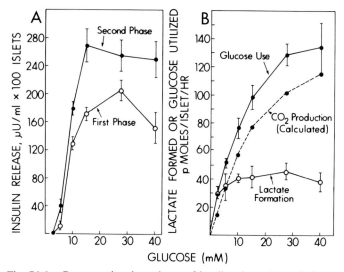

Fig. 76-6. Concentration dependency of insulin release (A) and glucose metabolism (B) by isolated pancreatic islets. Values described are from data shown in Fig. 76-5. (From Zawalich and Matschinsky: *Endocrinology 100:* 1, 1977.)

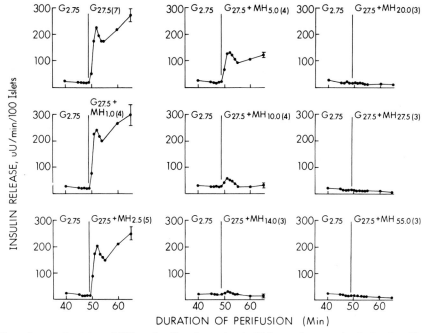

Fig. 76-7. Effect of mannoheptulose (MH) on insulin release due to 27.5 mM glucose using isolated perifused rat islets.[42]

ENZYMES OF GLUCOSE METABOLISM

reason to believe that this overall picture is not entirely correct. In one recent study, it was shown that the fraction of glucose converted to lactate varied as the glucose load increased, falling from 50 to 15 percent.[41] Considering this observation and the fact that the incubation medium serves as an artificial lactate sink, it seems reasonable to extrapolate that islet tissue has only limited or no aerobic glycolytic activity *in vivo*. In another recent study, evidence is presented which indicates that the pentose–phosphate shunt may be stimulated by exposure to high glucose concentrations and that the failure to demonstrate such stimulation might be due to the fact that high levels of insulin that accumulated during incubation blocked the pentose–phosphate shunt and insulin secretion in most previous studies.[48] The latter study exemplifies a growing concern that most measurements of metabolic flux have been performed under unphysiologic conditions, that is, in islets that secrete little or no insulin. New approaches have to be designed allowing a new look at these fundamental questions.

Corresponding studies of islet metabolism of amino acids, fatty acids, and ketone bodies are very limited, and some can be criticized methodologically. First, the capacity of islet tissue to metabolize amino acids was usually studied with individual amino acids at highly unphysiologic levels.[49] There is only one report in which the possible effect of a physiologic amino acid mixture on glucose utilization and lactate formation from glucose was investigated.[45] It was observed that in the presence of 10 mM of the amino acid mixture, glucose utilization and lactate formation were inhibited and that the glucose concentration–dependency curves of glucose utilization and lactate formation were hyperbolic. These data would seem to support the notion that physiologically the concentration-dependency curves are indeed hyperbolic. It is not known, however, to what extent the amino acids are actually consumed under such conditions. Corresponding studies with ketone bodies and fatty acids show that these substances serve as fuels in the islets of obese hyperglycemic mice.[51] Here again, little is known about the possible interactions between lipids and their metabolites on one hand and carbohydrate on the other. In addition, the relative contribution of the various cell types to amino acid and lipid metabolism is unknown.

In view of the observations just described, great efforts were made to elucidate the enzymatic steps involved in glucose metabolism of islet tissue. Studies on the nature of glucose penetration and glucose phosphorylation led to the recognition that the pancreatic β cells, like liver cells, are endowed with a very active glucose carrier, which allows for rapid adjustments of free intracellular glucose levels to altered blood glucose concentrations. Under

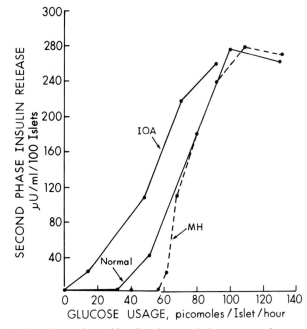

Fig. 76-8. Comparison of insulin release and glucose usage from normal and iodoacetate- and mannoheptulose-treated rat islets. The different rates were obtained by altering the glucose concentration of the medium (normal) or by including variable concentrations of iodoacetate (0.2–1.0 mM) or mannoheptulose (0.5–55 mM) in the medium containing 27.5 mM glucose as stimulus. (From Zawalich et al. *Endocrinology 100:* 1276, 1977.)

ordinary conditions, glucose entry is not a rate-limiting step in glucose metabolism of β cells. It was discovered that the pancreatic islets, like liver and intestinal mucosa, show evidence of the presence of at least two hexose phosphorylating enzymes, the classical low-K_m hexokinase and the high-K_m glucokinase. Kinetic evidence of the latter enzyme was first seen in suspensions of freeze-dried β cell islets of the ob/ob mouse,[52] and similar results were then obtained with homogenates of normal mouse islets[53] and, recently, of rat islets.[54] It is postulated that the high-K_m enzyme might also react with mannose, as shown to be true for the enzyme from liver.[55] There is functional evidence for the presence of a third hexose-phosphorylating system in islets,[43] fructokinase, which would result in the formation of fructose-1-phosphate. The presence of this enzyme would partly explain the apparent lack of glucose blockade of fructose use, and vice versa, by isolated islet tissue. It would seem that thorough studies of the hexose-phosphorylating enzymes in islets are needed to settle some of the questions just pointed out.

The usual complement of enzymes that metabolize glucose-6-phosphate has been demonstrated in islet tissue, as well as all the enzymes of the major pathways that branch off at the glucose-6-phosphate intersection.[39,56,57] Rather than presenting these enzyme patterns here, it seems more important to discuss some of the limitations of our current knowledge in this area. It would seem necessary to gather data on the fractions of enzyme capacities used under physiologic conditions of rest and secretory work. These capacities need to be estimated under conditions of physiologic intracellular pH, ionic environment, and physiologic levels of substrates, cofactors, and known modulators, and then related to metabolic flux data obtained under physiologic conditions. Such studies would help pinpoint where the control steps might be.

Judging from other tissues, it can be surmised that there may be numerous enzymatic steps in glucose and glycogen metabolism in islet tissue that are potential sites of metabolic regulation (Table 76-2). The details of the regulation of glucose and glycogen metabolism in islet tissue remain to be clarified; hence the significance of the characteristic pattern of their regulation in specific islet cells with regard to the secretory function of these cells is also unknown. For example, it has been claimed that β cells do not exhibit a Pasteur effect.[58] This provocative claim needs to be reassessed. It has also been proposed that the sequence leading from glyceraldehyde-3-phosphate to 3-phospho-glycerate might play an important regulatory function in the generation of the trigger for insulin release by glucose.[60] There is little hard evidence for this.

Of paramount importance seems to be the regulation of the monosaccharide transport and phosphorylating system. Because of the rapid sugar entry into β cells and the probable involvement of four different enzyme species in the metabolism of hexoses (hexokinase, glucokinase, fructokinase, and glucose-6-phophatase), it is difficult to predict the ways in which the first enzymatic step of glycolysis might be controlled. However, it seems that glucokinase might be the determinant enzyme, possibly explaining the hyperbolic nature of the concentration-dependency curve of glucose usage, with a half maximal rate at the K_m of that enzyme (10 mM). This would seem to indicate that the low-K_m enzyme is virtually completely blocked in such studies. The sigmoidal concentration-dependency curve seen under certain conditions might, however, be due to a contribution of hexokinase at the low glucose levels, with complete blockage ensuing at higher glucose levels. Since glucose exposure leads to elevation of ATP[61] and glucose-6-phosphate[47,52] and lowering of Pi[61] in islet tissue, such inhibition at high glucose levels would seem plausible. The energy potential, phosphate potential, and glucose-6-phosphate complement of the islet cells of the starting material might determine the shape of the dose–response curves—sigmoidal or hyperbolic. The physiologic significance of the complex monosaccharide phosphorylating system remains, however, speculative. Of the other potential regulatory enzymes of glycolysis, only phosphofructokinase has received some attention in islet tissue.[62] It was shown that ATP and citrate serve as inhibitors in a fashion seen in other tissues. Other known and probable points of control of carbohydrate are listed in Table 76-2 to underscore the limited knowledge concerning regulation of intermediary metabolism of pancreatic islets.

In the preceding discussion of carbohydrate metabolism in pancreatic islet tissue, the question of cellular heterogeneity of this tissue was neglected. Since as much as 25 percent of the tissue mass consists of cell types other than β cells, the interpretation of the biochemical information just presented is hampered. Indeed, recent studies have indicated that glucose metabolism of pancreatic α cells differs fundamentally from that of β cells:[63,64] First, glucose has only limited accessibility to α cells. It was found that the intracellular glucose space is only $\frac{1}{4}$–$\frac{1}{2}$ that observed for β cells. It was also found that maintenance of ATP levels in vitro is largely independent of extracellular glucose, in contrast to what is known about β cells. These two facts suggest that there might be essential differences in the enzyme pattern of the two major cell types of the pancreatic islets.

SIGNIFICANCE OF METABOLITE AND COFACTOR LEVEL MEASUREMENTS IN ISLETS AND ISLET TISSUE

In the preceding sections the capacities of islet cells to metabolize the various fuels were discussed as well as the enzymatic machinery serving these metabolic pathways. In an effort to evaluate the possible significance of intermediary metabolism and energy metabolism for the chemoreceptor function of pancreatic islet cells, it became necessary to study the metabolite and cofactor profiles. These measurements were conducted with the hope of detecting the hypothetical metabolic signals that might stimulate or inhibit hormone release. Since fuel-induced hormone release is graded in nature, it is reasonable to assume the existence of graded-level alterations of such critical metabolites and cofactors. For this biochemical approach it matters little whether the β-cell population is homogeneous or whether it is composed of cells with very different thresholds, as some electrophysiologic data suggest.

The studies to be described are technically difficult and in many instances methodologically far from optimal. Ideally, such

Table 76-2. Regulatory Enzymes of Pathways Involved in Glucose and Glycogen Metabolism

 1. Extracellular glucose → intracellular glucose
 2. Glucose → glucose-6-phosphate
 3. Glycogen → glucose-1-phosphate
 4. Glucose-6-phosphate → 6-phosphogluconate
 5. UDP-glucose → glycogen
 6. Fructose-6-phosphate → fructose-1,6-diphosphate
 7. Glyceraldehyde-3-phosphate → 1,3-diphosphoglycerate
 8. Phosphoenolpyruvate → pyruvate
 9. Pyruvate →→ citrate
10. Isocitrate →→→ α-ketoglutarate
11. Succinate → fumarate

metabolite and cofactor profiles should be determined in a well-controlled *in vitro* system, in which a graded stimulus can be applied via the circulation and the released hormone can be rapidly and efficiently removed from the extracellular space. In such a design possible artifacts due to delayed diffusion of the stimulus into, and of the hormone out of, the islets are avoided. For example, it can be calculated that in a large isolated islet (200 μm shortest diameter), as frequently employed, the insulin content in the center of the islet may be several μg/ml, a concentration known to block secretory activity. It is not unlikely that in many studies with isolated islets, only the outer shell of the β-cell material shows secretory activity, with the core of the islets at rest, which makes interpretation of the resulting data difficult, if not impossible. The isolated perfused pancreas is the ideal preparation avoiding such potential difficulties. Superfused monolayer cultures of pancreatic islets would seem equally well suited, but have not been used for this purpose. With isolated intact perifused pancreatic islets, at least some of the problems are overcome due to the rapid turnover of the medium. Difficulties are encountered with batches of islets incubated in small volumes since the insulin content of the medium may become large enough to block insulin release.[11]

There is considerable controversy as to what happens to the metabolite and cofactor profiles when islets are exposed to high levels of glucose.[56] Most investigators agree that prolonged exposure of islet tissue *in vivo* or *in vitro* leads to accumulation of intermediates and cofactors involved in glucose metabolism. Such changes include elevated levels of glucose-6-phosphate,[15,36,52,65,66] 6-phosphogluconate,[36,65] fructose-1,6-diphosphate,[36,52,66] phosphoglycerates,[37] sorbitol,[67] DPNH,[68,69] and ATP,[69] or a fall of ADP,[69] AMP,[69] and Pi.[61,69] Discrepancies arose when the early time courses following glucose exposure were studied. Everyone using mouse islet tissue *in vivo* or *in vitro* observed rapid elevations of glucose-6-phosphate.[36,66,70] However, in the rat striking differences exist between different preparations: rapid changes of glucose-6-phosphate and DPNH were observed in islets from fed rats using the isolated perfused pancreas (Fig. 76-9)[69] or isolated perifused islets,[69] but in anesthetized fed animals *in vivo*[36] there were only delayed metabolite changes. When the isolated perfused pancreas of fed animals is stimulated with high glucose, the rise of glucose-6-phosphate coincides with the rise of insulin release. The glucose-6-phosphate level doubles within 30 sec, and almost triples after 30 min of perfusion with 16 mM glucose. The rise of DPNH is somewhat delayed as compared to the onset of stimulated insulin release and it is clearly biphasic. After 30 min of exposure to high glucose, the DPNH level more than doubles. The concentration of fructose-1,6-diphosphate changes more sluggishly, with a delay of about 1 min, and reaches twice the zero time value after one-half hour with high glucose. Using the isolated perfused pancreas from animals fasted 12–16 h, there was little or no change of metabolite or cofactor levels unless perfusion continued for 45 min, and even then the changes were minor (Fig. 76-10).[37] The metabolic patterns are unaltered following 30 sec of exposure to high glucose at a time when insulin secretion has been initiated. Compared to the data with the pancreas from fed animals, the higher levels of glucose-6-phosphate are noteworthy. Since the fructose-1,6-diphosphate levels are comparable in the two sets of data, an inhibition at the phosphofructokinase step as a result of brief starvation might explain the results.

It is currently difficult to present a convincing interpretation of these apparently contradictory data. It seems constructive, however, to look at the mass of results obtained with monosaccharides and related compounds from two major vantage points: (1) Are

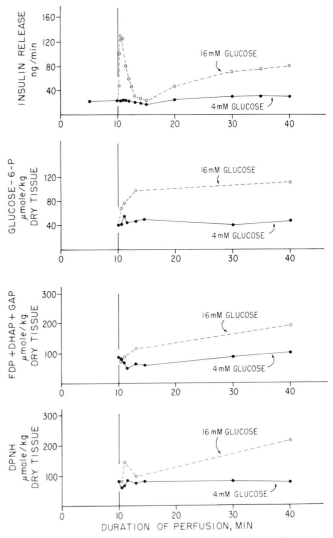

Fig. 76-9. Effect of high glucose on insulin release and metabolite patterns of islet tissue of the isolated perfused pancreas from rats fed ad libitum. Each value represents the mean of at least five perfusion experiments (Hintz and the authors, unpublished data).

there indications for the presence of specific trigger metabolites or cofactors? (2) Are there indications for the occurrence of more generalized metabolic alterations such as, for instance, the phosphate potential, the redox potential, or the pH of the cell? A rapid and graded level change consistently observed and tightly coupled with release would be sufficient grounds to consider a metabolite or cofactor as a trigger molecule. As it stands now, a trigger or trigger combination that might explain glucose-stimulated insulin release has not been identified. For the case of glucose-6-phosphate, the few instances of negative results[36,37] weigh heavier than the numerous sets of positive ones. The lack of change of glucose-6-phosphate in fed rats *in vivo* and in the isolated perfused rat pancreas following brief starvation (in both instances accompanied by active glucose-stimulated hormone secretion) seems to eliminate this metabolite as a trigger candidate. Fructose-1,6-diphosphate is changed too sluggishly *in vitro*[37,69] and has been found to rise in conditions not associated with insulin release.[36] Phosphoglycerates and phosphoenolpyruvate seemed to be little affected at early time points.[37] 6-Phosphogluconate responds too slowly.[71] ATP and ADP were found to be maintained at very constant levels.[37] DPNH measured directly[69] or judged from fluorescence changes[68] has been found to rise quickly in all experiments with glucose. The difficulty with DPNH is the fact that it does not change or falls when glyceraldehyde is employed.[72] A rapid fall of ADP, AMP, and inorganic phosphate was recently observed,[61,69] but it seems premature to call these processes trigger events, since so far they have been observed only under one set of special conditions. Obviously, there are numerous potential trigger metabolites not yet studied.

Although the search seems discouragingly difficult, it must be continued. Possible alterations of the phosphate potential, the redox potential, or the intracellular pH have received little attention in this connection. Such a mechanism would offer the advantage of explaining the action of other metabolizable fuels, e.g., amino acids, ketone bodies, and α-ketomonocarboxylic acids. Currently available data indicate that the phosphate potential[61,69] and the redox potential[68,69] are rapidly increased when insulin secretion is stimulated by glucose, and it can be conjectured that the pH might drop. More work has to be done to decide whether such changes are sufficient cause, an essential factor, or merely a consequence of stimulated insulin release.

Little work has been done with α cells using the approach of metabolite and cofactor level measurements.[63,64] The limited available data were obtained with pure α cell islets that result from β cell destruction with streptozotocin or alloxan. It seems that even after insulin treatment of the donor animals, α cell function was altered. A more reliable approach might be to cure streptozotocin-diabetic rats by islet transplantation and study the α cell islets of these normalized animals. Nevertheless, it was observed that response to glucose or to amino acids did not alter the levels of ATP, lactate, or cAMP in α cells.[63,64]

ANOMERIC SPECIFICITY OF GLUCOSE ACTION ON α AND β CELLS

It was discovered that the α anomers of glucose and 3-0-methylglucose are more powerful protectors of islet cells against alloxan poisoning than are the β anomers.[73] The possibility was considered that the interaction of hexose and alloxan might occur at the putative glucoreceptor site of the pancreatic islet cells. Other investigators performed the next logical experiment to test whether glucose stimulation of insulin release and glucose inhibition of glucagon secretion showed similar anomeric specificity. This was indeed the case. The α anomer was found to be more potent in both α and β cells.[13,14] Since in most tissues glycolysis shows no anomeric preference for glucose,[74] the results were taken as evidence for the presence of a glucoreceptor in islet cells.

Two groups of investigators have tested whether glycolysis in islet tissue discriminates between the two anomers of glucose. One group has published two meticulous studies indicating indiscriminate usage of α- and β-D-glucose by mouse islets.[75,76] The other has performed in vitro studies with rat islets suggesting that α-D-glucose may be preferentially used.[77] The rate-limiting step was located at the hexose isomerase step, which prefers α-D-glucose-6-phosphate as substrate. Consistent with this, it was found that the glucose-6-phosphate/fructosediphosphate ratios were high or low when β-D-glucose or α-D-glucose, respectively, were used. α-D-Glucose produced more lactate than did β-D-glucose. Currently, there is no way of reconciling these two sets of opposite data. One difficulty not considered in either study arises from the fact that the α anomer is the more powerful stimulus and that increased secre-

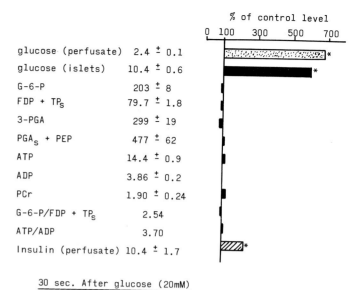

	% of control level 0 100 300 500 700
glucose (perfusate) 2.4 ± 0.1	
glucose (islets) 10.4 ± 0.6	
G-6-P 203 ± 8	
FDP + TP$_S$ 79.7 ± 1.8	
3-PGA 299 ± 19	
PGA$_S$ + PEP 477 ± 62	
ATP 14.4 ± 0.9	
ADP 3.86 ± 0.2	
PCr 1.90 ± 0.24	
G-6-P/FDP + TP$_S$ 2.54	
ATP/ADP 3.70	
Insulin (perfusate) 10.4 ± 1.7	

30 sec. After glucose (20mM)

Fig. 76-10. Metabolite pattern of islets of Langerhans and insulin release due to high glucose as seen in studies with the isolated perfused pancreas from rats fasted 12–18 h. The units of measurement for control values are as follows: mM for perfusate glucose; mmol/kg dry tissue for islet glucose, ATP, ADP, and phospho-creatine; μmol/kg dry tissue for glucose-6-phosphate (G-6-P), fructosediphosphate plus triosephosphates (FDP + TPs), 3-phosphoglycerate (3-PGA), phosphoglycerates plus phosphoenolpyruvate (PGA + PEP); and μU/ml for insulin. Perfusate and tissue were sampled 30 sec after the switch from 2.5 to 20 mM glucose in the perfusate. $N = 6$. (From Matschinsky et al. *Diabetes 21 (Suppl. 2):* 555, 1972.)

tory activity may enhance glycolysis, which might lead to an apparent preferential use of the α anomer. More work is needed to resolve these most intriguing issues.

ROLE OF THE cAMP SYSTEM AND OF Ca^{++} IN THE CHEMORECEPTOR FUNCTION OF α and β CELLS

Any hypothesis explaining the mechanism of stimulus–secretion coupling of islet cells has to integrate two additional basic facts: physiologic stimulation of α as well as β cells requires extracellular Ca^{++}, and activation of the adenyl cyclase system seems to potentiate insulin release as well as glucagon release.[16] Stimulation of islet cells by glucose increases the uptake of Ca^{++},[78] and it can be surmised that the intracellular Ca^{++} level is elevated, with the consequence that insulin release is stimulated. Adenyl cyclase activators (glucagon) and phosphodiesterase inhibitors (theophylline) potentiate glucose-stimulated insulin release.[79] Glucose itself elevates cAMP in isolated perifused pancreatic islets (Fig. 76-11).[80–82] The temporal profile of the cAMP response in islets is biphasic and closely parallels the insulin-release profile seen with high glucose. Even though there is evidence for the primary involvement of adenyl cyclase in this glucose-induced cAMP rise, the complexities of the system leave uncertain whether the diesterase might be involved. It is noteworthy that the glucose-induced cAMP rise is Ca^{++} dependent.[83] It is entirely unclear in molecular terms, how, the elevated cAMP potentiates insulin release. Efforts are being made to explain its action through altered phosphorylation and dephosphorylation of essential factors involved in the release process, but the data provided so far are far from convincing.[84]

MODEL SYSTEM OF SIGNAL RECOGNITION AND TRANSDUCTION IN PANCREATIC ISLETS

The theoretically possible explanations for the fuel recognition process in the stimulus–secretion coupling of pancreatic islet cells were introduced earlier. Having presented selected data related to that problem, an effort is now made to organize this information in the form of a model system. Three major possibilities were previously outlined: (1) the fuel receptor model, (2) the metabolism model, and (3) a model combining the features of these two. The following evidence (most of which was reviewed in preceding paragraphs) is usually cited in favor of the metabolism model of fuel recognition:

1. Many stimulators or inhibitors of pancreatic islet cells are substrates for intermediary metabolism (glucose, mannose, fructose, glucosamine, N-acetylglucosamine, xylitol, sorbitol, glyceraldehyde, amino acids, fatty acids, and ketone bodies).

2. The order of potencies for insulin release roughly parallels the order of suitability as fuel molecules [glucose (100) > mannose > N-acetylglucosamine, > fructose >> galactose = 3-0-methylglucose (0)].

3. Specific inhibition of fuel metabolism interferes with fuel stimulation or inhibition of hormone secretion. (Mannoheptulose, 2-desoxyglucose, and glucosamine interfere with glucose and mannose actions, in contrast to glyceraldehyde, which is not affected by these inhibitors. Iodoacetate blocks hexose and glyceraldehyde-induced insulin release).

4. For glucose, mannose, and glyceraldehyde, the concentration supporting half maximal metabolic flux and inducing half maximal stimulation of insulin release coincide.

5. There are rapid metabolite and cofactor changes in islet tissue following exposure to sugars and amino acids.

There are, however, exceptions regarding many of these points:

1. There are sugars and amino acids that cause hormone release without being fuels for islet tissue: galactose may, under certain conditions, serve as an activator of insulin release, and the nonmetabolizable amino acids (BCH, GPA, and α-aminoisobutyric acid) can serve as stimulators.

2. The parallelism of fuel and releasing functions is only limited: in contrast to fructose, D-glucosamine is a very poor substrate and can serve as a stimulus on its own. Mannoheptulose and 2-desoxyglucose may function as potentiators of tolbutamide-, α-ketoisocaproate-, and glyceraldehyde-induced insulin release.

3. The interpretation of the mannoheptulose, 2-desoxyglucose, and glucosamine inhibition of glucose and mannose actions is complicated by the theoretical possibility that they might prevent binding of these stimulatory sugars to the proposed receptors.

4. The dose-dependency curves of hexose-induced hormone release and hexose usage are not superimposable, as originally thought. The concentration-dependency curve of glucose metabolism is hyperbolic, and that for glucose-induced hormone release is sigmoidal. Furthermore, these relationships can be almost completely dissociated by various means.

5. Alterations of metabolite and cofactor profiles due to high levels of stimulants are not a consistent finding.

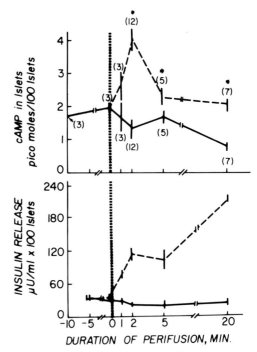

Fig. 76-11. Kinetics of insulin release and cAMP level changes in isolated perifused rat islets. At 0 time the basal solution containing 2.75 mM glucose was changed to a stimulating solution with 27.5 mM glucose. (From Zawalich et al.: *Diabetologia 11:* 231, 1975.

6. It was shown that the α anomer of glucose is more potent than the β anomer in α and β cells, with no apparent difference in the suitability of the anomers to serve as substrates for glycolysis.

7. The fuel and releasing function of secretagogues can be dissociated. Following brief fasting, for example, metabolism of glucose and glyceraldehyde by islet tissue proceeds unaltered, but glucose-stimulated insulin release is selectively impaired. Phenylpyruvate, a known inhibitor of glycolysis, and in all likelihood an unsuitable fuel molecule, is a powerful insulin releaser.

8. The hexose protection of α and β cells against alloxan damage suggests the presence of hexose receptor sites related to hormone release.

9. Glucose was found to stimulate insulin release, apparently without being metabolized, using a cell-free system comprised of a membrane fraction prepared from codfish islet tissue and of insulin granules fractionated from mouse islet homogenate.[91]

To explain these observations, a working hypothesis has been adopted which combines the features of the receptor model with those of the metabolism model of fuel molecule recognition (Fig. 76-12).

According to this hypothesis, fuel molecules themselves act as stimuli or inhibitors of hormone release at membrane-bound receptor sites. For simplicity, only hexoses, glyceraldehyde and α-ketoisocaproate are incorporated in the scheme. The list could be enlarged by amino acids, ketone bodies, and fatty acids. These sites are called *fuel receptors;* they may be part of substrate carrier systems or independent sites. The primary event set off by the fuel molecules per se is an alteration of ion conductivity with the consequence of cellular depolarization or hyperpolarization and opening or closing of a Ca^{++} gate controlled by the membrane

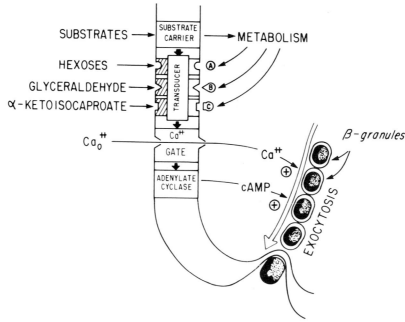

Fig. 76-12. Hypothetical fuel receptor mechanisms in pancreatic islets. The cell membrane of the islet cell contains five coupled systems: (1) the substrate carriers, which may or may not function as fuel receptors; (2) a receptor–transducer complex with fuel receptors (e.g., for hexoses, glyceraldehyde, and α-ketoisocaproate) on the outside and sites for various fuel-derived metabolites and cofactors (e.g., a, b, c) on the inside of the membrane; (3) a Ca^{++} gate that controls Ca^{++} entry; (4) the adenylate cyclase system; and (5) the secretory complex comprised of microtubule and secretory granules involved in the process of exocytosis driven by Ca^{++} and cAMP.

potential.[60] The change of the intracellular Ca^{++} level is the final sufficient signal for stimulation or inhibition of hormone release. The microtubule–microfilament system drives the process of exocytosis[85] when activated by elevated cytoplasmatic Ca^{++} levels. The basic process is controlled in an unknown way by the intermediary metabolism (i.e., alterations of the intermediate and/or cofactor level, the phosphate potential, the redox potential, or intracellular pH) and by the cAMP system. Under some conditions activation of intermediary metabolism or the cAMP system may be sufficient cause for hormone release to occur,[92] and in most instances it seems to be an essential factor in the fuel recognition process.[41,42]

METABOLISM AND FUNCTION OF α AND β CELLS IN THE DIABETIC STATE

It remains unresolved what goes wrong in the pancreatic β cells in diabetes. It is a monumental task to explore the molecular basis of the β cell impairment in human diabetes. The reasons for this lack of knowledge are obvious. A reasonable first step taken by many investigators is to study β cell involvement in various forms of experimental and genetic diabetes in animals. A few of these systems seem particularly promising: (1) the reversible β cell impairment in starvation;[86] (2) the islet cell disease of the genetically diabetic Chinese hamster;[87] and (3) the α cell involvement in streptozotocin- or alloxan-diabetic animals.[35,63,64]

The influence of food intake on β cell function is most impressive and has been clearly demonstrated by in vitro studies.[88] A 16-hour fast in the rat blunts insulin release induced by 8–10 mM glucose stimulus in vitro. After 24 hours of fasting, inhibition of release is more pronounced. The stimulation by higher glucose levels is unimpaired following short fasting. In other words, the dose–response curve for glucose-stimulated insulin release is shifted to the right. The defect is readily reversible on refeeding

with a half-time of 6–8 hours. This form of starvation diabetes seems to be relatively specific for the hexoses, glucose and mannose, but is not apparent with glyceraldehyde and α-ketoisocaproate. These tests are obviously not exhaustive. Extended starvation (72 hours) also reduces the β cell response to tolbutamide[31] and other stimulants.[89] There seems to be little alteration of the α cell function in starvation, as indicated by the magnitude of amino acid–induced glucagon release and by the efficient suppression of stimulated release by glucose or tolbutamide.[31] Glucose utilization by islets in vitro as measured by the formation of tritiated water from 5-^{3}H-glucose is not altered during the early periods of starvation (8–24 hours).[88] This observation of normal glycolytic flux does not preclude the existence of altered metabolite and cofactor patterns incapable of causing insulin release due to glucose. At later times there is some reduction of glycolysis.[54] This late consequence of starvation is also apparent in changes of the enzymatic machinery:[54] glucokinase and phosphofructokinase activities of islet tissue were decreased. The cAMP response of islet tissue to glucose is also reduced by starvation.[93]

These data indicate that glucose-induced insulin release involves a substrate-specific inducible fuel recognition system. Such a labile system could be an obvious site for dysregulation of islet cell function in disease. Corresponding data were obtained with islets from the genetically diabetic Chinese hamster.[90] The glucose sensitivity *in vitro* of islets isolated from diabetic animals was reduced, and the cAMP response was blunted. Similar studies with islets from another genetically diabetic animal, the spiny mouse, resulted in virtually the same defects.[94] The similarities between starvation-induced and genetic diabetes cannot be overlooked. A fruitful working hypothesis comes to mind: diabetes might be the result of a defect in fuel induction of the recognition system.

Information on the metabolism of diabetic α cells is even more limited. There is now little doubt that glucose suppressibility of stimulated glucagon release is reduced in chronic diabetes and that it can be remedied by insulin treatment in vivo.[63] Glucose metabo-

Glucose Metabolism and α-Cell Function in Vitro

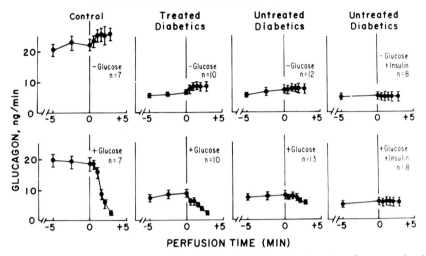

Fig. 76-13. Glucose suppression of amino acid–induced glucagon release in the isolated perfused pancreas from normal and diabetic rats. The amino acid mixture concentration was 10 mM, and 10 mM glucose was present from 0 time to 3 min, at which time the pancreas was sampled. Exogenous insulin was included at 1 μg/ml of perfusate. Insulin secretion due to glucose was seen only in the controls. In the perfusate of all diabetic pancreases insulin was virtually absent. (From Matschinsky et al. *J. Biol. Chem. 251:* 6053, 1976.)

lism of α cells might be governed by glucose transport, since it was found that a transmembranous glucose gradient exists in α cells.[13,64] Although there is currently no experimental evidence for an impaired glucose entry process in diabetic α cells, it seems fruitful to postulate that decreased sugar transport might arise as a result of insulin deficiency and might contribute to the diabetic α cell defect.

It has been proposed that there might be a primary α- and β-cell defect in human diabetes.[9] The results in animals with streptozotocin diabetes and in the genetically diabetic Chinese hamster indicate that it is unnecessary to postulate a primary α cell lesion since β cell destruction leads to the impairment of α cell function, which can be partially normalized by insulin treatment *in vivo* (Fig. 76-13). The diabetic impairment of α cell function manifested by hyperglucagonemia *in vivo* is apparent from a paradoxical decreased capacity to respond to an amino acid stimulus and from delayed glucose suppression of stimulated glucagon *in vitro*. Insulin treatment in vivo but not *in vitro* restores glucose suppressibility yet does not normalize the physiologic α cell secretory response. One explanation of the paradoxical hyposecretion of α_2 cells seen in vitro might be that the somatostatin-producing α_1 cells, which seem to increase in absolute number in the diabetic islet, curb glucagon secretion in the perfusion setting used in the cited studies.

These studies of α and β cell metabolism and function in diabetic animal models are just in a beginning stage. The results indicate that much can be learned from such studies, and it is hoped that the experience gained from working with the experimental material will be helpful in solving the mystery of the human β cell disease, diabetes.

REFERENCES

1. See Chapter MM by R. H. Unger and L. Orci. Glucagon (secretion, transport, metabolism, physiological regulation of secretion, and derangements in diabetes).
2. Woods, S. C., and Porte, D., Jr. Neural control of the endocrine pancreas. *Physiol. Rev. 54:* 596, 1974.
3. Matschinsky, F. M., Ellerman, J., Stillings, S., Raybaud, F., Pace, C., Zawalich, W. Hexoses and insulin secretion, in A. Hasselblatt and F. V. Bruchhausen, (eds): Insulin II. Berlin, Springer, 1975, pp. 79–109.
4. Pagliara, A. S., Stillings, S. N., Hover, B., Martin, D. M., and Matschinsky, F. M. Glucose modulation of amino acid induced glucagon and insulin release in the isolated perfused rat pancreas. *J. Clin. Invest. 54:* 819, 1974.
5. Unger, R. H., Ohneda, A., Aguillar-Parada, E. The role of aminogenic glucagon secretion in blood glucose homeostatis. *J. Clin. Invest. 48:* 810, 1969.
6. Lefebvre, P. J. Personal communication.
7. Matschinsky, F. M. Unpublished observations.
8. Gerich, J. E., Charles, M. A., and Grodsky, G. M. Characterization of the effects of arginine and glucose on glucagon and insulin release from the *in vitro* perfused rat pancreas. *J. Clin. Invest. 54:* 833, 1974.
9. Unger, R. H. Diabetes and the alpha cell. *Diabetes 25:* 136, 1976.
10. Grodsky, G. M. The kinetics of insulin release, in A. Hasselblatt and F. V. Bruchhausen (eds): *Insulin II.* Berlin, Springer, 1975, pp. 1–12.
11. Pace, C. S., Matschinsky, F. M., Lacy, P. E., and Conant, S. Electrophysiological evidence for the autoregulation of β-cell secretion by insulin. *Biochim. Biophys. Acta* (in press).
12. Norfleet, W. T., Pagliara, A. S., Haymond, M. W., Matschinsky, F. M. Comparison of α- and β-cell secretory responses in islets isolated with collagenase and in the isolated perfused pancreas of the rat. *Diabetes 24:* 961, 1975.
13. Matschinsky, F. M., Pagliara, A. S., Hover, B. A., Haymond, M. W., Stillings, S. N. Differential effects of α- and β-D-glucose on insulin and glucagon secretion from the isolated perfused rat pancreas. *Diabetes 24:* 369, 1975.
14. Grodsky, G. M., Fanska, R., West, L., Manning, M. Anomeric specificity of glucose stimulated insulin release: evidence for a glucoreceptor. *Science 186:* 536, 1974.
15. Ashcroft, S. J. H., Bassett, J. M., Randle, P. J. Insulin secretion mechanisms and glucose metabolism in isolated islets. *Diabetes 21:* 538, 1972.
16. Renold, A. E., Kanazawa, Y., Lambert, A., Orci, L., Burr, I., Balant, L., Beaven, D. W., Grodsky, G. M., Stauffacher, W., Jeanrenaud, B., and Roullier, C. Insulin biosynthesis and secretion—a still unsettled topic. *N. Engl. J. Med. 282:* 173, 1970.
17. Zawalich, W., and Matschinsky, F. M. Unpublished observations.
18. Ashcroft, S. J. H., and Randle, P. J. The pancreas and insulin release, in J. Vallance-Owen (ed): Diabetes, Its Physiological and Biochemical Basis. MTP Press, 1975, pp. 31–62.
19. Müller, W. A., Faloona, G. R., and Unger, R. H. The effect of experimental insulin deficiency on glucagon secretion. *J. Clin. Invest. 50:* 1972, 1971.
20. Matschinsky, F. M., Fertel, R., Kotler-Brajtburg, J., Stillings, S. N., Ellerman, J., Raybaud, F., and Holowach-Thurston, J. Factors governing the action of small calorigenic molecules on the islets of Langerhans, in X. J. Mussacchia and K. P. Breitenbach (eds): Pro-

ceedings of the 8th Midwest Conference on Endocrinology and Metabolism. Colombia, Univ. Missouri, 1973, pp. 63–86.

21. Panten, N. Amino acids and insulin secretion, in A. Hasselblatt and F. V. Bruchhausen (eds): Insulin II. Berlin, Springer, 1975, pp. 115–129.

22. Orci, L., Unger, R. H., and Renold, A. E. Structural coupling between pancreatic islet cells. *Experientia 29:* 1015, 1973.

23. Luft, R., Efendic, S., and Hokfelt, T. Immunohistochemical evidence for the location of somatostatin like immunoreactivity in a cell population of the pancreatic islets. *Med. Biol. 52:* 428, 1974.

24. Lacy, P. E., and Greider, M. H. Anatomy and ultrastructural characterization of pancreatic islets. Chapter MM.

25. Loubatieres-Mariani, M. M., Chapal, L., Alric, R., and Loubatieres, A. Studies of cholinergic receptors involved in secretion of insulin using the isolated perfused rat pancreas. *Diabetologia 9:* 439, 1973.

26. Burr, I. M., Balant, L., Stauffacher, W., and Renold, A. E., Adrenergic modification of glucose induced biphasic insulin release from perifused rat pancreas, *Europ. J. Clin. Invest. 1,* 216–224 (1971).

27. Sussman, K. E., and Vaughan, G. D. Insulin release after ACTH, glucagon and adenosine-3′,5′-phosphate (cyclic AMP) in the perfused isolated rat pancreas. *Diabetes 16:* 449, 1967.

28. Iversen, J. Adrenergic receptors and the secretion of glucagon and insulin from the isolated perfused canine pancreas. *J. Clin. Invest. 52:* 2102, 1973.

29. Grodsky, G. M., Bennett, L. L., Smith, D., and Nemechek, K. The effect of tolbutamide and glucose on the timed release of insulin from the isolated perfused pancreas, in W. J. H. Butterfield and W. van Westering (eds): Tolbutamide after Ten Years. Amsterdam, Excerpta Medica, 1967, pp. 11–21.

30. Loubatieres, A. The action of sulfonylurea on pancreatic islets, in D. Steiner and N. Freinkel (eds): Handbook of Physiology, section 7, Endocrinology, vol. I. Washington, D.C., American Physiological Society 1972, pp. 425–431.

31. Rujanavech, C., and Matschinsky, F. M. Unpublished observations.

32. Lenzen, S. The effect of hydrocortisone treatment and adrenalectomy on insulin and glucagon secretion from the perfused rat pancreas. *Endokrinologie 68:* 189, 1976.

33. Samols, E., and Harrison, J. Intraislet negative insulin–glucagon feedback. *Metabolism 25 [Suppl. 1]:* 1443, 1976.

34. Samols, E., Tyler, J. M., and Marks, V. Glucagon-insulin interrelationships, in P. J. Lefebvre and R. H. Unger (eds): Glucagon. New York, Pergamon, 1972, pp. 151–173.

35. Pagliara, A. S., Stillings, S. N. Haymond, M. W., Hover, B. A., and Matschinsky F. M. Insulin and glucose as modulators of the amino acid induced glucagon release in the isolated pancreas of alloxan and streptozotocin diabetic rats. *J. Clin. Invest. 55:* 244, 1975.

36. Matschinsky, F. M., Ellerman, J. E., Krzanowski, J., Jr., Kotler-Brajtburg, J., Landgraf, R., and Fertel, R. The dual function of glucose in islets of Langerhans. *J. Biol. Chem. 246:* 1007, 1971.

37. Matschinsky, F. M., Landgraf, R., Ellerman, J. E., and Kotler-Brajtburg, J. Glucoreceptor mechanisms in islets of Langerhans. *Diabetes 21 [Suppl. 2]:* 555, 1972.

38. Lambert, A. The regulation of insulin secretion. *Rev. Physiol. Bio. Chem. Pharmacol. 75:* 98, 1976.

39. Hellerström, C., and Brolin, S. E. Energy metabolism of the β-cell, in A. Hasselblatt and F. V. Bruchhausen (eds): Insulin II. Berlin, Springer, 1975, pp. 57–78.

40. Hellman, B., Idahl, L. A., Lernmark, A., Sehlin, J., and Taljedal, I. B. The pancreatic β-cell recognition of insulin secretagogue. Effect of calcium and sodium on glucose metabolism and insulin release. *Biochem. J. 138:* 33, 1974.

41. Zawalich, W. S., and Matschinsky, F. M. Sequential analysis of the releasing and fuel function of glucose in isolated perifused pancreatic islets. *Endocrinology 100:* 1, 1977.

42. Zawalich, W. S., Pagliara, A. S., and Matschinsky, F. M. Effects of Iodoacetate, mannoheptulose and 3-0-methyl glucose on the secretory function and metabolism of isolated pancreatic islets. *Endocrinology 100:* 1276, 1977.

43. Zawalich, W. S., Pagliara, A. S., and Matschinsky, F. M. In preparation.

44. Matschinsky, F. M., and Ellerman, J. E. Dissociation of insulin releasing and metabolic functions of hexoses in islets of Langerhans. *Biochem. Biophys. Res. Comm. 50:* 193, 1973.

45. Pace, C. S., Ellerman, J., Hover, B. A., and Matschinsky, F. M. Multiple metabolic functions of glucose in rat pancreatic islets. *Diabetes 24:* 476, 1976.

46. Ashcroft, S. J. H., Weerasinghe, L. C. C., Bassett, J. M., and Randle, P. J. The pentose cycle and insulin release in mouse pancreatic islets. *Biochem. J. 126:* 525, 1972.

47. Ashcroft, S. J. H., and Randle, P. J. Glucose metabolism in mouse pancreatic islets. *Biochem. J. 118:* 143, 1970.

48. Ammon, H. P. T. Personal communication.

49. Hellman, B., Sehlin, J., and Taljedal, I. B. Effects of glucose and other modifiers of insulin release on the oxidative metabolism of amino acids in microdissected pancreatic islets. *Biochem. J. 123:* 513, 1971.

50. Landau, B. R. Quantitation of pathways of carbohydrate metabolism, in D. Steiner and N. Freinkel (eds): Handbook of Physiology, section 7, Endocrinology, vol. I. Washington, D.C., American Physiological Society, 1972, pp. 215–218.

51. Berne, C. Oxidation of fatty acids and ketone bodies in isolated pancreatic islets. *Diabetologia 8:* 364, 1972.

52. Matschinsky, F. M., and Ellerman, J. E. Metabolism of glucose in islets of Langerhans. *J. Biol. Chem. 243:* 2730, 1968.

53. Ashcroft, S. J. H., and Randle, P. J. Enzymes of glucose metabolism in normal mouse pancreatic islets. *Biochem. J. 119:* 5, 1970.

54. Malaisse, W. J., Sener, A., and Levy, J. The stimulus–secretion coupling of glucose induced insulin release; fasting induced adaptation of key glycolytic enzymes in isolated islets. *J. Biol. Chem. 251:* 1731, 1976.

55. Coore, H. G., and Randle, P. J. Inhibition of glucose phosphorylation by mannoheptulose. *Biochem. J. 91:* 56, 1964.

56. Matschinsky, F. M. Enzymes, metabolites, and cofactors involved in intermediary metabolism of islets of Langerhans, in the endocrine pancreas, in D. Steiner and N. Freinkel (eds): Handbook of Physiology, Section 7. Baltimore, Williams & Williams, 1972, pp. 199–214.

57. Grodsky, G. M. Insulin and the Pancreas. *Vitam. Horm. 28:* 37, 1970.

58. Hellman, B., Idahl, L. A., Sehlin, J., and Taljedal, I. B. Influence of anoxia on glucose metabolism in pancreatic islets: lack of correlation between fructose-1,6-diphosphate and apparent glycolytic flux. *Diabetologia 11:* 495, 1975.

59. Fajans, S. S., Floyd, J. C., Jr., Knopf, R. F., and Conn, J. W. Effect of amino acids and proteins on insulin secretion in man. *Rec. Prog. Horm. Res. 23:* 617, 1976.

60. Mathews, E. K. Calcium and stimulus secretion coupling in pancreatic islet cells, in E. Carafoli et al. (eds): Calcium Transport in Contraction and Secretion. Amsterdam, North Holland, 1975, pp. 203–210.

61. Bukowiecki, L., Trus, M. D., Matschinsky, F. M., and Freinkel, N. Islet phosphate content during secretory stimulation. *Diabetes 25 [Suppl. 1]:* 346, 1976.

62. Matschinsky, F. M., Rutherford, C. K., and Ellerman, J. Accumulation of citrate in pancreatic islets of obese hyperglycemic mice. *Biochem. Biophys. Res. Commun. 33:* 855, 1968.

63. Matschinsky, F. M., Pagliara, A. S., Hover, B. A., Pace, C. S., Ferrendelli, J. A., and Williams, A. D. Hormone secretion and glucose metabolism in islets of Langerhans of the isolated perfused pancreas from normal and streptozotocin diabetic rats. *J. Biol. Chem. 251:* 6053, 1976.

64. Matschinsky, F. M., Pagliara, A. S., Stillings, S. N., and Hover, B. A. Glucose and ATP levels in pancreatic islet tissue of normal and diabetic rats. *J. Clin. Invest. 58:* 1193, 1976.

65. Montague, W., and Taylor, K. W. Islet cell metabolism during insulin release. Effects of glucose, citrate, octanoate, tolbutamide, glucagon, and theophylline. *Biochem. J. 115:* 257, 1969.

66. Idahl, L. A. Dynamics of the pancreatic β-cell response to glucose. *Diabetologia 9:* 403, 1973.

67. Malaisse, W. J., Sener, A., and Mahy, M. The stimulus secretion coupling of glucose induced insulin release. Sorbitol metabolism in isolated islets. *Eur. J. Biochem. 47:* 365, 1974.

68. Panten, N., Christians, J., Kriegstein, E. V., Poser, W., and Hasselblatt, A. Effects of carbohydrate upon fluorescence of reduced pryidine nucleotides from perfused isolted pancreatic islets. Naunyn Schmiedeberg's *Arch. Pharmacol. 276:* 55, 1973.

69. Trus, M., Woerner, H., and Matschinsky, F. M. In preparation.

70. Ashcroft, S. J. H., Capito, K., and Hedeskov, C. J. Time course of glucose induced changes in glucose-6-phosphate and fructose-1,6-diphosphate content of mouse and rat pancreatic islets. *Diabetologia 9:* 299, 1973.

71. Matschinsky, F. M., Kauffman, F. C., and Ellerman, J. E. Effect of hyperglycemia on the hexose monophosphate shunt in islets of Langerhans. *Diabetes 17:* 475, 1968.

72. Panten, N., Ishida, H., and Beckman, J. Effects of glyceraldehyde and 3-0-methyl glucose upon fluorescence of reduced pyridine nucleotides from perifused isolated pancreatic islets. *Horm. Res. 7:* 164, 1976.

73. Rossini, A. A., Berger, M., Schadden, J., and Cahill, G. F., Jr. Beta cell protection to alloxan necrosis by anomers of D-glucose. *Science 183:* 424, 1973.

74. Benkovic, S. J., and Schray, K. J. The anomeric specificity of glycolytic enzymes. *Adv. Enzymol. 44:* 139, 1976.

75. Idahl, L. A., Sehlin, J., and Taljedal, I. B. Metabolic and insulin releasing activities of D-glucose anomers. *Nature 254:* 75, 1975.

76. Idahl, L. A., Rahemtulla, F., Sehlin, J., and Taljedal, I. B. Further studies on the metabolism of D-glucose anomers in pancreatic islets. *Diabetes 25:* 450, 1976.

77. Malaisse, W. J., Sener, A., Koser, M., and Herchuelz, A. Stimulus secretion coupling of glucose induced insulin release. *J. Biol. Chem. 251:* 5936, 1976.

78. Hellman, B., Sehlin, J., and Taljedal, I. B. Calcium uptake by pancreatic β-cells as measured with the aid of $^{45}Ca^{++}$ and ^{3}H-mannitol. *Am. J. Physiol. 221:* 1795, 1971.

79. Malaisse, W. J. Participation of the adenylate cyclase system, in A. Hasselblatt and F. V. Bruchhausen (eds): Insulin II. Berlin, Springer, 1975.

80. Charles, M. A., Fanska, R., Schmid, F. G., Forsham, P. H., and Grodsky, G. M. Adenosine-3'5'-monophosphate in pancreatic islets: glucose induced insulin release. *Science 179:* 569, 1973.

81. Grill, V., and Cerasi, E. Stimulation by D-glucose of cyclic adenosin-3',5' monophosphate accumulation and insulin release in isolated pancreatic islets of the rat. *J. Biol. Chem. 249:* 4196, 1974.

82. Zawalich, W. S., Karl, R. C., Ferrendelli, J. A., and Matschinsky, F. M. Factors governing glucose induced elevation of cyclic −3',5'-AMP levels in pancreatic islets. *Diabetologia 11:* 231, 1975.

83. Karl, R. C., Zawalich, W. S., Ferrendelli, J. A., and Matschinsky, F. M. The role of Ca^{++} and cyclic adenosine-3', 5'-monophosphate in insulin release induced *in vitro* by the divalent cation ionophore A 23187. *J. Biol. Chem. 250:* 4575, 1975.

84. Sharp, G. W. G., Wollheim, C., and Müller, W. A., Gutzeit, A., Trueheart, P. A., Blondel, B., Orci, L., and Renold, A. E. Studies on the mechanism of insulin release. *Fed. Proc. 34:* 1537, 1975.

85. Malaisse, W. J., Malaisse-Lagae, F., Walker, M. O., and Lacy, P. E. The stimulus-secretion coupling of glucose-induced insulin release. The participation of a microtubular microfilamentous system. *Diabetes 20:* 257, 1971.

86. Grey, N. J., Goldring, S., and Kipnis, D. M. The effect of fasting, diet and actinomycin D on insulin secretion in the rat. *J. Clin. Invest. 49:* 881, 1970.

87. Frankel, B. J., Gerich, J. E., Hagura, K., Fanska, R. E., Gerritsen, G. C., and Grodsky, G. M. Abnormal secretion of insulin and glucagon by the *in vitro* perfused pancreas of the genetically diabetic Chinese hamster. *J. Clin. Invest. 53:* 1637, 1974.

88. Zawalich, W. S., Dye, E. S., Rognstad, R., Pagliara, A. S., and Matschinsky, F. M. Starvation induced alterations of islet cell sensitivity. *Diabetes 26 [Suppl. 1]:* 379, 1977.

89. Ashcroft, S. J. H. The control of insulin release by sugars, in: Polypeptide Hormones: Molecular and Cellular Aspects, Ciba Foundation Symposium 41 (new series). Amsterdam, Elsevier, 1976, pp. 117–139.

90. Rabinovitch, A., Renold, A. E., and Cerasi, E. Decreased cyclic AMP and insulin response to glucose in pancreatic islets of diabetic Chinese hamsters. *Diabetologia 12:* 581, 1976.

91. Davis, B., and Lazarus, N. R. An *in vitro* system for analyzing insulin release caused by secretory granules-plasma membrane interaction: definition of the system. *J. Physiol. 256:* 709, 1976.

92. Malaisse, W. J., Sener, A., Koser, M., Ravazolla, M., and Malaisse-Lagae, F. The stimulus–secretion coupling of glucose-induced insulin release. Insulin release due to glycogenolysis in glucose-deprived islets. *Biochem. J. 164:* 447, 1977.

93. Rabinovitch, A., Grill, V., Renold, A. E., and Cerasi, E. Insulin release and cyclic AMP accumulation in response to glucose in pancreatic islets of fed and starved rats. *J. Clin. Invest. 58:* 1209, 1976.

94. Cerasi, E. Mechanism of glucose stimulated insulin release in health and in diabetes: some reevaluations and proposals. *Diabetologia 11:* 1, 1975.

INSULIN METABOLISM

Insulin is distributed in a space considerably larger than the plasma volume and has a rapid half-life of 3 to 5 minutes. The hormone is found in the bile, lymph, and urine in low concentrations. Although many tissues may accumulate small amounts of insulin, its major sites of uptake and degradation are the liver[21] and kidneys.[22] The liver removes approximately 40 to 50 percent of the insulin reaching it by way of the portal vein. The hepatic uptake mechanism is saturable and may be modulated by fasting or nutrients stimulating insulin release. The renal arteriovenous difference is 40 percent, which indicates that both glomerular filtration and peritubular uptake are important mechanisms involved in insulin uptake. There is evidence that insulin is filtered through the glomerulus but is almost completely reabsorbed and degraded by the proximal convoluted tubules.

Two enzyme systems have been implicated in insulin degradation. The first involves a proteolytic enzyme, insulin specific protease, which is found predominantly in the cytosol of many tissues.[23] The greatest activities are present in the liver, pancreas, and kidney. The enzyme has been purified from skeletal muscle and shown to be sulfhydryl dependent with a pH optimum of 7.4. The second system is glutathione-insulin transhydrogenase,[24] which catalyzes the reductive cleavage of the insulin disulfide bonds by glutathione with liberation of the intact A and B chains. It is believed that the chains are subsequently rapidly degraded to small molecular weight peptides. Which of these mechanisms is active under physiologic conditions is unknown at present.

INSULIN SECRETION IN DIABETES

In ketosis-prone diabetic patients, the circulating plasma insulin level is low or undetectable. Although serum insulin may be measurable, the secretory response to glucose is characteristically absent. These findings are consistent with pathological observations of marked loss of beta cells in the islets of these subjects. It is of interest that patients with significant fasting hyperglycemia, but a less severe metabolic disturbance, maintain their basal insulin concentration close to or within the normal range. In patients with milder disorders, the plasma insulin response to glucose is delayed and subnormal in relation to carefully chosen age- and weight-matched controls.[25] In the glucose tolerance test there is both a quantitative decrease in total insulin secretion and a sluggish early response, with a tendency for the peak level to occur later than normal. The initial delay in secretion generally correlates well with the tendency in these tests for the blood sugar level to rise to abnormally high levels.

The nature of this defect has been a controversial question that has generated many theories. One of the most popular of these is the idea of an inherent secretory defect in the beta cells of diabetics, which might be regarded as a primary defect in the disease. An alternative hypothesis that is rapidly gaining favor is the concept that the islet cells may have an inherent or acquired alteration in their sensitivity, or ability to respond, to the stimulus of glucose. This is based on the findings in some laboratories that other stimuli to insulin secretion, such as certain amino acids and sulfonylurea compounds, elicit normal secretory responses in mild diabetics, while the response to glucose is impaired.[26] Recent studies have focused attention on the possible existence of a glucoreceptor that senses the blood glucose concentration and generates an intracellular signal for insulin secretion. The nature and location of this glucoreceptor and of the signal that it generates

are questions of obvious importance which are unanswered at the present time.

Studies of the pathological changes in the pancreatic islets in adult-onset diabetes in humans support the concept of a more generalized failure of islet responsiveness rather than a defect in the secretory mechanism per se. Gepts[27] has pointed out that there is almost invariably a decrease in total islet tissue mass in the diabetic pancreas, on average amounting to a reduction of about 50 percent. Moreover, there is a similar reduction of insulin stores in the remaining pancreatic beta cells of these individuals, as evidenced by some degree of degranulation of the islet tissue and by a decrease in the total amount of insulin that can be extracted from the pancreas. Clearly, these data point to a defect that involves the production of insulin and the regeneration of islet cells, as well as the ultimate secretion of insulin. Glucose unresponsiveness may also be implicated in these processes, as it is known that glucose is a potent stimulus to insulin biosynthesis. Indeed, it appears to be the most important stimulus, inasmuch as amino acids are much less active in this regard. There is also a growing body of evidence indicating that hyperglycemia plays a role in stimulating mitotic activity and hyperplasia of the beta cells in the islets of Langerhans. All these observations thus take on greater significance when viewed in the context of an altered glucoreceptor mechanism in the diabetic's beta cells. Such an alteration in the diabetic islet cells could account for the observed impairment of renewal of islet tissue through failure to adequately stimulate division and could account for decreased insulin biosynthesis and storage through failure to adequately maintain or stimulate these processes. Ultimately, all these effects in combination would lead to a reduced secretory response of the islet cells to glucose. It is important, therefore, to focus attention not only on the mechanisms involved in secretion but also on those that regulate insulin biosynthesis and islet cell growth and division.

While the concept of an intrinsic defect in the beta cells in most diabetics is an attractive working hypothesis, other factors also merit further consideration. Recent studies of the inheritance pattern of diabetes and its incidence, particularly in identical twins,[28] strongly suggest that other causes for diabetes may exist and account for a significant fraction of the total number of cases. Studies of pancreatic pathology, particularly in juvenile diabetics, indicate the occurrence of a complex destructive lesion in the islets of Langerhans that may be due to purely extrinsic causes acting upon a genetically favorable substratum. Among such possible causes are two of particular interest and concern: autoimmunity and viral infection. In juvenile diabetes of short duration, the islets often contain infiltrates of mononuclear cells. This "insulitis" is not unlike that seen in experimental animals exposed to viruses that are known to produce islet destruction.

CIRCULATING PROINSULIN-LIKE COMPONENTS

MEASUREMENT OF PROINSULIN IN SERUM

A number of studies of normal human plasma or urine samples have indicated the presence of small amounts of immunoreactive material similar in molecular weight to proinsulin.[29,30] Although it would be advantageous to measure human proinsulin and its intermediate fractions (proinsulin-like components, PLC) by direct immunoassay in unextracted serum, this has not been possible. The reasons lie in the cross-reactivity of proinsulin with insulin on the one hand and the C-peptide on the other. As all three of these peptides have been identified in the circulation, a preliminary step is required to separate them from each other. The most commonly used approach has involved gel filtration of serum followed by measurement of the column fractions in the insulin immunoassay. Another method for separating insulin from proinsulin has been described by Kitabchi and his co-workers.[31] These investigators have used an enzyme that is relatively specific for the proteolytic degradation of insulin, but not proinsulin. Measuring samples in an insulin assay before and after incubation with this enzyme (insulin specific protease, ISP) enables one to determine the relative concentrations of the two peptides.

CHARACTERIZATION OF CIRCULATING PROINSULIN-LIKE COMPONENTS

In most studies, PLC has been measured after gel filtration of sera on Sephadex or Bio-Gel columns equilibrated in acetic acid, borate, or veronal buffers. Because of its higher molecular weight, PLC elutes before insulin and may be identified in either the insulin or the human C-peptide immunoassays. However, these methods do not differentiate the two-chain proinsulin intermediates from the single chain precursor, and additional techniques are required to demonstrate their presence in the circulation. Lazarus et al.[32] have described the presence of a proinsulin intermediate, in addition to proinsulin, in the serum of a patient with a surgically documented carcinoma of the pancreatic islets. The fasting total immunoassayable insulin concentration was approximately 1000 μU/ml and the percentage of PLC was 85 percent. An acid alcohol extract of serum was electrophoresed on polyacrylamide gel, and three peaks were identified. Two of these had mobilities corresponding to insulin and proinsulin, while the third peak ran in an intermediate position. The authors suggested that the migration behavior of this peak was compatible with desdipeptide proinsulin.

CIRCULATING PROINSULIN LEVELS IN NORMAL SUBJECTS AND IN DISEASE STATES

The mean fasting proinsulin levels in normal subjects is 0.16 ± 0.2 ng/ml.[33] In studies using a human insulin standard for measurement of both proinsulin and insulin, PLC comprises 15 percent of the total immunoreactive insulin concentration (range 0 to 22 percent). After oral glucose, the levels of proinsulin rise slowly and peak later than those of insulin. When expressed as a percentage of the insulin concentration, a decline from the fasting value is observed during the first 15 to 60 minutes.[34] Thereafter, proinsulin contributes an increasing amount to the immunoreactive insulin level. Obese patients with hyperinsulinemia have raised fasting concentrations of proinsulin and a greater absolute increase after glucose than subjects of normal weight. However, the high levels of proinsulin coexist with raised insulin concentrations, so that the relative proportions of the two polypeptides are generally in the same range as that observed in healthy subjects.

Great interest has been expressed in the possibility that an altered proinsulin–insulin ratio might occur in patients with diabetes mellitus. Results in a limited number of both normal weight and obese patients with mild diabetes characterized only by glucose intolerance demonstrated basal and postglucose responses indistinguishable from control subjects. More recently, however, Duckworth et al.,[35] using the insulin-specific protease to measure proinsulin, reported that both obesity and carbohydrate intolerance were associated with slightly increased PLC levels but that the coexistence of the two conditions, especially in older diabetics, was marked by significantly elevated PLC concentrations and a rise in the PLC–insulin ratio. In contrast, children with mild diabetes and elevated immunoreactive insulin levels have proinsu-

lin values within the normal range in both the fasting and stimulated state.[36]

The major clinical significance of a raised serum proinsulin concentration has been in the diagnosis of pancreatic islet cell tumors (Fig. 77-1). For example, Sherman et al.[37] described 3 of 21 islet cell tumor patients with basal immunoreactive insulin concentrations within the normal range but only 1 with a normal proinsulin concentration. Four subjects had percentage PLC that overlapped their controls. These findings are representative of the conclusions in a number of other reports. The possibility that serum PLC estimations may be useful in differentiating benign beta-cell tumors from carcinomas has been considered. Most patients with malignant islet cell tumors do have a markedly elevated percentage PLC. However, a significant number of subjects with adenomas also fall into this high range. On the other hand, it seems that the finding of a low percentage PLC in a patient with an islet cell tumor does favor the diagnosis of a benign lesion.

Recently, a family with hyperproinsulinemia has been described.[38] Members of the kindred demonstrating hyperproinsulinemia were found in four generations and ranged from 2 to 69 years in age. The proportion of male and female affected and unaffected progeny was the same, and the abnormality was transmitted by both sexes. The pattern of inheritance indicates that familial hyperproinsulinemia is transmitted as an autosomal dominant defect. The serum proinsulin fraction in the affected members ranged from 74 to 92 percent of the total serum immunoreactive insulin concentration, despite wide variation in the levels of serum insulin.

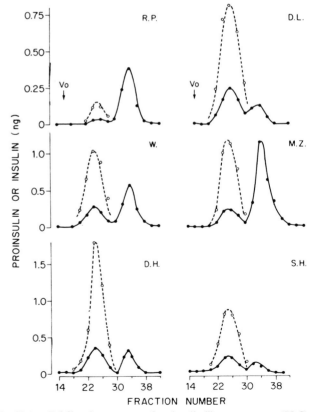

Fig. 77-1. Gel filtration patterns of proinsulin-like components (PLC) and insulin in a control subject (top left) and 5 patients with islet cell tumors. The sera were gel filtered on Bio-Gel P-30 columns equilibrated in a borate albumin buffer and measured in the insulin immunoassay. The dotted line represents the PLC value read from the human proinsulin standard. Note the different scales on the ordinate.

PERIPHERAL METABOLISM OF PROINSULIN

Proinsulin comprises 2 to 9 percent of the immunoreactive insulinlike material in normal pancreas, a value similar to that found in the portal vein of man[39] but much lower than that found in peripheral serum. This discrepancy can be explained by the slower metabolism of proinsulin compared to insulin. Sonksen et al.[40] showed a mean metabolic clearance rate (MCR) of 13.3 ml/kg/min for insulin and 3.1 ml/kg/min for proinsulin, with mean half-lives of 4.4 and 25.6 minutes, respectively, in healthy subjects. Similarly, the half disappearance time of endogenous proinsulin (18 to 25 minutes) was markedly slower than that of insulin (3 to 4 minutes). In contrast to the differences in their MCR, the renal disposition of insulin and proinsulin is similar, being characterized by high extraction and very low urinary clearance.[41] The renal arteriovenous differences of proinsulin and insulin averaged 36 and 40 percent, respectively, and were linearly related to their arterial concentrations. The fractional urinary clearance never exceeded 0.6 percent, indicating that more than 99 percent of the amount filtered was sequestered in the kidney. On the other hand, studies on the removal of proinsulin and insulin by the isolated perfused rat liver have shown that the hepatic extration of proinsulin is considerably slower than that of insulin, at both high and low concentrations.[43] It should also be noted that there is no evidence for conversion of proinsulin to insulin in the circulation.

CIRCULATING C-PEPTIDE

MEASUREMENT OF C-PEPTIDE IN SERUM

Although the insulin immunoassay has been widely applied to the study of circulating insulin levels in healthy subjects and in diabetics managed with diet or oral hypoglycemic agents, the method has proved less useful in insulin-treated diabetic patients. The reasons for this include the development of circulating insulin antibodies in response to repeated injections of bovine and/or porcine insulin and the immunologic similarity of these species of insulin compared to the human hormone. Although a number of investigators have devised ingenious methods to circumvent these problems, there is little information about the natural history of beta-cell function in insulin-treated diabetics. The development of an immunoassay for human C-peptide provided an alternative means of studying beta-cell secretory capacity in these patients. Proteolytic conversion of proinsulin results in the formation of equimolar concentrations of C-peptide and insulin, which are stored within the beta-cell granules and subsequently liberated together during exocytosis. Circulating levels of C-peptide thus reflect beta-cell secretory activity, and because neither insulin nor insulin antibodies interfere with the C-peptide immunoassay, its measurement has opened up new approaches for the study of beta-cell function in a variety of physiologic and pathological circumstances.

C-peptide, together with insulin and proinsulin, is secreted by the pancreatic beta cells into the portal circulation and must pass through the liver before entering the peripheral blood. In order to relate peripheral concentrations to beta-cell secretion, simultaneously determined portal and peripheral blood levels were compared in subjects whose portal blood was obtained by umbilical vein catheterization prior to operation.[39] In general, both portal and peripheral serum concentrations of C-peptide were greater than those of insulin on a molar basis, but at times of peak secretion, insulin and C-peptide were present in portal blood in

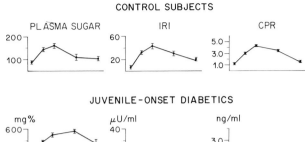

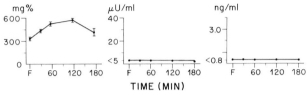

Fig. 77-2. Plasma sugar (mg/100 ml), immunoreactive insulin (IRI), and C-peptide (CPR) levels during an oral glucose tolerance test in control subjects (above) and 5 juvenile-onset diabetics at the time of diagnosis of their disease (below).

nearly equimolar quantities. These findings confirm that insulin and C-peptide are released by the beta cell in equimolar concentrations, but this relationship is not preserved in the peripheral circulation. Differences in the metabolic clearance rates of insulin and C-peptide account for the different ratio of these two peptides in peripheral blood. Thus the MCR of insulin is much faster than C-peptide in man and rats.[41]

Both insulin and C-peptide levels are very low or unmeasurable during episodes of ketoacidosis in adult-onset diabetics (Fig. 77-2). Similarly, C-peptide is undetectable or very low in newly diagnosed untreated juvenile-onset diabetics with fasting blood sugars above 200 mg/100 ml.[43] Following correction of the ketoacidosis or severe hyperglycemia by insulin therapy, partial recovery of beta-cell function occurs, as assessed by increases in serum C-peptide (Fig. 77-3). Sequential studies in insulin-treated diabetic patients show significant increases in serum C-peptide during the phase of clinical remission, while clinical relapse was again associated with decreasing serum C-peptide concentrations.[44] These studies indicate that beta-cell secretory ability may be temporarily

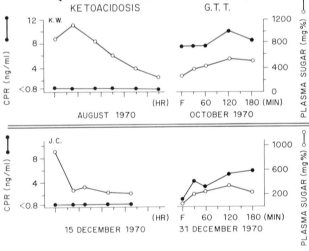

Fig. 77-3. Serum C-peptide and plasma sugars (mg/100 ml) during the initial 10 hours of therapy for ketoacidosis and 12 weeks (KW) and 2 weeks (JC) later during oral glucose tolerance test (GTT).

impaired and that partial recovery in their function may occur. At present, there is little information about the factors that may be important in affecting this process.

Measurement of serum C-peptide in patients with established diabetes has shown varying degrees of beta-cell secretory impairment. Ketosis-prone juvenile diabetics who had been treated with insulin for longer than 5 years have very low or unmeasurable C-peptide in the basal or poststimulatory state. However, C-peptide may be detected in many of these patients during the first years of their disease. This suggests that the loss of beta-cell secretory capacity in juvenile-onset diabetes is not abrupt, but continues for several years after the diabetes becomes clinically manifest.

The clinical significance of retention of a low level of beta-cell secretory ability in diabetic patients has been considered by a number of investigators who compared C-peptide levels in metabolically stable and unstable diabetics.[45] The stable group had greater C-peptide levels in both the basal state and following stimulation with either oral glucose or arginine. In the unstable group, basal C-peptide levels were at the lower limit of sensitivity of the assay, and no response to either glucose or arginine could be detected. It is of interest that these unstable diabetics also showed a severe alpha-cell defect as measured by minimal glucagon responses to hypoglycemia.

MEASUREMENT OF C-PEPTIDE IN URINE

Although peptide hormone concentrations in blood reflect most accurately the minute-to-minute changes in their secretion, measurement of urine levels may be advantageous in reflecting average serum values over a period of time. Furthermore, this approach may also be useful in situations where repeated blood sampling is difficult, such as in small children. While assay of insulin in urine has been shown to be feasible, its value is diminished because only a small fraction of the total amount of insulin secreted appears in the urine. Because the urinary clearance of C-peptide is much higher than that of insulin in animals, a number of investigators have considered the utility of measuring urine C-peptide in man.[46,47] In nondiabetic subjects with normal kidney function or various renal diseases, C-peptide clearance was independent of creatinine clearance. Urine C-peptide clearance was greater than that of insulin, and the total quantity of C-peptide excreted in the urine per day represented 5 percent of pancreatic secretion, as compared to only 0.1 percent in the case of insulin. Healthy subjects excreted 36 ± 4 μg C-peptide per 24 hours, while this value in juvenile-onset diabetics was only 1.1 ± 0.5 μg. Adult-onset diabetics excreted 24 ± 7 μg/24 hours, the range overlapping the excretory rates of both normal subjects and juvenile-onset diabetics.

REFERENCES

1. Lacy, P. E., Greider, M. H.: Ultrastructural organization of mammalian pancreatic islets, in Steiner D. F., Freinkel N. (eds): Handbook of Physiology. American Physiological Society, 1972, chap 4, sec 7, vol 1, p 77.
2. Randle, P. J., Hales, C. N.: Insulin release mechanisms, in Steiner D. F., Freinkel, N. (eds): Handbook of Physiology. American Physiological Society, 1972, chap 13, sec 7, vol 1, p 219.
3. Lacy, P. E., Howell, S. L., Young, D. A., et al: New hypothesis of insulin secretion. *Nature 219:* 1177–1179, 1968.
4. Malaisse, W., Malaisse-Lagae, F., Wright, P. H.: A new method for the measurement in vitro of pancreatic insulin secretion. *Endocrinology 80:* 99–108, 1967.
5. Curry, D. L., Bennett, L. L., Grodsky, G. M.: Requirement for calcium ion in insulin secretion by the perfused rat pancreas. *Am J Physiol 214:* 174–178, 1968.
6. Malaisse, W. J.: Insulin secretion: Multifactorial regulation for a single process of release. *Diabetologia 9:* 167–172, 1973.
7. Aschcroft, S. J. H., Randle, P. J.: The pancreas and insulin release, in J Vallance Owen (ed): Diabetes: Its Physiological and Biochemical Basis. MTP Press, 1975, chap 2, p 31.
8. Dean, P. M., Matthews, E. K.: Glucose-induced electrical activity in pancreatic islet cells. *J Physiol London 210:* 255–264, 1970.
9. Dean, P. M., Matthews, E. K.: Electrical activity in pancreatic islet cells: Effect of ions. *J Physiol London 210:* 265–275, 1970.
10. Rossini, A. A., Soeldner, J. S., Hiebert J. M., et al: The effect of glucose anomers upon insulin and glucagon secretion. *Diabetologia 10:* 795–799, 1974.
11. Fajans, S. S., Floyd, J. C.: Stimulation of islet cell secretion by nutrients and by gastrointestinal hormones released during digestion, in Steiner, D. F., Freinkel, N. (eds): Handbook of Physiology. American Physiological Society, 1972, chap 30, sec 7, vol 1, p 473.
12. Christensen, H. N., Hellman, B., Lernmark A., et al: In vitro stimulation of insulin release by non-metabolizable, transport specific amino acids. *Biochim Biophys Acta 241:* 341–348, 1971.
13. Malaisse, W. J.: Hormonal and environmental modification of islet activity, in Steiner D. F., Freinkel N. (eds): Handbook of Physiology. American Physiological Society, 1972, chap 14, sec 7, vol 1, p 237.
14. Porte, D. Jr.: A receptor mechanism for the inhibition of insulin release by epinephrine in man. *J Clin Invest 46:* 86–94, 1967.
15. Pederson, R. A., Schubert, H. E., Brown, J. C.: Gastric inhibitory polypeptide: Its physiological release and insulinotropic action in the dog. *Diabetes 24:* 1050–1056, 1975.
16. Ensinck, J. W., Williams, R. H.: Hormonal and nonhormonal factors modifying man's response to insulin, in Steiner D. F., Freinkel N. (eds): Handbook of Physiology. American Physiological Society, 1972, chap 43, sec 7, vol 1, p 665.
17. McIntyre, N., Holdsworth, C. D., Turner D. S.: New interpretation of oral glucose tolerance. *Lancet 2:* 20–21, 1964.
18. Goodner, C. J., Porte, D. Jr.: Determinants of basal islet secretion in man, in Steiner, D. F., Freinkel, N. (eds): Handbook of Physiology, American Physiological Society, 1972, chap 38, sec 7, vol 1, p 597.
19. Grodsky, G. M., Bennett, L. L., Smith, D. F. et al: Effect of pulse administration of glucose or glucagon on insulin secretion in vitro. *Metabolism 16:* 222–223, 1967.
20. Grodsky, G. M., Landahl, H., Curry, D.: In vitro studies suggesting a two-compartment model for insulin secretion, in Falkmer, S., Hellman, B., Taljedal, I-B (eds): Structure and Metabolism of the Pancreatic Islets. Oxford, Pergamon Press, 1970, p 409.
21. Kaden, M., Harding, P., Field, J. B.: Effect of intraduodenal glucose administration on hepatic extraction of insulin. *J Clin Invest 52:* 2016–2028, 1973.
22. Rubenstein, A. H., Mako, M. E., Horwitz, D. L.: Insulin and the kidney. *Nephron 15:* 306–332, 1975.
23. Burghen, G. A., Kitabchi, A. E., Brush, J. S.: Characterization of a rat liver protease with specificity for insulin. *Endocrinology 91:* 633–637, 1972.
24. Varandani, P. T.: Insulin degradation: I. Purification and properties of glutathione insulin transhydrogenase of rat liver. *Biochim Biophys Acta 286:* 126–135, 1972.
25. Kipnis, D. M.: Insulin secretion in diabetes mellitus. *Ann Intern Med 69:* 891–903, 1968.
26. Simpson, R. G., Benedetti, A., Grodsky, G. M., et al: Early phase of insulin release. *Diabetes 17:* 682–692, 1968.
27. Gepts, W.: Pathology of islet tissue in human diabetes, in Steiner D. F., Freinkel N. (eds): Handbook of Physiology. American Physiological Society, 1972, chap 17, sec 7, vol 1, p 289.
28. Tattersall, R. B., Pyke, D. A.: Diabetes in identical twins. *Lancet 2:* 1120–1122, 1972.
29. Rubenstein, A. H., Cho, S., Steiner, D. F.: Evidence for proinsulin in human urine and serum. *Lancet 1:* 1353–1355, 1968.
30. Roth, J., Gorden, P., Pastan, I.: "Big insulin": A new component of plasma insulin detected by immunoassay. *Proc Natl Acad Sci USA 61:* 138–145, 1968.
31. Kitabchi, A. E., Duckworth, W. C., Brush, J. S., et al: Direct measurement of proinsulin in human plasma by the use of an insulin-degrading enzyme. *J Clin Invest 50:* 1792–1799, 1971.

32. Lazarus, N. R., Gutman, R. A., Panhos, J. C., et al: Biologically active circulating proinsulin-like materials from an islet cell carcinoma patient. *Diabetologia 8:* 131–136, 1972.

33. Mako, M. E., Block, M., Starr, J., et al: Proinsulin in chronic renal and hepatic failure: A reflection of the relative contribution of the liver and kidney to its metabolism. *Clin Res 21:* 631, 1973.

34. Gorden, P., Roth, J.: Plasma insulin: Fluctuations in the "big" insulin component in man after glucose and other stimuli. *J Clin Invest 48:* 2225–2234, 1969.

35. Duckworth, W. C., Kitabchi, A. E., Heinemann, M.: Direct measurement of plasma proinsulin in normal and diabetic subjects. *Am J Med 53:* 418–427, 1972.

36. Rosenbloom, A., Starr, J. L., Juhn, D., et al: Serum proinsulin in children and adolescents with chemical diabetes. *Diabetes 24:* 753–757, 1975.

37. Sherman, B. M., Pek, S., Fajans, S. S., et al: Plasma proinsulin in patients with functioning pancreatic islet cell tumors. *J Clin Endocrinol 35:* 271–280, 1972.

38. Gabbay, K. H., DeLuca, K., Fisher, J. N., et al: Familial hyperproinsulinemia: An autosomal dominant defect. *N Engl J Med 294:* 911–915, 1976.

39. Horwitz, D. L., Starr, J. I., Mako, M. E., et al: Proinsulin, insulin and C-peptide concentrations in human portal and peripheral blood. *J Clin Invest 55:* 1278–1283, 1975.

40. Sonksen, P. H., Tompkins, C. V., Srivastava, M. C., et al: A comparative study on the metabolism of human insulin and porcine proinsulin in man. *Clin Sci Mol Med 45:* 633–654, 1973.

41. Katz, A. I., Rubenstein, A. H.: Metabolism of proinsulin, and C-peptide in the rat. *J. Clin Invest 52:* 1113–1121, 1973.

42. Rubenstein, A. H., Pottienger, L. A., Mako, M., et al: The metabolism of proinsulin and insulin by the liver. *J Clin Invest 51:* 912–921, 1972.

43. Block, M. B., Mako, M. E., Steiner, D. F., et al: Circulating C-peptide immunoreactivity. Studies in normals and diabetes patients. *Diabetes 21:* 1013–1026, 1972.

44. Block, M. B., Rosenfield, R. L., Mako, M. E., et al: Sequential changes in beta-cell function in insulin-treated diabetic patients assessed by C-peptide immunoreactivity. *N Engl J Med 288:* 1144–1148, 1973.

45. Reynolds, C., Molnar, G. D., Horwitz, D. L., et al: Abnormalities of endogenous glucagon and insulin in unstable diabetes. *Diabetes 26:* 36–45, 1977.

46. Kuzuya, T., Matsuda, A., Saito, T., et al: Human C-peptide immunoreactivity (CPR) in blood and urine: Evaluation of a radioimmunoassay method and its clinical applications. *Diabetologia 12:* 511–518, 1976.

47. Horwitz, D. L., Rubenstein, A. H., Katz, A. I.: Quantitation of human pancreatic beta-cell function by immunoassay of C-peptide in urine. *Diabetes 26:* 30–35, 1977.

78

Glucagon: Secretion, Transport, Metabolism, Physiologic Regulation of Secretion, and Derangements in Diabetes

Roger H. Unger

Lelio Orci

INTRODUCTION

Cytochemical differences between cells of the islets of Langerhans were first observed by Lane in 1907,[1] 15 years before the isolation of insulin[2] and glucagon,[3] and the terms α *cell* and β *cell* were first introduced. Lane was led to the conviction that the islet cells produced a "twofold substance," which, "when poured into the blood stream, has an effect on metabolism," a notion that now seems quite remarkable. Indeed, a reasonable interpretation of the ensuing seven decades of research is that the α cells and β cells (Fig. 78-1A) function as a coupled bihormonal secretory unit releasing appropriate mixtures of insulin and glucagon, not only to regulate moment-to-moment glucose flux with but minimal change in extracellular glucose concentration, but also to guide metabolic events toward anabolism or catabolism in accordance with need.[4] Under the primary and dominant control of ambient glucose concentration, this bicellular couple is also influenced by other nutrients, several stimulating or suppressing hormones, and neural and neuroendocrine signals.

SPECIAL ANATOMIC–FUNCTIONAL CONSIDERATIONS OF THE α–β CELL UNIT

The juxtaposed α and β cells enjoy an anatomic intimacy that may well be unique among heterogeneous endocrine tissues. Two types of membrane specializations, tight junctions (Fig. 78-2), points of fusion between the outer leaflets of the adjacent plasma membranes, and gap junctions (Figs. 78-2 and 78-3), low-resistance pathways permitting electrical and metabolic coupling of adjacent cells,[5] have recently been identified in the pancreatic islets[6–8] (Figs. 78-2–78-4). Although the exact function of both junctions in the islets of Langerhans is unknown, their presence has generated considerable speculation.

It is believed that tight junctions are not fixed components of an anatomically stable membrane, but rather are undergoing constant change as part of a process of continuous "remodeling" of the plasma membrane. Under certain circumstances, they may proliferate into a extensive network capable of "trapping" large quantities of secretory products[9] such as insulin within an area enclosed by the tight junction (Fig. 78-5); this evidence of hormone "trapping" raises the possibility that tight junctions may serve to compartmentalize the intercellular space between the islet cells, providing channels through which secretory products may reach the extracellular space without directly contacting specific sites in the surrounding cells. Conversely, tight junctional networks may be envisioned as delimiting certain areas of the cell membrane which could be isolated from, or specifically exposed to, certain external influences, such as high local concentrations of hormones released from adjacent cells.[10]

As far as gap junctions are concerned, if, as has been shown for certain other tissues,[5] these sites of intercellular communication between α and β cells permit molecules of under 500 mol wt to pass from one cell to another without entering the intercellular space, they may constitute important functional equipment. The remarkable secretory coordination of the α–β cell unit, which provides precisely the appropriate mixture of counterbalancing

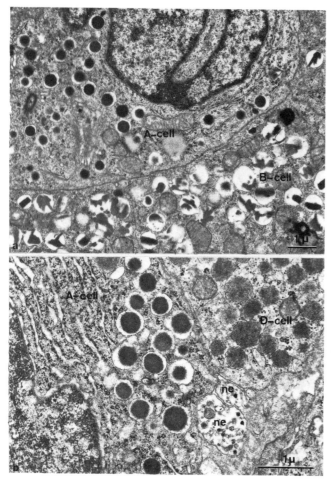

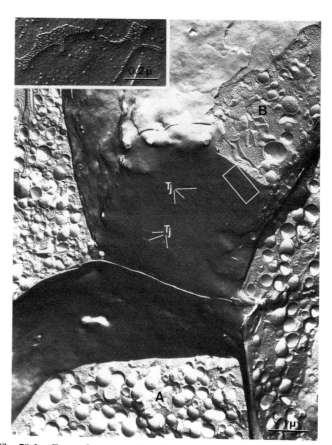

Fig. 78-1. Dog pancreatic islet. A. One sees the striking differences between the secretory granules of a glucagon-producing cell (α cell) and an insulin-producing cell (β cell). $\times$ 11,000. B. Nerve terminals are seen in close relationship with an α cell and a D cell. $\times$ 22,000.

Fig. 78-3. Freeze-fracture replica of an islet isolated from sulphonylurea-treated rat. The fracture process has split the plasma membranes of two adjacent cells: one (B) appears poorly granulated and is tentatively identified as a β cell, the other (A) is well granulated and is tentatively identified as an α cell.[7] The short fibrils (TJ) represent elements of a poorly developed tight junction. $\times$ 17,000. In the area outlined by the rectangle and seen at higher magnification in the inset, one sees aggregates of particles characteristic of gap junctions. $\times$ 79,000. (See also Fig. 78-4.)

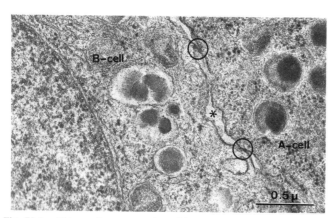

Fig. 78-2. Thin-section preparation of human islet. The field shows the intercellular space (asterisk) between an insulin-producing cell (β cell) and a glucagon-producing cell (α cell). The intercellular space is narrowed at the points in which the two cell membranes come into very close proximity. These regions may be the site of intercellular junctions of the tight or gap type. Because of the small area involved in a tight or gap junction (see Fig. 78-3), their exact nature cannot be clearly determined with this technique. $\times$ 46,000.

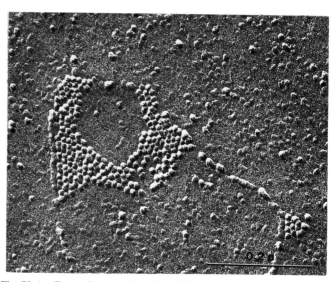

Fig. 78-4. Freeze-fracture of rat islet. This portion of the exposed face of an islet cell membrane shows aggregates of globular subunits or particles characteristic of gap junctions. Gap junctions are considered as specialized areas of cell membranes implicated in cell-to-cell transfer of ions and in cell-to-cell transfer of cellular metabolites (intercellular coupling).[5] $\times$ 201,000.

hormones, could well require an internal communication system. One can thus imagine the islets functioning as a synctium in which the net hormonal output is maintained through cell-to-cell communication, but in which individual cells secrete asynchronously.[7]

In considering morphologic features of α–β cell unit in such general terms, one should be aware of two recent developments which may prove to have important functional implications. The first of these concerns the identification of extrapancreatic α cells in the upper gastrointestinal tract of the dog (Fig. 78-6)[11–14] and man,[15] and the second, the demonstration by immunofluorescence[16–18] of somatostatin-containing cells (D cells) in the islets and in the gastrointestinal tract (Fig. 78-7).

GENERAL FUNCTIONAL CONCEPTS OF THE α–β CELL UNIT

As will be emphasized subsequently, the α and β cells are exquisitely perceptive glucose sensors. Although they also perceive and respond to changes in the concentration of other substrates and certain hormones, their responses to substances other than glucose is influenced most profoundly by the ambient concentration of glucose and by the antecedent carbohydrate intake. It is

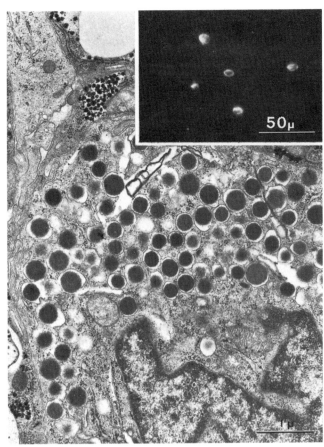

Fig. 78-6. Cell in the dog fundic mucosa resembling the pancreatic α cell (compare with Fig. 78-1). $\times$ 28,000. Inset: Indirect immunofluorescence technique showing fluorescent cells to antiglucagon (30K) in the dog fundic mucosa. $\times$ 450.

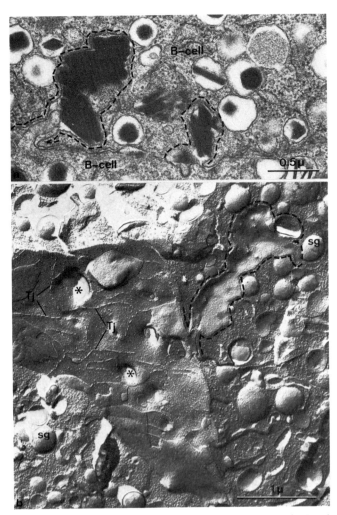

Fig. 78-5. A. Rat isolated islet treated with pronase (4 μg/ml) for 90 min, then exposed to a high glucose concentration (3.0 mg/ml) for 90 min. Large masses of electron-dense material (delineated by the dotted lines) are seen within the intercellular space between two β cells. These masses are formed by the coalescence of extruded granule cores. $\times$ 41,000. B. Replica of freeze-fractured islet treated as in A. The fracture plane has passed through two adjacent cells, revealing the cytoplasm containing secretory granules (SG) and exposing the cell membrane faces. Numerous fibrils (TJ) are disposed to form a well-developed tight junction network. Within this network, several concavities (two of which are labeled with the asterisks) are seen. These deformations are considered to represent the impresses of the extracellular accumulations of secretory product (see A). The membrane (delineated by dotted lines) is in continuity with the cell membrane and extends in the cytoplasm. It is possibly the result of the fusion of the membranes of several granules whose cores have been discharged in series through a single aperture in the cell membrane. $\times$ 31,000.

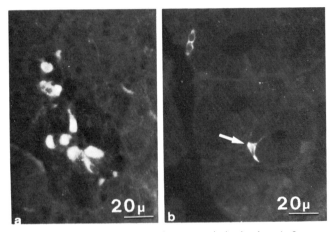

Fig. 78-7. Fluorescent cells to antisomatostatin in the dog. A. In a pancreatic islet. B. In the antral region of the stomach. $\times$500.

therefore reasonable to regard the regulation of glucose homeostasis as the overriding short-term functional concern of these cells.

A glucose-sensitive bihormonal system, which responds to glycemic change by reciprocal alterations in the output of two counterbalancing glucoregulatory hormones, must be assumed to subserve an important glucoregulatory function. Secretion of insulin facilitates the efflux of glucose from the extracellular space into insulin-responsive cells of the liver, muscle, and fat, while glucagon promotes glucose influx from hepatocytes into the extracellular space. Given these now well-established facts, it would appear that the important benefit of "push–pull" regulation of glucose flux by the α–β cell unit is to bring about or allow major changes in glucose flux without major perturbations of glucose concentration.[18] A prolonged fast will normally cause only a modest decline in glucose concentration because of a reduction in insulin, the regulator of glucose efflux from the extracellular space, and a modest increase in glucagon, the regulator of glucose influx. Thus, nonessential glucose utilization is reduced and hepatic glucose production is raised to meet essential glucose needs, i.e., the needs of the glucose-dependent central nervous system, at first largely through glycogenolysis but then via gluconeogenesis, until ketogenesis is sufficient to meet its fuel needs. At the other extreme, during vigorous exercise, glucose utilization by exercising muscle increases markedly. However, an equally marked increase in glucose influx from the liver,[19] mediated in large part by a fivefold increase in glucagon concentration,[20–22] together with diminished insulin secretion reducing glucose efflux into tissues such as fat and liver, maintains normoglycemia, an example of high glucose turnover without much change in glucose concentration. Finally, during the ingestion of carbohydrate, a marked increase in secretion of insulin minimizes hyperglycemia by accelerating the efflux of exogenous glucose, while the associated suppression of glucagon abolishes endogenous glucose production by the liver.[23] These relationships are schematized in Figure 78-8.

A second function of the bihormonal α–β unit is to permit appropriate regulation of the homeostasis of nutrients other than glucose by allowing increases in insulin secretion without danger of concomitant hypoglycemia. For example, the ingestion of protein requires an increase in insulin secretion for the incorporation of the amino acids into new protein.[24] The aminogenic insulin secretion required for this purpose would result in hypoglycemia were it not accompanied by an increase in glucagon secretion, which returns to the extracellular space precisely as much glucose as leaves the extracellular space as a consequence of the increased insulin levels.[25] Thus, as demonstrated by Cherrington and Vranic,[26] glucose turnover increases without changing glucose concentration. Similarly, this bihormonal system makes possible inhibition of lipolysis by insulin without a fall in glucose concentration.

IMMUNOREACTIVE GLUCAGON (IRG) OF TISSUE AND PLASMA GLUCAGON

Gel filtration of acid alcohol extracts of pancreatic tissue obtained from dogs, hog, beef, and man have disclosed two major peaks of immunoreactivity.[27] Approximately 95 percent of the immunoreactivity elutes with the glucagon marker and exhibits the same biologic activity as crystalline pancreatic glucagon. About 5 percent of the immunoreactivity in such extracts has a molecular weight in excess of 9000 and is devoid of biologic activity (Fig. 78-9). Mild tryptic digestion gives rise to an immunoreactive moiety slightly smaller than glucagon and lacking glucagon's biologic

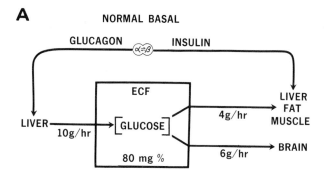

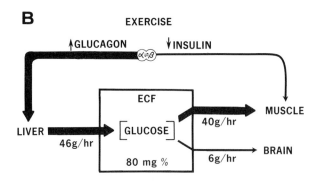

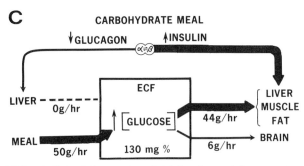

Fig. 78-8. A. Role of glucagon in maintaining glucose influx at a rate equal to glucose efflux into insulin-independent tissues, chiefly the brain, and insulin-dependent tissues such as liver, muscle, and fat, so as to maintain extracellular fluid (ECF) glucose concentration above a hypoglycemic range, thus providing for adequate cerebral glucose delivery. B. Role of glucagon in maintaining glucose influx equal to markedly increased glucose efflux into exercising muscle so as to maintain ECF glucose concentration above a hypoglycemic range and maintain cerebral glucose delivery. C. Role of insulin in increasing glucose efflux during the rapid influx of ingested glucose so as to prevent an abnormal rise in ECF glucose. Reduced glucagon secretion may facilitate this by helping to turn off hepatic glucose production. (From Unger: *Diabetes 25:* 136, 1976.)

activity.[27] This large glucagon immunoreactivity is now believed to represent proglucagon.[28,29]

Gel filtration of plasma also reveals both these fractions to be present, although in varying proportions.[30,31] The glucagon-sized plasma fraction changes promptly during stimulation and suppression. The proglucagon-sized moiety also changes during such acute maneuvers.[32] but generally to a lesser degree (Fig. 78-10). On the basis of animal studies, the proglucagon-sized IRG is estimated to have a disappearance time approximately five times that of true glucagon.[33] During chronic sustained hyperglucagonemia, as in phloridzin hypoglycemia or in uncontrolled diabetes, the proglucagon-sized fraction as well as glucagon levels are increased.[32]

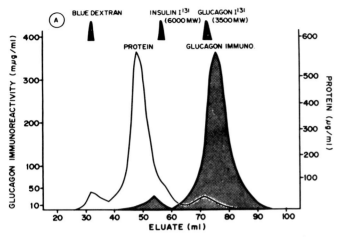

Fig. 78-9. Elution pattern of glucagon immunoreactivity in canine pancreatic extracts, showing an early appearing peak with a molecular weight greater than that of the insulin marker. It is considered to represent proglucagon. (From Rigopaulou et al. *J. Biol. Chem.* 245: 496, 1970).

Gel filtration studies also reveal the presence of a globulin-sized fraction in plasma.[31] This has been detected with antisera considered to be the most highly specific for pancreatic glucagon and has been referred to in the literature as *big plasma glucagon* (BPG). This is probably responsible for nonspecific interference attributed in the past to plasma globulin[34] and more recently

referred to as *interfering factor*.[35] When it is subjected to tryptic hydrolysis, an increase in glucagon immunoreactivity of a smaller molecular size is generated.[31] Inasmuch as it has been identified in aqueous extracts of isolated islets, it could represent a primitive precursor of glucagon, but it is widely regarded as glucagon bound to a large protein. Its presence to a variable degree in human plasma introduces a potential source of error in the glucagon assay when used for comparison of steady-state levels in groups,[35] prompting some workers to remove it by extraction[36] or to correct for it by other maneuvers.[35] However, its concentration appears to be extremely constant, at least over a short period of time, so that it is not a problem in experiments in which acute changes in plasma glucagon are measured.

In addition to BPG, proglucagon, and glucagon, there is a fourth immunoreactive peak of IRG of smaller molecular size than glucagon[31] and it is regarded as a derivative (Fig. 78-10). In the interest of nomenclatural simplicity, the four IRG fractions have been designated as *BPG* or $IRG^{150,000}$, *proglucagon*, or IRG^{9000} *glucagon*, and IRG^{2000}.

The same four fractions have been observed in the plasma of totally depancreatized dogs[32] (Fig. 78-11). Inasmuch as acid alcohol extracts of the canine stomach contain the same two immunoreactive fractions observed in pancreatic extracts,[14] it is likely that this represents gastrointestinal true glucagon. Indeed, studies of partially purified extracts of porcine duodenum reveal a polypeptide that is identical to purified beef or pork glucagon with respect to its immunometric properties, its isoelectric point, its affinity for

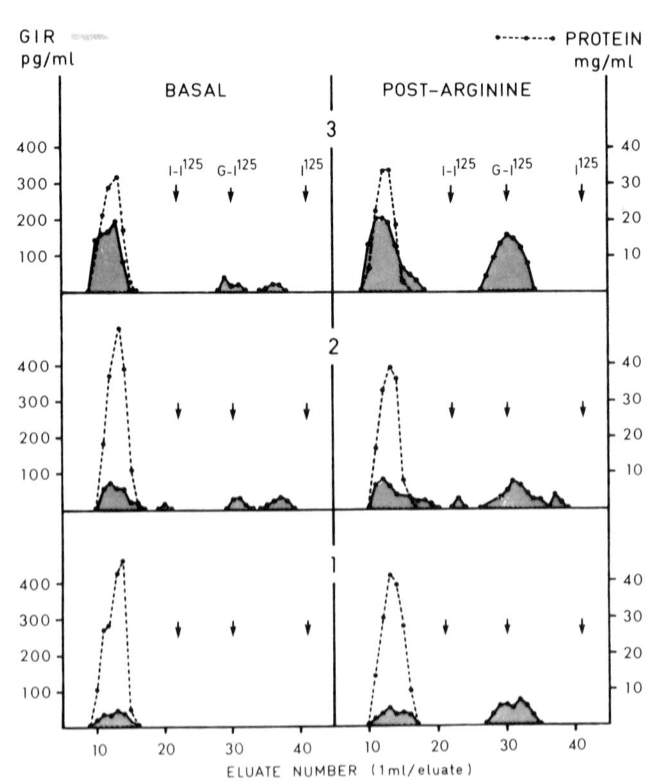

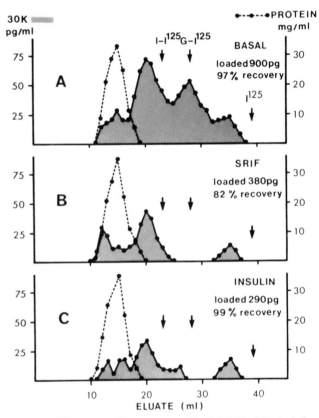

Fig. 78-10. Chromatographic pattern on Bio Gel P-30 of plasma obtained from three normal subjects in the basal state and after arginine stimulation of the α cell. The arrows indicate the elution volume of the radioactive markers [^{125}I-insulin (I-I^{125}) ^{125}I-glucagon (G-I^{125})]. The shaded area represents the glucagon immunoreactivity (GIR) and the broken line the protein content of the eluates. (From Valverde et al.: J. Clin. Endocrinol. Metab. *39:* 1092).

Fig. 78-11. Chromatographic pattern on Bio Gel P-10 of 4 ml of plasma from a depancreatized dog in the basal state and during somatostatin or insulin infusion. The shaded area represents the glucagon immunoreactivity and the broken line the protein content of the eluates. The arrows indicate the elution volume of the radioactive markers [^{125}I-insulin (I-I^{125}), ^{125}I-glucagon (G-I^{125})]. (From Valverde et al.: Metabolism *24:* 1021).

rat liver plasma membranes, and its adenylate cyclase–stimulating activity[14] (Table 78-1), and immunocytochemical studies at both light and electron microscopic levels reveal the presence of true α cells in the oxyntic tissue of the dog stomach[11-14] (Fig. 78-3).

GLUCAGON METABOLISM

GLUCAGON SECRETION

Glucagon is secreted by the α cells into the intercellular space. There is no clear evidence that glucagon in the plasma is bound to a plasma protein, although this possibility has been considered to explain the globulin-sized BPG, which could be a globulin with multiple glucagons attached to it, rather than a glucagon precursor.

Plasma contains glucagon-degrading substances, first noted by Mirsky et al.[37] Human and rat plasma are particularly glucagonolytic. Just how much circulating glucagon is degraded in the circulation is unknown. The disappearance of true glucagon from the circulation is rapid. When injected into the peripheral venous circulation crystalline glucagon has a half-time of disappearance of approximately 6 min,[38] slightly less than earlier estimates made with radioiodinated glucagon preparations. However, measurements of endogenous IRG in which the immunoreactive components were separated by chromatography in the plasma of a hyperglucagonemic phloridzinized dog have been made by Valverde et al: they estimate that the disappearance time of the true glucagon is about 3 min, while that of proglucagon-sized IRG is approximately 16 min.[33] Although not measured, the disappearance time of BPG must be considerably longer.

Glucagon in the portal blood has been estimated to range from 300 to 5000 pg/ml, entirely compatible with physiologic binding to hepatic receptors estimated by Rodbell et al. to have a K_m of 4.5×10^{-9}.[39] In anesthetized patients undergoing laparotomy, a basal concentration of about 160 pg/ml was measured in the portal blood with antiserum 30K, at a time when peripheral venous glucagon levels averaged 100 pg/ml.[40] With arginine stimulation glucagon rose above 1000 pg/ml in the portal vein before a change in peripheral venous glucagon was noted. Hepatic clearance of glucagon has not been as carefully studied as that of insulin. Hepatic clearance of insulin appears to increase in absolute terms with concentration, although the percent of the perfused insulin removed by the liver declines as the concentration rises. In the case of glucagon, however, the available data, sparse though it is, suggests a constant percentage of removal that is not altered by a rising concentration, at least within the range studied.

Once bound to the glucagon receptor, glucagon activates adenylate cyclase through mechanisms described in detail in Chapter 153, and presumably through the second messenger, cAMP, exerts its various hepatic effects. Glucagon-binding proteins of high ($K_A = 8.7 \times 10^9$/M) and low affinity have been partially purified from rat liver plasma membranes and been found to have a molecular weight of about 190,000.[41] They also bind ^{125}I-insulin (a fact which is teleologically provoking) but not ^{125}I-ACTH.

The portoperipheral venous plasma glucagon gradient varies, being minimal during suppression of secretion and increasing markedly immediately after secretory stimulation. Clearly, it is possible for glucagon to increase in the portal blood without a perceptible change in the peripheral plasma. The endoportal infusion of 30 ng/min in a conscious dog for 30 min can increase peripheral venous glucose levels without changing peripheral venous glucagon.

GLUCAGON REMOVAL

The glucagon molecule is largely destroyed by the liver and kidney. In the liver cell, the site of glucagon degradation is believed to be separate from the glucagon receptor.[41] A glucagon-degrading enzyme system has been purified from hepatic glutathione-insulin-transhydrogenase, and the site of cleavage with detachment of His-Ser-Glu-NH from the terminal fragment has been defined by Kakiuchi and Tomizawa.[42] More recently, however, Duckworth and Kitabchi[43] report that the so-called "insulin-specific protease" appears to be a glucagon-degrading enzyme, although their studies were done in muscle tissue rather than liver.

The kidneys are the major posthepatic site of glucagon clearance. In the presence of severe renal failure or bilateral nephrectomy, the disappearance curve of intravenously injected crystalline glucagon is markedly prolonged, as is the hyperglycemic action of the hormone. Lefebvre and Luyckx have shown that ligation of the renal vessels in dogs is accompanied by a prompt increase in plasma glucagon, entirely attributable to reduced clearance by the kidney.[44] It is believed that, under normal circumstances, glucagon is filtered by the glomerulus and reabsorbed by the proximal tubules, where it undergoes intrarenal degradation.

Glucagon is recovered in the bile following its intravenous injection in the rabbit and in man. Moreover, stimulation of endogenous glucagon secretion by pancreozymin or arginine is followed by a quick increase in biliary glucagon excretion and glucose infusion inhibits this. Approximately 0.5 mg/day is said to be excreted in the bile and biliary excretion is believed by Assan to reflect physiologic secretion by α cells.[38]

SECRETORY MECHANISMS OF THE α CELL

Although the molecular and morphologic events governing glucagon secretion have not as yet been as extensively studied as the secretion of insulin, exocytotic extrusion of secretory granules from the α cells into the extracellular space has been observed (Fig. 78-12).

FACTORS MODIFYING GLUCAGON SECRETION

Glucagon is a powerful glycogenolytic and gluconeogenic hormone (Chapter 79). As such, it is teleologically reasonable to regard its primary role as that of regulator of net hepatic glucose production for the purpose of maintaining adequate delivery of glucose to vital tissues such as the central nervous system, for which glucose serves as a primary fuel. The ability of the α cell to sense and respond to minor fluctuations in glucose concentration will determine the rate of glucose influx into the extracellular space. The normal α cell, like the normal β cell, is under the obligatory influence of the arterial glucose concentration. Although

Table 78-1. Comparison of Gastrointestinal Glucagon, Glucagon-like Immunoreactivity (GLI) and Pancreatic Glucagon

	Pancreatic Glucagon	GI Glucagon	GLI
Mol wt	3485	3500	2900
Isoelectric point	6.2	6.2	>10
Ratio 78J/30K	1.0	0.9	61
Glycogenolytic activity (% of 10 μg of glucagon)	100	100	50
70% of maximum adenylate cyclase stimulation M	10^{-8}	10^{-8}	10^{-7}
Affinity for rat liver membranes	4×10^{-9}	3×10^{-9}	5×10^{-8}

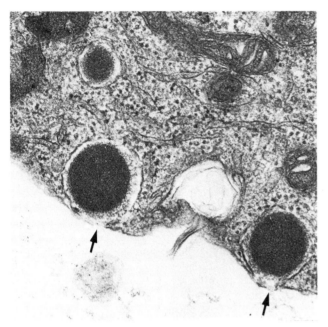

Fig. 78-12. Field from an α cell of rat pancreatic islet stimulated with arginine. The arrows point to two stages of exocytotic events of α granules. $\times$ 42,000.

the rates of insulin and glucagon secretion are influenced by many diverse factors, to be mentioned below, such influences normally will not prevail under circumstances in which either hypoglycemia or hyperglycemia would result. For example, insulin secretion does not respond to stimuli other than glucose during starvation[45] and glucagon is not stimulated during a glucose load.[46]

The primary dedication of the α and β cells to glycemic control enables the normal individual to maintain a glucose concentration within an extremely narrow range despite the extreme changes in availability of exogenous glucose and in the need for glucose.

BASAL GLUCAGON SECRETION

After an overnight fast, in normal individuals, the glucagon level is reported to average 75 pg/ml, depending on the antiserum and method of radioimmunoassay employed. Probably the level of true glucagon after substraction of nonglucagon IRG averages 25 pg/ml and ranges from 5 to 80 pg/ml. The function of the basal level of glucagon secretion is to maintain hepatic glucose production at a rate equal to glucose utilization, which in the basal state is largely confined to the central nervous system. The rarity of fasting hypoglycemia in normal individuals provides evidence of its remarkable effectiveness in this respect; if glucagon secretion is suppressed by infusing somatostatin, plasma glucose declines promptly.[47,48] This decline is believed to result from reduced glucagon-mediated hepatic glucose production in the face of continuing central nervous system glucose utilization.[49]

During total starvation[45] or carbohydrate restriction,[50] normal individuals exhibit a gradual rise in plasma glucagon, which, at approximately 48 hours, averages between 50 and 100 percent of the overnight fasting level. The rise in glucagon is accompanied by a decline in insulin, the insulin–glucagon molar ratio dropping to 0.4, a hormonal mixture which would maximize hepatic glucose production by means of increased glycogenolysis and, when glycogen stores are depleted, through increased gluconeogenesis. The metabolic extravagance, in terms of nitrogen wastage, of a high rate of gluconeogenesis is gradually reduced as plasma ketones rise

to provide an alternative energy source for the central nervous system, and then glucose turnover diminishes as glucagon levels decline. The resulting reduction in gluconeogenesis conserves nitrogen and, thus, increases the capacity to endure prolonged starvation.[51] There is now mounting evidence that glucagon plays an important and perhaps essential role in converting the liver into a ketogenic organ.[52–54]

Thus, the α cells, as well as the β cells, appear to play a central role in the response to both carbohydrate deprivation or total starvation. The decline in the insulin–glucagon molar ratio, from approximately 3.0 after an overnight fast to 0.4 after 48 hours of starvation, may be essential for the maintenance of euglycemia and for the development of alternative energy sources such as increased levels of FFA and ketones. The decline in insulin that increases lipolysis is limited by ketone-stimulated insulin secretion so that severe ketoacidosis can be avoided;[55] if, as proposed by McGarry et al.,[52] glucagon is necessary for hepatic conversion of FFA to ketones, then another example of bihormonal cooperation in regulation of nutrient flux is provided (Chapter 80).

RESPONSE TO HYPOGLYCEMIA

The function of the α cell is to prevent hypoglycemia. In normal individuals, hypoglycemia virtually never occurs, even after prolonged starvation or violent exercise, a testimony to the effectiveness of the hormonal safeguards.

Experimentally induced hypoglycemia is by its very nature an unphysiologic maneuver which has overwhelmed the elaborate defense system. Insulin-induced hypoglycemia is accompanied by a rapid rise in plasma glucagon, lasting for more than 60 minutes. However, despite continued profound hypoglycemia, glucagon levels return toward normal thereafter. The magnitude and the duration of the glucagon response to insulin-induced hypoglycemia is in sharp contrast with the glucagon response to hypoglycemia produced by means other than insulin, in all of which insulin levels are markedly reduced. In phloridzin-induced hypoglycemia, for example, even though glucose levels are higher than in insulin-induced hypoglycemia, the glucagon response far exceeds that of insulin-induced hypoglycemia, both in magnitude and in duration. Hyperglucagonemia in excess of 600 pg/ml can continue for many days.[56] In alcohol-induced hypoglycemia, in which insulin is also reduced, hyperglucagonemia is striking.[57] Finally, in hypoglycemia resulting from adrenal insufficiency, marked hyperglucagonemia is also observed.[58] It would appear that when hypoglycemia is accompanied by a low level of insulin, α cell secretion rises dramatically. When the insulin level is high, the hyperglucagonemia is less marked and more transient. In insulinoma patients, for example, elevated plasma levels of glucagon are uncommon. The infusion of insulin in dogs with phloridzin-induced hypoglycemia reduces the hyperglucagonemia.[59] These observations are of possible clinical importance. They suggest that the hypoglycemia observed in insulinoma patients may be in part the result of inadequate α cell sensing or response to the glucose concentration. Second, in insulin-treated diabetes the α cell may similarly be incapable of responding to hypoglycemia,[60] an irony in a disease in which the α cell appears to hyperrespond unnecessarily and probably deleteriously to other stimuli.

The mechanism by which insulin obtunds the α cell response to hypoglycemia is uncertain. There is evidence that insulin directly inhibits glucagon secretion by the α cell.[61] Alternatively, the effect of insulin could be to control glucose entry into the α cell, glucose in turn determining the rate of glucagon secretion. There is considerable evidence that, in the absence of insulin, glucose, at least in the intact alloxan-diabetic animal, does not suppress gluca-gon release and, if anything, tends to increase paradoxically the secretion of glucagon,[62] small quantities of insulin administered under these conditions cause an immediate precipitous fall in plasma glucagon, as if it were necessary to activate the glucose sensor or to permit the penetration of glucose into the α cell. Edwards and Taylor have provided evidence that the turning off of glucagon secretion is an energy-requiring process,[63] and it is there-fore possible that in the absence of insulin glucose penetration is insufficient to prevent glucagon secretion; agents which interfere with glucose metabolism, such as 2-deoxyglucose and mannuhep-tulose, cause increased glucagon secretion despite concomitant hyperglycemia.[64]

Thus, the mechanism involved in the glucose sensing and/or glucagon suppression may be a complex one, perhaps involving both a direct action of insulin on the α cell and an indirect action of insulin, permitting glucose entry into the cell to provide the neces-sary energy source.

THE α CELL RESPONSE TO NUTRIENTS

Carbohydrate Feeding

During a carbohydrate meal, an oral glucose tolerance test, or an intravenous infusion of glucose, plasma insulin levels increase and glucagon levels decline, so the molar ratio of insulin to gluca-gon rises (Fig. 78-13). The liver is thereby converted from a glucose-producing[65] organ to a glucose-storing organ. The decline in glucagon would, by itself, reduce net hepatic glucose production without a rise in insulin,[48,66] but in the circumstance of carbohy-drate loading, the rise in insulin secretion is by far the most important component of the islet cell response. Not only is glucose efflux from the extracellular space into the liver, muscle, and fat cells increased, but, at least when glucagon levels are low, insulin further inhibits hepatic glucose production directly.[66,67-69]

There is suggestive evidence that signals arising from the

GLUCAGON RESPONSE TO A CARBOHYDRATE MEAL IN 11 NORMAL SUBJECTS

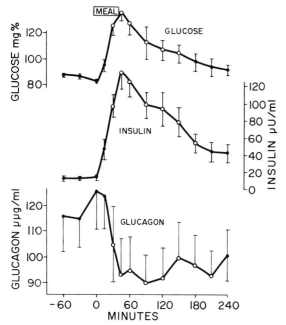

Fig. 78-13. Effect of a large carbohydrate meal on plasma insulin and glucagon in normal subjects. (From Müller et al. *N. Eng. J. Med. 283:* 109, 1970.)

gastrointestinal tract during the absorption of glucose provide for earlier and greater glucagon suppression than can be accounted for by the rise in arterial glucose concentration,[70] much as is believed to occur in the case of stimulation of the β cell by oral glucose. Although secretin and somatostatin are the only known hormones with glucagon-suppressing activity and both are present in the gastrointestinal tract, the nature of the glucagon-suppressing enter-oinsulinar signal to the α cell is as yet unidentified. Moreover, there is evidence that glucose absorption may cause the release of a glucagon-stimulating polypeptide hormone (GIP),[71] so that the net enteroinsular signal could be the summation of opposing influ-ences.

Protein Meal

The ingestion of a carbohydrate-free protein meal, such as ground beef, casein, amino acid mixtures, or casein hydrolysate, elicits a prompt and substantial increase in plasma glucagon. A carbohydrate-free meal is a form of glucose need, inasmuch as an anabolic disposition of the ingested amino acids into protein bio-synthesis requires that insulin be secreted, thereby enhancing glucose efflux from the extracellular space. There being no dietary source of glucose at that time, only by increasing hepatic glucose production can hypoglycemia be prevented.[72] The secretion of an appropriate quantity of glucagon increases hepatic glucose produc-tion sufficiently to maintain euglycemia despite the increased glu-cose efflux, an example of increased glucose turnover, which, during arginine infusion rises 70 percent[73] without a change of glucose concentration. If one suppresses glucagon during an influx of a glucogenic amino acid such as alanine, plasma glucose falls even in the absence of insulin secretion.

When a protein meal is ingested with an equal amount of glucose, there is no need for glucagon secretion and, indeed, the glucagon response is reduced during the hyperglycemic period and the insulin response is exaggerated, resulting in a considerably higher insulin–glucagon ratio (Fig. 78-14). The effect of a more rapid concomitant influx of exogenous glucose in suppressing the glucagon response and potentiating the insulin response to a pro-tein meal is even more dramatic; when a steak meal is ingested during an intravenous glucose influsion, the mean insulin–gluca-gon ratio rises to 400. It is believed that at such high insulin–glucagon ratios a much greater share of the ingested amino acids is captured for anabolic purposes. This probably explains the well-known protein-sparing effect of glucose and the efficacy of hyper-alimentation regimes in certain patients.

Conversely, during starvation or carbohydrate deprivation, the α–β cell response to protein ingestion or to arginine infusion is reversed. Basal glucagon levels are elevated and they rise to higher levels during the protein meal (Fig. 78-15); at such times, basal insulin values are low and exhibit little or no change in response to the protein. The insulin–glucagon ratio consequently remains in the low catabolic basal range or declines even further, preempting a larger share of the ingested amino acids for gluconeogenesis at the expense of protein biosynthesis; indeed, in the carbohydrate-deprived state, a steak meal or an alanine infusion is accompanied by a rise in plasma glucose (Fig. 78-15). It is thus clear that not only the concurrent availability of exogenous carbohydrate but also the antecedent availability of glucose exerts an extraordinary qualita-tive as well as quantitative influence upon the α cell and β cell responses to nonglucose nutrients, through which their own meta-bolic disposition may be mediated appropriately.

As in the case of glucose, it is believed that the absorption of amino acids is accompanied by the release of a signal or signals to the islets of Langerhans which result in early secretion of insulin

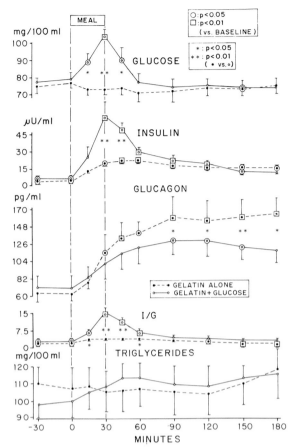

Fig. 78-14. Comparison of the effect of a protein meal ingested alone or with an equal amount of glucose upon insulin, glucagon, and insulin–glucagon ratio (I/G) in normal subjects. Glucose and triglycerides are also shown. (From Fujita et al. *Diabetes 24:* 552, 1975.)

and glucagon prior to the increase in arterial α-amino nitrogen levels. Although the signal has not as yet been identified, it is well established that many of the gastrointestinal hormones released following the ingestion of a protein meal, such as gastrin, pancreo-

zymin-cholecystokinin, and GIP, have insulin-stimulating properties.[71,74,75] In addition, the administration of atropine reduces the glucagon response to a protein meal, suggesting that at some level, cholinergic signals are involved.[76]

Fat Meal

In man, the ingestion of a meal consisting entirely of fat seldom if ever occurs, and the effect of a pure long-chain triglyceride load on the secretion of islet cell hormones has only rarely been tested.[77–79] Orally ingested peanut oil appears to cause a slight rise in plasma glucagon levels, but the accompanying nausea and feeling of fullness suggests marked inhibition of gastric emptying. When long-chain triglycerides are administered intraduodenally in conscious dogs, a substantial increase in plasma glucagon is observed (Fig. 78-16). The increase in glucagon secretion that accompanies the absorption of long-chain triglycerides is believed to be entirely the result of an enteric signal to the α cells.[79] Chyle, collected from dogs with thoracic fistula following an intraduodenal fat meal, does not increase plasma glucagon when it is infused intravenously into other dogs; however, glucagon does rise in the plasma of fat-fed dogs with a thoracic duct fistula even though the absorbed triglycerides have been excluded from the circulation.[79] The enteric signal to the α cell released during fat absorption has not been identified; however, inasmuch as both pancreozymin-cholecystokinin and GIP have glucagon-stimulating activity and both are known to increase during the absorption of fat, they are candidate hormones for this role. Again, cholinergic activity may somehow be involved because of the fact that atropine reduces this response.[76]

As in the case of protein or other nonglucose stimuli of islet cell hormone secretion, glucose availability markedly influences the α cell and β cell responses to fat absorption. As shown in Figure 78-16, an intraduodenal fat meal given during the intravenous administration of glucose completely changes the pattern of response of the islet cell hormones from that which occurs during normoglycemia; fat-induced glucagon secretion is completely abolished by hyperglycemia, while an enormous insulin response, considerably greater than that elicited by intravenous glucose

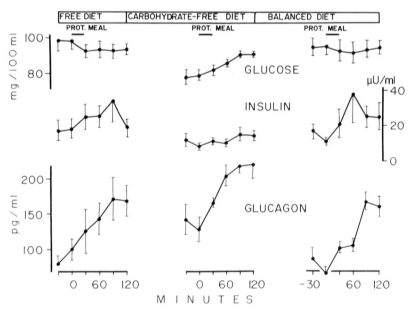

Fig. 78-15. Effect of carbohydrate restriction upon the response of glucose, insulin, and glucagon to a beef meal in normal individuals. During carbohydrate restriction the attenuated insulin response, together with high glucagon levels, is believed to account for the associated rise in plasma glucose levels. (From Müller et al. *N. Eng. J. Med. 285:* 1450, 1971.

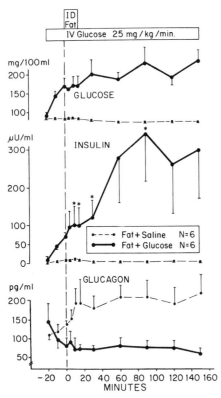

Fig. 78-16. Intraduodenal administration of a fat meal to conscious dogs is accompanied by a rise in glucagon. If the fat meal is administered during the intravenous infusion of glucose, however, the rise in glucagon does not occur; instead a marked increase in insulin, which was not observed in the absence of the glucose infusion, is present. (From Dobbs et al. *Metabolism* 24: 69, 1975.)

alone, is now observed. It is therefore considered likely that the enteric signal or signals released during the absorption of fat must interact with both α cell and β cells, but that glucagon secretion cannot be stimulated during hyperglycemia, and insulin secretion cannot be stimulated except in the presence of hyperglycemia.

RELATIONSHIP OF THE ISLETS OF LANGERHANS TO CARBOHYDRATE-INDUCED CHANGES IN TRIGLYCERIDES

It has been postulated that glucagon, a hormone that reduces hepatic very low density lipoprotein (VLDL) secretion, and insulin, one that promotes VLDL secretion, might mediate carbohydrate-induced changes in triglyceride levels.[80] Normal subjects fed a diet low in carbohydrate exhibit a decline in the basal and protein-stimulated insulin levels and an increase in the basal and protein-stimulated glucagon levels.[81] This reduction in the insulin–glucagon ratio is accompanied by a marked decrease in triglycerides. By contrast, a high-carbohydrate diet is associated with high basal and protein-stimulated insulin levels and lowered basal and protein-stimulated glucagon levels. This high insulin–glucagon ratio is accompanied by high plasma triglyceride levels.[81] Although such correlations between insulin–glucagon ratios and triglyceride levels do not necessarily indicate a cause and effect relationship, they are compatible with the thesis that, at least in normal subjects, the effect of carbohydrate intake upon triglyceride levels is mediated by the relative concentrations of insulin and glucagon— perhaps another example of their influence in anabolic–catabolic events.

GLUCAGON RESISTANCE

Glucagon resistance may ultimately be shown to play a role in certain metabolic states that can be characterized as "hyperanabolic" in the sense that biosynthetic processes are accelerated. Eaton et al. have proposed that certain hyperlipidemic disorders may be the result of hepatic glucagon resistance.[82] Recently, it has been demonstrated that enlarged fat-laden adipocytes exhibit a reduced sensitivity to glucagon,[83] resulting from reduced binding of glucagon to the plasma membrane receptors, which suggests that glucagon resistance could be implicated in certain forms of obesity. Physiologic glucagon resistance appears to be present during fetal development, a period when accelerated anabolism is obviously required.[84] Despite the fact that glucagon is present in the fetal circulation in the same concentration as in the adult, the fetal liver accumulates large quantities of glycogen and, obviously, is undergoing rapid DNA synthesis. The failure of fetal glucagon to oppose these anabolic processes is probably the consequence of the fact that glucagon binding to the plasma membrane of fetal hepatocytes is extremely low and the adenylate cyclase response to glucagon is proportionately reduced; by contrast, insulin-binding during fetal life is only slightly below adult levels (Fig. 78-17). Fetal hepatocytes, therefore, seem primed to respond to the anabolic hormone, insulin, but not to the catabolic hormone, glucagon, irrespective of the concentration of glucagon that may be present in the portal blood. In the rat, glucagon binding by hepatocyte membranes reaches the adult level only after the first postnatal month, but, at the time of birth, glucagon binding and adenylate cyclase response have risen to about 60 percent of the adult level, thus allowing for hormonal control of hepatic glucagon production following separation of the newborn from the maternal glucose supply.[84]

EXERCISE

Perhaps no biologic function is as vital to survival as the appropriate distribution of fuels during "fight and flight" situations. In exercising dogs and humans, the normal islet cell response consists of an increase in glucagon and a decline in insulin. In the dog exercised to the point of collapse, plasma glucagon may

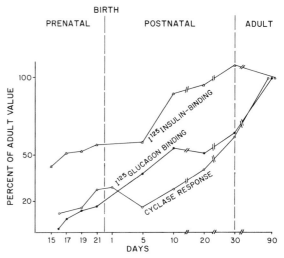

Fig. 78-17. Comparison of the response of adenylate cyclase activity to glucagon and of the binding of ^{125}I-glucagon and ^{125}I-insulin to the isolated hepatocyte membranes of prenatal and postnatal rats expressed as percentage of adult values. Note the low level of glucagon binding and glucagon response during prenatal life.

rise to six times the basal value and the insulin–glucagon ratio may decline below 0.4, the nadir observed during starvation. This hormonal mixture would be expected to increase greatly the rate of hepatic glucose production so as to meet the enormous increase in glucose utilization by muscle without reducing arterial glucose concentration and thereby depriving the brain of sufficient fuel (Fig. 78-18). Again, this bihormonal system makes possible a major increase in glucose turnover while maintaining glucose concentration within the normal range. This islet cell response to strenuous exercise, while always influenced by glucose concentration, is believed to be under adrenergic control and, in rats, adrenergic blocking agents reportedly abolish exercise-induced hyperglucagonemia and hypoinsulinemia.[21,22] If glucose is infused during the exercise, increased hepatic glucose production is rendered unnecessary and the rise in glucagon no longer develops.

The importance of glucagon during exercise is difficult to evaluate. Blockade of glucagon secretion with somatostatin during strenuous treadmill exercise in dogs results in lower glucose concentrations than in hyperglucagonemic dogs and seems to decrease the running time prior to collapse; but severe hypoglycemia does not occur, presumably because the high levels of circulating levels of catecholamines and direct sympathetic innervation of the liver result in sufficient glucose production to meet the glucose needs.

STRESS

"Acute stress" is defined as a sudden event that poses an actual or potential threat to life or well-being, or is so perceived by the organism. When the stress is the result of actual injury, be it traumatic, thermal, ischemic, or inflammatory, it is accompanied by a resetting of the glucose concentration to higher levels. This is

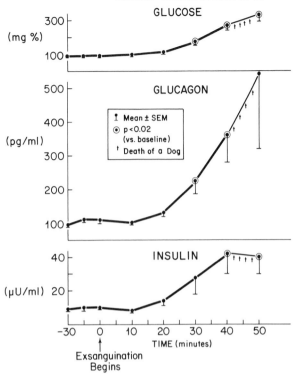

Fig. 78-19. Effect of exsanguination on plasma glucagon, insulin, and glucose levels in conscious dogs. (From Lindsey et al. *Diabetes 24:* 313, 1975.)

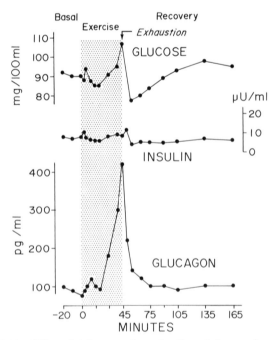

Fig. 78-18. Effect of violent exercise on insulin and glucagon levels in the dog. Stippled area represents the period of treadmill exercise to the point of collapse. Plasma glucose levels are maintained, presumably in large part because of the rise in glucagon accompanied by an increase in insulin despite the marked efflux of glucose into exercising muscle. (From Unger, R. H., and Lefebvre, P. J. Glucagon Physiology. In Glucagon Molecular Physiology, Clinical and Therapeutic Implications. Edited by P. J. Lefebvre and R. H. Unger. Amsterdam, Pergamon, 1972, p. 220.)

particularly apparent when shock is present or imminent, whether due to trauma,[85] exsanguination (Fig. 78-19),[86] depletion of extracellular fluid volume, endotoxinemia,[87] or myocardial damage.[88] Teleologically, the high arterial glucose levels observed in these circumstances in nondiabetic subjects constitute the only device whereby glucose delivery to the brain can be maintained in the face of a declining cerebral blood flow. Conditions of severe stress are accompanied by absolute hyperglucagonemia and absolute or relative hypoinsulinemia,[85–91] a bihormonal setting that would increase glucose production and minimize glucose utilization by muscle and fat and thus conserve endogenously produced glucose for the brain. The magnitude of "stress hyperglycemia" seems to vary with the magnitude of the stress and the depths of the accompanying shock. In uncomplicated major surgical procedures, if blood pressure and extracellular fluid volume are well maintained, the hormonal changes are minimal.[85] However, even in relatively mild stress as, for example, in moderately severe infection, glucagon levels are significantly above normal[87] and the insulin response to a glucose load is somewhat attenuated, thus accounting for the impaired glucose tolerance observed in nondiabetics during infection and other forms of organic stress such as acute myocardial infarction. In the diabetic, stress induces at least as much hyperglucagonemia as in the nondiabetic, but the capacity of the β cell to compensate is impaired or lacking; if insulin levels are thus fixed, the hyperglucagonemia precipitated by infection or by other stress will cause metabolic decompensation,[87] a familiar event to clinicians who treat diabetic patients.

While the mechanism of stress hyperglycemia has not been finally elucidated, stimulation of the ventromedial nucleus of the hypothalamus increases glucagon secretion,[92] as does electrical stimulation of the sympathetic nerve to the pancreas.[93] It seems reasonable that afferent impulses to the hypothalamus may initiate neural impulses through fibers crossing through the floor of the fourth ventricle, presumably encountered by Claude Bernard in his classic piqûre experiments, and ultimately signaling the islet cells through sympathetic fibers. In addition, circulating catecholamines clearly influence the islets of Langerhans, stimulating glucagon secretion via beta-adrenergic receptors[94] and inhibiting insulin secretion via alpha-adrenergic receptors.[95] Cortisol increases α cell sensitivity to certain stimuli[96] while enhancing hepatic sensitivity to glucagon.[97] Finally, direct sympathetic influence on the hepatocytes themselves, either via the sympathetic nervous system or circulating catecholamines, may provide a failsafe for glucose production in critical emergency situations.

It is important therapeutically to recognize that stress hyperglycemia may be a compensatory device to provide adequate fuel delivery to the brain, and not an abnormality requiring correction with insulin. In the presence of a volume deficit, efforts to reduce the hyperglycemia, which in nondiabetic subjects seldom exceeds 350 mg/100 ml unless exogenous glucose is being administered, is ill-advised unless hyperosmolality is present. Rather, the therapeutic effort should be directed toward correction of the volume deficit as promptly as possible, in which case the stress hyperglycemia will recede spontaneously. However, when the underlying cause of the stress involves substantial damage to tissue, as in burns, infection, trauma, etc., the low insulin–glucagon ratio may persist long after the volume deficit has been corrected. The possible influence of this alteration in the hormonal setting on the negative nitrogen balance of such disorders will be discussed in more detail in the section on catabolic diseases.

Our understanding of neuroendocrine control of the pancreas is in its infancy (Fig. 78-1B).[97a] It seems likely that the sympathetic nervous system and circulating catecholamines mediate the almost instantaneous decline in the insulin–glucagon ratio that accompanies stress.

Recent observations, which in our present state of ignorance, cannot as yet be organized into any rational control scheme, perhaps deserve passing mention. The human pancreas contains considerable amounts of adrenaline, the release of which is increased in the perfused canine pancreas by hypoglycemia.[98] Cholinergic nerve endings are also abundant in the pancreas and, when stimulated, increase the release of both insulin and glucagon. Atropine appears to inhibit the response of the α cells and β cells to nutrient stimulation; however, the precise role of the cholinergic system in the islet cell response is uncertain. Other substances such as serotonin and somatostatin, recently identified in islet cells, may participate in "turning off" the secretion of these hormones.

DIABETES MELLITUS

GENERAL PRINCIPLES AND THEORY

There is mounting evidence that the pancreatic and gastroduodenal α cells, the source of true glucagon, function abnormally in all forms of diabetes mellitus. It can be argued that diabetes in its overt form is a double disorder of islet cell function and that insulin deficiency by itself, believed from the time of von Mering and Minkowski to explain all metabolic manifestations of the condition, cannot account for the full spectrum of metabolic change. It has been proposed[99] that the principal consequence of the insulin deficiency is the underutilization of glucose and that the overproduction of glucose by the liver is largely the consequence of the absolute or relative excess of pancreatic and/or gastroduodenal glucagon that is invariably present when insulin is deficient. While insulin directly inhibits hepatic glucose production;[67–69] the major influence responsible for the glucose overproduction of uncontrolled diabetes is the hyperglucagonemia.[100]

The bihormonal abnormality hypothesis of diabetes may also extend to the syndrome of diabetic ketoacidosis. Recent studies by McGarry et al.[52] suggest that insulin deficiency contributes to ketoacidosis by permitting hyperlipolysis, thus presenting the liver with increased quantities of free fatty acids for conversion to ketoacids, but that the presence of glucagon is required to convert the liver to a ketogenic organ capable of producing large quantities of ketones. Their proposal is supported by clinical studies demonstrating that glucagon rises promptly following insulin withdrawal in juvenile diabetics and is correlated with the rise in blood ketones,[54] which can be prevented by suppressing glucagon with somatostatin.[53]

If, indeed, α cell dysfunction plays an essential mediating role in important aspects of the metabolic derangement of diabetes mellitus, substantial revision of pathophysiologic concepts are required and new approaches to therapy of the disease become possible.

FASTING PLASMA GLUCAGON IN DIABETES

Fasting plasma glucagon levels in diabetics of both the adult onset and the juvenile onset type, measured by radioimmunoassays employing the most specific antiserum available, have not revealed important differences from nondiabetics. In some series, small statistically significant elevations in mean fasting plasma glucagon have been reported in diabetics, but these differences are minor in absolute biologic terms. The major difference between diabetics and nondiabetics in the basal state is that, despite the hyperglycemia, glucagon levels of diabetics remain in or slightly above the range of normoglycemic nondiabetics. In nondiabetics the infusion of glucose to produce comparable levels of hyperglycemia reduces glucagon levels an average of about 25 pg/ml below the mean basal level. However, such maneuvers in normals are invariably accompanied by a rise in insulin and it seems likely that the decline in glucagon thus induced is the result of both the increase in glucose and the increase in insulin.

This probability is based on several experimental observations: First, in alloxan-dibetic dogs incapable of increasing insulin secretion, hyperglycemia induced by glucose infusion does not decrease plasma glucagon but, in fact, increases it[62] unless additional exogenous insulin is provided concurrently (Fig. 78-20). Second, in normal subjects, if hypoglycemia is prevented during the infusion of insulin by a concomitant glucose infusion, glucagon declines dramatically in the absence of hyperglycemia,[19] suggesting a direct action of insulin (Fig. 78-21). Thus, it seems that an increase in plasma insulin secretion is essential for glucagon suppression. In diabetics, the infusion of insulin, even in very low doses, together with sufficient glucose to prevent a fall in plasma glucose, will effectively reduce plasma glucagon to near normal levels in both adult and juvenile-type diabetics.[101] Thus. in human diabetes, the α cell does respond to plasma insulin, even in concentrations of only 40 μU/ml, but plasma glucagon does not decline to levels as low as those to which nondiabetics can be suppressed when similar insulin levels are maintained in the presence of only slight hyperglycemia (Table 78-2). When diabetic insulin levels are raised to about 300 μU/ml their glucagon levels descend into the range of suppressed nondiabetics. Moreover, in insulin-treated juvenile-type diabetics, the doses of insulin required to reduce

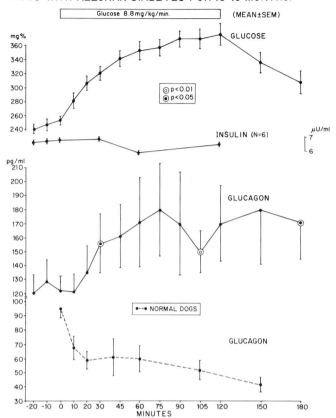

Fig. 78-20. Paradoxical effect of hyperglycemia induced by glucose infusion upon glucagon levels in conscious alloxan-diabetic dogs. The normal glucagon response to the same glucose infusion is indicated by the broken lines. (From Braaten et al. *J. Clin. Invest. 53:* 1017, 1974.)

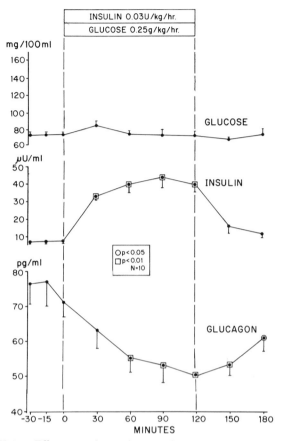

Fig. 78-21. Effect upon plasma glucagon of normal humans of insulin and glucose infused at a rate which raises insulin to 30–50 μU/ml but maintains constant plasma glucose levels. There is a significant reduction of glucagon in the absence of hyperglycemia. (From Raskin et al. *J. Clin. Invest. 56:* 1132, 1975.)

fasting glucagon levels into the normal fasting range relative to the glucose levels are in excess of 90 U/day,[102] suggesting that in such patients the α cell is normalized with difficulty by supraphysiologic doses of insulin. Whether more appropriate insulin delivery systems via some type of "artificial pancreas" would correct the hyperglucagonemia remains to be determined. However, somatostatin promptly suppresses glucagon even in the total absence of insulin, both in experimental diabetes[49] and in human diabetes.[53]

Plasma glucose levels decline when glucagon is suppressed by somatostatin (Fig. 78-22) in the absence of any insulin. This signifies that the rate of hepatic glucose production has fallen below the rate of glucose utilization by insulin-independent tissues such as the central nervous system, and reveals the importance of glucagon's contribution to the fasting hyperglycemia. The effect of somatostatin-induced glucagon suppression on plasma glucose is even more impressive in the presence of insulin (Fig. 78-23). The difficulty in suppressing fasting glucagon levels in some diabetics with insulin injections may account for difficulties in normalizing their blood glucose levels.

CARBOHYDRATE MEAL

In nondiabetics the ingestion of a carbohydrate meal is reported to result in a decline in plasma glucagon levels.[103] In both adult-type and juvenile-type diabetics, however, the ingestion of

carbohydrate fails to lower plasma glucagon (Fig. 78-24). In fact, in many patients, a paradoxical increase in glucagon may occur.[104] Moreover, the concomitant infusion of insulin to diabetics during such a meal, so as to produce rapid and supraphysiologic elevations of plasma insulin, fails to restore the normal downward response of plasma glucagon (Fig. 78-25),[105] in apparent contrast with the ability of small doses of insulin to lower glucagon in fasting diabetics.[101] Although the precise mechanisms involved are not clear, it has been reported that GIP is released during a glucose load and that it has glucagon-stimulating activity.[71] Perhaps in the nondiabetic the glucagon-suppressing effects of the carbohydrate load—namely, the rising insulin and glucose levels plus the release of an enteric glucagon-suppressing signal—outweigh the glucagon-stimulating effects of α-cytotropin release from the gut. In the diabetic, however, even much higher hyperglycemia and hyperinsulinemia seem incapable of blocking the glucagon-stimulating influence of the meal. While the explanation is still conjectural, the

Table 78-2. Comparison of Mean Nadirs of Plasma Glucagon During iv Insulin

Hyperglycemia Nondiabetics ($N=5$)	Adult-Type Diabetics ($N=10$)	Juvenile-Type Diabetics ($N=7$)
A. 39 ± 2	B. 54 ± 1	C. 53 ± 4

A versus B, $p < 0.001$. A versus C, $p < 0.05$.

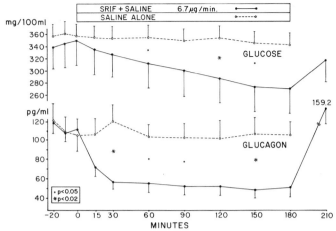

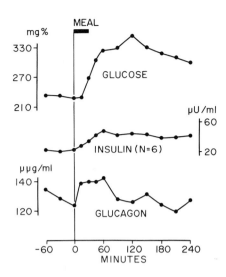

Fig. 78-22. Suppression of hyperglucagonemia by means of somatostatin infusion causes a gradual decline in plasma glucose, even in insulin-deprived alloxan-diabetic dogs. This is attributed to a decrease in the rate of hepatic glucose production to below the rate of glucose utilization by insulin-independent tissues such as the brain. When the glucagon blockade is terminated and hyperglucagonemia returns, plasma glucose rises promptly. (From Sukurai et al. *Metabolism 24:* 1287, 1975.)

Fig. 78-24. Effect of a large carbohydrate meal on plasma insulin, glucagon, and glucose of adult-type diabetics. Not only is normal suppression of plasma glucagon absent, but a paradoxical rise is frequently observed during the first hour after the ingestion of the meal. Juvenile-type diabetics generally exhibit a similar pattern. (From Müller et al. *N. Engl. J. Med. 283:* 109, 1970.)

clinical importance of this glucagon-stimulating effect of a carbohydrate load may be significant. As shown in Figure 78-23, when glucagon is reduced during a meal by somatostatin injection, the postprandial hyperglycemia that occurs in juvenile diabetics given 15 U of regular insulin subcutaneously together with breakfast is not only prevented, but plasma glucose is lowered. One can interpret this important finding as evidence that, in the absence of glucagon, first circulation hepatic uptake of glucose is far greater than during glucagon secretion, although an inhibitory effect of somatostatin on glucose absorption must also be considered.

As shown in Figure 78-26, while glucagon levels are lowered by increasing the doses of insulin, bursts of glucagon continue to occur throughout the day in some juvenile diabetics and even

massive doses of over 210 U/day may not reduce this. In some juvenile diabetics, however, a relatively normal glucagon response is observed when sufficient insulin is given. The daytime glucagon surges appear to coincide in general with the elevations in plasma glucose that occur in spite of the large doses of insulin which must be causing an abnormally high rate of glucose utilization; yet, plasma glucose levels rise during meals. The labile hyperglycemia may be the result of sudden glucagon-induced increases in hepatic glucose production; as was shown in Figure 78-23, somatostatin blockade of glucagon during a meal abolished the postprandial glucose rise that occurs when insulin alone is given.

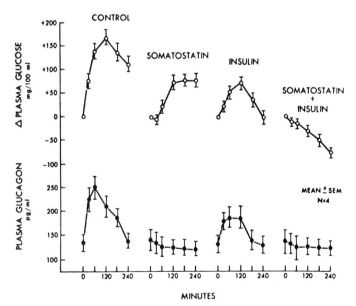

Fig. 78-23. Plasma glucose and the glucagon changes after a standard (500-calorie) breakfast in four insulin-dependent diabetic subjects, showing the effect of somatostatin infusion (500 μg/h), crystalline insulin (15 U subcutaneously, one-half hour before the meal), and a combination of somatostatin infusion and subcutaneous crystalline insulin (mean ± SEM). (From Gerich et al.: N. Engl. J. Med. 29: 555, 1974)

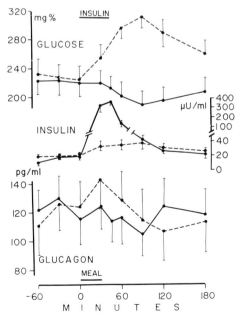

Fig. 78-25. Effect in adult-type diabetics of a large carbohydrate meal during the concomitant infusion of exogenous insulin upon plasma glucagon (solid lines). Despite marked insulinemia, mean plasma glucagon does not differ significantly from that observed in the same individuals given the same meal of exogenous glucagon without insulin (broken lines). (From Unger et al. *Diabetes 21:* 301, 1972.)

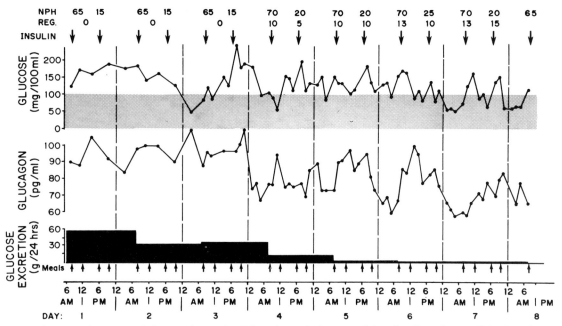

Fig. 78-26. Pattern of plasma glucagon and glucose observed at 2-hour intervals for several days in a juvenile-type diabetic during improving blood glucose control through increasing doses of insulin. Arrows at the top indicate the time of subcutaneous administration of insulin. Arrows at the bottom represent meal times. Note the failure to abolish daytime rises in glucagon despite an overall reduction of basal and daytime glucagon levels.

PROTEIN MEAL AND AMINO ACID INFUSION

In normal subjects, a protein meal is accompanied by a rise in glucagon, the function of which is to prevent aminogenic hypoglycemia as a result of aminogenic insulin secretion. In the diabetic, however, hyperglycemia is present and insulin secretion is diminished or absent, so a rise in glucagon secretion is obviously purposeless. However, glucagon does increase in the diabetic during a protein meal (Fig. 78-27) and may further augment the hyperglycemia. As shown in Figure 78-28, the infusion of arginine in juvenile diabetics causes an exaggerated rise in glucagon despite the hyperglycemia, and plasma glucose rises an average of 65 mg/100 ml in 70 min. Aminogenic stimulation may be an important factor in the mealtime rises in plasma glucagon observed in juvenile-type diabetics, and may well contribute to the labile plasma glucose pattern.

MECHANISM OF DIABETIC HYPERGLUCAGONEMIA

It is not clear whether or not the α cell abnormalities described are secondary to abnormal insulin secretion or whether the α cell and β cell derangements represent independent abnormalities which may begin at different times or at the same time. In favor of the view that the α cell abnormality is secondary to insulin lack is the fact that it can be diminished, although not to normal, by the infusion of insulin in doses which produce only small elevations in plasma insulin.[101] On the other hand, independence of the α cell abnormality is favored by the fact that even supraphysiologic rates of insulin infusion fail to restore to normal the α cell response to a carbohydrate meal[105] and that chronic high-dose insulin therapy frequently fails to normalize glucagon in juvenile diabetics. An increase in glucagon-containing cells has been observed in such patients (Fig. 78-29).

More impressive evidence favoring an independent α cell defect is derived from the fact that in Pima Indians both hyperinsulinemic and hypoinsulinemic diabetics have an exaggerated glucagon response to arginine infusion compared to nondiabetic Indian controls with intermediate levels of insulin[106] (Fig. 78-30). At least

in this group of patients, the α cell abnormality seems unrelated to the level of plasma insulin. In nondiabetic offspring of two diabetic parents, presumed to have a high risk of future diabetes, a significant exaggeration of the glucagon response to arginine was ob-

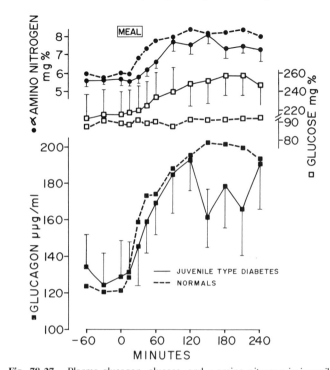

Fig. 78-27. Plasma glucagon, glucose, and α-amino nitrogen in juvenile-type diabetics (solid line) and nondiabetics (broken line) during a large protein meal. Despite a level of hyperglycemia, which in nondiabetics would completely abolish the protein-induced increase in glucagon, the glucagon levels of diabetics respond as if hyperglycemia were not present. This rise in glucagon without a rise in insulin may explain the 40 mg/100 ml increase in plasma glucose observed in the diabetic group. (From Müller et al. *N. Eng. J. Med.* 283: 109, 1970.)

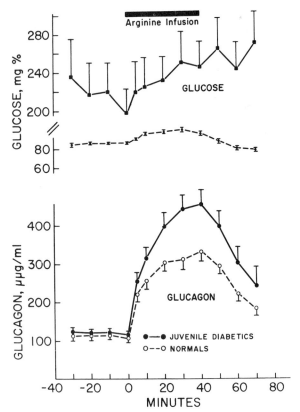

Fig. 78-28. Effect of arginine infusion in juvenile-type diabetics compared to nondiabetics. The exaggerated rise in glucagon is accompanied by a 65 mg/100 ml increase in mean plasma glucose in 70 min. Aminogenic stimulation may therefore be an important factor in the mealtime rises of plasma glucagon in diabetic patients with fixed insulin levels. (From Unger et al. *J. Clin. Invest. 49:* 837, 1970.)

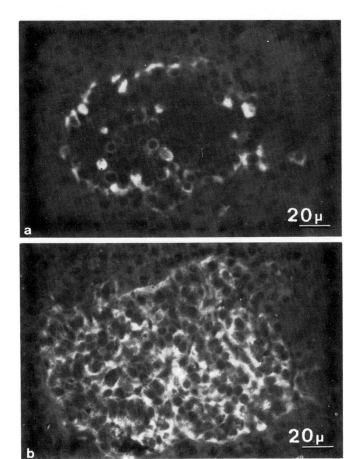

Fig. 78-29. Indirect immunofluorescence technique showing fluorescent cells to antiglucagon (30K) in the pancreatic islet. A. From an adult nondiabetic human. B. From a 32-year-old white male with severe juvenile-type diabetics of 18 years' duration.

served at a time when insulin levels and glucose tolerance were normal;[107] in first-degree relatives of diabetic patients, nonsuppressibility of plasma glucagon by hyperglycemia has been reported.[108] In view of the fact that α and β cells originate from a common anlage, it would not be surprising if both were afflicted with a common defect, at least in the genetic forms of this disease.

GASTRIC GLUCAGON

The contribution of gastric glucagon to hyperglucagonemia of human diabetes is not clear. If the pancreas is destroyed or extirpated, all plasma glucagon is obviously of extrapancreatic origin. In some chronic juvenile diabetics, islets are still present although in decreased number. They consist of α cells, which stain for glucagon immunoreactivity (Fig. 78-29), and D cells, which stain for somatostatin or a somatostatinlike immunoreactive material, but are virtually devoid of β cells.[109] In addition, a few scattered α and D cells are identified among the exocrine cells; in such patients, the pancreas could be a major source of circulating glucagon.

In experimental diabetes in laboratory animals, it is possible to compare the contribution of pancreatic and extrapancreatic glucagon to plasma glucagon in the diabetic and nondiabetic state. In nondiabetic dogs, during an arginine infusion, virtually all plasma glucagon comes from the pancreas. In the totally depancreatized, insulin-deprived dog, plasma glucagon is derived largely from the fundus; gastroepiploic vein glucagon levels may be 150 pg/ml above the vena caval concentrations and this difference increases 1000 pg/ml during intravenous arginine infusion (Fig. 78-

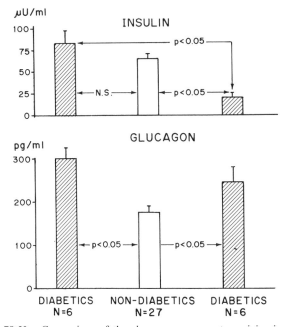

Fig. 78-30. Comparison of the glucagon response to arginine in nondiabetic Pima Indians (open bars) and diabetic Pima Indians (hatched bars) with hyperinsulinemia and hypoinsulinemia. In both diabetic groups the glucagon response was significantly greater than that of nondiabetic Indians with intermediate levels of insulin.

31). Administration of insulin stops gastric glucagon secretion within 30 min in such dogs and peripheral glucagon becomes unmeasurable.

In the insulin-deprived, alloxan-diabetic dog, the peripheral hyperglucagonemia is derived from both the pancreas and the stomach.[110] As shown in Figure 78-32, basal levels in both pancreaticoduodenal and gastroepiploic veins are considerably greater than the levels in the inferior vena cava and, when arginine is administered, a marked rise in glucagon is observed in the venous effluent of both organs.

The role of nonpancreatic glucagon in the aminogenic hyperglucagonemia of human diabetics is uncertain. One can imagine that the ingestion of protein might elicit, particularly in the poorly controlled diabetic, an outpouring of gastrointestinal glucagon that would increase hepatic glucose production and capture a disproportionate share of the ingested amino acids for unnecessary gluconeogenesis at the expense of protein synthesis. In the only two totally depancreatized patients thus far examined, both of whom were well controlled on insulin, the infusion of arginine failed to cause a rise in plasma glucagon above the basal level.[111] However, this would not be unexpected in well-insulinized diabetics since insulin is such a powerful suppressant of gastric glucagon secretion. The status of extra-pancreatic glucagon in humans is uncertain.

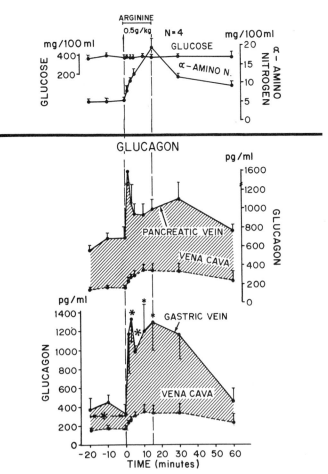

Fig. 78-32. Simultaneous measurements of basal and arginine-stimulated plasma glucagon levels in the pancreatic vein, a gastric vein draining the fundus of the stomach, and the inferior vena cava in insulin-deprived, conscious, alloxan-diabetic dogs. Note the gradient of glucagon immunoreactivity across the stomach as well as across the pancreas. The administration of insulin virtually abolishes the gastric gradient of glucagon and reduces the glucagon gradient across the pancreas to the normal range. (From Blazquez et al. *J. Lab. Clin. Med. 89:* 971, 1977.)

When insulin is given to insulin-deprived, alloxan-diabetic dogs, gastric secretion of glucagon stops completely within 30 min, as in depancreatized dogs; pancreatic glucagon secretion declines sharply but does not stop. The greater insulin sensitivity exhibited by depancreatized diabetics would appear to be the result of the lack of this continuing pancreatic glucagon secretion after extrapancreatic glucagon secretion by the exquisitely insulin-sensitive gastroduodenal α cells is extinguished by insulin.

GLUCAGON IN UNCONTROLLED DIABETES

Mean glucagon levels in patients with diabetic ketoacidosis or with nonketotic extreme hyperglycemia hyperosmolality are many times greater than the fasting levels of nondiabetics and of diabetics under ordinary conditions. Thus, despite the accompanying marked hyperglycemia, plasma glucagon levels are enormously increased (Fig. 78-33).

The hyperglucagonemia in such circumstances is quite probably the result of several factors. Total deficiency of insulin, whether induced by neutralization of circulating insulin, antiinsulin serum, blockade of insulin release by diazoxide or mannoheptulose,[64] or destruction of β cells by alloxan[64] or streptozotocin,[112] results in rapid development of absolute or relative hyperglucago-

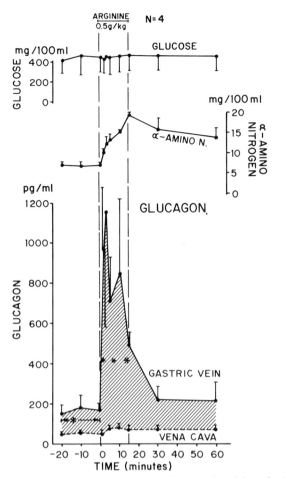

Fig. 78-31. Simultaneous measurements of basal and arginine-stimulated plasma glucagon levels in a gastric vein draining the gastric fundus and in the inferior vena cava of insulin-deprived, conscious, totally depancreatized dogs. A marked gradient across this portion of the stomach suggests that it is a major source of the hyperglucagonemia observed in insulin-deprived depancreatized animals. (From Blazquez et al. *Endocrinology 99:* 1182, 1976.)

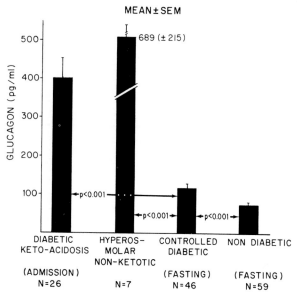

Fig. 78-33. Plasma glucagon levels in poorly controlled diabetic patients with diabetic ketoacidosis or nonketotic hyperosmolar syndrome compared to well-controlled diabetic patients and nondiabetics. (From Unger and Orci. *Physiol. Rev. 556: 778*, 1976.)

nemia. In the untreated alloxan-diabetic or depancreatized dog, even small quantities of insulin result in an immediate and rapid decline in plasma glucagon, suggesting that the α cell is an insulin-requiring cell and that, in the absence of insulin, it cannot function properly as a glucose sensor.

However, other factors must certainly play an important role. Extracellular fluid volume depletion, irrespective of its cause, causes marked hyperglucagonemia even in nondiabetics, presumably via β-adrenergic stimulation. Virtually all patients with diabetic ketoacidosis or with extreme nonketotic hyperglycemia are severely volume-depleted; one must consider this mechanism as an important cause of the increased glucagon secretion that uniformly occurs in these situations. Furthermore, it is now quite clear that the kidney is a major site of glucagon degradation and that ligation of the renal blood vessels will, in an otherwise healthy dog, result in a rapid rise in plasma glucagon.[113] Inasmuch as severely ill, volume-depleted diabetics have reduced glomerular filtration, this mechanism can contribute to hyperglucagonemia by lowering the metabolic clearance of the hormone.

Stress, as defined earlier, can induce marked hyperglucagonemia in nondiabetic subjects. Even in nondiabetics, stress-induced discharge of catacholamines and direct sympathetic nervous control of β cells may so inhibit insulin secretion that the associated hyperglucagonemia brings about stress hyperglycemia. In a diabetic patient, β cell function is compromised even in the unstressed state and stress will result in more marked hyperglucagonemia. The net result is marked endogenous hyperglycemia as the hyperglucagonemia increases hepatic glucose production to a rate exceeding glucose utilization, and deterioration in metabolic control ensues. In well-controlled insulin-treated dogs, when long-acting zinc glucagon is injected so as to produce hyperglycagonemia of the magnitude associated with severe stress, hyperglycemia, glycosuria, increased urea excretion, and weight loss develop despite continued administration of doses of insulin that previously maintained an excellent level of diabetic control (Fig. 78-34). This suggests that hyperglucagonemia by itself, unless accompanied by an increase in insulin, can generate the full syndrome of diabetic decompensation. Infection, trauma, and other

severe stresses all cause hyperglucagonemia in the nondiabetic, which can explain the metabolic deterioration, including the ketoacidosis, that they induce in the diabetic patient.

CATABOLIC DISEASES

An increased concentration of glucagon relative to insulin is believed to change metabolic processes toward catabolism and away from anabolism. By that, it is meant that breakdown of macromolecules such as glycogen, triglycerides, and protein is accelerated to provide a source of fuels and the biosynthesis of macromolecules from energy-yielding precurser components is reduced. Thus, glycogenolysis is accelerated and glycogenesis decreases, amino acids are preferentially diverted to gluconeogenesis at the expense of protein synthesis, lipolysis increases, and lipogenesis decreases. Lipoprotein synthesis and secretion by the liver is reduced, hepatic DNA synthesis is reduced, and hepatic lysosomes increase. A catabolic mode is appropriate in life situations when fuels are urgently needed and no alternatives to endogenous sources are available, as for example, in fasting and prolonged exercise, but it is highly inappropriate in circumstances in which increased anabolism is vital to survival. However, in a variety of serious illnesses, the insulin–glucagon ratio is low and the nitrogen balance is negative and there is loss of weight. Inasmuch as exogenous hyperglucagonemia can induce a catabolic

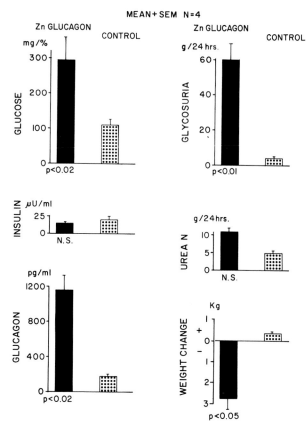

Fig. 78-34. Effect of hyperglucagonemia induced by injections of zinc glucagon (closed bars) upon plasma glucose, insulin, and glucagon, daily excretion of glucose and urea, and body weight in four dogs receiving their usual dose of NPH insulin. The control values of all measurements are represented by the stippled bars. Note that the induction of hyperglucagonemia causes marked deterioriation in diabetic control and weight loss. (From Rocha et al. *N. Eng. J. Med. 288: 700*, 1973.)

state when insulin is fixed,[87] it has been proposed that the low insulin–glucagon ratio mediates these manifestations of severe illness. Severe infection and traumatic or thermal injury are notable examples of the catabolic state.[114] At a time when increased DNA synthesis and immunoglobulin synthesis would seem to call for an increasingly anabolic hormonal setting, precisely the opposite setting prevails. In support of a key role of the low insulin–high glucagon setting in the hypercatabolic state, is the fact that hyperalimentation regimens, in which insulin–glucagon molar ratios are elevated by the administration of insulin and glucose, seem to reverse the negative nitrogen balance and promote more rapid healing.[115] In addition, spontaneous increases in the insulin–glucagon ratio appear to coincide with reversal of the negative nitrogen balance in burn patients and with the onset of wound healing[114] (Fig. 78-35). It is a clinical fact that whenever the insulin–glucagon molar ratio is low, as in starvation or uncontrolled diabetes, negative nitrogen balance and weight loss develop and these are reversed by any measure which increases the insulin–glucagon ratio.

In view of the foregoing hormonal differences in catabolic patients, the premise that a positive nitrogen balance requires a basal insulin–glucagon ratio above 2 or 3 and a rise to 5–20 times above the basal level during an influx of exogenous nutrients is probably reasonable. Seriously ill individuals are unable to generate such a rise when presented with exogenous nutrients. Intravenous administration of glucose may therefore result in hyperglycemia and glycosuria even to the point of extreme hyperglycemia with coma. Exogenous insulin may be required to correct the low insulin–glucagon ratio in such patients. The mechanism of the unresponsiveness to glucose of the low insulin–glucagon ratio in catabolic situations is unknown but is assumed to be via the sympathetic nervous system.

Patients with severe chronic liver disease also exhibit high glucagon levels[116] and their insulin–glucagon ratios tend to be on the low side.[117] It has been reported that oral hyperalimentation, i.e., the simple addition to the diet of 20 g of glucose loads at frequent intervals, will greatly enhance the rise in insulin–glucagon ratio in response to a protein meal. In cirrhotics, a protein-containing meal without the added glucose caused a rise in blood ammonia, but when the glucose supplements were given the rise in blood ammonia was prevented and, in fact, a decline was noted.[117] It has been proposed that this results from greater utilization of the ingested amino acids for protein biosynthesis, thereby reducing the quantity of amino acids available for urea production and the generation of ammonia.

HYPERANABOLIC STATES

A positive nitrogen balance and rapid macromolecular synthesis is a normal prerequisite during fetal development or during regeneration of tissues. It is worth noting once again that in the fetal liver during the phase of rapid growth the sensitivity of the adenylate cyclase response to glucagon is markedly reduced. This glucagon resistance, which persists until 30 days after birth, is believed to ensure an anabolic mode that cannot be altered by changing maternal nutrient needs. Thus, with an unchanging "environment," i.e. the uterus, and unchanging metabolic demands, i.e., growth, the fetal insensitivity to glucagon and its presumed sensitivity to insulin guarantee secure and uninterrupted anabolism. This "glucagon resistance" may be vital to normal growth and development. In partially hepatectomized rats in whom plasma glucagon levels are also increased but hepatic regeneration, nevertheless, is accelerated, again glucagon resistance seems to be present;[118] glucagon binding by liver membranes is significantly reduced under these circumstances, while insulin binding remains unaffected and DNA synthesis can increase and rapid regeneration can occur despite the associated hyperglucagonemia.

The synthesis of lipoproteins by the liver is also promoted by insulin[119] and VLDL release is blocked by glucagon, presumably by preventing apoprotein synthesis. It was first suggested by Eaton and Kipnis[80] that glucagon suppression by a high-carbohydrate intake might account for increased endogenous lipoprotein production induced by a high-carbohydrate intake. Recent studies in man are compatible with this concept in that a significant relationship between the carbohydrate-induced change in the insulin–glucagon ratio and the triglyceride level of normal subjects has been demonstrated.[81] This may mean that VLDL production in response to changes in carbohydrate intake is mediated by changes in the concentrations of insulin and glucagon that perfuse the liver.

GLUCAGONOMA

The first recognized case of glucagonoma was probably that of Gussner and Corting in 1960, but it was not until 1966 that positive laboratory proof of the existence of a glucagon-producing tumor of the islets of Langerhans was recorded by McGavran et al.[120] Mallinson and co-workers have recently collected several additional cases and have attempted to characterize the glucagonoma syndrome.[121] Of the 9 patients they described, 8 were postmenopausal females and all were under treatment for "necrolytic migratory erythema" and stomatitis. All patients exhibited weight loss and 7 were said to have diabetes. In 4 patients, high plasma glucagon levels were noted, together with low plasma amino acid

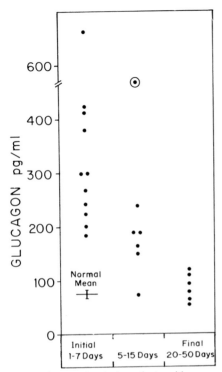

Fig. 78-35. Plasma glucagon levels in patients with severe burns. Note that in the surviving patients glucagon is lower in the second week, except for 1 patient who had a severe infection (circle). During the period of healing after the 20th day, plasma glucagon has returned to the normal range. (From J.A.M.A.)

levels. Weight loss was prominent in these patients. Circumoral crusting and painful glossitis was frequent. The skin lesions were most severe in the lower abdomen, groin, and perineum. They began as erythematous lesions which subsequently became papular with superficial central blistering and soon ruptured to leave crusts or weeping surfaces. These tended to heal in the center and spread peripherally with a well-defined margin. Healing was associated with hyperpigmentation, the entire cycle taking approximately 1–2 weeks, during which time new lesions appeared, coalescing into angular or linear lesions in otherwise normal skin. Skin biopsies showed necrolysis leading to bullous disruption of the upper epidermis. Although 7 of the 9 patients reported by Mallinson et al. were diabetic, none had a family history of diabetes. Weight loss was generally pronounced; it was attributable to malignancy or to anorexia in 3 of the patients, but not in the others. Glucagon levels in this group ranged from 850 to 3500 pg/ml.

In the first proven glucagonoma patient described by Mac-Gavran et al., glucagon levels as high as 50,000 pg/ml were recorded. This patient also was under treatment for skin disease. Despite the use of steroids, she exhibited only very mild diabetes. She was otherwise asymptomatic until she developed right-sided pleuritic pain resulting from massive enlargement of the liver due to hepatic metastases. A pancreatic tumor was removed from the patient, but the extent of the hepatic metastases precluded subtotal hepatectomy. Although the original diagnosis was adenocarcinoma of the pancreas, the postoperative course was too benign and protracted for a carcinoma of the exocrine pancreas. Reexamination of the tissue specimen suggested a tumor of endocrine origin and prompted extensive histochemical and electronmicroscopic studies, which strongly suggested a primary α cell tumor. Extracts of the hepatic metastases, obtained postmortem, demonstrated an enormous concentration of glucagon which was immunologically and biologically indistinguishable from purified pancreatic glucagon.

Diabetes is not a common or striking feature of this disorder when insulin secretion is relatively normal. However, in a patient reported by Yoshinago et al. the tumor had replaced most of the normal pancreas and large doses of exogenous insulin were required.[122]

The diagnosis of glucagonoma should be considered in all patients with unexplained skin lesions and in individuals with extensive hepatic metastases in whom the relative indolence of the condition seems incompatible with metastatic disease of nonendocrine origin. Marked hyperglucagonemia is pathognomonic, but it should be kept in mind that any sick patient under stress may exhibit glucagon levels of up to 1500 pg/ml. Patients who are seriously ill but who exhibit glucagon levels in excess of 1500 pg/ml should be suspected of having glucagonoma. In the unstressed patient who is not a poorly controlled diabetic, levels of more than 750 pg/ml are strongly suggestive of the disease, provided there is no cirrhosis or portal vein shunting. Spuriously high measurements of plasma glucagon may occur rarely in perfectly healthy patients with hypermacroglucagonemia (excess BPG), and the significance of this is unknown. In the only glucagonoma patient in whom the plasma was subjected to gel filtration, the BPG was not elevated; proglucagon and glucagon were the cause of the high plasma IRG.

REFERENCES

1. Lane, M. A. The cytological characters of the areas of Langerhans. *Am. J. Anat. 7:* 409, 1907.
2. Banting, F. G., and Best, C. H. The internal secretion of the pancreas. *J. Lab. Clin. Med. 7:* 251, 1922.
3. Kimball, C. P., and Murlin, J. R. Aqueous extracts of pancreas. III. Some precipitation reactions of insulin. *J. Biol. Chem. 58:* 337, 1923.
4. Unger, R. H. Glucagon and the insulin: glucagon ratio in diabetes and other catabolic illnesses. *Diabetes 20:* 834, 1971.
5. Staehelin, L. A. Structure and function of intercellular junctions. *Int. Rev. Cytol. 39:* 191, 1963.
6. Orci, L., Unger, R. H., and Renold, A. E. Structural coupling between pancreatic islet cells. *Experientia 29:* 1015, 1973.
7. Orci, L., Malaisse-Lagae, G., Ravazzola, M., et al. The morphologic basis for intercellular communication between pancreatic alpha and beta cells. *J. Clin. Invest. 56:* 1066, 1975.
8. Orci, L., Malaisse-Lagae, F., Amherdt, M., et al. Cell contacts in human islets of Langerhans. *J. Clin. Endocrinol. Metab. 41:* 841, 1975.
9. Orci, L., Amherdt, M., Henquin, J. C., et al. Pronase effect of pancreatic beta cell secretion and morphology. *Science 180:* 647, 1973.
10. Samols, E., Marri, G., and Marks, V. Promotion of insulin secretion by glucagon. *Lancet 2:* 415, 1965.
11. Orci, L., Pictet, R., Forssmann, W. G., et al. Structural evidence for glucagon producing cells in the intestinal mucosa of the rat *Diabetologia 4:* 56, 1968.
12. Bussolati, G., Capella, C., Solcia, E., et al. Ultrastructural and immunofluorescent investigations on the secretin cell in the dog intestinal mucosa. *Histochemie 26:* 218, 1971.
13. Sasagawa, T., Kobayashi, S., and Fujita, T. Electron microscopy of human GEP endocrine cells. In: Gastro-Entero-Pancreatic Endocrine System. Edited by T. Fujita. Tokyo, Igaku Shoin, 1973, p. 31.
14. Sasaki, H., Rubalcava, B., Baetens, D., et al. Identification of glucagon in the gastrointestinal tract. *J. Clin. Invest. 56:* 135, 1975.
15. Baetens, D., Loeb, P., Unger, R. H., et al. Unpublished observations.
16. Luft, R., Efendic, S., Hokfelt, T., et al. Immunohistochemical evidence for the location of somatostatin-like immunoreactivity in a cell population of the pancreatic islets. *Med. Biol. 52:* 428, 1974.
17. Dubois, M. P. Immunoreactive somatostatin is present in discrete cells of the endocrine pancreas. *Proc. Natl. Acad. Sci. U.S.A. 72:* 1340, 1975.
17a. Rufener, C., Dubois, M. P., Malaisse-Lagae, F., and Orci, L. Immunofluorescent reactivity to antisomatostatin in the gastrointestinal mucosa of the dog. *Diabetologia II:* 321, 1975.
17b. Orci, L. Somatostatin-containing cells in the pancreas and the gastrointestinal tract. Ciba Foundation Symposium 41, 1975.
18. Unger, R. H. Diabetes and the alpha cell. 1975 Banting Memorial Lecture. *Diabetes* (in press).
19. Reichard, G. A., Issekutz, B., Jr., Kimbel, P., et al. Blood glucose metabolism in man during muscular work. *J. Appl. Physiol. 16:* 1001, 1961.
20. Bottger, I., Schlein, E., Faloona, G. R., et al. The effect of exercise on glucagon secretion. *J. Clin. Endocrinol. Metab. 35:* 117, 1972.
21. Luyckx, A. S., and Lefebvre, P. J. Mechanisms involved in the exercise-induced increase in glucagon secretion in rats. *Diabetes 23:* 81, 1974.
22. Harvey, D., Faloona, G. R., and Unger, R. H. The effect of adrenergic blockade on exercise-induced hyperglucagonemia. *Endocrinology 94:* 1254, 1974.
23. Combes, B., Adams, R. H., Strickland, W., et al. The physiological significance of the secretion of insulin into the portal circulation. IV. Hepatic uptake of glucose during glucose infusion in nondiabetic dogs. *J. Clin. Invest. 40:* 1706, 1961.
24. Wool, I. G., and Krahl, M. E. Incorporation of C^{14}-histidine into protein of isolated diaphragms: interactions of fasting, glucose and insulin. *Am. J. Physiol. 197:* 367, 1959.
25. Unger, R. H., Ohneda, A., Aguilar-Parada, E., et al. The role of aminogenic glucagon secretion in blood glucose homeostasis. *J. Clin. Invest. 48:* 810, 1969.
26. Cherrington, A. D., and Vranic, M. Effect of arginine on glucose turnover and plasma free fatty acids in normal dogs. *Diabetes 22:* 537, 1973.
27. Rigopoulou, D., Valverde, I., Marco, J., et al. Large glucagon immunoreactivity in extracts of pancreas. *J. Biol. Chem. 245:* 496, 1970.
28. Noe, B. D., and Bauer, G. E. Evidence for glucagon biosynthesis involving a protein intermediate in islets of the anglerfish (lophius amencauus). *Endocrinology 89:* 642, 1971.
29. Tager, H. S., and Steiner, D. F. Isolation of a glucagon-containing peptide: Primary structure of a possible fragment of proglucagon. *Proc. Natl. Acad. Sci. U.S.A. 70:* 2321, 1973.

30. Valverde, I., Rigopoulou, D., Marco, J., et al. Characterization of glucagon-like immunoreactivity (GLI). *Diabetes 19:* 614, 1970.

31. Valverde, I., Villamer, M. L., Lazano, I., et al. Presence of glucagon immunoreactivity in the globulin fraction of human plasma ("big plasma glucagon"). *J. Clin. Endocrinol. Metab. 39:* 1090, 1974.

32. Valverde, I., Dobbs, R., and Unger, R. H. Heterogenity of plasma glucagon immunoreactivity in normal, depancreatized and alloxan diabetic dogs. *Metabolism 24:* 1021, 1975.

33. Valverde, I., Roman, D., and Dobbs, R. Heterogenity of plasma glucagon in depancreatized alloxanized and ploridzinized dogs. *Diabetes 24 [Suppl. 2]:* 412, 1975, (abstract 77).

34. Unger, R. H., and Eisentraut, A. New aspects of glucagon pathology and pathophysiology. In: Internatl. Congress Series #312, Diabetes. Proc. 8th Congress Internatl. Diabetes Federation, Brussels, Belgium, July 15–20, 1974. Editors W. J. Malaisse and J. Pirart. Amsterdam. Excerpta Medica, 1974, pp. 137.

35. Weir, G. C., Turner, R. C., and Martin, D. B. Glucagon radioimmunoassay using antiserum 30K: Interference by plasma. *Horm. Metab. Res. 5:* 241, 1973.

36. Walter, R. M., Dudl, R. J., Palmer, J. P., et al. The effect of adrenergic blockade on the glucagon responses to starvation and hypoglycemia in man. *J. Clin. Invest. 54:* 1214, 1974.

37. Mirsky, I. A., Perisutti, G., and Davis, N. C. The destruction of glucagon, adrenocorticotropin and somatotropin by human blood plasma. *J. Clin. Invest. 38:* 14, 1959.

38. Assan, R. In vivo metabolism of glucagon. In: Glucagon Molecular Physiology, Clinical and Therapeutic Implications. Edited by P. J. Lefebvre and R. H. Unger, Amsterdam, Pergamon, 1972, p. 53.

39. Rodbell, M., Krans, H. M. J., Pohl, S.L., et al. Glucagon sensitive adenyl cyclase system in plasma membranes of rat liver. III. Binding of glucagon: method of assay specificity. *J. Biol. Chem. 246:* 1861, 1971.

40. Blackard, W. G., Nelson, N. C., and Andrews, S. S. Portal and peripheral vein immunoreactive glucagon concentrations after arginine or glucose infusions. *Diabetes 23:* 199, 1974.

41. Giorgio, N. A., Johnson, C. B., and Blericher, M. Hormone receptors. III. Properties of glucagon-binding proteins isolated from liver plasma membranes. *J. Biol. Chem. 249:* 428, 1974.

42. Kakiuchi, S., and Tomazawa, H. H. Properties of a glucagon-degrading enzyme of beef liver. *J. Biol. Chem. 239:* 2160, 1964.

43. Duckworth, W. C., and Kitabchi, A. E. Insulin and glucagon degradation by the same enzyme. *Diabetes 23:* 536, 1974.

44. Lefebvre, P., and Luyckx, A. Effect of acute kidney exclusion by ligation of renal arteries on peripheral plasma glucagon levels and pancreatic glucagon production in the anesthetized dog. *Metabolism* (in press).

45. Aguilar-Parada, E., Eisentraut, A. M., and Unger, R. H. Effects of starvation on plasma pancreatic glucagon in normal man. *Diabetes 18:* 717, 1969.

46. Muller, W. A., Faloona, G. F., and Unger, R. H. The effect of alanine on glucagon secretion. *J. Clin. Invest. 50:* 2215, 1971.

47. Mortimer, C. H., Turnbridge, W. M. G., Carr, D., et al. Effects of growth-hormone release-inhibiting hormone on circulating glucagon, insulin, and growth hormone in normal, diabetic, acromegalic, and hypopituitary patients. *Lancet 1:* 697, 1974.

48. Koerker, D. J., Ruch, W., Chideckel, E., et al. Somatostatin: hypothalamic inhibitor of the endocrine pancreas. *Science 184:* 482, 1974.

49. Sakurai, H., Dobbs, R., and Unger, R. H. Somatostatin-induced changes in insulin and glucagon secretion in normal and diabetic dogs. . *Clin. Invest. 54:* 1395, 1974.

50. Muller, W. A., Faloona, G. R., and Unger, R. H. The influence of the antecedent diet upon glucagon and insulin secretion. *N. Engl. J. Med. 285:* 1450, 1971.

51. Cahill, G. F., Jr., Herrera, M. G., Morgan, A. P., et al. Hormone fuel interrelationships during fasting. *J. Clin. Invest. 45:* 1751, 1966.

52. McGarry, J. D., Wright, P., and Foster, D. Hormonal control of ketogenesis: Rapid activation of hepatic ketogenic capacity in fed rats by anti-insulin serum and glucagon. *J. Clin. Invest. 55:* 1202, 1975.

53. Gerich, J. E., Lorenzi, M., Bier, D. M., et al. Prevention of human diabetic ketoacidosis by somatostatin. Evidence for an essential role of glucagon. *N. Eng. J. Med. 292:* 985, 1975.

54. Alberti, K. G. M. M., Christensen, N. J., Iversen, J., et al. Role of glucagon in other hormones in development of diabetic ketoacidosis. *Lancet 1:* 1307, 1975.

55. Madison, L. L., Mebane, D., Unger, R. H., et al. The hypoglycemia actions of ketones. II. Evidence for a stimulatory feedback of ketones on the pancreatic beta cells. *J. Clin. Invest. 43:* 408, 1964.

56. Unger, R. H., Eisentraut, A. M., McCall, M. S., et al. Measurements of endogenous glucagon in plasma and the influence of blood glucose concentration upon its secretion. *J. Clin. Invest. 41:* 682, 1962.

57. Palmer, J. P., and Ensinck, J. W. Stimulation of glucagon secretion hypoglycemia by ethanol in man. *Diabetes 24:* 295, 1975.

58. Dobbs, R., and Unger, R. H. Unpublished observations.

59. Braaten, J., and Unger, R. H. Unpublished observations.

60. Gerich, J. E., Langlois, M., Noacco, C., et al. Lack of glucagon responses to hypoglycemia in diabetes: Evidence for an intrinsic pancreatic alpha cell defect. *Science 182:* 171, 1973.

61. Samols, E., Tyler, J. M., and Marks, V. Glucagon–insulin interrelationships. In: Glucagon Molecular Physiology, Clinical and Therapeutic Implications. Edited by P. J. Lefebvre and R. H. Unger, Amsterdam, Pergamon, 1972, pp. 151.

62. Braaten, J. T., Faloona, G. R., and Unger, R. H. Effect of insulin on the alpha cell response to hyperglycemia in long-standing alloxan diabetes. *J. Clin. Invest. 53:* 1017, 1974.

63. Edwards, J. C., and Taylor, K. W. Radioimmunoassay of glucagon released from isolated guinea pig islets of Langerhans incubated in vitro. *Biochem. Biophys. Acta. 215:* 297, 1970.

64. Muller, W. A., Faloona, G. R., and Unger, R. H. The effect of experimental insulin deficiency on glucagon secretion. *J. Clin. Invest. 50:* 1992, 1971.

65. Eaton, R. P., Kipnis, D. M., Karl, I., and Eisenstein, A. B. Effects of glucose feeding on insulin and glucagon secretion and hepatic gluconeogenesis in the rat. *Clin. J. Phys. 227:* 101, 1974.

66. Jennings, A. S., Cherrington, A. D., Chiasson, J. L., et al. The fine regulation of basal hepatic glucose production. *Clin. Res. 23:* 323-A, 1975, (Abstract).

67. Madison, L. L., Mebane, D., Lecosq, G., et al. Insulin's control of the role of the liver in the disposition of glucose loads. Proc. Fourth Congress Internat'l. Diabetes Federation. Geneva, Medicine and Hygiene, 1961, pp. 598–601.

68. Park, C. R., and Exton, J. H. Glucagon and the metabolism of glucose. In: Glucagon Molecular Physiology, Clinical and Therapeutic Implications. Edited by P. J. Lefebvre and R. H. Unger, Amsterdam, Pergamon, 1972, pp. 77.

69. Cherrington, A. D., and Vranic, M. Effect of interaction between insulin and glucagon on glucose turnover and FFA concentration in normal and depancreatized dogs. *Metabolism 23:* 729, 1974.

70. Santeusanio, F., Faloona, G. R., and Unger, R. H. Suppressive effect of secretin upon pancreatic alpha cell function. *J. Clin. Invest. 51:* 1743, 1972.

71. Rabinovitch, A., and Dupre, J. Effects of gastric inhibitory polypeptide present in impure pancreozymin-cholecystokinin on plasma insulin and glucagon in the rat. *Endocrinology 94:* 1139, 1974.

72. Unger, R. H., Ohneda, A., Aguilar-Parada, E., et al. Role of aminogenic glucagon secretion in blood glucose homeostasis. *J. Clin. Invest. 48:* 810, 1969.

73. Cherrington, A. D., Kawamori, R., Pek, S., et al. Arginine infusion in dogs: Model for the roles of insulin and glucagon in regulatory glucose turnover and FFA levels. *Diabetes 23:* 805, 1974.

74. Kaneto, A., Mizuno, Y., Tasaka, Y., et al. Stimulation of glucagon secretion by tetragastrin. *Endocrinology 86:* 1175, 1970.

75. Unger, R. H., Ketterer, H., Dupre, J., et al. The effects of secretin, pancreozymin and gastrin upon insulin and glucagon secretion in anesthetized dogs. *J. Clin. Invest. 46:* 630, 1967.

76. Dobbs, R., and Unger, R. H. Unpublished observations.

77. Balasse, E., and Ooms, H. A. Effet d'une elevation aigue du taux des acides gras libres (NEFA) sur la tolerance glucidique et la reponse insulinique a l'hyperglycemie chez l'homme normal. Rev. Fr. Etudes *Clin. Biol. 13:* 62, 1968.

78. Pi-Sunyer, F. X., Hashim, S. A., and Van Itallie, T. B. Insulin and ketone responses to ingestion of medium and long-chain triglycerides in man. *Diabetes 18:* 96, 1969.

79. Bottger, I., Dobbs, R., Faloona, G. R., et al. The effects of triglyceride absorption upon glucagon, insulin and gut glucagon-like immunoreactivity. *J. Clin. Invest. 52:* 2532, 1973.

80. Eaton, R. P., and Kipnis, D. M. Effect of glucose feeding on lipoprotein synthesis in the rat. *Am. J. Physiol. 217:* 1153, 1969.

81. Fujita, Y., Gotto, A., and Unger, R. H. Relationships of insulin and glucagon to triglyceride levels during a high and low carbohydrate intake. *Diabetes 24:* 552, 1975.

82. Eaton, R. P., Schade, D. S., and Conway, M. Decreased glucagon activity: A mechanism for genetic and acquired endogenous hyperlipaemia. *Lancet 2:* 1545, 1974.

83. Livingston, J. M., Cuatrecasas, P., and Lockwood, D. H. Studies of glucagon resistance in large rat adipocytes. ^{125}I-labelled glucagon binding and lipolytic capacity. *J. Lipid Res. 15:* 26, 1974.

84. Blazquez, E., Rubalcava, B., Montesano, R., et al. Development of insulin and glucagon binding and the adenylate cyclase response in liver membranes of the prenatal, postnatal and adult rat: Evidence of glucagon "resistance". *Endocrinology 98:* 1014, 1976.

85. Lindsey, C. A., Santeusanio, F., Braaten, J., et al. Pancreatic alpha cell function in trauma. *J.A.M.A. 227:* 757, 1974.

86. Lindsey, C. A., Faloona, G. R., and Unger, R. H. Plasma glucagon levels during rapid exsanguination with and without adrenergic blockade. *Diabetes 24:* 313, 1975.

87. Rocha, D. M., Santeusanio, F., Faloona, G. R., et al. Abnormal pancreatic alpha cell function in bacterial infections. *N. Engl. J. Med. 288:* 700, 1973.

88. Willerson, J. T., Hutcheson, D., Leshin, S. J., et al. Serum glucagon and insulin levels and their relationship to blood glucose values in patients with acute myocardial infarction and acute coronary insufficiency. *Am. J. Med. 27:* 747, 1974.

89. Corey, L. C., Lowery, B. D., and Clautier, C. T. Blood sugar and insulin response in humans in shock. *Ann. Surg. 172:* 342, 1970.

90. Bauer, W. E., Vigas, S. N. M., Haist, R. E., et al. Insulin response during hypovolemic shock. *Surgery 66:* 80, 1969.

91. Moss, G. S., Cerchio, G. M., Siegel, D. C., et al. Serum insulin response in hemorrhagic shock in baboons. *Surgery 68:* 34, 1970.

92. Frohman, L. A., and Bernardis, L. L. Effect of hypothalamic stimulation on plasma glucose, insulin and glucagon levels. *Am. J. Physiol. 221:* 1596, 1971.

93. Marliss, E. B., Girardier, L., Seydoux, J., et al. Glucagon release induced by pancreatic nerve stimulation in the dog. *J. Clin. Invest. 52:* 1246, 1973.

94. Iversen, J. Adrenergic receptors in the secretion of glucagon and insulin from the isolated perfused canine pancreas. *J. Clin. Invest. 52:* 2102, 1973.

95. Porte, D., Jr., Graber, A. L. Kuzuya, T., et al. The effect of epinephrine on immunoreactive insulin levels in man. *J. Clin. Invest. 42:* 228, 1966.

96. Marco, J., Calle, C., Roman, D., et al. Hyperglucagonism induced by glucocortocoid treatment in man. *N. Engl. J. Med. 288:* 128, 1973.

97. Exton, J. H., Jefferson, L. S., Butcher, R. W., et al. Gluconeogenesis in the perfused liver. The effects of fasting, alloxan diabetes, glucagon, epinephrine, adenosine 3'5'-monophosphate and insulin. *Am. J. Med. 40:* 709, 1966.

97a. Woods, S. C., and Porte, D., Jr. Neural control of the endocrine pancreas. *Physiol. Rev. 54:* 596, 1974.

98. Christensen, N. J. Proceedings of the Symposium of the Kroc Foundation, Santa Ynez, California, March 1975.

99. Unger, R. H., and Orci, L. The essential role of glucagon in the pathogenesis of diabetes mellitus. *Lancet 1:* 14, 1975.

100. Sakurai, H., Dobbs, R., and Unger, R. H. The role of glucagon in the pathogenesis of the endogenous hyperglycemia of diabetes mellitus. *Metabolism* (in press).

101. Raskin, R., Fujita, Y., and Unger, R. H. Effect of insulin–glucose infusions on plasma glucagon levels in fasting diabetics and nondiabetics. *J. Clin. Invest. 56:* 1132, 1975.

102. Raskin, P., and Unger, R. H. Unpublished observations.

103. Muller, W. A., Faloona, G. R., Aguilar-Parada, E., et al. Abnormal alpha cell function in diabetes: Response to carbohydrate and protein ingestion. *N. Engl. J. Med. 283:* 109, 1970.

104. Buchanan, K. D., and McCarroll, A. M. Abnormalities of glucagon metabolism in untreated diabetes mellitus. *Lancet 2:* 1394, 1972.

105. Unger, R. H., Madison, L. L., and Muller, W. A. Abnormal alpha cell function in diabetics: Response to insulin. *Diabetes 21:* 301, 1972.

106. Aronoff, S., Bennett, P., Miller, M., et al. Evidence for the independence of the A-cell and B-cell dysfunction in human diabetes. *N. Engl. J. Med.* (submitted for publication).

107. Tan, M. H., Bottger, I., Unger, R. H., et al. Alpha cell function in genetic prediabetics. *Diabetes* (submitted for publication).

108. Kirk, R. D., Dunn, P. J., Smith, J. R., et al. Abnormal pancreatic alpha cell function in first-degree relatives of known diabetics. *J. Clin. Endocrinol. Metab. 40:* 913, 1975.

109. Orci, L., Bactens, D., Rufener, C., Amherdt, M., Ravazzola, M., Studer, P., Malaisse-Lagae, F., and Unger, R. H. Hypertrophy and hyperplasia of somatostatin-containing D-cells in diabetes. *Proc. Nat. Acad. Sci. 73:* 1338, 1976.

110. Munoz, L., Blazques, E., and Unger, R. H. Gastric A-cell function in normal and diabetic dogs. Diabetes *24 [Suppl. 2]:* 411, 1975.

111. Muller, W. A., Brennan, M. F., Tan, M. H., et al. Studies of glucagon secretion in pancreatectomized patients. *Diabetes 23:* 512, 1974.

112. Katsilambros, N., Rahman, Y. A., Fussganger, K. E., et al. Action of streptozotocin on insulin and glucagon response of rat islets. *Horm. Metab. Res. 2:* 268, 1970.

113. Lefebvre, P. J., and Luyckx, A. Effect of acute kidney exclusion by ligation of renal arteries on peripheral plasma glucagon levels and pancreatic glucagon production in the anesthetized dog. *Metabolism* (in press).

114. Wilmore, D. W., Lindsey, C. A., Faloona, G. R., et al. Hyperglucagonemia after burns. *Lancet 1:* 73, 1974.

115. Allison, S. P., Hinton, P., and Chamberlain, M. J. Intravenous glucose tolerance, insulin and free-fatty-acid levels in burned patients. *Lancet 2:* 1113, 1968.

116. Marco, J., Diego, J., and Villanueva, M. L. Elevated plasma glucagon levels in cirrhosis of the liver. *N. Engl. J. Med. 289:* 1107, 1973.

117. Walker, C., Peterson, W., Jr., and Unger, R. H. Blood ammonia levels in advanced cirrhotics during therapeutic elevation of the insulin: glucagon ratio. *N. Engl. J. Med. 291:* 168, 1974.

118. Leffert, H., Rubalcava, B., Blazquez, E., et al. Hormonal changes during liver regeneration. *Proc. Natl. Acad. Sci. USA 72:* 4033, 1975.

119. Reaven, G. M., Lerner, R. L., Stern, M. P., et al. Role of insulin in endogenous hypertriglyceridemia. *J. Clin. Invest. 46:* 1756, 1967.

120. McGavran, M. H., Unger, R. H., Recant, L., et al. A glucagon-secreting alpha cell carcinoma of the pancreas. *N. Engl. J. Med. 274:* 1408, 1966.

121. Mallinson, C. N., Bloom, S. R., Warin, A. P., et al. A glucagonoma syndrome. *Lancet 2:* 7871, 1974.

122. Yoshinega, T., Okuno, G., Shinji, Y., Tsujii, T., and Nishikawa, M. Pancreatic A-cell tumor associated with severe diabetes. *Diabetes 15:* 709, 1966.

79

Insulin and Glucagon Actions and Consequences of Derangements in Secretion

John E. Liljenquist
Ulrich Keller
Jean-Louis Chiasson
Alan D. Cherrington

INTRODUCTION

The human body is equipped with regulatory mechanisms designed to ensure an adequate supply of fuel to its various tissues in times of either feast or famine. The design is such that ingested substrates (carbohydrate, lipid, and protein) are diverted to storage (liver, fat, and muscle) during periods of feeding and are later utilized (glycogenolysis, gluconeogenesis, and ketogenesis) during periods of food deprivation. Two of the most important determinants of the flux of fuels into and out of storage forms are the pancreatic hormones insulin and glucagon. In most situations these two hormones are antagonistic and thereby play a role in the fine regulation of many metabolic processes. It is the purpose of this chapter to demonstrate the metabolic effects each hormone can have, to point out those actions which occur with physiologic amounts of either hormone, to illustrate the consequences of a deficiency of either hormone, and finally to examine the interac-

tions between the two hormones in metabolic regulation. The emphasis will be on in vivo data in an attempt to understand normal physiology as it occurs in intact animals and man. With an understanding of the normal situation, pathophysiologic states will then be examined. The reader is referred to recent review articles for a more exhaustive review of the in vitro evidence bearing on the material to be discussed.[1,2]

ACTIONS AND INTERACTIONS OF GLUCAGON AND INSULIN IN REGULATING HEPATIC GLUCOSE PRODUCTION

EFFECTS OF GLUCAGON ON HEPATIC GLYCOGEN METABOLISM

In 1923, Murlin et al.[3] hypothesized the existence of a pancreatic hormone which raised the blood sugar instead of lowering it, as did insulin, and called this hormone *glucagon* (although for many years it was simply referred to as *hyperglycemic glycogenolytic factor*). It was not until 1953 that glucagon was isolated and crystallized.[4,5] The elucidation of its amino acid sequence[6] in 1956 and the establishment of an immunoassay for determination of its plasma concentration[7] in 1959 did much to promote investigation into glucagon's metabolic actions, particularly its stimulatory effect on hepatic glucose output. Glucagon is now known to increase glucose production through stimulatory effects on both glycogenolysis and gluconeogenesis.[8,9] Since glucose production in the postabsorptive state is primarily attributable to glycogenolysis,[9,10] this aspect of the hormone's actions will be discussed first.

The stimulatory effect of glucagon on glycogen breakdown is thought to be mediated by an increase in the intracellular level of cAMP.[1,2] Indeed, glucagon has been shown to elevate cAMP levels in the livers of various mammals,[11] in perfused rat liver,[12] and in isolated rat liver cells.[13,14] In addition, it has been shown to increase the release of cAMP from the liver in man.[15] The mechanism by which increased cAMP levels stimulate glycogenolysis has at least been partially clarified. The cyclic nucleotide enhances the process through a complex activation of phosphorylase. The first step in the sequence appears to be the allosteric activation of cAMP-dependent protein kinase, which then activates phosphorylase kinase.[14,16,17] This enzyme in turn catalyzes the conversion of inactive phosphorylase b to active phosphorylase a.[16,17] The activated form of phosphorylase then causes the breakdown of glycogen, yielding glucose-1-phosphate and, ultimately, glucose.

It is noteworthy that the protein kinase which catalyzes the phosphorylation of phosphorylase b also catalyzes the phosphorylation of glycogen synthase.[18,19] Although phosphorylation occurs in both cases, it results in activation of phosphorylase but in inactivation of glycogen synthase.[20,21] Recent studies have shown that the enzymes regulating glycogen synthesis and breakdown are themselves directly interrelated in a complex manner such that a change in the activity of phosphorylase per se alters the activity of the synthase.[22-24] Data have also recently accumulated indicating that a rise in cytosolic calcium can cause activation of phosphorylase and promote glycogen breakdown.[25,26] It has been suggested in fact that this ion may be the intracellular mediator involved in the stimulation of glycogenolysis by α-adrenergic agents, and by vasopressin and angiotensin.[25] Evidence currently available suggests that modification of intracellular calcium levels plays little or no role in the effects of glucagon on glycogenolysis.[25,26]

Glucagon's glycogenolytic action in vivo was clearly demonstrated as early as 1964, when it was shown to stimulate hepatic glucose production in man.[27] Note the widening of the hepatic vein–arterial glucose concentration difference and the rapid development of hyperglycemia in four human subjects receiving constant infusions of the hormone depicted in Figure 79-1. It should again be pointed out that glycogenolysis is responsible for 75–85 percent of glucose production after an overnight fast, and thus the increase in glucose production observed under such conditions is primarily attributable to stimulation of glycogenolysis.[8,10] Studies by DeBodo et al.,[28] in which glucose production was measured using a tracer method, also demonstrated glucagon's ability to stimulate glucose output in vivo. In both of these studies, however, the amounts of glucagon used were large, undoubtedly resulting in circulating glucagon levels far in excess of those normally found in plasma. More recently, physiologic amounts of glucagon

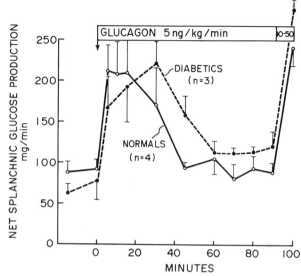

Fig. 79-2. Effect of glucagon infusions (5 ng/kg/min) on net splanchnic glucose production in 4 normal (○——○) and 3 diabetic (●——●) men. Data are expressed as means ± SE. The infusion rates were increased between 90 and 100 min to 10–50 ng/kg/min. (From Bomboy et al. *Diabetes 26:* 180, 1977.

have been shown to elicit glycogenolytic responses in vivo. Using measurements of splanchnic arteriovenous differences, Bomboy et al.[29] and Felig et al.[30] demonstrated that in man plasma glucagon levels of 500 pg/ml, which are within the range found in portal venous plasma,[31,32] resulted in a greater than twofold increase in the rate of glucose production. Similar results were obtained by Cherrington et al.[33] using a tracer method in dogs.

While glucagon's effect on glycogenolysis is potent and rapid in onset, it does not seem to persist for long periods of time.[29,30,34] Studies in normal and insulin-dependent diabetic man by Bomboy et al.[29] showed that while administration of glucagon at 5 ng/kg/min caused a prompt increase in splanchnic glucose production, its effect had disappeared within 45–60 min despite persisting hyperglucagonemia and despite the inability of the diabetics to secrete insulin (Fig. 79-2). These data thus suggest the existence of a non–insulin-mediated mechanism which limits glucagon-stimulated hepatic glucose production. Similarly, the glucagon-induced hepatic release of cAMP in man also follows a spike-decline pattern.[15] The mechanism by which this "down regulation" occurs is not known, but its importance to the concept of the insulin–glucagon molar ratio is obvious and will be discussed later.

In summary, glucagon is a potent stimulator of hepatic glucose production (glycogenolysis) in postabsorptive animals, including man. It is effective at concentrations well within the range of those found in the portal vein under various physiologic circumstances. The effect of elevated glucagon levels on glycogenolysis is manifest very quickly but wanes with time both in the presence and absence of counterregulatory changes in insulin secretion.

EFFECTS OF INSULIN ON HEPATIC GLYCOGEN METABOLISM

In the 30 years following the discovery of insulin, no direct effects of the hormone on hepatic glucose metabolism were convincingly demonstrated. By 1958, Haft and Miller had developed a liver perfusion system sufficiently sensitive to demonstrate the now classical action of insulin to convert the liver from a glucose-producing organ to a glucose-consuming organ.[35] Mortimore, in

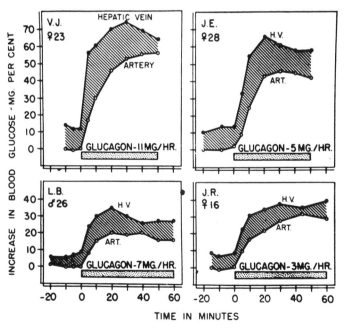

Fig. 79-1. Increases in arterial and hepatic venous glucose concentrations during continuous, 1-hour iv infusion of glucagon in four control subjects. Shaded areas represent hepatic vein–arterial glucose differences (From Kibler et al. J. Clin. Invest.)

1963, reported studies which verified the ability of insulin to decrease hepatic glucose production,[36] and later he and co-workers showed that this effect was associated with an inhibition of glycogenolysis.[37]

The mechanism by which insulin inhibits glycogenolysis is not completely understood. The hormone has been shown to lower cAMP levels in perfused liver[38] and in isolated rat liver cells.[39] The result of this, as one would expect, is a reduction in cAMP-dependent protein kinase activity and in phosphorylase activity. The mechanism by which insulin alters the hepatic cAMP concentration remains uncertain. Increased hepatic phosphodiesterase activity may contribute to this effect. In a recent study physiologic insulin concentrations markedly increased hepatic phosphodiesterase activity,[39] although this effect was not observed in previous studies.[40] Stimulation of this enzyme would enhance hydrolysis of cAMP and, in the face of unchanged adenylate cyclase activity, would result in a reduction in the cAMP level. This reduction would of course reverse the sequence of events previously described when the effect of glucagon on the glycogenolytic cascade was discussed.

Insulin's ability to lower cAMP concentrations may, however, only partly explain the action of the hormone on glycogen metabolism. Work by Shen et al.[41] suggests that insulin may also inhibit glycogenolysis by inhibiting the action of cAMP on protein kinase. (As discussed later in this chapter, insulin infusion in the intact dog not only results in a rapid inactivation of hepatic phosphorylase, but also in a rapid activation of hepatic glycogen synthetase, i.e., an increase in the I form of the enzyme. Bishop[42] has presented data suggesting that insulin may activate a phosphatase that catalyzes the dephosphorylation of the D form of glycogen synthetase to the I form.)

Even before in vitro evidence accumulated with regard to the hepatic effects of insulin on glucose metabolism, a study in vivo had suggested its inhibitory effect on glucose output. In 1952, Bearn et al.[43] administered insulin to human subjects who had undergone hepatic vein catheterization and noted a decrease in the release of glucose from the liver. Further evidence concerning the role of insulin in the regulation of hepatic glucose production in vivo has come from the work of Madison and co-workers.[44] They demonstrated the ability of insulin to reduce hepatic glucose output in dogs by infusing insulin concomitantly with glucose to prevent hypoglycemia and the counterregulatory changes which would otherwise have occurred (Fig. 79-3). This finding was later confirmed by Starzl et al.,[45,46] Steele et al.,[47] and Bishop et al.[48]

While the potential of insulin to inhibit glucose production was established in the 1960s, it was not until the early 1970s that physiologic levels of the hormone were shown to be effective. Long et al.,[49] using an isotope dilution technique in man, demonstrated that a modest rise in insulin induced by a glucose infusion resulted in a 75 percent decrease in glucose production without changing peripheral glucose oxidation, suggesting that the liver was the major site of action of small increments in circulating insulin. This study, however, failed to take into account any alterations in the plasma glucagon or glucose level per se. Similar results have been obtained by Felig et al.[50,51] in experiments in man using the hepatic vein catheterization technique. In these studies, a low-dose glucose infusion (2mg/kg/min) produced modest hyperglycemia and hyperinsulinemia, no change in the plasma glucagon levels, and an 85 percent decline in splanchnic glucose production. When the same glucose infusion was administered to diabetic men, no decrease in splanchnic glucose production was noted. Thus, a change in plasma glucose per se was not capable of altering hepatic glucose production unless accompanied by a rise in insulin. These

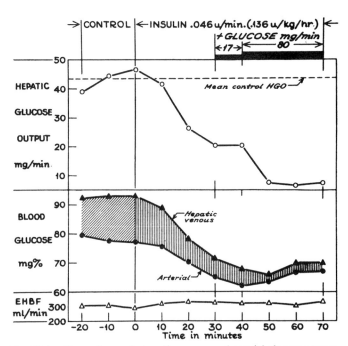

Fig. 79-3. Mean changes in hepatic venous and arterial glucose concentrations, hepatic blood flow, and the hepatic glucose output during the slow infusion of glucagon-free insulin plus glucose. (From Madison et al. *J. Clin. Invest. 39:* 513, 1960.)

data indicated that small increments in plasma insulin are capable of exerting potent inhibitory effects on hepatic glucose production. In other studies, Chiasson et al.[52] raised circulating insulin levels to 73 μU/ml in the dog while maintaining euglycemia by glucose infusion and observed a virtual abolition of splanchnic glucose production. While this study seems to demonstrate a direct effect of insulin on hepatic glucose production in vivo, a 30 pg/ml fall in circulating glucagon was observed, making interpretation somewhat difficult. Similar studies have been performed in man.[53]

Not only does insulin inhibit glucose production (glycogenolysis), it also stimulates hepatic glucose storage. In studies in the dog, Bishop et al.[48] administered insulin along with sufficient glucose to maintain normoglycemia. Under these conditions, insulin stimulated the incorporation of ^{14}C-glucose into glycogen. This action of insulin to stimulate glycogen synthesis, however, is highly dependent on the prevailing plasma glucose concentration. Chiasson et al.[52] have shown that net splanchnic glucose storage did not occur in the presence of hyperinsulinemia when the plasma glucose concentration was held at basal levels by concomitant glucose infusion. In order to achieve net hepatic glucose uptake, Madison et al.[54] have shown that hyperinsulinemia must be accompanied by hyperglycemia (Fig. 79-4). On the other hand, if hyperglycemia is not accompanied by hyperinsulinemia, as in diabetes, no net glucose storage as glycogen occurs until insulin is added.[55]

These studies suggest that in the whole animal insulin has a definite role in stimulating glycogen synthesis. This hypothesis, however, appears to contradict a large body of evidence from in vitro studies which suggests that it is the glucose level per se rather than the insulin level which is the major determinant of the rate of glycogen synthesis, as discussed by Hers,[23] a concept initially proposed by Soskin and Levine[55a] and supported by recent studies of Glinsmann et al.[56] and Bucolo et al.[57] The reason for this apparent discrepancy between these in vivo and in vitro studies is unclear. One factor which may minimize the in vivo actions of glucose to inactive phosphorylase a is glucagon, which in basal

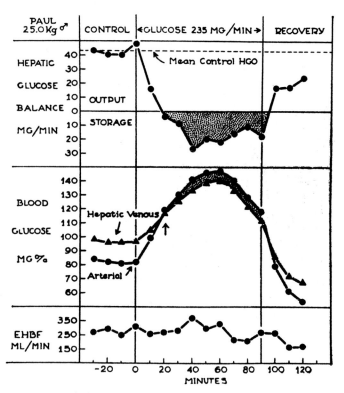

Fig. 79-4. Typical example of change in hepatic metabolism from output of glucose to uptake of glucose during glucose infusions in nondiabetic dogs. Liver changed from organ of glucose output to one of glucose uptake when arterial glucose concentration was raised to 120 mg/100 ml. EHBF, estimated hepatic blood flow. Reprinted from Madison, L. *The Archives of Internal Medicine,* March 1969, Volume 123: 284, copyright 1969, American Medical Association.

concentrations has been shown to play an important role in maintaining hepatic glucose production.[31]

In summary, physiologic increments in circulating insulin can decrease hepatic glucose output by inhibiting glycogenolysis. This effect of insulin does not require hyperglycemia. The effects of insulin on glycogen synthesis, however, are closely related to the circulating glucose concentration. Contrary to in vitro reports suggesting that glucose is more important than insulin in regulating hepatic glucose balance, the data in whole animals and man suggest that both are important and that it is the interaction of insulin and glucose which determines the rate of glycogen storage. While the plasma glucose concentration influences the amount of glucose to be stored in the liver, the plasma insulin level determines whether there will be storage or not.

EFFECTS OF GLUCAGON ON HEPATIC GLUCONEOGENESIS AND GLUCONEOGENIC SUBSTRATE SUPPLY

The first evidence that glucagon influenced amino acid metabolism was obtained in 1953 when Tyberheim increased urea excretion in rabbits by treating them with glucagon.[58] Similar results were soon obtained in man.[59] It is now thought that glucagon exerts its effect on amino acid metabolism primarily by affecting the metabolic fate of amino acids within the liver.[9] The hormone enhances their conversion into glucose; in other words, glucagon modifies amino acid metabolism primarily by stimulating hepatic gluconeogenesis. While the process of gluconeogenesis is of minor importance to overall glucose production after an overnight fast, it

becomes important during prolonged periods of fasting, in exercise, and in neonatal life as well as under certain pathologic conditions such as diabetes and adrenal insufficiency.[10]

Glucagon has been shown to rapidly enhance gluconeogenesis from lactate, pyruvate, alanine, and glycerol in the perfused rat liver and in isolated hepatocytes.[60-63] Since these effects can be mimicked by exogenous cAMP and are preceded by a rise in the intracellular level of the nucleotide and activation of cAMP-dependent protein kinase,[14] it is considered that they are mediated via this nucleotide. However, efforts to link cAMP or protein kinase to the phosphorylation or activation of specific gluconeogenic enzymes in vivo or in vitro have not been successful and the precise site(s) of action of glucagon in this process remains unknown.

Various studies in which the effects of glucagon on the levels of metabolic intermediates within the liver and on the fate of isotopic precursors have identified two points in the gluconeogenic pathway as probable sites of glucagon and/or cAMP action. These are between pyruvate and phosphoenolpyruvate and between fructose-1,6-diphosphate and glucose-6-phosphate.[61] A more detailed description of the postulated mechanisms by which glucagon could act at these sites can be found elsewhere.[64] It should be noted that glucagon is now also thought to inhibit glycolysis.[65,66] Pilkis et al.[65] have shown that the hormone reduces the conversion of labeled dihydroxyacetone into lactate in hepatocytes from fed rats. This effect is probably the result of a cAMP-induced phosphorylation of pyruvate kinase which results in inactivation of the enzyme.[67-69] This could contribute to the enhancement of gluconeogenesis since recycling of substrate through pyruvate kinase is substantial in liver.[70] Lastly, it has been suggested that glucagon might affect gluconeogenesis by enhancing the transport of alanine and other amino acids across the hepatocyte membrane.[67,71] In studies in vivo,[9] however, glucagon infusions resulting in levels of up to 5000 pg/ml did not result in increased splanchnic extraction of alanine.[9]

Despite the original observation in vivo of increased ureogenesis after glucagon administration and plentiful evidence from in vitro studies all suggesting that glucagon indeed promotes gluconeogenesis,[72] studies in vivo directly establishing glucagon as a gluconeogenic hormone have only recently been performed. In 1974, Cherrington and Vranic[34] showed that large increments in plasma glucagon resulted in increased recycling of glucose in the dog, a finding which was explained by a stimulation of gluconeogenesis. In the same year, Chiasson et al.[73] published data demonstrating the ability of glucagon at high but still physiologic levels to stimulate the conversion of ^{14}C-alanine to ^{14}C-glucose in the dog. Figure 79-5 illustrates data from similar studies by the same group[9] which showed that physiologic levels of glucagon are also capable of enhancing gluconeogenesis in man. In this study, ^{14}C-alanine was administered as a constant infusion and its conversion into ^{14}C-glucose by the liver was determined. Infusion of glucagon at 15–50 ng/kg/min resulted in a 93 percent increase in the net splanchnic production of ^{14}C-glucose. This gluconeogenic effect of glucagon was exerted in the absence of any increase in net splanchnic alanine extraction. Thus glucagon was shown to exert its gluconeogenic effect on an intrahepatic step rather than on membrane transport.

While glucagon has potent stimulatory effects on hepatic gluconeogenesis, its role in regulating gluconeogenic substrate supply appears to be limited. Haas et al.[74] could demonstrate no effect of glucagon on alanine release from rat skeletal muscle, while Ruderman and Berger[75] found glucagon to be without effect on glutamine and alanine formation in the same tissue. Pozefsky et al.,[76] in human forearm studies, noted that the flux of amino acids and lactate across skeletal muscle was not affected by increasing con-

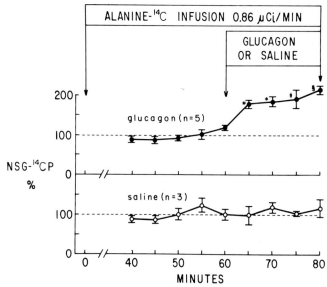

Fig. 79-5. Effects of glucagon (●——●) and saline (○——○) on the net splanchnic ^{14}C-glucose production (NSG-^{14}CP) expressed as a percent of mean baseline value. Values are means ± SEM. The following p values are indicated: *, < 0.02; ‡, < 0.05; §, < 0.01. (From Chiasson et al. *Diabetes 24*: 580, 1975.

centrations of glucagon. While glucagon has not been shown in isolated skeletal muscle preparations to affect amino acid flux, glucagon administration in the intact animal and man does result in declines in several plasma amino acids, especially alanine, the major gluconeogenic amino acid.[10] This decline in circulating alanine in response to glucagon occurs without an increase in splanchnic alanine uptake[9] and occurs in diabetic man, who secretes no insulin in response to the glucagon, as indicated by no rise in circulating C-peptide reactivity.[77] Marliss et al. have also described a hypoaminoacidemic effect of low doses of glucagon administered during prolonged fasting and showed that it was not associated with increased urea production or increased insulin secretion.[78] These findings suggest that glucagon may have a modest effect in regulating the circulating levels of various amino acids; the site of this action remains unknown.

In summary, glucagon has been shown to stimulate the conversion of lactate, pyruvate, alanine, and glycerol into glucose. It does so primarily by affecting enzymes in the gluconeogenic and glycolytic pathways within the liver in a manner not yet completely understood but apparently involving cAMP. The effects of glucagon on substrate supply and amino acid membrane transport appear to be small in magnitude and probably are of little or no significance in man. Glucagon exerts its effects on gluconeogenesis rapidly and does so at concentrations well within the physiologic range.

EFFECTS OF INSULIN ON HEPATIC GLUCONEOGENESIS AND GLUCONEOGENIC SUBSTRATE SUPPLY

Diabetes mellitus had been known for centuries to be a disease that may be associated with muscle wasting. Studies performed soon after the discovery of insulin indicated that insulin administration could reverse the negative nitrogen balance so characteristic of this disease. It is now known from a variety of in vitro studies that insulin can inhibit the action of glucagon or catecholamines on gluconeogenesis.[13,38,66] This effect is probably in part

due to the ability of insulin to lower cAMP levels, as discussed earlier. Evidence is also available, however, to suggest that this hormone may work in other ways. For example, insulin can inhibit the stimulation of gluconeogenesis by the α-adrenergic agonist phenylephrine, which does not alter cAMP levels.[79] It can also suppress the stimulatory effect of glucagon on liver cells incubated in the absence of extracellular Ca^{++} even though it apparently does not lower cAMP levels under those conditions.[38] The nature of the cAMP-independent mechanism by which insulin may reduce gluconeogenesis is unknown.

Despite abundant in vitro evidence for insulin's inhibitory action on gluconeogenesis, there is a paucity of such data in vivo. DeMeutter et al.[80] showed that insulin could suppress the accelerated ^{14}C-glucose production which was observed during labeled lactate administration in diabetic man. These results, however, could be interpreted to mean that the insulin effect was either due to inhibition of gluconeogenesis, increased storage of ^{14}C-glucose as glycogen, or accelerated peripheral glucose uptake. Nadkarni and Chitnis[81] administered ^{14}C-glycine to rats and noted decreased ^{14}C-glucose accumulation in liver glycogen, blood glucose, and muscle glycogen after insulin administration, suggesting inhibition of gluconeogenesis from glycine. More recently, Chiasson et al.[52,53] have demonstrated that insulin at plasma levels within the physiologic range could markedly suppress the conversion of ^{14}C-alanine into ^{14}C-glucose in both the dog and man. Furthermore, these authors showed that the drop in splanchnic ^{14}C-glucose production could not be explained by an intrahepatic diversion of the newly synthesized glucose into glycogen.

Unlike glucagon, insulin exerts a marked peripheral effect, thereby regulating gluconeogenic substrate supply to the liver as well as the intrahepatic fate of the extracted precursors. Insulin lowers plasma amino acid levels[82] and has been shown to decrease forearm release of certain amino acids.[83] Since the hormone is antilipolytic it also tends to reduce the level of glycerol in plasma.[84]

In addition, it has also been suggested that insulin may inhibit gluconeogenesis by decreasing the hepatic extraction of various gluconeogenic precursors. Infusion of glucose into man resulted in hyperglycemia, hyperinsulinemia, and a 30–60 percent decline in the splanchnic uptake of various amino acids.[50] Similar results were obtained in experiments in which oral glucose tolerance tests were given to men with hepatic vein catheters in place.[85] Chiasson et al., however, demonstrated that raising the insulin to over 200 μU/ml failed to alter splanchnic extraction of alanine.[52] Since the latter result was obtained in an experiment where normoglycemia was maintained, the question is raised as to whether it is the glucose rather than the insulin or a combination of the two which is modifying splanchnic amino acid uptake.

Insulin thus appears to exert its inhibitory effects on hepatic gluconeogenesis in two ways: (1) by decreasing the flow of gluconeogenic substrates from the periphery, and (2) by directly inhibiting their conversion into glucose within the liver. It seems unlikely that modification of precursor uptake by the liver plays a major role in the effect of the hormone on gluconeogenesis. It is also clear that insulin can exert its effects at plasma concentrations found under a variety of physiologic conditions.

INTERACTION OF GLUCAGON AND INSULIN IN THE REGULATION OF HEPATIC GLYCOGENOLYSIS AND GLUCONEOGENESIS

In the preceding sections, we have described the separate actions of insulin and glucagon in regulating glycogenolysis and gluconeogenesis. At this point, we shall present evidence to sug-

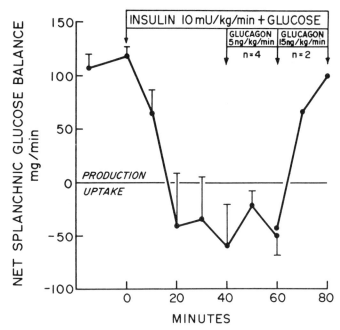

Fig. 79-6. Effect of a 10 mU/kg/min insulin infusion on splanchnic glucose balance before and during infusions of glucagon at 5 and 15 ng/kg/min. Sufficient glucose was infused to prevent hypoglycemia. (From Bomboy et al. *J. Clin. Endocrinol. Metab. 44:* 476, 1977.)

gest that a dynamic interaction exists between these two hormones which results in the fine regulation of glycogenolysis and gluconeogenesis in vivo.

Several studies in vitro have examined this interaction. Jefferson et al.[86] and Glinsmann and Mortimore,[87] using perfused rat liver, and Wagle,[88] using isolated hepatocytes, have shown that insulin can inhibit glucagon-stimulated glycogenolysis. Furthermore, Mackrell and Sokal[89] have shown that insulin can inhibit glucagon-induced activation of hepatic phosphorylase. Several groups[35,87,89,90] have shown that low levels of insulin can markedly inhibit ureogenesis stimulated by glucagon. In addition, Pilkis et al.[13] have recently reported that insulin can inhibit glucagon-stimulated gluconeogenesis in isolated hepatocytes.

In vivo studies demonstrating the interaction of insulin and glucagon in regulating hepatic glucose production have been more difficult to perform. Bomboy et al.[91] demonstrated the potential ability of insulin to inhibit the glycogenolytic response to glucagon in man. In this study (Fig. 79-6) supraphysiologic levels of insulin (1500 μU/ml) were maintained by constant infusion of the hormone and glucose was infused to avoid hypoglycemia. Under such conditions, infusion of glucagon at 5 ng/kg/min had no effect on splanchnic glucose production. Increasing the glucagon infusion to 15 ng/kg/min, on the other hand, increased splanchnic glucose production, thus overcoming insulin's inhibitory effect. While this study demonstrated an ability of the two hormones to interact in vivo, it was not until recently that the interaction of physiologic amounts of insulin and glucagon in the regulation of hepatic glucose production has been examined in vivo. Felig et al.[30] infused glucose (2 mg/kg/min) into normal men such that small increments in plasma glucose and insulin occurred and resulted in an 85–100 percent inhibition of splanchnic glucose output. The addition of glucagon (3 ng/kg/min), which raised plasma glucagon levels by 272 ± 30 pg/ml, resulted in an intermediate reversal of this inhibition of splanchnic glucose production. These data point out the ability of an increment in circulating glucagon within the physiologic range to reverse an inhibition of glucose production by physiologic increases in insulin and glucose.

The importance of the interaction of basal levels of insulin and glucagon in regulating hepatic glucose production after an overnight fast has been examined by Cherrington et al.[31] In these studies performed in dogs, somatostatin,[92] a recently discovered polypeptide hormone which inhibits insulin and glucagon secretion when administered systemically,[93] was used as a tool to dissect the individual roles of each hormone in the control of glucose output. Figure 79-7 outlines the results from these studies. When somatostatin alone was administered, resulting in combined insulin and glucagon deficiency, glucose production measured by either isotopic dilution or arteriovenous difference techniques fell by 40 percent over a 60-min period. When somatostatin was administered along with an intraportal replacement infusion of insulin so as to maintain normal plasma insulin levels, a state of selective glucagon deficiency was produced which also resulted in a 40 percent decline in glucose production. When isolated insulin deficiency was produced by infusing somatostatin plus an intraportal replacement infusion of glucagon, glucose production rose by 60 percent. When both hormones were replaced intraportally during somatostatin infusion, glucose production remained unchanged, indicating that somatostatin was exerting its effects on glucose production only through its inhibition of pancreatic islet cell secretion. Virtually identical results were obtained by Jennings et al.[94] for the regulation of gluconeogenesis in the postabsorptive state as assessed by the conversion of ^{14}C-alanine to ^{14}C-glucose across the splanchnic bed. These results suggest that basal glucagon plays an important role in the maintenance of hepatic glucose production in vivo and that a lack of glucagon results in hypoglycemia. Furthermore, they show that the role of basal insulin is to restrain the stimulatory effects of glucagon on this process and that an acute deficiency of insulin results in hyperglycemia. Thus, the fine regulation of basal hepatic glucose production is the result of the ongoing interaction between the basal amounts of these two hormones.

We have performed similar studies in man.[95] Infusion of somatostatin plus insulin in sufficient amounts to maintain arterial insulin levels of 10–14 μU/ml produced a state of selective hypoglucagonemia. Under these conditions, splanchnic glucose produc-

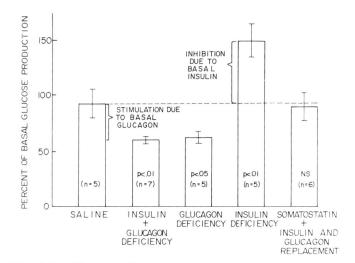

Fig. 79-7. Effects of saline, somatostatin, somatostatin + intraportal insulin, somatostatin + intraportal glucagon, and somatostatin + intraportal insulin and glucagon infusion in overnight fasted anesthetized dogs. Each bar represents the mean ± SEM percent change in the rate of glucose production (isotopically determined) during the last 50 min of the treatment period. The *p* values were obtained (nonpaired *t* test) by comparing the response in the treatment group to the saline-infused group. (From Cherrington et al. *J. Clin. Invest. 58:* 1415, 1976.)

tion fell by 75 percent and remained suppressed for the duration of the study. These data suggest that glucagon plays an important role in man in maintaining hepatic glucose production and that the body is not able to quickly compensate for its lack.

Some years ago it was suggested by Unger[96] that, since insulin and glucagon exert opposing effects on hepatic glucose flux, the circulating molar ratio of insulin to glucagon (I/G ratio) might most appropriately express the net metabolic effect to be expected of these two antagonistic hormones in a given situation. Recently, however, data have indicated that a given I/G ratio can be associated with quite different hepatic effects. Cherrington et al.[34] examined the relevance of the I/G ratio in vivo in studies in depancreatized dogs maintained on constant basal intraportal insulin infusions. In these dogs which could not mobilize extra insulin, glucagon administration caused glucose production to rise and then fall despite continuing hyperglucagonemia (i.e., despite a constant I/G ratio). In other similar studies glucose production could be maintained during glucagon infusion but only when the glucagon infusion rate was increased progressively.[97] These data in the dog suggested that the stimulatory effects of glucagon on hepatic glucose production waned with time. This hypothesis was tested and verified in man, as described earlier in this chapter,[29] by infusing glucagon in normal and diabetic man and noting that glucose production was stimulated only transiently despite continuing hyperglucagonemia. These findings indicated that a lowering of the I/G ratio can be associated with either basal or elevated rates of glucose production depending on when the observation was made.

Vranic et al.[98] have shown that the normally observed fall in circulating insulin and rise in circulating glucagon which accompany exercise in normal dogs are not necessary for the mediation of the increase in glucose production noted during exercise. These findings indicate that while the response of hepatic glucose production to exercise may conform to that predicted by changes in the I/G ratio (i.e., insulin decreased, glucagon increased, glucose production increased), in reality the increase in glucose production was not due to this alteration in I/G ratio. Thus, when changes in the circulating levels of glucagon and insulin occur, the metabolic results observed often do not conform to that predicted by the observed change in the I/G ratio or are not the consequence of the hormonal changes noted. Therefore, the original hope of those who proposed the concept of the I/G ratio as an expression of the net metabolic effect to be expected from the antagonism between circulating insulin and glucagon has not been realized.

In summary, a dynamic hepatic interaction exists between insulin and glucagon in the basal state. Basal glucagon stimulates glycogenolysis and gluconeogenesis and thus is important in the maintenance of the basal rate of hepatic glucose output. Basal insulin, on the other hand, exerts an inhibitory action on these processes, restraining the stimulatory effects of glucagon. The result of this interaction is the fine regulation of hepatic glucose production.

INTERACTION OF GLUCAGON AND INSULIN IN REGULATING GLUCOSE HOMEOSTASIS

It is the regulation of glucose homeostasis which is ultimately important to the well-being of the organism. Since glucose is such an important fuel for the brain and other tissues, it is crucial that the body handle it judiciously. Glucose homeostasis implies the maintenance of the circulating glucose concentration in a narrow concentration range under a wide variety of conditions. It is the purpose of this section to describe how synchronized changes in the concentrations of insulin and glucagon result in such a tight control of the glucose level.

A constant glucose level can only be maintained when the production of glucose (from liver or gut) and the removal of glucose (utilization by various tissues) from the circulation are balanced. When either the rate of production or utilization exceeds the other, a state of glucose disequilibrium will exist, resulting in hyperglycemia or hypoglycemia, either of which can be harmful. A regulatory system is present which stores glucose when it is in excess and which releases it for combustion during fasting and other times of need. In the preceding sections, we have described the actions and interactions of insulin and glucagon on hepatic glucose production. At this point, we shall attempt to demonstrate how the hepatic effects of these hormones on glucose production and their effects on peripheral glucose utilization interact in the whole animal to achieve glucose homeostasis.

It should be stated at the outset that little if any interaction occurs between insulin and glucagon in the regulation of peripheral glucose utilization. Insulin has been shown to have major effects in promoting glucose utilization in muscle and fat.[99] Studies in the perfused hind limb of the rat[74,75] and in human forearm[76] have suggested that glucagon has no effect on glucose utilization by muscle. Furthermore, studies in vivo in depancreatized dogs maintained on constant basal intraportal insulin infusions have shown that glucagon failed to alter peripheral glucose clearance.[34]

We shall now examine three metabolic situations in which the levels of insulin and glucagon change in various ways and will attempt to relate these changes to the control of glucose homeostasis. These situations are (1) protein ingestion (levels of both hormones increased), (2) strenuous exercise (insulin level diminished, glucagon level increased), and (3) carbohydrate ingestion (insulin level increased, glucagon level decreased).

Unger et al.[100] initially proposed that the stimulation of glucagon secretion which occurs during protein ingestion might be necessary to prevent hypoglycemia that might otherwise ensue due to the concomitant stimulation of insulin secretion. Cherrington et al.[97,101] in studies in dogs, delineated the roles of insulin and glucagon in maintaining glucose homeostasis during aminogenic stimulation of pancreatic hormone release.

In the first part of this study, arginine was infused intravenously into normal dogs. Endogenous insulin and glucagon secretion were both stimulated by the amino acid, as were the rates of glucose production and utilization. Since the increase in glucose production equaled the increase in glucose utilization the plasma glucose concentration remained unchanged. These authors then undertook another series of experiments to determine the role that the rises in circulating insulin and glucagon play in bringing about the increased glucose turnover. Dogs underwent pancreatectomy and simultaneous intraportal basal insulin replacement. Despite having persistent basal glucagon levels (derived from gastrointestinal α cells), these animals did not increase either insulin or glucagon secretion in response to arginine; as a result, they exhibited no increase in glucose production or utilization. Subsequently, arginine was again given, this time along with replacement infusions of insulin and glucagon at rates designed to achieve the same circulating insulin and glucagon levels as seen in normal dogs during arginine infusion. Restitution of the pancreatic hormone response restored the normal increases in glucose production and utilization and normoglycemia was again maintained. Inadequate replacement of insulin resulted in hyperglycemia, while inadequate replacement of glucagon resulted in hypoglycemia. These data represent the best example of a situation in which the interaction of these hormones at the liver results in a stimulation of glucose production which is balanced by an insulin-stimulated enhancement of peripheral glucose uptake so that glucose can be moved from its storage site in the liver to the periphery with minimal alteration of the plasma glucose concentration.

Wahren et al.[102] have performed similar studies involving protein ingestion in normal and diabetic men. When normal men ingest a pure protein meal, modest increases in plasma insulin and glucagon occur, yet the plasma glucose level remains unchanged. The rise in insulin is not sufficient to increase peripheral glucose utilization. Thus, the achievement of glucose homeostasis under these conditions occurs at the liver. Despite increases in both insulin and glucagon concentrations, splanchnic glucose output remains unchanged, thus indicating that the increases in insulin and glucagon offset each other in their action on glucose production. This was clearly shown to be the case when diabetics ingested the same protein meal. In these studies, plasma glucagon rose, but was not counteracted by a rise in insulin, and a result splanchnic glucose output increased and the plasma glucose rose.

These studies concerning aminogenic pancreatic hormone stimulation demonstrate clearly how glucose homeostasis can be maintained in situations in which both insulin and glucagon increase. In other situations, the hormone levels change in divergent directions and we will now examine the role of these changes in the maintenance of glucose homeostasis.

Vranic et al.[98] have attempted to define the roles of insulin and glucagon in regulating glucose production and utilization during strenuous exercise in dogs. Their data indicate that strenuous exercise is characterized by a threefold rise in the circulating glucagon level, a 50 percent decline in plasma insulin concentration, and a threefold increase in glucose production and utilization. Once again, however, since these changes occurred synchronously, euglycemia was maintained. The effects of similar exercise were then studied in depancreatized dogs whose basal insulin secretion was replaced by exogenous infusion. Although these animals could not mobilize extra insulin or glucagon in response to the stimulus of exercise, they exhibited near normal increases in glucose production and utilization. These data thus indicate that the increased glucose production and utilization seen during exercise are mediated in large measure by factors other than glucagon and insulin and that the body has other means to safeguard the plasma glucose level. When basal insulin was not supplied during the period of exercise, however, glucose utilization did not increase normally and hyperglycemia developed. Thus, while insulin does not appear to play the primary role in the increased glucose utilization of exercise, it does play a permissive role.

Another situation in which divergent changes in the levels of insulin and glucagon occur is that of carbohydrate ingestion. During ingestion of a carbohydrate load, the level of insulin in plasma increases while that of glucagon declines. These changes would be appropriate to minimize the alteration in the blood glucose level. It would appear, however, that it is the action of insulin which is the primary determinant of glucose homeostasis under these conditions and that the observed decline in circulating glucagon is not essential in maintaining glucose homeostasis. Felig et al.[50,51] administered small amounts of glucose intravenously in normal men, resulting in modest increments in plasma glucose and insulin, no change in plasma glucagon, and an 85 percent diminution in splanchnic glucose output. Sherwin et al.[103] infused glucagon (3 ng/kg/min) for 3 hours prior to and during oral glucose tolerance tests and noted no difference in glucose tolerance as compared to controls. These data indicate that the handling of a carbohydrate load appears to be determined in large measure by the interaction between insulin and glucose and is not dependent on the fall in circulating glucagon which usually accompanies the ingestion of carbohydrate meals.

In summary, glucose homeostasis is so important that the body has several mechanisms through which it regulates the glucose level. During protein ingestion, the hepatic interaction of insulin and glucagon plays a crucial role in maintaining euglycemia. After carbohydrate ingestion, however, the interaction of insulin and glucose rather than glucagon appears to be the major determinant of the rate of carbohydrate disposal. In strenuous exercise, in addition to insulin, other factors, perhaps involving the adrenergic nervous system, apparently play key roles in producing glucose homeostasis.

ACTIONS AND INTERACTIONS OF INSULIN AND GLUCAGON IN THE REGULATION OF LIPOLYSIS AND KETOGENESIS

Fat is stored in the body in adipocytes in the form of triglycerides. In situations of fuel need such as starvation the body becomes dependent on energy supply through mobilization of the stored fat. The hydrolysis of triglycerides yields free fatty acids (FFA) and glycerol. The FFA may be utilized in extrahepatic tissues or travel to the liver, where they are either oxidized or esterified into large molecules (triglycerides, phospholipids, etc.).[104]

FFA are also the precursors of the ketone bodies acetoacetate and β-hydroxybutyrate which can serve as fuels for most extrahepatic tissues. Increased fat mobilization and ketogenesis are characteristic features of insulin-deficient diabetes. There is now ample evidence that many metabolic processes in the adipocyte and in the liver are in large measure controlled through the actions and interactions of insulin and glucagon.

EFFECTS OF INSULIN ON LIPOLYSIS AND KETOGENESIS

Insulin can suppress ketogenesis through two major mechanisms: first, by inhibiting peripheral lipolysis and, thus, decreasing the flow of FFA to the liver; and, second, by a direct effect on the liver itself. It is well established that increasing the FFA flow to the liver will increase the ketone body production by that organ and vice versa.[105,106] Since insulin is known to be a potent inhibitor of lipolysis,[107-109] its antiketogenic action in vivo is at least in part the result of its ability to reduce the circulating FFA levels. FFA are the main precursor substrates for ketogenesis and the hepatic FFA extraction rate is known to be proportional to the circulating FFA concentration.[110] On the other hand, evidence has also been presented to show that insulin has a direct antiketogenic effect on the liver itself. Haft and Miller[111] demonstrated the ability of insulin to suppress ketogenesis in isolated livers of diabetic rats, and Foster[112] has reported similar findings in fasting rats in vivo. Bieberdorf et al.[113] maintained circulating FFA in the rat via an infusion of chylomicrons and heparin while administering insulin and, despite the absence of changes in FFA level, hepatic ketogenesis was markedly suppressed. Studies by Woodside and Heimberg[114] suggested that insulin decreases hepatic fatty acid oxidation and enhances entry of FFA into synthetic pathways. They showed that insulin, when given in vivo, decreases hepatic ketone output and increases triglyceride synthesis in livers of rats made acutely diabetic with antiinsulin serum.

It should also be pointed out that the circulating ketone level is not solely determined by ketone production but also by ketone utilization. Söling et al.[115] have demonstrated in vitro that insulin is capable of enhancing peripheral uptake of ketone bodies. Such an action of insulin in vivo would serve to lower circulating ketone levels. In that regard, Balasse and Havel[116] have demonstrated that ketone body utilization is impaired in diabetic dogs.

Of all these actions of insulin, the potent antipolytic effect of the hormone probably plays the dominant role in normal man to control ketogenesis, as there can be only little ketone production when a limited amount of ketone substrate (FFA) is provided. As detailed in Chapter 80, insulin plays a major role in the regulation of hepatic ketogenesis that appears to be localized at the reactions concerned with the transfer of long-chain fatty acids across the inner mitochondrial membrane, and there is little doubt that increased hepatic ketogenesis is a major determinant of the hyperketonemia associated with fasting and diabetes.

EFFECTS OF GLUCAGON ON LIPOLYSIS AND KETOGENESIS

Glucagon has been shown to be lipolytic in many animal species.[117-120] In man, however, its effect has been difficult to demonstrate. In studies utilizing human adipocytes glucagon had only a modest lipolytic effect.[121-124] Studies performed in intact man have demonstrated only transient lipolytic responses to large doses of glucagon.[125-126] Indeed, early studies in vivo in various species, including man, showed a marked decline in circulating FFA after glucagon administration,[127-130] but this was attributed to the glucagon-induced rise in plasma insulin[131] and the antilipolytic effects of the latter.

As insulin is such a potent inhibitor and glucagon a weak stimulator of lipolysis in man, any effect of glucagon on lipolysis will most likely be noted only when insulin is low or absent. In this regard, recent studies in diabetic man demonstrated that glucagon administration results in an increase in plasma glycerol, which is an index of lipolysis (Fig. 79-8).[132] The ability of glucagon to stimulate lipolysis in man has also been demonstrated by Gerich et al.,[133] who withdrew insulin from diabetic subjects and allowed ketosis to develop. One group of such subjects received a somatostatin infusion at the same time as insulin was withdrawn in order to markedly suppress endogenous glucagon secretion. In this group, the circulating FFA and glycerol rose much more slowly than in the diabetics in whom glucagon was not suppressed, suggesting a

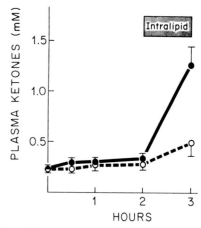

Fig. 79-9. Effects of acute elevation of plasma free fatty acid concentration on plasma ketone levels in rats receiving a glucagon infusion. Fed animals received guinea pig serum with (•) or without (o) glucagon for a period of 3 h. At the 2-h time point another 50 U of heparin was given and an infusion of Intralipid was started at a rate of 20 μl/min. A further 50 U of heparin was given after 2.5 h. Values represent means ± SEM for four animals in each group. (From McGarry et al. J. *Clin. Invest.* 55: 1205, 1975.)

definite lipolytic role for endogenous glucagon in this setting of hypoinsulinemia. As mentioned before, the rate of ketone body synthesis by the liver is determined in part by the amount of FFA delivery to the liver. Thus, any increase in FFA supply to the liver induced by glucagon-stimulated lipolysis would lead to enhanced ketogenesis. In addition to its lipolytic action in various animal species, glucagon has been shown to have a direct ketogenic effect in rat liver.[90,134-136] Similar effects were observed after glucagon injection in normal men.[126] This action appears to be mediated within the liver by shunting extracted FFA away from pathways of triglyceride synthesis toward oxidative pathways (i.e., ketogenesis and Krebs cyclic oxidation).[137,138]

INTERACTION OF INSULIN AND GLUCAGON IN THE REGULATION OF LIPOLYSIS AND KETOGENESIS

Evidence has accumulated during the past years that ketotic states such as fasting or diabetes are characterized not only by accelerated FFA mobilization but also by an enhanced capacity of the liver to oxidize FFA.[139] McGarry and Foster have suggested that hepatic ketogenesis is under bihormonal control and is turned "on–off" by the relative blood concentrations of insulin and glucagon.[136] These investigators noted that the rat liver develops an enhanced capacity for long-chain fatty acid oxidation and ketogenesis after 6–9 hours of fasting. During fasting, insulin levels fall and glucagon levels rise. When similar hormonal changes were induced by infusing glucagon or antiinsulin serum into fed rats, the liver in both cases switched from a nonketogenic to a ketogenic profile within 1 hour; that is, the liver developed the capacity to rapidly oxidize long-chain fatty acids. However, the infusion of glucagon into fed rats increased ketone levels only when FFA were elevated by simultaneous infusion of Intralipid and heparin (Fig. 79-9).[136] Thus, significant stimulation of ketogenesis by glucagon in vivo requires increased FFA supply and enhanced hepatic capacity for long-chain FFA oxidation, neither of which are seen in a physiologic setting when insulin levels are elevated.

Liljenquist et al.[132] and Gerich et al.[133] have shown in studies in diabetic man that glucagon can accelerate ketogenesis. Whether this was a direct hepatic effect of glucagon, however, could not be answered in these studies as glucagon markedly augmented lipoly-

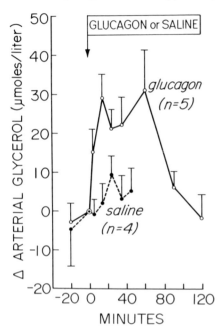

Fig. 79-8. Effect of glucagon and saline on the change in arterial glycerol concentration in diabetic men. Mean values ± SE are shown. (From Lilijenquist et al. *J. Clin. Invest.* 53: 192, 1974.)

sis in both studies, thus providing increased ketogenic substrate for the liver. Thus, it remained to be established whether glucagon in physiologic concentrations could stimulate ketogenesis directly during states of insulin deficiency. Furthermore, it had not been clarified if basal levels of glucagon stimulate ketogenesis in the nondiabetic state. Answers to these questions can be obtained from the studies of Keller et al.[140] in which the interactions of basal insulin, glucagon, and FFA on the hepatic production of ketone bodies in fasting anesthetized dogs were studied. Somatostatin was used to produce an acute deficiency of both insulin and glucagon. The metabolic effects were compared to those obtained in two groups of dogs receiving somatostatin in combination with an intraportal replacement of glucagon or insulin, resulting in selective deficiencies of glucagon or insulin. In all experiments FFA were acutely elevated by infusion of Intralipid and heparin in the second part of the study in order to assess the combined effect of substrate elevation and altered pancreatic hormone levels on ketogenesis.

Figure 79-10 demonstrates the results of this study. In saline controls (Fig. 79-10A), hepatic ketone production increased during Intralipid and heparin infusion. Deficiency of both insulin and glucagon induced by somatostatin infusion (Fig. 79-10B) resulted in a slight but insignificant increase in ketone production at both low and high FFA levels. In contrast, maintenance of glucagon at basal levels during somatostatin-induced insulinopenia (Fig. 79-10C) was associated with a significant rise of hepatic ketone output at both FFA levels. The highest rate of ketogenesis was observed with the combination of insulin deficiency, basal levels of glucagon, and FFA elevation. Isolated glucagon deficiency (Fig. 79-10D) did not alter the rate of ketone production, which indicates that the restraining effect of basal insulin completely overrides the ketogenic potential of basal glucagon. Of particular interest was the finding that the stimulatory effect of glucagon on ketogenesis could be exerted without increased lipolysis or enhanced hepatic FFA uptake. From these data it was concluded that basal levels of glucagon exert a powerful ketogenic action during acute insulin deficiency. This effect was due to an intrahepatic effect since FFA uptake was not affected. A maximal ketogenic rate ensued following abundant FFA supply, and an altered metabolic set of the liver was induced by glucagon when accompanied by insulin deficiency.

Evidence has now accumulated suggesting that the control site of hepatic ketogenesis resides in the carnitine acyltransferase enzyme system.[141,142] This enzyme promotes the reversible coupling of long-chain fatty acids to carnitine, which is required for the translocation of the fatty acid to the mitochondrial oxidation site. In studies using the medium-chain fatty acid octanoate and (−)-octanolycarnitine, McGarry et al.[142] demonstrated that the activity of this enzyme is increased in ketotic rat liver. Since fatty acid β-oxidation is a rate-limiting step in hepatic ketone body production, enhanced fatty acid oxidation results in increased ketogenesis. In recent studies the same authors provided further insight into the relationship between glucagon and accelerated ketogenic capacity of the liver.[143] It had previously been noted that glucagon, when given in vitro failed to activate ketogenesis despite a marked activation of glycogenolysis.[136] These data suggested that an extrahepatic factor present in vivo might mediate the glucagon effect. Determination of carnitine content in rat livers demonstrated a positive correlation with hepatic ketogenic capacity. In addition, perfusion of rat livers with carnitine induced stimulation of ketogenesis. It was hypothesized from these studies, therefore, that increased hepatic carnitine content observed during glucagon administration was the result of increased carnitine mobilization from peripheral tissues.[143] There is also evidence to suggest that glyco-

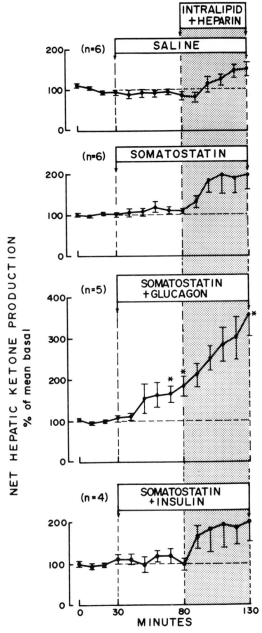

Fig. 79-10. Effects of various infusions on net hepatic ketone production. A. Saline. B. Somatostatin. C. Somatostatin with intraportal replacement of glucagon. D. Somatostatin with intraportal replacement of insulin. During acute free fatty acid elevation induced by infusion of Intralipid and heparin, net hepatic ketone production increased significantly after 100 min in all animals compared to the preinfusion value ($p < 0.01$). In the group treated with somatostatin and glucagon, net hepatic ketone production was significantly higher than in saline controls ($p < 0.01$) and dogs treated with somatostatin alone ($p < 0.05$). Values are means ± SE. (From Keller et al. *Diabetes 26:* 1040, 1977.)

gen depletion plays a contributing role in the glucagon-mediated stimulation of ketogenesis.[134,144]

In summary, while both insulin and glucagon have been demonstrated to exert effects on lipolysis and ketogenesis in vivo, and to do so at physiologic concentrations, insulin must be assigned the predominant role in normal man in regulating ketogenesis, both by its powerful restraining effect on lipolysis at the adipocyte and on FFA oxidation at the liver. Only in states of hypoinsulinemia does it appear that the actions of glucagon on both lipolysis and ketogenesis become manifest. Data will be presented in the next section which suggest that under such circumstances (diabetes mellitus), glucagon may play a significant role in stimulating ketogenesis.

CONSEQUENCES OF DERANGEMENTS IN SECRETION OF INSULIN AND GLUCAGON

In the previous sections, we have tried to present an integrated picture of the actions and interactions of insulin and glucagon in the regulation of glucose homeostasis, lipolysis, and ketogenesis. In the final section, we will examine the consequences of derangements in secretion of these two hormones in intact animals and man. Based on the material previously presented, we should be able to predict the nature of the metabolic abnormalities that occur when hormonal secretion is altered.

DIABETES MELLITUS

Certainly the classic disease state to be included in such a discussion is diabetes mellitus. Not only does insulinopenia exist, but hyperglucagonemia also frequently is present, possibly as an inherent part of the disease.[145,146] Until recently, the metabolic sequelae of diabetes have been attributed to the lack of insulin alone, glucagon being felt to play little or no role in the pathogenesis of this condition.[147] It was felt that insulin lack alone resulted in lipolysis, elevated circulating FFA levels, accelerated ketogenesis, and hyperglycemia. Since insulin replacement resulted in a disappearance of all these abnormalities, it was felt unnecessary to postulate a role for glucagon in their pathogenesis. While it has been possible to withdraw insulin from diabetic subjects to determine the effects of its absence, until recently there was no way to selectively withdraw glucagon and to determine the effects of its absence. While pancreatectomy in the dog produces total insulin lack, Cherrington et al. initially noted that plasma glucagon levels were present at their basal concentration.[97] This observation led to the discovery of glucagon-secreting cells in the gastrointestinal tract[148] which are capable of maintaining basal plasma glucagon concentrations after pancreatectomy.[149–151] Whether this is the case in depancreatized man remains unclear, although two studies have failed to find significant amounts of glucagon in depancreatized man.[152,153] It should be pointed out, however, that these patients were receiving daily insulin injections and full expression of gastrointestinal α-cell activity may only be manifested in insulin-deprived states.[151] Regardless of whether depancreatized humans have significant glucagon levels, virtually all diabetics exhibit normal or elevated glucagon levels.[96,145] The recent availability of somatostatin, however, has allowed for the acute induction of glucagon deficiency, as this agent is capable of suppressing glucagon secretion from α cells both in the pancreas and gut,[154] thus opening a new era of investigation into the effects of glucagon.

The studies of Cherrington et al.[155] suggest that glucagon could in fact contribute to the hyperglycemia which occurs in diabetes. In these studies (Fig. 79-11), somatostatin was infused into dogs to inhibit endogenous insulin and glucagon secretion, but the glucagon level was maintained by infusing glucagon intraportally in basal amounts (0.8 ng/kg/min). Removal of insulin's inhibitory effect resulted in a rapid glucagon-induced increase in glucose production. Since the rate of glucose production initially exceeded the rate of utilization, glucose accumulated in the blood, resulting in hyperglycemia. As with absolute elevations of glucagon, the effects of a relative hyperglucagonemia also waned with time, such

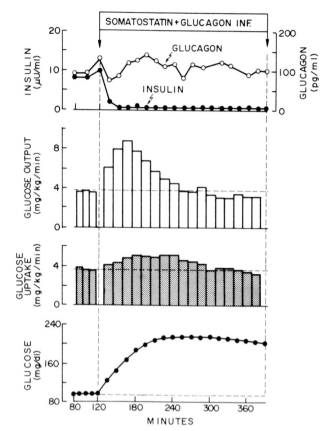

Fig. 79-11. Effects of an intravenous infusion of somatostatin and an intraportal infusion of glucagon at 0.8 ng/kg/min. A. Effect on plasma insulin and glucagon levels. B. Effect on glucose output. C. Effect on glucose uptake. D. Effect on plasma glucose concentration. Glucose output and uptake were measured by an isotopic dilution technique using ^{3}H-glucose. (From Cherrington et al. Unpublished observations.)

that within 2 hours the rate of glucose production was again basal and almost equivalent to the rate of glucose utilization. Once this balance was reestablished, the glucose remaining in the vascular compartments was trapped. Normally, insulin release would have returned the glucose levels to normal, but in this somatostatin-treated animal, insulin could not be mobilized. Interestingly, glucose utilization was normal in the face of insulin lack, but only because the plasma glucose level was twice normal and was thereby compensating for insulin lack by increasing the glucose gradient across the cell membrane. This study shows clearly that in times of hypoinsulinemia a burst of glucagon-induced glucose production, even if evanescent, can contribute to a prolonged period of hyperglycemia.

Gerich et al.[156] have reported data in diabetic man which suggest that inhibition of glucagon secretion by somatostatin during food ingestion results in a lessening of the postprandial plasma glucose rise. Although the rise in plasma glucose was less when somatostatin was administered and glucagon secretion was diminished, more recent studies suggest that somatostatin blunts gastrointestinal carbohydrate absorption, thus possibly explaining the blunted plasma glucose rise.[157]

Gluconeogenesis is also accelerated in diabetes mellitus. Bondy et al.[158] catheterized diabetic patients in ketoacidosis and noted not only accelerated glucose production across the splanchnic bed, but also a markedly increased rate of urea production, which was restored to normal by insulin administration. Wahren et al.[51] have demonstrated that the splanchnic uptake of several gluconeogenic amino acids is increased in diabetes. Furthermore, DeMeutter and Shreeve[80] demonstrated that ^{14}C-glucose derived from labeled pyruvate or lactate reached higher plasma levels in diabetic than in normal men. The studies of Jennings et al.,[94] noted earlier, demonstrated that gluconeogenesis was markedly stimulated when hypoinsulinemia and normoglucagonemia existed simultaneously. These data all indicate that gluconeogenesis is accelerated in diabetes and suggest that this increase in gluconeogenic rate is in large measure due to glucagon acting on this process unopposed by insulin.

The most dangerous acute complication of diabetes mellitus, ketoacidosis, was felt for many years to be essentially the result of insulin lack alone. It was believed that insulinopenia led to accelerated peripheral lipolysis, increased FFA delivery to the liver, and accelerated ketogenesis. The studies of Gerich et al.[133] however, concerning the roles of insulin and glucagon in the development of ketoacidosis in diabetic man, have provided additional insight into this question. In these studies, diabetic subjects received a 14-hour insulin infusion, which resulted in normal plasma levels of β-hydroxybutyrate, glucose, and glucagon (Fig. 79-12). Insulin was then withdrawn and an infusion of somatostatin or saline begun. In the saline-treated patients, all three parameters rose rapidly after insulin withdrawal, while in the somatostatin-treated subjects, in whom glucagon was markedly suppressed, there was only a modest rise in plasma glucose and β-hydroxybutyrate. Not only was the hyperglycemia and hyperketonemia less in the patients in whom glucagon was suppressed, but the plasma FFA and glycerol concentrations were also less in these patients, suggesting that glucagon does have physiologic lipolytic as well as ketogenic and glycogenolytic actions in man when insulin is deficient. This study raises the question as to whether the therapeutic use of somatostatin might prove beneficial to human diabetics. While somatostatin

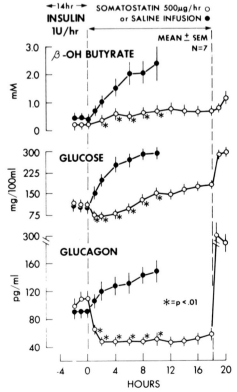

Fig. 79-12. Effect of somatostatin on plasma β-hydroxybutyrate (β-OH butyrate), glucose, and glucagon levels after acute withdrawal of insulin in seven patients with juvenile-type diabetes. (By permission, from Gerich et al. *The New England Journal of Medicine* 292: 986, 1975.

administration has been reported to diminish insulin requirements in diabetic patients,[159] the undesirable ability of somatostatin to inhibit growth hormone secretion might limit the usefulness of this agent in juvenile diabetics who are still growing. Should an analogue become available which specifically inhibited glucagon secretion, it might prove helpful. On the other hand, human patients who are diabetic secondary to pancreatic disease (pancreatitis, pancreatectomy) and are deficient in both insulin and pancreatic glucagon have been reported to be more susceptible to hypoglycemia.[160] Therapeutic use of an agent to inhibit glucagon secretion in diabetics might have a similar result.

The study of Gerich et al.[133] throws significant light on the bihormonal regulatory system which controls these processes of glycogenolysis, lipolysis, and ketogenesis in man. Of the two hormones, insulin certainly plays the more important role, as it has the ability to suppress glucagon secretion, and when insulin is present its antilipolytic and antiketogenic effects predominate. In its absence, however, glucagon does exert effects on these processes which accelerate the rate of development and magnify the amplitude of the metabolic abnormalities characteristic of uncontrolled diabetes mellitus.

The data presented above taken as a whole suggest strongly that the metabolic derangements characteristic of diabetes mellitus are indeed bihormonal in origin and that we are no longer justified in believing that insulin lack is the sole cause of these metabolic abnormalities.

OTHER CONDITIONS ASSOCIATED WITH ABNORMAL LEVELS OF GLUCAGON AND INSULIN

Only recently has the syndrome of hyperglucagonemia secondary to a glucagon-secreting α-cell tumor of the pancreas been described.[161] The syndrome is characterized by anemia, weight loss, stomatitis, diabetes, and a peculiar skin rash termed *necrolytic migratory erythema*. Based on the knowledge of the actions of glucagon outlined in this chapter, what should we expect to find in a patient with chronic pharmacologic levels of plasma glucagon? The syndrome has not been fully studied as yet, but certain abnormalities have been described. The most striking metabolic abnormality noted is the marked hypoaminoacidemia (Fig. 79-13). The hypoaminoacidemia is much more severe than in diabetes mellitus or in dietary protein deficiency. The mechanism for the development of the anemia, skin rash, weight loss, and hyperglycemia is not known but seems clearly associated with the hyperglucagonemia. It has been postulated that the skin lesion is due to the hypoaminoacidemia as the skin normally contains a high concentration of free amino acids.

There are many catabolic conditions, such as renal failure,[162] severe burns,[163] bacterial infections,[164] and hepatic cirrhosis[165] in which elevated glucagon levels have been reported. The role which glucagon plays in the catabolism of these disorders remains to be defined.

Persistently elevated levels of insulin have been reported in patients with insulin-producing β-cell tumors of the pancreas.[166] Fasting hypoglycemia is the most frequently occurring sign of this condition.[167] Suppression of hepatic glucose production probably plays a major role in the induction of the hypoglycemia associated with this condition. Amino acid metabolism and the process of gluconeogenesis have not been studied definitively in this condition.

Symptomatic hypoglycemia occurs in many clinical conditions besides insulinoma and may be the result of inappropriate insulin secretion.[168,169] A discussion of the many clinical entities

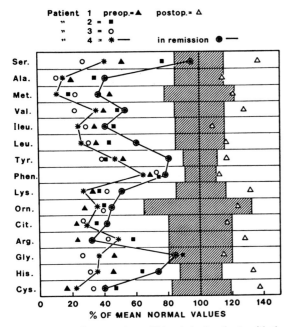

Fig. 79-13. Fasting plasma amino acid levels in 4 patients with the glucagonoma syndrome. Shaded area is mean ± 2 SD of normal values. (From Mallinson et al. Lancet ii 4, 1974.)

associated with hypoglycemia is beyond the scope of this chapter. For further information the reader is referred to appropriate reviews.[168,169]

SUMMARY

The data presented in this chapter provide strong evidence for the existence of a dynamic interaction between the two pancreatic hormones, insulin and glucagon, resulting in a fine regulation in vivo of several important metabolic processes. The emerging importance of glucagon as a participant rather than as a bystander in the regulation of hepatic glycogenolysis, gluconeogenesis, lipolysis, and ketogenesis is stressed. The major role of insulin in regulating these processes is redefined to make a place for the prominent role of glucagon. To insulin must be ascribed the more important role in regulating these processes, because it is able to suppress glucagon secretion and its inhibitory effects on peripheral release of substrate (FFA and amino acids) are not effectively counteracted by glucagon. Nonetheless, where insulin is low, glucagon is ready to exert its effects until overriden by insulin again. In diabetes mellitus, in which hypoinsulinemia and hyperglucagonemia are major characteristics of the disease state, the lack of glucose and ketone body homeostasis may in large measure be due to glucagon accelerating glucose production and ketogenesis unopposed by insulin. Thus, the metabolic derangements noted when an imbalance exists between insulin and glucagon are in large measure accounted for by the imbalance in hormone concentration.

REFERENCES

1. Exton, J. H., Park, C. R., Interaction of insulin and glucagon in the control of liver metabolism, in Greep, R. O., and Astwood, E. B. (eds): Handbook of Physiology, section 7, Endocrinology. Baltimore, Waverly, 1972, pp. 437–455.
2. Park, C. R., Exton, J. H., Glucagon and the metabolism of glucose, in Lefebvre, P. J., and Unger, R. H. (eds): Glucagon: Molecular Physiology, Clinical and Therapeutic Implications. Oxford, Pergamon, 1972, pp. 77–108.
3. Murlin, J. R., Clough, H. D., Gibbs, C. B. F., et al., Aqueous extracts of pancreas I. Influence on the carbohydrate metabolism of depancreatized animals. J. Biol. Chem. 56: 253, 1923.
4. Staub, A., Sinn, L., Behrens, O. K., Purification and crystallization of hyperglycemic glycogenolytic factor (HGF). Science 117: 628, 1953.
5. Staub, A., Sinn, L., Behrens, O. K., Purification and crystallization of glucagon. J. Biol. Chem. 214: 619, 1955.
6. Bromer, W. W., Sinn, L., Staub, L. G., et al., The amino acid sequence of glucagon. J. Am. Chem. Soc. 78: 3858, 1956.
7. Unger, R. H., Eisentraut, A. M., Keller, S., et al., Glucagon antibodies and their use for immunoassay for glucagon. Proc. Soc. Exp. Biol. Med. 102: 621, 1959.
8. Sutherland, E. W., Cori, C. F., Influence of insulin preparations on glycogenolysis in liver slices. J. Biol. Chem. 172: 737, 1948.
9. Chiasson, J. L., Liljenquist, J. E., Sinclair-Smith, B. C., et al., Gluconeogenesis from alanine in normal postabsorptive man. Intrahepatic stimulatory effect of glucagon. Diabetes 24: 574, 1975.
10. Felig, P., The glucose-alanine cycle. Metabolism 22: 179, 1973.
11. Goldberg, N. D., Dietz, S. B., O'Toole, A. G., Cyclic guanosine 3',5'-monophosphate in mammalian tissues and urine. J. Biol. Chem. 244: 4458, 1969.
12. Exton, J. H., Robison, G. A., Sutherland, E. W., et al., Studies on the role of adenosine 3',5'-monophosphate in the hepatic actions of glucagon and catecholamines. J. Biol. Chem. 246: 6166, 1971.
13. Pilkis, S. J., Claus, T. H., Johnson, R. A., et al., Hormonal control of cyclic 3',5'-AMP levels and gluconeogenesis in isolated hepatocytes from fed rats. J. Biol. Chem. 250: 6328, 1975.
14. Cherrington, A. D., Exton, J. H., Studies on the role of cyclic AMP-dependent protein kinase in the actions of glucagon and catecholamines on liver glycogen metabolism. Metabolism 25: 1351, 1976.
15. Liljenquist, J. E., Bomboy, J. D., Lewis, S. B., et al., Effect of glucagon on net splanchnic cyclic AMP production in normal and diabetic men. J. Clin. Invest. 53: 198, 1974.
16. Krebs, E. G., DeLange, R. J., Kemp, D. G., et al., Activation of skeletal muscle phosphorylase. Pharmacol. Rev. 18: 163, 1966.
17. Vandenheede, J. R., Keppens, S., DeWulf, H., The activation of liver phosphorylase b kinase by glucagon. FEBS Lett. 61: 213, 1976.
18. Soderling, T. R., Hickenbottom, J. P., Inactivation of glycogen synthetase and activation of phosphorylase b kinase by the same cyclic 3',5'-AMP-dependent kinase. Fed. Proc. 29: 601A, 1970.
19. Walsh, D. A., Krebs, E. G., Reimann, E. M., et al., The receptor protein for cyclic AMP in the control of glycogenolysis, in Greengard, P., and Costa, E. (eds): Role of Cyclic AMP in Cell Function. New York, Raven, 1970, p. 265.
20. DeWulf, H., and Hers, H. G., The interconversion of liver glycogen synthetase a and b in vitro. Eur. J. Biochem. 6: 552, 1968.
21. Larner J., Villar-Palasi, C., Goldberg, N. D., et al., Hormonal and nonhormonal control of glycogen synthesis. Control of transferase phosphatase and transferase I kinase. Adv. Enzyme Reg. 6: 409, 1968.
22. Hue, L., Bontemps, F., Hers, H. G., The effect of glucose and of potassium ions on the interconversion of the two forms of glycogen phosphorylase and of glycogen synthetase in isolated rat liver preparations. Biochem. J. 152: 105, 1975.
23. Hers, H. G., The control of glycogen metabolism in the liver. Annu. Rev. Biochem. 45: 167, 1976.
24. Hutson, N. J., Brumley, F. T., Assimacopoulos, F. D., et al., Studies on the α-adrenergic activation of hepatic glucose output. I. Studies on the α-adrenergic activation of phosphorylase and gluconeogenesis and inactivation of glycogen synthase in isolated rat liver parenchymal cells. J. Biol. Chem. 25: 5200, 1976.
25. DeWulf, H., Keppens, S., Is calcium the second messenger in liver for cyclic AMP-independent glycogenolytic hormones? Arch. Intern. Physiol. Biochim. 84: 159, 1976.
26. Assimacopoulos-Jeannet, F. D., Blackmore, P. F., Exton, J. H., Studies on the α-adrenergic activation of hepatic glucose output. III. Studies on the role of calcium in the α-adrenergic activation of phosphorylase. J. Biol. Chem. 252: 2662, 1977.
27. Kibler, R. F., Taylor, W. J., Myers, J. D., The effect of glucagon on net splanchnic balances of glucose, amino acid nitrogen, urea, ketones and oxygen in man. J. Clin. Invest. 43: 904, 1964.
28. DeBodo, R. C., Steele, R., Altszuler, N., et al., On the hormonal regulation of carbohydrate metabolism: Studies with ^{14}C-glucose. Recent Prog. Horm. Res. 19: 445, 1963.
29. Bomboy, J. D., Jr., Lewis, S. B., Lacy, W. W., et al., Transient

stimulatory effect of sustained hyperglucagonemia on splanchnic glucose production in normal and diabetic man. *Diabetes 26:* 177, 1977.

30. Felig, P., Wahren, J., Hendler, R., Influence of physiologic hyperglucagonemia on basal and insulin-inhibited splanchnic glucose output in normal man. *J. Clin. Invest. 58:* 761, 1976.

31. Cherrington, A. D., Chiasson, J. L., Liljenquist, J. E., et al., The role of insulin and glucagon in the regulation of basal glucose production in the post absorptive dog. *J. Clin. Invest. 58* 1407, 1976.

32. Blackard. W. G., Nelson, N. C., Andrews. S. S., Portal and peripheral vein immunoreactive glucagon concentrations after arginine or glucose infusions. *Diabetes 23:* 199, 1974.

33. Cherrington, A. D., Vranic, M., Fono, P., et al., Effect of glucagon on glucose turnover and plasma free fatty acids in depancreatized dogs maintained on matched insulin infusions. *Can J. Physiol. Pharm. 50:* 946, 1972.

34. Cherrington, A. D., Vranic, M., Effect of interaction between insulin and glucagon on glucose turnover and FFA concentration in normal and depancreatized dogs. *Metabolism 23:* 729, 1974.

35. Miller, L. L., Some direct actions of insulin, glucagon and hydrocortisone on the perfused rat liver. *Recent Prog. Horm. Res. 17:* 539, 1961.

36. Mortimore, G. E., Effect of insulin on release of glucose and urea by isolated rat liver. *Am. J. Physiol. 204:* 699, 1963.

37. Mortimore, G. E., King, E., Jr., Mondon, C. D., et al., Effects of insulin on net carbohydrate alterations in perfused rat liver. *Am. J. Physiol. 212:* 179, 1967.

38. Claus, T. H., Pilkis, S. J., Regulation by insulin of gluconeogenesis in isolated rat hepatocytes. *Biochem. Biophys. Acta. 421:* 246, 1976.

39. Loten, E. G., Unpublished observations.

40. Menahan, L. A., Hepp, K. D., Wieland, O., Liver 3',5'-nucleotide phosphodiesterase and its activity in rat livers perfused with insulin. *Eur. J. Biochem. 8:* 435, 1969.

41. Shen, L. C., Villar-Palasi, C., Larner, J., Hormonal alteration of protein kinase sensitivity to 3',5'-cyclic AMP. *Physiol. Chem. Phys. 2:* 536, 1970.

42. Bishop, J. S., Inability of insulin to activate liver glycogen transferase D phosphatase in the diabetic pancreatectomized dog. *Biochim. Biophys. Acta. 208:* 208, 1970.

43. Bearn, A. G., Billings, B. H., Sherlock, S., The response of the liver to insulin in normal subjects and in diabetes mellitus. *Clin. Sci. 11:* 151, 1952.

44. Madison, L. L., Coombes, B., Adams, R., et al., III. The physiological significance of the secretion of insulin into the portal circulation. *J. Clin. Invest. 39:* 507, 1960.

45. Starzl, T. E., Butz, G. W., Meyer, W. H., et al., Effect in dogs of various portal vein shunts on response to insulin. *Am. J. Physiol. 203:* 275, 1962.

46. Starzl. T. E., Scanlan, W. A., Thornton, F. H., et al., Effect of insulin on glucose metabolism in the dog after portacaval transposition. *Am. J. Physiol. 209:* 221, 1965.

47. Steele, R., Bishop, J. S., Dunn, A., et al., Inhibition by insulin of hepatic glucose production in the normal dog. *Am. J. Physiol. 208:* 301, 1965.

48. Bishop, J. S., Steele, R. Altszuler, N., et al., Effects of insulin on liver glycogen synthesis and breakdown in the dog. *Am. J. Physiol. 208:* 307, 1965.

49. Long. C. L., Spencer, J. L., Kinney, J. M., et al., Carbohydrate metabolism in normal man and effect of glucose infusion. *J. Appl. Physiol. 31:* 102, 1971.

50. Felig. P., Wahren, J., Influence of endogenous insulin secretion on splanchnic glucose and amino acid metabolism in man. *J. Clin. Invest. 50:* 1702, 1971.

51. Wahren, J., Felig. P., Cerasi, E., et al., Splanchnic and peripheral glucose and amino acid metabolism in diabetes mellitus. *J. Clin. Invest. 51:* 1870, 1972.

52. Chiasson, J. L., Liljenquist, J. E., Finger, F. E., et al., Differential sensitivity of glycogenolysis and gluconeogenesis to insulin infusions in dogs. *Diabetes 25:* 283, 1976.

53. Chiasson, J. L., Liljenquist, J. E., Cherrington, A. D., et al., The suppressive effect of insulin infusions on gluconeogenesis from alanine in normal man. (submitted for publication).

54. Madison, L. L., Role of insulin in the hepatic handling of glucose. *Arch. Intern. Med. 123:* 284, 1969.

55. Madison, L. L., Mebane, D., Lecocq, F., et al., Physiological signifiance of the secretion of endogenous insulin into the portal circulation. V. The quantitative importance of the liver in the disposition of glucose loads. *Diabetes 12:* 8, 1963.

55a. Soskin, S., Levine, R., Carbohydrate Metabolism. Chicago, Univ. Chicago Press, 1946, p. 315.

56. Glinsmann, W. H., Hern, E. P., Lynch, A., Intrinsic regulation of glucose output by rat liver. *Am. J. Physiol. 216:* 698, 1969.

57. Bucolo, R. J., Bergman, R. N., Marsh, D. J., et al., Dynamics of glucose autoregulation in the isolated blood-perfused canine liver. *Am. J. Physiol. 227:* 209, 1974.

58. Tyberghein, J., Action du glucagon sur le métabolisme des protéines. *Arch. Int. Physiol. 61:* 104, 1953.

59. Salter, J. M., Ezrin, C., Laidlaw, J. C., et al., Metabolic effects of glucagon in human subjects. *Metabolism 9:* 753, 1960.

60. Exton, J. H., Park, C. R., Control of gluconeogenesis in liver. II. Effects of glucagon, catecholamines, and adenosine 3',5'-monophosphate on gluconeogenesis in the perfused rat liver. *J. Biol. Chem. 243:* 4189, 1968.

61. Exton, J. H., Park, C. R., Control of gluconeogenesis in liver. III. Effects of L-lactate, pyruvate, fructose, glucagon, epinephrine and adenosine 3',5'-monophosphate on gluconeogenic intermediates in perfused rat liver. *J. Biol. Chem. 244:* 1424, 1969.

62. Mallette, L. E., Exton, J. H., Park, C. R., Control of gluconeogenesis from amino acids in perfused rat liver. *J. Biol. Chem. 244:* 5713, 1969.

63. Claus, T. H., Pilkis, S. J., Park, C. R., Stimulation by glucagon of the incorporation of U-^{14}C substrates into glucose by isolated hepatocytes from fed rats. *Biochim. Biophy. Acta. 404:* 110, 1975.

64. Exton, J. H., Vi, M., Lewis, S. B., et al., Mechanism of glucagon activation of gluconeogenesis, in Soling, H. D., and Willons, B. (eds): Regulation of Gluconeogenesis. New York, Academic, 1971, pp. 160–178.

65. Pilkis, S. J., Riou, J. P., Claus, T. H., Hormonal control of (^{14}C)-glucose synthesis from (U-^{14}C)-dihydroxyacetone and glycerol in isolated rat hepatocytes. *J. Biol. Chem.* (in press).

66. Felui, J. E., Hue, L., Hers, H. G., Hormonal control of pyruvate kinase activity and of gluconeogenesis in isolated hepatocytes. *Proc. Natl. Acad. Sci. U.S.A. 73:* 2762, 1976.

67. Lyungstrom, O., Helimquist, G., Engstrom. L., Phosphorylation of purfied rat liver pyruvate kinase by cyclic 3',5'-AMP-stimulated protein kinase. *Biochim. Biophys. Acta. 358:* 289, 1974.

68. Titanji, V. P. K., Zetterquist, O., Engstrom, L., Regulation *in vitro* of rat liver pyruvate kinase by phosphorylation-dephosphorylation reactions, catalyzed by cyclic AMP-dependent protein kinases and a histone phosphatase. *Biochim. Biophys. Acta. 422:* 98, 1976.

69. Ekman, P., Dahlquist, U., Humble, E., et al., Comparative studies on the L-type pyruvate kinase from rat liver and the enzyme phosphorylated by cyclic 3',5'-AMP-stimulated protein kinase. *Biochim. Biophys. Acta. 429:* 374, 1976.

70. Friedmann, B., Goodman, E. H., Jr., Saunders, H. L., et al., Regulation of metabolism in the liver. Estimation of pyruvate recycling during gluconeogenesis in perfused rat liver. *Metabolism 20:* 2, 1971.

71. Mallette, L. E., Exton, J. H., Park, C. R., Effects of glucagon on amino acid transport and utilization in the perfused rat liver. *J. Biol. Chem. 244:* 5724, 1969.

72. Garcia, A., Williamson, J. R., Cahill, G. F., Jr., Studies on the perfused rat liver. II. Effect of glucagon on gluconeogenesis. *Diabetes 15:* 188, 1966.

73. Chiasson, J. L., Cook, J., Liljenquist, J. E., et al., Glucagon stimulation of gluconeogenesis from alanine in the intact dog. *Am. J. Physiol. 227:* 19, 1974.

74. Haas, R., Clausen, E., Wood, C., et al., Effect of somatostatin, insulin and glucagon on glucose uptake and alanine release by the isolated perfused rat hindlimb. *Clin. Res. 23:* 110A, 1975.

75. Ruderman, N. B., Berger, M., The formation of glutamine or alanine in skeletal muscle. *J. Biol. Chem. 249:* 5500, 1974.

76. Pozefsky, T., Tancredi, R. G., Moxley, R. T., et al., Metabolism in forearm tissues in man. Studies with glucagon. *Diabetes 25:* 128, 1976.

77. Lacy, W. W., Lewis, S. B., Liljenquist, J. E., et al., Control of plasma amino acids by glucagon and insulin. *Diabetes 21:* 340, 1972 (Abstract).

78. Marliss. E. B., Aoki, T. T., Unger, R. H., et al., Glucagon levels and metabolic effects in fasting man. *J. Clin. Invest. 49:* 2256, 1970.

79. Cherrington, A. D., Assimacopoulos, F. D., Harper, S. C., et al., Studies on the α-adrenergic activation of hepatic glucose output. II. Investigation of the role of adenosine 3',5'-monophosphate and adenosine 3',5'-monophosphate-dependent protein kinase in the actions of phenylephrine in isolated hepatocytes. *J. Biol. Chem. 251:* 5209, 1976.

80. DeMeutter, R. C., Shreeve, W. W., Conversion of DL-Lactate-2-C[14] or 3-C[14] or pyruvate-2-C[14] to blood glucose in humans: Effects of diabetes, insulin tolbutamide and glucose load. *J. Clin. Invest.* 42: 525, 1963.

81. Nadkarni, G. B., Chitnis, K. E., Effect of insulin on gluconeogenesis from glycine-2-C[14]. *Arch. Biochem, Biophys.* 101: 466, 1973.

82. DeBarnola, F. V., The effect on insulin on plasma free amino acids. *Acta Physiol. Lat. Am.* 15: 260, 1965.

83. Pozefsky, T., Felig, P., Tobin, J. D., et al., Amino balance across tissues of the forearm in postabsorptive man. Effects of insulin at two dose levels. *J. Clin. Invest.* 48: 2273, 1969.

84. Hagen, J. H., The effect of insulin on concentration of plasma glycerol. *J. Lipid Res.* 4: 46, 1963.

85. Felig, P., Wahren, J., Hendler, R., Influence of oral glucose ingestion on splanchnic glucose and gluconeogenic substrate metabolism in man. *Diabetes* 24: 468, 1975.

86. Jefferson, L. S., Exton, J. H., Butcher, R. W., et al., Role of adenosine 3',5'-monophosphate in the effects of insulin and antiinsulin serum on liver metabolism. *J. Biol. Chem.* 243: 1031, 1968.

87. Glinsmann, W. H., Mortimore, G. E., Influence of glucagon and 3',5'-AMP on insulin responsiveness of the perfused rat liver. *Am. J. Physiol.* 215: 553, 1968.

88. Wagle, S. R., Interrelationship of insulin and glucagon ratios on carbohydrate metabolism in isolated hepatocytes containing high glucagon. *Biochem. Biophys. Res. Commun.* 67: 1019, 1975.

89. Mackrell, D. J., Sokal, J. E., Antagonism between the effects of insulin and glucagon on the isolated liver. *Diabetes* 18: 724, 1968.

90. Menahan, L. A., Wieland, O., Interactions of glucagon and insulin on the metabolism of perfused livers from fasted rats. *Eur. J. Biochem.* 9: 55, 1969.

91. Bomboy, J. D., Lewis, S. B., Sinclair-Smith, B. C., et al., Insulin–glucagon interaction in controlling splanchnic glucose production in normal man. *J. Clin. Endocrinol. Metab.* 44: 474, 1977.

92. Brazeau, P., Vale, W., Burgus, R., et al., Hypothalamic peptide that inhibits the secretion of immunoreactive pituitary growth hormone. *Science* 179: 77, 1973.

93. Koerker, D. J., Ruch, W., Chideckel, E., et al., Somatostatin: Hypothalamic inhibitor of the endocrine pancreas. *Science* 184: 482, 1974.

94. Jennings, A. S., Cherrington, A. D., Liljenquist, J. E., et al., The role of insulin and glucagon in the regulation of gluconeogenesis in the postabsorptive dog. *Diabetes* 26: 847, 1977.

95. Liljenquist, J. E., Mueller, G. L., Cherrington, A. D., et al., Evidence for an important role of glucagon in the regulation of hepatic glucose production in normal man. *J. Clin. Invest.* 59: 369, 1977.

96. Unger. R. H., Glucagon and the insulin:glucagon ratio in diabetes and other catabolic illnesses. *Diabetes* 20: 834, 1971.

97. Cherrington, A. D., Kawamori, R., Pek, S., et al., Arginine infusions in dogs: Model for the roles of insulin and glucagon in regulating glucose turnover and free fatty acid levels. *Diabetes* 23: 805, 1974.

98. Vranic, M., Kawamori, R., Pek, S., et al., The essentiality of insulin and the role of glucagon in regulating glucose utilization and production during utilization and production during strenous exercise in dogs. *J. Clin. Invest.* 57: 245, 1976.

99. Park, C. R., The transport of glucose and other sugars across cell membranes and the effect of insulin, in Wolstenholme, G. E. W., and O'Connor, C. M. (eds): Ciba Foundation Colloquia on Endocrinology, vol. 9, Internal Secretion of the Pancreas. Boston, Little, Brown, 1956, pp. 240–265.

100. Unger, R. H., Ohneda, A., Aguilar-Parada, E., et al., The role of aminogenic glucagon secretion in blood glucose homeostasis. *J. Clin. Invest.* 48: 810, 1969.

101. Cherrington, A. D., Vranic, M., Effect of arginine on glucose turnover and plasma free fatty acids in normal dogs. *Diabetes* 22: 537, 1973.

102. Wahren, J., Felig, P., Hagenfeldt, L., Effect of protein ingestion on splanchnic and leg metabolism in normal man and in patients with diabetes mellitus. *J. Clin. Invest.* 57: 987, 1976.

103. Sherwin, R. S., Fisher, M., Hendler, R., et al., Hyperglucagonemia and blood glucose regulation in normal, obese and diabetic subjects. *N. Engl. J. Med.* 294: 455, 1976.

104. Ontko, J. A., Metabolism of free fatty acids in isolated liver cells. Factors affecting the partition between esterification and oxidation. *J. Biol. Chem.* 247: 1788, 1972.

105. Mayes, P. A., Studies on the major pathways of hepatic lipid metabolism using the perfused liver, in Jeanrenaud, B., and Hepp, D. (eds): Adipose Tissue, Regulation and Metabolic Functions. New York, Academic, 1970, p. 186.

106. Exton, J. H., Corbin, J. G., Park, C. R., Control of gluconeogenesis in liver. IV. Differential effect of fatty acids and glucagon on ketogenesis and gluconeogenesis in the perfused rat liver. *J. Biol. Chem.* 244: 4095, 1969.

107. Mahler, R., Stafford, W. S., Tarrant, M. E., et al., The effect of insulin on lipolysis. *Diabetes* 18: 297, 1964.

108. Khoo, J. C., Steinberg, D., Thompson, B., et al., Hormonal regulation of adipocyte enzymes. The effects of epinephrine and insulin on the control of lipase, phosphorylase kinase, phosphorylase and glycogen synthetase. *J. Biol. Chem.* 248: 3823, 1973.

109. Zierler, K. L., Rabinowitz, D., Effect of very small concentrations of insulin on forearm metabolism. Persistence of its actions on potassium and free fatty acids without an effect on glucose. *J. Clin. Invest.* 43: 950, 1964.

110. Aydin, A., Sokal, J. E., Uptake of plasma free fatty acids by the isolated rat liver: Effect of glucagon. *Am. J. Physiol.* 205: 667, 1963.

111. Haft, D. E., Miller, L. L., Alloxan diabetes and demonstrated direct action of insulin on metabolism of isolated perfused rat liver. *Am. J. Physiol.* 192: 33, 1958.

112. Foster, D. W., Studies in the ketosis of fasting. *J. Clin. Invest.* 46: 1283, 1967.

113. Bieberdorf, F. A., Chernick, S. S., Scow, R. O., Effect of insulin and acute diabetes on plasma FFA and ketone bodies in the fasting rat. *J. Clin. Invest.* 49: 1685, 1970.

114. Woodside, W. F., Heimberg, M., Effects of anti-insulin serum, insulin and glucose on output of triglycerides and on ketogenesis by the perfused rat liver. *J. Biol. Chem.* 251: 13, 1976.

115. Söling, H. D., Garlepp, H. J., Creutzfeldt, W., Die wirkung von insulin und glukose und die Ketokörperanfnahme total eviszerierter, normaler, hungernder und alloxandiabetischer Ratten. *Biochim. Biophys. Acta* 100: 530, 1965.

116. Balasse, E. O., Havel, R. J., Evidence for an effect of insulin on the peripheral utilization of ketone bodies in the dog. *J. Clin. Invest.* 50: 801, 1971.

117. Lewis, G. P., Matthews, J., The mobilization of free fatty acids from rabbit adipose tissue *in situ. Br. J. Pharmacol.* 34: 564, 1968.

118. Goodrich, A. G., Ball, E. G., Studies on the metabolism of adipose tissue. XVIII. *In vitro* effects of insulin, epinephrine and glucagon on lipolysis and glycolysis in pigeon adipose tissue. *Comp. Biochem. Physiol.* 16: 367, 1965.

119. Grande, F., Lack of insulin effect on free fatty acid mobilization produced by glucagon in birds. *Proc. Soc. Exp. Biol. Med.* 130: 711, 1969.

120. Lefebvre, P., The physiological effect of glucagon on fat mobilization. *Diabetologia* 2: 130, 1966.

121. Bjorntorp, P., Karlsson, M., Hovden, A., Quantitative aspects of lipolysis and reesterification in human adipose tissue *in vitro. Acta Med. Scand.* 185: 89, 1969.

122. Gries, F. A., Hormonal control of human adipose tissue metabolism *in vitro,* in Jeanrenaud, B., and Hepp, D. (eds): Adipose Tissue, Regulation and Metabolic Functions. New York, Academic, 1970, p. 167.

123. Burns, T. W., Langley, P. E., Adrenergic receptors and cyclic AMP in the regulation of human adipose tissue lipolysis. *Ann. N.Y. Acad. Sci.* 185: 115, 1971.

124. Mosinger, B., Kuhn, E., Kujalová, V., Action of adipokinetic hormones on human adipose tissue *in vitro. J. Lab. Clin. Med.* 66: 380, 1965.

125. Pozza, G., Pappalettera, A., Melogli, O., et al., Lipolytic effect of intraarterial injection of glucagon in man. *Horm. Metab. Res.* 3: 291, 1971.

126. Schade, D. S., Eaton, R. P., Modulation of fatty acid metabolism by glucagon in man. I. Effects in normal subjects. *Diabetes* 24: 502, 1975.

127. Dreiling, D. A., Bierman, E. L., Debons, A. F., et al., Effect of ACTH, hydrocortisone, and glucagon on plasma nonesterified fatty acid concentration (NEFA) in normal subjects and in patients with liver disease. *Metabolism* 11: 572, 1962.

128. Lipsett, M. B., Engel, H. R., Bergenstal, D. M., Effects of glucagon on plasma unesterified fatty acids and on nitrogen metabolism. *J. Lab. Clin. Med.* 56: 342, 1960.

129. Warembourg, H., Biserte, G., Jaillard, T., et al., Variations quantitatives et qualitatives des acides gras non estérifiés et des triglycerides circulants induites par le glucagon. *Clin. Chim. Acta.* 28: 103, 1970.

130. Lefebvre, P., Glucagon et taux sanguin des acides gras non estérifiés chez l'homme. *Ann. Endocrinol.* 26: 602, 1965.

131. Samols, E., Marri, G., Marks, V., Promotion of insulin secretion by glucagon. *Lancet 2:* 415, 1965.

132. Liljenquist, J. E., Bomboy, J. D., Lewis, S. B., et al., Effects of glucagon on lipolysis and ketogenesis in normal and diabetic man. *J. Clin. Invest. 52:* 190, 1974.

133. Gerich, J. E., Lorenzi, M., Bier, D. M., et al., Prevention of human diabetic ketoacidosis by somatostatin. Evidence for an essential role of glucagon. *N. Engl. J. Med. 292:* 985, 1975.

134. Haugaard, E. S., Haugaard, N., The effect of hyperglycemic–glycogenolytic factor on fat metabolism of liver. *J. Biol. Chem. 206: 641, 1954.*

135. Williamson, J. R., Effects of fatty acids, glucagon and anti-insulin serum on the control of gluconeogenesis and ketogenesis in rat liver. *Adv. Enzymol. Reg. 5:* 229, 1967.

136. McGarry, J. D., Wright, P. H., Foster, D. W., Hormonal control of ketogenesis. Rapid activation of hepatic ketogenic capacity in fed rats by anti-insulin serum and glucagon. *J. Clin. Invest. 55:* 1202, 1975.

137. Heimberg, M., Weinstein, I., Kohout, M., The effects of glucagon, dibutyryl cyclic adenosine 3′,5′-monophosphate and concentration of free fatty acid on hepatic lipid metabolism. *J. Biol. Chem. 244:* 5131, 1969.

138. Poledne, R., Mayes, P. A., Lipolysis and the regulation and fatty acid metabolism in the liver. *Biochem. J. 119:* 47P, 1970.

139. McGarry, J. D., Foster, D. W., Regulation of ketogenesis and clinical aspects of the ketotic state. *Metabolism 21:* 471, 1972.

140. Keller, U., Chiasson, J. L., Liljenquist, J. E., et al., The roles of insulin, glucagon and free fatty acids in the regulation of ketogenesis in dogs. *Diabetes 26:* 1040, 1977.

141. Fritz, I. B., An hypothesis concerning the role of carnitine in the control of interrelationships between fatty acid and carbohydrate metabolism. *Perspect. Biol. Med. 10:* 643, 1967.

142. McGarry, J. D., Foster, D. W., The metabolism of (−)-octanoylcarnitine in perfused livers from fed and fasted rats. Evidence for a possible regulatory role of carnitine acyltransferase in the control of ketogenesis. *J. Biol. Chem. 249:* 7984, 1974.

143. McGarry, J. D., Robles-Valden, C., Foster, D. W., The role of carnitine in hepatic ketogenesis. *Proc. Natl. Acad. Sci. USA 72:* 4385, 1975.

144. Blixenkrone-Møller, N., Respiratorischer Stoffwechsel und Ketonbildung der Leber. *Z. Physiol. Chem. 252:* 117, 1938.

145. Müller, W. A., Faloona, G. R., Aguilar-Parada, E., et al., Abnormal alpha-cell function in diabetes. Response to carbohydrate and protein ingestion. *N. Engl. J. Med. 283:* 109, 1970.

146. Gerich, J. E., Langlois, M., Noacco, C., et al., Comparison of the suppressive effects of elevated plasma glucose and free fatty acid levels on glucagon secretion in normal and insulin-dependent diabetic subjects. Evidence for selective alpha-cell insensitivity to glucose in diabetes mellitus. *J. Clin. Invest. 58:* 320, 1976.

147. Cahill, G. F., Jr., Physiology of insulin in man. *Diabetes 20:* 785, 1971.

148. Sasaki, H., Rubalcava, B., Baetens, D., et al., Identification of glucagon in the gastrointestinal tract. *J. Clin. Invest. 56:* 135, 1975.

149. Vranic, M., Pek, S. Kawamori, R., Increased "glucagon immunoreactivity" in plasma of totally depancreatized dogs. *Diabetes 23:* 905, 1974.

150. Matsuyama, T., Foa, P., Plasma glucose, insulin, pancreatic and enteroglucagon levels in normal and depancreatized dogs. *Proc. Soc. Exp. Biol. Med. 147:* 97, 1975.

151. Mashiter, K., Harding, P. E., Chou, M., et al., Persistent pancreatic glucagon but not insulin response to arginine in pancreatectomized dogs. *Endocrinology 96:* 678, 1975.

152. Müller, W. A., Brennan, M. F., Tan, M. H., et al., Studies of glucagon secretion in pancreatectomized patients. *Diabetes 23:* 512, 1974.

153. Barnes, A. J., Bloom, S. R., Pancreatectomized man: A model for diabetes without glucagon. *Lancet 1:* 219, 1976.

154. Sakurai, H., Dobbs, R. E., Unger, R. H., The role of glucagon in the pathogenesis of the endogenous hyperglycemia of diabetes mellitus. *Metabolism 24:* 1287, 1975.

155. Cherrington, A. D., Chiasson, J. L., Liljenquist, J. E., et al., Unpublished observations.

156. Gerich, J. E., Lorenzi, M., Schneider, V., et al., Effects of somatostatin on plasma glucose and glucagon levels in diabetes mellitus. *N. Engl. J. Med. 291:* 544, 1974.

157. Wahren, J., Felig, P., Somatostatin (SRIF) and glucagon in diabetes: Failure of glucagon suppression to improve i.v. glucose tolerance and evidence of an effect of SRIF on glucose absorption. *Clin. Res. 24:* 461A, 1976.

158. Bondy, P. K., Bloom, W. L., Whitner, V. S., et al., Studies on the role of the liver in human carbohydrate metabolism by the venous catheter technique. II. Patients with diabetic ketosis before and after the administration of insulin. *J. Clin. Invest. 28:* 1126, 1949.

159. Gerich, J., Lorenzi, M., Tsalikian, E., et al., Prolonged intravenous and subcutaneous somatostatin in treatment of human diabetes. *Diabetes 25 [Suppl. 1]:* 340, 1976.

160. Bank, S., The management of diabetes in the underprivileged with special reference to pancreatic diabetes. *S. Afr. Med. J. 40:* 342, 1966.

161. Mallinson, C. N., Bloom, S. R., Warin, A. P., et al., A glucagonoma syndrome. *Lancet 2:* 1, 1974.

162. Bilbrey, G. L., Faloona, G. R., White, M. G., et al., Hyperglucagonemia of renal failure. *J. Clin. Invest. 53:* 841, 1974.

163. Wilmore, D. W., Moylan, J. A., Pruitt, B. A., et al., Hyperglucagonemia after burns. *Lancet 1:* 73, 1974.

164. Rocha, D. M., Santeusanio, F., Faloona, G. R., Abnormal pancreatic alpha-cell function in bacterial infections. *N. Engl. J. Med. 288:* 700, 1973.

165. Marco, J., Diego, J., Villaneuva, M. L., et al., Elevated plasma glucagon levels in cirrhosis of the liver. *N. Engl. J. Med. 289:* 1107, 1973.

166. Scholz, D. A., Remine, W. H., Priestly, J. T., et al., Clinics on endocrine and metabolic diseases. Hyperinsulinism: review of 95 cases of functioning pancreatic islet cell tumors. *Proc. Staff Meet. Mayo Clin. 35:* 545, 1960.

167. Service, F. J., Dale, A. J. D., Elveback, L. R., et al., Insulinoma. Clinical and diagnostic features of 60 consecutive cases. *Mayo Clin. Proc. 51:* 417, 1976.

168. Arky, R. A., Pathophysiology and therapy of the fasting hypoglycemias. *DM,* February, 1968.

169. Hofeldt, F. D., Reactive hypoglycemia. *Metabolism 24:* 1193, 1975.

80

Regulation of Hepatic Ketogenesis

J. Denis McGarry
Daniel W. Foster

The ketone bodies, acetoacetate and β-hydroxybutyrate, accumulate in the blood of man under both physiological and pathological conditions. In the former they function to assure survival of the organism; in the latter they may cause its death. The regulation of hepatic ketogenesis, in which the endocrine system plays a significant role, and the relationship of the control of ketone body synthesis to the overall metabolic changes that accompany starvation and uncontrolled diabetes mellitus are the focus of this chapter.

PHYSIOLOGICAL PERSPECTIVE

The overall role of the ketone bodies* in normal physiology is now reasonably well understood.[1] In the fed state their rate of production by the liver is minimal and circulating plasma concentrations are low. When food is unavailable, on the other hand, rapid changes occur in body metabolism that cause a dramatic acceleration in the hepatic synthesis of acetoacetic and β-hydroxybutyric acids. In teleological terms the adaptive responses that occur during fasting can be considered to have as a primary purpose the provision of adequate substrate for energy production and for the maintenance of structural integrity of body tissues when glucose availability is limited. Of all these tissues the central nervous system appears to be most vulnerable to substrate deficiency. Under ordinary circumstances the brain utilizes glucose as an essentially exclusive substrate and does so in large amounts.[2,3] With the onset of fasting, as glucose derived from the diet disappears, two protective processes become operative. First, hepatic glucose output increases. This occurs initially via glycogen breakdown and subsequently by enhanced gluconeogenesis. Second, alternative substrate is provided through mobilization of free fatty acids from peripheral adipose tissue stores. A peculiarity of this

metabolic adaptation is that fatty acids are efficient fuels for respiration in almost all tissues, including heart, kidney, muscle, liver, and gut, while their direct oxidation by the brain in vivo occurs to only negligible degree.[4,5] The latter is true despite the fact that oxidation of isotopic fatty acids to CO_2 can be demonstrated by brain preparations in vitro.[6] In contrast, the ketone bodies can be efficiently utilized by the brain, both in vitro[6–8] and in vivo[9]; indeed, after prolonged starvation in man acetoacetate and β-hydroxybutyrate supply well over half the energy requirements of the central nervous system.[9] In adults the rate of ketone body utilization in the brain is likely concentration dependent[1,10] and, contrary to earlier impressions,[11] does not require induction of the enzymes of ketone utilization.[12] In the early phases of fasting in man ketone body oxidation by tissues other than the central nervous system, particularly skeletal muscle, appears to be brisk, but as the period of food deprivation extends beyond 3 days fatty acids become the predominant substrate.[13–15] The consequence of this change is that overall ketone utilization is diminished and plasma concentrations rise out of proportion to increased hepatic production, assuring an adequate supply of utilizable substrate for the central nervous system in the face of potential glucose deficiency. The importance of this protective adaptation is emphasized by the demonstration that only modest elevation in the concentration of plasma ketones blunts the response to insulin-induced hypoglycemia in both dog[16] and man.[17]

It is obvious from the preceding formulation that the accumulation of ketone bodies in the blood during starvation subserves a useful function. It must be remembered, however, that both acetoacetate and β-hydroxybutyrate are strong organic acids. (The pKa of acetoacetic acid is 3.58.) It is imperative, therefore, that the rate of production of ketone bodies be modulated if severe metabolic acidosis is to be avoided. In normal man and animals this is accomplished by the operation of a feedback system involving the pancreas, liver, and adipose tissue. While the hormonal changes that function to control ketogenesis are complicated, it seems clear that insulin plays a central role. This conclusion is based on the fact that insulin values fall with starvation[13,18,19] and that extremely small quantities of the hormone can reverse fasting ketosis even in the absence of exogenous glucose.[20,21] Recognition of the feedback system followed the discovery that ketones were able to stimulate insulin release from the pancreas in the dog[22] and in man.[14] It has also been found that free fatty acids stimulate insulin release, but this effect is not as marked.[23,24] The simplest description of the system, derived from these studies, would be as follows. When starvation begins, plasma glucose concentrations fall over a several hour period resulting in diminished insulin release from the

---

*In this chapter "ketones" and "ketone bodies" are used interchangeably to indicate both acetoacetate and β-hydroxybutyrate. Although chemically incorrect, this terminology has seen long usage in both the biochemical and clinical literature.

pancreas. As a consequence free fatty acids are mobilized from adipose tissue for direct oxidation in extrahepatic tissues and for conversion into ketone bodies in the liver, the latter process providing a utilizable substrate to substitute for glucose in the central nervous system. When ketone (and fatty acid) concentrations reach a given level insulin secretion from the pancreas is stimulated. The newly released insulin then acts to modulate hepatic production of acetoacetate and β-hydroxybutyrate, primarily by diminishing lipolysis and free fatty acid delivery from fat stores but possibly also by directly altering the metabolic pattern of the liver itself (see below). The end result is a modest elevation of free fatty acids (to about 0.7 mM) and total ketones (to about 4 mM) that is sufficient to supply adequate substrate for all body tissues but insufficient to cause a major acidosis.

In uncontrolled diabetes (genetic or acquired), the absence of insulin (or inhibition of its release from diminished pancreatic stores by stress-induced secretion of epinephrine[25,26]) activates a process qualitatively similar to starvation with the exception that the insulin segment of the feedback loop is missing. As a consequence, free fatty acid and ketone body concentrations rise in uncontrolled fashion (free fatty acids about 2 mM, total ketones about 20 mM), producing profound acidosis, coma, and death.[27,28]

As will be discussed subsequently this formulation now requires modification to include the role of glucagon and possibly other hormones. Its basic structure, however, will almost certainly remain intact.

REQUIREMENTS FOR KETOGENESIS

Current concepts of the nature of the ketogenic process emphasize that two requirements must be met before maximal ketogenesis can occur. These prerequisites are as follows:

1. There must be a sufficient rate of delivery of free fatty acids from adipose tissue stores to the liver to assure adequate substrate for acetoacetate and β-hydroxybutyrate synthesis.
2. There must be a change in the metabolic "set" of the liver such that an increased fraction of the incoming fatty acids enter the β-oxidative pathway for ketone body formation rather than being esterified to form triglycerides and phospholipids.

Fasting and uncontrolled diabetes, the two most common conditions leading to the development of ketosis, are accompanied by increased concentrations of free fatty acids in the plasma. Since acetoacetate and β-hydroxybutyrate are derived almost exclusively from the oxidation of long chain fatty acids in the liver, many authors have assumed that the enhanced production of ketone bodies in ketotic states results simply from the increased delivery of fatty acids to the liver.[29–31] (Increased uptake of fatty acids would be the automatic consequence of higher plasma concentrations because the hepatic extraction fraction for fatty acids is fixed.[31,32]) According to this viewpoint ketogenesis would be primarily a substrate-regulated phenomenon, an interpretation attractive for its simplicity and backed by considerable experimental evidence. For example, if fatty acid concentrations are increased, acetoacetate production in liver homogenates taken from nonketotic (fed) animals is stimulated.[33,34] Moreover, systematic semi-starvation of pancreatectomized diabetic rats, which depletes adipose tissue and liver triglycerides, causes a diminution in blood ketone concentrations and a reduction of acetoacetate and β-hydroxybutyrate synthesis by liver slices taken from the same animals.[35] The interpretation given to the latter experiment, which

Table 80-1. Rates of Ketone Body Production in Perfused Livers from Fed, Fasted, and Alloxan Diabetic Rats

Experimental Condition	Total Ketone Body Production*	
	Minus Oleate	1.25 mM Oleate
	(μmol $\cdot$ 100 g body wt$^{-1} \cdot$ 60 min^{-1})	
Fed	29 $\pm$ 3	54 $\pm$ 7
Fasted	125 $\pm$ 9	248 $\pm$ 12
Alloxan diabetic	251 $\pm$ 10	260 $\pm$ 18

*Acetoacetate + β-hydroxybutyrate

appears to be entirely reasonable, was that ketogenesis was limited by substrate depletion; i.e., when no adipose tissue triglyceride is available to supply fatty acids for oxidation in the liver, ketone body production stops. Along the same lines, blockade of free fatty acid release from the periphery by nicotinic acid can, under certain circumstances, be shown to lower plasma ketone concentrations in ketotic states.[30,36] Additional insight into the role of substrate availability in the regulation of ketogenesis came from studies in the isolated perfused liver of the alloxan diabetic rat which showed that rates of acetoacetate and β-hydroxybutyrate formation were initially independent of exogenous fatty acids, but that after prolonged perfusion, during which hepatic triglyceride concentrations fell, exogenous fatty acids were required to sustain rapid ketone synthesis.[37] *It is thus apparent that adequate provision of free fatty acids is a sine qua non for ketogenesis to occur at any significant rate.*

On the other hand, it is now equally clear that accelerated peripheral lipolysis, elevated plasma fatty acid concentrations, and increased uptake of fatty acids by the liver are not sufficient in themselves to induce major hepatic ketogenesis. Acute elevations of free fatty acids do not increase blood ketone body levels in normal dogs.[24,38] Moreover, starvation ketosis in the rat is reversed by administering dihydroxyacetone or glycerol without causing a fall in the elevated free fatty acid concentrations present before treatment.[39] Similarly, Bieberdorf et al.[40] reversed starvation ketosis in rats with small amounts of insulin, then raised plasma free fatty acids by infusing chylomicrons and heparin; despite this maneuver plasma ketone bodies remained low. Finally, distinct differences in ketogenic capacity can be demonstrated in isolated perfused livers from fed (nonketotic) rats and those from starved or diabetic animals in the presence of the same high fatty acid concentration in the media.[41,42] As shown in Table 80-1, diabetic livers produced ketones at maximum rates in the presence or absence of exogenous fatty acids due to the availability of excess hepatic triglyceride stores.[37] When livers from fasted animals were perfused with high oleate concentrations, production of ketones could be raised to the diabetic rate. On the other hand, despite the provision of exogenous fatty acid, livers from fed rats were incapable of producing acetoacetate and β-hydroxybutyrate at rapid rates; indeed, synthesis in the presence of added oleate was lower than the endogenous rate in livers from fasted animals. *Clearly, therefore, a change in intrahepatic metabolism is required if rapid production of ketone bodies is to occur.*

HEPATIC METABOLISM IN KETOTIC STATES

Two questions arise from consideration of the data indicating the necessity for a change in hepatic fatty acid metabolism in order for ketogenesis to supervene:

1. What is the locus of the primary control site in the ketogenic process?

2. What is the nature of the regulation exerted at this site? Evidence bearing on these two questions is now reviewed in sequence.

SITE OF REGULATION FOR KETOGENESIS

The immediate substrate for ketone body formation is acetyl CoA and its conversion into acetoacetate is accomplished via operation of the HMG CoA cycle.[43] Almost all early speculation as to the site of regulation centered about pathways of utilization of acetyl CoA in the cell. Major emphasis was placed on the possibility that diminished Krebs cycle activity might account for a diversion of acetyl CoA into ketones secondary to a deficiency of oxalacetate, a consideration based primarily on the studies of Lehninger.[44] Details of this theory and of the potential mechanisms whereby tissue concentrations of oxalacetate might be depressed have been discussed in detail[1,45] and need not be covered here. In an attempt to assess the role of the Krebs cycle in ketogenic states we carried out a series of experiments in the isolated perfused liver using radioactive octanoate as substrate.[41] The medium chain fatty acid was chosen because, in contrast to physiological long chain homologs, it is not utilized for triglyceride synthesis and it does not require a transport system for entry into the mitochondrion, the site of fatty acid oxidation. By measuring the specific activity of the ketone bodies produced from ^{14}C-labeled octanoate it was possible to estimate the specific activity of the intramitochondrial acetyl CoA pool and thus directly measure the flux of acetyl CoA through the tricarboxylic acid cycle. It was found that when ketogenic rates were high, as in livers from fasted animals, 2-carbon flow through the cycle was, in fact, depressed. By varying the concentration of octanoate in the media, however, it was noted that the relationship between the two pathways was not a simple one. At low concentrations of fatty acid the absolute rates of ketone body production and tricarboxylic acid cycle activity both increased. As substrate load was elevated carbon flow through the two pathways diverged, ketone production continuing to increase while 2-carbon flux through the cycle began to decline, ultimately falling below control rates. *These data indicated that a depression of acetyl CoA entry into the Krebs cycle was not required for accelerated rates of acetoacetate and β-hydroxybutyrate synthesis to occur.* It is likely that the reverse sequence is operative, i.e., that high rates of fatty acid oxidation and ketogenesis diminish Krebs cycle flux rather than vice versa. In the cited study acetyl CoA entry into the fatty acid synthetic pathway was also measured. The rates of fatty acid synthesis in the perfused liver were much higher than those estimated from all previous in vitro studies, and acetyl CoA flux into lipogenesis was similar in magnitude to that through the Krebs cycle. In livers from ketotic animals diminished 2-carbon unit movement into fatty acids accounted for a greater proportion of the shift of acetyl CoA into ketone synthesis than did diminished tricarboxylic acid cycle activity. These conclusions were in accord with the calculations of Williamson et al.[46] regarding Krebs cycle activity during ketogenesis and the assessment by Regen and Terrell[47] that underutilization of acetyl CoA for lipogenesis contributes to enhanced ketone body formation in starvation. *To recapitulate, in the fasting state there is a diversion of acetyl CoA from oxidative and lipogenic pathways into ketone body production with the lipogenic defect predominating.* As can be seen from Table 80-2, diminished flux into the tricarboxylic acid and fatty acid synthesizing pathways, matched almost precisely the increased incorporation into acetoacetate and β-hydroxybutyrate. It is pertinent to note at this point that despite earlier speculation that the enzymes of the HMG CoA cycle might be activated in ketotic states,[21] subsequent experiments have

Table 80-2. The Incorporation of [1-14C]Octanoic Acid into CO_2, Fatty Acids, and Ketone Bodies in Perfused Livers from Normal and Fasted Rats*

Condition	Labeled C_2 Units Incorporated into		
	Ketones	CO_2	Fatty Acids
	(μmol $\cdot$ 60 min^{-1} $\cdot$ 100 g body wt^{-1})		
Normal	111 ± 4.1	87 ± 5.5	92 ± 13
Fasted	243 ± 11.4	41 ± 3.2	9 ± 1.1
Δ	+132	−46	−81

*50 μmol of [1-14C]octanoate was given as a priming dose (into 80 ml of perfusion media) and followed by an infusion at the rate of 2 μmol/min. Results are given as micromoles of octanoate-derived 2-carbon units incorporated into the indicated product. Values are expressed as means ± SEM for 5 animals in each group.
Data taken from McGarry and Foster.[41]

shown this not to be the case. Equivalent maximum rates of ketogenesis occur in homogenates of livers from fed, fasted, and alloxan diabetic animals provided the generation of acetyl CoA is not limiting.[48,49]

Although these studies indicated that alterations in the utilization pattern of acetyl CoA are of primary importance in determining rates of ketone formation from octanoic acid in starvation ketosis, there was good evidence to suggest that *the rate of generation of acetyl CoA is the key determinant of the rate of ketogenesis when physiological fatty acids served as substrates.* For example, the early work of Soskin and Levine[50] and Lossow et al.[51–53] demonstrated that long chain fatty acid oxidation and ketogenesis were enhanced in livers from fasted and diabetic animals and were restricted or returned to normal by refeeding or insulin treatment. It can now be concluded that under physiological conditions the rate of fatty acid oxidation, and thus the generation of acetyl CoA, is far more important than disposal of the latter in determining ultimate rates of ketogenesis. This can be seen from a comparison of the metabolism of isotopic octanoic and oleic acids in livers from normal and ketotic animals. We showed[41] that [1-14C] octanoate was oxidized to acetyl CoA at identical rates in livers from fed, fasted, and diabetic rats (290, 293, and 302 μmol of C_2 units $\cdot$ 60 min^{-1} $\cdot$ 100 g body weight^{-1}, calculated from the recovery of isotope in ketones, CO_2, and fatty acids). Since the incorporation of C_2 units derived from octanoate into acetoacetate and β-hydroxybutyrate occurred at a rate of 111 μmol $\cdot$ h^{-1} $\cdot$ 100 g body weight^{-1} in the fed state and 243 and 273 μmol $\cdot$ h^{-1} $\cdot$ 100 g body weight^{-1} in fasting and diabetes, respectively,[41] it can be seen that underutilization of acetyl CoA in alternative pathways at most could account for a 2.5-fold increase in ketogenesis in the ketotic livers. When similar experiments were done utilizing oleate (a physiological long chain fatty acid) as substrate the difference in rates of ketogenesis in livers from fed and fasted rats was 12-fold.[42] It seemed likely that in this case the rate of ketogenesis was determined primarily by the rate of acetyl CoA generation. High rates of fatty acid oxidation increase the acetyl CoA concentration and, more importantly, the acetyl CoA:CoA ratio at the ketogenic site,[54] the latter ratio presumably setting the synthetic rate.* It is of interest that, in rats at least, the maximal capacity for ketone body production determined in vitro appears to correlate closely with

---

*The relationship between acetyl CoA concentrations in the liver and ketone body production is not a simple one as is evidenced by the fact that ketosis can be reversed under circumstances in which total hepatic acetyl CoA levels do not change.[21,39] This doubtless reflects the fact that acetyl CoA pools are compartmentalized such that changes in the "ketogenic pool" are not reflected in whole tissue measurements.[55,56]

acetoacetate and β-hydroxybutyrate synthesis occurring in vivo in severely ketotic alloxan diabetic animals.[57]

If the rate of acetyl CoA generation does in reality represent the single most important feature in the control of ketone body synthesis, it follows that an understanding of the factors that regulate rates of fatty acid oxidation is of fundamental importance in dissecting control of the overall ketogenic pathway. It was recognized early that long chain fatty acids taken up by the liver had only two major paths of metabolism available to them: they could either be esterified to form triglycerides and phospholipids (and to a lesser extent cholesterol esters) or they could be oxidized to acetyl CoA. The importance of partitioning of fatty acids between oxidative and esterification pathways was emphasized by Fritz[58] and substantiated by the important observation of Mayes and Felts[59] that in the fasted state oleic acid incorporation into triglycerides decreased simultaneously with an enhanced conversion of the fatty acid into ketone bodies. The initial interpretation of the data was that fatty acids were shunted into the oxidative pathway with increased generation of acetyl CoA and ketone bodies because of diminished triglyceride synthesis. Since it was commonly believed that the rate of triglyceride synthesis was determined by the available concentration of free sn-glycero-3-phosphate,[58,60,61] it was natural to assume that the latter intermediate was depressed in starvation and that this accounted for the diminution in triglyceride formation. This formulation subsequently proved untenable. Measurements of sn-glycero-3-phosphate showed that its concentration was actually higher in livers from fasted animals than in those from fed controls.[42,62] In addition, no correlation could be shown between sn-glycero-3-phosphate levels and ketosis in vivo when antiketogenic agents were given,[39] a result which also held in studies with the isolated perfused liver.[42] Most important, it was shown that acute blockade of fatty acid oxidation with the inhibitor (+)-decanoylcarnitine in isolated perfused livers from fasted animals resulted in an immediate resumption of triglyceride synthesis.[19] Similar observations have been made in livers from severely ketotic alloxan diabetic rats.[63] It was thus apparent that no defect existed in the triglyceride synthetic machinery, a fact which suggested that rates of fatty acid oxidation determined the availability of fatty acids for esterification processes rather than the reverse sequence. Studies from other laboratories were entirely compatible with this viewpoint.[64-66]

Once this conclusion was reached it was possible to infer the control site for fatty acid oxidation on the basis of the studies with octanoic and oleic acids mentioned earlier.[41,42] Since octanoate was oxidized to acetyl-CoA at the same rate in livers from normal, fasted, and diabetic rats (whose blood ketones varied from less than 1 to over 20 mM) it was possible to deduce that the capacity for β-oxidation in the mitochondrion was fixed, large, and probably invariant in normal and ketotic states. Direct experimental proof that this deduction was correct has recently been provided.[67] *It can, therefore, be concluded that entry of a fatty acid into the mitochondrion is followed by rapid oxidation to acetyl CoA at a rate determined by the substrate concentration. Since oxidation of oleic acid was markedly restricted in the fed state (or enhanced during fasting or diabetes) it seemed reasonable to conclude that the regulatory site must be at the transfer step for long chain fatty acids across the mitochondrial membrane, a reaction that is not required for the oxidation of the medium chain homologs.*[55,58] Evidence compatible with this formulation was also available from in vivo studies. As noted earlier, when starvation ketosis was reversed with insulin in the rat, experimental elevation of long chain free fatty acid levels was not accompanied by reappearance

of the ketotic state.[40] However, when similar experiments were carried out with octanoic acid infusion substituting for long chain fatty acids, plasma ketones briskly increased to the control level or higher,[41] indicating that the antiketogenic effect of insulin was inoperative against octanoate.

Proof that the regulatory site for fatty acid oxidation and ketogenesis was at the transfer reaction for long chain fatty acids across the mitochondrial membrane was difficult to obtain. It has long been known that the translocation of physiological fatty acids into the mitochondrion involves a reversible transacylation between coenzyme A and carnitine.[55,68] Recent evidence suggests that the sequence involves two enzymes: carnitine acyltransferase I, which is loosely attached to the outer aspect of the inner mitochondrial membrane and catalyzes the formation of palmityl (or oleyl) carnitine from palmityl (or oleyl) CoA, and carnitine acyltransferase II, which is tightly bound to the inner aspect of the inner mitochondrial membrane and catalyzes the re-formation of long chain fatty acyl CoA from long chain fatty acyl carnitine.[69-71] In view of the proposed role of mitochondrial transport in determining the rates of fatty acid oxidation, the logical supposition would be that increased activity of this enzyme system would be found in ketotic states. While modest elevation of carnitine acyltransferase activity has been reported in broken-cell preparations of livers from ketotic rats,[72-74] the extent of activation was small compared to the increase in ketogenesis known to occur in these conditions. In our own hands, when examined under V_{max} conditions with mitochondria intact, ketogenesis from oleic acid occurs to an equal extent in *homogenates* of livers from fed and fasted rats. Surprisingly, this rate surpasses that occurring in perfused livers from alloxan diabetic rats with ketoacidosis severe enough to ultimately kill the animals.[75] It has also been reported that the activity of carnitine acyltransferases in rat liver mitochondria was higher than the maximal activities of the enzymes of fatty acid oxidation,[76,77] findings that cast doubt on a regulatory role for the former. However, it has been emphasized repeatedly that findings obtained from enzyme studies in vitro may prove misleading as guidelines to the metabolism of the intact cell.[78] For this reason we decided to try another approach to the problem. Using the isolated perfused liver system we compared the metabolism of oleate, octanoate, and (−)-octanoylcarnitine in livers from fed and fasted rats. The rationale was as follows. Octanoic acid is oxidized rapidly and at equal rates in livers from ketotic and nonketotic animals, presumably because of unrestricted access into the mitochondrion and to the enzymes of β-oxidation. If octanoate were now esterified to (−)-carnitine, requiring carnitine acyltransferase II activity for further metabolism, and if the latter enzyme were rate limiting for fatty acid oxidation in the intact liver, then ketogenesis from (−)-octanoylcarnitine, in contrast to octanoate, should be low in livers from fed animals and relatively much higher in those from fasted rats. As shown in Table 80-3, this turned out to be the case.[79] In essence the pattern of (−)-octanoylcarnitine metabolism was identical with that of oleate, the physiological fatty acid, a finding which strongly supports a major role for carnitine acyltransferase II in the regulation of ketone body synthesis in the intact liver. The experiments do not allow a conclusion to be drawn about transferase I since (−)-octanoylcarnitine would bypass this step. Additional evidence that carnitine acyltransferase is the primary site for controlling ketogenesis came from studies with (+)-octanoylcarnitine, a potent inhibitor of the transferase enzymes. When added at a concentration of 0.5 mM, ketone production from (−)-octanoylcarnitine was initially inhibited as would be predicted from the operating hypothesis. In contrast to the situation with long chain fatty acids, however, this

Table 80-3. Ketone Body Production from (−)-Octanoylcarnitine and Endogenous Fatty Acids*

Substrate	Condition	Specific Activity	Ketones Produced (μmol·100 g body wt^{-1}·h^{-1})	Enhancement by Fasting
(−)-OC	Fed	0.20	6.6 ± 1.0	
	Fasted	0.23	46 ± 1.4	7.0
Endogenous	Fed	—	27 ± 4.4	
fatty acids†	Fasted	—	154 ± 2.1	5.7

*Livers from fed and fasted rats were perfused with 1.25 mM (−)-[1-^{14}C] octanoylcarnitine [(−)OC]. Endogenous (long chain) fatty acid oxidation to total ketones (acetoacetate + β-hydroxybutyrate) was calculated from the specific activity of the isolated ketone bodies. A specific activity of 1.0 would indicate that all of the newly formed ketones came from the radioactive substrate. Results are given as means ± SEM for 5 animals in each group.
†Free fatty acids derived from hepatic triglyceride stores.

inhibition was transient. As the perfusion continued ketogenic rates began to increase and it could be shown that acetoacetate and β-hydroxybutyrate were being formed from both (−)-octanoylcarnitine and endogenous fatty acids. With 2 mM (+)-octanoylcarnitine present the same sequence occurred, but the reinitiation of ketone synthesis was delayed. It was then shown that free (−)-carnitine added to the media also relieved the inhibition produced by (+)-octanoylcarnitine. The interpretation was as follows: The inhibition of carnitine acyltransferase caused by (+)-octanoylcarnitine, even at 2 mM, was incomplete. As (−)-octanoylcarnitine was metabolized, free (−)-carnitine was released and acted to overcome the (+)-octanoylcarnitine block in competitive fashion, a sequence which was entirely compatible with the postulate that the carnitine acyltransferase system is the critical site for regulation of ketogenesis. Why carnitine acyltransferase activity becomes nonlimiting (activated) in homogenates or isolated mitochondria from the same livers is not yet known.

To summarize, while alterations in tricarboxylic acid cycle activity and fatty acid synthesis can affect final rates of ketogenesis by altering the disposal of acetyl CoA generated in the mitochondria, it is the rate of generation of acetyl CoA that is of primary importance. In the intact liver the enzymes of fatty acid oxidation appear to be present in excess under all conditions so far studied. The evidence is convincing that rates of fatty acid oxidation and, consequently, rates of ketogenesis will be determined by the activity of the carnitine acyltransferase system. Relative activity at this site likewise determines the distribution of fatty acids between esterifying and oxidative pathways. These concepts are shown schematically in Figure 80-1. In the fed state, where fatty acid delivery to the liver is low, carnitine acyltransferase activity is restricted and the bulk of the fatty acids taken up is esterified. In starvation and diabetes fatty acid delivery is enhanced and the carnitine acyltransferase system is activated with resultant overproduction of acetoacetate and β-hydroxybutyrate. Although not shown in the figure, if fatty acid uptake by the liver becomes sufficiently great, the oxidative pathway appears to become saturated and triglyceride synthesis also increases, with production of a fatty liver.[27,80] This is not an infrequent finding in uncontrolled diabetes.

NATURE OF THE "OFF–ON" SIGNAL FOR FATTY ACID OXIDATION AND KETOGENESIS

While the primary site for the control of fatty acid oxidation and ketogenesis now seems fairly securely localized to the carnitine acyltransferase reaction, the nature of the regulation exerted

at this locus requires clarification. Whatever the mediators of control may be, it is obvious that the activation–inactivation process can occur quickly. Hepatic metabolism in the rat is altered to a "ketogenic set," meaning that incoming fatty acids are preferentially oxidized at the expense of esterification reactions, by as little as 6 h of fasting, and can be reversed by carbohydrate feeding even more rapidly.[19] Since the altered metabolism and changing pattern of circulating fuels that characterize the adaptation to starvation in both man and animals are accompanied (and probably mediated) by major alterations in endocrine gland activity, we assumed that the changes occurring in the liver that lead to accelerated ketone production would be hormonally induced. Evidence compatible with this assumption has recently been obtained.[81] When anti-insulin serum (AIS) was administered intravenously to fed rats, plasma glucose, total ketones, and free fatty acids began to rise within 1 h in the pattern typical of antibody-induced diabetes.[82,83] When livers from these animals were perfused with oleic acid it was clear that fatty acid oxidation had already been "turned on," with ketogenic rates intermediate between those of livers from control and fasted animals. Three hours of treatment with AIS further increased the ketogenic capacity to a level approximately 75 percent of that in the fasted state. When fed rats were given glucagon in high doses, treatment for 1 to 3 h resulted in only slight increases in the plasma glucose and no change in plasma ketones or free fatty acids. Surprisingly, however, when livers from these nonketotic rats were perfused with oleate they behaved exactly as did the livers taken from the AIS-treated animals; i.e., fatty acid oxidation and ketogenesis were activated. These points are illustrated in Figures 80-2 and 80-3. The glucagon experiments were then repeated at a dosage schedule 1/200 of that used in the original group of animals. Plasma insulin and glucagon concentrations were measured at the end of the infusions; the former were in the normal range for fed animals (34 μU/ml) while the latter were about twice

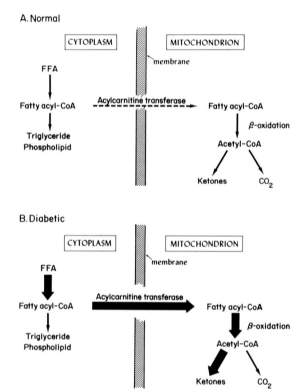

Fig. 80-1. Schematic representation of the control of ketogenesis. (Reprinted from McGarry and Foster,[105] by permission of the *Journal of Clinical Investigation*.)

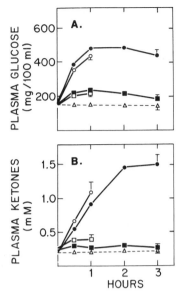

Fig. 80-2. Effects of anti-insulin serum and glucagon on plasma glucose and ketone levels in fed rats. Animals were fitted with arterial and venous catheters and placed in restraining cages. After the injection of 100 U of heparin and collection of a zero time arterial blood sample (0.2 ml) an infusion of guinea pig serum containing 1.6–2.1 U of insulin antibody/ml (○, 1 h; ●, 3 h), 100 μg of glucagon/ml (□, 1 h; ■, 3 h), or neither agent (△) was given through the venous catheter at a rate of 200 μl/min for 5 min, followed by 10 μl/min for the remainder of the experiment. Further arterial blood samples were taken at the indicated times for analysis of plasma glucose and ketone concentrations. Values represent means for 8 animals in each group. For purposes of clarity standard errors of the means are shown only for the final time point but in every case were smaller than this at earlier times. (Reprinted from McGarry et al.,[81] by permission of the *Journal of Clinical Investigation.*)

normal values (231 pg/ml). Once again perfusion of the livers indicated a switch in metabolism to a ketogenic profile. Thus a ketogenic liver had been produced in an animal that was neither insulin deficient nor ketotic. The findings appear to be compatible with the view that the change in hepatic metabolism leading to accelerated ketogenesis is hormonally induced and that it probably is mediated bihormonally through a change in the glucagon–insulin ratio. Considerable evidence has accrued that this is the case for hepatic glucose production via glycogenolysis and gluconeogenesis.[84–88*] Anti-insulin serum would alter the ratio by both decreasing portal vein insulin and increasing portal vein glucagon concentrations,[89] while glucagon infusion would change the ratio unilaterally by elevating circulating levels of the alpha cell hormone without blocking insulin release. The failure of ketosis to develop in the glucagon-treated rats despite the presence of a liver activated for ketogenesis was due to the fact that plasma free fatty acid levels remained low (a consequence of sufficient insulin to inhibit peripheral lipolysis), as was shown by the fact that acute elevation of free fatty acids experimentally in vivo resulted in a prompt rise in plasma acetoacetate and β-hydroxybutyrate concentrations.[81] No significant increase was produced in control rats despite equivalent elevation of free fatty acids. On the basis of these findings it can be concluded that insulin deficiency is required for the development of ketosis but not for the alteration in liver metabolism which will allow incoming fatty acids to be diverted to ketone production. An analogous situation holds in

man as illustrated by the experiments of Liljenquist et al.[90] who infused glucagon in normal controls and diabetic patients. The former had no rise in plasma ketones because insulin secretion was stimulated by glucagon,[91] whereas the latter, deficient in insulin, demonstrated increased fatty acid mobilization and ketonemia.

It is important to note that current evidence suggests that absolute concentrations of glucagon and insulin are much less important in regulatory terms than their values relative to each other and that changes in these parameters need not be large to effect major changes in metabolism.[85] This point is well illustrated in time sequence studies of the development of diabetic acidosis in the rat treated with alloxan.[80] In the first 12 h the appearance of hyperglycemia, elevated free fatty acid levels, and ketosis was accompanied by a fall in circulating insulin but no change in plasma glucagon; in other words, absolute hyperglucagonemia was not required for hyperglycemia to develop. On the other hand, in the second 24 h insulin concentrations reached their nadir and glucagon concentrations rose dramatically as hyperglycemia and ketoacidosis approached fatal levels. The key role of glucagon has been emphasized by Gerich et al.[92] who used somatostatin to suppress secretion of the alpha cell hormone in insulin-requiring diabetic patients. Compared with controls not receiving somatostatin the induction of ketosis following insulin withdrawal was significantly blunted. This study provides strong support for the role of glucagon in converting liver metabolism into a ketogenic mode. Schade and Eaton,[93] approaching the problem from the opposite side, showed that administration of glucagon increased the conversion of fatty acids into ketones in diabetic man exactly as was the case in the rat experiments described earlier. Both experiments are compatible with the view that glucagon functions as the primary hormonal regulator for hepatic ketogenesis whereas insulin acts predominantly at the periphery to control the delivery of the fatty acid substrate to the liver.

It was clearly established that both anti-insulin serum and glucagon activated (−)-octanoylcarnitine oxidation in parallel with increased oleate oxidation, suggesting that the control site in both natural and induced ketogenesis is the carnitine acyltransferase reaction.[81] However, concentrations of anti-insulin serum or gluca-

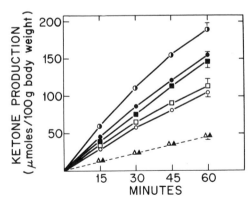

Fig. 80-3. Comparison of the effects of anti-insulin serum (AIS), glucagon, and fasting on ketogenesis from oleate in the perfused rat liver. Fed animals were treated as described in the legend to Figure 80-2 or were fasted for 24 h. The livers were then perfused with recirculating medium containing oleic acid at an initial concentration of 0.7 mM and rates of ketone production were determined. Treatment of rats was as follows: ▲, none; △, control serum, 3 h; ○, AIS, 1 h; ●, AIS, 3 h; □, glucagon, 1 h; ■, glucagon, 3 h; ◑, fasted 24 h. Values represent means for 4 animals in each group. For purposes of clarity standard errors are shown only for the 60-min point but in every case were smaller than this at earlier times. (Reprinted from McGarry et al.,[81] by permission of the *Journal of Clinical Investigation.*)

*This hypothesis has been formally presented recently by Unger and Orci.[108]

gon that rapidly induced a ketogenic "set" in the liver when administered in vivo to fed animals did not have this effect when livers removed from fed animals were perfused with similar concentrations,[63] and it appears possible that factors other than or in addition to an elevation of the glucagon–insulin ratio might be required to initiate the alterations in hepatic fatty acid metabolism characteristic of the ketotic state.

Recent studies from our laboratory[94] have provided some insight as to how the hormones might exert their effect in vivo. We have shown that fasting and diabetes are both accompanied by major increases in hepatic carnitine content. Moreover, carnitine levels in the liver can be acutely increased by administration of glucagon and anti-insulin serum to fed, nonketotic rats. Finally, carnitine can enhance the capacity of the liver to convert fatty acids into ketone bodies when added directly to the isolated perfused liver system. It is the only compound known to produce this change. In this regard, it is of interest that in 1955 Fritz[95] showed that extracts of muscle could stimulate fatty acid oxidation when added to rat liver slices and homogenates. He identified the stimulatory material in the extracts as carnitine.

While much additional work will be required to fill in the details, the current working model can be formulated as follows: *Ketosis is initiated by a relative or absolute excess of glucagon and a relative or absolute deficiency of insulin. One effect of the former is to bring about an increase in hepatic carnitine content which in turn activates the carnitine acyltransferase system and the potential for accelerated fatty acid oxidation. The latter causes increased lipolysis and mobilization of fatty acids to the liver where they are efficiently utilized for ketone production via the activated β-oxidation sequence.*

How carnitine levels in liver are increased (mobilization from muscle? increased hepatic synthesis?) remains an open question. Also at issue is whether carnitine acts directly and alone or whether some other change in hepatic metabolism is additionally required. It has long been known that ketotic states are accompanied by hepatic glycogen depletion.[96–99] There is, under widely varying experimental conditions, an excellent reciprocal correlation between glycogen content and capacity for ketogenesis in the liver.[19,81] Whether glycogen plays a direct role in regulating fatty acid oxidation or whether it simply changes concomitantly with some other process, effectively serving as a marker for the regulatory system, is unknown.

Additional evidence that the "off–on" signal for ketogenesis has something to do with carbohydrate metabolism in the liver comes from the many studies which show that carbohydrate feeding rapidly reverses starvation ketosis in vivo.[19,21,50–52,100] More importantly, such compounds as fructose, dihydroxyacetone, glycerol, and lactate have definite antiketogenic potential in the isolated perfused liver (Table 80-4).[4,39,42,60] All of these compounds are intermediates of the gluconeogenic–glycolytic cycle or precursors thereof. All of them likewise divert long chain fatty acids from the oxidative pathway into triglyceride synthesis and simultaneously depress the rate of oxidation of (−)-octanoylcarnitine.[63] It is, therefore, possible that both an increase in carnitine content and glycogen depletion are required to initiate the ketogenic change.

It has recently been discovered that malonyl-CoA, the first committed intermediate in the conversion of glucose into fat, is a potent inhibitor of carnitine acyltransferase I (Ki about 1-2 μM), the first step specific to the opposing pathway of fatty acid oxidation.[100a] Malonyl-CoA is the only physiological compound known to have this effect. This finding, coupled with the fact that hepatic malonyl-CoA levels fall under conditions of insulin deficiency and glucagon excess,[100b,b] strongly suggests that malonyl-CoA repre-

Table 80-4. Ketone Body Production in the Isolated Perfused Liver. Effect of Antiketogenic Agents*

State of Animals	Antiketogenic Agent	Total Ketones
Normal (6)	None	29 ± 3
Fasted (6)	None	173 ± 12
Fasted (6)	Glucose (11mM) + insulin (40mU/ml)	161 ± 7
Fasted (6)	Fructose (11 mM)	74 ± 7
Fasted (6)	Glycerol (11 mM)	81 ± 8
Fasted (6)	L-Lactate (10 mM)	77 ± 4

*Results are given as means ± SEM for the number of experiments shown in parentheses and refer to micromoles of acetoacetate and β-hydroxybutyrate produced per 100 g body weight per hour. Oleate concentration was maintained at approximately 0.5 mM. Data taken from McGarry and Foster.[42]

sents an important element in the long sought for "carbohydrate key" to the control of ketogenesis. Moreover, its strategic location in the metabolism of glucose confers upon malonyl-CoA a central role in the coordination of heptic fatty acid synthesis and oxidation. Since malonyl-CoA had no effect on carnitine acyltransferase II, the question arises as to why the ability of perfused rat liver to oxidize octanoylcarnitine (which requires only carnitine acyltransferase II for entry into the mitochondrion) was found to be directly related to its capacity for long chain fatty acid oxidation, as detailed in the text. One possibility would be that Transferase I and Transferase II are subject to coordinate metabolic control, but by different mechanisms. Alternatively, it is conceivable that the enhanced oxidation of octanoylcarnitine in livers from ketotic animals reflects increased permeability of the liver cell to this substrate, rather than activation of Transferase II.

REVERSAL OF EXPERIMENTAL DIABETIC KETOACIDOSIS

As already noted, following the studies of Fritz and co-workers[101,102] and Williamson et al.[103,104] we utilized the nonphysiological carnitine ester of decanoic acid in experiments designed to determine the relationship between fatty acid esterification and oxidation in ketotic states.[19] The capacity of this competitive inhibitor of carnitine acyltransferase to block ketone production in perfused livers from fasting and diabetic animals was remarkable and ketogenic rates fell almost to zero soon after the introduction of the compound into the medium. When the inhibitor was given intravenously to severely ketotic rats, the results were also impressive, as illustrated in Figure 80-4.[105] The data of panel B indicate that (+)-decanoylcarnitine was more effective than large doses of insulin in reversing ketosis. When insulin was given simultaneously with the (+)-carnitine ester a synergistic effect was noted. (+)-Decanoylcarnitine was equally effective whether given by constant infusion or as a single bolus. In anesthetized animals (+)-decanoylcarnitine also accentuated the hypoglycemic effect of insulin (panel A); it did not do so in nonanesthetized rats, which exhibited a much greater sensitivity to the hormone. The presumption was that in the former group peripheral blockade of fatty acid oxidation was necessary to enhance the capacity of insulin to transport glucose into muscle at a rate equivalent to that seen in the awake (exercising) animals receiving insulin alone.[105] While the effects of (+)-decanoylcarnitine were reversible both in vivo and in vitro and while no toxic effects were noted either short or long

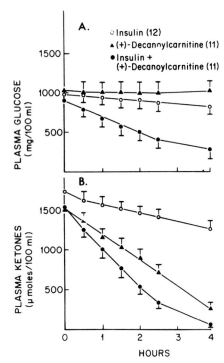

Fig. 80-4. The effect of intravenous administration of insulin and (+)-decanoylcarnitine in anesthetized diabetic rats. Animals that were still under pentobarbital anesthesia after the placement of arterial and venous catheters were placed in restraining cages and received 100 U of heparin at zero time. After collection of an arterial blood sample (0.1 ml) an infusion of 5 percent albumin in 0.9 percent sodium chloride, pH 7.4, containing insulin (1 U/ml), (+)-decanoylcarnitine (20 mg/ml), or both agents was given through the venous catheter at a rate of 75 μl/min for 10 min followed by 10 μl/min until the 2-h time point. Further arterial blood samples were collected at the indicated times for analysis of plasma glucose and ketone body concentrations. Values represent means ± SEM for the number of animals shown in parentheses. (Reprinted from McGarry and Foster,[105] by permission of the *Journal of Clinical Investigation*.)

term, it was clear that the compound had surface active properties which were potentially harmful to cell membranes. We were particularly concerned about the possibility of hemolysis during intravenous infusion. As a consequence, 6- and 8-carbon homologs of (+)-decanoylcarnitine were synthesized and tested for antiketogenic activity.[106] In these studies (+)-octanoylcarnitine proved to be as potent as (+)-decanoylcarnitine in blocking ketone production in the perfused liver and in reversing ketoacidosis in rats rendered diabetic by alloxan. Importantly, shortening the fatty acid chain length by two carbons essentially removed the hemolytic potential seen with (+)-decanoylcarnitine. (+)-Octanoylcarnitine was not metabolized in the body and was excreted unchanged into the urine. with up to 75 percent of the injected material being cleared in 1 h. Following entry into the logarithmic descent phase in plasma the half-life was approximately 4.5 h. Finally it was shown that (+)-octanoylcarnitine was effective in reversing ketosis when given orally, though considerably larger doses were required than when it was given by the intravenous route. Reversal of starvation and diabetic ketosis in cats and dogs has subsequently been shown using (+)-octanoylcarnitine given intravenously.[63]

We are uncertain about the clinical implications of these findings. Human diabetic ketoacidosis is a common problem[107] with the potential to cause death, though with careful treatment using intravenous fluids and insulin overall mortality should be low.[27] Under certain circumstances, however, it may be desirable

or necessary to reverse ketoacidosis more rapidly than can be accomplished by current therapy, which usually requires 7 to 9 h for significant reduction of blood ketone concentrations in severe cases.[27] Examples would be patients in ketoacidosis requiring surgery or those in deep and unresponsive coma. It seems possible that (+)-octanoylcarnitine would be a useful therapeutic adjunct in such situations, and clinical trials may, therefore, be warranted at a future date. Entirely in the realm of speculation is a second possible use of the compound. Since (+)-octanoylcarnitine is effective orally, at least in the rat, it is barely conceivable that it may have a role in prophylaxis of ketoacidosis; i.e., it is possible that the ketoacidosis-prone patient could be protected in stressful situations such as intercurrent infection or when facing surgery by the oral administration of (+)-octanoylcarnitine to prevent activation of the ketogenic process.

ACKNOWLEDGEMENTS

The authors' studies referred to in this chapter have been supported by U.S. Public Health Service Grant AM18573. Dr. McGarry is the recipient of USPHS Research Career Development Award 5-KO4 AM 70763.

REFERENCES

1. Williamson, D. H., and R. Hems. 1970. Metabolism and function of ketone bodies. In Essays in Cell Metabolism. W. Bartley, H. L. Kornberg, and J. R. Quayle, eds. Wiley-Interscience, New York, pp. 257–281.
2. Kety, S. S. 1957. The general metabolism of the brain in vivo. In Metabolism of the Nervous System. D. Richter, ed. Pergamon Press, New York, pp. 221–237.
3. Reinmuth, O. M., P. Scheinberg, and B. Bourne. 1965. Total cerebral blood flow and metabolism. Arch. Neurol. 12: 49–66.
4. Gordon, R. S., Jr., and A. Cherkes. 1956. Unesterified fatty acid in human blood plasma. J. Clin. Invest. 35: 206–212.
5. Allweis, C., T. Landau, M. Abeles, and J. Magues. 1966. The oxidation of uniformly labelled albumin-bound palmitic acid to CO₂ by the perfused cat brain. J. Neurochem. 13: 795–804.
6. Openshaw, H., and W. M. Bortz. 1968. Oxidation of glucose, acetoacetate and palmitate in brain mince of normal and ketotic rats. Diabetes 17: 90–95.
7. Rolleston, F. A., and E. A. Newsholme. 1967. Effects of fatty acids, ketone bodies, lactate and pyruvate on glucose utilization by guinea pig cerebral cortex slices. Biochem. J. 104: 519–523.
8. Itoh, T., and J. H. Quastel. 1970. Acetoacetate metabolism in infant and adult rat brain in vitro. Biochem. J. 116: 641–655.
9. Owen, O. E., A. P. Morgan, H. G. Kemp, J. M. Sullivan, M. G. Herrera, and G. F. Cahill, Jr. 1967. Brain metabolism during fasting. J. Clin. Invest. 46: 1589–1595.
10. Bates, M. W., H. A. Krebs, and D. H. Williamson. 1968. Turnover rates of ketone bodies in normal, starved, and alloxan diabetic rats. Biochem. J. 110: 655–661.
11. Smith, A. L., H. S. Satterthwaite, and L. Sokoloff. 1969. Induction of brain D(−)-β-hydroxybutyrate dehydrogenase activity by fasting. Science 163: 79–81.
12. Williamson, D. H., M. W. Bates, M. A. Page, and H. A. Krebs. 1971. Activities of enzymes involved in acetoacetate utilization in adult mammalian tissues. Biochem. J. 121: 41–47.
13. Owen, O. E., and G. A. Reichard, Jr. 1971. Human forearm metabolism during progressive starvation. J. Clin. Invest. 50: 1536–1545.
14. Owen, O. E., G. A. Reichard, Jr., H. Markus, G. Boden, M. A. Mozzoli, and C. R. Shuman. 1973. Rapid intravenous sodium acetoacetate infusion in man. Metabolic and kinetic responses. J. Clin. Invest. 52: 2606–2616.
15. Garber, A. J., P. H. Menzel, G. Boden, and O. E. Owen. 1974. Hepatic ketogenesis and gluconeogenesis in humans. J. Clin. Invest. 54: 981–989.

16. Flatt, J. P., G. L. Blackburn, G. Randers, and J. B. Stanbury. 1974. Effects of ketone body infusion and hypoglycemic reaction in postabsorptive dogs. *Metabolism 23:* 151–158.

17. Drenick, E. J., L. C. Alvarez, G. C. Tamasi, and A. S. Brickman. 1972. Resistance to symptomatic insulin reactions after fasting. *J. Clin. Invest. 51:* 2757–2762.

18. Owen, O. E., P. Felig, A. P. Morgan, J. Wahren, and G. F. Cahill, Jr. 1969. Liver and kidney metabolism during prolonged starvation. *J. Clin. Invest. 48:* 574–583.

19. McGarry, J. D., J. M. Meier, and D. W. Foster. 1973. The effects of starvation and refeeding on carbohydrate and lipid metabolism in vivo and in the perfused rat liver. *J. Biol. Chem. 248:* 270–278.

20. Amatruda, T. T., and F. L. Engel. 1959. The role of the endocrine glands in ketosis. I. The ketosis of fasting. *Yale J. Biol. Med. 31:* 303–323.

21. Foster, D. W. 1967. Studies in the ketosis of fasting. *J. Clin. Invest. 14:* 1283–1296.

22. Madison, L. L., D. Mebane, R. H. Unger, and A. Lochner. 1964. The hypoglycemic action of ketones. II. Evidence for a stimulatory feedback of ketones on the pancreatic beta cells. *J. Clin. Invest. 43:* 408–415.

23. Madison, L. L., W. A. Seyffert, Jr., R. H. Unger, and B. Barker. 1968. Effect of plasma free fatty acids on plasma glucagon and serum insulin concentrations. *Metabolism 17:* 301–304.

24. Seyffert, W. A., Jr., and L. L. Madison. 1967. Physiologic effects of metabolic fuels on carbohydrate metabolism. I. Acute effect of elevation of plasma free fatty acids on hepatic glucose output, peripheral glucose utilization, serum insulin, and plasma glucagon levels. *Diabetes 16:* 765–776.

25. Porte, D., Jr., A. L. Graber, T. Kuzuya, and R. H. Williams. 1966. The effect of epinephrine on immunoreactive insulin levels in man. *J. Clin. Invest. 45:* 228–236.

26. Block, M. B., R. L. Rosenfield, M. E. Mako, D. F. Steiner, and A. H. Rubenstein. 1973. Sequential changes in beta-cell function in insulin-treated diabetic patients assessed by C-peptide immunoreactivity. *N. Engl. J. Med. 288:* 1144–1148.

27. McGarry, J. D., and D. W. Foster. 1972. Regulation of ketogenesis and clinical aspects of the ketotic state. *Metabolism 21:* 471–489.

28. Foster, D. W. 1974. Insulin deficiency and hyperosmolar coma. *Adv. Intern. Med. 19:* 159–173.

29. Hanson, P. G., R. E. Johnson, and D. S. Zaharko. 1965. Correlation between ketone body and free fatty acid concentrations in the plasma during early starvation in man. *Metabolism 14:* 1037–1040.

30. Carlson, L. A. 1969. Antilipolysis as a tool in the study of clinical and experimental diabetes. *Diabetologia 5:* 361–365.

31. Basso, L. V., and R. J. Havel. 1970. Hepatic metabolism of free fatty acids in normal and diabetic dogs. *J. Clin. Invest. 49:* 537–547.

32. Heimberg, M., I. Weinstein, and M. Kohout. 1969. The effects of glucagon, dibutyryl cyclic adenosine 3′,5′-monophosphate, and concentration of free fatty acid on hepatic lipid metabolism. *J. Biol. Chem. 244:* 5131–5139.

33. Ontko, J. A. 1964. On the biochemical etiology of ketosis. *Life Sci. 3:* 573–578.

34. Ontko, J. A. 1967. Chylomicron, free fatty acid and ketone body metabolism of isolated liver cells and liver homogenates. *Biochim. Biophys. Acta 137:* 13–22.

35. Scow, R. O., and S. S. Chernick. 1960. Hormonal control of protein and fat metabolism in the pancreatectomized rat. *Recent Prog. Horm. Res. 16:* 497–545.

36. Rooth, G., B. Kågedal, and S. Carlström. 1969. The effect of inhibition of lipolysis on blood concentration of 3-hydroxybutyrate and acetoacetate. *Clin. Sci. 37:* 143–150.

37. Van Harken, D. R., C. W. Dixon, and M. Heimberg. 1969. Hepatic lipid metabolism in experimental diabetes. *J. Biol. Chem. 244:* 2278–2285.

38. Crespin, S. R., W. B. Greenough, III, and D. Steinberg. 1969. Stimulation of insulin secretion by infusion of free fatty acid. *J. Clin. Invest. 48:* 1934–1943.

39. Williamson, D. H., D. Veloso, E. V. Ellington, and H. A. Krebs. 1969. Changes in the concentrations of hepatic metabolites on administration of dihydroxyacetone or glycerol to starved rats and their relationship to the control of ketogenesis. *Biochem. J. 114:* 575–584.

40. Bieberdorf, F. A., S. S. Chernick, and R. O. Scow. 1970. Effect of insulin and acute diabetes on plasma FFA and ketone bodies in the fasting rat. *J. Clin. Invest. 49:* 1685–1693.

41. McGarry, J. D., and D. W. Foster. 1971. The regulation of ketogenesis from octanoic acid. The role of the tricarboxylic acid cycle and fatty acid synthesis. *J. Biol. Chem. 246:* 1149–1159.

42. McGarry, J. D., and D. W. Foster. 1971. The regulation of ketogenesis from oleic acid and the influence of antiketogenic agents. *J. Biol. Chem. 246:* 6247–6253.

43. Lynen, F., V. Henning, C. Bublitz, B. Sorbo, and L. Kroplin-Reuff. 1958. Der chemische Mechanismus der Acetessigsäurebildung in der Leber. *Biochem. Z. 330:* 269–295.

44. Lehninger, A. L. 1946. A quantitative study of the products of fatty acid oxidation in liver suspensions. *J. Biol. Chem. 164:* 291–306.

45. Wieland, O. 1968. Ketogenesis and its regulation. *Adv. Metab. Dis. 3:* 1–47.

46. Williamson, J. R., E. T. Browning, R. G. Thurman, and R. Scholz. 1969. Inhibition of glucagon effects in perfused liver by (+)-decanoylcarnitine. *J. Biol. Chem. 244:* 5055–5064.

47. Regen, D. M., and E. B. Terrell. 1968. Effects of glucagon and fasting on acetate metabolism in perfused rat liver. *Biochim. Biophys. Acta 170:* 95–111.

48. Williamson, D. H., M. Bates, and H. A. Krebs. 1968. Activity and intracellular distribution of enzymes of ketone body metabolism in rat liver. *Biochem. J. 108:* 353–361.

49. McGarry, J. D., and D. W. Foster. 1969. Ketogenesis in vitro. *Biochim. Biophys. Acta 177:* 35–41.

50. Soskin, S., and R. Levine. 1941. Origin of ketone bodies from fat and their regulation. *Arch. Intern. Med. 68:* 674–686.

51. Lossow, W. J., and I. L. Chaikoff. 1954. Carbohydrate sparing of fatty acid oxidation. I. The relation of fatty acid chain length to the degree of sparing. II. The mechanism by which carbohydrate spares the oxidation of palmitic acid. *Arch. Biochem. Biophys. 57:* 23–40.

52. Lossow, W. J., G. W. Brown, Jr., and I. L. Chaikoff. 1956. Sparing of palmitic acid oxidation by carbohydrate: Prefeeding versus addition to medium. *J. Biol. Chem. 222:* 531–535.

53. Lossow, W. J., G. W. Brown, Jr., and I. L. Chaikoff. 1956. The action of insulin in sparing fatty acid oxidation: A study with palmitic acid-1-C^{14} and octanoate-1-C^{14}. *J. Biol. Chem. 220:* 839–849.

54. Sauer, F., and J. D. Erfle. 1966. On the mechanism of acetoacetate synthesis by guinea pig liver fractions. *J. Biol. Chem. 241:* 30–37.

55. Fritz, I. B. 1967. An hypothesis concerning the role of carnitine in the control of interrelations between fatty acid and carbohydrate metabolism. *Perspect. Biol. Med. 10:* 643–677.

56. Dietschy, J. M., and J. D. McGarry. 1974. Limitations of acetate as substrate for measuring cholesterol synthesis in liver. *J. Biol. Chem. 249:* 52–58.

57. McGarry, J. D., M. J. Guest, and D. W. Foster. 1970. Ketone body metabolism in the ketosis of starvation and alloxan diabetes. *J. Biol. Chem. 245:* 4382–4390.

58. Fritz, I. B. 1961. Factors influencing the rates of long chain fatty acid oxidation and synthesis in mammalian systems. *Physiol. Rev. 41:* 52–129.

59. Mayes, P. A., and J. M. Felts. 1967. Regulation of fat metabolism in the liver. *Nature 215:* 716–718.

60. Wieland, O., and F. Matschinsky. 1962. Zur Natur der antiketogenen Wirkung von Glycerin und Fructose. *Life Sci. 2:* 49–54.

61. Tzur, R., E. Tal, and B. Shapiro. 1964. α-Glycerophosphate as regulatory factor in fatty acid esterification. *Biochim. Biophys. Acta 84:* 18–23.

62. Veech, R. L., L. Raijman, and H. A. Krebs. 1970. Equilibrium relations between the cytoplasmic adenine nucleotide system and nicotinamide-adenine nucleotide system in rat liver. *Biochem. J. 117:* 499–503.

63. McGarry, J. D., and D. W. Foster. Unpublished observations.

64. Ontko, J. A. 1972. Metabolism of free fatty acids in isolated liver cells. *J. Biol. Chem. 247:* 1788–1800.

65. Ontko, J. A. 1973. Effects of ethanol on the metabolism of free fatty acids in isolated liver cells. *J. Lipid Res. 14:* 78–86.

66. Woodside, W. F., and M. Heimberg. 1972. Hepatic metabolism of free fatty acids in experimental diabetes. *Israel J. Med. Sci. 8:* 309–316.

67. DiMarco, J. P., and C. Hoppel. 1975. Hepatic mitochondrial function in ketogenic states. Diabetes, starvation and after growth hormone. *J. Clin. Invest. 55:* 1237–1244.

68. Shepherd, D., D. W. Yates, and P. B. Garland. 1965. The relationship between the rates of conversion of palmitate into citrate or acetoacetate and the acetyl-coenzyme A content of rat liver mitochondria. *Biochem. J. 97:* 38C–40C.

69. Hoppel, C. L., and R. J. Tomec. 1972. Carnitine palmityltransferase.

Location of two enzymatic activities in rat liver mitochondria. *J. Biol. Chem. 247:* 832–841.

70. Kopec, B., and I. B. Fritz. 1973. Comparison of properties of carnitine palmitoyltransferase I with those of carnitine palmitoyltransferase II, and preparation of antibodies to carnitine palmitoyltransferases. *J. Biol. Chem. 248:* 4069–4074.

71. Brosnan, J. T., B. Kopec, and I. B. Fritz. 1973. The localization of carnitine palmitoyltransferase on the inner membrane of bovine liver mitochondria. *J. Biol. Chem. 248:* 4075–4082.

72. Norum, K. R. 1965. Activation of palmityl-CoA carnitine palmityl transferase in livers from fasted, fat fed, or diabetic rats. *Biochim. Biophys. Acta 98:* 652–654.

73. Aas, M., and L. N. W. Daae. 1971. Fatty acid activation and acyl transfer in organs from rats in different nutritional states. *Biochim. Biophys. Acta 239:* 208–216.

74. Harano, Y., J. Kowal, R. Yanazaki, L. Lavine, and M. Miller. 1972. Carnitine palmitoyltransferase activities (1 and 2) and the rate of palmitate oxidation in liver mitochondria from diabetic rats. *Arch Biochem. Biophys. 153:* 426–437.

75. Davis, R. M., J. D. McGarry, and D. W. Foster. Unpublished observations.

76. Van Tol, A., and W. C. Hülsmann. 1969. The localization of palmitoyl-CoA: Carnitine palmitoyltransferase in rat liver. *Biochim. Biophys. Acta 189:* 342–353.

77. Pande, S. V. 1971. On rate-controlling factors of long chain fatty acid oxidation. *J. Biol. Chem. 246:* 5384–5390.

78. Srere, P. A. 1969. Some complexities of metabolic regulation. *Biochem. Med. 3:* 61–72.

79. McGarry, J. D., and D. W. Foster. 1974. The metabolism of (−)-octanoylcarnitine in perfused livers from fed and fasted rats. Evidence for a possible regulatory role of carnitine acyltransferase in the control of ketogenesis. *J. Biol. Chem. 249:* 7984–7990.

80. Meier, J. M., J. D. McGarry, G. R. Faloona, R. H. Unger, and D. W. Foster. 1972. Studies of the development of diabetic ketosis in the rat. *J. Lipid Res. 13:* 228–233.

81. McGarry, J. D., P. H. Wright, and D. W. Foster. 1975. Hormonal control of ketogenesis. Rapid activation of hepatic ketogenic capacity in fed rats by anti-insulin serum and glucagon. *J. Clin. Invest. 55:* 1202–1209.

82. Armin, J., R. T. Grant, and P. H. Wright. 1960. Acute insulin deficiency provoked by single injections of anti-insulin serum. *J. Physiol. 153:* 131–145.

83. Balasse, E. O., D. M. Bier, and R. J. Havel. 1972. Early effects of anti-insulin serum on hepatic metabolism of plasma free fatty acids in dogs. *Diabetes 21:* 280–288.

84. Unger, R. H. 1974. Alpha- and beta-cell interrelationships in health and disease. *Metabolism 23:* 581–593.

85. Parilla, R., M. N. Goodman, and C. J. Toews. 1974. Effect of glucagon: insulin ratios on hepatic metabolism. *Diabetes 23:* 725–731.

86. Cherrington, A. D., R. Kawamoi, S. Pek, and M. Vranic. 1974. Arginine infusion in dogs. Model for the roles of insulin and glucagon in regulating glucose turnover and free fatty acid levels. *Diabetes 23:* 805–815.

87. Sakurai, H., R. Dobbs, and R. H. Unger. 1974. Somatostatin-induced changes in insulin and glucagon secretion in normal and diabetic dogs. *J. Clin. Invest. 54:* 1395–1402.

88. Gerich, J. E., M. Lorenzi, V. Schneider, C. W. Kwan, J. H. Karam, R. Guillemin, and P. H. Forsham. 1974. Inhibition of pancreatic glucagon responses to arginine by somatostatin in normal man and in insulin-dependent diabetics. *Diabetes 23:* 876–880.

89. Müller, W. A., G. R. Faloona, and R. H. Unger. 1971. The effect of experimental insulin deficiency on glucagon secretion. *J. Clin. Invest. 50:* 1992–1999.

90. Liljenquist, J. E., J. D. Bomboy, S. B. Lewis, B. C. Sinclair-Smith,

P. W. Felts, W. W. Lacy, O. B. Crofford, and G. W. Liddle. 1974. Effects of glucagon on lipolysis and ketogenesis in normal and diabetic man. *J. Clin. Invest. 53:* 190–197.

91. Liljenquist, J. E., J. D. Bomboy, S. B. Lewis, B. C. Sinclair-Smith, P. W. Felts, W. W. Lacy, O. B. Crofford, and G. W. Liddle. 1974. Effect of glucagon on net splanchnic cyclic AMP production in normal and diabetic men. *J. Clin. Invest. 53:* 198–204.

92. Gerich, J. E., M. Lorenzi, D. M. Bier, V. Schneider, E. Tsalikian, J. H. Karam, and P. H. Forsham. 1975. Prevention of human diabetic ketoacidosis by somatostatin. *N. Engl. J. Med. 292:* 985–989.

93. Schade, D. S., and R. P. Eaton. 1975. Glucagon regulation of plasma ketone body concentration in human diabetes. *J. Clin. Invest. 56:* 1340–1344.

94. McGarry, J. D., C. Robles-Valdes, and D. W. Foster. 1975. The role of carnitine in hepatic ketogenesis. *Proc. Natl. Acad. Sci. U.S.A. 72:* 4385–4388.

95. Fritz, I. B. 1955. The effects of muscle extracts on the oxidation of palmitic acid by liver slices and homogenates. *Acta Physiol. Scand. 34:* 367–385.

96. Embden, G., and F. Kalberlah. 1906. Über Acetonbildung in der Leber. *Beitr. Z. Chan. Physiol. Pathol. 8:* 121–128.

97. Embden, G., and J. Wirth. 1910. Über Hemmung der Acetessigsaurebildung in der Leber. *Biochem. Z. 27:* 1–19.

98. Blixenkrone-Møller, N. 1938. Respiratorischer Stoffwechsel und Ketonbildung der Leber. *Z. Physiol. Chem. 252:* 117–136.

99. Mirsky, I. A. 1942. The etiology of diabetic acidosis. *JAMA 118:* 690–694.

100. Weinhouse, S., R. H. Millington, and B. Friedman. 1949. The effect of carbohydrate on the oxidation of fatty acids by liver slices. *J. Biol. Chem. 181:* 489–498.

100a. McGarry, J.D., Mannaerts, G.P., and Foster, D.W. A possible role for malonyl-CoA in the regulation of heptic fatty oxidation and ketogenesis. *J. Clin. Invest. 60:*265–270, 1977.

100b. Guynn, R.W., Veloso, D., and Veech, R.L. The concentration of malonyl-coenzyme A and the control of fatty acid synthesis *in vivo*. *J. Biol. Chem. 247:*7325–7331, 1972.

100c. Cook, G.A., Nielsen, R.C., Hawkins, R.A., Mehlman, M.A., Lakshmanan, M.R., and Veech, R.L. Effect of glucagon on heptic malonyl coenzyme A concentration and on lipid synthesis. *J. Biol. Chem. 252:*4421–4424, 1977.

101. Fritz, I. B., and S. K. Schultz. 1965. Carnitine acyltransferase. II. Inhibition by carnitine analogues and by sulfhydryl reagents. *J. Biol. Chem. 240:* 2188–2192.

102. Delisle, G., and I. B. Fritz. 1967. Interrelations between hepatic fatty acid oxidation and gluconeogenesis: A possible regulatory role of carnitine palmityltransferase. *Proc. Natl. Acad. Sci. U.S.A. 58:* 790–797.

103. Williamson, J. R., E. R. Browning, R. Scholz, R. H. Kreisberg, and I. B. Fritz. 1968. Inhibition of fatty acid stimulation of gluconeogenesis by (+)-decanoylcarnitine in perfused rat liver. *Diabetes 17:* 194–207.

104. Williamson, J. R., E. T. Browning, R. G. Thurman, and R. Scholz. 1969. Inhibition of glucagon effects in perfused rat liver by (+)-decanoylcarnitine. *J. Biol. Chem. 244:* 5055–5064.

105. McGarry, J. D., and D. W. Foster. 1973. Acute reversal of experimental diabetic ketoacidosis in the rat with (+)-decanoylcarnitine. *J. Clin. Invest. 52:* 877–884.

106. McGarry, J. D., and D. W. Foster. 1974. Studies with (+)-octanoylcarnitine in experimental diabetic ketoacidosis. *Diabetes 23:* 485–493.

107. Beigelman, P. M. 1971. Severe diabetic ketoacidosis (diabetic "coma"). 482 episodes in 257 patients; experience of 3 years. *Diabetes 20:* 490–500.

108. Unger, R. H., and L. Orci. 1975. The essential role of glucagon in the pathogenesis of diabetes mellitus. *Lancet 1:* 14–16.

Diabetes Mellitus: Description, Etiology and Pathogenesis, Natural History, and Testing Procedures

Stefan S. Fajans

INTRODUCTION AND DESCRIPTION

"Idiopathic" or primary diabetes mellitus is a genetically determined disorder of metabolism associated with relative or absolute insufficiency of insulin. In its fully developed clinical expression, it is characterized by fasting hyperglycemia, atherosclerotic and microangiopathic vascular disease, and neuropathy. It is distinguished from secondary types of diabetes or carbohydrate intolerance resulting from (1) destruction of the pancreas by disease or surgical excision of pancreatic tissue, (2) endocrine disease with excessive secretion of growth hormone, hydrocortisone, aldosterone, catecholamines, glucagon, or somatostatin, (3) administration of steroids or drugs, and (4) central nervous system disease; and carbohydrate intolerance associated with a variety of well-defined genetic syndromes.[1] Only a few decades ago a generally accepted definition of diabetes mellitus would have stressed the presence of continuous hyperglycemia and glycosuria. Even today a few investigators and clinicians are hesitant to accept a definite diagnosis of diabetes in the absence of fasting hyperglycemia (i.e., continuous hyperglycemia). However, the majority agree that diabetes mellitus may present clinically in a mild or asymptomatic form without fasting hyperglycemia. The typical vascular and neuropathic manifestations may occur in patients with a genetic predisposition to the disease who have relatively mild carbohydrate intolerance and fasting blood glucose levels within the "normal" range. The complications of the disease may bring the patient to medical attention for the first time, even though hyperglycemia is asymptomatic and may have been present for a prolonged period of time. A definition of "carbohydrate intolerance" is difficult, since there is no strict separation between normal and abnormal carbohydrate tolerance even in healthy, ambulatory individuals. The definition is based on statistical rather than biological considerations. Examining carbohydrate tolerance in most groups of first-degree relatives of diabetes patients (with the exception of the Pima Indians, who have an extremely high prevalence of diabetes[2]) there is no bimodality but a continuum between normal and abnormal carbohydrate metabolism.[3] The selection of useful diagnostic tests and criteria depends on an understanding of (1) the heterogeneous nature of diabetes mellitus in terms of etiology and pathogenesis, and (2) the fact that the natural history of diabetes mellitus may show great variability within the various types of the disease.

Clinically we recognize two major types of "primary or idiopathic" diabetes mellitus. One is the *juvenile-onset* type in which there is complete insulin insufficiency. The patient is ketosis-prone and is dependent on exogenous insulin for survival. Classically, the juvenile-onset type of diabetes is first recognized during childhood or adolescence. However, this type of diabetes can make its clinical appearance at any age. When untreated, it is associated with the acute symptoms secondary to insulin insufficiency (polyuria, polydipsia, polyphagia, weight loss, fatigue). The second major type is *maturity-onset* diabetes. This diabetes is "insulin-independent," since the patient does not develop ketosis without insulin therapy and is termed to be "ketosis-resistant." Nevertheless, a maturity-onset-type diabetic may require insulin for correction of fasting hyperglycemia. In others, this therapeutic goal can be accomplished without insulin by therapy with diet or diet plus oral drugs. Maturity-onset-type diabetes is usually not associated with symptoms of insulin insufficiency and is diagnosed most frequently in individuals in middle age or older age groups. However, since 1960 it has been recognized that typical maturity-onset-type diabetes can be recognized in asymptomatic young people, particularly if it is looked for in first-degree relatives of maturity-onset-type diabetic patients (as reviewed in ref. 4).

The biochemical and clinical manifestations of diabetes span a spectrum from the recognizable but asymptomatic form of the disease to symptomatic diabetes with acute metabolic decompensation (ketoacidosis, hyperosmolar coma) or with chronic complications or associations (complications of pregnancy, cataracts, neuropathy, atherosclerosis, microangiopathy). Since hyperglycemia and the chronic complications are found in both juvenile-onset-type and maturity-onset-type diabetes, and since both types occasionally occur in the same families, these two types of diabetes usually have been thought to represent only a quantitative difference in the defect in insulin secretion or action and attendant sequelae. However, evidence has accumulated to suggest the existence of heterogeneity of "idiopathic diabetes mellitus" in terms of (1) inheritance, (2) environmental factors, (3) insulin responses to glucose in maturity-onset-type diabetes, and (4) prevalence of vascular disease. It appears that "idiopathic" diabetes mellitus is not a single specific disease entity but a syndrome comprised of a number of diseases. In that respect, diabetes may be likened to hypertension, which is caused by a variety of pathogenetic mechanisms, but each entity may be associated with similar vascular complications.

ETIOLOGY AND PATHOGENESIS OF DIABETES MELLITUS

HETEROGENEITY OF INHERITANCE

In primary diabetes mellitus, genetic as well as environmental factors appear to be involved in its evolution. Differing environmental factors, superimposed on differences in genetic susceptibility, may be important in the pathogenesis of various forms of the disease. Evidence supporting the presence of genetic heterogeneity, reviewed to a major extent at an International Workshop on the Genetics of Diabetes Mellitus[5] and by Zonana and Rimoin,[6] consists of five different lines of evidence. These include (1) pedigree analysis of two forms of diabetes in young people, (2) histocompatibility (HLA) studies, (3) analysis of prevalence of diabetes and HLA types in identical twins, (4) evidence of autoimmune abnormalities as expressed by the finding of cell-mediated immunity, and (5) evidence of autoimmune phenomena as expressed in the finding of circulating pancreatic islet cell antibodies.

Pedigree Analysis of Two Forms of Diabetes in Young People

A difference in the pattern of inheritance of diabetes has been shown between families of 26 propositi with *maturity-onset-type diabetes in young people* (MODY) and families of 35 propositi with classical *juvenile-onset-type diabetes* (JOD).[7] In the families of MODY (1) 85 percent of propositi had a diabetic parent, (2) 46 percent of families showed direct vertical transmission of diabetes through three generations, (3) 53 percent of tested siblings had

latent diabetes, and (4) the diabetic phenotype in the families was consistent, most affected individuals having a non-insulin-requiring type of diabetes. These findings are compatible with autosomal dominant inheritance of MODY, although they do not exclude multifactorial inheritance. In contrast, in the families of JOD, only 11 percent of propositi had a diabetic parent, and three-generation inheritance was found in only 6 percent of JOD families. Of 74 tested siblings, 6 (8 percent) had JOD-type diabetes and only 2 (3 percent had latent diabetes. These observations not only provide evidence of genetic heterogeneity but also further indicate the need for careful definition of the phenotype of diabetes in populations in which the genetics of diabetes is to be analyzed.

In contrast to the high prevalence of maturity-onset-type diabetes (MOD) among the parents and grandparents of MODY propositi, there is an equal incidence of adult-onset-type diabetes among ancestors of juvenile diabetics and nondiabetics.[8] This has been interpreted as evidence that juvenile and adult-onset diabetes have different genetic origins.

The Histocompatibility System (HLA) and Genetic Susceptibility to Diabetes Mellitus

A difference in the inheritance between juvenile-onset and maturity-onset types of diabetes may be associated with a difference in the frequency of occurrence of certain histocompatibility types or HLA antigens and a difference in the frequency with which viral and/or autoimmune processes may be involved. Following the recent studies of the major histocompatibility (HLA) system in man, it was found that in classical JOD, the major genetic susceptibility is HLA-linked. A search for an association between the HLA system and a particular disease is more likely to be productive when there is familial aggregation and where virus and autoimmunity seem to be involved. In JOD there is evidence for the existence of all these possible pathogenetic factors. The HLA system probably contains the so-called immune response (Ir) genes or determinants.[9] If this is true, the associations observed with four types of cell surface antigens, HLA-A, B, C, and D of chromosome #6 must be considered secondary to primary associations with Ir determinants in linkage disequilibrium with unknown HLA markers.

HLA-B8, BW15, B18, A1, CW3, DW3, and DW4 have been found with increased frequency in JOD but not in MOD. In subjects who possess two of these antigens, the risk appears to be additive, suggesting that they may be operating through different pathogenetic mechanisms.[10,11] B7 and B5 have been found with decreased frequency in JOD but not in MOD. These findings support the concept that insulin-dependent and insulin-independent diabetes are two different disease entities. It is likely that in insulin-dependent diabetes, irrespective of age of onset, there are one or more immune response genes in linkage disequilibrium with HLA antigens that may impart increased susceptibility to beta cell damage by permitting interaction of a virus with specific cell membrane antigens. If this interaction fails to eliminate an infective virus, there may result direct viral invasion and destruction of the beta cells. Alternately, this interaction between the virus and the membrane receptor may modify adversely an immune response, resulting in an autoimmune process and cell-mediated beta cell destruction. On the other hand, B7 and B5 antigens may impart a protective effect against islet cell damage.

Analysis of Prevalence of Diabetes and HLA Types in Identical Twins

Genetic heterogeneity has been found among sets of identical twins of whom at least one had diabetes mellitus.[12] Concordance of diabetes among pairs of identical twins was very high (92 percent) among those in whom the age of onset of diabetes in the index twin was 40 years or more (mostly maturity-onset type), while concordance was found with a frequency of only 53 percent in those in whom diabetes was diagnosed under 40 years of age in one twin (mostly juvenile-onset type). This suggests that there is a difference in genetic as well as environmental factors in the etiology and pathogenesis of diabetes between these two groups of identical twins.

Histocompatibility typing performed in 84 pairs of identical twins of whom at least one was diabetic[13] has also suggested that there are possible differences in a hereditary predisposition to diabetes. Twenty-two pairs of identical twins were maturity-onset diabetics; all were concordant, and they showed no disturbance of HLA frequencies. Of the remaining 62 pairs of juvenile-onset diabetics, 31 were discordant and 31 concordant. Frequency of the BW15 antigen was equally increased in both the concordant and discordant pairs. The fact that BW15 is increased in the discordant pairs shows that there is a genetic predisposition to diabetes even in a nondiabetic twin. HLA-B8 was increased only in the concordant pairs. The fact that HLA-B8 is not increased in the discordant pairs suggests that different alleles may underlie susceptibility in the two groups of twins.

Autoimmune Abnormality as Expressed by the Finding of Cell-mediated Immunity

Autoimmunity has been linked to insulin-dependent juvenile-onset-type diabetes.[14] The evidence supporting such an association can be summarized as follows: (1) the clinical association with other diseases that have autoimmune features, including antibody-positive thyroid disorders (Hashimoto thyroiditis and Graves disease), pernicious anemia, Addison's disease, hypoparathyroidism, and the coexistence of diabetes with multiple autoimmune disorders; (2) the finding of increased incidence of organ-specific humoral antithyroid, gastric-parietal cell and adrenal antibodies; (3) the demonstration of insulitis in patients dying soon after the onset of diabetes, suggesting a cellular immune response; (4) demonstration of antipancreatic cell-mediated immunity by leukocyte migration inhibition and lymphocyte transformation tests; and (5) detection by immunofluorescence of humoral islet cell antibodies in patients with juvenile-onset diabetes.

Cell-mediated Immunity. Organ-specific cell-mediated autoimmunity has been detected in diabetes mellitus by two in vitro techniques.[15] One is the leukocyte migration-inhibition test. Positive leukocyte migration-inhibition tests have been shown in JOD, using extracts of porcine, calf, and normal human pancreas (as well as insulinoma cells) as antigen. The same prevalence of positive migration-inhibition tests occurs irrespective of whether or not there are pancreatic islet cell antibodies in the patient's serum and whether or not the patient has ever received insulin. A second is the lymphocyte transformation test. Mitogen- or antigen-induced transformation of lymphocytes to blast cells are alternative in vitro tests of cellular immune function.

Using human insulinoma cells as model beta cells, Huang and McLaren[16] have developed an in vitro assay of lymphocyte-mediated cytotoxicity. Lymphocytes from 23 JOD patients demonstrated significant cytoadherence and cytotoxicity against human insulinoma cells in vitro as compared to lymphocytes from normal subjects. Serum antibodies failed to show any cytotoxicity with the cell suspension. Thus, cell-mediated immunity against cell surface components of beta cells was postulated to play an important role in the pathogenesis of juvenile-onset diabetes. This occurred before insulin therapy, which implies that sensitization to insulin is not a primary factor. The findings suggested to the authors that insulin-dependent diabetes may be a disease of autoaggression.

They also postulated that infectious agents, particularly viruses, might trigger this process of autoimmune beta cell destruction in a genetically predisposed individual.

A new model of diabetes mellitus has been described with a suggested pathogenesis of a chemically initiated cell-mediated immune reaction.[17] Multiple small injections of streptozotocin in mice produced pancreatic insulitis characterized by mononuclear inflammatory cells in and around the pancreatic islets. This was in contrast to the virtually inflammatory-free islet lesions observed after a single large injection. The time required for the first appearance of inflammatory cells was 5 to 6 days after the last injection and is compatible with a cell-mediated immune reaction conceivably directed against beta cells modified by administration of streptozotocin. The reduction in beta cell numbers and elevation of plasma glucose became progressively more pronounced during the 10 to 25 days after the last injection, long after streptozotocin is cleared from the bloodstream. The authors speculate that the mononuclear inflammatory cells are responsible for the progressive beta cell destruction and the resulting increasingly severe hyperglycemia. Ultrastructural evidence of abundant type C virus within the beta cells of the streptozotocin-treated mice suggested that streptozotocin may activate murine leukemia virus in susceptible hosts.

Autoimmune Phenomena as Expressed by the Finding of Circulating Pancreatic Islet Cell Antibodies (PICA or ICA)

Humoral antibodies in diabetes reacting specifically with pancreatic islet cells were first demonstrated only in diabetic patients with insulin-dependent diabetes plus coexisting evidence of autoimmunity.[18,19] Subsequently, islet cell antibodies have been found in insulin-dependent diabetics without other coexistent autoimmune disease.

Circulating antibodies to live, tissue-cultured human insulinoma cells were identified in 34 of 39 insulin-dependent diabetic patients by an indirect immunofluorescent technique.[20] The antibodies were not related to therapy with exogenous insulin. The antibodies were of the IgM and IgG classes. In another study, antibodies reacting with human pancreatic islet cells were found by immunofluorescence in the serum of 51 to 105 children with diabetes mellitus of recent onset.[21] These patients had no other evidence of autoimmune disease. It seems likely, therefore, that there may be autoimmune activity directed against islet cells in a substantial proportion, if not in the majority, of cases of childhood diabetes of recent onset. The age distribution and seasonal variation in onset that occurs in juvenile diabetes suggests that autoimmune damage may be combined with a seasonal factor, e.g., viral.

Irvine et al.[22] found that the prevalence of ICA was 0.5 percent in the general population but 70 percent at the time of clinical diagnosis of JOD. ICA occurred irrespective of age at diagnosis in insulin-dependent patients. In insulin-independent diabetics requiring oral hypoglycemic agents, there was an 8 percent overall prevalence of ICA with a 20 percent prevalence at the time of progression. Those subjects who were ICA-positive had a strong tendency to develop insulin-dependent diabetes in subsequent years, suggesting different grades of disease severity.

Another study[23] has confirmed the strong association of ICA with insulin-dependent diabetes. The prevalence of ICA declined as the duration of the disease increased. This decline was particularly rapid during the first 5 weeks of clinical disease, falling from 85 to 50 percent. Subsequently, the prevalence remained steady until the end of the first year. Over the next few years, the prevalence fell to between 10 and 20 percent, after which no further decline was observed. The decrease in antibody prevalence was independent of the age of patients. The initially high prevalence of ICA was undoubtedly due to selection of patients who had symptoms for only a short time; patients with symptomatic onset within 1 week of testing probably had undergone very recent islet cell destruction. Others, in whom symptoms appeared more gradually, may have had more insidious damage going on for longer periods of time, and their antibodies may have already disappeared. In some nondiabetic subjects who were first-degree relatives of an insulin-dependent diabetic, overt diabetes developed years after detection of ICA. This suggests that the event that leads to diabetes occurs months or years before clinical features develop.

A rare form of insulin-resistant diabetes mellitus associated with acanthosis nigricans has been reported. Insulin resistance in these patients results from marked decrease in insulin binding to its membrane receptors. In some patients (type A), the defect is due to a primary decrease in the number of insulin receptors, not secondary to hyperinsulinemia. In the second group of patients (type B), there is a decreased affinity of the receptor for insulin. In this condition, insulin resistance results from circulating antibodies to the insulin receptor.[24] The circulating antibody or inhibitor of insulin receptors has been characterized as an immunoglobulin that is polyclonal in nature. These antibodies are directed at determinants on or near the insulin receptor and are responsible for the observed insulin resistance.[25]

Relation of HLA to ICA. There is still a difference of opinion as to whether there is an increased association between the increased prevalence of HLA antigens in JOD and that of pancreatic islet cell antibodies. Frequency of HLA-B8 was significantly increased in pancreatic ICA-positive patients (61 percent) compared with ICA-negative patients (35 percent) and the control population (28 percent).[26] This increased frequency of HLA-B8 was even more striking in diabetics in whom ICA persisted for more than 5 years (73 percent). These findings appear to link the genetic marker for JOD and antipancreatic autoimmunity.

HETEROGENEITY OF ENVIRONMENTAL FACTORS

Environmental factors superimposed on an inherited predisposition may be essential for the development of recognizable or clinical diabetes. A variety of environmental factors may precipitate or cause the emergence of the disease. Recently, viruses have been implicated in the pathogenesis of juvenile-onset-type diabetes, while nutritional factors have been thought to play a role in the pathogenesis of maturity-onset-type diabetes.

A seasonal variation in the incidence of JOD has been reported, implying the presence of seasonal, environmental etiological factors, and virus infection seems a likely candidate.[27] Infective agents that have been implicated have included Coxsackie virus B4, mumps, hepatitis, congenital rubella, and other viruses. Some of this evidence is contradictory and inconclusive. If, in fact, viruses are involved in the pathogenesis of JOD, it is likely that they can initiate pancreatic damage primarily in individuals who are genetically predisposed to such damage. As reviewed above, the juvenile form of diabetes appears to be linked to histocompatibility antigens that may be associated with certain genes controlling immune responses.

Diabetes could result also from a series of infections producing cumulative pancreatic damage. Alternatively, a viral infection may set up an autoimmune reaction which, once triggered, would sustain continuing beta cell damage.

Although there is as yet little direct evidence for a viral etiology of diabetes in man, studies of virus-induced diabetes in animals produce circumstantial support for the virus theory in

man. Craighead[28] has shown that a diabeteslike disease can be produced in certain strains of mice by the M variant of the encephalomyocarditis (EMC) virus. After inoculation, viremia is relatively transient and is followed by the abrupt appearance of circulating neutralizing antibody in the serum. Immunofluorescence studies of the pancreas have demonstrated viral antigens exclusively in the insular tissue. The severity of the diabetic syndrome is directly related to the amount of necrosis of beta cells. The most important factor in the development of diabetes in mice seems to be a genetic susceptibility to pancreatic damage resulting from the infection. Genetic studies showed that several strains of mice regularly develop hyperglycemia during the acute stages of infection, whereas other strains infrequently exhibit evidence of abnormal carbohydrate metabolism. Other investigators have shown also that some strains of mice are susceptible while others are resistant to the diabetogenic effects of EMC virus.[29]

There may be variation in etiologic and pathogenic factors in JOD. As discussed, in the majority, a viral agent superimposed on a genetic susceptibility of the beta cells and ensuing autoimmunity, may lead to beta cell damage and insulin insufficiency. In a few patients, an overwhelming viral insulitis may lead to insulin insufficiency even without underlying genetic susceptibility or without any evidence of autoimmunity, and this might account for patients who do not have ICA even at diagnosis. In another small group, a strong predisposition to organ-specific endocrine autoimmunity (autoimmune polyendocrinopathies), including the islets, may lead to beta cell insufficiency without a superimposed environmental factor, such as a viral infection.

In maturity-onset-type diabetes, representing a different type of genetic predisposition (no disturbance of HLA frequencies), other environmental factors such as overnutrition, obesity,[30,31] or pregnancy may lead to hyperglycemia.

HETEROGENEITY OF INSULIN RESPONSE TO GLUCOSE IN MATURITY-ONSET-TYPE DIABETES

Although juvenile-onset-type diabetes is characterized by a grossly subnormal or by absent insulin secretory response to glucose, insulin responses in the early stages of maturity-onset-type diabetes are quite variable. Diminished initial rapid release of insulin followed by either a subnormal later response or by a normal or even higher than normal insulin response has been reported.[4,32a,32b] Figure 81-1 shows the mean glucose tolerance test

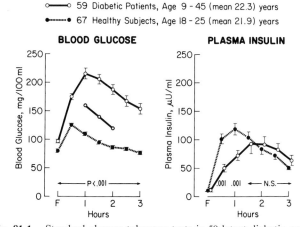

Fig. 81-1. Standard glucose tolerance tests in 59 latent diabetic patients and in 67 healthy control subjects (1.75 g glucose orally per kilogram of ideal body weight). All points are mean ± SEM. (Reproduced by permission of *Transactions of Association of American Physicians*, Fajans et al., 87:83, 1974.)

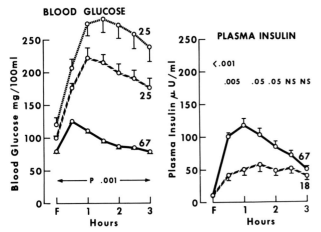

Fig. 81-2. Initial diagnostic standard glucose tolerance tests (1.75 g of glucose orally per kilogram of ideal body weight), glucose tolerance test with highest increases in blood glucose levels in patients with latent diabetes (ages 9 to 17 years at diagnosis), and glucose tolerance tests in healthy control subjects. All points are mean ± SEM. (Reproduced by permission of *Archives of Internal Medicine,* Fajans et al., 136:194, 1976.)

and the insulin response to glucose of 59 diabetic patients aged 9 to 45 years at diagnosis (mean age 22.3 years) and those of 67 healthy control subjects with a mean age of 21.9 years. In the diabetic patients, both the fasting and postglucose blood glucose levels during the glucose tolerance test were significantly higher than those of the control subjects. In the diabetic patients, increases in plasma levels of insulin after the administration of glucose were significantly delayed, while the levels were similar after 90 minutes in spite of the disparate blood glucose levels. Figure 81-2 shows glucose tolerance tests and insulin responses to glucose for 25 diabetic patients aged 9 to 17 years at diagnosis. Again, the means of the initial fasting blood glucose levels and blood glucose levels after the administration of glucose were significantly higher (p<.001) than in the control subjects. Plasma levels of insulin for 18 of the nonobese diabetic patients show a greatly delayed and subnormal insulin response to glucose.

On the other hand, a normal or higher than normal initial response followed by a later supernormal insulin response in latent diabetes has also been reported.[4,32b,33] The finding of normal or even high insulin levels in mild diabetes has given rise to the concept of insulin resistance as the initial lesion in early MOD.[33] Decreased binding of insulin to its receptors may be related to insulin resistance in latent diabetes.[34]

Figure 81-3 examines the insulin responses to glucose of the patients with the lowest and those with the highest insulin responses during the glucose tolerance test. Sixteen of the 59 patients shown in Figure 81-1 had low total increments in insulin defined as "low response." Eight patients had high total increments in relation to the control subjects, which are defined as "high responses."[4,32b] The differences in the plasma levels of insulin in these latent diabetic patients classified as having low and high insulin responses to glucose, respectively, are striking (Fig. 81-3), although blood levels for the corresponding groups were significantly different only at 2½ and 3 hours during the initial glucose tolerance test on which the diagnosis of diabetes was first made.[4] From prolonged prospective longitudinal studies, two additional observations have emerged which indicate that we are dealing with true heterogeneity of insulin responses and not with a

spectrum of insulin responses. When glucose tolerance improved in those patients with initially low insulin responses, insulin responses to administered glucose increased significantly, suggesting that greatly decreased insulin responses appear to be the determinant, at least in part, of abnormal carbohydrate tolerance. On the other hand, when glucose tolerance improved in those patients with high insulin responses, plasma levels of insulin decreased concomitantly. This suggests that in these latter patients, hyperinsulinemia is secondary or compensatory to factors that cause glucose intolerance. Furthermore, progression to diabetes requiring insulin injections to control fasting hyperglycemia occurred only in individuals who had insulin responses that were delayed and lower than the mean response of the control subjects. Such an insulin response appears to be a more reliable prognostic indicator of decompensation to requirement of insulin at a later date than the degree of abnormality of carbohydrate intolerance. In contrast, none of the patients with "high" insulin responses, or whose responses exceeded the mean of the control subjects, have progressed to diabetes that required insulin injections.[4] The data of Johansen indicate also that young latent diabetics who progressed to insulin-requiring diabetes had had delayed and subnormal insulin responses to orally given glucose.[35] Among patients reported by various investigators, only those patients with low insulin responses progressed to diabetes that required insulin injections. None of the children with elevated insulin responses were said to have progressed to diabetes that required insulin.[36]

HETEROGENEITY OF VASCULAR DISEASE

Variations in occurrence of significant vascular disease in diabetes also suggest that we are dealing with a syndrome that includes entities in which different pathogenetic factors (genetic, environmental) are at play. Among a group of patients with classical juvenile-onset-type, ketoacidosis-prone diabetes of more than 30 years' duration and with continuous hyperglycemia ("poorly controlled"), 20 percent do not have clinically significant retinopathy or nephropathy.[37] As reported from at least six clinics in five different countries, among insulin-requiring ketosis-prone patients who have survived diabetes for 20 to 40 years or more, clinical

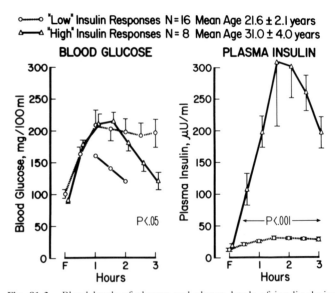

Fig. 81-3. Blood levels of glucose and plasma levels of insulin during glucose tolerance tests in which first insulin determinations were made in latent diabetic patients with low and high insulin responses to glucose. All points are mean ± SEM. (Reproduced by permission of *Archives of Internal Medicine,* Fajans, et al., 136:194, 1976.)

evidence of microvascular disease, atherosclerosis, or neuropathy has been found in only 20 to 40 percent.[38] In a further report, 73 patients with juvenile diabetes mellitus of 40 years' or more duration were studied retrospectively.[39] Diabetic retinal changes on fundoscopic examination were not demonstrable in about one-quarter of the patients. Fifty-nine percent were free of renal involvement and were normotensive. Seventy-nine percent had no coronary artery disease. Thus, JOD can be compatible with long survival and minor complications. There may be genetic differences in the vulnerability of vascular tissue to the environmental metabolic abnormalities accompanying the diabetic state such as hyperglycemia, hyperlipidemia, alterations in amino acid metabolism, and other disturbances in metabolism or hormonal release.

SUMMARY OF ETIOLOGIC AND PATHOGENETIC FACTORS IN DIABETES MELLITUS

Table 81-1 summarizes some of the proposed and possible factors important in the etiology and pathogenesis of diabetes mellitus discussed in this chapter and in preceding chapters on the pancreatic islet cells. Only a few additional comments will be made in regard to the factors not mentioned before.

There is little or no evidence that an abnormality in conversion of proinsulin to insulin or synthesis of an abnormal insulin

Table 81-1. Proposed Etiologic and Pathogenetic Factors in Diabetes Mellitus (Heterogeneous)

A. Genetically determined abnormality of beta cell function (stimulus recognition–message propagation–secretion) or number
  1. Delayed and decreased insulin secretory response to nutrients (glucose and amino acids)
    a. Decreased number of beta cell receptor sites to glucose or amino acids
    b. Decreased affinity of receptor sites
    c. Altered microtubular response
    d. Altered microfilamentous activity
    e. Altered cation shifts
    f. Abnormality in cAMP
  2. Decreased insulin biosynthesis
  3. Abnormality in conversion of proinsulin to insulin
  4. Synthesis of an abnormal insulin with impaired biological activity
  5. Decrease in beta cell replication rate—early senescence
  6. Increased susceptibility of beta cells to environmental factors linked to HLA system
B. Environmental factors altering beta cell integrity and function
  1. Infective agents—viruses
  2. Autoimmunity—antipancreatic cell-mediated immunity; increased susceptibility to beta cell damage by viral agents due to defective immune response influenced by genes in the HLA chromosomal region (associated with HLA-B8 and/or BWl5 or CW3 or DW3 and DW4 antigens) and leading to an autoimmune process (in proportion of juvenile-onset-type diabetes)
  3. Diet (calories) leading to obesity; pregnancy (maturity-onset type)
  4. Autonomic nervous system—increased adrenergic activity
C. Abnormality of insulin action
  1. Insensitivity to endogenous insulin
    a. Release of insulin with impaired biological activity
    b. Decreased number of insulin receptor sites
    c. Interference with binding of insulin to its receptor sites—antibodies to insulin receptors
    d. Decreased activity of key enzyme(s)
D. Abnormality in glucagon secretion
  1. Secondary to insulin insufficiency
  2. Primary abnormality
E. Abnormal formation or degradation of basement membrane
  1. Primary abnormality on genetic basis
  2. Secondary to insulin insufficiency

with impaired biological activity plays a significant role. In regard to A.5., it has been postulated that one of the basic tissue abnormalities that characterize the human diabetic state and its complications is accelerated aging or senescence.[40] It may be on a genetic basis, and it may be exacerbated by hyperglycemia. This accelerated senescence of tissues may be manifested by a decreased replication rate of beta cells of the pancreatic islets in response to injury, an accelerated rate of cell death in basal lamina, and a decreased replication rate of cultured fibroblasts from diabetic patients,[41] and it may be responsible for the increased incidence of senile cataracts and osteoporosis and the accelerated atherosclerosis found in diabetic patients. The width of muscle capillary basement membrane increases with age in healthy subjects, and this thickening is accelerated in diabetes.[42]

Increased adrenergic activity may play a role in defective insulin release. In nonketotic hyperglycemic diabetic patients, alpha-adrenergic blockade increased basal insulin levels to a greater extent than in normal subjects and also partially restored the acute insulin response to intravenous glucose stimulation in diabetics.[43] The data also demonstrated that circulating catecholamine levels, both in the basal state and immediately after glucose stimulation, were greater in diabetic than in normal subjects, providing a possible hormonal mediator for the observed increases in endogenous alpha-adrenergic activity in these nonketotic diabetic patients.

THE NATURAL HISTORY OF DIABETES MELLITUS

As reviewed above, "idiopathic" diabetes is a disease in which an inherited susceptibility plays an important part. This susceptibility has its origin at conception and may exist for prolonged periods before additional pathogenetic factors of environmental origin cause the emergence of a recognizable abnormality of carbohydrate metabolism. The genetic defect may remain without clinical expression indefinitely. Thus, a definition of genetic or "idiopathic" diabetes mellitus should include stages in the natural history of the disease which presently cannot be recognized, since we lack reliable markers for the various types of "genetic diabetes." An arbitrary definition of steps in the natural history of diabetes has been based on the absence or presence and on the degree of abnormality of glucose metabolism. Table 81-2 presents a scheme depicting the natural history of diabetes divided into four stages. The terminology employed in this table includes the definitions used by our group and that employed by the British Diabetic Association and the World Health Organization.[44]

Overt (or clinical) diabetes is the most advanced of these stages. Classical symptoms may be present; there is gross fasting hyperglycemia; there is no insulin secretory response to administered glucose. This stage can be divided further into the ketotic and nonketotic forms of the disease which, at least in part, may differ in etiology and pathogenesis.

The preceding stage is latent (or asymptomatic, chemical) but clinically detectable diabetes. A latent diabetic is an individual who has no symptoms, signs, or complications referable to the disease (except for reactive hypoglycemia in some patients) but in whom a diagnosis of diabetes can be established by presently accepted laboratory procedures. This stage may also be characterized by an elevated fasting blood glucose level but of lesser severity than in overt diabetes. When the fasting level of blood glucose is below diagnostic levels, this stage can be recognized by a definitely abnormal glucose tolerance test. The heterogeneous nature of the plasma insulin response to administered glucose in this stage has been discussed.

Table 81-2. Stages in the Natural History of Diabetes Mellitus

Terminology by: Author	Prediabetes ⟶ ⟵	Subclinical diabetes ⟶ ⟵	Latent diabetes ⟶ ⟵	Overt diabetes
World Health Organization	Potential diabetes	Latent diabetes	Asymptomatic diabetes (subclinical or chemical)	Clinical diabetes
FBS	Normal	Normal	Normal or ↑	↑
GTT	Normal	Normal / Abnormal during pregnancy, stress	Abnormal	Not necessary for diagnosis
Cortisone-GTT	Normal	Abnormal	Not necessary	—

Progression *or* regression from one stage to the next stage (1) may never occur, or (2) may occur very slowly over many years, or (3) may be rapid or even explosive. See text.

An earlier stage is subclinical diabetes or latent diabetes by the World Health Organization definition. In this stage, not only the fasting blood glucose level but also the glucose tolerance test is normal under usual circumstances. However, diabetes may be suspected because of evidence of insufficient functional reserve of the islet cells under stress. An example would be a woman who has a normal glucose tolerance test but who has a history of abnormality of glucose tolerance during pregnancy. The latter has been termed pregnancy or gestational diabetes. A high proportion of such women develop latent or overt diabetes in the years that follow. A delayed and subnormal insulin secretory response to glucose has been demonstrated in some patients with gestational diabetes.[45] Another example of subclinical diabetes may be an individual with a normal glucose tolerance test but an abnormal cortisone-glucose tolerance test in the nonpregnant state. The plasma insulin response in groups of subjects with abnormal steroid-glucose tolerance tests is delayed and lower as compared to those found in subjects with normal steroid-glucose tolerance tests.[46,47]

The earliest stage is prediabetes or potential diabetes (WHO). This stage exists prior to the onset of identifiable diabetes mellitus whether it be overt, latent, or subclinical. It identifies the interval of time from conception until the demonstration of impaired glucose tolerance in an individual predisposed to diabetes on genetic grounds. This period can be identified only *retrospectively*. Prediabetes or potential diabetes can be *suspected* to be present in individuals who have an increased probability of developing diabetes on genetic grounds, such as in some nondiabetic identical twins of diabetic patients (particularly of MOD or MODY or in HLA- and ICA-positive siblings) or in some nondiabetic offspring of two MOD patients (not all will develop diabetes). During the prediabetic period, glucose tolerance and cortisone-glucose tolerance tests are normal; thus an individual cannot be identified as "prediabetic" by present techniques.

Recent evidence would suggest that there is more than one form of "genetic prediabetes." Among young nondiabetic monozygotic twins of JOD patients,[12,48,49] a normal insulin secretory response to glucose has been found. Also, as reviewed earlier, discordance of diabetes in monozygotic twins has been found to be relatively high in those pairs where the index twin developed diabetes under the age of 40 years. This suggests that in these twins, diabetes evolves from "prediabetes" only with the superimposition of a specific environmental factor such as a viral infection and/or development of autoimmunity. Furthermore, a genetic difference may exist between the JOD twin pairs that are concordant and discordant for diabetes.

Still another form of genetic prediabetes may be found in offspring of MOD parents. These prediabetics may have a reduced insulin secretory response to glucose,[48] a defect demonstrated in the majority of patients with subclinical or latent diabetes.[46,50] These offspring of two diabetic parents develop MOD more frequently than the younger monozygotic twins[49,51] and probably resemble the older monozygotic twins with a type of genetic predisposition (no disturbance of HLA frequencies) different from the prediabetic who will develop juvenile-onset-type diabetes. In a study of offspring of concordant MOD parents, it was estimated that 60 percent will have abnormal glucose tolerance at the age of 60 years.[30] In maturity-onset-type diabetes in general, different environmental factors, such as overnutrition and resulting obesity, or pregnancy, may lead from prediabetes to hyperglycemia.

In the natural history of diabetes, progression *or* regression from one stage to the next stage (1) may never occur, or (2) may occur very slowly over many years, or (3) may be rapid or even explosive,[44] depending on the type of the genetic predisposition (type of "prediabetes") and the type of environmental factor involved. For example, a patient with a genetic susceptibility to juvenile-onset-type, ketosis-prone diabetes may remain a "prediabetic" for life if the necessary viral and/or autoimmune factors do not supervene. When clinical diabetes does occur, it is usually manifested by an abrupt onset of insulin insufficiency without previously known abnormality of carbohydrate intolerance. Thus, there is rapid progression from "prediabetes" to overt diabetes without recognition of subclinical or latent diabetes. An example is given in Table 81-3. Occasionally by prospective testing in siblings of patients with JOD, carbohydrate intolerance can be recognized before decompensation to insulin-requiring ketotic disease (Fig. 81-4).

During a prospective study of the natural history of latent or chemical diabetes in young people (for up to 22 years), it was found that at recognition of carbohydrate intolerance, JOD and MODY patients may have identical abnormal glucose tolerance tests. However, individuals who are in the early stages of JOD usually progressed to insulin-requiring diabetes within 2 years of diagnosis, although longer intervals have been recorded.[4] As reviewed above, progression to diabetes that required insulin injections (some to ketosis-prone type) occurred only in those individuals who initially had very low insulin responses to glucose or had

Table 81-3. Rapid Progression from "Prediabetes" to Overt Diabetes

K. B.: male, height 5'9", weight 175 lb
Family history—father, mother, 2 siblings with diabetes mellitus

Date	Age	Test	F	½	1	1½	2	2½	3
						(in mg/dl)			
12/2/54	16	GTT	82	106	88	85	74	85	79
12/3/54	16	Cort-GTT	81	121	91	84	90	98	67
Nov. 1955	17		350—7 weeks of polyuria, polydipsia, 30-pound weight loss, fatigue						

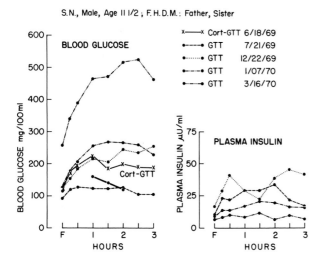

Fig. 81-4. Decompensation from subclinical diabetes to latent diabetes and to overt insulin-requiring ketotic diabetes within 9 months in an 11 1/2-year-old brother of a juvenile-onset-type, ketotic diabetic sister.

insulin responses that were delayed and lower than the mean response of the control subjects. Some of these patients had circulating islet cell antibodies at recognition of mild carbohydrate intolerance, indicating that they had JOD. On the other hand, in

young maturity-onset-type diabetic patients (MOD or MODY), with a different genetic susceptibility, we have recorded intervals of time up to 18 years before progression to fasting hyperglycemia or to insulin-requiring but nonketotic diabetes.[4,52] An example is shown in Table 81-4. Among young people (under age 25 years at diagnosis) with asymptomatic MOD, glucose intolerance does not progress in severity in approximately 80 percent of patients followed for as long as 22 years.[4,52] This can also be observed in nonobese patients with extremely low insulin responses to glucose that have not decreased further over periods of up to 16 years.[4] These patients have been negative for islet cell antibodies. In these patients, asymptomatic diabetes, some with mild fasting hyperglycemia, might still be undiscovered if they had not been tested as first-degree relatives of diabetic patients. It is in this population group that recognition of asymptomatic diabetes appears to be of greatest usefulness.

The concept that there may be fluctuations in either direction in the expression of the carbohydrate aspect of the disease is an important one in genetic studies or in studies attempting to ascertain a relationship between duration of "known" carbohydrate intolerance and recognition of vascular disease. Such fluctuations are particularly common when carbohydrate intolerance is mild,[51,53] as in maturity-onset-type diabetes. Table 81-5 shows fluctuations in glucose tolerance from abnormal to normal to abnormal over a period of 19 years in a patient in whom the diagnosis

Table 81-4. "Maturity-Onset-Type" Diabetes in Childhood

A. P. S.: female
Family history—Diabetes: (1) father, died of vascular disease; (2) mother, died of vascular disease; (3) Two brothers (one died of vascular disease) and one sister

Date	Age	Glucose Tolerance Test							Height	Weight (lb)
		F	1/2	1	1 1/2	2	2 1/2	3		
					(in mg/dl)					
1/12/54	10	94	146	214	207	161	160	135	4'9" 1400-calorie diet	118
11/29/54	10	85	—	129	146	100	118	104		110
5/8/58	14	82	105	136	142	150	105	—	5'2 1/2"	177
5/19/59	15	92	144	185	157	156	164	133	5'2 1/4"	178
11/23/59	15	91	125	132	106	136	120	102	1400-calorie diet	160
1/16/61	17	Delivery: M, 8 lb, 6 oz								
3/6/62	18	Delivery: F, 11 lb, 8 oz								
3/4/63	19	88	—	224	—	207	162	—	5'3"	205
7/4/66	22	Delivery: M, 10 lb, 8 oz								
1/11/68	24	87	169	—	182	168			5'3"	185
11/12/69	26	85	149	207	222	212	161	131		170
11/30/70	27	101	210	269	238	246	227	165		199
5/11/72	28	134		258	274	288	288	248		208
7/5/72	29	118								198
1/4/73	29	191								204
7/27/73	30	117								189
8/12/74	31	274								205
9/6/74	31	109							Chlorpropamide 500 mg q.d.	
11/22/74	31	222							No medication	200
5/7/75	32	114							Chlorpropamide, 500 mg q.d.	200
8/13/76	33	319							Off diet and medicine for 1 year	202
10/21/76	33	97							Diet and chlorpropamide 500 mg q.d.	191
3/3/77	33	153							Diet and chlorpropamide 500 mg q.d.	179

Table 81-5. Spontaneous Variations in Glucose Tolerance in Patient with Maturity-Onset-Type Diabetes, with and Without Changes in Weight

R. O.: male, born 11/9/19, height 5'10"
Family history—father with MOD

Date	GTT							Weight (lb)
	F	½	1	1 ½	2	2 ½	3	
				(in mg/dl)				
3/10/58	102	187	244	228	222	195	100	187
4/28/58	85	124	166	151	109	105	119	170
9/15/60	95	167	210	174	186	114	86	168
9/18/67	83	131	203	210	153	120	88	170
11/10/69	81	135	158	108	93	185	82	168
11/29/72	98	165	234	230	188	129	87	168
9/20/74	84	132	205	218	181	145	130	166
2/6/76	109	167	139	132	112	97	88	168
11/3/76	110	191	246	253	178	140	93	174
6/20/77	144	232	—	293	247	177	118	166

of diabetes was made at age 38. At age 58, he manifested fasting hyperglycemia for the first time. However, even the overt stage of the disease may regress. Extreme examples, such as regression from overt ketotic diabetes to prediabetes, have been reported in individuals who have been in diabetic coma and who have subsequently exhibited normal standard and normal cortisone-glucose tolerance tests.[54] Remission of overt diabetes with ketoacidosis to latent (chemical, asymptomatic) diabetes after a period of therapy with insulin has been documented more frequently.[55] This has been shown to be associated with improvement of beta-cell secretory activity.[56] However, as we have reported previously, in individual patients there may be no consistent relationship between glucose tolerance and the insulin response to glucose as measured by plasma levels of insulin in peripheral blood by conventional radioimmunoassay.[57] These findings suggest that factors in addition to the abnormal pancreatic insulin response to glucose may determine normality or abnormality of glucose tolerance.

Fluctuations in glucose tolerance can be observed in obese patients with weight loss or weight gain (Table 81-4). They are also seen in nonobese patients with consistently subnormal levels of plasma insulin after the administration of glucose. The nonprogressive course of asymptomatic diabetes in many young individuals suggests that in middle-aged individuals in whom the occurrence of microangiopathy, occlusive vascular disease, or neuropathy may have led to a diagnosis of diabetes for the first time, the abnormality of carbohydrate metabolism may have been present for a long time. Thus the "duration" of diabetes as manifested by glucose intolerance cannot be determined in most individuals (1) since a recognizable abnormality in glucose tolerance may precede the diagnosis by decades and (2) because of the possible intermittent nature of glucose intolerance.

TESTING PROCEDURES

The diagnosis of diabetes depends upon the proper use and interpretation of laboratory procedures. When classic symptoms or complications of diabetes are present, the diagnosis is usually suspected and confirmed. However, in the early, mild, or nonprogressive forms of the disease, when the patient is asymptomatic, the diagnosis may be delayed for many years or missed unless laboratory tests are freely employed. In some cases, the presence of asymptomatic or latent diabetes will be suspected by routine performance of urinalysis and determination of fasting blood glucose levels. In the mildest form of the disease, the fasting level of

blood glucose may be within the normal range, and the only recognizable abnormality will be a diminished ability to utilize a carbohydrate load at a normal rate, as demonstrated by a glucose tolerance test or by a postglucose plasma glucose screening procedure. The oral glucose tolerance test remains the most sensitive and practical test for the early recognition of asymptomatic (latent or chemical) diabetes without fasting hyperglycemia, even if it is a nonspecific test and has been used and interpreted inappropriately by some.

There is no consensus concerning techniques for performance or interpretation of the standard oral glucose tolerance test. Before one can interpret the results of blood glucose determinations and glucose tolerance tests, one must be familiar with the procedures and chemical methods in general use, including technical variables and host variables.

TECHNICAL VARIABLES

Venous Blood versus Capillary Blood

In the adult, venous blood from an anticubital vein is usually employed for analysis and is recommended, since diagnostic criteria are based upon analysis of venous samples from healthy subjects. Blood should be obtained with minimum stasis. Capillary blood may be used, but results are less reproducible. Capillary blood glucose approximates that of arterial blood. In the fasting state, levels of blood glucose in arterial blood are only 2–3 mg/dl above those of venous blood. However, after the ingestion or injection of glucose, glucose values may be 20–70 mg/dl higher in capillary than in venous blood.

Fluid Analyzed. Plasma or Serum versus Whole Blood

With the use of automated methods, plasma or serum rather than whole blood is generally employed. Plasma or serum are preferable because they provide more stable values for glucose determination, are independent of hematocrit, and reflect extracellular glucose concentration more accurately. Since the concentration of glucose in plasma or serum is higher than in whole blood (containing water from laked red blood cells), results obtained cannot be used interchangeably. Levels of glucose in plasma or serum are approximately 15 percent higher (not 15 mg/dl) than in whole blood. A conversion of glucose values from whole blood to plasma may be made, when the hematocrit is normal, by multiplying the whole blood value by 1.15. In the preparation of plasma or serum, the blood sample should be chilled or refrigerated to prevent glycolysis of glucose by formed blood cells, resulting in lowering of plasma glucose values. Fluoride in the collection tube will inhibit glycolysis but cannot be used when enzymatic methods for glucose determination are employed.

Methods for Determining Blood Glucose

The most common methods for determination of levels of glucose are the Hoffman ferricyanide reduction method frequently used by Auto-Analyzer and other automated procedures and glucose-specific enzymatic methods, which give results that are about 10 mg/dl lower than those given by copper reduction methods.

Glucose Dose and Concentration Used for Glucose Tolerance Tests

The glucose dose employed has varied from a 50-g glucose load (Great Britain) to 75, 100, or 40 g/m² body surface. The load employed at the University of Michigan is 1.75 g/kg ideal body weight. Ideal body weight is calculated from the subject's height and age. All ages above 25 are equated at 25 years, since according to life insurance tables, ideal body weight stays constant for a given height after this age. In most females, the load will approximate 100 g of glucose. Most males will receive 120–140 g according to this method. The higher the glucose load, the more reproducible[58] and sensitive is the test, particularly in patients with borderline abnormalities. If test results are normal or definitely abnormal, the size of the glucose load is of little importance. On the other hand, the higher the glucose load, the greater is the likelihood that the patient may become nauseated during glucose ingestion. To avoid nausea, the glucose or carbohydrate load should not be given in a solution exceeding 25 percent in concentration. It is usually flavored with lemon juice and chilled for palatability. Various cola-flavored solutions of glucose and partially digested polysaccharides have been proposed as an equipotent challenge of ability to dispose of the carbohydrate load, usually in 75-g amounts. As noted above, such loads are adequate for screening and for most diagnostic tests, although the sensitivity of the test, particularly for borderline abnormalities, is slightly decreased as compared to loads containing 100 g of glucose or 1.75 g/kg body weight. Timing of the glucose tolerance test is begun after the first swallow of the glucose solution. Samples obtained should include fasting blood glucose, ½, 1, 1½ (particularly for borderline tests), 2, 2½, and 3 hours after the beginning of glucose ingestion. If a history of symptoms of reactive hypoglycemia 3 or more hours after a meal can be obtained, the test is prolonged to 5 hours.

HOST VARIABLES THAT MAY OR DO ALTER THE INTERPRETATION OF GLUCOSE TOLERANCE TEST

High-Carbohydrate Preparatory Diet

The patient should consume a diet containing 250–300 g of carbohydrate, and calories for maintenance of weight, for at least 3 days before the test to obtain the best reproducibility of the test and to minimize falsely abnormal results. Although ingestion of smaller amounts of carbohydrate (150 g or more) is probably sufficient to prevent plateau or diabetic-type curves in healthy young subjects, a standardized high-carbohydrate preparation diet is advisable to ensure reproducibility of the test. When the glucose tolerance test preparation diet is omitted as unpractical, normal results can be accepted, but an abnormal test has to be repeated after proper dietary preparation. The diet eliminates both falsely positive results and nonreproducibility of several tests done in the same subject without using the preparatory diet. Seltzer[59] has demonstrated the importance of the glucose tolerance preparation diet, particularly in elderly subjects. "Abnormal" glucose tolerance tests on an ad lib diet were normal after ingestion of a high-carbohydrate preparatory diet. A low-carbohydrate intake for several days preceding the glucose tolerance test obliterates the first phase immediate insulin response to administered glucose that is most important in determining normal glucose tolerance. In subjects who have been on reduction diets or have a decreased carbohydrate and caloric intake because of anorexia or other reasons, the preparatory diet must be taken for longer periods of time to assure maximal glucose utilization during the glucose tolerance test. Coffee or smoking before or during the test is not allowed.

Physical Activity Before and During Test

The test should be performed on ambulatory patients rather than on patients at bed rest or hospitalized for other conditions. Walking during the test from the waiting room to the blood-drawing room is permitted, as this is the testing condition in control subjects. Undue exercise should be prohibited. Patients should be seated comfortably during the test. Physical inactivity or immobilization owing to any cause in the preceding days will decrease glucose tolerance.

Time of Day

Standard glucose tolerance tests should be performed in the morning after a minimum of 10 hours of fasting. There is a diurnal variation in glucose tolerance. It deteriorates in the afternoon. Also, 5 to 10 hours after a meal, glucose tolerance is not as good as after longer fasts, while it improves 1 to 5 hours after a meal.[60]

Acute or Chronic Illness

Criteria for the interpretation of the glucose tolerance test, separating normal from abnormal or signifying diabetes, apply only to otherwise healthy, ambulatory subjects under the age of 50 years and do not apply to individuals with acute or chronic disease. In particular, they do not apply to patients with acute cardiovascular and cerebrovascular disease; patients with active endocrine diseases such as acromegaly, Cushing's syndrome, pheochromocytoma, primary aldosteronism, glucagonoma, and thyrotoxicosis; patients with hepatic, renal, or central nervous system disease or infection; patients with a poor nutritional intake or potassium depletion; patients under emotional stress; individuals who are confined to bed; and individuals being treated with a variety of drugs (thiazides, nicotinic acid, Dilantin, glucocorticoids, salicylates, oral hypoglycemic agents). Synthetic estrogen (mestranol) contained in birth control pills may have the same effect as pregnancy in producing a state similar to gestational diabetes. Carbohydrate abnormality associated with hyperlipoproteinemia may also not signify the presence of genetic diabetes mellitus. It is important to prepare the patient psychologically for the oral glucose tolerance test. If autonomic nervous responses (pallor, sweating, nausea, fainting) develop during the first 2 hours of the test, the procedure should be discontinued and repeated another time.

Age

It has been reported repeatedly that tolerance to glucose diminishes with advancing age. The magnitude of the increases suggest that the diagnostic criteria employed for the interpretation of the glucose tolerance test in the younger age group may have to be modified for those with advancing age. Unfortunately, no good data exist regarding reliable minimal diagnostic criteria for individuals over the age of 50.[3,44,61] What is presently unknown is whether a decrease in tolerance to glucose with advancing age is (1) due to age-related physiological decrease in glucose tolerance in nondiabetic subjects, or (2) due to an increasing incidence of latent or asymptomatic diabetes with increasing age, or (3) a combination of both factors. Data in support of both of the first two possibilities have been presented.[61,62] Further discussion of the effect of age will be given during the discussion of interpretation.

CRITERIA EMPLOYED FOR THE INTERPRETATION OF LEVELS OF FASTING PLASMA OR BLOOD GLUCOSE AND OF THE STANDARD ORAL GLUCOSE TOLERANCE TEST

Fasting Blood Glucose

The determination of levels of glucose in fasting blood is the most specific but least sensitive method for the diagnosis of diabetes mellitus. A value of 140 mg/dl or greater in plasma or serum, or of 120 mg/dl or greater in whole blood, establishes a diagnosis of diabetes. A level between 115 and 140 mg/dl in plasma or serum, or 100–120 mg/dl for whole blood, is also of significance but should

glucose tolerance.[66] Thus, an abnormal glucose tolerance test in an obese subject, even in the absence of fasting hyperglycemia, can be interpreted as indicating the presence of diabetes in addition to obesity.

It has been stated[68] that the U.S. Public Health Service (USPHS) criteria appear to be more reliable, since a larger proportion of individuals classified as abnormal by these criteria (52 percent) progressed to overt diabetes than did individuals so classified by the Michigan criteria (32 percent). However, even in young people who were between the ages of 9 to 25 years, when a diagnosis of latent diabetes was made that satisfied both sets of diagnostic criteria, there was no progression of the disease (further deterioration of carbohydrate tolerance) in the large majority of patients for periods up to 16 years.[4] Thus, validation of diagnostic criteria for the interpretation of the glucose tolerance test need not depend on the demonstration of a high rate of progression to overt diabetes. In one study, the USPHS criteria were found to be less sensitive than the other criteria in detecting abnormality of carbohydrate tolerance in first-degree relatives of diabetic patients.[69]

If diabetes mellitus can exist without an elevation of the fasting blood sugar level, the fasting level should not be one of the criteria for the interpretation of the glucose tolerance test. Furthermore, if one considers diagnostic criteria for the glucose tolerance test that include an elevated 3-hour level, one would eliminate from consideration glucose tolerance tests characteristic of diabetes within the first 2 hours and in which the 3-hour level is not elevated because of subsequent reactive hypoglycemia. Reactive hypoglycemia 3 to 5 hours after ingestion of glucose occurs in individuals whose glucose tolerance tests disclose mild diabetes mellitus. Symptoms of spontaneous hypoglycemia may indeed be one of the earliest clinical manifestations of the disease. There is a delay in insulin release after administration of glucose, and the resulting hyperglycemia causes a delayed but supernormal release of insulin followed by hypoglycemia.

The criteria discussed above have been criticized for giving too high an incidence of abnormality or diabetes.[70] Siperstein suggests that a diagnosis of diabetes mellitus should be made only on the basis of fasting hyperglycemia, but if a glucose tolerance test is to be used, he proposes diagnostic levels of over 260 mg/dl at 1 hour and over 220 mg/dl at 2 hours. This suggestion is based on (1) a publication of Unger of 1957,[71] (2) a publication of Andres,[61] and (3) population studies.

Unger studied 152 food handlers who on screening had 1½-hour postprandial blood sugar levels below 130 mg/dl. The subjects were 17 to 71 years of age, with a mean age of 39.4 years. A family history was not obtained. The Somogyi-Nelson blood glucose method was used, and it was stated that the "technical accuracy of the data seemed beyond reproach." However, 20 subjects had fasting blood sugars below 67 mg/dl, which is below the mean −2 standard deviations of fasting blood sugars of our control subjects by the same method. Fourteen subjects had fasting blood sugar levels between 42 and 61 mg/dl. The published estimated minimal daily carbohydrate intake was below 125 g/day in 18 subjects. If 1-hour and 2-hour blood glucose levels above 160 and 120 mg/dl are used as cutoff points, 33 of 152, or 21 percent, had "abnormal tests." The highest abnormal test had the following values: fasting, 70; 1 hour, 248; 2 hours, 231 mg/dl. In view of the relatively low fasting blood sugar levels, starvation diabetes cannot be ruled out. The lowest "abnormal test" had a fasting level of 80, a 1-hour level of 161, and a 2-hour level of 125 mg/dl. Even by our former criteria (1-hour level, 160 mg/dl), this would not be an abnormal test without a 1½-hour level to rule out a rebound curve. Thus, there is little justification for using these data as supporting the levels

proposed by Siperstein as representing the upper limits of normal. Unger also performed duplicate tests in 49 of the "normal control subjects" and commented on "erratic results or capriciousness of the oral glucose tolerance test." Utilizing the same 160 and 120 mg/dl criteria, 40 tests were normal on both tests, 8 were abnormal on both tests, and 1 subject gave an abnormal result on the first test and a normal one on the second test. Thus, only 1 of 49 test pairs was "not reproducible."

Andres performed oral glucose tolerance tests on an aging population and discussed the problem of aging and glucose tolerance.[61] All subjects were hospitalized overnight, and the glucose tolerance test was performed at bed rest. Glucose tolerance preparation diets were not used. He found an increase in the mean 2-hour blood glucose level of 6 mg/dl per decade. On the basis of the data obtained, he constructed a nomogram for oral glucose tolerance tests. This nomogram gives arbitrary percentile cutoff points of "abnormal" or "borderline" tests for each age group and increasing with age. According to Andres, this nomogram can be used to rank an individual in relation to his age-matched cohorts but not to evaluate whether a test is normal or abnormal.

Various other proposals have been made in regard to age adjustments of blood glucose standards. Computing the mean +2 standard deviation for each age decade would give the distressing results that the prevalence of diabetes would be the same at all stages of the life span.[61] We have used the arbitrary scheme of adding 10 mg/dl for each decade over the 50-year age group. O'Sullivan advocates no age adjustment and gives plausible reasons,[62] and several investigators have found no or only a small effect of age on glucose tolerance in healthy subjects, at least up to 45 years of age. The decision of whether or not to adjust for age cannot be made with confidence at this time, and statistical manipulation of survey data are unlikely to resolve this dilemma.[61]

Population studies utilizing determination of postglucose blood sugar levels cannot be used to establish criteria for normal glucose tolerance. In such surveys, diabetics are frequently not excluded nor are the first-degree relatives of diabetics. Ambulatory patients with chronic illness or those taking various drugs are frequently included. Such tests are commonly not done in the fasting or basal condition and are done at any time during the day, such as in the afternoon or evening and at variable intervals after the last meal. Abnormality is frequently judged on the basis of a single postglucose determination. In one study, there was a 13.8 percent abnormality on the basis of a single postglucose elevation but a 1.2 percent abnormality when three plasma glucose levels were used.[62]

Standards have been developed for diabetes detection (and treatment) in Indian populations so that diabetes diagnosis is limited to persons with high probabilities of having the disease or to high-risk groups.[72] In nonpregnant individuals, the criterion selected for making a diagnosis of diabetes on a modified glucose tolerance test is a 2-hour postglucose plasma glucose level (a screening procedure) of greater than 200 mg/dl. The rationale for selecting this level includes the bimodal distribution of 2-hour postglucose plasma glucose levels found in Pima Indians in all decades, age 25 years or over.[2] The presence of two components in the distribution indicated to the authors that there is biological heterogeneity of glucose tolerance with two subgroups in that population. Because of the finding of bimodality, the authors believe that these cutoff points differentiate between "nondiabetes" and "diabetes." They support their argument by noting that the frequency of diabetic retinopathy was low among subjects within the first component of the glucose distribution curve and high, reaching a plateau between 18 and 23 percent, in the patients at the beginning of the second component of the glucose distribution. There was an abrupt increase of specific diabetic complications (retinopathy, nephropathy) on follow-up evaluation of Pimas whose 2-hour postglucose plasma glucose levels were greater than 200 mg/dl. On the other hand, in pregnant women during the first or second trimester, a 2-hour postglucose plasma glucose level of greater than 140 mg/dl was considered diagnostic for diabetes and had prognostic implications for the complications of diabetic pregnancies.[2,72] In other words, for the pregnant patient, the Indian Health Service physicians do not accept the dividing line of 200 mg/dl derived from the bimodal distribution and the increased prevalence of specific diabetic complications as being the best criterion for separating nondiabetes from diabetes. Since pregnancy has a tendency to elevate 2-hour postglucose plasma glucose levels in nondiabetic and diabetic patients, it is likely that a level of 140 mg/dl would also separate normal from abnormal in the nonpregnant individual.

INDICATIONS FOR PERFORMANCE OF THE ORAL GLUCOSE TOLERANCE TEST

1. Abnormal or borderline glucose values during screening procedures. Examples are borderline fasting plasma glucose values, borderline or abnormal postglucose or postprandial glucose values, or high random values in the nonfasting state. Glycosuria without diagnostic fasting hyperglycemia is another indication.

2. To identify or rule out gestational diabetes. Gestational diabetes should be suspected in obstetrical patients with a history of previous pregnancies productive of stillbirths, neonatal deaths, large newborn babies (over 9 pounds), or toxemia of pregnancy, glycosuria, obesity, or strong family history of diabetes. Gestational diabetes increases perinatal morbidity. Glycosuria found for the first time during pregnancy should not be assumed to be due to a lowering of the renal threshold. The glucose tolerance test should be performed during pregnancy rather than waiting for the postpartum period. Fifty percent of gestational diabetics progress to overt diabetes within 5 to 7 years. Gestational diabetes is associated with an increase in hemoglobin A_{1c}, decreased oxygen dissociation, and possible decreased tissue oxygenation. By achieving normal postprandial blood glucose levels, increased perinatal morbidity and an increase in hemoglobin A_{1c} can be prevented or ameliorated, and progression to overt diabetes may be attenuated.

3. Identification of asymptomatic maturity-onset-type diabetes associated with obesity, particularly in patients with a close family history of diabetes. Diagnosis of maturity-onset-type diabetes provides greater motivation for weight reduction.

4. Individuals under age 50 with a first-degree family history of diabetes, particularly of maturity-onset type.

5. Patients with otherwise unexplained neuropathy, atherosclerosis, coronary artery disease, peripheral vascular disease, retinopathy, or nephropathy, particularly those under 50 years of age.

6. Patients with transitory glycosuria or nondiagnostic hyperglycemia found in the course of surgical procedures, trauma, emotional stress, myocardial infarction, cerebrovascular accident, or administration of adrenal steroids. The test should be performed after recovery from acute illness or stress.

7. Patients with symptoms of spontaneous hypoglycemia, particularly those with a family history of diabetes.

8. To differentiate between patients with "low" and "high" insulin responses to administered glucose when abnormality of glucose tolerance is established. The nature of the insulin response has prognostic implications. Patients with low insulin responses may progress to insulin-requiring diabetes; those with high insulin responses do not.

LEVELS OF PLASMA INSULIN

The heterogeneity of insulin responses in MOD and MODY patients demonstrates that plasma insulin levels during the glucose tolerance test are not of diagnostic value, although they may be of prognostic significance (see p. 953).

SCREENING TESTS

The best procedure for routine screening for diabetes is a single blood glucose determination 2 hours after the ingestion of a 75–100 g glucose load. This screening procedure is more sensitive than blood glucose determinations after a meal high in carbohydrates or a mixed meal of carbohydrates and protein. After a mixed meal, postprandial insulin levels are higher and blood glucose levels are lower than after a glucose meal, since glucose and amino acids potentiate each other in respect to insulin release.[73] A 2-hour postglucose blood sugar level is a screening procedure and not a diagnostic procedure for diabetes mellitus. In the diagnosis of diabetes, one depends on the magnitude of hyperglycemia as well as on its duration. Plateau curves without a peak blood sugar elevation but with an elevated 2-hour level are neither normal nor diagnostic. Better discrimination between diabetic and nondiabetic values of the oral glucose tolerance test is given by the 2-hour than by the 1-hour blood glucose value when a single value is used.[74,75] When a 2-hour criterion of 140 mg/dl (capillary blood, 75-g carbohydrate load) was used as a cutoff point in a mass screening program for diabetes mellitus in Cleveland, an overall positive rate of 4.1 percent was found.[76] If this rate was corrected for those who failed to retest positive, only 2.6 percent of Cleveland's screenees had firmly abnormal tests. These figures are very close to the most conservative perception of the expected prevalence of diabetes.[76]

TESTING OF URINE

Testing of urine for glucose is utilized primarily for following diabetic control and for screening. A positive urinary glucose test should alert the physician for further screening or diagnostic procedures, while a negative test does not rule out the presence of diabetes even with fasting hyperglycemia. Methods of urine testing are described in standard manuals of laboratory procedures.

INTRAVENOUS GLUCOSE TOLERANCE TEST (IV GTT)

For satisfactory results with the iv GTT, the same precautions must be considered as for the performance of the oral glucose tolerance test. It is generally used for research purposes or for patients with significant gastrointestinal disturbances that interfere with normal absorption of glucose. The test has the following advantages: (1) avoidance of the variables of gastrointestinal absorption, (2) evaluation of the test by a single figure (K value), (3) the test can be performed within 1 hour, and (4) nausea can be avoided. The intravenous glucose tolerance test also has disadvantages. The iv GTT is a less physiological test than the oral glucose tolerance test. The oral route is the usual one of ingress of food. It stimulates the secretion of several gastrointestinal hormones, which in turn have a highly significant effect on the secretion and action of insulin.

Second, with the usual load used, 50 cc of 50 percent glucose or 25 g of glucose, this test is less sensitive than the oral test in patients with mild diabetes. When carbohydrate utilization is only mildly diminished, a small load given may be removed in a normal fashion. On the other hand, for the oral test, a larger load is given with persistent absorption over hours, necessitating the removal of a continuing influx of glucose. The sensitivity of the intravenous glucose tolerance test can be improved by giving larger amounts of glucose than those usually used.[64a]

The test is generally performed with a rapid injection of glucose. The results are expressed by plotting the rate of fall of blood glucose per unit time on semilogarithmic paper, derivation of a single K value, which expresses the decrease of glood glucose in percent per minute, representing glucose utilization.[64b]

ORAL CORTISONE- OR STEROID-GLUCOSE TOLERANCE TEST

It has been reported that a subclinical defect in carbohydrate metabolism can be uncovered in some healthy relatives of diabetic patients with normal standard glucose tolerance tests by the use of a standardized dose of cortisone or other steroid.[3] In general, these tests should be thought of, not as diagnostic tests, but as research procedures. The results obtained with the cortisone–glucose tolerance test permitted the separation of nondiabetic first-degree relatives of diabetic patients into two groups. Those with a "positive response" to the test responded as did the majority of mildly diabetic patients, while those exhibiting a "negative response" reacted as did the majority of control subjects who had been selected because they had no family history of diabetes. Long-term follow-up studies of both groups have shown that 26 percent of individuals with positive response have progressed in subsequent years to latent or clinical diabetes, while over the same period of time this course occurred in only 3.6 percent of subjects with negative responses. Nondiabetic relatives of diabetic patients who have positive tests (subclinical diabetes) exhibited a defect in the secretion of insulin that distinguished them from subjects with negative tests.[46] This defect is similar in pattern to that observed in mild maturity-onset-type diabetic patients during the standard test. This deficiency in the secretion of insulin represents an important part of the mechanism that induces a positive cortisone–glucose tolerance test. It is likely that the cortisone–glucose tolerance test will uncover subclinical diabetes in a much greater proportion of future diabetics with maturity-onset-type diabetes than in individuals who subsequently will develop juvenile-onset-type diabetes.

HEMOGLOBIN A_{1c} (GLYCOSYLATED HEMOGLOBIN)

Hemoglobin A_{1c}, the most abundant minor hemoglobin component in human erythrocytes, is increased in diabetes and is formed by having a hexose group attached as a ketamine to the N-terminal valines of the normal beta chains of hemoglobin A.[77] The rate of formation of hemoglobin A_{1c} should be directly proportional to the time-average concentration of glucose within the erythrocyte.[77] It has also been shown that there is a highly significant correlation between hemoglobin A_{1c} concentration and response to an oral glucose tolerance test in diabetic patients, independent of fasting blood sugar levels.[78] When diabetic patients are hospitalized and the blood glucose is optimally and carefully regulated, the hemoglobin A_{1c} levels are reduced to or toward normal with a lag time of 5 to 6 weeks.[79] This work suggests that by measurement of the concentration of hemoglobin A_{1c}, long-term blood glucose regulation can be assessed objectively in the diabetic patient. However, insufficient information is available presently to indicate whether the concentration of hemoglobin A_{1c} can be used in the diagnosis of chemical diabetes. This is possible, since a group of 13 children with moderate impairment of glucose tolerance (mean fasting plasma glucose level of 97 mg/dl, maximum level of 206 mg/dl, and 2-hour level of 155 mg/dl) had significantly elevated hemoglobin A_{1c} levels.[65]

A rapid method for determining hemoglobin A_{1c} concentration might be useful in screening populations for diabetes.

MEASUREMENT OF CAPILLARY BASEMENT MEMBRANE WIDTH

It has been noted that there is a thickening of the basement membrane of capillaries of a variety of tissues in diabetic patients. Siperstein et al. reported on a morphometric electron-microscopic technique for quantitating the thickness of basement membrane of muscle capillaries obtained by muscle biopsy of the quadraceps femoris.[80] They reported that muscle capillary basement membrane width is thickened in 92 to 98 percent of diabetic patients as compared to 2 to 8 percent in control subjects. These investigators also reported that basement membrane thickening in diabetes is unrelated to age, sex, or duration and degree of hyperglycemia. Utilizing a different technique of fixation and estimation of width,[81] Kilo et al. found an overall incidence of approximately 60 percent of basement membrane thickening in diabetic patients.[42] They also reported a significant increase with age in basement membrane width in normal and diabetic males and females. In addition, among insulin-requiring diabetics, they found an increase in prevalence of basement membrane thickening with increasing duration of known diabetes that was highly significant statistically. Controversy continues about different methods of fixation and of estimation of capillary basement membrane width and their relation to the differences in results obtained.[82,83] More recently, Raskin et al.[84] have reported that muscle capillary basement membrane thickening is present in only 40 percent of insulin-requiring juvenile-onset diabetic patients below the age of 20 years. In a study of latent diabetic patients,[4] utilizing the Williamson technique,[81] 26 percent had basement membrane thickening (36 percent of patients when those under 20 years of age are excluded). In addition, there was also a significant correlation between basement membrane width and known duration of carbohydrate intolerance.[4] In Pima Indians, a significant correlation between duration of diabetes and basement membrane thickening was also found.[85]

At the present time, it would appear that thickening of muscle capillary basement membrane width may be of value in detecting early evidence of the presence of microangiopathy in genetic diabetes and in confirming the presence of genetic diabetes in subjects with hyperglycemia. Estimation of capillary basement membrane width appears to be an insensitive method of diagnosing diabetes either in individuals under 20 years of age or in older individuals with mild diabetes of relatively short duration. Basement membrane thickening is not entirely specific for diabetes.

REFERENCES

1. Rimoin, D. L.: Inheritance of diabetes mellitus. *Med. Clin. North Am.*, 55: 807, 1971.
2. Bennett, P. H., Rushforth, N. M., Miller, M., and LeCompte, P. M.:

Epidemiologic studies of diabetes in the Pima Indians. *Recent Prog. Horm. Res., 32:* 333, 1976.

3. Fajans, S. S., and Conn, J. W.: Prediabetes, subclinical diabetes and latent clinical diabetes: Interpretation, diagnosis and treatment, In: On the Nature and Treatment of Diabetes, B. S. Leibel and G. A. Wrenshall (eds.). Excerpta Medica, Int'l Cong. Ser. 84, New York, 1965, p. 641.

4. Fajans, S. S., Floyd, J. C., Jr., Tattersall, R. B., Williamson, J. R., Pek, S., and Taylor, C. I.: The Various faces of diabetes in the young—changing concepts. *Arch. Intern. Med., 136:* 194, 1976.

5. Creutzfeldt, W., Köbberling, J., and Neel, J. V. (eds.), The Genetics of Diabetes Mellitus. Springer-Verlag, Heidelberg, 1976.

6. Zonana, J., and Rimoin, D. L.: Current concepts in genetics: Inheritance of diabetes mellitus. *N. Engl. J. Med., 295:* 603, 1976.

7. Tattersall, R. B., and Fajans, S. S.: A difference between the inheritance of classical juvenile-onset and maturity-onset type diabetes of young people. *Diabetes, 24:* 44, 1975.

8. MacDonald, M. J.: Equal incidence of adult-onset diabetes among ancestors of juvenile diabetics and nondiabetics. *Diabetologia, 10:* 767, 1974.

9. Svejgaard, A.: HLA factors and immune function. *Acta Endocrinol. (KBH), 83:* 77, 1976.

10. Cudworth, A. G., and Woodrow, J. C.: Genetic susceptibility in diabetes mellitus: Analysis of HLA association. *Br. Med. J., 2:* 846, 1976.

11. Nerup, J., Ortved-Anderson, O., Christy, M., Platz, P., Ryder, L., Thomsen, M., and Svejgaard, A.: HLA, autoimmunity, virus and the pathogenesis of juvenile diabetes mellitus. *Acta Endocrinol. (KBH), Suppl. 205:* 167, 1976.

12. Tattersall, R. B., and Pyke, D. A.: Diabetes in identical twins. *Lancet, 2:* 1120, 1972.

13. Nelson, P. G., Pyke, D. A., Cudworth, A. G., Woodrow, J. C., and Batchelor, J. R.: Histocompatibility antigens in diabetic identical twins. *Lancet, 2:* 193, 1975.

14. Editorial: Autoimmune diabetes mellitus. *Lancet, 2:* 1549, 1974.

15. Irvine, W. J., MacCuish, A. C., Campbell, J., and Duncan, L. J. P.: Organ-specific cell-mediated autoimmunity in diabetes mellitus. *Acta Endocrinol. (KBH), Suppl. 205:* 65, 1976.

16. Huang, S.-W., MacLaren, N. K.: Insulin-dependent diabetes: A disease of autoaggression. *Science, 192:* 65, 1976.

17. Like, A. A., Rossini, A.A.: Streptozotocin-induced pancreatic insulitis: New model of diabetes mellitus. *Science, 193:* 415, 1976.

18. Bottazzo, G. F., Florin-Christensen, A., Doniach, D.: Islet-cell antibodies in diabetes mellitus with autoimmune polyendocrine deficiencies. *Lancet, 2:* 1279, 1974.

19. MacCuish, A. C., Irvine, W. J., Barnes, E. W., and Duncan, L. H.: Antibodies to pancreatic islet cells in insulin-dependent diabetics with coexistent autoimmune disease. *Lancet, 2:* 1529, 1974.

20. MacLaren, N. K., Huang, S.-W., and Fogh, J.: Antibody to cultured human insulinoma cells in insulin-dependent diabetes. *Lancet, 1:* 997, 1975.

21. Lendrum, R., Walker, G., and Gamble, D. R.: Islet-cell antibodies in juvenile diabetes mellitus of recent onset. *Lancet, 1:* 880, 1975.

22. Irvine, W. J., McCallum, C. J., Gray, R. S., Campbell, C. J., Duncan, L. J. P., Farquhar, J. W., Vaughan, H., and Morris, P. J.: Pancreatic islet-cell antibodies in diabetes mellitus correlated with the duration and type of diabetes, Coexistent autoimmune disease, and HLA type. *Diabetes, 26:* 138, 1977.

23. Lendrum, R., Walker, G., Cudworth, A. G., Theophanides, C., Pyke, D. A., Bloom, A., and Gamble, R. F.: Islet-cell antibodies in diabetes mellitus. *Lancet, 2:* 1273, 1976.

24. Kahn, C. R., Flier, J. S., Bar, R. S., Archer, J. A., Gorden, P., Martin, M. M., and Roth, J.: The syndromes of insulin resistance and acanthosis nigricans. Insulin-receptor disorders in man. *N. Engl. J. Med., 294:* 739, 1976.

25. Flier, J. S., Kahn, R., Jarrett, D. B., and Roth, J.: Characterization of antibodies to the insulin receptor. *J. Clin. Invest., 58:* 1442, 1976.

26. Morris, P. J., Irvine, W. J., Gray, R. S., Duncan, L. J. P., Vaughan, H., McCallum, F. J., Campbell, C. J., and Farquhar, J. W.: HLA and pancreatic islet cell antibodies in diabetes. *Lancet, 2:* 652, 1976.

27. Craighead, J. E.: The role of viruses in the pathogenesis of pancreatic disease and diabetes mellitus. *Prog. Med. Virol., 19:* 161, 1975.

28. Craighead, J. E.: Animal model of human disease: Diabetes mellitus (juvenile- and maturity-onset types). *Am. J. Pathol., 78:* 537, 1975.

29. Ross, M. E., Onodera, T., Brown, K. S., and Notkins, A. L.: Virus-induced diabetes mellitus. IV. Genetic and environmental factors influencing the development of diabetes after infection with the M variant of encephalomyocarditis virus. *Diabetes, 25:* 190, 1976.

30. Tattersall, R. B., and Fajans, S.S.: Prevalence of diabetes and glucose intolerance in 199 offspring of thirty-seven conjugal diabetic parents. *Diabetes, 24:* 452, 1975.

31. Radder, J. K., and Terpstra, J.: The incidence of diabetes mellitus in the offspring of diabetic couples. Investigation based on the oral glucose tolerance test. *Diabetologia, 11:* 135, 1975.

32a. Fujita, Y., Herron, A. L., and Seltzer, H. S.: Confirmation of impaired early insulin response to glycemic stimulus in nonobese mild diabetics. *Diabetes, 24:* 17, 1975.

32b. Fajans, S. S., Floyd, J. C., Jr., Taylor, C. I., and Pek, S.: Heterogeneity of insulin responses in latent diabetes. *Trans. Assoc. Am. Phys., 87:* 83, 1974.

33. Reaven, G. M., Bernstein, R., David, B., and Olefsky, J. M.: Nonketotic diabetes mellitus: Insulin deficiency or insulin resistance? *Am. J. Med., 60:* 80, 1976.

34. Olefsky, J. M.: The Insulin receptor: Its role in insulin resistance of obesity and diabetes. *Diabetes, 25:* 1154, 1976.

35. Johansen, K.: Mild carbohydrate intolerance developing into classical juvenile diabetes. *Acta Med. Scand., 189:* 337, 1971.

36. Rosenbloom, A. L., Drash, A., and Guthrie, R. A. (eds): Workshop on chemical diabetes in childhood. *Metabolism 22:* 211, 1973.

37. Knowles, H.: Long-term juvenile diabetes treated with unmeasured diet. *Trans. Assoc. Am. Phys., 85:* 95, 1971.

38. Oakley, W. G., Pyke, D. A., Tattersall, R. B., and Watkins, P. J.: Long-term diabetes. A clinical study of 92 patients after 40 years. *Q. J. Med., 43:* 145, 1974.

39. Paz-Guevara, A. T., Hsu, T.-H., and White, P.: Juvenile diabetes mellitus after forty years. *Diabetes, 24:* 559, 1975.

40. Vracko, R., and Benditt, E. P.: Manifestations of diabetes mellitus—their possible relationships to an underlying cell defect. *Am. J. Pathol., 75:* 204, 1974.

41. Goldstein, S., Niewiarowski, S., and Singal, D. P.: Pathological implications of cell aging in vitro. *Fed. Proc., 34:* 56, 1975.

42. Kilo, C., Vogler, N., and Williamson, J. R.: Muscle capillary basement membrane changes related to aging and to diabetes mellitus. *Diabetes, 21:* 881, 1972.

43. Robertson, R. P., Halter, J. B., and Porte, D., Jr.: A role for alpha-adrenergic receptors in abnormal insulin secretion in diabetes mellitus. *J. Clin. Invest., 57:* 791, 1976.

44. Fajans, S. S.: What is diabetes: Definition, diagnosis and course. *Med. Clin. North Am., 55:* 793, 1971.

45. Metzger, B. E., Nitzan, M., and Freinkel, N.: The beta cell in gestational diabetes: Victim or culprit? *Clin. Res., 22:* 651A, 1974.

46. Rull, J. A., Conn, J. W., Floyd, J. C., Jr., and Fajans, S. S.: Levels of plasma insulin during cortisone glucose tolerance tests in "nondiabetic" relatives of diabetic patients. *Diabetes, 19:* 1, 1970.

47. Kalkhoff, R. K., Richardson, B. L., and Stoddard, J. F.: Defective plasma insulin response during prednisolone glucose tolerance tests in subclinical diabetic mothers of heavy infants. *Diabetes, 17:* 37, 1968.

48. Johansen, K., Soeldner, J. S., and Gleason, R. E.: Insulin, growth hormone and glucagon in prediabetes—a review. *Metabolism, 23:* 1185, 1974.

49. Johansen, K., Soeldner, J. S., Gleason, R. E., Gottlieb, M. S., Park, B. N., Kaufman, R. L., and Tan, M. H.: Serum insulin and growth hormone response patterns in monozygotic twin siblings of patients with juvenile-onset diabetes. *N. Engl. J. Med., 293:* 57, 1975.

50. Floyd, J. F., Jr., Fajans, S. S., Conn, J. W., Thiffault, C., Knopf, R. F., and Gunthsche, E.: Secretion of insulin induced by amino acids and glucose in diabetes mellitus. *J. Clin. Endocrinol. Metab., 28:* 266, 1968.

51. Kahn, C. B., Soeldner, J. S., Gleason, R. E., Rojas, L., Camerini-Davalos, R., and Marble, A.: Clinical and chemical diabetes in offspring of diabetic couples. *N. Engl. J. Med., 281:* 343, 1969.

52. Fajans, S. S., Taylor, C. I., Floyd, J. C., Jr., and Conn, J. W.: Some aspects of the natural history of diabetes mellitus. In: Diabetes: Proceedings of the 8th Cong. IDF. Excerpta Medica, Int'l. Cong. Series 312, New York, 1974, p. 329.

53. O'Sullivan, J. B., and Hurwitz, D.: Spontaneous remissions in early diabetes mellitus. *Arch. Intern. Med., 117:* 769, 1977.

54. Peck, F. B., Jr., Kirtley, W. R., and Peck, F. B., Sr.: Complete remission of severe diabetes. *Diabetes, 7:* 93, 1958.

55. Pirart, J., and Lauvaux, J. P.: Remission in diabetes. In: Handbook

of Diabetes, vol. 2, E. Pfeiffer (ed.). Lehmanns, Munich, 1971, p. 443.

56. Block, M. B., Rosenfield, R. L., Mako, M. E., Steiner, D. F., and Rubenstein, A. H.: Sequential changes in beta-cell function in insulin-treated diabetic patients assessed by C-peptide immunoreactivity. *N. Engl. J. Med., 288:* 1144, 1973.

57. Fajans, S. S., Floyd, J. C., Jr., Pek, S., and Conn, J. W.: Studies on the natural history of asymptomatic diabetes in young people. *Metabolism, 22:* 327, 1972.

58. Toeller, M., and Knubmann, R.: Reproducibility of oral glucose tolerance tests with three different loads. *Diabetologia, 9:* 102, 1973.

59. Seltzer, H. S.: Diagnosis of diabetes. In: Diabetes Mellitus, Theory and Practice, M. Ellenberg and H. Rifkin (eds.). McGraw-Hill Book Co., New York, 1970, chap. 18, pp. 436–507.

60. Mayer, K. H., Stamler, J., Dyer, A., Freinkel, N., Stamler, R., Berkson, D. M., and Farger, B.: Epidemiologic findings on the relationship of time of day and time since last meal to glucose tolerance. *Diabetes, 25:* 936, 1976.

61. Andres, R.: Aging and diabetes. *Med. Clin. North Am., 55:* 835, 1971.

62. O'Sullivan, J. B.: Age gradient in blood glucose levels. Magnitude and clinical implications. *Diabetes, 23:* 713, 1974.

63. Felig, P., Wahren, J., and Hendler, R.: Influence of oral glucose ingestion on splanchnic glucose and gluconeogenic substrate metabolism in man. *Diabetes, 24:* 468, 1975.

64a. Moorhouse, J. A.: Intravenous glucose tolerance tests. In: Diabetes Mellitus: Diagnosis and Treatment, G. J. Hamwi and T. S. Danowski (eds.). ADA, New York, 1967, chap. 10, pp. 51–54.

64b. Soeldner, J. S.: The intravenous glucose tolerance test. In: Diabetes Mellitus: Diagnosis and Treatment, S. S. Fajans and K. E. Sussman (eds.). ADA, Inc., New York, 1971, chap. 19, pp. 107–113.

65. Paulsen, E. P., and Koury, M.: Hemoglobin A_{1c} levels in insulin-dependent and -independent diabetes mellitus. *Diabetes, 25:* 890, 1976.

66. LeFebvre, P., Mosora, F., Lacroix, M., Luyckx, A., Lopez-Habib, G., and Duchesne, J.: Naturally labeled ^{13}C-glucose. Metabolic studies in human diabetes and obesity. *Diabetes, 24:* 185, 1975.

67. Report of the Birmingham Diabetes Survey Working Party: Ten-year follow-up report on Birmingham Diabetes Survey. *Br. Med. J., 2:* 35, 1976.

68. O'Sullivan, J. B., and Mahan, C. M.: Prospective study of 352 young patients with chemical diabetes. *N. Engl. J. Med., 278:* 1036, 1968.

69. Köbberling, J., and Creutzfeldt, W.: Comparison of different methods for the evaluation of the oral glucose tolerance test. *Diabetes, 19:* 870, 1970.

70. Siperstein, M. D.: The glucose tolerance test: A pitfall in the diagnosis of diabetes mellitus. *Adv. Intern. Med., 20:* 297, 1975.

71. Unger, R. H.: The standard 2-hour oral glucose tolerance test in diagnosis of diabetes mellitus in subjects without fasting hyperglycemia. *Ann. Intern. Med., 47:* 113, 1957.

72. Sievers, M. L.: Diabetes mellitus in American Indians—standards for diagnosis and management. *Diabetes, 25:* 528, 1976.

73. Floyd, J. C., Jr., Fajans, S. S., Pek, S., Thiffault, C. A., Knopf, R. F., and Conn, J. W.: Synergistic effect of essential amino acids and glucose upon insulin secretion in man. *Diabetes, 19:* 109, 1970.

74. Rushforth, N. B., Bennett, D. H., Steinberg, A. G., and Miller, M.: Comparison of the value of the two- and one-hour glucose levels of the oral glucose tolerance test in the diagnosis of diabetes in Pima Indians. *Diabetes, 24:* 538, 1975.

75. Valleron, A. J., Eschwege, E., Papoz, L., and Rosselin, G. E.: Agreement and discrepancy in the evaluation of normal and diabetic oral glucose tolerance test. *Diabetes, 24:* 585, 1975.

76. Genuth, S. M., Houser, H. B., Carter, J. R., Jr., Merkatz, I., Price, J. W., Schumacker, O. P., and Wieland, R. G.: Community screening for diabetes by blood glucose measurement. *Diabetes, 25:* 1110, 1976.

77. Bunn, H. F., Haney, D. N., Kamin, S., Gabbay, K. H., and Gallop, P. M.: The biosynthesis of human hemoglobin A_{1c}. *J. Clin. Invest., 57:* 1652, 1976.

78. Koenig, R. J., Peterson, C. M., Kilo, C., Cerami, A., and Williamson, J. R.: Hemoglobin A_{1c} as an indicator of the degree of glucose intolerance in diabetes. *Diabetes, 25:* 230, 1976.

79. Koenig, R. J., Peterson, C. M., Jones, R. L., Saudek, C., Lehrman, M., and Cerami, A.: Correlation of glucose regulation and hemoglobin A_{1c} in diabetes mellitus. *N. Engl. J. Med., 295:* 417, 1976.

80. Siperstein, D. M., Unger, R. H., and Madison, L. L.: Studies of muscle capillary basement membranes in normal subjects, diabetic and prediabetic patients. *J. Clin. Invest., 47:* 1973, 1968.

81. Williamson, J. R., Vogler, N. J., and Kilo, C.: Estimation of vascular basement membrane thickness. *Diabetes, 18:* 567, 1969.

82. Siperstein, M. D., Raskin, P., and Burns, H.: Electron microscopic quantification of diabetic microangiopathy. *Diabetes, 22:* 514, 1973.

83. Williamson, J. R., Rowold, E., Hoffman, P., and Kilo, C.: Influence of fixation and morphometric technics on capillary basement-membrane thickening prevalence data in diabetes. *Diabetes, 25:* 604, 1976.

84. Raskin, P., Marks, J. F., Burns, H., Jr., Plumer, M. E., and Siperstein, M. D.: Capillary basement membrane width in diabetic children, *Am. J. Med., 58:* 365, 1975.

85. Aronoff, S. L., Bennett, P. H., Williamson, J. R., Siperstein, M. D., Plumer, M. E., and Miller, M.: Muscle capillary basement membrane (MCBM) measurements in prediabetic, diabetic, and normal Pima Indians and normal Caucasians. *Clin. Res., 24:* 455A, 1976.

86. Fajans, S. S., and Conn, J. W.: The approach to the prediction of diabetes mellitus by modification of the glucose tolerance test with cortisone. *Diabetes, 3:* 296, 1954.

87. Fajans, S. S., and Conn, J. W.: The early recognition of diabetes mellitus. *Ann. N. Y. Acad. Sci., 82:* 208, 1959.

82

Diabetic Ketoacidosis, Nonketotic Hyperosmolar Coma, and Lactic Acidosis

Albert I. Winegrad
Anthony D. Morrison

DIABETIC KETOACIDOSIS

INTRODUCTION

Diabetic ketoacidosis is a clinical condition with greatly varying presentations characterized by hyperglycemia, hyperketonemia, and a metabolic acidosis that can be attributed in major part to elevated plasma levels of acetoacetate and β-hydroxybutyrate. The term is restricted to episodes occurring in known or previously undiagnosed diabetics, and in these instances deficient insulin modulation of metabolism is the primary factor in the pathogenesis of the disorder. A propensity to diabetic ketoacidosis is the essential basis for the clinical classification of patients as juvenile (i.e., ketosis-prone) diabetics irrespective of age, and its prevention is the overriding therapeutic consideration in the long-term management of such patients. The essential characteristics of diabetic ketoacidosis are rapidly induced in experimental animals by acute, severe, deficiency of circulating insulin such as that resulting from the injection of anti-insulin serum into rats.[1] However, the metabolic derangements resulting from marked insulin deficiency may reflect, in part, secondary hormonal alterations and are subject to modification by a host of factors. These include deficiencies of growth hormone or glucocorticoids, somatostatin-induced inhibition of glucagon secretion, and in laboratory animals marked depletion of adipose tissue triglyceride stores resulting from prior starvation. Most of the clinical manifestations of diabetic ketoacidosis are explicable as the consequences of persistent hyperglycemia and its associated osmotic diuresis and of the hyperketonemic metabolic acidosis. However, there is, as yet, no adequate explanation for the development of impaired consciousness or coma in some patients. Moreover, there is no good correlation between the patient's clinical condition on presentation and the severity of the hyperglycemia, hyperketonemia, or metabolic acidosis observed. The marked variation in clinical status on presentation may reflect the duration as well as the severity of the metabolic derangements resulting from inadequate insulin modulation of metabolism, but a number of other factors appear to be operative. These include the manifestations of independent disease processes such as infection, disorders that may restrict the capacity for cardiovascular, renal, or pulmonary adaptations to the metabolic derangements, and exposure to drugs (e.g., diuretics, alcohol, phenoformin, propranalol). As a consequence of this situation the use of arbitrary criteria for the subclassification of patients with diabetic ketoacidosis based primarily upon the initial degree of hyperglycemia, hyperketonemia, and metabolic acidosis is of restricted value and tends to obscure the diverse factors that may contribute to the clinical condition and prognosis in any given patient. Diabetic ketoacidosis is an acute life-threatening emergency, and errors in its management, such as failure to anticipate and prevent hypokalemia or cardiovascular collapse, all too frequently contribute to mortality. The recent Report of the National Committee on Diabetes[2] notes that 5 to 13 percent of ketoacidosis episodes end fatally, and this condition is currently responsible for approximately 10 percent of all deaths in diabetic patients in U.S. hospitals. Diabetic ketoacidosis accounts for 65 percent of all admissions due to diabetes in the 0–19 age group, and 40 percent in the 20–34 age group. The incidence of diabetic ketoacidosis in the United States remained stable over a recent 5-year period from 1968 to 1973, and the National Committee on Diabetes concluded that current health education and delivery of care appear to be inadequate insofar as the prevention and treatment of diabetic ketoacidosis are concerned.

CLINICAL MANIFESTATIONS

Even in the absence of specific precipitating illness, malaise and "tiredness" are frequent initial complaints. Polyuria and polydipsia are almost invariably present but their duration prior to presentation may vary from several hours to several weeks. The significance of the polyuria and polydipsia may be obscured either by symptoms arising from an acute febrile illness, or by the nonspecific gastrointestinal complaints that ultimately develop in the majority of patients and which are quite marked in children. These include anorexia, nausea, vomiting, and varying forms of abdominal pain; these symptoms may be misinterpreted as those of an intercurrent gastorenteritis, and in children particularly may raise the question of an acute intraabdominal emergency. (Although leukocytosis, abdominal tenderness, guarding, and decreased bowel sounds may be present, rebound tenderness is usually absent. It is inexcusable for the presence of glucosuria and ketonuria to go undetected in such instances, and with proper treatment for ketoacidosis these symptoms and findings resolve over a period of several hours in most patients.) Serious errors in the evaluation of the initial manifestations of diabetic ketoacidosis occur most frequently in previously undiagnosed ketosis-prone diabetics. The development of alterations in consciousness is not an invariable concomitant of diabetic ketoacidosis, and patients with marked hyperglycemia and hyperketonemic metabolic acidosis may walk into an emergency ward unassisted and give a lucid history. Drowsiness is, however, common and is the initial manifestation of impaired consciousness in those patients who subsequently progress to stupor and finally to coma. Focal neurological findings or seizures should not be attributed to diabetic ketoacidosis. Impaired consciousness of some degree is usually present in the minority of patients who present with circulatory collapse. Respiration is usually rapid, and particularly in patients with significant impairment of consciousness, deep and sighing. Evidence of dehydration on physical examination is usually present but quite variable, and the ability of modern physicians to detect acetone in the breath (without the assistance of a gas-liquid chromatograph) seems to be restricted to a fraction of the patients admitted with diabetic ketoacidosis.

Diagnosis

Once considered, the diagnosis of diabetic ketoacidosis can usually be evaluated with great rapidity. The diagnosis of diabetic ketoacidosis rests upon the demonstration of a combination of hyperglycemia, hyperketonemia, and a metabolic acidosis that can be attributed in major part to the hyperketonemia; this pattern of metabolic derangement is, of course, the common and consistent consequence of acute severe insulin deficiency in man and experimental animals. Patients with alcoholic ketoacidosis in whom there is characteristically a history of symptoms suggestive of alcohol withdrawal prior to the development of impaired consciousness also exhibit hyperglycemia, hyperketonemia, and a metabolic acidosis attributable in major part to hyperketonemia.[3] However, there is at present no firm basis for differentiating diabetic ketoacidosis and alcoholic ketoacidosis insofar as the management of the acute episode is concerned (vide infra). In contrast there are a host of conditions in which hyperketonemia and metabolic acidosis due in part to elevated lactate levels occur in association with a *low* plasma glucose concentration. These include diseases which predispose to fasting hypoglycemia with reduced plasma insulin concentrations such as glycogen storage disease types I and III, inherited defects in hepatic gluconeogenesis (e.g., hereditary fructose-1,6-diphosphatase deficiency), the syndrome of hypoglycemia associated with large mesenchymal tumors, alcoholic hypoglycemia, and Jamaican vomiting sickness.[4,5] These disorders are distinguished from diabetic ketoacidosis by the presence of a low plasma glucose level, and the relief of hypoglycemia is essential to the reversal of the acute metabolic acidosis.

Hyperglycemia, hyperketonemia, and a metabolic acidosis may also be present in patients who otherwise fit the diagnostic criteria for the syndromes of hyperglycemic nonketotic "coma" or lactic acidosis which in the past had not been clearly distinguished from diabetic ketoacidosis. To establish the existence of these entities it was necessary to use somewhat arbitrary criteria to select patients in whom the clinical condition could clearly be distinguished from the common form of diabetic ketoacidosis. The diagnosis of these entities is considered later, but it must be noted that in specific patients with diabetic ketoacidosis the metabolic derangements observed may include the extreme hyperglycemia observed in hyperglycemic nonketotic "coma" and that diabetics with lactic acidosis not infrequently have a significant degree of hyperketonemia and benefit from insulin treatment.[6]

The degrees of hyperglycemia, hyperketonemia, and metabolic acidosis in individual patients presenting with diabetic ketoacidosis (DKA) vary markedly[6]; but for the comparison of treatment most workers set arbitrary requirements particularly with regard to the degree of metabolic acidosis as reflected by the plasma bicarbonate (frequently 8–10 meq/liter or less) or plasma pH. This unfortunately obscures the true range of variation and in some instances the extent to which the hyperglycemia and hyperketonemic metabolic acidosis may vary independently for a variety of reasons. In a recent series of 70 episodes of DKA, plasma glucose concentration ranged from 200 to 2000 mg/dl in patients in whom a pH less than 7.37 and a positive serum nitroprusside test was present.[7] While it is likely that this series contained a number of patients with diabetic ketoacidosis of relatively brief duration and patients who could have been classified as hyperglycemic nonketotic "coma," marked degrees of hyperketonemic metabolic acidosis may occur in the presence of modest degrees of hyperglycemia, and values as low as 200 mg/dl are not that unusual. In some instances this can be explained as the consequence of prior administration of insulin, since the rapidity with which the metabolic acidosis and elevated plasma levels of acetoacetate and acetone (which are responsible for the positive plasma nitroprusside reaction) respond to insulin is often much slower than the fall in plasma glucose concentration. Markedly positive reactions for glucose and ketones in the urine are helpful initial indications of hyperglycemia and hyperketonemia at some time in the recent past, but are unreliable guides to the actual levels in plasma.

The presence of hyperglycemia is usually readily demonstrated by means of commercially available paper strips impregnated with glucose oxidase and an appropriate indicator, such as Dextrostix. However, errors due to improperly stored materials are frequent and the use of a standard to control for inactivated enzyme is desirable. The quantification of plasma glucose can now be achieved within a few minutes in small samples by means of a microcentrifuge and a variety of commercially available glucose analyzers which detect the oxygen uptake associated with the glucose oxidase reaction.

Quantitative estimates of the plasma levels of acetoacetate and β-hydroxybutyrate are unfortunately not available to most physicians with sufficient rapidity to be of value in the initial diagnosis or management of patients with diabetic ketoacidosis. As a consequence, the demonstration of hyperketonemia rests almost invariably on the presence of a positive reaction with commercially available powders (Acetest tablets which must be crushed for use with plasma, or impregnated paper strips, Ketostix). These reagents, which provide a convenient method for carrying out the nitroprusside test, do not give a positive test with the predominant plasma ketone body, β-hydroxybutyrate. The positive reaction (i.e., the development of a purple color) reflects the presence of elevated concentrations of acetoacetate and to varying degrees of acetone in the plasma or urine of patients with DKA. These tests provide a convenient rapid method for the demonstration of elevated plasma levels of acetoacetate but are not quantitative under the best of circumstances. Alberti and Hockaday documented the wide range of acetoacetate levels found by a quantitative enzymatic assay in plasma samples from patients with DKA giving a +, ++, or +++ reaction with Ketostix. With a ++ reaction the acetoacetate levels were found to vary from 0.5 mM to more than 5.0 mM with a mean less than 3 mM. With a +++ reaction the mean acetoacetate concentration was found to be 3 mM but the range was from 1.6 to 5.5 mM.[8] The contribution of acetone to the positive test observed in the plasma of a given patient with DKA cannot be assessed except in those institutions prepared to perform rapid gas-liquid chromatographic analysis of plasma or expired air for clinical purposes. Acetone has recently been found to be present in the plasma of patients with DKA in concentrations of 2.5–12.9 mM, and in Sulway's experience was present in higher concentrations than acetoacetate.[9] Acetone does not give as intense a color reaction in the nitroprusside test as equimolar concentrations of acetoacetate; the intensity has been reported to vary from 1/4th to 1/20th that observed with acetoacetate with different commercial reagents. For practical purposes a moderately to strongly positive plasma nitroprusside reaction is present in the vast majority of patients in whom the metabolic acidosis ultimately proves to be primarily due to hyperketonemia, and it is extremely helpful in confirming the presence of a pattern consistent with the metabolic consequences of marked deficiency in insulin in a patient with hyperglycemia and metabolic acidosis. It must be noted that the ratio of β-hydroxybutyrate to acetoacetate in plasma, while normally on the order of 2:1, has been found to vary markedly in patients presenting in diabetic ketoacidosis and may be as high as 32:1.[6] Consequently the plasma nitroprusside reaction gives a poor indication of total plasma acetoacetate and β-hydroxybutyrate concentrations. As discussed in other sections of this text, the circulating plasma–β-hydroxybutyrate–acetoacetate concentrations tend to reflect the hepatic β-hydroxybutyrate/acetoacetate ratio resulting from the maintenance of near equilibrium in the interconversion of β-hydroxybutyrate and acetoacetate by mitochondrial β-hydroxybutyrate dehydrogenase and the redox state* of the free $NAD^+/NADH$ couple in hepatic mitochondria. Thus it is difficult to assess the plasma total ketone body concentration from the plasma nitroprusside reaction, and while markedly elevated levels are usually associated with strongly positive reactions for acetoacetate (and acetone) out to several dilutions, this is not always the case. A number of instances have been reported in which the magnitude of the hyperketonemia in patients with hyperglycemia and severe metabolic acidosis has been underestimated because of a marked increase in the β-hydroxybutyrate/acetoacetate ratio (in one case an acetoacetate of 0.33 mM was associated with a β-hydroxybutyrate of over 7 mM) usually in association with an increase in plasma lactate concentration. The same mechanism has helped to obscure the frequent occurrence of significant elevations of total plasma ketone concentrations in diabetics with lactic acidosis. Another point that frequently leads to confusion is that alterations in a markedly elevated plasma β-hydroxybutyrate/acetoacetate ratio commonly occur in the course of treatment for diabetic ketoacidosis and on occasion in successful treatment for lactic acidosis in diabetics; this may result in an increase in plasma acetoacetate concentration at a time when total plasma ketone

---

*The redox state of the pyridine nucleotides is used as an abbreviation for the value of the ratio of the concentrations of the free oxidized and reduced forms of a specific pyridine nucleotide in a given subcellular compartment.

concentration is decreasing.[6] These points underscore the limitations of the nitroprusside test as commonly employed, particularly with regard to evaluating the degree of hyperketonemia and the response to treatment. It is obvious that it is extremely difficult to judge the degree to which plasma ketones are responsible for an associated metabolic acidosis, by comparing the unmeasured anion gap and comparing it with the nitroprusside reaction in serial dilutions. The practical point is that the presence of a positive nitroprusside reaction of more than a trace in a diabetic with hyperglycemia and a metabolic acidosis is an indication for exogenous insulin treatment, even though in retrospect another anion (e.g., lactate) may prove to be a major factor.

The presence of a metabolic acidosis is indicated by an increase in undetermined plasma anions as estimated by the anion gap (the Δ between the serum Na^+ and the sum of the serum Cl^- and total CO_2 concentrations, the normal being 5–15 meq/liter), and by the demonstration of decreased blood pH with a decreased pCO_2 and a reduction in the calculated HCO_3 concentration. In most instances the respiratory compensation for the metabolic acidosis in patients with diabetic ketoacidosis appears to be appropriate when their "pCO_2–bicarbonate plot" is examined. The importance of respiratory compensation underscores the possible adverse effects of the diminished pulmonary ventilation observed by Kety et al.[10] in patients whose pH was below 7.0, or of the presence of drugs (e.g., alcohol) in concentrations sufficient to impair respiration. In one-third of the cases studied by Hockaday and Alberti the arterial pO_2 was found to be less than 80 mm Hg.[6]

PATHOGENESIS

Specific details of the alterations in insulin and glucagon secretion associated with diabetic ketoacidosis, and the mechanisms of the hyperglycemia and hyperketonemia found in this condition are given in Chapters 77 through 80.

Acute severe insulin deficiency in experimental animals or man, when induced by mechanisms that do not directly modify the secretion of glucagon, growth hormone, or glucocorticoids, reproducibly results in the characteristic manifestations of diabetic ketoacidosis. The presence of very low or undetectable concentrations of plasma insulin in patients in diabetic ketoacidosis, and of an absent or markedly restricted capacity for insulin secretion as assessed by C-peptide assays is now well documented (see Chapter 77). There is at present no convincing evidence for the role of insulin antagonists in the plasma of most patients with diabetic ketoacidosis. While the manifestations of severe insulin deficiency can be modified or delayed by the inhibition of glucagon secretion with somatostatin, or by the presence of growth hormone or cortisol deficiency, evidence that DKA primarily results from an excess of these hormones is lacking.

As noted elsewhere, acute severe insulin deficiency may induce secondary alterations in pancreatic glucagon secretion, and in some species apparently in glucagon secretion by cells in the gastrointestinal tract, and elevated plasma glucagon levels are found in most patients with diabetic ketoacidosis (see Chapter 78). However, diabetic ketoacidosis can occur in the depancreatectomized man, and there is still no convincing evidence for elevated plasma glucagon levels in such individuals. Consequently it seems fair to conclude that in most instances the primary hormonal abnormality required for the development of diabetic ketoacidosis is a derangement in insulin secretion. This is well supported by the efficacy of exogenous insulin in reversing the metabolic derangement. With infrequent exception the development of acute diabetic ketoacidosis in a previously undiagnosed diabetic is followed by a persistent requirement for exogenous insulin to prevent the development of ketoacidosis. This presumably reflects the acute processes affecting the pancreatic beta cells reflected in the pathological changes found in these patients (see Chapter 74). The nature of these processes may be diverse, but in a few instances the development of ketoacidosis and a marked impairment in endogenous insulin secretion have been correlated with evidence of an acute viral infection such as mumps.[11] Rubenstein (see Chapter 77) has documented the presence of some residual insulin secretion in individual juvenile diabetics by C-peptide assays of plasma, and demonstrated a correlation between variations in this residual secretion and propensity to ketoacidosis and "brittleness." Obviously factors such as drugs and α-adrenergic stimulation may potentially remove the buffering capacity of this residual endogenous secretion and modify the effectiveness of any fixed regimen of exogenous insulin in maintaining adequate regulation of carbohydrate and lipid metabolism to prevent the development of DKA. Autonomic stimuli affecting insulin secretion, the rate of FFA release from adipose tissue, and hepatic glycogenolysis in a manner opposing the effects of insulin in the latter tissues can be a significant factor in the development of DKA and its progression. This has been clearly demonstrated by controlled studies in juvenile diabetics in whom frequent episodes of ketoacidosis were precipitated by emotional upsets. When given tasks to perform which were beyond their expected capacities, these patients rapidly developed increasing hyperglycemia, elevations of plasma FFA, and hyperketonemia which best correlated with evidence of increased urinary catecholamine excretion.[12] The manner in which acute febrile illness induces acute DKA in known diabetics on a fixed exogenous insulin regimen is still unclear; the possibility that alterations in autonomic discharge or in cortisol and growth hormone secretion play a role is frequently cited. However, acute illness frequently leads to omission or decreases in insulin administration by patients, and the extent to which intercurrent undiagnosed illness directly affects residual insulin secretion is usually not assessed.

The pathogenesis of the fasting hyperglycemia found in patients with DKA can be explained in major part by the known role of a normal insulin secretory mechanism in the regulation of hepatic glycogenolysis and gluconeogenesis, and only to a lesser extent by decreases in glucose utilization in tissues in which it is subject to insulin regulation since fasting is normally associated with a relatively low rate of glucose utilization in these tissues (see Chapter 79). The studies of McGarry and Foster (Chapter 80) have helped to clarify the role of insulin in the regulation of hepatic ketogenesis and the pathogenesis of the hyperketonemia characteristic of DKA. Their formulation notes that the markedly increased hepatic ketogenesis which is the primary determinant of the hyperketonemia is a consequence of both an increased uptake of long chain free fatty acids by the liver and an alteration in the regulation of the transport of the CoA derivatives of these fatty acids across the inner mitochondrial membrane. The latter process, mediated by the components of the palmitoyl CoA carnitine acyltransferase reactions, appears to be the major site of regulation of hepatic long chain fatty acid oxidation, and of the partition of fatty acid metabolism between oxidation and triglyceride and phospholipid synthesis in the liver. A markedly accelerated rate of hepatic long chain fatty acid oxidation now appears to be the major determinant of the accelerated rate of hepatic ketogenesis, and increases in the mitochondrial concentration of acetyl CoA and its concentration relative to that of free CoA result in increased ketogenesis as a consequence of the kinetic characteristics of the enzymes concerned with the synthesis of free acetoacetate, the parent ketone body.

From present formulations insulin deficiency operates at two major sites in the pathogenesis of the hyperketonemia of DKA. In adipose tissue the loss of insulin modulation of the net production of long chain free fatty acids from adipose tissue triglycerides results in an accelerated rate of release of FFA and is responsible for the elevated plasma FFA characteristically present in the plasma of patients with DKA (see Chapters 79 and 144). The plasma FFA concentration is the major determinant of the uptake of FFA by the liver, and there is ample documentation of an increased transfer of long chain fatty acids from adipose to liver in experimental DKA. As detailed in Chapter 80, insulin deficiency appears to increase the activity of the system for the transport of the activated derivatives of the long chain fatty acids (or at least their acyl moiety) across the inner mitochondrial membrane and their access to the enzymes of the fatty acid oxidation system which quantitatively oxidize them to acetyl CoA. Evidence that the activity of the palmitoyl CoA carnitine acyl transferase reactions is directly affected by insulin is still lacking, but both the increase in hepatic carnitine concentrations and the decrease in liver glycogen which correlate with the activation of this system in acute severe insulin deficiency are corrected by exogenous insulin (Chapter 80). If the secondary rise in plasma glucagon that results from acute severe insulin deficiency is accepted as essential for the increase in the ketogenic capacity of the liver, a view that is still in dispute, this effect would suggest an additional site at which insulin deficiency operates in the pathogenesis of the hyperketonemia of DKA (see Chapters 76 and 78). The bulk of the evidence available indicates that the hyperketonemia found in human and experimental diabetic ketoacidosis is dependent on and primarily a consequence of increased hepatic ketogenesis. However, it has been suggested that "impaired" peripheral utilization may contribute and may be essential to the production of severe ketoacidosis.[13] "Impaired" utilization in this context refers to an alteration in the usual regulatory relationships between plasma acetoacetate and β-hydroxybutyrate concentrations and estimates of ketone body uptake and utilization. Constant intravenous infusions of acetoacetate of a given rate result in higher steady state ketone body concentrations and lower estimated rates of ketone body utilization in rats or dogs with experimental diabetes than in normal animals[14,15]; in rats these alterations are not acutely corrected by insulin but improve after several days of treatment. In normal dogs infused with [^{14}C]acetoacetate at a constant rate insulin decreased both plasma ketone body and FFA concentrations, and increased the efflux rate of expired $^{14}CO_2$.[15] It has been suggested that long chain fatty acids may be utilized in preference to ketone bodies in prolonged starvation, that a similar situation may obtain in the perfused hindlimb of diabetic rats, and that the effects of insulin may be related to alterations in the plasma or local tissue concentrations of FFA.[16] Owen and Reichard found a mean estimated hepatic ketone body production rate of 131 g/24 h in a group of patients in diabetic ketoacidosis. This value was similar to that found in normal obese subjects after a 3-day fast but was associated with much higher blood acetoacetate and β-hydroxybutyrate concentrations.[13]

The origin of the apparent alterations in peripheral ketone body utilization in human and experimental diabetic ketoacidosis and the time course of their development require clarification. There is no convincing evidence that insulin directly regulates ketone body utilization in brain, skeletal muscle, kidney, or other quantitatively important potential sites of utilization; it seems likely that the alterations observed are secondary phenomena. Detailed studies have not been carried out to define the extent to which the apparent alterations in peripheral ketone body utilization may reflect alterations in circulation, in the total energy requirements of specific tissues (e.g., brain, muscle) in DKA, in the activation of acetoacetate to acetoacetyl CoA, in the conversion of β-hydroxybutyrate to acetoacetate as the result of possible alterations in the redox state of the mitochondrial $NAD^+/NADH$ couple in peripheral tissues, or in the concentrations of alternative substrates such as glucose and FFA. It should be emphasized that total ketone body production and utilization are increased in diabetic ketoacidosis, and that a primary role for increased hepatic ketogenesis in the pathogenesis of the hyperketonemia has been clearly established.

TREATMENT

The details of treatment must be individualized, but there are essential considerations that pertain to the treatment of all patients with diabetic ketoacidosis. The restoration and preservation of an adequate circulation and renal function, as reflected in urine volume, usually require rapid correction of the deficits in intravascular volume; the correction of total water deficits which may be on the order of 10 to 15 percent of previous body weight[17] is then accomplished more gradually. The administration of rapidly acting insulin in doses adequate to initiate and maintain progressive improvement in the degree of hyperglycemia and hyperketonemia obviates the factors primarily responsible for the osmotic diuresis and metabolic acidosis; *therapy designed to directly affect plasma pH is not required in most instances.* Hypokalemia is a potential source of morbidity and mortality during treatment and its prevention is an important consideration.[18] A thorough search for specific precipitating or complicating illness is indicated since their prompt identification and treatment may critically affect the patient's course. With these general considerations in mind the details of treatment must be modified to fit the conditions found initially in any given patient and on subsequent frequent reassessments of their response to treatment.

While it is common practice for the purposes of reporting to restrict the diagnosis of "true diabetic ketoacidosis" to patients meeting arbitrary criteria with regard to the degree of metabolic acidosis (e.g., bicarbonate of 10 meq/liter or less) or of hyperketonemia (e.g., total ketones of 3.0 nmol/liter or greater), these criteria do not adequately reflect the potential seriousness of the patient's clinical condition and obscure the necessity for prompt and intensive medical attention to patients with hyperglycemia, hyperketonemia, and metabolic acidosis who do not meet these criteria. Controlled clinical trials of specific aspects of the treatment of diabetic ketoacidosis are relatively rare. Almost every aspect of treatment remains a matter of some controversy. The bases of the authors' general recommendations are thus noted in the following.

Intravenous Fluids and Electrolyte

The restoration and preservation of an adequate circulation and urine output are prime initial considerations; the presence of shock on admission or its development during treatment is recognized to be associated with an increased mortality.[19] It has been well documented that in experimentally induced hyperglycemia and osmotic diuresis the urinary sodium concentration is lower than that in plasma, being on the order of 30 to 80 meq/liter,[20] and that during the recovery from diabetic acidosis the reconstitution of normal body electrolyte composition requires replacement of water in a ratio to sodium greater than that found in plasma. However, it does not follow that the aims of initial intravenous fluid therapy are best achieved by the administration of large volumes of hypotonic sodium chloride solutions. As noted by McCurdy,[20] the administration of isotonic (i.e., 0.9 percent NaCl) is more effective in achieving rapid expansion of extracellular and

intravascular volume than equal volumes of hypotonic solutions in patients with dehydration resulting from osmotic diuresis associated with hyperglycemia. Consequently, we recommend that at the outset of treatment isotonic saline should be infused rapidly, at the rate of approximately 1 liter/h in adults without cardiac disease, until the blood pressure is stable and a urine flow of at least 1–2 ml/min is documented. Whenever possible the use of a catheter should be avoided (it is rarely justified in patients who are not comatose), but the assessment of urine flow is important since persistent oliguria may reflect inadequate expansion of intravascular volume, or may be the initial manifestation of the syndrome of acute tubular necrosis complicating diabetic ketoacidosis. In some instances in which there is an inadvertent delay in the initiation of insulin treatment rapid expansion of the extracellular fluid volume with intravenous normal saline may result in significant decreases in the degree of hyperglycemia. This is naturally more commonly observed with severe dehydration and higher initial plasma glucose concentrations.

The threat of symptomatic hypokalemia is inherent in the treatment of diabetic ketoacidosis and may be significantly increased when the plasma pH is acutely raised by the administration of sodium bicarbonate intravenously. Total body K^+ deficits have been estimated to be on the order of 5 meq/kg body weight,[17] but significantly greater deficits have been documented in balance studies of individual patients recovering from the acute episode. The magnitude of these deficits is not accurately reflected in the initial serum K^+ concentration which is commonly normal or elevated, averaging 4.4 meq/liter in one recently reported series.[6] This reflects the effects of a variety of factors including the known tendency of a metabolic acidosis to increase plasma K^+ concentration in association with a decrease in tissue K^+ concentrations. The presence of a serum K^+ that is low or low normal in the face of significant metabolic acidosis in a patient with diabetic ketoacidosis usually reflects an extreme degree of K^+ depletion and an increased risk of severe symptomatic hypokalemia during treatment unless it is prevented by prompt and vigorous K^+ replacement. Irrespective of the initial serum K^+ concentration, it invariably falls during the course of treatment. A fall to low levels associated with manifestations of hypokalemia may occur rapidly, or after a period of hours, in any given patient. The decrease in serum K^+ reflects a variety of factors: the effects of insulin on K^+ uptake by tissues such as skeletal muscle and liver; the uptake of K^+ and release of H^+ by cells associated with the correction of a metabolic acidosis, expansion of the extracellular fluid volume with non-K^+-containing solutions, and persistent urinary K^+ loss, which Hockaday and Alberti estimated to be at least on the order of 50–100 meq during the first 24 h of treatment irrespective of the amount of K^+ infused.[6] Hypokalemia may be asymptomatic, but abdominal distension, ileus, muscle weakness, cardiac dysrhythmia, and acute respiratory paralysis are well-recognized manifestations of hypokalemia in patients treated for diabetic ketoacidosis. In deaths attributed to hypokalemia acute respiratory failure is common.

The propensity to hypokalemia requires consideration in every patient irrespective of the initial serum K^+ concentration, but an increased mortality from hypokalemia has been particularly associated with an initially low normal or low serum K^+ concentration. In such patients and in those with a history of protracted vomiting, diarrhea, or polyuria the initiation of replacement therapy is a particularly urgent requirement. Although the electrocardiogram may not accurately reflect the serum K^+, it should be examined prior to the start of intravenous K^+ replacement, and monitored continuously in patients in whom very vigorous replacement is likely to be required since serum K^+ determinations can only be obtained at intervals and the development of hyperkalemia is the risk that limits the rate of K^+ infusion. It is our practice to initiate K^+ replacement as soon as a stable blood pressure and an adequate rate of urine production has been achieved by the infusion of 1–2 liters of isotonic saline. This is done by switching to a solution containing 0.5 N saline and 40 meq of K^+ (preferably as the buffered phosphate), which in most instances can be safely administered at an initial rate not exceeding 1 liter/h; 40 meq k^+/liter is included in all of the subsequent intravenous fluids administered during the first 12 h unless specific contraindications are present. There have been a number of reported instances in which unusually high rates of intravenous K^+ replacement (as high as 80 meq/h) were required to alleviate severe hypokalemia that developed during treatment for diabetic ketoacidosis.[6] In patients in whom there appears to be an unusually high risk of symptomatic hypokalemia (e.g., initial K^+ or 3.5 meq/liter or less in the face of a marked metabolic acidosis) it may be appropriate to initiate K^+ replacement with a solution containing 60 meq/liter in 0.5 N saline. In such patients the response of the serum K^+ and ECG should be monitored carefully and the K^+ concentration in the administered intravenous fluids adjusted accordingly, usually over the range of 40–60 meq/liter. The risk of hypokalemia remains significant in such patients for a prolonged period, and inclusion of K^+ in the intravenous fluids administered over the first 24 h, with appropriate control, seems warranted. The aim of K^+ replacement therapy is to prevent the development of hypokalemia and not to replace an estimated total deficit or merely the observed urinary loss. When the patient is capable of retaining oral fluids the repletion of total K^+ deficits may be assisted in this manner (e.g., orange juice contains approximately 5 meq/100 ml).

The value of administering sodium bicarbonate intravenously to acutely increase the arterial pH has not been documented; this practice may have adverse effects under certain circumstances and consequently its routine use has been abandoned in most centers. The methods for the estimation of the quantities of sodium bicarbonate required to raise the plasma bicarbonate to nearly normal levels frequently result in the administration of doses that induce alkalosis and increase the risk of symptomatic hypokalemia. Posner and Plum reported that the administration of large doses of bicarbonate (on the order of 180 meq) to a group of patients with metabolic acidosis, including some with diabetic ketoacidosis, was followed by marked deterioration in mental status; they suggested that this might be related to an associated paradoxical fall in CSF pH which was higher than that in plasma prior to treatment.[21] The bicarbonate concentration in CSF is regulated independently of that in plasma and only slowly reflects changes in plasma concentration, whereas there appears to be rapid equilibration of pCO_2 between arterial blood and CSF. The administration of bicarbonate increases arterial pH, alters respiratory compensation for acidosis, and results in a rise in CSF pCO_2 before a significant increase in CSF bicarbonate occurs resulting in a decrease in CSF pH. Other workers have confirmed the development of a paradoxical decrease in CSF pH under these conditions, but its significance with regard to alterations in mental status has not been firmly established.

Significant losses of inorganic phosphate occur during the development of diabetic ketoacidosis but on presentation levels are normal or somewhat elevated. In normal subjects glucose ingestion or the injection of insulin tends to decrease the plasma inorganic phosphate levels, and in the course of diabetic ketoacidosis the plasma phosphate levels tend to fall, presumably due to intracellular sequestration as organic phosphate. Hockaday and Alberti reported that several of their patients had plasma inorganic phos-

phate levels as low as 1 mg/dl after 24 h and sometimes required several days before returning to normal levels.[6] However, there are as yet no well-documented clinical consequences of this hypophosphatemia, and a specific indication for the administration of intravenous phosphate has not been established. It has been suggested that hypophosphatemia could contribute to impaired tissue oxygenation as the result of the relationship between low plasma inorganic phosphate and low erythrocyte 2,3-diphosphoglycerate (2,3-DPG) concentrations.[22] The affinity of hemoglobin for oxygen is subject to immediate modification by pH, and acidosis tends to decrease its affinity. In diabetic ketoacidosis, as well as in experimental acidosis in man, there is a compensatory decrease in the concentrations of 2,3-DPG, an allosteric modifier of the affinity of hemoglobin for oxygen, such that an apparently normal in vivo oxygen affinity is preserved despite the acidosis. Following rapid correction of the acidosis by bicarbonate infusion the rise in erythrocyte 2,3-DPG may be delayed. It has been suggested that this may cause a left shift of the in vivo oxygen dissociation curve with impaired tissue oxygen availability unless there is a marked increase in cardiac output or a marked reduction in mixed venous oxygen tension.[22] Erythrocyte 2,3-DPG concentration is also subject to regulation by plasma inorganic phosphate level, persistently low plasma phosphate levels being associated with low erythrocyte 2,3-DPG levels that rapidly rise in response to phosphate administration. It has been suggested that the low plasma phosphate levels in patients treated for diabetic ketoacidosis may further retard the normal restoration of normal erythrocyte 2,3-DPG concentrations and a normal oxygen–hemoglobin dissociation curve. Hockaday and Alberti reported that it could take as long as 96 h for 2,3-DPG to return to normal, although plasma pH was usually normal within 24 h.[6] Whether this has significant clinical consequences in most patients treated for diabetic ketoacidosis is still unclear, and the value of phosphate administration has not been studied under controlled conditions. However, since patients treated for diabetic acidosis may show a persistent hyperchloremia attributable in part to the administration of NaCl in large quantities, we have long felt it preferable to administer K^+ as the buffered phosphate(s), particularly in view of the documented phosphate deficiency and the fall in plasma phosphate that occurs in association with treatment. The value of this practice has not been subjected to controlled studies. The necessity for frequent plasma inorganic phosphate determinations has not been established, but merits further study.

Kassirer notes that extreme acidosis can usually be alleviated over a period of several hours merely by raising plasma bicarbonate concentration 4–6 meq/liter[23]; this eliminates the danger of extreme acidosis but averts the development of posttreatment respiratory alkalosis if the low pCO_2 persists for some time after alkali therapy. When the quantity of alkali needed to raise plasma bicarbonate is being calculated, the volume of distribution should be assumed to be approximately 50 percent of body weight. Thus

$$\text{amount of alkali (meq)} = \text{body wt (kg)} \times 0.5 \\ \times \text{ desired increment in} \\ \text{bicarbonate concentration (meq/liter)}$$

By the formulation of Kassirer an ampule of sodium bicarbonate containing 44.6 meq might be expected to induce a rise in plasma bicarbonate on the order of 1.3 meq/liter, but significant deviations from the predicted change may occur and the process must be considered one of titration. The administration of large doses of bicarbonate and the resulting alteration in pH may significantly increase the quantity of exogenous K^+ required to prevent hypokalemia. The ECG and serum K^+ should be monitored at frequent intervals; it is preferable to administer the bicarbonate in a separate drip (in 0.5 N saline) so that the administration of the solution containing 0.5 N NaCl and K$^+$ 40 mM can be varied independently if required.

Insulin Therapy

Rapidly acting insulin preparations suitable for intravenous administration (if required) are the only preparations suitable for the treatment of diabetic ketoacidosis. In recent years the dosage and mode of administration have been subjects of renewed interest and controversy. The aims of insulin therapy are to modify the metabolic derangements responsible for the hyperglycemia, hyperketonemia, and metabolic acidosis; the evaluation of the efficacy of insulin treatment has been a subject of controversy and is hampered by the frequent lack of a capacity to obtain rapid, accurate determinations of plasma free fatty acid, acetoacetate, and β-hydroxybutyrate concentrations in time to apply these to a clinical situation. The pattern of response observed in successfully treated patients is a fall in plasma glucose concentration that is usually roughly paralleled by a decrease in plasma free fatty acid concentration.[24] It must be remembered that rapid expansion of the extracellular fluid volume and improved renal function in severely dehydrated patients may contribute to an initial fall in plasma glucose concentration. A number of workers have observed that the β-hydroxybutyrate and total plasma ketone body concentrations begin to fall at approximately the same time as the plasma glucose and FFA concentrations. However, the plasma acetoacetate not uncommonly rises initially before declining at a rate slower than that of the total plasma ketone body concentration.[25] Since the liver can rapidly achieve the equilibration of exogenously administered D-β-hydroxybutyrate and acetoacetate in plasma, the rise in plasma acetoacetate during insulin treatment for diabetic ketoacidosis probably reflects in part a change in the ratio of β-hydroxybutyrate/acetoacetate imposed by the near equilibrium of the hepatic mitochondrial β-hydroxybutyrate dehydrogenase reaction as the result of a change in the redox state of the free NAD$^+$/NADH couple in hepatic mitochondria. As a consequence, strongly positive plasma and urinary reactions for "ketones" using the nitroprusside reaction may persist for prolonged periods after insulin administration has resulted in significant decreases in plasma glucose, FFA, and total ketone body concentration. Moreover, in some instances associated with a markedly elevated initial plasma β-hydroxybutyrate/acetoacetate ratio, uncritical evaluation of the nitroprusside reactions obtained with serial dilutions of plasma may erroneously suggest a rise in total plasma ketone body concentration. The plasma acetone concentration, which may be high enough to contribute significantly to the plasma nitroprusside reaction initially, falls at a very slow rate, reflecting its slow disposition in expired air. Significantly elevated plasma acetone concentrations may persist for as long as 24 h after recovery from ketoacidosis.[9] As a consequence of the points just cited, the use of plasma or urine nitroprusside reactions to assess the efficacy of exogenous insulin given to patients with diabetic ketoacidosis is of limited value, and can lead to serious errors (e.g., hypoglycemia) if the plasma gluclose is not monitored. In the majority of patients who do not receive sodium bicarbonate significant improvement in plasma bicarbonate and pH tends to lag significantly behind the initial decreases in plasma glucose and total ketone body concentrations. In one recent series treated with large doses of insulin given intravenously plasma glucose was reduced to 250 mg/dl or below within 2.2–5.5 h, but 4.2–11.5 h was required for the plasma bicarbonate to reach 20 meq/liter or above.[26] In some instances the plasma bicarbonate may remain below normal for 24 h or more, usually associated with a persistent

hyperchloremia. Although this has usually been attributed to the administration of large quantities of NaCl and KCl, one recent study suggests that in some instances a transient defect in renal tubular bicarbonate reabsorption may contribute.[27]

An understanding of the patterns and time courses of the changes in plasma glucose, FFA, β-hydroxybutyrate, acetoacetate, and in plasma pH and bicarbonate concentrations is a relatively recent development, and has helped to clarify the choice of an appropriate index for assessing the efficacy of exogenous insulin under clinical conditions. Although the initial expansion of extracellular fluid volume and improved renal perfusion may contribute to the initial decline in plasma glucose concentration, *insulin therapy that initiates and sustains a progressive fall in plasma glucose has been almost invariably found to initiate a fall in plasma FFA and total ketone body concentrations when the latter data were finally available, and to have initiated the processes that will eventuate in correction of the metabolic acidosis.*

Although the aims of insulin treatment in diabetic ketoacidosis are readily achieved by a variety of regimens, the appropriate dosages and routes of administration have been the subjects of recent controversy. However, the major errors in the use of insulin are (1) failure to monitor plasma glucose at frequent intervals to assess the efficacy of the doses administered; the use of glucose-containing solutions at the outset deprives the physician of this valuable indicator and has no established basis. (2) Failure to adjust insulin dosage appropriately when a significant decrease in plasma glucose is delayed for more than 1–2 h or when it falls precipitously and threatens hypoglycemia. (3) Failure to continue the administration of insulin at frequent intervals (4–6 h) following recovery and thus permitting a recrudescence of hyperglycemia and hyperketonemia.

The present controversy concerning the use of insulin must be viewed in perspective. Clinical practice was strongly influenced for many years by the report of Root in 1945, which attributed a marked reduction in the mortality experience at the Joslin Clinic (from 12 to 1.6 percent) to the administration of large doses of insulin within the first 3 h after admission in ketoacidosis; the average dose given in this study was 216 U.[28] This observation antedated the general recognition of the importance of hypokalemia as a cause of death, and present knowledge of the pattern and temporal course of the reversal of the metabolic derangements in diabetic ketoacidosis. Moreover, during the subsequent decade it was widely held that a circulating insulin "antagonist" played a significant role in the pathogenesis of most cases of diabetic ketoacidosis, a view that has now been generally abandoned.

There are at present at least three commonly used approaches to insulin treatment for diabetic ketoacidosis, which if used appropriately are (in the authors' views) equally effective.

Continuous Intravenous Infusion. Regular insulin is diluted with physiological saline to provide a solution with approximately 0.50 U/ml and infused at a rate of 4–8 U/h by means of a constant infusion pump. (Some workers add 1 to 2 percent albumin to minimize insulin binding to glass.) Some workers give an initial priming dose of 0.5–12 U. In patients previously untreated with insulin plasma levels of 20–200 μU/ml have been achieved.[29] The clinical response to this regimen has generally been similar to that observed with other regimens, although the total insulin administered over the initial 24 h is significantly lower than that previously employed to treat DKA. Studies of this form of insulin treatment have helped to dispel the existence of "insulin resistance" in most patients with diabetic ketoacidosis and the need for very large insulin doses. However, the need for monitoring the effectiveness of the insulin administered remains, as does the need to modify the rate of insulin administration in some patients to prevent undue delay in lowering plasma glucose. As in other treatment regimens 5 percent glucose should be added to the electrolyte solutions when the plasma glucose approaches 200–250 mg/dl, and the rate of insulin infusion modified to prevent hypoglycemia, or replaced by subcutaneous injections of small doses of regular insulin at intervals of 2–4 h. Claims for the superiority of this regiment are disputed; the same degree of physician supervision is required, and in some instances the use of a constant infusion pump proves to be a nuisance in efforts to provide appropriate care for a seriously ill patient.

Repeated Intramuscular Injections of Small Doses of Insulin. The patients are given an intramuscular injection of 20 U of regular insulin initially (intravenously if in shock) and they are given 10 U im at hourly intervals.[26] Again 5 percent glucose is administered when the plasma glucose approaches 200–250 mg/dl, and insulin administration is modified usually by switching to subcutaneous administration at longer intervals. Plasma glucose response must be monitored to permit alterations in dosage, and the same degree of physician attention is required as in other regimens. The method is simple and effective, provided the patient's plasma glucose response is carefully monitored. The introduction of this regimen was based on the premise that the effectiveness of an intravenously administered bolus of insulin was restricted to the short half-life of labeled insulin administered intravenously to patients not previously treated with insulin, i.e., a few minutes. This premise is erroneous, but the use of intramuscular injections may obviate variable absorption of small doses of insulin given subcutaneously.

Repeated Injections of Insulin Intravenously. Regular insulin is injected as a bolus intravenously in doses ranging from 10 to 100 U at intervals of 1 to 2 or 3 h.[26] Most commonly workers using this method give doses of 50–100 U at intervals of 1–3 h. The authors commonly use an initial dose of 25 U, determine plasma glucose at 1 h, and give the second injection intravenously within 1.5–2 h in doses determined by the observed response in plasma glucose. Doses of regular insulin are continued at intervals of 1.5–2 h until the plasma glucose approaches 200–250 mg/dl, at which point 5 percent glucose is administered, and the patient switched to treatment with small doses (5–20 U) of regular insulin subcutaneously at intervals not exceeding 4 h with continued frequent monitoring of plasma glucose. The regimen is relatively simple, the unusual patient requiring larger doses of insulin is usually quickly identified, and the need for a conscious evaluation of the effectiveness of insulin treatment in all patients is emphasized.

Prior to the introduction of the constant intravenous infusion and repeated intramuscular injection regimens it was well recognized that in most patients the total dose of insulin administered reflected arbitrary judgments by the physician. In 1954 Smith and Martin failed to demonstrate significant differences in the rapidity of plasma glucose or serum bicarbonate responses in patients treated with 80, 160, or 240 U given intravenously at 2-h intervals.[30] There is no evidence that any of the regimens just cited are inherently superior either in theory or in practice. The latter point was documented in a recent study by Soler et al.[26] Madison has properly pointed out that there is a tendency to exaggerate the importance of using very small doses of insulin in the treatment of DKA and thereby a risk of unduly delaying effective treatment in some patients.[31]

The recognition that diabetic ketoacidosis frequently responds to treatment with repeated small doses of exogenous insulin along with appropriate intravenous fluid therapy has particular relevance to a large group of patients usually excluded from published series. These patients present with hyperglycemia, hyperketonemia, and a metabolic acidosis that is of a mild to modest degree; this often reflects a presentation at a relatively early stage of diabetic ketoacidosis or modification of the clinical manifestations by previous inadequate insulin administration. This is a common occurrence in previously known insulin-requiring diabetics who omit or fail to increase their exogenous insulin dosage in association with an intercurrent infection, emotional upset, or the use of drugs that may significantly modify the effectiveness of insulin or the patient's residual insulin secretory capacity. While many of these patients respond rapidly to rehydration and the administration of small doses of exogenous insulin and can be appropriately managed in a holding unit, their course is not predictable and they deserve careful evaluation and monitoring during treatment.

In patients who had previously been treated with diet and arylsulfonyureas or phenformin as adjuvants, the development of diabetic ketoacidosis requires the discontinuation of these pharmacological agents. After recovery from the acute episode, treatment with exogenous insulin should be continued. It is wise to consider such patients as potentially ketosis-prone for the rest of their life even though some acute event (e.g., acute infection, myocardial infarction, or the use of drugs affecting insulin secretion) may provide an apparent explanation for the acute deterioration in their ability to maintain sufficient endogenous insulin secretion to obviate ketoacidosis. If efforts to withdraw insulin treatment are made, they should be instituted only after complete recovery from the acute episode and contributing illness and under conditions in which the patient can be carefully observed.

Complications

Common complications of diabetic ketoacidosis, or more correctly of its treatment, are hypoglycemia and hypokalemia as noted previously. In earlier series the development of acute vascular insufficiency during treatment was a significant cause of death; as noted in the discussion of hyperglycemic nonketotic coma (vide infra) this might have been conditioned in some instances by failure to rapidly and adequately replace Na^+ deficits in patients with marked hyponatremia and marked hyperglycemia in whom a rapid decline in plasma glucose resulted from insulin administration. However, the development of shock also requires consideration of pulmonary embolus, myocardial infarction, acute pancreatitis, and septicemia along with other causes, as well as the superimposition of acute lactic acidosis related to these complications. On occasion the course of diabetic ketoacidosis may be modified by the development of clinical and laboratory evidence of acute pancreatitis in patients with no previous history of pancreatitis; this occurs in both known and previously unknown diabetics. The causes of this complication have not been adequately studied. It is frequently associated with shock and has a high mortality; this is not the case in patients in whom a mild elevation of amylase is the only possible intimation of an associated pancreatitis. Patients with erythrocyte glucose-6-phosphate deficiency may have an acute hemolytic episode in association with diabetic ketoacidosis, and this disorder may be first diagnosed by studies carried out to explain the development of anemia during treatment for DKA.

In the 1960s centers throughout the world reported the development of acute cerebral edema in children and young adults treated for diabetic ketoacidosis. Although uncommon, this edema was a major source of mortality in a population with a good prognosis for recovery from diabetic ketoacidosis.[32] The reported cases were frequently individuals who did not appear seriously ill on admission. They were generally alert or only mildly drowsy, and they usually had no initial evidence of shock or of a serious complicating illness. As a group they exhibited a very prompt fall in plasma glucose following the initiation of therapy, and in most instances there was also significant improvement in the degree of metabolic acidosis without evidence of hypokalemia before CNS symptoms developed. After 4–6 h of treatment these patients developed acute impairment of consciousness which was preceded in some instances by complaints of headache. The development of increased CSF pressure or papilledema was documented in some of these patients; the majority of these patients died and in a number of instances the presence of antemortem cerebral edema was documented at autopsy. The majority of the reported cases were children or adolescents who were treated with the relatively large quantities of hypotonic saline and the large doses of insulin then commonly employed. The syndrome is now extremely rare, even in institutions in which it previously was an important cause of death in patients of this age group.

The causes of this syndrome has not been clearly established and may be multiple. We observed one patient in her twenties who developed diabetic ketoacidosis over a period of 48 h without any prior evidence of diabetic ketoacidosis. Her mental status deteriorated despite relatively rapid improvement in her hyperglycemia and metabolic acidosis, and she remained in a deep coma with evidence of increased intracranial pressure before expiring. At autopsy the brain had alterations consistent with antemortem cerebral edema, but on microscopic examination there were changes consistent with an acute hemorrhagic leukoencephalitis, a condition usually associated with an acute immunologic or viral process. Her pancreatic islets had the expected alterations, and there was also evidence of a mild parenchymal pancreatitis. It is possible that in this instance the process affecting the pancreatic beta cells may have directly contributed to the cerebral alterations and the death of this patient.

In normal dogs the induction of persistent hyperglycemia by the infusion of glucose for 4 h, followed by rapid rehydration with isotonic saline, reproducibly induces increased intracisternal pressure and evidence of brain swelling; this is not observed when rehydration is carried out in dogs exposed to comparable degrees of persistent osmotic diuresis induced by mannitol infusion.[33] These observations have been confirmed in rabbits.[34] A tendency for the CSF pressure to rise to abnormally high levels has been observed in patients treated for diabetic ketoacidosis in whom the pressure was continuously monitored by means of an in-dwelling catheter in the lumbar subarachnoid space.[35] This has not been observed when repeated observations of CSF pressure have been attempted by repeated lumbar punctures but may be related to the timing of observations and to the effects of the persistent leak of CSF fluid from the site of the initial spinal tap. The data in rabbits suggest the possibility that the brain water content tends to fall and then rise during severe persistent hyperglycemia and dehydration induced by glucose infusion.[34] The rise may reflect the development of mild degrees of brain edema, a common response to cerebral injury of many types; it is possible that under these circumstances the rapidity with which the osmolality of the plasma is lowered during rehydration and the level to which it is reduced may condition the development of marked swelling. The mechanisms responsible for this experimentally induced increased intracranial pressure are still obscure; the cerebral electrolyte and metabolite composition has not been studied in small animals in which the brain can be frozen with sufficient rapidity to permit meaningful compositional studies. The authors have the impression that the extreme rarity of acute cerebral edema in children and young adults now treated for diabetic ketoacidosis in contrast to its occurrence in isolated instances in most large centers during the 1960s may be related to the fact that the treatment of DKA has changed. Most centers shifted from the use of large quantities of rapidly infused hypotonic solutions as initial treatment for diabetic ketoacidosis and now tend to avoid precipitous falls in plasma glucose in children who have had persistent hyperglycemia and marked dehydration. This difference is noted in the report of two successive series from the group in Birmingham, England, acute cerebral edema being a common cause of death in children in the first series but totally absent in the second.[36]

HYPERGLYCEMIC DEHYDRATION SYNDROME

INTRODUCTION

The older literature contains isolated reports of patients with diabetic ketoacidosis who presented with marked hyperglycemia, dehydration, and alterations in consciousness but in whom marked hyperketonemia and metabolic acidosis were absent. However, it was the report of Sament and Schwartz in 1957 that led to the clear distinction of this syndrome from diabetic ketoacidosis.[37] The syndrome was originally referred to as hyperosmolar coma. However, it is now recognized that coma is not an invariable manifestation, and while hyperosmolarity is usually present, its role in the pathogenesis of the disturbances in consciousness that may occur is still a matter of dispute. Moreover, the use of the term hyperosmolar coma has served to perpetuate the misconception that rapid reduction in plasma osmolality is the critical consideration in the treatment of this syndrome. Depending on the diagnostic criteria employed the frequency of this syndrome ranges from one-sixth that of diabetic ketoacidosis to one rivaling that of the latter syndrome in adult populations. The essential characteristics of the syndrome are best appreciated from a consideration of the usual clinical course.

The hyperglycemia dehydration syndrome is an inherent risk of non-ketosis-prone diabetes, and is most frequently observed in middle-aged patients with no previous diagnosis of diabetes. A high percentage of these patients have a family history of diabetes mellitus and are under medical care for some significant illness which may occasion the institution of therapy with a variety of drugs that may impair carbohydrate tolerance or predispose to dehydration, e.g., glucocorticoids, diphenylhydantoin, diuretics (thiazides, furosemide). However, the syndrome may develop in the absence of drug administration. The patients characteristically develop the classic manifestations of symptomatic hyperglycemia, polyuria, and polydipsia which increase in intensity and persist for several days to weeks before they seek medical attention or before the significance of their symptoms is appreciated. This is frequently the result of the confusion occasioned by associated illness. In a recent series the average duration of symptoms was 12 days. The patients may be recognized prior to the development of other manifestations despite severe dehydration although weakness is an almost invariable complaint. Most of the reported cases were not seen until after the development of neurological manifestations. These may be alterations in consciousness, e.g., drowziness, stupor, or frank coma as in diabetic ketoacidosis. However, in contrast to the latter syndrome the patients may present with minimal impairment of consciousness and focal neurological findings including focal seizures and transient hemiparesis. The disappearance of these focal manifestations after recovery from the hyperglycemic dehydration syndrome is the basis for the assumed association, but exclusion of independent contributing causes is required. (It is well recognized that cerebrovascular accidents may result in elevations in plasma glucose and that inadequate attention to the fluid requirements of unconscious patients may result in marked dehydration resulting in some instances in alterations in plasma composition resembling those found in the hyperglycemic dehydration syndrome.) In some instances the development of impaired consciousness appears to follow the onset of vomiting, which may impair the retention of oral fluids; in others it develops despite large fluid intakes but often of drinks containing large quantities of sucrose. The development of impaired consciousness or focal neurological findings was the impetus to seek medical attention in most of the earlier reported cases. In addition approximately 30 percent of these earlier cases presented with shock. In some series there is also a high frequency of associated infection (pneumonia, gram negative bacterial infection). Autopsy of these earlier cases also indicated an increased frequency of pancreatitis, pulmonary embolus, and thromboembolic phenomena.

The criteria that have been employed for the diagnosis of the hyperglycemia dehydration syndrome with or without associated alterations in consciousness or focal neurological findings differ in detail. However, the essential characteristics are the presence of hyperglycemia, dehydration, and hyperosmolality in the absence of a markedly elevated plasma ketone body concentration or a significant degree of metabolic acidosis. For practical purposes these criteria serve to distinguish this syndrome from most cases of diabetic ketoacidosis, lactic acidosis, or alcoholic ketoacidosis. (As noted previously in some patients the marked hyperglycemia and dehydration associated with the hyperglycemic dehydration syndrome may be found in association with evidence of lactic acidosis or hyperketonemic metabolic acidosis.) In 84 patients reviewed by McCurdy,[20] the blood glucose averaged 1096 mg/dl but ranged from 400 to 2760 mg/dl; thus although the plasma glucose concentration in recently reported series tends to average 1000 mg/dl and be higher than that found in most patients with diabetic ketoacidosis there is considerable overlap. The blood urea nitrogen is elevated, averaging 87 and 65 mg/dl in two large series.[38,39] As noted by McCurdy the BUN/creatinine ratio may exceed 30:1 compared with the usual ratio of 10:1 in normals, reflecting the effect of marked volume depletion on renal function, and in some instances probably the effect of specific agents (e.g., steroids) on BUN. However, in some cases markedly elevated serum creatinines reflecting renal parenchymal disease (acute tubular necrosis, etc.) have been observed. The plasma osmolality as determined by freezing point depression is usually markedly elevated, averaging 384 mosmol/kg water in one series. Calculated plasma osmolarity [(mosmol/liter) = 2(Na + K) + plasma glucose (mg/dl)/18 + BUN/28] was found to average 373 in the series reported by Gerich as compared with 331 in a series of patients with diabetic ketoacidosis.[39] However, while the plasma osmolarity tends to be higher than that observed in patients with diabetic ketoacidosis, there is also considerable overlap. (McCurdy prefers to estimate effective plasma osmolality for clinical purposes by omitting the minor contribution of K^+ and the effect of the serum BUN since urea equilibrates in total body water; the normal range by this calculation is 280–300 mosmol/liter. In 84 patients with the hyperglycemic dehydration syndrome the values on admission ranged from 268 to 465, and as noted in McCurdy's review six of these patients actually had calculated values below 300.) The reported values for plasma bicarbonate reflect in part differing criteria for diagnosis; it averaged 17 and 22 meq/liter in two large series.[38,39] As required by the criteria employed the arterial pH

when determined is usually slightly decreased but not to a degree indicative of significant metabolic acidosis. Quantitative data on the levels of acetoacetate and β-hydroxybutyrate in plasma in such patients are rather fragmentary, but in most instances, there is not a strongly positive plasma reaction with the nitroprusside reagent, or a large calculated "anion gap."

PATHOGENESIS

Patients with hyperglycemic dehydration are an extremely heterogeneous group despite the use of criteria to select patients for publication which probably results in selection of the extreme examples of this syndrome. This selection served, however, to demonstrate that impaired consciousness, including coma, and shock could occur in association with marked hyperglycemia and dehydration in the absence of marked hyperketonemia and metabolic acidosis, and that mortality in such patients was on the order of 40 to 50 percent. The syndrome occurs most commonly in known adult onset diabetics or in patients who meet the diagnostic criteria for non-ketosis-prone diabetes after recovery from the acute episode. It is likely that the diverse factors speculated to contribute to an impaired insulin secretory mechanism and the development of overt non-ketosis-prone diabetes lie at the basis of this syndrome. There is general agreement that in these patients hyperglycemia results in a persistent osmotic diuresis that eventuates in marked dehydration with significant deficits of Na^+ and K^+ and marked contraction of total body water and circulating extracellular fluid volume. The marked degree of dehydration can be explained in part as the result of concomitant illness or drugs that may independently predispose to dehydration (e.g., fever, vomiting, diarrhea, diuretics) and by delays in the recognition and treatment of the symptomatic hyperglycemia. It seems likely that the extreme degrees of hyperglycemia seen in some patients reflect not only extreme degrees of dehydration but the effects of a markedly reduced glomerular filtration rate on the capacity of the kidneys to moderate hyperglycemia by increased urinary excretion. A propensity to the development of shock under these conditions, particularly in association with infection, pancreatitis, or vascular thrombosis, is not unexpected. The presence of detectable concentrations of plasma IRI has been documented in most of the patients with hyperglycemic dehydration in whom it has been examined, but the absolute levels are clearly inappropriate for the associated degree of hyperglycemia, averaging 17.2 and 7.5 ± 1.9 μU/ml in two series,[38,39] and ranging from undetectable to 50 μU/ml in another.[40] In efforts to explain the absence of marked hyperketonemia it must be noted that in most of the reported cases the plasma levels of FFA, although elevated (958 ± 126 in one recent series), were usually not as elevated as those observed in a series of patients with diabetic ketoacidosis studied by the same workers (2256 ± 250).[39] More significant elevations of plasma FFA were observed by Vinik et al. who also noted elevated plasma triglyceride concentrations.[40] The most likely explanation for the lack of marked hyperketonemia is that insulin modulation of lipolysis and hepatic ketogenesis is preserved to a considerable degree despite the gross derangement in plasma glucose regulation. This is disputed by workers who note a considerable overlap between the plasma insulin levels in patients with diabetic ketoacidosis and those with hyperglycemic dehydration. However, the adequacy of these levels cannot be assessed without knowledge of the countervailing factors affecting lipolysis and hepatic fatty acid metabolism which may not be adequately reflected in plasma constituents. Although lower levels of growth hormone and cortisol have been found in patients with the hyperglycemic dehydration syndrome than in DKA,[39] there is no evidence that increased growth hormone or cortisol concentrations are required to initiate severe hyperketonemia with marked insulin deficiency. Given the recent formulation of the regulation of hepatic ketogenesis presented by McGarry and Foster (see Chapter 80) it seems reasonable to speculate that throughout most of the period of the development of the hyperglycemic dehydration syndrome, the levels of insulin available remain adequate to regulate hepatic fatty acid oxidation and hence ketogenesis. The extent to which this may reflect lack of changes in pancreatic glucagon secretion and in hepatic carnitine and glycogen concentrations which appear to contribute to the markedly increased hepatic ketogenesis of experimental diabetic ketoacidosis remains to be examined. As noted by Foster, comparisons of peripheral plasma IRI concentrations in diabetic dehydration and diabetic ketoacidosis may not reflect significant differences in portal venous IRI concentrations in these two conditions,[41] and it is the later concentrations which are important with regard to the regulation of hepatic ketogenesis.

The mechanisms responsible for the alterations in consciousness or the focal neurological findings found in some patients with hyperglycemic dehydration are unknown, and there is no compelling evidence that a single common mechanism is responsible. Although it is commonly assumed that there is a good correlation between plasma osmolality and mental status in such patients, the frequent observation of unimpaired mental status with marked degree of hyperglycemia and hyperosmolality, and the poor correlation between decreasing plasma osmolality during treatment and improvement in mental status in unconscious patients, have resulted in controversy over the validity of this assumption. The brain pathology associated with fatal hyperglycemic dehydration and coma still requires detailed examination. In a few instances localized brain infarcts have been observed; but the large subdural hemorrhages and rupture of connecting veins associated with hypernatremia in children have not been reported, although the latter is frequently cited as a model for altered consciousness associated with hyperosmolality. Obvious considerations are altered cerebral perfusion resulting from the marked dehydration as well as effects related to the specific drugs and illnesses present in any given patient. Cerebral edema is a common response to a variety of injuries. However, in the absence of herniation it is difficult to document the existence of antemortem cerebral edema at autopsy. Many of these patients have been subjected to artificial respiration which can induce alterations in the appearance of the brain at autopsy.

TREATMENT AND PREVENTION

The reported series of patients with "hyperosmolar coma" are extremely heterogeneous with regard to clinical manifestations (including the state of consciousness) and laboratory findings on presentation, as well as with regard to the presence and nature of precipitating or coexistent severe illness and exposure to pharmacological hazards. Consequently it is difficult to evaluate the benefit of current therapy from the mortality experiences. In most reported series approximately 40 to 50 percent of these episodes end fatally, but mortalities as low as 15 to 25 percent have been reported. The attribution of the cause of death is frequently difficult in complicated clinical problems. Infection, pulmonary embolism, thrombosis of pelvic and leg veins, and pancreatitis have appeared to be significant factors. In the 84 cases included in the review by McCurdy,[20] approximately one-third were febrile and in shock on admission, although this experience is not reflected in all series. Of particular concern are the significant number of deaths

attributed to the development of shock in patients who were not hypotensive on admission but in whom it developed during treatment as the blood sugar fell. Deaths associated with hypokalemia, and deaths that were related to the development of oliguria and evidence of the syndrome of acute tubular necrosis during treatment have also been reported. Although the development of acute cerebral edema during treatment has been reported,[42] this does not appear to be a significant cause of mortality.

Given the limitations of any present recommendations for the treatment of the hyperglycemic dehydration syndrome, the primary aims should be the rapid correction of the severe dehydration and contracted extracellular fluid volume and the prevention of shock and hypokalemia developing during treatment. In addition, in each patient it is obvious that the identification and treatment of specific complicating illnesses are required. It should be noted that there is no evidence that the patient's clinical condition and likelihood of survival are materially improved by efforts to achieve the rapid reduction of plasma osmolality to normal levels or by the rapid correction of the total water deficits. As noted by McCurdy there is a strong suggestion that such therapy may be hazardous.[20] Unless specific contraindications exist isotonic saline should be infused rapidly until the blood pressure is stable and urine volume is adequate; given the magnitude of the sodium deficit in most patients the administration of 2 liters (310 meq Na^+) over the first 1.5 h is usually appropriate. Despite the presence of hyperosmolality the more immediate threat to the patient is the development of hypovolemic shock. Isotonic saline is more effective than hypotonic saline in rapidly expanding the extracellular fluid volume. As noted by McCurdy in her review,[20] although the serum Na^+ averages 141/meq/liter, it ranges from 119 to 188 meq/liter. If the Na^+ concentration is low, and the calculated effective plasma osmolality [$2Na^+$ + glucose (mg/dl)/18 is low or low normal (normal 280–300), the osmotic contribution of glucose to the maintenance of extracellular fluid volume may be of considerable import. The ritualistic use of rapidly infused hypotonic saline combined with large doses of insulin which results in rapid falls in plasma glucose may contribute to the development of water intoxication and shock in such patients. (If the infusion of isotonic saline results in stabilization of blood pressure but oliguria persists, it may be necessary to consider a trial of diuretics such as ethycrynic acid or furosemide. The subsequent fluid therapy should be adjusted appropriately if it appears that significant renal damage has occurred.)

During the second phase of fluid replacement the patient should receive 0.50 N saline containing 30 meq/liter of K^+ as the phosphate(s). The aim of therapy is rapid *partial* correction of water deficits, continued replacement of sodium deficits, and the prevention of hypokalemia. Initial hyperkalemia is unusual in patients with the hyperglycemic dehydration syndrome, the initial values averaging 5.0 meq/liter, but 20 of the 66 cases included in McCurdy's review in whom this point was documented had plasma levels below 4.0 meq/liter[20] and deaths related to hypokalemia have been observed. The rates of administration must be modified on an individual basis with careful monitoring of the fluid intake and output and apparent net retention, as well as of the plasma electrolytes, glucose, and calculated or determined osmolality. The initial rate of infusion should be on the order of 1 liter/h and reduced in successive phases as the patient recovers.

The methods of insulin administration and means for assessing its effectiveness from the sequential changes in the plasma glucose concentration described for the treatment of diabetic ketoacidosis may be applied to the treatment of the hyperglycemic dehydration syndrome with one caveat. In patients with marked sodium deficiency it may be undesirable to induce precipitous falls in plasma glucose. Since the initial effects of volume expansion combined with a large intravenous dose of insulin in any given patient cannot be predicted, it is probably preferable to initiate treatment by the intravenous or intramuscular route with doses on the order of 20–25 U. The aim of therapy is to assure a sustained decline in plasma glucose to normal levels over a period of several hours, but it is important to reassess plasma glucose at frequent intervals to assure the adequacy of the insulin doses administered. Obviously the presence of infection, or prior administration of steroids or other agents may affect the doses required. A few instances have been reported in which very large doses of insulin appeared to be required, and this possibility must be considered.

The use of 5 percent glucose as a means of replacing water deficits should be avoided until the plasma glucose has been reduced to the level of 200–250 mg/dl, but continued attention to the replacement of urinary Na$^+$ and K$^+$ loss during this period is appropriate. Following stabilization, the patient should be maintained on exogenous insulin treatment at 4- to 6-h intervals, and ultimately transferred to treatment with appropriate mixtures of rapidly and more slowly acting insulin preparations. Although some patients subsequently can be maintained free of symptomatic hyperglycemia without the use of insulin, this is usually not the case immediately after recovery from the acute episode and in the face of a contributing illness or need for continued glucocorticoid administration. It is preferable to delay efforts to stop insulin treatment until the patient has been observed for a period of at least several weeks.

Delay in seeking medical attention, and physician error are important contributing factors in the development of the hyperglycemic dehydration syndrome. Appropriate patient and physician education should materially decrease the incidence of this syndrome. Patients with a family history of diabetes should be taught the significance of polyuria and polydipsia, and physicians should pay increased attention to a family history of diabetes when considering treatment with drugs that may impair insulin secretion or its effectiveness in regulating plasma glucose concentration.

ALCOHOLIC KETOACIDOSIS

DEFINITION

Although alcoholic ketoacidosis was originally described by Dillon and co-workers in 1940,[43] it was not until 1971 that a report of three well-studied cases by Jenkins et al.[3] clearly established its existence as a distinct syndrome. It has subsequently been observed in most medical centers and does not appear to be a rarity, although both its true incidence and mortality remain to be clarified. The patients have been chronic alcoholics in whom a characteristic sequence of events precedes their presentation with severe dehydration, mental obtundation, and a marked metabolic acidosis that is primarily attributable to hyperketonemia, although some elevation in plasma lactate concentration is frequently present. The plasma glucose concentration, however, is normal or only moderately elevated. In one patient who had 18 episodes of alcoholic ketoacidosis reported by Jenkins et al. the admission blood glucose concentrations ranged from 57 to 330 mg/dl.[3] The diagnosis of alcoholic ketoacidosis can frequently be established with certainty only after the patient has recovered from the acute episode, when all of the pertinent historical and laboratory data are available, and the patient's subsequent course is defined. There appears to be a characteristic pattern in the development of this syndrome. The patient who is a chronic alcoholic goes on a binge which lasts

for several days or longer; anorexia develops and food intake ceases although the alcohol consumption continues. (Although these conditions are ideal for the precipitation of alcohol hypoglycemia its appearance in the development of this syndrome has not been documented.) The patient then develops persistent vomiting which leads to the cessation of alcohol intake. Characteristically the patients present 12–96 h after their last alcohol intake, and the accuracy of this portion of the history has been confirmed by the blood ethanol concentration in those patients in whom it has been determined. The ingestion of methanol or ethylene glycol has been excluded in a sufficient number of cases to exclude their contribution to the development of this syndrome. There is a striking tendency for episodes of alcoholic ketoacidosis to recur in the same patient; we observed one patient who had 16 episodes over a 3-year period.

The composite data that permitted the distinction of alcoholic ketoacidosis as a syndrome distinct from diabetic ketoacidosis include the following. The plasma glucose on presentation may be normal, although in many instances it overlaps the lower range of that observed in patients with diabetic ketoacidosis. The patients are not known, insulin-dependent, ketosis-prone diabetics, and following recovery from the acute episode they do not exhibit a requirement for exogenous insulin to prevent hyperketonemia. Most patients exhibit abnormalities in their oral and intravenous glucose tolerance tests shortly after recovery from the acute episode which improve to varying degrees following more prolonged convalescence, abstinence from alcohol, and improved nutrition. However, a number of patients exhibit persistent abnormalities in glucose tolerance which might be classified as "chemical diabetes." In a number of well-documented instances, beginning with the cases observed by Dillon et al.,[43] the metabolic acidosis and hyperketonemia have responded to rehydration with fluids containing glucose without the administration of exogenous insulin. In conjunction with the characteristic history of the events preceding the acute episode, these data provide convincing evidence for the existence of alcoholic ketoacidosis as a distinct syndrome. Although most of the well-documented cases have recovered from the acute episode, a number of fatalities have been observed, and the syndrome must be considered potentially lethal.

PATHOGENESIS

The pathogenesis of alcoholic ketoacidosis has not been clearly established. However, in the authors' view, the limited existing data provide the basis for a plausible working hypothesis that has therapeutic implications. The usual history in these patients suggests that the development of the marked hyperketonemia and metabolic acidosis occurs under circumstances in which the manifestations of the alcohol withdrawal syndrome would be anticipated, and indeed have been present in a number of the reported patients. Alcohol withdrawal is preceded by a period in which the regulation of hepatic ketogenesis (i.e., the ketogenic capacity of the liver—see Chapter 80) would be expected to be modified as the consequence of both chronic alcohol ingestion and starvation. The plasma FFA concentration is elevated in patients with alcoholic ketoacidosis on admission and falls during successful therapy. The syndrome rapidly responds to treatment appropriate for diabetic ketoacidosis, or in some well-documented instances to fluid replacement with solutions containing glucose. Although the plasma contains detectable concentrations of immunoreactive insulin on admission in most of the reported cases, in many instances the concentrations are low relative to the plasma glucose concentrations.[44] In at least one instance it has been documented that the infusion of a glucose-containing solution during treatment without exogenous insulin resulted in small but significant increases in plasma insulin concentrations.[45] There is little reason to doubt that inadequate insulin regulation of adipose tissue lipolysis and hepatic fatty acid oxidation relative to other factors tending to stimulate these processes plays a role in the pathogenesis of this syndrome. Administering alcohol to rats for several days results in a marked increase in the rate at which slices of their liver convert palmitate to acetoacetate during in vitro incubation; this effect is not reproduced by the addition of alcohol to liver slices from control rats.[46] Alcohol administration also results in a significant increase in hepatic carnitine concentration.[47] However, the factors responsible for the increase in the ketogenic capacity of the liver in rats exposed to alcohol for several days have not been thoroughly explored. In humans fed a calorically adequate diet Lefevre et al. found that the substitution of alcohol for dietary carbohydrate resulted in a 30-fold increase in plasma ketone body concentration over a period of several days; in contrast, the substitution of fat for carbohydrate resulted in only an eight- to ten-fold increase.[46] Careful examination of the data of Lefevre et al. suggests that the effects of a high ethanol intake on plasma ketone body concentration in man are subject to modification by dietary carbohydrate intake. Alcohol is known to inhibit the response of the pancreatic beta cell to increased glucose concentrations (see Chapters 76 and 77).

The limited data available suggest that the following may be a plausible outline of the pathogenesis of alcoholic ketoacidosis: Binge drinking in a chronic alcoholic would be expected to induce some elevation of plasma ketone body concentration which would be exaggerated by the superimposition of starvation. The effects of alcohol, decreased carbohydrate intake, and subsequently starvation as well as modifications in autonomic nervous system activity associated with chronic alcohol ingestion might be expected to decrease plasma insulin relative to the activity of other factors that tend to increase adipose tissue FFA release and alter the regulation of long chain fatty acid oxidation in the liver. The possibility that increases in plasma glucagon resulting from starvation or local effects of alcohol on the intestinal mucosa contribute to the alterations in hepatic ketogenic capacity merits examination. Under these circumstances plasma insulin is probably the determining factor in modulating the magnitude of the resultant hyperketonemia. If vomiting, dehydration, marked alterations in autonomic nervous system activity, and secondary alterations in adrenocortical function which are associated with the alcohol withdrawal syndrome are then superimposed, the development of a fulminant metabolic acidosis due to hyperketonemia would scarcely be surprising. Plasma and urinary catecholamine levels are elevated during alcohol withdrawal and may reflect increased adrenergic stimulation that could stimulate adipose tissue lipolysis and further impair insulin secretion. The major value of this information, aside from providing a hypothesis for evaluation, is that it emphasizes the likelihood that an increase in endogenous insulin secretion or the administration of exogenous insulin is probably critical for the reversal of the syndrome. Further, it suggests that the extent to which alcohol withdrawal may contribute to the clinical manifestations of the syndrome merits closer examination.

It has been argued that the apparent rarity of alcoholic ketoacidosis in chronic alcoholics, and the tendency for recurrent episodes in the affected patients may reflect the need for some unique, possibly genetic predisposition. However, the true incidence of this syndrome, particularly in less fulminant form, remains to be established. Moreover, in the published cases the frequency with which some abnormality in glucose tolerance persists following recovery from the syndrome raises the possibility that mild, inherent abnormalities in insulin secretion may be a factor that increases the likelihood of the development of alcoholic ketoacidosis.

In the reported cases the levels of plasma glucose appear to vary markedly from episode to episode, and in some instances are similar to those observed in some patients with diabetic ketoacidosis. The source of this variation remains to be clarified, but given the complex nature of the probable pathogenesis of this syndrome and the real possibility for varying degrees of initial nutritional deficiencies this is not incompatible with the suggested pathogenesis.

It should be noted that varying degrees of hyperketonemia and lactate acidosis may be present in patients who present with alcoholic hypoglycemia. Although a discussion of this problem is beyond the scope of this chapter it should be noted that alcoholic hypoglycemia is dependent on the presence of elevated blood alcohol concentrations and fasting. The possibility that patients with alcoholic ketoacidosis may in some instances present after an earlier episode of alcoholic hypoglycemia must be considered, but in the reported cases the historical data do not suggest this sequence.

TREATMENT

The fluid and electrolyte therapy outline for the treatment of diabetic ketoacidosis can be applied with equal validity to patients with alcoholic ketoacidosis. The prevention of both shock and symptomatic hypokalemia during treatment is an essential consideration. There is no established indication for efforts to rapidly alter plasma pH, which usually responds as the hyperketonemia and dehydration are corrected. However, as in diabetic ketoacidosis the use of bicarbonate in doses designed to produce small increments in plasma bicarbonate concentration may be an appropriate prophylactic measure in patients with very low plasma pH and bicarbonate concentrations (see treatment of diabetic ketoacidosis).

The inclusion of 5 percent glucose in the intravenous fluids administered to patients with alcoholic ketoacidosis who recovered without the use of exogenous insulin is probably essential to the success of this form of treatment. However, the clinical experience with this syndrome is still limited, and its full spectrum may not have been documented in the reported patients. In our own view the effect of glucose in this condition is probably due in large part to the stimulation of endogenous insulin secretion, and possibly to a decrease in glucagon secretion (which remains to be examined). This effect and the decreased autonomic stimulation of lipolysis resulting from other aspects of the patient's treatment are probably responsible for the reversal of the metabolic derangement. Consequently there is no contraindication to the use of exogenous insulin, and in fact some of reported patients were initially treated in this manner. Whenever there is any question about the differentiation of alcoholic ketoacidosis and diabetic ketoacidosis exogenous insulin should be used to avoid any possible delay in providing effective therapy for a patient with diabetic ketoacidosis. In addition, in severely ill patients with an unquestioned diagnosis of alcoholic ketoacidosis in which the response to therapy with 5 percent glucose-containing solutions is delayed despite significant initial rises in plasma glucose concentration, the use of small doses of exogenous insulin (2–4 U) at intervals of 2–4 h should be considered. Although controlled studies are not available, in such circumstances the use of exogenous insulin appears to speed the reversal of the metabolic derangement.

The patient with alcoholic ketoacidosis also merits treatment appropriate for any patient with threatening or overt alcohol withdrawal reaction. Although specific value for the use of multivitamin preparations is lacking, the administration of a single injection of 50–100 mg of thiamine im, or by slow intravenous infusion, is considered judicious. In a few patients chlordiazepoxide was employed to control overt manifestations of alcohol withdrawl; it appears important to assess the extent to which such manifestations may contribute to the clinical status of any given patient and determine whether the use of this agent may be indicated. The possibility of a complicating and possibly contributing illness (e.g., pneumonia) should also be excluded.

LACTIC ACIDOSIS IN DIABETICS

INTRODUCTION

Severe metabolic acidosis primarily attributable to elevated plasma (extracellular fluid) concentrations of lactate occurs in both nondiabetics and diabetics under a variety of circumstances which appear to be contributory or causal. However, approximately 50 percent of the reported cases of idiopathic lactic acidosis occurred in diabetics and the basis of this association has not been established[48] In diabetics, as in nondiabetics, lactic acidosis most commonly occurs in association with some form of shock (cardiogenic, hypovolemic, or septic). Alcohol may be a significant contributory factor in the development of lactic acidosis in some diabetics; lactic acidosis has been observed in alcoholic diabetics following binge drinking and starvation.[49] The latter conditions are similar to those that may precipitate alcoholic hypoglycemia in nondiabetics, a condition that may be associated with a significant degree of lactic acidosis.[50] Phenformin appears to be a significant factor in some instances; this appears to be particularly true in older diabetics with some degree of renal impairment and phenformin may be a pharmacological hazard in the face of acute cardiovascular or pulmonary disease that threatens shock or severe hypoxemia.[51] While there are a host of other conditions and agents that may condition the development of lactic acidosis in nondiabetics there is at present no evidence that they have special significance with regard to the development of lactic acidosis in diabetics. These conditions include leukemia[48]; large mesenchymal tumors; metastatic carcinoma[52]; hepatic glucose-6-phosphatase deficiency or hepatic fructose-1,6-diphosphatase deficiency, both of which predispose to fasting hypoglycemia and a metabolic acidosis with elevated lactate levels[4]; and inherited defects in the hepatic metabolism of fructose or galactose (hereditary fructose intolerance, galactosemia) in which large loads of the offending sugar precipitate hypoglycemia and lactic acidosis.[53]

Idiopathic lactic acidosis is diagnosed by exclusion; the term implies that the episode developed in the absence of initial evidence of shock, severe hypoxemia, exposure to potentially contributing drugs, or of any illness known to condition the development of lactic acidosis.

Elevated plasma lactate concentrations may contribute significantly to the metabolic acidosis in some patients with diabetic ketoacidosis, although this is not a common occurrence; in 55 patients studied by Hockaday and Alberti, 4 had blood lactate concentrations greater than 7 mM.[6] Although a severe metabolic acidosis is unusual in patients with the hyperglycemic dehydration syndrome the development of lactic acidosis has been observed. Recently it has been recognized that older diabetics who have not previously exhibited a propensity to ketoacidosis may present with a severe metabolic acidosis primarily attributable to lactic acidosis but with a significant degree of hyperketonemia whose magnitude

may be obscured by a markedly elevated plasma β-hydroxybutyrate/acetoacetate ratio, and a plasma nitroprusside reaction that fails to accurately reflect the degree of hyperketonemia.

PATHOGENESIS

Lactate is a normal constituent of blood, plasma, and all mammalian cells. In normal fasting subjects at rest the arterial blood concentration is approximately 0.4–0.8 mM, and the plasma concentration is approximately 20 percent higher. Venous lactate concentrations reflect local tissue metabolism and vary from site to site. In clinical samples drawn from the usual venopuncture sites without stasis the blood lactate concentration is usually in the range of 1 mM. Lactic acid has a pKa of 3.86 and, like the closely related compound pyruvic acid, is a strong organic acid. In diabetics with lactic acidosis the concentrations of blood lactate (usually venous) are reported to vary from 7 to 31 mM; however, the lower limit reflects an arbitrary cutoff value used for some workers in selecting patients for analysis. As would be expected from their biochemical relationship, blood pyruvate, which is normally on the order of 0.1–0.2 mM, is also elevated in diabetics with lactic acidosis. However, the concentration of pyruvate is usually on the order of one-tenth or less that of lactate.

Pyruvate is the product of glycolysis in mammalian cells, but the cytoplasmic lactic dehydrogenase activity, which catalyzes the reaction pyruvate + NADH + H$^+$ $\leftrightarrows$ lactate + NAD$^+$, appears to maintain a near equilibrium between the substrates and products of this reaction. The concentration ratios of lactate/pyruvate closely approximate those predicted by the equilibrium constant for this reaction at intracellular pH and by the redox state of the free NAD$^+$/NADH couple in the cytoplasm. The equilibrium of the reaction favors the reduction of pyruvate to lactate, and in livers from normal fed rats the redox state of the cytoplasmic NAD$^+$/NADH couple is such that the lactate/pyruvate ratio is approximately 8. In cells that lack mitochondria (mature erythrocytes) and in a few tissues which appear to derive the major fraction of their energy requirements from glycolysis (e.g., renal medulla) the release of lactate accounts for a major fraction of the glucose uptake. Lactate release by these tissues serves to dispose of metabolic hydrogen generated by the one dehydrogenation reaction of glycolysis (glyceraldehyde-3-phosphate dehydrogenase) and permits effective operation of this reaction and the substrate level phosphorylation that is essential for the ultimate generation of ATP as a consequence of glycolysis. The lactate released retains the major fraction of the energy potentially available from the oxidation of glucose to CO$_2$ and H$_2$O and can be utilized for oxidation in a number of tissues including the liver and heart; this requires the initial conversion of lactate to pyruvate by cytoplasmic lactic dehydrogenase activities. In most mammalian tissues the observed rates of lactate production under physiological conditions represent only a very small fraction of the total enzymatic capacity for the conversion of glucose or glycogen to pyruvate (i.e., glycolysis). The energy requirements of these cells are primarily derived from the mitochondrial oxidation of pyruvate, fatty acids, or ketones to CO$_2$ and H$_2$O and the synthesis of ATP by oxidative phosphorylation. A variety of mechanisms exist by which the rate of glycolysis in these cells is regulated and maintained at rates appropriate to the cells requirements for pyruvate for mitochondrial oxidation and synthetic reactions. These mechanisms include the ability of changes in the relative concentrations of the components of the cytoplasmic adenylate nucleotide pool (ATP, ADP, AMP) and inorganic phosphate that result from alterations in the balance between ATP synthesis and utilization to modify the activity of key glycolytic enzymes and increase or decrease glycolytic flux in an appropriate manner. This mechanism explains in major part the marked increase in glycolysis that occurs with anoxic inhibition of respiration and mitochondrial ATP synthesis (the Pasteur effect).[54] Glycolysis yields only a small fraction of the ATP potentially available from the mitochondrial oxidation of pyruvate (and other substrates) and through shuttles of the NADH generated by glycolysis. During anoxia marked increases in glycolysis are thus required to meet the cell's energy requirements for survival and to restore and maintain the "energy charge" of the cytoplasmic adenylate nucleotide pool in a normal range. The marked increase in lactate production reflects both a marked increase in glycolysis and the more reduced redox state of the cytoplasmic $NAD^+/NADH$ couple in these tissues. While anoxia can markedly increase lactate production by many tissues, the marked increases in lactate production that occur when the blood supply to a tissue is interrupted or with tissue injury probably reflect a multitude of additional factors including local autonomic and hormonal effects. (It is of interest that many tissues that do not exhibit significant rates of lactate production in situ frequently exhibit high rates of aerobic lactate production when studied in vitro because of tissue injury.[55]

Although increasing blood lactate concentration may result in increased hepatic extraction of lactate over a significant range, the utilization of lactate by the liver is dependent on its conversion to pyruvate by the lactic dehydrogenase reaction. The latter may be impaired by marked alterations in production associated with impaired disposition and provides a ready explanation for the rapidity with which lactic acidosis may develop in conditions such as shock, in which a complex interaction of impaired tissue perfusion, injury, hormonal, and neural effects seems to predispose to these derangements. Thus the presence of shock in most of the reported diabetic patients with lactic acidosis provides a plausible explanation for the syndrome. However, there is at the moment no adequate explanation for the increased frequency of idiopathic lactic acidosis in diabetics.

The role of phenformin in the development of lactic acidosis is still a subject of controversy. The ability of this drug to induce lactic acidosis in humans when ingested in suicidal doses is well documented. Kreisberg has recently reported that there were approximately 200 documented cases of lactic acidosis occurring in diabetics treated with phenformin in doses of 100–150 mg/day; in approximately 30 percent of these cases no other known or contributing cause for lactic acidosis was present.[56] However, the true incidence of lactic acidosis in phenformin-treated diabetics is still unknown. The pharmacology and use of phenformin in the treatment of non-ketosis-prone diabetes mellitus are discussed in Chapter 85. In the authors' view, the data in animals cannot be readily transposed to conditions in human diabetics. However, it appears that at adequate doses this drug can predispose to lactic acidosis by a variety of mechanisms, including impaired hepatic disposition of lactate for gluconeogenesis and increased peripheral lactate production; these effects might constitute a pharmacological hazard in older diabetics who have a greater risk of acute clinical events (e.g., myocardial infarction, shock) which are in themselves causes of lactic acidosis.

DIAGNOSIS

As previously noted the majority of cases of lactic acidosis in diabetics occur in association with some known predisposing cause to shock, e.g., cardiac disease, septicemia. In hospitalized older diabetic patients the onset of lactic acidosis is frequently suggested by the sudden development of hypernea and impaired consciousness in association with a history of some predisposing

disease. However, a number of diabetics presenting with idiopathic or phenformin-related lactic acidosis may have nonspecific prodromal symptoms for several days, and a change in the usual state of health in an older diabetic, particularly when there is a history of alcoholism or phenformin, merits careful evaluation. A presumptive diagnosis is based upon the presence of a metabolic acidosis with an increased anion gap that cannot be attributed to uremia, salicylate intoxication, methanol or ethylene glycol ingestion, or hyperketonemia. Even in the absence of previous episodes of diabetic ketoacidosis the possibility of a significant degree of associated hyperketonemia cannot be excluded on the basis of a weak or moderately positive plasma nitroprusside test in a diabetic with a severe metabolic acidosis and a large anion gap. A markedly elevated plasma β-hydroxybutyrate/acetoacetate ratio has been observed in cases of lactic acidosis in diabetics with a significant degree of associated hyperketonemia as ultimately demonstrated by quantitative determinations of plasma acetoacetate and β-hydroxybutyrate concentrations.[57] There are no generally accepted criteria for the diagnosis; venous lactate concentrations ranging from 1.3 to 7.0 mM and arterial pH values as high as 7.37 have been employed in assembling patients for study. Relman has noted that in lactic acidosis the degree of respiratory compensation is usually disproportionate for the degree of metabolic acidosis.[58] In a series of cases of lactic acidosis he found that for any given bicarbonate concentration the arterial pCO_2 tended to be as much as 8 mm Hg lower than that observed in patients with diabetic ketoacidosis.

TREATMENT

In the absence of controlled clinical trials recommendations for treatment must be considered tentative. The treatment of any known predisposing cause (e.g., shock, septicemia) and a search for such causes are obviously overriding considerations. The use of bicarbonate given intravenously to moderate the degree of metabolic acidosis in the hope that the syndrome is reversible is commonly employed. The general considerations in its use are similar to those outlined in the treatment of diabetic ketoacidosis; however, in lactic acidosis the efficacy of doses calculated to raise the plasma bicarbonate by 4–6 mM is frequently less than that observed in diabetic ketoacidosis, and problems resulting from the administration of large quantities of $NaHCO_3$ frequently include the problem of excess sodium administration. Despite the absence of controlled trial, we recommend the use of insulin in diabetics with lactic acidosis with plasma glucose concentrations in excess of 250 mg/dl, particularly when there is no obvious precipitating cause (e.g., shock or when alcohol or phenformin appears to be a contributing factor). This recommendation is based both on the difficulty in rapidly documenting the degree of associated hyperketonemia that may be present even in patients who have previously not been ketosis-prone, and on the unexpected improvement and recovery of a number of elderly diabetic patients with severe metabolic acidosis primarily attributable to lactate when insulin is added to the treatment regimen. Care must be exercised to obviate hypoglycemia, and relatively small doses of insulin (5–10 U im or iv) at intervals of 2–4 h are usually employed. In our present state of ignorance of the factors that predispose diabetics to idiopathic lactic acidosis further evaluation of this practice appears warranted.

REFERENCES

1. Wright, P. H.: Experimental diabetes induced by insulin antibodies. In Liebel, S. B. and Wrenshall, G. A. (eds): On the Nature and

Treatment of Diabetes. Amsterdam, Excerpta Medica Foundation, 1965, pp. 354–360.

2. Crofford, O.: Reports to Congress of the National Commission on Diabetes (DHEW Publication No (NIH) 76-1018). Washington, D.C., U.S. Govt. Printing Office, 1975.

3. Jenkins, D. W., Eckel, R. E., and Craig, J. W.: Alcoholic Ketoacidosis. *JAMA 217:* 177–183, 1971.

4. Pagliara, A. S., Karl, I. E., Haymond E., and Kipnis, D. M.: Hypoglycemia in infancy and childhood, Part II. *J Pediatr 82:* 558–577, 1973.

5. Fajans, S. S. and Floyd, J. C., Jr.: Fasting hypoglycemia in adults. *N Engl J Med 294:* 766–772, 1976.

6. Hockaday, T. D. R. and Alberti, K. G. M. M.: Diabetic coma. *Clin Endocrinol Metab 1:* 751–788, 1972.

7. Fulop, M., Tannenbaum, H., and Dreyer., N.: Ketotic hyperosmolar coma. *Lancet 2:* 635–639, 1973.

8. Alberti, K. G. M. M. and Hockaday, T. D. R.: Rapid blood ketone body estimation in the diagnosis of diabetic ketoacidosis. *Br Med J 2:* 565–568, 1972.

9. Sulway, M. J. and Malins, J. M.: Acetone in diabetic ketoacidosis. *Lancet 2:* 736–740, 1970.

10. Kety, S. S., Polis, B. D., Nadler, C. S., and Schmidt, C. F.: The blood flow and oxygen consumption of the human brain in diabetic acidosis and coma. *J Clin Invest 27:* 500–510, 1948.

11. Block, M. B., Berk, J. E., Fridhandler, L. S., Steiner, D. F., and Rubenstein, A. H.: Diabetic Ketoacidosis associated with mumps virus infection. *Ann Intern Med 78:* 663–667, 1973.

12. Baker, L., Barcai, A., Kaye, R., and Haque, N.: β-Adrenergic blockade and juvenile diabetes: Acute studies and long-term therapeutic trial. *J Pediatr 75:* 19–29, 1969.

13. Owen, O. E. and Reichard, G. A., Jr.: Ketone body metabolism in normal, obese and diabetic subjects. *Israel J Med Sci 11:* 560–570, 1975.

14. Bässler, K. H., Horback, L., and Wagner, K.: Dynamics of ketone body metabolism in diabetic rats. *Diabetologia 8:* 211–214, 1972.

15. Balasse, E. O., and Havel, R. J.: Evidence for an effect of insulin on the peripheral utilization of ketone bodies in dogs. *J Clin Invest 50:* 801–813, 1971.

16. Ruderman, N. B., and Goodman, M. N.: Inhibition of muscle acetoacetate utilization during diabetic ketoacidosis. *Am J Physiol 226:* 136–143, 1974.

17. Nabarro, J. D. N., Spencer, A. G., and Stowers, J. M.: Metabolic studies in severe diabetic ketosis. *Q J Med 21:* 225–248, 1952.

18. Winegrad, A. I. and Clements, R. S., Jr.: Diabetic ketoacidosis. *Med Clin North Am 54:* 899–911, 1971.

19. Martin, H. E., Smith, K., and Wilson, M. L.: The fluid and electrolyte therapy of severe diabetic acidosis and ketosis. *Am J Med 24:* 376–389, 1958.

20. McCurdy, D. K.: Hyperosmolar, hyperglycemic nonketotic diabetic coma. *Med Clin North Am 54:* 683–699, 1970.

21. Posner, J. B. and Plum, F: Spinal fluid pH and neurologic symptoms in systemic acidosis. *N Engl J Med 277:* 605–613, 1967.

22. Alberti, K. G. M. M., Darley, J. H., Emerson, P. M., and Hockaday, T. D. R.: 2,3-Diphosphoglycerate and tissue oxygenation in uncontrolled diabetes mellitus. *Lancet 2:* 391–395, 1972.

23. Kassirer, J. P.: Serious acid–base disorders. *N Engl J Med 291:* 773–776, 1974.

24. Bierman, E. L., Dole, V. P., and Roberts, T. N.: An abnormality of nonesterified fatty acid metabolism in diabetes mellitus. *Diabetes 6:* 475–479, 1957.

25. Stephens, J. M., Sulway, M. J., and Watkins, P. J.: Relationship of blood acetoacetate and 3-hydroxybutyrate in diabetes. *Diabetes 20:* 485–489, 1971.

26. Soler, N. G., Wright, A. D., Fitzgerald, M. G., and Malins, J. M.: Comparative study of different insulin regimens in management of diabetic ketoacidosis. *Lancet 2:* 1221–1224, 1975.

27. Giammarco, R., Goldstein, M. B., Halperin, M. L., and Stinebaugh, B. J.: Renal tubular acidosis during therapy for diabetic ketoacidosis. *Can Med Assoc J 112:* 463–466, 1975.

28. Root, H. F.: The use of insulin and the abuse of glucose in the treatment of diabetic coma. *JAMA 127:* 557–564, 1945.

29. Page, M. McB., Alberti, K. G. M. M., Greenwood, R., Gumaa, K. A., Hockaday, T. D. R., Lowy, C., Nabarro, J. D. N., Pyde, D. A.,

30. Sönkson, P. H., Watkins, P. J., and West, T. E. T.: Treatment of diabetic coma with continuous low-dose infusion of insulin. *Br Med J 2:* 687–690, 1974.

31. Smith, K. and Martin, H. E.: Response of diabetic coma to various insulin dosages. *Diabetes 3:* 287–295, 1954.

32. Madison, L. L.: Low-dose insulin: A plea for caution. *N Eng J Med 294:* 393–394, 1976.

33. Young, E. and Bradley, R. F.: Cerebral edema with irreversible coma in severe diabetic ketoacidosis. *N Engl J Med 276:* 665–669, 1967.

34. Clements, R. S., Jr., Prockop, L. D., and Winegrad, A. I.: Acute cerebral edema during treatment of hyperglycemia. *Lancet 2:* 384–386, 1968.

35. Arieff, A. I. and Kleeman, C. R.: Studies on mechanisms of cerebral edema in diabetic comas. *J Clin Invest 52:* 571–583, 1973.

36. Clements, R. S., Jr., Blumenthal, S. A., Morrison, A. D., and Winegrad, A. I.: Increased cerebrospinal-fluid pressure during treatment of diabetic ketosis. *Lancet 2:* 671–675, 1971.

37. Soler, N. G., Bennett, M. A., FitzGerald, M. G., and Malins, J. M.: Intensive care in the management of diabetic ketoacidosis. *Lancet 1:* 951–954, 1973.

38. Sament, S. and Schwartz, M. B.: Severe diabetic stupor without ketosis. *S Afr Med J 31:* 893–894, 1957.

39. Arieff, A. I. and Carroll, H. J.: Nonketotic hyperosmolar coma with hyperglycemia: Clinical features, pathophysiology, renal function, acid-base balance, plasma-cerebrospinal fluid equilibria and the effects of therapy in 37 cases. *Medicine 51:* 73–94, 1972.

40. Gerich, J. E., Martin, M. M., and Recant, L.: Clinical and metabolic characteristics of hyperosmolar nonketotic coma. *Diabetes 20:* 228–238, 1971.

41. Vinik, A., Seftel, H., and Joffe, B. I.: Metabolic findings in hyperosmolar, nonketotic diabetic stupor. *Lancet 2:* 797–799, 1970.

42. Foster, D. W.: Insulin deficiency and hyperosmolar coma. *Adv Intern Med 19:* 159–173, 1973.

43. Maccario, M. and Messis, C. P.: Cerebral edema complicating treated nonketotic hyperglycemia. *Lancet 2:* 352–353, 1969.

44. Dillon, E. S., Dyer, W. W., and Smelo, L. S.: Ketone acidosis of nondiabetic adults. *Med Clin North Am 24:* 1813–1822, 1940.

45. Levy, L. J., Duga, J., Girgis, M., and Gordon, E. E.: Ketoacidosis associated with alcoholism in nondiabetic subjects. *Ann Intern Med 78:* 213–219, 1973.

46. Cooperman, M. T., Davidoff, F., Spark, R., and Pallotta, J.: Clinical studies of alcoholic ketoacidosis. *Diabetes 23:* 433–439, 1974.

47. Lefevre, A., Adler, H., and Lieber, C. S.: Effect of ethanol on ketone metabolism. *J Clin Invest 49:* 1775–1782, 1970.

48. Kondrup, J. and Grunnet, N.: The effect of acute and prolonged ethanol of treatment on the contents of coenzyme A, carnitine and their derivatives in rat liver. *Biochem J 132:* 373–379, 1973.

49. Oliva, P. B.: Lactic acidosis. *Am J Med 48:* 209–225, 1970.

50. Fulop, M. and Hoberman, H. D.: Alcoholic ketosis. *Diabetes 24:* 785–790, 1975.

51. Madison, L. L.: Ethanol-induced hypoglycemia. *Adv Metab Dis 3:* 85–108, 1968.

52. Assan, R., Heuclin, C., Girard, J. R., LeMaire, F., and Attali, J. R.: Phenformin-induced lactic acidosis in diabetic patients. *Diabetes 24:* 791–800, 1975.

53. Nissan, S., Bar-Maor, A., and Shafrir, E.: Hypoglycemia associated with extrapancreatic tumors. *N Engl J Med 278:* 177–183, 1968.

54. Kogut, M. D., Roe, T. F., Ng, W., and Donnel, G. N.: Fructose-induced hyperuricemia: Observations in normal children and in patients with hereditary fructose intolerance and galactosemia. *Pediatr Res 9:* 774–448, 1975.

55. Krebs, H. A.: The Pasteur effect and the relations between respiration and fermentation. *Essays Biochem 8:* 1–34, 1972.

56. Elkin, A. R. and Kuhn, N. J.: Aerobic lactate production by mammary tissue. *Biochem J 146:* 273–275, 1975.

57. Kreisberg, R. A.: Lactic acidosis interrelationships with diabetes mellitus and phenformin. In Fajans, S. S. (ed): *Diabetes Mellitus* (DHEW Publication No (NIH) 76-854). Washington, D.C., U.S. Govt. Printing Office, 1976, pp. 142–153.

58. Marliss, E. B., Ohman, J. L., Jr., Aoki, T. T., and Kozak, G. P.: Altered redox state obscuring ketoacidosis in diabetic patients with lactic acidosis. *N Engl J Med 283:* 978–980, 1970.

59. Relman, A. S.: Lactic acidosis. *Trans Am Clin Clinatol Assoc 82:* 70–76, 1970.

83

Late Complications of Diabetes

Albert I. Winegrad
Anthony D. Morrison
Douglas A. Greene

INTRODUCTION

There is a heterogeneous group of clinical syndromes reflecting dysfunction and pathology in specific organs or tissue systems that occur in association with chronic diabetes mellitus: Their development either singly or in any combination, in a given patient is at present unpredictable, and they are appropriately referred to collectively as the late complications of diabetes. These syndromes do not have a common pathological basis, and in specific instances they occur in nondiabetics without any apparent difference in their underlying pathology. Moreover, no simplistic classification, such as efforts to divide them all into those that result from what is termed "macroangiopathy" and those that result from "diabetic microangiopathy," is justified on the basis of existing data, and the terms themselves have not been precisely defined.

This chapter considers the major complications of diabetes as syndromes arising from dysfunction of specific organs: it attempts to review briefly the information available concerning their pathological basis, and efforts to understand their pathogenesis. Certain limitations are obvious at the outset. We cannot at present distinguish between possibly different etiologic forms of juvenile or adult

onset diabetes and must consider together the late complications of what may prove to be quite diverse disease entities, whose only common characteristic is the development of alterations in the regulation of plasma glucose concentration, which meet our present diagnostic criteria. Our information concerning the normal biology and biochemistry of the vascular system and regional differences in vessels of the same type (e.g., capillaries) is fragmentary, as is our understanding of how they may be affected by specific disease processes. Patients with diabetes mellitus are heterogeneous, and our ability to assess the presence of independent genetic or environmental factors that may adversely affect specific organs or tissues in a manner that might help explain the unpredictable development of specific late complications of diabetes is limited. Despite these limitations emphasis on the development and assessment of information concerning specific late complications of diabetes is valuable clinically, and in the development of new approaches to their understanding and treatment.

DIABETIC NEUROPATHY

INTRODUCTION

The diverse syndromes resulting from dysfunction of the peripheral or autonomic nervous system which occur in association with diabetes mellitus are collectively referred to as diabetic neuroapthy. Estimates of the incidence of diabetic neuropathy vary from 5 to 60 percent. However, the true incidence is unknown since the observed incidence appears to be markedly affected by the specific diagnostic criteria employed and by the age and duration of diabetes in the patients studied. The development of overt diabetic neuropathy in any given patient is at present quite unpredictable. The simplified classification of diabetic neuropathy given in Table 83-1 has been adapted from several now in common use. Although mixed syndromes frequently occur, the endocrinologist should recognize that there are a number of relatively well-defined syndromes which differ in their prognosis, their associated pathology, and probably in their mode of pathogenesis.

ASYMMETRICAL DIABETIC NEUROPATHY

A mononeuropathy is a syndrome in which the symptoms and objective findings can be clearly related to dysfunction of a single nerve trunk. Mononeuropathy multiplex is characterized by the simultaneous or successive dysfunction of several nerve trunks under conditions that permit a clear delineation of the specific nerve trunks affected. This is in contrast to polyneuropathy which

Table 83-1. Classification of Diabetic Neuropathy

A. Asymmetrical diabetic neuropathy
  1. Cranial mononeuropathy and mononeuropathy multiplex
  2. Peripheral mononeuropathy and mononeuropathy multiplex
B. Symmetrical distal polyneuropathy
C. Autonomic neuropathy

implies a more diffuse symmetrical disorder. Asymmetrical diabetic neuropathy is characterized by mononeuropathy or mononeuropathy multiplex affecting cranial or spinal nerves.

Cranial Mononeuropathy and Mononeuropathy Multiplex

Isolated and multiple palsies of the nerves to the extraocular muscles occur more frequently in diabetics than in nondiabetics. They usually occur in patients over the age of 50, and frequently in patients who have no other evidence of overt diabetic neuropathy. The most common syndrome is an isolated third nerve palsy that spares the pupillary reflexes in most instances.[1] The sixth nerve is less commonly affected, and the fourth nerve is rarely affected alone, but may be involved in combination. The onset is usually acute, and in approximately 50 percent of cases is associated with pain behind or above the eye, which may be intense. There is still disagreement as to whether the pain results from involvement of the first two branches of the trigeminal nerve within the cavernous sinus. The cranial nerve palsies associated with diabetes mellitus exhibit a tendency for spontaneous improvement over a period of months. However, recurrent lesions and involvement of the contralateral third nerve may occur. The relationship of diabetes mellitus to other cranial nerve palsies is less firmly established, although it has been suggested that there is an association with Bell's palsy[2] and with nerve deafness.[3]

Information concerning the pathological basis of the cranial nerve palsies associated with diabetes mellitus is still fragmentary. In an elderly diabetic who developed a third nerve palsy 1 month prior to death Asbury et al. found a focal demyelinating lesion in the intracavernous portion of the third nerve which was interpreted as being ischemic in nature.[4] The patient had had a third palsy on the opposite side 3 years previously from which she had recovered, and no residual lesion was detected in that nerve. Severe hyaline thickening with luminal encroachment was present in many of the small arteries and arterioles within both nerves, but arterioles supplying other cranial nerves in the cavernous sinus and arterioles in other tissues were only minimally affected. In tracing out the nutrient circulation to both third nerves only a single occluded epineural arteriole was found in the more recently affected nerve. However, this appeared to be unrelated to the intracavernous lesion.

Peripheral Mononeuropathy and Mononeuropathy Multiplex

Syndromes resulting from dysfunction of an isolated peripheral nerve or of a number of peripheral nerves occur in association with diabetes mellitus. However, attribution to diabetes mellitus is frequently the result of a process of exclusion. The isolated peripheral nerve lesions often occur at the common sites for external pressure palsies (the radial nerve in the upper arm, the common peroneal at the neck of the fibula) or at site of entrapment (the medial nerve in the carpal tunnel, and the ulnar nerve in the cubital tunnel). In addition isolated involvement of the femoral nerve is much more common in diabetics than in nondiabetics. In cases of peripheral mononeuropathy multiplex observed in older diabetics the proximal nerves of the lower extremity (i.e., the femoral, sciatic, and obturator) are frequently involved; in these instances there is striking tendency for the neuropathy to affect one limb and then, after a variable period of time, to affect the other. The onset of isolated peripheral nerve palsies and of mononeuropathy multiplex associated with diabetes mellitus is characteristically abrupt and is frequently associated with pain, although it may be insidious.[5] The major manifestation is muscle weakness which may eventuate in muscle wasting; the sensory deficits are frequently less marked. As in other forms of diabetic neuropathy affecting the peripheral nerves the CSF protein tends to be moderately elevated. The term diabetic amyotrophy[6] has been used to refer to a syndrome occurring in older diabetics in which asymmetrical weakness and wasting of the proximal muscle of the leg occurs without conspicuous sensory loss, although the knee jerk is depressed or absent. This is commonly associated with pain in the thigh muscles, and sometimes in the lumbar region and perineum. Most of the cases recently studied appear to represent a form of peripheral mononeuropathy multiplex.

There is no consistent relationship between the development of these asymmetrical diabetic neuropathies and the presence of symptomatic hyperglycemia, and little evidence of a consistent response to efforts to achieve better "diabetic control" (i.e., a lesser degree of hyperglycemia). However, these are probably a heterogeneous group of disorders, since in specific instances it appears that external pressure or nerve entrapment is a significant factor in precipitating clinical manifestations, whereas in others, as noted later, there is reason to believe that acute ischemia is the precipitating event. Thus in one well-studied case of mononeuropathy multiplex in an elderly diabetic Raff and Asbury found multiple small infarcts scattered throughout the obturator, femoral, sciatic, and posterior tibial nerves.[7] However, in over 4000 serial sections of the affected portion of the obturator nerve only one small artery was occluded by a thrombus and its wall appeared normal. Endothelial and perithelial cell proliferation was observed in arterioles and capillaries primarily within the area of infarction, but the nature of the vascular disease responsible for the nerve infarcts remains obscure. It should be noted that in experimental animals the occlusion of single or multiple nutrient arteries to a nerve, or stripping its epineurium for long distances may be carried out without significantly altering nerve function or morphology. While it appears likely that acute ischemia may be a major factor in the pathogenesis of cranial nerve palsies associated with diabetes mellitus and of peripheral mononeuropathy multiplex in elderly diabetics, the present uncertainties concerning the pathogenesis of the clinical manifestations of these and other asymmetrical diabetic neuropathies do not permit the assumption that they are primarily the consequence of "diabetic microangiopathy." Moreover, as discussed later the definition of this term as it applies to the vascular supply of cranial and peripheral nerves has not been established.

SYMMETRICAL DISTAL POLYNEUROPATHY

The most common form of diabetic neuropathy is characterized by the development of a symmetrical sensory loss which first affects the distal portions of the lower extremities. Motor weakness is usually less prominent, but when detectable it is bilateral and chiefly distal. In some cases the upper extremities may be affected in a similar fashion. The onset of diabetic polyneuropathy is usually insidious and the majority of patients have minimal symptoms. This may account for the frequency with which the diagnosis is first made in patients who present with foot ulcers or diabetic Charcot joints, whose development is conditioned by the sensory deficits. When symptoms are present, numbness and tingling in the feet are common. There may also be burning, or cramping pain which tends to be more intense at night. The clinical manifestations and objective findings vary. This may reflect the stage at which the diagnosis is considered and the sensitivity of the methods employed to assess the neurological deficits, but some workers have also attempted to identify subgroups with manifestations that reflect predominantly small or large peripheral nerve fiber involvement. On standard neurological examination depression or loss of ankle jerks and impairment or loss of vibration sense in the feet are common early findings. The development of impaired perception of vibration, touch, pain, and position sense with a "stocking" distribution is also characteristic.

In patients with symmetrical diabetic neuropathy the most prominent lesions are found in the distal portions of the peripheral nerves, and it is currently believed that the occasional changes observed in the anterior horn cells and posterior root ganglia are secondary to changes in the nerve processes. The peripheral nerves exhibit a loss of myelinated nerve fibers with an increase in the connective tissue elements of the nerve bundle; in addition, there is often a proliferation of Schwann cells which have lost their usual relationship to an axon. In most recent neuropathological studies significant disease of the vasa nervorum has been absent, and most workers believe that the lesions observed are conditioned by some chronic metabolic derangement. Studies of teased single myelinated nerve fibers from patients with symmetrical diabetic neuropathy by Thomas and Lascelles demonstrated the presence of segmental demyelination with initial preservation of the axon.[8] In addition the loss of regular spacing of the nodes of Ranvier, and of the usual relationship between axon diameter and internode distance suggests that the nerves may have been subjected to repeated episodes of demyelination and remyelination; however, the process may also progress and lead to axonal loss. Since the myelin sheath is derived from the Schwann cell membrane it has been suggested that the process may initially affect this cell type. However, segmental demyelination may also occur secondary to alterations in the axon, and some workers believe that the lesions are compatible with a "dying back" of the axonal process.[9] Sural nerve biopsies from patients with adult onset diabetes of several years' duration who had no neurological symptoms and no evidence of overt neuropathy, on standard neurological examination, have been found to contain lesions similar to those found in the peripheral nerves of patients with overt polyneuropathy; however, these lesions are usually less marked.[10] This suggests that the development of overt diabetic polyneuropathy may usually be preceded by a period in which inapparent but irreversible alterations occur in the peripheral nerve.

The natural history of diabetic polyneuropathy requires clarification. In newly diagnosed juvenile diabetics with no objective findings on standard neurological examination the application of sensitive techniques has demonstrated the presence of widespread alterations in sensory perception, and alterations in the electrophysiological properties of peripheral motor and sensory nerves.[11,12] The latter include decreased peripheral motor and sensory nerve conduction velocities; these have been reported to improve following the initiation of insulin treatment but tend to decline with increasing duration of disease.[11,13] It is thought that these alterations may represent a subclinical phase of diabetic polyneuropathy but the associated pathology, if any, has not been established. Patients with overt diabetic polyneuropathy, and long-standing diabetics without overt evidence of polyneuropathy characteristically exhibit decreased peripheral motor and sensory nerve conduction velocities that have been attributed to the pathological lesions present in their peripheral nerves, the alterations being compatible with the expected effects of segmental demyelination.[10]

Most endocrinologists agree that the diagnosis of overt diabetic polyneuropathy is an indication for efforts to achieve a closer approximation of normal diurnal plasma glucose fluctuations, and that insulin is the preferred agent to be used in combination with weight reduction where the latter is indicated. We subscribe to this view, even though the limitations of present therapy, and the lack of appropriate controlled studies of age- and sex-matched patients with diabetic polyneuropathy of similar clinical severity and similar peripheral nerve pathology must be acknowledged. There are numerous well-documented instances in which the institution or modification of insulin treatment has been followed by improvement in symptoms, sometimes following an initial exacerbation, and improvement in objective neurological findings over a period of time. Unfortunately this response is neither consistent or predictable in any given patient, and the need for improved methods for the prevention and treatment of diabetic polyneuropathy is well recognized. No consistent relationship to deficiencies of thiamine or B_{12} have been established for diabetic polyneuropathy. However, efforts to identify nutritional deficiencies, drugs (e.g., alcohol), physical factors, and unrelated diseases which might contribute to the neurological manifestations in patients with diabetic polyneuropathy are indicated since they suggest additional therapeutic approaches.

The evidence suggesting that the development of diabetic polyneuropathy is conditioned by some chronic metabolic disturbance has spurred renewed efforts to study its pathogenesis in experimental animals. Thus far there is no animal model for overt diabetic polyneuropathy. However, Chinese hamsters with hyperglycemia and particularly with hyperglycemia and ketonuria of several years' duration have been found to develop lesions in their peripheral nerves similar to those found in long-standing human diabetics.[14] In rats experimental diabetes induced by pancreatectomy,[15] alloxan,[15] or streptozotocin[16] results in the rapid development of impaired peripheral motor and sensory nerve conduction velocity but only in animals who become persistently hyperglycemic. The relationship of insulin deficiency and possibly hyperglycemia to the development of this alteration has been established since it can be prevented by insulin treatment but only under conditions which obviate any prolonged period of hyperglycemia. Treatment that results only in a decrease in the degree of hyperglycemia and normal weight gain is not consistently effective.[16] Matschinsky and his co-workers have also observed that experimental diabetes in the rat results in impaired axonal transport and that this can be corrected by insulin treatment[17]; impaired axonal transport is a mechanism commonly invoked in the pathogenesis of "dying back" peripheral neuropathies. In addition, evidence has been presented for the impaired incorporation of labeled amino acids into myelin protein by isolated segments of peripheral nerve from diabetic rats.[18] However, the manner in which insulin deficiency and/or hyperglycemia may affect the metabolism and function of specific cellular components of the peripheral nerve remains to be clarified, and major technical obstacles remain to be solved in approaching the normal metabolism of the peripheral nerve. The presence of polyol pathway activity has been demonstrated in rat, rabbit, and human peripheral nerve, and elevated levels of glucose, sorbitol, and fructose have been demonstrated in tissue from hyperglycemic animals and humans.[19,21] The data of Stewart et al. suggest that these levels fluctuate rapidly in response to an alteration in plasma glucose concentration,[19] but there is no direct evidence that they induce osmotic swelling in components of the peripheral nerve. In rats with experimental diabetes the development of impaired motor nerve conduction velocity and its prevention by insulin treatment are correlated with changes in the nerve free myoinositol content.[16] Myoinositol, a cyclic polyol which is a normal dietary component and a constituent of the inositol-containing phospholipids, is known to be excreted in increased quantities in the urine in human and experimental diabetes.[22] It is present in high concentrations in mammalian cells but the extent to which this reflects synthesis in situ or active concentration is unknown in most tissues. It has been reported that increased dietary myoinositol intake in rats with experimental diabetes will prevent the usual decrease in nerve free myoinositol content and the development of impaired motor nerve conduction velocity despite persistent hyperglycemia and high tissue concentrations of sorbitol and fructose.[16] The relationship of these observations to the impaired nerve conduction velocities observed in newly diagnosed juvenile diabetics remains to be examined.

Recent studies have failed to demonstrate any significant alterations in the pattern of the major lipid and protein components of purified myelin prepared from the peripheral nerves of diabetic patients.[23] However, the isolation and characterization of the diverse intrinsic proteins of peripheral nerve myelin are still in an early phase.

AUTONOMIC NEUROPATHY

Systematic evaluations of autonomic nervous function in patients with diabetes mellitus by sensitive objective techniques are infrequently carried out. However, from studies in which selected aspects of autonomic function were examined it appears that most long-standing diabetics have widespread alterations in autonomic nervous function which are subclinical and are usually ignored until the development of symptoms.[24] The latter remains an essentially unpredictable event although some workers maintain the existence of a relationship to an antecedent period of "poor control."

Sympathetic denervation of peripheral blood vessels particularly affecting the lower extremity occurs in many long-standing diabetics, and in approximately 50 percent of a group with peripheral neuropathy reported by Martin.[25] This results in a modification of central vasomotor reflexes and makes the patient subject to prolonged vasospasm of surface vessels as a result of local cooling. This may be associated with altered sudomotor activity and result in cold extremities with increased sweating in the affected area. In some instances the impaired vasomotor function may progress and result in orthostatic hypotension which may be subclinical or a source of dizziness and syncopal episodes.

Excessive sweating in the upper half of the body with decreased sweating below the waist and heat intolerance have been reported to occur in some diabetic patients with peripheral neuropathy and evidence of altered vasomotor function, and are attributed to altered sudomotor function.

Retrograde ejaculation resulting from incompetence of the internal vesicle sphincter due to involvement of the pelvic autonomic system occurs in association with impotence; the latter alone or in combination has been estimated to occur in 25 to 30 percent of diabetic males under the age of 40.[26] Urinary incontinence can rarely be ascribed to diabetes. However, increasing

significance has been attributed to the impaired or absent sense of bladder filling with low expulsive force and an increased bladder capacity, which is demonstrable by cystomanometric studies in a significant number of long-standing male and female diabetics.[1] This dysfunction is rarely assessed in asymptomatic diabetics unless it becomes a significant factor in the pathogenesis of chronic urinary tract infection.

There is a discrepancy between the frequency with which alterations in pharyngeal and esophageal motility are observed in cineradiographic studies in diabetics and the rarity with which this is associated with symptoms. Similarly, gastric motor abnormalities occur in 20 to 30 percent of diabetics often without clinical manifestations. Gastric motor abnormalities are infrequently invoked as a cause of nausea and vomiting in diabetics, but there is the clinical impression that they may be significant factors in the difficulty encountered in treating some "brittle diabetics." Diabetic diarrhea is a diagnosis by exclusion (infections, celiac disease, chronic pancreatitis, etc.) but is frequently associated with the presence of manifestations of autonomic neuropathy in other organs and of motor abnormalities of the small bowel. Small bowel transit time is usually rapid, but may be delayed; it is in the latter instances that bacterial overgrowth in the small bowel may lead to a "blind loop" syndrome with diarrhea and steatorrhea.[1] Fecal incontinence may be expressed as sudden uncontrolled bowel movements occurring during sleep (nocturnal diarrhea) or when the patient is awake. The attribution of constipation in diabetes to autonomic neuropathy is usually extremely difficult. However, massive colonic distension resulting from atony and dilatation of the colon is occasionally observed in patients with other manifestations of autonomic neuropathy.

It is apparent that significant manifestations of autonomic neuropathy may be undetected until symptoms arising from a specific organ stimulate systematic study of autonomic function. Moreover, with regard to a number of the manifestations of autonomic neuropathy, independent factors (e.g., urinary tract infection, bacterial overgrowth of the small bowel, dehydration resulting from exposure to a hot climate) may play a significant factor in the precipitation of acute clinical manifestations.

It is a common clinical impression that clinical manifestations of autonomic neuropathy usually occur in association with objective evidence of diabetic polyneuroapthy. However, precise data are not available. The treatment of specific manifestations of autonomic neuropathy cannot be considered in detail. There are a number of well-studied cases in which efforts at more rigorous diabetic "control" were associated with improvement in the symptoms and objective findings in patients with a variety of manifestations of autonomic neuropathy; however, this response is not consistent or predictable and some manifestations such as impotence are rarely affected. The institution of insulin and diet therapy in such patients remains good medical practice, and the limitations of such therapy must be viewed in light of what appears to be the natural history of these syndromes with a long period of asymptomatic alteration in function, and the probability that unrelated factors can contribute to the severity of symptoms. The pathology associated with autonomic neuropathy has been neglected and the data are fragmentary. There is evidence that nonmyelinated fibers in peripheral nerves are quantitatively more affected in early diabetes, and are decreased in peripheral nerves from long-standing diabetics.[27] Swelling and degenerative changes in the ganglion cells of the sympathetic trunk have been reported to occur in patients with diabetic autonomic neuropathy, and one group has reported that degenerative changes frequently occur in the bladder intramural fibers and in hypogastric nerve fibers in diabetes.[28]

ATHEROSCLEROTIC HEART DISEASE IN DIABETICS

CLINICAL DATA

The clinical manifestations and pathological findings associated with ASHD do not differ in diabetic and nondiabetic subjects. However, in the United States and Western Europe ASHD accounts for a major fraction of the excess morbidity and mortality among diabetics.[29] In these regions there is a greater frequency and higher mortality of ASHD in diabetics, and the manifestations appear at an earlier age. Moreover, in patients with diabetes mellitus the usual sex difference in the incidence and prevalence of myocardial infarction is virtually abolished. The association between diabetes mellitus and ASHD is not uniformly apparent in different regions of the world. In the past there was a very low prevalence of ASHD in Japan; during that period ASHD was not a significant cause of excess morbidity and mortality in diabetics in Japan.[30] However, more recent data suggest that there has been an increased prevalence of ASHD in Japan, and that a difference between diabetic and nondiabetics, in this regard, is now emerging.[31]

The basis for the association between diabetes mellitus and ASHD in this country and Western Europe is still unclear. Although diabetics have a higher prevalence of hypertension recent epidemiological studies suggest that the increased incidence of fatal and nonfatal coronary events associated with hyperglycemia is independent of hypertension.[32] Moreover, a recent prospective study of mortality in normotensive subjects demonstrated a higher incidence of cardiovascular deaths in normotensive diabetics.[33] As discussed in Chapter 144, mechanisms exist by which an impaired insulin secretory mechanism may result in hyperlipidemia in diabetics. However, Bierman and Porte found that only 30 to 35 percent of diabetics had either hypertriglyceridemia or hypercholesterolemia when compared with normal sex-matched controls.[34] The relationship between diabetes mellitus and hyperlipidemia has been a subject of controversy and confusion. When plasma lipoprotein electrophoresis was used in an effort to define the phenotypic expression of inherited lipid abnormalities, types III, IV, and V were usually found to be associated with hyperglycemia, but there was no firm basis for excluding the presence of diabetes mellitus as an independent disorder in these patients. Recent studies by Goldstein and his collaborators represent a major advance.[35] They examined the fasting plasma triglyceride and cholesterol concentrations in 500 survivors of a myocardial infarction and their spouses (who were used as unrelated controls exposed to the same environmental factors). These authors also carried out an analysis of lipid concentrations in the families of the survivors who were found to have an abnormally elevated plasma triglyceride or cholesterol concentration. Goldstein et al. found that 20 percent of the survivors less than 60 years of age and 7 percent of the older survivors had one of three inherited lipid disorders, which from their studies appeared to represent the dominant expression of three different autosomal genes. The presence of these disorders—familial hypercholesterolemia, familial hypertriglyceridemia, and a newly defined entity, familial combined hyperlipidemia—could not be established in any given hyperlipidemic subject on the basis of their plasma lipoprotein electrophoretic pattern, for in these studies it was found that no pattern was specific for any specific genetic lipid disorder. (At the moment the firm diagnosis of these inherited disorders requires family studies.) Using rigorous criteria for the diagnosis of diabetes mellitus that would exclude many adult onset diabetics (i.e., fasting blood sugar greater than 120 mg/dl or treat-ment with insulin or an oral hypoglycemia agent), Goldstein et al. found that 12 percent of the survivors of a myocardial infarction were diabetic; 22 percent of the survivors with familial hypertriglyceridemia were diabetic; 15 percent of the survivors with familial combined hyperlipidemia were diabetic; but only 6 percent of the survivors with familial hypercholesterolemia were diabetic.[36] In a follow-up Brunzell et al. found that diabetes mellitus and hypertriglyceridemia segregated independently in a large group of first-degree relatives of survivors of a myocardial infarction with both diabetes and an elevated triglyceride concentration.[37] These workers suggested that the frequently reported association between diabetes mellitus and hypertriglyceridemia may reflect, in part, preferential selection of patients with both diabetes and an inherited form of hyperlipidemia since it appears that the combination may be more commonly associated with symptoms (i.e., of ASHD). Preliminary estimates suggest that the genes for familial hypertriglyceridemia and for familial combined hyperlipidemia occur with great frequency in the general population.

EXPERIMENTAL STUDIES

The manner in which diabetes mellitus may alter the likelihood of developing ASHD in any given patient must ultimately be explained in terms of the pathogenesis of the atherosclerotic lesion. Although hypertension, smoking, and alterations in plasma lipid concentrations have been identified as risk factors, along with hyperglycemia, the manner in which these may interact in the pathogenesis of atherosclerotic lesions or subsequent thrombosis remains a matter of speculation. The multifactorial origin of atherosclerotic lesions is accepted in most present formulations of the processes that occur in the inner arterial wall; these are well represented by the recent hypothesis presented by Ross and Glomset.[38] These workers suggest that the migration of the vascular smooth muscle cells into the subintimal space and their proliferation in that region is the cardinal factor in the development of the atherosclerotic lesion. They suggest that the endothelial cell influences the behavior of the arterial smooth muscle cells by normally providing a barrier to the passage of plasma proteins, and that factors that injure the endothelium alter this barrier. According to this formulation endothelial cell injury alters the environment of the vascular smooth muscle cells and alters the concentrations of plasma lipoproteins to which they are exposed; in response to these alterations some of the smooth muscle cells migrate into the intima and proliferate. The arterial smooth muscle cells are the principal cells that accumulate in arterial lesions that result from a variety of experimental injuries and in the earliest stages of the atherosclerotic process. They synthesize the extracellular connective tissue elements found in these lesions. The response of these cells to increased concentrations of cholesterol-rich lipoproteins (β-lipoproteins) is a subject of active investigation; recent studies by Goldstein, Brown, and their co-workers suggest that if the regulation of β-lipoprotein uptake by cultured arterial smooth muscle cells at the level of specific cell receptors is bypassed by altering the charge on the surface of the lipoprotein, the cells accumulate large quantities of lipid and develop into the "foam cells" characteristic of a latter stage in the atherosclerotic process. However, present formulations of the atherosclerotic process suggest that if the endothelial cell barrier is reestablished after injury, the resulting intimal lesions may be self-limited and regress. Regression or progression may be dependent on the balance between factors regulating the proliferation and regression of smooth muscle cells; it is at this level that Ross and Glomset believe that hormonal imbalances may have their greatest effect.

Viewed from the perspective of present formulations of the pathogenesis of the atherosclerotic lesion, diabetes could contribute in a number of ways which are currently being investigated. Diabetes could alter the metabolism of arterial endothelial cells in a manner that decreases their barrier function or increases the likelihood of endothelial cell injury. In this regard it has been suggested that platelet function is altered in diabetics in a manner that could contribute to endothelial cell injury.[39] Diabetes could contribute to elevated plasma concentrations of very low density or low-density lipoproteins at the time of endothelial injury. Recent studies have suggested a relationship between the relative concentrations of plasma cholesterol in low-density and high-density lipoproteins and ASHD, leading to the suggestion that increased concentrations of high-density lipoproteins are protective. Other workers have reported that high-density lipoproteins decrease the uptake of low-density β-lipoproteins by cultured arterial smooth muscle cells. There are some data to suggest that diabetes may be associated with a relative reduction in plasma high-density lipoprotein concentrations. Diabetes may directly or indirectly alter the metabolism of the vascular smooth muscle cells in a manner which potentiates the formation of irreversible vascular lesions by modifying its response to factors that tend to affect their proliferation or regression, including their handling of lipoproteins that enter the intima–media preparations in vitro, are suspect. It appears that the the proliferation of vascular smooth muscle cells in tissue culture[40] in a manner similar to that reported for other cell types.[41] Some workers speculate that the high plasma insulin concentrations found in association with hyperglycemia in some adult onset diabetics might contribute to atherogenesis in this manner. The manner in which insulin deficiency and/or hyperglycemia may affect the arterial metabolism is unknown, since most of the available data on this point, which were derived from studies of aortic intima–media preparations in vitro, are suspect. It appears that the methods previously employed to study this tissue result in preparations with extensive endothelial cell injury at the outset.[42]

RENAL DISEASE IN DIABETES MELLITUS— "DIABETIC NEPHROPATHY"

CLINICAL DATA

The attribution of a primary cause of death in a uremic diabetic who may also have hypertension and ASHD can be difficult. However, there is general agreement that renal disease is a significant source of excess morbidity and mortality in patients with long-standing diabetes mellitus. In studies reported from the Joslin Clinic in the mid 1960s deaths attributed to "renal vascular disease" were 17 times greater in diabetics than in the general population.[43] In addition it was noted that almost half of the deaths occurring in patients with diabetes mellitus diagnosed prior to age 20 were attributable to some form of renal disease. Both the classification of renal disease in long-standing diabetics who present with chronic renal failure and the natural history of what is commonly called diabetic nephropathy require clarification.

There are a variety of possible causes for the development of chronic renal disease in diabetics, but it was not until 1936 that the studies of Kimmelstiel and Wilson suggested the existence of pathological processes uniquely associated with diabetes mellitus.[44] The Kimmelstiel–Wilson lesion has only rarely been observed in patients who were not known to be diabetic during life, but is found at autopsy in only approximately 25 percent of dia-

betics. It appears as a nearly spherical hyaline mass, characteristically occupying the center of a peripheral glomerular lobule, and having an apparently patent capillary running over its surface; the mass is acidophilic and is PAS positive. This specific lesion has proven to be of diagnostic rather than clinical significance, for there is no correlation between the presence or severity of these nodules and the clinical manifestations or degree of functional renal impairment in individual patients. The pathological process in the kidney associated with diabetes mellitus that may be of greater clinical significance is what appears as a diffuse hyaline thickening of the glomerular capillary basement membrane (GBM) on light microscopy, the material also being PAS positive. On electron microscopic examination the diffuse lesion has two major components: thickening of the peripheral GBM, and an increase in the area of the interstitial tissue lying between the glomerular capillaries (i.e., the mesangium).[45] Varying degrees of the diffuse lesion are common in patients with long-standing diabetes, and the specific nodular lesion is invariably accompanied by the diffuse lesion. The natural history of these lesions is still a matter of dispute, but the quantitative studies of Ruth Østerby suggest that both the GBM and the mesangial regions are normal in juvenile diabetics at the time of diagnosis.[46] In diabetics dying in uremia, the majority have pathological alterations in the kidney in addition to those just described; these include interstitial cellular infiltration (frequently referred to as "pyelonephritis") and arteriolar sclerosis with hyalinization of both the efferent and afferent glomerular arterioles. The development of clinical manifestations of diabetic nephropathy and the subsequent course are unpredictable. The mortality attributed to this syndrome appears to peak between 10 and 19 years after the diagnosis of diabetes in young patients with juvenile diabetes and then declines. In patients in whom the diagnosis of diabetes was made between the ages of 40 and 59 years only 2.5 percent of the deaths in the Joslin series were attributed to diabetic nephropathy, and other renal disease accounted for 3.0 percent of the deaths.[43]

In a recent study renal biopsies were examined by light microscopy in 31 diabetics who were then followed for a period of 8–12 years.[47] At the time of biopsy neither renal function nor proteinuria was closely related to the histological changes observed in the biopsy. Although all those with heavy proteinuria (more than 3.0 g/day) had advanced renal changes, some patients with serious biopsy lesions had no proteinuria and normal serum creatinine concentrations. All of the patients with marked proteinuria (and marked biopsy changes) died during the follow-up period, usually from renal failure. However, when proteinuria was smaller in amount the prognosis was variable, irrespective of the initial histological changes, and in some instances renal function remained unaltered over a period of many years. In this series hypertension was a late feature and usually did not appear until renal failure was quite advanced. The data on the natural history of diabetic nephropathy are still fragmentary, and do not include long-term prospective studies with repeated renal biopsies studied by electron microscopy.

The clinical manifestations of diabetic nephropathy are quite variable. As indicated earlier, asymptomatic proteinuria of a mild degree may persist for years without deterioration in renal function. In other instances the severity of the asymptomatic proteinuria may rapidly progress to the point at which the patient persistently excretes 3–5 g/day or more; this has an ominous prognosis.[47] Although the development of the nephrotic syndrome is a characteristic phase in the subsequent progression of diabetic nephropathy it does not appear to be an invariable event. Ultimately evidence of progressive deterioration in glomerular and tubular function ensues with the development of chronic uremia; at this stage there is almost invariable evidence of diabetic retinopathy and the clinical manifestations may also be modified by the presence of hypertension (which is present in 80 percent of cases), as well as by the coexistence of ASHD. Death usually occurs within 2 to 5 years following the development of marked, persistent proteinuria.

In some insulin-requiring diabetics the development of renal failure may be associated with a marked reduction in their exogenous insulin requirements; however, this is not a consistent event. A variety of factors have been suggested to contribute to this phenomenon; these include decreased caloric intake and the decrease in renal insulin extraction which occurs in association with chronic renal failure.[43]

The symptomatic treatment of chronic renal failure attributed to diabetic nephropathy is similar to that currently employed in the management of other forms of chronic renal disease.

The role of chronic hemodialysis in the management of diabetics with chronic uremia is currently undergoing reevaluation. Shapiro et al. treated 58 patients over a 7½-year interval.[48] Of these, 27 patients died, 6 within the first 3 months of treatment, and 23 continued to be maintained on dialysis. The mortality and morbidity were poorer than those observed in nondiabetic uremics, even when compared with those over 60 years of age. Cardiac disease, acute myocardial infarction in most instances, was the most common cause of death. Coexisting blindness and neuropathy are problems in the management and rehabilitation of these patients. Of the 58 patients, 25 were blind in one or both eyes at the outset of hemodialysis, and all of the 5 patients in whom treatment was discontinued became blind during dialysis. The clinical manifestations of uremic neuropathy and diabetic polyneuropathy are impossible to differentiate in such patients, and in a group study by Blagg et al. the manifestations improved and progressed in equal numbers during chronic hemodialysis.[49]

Renal transplantation is also being evaluated in a number of centers. Najarian and co-workers carried out 68 kidney transplants in 63 patients between 1969 and 1974.[50] The cumulative 3-year survival was 30 percent in diabetics receiving a cadaver kidney as compared with 80 percent in nondiabetic-matched controls. In diabetics receiving a kidney from a related donor the cumulative 5-year survival was 53 percent as compared with 68 percent in nondiabetic controls. Infection and myocardial infarction were the major causes of death. There was a high incidence of urological complications, including ureteral necrosis. In the patients with functioning kidneys visual acuity stabilized during the first 2 years after transplantation. These workers observed a vary rapid progression of diabetic retinopathy in patients being evaluated for renal transplantation over a 1- to 2-year period and currently accept patients when the serum creatinine is 6–8 mg/dl rather than 12–15 mg/dl as in nondiabetics.

Mauer et al. recently reported that 10 of 12 kidneys transplanted into diabetics developed PAS-positive hyalinization of the glomerular arterioles within 2 to 5 years and that in six instances both the afferent and efferent arterioles were affected in a manner characteristic of diabetic nephropathy.[51] In one instance nodular glomerularsclerosis was observed. Comparable changes were said to be absent in kidneys transplanted into nondiabetics within the first 5 years; and although hyalinization of the glomerular arterioles was subsequently observed in infrequent instances, involvement of both afferent and efferent arterioles was not seen. While this approach may ultimately provide evidence that the development of

renal lesions is a consequence of transplantation into a diabetic, most of the kidneys were donated by parents or siblings of the diabetics, and alterations attributable to rejection in the glomeruli of most of the kidneys prevented comparison of the glomeruli of the diabetics and nondiabetics.

THE GLOMERULUS AND THE GLOMERULAR CAPILLARY BASEMENT MEMBRANE IN DIABETES MELLITUS

As indicated previously it appears likely that the development of clinically significant diabetic nephropathy may be critically influenced by processes unrelated to those reflected in the pathological lesions in the glomerulus that are characteristic of diabetes mellitus. However, the attention focused on the increased GBM thickness, the accumulation of GBM-like material in the mesangial regions, and the Kimmelstiel–Wilson nodule is understandable, for these lesions have been considered the manifestations of a widespread disease of small blood vessels (diabetic microangiopathy) that is uniquely associated with diabetes mellitus. This concept arose from the observation of certain similarities in the alterations in the glomerular and retinal vasculature found in long-standing diabetics when sections stained with PAS were examined by light microscopy. Increased PAS staining was subsequently found in the walls of small blood vessels of varying sizes and structure in many organs. The PAS stain is now known to indicate the presence of neutral polysaccharide that is covalently bound to protein (i.e., glycoprotein). In the glomerulus, the PAS-positive material corresponds to the thickened GBM and the GBM-like material in the mesangium observed on EM examination. It should be noted, however, that there are significant differences in the lesions observed in the retinal and glomerular capillary circulations in long-standing diabetics aside from the similarities noted, and the primary nature of the vascular disease affecting these organs in the diabetic is unknown. Although there is much evidence that the structural appearance of small blood vessels in many organs is altered in association with long-standing diabetic mellitus, the term microangiopathy is badly in need of redefinition. It is frequently used at present to indicate the presence of capillary basement membrane thickening not only in the glomerulus and retina but in muscle and other organs. However, it remains to be demonstrated whether capillary basement membrane thickening is the primary or really significant aspect of the alterations that occur in the retinal and capillary circulations in diabetics. Furthermore, the circumstances under which capillary basement membrane thickening in other organs truly reflects the same primary processes operative in the retinal and glomerular circulations remain to be established.

Østerby examined renal biopsies by quantitative electron microscopic methods and demonstrated that the appearance and width of the glomerular capillary basement membrane (GBM) and the appearance and area of the mesangial regions are normal at the outset of juvenile diabetes.[46] In repeat biopsies obtained 1½ to 2½ years after the onset of disease she found evidence of significant thickening of the peripheral glomerular capillary basement membrane with a parallel increase in the quantity of base-membrane-like material in the mesangium. However, the area of the mesangial regions, the number of cells in the glomerulus, and the percentage of mesangial, endothelial, and epithelial cells were not significantly altered during the first 5 years of juvenile diabetes.[52] Thus there is no evidence of an alteration in GBM or in GBM-like material in the mesangium which antedates the development of a detectable abnormality in plasma glucose regulation in these patients. Recent studies have demonstrated that the glomerular filtration rate, renal plasma flow, and kidney size as measured by x-ray tend to be increased in newly diagnosed juvenile diabetics, and that both GFR and kidney size fall significantly after insulin treatment for a few months.[53] Østerby observed that the volume of the glomerular tuft, both of the capillary lumina and the individual glomerular cells, is increased in newly diagnosed juvenile diabetics without any increase in cell number. A partial normalization of these alterations was apparent in biopsies obtained after 1–6 years of disease. Østerby has suggested that these changes could reflect a pressure-induced unfolding which may have a relationship to the increased GFR.`

Basement membranes are extracellular matrices which are widely distributed in both vascular and avascular tissues. The cells responsible for the synthesis of GBM are currently believed to be the epithelial cells, but the supporting evidence is far from conclusive. In recent years it has been possible to isolate relatively intact glomeruli from mammalian and human kidneys, to remove the cellular components by sonification, and to obtain preparations of GBM for analysis. Studies of the amino acids and carbohydrate composition of bovine GBM by Spiro[54,55] and of human GBM by Beisswenger and Spiro[56] indicate a relationship between GBM and the collagen family of proteins despite the amorphous appearance of the GBM on EM examination. These workers found that glycine accounted for 22 percent of the amino acid residues in human GBM, and that the GBM contained significant quantities of hydroxyproline (8.4 percent) and hydroxylysine (2.1 percent). However, there are important differences between the compositions of human and bovine GM and that of fibrillar collagen: there is a much higher hydroxylysine content in the GBM, a significant number of half-cystine residues (2.1 percent) which are absent from tropocollagen, and sugar residues account for approximately 7 percent of the dry weight of the GBM, but less than 1 percent in tropocollagen.[55] (Westberg and Michael also noted that in common with other basement membranes, in human GBM a significant proportion of the hydroxyproline has a hydroxyl group in the 3 position of the pyrrolidine ring instead of the 4 position.[57]

Studies of bovine and human GBM indicate that the carbohydrate is present in two distinct units, one being a disaccharide of glucose and galactose linked to the hydroxyl group of hydroxylysine (2-O-α-D-glucopyranosyl-5-O-β-D-galactopyranosylhydroxylysine). The higher molecular weight carbohydrate unit is a branched heteropolysaccharide containing sialic acid, fucose, galactose, glucosamine, and mannose which are linked to asparagine units. The carbohydrate is equally distributed by weight between these two types of units with 10 disaccharides for every heteropolysaccharide.[55,56] Beisswenger and Spiro compared the composition of GBM isolated from the kidneys of 8 insulin-requiring diabetics who had moderate to severe glomerular changes on histologic examination after 6 to 20 or more years of disease, with that of GBM from nondiabetics of a comparable age span.[56] They found that GBM isolated from the diabetics' kidneys contained an increased hydroxylysine content and a proportionally decreased lysine content; the sum of the lysine and hydroxylysine residues/1000 amino acid residues was the same in normal and diabetic GBM. These authors also observed an increase in the glucose and galactose content of the diabetic GBM, and an increase in the ratio of disaccharide to heteropolysaccharide units. The percentage of hydroxylysine residues which were glucosylated was the same in the normal and diabetic GBM. Less significant differences were observed in hydroxyproline and glycine, which were increased in the diabetic GBM. Beisswenger and Spiro suggested that in addi-

tion to the increased quantity of GBM associated with individual glomeruli there appeared to be a specific alteration in the chemical composition of the GBM in patients with long-standing diabetes mellitus, and that their findings were compatible with an overproduction in the diabetics of those subunits of the basement membrane that are rich in hydroxylysine and its linked disaccharide unit. Westberg and Michael[57] and Kefalides[58] have independently reported that they could not detect alterations in the composition of GBM isolated from the kidneys of long-standing diabetics similar to those described by Beisswenger and Sprio, although Westberg and Michael did note a decrease in half-cystine residues. The extent to which these discrepant observations may have resulted from the differences in methodology and in the populations examined in these studies has not been clarified. Beisswenger reported that GBMs isolated from the kidneys of nondiabetics with a variety of diseases affecting the glomerulus did not differ in their amino acid and carbohydrate composition from that of GBM isolated from age-matched controls.[59] The resolution of this controversy will probably require further clarification of the structure of GBM and of the processes involved in its synthesis, extracellular assembly, and degradation, Studies by Hudson and Spiro suggest that disulfide bonds are the major cross-links in GBM, and about 80 percent of the reduced alkylated bovine GBM is soluble in sodium dodecyl sulfate. These workers have separated and identified a number of subunits from such preparations which exhibit a marked heterogeneity unrelated to molecular weight.[60,61] It has been suggested that this may result from postribosomal steps in biosynthesis, and from physiological degradative processes. Bornstein has reviewed the data which suggest that genetically distinct procollagens exist in different tissues of the same animal, and that several genetically distinct "collagens," including chick lens basement membrane, are synthesized as higher molecular weight precursors.[62] There has been an explosive development of information concerning the precursor of fibrillar collagen, procollagen, and its extracellular conversion to collagen; however, comparable data concerning the synthesis of a vascular basement membrane are still lacking.

Thus at present there is general agreement that there is an increase in GBM thickness in association with diabetes mellitus, but controversy concerning the changes in composition and structure which may occur in association with long-standing diabetes. However, none of the workers in this field have found evidence of an inherited abnormality in GBM composition in diabetics. Since the cells responsible for GBM synthesis, extracellular modification, and degradation have not been clearly identified the specific site or sites of the primary disturbance responsible for the development of a thickened GBM, or for the accumulation of GBM-like material in the mesangial regions, cannot be discerned. It is possible that the recently developed methods for the culture of human endothelial cells may provide a means of approaching this problem.

EXPERIMENTAL DATA

Efforts to study the pathogenesis of the alterations in GBM associated with long-standing human diabetes in animals with experimental diabetes have been hampered by the lack of a well-accepted model. There is considerable controversy concerning the relationship of the pathological changes found in the glomeruli of rats and rabbits with long-standing alloxan or streptozotocin diabetes (both of which are also renal toxins) and those occurring in human diabetics. Bloodworth et al. have reported the development of nodular glomerular sclerosis in dogs with long-term alloxan diabetes,[63] and in experimental diabetes induced by the administration of bovine growth hormone.[64] These workers have reported the development of diffuse glomerulosclerosis in monkeys with chronic alloxan diabetes (in excess of 7 years) and in isolated instances a nodular lesion.[65] The source of the controversy concerning these observations has invariably been the degree of similarity of the lesions observed to those occurring in humans, and the specificity of the changes; in this regard the occasional development of nodular lesions not associated with other forms of renal disease in these animals is of interest. Pending the clarification of a suitable animal model, the significance of studies of the effects of acute or chronic experimental diabetes on the incorporation of labeled amino acids into total protein or protein recovered with ''purified'' GBM following in vitro incubation of isolated glomeruli is difficult to evalute. Although some workers have reported increased incorporation of labeled proline or lysine into GBM protein,[66] Beisswenger recently reported that acute and chronic streptozotocin diabetes did not significantly alter the apparent rates of incorporation of lysine into lysine or hydroxylysine residues in GBM following incubation of glomeruli from these animals.[67] Moreover, he found no significant difference in the amino acid or carbohydrate composition of GBM from animals with streptozotocin diabetes of 14 months duration and normal controls. Hence, the significance of the observation that the enzyme catalyzing the glucosylation of galactosylhydroxylysine in rat kidney cortex is increased by alloxan diabetes and subject to modification by insulin treatment, which was interpreted as reflecting increased GBM synthesis in diabetes, is currently unresolved. Similarly, the significance of the provocative report by Mauer et al.[68] that rats with streptozotocin diabetes develop mesangial thickening with the deposition of large quantitites of immunoglobulins in the mesangium, and that successful pancreatic islet transplantation results in a reduction in mesangial thickening and in mesangial staining for IgG, IgM, and C3, has not been firmly established. Given the present stage of knowledge concerning the normal function and metabolism of the diverse cell types found in the renal glomeruli, it is difficult to attribute great significance to the difficulties encountered in developing appropriate animal models for human diabetic nephropathy.

There are numerous well-documented cases in which nodular glomerulosclerosis has been observed in patients with chronic pancreatitis or homochromatosis who lack a family history of diabetes. However, in the absence of a biochemical marker for genetically determined diabetes mellitus, some workers remain unconvinced of the significance of these observations.

OTHER FORMS OF RENAL DISEASE IN DIABETICS

As noted in the section on autonomic neuropathy the development of an increased residual bladder volume occurs in association with autonomic neuropathy in some patients[1] and may be a major factor in predisposing to chronic urinary tract infection which eventuates in uremia. In addition there is an association between diabetes mellitus and papillary necrosis.[43] Although classically this has been considered in cases with fever, renal colic, hematuria, and the passage of bits of tissue in the urine, it is more frequently demonstrated by radiological study in patients who are asymptomatic. On occasion rapidly progressive renal insufficiency results from papillary necrosis in diabetics. The mechanisms involved remain obscure but sclerosis of the intrarenal arteries, infection, and in some cases uretheral dilation and reflux due to altered bladder function resulting from diabetic neuropathy are considered significant factors.

OCULAR COMPLICATIONS OF DIABETES MELLITUS

DIABETIC RETINOPATHY

Introduction

Impaired vision in patients with diabetes mellitus can result from cataracts, refractive errors, and glaucoma. However, the most important ocular complications giving rise to blindness are the pathological alterations in the retina which are collectively referred to as diabetic retinopathy. Caird et al., using data derived from studies in Great Britain, estimate that 2 percent of the diabetic population in that country is blind, a figure which is 10 times that for the general population.[69] He noted that the diabetic is at least 10 times, and probably nearer 20 times, more likely to become blind from retinopathy than a nondiabetic from all other causes of blindness put together. Clinically detectable retinopathy is virtually unknown under age 10, and is very rare under age 15. It then increases steadily in frequency until about age 40 and then remains roughly constant at about 30 to 35 percent. Retinopathy is rarely observed at the time of diagnosis in patients who are under 40, but the frequency of retinopathy at the time of diagnosis increases with age, reaching 10 percent in patients age 61–70. In patients diagnosed before age 30 retinopathy is relatively unusual during the initial 5 years, but the frequency rises rapidly to 50 percent after 12 years and 75 percent or more after 20 years. Irrespective of the age at diagnosis, diabetics have a 50 percent chance of having clinically detectable retinopathy 10–15 years after diagnosis. The British workers classify patients with more severely affected eyes (preretinal hemorrhage, new vessel formation, and glial proliferation) as having ''malignant retinopathy.''[69] In their experience in patients diagnosed before age 30 malignant retinopathy is rare during the first 15 years. Caird found no definite evidence of any particular racial susceptibility to diabetic retinopathy, although the literature is confusing since age at diagnosis and duration of disease are frequently ignored. The possibility of independent genetic factors modifying the frequency of diabetic retinopathy in patients with diabetes mellitus has not been excluded. However, a study of 75 families, each with more than one diabetic member, failed to demonstrate any aggregation of patients with retinopathy within families.[69]

The diagnosis of diabetic retinopathy, its classification, and the information available concerning its course are based on ophthalmoscopic examination, supplemented in some instances by slit lamp examination of the retina, and fluorescein angiography of the retina. Davis and co-workers have noted that while there is general agreement about the ophthalmoscopic appearance of diabetic retinopathy, it is difficult or impossible to define it in such a way as to exclude the similar fundus appearance sometimes seen in hypertension, ''severe arteriosclerosis,'' branch vein occlusion, dysproteinemias, and rare retinal vascular anomalies.[70] (This candor is not always evident in discussions of diabetic retinopathy by endocrinologists.)

Ophthalmologists conventionally classify diabetic retinopathy into two major stages: nonproliferative and proliferative. This classification is incorporated into the Airlie House classification based on photographic and ophthalmoscopic findings which was formulated to provide a framework for prospective studies.[70]

Nonproliferative Diabetic Retinopathy

It is first manifested by microaneurysms which can be seen by routine ophthalmoscopy, but their recognition is greatly facilitated by fluoroscein angiography. These are globular or fusiform outpouchings varying in color from purple-red to yellow-white, ranging in size from 10 to 200 μm and arising from one side of the capillary wall. Fluoroscein angiography has shown that microaneurysms are particularly prominent around the edges of areas of nonperfused obliterated capillaries.[71] Endocrinologists customarily describe small red dots in the posterior fundus of a diabetic on routine ophthalmoscopic examination as *microaneurysms,* ignoring the lack of pathological precision required for this diagnosis and the fact that many ophthalmologists confess their inability to distinguish some of these dots from punctate hemorrhages. The dots vary in size from just visible pinpoints to those whose diameter approximates a width of a retinal arteriole. They sometimes lie alongside larger vessels, but are usually away from them. Their numbers vary and they may be present in small groups of clusters.

In the experience at the Radcliffe Infirmary Diabetic Clinic from 1949 to 1965 microaneurysms were the only or earliest evidence of diabetic retinopathy in 24 percent of patients, this being most commonly the case in younger patients. However, in most patients microaneurysms are accompanied by hemorrhages or exudates.[69] It must be noted that true microaneurysms have been observed in association with a variety of other diseases; however, in some instances their distribution in the retina characteristically differs. These conditions include malignant hypertension, retinal vein thrombosis, Eales' disease, macroglobulinemia, multiple myeloma, pulseless disease, and sickle cell anemia.[69] Studies by light microscopy of trypsin-digested preparations of the retinas from patients with early diabetic retinopathy have demonstrated that the microaneurysms tend to occur around the margins of a region in which the cellular components of the capillary (the endothelial cells and pericytes) are no longer distinguishable, suggesting an area of capillary occlusion. The microaneurysms in these preparations vary in appearance, some being highly cellular, and others having very thickened walls which stain intensely with PAS; the latter are considered by some workers to be a later stage in the same process. Cogan and Kuwabara have called attention to the presence of larger caliber, dilated, hypercellular capillaries (shunt vessels) which tend to occur in association with areas of occluded capillaries.[72] These investigators have suggested that the initial lesion is a loss of capillary pericytes resulting in loss of capillary tone, microaneurysm formation, and dilatation of some capillaries which shunt blood leading to obliteration of adjacent capillaries. Other workers feel that the sequence is just the reverse, and that capillary obliteration results in secondary dilatation of some vascular channels.[73] Smith and Becker conclude that regardless of the precise initial sequence, retinal capillary closure occurs early in the natural history of diabetic retinopathy, inducing tissue hypoxia which can be demonstrated by clinical and pathological techniques.[71]

Retinal edema is common in both nonproliferative and proliferative diabetic retinopathy. It often involves the macula and is the most common cause of reduced vision in nonproliferative retinopathy. On ophthalmoscopic examination (or less commonly on slit lamp examination of the retina) the macula appears swollen; in these circumstances fluoroscein angiograms show diffuse intraretinal leakage of fluoroscein which is thought to reflect an altered permeability of the surrounding capillaries.[74]

Retinal edema is commonly found in association with microaneurysms in nonproliferative diabetic retinopathy. It is now recognized that soft exudates ("cotton wool spots") are very common in relatively early diabetic retinopathy and seem to be unrelated to the presence of hypertension. These grayish-white lesions with indistinct borders have been shown to result from microinfarctions in the superficial nerve fiber layer; this has been interpreted as

supporting the fundamental role of closure of capillaries and/or terminal arterioles in early diabetic retinopathy.

Another ophthalmoscopic manifestation of nonproliferative diabetic retinopathy is the presence of "hard or "waxy" exudates. These are discrete yellow-white flecks usually occurring near areas of abnormal capillaries and microaneurysms; they may form a partial or complete circle around an edematous macula. Pathologically these are pockets of protein and lipid presumably extravasated in the deep layers of the retina.[71]

Abnormalities of the retinal veins consisting of uniform dilatation, irregular construction, and increased tortuosity have been described in diabetics. Clinically, uniform dilatation is difficult to assess, but in younger diabetics Kohner et al. have demonstrated an increase in the caliber of the retinal veins which tends to increase with increasing duration of disease[75]; there have been reports that this can disappear in association with modifications in hyperglycemic treatment.

Retinal hemorrhages are commonly round or "blot" hemorrhages in the deeper retinal layers. However, flame-shaped hemorrhages in the superficial layers also occur. Hemorrhages tend to occur in the posterior pole, and when attributed to diabetic retinopathy are almost always accompanied by exudates or microaneurysms.

The presence of nonproliferative diabetic retinopathy does not necessarily portend a visual handicap or the development of blindness. At present the course of nonproliferative diabetic retinopathy in any given patient is quite unpredictable, although there appears to be some relationship to visual acuity at the time of diagnosis and also to the duration of diabetes. Sequential ophthalmologic examination of patients with early diabetic retinopathy has demonstrated that over a period of months individual "microaneurysms" may remain unaltered, may disappear, or may be replaced by hemorrhage, a small white dot, or exudate.

Proliferative Diabetic Retinopathy

This is characterized by the appearance of neovascularization which first appears as a "brush" of fine capillaries in an area where the normal capillary bed has been damaged or destroyed. The sites of predelection are the optic disc, along the course of main vessels, and in the equatorial region. The appearance of neovascularization drastically changes the clinical picture and prognosis. The new vessels form networks along the inner surface of the retina and follow a cycle of proliferation and regression. They first appear as fine-walled vessels; after a period of time there appears to be an increase in the size of the vessels with evidence of the formation of surrounding connective tissue. Over a period of 1–2 years there is usually regression and scarring with the formation of an avascular connective tissue mass over the retina and disc associated with an attenuation of the normal retinal arterioles. Adhesions form between this network of fibrovascular tissue and the vitreous body. When the vitreous contracts these fragile vessels are pulled forward, resulting in vitreous hemorrhage and/or retinal detachment which are the two major causes of blindness.[71]

The rate of progression of proliferative diabetic retinopathy is variable. Occasionally it will go into remission, during which the vitreous contraction and recurrent hemorrhages stop, and there is overall ischemia of the retina. The therapy of diabetic retinopathy is less than satisfactory at this time. No proven medical therapy exists and there is still controversy concerning the relationship of the development or progression of significant diabetic retinopathy to the arbitrary standards of control now in common use.

The observation that postpartum pituitary insufficiency was associated with a dramatic improvement in diabetic retinopathy in a young diabetic[76] led to the introduction of hypophysectomy and pituitary ablation, by a variety of means, for the treatment of rapidly advancing proliferative retinopathy. Kohner has reviewed the results of a controlled, randomized study of pituitary ablation carried out at Hammersmith Hospital in London by means of transphenoidal yttrium-90 implantation.[77] Although the procedure appeared to have some value, the significant mortality associated with pituitary ablation and the development of photocoagulation subsequently led that group to restrict pituitary ablation to patients with new vessels on the disc.

Photocoagulation employs the use of high intensity light from a xenon arc or laser to produce a "burn" with subsequent scarring in the posterior part of the eye. Photocoagulation is used primarily in proliferative retinopathy but has also been employed in nonproliferative retinopathy when vision is impaired due to mascular edema; in this instance the therapy is thought to aid in sealing leaks demonstrated by fluoroscein angiography. In proliferative retinopathy photocoagulation is thought to decrease the stimulus to neovascularization by destroying areas of critical ischemia, by destroying new vessels which might hemorrhage, by decreasing leakage from permeable capillaries, and by inducing chorioretinal adhesions and thus limiting the ease of retinal detachment and by diminishing metabolic requirements of the retina.[71]

The Diabetic Retinopathy Study is a randomized, controlled clinical trial being carried out in 15 centers in the U. S. to evaluate the benefit of photocoagulation in preventing severe visual loss in eyes with proliferative retinopathy. A preliminary, 2-year report documented the high risk of severe visual loss when neovascularization was classified as moderate or severe on entry into the study, particularly when it involved the optic disc, and most particulary when accompanied by fresh hemorrhage. The effects of treating one randomly selected eye with zenon arc or argon laser photocoagulation in these high risk patients were so striking that the trial organizers felt constrained to modify the protocol and recommend treatment for the control eyes.[78] Vitrectomy is just now being evaluated in a randomized controlled trial. As noted previously some degree of retinopathy is almost invariably present in patients with renal failure attributed to diabetic nephropathy. The frequent coexistence of ASHD and renal disease in patients in whom blindness results from diabetic retinopathy undoubtedly accounts for the mortality of about 15 percent per year regardless of age. This is about 20 times that mortality of diabetics age 25, and twice that of diabetics at age 70. The median survival is less than 5 years.

Pathogenesis

The pathogenesis of diabetic retinopathy is at present largely a matter of speculation. Although it is commonly considered a manifestation of diabetic microangiopathy the meaning of this term as applied to the retinal circulation has not been clearly defined. If the initial event is the loss of the capillary pericyte, as suggested by Cogan and Kuwabara,[72] it must be noted that, as yet, there is no evidence that a similar process occurs in the renal glomerular capillaries, or in skeletal muscle capillaries, in diabetics. If retinal capillary obliteration is the initial event,[73] the presence of PAS-positive material in the remnants provides little indication of the nature of the primary process. Although alterations in capillary permeability could contribute to retinal edema and subsequent closure of retinal capillaries, this remains to be evaluated. The nature of the microaneurysms also requires clarification. Most diabetic microaneurysms are thin-walled, but some have a thick wall which stains intensely with PAS. Endothelial cell degeneration and proliferation, plus basement membrane thickening with vacuolization, are also observed. Ashton has suggested that micro-

aneurysms may represent abortive attempts at neovascularization.[73] The stimulus for neovascularization is unknown, although it is frequently suggested that hypoxia either directly or through the mediation of tissue factors released in response to hypoxia, is important. Explanation is also required for the evidence that impaired color vision alterations in electrooculography and electroretinopathy, decreased flicker fusion response, and small blind spots identified by scotometry may be present in newly diagnosed diabetics without evidence of ophthalmoscopically apparent retinopathy.[71]

Limited information concerning the pathogenesis of diabetic retinopathy can be derived from studies attempting to relate the degree of "control" with the frequency or progression of diabetic retinopathy, or from the observation that retinopathy of similar appearance occurs in patients with diabetes that is apparently nongenetic in origin. Reports of "diabetic retinopathy" in patients with normal glucose tolerance tests and increased muscle capillary basement thickening are difficult to evaluate since the validity of the latter as a marker for genetically determined diabetes is not firmly established, and the ophthalmoscopic findings are not necessarily unique to diabetic retinopathy. Efforts to develop suitable animal models for studies of diabetic retinopathy still lag. The existence of significant species differences in the retinal circulation and in other aspects of retinal and ocular structure is now well recognized. The occurrence of lesions resembling those found in human diabetics has been reported in a number of spontaneous forms of diabetes in rodents and fish, and the development of microaneurysms has been reported to occur in rats with chronic streptozotocin diabetes.

CATARACTS

Under the age of 40 lens opacities are rare enough in the general population for their occurrence in a diabetic to be at least presumptively attributed to diabetes. Over the age of 40 there must always be some doubt about the relationship between lens opacity and diabetes in the individual patient regardless of the morphological type of cataract. There is no doubt that cataract extraction is more common in diabetics (Caird et al.[79] found that 8.8 percent of patients having their first extraction of a senile cataract were known diabetics and a further 4.2 percent were found to be diabetics). However, the common assumption that cataracts occur more frequently in diabetics than nondiabetics is not as well documented. Only one form of cataract is considered characteristic of diabetes mellitus, the "snowflake" pattern of opacity. Most of the reported cases have been in adolescents or infants and have usually been associated with symptomatic hyperglycemia. These cataracts may progress rapidly, and there are well-documented reports of regression in response to therapy that decreases the degree of hyperglycemia.[69]

Rats with experimental diabetes develop cataracts with great regularity, and with a rapidity which is related to the degree of hyperglycemia.[80] In these animals cataract formation can be prevented or delayed by lowering the plasma glucose by insulin treatment[80] or by the administration of phloridzin.[81] When rabbit lenses are maintained in organ culture high concentrations of glucose increase the rapidity with which lens opacities develop.[82] The development of experimental "sugar cataracts" has been shown to be related to increased polyol pathway activity in the lens as originally suggested by van Heyningen.[83] Hyperglycemia results in an increased glucose concentration in aqueous humor, and since the intracellular transport of glucose is not rate limiting for glucose phosphorylation in lens, there is a rise in the free intracellular glucose concentration in the lens. The lens and many other mammalian tissues contain alditol:NADP oxidoreductase, an enzyme that catalyzes the reduction of glucose to its polyhydric alcohol or polyol derivative, sorbitol. This enzyme has a high apparent K_m for glucose and its activity appears to be regulated by the intracellular glucose concentration.[84] Although sorbitol is a normal constituent of rat and human lens, greatly elevated concentrations are found in the lens in hyperglycemic rats and humans. The increased concentrations of sorbitol are probably the explanation for the associated increase in tissue free fructose concentration which results from the oxidation of sorbitol by an NAD:polyol dehydrogenase, which resembles liver sorbitol dehydrogenase. Mutant mice that lack lens alditol:NADP oxidoreductase do not develop cataracts after the induction of experimental diabetes, whereas related strains who have the lens enzyme develop cataracts with great regularily.[85] Chylack and Kinoshita have also demonstrated that the development of opacities in cultured lenses exposed to high glucose concentrations can be prevented by the addition of an inhibitor of lens alditol:NADP oxidoreductase to the medium.[82] Kinoshita attributes the relationship between increased polyol pathway activity and the development of "sugar cataracts" to the osmotic effects of the increased lens sorbitol concentrations.[86] Most mammalian cells lack systems for the facilitated transport of sorbitol across the cell membrane (the liver being an obvious exception), and despite an apparent increase in the rate of sorbitol oxidation to fructose the increases in lens sorbitol that occur in experimental diabetes are sufficient to exert a significant osmotic effect. Support for this "osmotic hypothesis" is provided by the fact that the alterations in the active concentration of amino acid and free myoinositol and in the regulation of the ion composition of the lens which occur when lenses are maintained in organ culture with high concentrations of glucose or galactose, can be modified by increasing the osmolality of the medium.[87-89] The "osmotic hypothesis" was initially an outgrowth of early light microscopic studies which suggested that the development of "sugar cataracts" results from hydropic swelling of the lens fibers which progressed to rupture of the lens fibers and local deposition of a proteinaceous debris. However, recent EM studies indicate that this is not the case.[90] An early event in the formation of "sugar cataracts" is a marked proliferation of the rough endoplasmic reticulum in the anterior lens epithelial cells which normally consist of a single cell layer; these cells subsequently proliferate and form a multicell layer. While cytoplasmic vacuoles appear in the course of cataract formation, a more striking early change is the appearance of large fluid-filled spaces outside the lens fibers. The relationship of these alterations to the "osmotic hypothesis" remain to be clarified. Increased polyol pathway activity is believed to play a role in the pathogenesis of "snowflake" cataracts and possibly of the transient myopia which so often occurs in diabetics; its contribution to the development of senile cataracts has not been established.

GLAUCOMA

In diabetics glaucoma may develop in association with neovascularization of the iris (rubeosis iridis), which in diabetics is almost invariably associated with severe proliferative retinopathy. In addition Becker has shown that primary open angle glaucoma, which is believed to result from some unexplained change in the channels which permit egress of aqueous humor, is more prevalent in diabetics than nondiabetics.[91] Diabetics with wide angle glaucoma appear to be more susceptible to glaucomatous visual field loss, although proliferative retinopathy appears to occur less frequently in these patients.

DISEASE OF THE FOOT AND LEG IN DIABETICS

INTRODUCTION

Diabetes mellitus is associated wth an increased morbidity and mortality from syndromes affecting the foot and leg whose development is conditioned by alterations in the circulation and/or innervation of the lower extremity. The frequency of intermittent claudication, foot ulcer, osteomyelitis, infections including gangrene, and amputations in adult diabetics is so excessive in comparison with nondiabetics that the association is generally accepted although the statistical data are still inadequate. Present evidence suggests that approximately 50 percent of amputations of portions of the lower extremities in the United States are performed on patients with clinically evident diabetes mellitus. The frequency of gangrene of the foot or leg has been estimated to be 50 to 70 times greater in diabetics than in nondiabetics,[92] and Wahlberg has reported that approximately one-third of a series of patients with intermittent claudication had impaired glucose tolerance.[93]

ISCHEMIC DISEASE OF THE LOWER EXTREMITY IN DIABETICS

Atherosclerosis is the pathological process that conditions the development of intermittent claudication and of acute arterial occlusions that result in acute ischemia. Chronic or acute arterial occlusion and ischemia condition the development of foot ulcers in specific diabetics, and the development of gangrene affecting a large segment of the lower extremity in diabetics is primarily associated with occlusive atherosclerotic lesions. The locations of the atherosclerotic lesions resulting in clinical manifestations in the lower extremities of diabetics appear to differ from the usual locations in nondiabetics. In the diabetics the tibial and popliteal arteries are most frequently involved, whereas in nondiabetics lesions in the aorta, iliac, or femoral arteries are more frequently responsible for clinical manifestations. Moreover, in the diabetic multisegmental occlusions with diffuse mural change proximal and distal are more frequently observed in the affected arteries, and the frequency with which significant occlusions are present in both lower extremities is also greater. As noted by Levin,[94] these characteristics result in a much poorer prognosis for reconstructive vascular surgery in the diabetic since the affected vessels are smaller, the affected segment is longer, and the vessels above and below the occlusion are more likely to be diseased.

The development of foot ulcer in certain diabetics can be attributed primarily either to vascular insufficiency or to diabetic polyneuropathy, but in many instances the two processes coexist and a clear distinction is impossible. An effort to distinguish the primary factor is important since the risk of rapidly progressive infection which may threaten the life of the patient is usually associated with ulcers occurring in limbs with severe vascular insufficiency. A history of intermittent claudication or rest pain, the presence of cold feet that blanch on elevation and exhibit a delayed return of dependent rubor when lowered, and absent pedal pulses would strongly suggest the presence of arterial occlusive disease and vascular insufficiency. Because of the attendant risk, arteriography is primarily employed as a preoperative technique in such patients, but noninvasive methods for assessing blood flow have been found useful in some centers. The presence of gas in an infected foot lesion in the diabetic, irrespective of the primary conditioning process, does not necessarily indicate a clostridial infection, although this does occur; in the diabetic, anaerobic streptococci, *Escherichia,* and *Bacteroides* are frequently associated with gas-forming infections of the lower extremity, and mixed infections are not uncommon. In patients with severe vascular insufficiency of the leg or foot the development of a foot ulcer is potentially lifethreatening because of the risk of rapidly progressive infection and toxemia. This consideration dictates the hospitalization of these patients and the active participation of a skilled surgical consultant in the patient's management from the outset. Even if healing occurs with the relief of the pressure of weight bearing, appropriate antibiotics, and local wound care, the risk of recurrence is high unless the vascular insufficiency is transient or can be corrected by surgery. Even though the affected area may appear to be restricted, if surgery is required, it is more likely to involve an extensive amputation because of the necessity to avoid a surgical wound in ischemic tissue.

It is frequently stated that the development of ischemic foot ulcer in the diabetic may be significantly influenced by the presence of "small blood vessel disease" and may occur in the presence of good pulses and in the absence of evidence of significant occlusive arterial disease. However, the validity of this view remains to be documented. Hyalinization of arterioles and "proliferative" changes in arteriolar endothelium have been reported to be more pronounced in the limbs of diabetics than in nondiabetics,[95] but both the nature of the "proliferative" changes and the significance of arteriolosclerosis in the pathogenesis of peripheral vascular complications in the diabetic are matters of dispute. Skin capillaries from the big toes of diabetics have been reported to have an increased width of their basement membranes when compared with skin capillaries in nondiabetics.[96] The quantitative assessment of skin capillary basement membrane width presents technical problems because it consists of many lamellae separated by spaces of variable width. There is no firm evidence of widespread occlusive capillary disease in the skin or other tissues of the foot in chronic diabetics. Moreover, there is as yet no evidence that increased capillary basement membrane width significantly impairs the transcapillary exchange of nutrients, oxygen, or CO_2. It is possible that the role of the capillary endothelium as a selective diffusion barrier is modified in the feet of the diabetic as appears to occur in the retina, but this remains to be demonstrated and its pathological potential in the foot established. Medial calcification of the muscular arteries of the leg appears to occur at an earlier age and with increased severity in diabetics. However, this process is independent of atherosclerosis affecting the intima, and as is the case with "small blood vessel disease" there is no firm evidence that it contributes to the peripheral vascular complications in the lower extremities of diabetics.

FOOT ULCER ASSOCIATED WITH DIABETIC POLYNEUROPATHY

In some diabetics the development of foot ulcer appears to be primarily conditioned by the consequences of distal symmetrical diabetic polyneuropathy. Atrophic changes in the skin of the feet similar to those observed with occlusive arterial disease are frequently associated with diabetic polyneuroapthy. Impaired pain, temperature, position, and vibration sensation may permit patients with diabetic polyneuropathy to suffer mechanical, thermal, or chemical trauma (keratolytic agents) to their feet without discomfort. This may result in ulceration which is most commonly plantar and occurs over a pressure point, but may occur at other sites of trauma. In some patients the development of an ulcer is conditioned by changes in the shape of the foot that may create new pressure points. Neuropathic atrophy of the interosseus muscles may thus result in pressure on the metatarsal heads. Diabetic polyneuropathy may condition the development of Charcot joints affecting the tarsal or metatarsal–phalangeal joints (usually unilaterally) which may also alter the conformation of the foot and lead to ulcers at the new pressure points. Local infection of neuropathic ulcers is common, and osteomyelitis may occur if bone is exposed or penetrated by the ulcer. However, rapidly progressive infection with toxemia is not the imminent threat that it is in patients with ulcers associated with severe vascular insufficiency. Appropriate attention to the bacteriology of the wound infection is essential, for infection with nonclostridial gasforming organisms has on occasion resulted in unnecessary or excessively mutilating amputations. Evidence of osteolysis affecting the metatarsals and phalanges may occur in the foot of the diabetic in the absence of osteomyelitis; these changes are more commonly encountered when evidence of vascular insufficiency is absent, and are used by some workers as a guide in efforts to determine the primary factor in the development of a foot ulcer. The prognosis for foot ulcers that appear to be primarily conditioned by diabetic polyneuropathy is better than for those primarily conditioned by occlusive arterial disease, although recurrence is common and restricted amputations are all too frequently required. The management of patients with neuropathic foot ulcers requires relief from weight bearing on the foot, and wound care with appropriate bacteriological and surgical consultation. Adequate attention to the prevention of subsequent mechanical, thermal, or chemical trauma to the feet is an essential factor in reducing the risk of recurrence. In some patients weight reduction, changes in occupation, or in patterns of activity may be required to minimize the risk of trauma to the feet. However, in the absence of consistently effective treatment for diabetic polyneuropathy the patient remains at risk for recurrent ulcer throughout his or her life.

GENERAL THEORIES OF PATHOGENESIS

The foregoing account of the diverse clinical syndromes associated with chronic diabetes mellitus should make clear the obstacles to the formulation or acceptance of any simple general theory for their pathogenesis. These syndromes are not inexorable consequences of diabetes mellitus, as currently diagnosed, but are true complications whose development in any given patient is unpredictable. Their manifestations reflect disease of diverse organs and cell types, and their pathological basis is diverse and complex. In many instances the normal biology and biochemistry of the affected tissue or cell type are very poorly understood. There is no means, at present, for distinguishing patients with diabetes mellitus according to the specific etiology of the syndrome, and the possibility that the process responsible for beta-cell dysfunction and pathology may directly affect other cell types in specific forms of diabetes cannot be evaluated. The heterogeneity of the diabetic population raises the likely possibility of the existence of independently determined genetic and environmental factors that can alter the likelihood of developing a specific complication. This can be illustrated by the data suggesting that the association between diabetes and hypertriglyceridemia in survivors of a myocardial infarction reflects the increased risk of this complication in patients who have both diabetes mellitus and familial hypertriglyceridemia or familial combined hyperlipidemia. Similarly, in specific patients the development of overt diabetic neuropathy may be related to the additive effects of neurotoxins (e.g., alcohol) and pressure injuries. In many instances the overt clinical manifestations of a diabetic complication occur at a late stage in the underlying pathological process, and in tissues in which the degree of subclinical pathology cannot be accurately evaluated without invasive techniques. Because of these considerations, the problem of assembling appropriately characterized groups for studies designed to derive information concerning pathogenesis of even a single specific complication from clinical trials is a formidable task.

Despite these obstacles the controversy concerning the value of currently available treatment with regard to preventing the complications of diabetes mellitus has become linked in most physicians' minds to a controversy over the validity of two general theories for their pathogenesis. In their simplest forms these theories can be stated as follows: (1) All of the currently recognized forms of diabetes mellitus are characterized by hyperglycemia and an abnormality in insulin secretion; metabolic derangements resulting from hyperglycemia and/or insulin deficiency are the primary factors in the development of the complications of diabetes. (2) Genetically determined diabetes mellitus is characterized by an inherited abnormality affecting capillaries in a wide range of tissues that is reflected in the development of increased capillary basement membrane thickness; this diabetic microangiopathy is unrelated to hyperglycemia and/or alterations in insulin secretion, and is the pathological basis for the development of diabetic retinopathy and nephropathy. (Some workers would still support the importance of this process in the pathogenesis of some foot ulcers, and of a specific form of cardiac disease with involvement of "small blood vessels.") Neither theory suffices to explain all the diverse clinical syndromes that constitute the late complications without significant modifications or exclusions. Thus the inherited diabetic micrangiopathy theory does not attempt to explain the increased incidence of myocardial infarction and peripheral arterial occlusions in diabetics, or in recent years the most common form of diabetic peripheral neuroapthy. Both of these hypotheses await convincing evidence of their general applicability. No firm conclusions can be drawn from clinical trials until means are developed that permit the prolonged maintenance in diabetics of the pattern of metabolic regulation that is dependent on a normal insulin secretory mechanism. (This is, of course, one of the rationales for efforts to examine the feasibility of islet transplantation and of developing an "artificial pancreas.") The successful development of appropriate models for specific complications in animals with experimental diabetes is still a matter of dispute, but may provide support for the "metabolic hypothesis" with regard to these complications. In general these efforts have not included serious consideration of the possible effects of independent genetic and environmental factors in determining the consequences of experimental diabetes in a given tissue or cell type.

The existence of widespread alterations in the ultrastructure of capillaries in long-standing diabetics, and their possible importance with regard to specific complications is not disputed. The relationship of these changes to overt evidence of hyperglycemia and other metabolic derangements resulting from an altered insulin secretory mechanism is the crux of the dispute over the "inherited microangiopathy hypothesis." The basic data in dispute do not concern the capillaries in organs where this process is believed to have its major significance with regard to the complications of diabetes, i.e., the renal glomerulus and the retina. Rather the controversy concerns the thickness of skeletal muscle capillary basement membrane, as quantitatively assessed in biopsies of the quadriceps femoris. Siperstein and his co-workers introduced the use of this technique to obtain quantitative data on the structure of capillaries in a tissue in which capillary structure lent itself to such methods and which could be biopsied in patients without undue

risk. Siperstein has reported that (using an upper limit of normal of 1600 Å) 91 percent of diabetic subjects over age 19 have thickened skeletal muscle capillary basement membranes, with a false positive error in nondiabetics of 2 percent, and concluded that thickening of muscle capillary BM is a remarkably constant feature of genetic diabetes.[97] His studies have failed to show any significant correlation between skeletal capillary BM width and such factors as the age of the diabetic subject, weight, or the severity of his carbohydrate abnormalities; nor did this author observe any relationship between glucose tolerance or insulin levels in normal subjects and skeletal muscle BM width. In 30 subjects considered to be "prediabetic" (because both of their parents were overt diabetics but who themselves had normal glucose tolerance tests and normal plasma insulin responses to glucose) Siperstein found that by variance analysis over 74 percent had increased skeletal muscle capillary BM width. On the basis of this and related data he concluded that his findings "would strongly suggest that diabetic vascular disease represents an independent and, conceivably, even a primary lesion of the diabetic syndrome."

These provocative observations are the subject of a continuing controversy. Williamson, Kilo, and their co-workers,[98] have reported that skeletal muscle capillary BM width significantly increases with age, and that the apparent rate of thickening with age differs in males and females. These workers reported that skeletal muscle capillary BM thickness increased with age more dramatically in diabetics than in nondiabetics and that on the average it is thicker in diabetics at all ages than in controls. However, the difference in capillary BM width was found to be minimal in the youngest diabetic subject and increased with the age of the patients studied. They stated that "this may be related to a longer known duration of diabetes, which in older subjects is very likely coupled with a longer duration of undetected asymptomatic carbohydrate intolerance." Their data also indicated a highly significant correlation between known duration of diabetes and the prevalence and magnitude of skeletal muscle capillary basement membrane thickening. The basis of these discrepant findings has been the subject of heated controversy. Differences in the techniques utilized to fix the tissue, to quantitatively assess BM width, and in the criteria used for the selection of subjects for study have been debated at length as possible explanations. The data of Siperstein indicate that the increase in skeletal capillary BM width plateaus by the onset of detectable hyperglycemia,[97] and his formualtion does not imply that changes in skeletal capillary BM width parallel in time those in the retinal or renal glomerular circulations. Indeed, he notes "it is unlikely that capillary basement membrane width in muscle will provide an accurate indication of this lesion in tissues such as the kidney or eye, where basement membrane thickness is probably related to the duration of overt diabetes."[97]

Without any judgment on the validity of the observations in skeletal capillary basement membrane, if it is agreed that the alterations in retinal and glomerular capillary structure appear to be related to duration of overt diabetes, as are the development of overt diabetic retinopathy and nephropathy, the basis for assuming that the alterations in capillary structure in these organs reflect an inherited abnormality that is independent of hyperglycemia and other metabolic derangements resulting from an altered insulin secretory mechanism is difficult to grasp.

The clarification of the pathogenesis of specific late complications will probably require less emphasis on efforts to develop general theories and more on an evaluation of the multiple factors that might contribute to the development of clinically significant pathology in the specific tissues affected in chronic diabetics. A multifactorial basis for many of these complications is strongly suggested by the very unpredictable nature of their occurrence in the diabetic population.

REFERENCES

1. Ellenberg, M.: Diabetic neuropathy. In Ellenberg, M. and Rifkin, H. (eds): Diabetes Mellitus: Theory and Practice. New York, McGraw-Hill, 1970, pp 822–847.
2. Adour, K. K., Winerd, J., and Doty, H. E.: Prevalence of concurrent diabetes mellitus and idiopathic facial paralysis (Bell's palsy). *Diabetes 24:* 449–451, 1971.
3. Friedman, S. A., and Schulman, R. H.: Hearing and diabetic neuropathy. *Arch Intern Med 135:* 573–576, 1975.
4. Asbury, A. K., Aldredge, H., Hershberg, R., and Fisher, C. M.: Oculomotor palsy in diabetes mellitus: A clinico-pathologic study. *Brain 93:* 555–566, 1960.
5. Locke, S.: The nervous system and diabetes. In Marble, A., White, P., Bradley, R. F., and Krall, L. P. (eds): Joslin's Diabetes Mellitus, 11th ed. Philadelphia, Lea & Febiger, 1971, pp 562–580.
6. Garland, H.: Diabetic amyotrophy. *Br Med J 2:* 1287–1290, 1955.
7. Raff, M. C. and Asbury, A. K.: Ischemic mononeuropathy and mononeuropathy multiplex in diabetes mellitus. *N Engl J Med 279:* 17–22, 1968.
8. Thomas, P. K. and Lascelles, R. G.: Schwann-cell abnormalities in diabetic neuropathy. *Lancet 1:* 1355–1357, 1965.
9. Dyck, P. J., Johnson, W. J., Lambert, E. H., and O'Brien P. C.: Segmental demyelination secondary to axonal degeneration in uremic neuropathy. *Mayo Clin Proc 46:* 400–431, 1971.
10. Chopra, J. S., Hurwitz, L. J., and Montgomery, D. A. D.: The pathogenesis of sural nerve changes in diabetes mellitus. *Brain 92:* 391–418, 1969.
11. Gregerson, G.: Variations in motor conduction velocity produced by acute changes of the metabolic state in diabetic patients. *Diabetologia 4:* 273–277, 1968.
12. Terkildsen, A. B. and Christensen, N. J.: Reversible nervous abnormalities in juvenile diabetics with recently diagnosed diabetes. *Diabetologia 7:* 113–117, 1971.
13. Gergerson, G.: Diabetic neuropathy: Influence of age, sex, metabolic control, and duration of diabetes on motor conduction velocity. *Neurology 17:* 972–980, 1967.
14. Schlaepfer, W. W., Gerritsen, G. C., and Dulin W. E.: Segmental demyelination in the distal peripheral nerves of chronically diabetic Chinese hamsters. *Diabetologia 10:* 541–548, 1974.
15. Eliasson, S. G.: Nerve conduction changes in experimental diabetes. *J Clin Invest 43:* 2353–2358, 1964.
16. Greene, D. A., DeJesus, P. V., Jr., and Winegrad, A. I.: Effects of insulin and dietary myoinositol on impaired peripheral motor nerve conduction velocity in acute streptozotocin diabetes. *J Clin Invest 55:* 1326–1336, 1975.
17. Schmidt, R. E., Matschinsky, F. M., Godfrey, D. A., Williams, A. D., and McDougal, D. B., Jr: Fast and slow axoplasmic flow in sciatic nerve of diabetic rats. *Diabetes 24:* 1081–1085, 1975.
18. Spritz, N., Singh, H., and Marinan, B.: Metabolism of peripheral nerve myelin in experimental diabetes. *J Clin Invest 55:* 1049–1056, 1975.
19. Stewart, M. A., Sherman W. R., Kurien, M. M., Moonsammy, G. I., and Wisgerhof, M.: Polyol accumulations in nervous tissue of rats with experimental diabetes and galactosemia. *J Neurochem 14:* 1057–1066, 1967.
20. Sherman, W. R., and Stewart, M. A.: Identification of sorbitol in mammalian nerve. *Biochem Biophys Res Commun 22:* 492–497, 1966.
21. Ward, J. D.: The polyol pathway in the neuropathy of early diabetes. In Camerini-Davalos, R. A. and Cole, H. S. (eds): Vascular and Neurological Changes in Early Diabetes. New York, Academic Press, 1973, pp 425–430.
22. Daughaday, W. H., Larner, J., and Houghton, E.: The renal excretion of inositol in normal and diabetic human beings. *J Clin Invest 33:* 326–332, 1954.
23. Palo, J., Savolainen, H., and Haltia, M.: Proteins of peripheral nerve myelin in diabetic neuropathy. *J Neurol Sci 16:* 193–199, 1972.
24. Murray, A., Ewing, D. J., Campbell, I. W., Neilson, J. M. M., and Clarke, B. F.: RR interval variations in young male diabetics. *Br Heart J 37:* 882–885, 1975.
25. Martin, M. M.: Involvement of autonomic nerve fibres in diabetic neuropathy. *Lancet 1:* 560–565, 1953.
26. Ellenberg, M. and Weber, H.: Retrograde ejaculation in diabetic neuropathy. *Ann Intern Med 65:* 1237–1246, 1966.
27. Brown, M. J., Martin, J. R., and Asbury, A. K.: Painful diabetic neuropathy. *Arch Neurol 33:* 164–171, 1976.
28. Faerman, I., Glocer, L., Celener, D., Jadzinsky, M., Fox, D., Maler, M., and Alvarez, E.: Autonomic nervous system and diabetes. *Diabetes 22:* 225–237, 1973.
29. Ostrander, L. D., Jr., and Epstein, F. H.: Diabetes, hyperglycemia and atherosclerosis: New research directions. In Fajans, S. S. (ed): Diabetes Mellitus (DHEW Publication No. (NIH) 76-854). Washington, D.C., U.S. Gov. Printing Office, 1976, pp 194–212.
30. Blackard, W. G., Omori, Y., and Freedman, L. R.: Epidemiology of diabetes mellitus in Japan. *J Chronic Dis 18:* 415–427, 1965.
31. Sasaki, A., Kamado, K., and Horiuchi, N.: A changing pattern of causes of death in Japanese diabetics: Observations over 14 years. In Baba, S., Goto, Y., and Fukui, I. (eds): Diabetes Mellitus in Asia. Amsterdam, Excerpta Medica, 1976, pp 98–108.
32. Garcia, M. J., McNamara, P. M., Gordon, T., and Kannell, W. B.: Morbidity and mortality in diabetics in the Framingham population. *Diabetes 23:* 105–111, 1974.
33. Pell, S., and D'Alonzo, C. A.: Factors associated with long-term survival of diabetics. *JAMA 214:* 1833–1840, 1970.
34. Bierman, E. L. and Porte, D., Jr: Carbohydrate intolerance and lipemia. *Ann Intern Med 68:* 926–933, 1968.
35. Goldstein, J. L., Hazzard, W. R., Schrott, H. G., Bierman, E. L., and Motulsky, A. G.: Hyperlipidemia in coronary heart disease. *J Clin Invest 52:* 1533–1577, 1973.
36. Goldstein, J. L., Hazzard, W. R., Schrott, H. G., Bierman, E. L., and Motulsky, A. G.: Genetics of hyperlipidemia in coronary heart disease. *Trans Assoc Am Physicians 85:* 120–138, 1972.
37. Brunzell, J. D., Hazzard, W. R., Motulsky, A. G., and Bierman, E. L.: Evidence for diabetes mellitus and genetic forms of hypertriglyceridemia as independent entities. *Metab Clin Exp 24:* 1115–1121, 1975.
38. Ross, R. and Glomset, J. A.: The pathogenesis of atherosclerosis. *N Engl J Med 295:* 369–377, 420–425, 1976.
39. Sagel, J., Colwell, J. A., Crook, L., and Laimins, M.: Increased platelet aggregation in early diabetes mellitus. *Ann Intern Med 82:* 733–738, 1975.
40. Stout, R. W., Bierman, E. L., and Ross, R.: Effect of insulin on the proliferation of cultured primate arterial smooth muscle cells. *Circ Res 36:* 319–327, 1975.
41. Evans, R. R., Morhenn, V., Jones, A. L., and Tomkins, G. M.: Concomitant effects of insulin on surface membrane conformation and polysome profiles of serum-starved Balb/c 3T3 fibroblasts. *J Cell Biol 61:* 95–106, 1974.
42. Morrison, A. D., Berwick, L., Orci, L., and Winegrad, A. I.: Morphology and metabolism of an aortic intima-media preparation in which an intact endothelium is preserved. *J Clin Invest 57:* 650–660, 1976.
43. Balodimos, M. C.: Diabetic nephropathy. In Marble, A., White, P., Bradley, R. F., and Krall, L. P. (eds): Joslin's Diabetes Mellitus, 11th ed. Philadelphia, Lea & Febiger, 1971, pp 526–561.
44. Kimmelstiel, P. and Wilson, C.: Intercapillary lesions in the glomeruli of the kidney. *Am J Pathol 12:* 83–97, 1936.
45. Østerby, R.: The number of glomerular cells and substructures in early juvenile diabetes. *Acta Pathol Microbiol Scand, Sec A 80:* 785–800, 1972.
46. Østerby, R.: Morphometric studies of the peripheral glomerular basement membrane in early juvenile diabetes. I. Development of initial basement membrane thickening. *Diabetologia 8:* 84–92, 1972.
47. Watkins, P. J., Blainey, J. D., Brewer, D. B., FitzGerald, M. G., Malins, J. M., O'Sullivan, D. J., and Pinto, J. A.: The natural history of diabetic renal disease. *Q J Med 41:* 437–456, 1972.
48. Shapiro, F. L., Leonard, A., and Comty, C. M.: Mortality, morbidity and rehabilitation results in regularly dialyzed patients with diabetes mellitus. *Kidney Int 6:* S8–S14, 1974.
49. Blagg, C. R., Eschbach, J. W., Sawyer, T. K., and Casaretto, A. A.: Dialysis for end-stage diabetic nephropathy. *Proc Clin Dial Transplant Forum 1:* 133–135, 1971.
50. Kjellstrand, C. M., Shideman, J. R., Simmons, R. L., Buselmeier, T. J., vonHartitzsch, B., Goetz, F. C., and Najarian, J. S.: Renal transplantation in insulin-dependent diabetic patients. *Kidney Int 6:* S15–S20, 1974.

51. Mauer, S. M., Barbosa, J., Vernier, R. L., Kjellstrand, C. M., Buselmeier, T. J., Simmons, R. L., Najarian, J. S., and Goetz, F. C.: Development of diabetic vascular lesions in normal kidneys transplanted into patients with diabetes mellitus. *N Engl J Med 295:* 916–920, 1976.

52. Lundbaek, K. and Østerby, R.: Renal disease in diabetes mellitus. In Fajans, S. S. (ed): Diabetes Mellitus (DHEW Publication No. (NIH) 76-854). Washington, D.C., U.S. Gov. Printing Office, 1976, pp 227–242.

53. Mogensen, C. E., and Andersen, M. J. F.: Increased kidney size and glomerular filtration rate in untreated juvenile diabetes: Normalization by insulin treatment. *Diabetologia 11:* 221–224, 1975.

54. Spiro, R. G.: Studies on the renal glomerular basement membrane: Preparation and chemical composition. *J Biol Chem 242:* 1915–1922, 1967.

55. Spiro, R. G.: Studies on the renal glomerular basement membrane: Nature of the carbohydrate units and their attachment to the peptide portion. *J Biol Chem 242:* 1923–1932, 1967.

56. Beisswenger, P. J. and Spiro, R. G.: Studies on the human glomerular basement membrane: Composition, nature of the carbohydrate units and chemical changes in diabetes mellitus. *Diabetes 22:* 180–193, 1973.

57. Westberg, N. G. and Michael, A. F.: Human glomerular basement membrane: Chemical composition in diabetes mellitus. *Acta Med Scand 194:* 34–47, 1973.

58. Kefalides, N. A.: Biochemical properties of human glomerular basement membrane in normal and diabetic kidneys. *J Clin Invest 53:* 403–407, 1974.

59. Beisswenger, P. J.: Specificity of the chemical alteration in the diabetic glomerular basement membrane. *Diabetes 22:* 744–750, 1973.

60. Hudson, B. G. and Spiro, R. G.: Studies on the native and reduced alkylated renal glomerular basement membrane. *J Biol Chem 247:* 4229–4238, 1972.

61. Hudson, B. G. and Spiro, R. G.: Fractionation of glycoprotein components of the reduced alkylated renal glomerular basement membrane. *J Biol Chem 247:* 4239–4247, 1972.

62. Bornstein, P.: The biosynthesis of collagen. *Annu Rev Biochem 43:* 567–603, 1974.

63. Bloodworth, J. M. B., Jr., Engerman, R. L., and Powers, K. L.: Experimental diabetic microangiopathy. 1. Basement membrane statistics in the dog. *Diabetes 18:* 455–458, 1969.

64. Bloodworth, J. M. B., Jr.: Experimental diabetic glomerulosclerosis, II. The dog. *Arch Pathol 79:* 113–125, 1965.

65. Bloodworth, J. M. B., Jr., Engerman, R. L., and Anderson, P. J.: Microangiopathy in the experimentally diabetic animal. In Camerini-Davalos, R. A. and Cole, H. S. (eds): Vascular and Neurological Changes in Early Diabetes. New York, Academic Press, 1973, pp 245–250.

66. Khalifa, A. and Cohen, M. P.: Golmerular protocollagen lysylhydroxylase activity in streptozotocin diabetes. *Biochim Biophys Acta 386:* 332–339, 1975.

67. Beisswenger, P. J.: Glomerular basement membrane. Biosynthesis and chemical composition in the streptozotocin diabetic rat. *J Clin Invest 58:* 844–852, 1976.

68. Mauer, S. M., Steffes, M. W., Sutherland, D. E. R., Najarian, J. S., Michael, A. F., and Brown, D. M.: Studies of the rate of regression of the glomerular lesions in diabetic rats treated with pancreatic islet transplantation. *Diabetes 24:* 280–285, 1975.

69. Caird, F. I., Pirie, A., and Ramsell, T. G.: Diabetes and the Eye, Oxford and Edinburgh, Blackwell, 1969.

70. Davis, M. D., Norton, E., and Myers, F. L.: The Airlie classification of diabetic retinopathy. In Goldberg, M. F. and Fine, S. (eds): Symposium on the Treatment of Diabetic Retinopathy (PHS Publication No. 1890). Washington, D.C., U.S. Gov. Printing Office, 1969, pp 7–22.

71. Smith, M. E. and Becker, B.: Ocular complications in diabetes. In Fajans, S. S. (ed): Diabetes Mellitus (DHEW Publication No (NIH)

76-854). Washington, D.C., U.S. Gov. Printing Office, 1976, pp 213–226.

72. Cogan, D. G. and Kuwabara, T.: Capillary shunts in the pathogenesis of diabetic retinopathy. *Diabetes 12:* 293–300, 1963.

73. Ashton, N.: Studies of the retinal capillaries in relation to diabetic and other retinopathies. *Br J Ophthalmol 47:* 521–538, 1963.

74. Ticho, V. and Patz, A.: The role of capillary perfusion in the management of diabetic macular edema. *Am J Ophthalmol 76:* 880–886, 1973.

75. Kohner, E. M., Saunders, S., Sutcliffe, B. A., and Dollery, C. T.: Retinal blood flow in diabetes. *Diabetologia 9:* 75 (abstract), 1973.

76. Poulsen, J. E.: Recovery from retinopathy in a case of diabetes with Simmonds disease. *Diabetes 2:* 7–12, 1953.

77. Kohner, E. M., Joplin, G. F., Cheng, H., Black, R., and Fraser, T. R.: Pituitary ablation in the treatment of diabetic retinopathy: A randomised trial. *Trans Ophthalmol Soc UK 92:* 79–90, 1972.

78. Diabetic Retinopathy Study Research Group: Preliminary report on effects of photocoagulation therapy. *Am J Ophthalmol 81:* 383–396, 1976.

79. Caird, F. I., Hutchinson, M., and Pirie, A.: Cataract and diabetes. *Br Med J 2:* 665–668, 1964.

80. Patterson, J. W.: Development of diabetic cataracts. *Am J Ophthalmol 35:* 68–72, 1952.

81. Patterson, J. W.: Effect of lowered blood sugar on development of diabetic cataracts. *Am J Physiol 172:* 77–82, 1953.

82. Chylack, L. T., Jr., and Kinoshita, J. H.: A biochemical evaluation of a cataract induced in a high glucose medium. *Invest Ophthalmol 8:* 401–412, 1969.

83. van Heyningen, R.: Formation of polyols by the lens of the rat with "sugar" cataract. *Nature 184:* 194–195, 1959.

84. Hayman, S. and Kinoshita, J. H.: Isolation and properties of lens aldose reductase. *J Biol Chem 240:* 877–882, 1965.

85. Kuck, J. F. R., Jr.: Response of the mouse lens to high concentrations of glucose or galactose. *Ophthalmol Res 1:* 166–174, 1970.

86. Kinoshita, J. H.: Cataracts in galactosemia. *Invest Ophthalmol 4:* 786–799, 1965.

87. Kinoshita, J. H., Merola, L. O., and Hayman, S.: Osmotic effects on the amino acid concentrating mechanism in the rabbit lens. *J Biol Chem 240:* 310–315, 1965.

88. Kinoshita, J. H., Merola, L. O., and Tung, B.: Changes in cation permeability in the galactose-exposed rabbit lens. *Exp Eye Res 7:* 80–90, 1968.

89. Kinoshita, J. H., Barber, G. W., Merola, L. O., and Tung, B.: Changes in the levels of free amino acids and myoinositol in the galactose-exposed lens. *Invest Ophthalmol 8:* 625–632, 1969.

90. Kuwabara, T., Kinoshita, J. H., and Cogan, D. G.: Electron microscopic study of galactose-induced cataract. *Invest Ophthalmol 8:* 133–149, 1969.

91. Becker, B.: Diabetes mellitus and primary open angle glaucoma. *Am J Ophthalmol 71:* 1–16, 1971.

92. Bell, E. T.: Atherosclerotic gangrene of the lower extremities in diabetic and nondiabetic persons. *Am J Clin Pathol 28:* 27–36, 1957.

93. Wahlberg, F.: Intravenous glucose tolerance in myocardial infarction, angina pectoris, and intermittent claudication. *Acta Med Scand Suppl 453:* 1966.

94. Levin, M. E.: Medical evaluation and treatment. In Levin, M. E. and O'Neal, L. W. (eds): The Diabetic Foot. St. Louis, Mosby, 1973, pp 1–39.

95. Goldenberg, M. D., Alex, M., Joshi, R. A., and Blumenthal, H. T.: Nonatheromatous peripheral vascular disease of the lower extremity in diabetes mellitus. *Diabetes 8:* 261–273, 1959.

96. Banson, B. B. and Lacy, P. E.: Diabetic microangiopathy in human toes, with emphasis on the ultrastructural change in dermal capillaries. *Am J Pathol 45:* 41–58, 1964.

97. Siperstein, M. D.: Capillary basement membranes and diabetic microangiopathy. *Adv Intern Med 18:* 325–344, 1972.

98. Kilo, C., Vogler, N., and Williamson, J. F.: Muscle capillary basement membrane changes related to aging and to diabetes mellitus. *Diabetes 21:* 881–905, 1972.

84

Diabetes in Childhood

Lester Baker
Charles A. Stanley

Nearly all children with diabetes have the characteristics of insulin dependence, proneness to ketosis, and marked metabolic lability. These constitute the profile of juvenile diabetes. In this chapter, causes of the marked metabolic lability seen in juvenile diabetes will be reviewed. The clinical corollaries imposed by this lability on those physicians concerned with the care of the child with diabetes will also be discussed.

Lability, in this chapter, is defined as those daily and day-to-day fluctuations of plasma glucose concentration that are not readily explicable in terms of dietary intake, exercise, or insulin dosage. In the nondiabetic individual (Fig. 84-1), there exists a tight sequence between the sensing of an insulin requirement, the secretion of insulin, and the monitoring of the effect of the secreted insulin. This feedback loop is closed by the beta cell which functions both to release insulin and to monitor the effect. In the individual with diabetes, this sequence is completely disrupted. Not only is the insulin secretory capacity of the islet cell destroyed, but the tight feedback loop between the sensing of an insulin requirement and the monitoring of its effect is also disrupted. Thus the most important cause for lability in the juvenile diabetic is the destruction of the beta cells. At the time of diagnosis, the child with diabetes characteristically has low levels of plasma insulin which are clearly inappropriate for the levels of plasma glucose. These low levels of plasma insulin would appear to represent the maximum secretory capacity of the compromised beta cells at that point. Direct challenges by insulin secretagogues, such as glucose, tolbutamide, arginine, or glucagon, result in little or no change in these low plasma insulin levels.[1,2] The marked deficiency of endogenous insulin present at the onset of the disease then progresses, after a variable period of partial recovery known as the remission or "honeymoon" phase, to one of absolute insulin deficiency. In some individuals, the remission may be complete. These children may maintain acceptable plasma glucose levels throughout the day without the need for exogenous insulin. An oral glucose tolerance test performed on such a patient will reveal a diabetic curve, however, and the insulin response will also be abnormal, being low in magnitude and delayed in its time course. The studies of Block et al.,[3] utilizing C-peptide to assay for endogenous insulin in the presence of anti-insulin antibodies, clearly demonstrate that beta-cell activity is responsible for the remission phase. The remission period may range from weeks to as long as 2 to 3 years. Factors that contribute to the ending of the remission phase are not known. Continued destruction by an inflammatory process, related either to viral insult or to an autoimmune phenomenon, is currently favored as a speculative cause.

Pathological examination of the pancreas at various stages of the disease corroborates the clinical picture. Ketosis-prone diabetic patients who die within a few months of diagnosis are found at autopsy to have beta cells reduced in number to approximately 10 percent of the expected normal.[4] The amount of extractable insulin at that time is extremely small.[5] In patients who die after chronic juvenile diabetes of more than several years' duration, beta cells are completely absent from the pancreas on histological examination, and no insulin can be extracted from the pancreas itself.[4,5]

This state of absolute insulin deficiency results in the classic labile juvenile diabetic. The papers of Molnar and co-workers[6–9] provide excellent documentation of this lability. Patients were studied in a metabolic ward setting. Glucose levels were monitored continuously while the patient was ambulatory. For several days, diabetic management was adjusted to achieve what was considered optimal control. When the patient appeared clinically stable, the actual studies were begun. Diet and exercise regimens were kept constant within and between days. Figure 84-2 shows the glucose curve obtained on a patient who was receiving one injection of intermediate-duration insulin daily. Glucose concentrations ranged from greater than 400 mg/dl to less than 40 mg/dl over the 2-day period of study despite the constancy of insulin dose, diet, and exercise. In addition, the pattern of glucose was different on the 2 days of study. Figure 84-3 demonstrates the picture seen in the same patient when multiple doses of short-acting insulin were used in an attempt to achieve a better approximation of normoglycemia. Once again, the striking features of this curve are the amplitude of the glycemic excursions and the lack of reproducibility of the day-to-day glucose pattern while on a regimen that had been held constant.

Thus, in the child with diabetes, with the destruction of the beta cells, the concise picture of Figure 84-1 is replaced by the complicated system outlined in Figure 84-4. The insulin requirement is no longer automatically sensed within the islet of Langerhans. Instead, it must be perceived by the child and/or the parents in the light of the factors that may affect insulin requirement. Several of these are potentially under the control of the patient, such as diet and exercise, but the "controllability" of these factors is age-dependent. Other important components that have implications with regard to insulin requirement are clearly not under the direct control of the child or his family. These include physical growth and development, emotions, infections, and the action of noninsulin hormones. By attempting to integrate the potential effects of these components with the need for insulin, the child and/or the parents choose an insulin dosage for the day. Clearly, the projected needs may not be matched by the actual events. In addition, the monitoring of the effect of insulin, done so efficiently by the glucose sensors in the beta cells, is now more remote and more inaccurate. Urine testing or the presence of symptoms tend to give information only when plasma glucose concentrations are

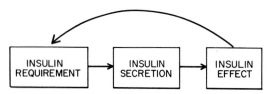

Fig. 84-1. A schematic representation of the tight feedback loop within the beta cell.

over 180–200 mg/dl (allowing for glucosuria to be detected) or when plasma glucose levels fall to less than 40–50 mg/dl (when central nervous system or autonomic nervous system symptoms are elicited because of hypoglycemia). Despite their inaccuracy, these measures of insulin effect are then interpreted by the child and/or the parents to infer necessary changes in one of the factors affecting insulin requirement or in the adjustment of the insulin dosage itself.

The complicated scheme of Figure 84-4 indicates the theoretical difficulty of achieving normoglycemia in the juvenile diabetic, and the previously cited figures (Fig. 84-2 and 84-3) indicate its practical impossibility, even in a metabolic ward setting, given the clinical tools currently available. Despite increasing evidence that hyperglycemia may be a key factor in the production of the microvascular complications of diabetes (recently emphasized by the ADA policy statement 11), the avoidance of hyperglycemia is impossible in the young patient with juvenile diabetes. Therapy in juvenile diabetes is therefore a series of compromises with the ideal goal of avoiding diabetic complications. Additional compromises in the therapeutic program are imposed by the age and developmental status of the child.

The use of the scheme shown in Figure 84-4 makes it easier to conceptualize the goals of treatment in juvenile diabetes, particularly as they relate to key phases of growth and development. The purpose of this section is to place these goals on a realistic and achievable plane.

The care of the child with diabetes can be related to four different stages of growth and development: (1) the preschool years (under age 5); (2) the middle childhood years (ages 5 through 10); (3) the preadolescent and adolescent years (ages 11 through 17); and (4) the young adult (age 17 onward). Each stage can be viewed with regard to those factors that affect insulin requirements, to the difficulty of monitoring the effects of insulin (the degree of diabetic "control"), and to the responsibilities of the child and the parents for diabetic management.

The infant under 5 years of age is an individual whose homeostasis is more unstable than in later life. Infections tend to provoke greater changes in metabolism, and fluid balance is more easily

upset. When diabetes is added to this setting, the changes become even greater; infection in the diabetic infant can result in rapid and major alterations in diabetic control. Similarly, the daily routine of the young infant tends to be an area of parent–child "conflict" as the child struggles to assert himself and the parents seek to define limits. Since many of the issues around which this dialogue takes place involve food and activity, it is clear that these will have repercussions with regard to diabetes management. A temper tantrum that results in the missing of a meal or a snack has direct consequences on diabetic control. The manner in which this problem is handled by the parents has implications not only for diabetes management but also for the emotional growth of the child and for family homeostasis in general.

In this age group, the assessments of the effects of insulin are relatively remote and insensitive. One has only to try to interpret irritability in a 2 year old (the "terrible two" stage) as a possible symptom of hypoglycemia to appreciate the difficulties involved. The child cannot aid in interpreting for the parents any symptoms that might be suggestive of hypoglycemia or hyperglycemia. Even the collection and evaluation of urine glucose patterns are difficult. The infant urinates into a diaper; collection of urine specimens that relate to a specific time are impossible, and attempts to use urine collecting bags quickly lead to skin excoriation. The scant improvement in the quality of the information thus obtained is clearly not worth the effort and the discomfort to the child.

Although the child has the disease, in this age group the parents must bear the entire burden of assessing the needs for insulin, determining the dosage, administering the insulin, and then monitoring its effect. This task is enormous, and it is not surprising that it may have repercussions on the parent–child relationship. The husband–wife relationship may also suffer. Frequently, the mother carries the major responsibility for the diabetic management, with the father in a peripheral and sometimes nonsupportive role.

The goals of diabetic management in this age group, not surprisingly, are relatively modest: (1) avoidance of extremes of hypoglycemia and hyperglycemia which will produce obvious symptoms; (2) quick correction of metabolic abnormalities during infection so as to prevent the appearance of diabetic ketoacidosis and the need for hospitalization; and (3) maintenance of normal growth, both physical and emotional. These goals involve the physician as a teacher. Parents must be sufficiently knowledgeable about the pathophysiology of diabetes and its treatment so that they can provide the primary diabetic care to their infant. The physician must also act as a counselor, since the family requires support and guidance in dealing with the psychological needs of the child and the rest of the family. The manner in which these

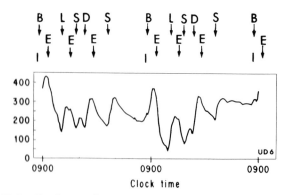

Fig. 84-2. Continuous glucose concentrations in a patient under "optimal" diabetic control on a constant regimen of once daily long-acting insulin (I), exercise (E), and diet (B = breakfast, L = lunch, D = dinner, and S = snack). (From F. J. Service et al: Diabetes *19*:644, 1970.)

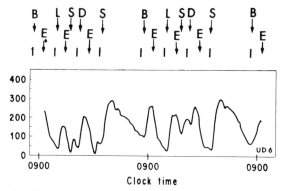

Fig. 84-3. Continuous glucose concentrations in the same patient when placed on regular insulin injections before each meal and the late evening snack in an attempt to produce better diabetic control. Abbreviations as in Figure 84-2. (From F. J. Service et al: Diabetes *19*:644, 1970.)

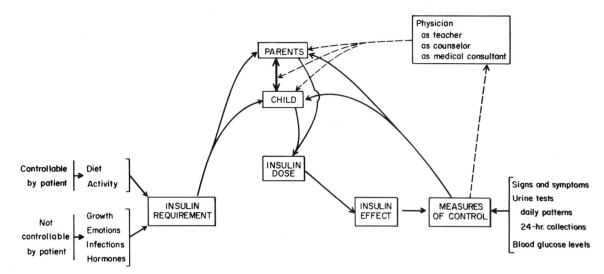

Fig. 84-4. A schematic representation of the complicated relationships existing in the child with diabetes. See text for amplification.

psychological issues are met has a major influence on the ability of the family to carry out a reasonable medical regimen for diabetic management.

The middle years of childhood (ages 5 through 10) provide a calmer background. The start of formal schooling imposes a more reproducible routine on the child. Meals and appetite tend to be more predictable. Although infections may become more numerous as the child enters a larger circle of contacts through school, the metabolic response is less than in infancy. Physical growth is steady and relatively slow in comparison to the periods before and after this time. Similarly, the middle childhood years are a relatively tranquil time with respect to emotions. Testing of parental authority still occurs as part of the emotional growth of the child, but this tends to be nonconfrontational. The child gains increasing abilities to discuss and verbalize his needs, both physical and emotional.

The characteristics of this age group have corollaries with respect to the child with diabetes. Diet and activity vary less than in infancy and become more consciously regulated by the child and the family. The impact of infections on diabetic control is somewhat less, and the steady but slow growth does not cause rapid changes in diabetic control. The enhanced skills of the child now make him a more cooperative partner in his management. He can help in deciphering whether his headache might be caused by hypoglycemia or by a bump on the head at school. He can bring attention to his increasing thirst before the lack of diabetic control is reflected in massive polyuria and glucosuria. He can also provide records of urine tests and timed urine collections. In this setting, there is more of a shared responsibility between the child and the parents for diabetic management, with the child performing some of the tasks of testing and reporting. The goals of diabetic management can therefore be expanded. Severe hypoglycemia should be avoided, particularly at night, but it is appropriate to strive for stricter regulation and as much modulation of the hyperglycemic swings as possible. Mild insulin reactions can be accepted if the child is trained to use his growing capabilities in order to recognize and report these early. Emphasis is still placed on the maintenance of normal physical and psychological growth.

The preadolescent and adolescent years bring with them major changes. The sense of order and routine in daily living that was present in the middle childhood years now gives way to a sense of constant change as the child gets more involved with athletics, school activities, and social events. The schedule of an adolescent is extremely variable and sometimes unpredictable. Peer pressures

affect eating habits (especially snacks) and activities. The adolescent becomes more involved in establishing his identity and independence outside the family, so that he is out of home for longer and longer intervals. In addition to the rapid changes in the psychosocial area, dramatic changes occur in physical growth and sexual maturation.

Diabetes in an adolescent can be a difficult management problem. Diet and activity become even more variable and unpredictable than in the infant. Rapid physical growth and sexual maturation place a constantly changing demand on insulin requirements. Despite an increased need for monitoring in order to judge insulin dosage, there is often an increasing lack of compliance with the medical regimen. In the infant, unpredictability and lack of cooperation with the diabetic program necessitates that the parents take over the tasks of urine testing and choice of insulin dose. In the adolescent, the parents cannot easily assume this responsibility, since the adolescent is less under the direct observation and control of his parents.

Psychological issues tend to dominate normal adolescent development, and this is no less so in adolescents with diabetes. In addition to the problems of noncompliance mentioned above, this is reflected in several other ways that represent a full spectrum of the interplay between emotions and diabetes. In some children, behavioral problems may lead to various stages of abandonment of the diabetic regimen (no urine testing, no dietary rules, sometimes no insulin) with loss of diabetic control. The disease may also be "used" for emotional reasons by the child or the parents; in these instances, diabetic control suffers as well as the psychological growth of the child. There also exists a small group of preadolescents and adolescents in whom emotional arousal leads to repeated bouts of diabetic ketoacidosis, even in the face of conscientiously administered supplemental insulin. For these individuals, recurrent diabetic acidosis appears to represent a psychosomatic disease.[12] These children clinically present as repeated episodes of diabetic ketoacidosis requiring hospitalization. Alternatively the clinical presentation will feature poor school attendance. The frequent episodes of ketosis may be severe enough to cause nausea, vomiting, and anorexia, which will impair the child's ability to attend school on a regular basis but will not be sufficiently severe to require repeated hospitalizations. Studies assessing the inherent diabetic lability of these patients have shown that it is not different from other children with diabetes.[12] In the context of family conflict, however, emotional arousal quickly leads to a rise in free fatty acids and ketosis. Endogenous catecholamines, presumably released in response to the emotional stress, appear to play a key role in the causation of the ketoacidosis. It is also likely that catecholamines are responsible for the state of temporary insulin resistance seen in these individuals, manifested clinically by the lack of response of these patients to the supplemental doses of insulin administered at home. Therapy with beta-adrenergic blocking agents has been found successful in some instances.[12] However, family therapy is now the recommended treatment of choice. These families appear to possess, in excess, certain specific qualities of interaction. The role of the child in these families is also a key factor. Therapy is thus directed at changing these interactional characteristics and changing the role of the child within the family.[13] This disease entity would appear to represent a specific expression of how problems at the parent–child level directly affect diabetic management and control.

Balanced against the well-known difficulties in the adolescent is the fact that the patient's cognitive capabilities have now matured to the point where he can be an active partner in the diabetic regimen. Although diet and activity may vary widely from day to day, the adolescent diabetic can be sufficiently trained in the physiological relationships between diet, activity, and insulin so as to provide excellent diabetic control without sacrificing the flexibility of his schedule. The adolescent can also be more aware of the effects of insulin. He can train himself to note very subtle signs and symptoms suggestive of unacceptable glucose levels and to take appropriate measures to counteract this. He is also able to provide more urine specimens for testing, along with aliquots of 24-hour collections as deemed necessary for adjusting the diabetic regimen. The goals of diabetic management in the adolescent are thus more demanding, not less. In addition to the continuing need to promote normal physical growth during the rapid phase of growth and sexual maturation, the physician can aim for as close an approximation of normoglycemia as possible. Plasma glucose levels taken at the peak of action of the patient's insulin should be within the normoglycemic range or only slightly above it. Since most of the issues that cause adolescent diabetic management to fall short of this goal are not medical, the role of the physician at this time is to deal with the emotional and behavioral problems that impede adequate management. He must provide the education and training concerning the physiological relationships between activity, food, and insulin. As medical consultant, he can provide answers to such questions as the need for two injections and the possible presence of a Somogyi effect. He monitors the overall goals of growth and good diabetic control. As the adolescent becomes more and more responsible for his own disease, it is critically important that the parents stay involved by giving them the task of supervising the implementation of the diabetic management program by the adolescent. This separates the parents from a policing role and places them in a more realistic parenting situation, where they teach, train, and guide the child in the important issues of diabetes, just as they monitor other adolescent areas of behavior (such as school performance and choice of friends).

Management of the young adult builds upon the principles outlined for the adolescent. The young adult now is completely responsible for his diabetic regulation and should aim for good control with every attempt to achieve as close an approximation of normoglycemia as possible.

A review of Figure 84-4 reemphasizes the role of the physician. He is clearly too peripheral to "manage" the diabetes; that is the daily responsibility of the child and the family. The sharing and separation of that responsibility between parent and child depends, as has been outlined, on the developmental stage of the child. The physician's medical role is to act as a consultant to the primary caretakers (parents/child). He defines the goals and provides the expert monitoring of the effectiveness of the program. He makes recommendations for further modifications in the management based on the family's therapeutic trials.

The other roles of the physician caring for a child with diabetes are those of educator and counselor. In the former, he provides the in-depth education, based on physiological principles and relationships, which will allow the parents and child to deal with each daily situation in a manner permitting the best diabetic control possible at that developmental stage. As counselor, he provides the psychological support and guidance that will also allow for the best possible diabetic management. The need to provide emotional guidance and counseling to the family with a diabetic child derives from pragmatic as well as idealistic considerations. The ability of the family and child to carry through a well-planned medical program relates more often to psychological factors than to metabolic ones. These involve the acceptance and understanding of the disease, the organization (appropriate or inappropriate) around the diabetes, and the impact of the diabetes on the affected child and other members of the family. An understanding of these relationships is as important for the physician caring for a diabetic child as is the knowledge of the duration of NPH insulin. It is only by combining the roles of consultant, educator, and counselor that the physician can be effective in the management of the child with diabetes.

REFERENCES

1. Parker, M. L., Pildes, R. S., Chao, K. L., Cornblath, M., and Kipnis, D. M. Juvenile diabetes mellitus, a deficiency in insulin. *Diabetes 17:* 27, 1968.
2. Drash, A., Field, J. B., Garces, L. Y., Kenny, F. M., Mintz, D., and Vazquez, A. M. Endogenous insulin and growth hormone response in children with newly diagnosed diabetes mellitus. *Ped. Res. 2:* 94, 1968.
3. Block, M. B., Rosenfield, R. L., Mako, M. E., Steiner, D. F., and Rubenstein, A. H. Sequential changes in beta-cell function in insulin-treated diabetic patients assessed by C-peptide immunoreactivity. *N. Engl. J. Med. 288:* 1144, 1973.
4. Gepts, W. Pathologic anatomy of the pancreas in juvenile diabetes mellitus. *Diabetes 14:* 691, 1965.
5. Wrenshall, G. A. Assays for insulin in the pancreas, in Williams, R. H. (ed): *Diabetes.* New York, Hoeber, 1960.
6. Molnar, G. D., Gastineau, C. F., Rosevear, J. W. and Moxness, K. E. Quantitative aspects of labile diabetes. *Diabetes 14:* 279, 1965.
7. Service, F. J., Molnar, G. E., Rosevear, J. W., Ackerman, E., Gatewood, L. C. and Taylor, W. F. Mean amplitude of glycemic excursions, a measure of diabetic instability. *Diabetes 19:* 644, 1970.
8. Cremer, G. M., Molnar, G. D., Taylor, W. F., Moxness, K. E., Service, F. J., Gatewood, L. C., Ackerman, E. and Rosevear, J. W. Studies of diabetic instability. Tests of insulinogenic reserve with infusions of arginine glucagon, epinephrine and saline. *Metabolism 20:* 1083, 1971.
9. Molnar, G. D., Taylor, W. F., and Langworthy, A. On measuring the adequacy of diabetes regulation: comparison of continuously monitored blood glucose patterns with values at selected time points. *Diabetelogia 10:* 139, 1974.
10. Molnar, G. D., Taylor, W. F., and HO, M. M. A Day-to-day variation of continuously monitored glycemia: A further measure of diabetic instability. *Diabetologia 8:* 342, 1972.
11. Cahill, G. J., Jr., Etzwiler, D. D., and Freinkel, N. Blood glucose control in diabetes. *Diabetes 25:* 237, 1976.
12. Baker, L., Minuchin, S., Rosman, B. The use of beta-adrenergic blockade in the treatment of psychosomatic aspects of juvenile diabetes mellitus, in Snart, A. G. (ed): Advances in Beta-adrenergic Blocking Therapy, vol. 5. Amsterdam, Excerpta Medica, 1974.
13. Minuchin, S., Baker, L., Rosman, B., Liebman, R., Milman, L., and Todd, T.: A conceptual model of psychosomatic illness in children. *Arch Gen. Psychiatry 32:* 1031, 1975.

85

Treatment of Diabetes Mellitus

Robert Sherwin
Philip Felig

INTRODUCTION

It is generally accepted that in all forms of diabetes an imbalance exists between the availability of insulin from endogenous sources (i.e., beta cell secretion) and the amount of insulin required by target tissues to maintain normal disposal and mobilization of glucose, fat, and protein. Normalization of these metabolic processes requires equalization of the supply of and demand for insulin. In the maturity onset diabetic, in whom obesity and resistance to insulin are present in 80 percent or more of cases, the demand for insulin is increased in the face of a diminished (but not exhausted) capacity for beta cell secretion. Treatment is thus directed at reducing the demand for insulin by dietary management involving a hypocaloric intake. In circumstances in which dietary measures fail or are insufficient in such patients, stimulation of endogenous insulin secretion by sulfonylurea agents may, in limited cases, be helpful. In contrast, the juvenile-onset, ketosis-prone, nonobese type of diabetic is characterized by an absolute deficiency of insulin which will not be improved by sulfonylurea administration nor substantially mitigated by dietary management. In such patients treatment with insulin is the mainstay of management. It is the purpose of this chapter to review each of these treatment modalities, focusing on the techniques as well as the goals of management.

DIET THERAPY

Dietary management forms the cornerstone of treatment of all diabetic patients. This is true in circumstances in which insulin or oral hypoglycemic agents are used as well as in the patients in whom dietary measures are the sole form of therapy. Despite its paramount importance, successful implementation of dietary management is achieved in only occasional patients.[1] The reasons for these frequent failures largely relate to a failure on the part of the physician and the patient to understand the goals, principles, and specific strategies of treatment.

Whereas the goal of insulin and oral agent treatment involves primarily the normalization of blood glucose, in the case of diet therapy the aim is twofold: normoglycemia and achievement of ideal body weight. These aims are achieved on the basis of three principles: (1) regulation of caloric intake; (2) avoidance of concentrated sweets without reducing total carbohydrate content; and (3) regularity of food intake.

Regulation of total caloric intake is directed at achievement of ideal body weight. For the maturity-onset diabetic in whom the incidence of obesity is as high as 80 percent, this generally entails a reduction in caloric intake. The importance of weight reduction in these patients is based on the fact that obesity results in resistance to endogenous insulin which is reversed by a return to ideal weight.[2] With restoration to normal weight, the demand for endogenous insulin is reduced and an improvement in glucose tolerance will ensue. In contrast to the obese, maturity-onset diabetic, a hypercaloric intake is indicated in the thin, wasted insulin-dependent diabetic, particularly in childhood. Such patients require an increase in calories to restore body fat and protein and to permit normal growth.

The total carbohydrate content of the diet should not be disproportionately restricted, but the intake of concentrated sweets (candies, table sugar, pastries) should be limited. There is no compelling evidence that isocaloric reduction in the carbohydrate content to 30 percent results in improvement of the diabetic state. Such an approach may in the long run be deleterious since the calories not taken as carbohydrate are generally made up in the form of a high fat intake which may have an adverse effect in accelerating atherosclerosis. Furthermore, an increase in the proportion of carbohydrate may improve glucose tolerance.[3] Once the appropriate caloric intake has been determined, approximately 45 percent of the calories should be provided in the form of carbohydrate. An exception is the diabetic with a carbohydrate-inducible (type III or IV) form of hyperlipidemia, in whom a low carbohydrate, low calorie intake is indicated. To avoid marked swings in the blood glucose concentration, particularly in insulin-dependent diabetics, simple sugars in the form of concentrated sweets should be avoided. Instead the carbohydrate in the diet should be primarily in the form of complex carbohydrates or starches (such as potatoes, beans, bread, noodle products) because the glucose contained in these foods is more slowly released into the bloodstream.

Day to day regularity of food intake with respect to total consumption of calories and carbohydrates and with regard to the timing of meals is of importance in insulin-dependent diabetics so as to prevent insulin-induced hypoglycemia. An increase in the number and frequency of feedings in the form of a midafternoon and bedtime snack is also helpful in this regard. The regularity and frequency of feedings are predicated on the fact that in contrast to the normal subject in whom insulin secretion is dictated by food ingestion, the insulin-dependent diabetic must match his food intake to the continuing action of injected insulin. The consistency in the pattern of food ingestion does not apply on those days in which there is a marked increase in caloric expenditure as a consequence of moderate to severe exercise. In normal subjects exercise causes a fall in endogenous insulin levels which permits an increase in hepatic glucose output. In the diabetic subject receiving insulin injections such homeostatic changes in circulating insulin levels will not occur in response to exercise. In such circumstances extra food should be taken so as to meet the needs of contracting muscles and to prevent hypoglycemia.

Despite the simplicity of these principles, less than 50 percent of the diabetic population adheres to the recommended dietary regimen.[1] Poor understanding on the part of the patient as well as the physician with respect to dietary goals and tactics is frequently responsible for failures. Often the basic prescription is clearly in error and unsuitable for the specific patient. For example, to many physicians a ''diabetic diet'' almost by definition means an 1800-cal intake. Such a diet in a vigorous, nonobese 160-lb insulin-dependent diabetic is obviously too restrictive and is likely to have one of the following adverse consequences: (1) the patient will not follow the diet and will supplement his intake, generally with concentrated sweets resulting in marked swings in the blood glucose; or (2) the patient may stick to the diet but will develop hypoglycemic episodes and/or lose weight. An 1800-cal diet is equally inappropriate in the 180-lb, 5-ft 2-in, 50-year-old, sedentary, noninsulin-dependent diabetic woman in whom the major objective should be weight reduction by means of a more limited caloric intake.

Dietary management thus must begin with a precise diet prescription which is meaningful to the patient as well as to the dietician. This necessarily involves tailoring the diet to the individual patient. For example, in the maturity-onset diabetic the most important consideration is caloric restriction. This should be emphasized to the patient and communicated to the dietician in terms of total caloric content. In contrast, in the nonobese insulin-dependent diabetic, regularity of food intake, use of between-meal snacks, and avoidance of concentrated sweets are of greater priority than is total caloric intake.

In both forms of diabetes (juvenile and maturity onset) the importance of patient education in implementation of dietary management cannot be overstated.[4] The use of exchange lists in which foods are broken down into six basic categories (milk, bread, vegetables, fruit, meat, and fat) is helpful. However, of greater importance is making certain that the patient understands the goals and strategies of the diet and that the dietary prescription takes into account the mores, behavior, and specific requirements of the individual patient.

ORAL HYPOGLYCEMIC AGENTS

The role of oral hypoglycemic agents in the management of adult-onset diabetes mellitus has undergone extensive reappraisal since the initial report of the University Group Diabetes Program (UGDP) in 1970.[5,6] During the decade prior to the UGDP report, the oral hypoglycemic drugs (particularly sulfonylureas) had become established as moderately effective agents in the control of hyperglycemia in many maturity-onset diabetics with significant residual insulin secretion. Since this group constitutes the major portion of diabetic patients and in view of the ease of administration and lack of frequent side effects, oral hypoglycemic agents gained widespread popularity among medical practitioners. Despite the UGDP findings, use of the oral hypoglycemic agents continues in many centers. It is therefore of interest to examine the pharmacology and clinical use of these drugs.

SULFONYLUREA AGENTS

The two classes of hypoglycemic drugs currently employed in diabetic management are the sulfonylurea and biguanide compounds (see Table 85-1). These compounds differ with regard to structure, action, and clinical usefulness.

The sulfonylurea drugs share a common molecular structure, but differ by the addition of substitutions on the benzene and urea groups. These substitutions account for differences in the potency, metabolism, and duration of action of the sulfonylureas. It is believed that sulfonylureas reduce blood glucose by augmenting the release of endogenous insulin by a direct effect on pancreatic islets. Numerous studies have demonstrated that intravenous administration of sulfonylureas produces acute release of insulin in man[7,8] and that the insulin response to feeding is increased after short-term sulfonylurea therapy.[9] This concept was further supported by evidence that these drugs failed to reduce blood glucose in depancreatized animals,[10] or in diabetics without residual endogenous insulin, and produced rapid release of insulin from isolated islet cell systems.[11] While these data convincingly demonstrate that sulfonylureas are potent insulin secretagogues under acute conditions, the chronic hypoglycemic action of these drugs may not be solely mediated via changes in insulin secretion. In fact, insulin secretion is actually reduced after several months of treatment despite improvement in glucose tolerance.[9] Although these findings may only reflect the reduced glucose levels achieved, recent studies by Olefsky and Reaven[12] provide an alternative explanation for these findings. These investigators demonstrated that insulin binding to circulating monocytes is reduced in nonobese maturity-onset diabetics and returns toward normal after chronic chlorpropamide therapy. Thus, augmented insulin sensitivity after sulfonylurea treatment may account for improved glucose tolerance without hyperinsulinemia. In addition, it has been suggested that sulfonylureas may have a direct inhibitory effect on hepatic glucose production.[13] However, the significance of these findings with respect to the usual clinical doses remains to be determined.

Differences in the duration of action of the sulfonylurea compounds reflect differences in drug metabolism. Tolbutamide, the shortest acting drug, is metabolized by the liver to metabolically inert products. In contrast, while acetohexamide and tolazimide are also metabolized by the liver, their metabolic products retain hypoglycemic action which may account for the more prolonged action of these drugs. The principal metabolic product of acetohexamide metabolism, hydroxyhexamide, is a particularly potent hy-

Table 85-1. Oral Hypoglycemic Agents

Generic Name	Trade Name	Dosage (g/day)		Duration of Action (h)
		Usual	Range	
Sulfonylureas				
Tolbutamide	Orinase	1.5	0.5–3.0	6–12
Acetohexamide	Dymelor	0.75	0.25–1.5	10–24
Tolazamide	Tolinase	0.25–0.5	0.1–1.0	10–24
Chlorpropamide	Diabinese	0.25	0.1–0.5	24–60
Biguanides				
Phenformin	DBI-TD	0.1	0.05–0.15	8–12

poglycemic agent, and like other active metabolites, is removed by the kidney.[14] On the other hand, chlorpropamide is bound to plasma proteins (a property which likely accounts for its long duration of action) and is excreted unchanged via the kidney.

Unlike phenformin, sulfonylureas may on occasion induce profound and sustained hypoglycemia. These hypoglycemic episodes are generally associated with a condition or drug which delays the metabolism of the sulfonylurea agent. Thus, sulfonylureas must be used with caution in the presence of liver and/or renal dysfunction, the latter being particularly common in the elderly diabetic patient. In addition, certain drugs have been shown to potentiate the effects of sulonylureas either by: (1) interfering with hepatic metabolism, e.g., sulfisoxazole,[15] bishydroxycoumarin[16]; (2) reducing urinary exertion, e.g., phenylbutazone[17]; or (3) possessing an additive hypoglycemic action, e.g., salicylates.[18]

Another complication of sulfonylurea treatment is the development of hyponatremia.[19] Although other sulfonylureas (except tolazimide) are capable of impairing water excretion,[20] clinically this syndrome is almost exclusively observed with chlorpropamide treatment. This is probably a consequence of its long half-life (and lack of escape from its effects). The hyponatremia is believed to result from chlorpropamide's ability to enhance the action of ADH.[21] An additional factor may be the failure of these patients to completely suppress ADH secretion in the face of a decline in serum osmolarity.[19]

The most important aspect of toxcity of the sulfonylurea drugs relates to the findings of the UGDP study. The UGDP study, originally conceived to evaluate the relative effectiveness of tolbutamide, phenformin, and insulin in reducing vascular complications in maturity-onset diabetes, led to the unexpected observation that cardiovascular mortality was actually increased in subjects receiving tolbutamide and phenformin when compared to placebo-and-insulin-treated groups.[5,6] These results were greeted by extensive debate among diabetologists and statisticians.[22-24] It was suggested that (1) the mortality was concentrated in only a few of the treatment centers; (2) cardiovascular risk factors were not adequately evaluated (smoking and drug histories were not adequately obtained); (3) the treatment schedule for oral agents was fixed and therefore no attempt was made to adjust the dose of the drug to the prevailing hyperglycemia (as is done in practice); and (4) the standards utilized to diagnose diabetes were inadequate, thereby including subjects with age-induced glucose intolerance. These and other cirticisms were extensively evaluated by a committee of the Biometric Society which upheld the conclusions of the UGDP study.[25] Whereas the Biometric Society report concluded that all possible cardiovascular risk factors were not in fact considered, the observation regarding cardiovascular toxicity was valid regardless of whether therapeutic doses were employed or nondiabetic subjects were included in the study. Furthermore, the Biometric Society report concluded that studies conducted in England[26] and Sweden[27] purporting to demonstrate a beneficial effect of tolbutamide on cardiovascular mortality were limited in scope and different in design, thereby precluding their usefulness in refuting the UGDP study.

It is of interest that the overall mortality in the groups receiving oral hypoglycemic agents (tolbutamide and phenformin) was slightly, but not significantly, different from the control or insulin-treated groups. While this observation does not preclude the findings regarding cardiovascular toxicity, it raises questions concerning the magnitude of the medical risks involved in treatment with these drugs. Furthermore, although these studies strongly suggest that other sulfonylurea drugs have similar toxic effects, conclusions regarding all drugs in this group cannot be established with

certainty at the present time. The UGDP study does, however, clearly establish that treatment with oral hypoglycemic agents offers no potential benefit in reducing mortality or vascular complications in the diabetic patient. These observations indicate that the oral hypoglycemic agents have limited usefulness in the treatment of maturity-onset diabetes, other than in the control of symptoms referable to hyperglycemia. Thus, in patients with fasting hyperglycemia, but without significant polyuria, polydipsia, and nitrogen wasting, these drugs have no place in diabetic management. Furthermore, in view of the possibility of significant cardiovascular toxicity, the oral hypoglycemic agents should be reserved for those *symptomatic* maturity-onset diabetics in whom dietary management is not successful and in whom insulin is not suitable because of patient unwillingness or physical and/or mental limitations.

PHENFORMIN

The mechanism for the hypoglycemic action of phenformin, while not established, is clearly independent of altered insulin secretion. It has been suggested that phenformin acts via stimulation of anaerobic glycolysis[28] and inhibition of gluconeogenesis.[29] However, the doses required to produce these effects in vitro generally exceed those used in clinical practice. More recently it has been demonstrated that phenformin inhibits gastrointestinal absorption of glucose.[30] This effect coupled with its anorexigenic properties may largely account for the drug's weak hypoglycemic action.

With respect to toxicity, phenformin is unique in its ability to enhance the risk of lactic acidosis in the diabetic patient.[31] This rare but frequently fatal complication of phenformin treatment may derive from the drug's stimulatory effect on anaerobic glycolysis (thereby augmenting the production of lactate), as well as from its inhibition of gluconeogenesis (thereby reducing lactate utilization). These effects are dose related. Thus lactic acidosis is particularly likely to occur in circumstances leading to reduced drug metabolism. The presence of renal and/or hepatic disease (phenformin is both excreted unchanged in the urine and metabolized by the liver) markedly increases the risk of lactic acidosis. Patients receiving phenformin are also particularly susceptible to lacticacidemia in the presence of conditions known to augment lactic acid production (hypoxia) or reduce lactate utilization (alcohol). Thus, phenformin is contraindicated in the presence of congestive heart failure, pulmonary insufficiency, and in the alcoholic. The risk of lactic acidosis in subjects receiving phenformin is demonstrated by the 1 to 2 percent incidence observed during the UGDP trials.[32]

The use of phenformin is also frequently associated with gastrointestinal symptoms such as anorexia and nausea. It is generally not as well tolerated as the sulfonylureas. Patients also complain of a peculiar metallic taste sensation. While the UGDP study indicated that both sulfonylureas and phenformin possess similar cardiovascular toxicity, the risk of lactic acidosis, the more significant gastrointestinal symptoms, the adverse effect on carbohydrate absorption, and the generally poorer effect (as compared to sulfonylureas) in lowering blood glucose markedly reduce the clinical usefulness of phenformin. Since the hazards of phenformin treatment generally exceed its therapeutic benefits, this drug should be prescribed only in the most unusual circumstances. We reserve its use for maturity-onset patients with symptomatic diabetes (polydipsia and polyuria) in whom (a) diet has been unsuccessful; (b) insulin treatment is refused or impractical; and (c) symptoms persist in the face of treatment with a sulfonylurea agent. Careful monitoring of renal and hepatic function should be obtained in patients given phenformin. In the face of evidence of a decrease in renal or hepatic function, the dose of phenformin should be reduced so as to avoid accumulation in plasma to toxic levels leading to the development of lactic acidosis. Phenformin is no longer licensed for sale in the United States.

INSULIN TREATMENT

Of the total population of diabetic patients only a small minority (15 to 25 percent) require insulin treatment. This category includes juvenile-onset diabetics, nonobese, ketosis-prone, adult-onset diabetics, obese patients with symptomatic diabetes in whom dietary measures have failed, and relatively mild diabetics during periods of intercurrent "stress" (e.g., surgery, acute inflammation) during which a transient deterioration in diabetic control is observed. Proper management of such patients requires familiarity with the types of insulin preparations available as well as individualization of treatment so as to meet the overall organic, psychic, as well as social needs of the patient.

INSULIN PREPARATIONS

Insulin therapy in the individual patient requires a knowledge of the time activities of the available insulin preparations as well as the individual response of the patient to the insulin preparation selected. The most widely used insulin preparations are the intermediate-acting NPH and Lente insulins and the rapid-acting Regular and Semilente insulins. In addition, long-acting Ultralente insulin is occasionally used to prolong the action of Lente insulin. These insulins used singly or in combination can generally be utilized to treat all insulin-dependent diabetics. (Protamine zinc and Globin insulin, though still commercially available, have little use in current clinical practice.)

Improvements in the preparation of commercially available insulin by fractionation techniques have significantly increased the purity of all insulin preparations. Single peak insulin (currently produced in North America) is greater than 98 percent pure insulin, whereas monocomponent insulin (available in Europe) is greater than 99 percent pure insulin. The use of purified insulins has proved particularly beneficial in patients with insulin allergy[33] and lipoatrophy.[34] The insulin preparations generally used consist of a beef–pork mixture; however, monospecies insulin is also available for special circumstances (in the presence of insulin allergy or resistance).

The approximate time course of activity of the various insulin preparations currently utilized is shown in Table 85-2. It should be noted, however, that it is not uncommon for diabetic patients to demonstrate a slower onset and longer duration of action than expected. This effect is at least in part a consequence of the development of insulin antibodies.[35] Thus, the time activity values for a particular preparation should be estimated on an individual basis. Furthermore, the duration of action of insulin will vary according to the insulin dose employed. The duration of action is prolonged as insulin dosage is increased. The larger the quantity of

insulin administered, the longer the critical levels of insulin necessary for glucose transport will be present at receptor sites.

Regular insulin (zinc–insulin crystals in a clear solution) until recently was prepared as an acid solution (pH 2.8–3.5) in order to maintain solubility. However, improved methods of insulin preparation have led to the introduction of Neutral Regular insulin (unbuffered Regular insulin with pH adjusted to neutrality) which demonstrates enhanced stability and permits greater flexibility in the use of mixtures with intermediate-acting insulins. After subcutaneous injection of Neutral Regular insulin the peak hypoglycemic effect (and peak serum levels of immunoreactive insulin) is observed in 1–3 h and blood glucose returns to baseline within 5–7 h.[33] Semilente insulin has a time course of activity similar to that of Neutral Regular insulin, although its peak effect (3–4 h) and duration of action tend to be more delayed. Semilente insulin consists of zinc–insulin microcrystals in an acetate buffer. The microcrystalline structure is responsible for the rapid absorption characteristics of the preparation. Since use of short-acting insulin alone would require frequent daily injections it was necessary to develop insulin preparations with more prolonged action.

The need for practical sustained-release preparations led to the important discovery by the Hagedorn Laboratory that mixtures of Regular and Protamine Zinc insulin in stoichiometric proportions (no free protamine and insulin) could enhance the action of Protamine Zinc insulin during the day and generally provide adequate circulating insulin at night to prevent severe fasting hyperglycemia the following day. This preparation, NPH insulin, demonstrated a peak activity of approximately 6–14 h and was readily mixed with Regular insulin (not so with PZI). Lente insulin, which was later introduced, provided a virtually identical time course of action and similar advantages regarding insulin mixtures. Lente insulin constitutes a mixture of the rapid-acting Semilente insulin (30 percent) with a long-acting Ultralente insulin (70 percent). The delayed absorption and action of Ultralente results from the fact that larger crystals are produced by careful adjustment of the pH of the preparation. With Lente insulin it is possible to prolong insulin action by addition of Ultralente as well as to increase its early effect by addition of Regular or Semilente insulin. While Lente insulin also offers a theoretical advantage in that it does not contain a foreign protein (Protamine), this has not proved to be of practical significance.

Whereas the intermediate-acting insulins are generally capable of preventing severe hyperglycemia and hyperketonemia throughout the day, their peak action does not coincide with the increases in blood glucose occurring with meals, thereby precluding optimal control of postprandial hyperglycemia. Blood glucose control can be improved in some patients by the use of insulin mixtures (short and intermediate acting), split doses, or combined-split doses. Despite all these possible combinations, however, it is rarely possible to achieve normalization of blood glucose throughout the day, except in only the mildest of diabetic patients.[36]

INITIATION AND ADJUSTMENT OF TREATMENT

Insulin therapy may be initiated in the hospital or in an outpatient setting, depending on the severity of the metabolic disorder and on the prior medical condition of the patient. Care should be taken at that time to (1) rule out factors which might precipitate diabetes and whose correction might obviate the need for insulin, e.g., Cushing's disease, pheochromocytoma, acromegaly, hypokalemia; and (2) determine the renal threshold of the patient in order to assess the future value of urinary glucose measurements (particularly in the elderly). Patients with stable

Table 85-2. Insulin Preparations

Action	Insulin Preparation	Peak Activity (h)	Duration (h)
Rapid	Regular (neutral)	1–3	5–7
	Semilente	3–4	10–16
Intermediate	NPH	6–14	18–28
	Lente	6–14	18–28
Prolonged	Ultralente	18–24	30–40

hyperglycemia (without acidosis) may be started on 10–20 U of intermediate-acting insulin (NPH or Lente). In patients with severe hyperglycemia or ketosis, supplementary short-acting insulin should be given in the morning and evening until adequate doses of intermediate-acting insulin are reached. Urine is tested for glucose (preferably by a copper reduction method) and ketones before meals and at bedtime (before snack), and blood glucose measured before breakfast and dinner meals in hospitalized patients. Urine specimens should be collected after the patient has emptied his bladder and then waited 30 min before voiding. Under these circumstances the urine sample reflects the blood sugar during the previous 30 min. The dose of intermediate-acting insulin is increased approximately 4–5 U every other day until urinary glucose values approach negative and blood glucose levels remain consistently below 200 mg/100 ml. Optimal doses of intermediate-acting insulin are eventually achieved by gradual dosage adjustment at a time when the patient has resumed his or her daily activities (outside of the hospital).

When the maximal hypoglycemic effect is achieved during the daytime, it is important to determine whether a single dose of intermediate-acting insulin is capable of sustaining the effect throughout the night. Patients in whom nighttime and morning hyperglycemia cannot be controlled without afternoon or early evening hypoglycemic reactions should receive a split dose schedule. NPH or Lente insulin is given before breakfast (65 to 90 percent of the total dose), and 10 to 35 percent is given as a second dose before the evening meal. Split doses are generally used in ketosis-prone diabetics, particularly during pregnancy. Finally, urinary and blood glucose concentrations are evaluated in the late morning to determine the need for supplementary short-acting insulin (combined dose). Usually approximately 6–15 U of regular insulin is added and the dose of intermediate-acting insulin is reduced by 4–8 U. Generally patients without significant residual insulin secretion will require the combined dose schedule. Rarely combined doses are required twice daily in unusually brittle patients.

Once the dose of insulin is established it is important that the patient continue urine testing (the frequency of testing will depend on the severity of the diabetes and on insulin preparations used) and that blood glucose is checked as an outpatient (1–4 month intervals). Generally the patient's insulin needs are not fixed, so periodic reevaluation is essential. Unfortunately the clinician's ability to assess the adequacy of diabetic control with random urine and blood measurements can only give small glimpses of the actual metabolic status of the patient. Hopefully new methods, e.g., assay of hemoglobin A_{1c},[37] will permit a more complete assessment of blood glucose regulation and improved control of hyperglycemia.

Initiation of insulin therapy is not complete without an intensive effort toward patient education. Instruction by a nurse trained in the technical and medical aspects of diabetes as well as by a dietician is particularly useful at this time. Insulin treatment will not be successful if dietary intake is haphazard or if faulty injection techniques are employed. Periodic instruction is strongly advisable, even in those patients who are seemingly knowledgeable.

COMPLICATIONS OF INSULIN THERAPY

Hypoglycemia

In view of the relatively small margin between optimal insulin treatment and hypoglycemia in some diabetic patients, it is not surprising that hypoglycemia is a major complication of insulin therapy. The frequency of hypoglycemia is generally greater in patients without residual insulin secretion (juvenile onset) and least in maturity-onset obese subjects in whom insulin resistance precludes effective insulin action. In the former group failure to secrete insulin in response to meals results in wide fluctuations in glucose concentration. Attempts to reduce these excursions in blood glucose may lead to excessive insulin doses between meals or during strenuous exercise. These episodes are generally minimized in such patients by split and combined dose schedules.

The most common causes of recurrent hypoglycemia are (1) chronic insulin overdose; (2) omission or delay of meals; (3) unusually heavy exercise; and (4) errors in injection technique. These problems are generally easily handled by careful history and proper education. Patients with a propensity for exercise-induced hypoglycemia may be taught to inject insulin in a non-exercised site (e.g. the abdomen)[37a] and to consume approximately 20 g of glucose when the urine is nonreactive. Faulty injection technique, e.g., failure to agitate the insulin vial properly before use, errors in the preparation of insulin mixtures, accidental injection into muscle, or injection into sites where insulin absorption is irregular, may be uncovered by regular instruction by a trained nurse. On the other hand, the sudden onset of frequent hypoglycemic episodes may result from (1) the development of renal insufficiency; (2) failure to reduce insulin dosage after resolution of stress or illness; (3) onset of diseases associated with hypoglycemia (adrenal or pituitary insufficiency, acute liver injury); (4) initiation of weight reduction program; and (5) the onset of pregnancy. Hypoglycemia may also occur during the course of pregnancy as a consequence of overzealous treatment of renal glycosuria (the renal threshold for glucose in pregnancy invariably declines). In addition, the severity and duration of hypoglycemic episodes may be increased in certain diabetics due to defective counterregulatory responses as a result of autonomic neuropathy or drugs (propranalol). Propranalol has assumed particular importance in view of its recent use in the treatment of anginal syndromes and hypertension. In the former circumstance profound hypoglycemia resulting from propranalol treatment could induce severe coronary insufficiency, while in the latter the presence of concomitant cerebrovascular disease could increase the sequelae of the hypoglycemic episode. Mental obtundation and coma resulting from prolonged hypoglycemia, particularly in elderly patients with cerebrovascular disease, is poorly responsive to correction by glucose and may be required several weeks for restoration of cerebral function or result in permanent brain damage.

Insulin-dependent diabetics should be instructed to have immediate access to a source of carbohydrate and to carry identification denoting their diabetic status. They should become familiar with symptoms resulting from the gradual onset of hypoglycemia (loss of ability to concentrate, aberrant behavior, or other mental dysfunction) and the signs of hypoglycemia while asleep (nightmares, morning headache, or wet bedsheets) in addition to the more commonly appreciated autonomic symptoms resulting from acute hypoglycemia. Finally, the patient's family and close friends should be instructed in the use of glucagon in the event of hypoglycemic coma and made aware that therapy must be instituted early, prior to seeking medical treatment.

Somogyi Phenomenon

Whereas excessive food intake or inadequate insulin administration are the most common causes of poor diabetic control, it is important to recognize that hyperglycemia and ketonuria may paradoxically occur after excessive insulin administration. Rebound hyperglycemia or the Somogyi phenomenon results from the release of catecholamines, cortisol, growth hormone, and glucagon in response to acute hypoglycemia and may cause a form of brittle diabetes. The magnitude of the rebound hyperglycemia is further aggravated by excessive food intake which generally accompanies the hypoglycemia. Patients exhibiting the Somogyi phenomenon are usually nonobese juvenile-onset diabetics who are difficult to control on single doses of insulin. Clinical clues suggesting rebound hyperglycemia are (1) the presence of widely varying urinary fractionals, ranging from negative to strong reactions for glucose and ketones; and (2) the development of weight gain despite the presence of heavy glycosuria. Rebound hyperglycemia may also be detected by the measurement of 24-h urinary glucose in 3–4 divided collection periods. This procedure is particularly useful in young diabetics in whom frequent blood sampling to detect wide fluctuations in blood glucose regulation is not feasible. If the Somogyi phenomenon is suspected, the patient's insulin dose may be reduced by 10 to 20 percent under careful supervision. Improvement in control despite reduction in insulin administration is strong presumptive evidence of the Somogyi phenomenon. In patients particularly prone to the development of ketoacidosis, the diagnosis should be made in the hospital by frequent blood sampling so that blood glucose regulation is carefully monitored as the dose of insulin is reduced.

Insulin Lipodystrophy

This distressing although benign complication of insulin treatment may take the form of hypertrophy or atrophy of subcutaneous tissues.

Lipohypertrophy is generally observed in patients who repeatedly use the same injection site for insulin injections. The fibrous masses that develop are hypoanesthetic and therefore the problem is often perpetuated (particularly in young diabetics) since these sites are favored for injection. Unfortunately the absorption of insulin from these sites is often erratic and incomplete, thereby leading to a deterioration in diabetic control. The mechanism for this phenomenon is not understood. However, the masses may slowly regress (or at least not increase) when insulin injection into the affected sites is avoided.

Lipoatrophy also generally develops at sites of insulin injection. However, a history of repeated injection into the site is usually not present. The condition usually develops within several months of initiation of insulin therapy and tends to regress or remain stationary after 1–2 years. Children (of both sexes) and adult females are particularly prone to lipoatrophy, whereas adult males are rarely affected. Recent evidence suggests that lipoatrophy may result from an undetermined contaminant in the manufacture of commercially produced insulins. The development of insulin preparations which are greater than 98 percent pure insulin (single peak) and 99 percent pure insulin (monocomponent) appears to have markedly reduced the incidence of this complication.[34]

Insulin-Induced Edema

This generally unappreciated complication is usually observed in poorly regulated diabetic patients in whom glycemic control is restored by insulin.[38] While sodium and fluid retention may in part be related to correction of volume depletion induced by glycosuria, recent evidence suggests insulin has a direct effect on urinary sodium excretion. Infusions of insulin in the upper physiologic range (without changes in blood glucose) markedly reduce urinary sodium excretion in the absence of changes in the filtered load of glucose, GFR, renal blood flow, or aldosterone.[39] While the possibility exists that a fall in circulating glucagon[40] during insulin replacement in the diabetic contributes to the antinatriuresis,[41] it is

likely that the primary factor is insulin itself since physiological hyperglucagonemia does not significantly alter urinary sodium excretion in diabetic patients when exogenous or endogenous insulin is available.[42]

GOALS OF THERAPY

Optimal management of the diabetic patient has as its goals: (a) normalization of carbohydrate, fat, and protein metabolism; (b) prevention of long-term degenerative complications (e.g., microangiopathy, neuropathy); (c) normal psychosocial adaptation; and (d) avoidance of hypoglycemia or other complications of therapy. At the present time, despite an experience with insulin therapy that exceeds more than 50 years, these goals remain elusive in their complete attainment. In fact, since the advent of insulin therapy, the morbidity and mortality attributable to the long-term chronic complications of diabetes have progressively increased. The failure to achieve optimal success with insulin (i.e., to effect a cure of diabetes) is responsible in part for the on-going dispute among diabetologists regarding the "tightness" of diabetic control. In simplistic terms the approaches to the management of diabetes have generally been divided into two camps, "loose" control and "tight" control.

Proponents of "loose" control advocate the use of insulin in amounts necessary to control symptoms (polydipsia, polyuria, weight loss) but without making any substantial effort at normalizing blood glucose levels. This philosophy has as its basis the belief that a causal relationship between the metabolic abnormalities of diabetes, notably hyperglycemia, and the long-term complications of this disorder has not been established. Evidence supporting this conclusion is the demonstration of basement membrane thickening (the earliest sign of microangiopathy) in "prediabetic subjects"[43] and the failure to observe a direct correlation between clinical control of diabetes and the prevention of complications.[44–46] Loose control is thus advocated so as to avoid the dangers of iatrogenic hypoglycemia incident to overzealous treatment with insulin.

Advocates of "tight" control of diabetes have in the past pointed to clinical studies purporting to demonstrate that rigid regulation of diabetes is associated with a decrease in complications.[47–50] As noted earlier, the opposite conclusion may be derived from at least some of such clinical studies[44–46] More recent arguments have focused on the evidence of metabolic alterations in target tissues which may be related to insulin deficiency. In the diabetic glomerular basement membrane, increased glucose deposition has been demonstrated.[51] In nerve tissue, accumulation of polyols derived from glucose via noninsulin-dependent pathways has been observed.[52] Most recently, increased glucose deposition in hemoglobin has been reported[53] and has been shown to correlate with the magnitude of hyperglycemia.[37,54,55] Finally, in contrast to the initial reports in prediabetics,[43] other studies have shown that basement membrane thickening is a function of the duration of clinically manifest diabetes.[56]

In addition to the evidence of metabolic changes in target tissues, there has been an increased awareness of the failure of any form of currently available exogenous insulin therapy to fully normalize the blood sugar. In healthy subjects, the blood glucose concentration is among the most tightly regulated metabolic parameters, varying by less than 50 percent throughout the course of the day. These minimal excursions in blood glucose reflect the exquisite sensitivity of the feedback regulation between glucose concentration and insulin secretion as well as the marked sensitivity of target tissues, particularly the liver, to small fluctuations in insulin.[57] In contrast, in the diabetic, even under optimal conditions of regulated food intake and activity and multiple daily injections of regular insulin, excursions in blood glucose above 200 mg/100 ml and below 50 mg/100 ml are frequently observed.[36,58] The failure to demonstrate a consistent relationship between the seeming control of blood sugar and the prevention of complications thus may reflect the inadequacy of currently available therapeutic regimens rather than the lack of a causal relationship. Noteworthy in this regard is the recent report of a prospective study in which attempts at scrupulous control with multiple injections of insulin were associated with less retinopathy.[59]

The bulk of the evidence at the present time thus suggests that the complications of diabetes are a consequence of metabolic abnormalities in target tissues resulting from insulin deficiency rather than the expression of some independent genetic input. Definitive data relative to this conclusion based on treatment studies are unlikely to be available until the normal feedback relationship between insulin and glucose can be achieved with islet cell transplants or an artificial pancreas (see later). Until such modes of therapy are available, we recommend that the goal of treatment be normalization of blood sugar (i.e., maintenance of random and fasting blood glucose below 150 mg/100 ml) with single or where necessary split doses of insulin to the extent that hypoglycemia can be avoided and pychosocial adaptation can be achieved. Obviously, individualization of treatment is necessary, not only in preventing hypoglycemia but in determining the psychic and social impact of a second daily injection of insulin.

FUTURE TREATMENT

As noted earlier, even under optimal conditions complete normalization of blood glucose levels by conventional administration of exogenous insulin is almost never achieved. Recognition of the inadequacy of current treatment regimens with respect to the metabolic abnormalities as well as the long-term complications of diabetes has led to a search for newer approaches to treatment. Current investigative efforts are directed at three possible modalities: (1) transplantation of islet cells; (2) development of an automatic insulin-delivery, glucose-sensing device ("artificial pancreas"); and (3) use of glucagon-suppressing agents (somatostatin).

The efficacy of islet transplantation in a variety of forms of experimental diabetes has been documented with isogenic transplants.[60,61] Reversion of histopathologic changes in the renal glomeruli of successfully transplanted rats has also been observed.[62] The major problem with this form of treatment remains immune rejection, thus precluding its ultilization at the present time in human diabetes.

Successful normalization of blood glucose levels has been achieved in insulin-dependent patients by means of an "artificial pancreas".[63] This device involves continuous withdrawal of minimal amounts of blood for glucose measurement on the basis of which a variable rate of insulin and/or glucose is delivered. The short-term efficacy of this type of insulin delivery in a small group of hospitalized patients has been demonstrated.[63] The major problem remains the development of a glucose sensor which may be implanted under the skin.

The evidence implicating glucagon in the pathogenesis of diabetes[64] has led to the hope that suppression of alpha cell function would improve diabetic control. Somatostatin, a tetradecapeptide isolated from the hypothalamus, effectively reduces plasma glucagon levels and decreases fasting and postprandial blood glucose levels in the diabetic.[65] However, recent data indicate that the postprandial effectiveness of this agent is largely a consequence of inhibition of carbohydrate absorption rather than improvement in glucose disposal.[66] Furthermore, this agent may worsen hyperglycemia in patients with residual endogenous insulin secretion. In normal subjects, following an initial fall in fasting blood glucose levels, a delayed rise in blood sugar to hyperglycemic levels is observed during prolonged administration of somatostatin.[67] This delayed hyperglycemia is due to the fall in plasma insulin which accompanies the hypoglucagonemia. Thus, in view of its gastrointestinal effects as well as its insulin-suppressant action it is unlikely that somatostatin will materially improve the management of the diabetic.

REFERENCES

1. West, K.: Diet therapy of diabetes: An analysis of failure. *Ann Intern Med 79:* 425–434, 1973.
2. Salans, L., Knittle, J. L., Hirsch, J.: The role of adipose cell size and adipose tissue insulin sensitivity in the carbohydrate intolerance of human obesity. *J Clin Invest 47:* 153–160, 1968.
3. Brunzell, J. D., Lerner, R. L., Hazzard, W. R., et al: Improved glucose tolerance with high carbohydrate feeding in mild diabetes. *N Engl J Med 284:* 521–524, 1971.
4. Davidson, J. K.: Controlling diabetes mellitus with diet therapy. *Postgrad Med 59:* 114–122, 1976.
5. Klimt, C. R., Knatterud, G. L., Meinert, C. L., et al: A study of the effects of hypoglycemic agents on vascular complications in patients with adult-onset diabetes. I. Design, methods and baseline results. *Diabetes 19* (Suppl 2): 747–783, 1970.
6. Meinert, C. L., Knatterud, G. L., Prout, T. E., et al: A study of the effects of hypoglycemic agents on vascular complications in patients with adult-onset diabetes. II. Mortality results. *Diabetes 19* (Suppl 2): 787–830, 1970.
7. Blackard, W. G., Nelson, N. C.: Portal and peripheral insulin concentrations following tolbutamide administration. *Diabetes 20:* 168–170, 1971.
8. Ganda, O. P., Kahn, C. B., Soeldner, J. S., et al: Dynamics of tolbutamide, glucose, and insulin interrelationships following varying doses of intravenous tolbutamide in normal subjects. *Diabetes 24:* 354–361, 1975.
9. Chu, P., Conway, M. J., Krouse, H. A., et al: The pattern of response of plasma insulin and glucose to meals and fasting during chlorpropamide therapy. *Ann Intern Med 68:* 757–769, 1968.
10. Loubatières, A.: Étude physiologique et pharmacodynamique de certains dérivés sulfamidés hypoglycémiants. *Arch Int Physiol 54:* 174–177, 1946.
11. Lacy, P. E., Walker, M. M., Fink, C. J.: Perfusion of isolated rat islets in vitro. Participation of the microtubular system in the biphasic release of insulin. *Diabetes 21:* 987–998, 1972.
12. Olefsky, J. M., Reaven, G. M.: Effects of sulfonylurea therapy on insulin binding to mononuclear leukocytes of diabetic patients. *Am J Med 60:* 89–95, 1976.
13. Ashmore, J., Cahill, G. E., Jr., Hastings, A. B.: Inhibition of glucose 6-phosphatase by hypoglycemia sulfonylureas. *Metabolism* (Clin Exp) *5:* 774–777, 1956.
14. Galloway, J. A., McMahon, R. E., Culp, H. W., et al: Metabolism, blood levels and rate of excretion of acetohexamide in human subjects. *Diabetes 16:* 118–127, 1967.
15. Christensen, L. K., Hansen, J. M., Kristensen, M.: Sulphaphenazole-induced hypoglycemic attacks in tolbutamide-treated diabetics. *Lancet 2:* 1298–1301, 1963.
16. Kristensen, M., Hansen, J. M.: Potentiation of the tolbutamide effect of dicoumarol. *Diabetes 16:* 211–214, 1967.
17. Field, J. B., Ohta, M., Boyle, C., et al: Potentiation of acetohexamide hypoglycemia by phenylbutazone. *N Engl J Med 277:* 889–894, 1967.
18. Seltzer, H. S.: Drug-induced hypoglycemia. A review based on 473 cases. *Diabetes 21:* 955–966, 1972.
19. Weissman, P. N., Shenkman, L., Gregerman, R. I.: Chlorpropamide hyponatremia. Drug-induced inappropriate antidiuretic-hormone activity. *N Engl J Med 284:* 65–71, 1971.
20. Hagan, G. A., Frawley, T. F.: Hyponatremia due to sulfonylurea compounds. *J Clin Endocrinol Metab 31:* 570–575, 1970.

21. Ingelfinger, J. R., Hays, R. M.: Evidence that chlorpropamide and vasopressin share a common site of action. *J Clin Endocrinol Metab 29:* 738–740, 1969.

22. Feinstein, A. R.: An analytic appraisal of the University Group Diabetes Program (UGDP) study. *Clin Pharmacol Ther 12:* 167–191, 1971.

23. Seltzer, H. S.: Avoiding the pitfalls of long-term therapeutic trials: Lessons learned from the UGDP study. *J Clin Pharmacol 12:* 393–398, 1972.

24. Cornfield, J.: The University Group Diabetes Program. A further statistical analysis of the mortality findings. *JAMA 217:* 1676–1687, 1971.

25. Report of the Committee for the Assessment of Biometric Aspects of Controlled Trials of Hypoglycemic Agents. *JAMA 231:* 583–608, 1975.

26. Keen, H., Jarrett, R. J., Ward, J. D., et al: Effect of treatment with oral compounds. In Camerini-Dávalos, R. A., Cole, H. S. (eds): Vascular and Neurological Changes in Early Diabetes. New York, Academic Press, 1973, p 521.

27. Paasikivi, J.: Long-term treatment of patients with abnormal intravenous glucose tolerance and myocardial infarction. In Camerini-Dávalos, R. A., Cole, H. S. (eds): Vascular and Neurological Changes in Early Diabetes. New York, Academic Press, 1973, p 533.

28. Steiner, D. F., Williams, R. H.: Actions of phenethylbiguanide and related compounds. *Diabetes 8:* 154–157, 1959.

29. Meyer, F., Ipaktchi, M., Clauser, H.: Specific inhibition of gluconeogenesis by biguanides. *Nature* (London) *213:* 203–204, 1967.

30. Kruger, F. A., Altschuld, R. A., Hollobaugh, S. L., et al: Studies on the site and mechanism of action of phenformin. II. Phenformin inhibition of glucose transport by rat intestine. *Diabetes 19:* 50–52, 1970.

31. Oliva, P. B.: Lactic acidosis. *Am J Med 48:* 209–225, 1970.

32. Knatterud, G. L., Klimt, C. R., Osborne, R. K., et al: A study of the effects of hypoglycemic agents on vascular complications in patients with adult-onset diabetes. V. Evaluation of phenformin therapy. *Diabetes 24* (Suppl 1): 65–184, 1975.

33. Galloway, J. A., Root, M. A.: New forms of insulin. *Diabetes 21* (Suppl 2): 637–648, 1971.

34. Wentworth, S. M., Galloway, J. A., Davidson, J. A., et al: An update of results of the use of "single peak" and "single component" insulin in patients with complications of insulin therapy. *Diabetes 25* (Suppl 1): 326, 1976.

35. Berson, S. A., Yalow, R. S., Bauman, A., et al: Insulin-^{131}I metabolism in human subjects. *J Clin Invest 35:* 170–190, 1956.

36. Service, F. J., Molnar, G. D., Rosevear, J. M., et al: Mean amplitude of glycemic excursions, a measure of diabetic instability. *Diabetes 19:* 644–655, 1970.

37. Koenig, R. J., Peterson, C. M., Jones, R. L., et al: Correlation of glucose regulation and hemoglobin A$_{ic}$ in diabetes mellitus. *N Engl J Med 295:* 417–420, 1976.

37a. Koivisto, V., and Felig, P.: Effects of leg exercise on insulin absorption in diabetic patients. *N. Eng. J. Med. 298:* 79–83, 1978.

38. Saudek, C. D., Boulter, P. R., Knopp, R. H., et al: Sodium retention accompanying insulin treatment of diabetes mellitus. *Diabetes 23:* 240–246, 1974.

39. DeFronzo, R. A., Cooke, C. R., Andres, R., et al: The effect of insulin on renal handling of sodium, potassium, calcium, and phosphate in man. *J Clin Invest 55:* 845–855, 1975.

40. Gerich, J. E., Tsalikian, E., Lorenzi, M., et al: Normalization of fasting hyperglucagonemia and excessive glucagon responses to intravenous arginine in human diabetes mellitus by prolonged infusion of insulin. *J Clin Endocrinol Metab 41:* 1178–1180, 1975.

41. Saudek, C. D., Boulter, P. R., Arky, R. A.: The natriuretic effect of glucagon and its role in starvation. *J Clin Endocrinol Metab 36:* 761–765, 1973.

42. Sherwin, R. S., Hendler, R., Felig, P.: Influnce of physiologic hyperglucagonemia on urinary glucose, nitrogen, and electrolyte excretion in diabetes. *Metabolism* (Clin Exp) *26:* 53–58, 1977.

43. Siperstein, M. D., Unger, R. H., Madison, L. L.: Studies of muscle capillary basement membranes in normal subjects, diabetic and prediabetic patients. *J Clin Invest 47:* 1973–1999, 1968.

44. Dolger, H.: Clinical evaluation of vascular damage in diabetes mellitus. *JAMA 134:* 1289–1291, 1947.

45. Howells, L. H.: Ocular complications of diabetes mellitus. *Br J Ophthalmol 37:* 716–724, 1953.

46. Knowles, H. C., Guest, G. H., Kessler, M., et al: The course of juvenile diabetes treated with unmeasured diet. *Diabetes 14:* 239–273, 1965.

47. Dunlop, D. M.: Are diabetes degenerative complications preventable? *Br Med J 2:* 383–385, 1954.

48. Johnsson, S.: Retinopathy and nephropathy in diabetes mellitus. Comparison of the effects of two forms of treatment. *Diabetes 9:* 1–8, 1960.

49. Colwell, J. A.: Effect of diabetic control on retinopathy. *Diabetes 15:* 497–499, 1966.

50. Chazan, B. I., Balodimos, M. C., Ryan, J. R., et al: Twenty-five to forty-five years of diabetes with and without vascular complications. *Diabetologia 6:* 565–569, 1970.

51. Spiro, R. G.: Biochemistry of the renal glomerular basement membrane and its alterations in diabetes mellitus. *N Engl J Med 288:* 1337–1342, 1973.

52. Gabbay, K. H., Merola, L. O., Field, R. A.: The sorbital pathway: Presence in sciatic nerve and spinal cord accumulation of products in diabetes. *Science 151:* 209–210, 1966.

53. Bunn, H. F., Haney, D. N., Gabbay, K. H., et al: Further identification of the nature and linkage of the carbohydrate in hemoglobin A$_{ic}$. *Biochem Biophys Res Commun 67:* 103–109, 1975.

54. Trivelli, L. A., Ranney, H. N., Lai, H. T.: Hemoglobin components in patients with diabetes mellitus. *N Engl J Med 284:* 353–357, 1971.

55. Koenig, R. J., Peterson, C. M., Kilo, C., et al: Hemoglobin A$_{ic}$ as an indicator of the degree of glucose intolerance in diabetes. *Diabetes 25:* 230–232, 1976.

56. Kilo, C., Vogler, N., Williamson, J. R.: Muscle capillary basement membrane changes related to aging and diabetes mellitus. *Diabetes 21:* 881–905, 1972.

57. Felig, P., Wahren, J.: Influence of endogenous insulin secretion on splanchnic glucose and amino acid metabolism in man. *J Clin Invest 50:* 1702–1711, 1971.

58. Molnar, G. D., Taylor, W. F., Ho, M. M.: Day-to-day variation of continuously monitored glycemia: A further measure of diabetic instability. *Diabetologia 8:* 342–348, 1972.

59. Job, D., Eschwege, E., Guyot, C., et al: Effect of multiple daily insulin injections on the course of diabetic retinopathy. *Diabetes 25:* 463–469, 1976.

60. Goetz, F. C.: Conference on beta cell function, transplantation, and implantable glucose sensors: A summary. *Metabolism* (Clin Exp) *23:* 875–884, 1974.

61. Matas, A. J., Sutherland, D. E. R., Najarian, J. S.: Current studies of islet and pancreas transplantation in diabetes. *Diabetes 25:* 785–795, 1976.

62. Mauer, S. M., Steffes, M. W., Sutherland, D. E. R., et al: Studies of the rate of regression of the glomerular lesions in diabetic rats treated with pancreatic islet transplantation. *Diabetes 24:* 280–285, 1975.

63. Albisser, A. M., Leibel, B. S., Ewart, T. G., et al: Clinical control of diabetes by the artificial pancreas. *Diabetes 23:* 397–404, 1974.

64. Unger, R. H.: Diabetes and the alpha cell. *Diabetes 25:* 136–151, 1976.

65. Gerich, J. E., Lorenzi, M., Schneider, V., et al: Effects of somatostatin on plasma glucose and glucagon levels in human diabetes mellitus. *N Engl J Med 291:* 544–547, 1974.

66. Wahren, J., Felig, P.: Influence of somatostatin on carbohydrate disposal and absorption in diabetes mellitus. *Lancet 2:* 1213–1216, 1976.

67. Sherwin, R. S., Hendler, R., DeFronzo, R. A., et al: Glucose homeostasis during prolonged suppression of glucagon and insulin secretion by somatostatin. *Proc Natl Acad Sci USA 74:* 348–352, 1977.

86

Insulin Allergy and Resistance

James B. Field

ANTIGENICITY OF INSULIN

The administration of protein of nonhuman origin to humans induces antibodies to such material. Thus the demonstration of antibodies to insulin in diabetic and nondiabetic patients receiving the hormone is not unexpected. Until 1956, insulin antibodies were usually demonstrated only in patients who manifested either allergy or resistance to insulin administration. The existence of insulin antibodies in all patients given the hormone for a period of several weeks to months was unequivocally established by the studies of Berson and Yalow.[1] Although all patients receiving insulin had antibodies to insulin, in the majority of them, such antibodies were of minimal clinical significance, since they were not associated with allergic manifestations nor did they correlate with the patient's insulin requirement.[2-4]

Both the species of origin and the purity of insulin are important determinants of antibody production. However, even injections of homologous insulin induce antibody formation, suggesting that the extraction and processing procedures have altered the molecule as compared to what is secreted endogenously.[5] Until recently, commercial insulin preparations contained significant amounts of other substances, such as proinsulin, desamidoinsulin, arginine insulin, and polymers of insulin.[6] These substances and other contaminating proteins may have been primarily responsible for eliciting antibodies to insulin, since the administration of monocomponent insulin, which contains over 99 percent insulin, induces very little, if any, insulin antibodies.[7-10] Thirteen diabetic patients treated by Schlichtkrull et al. with monocomponent insulin for up to 2 years had less than 0.5 mU insulin binding per milliliter, although some of them transiently developed antibodies.[7] In another series, only 4 of 12 patients receiving monocomponent insulin for 6 to 23 months developed significant antibody titers.[9] In 3, this was associated with hepatitis, and in the fourth, antibodies developed following influenza. Patients treated previously with commercial insulin usually had a significant reduction in antibody titers when treated with monocomponent insulin, but this was not always associated with a reduction in insulin dosage.[8-10] Sometimes,[9] but not always,[10] antibody titers began to rise again despite continued use of monocomponent insulin. Yue and Turtle attributed the development of insulin antibodies in previously untreated diabetic patients receiving monocomponent insulin to the variable purity of the preparations, which contained up to 18 percent monodesamidoinsulin and higher molecular weight contaminants.[8] Single-peak insulin appears to be more antigenic than monocomponent insulin, although some patients have received single-peak insulin for over a year without any evidence of antibody formation.[3] Administration of single-peak insulin to patients previously treated with commercial insulin was not associated with any reduction in insulin antibody titers.

Although there are individual variations, pork insulin tends to elicit less of an antibody response than does beef insulin.[9,11] Some patients have received recrystallized pork insulin several times for over 1 year without evidence of insulin antibodies.[2,9] Patients who develop antibodies to commercial insulin tend to have increasing titers up until 6 to 9 months of treatment with no subsequent increase.[2,10,11] Younger patients developed higher antibody titers than did older patients, but there was no sex difference nor any acceleration with infections.[2] In this series of patients, reinstitution of insulin treatment raised antibodies levels to those present prior to discontinuation of insulin treatment. As will be mentioned later, this is not true of patients who develop insulin resistance under this circumstance.

INSULIN ALLERGY

FREQUENCY AND CLASSIFICATION

Since insulin administration represents daily injections of a protein from an animal source, the presence of allergic reactions is not surprising. The incidence of such reactions has varied from 1 percent[12] to 56 percent[13] but has usually been between 5 and 30 percent as reviewed by Kreines.[14] Allergic reactions are more common in females and with the use of protamine zinc insulin as compared to crystalline insuline.[13] A history of previous allergy does not seem to predispose patients to the development of allergy to insulin. Such allergic manifestations can be divided into three types: mild local, severe local, and generalized.

MILD AND SEVERE LOCAL REACTIONS

More than 80 percent of the allergic reactions can be classified as mild local reactions.[13,15] They consist of stinging, redness, heat, pain, pruritis, or induration at the site of injection and begin during the first or second week of treatment with insulin.[13,16] The symptoms may begin within 30 minutes after injection but may not achieve their maximum intensity for 12 to 24 hours.[13,15,16] In most patients, such reactions spontaneously stop after 10 days to 2 weeks despite the continued use of insulin. In about 15 percent of these patients, severe local reactions to insulin develop. This is associated with extreme pain, marked induration, urticaria, erythema, maculopapular rash, or localized purpura without thrombocytopenia.[15] Symptoms are usually present within 1 hour of injection and may persist for up to a week in the absence of treatment.

GENERALIZED REACTIONS

Generalized reactions to insulin represent less than 1 percent of all allergic manifestations.[13,15,16] Most of these patients have previously demonstrated local allergic reactions to insulin. Such patients have severe pruritis, rash, paresthesias, and generalized urticaria that may also involve mucous membranes. The clinical picture may resemble serum sickness with joint pains, headache, and fever. Gastrointestinal symptoms of nausea, vomiting, abdominal cramps, and diarrhea are frequently present. Circulatory symptoms of pallor, flushing, palpitations, and even circulatory collapse and pulmonary difficulties may ensue. Fortunately, such instances of anaphylactic shock are the least common manifestations of insulin allergy.[15] In such patients, symptoms have occurred in a few to 45 minutes after administration of insulin. Only 3 of the 8 cases of anaphylactic shock reviewed by Hanauer and Batson were diabetics.[15] None of the 4 nondiabetics had a previous history of insulin allergy, while 2 of the diabetics had earlier episodes of urticaria. A history of interrupted therapy with insulin was obtained from most of the patients.[15–17] Generalized reactions to insulin usually developed immediately or soon thereafter upon reinstitution of insulin treatment.[16,17] Although some of these patients have also had insulin resistance, this is certainly not the usual finding.[16,18–20] Thrombocytopenic purpura has also been reported as an allergic manifestation to insulin.[21]

SKIN TESTS WITH INSULIN

Patients with allergic reactions to insulin have almost always had positive skin tests to insulin and demonstrated passive cutaneous anaphylaxis (Prausnitz-Kustner test).[14,16–18] Such tests were positive not only to the type of insulin that the patient was using but also to insulin obtained from other species, including human and synthetic insulin.[16,17] The degree of reactivity tends to vary with the species of insulin, with bovine insulin being the most positive.[17] Such positive skin tests are not restricted to patients with clinical manifestations of insulin allergy. Up to 40 to 50 percent of random diabetics treated with insulin for at least 6 months had positive skin tests for insulin.[17,22] The more purified the insulin, the less frequent were positive skin tests. The incidence was significantly decreased in 43 diabetics who had received no insulin in the prior year.[22] Fractionation of gamma globulins has indicated that an IgE is responsible for the allergic reactions to insulin,[17,18] although such patients have also had IgA and IgM insulin antibodies.[18,23] In contrast, IgG antibodies have been implicated in insulin resistance.[18]

TREATMENT OF INSULIN ALLERGY

Since the mild local allergic responses to insulin usually disappear despite the continued injection of the hormone, no treatment may be necessary. Use of insulin from another species may be associated with the disappearance of local allergic reactions. Monocomponent insulin is sometimes beneficial in patients with allergy to insulin.[10] If the allergic reactions become more severe or generalized, treatment is mandatory, as such patients have the potential

of developing anaphylactic reactions. Systemic antihistamines have sometimes,[24,25] but not always,[26,27] controlled the allergic reactions to insulin. Steroid or ACTH administration has usually alleviated the manifestation of insulin allergy.[15,25,26] In some cases, a smaller dose of steroids can be used if it is injected with the insulin.[26] The boiling of insulin has been reported to permit its use without provoking allergic responses while still preserving its hypoglycemic effect.[13,27] This procedure apparently only works with crystalline insulin.[27] Chemical modifications of insulin, such as phenylated insulin, have been successfully utilized in patients with insulin allergy.[28] After several daily injections of this modified insulin, the patients were able to return to their usual insulin preparation without any further problems. If none of these maneuvers are successful, the patient should be desensitized to insulin by injecting very small amounts of the hormone intradermally.[15–17] Pork monocomponent insulin should be used for desensitization unless it is demonstrated that the patient is less allergic to insulin from another species.[29] Desensitization should begin with 1/1000 of a unit, with subsequent injections every 30 to 45 minutes using twice as much insulin. If an allergic reaction occurs, the dilution of insulin should be increased by four. A syringe containing epinephrine should be available in case the patient develops a generalized reaction. The more concentrated insulin injections can be given subcutaneously. Once the patient has been desensitized, it is important to maintain insulin injections. Occasionally, crystalline insulin is necessary to maintain the desensitized state. Patients who have been desensitized usually have a marked reduction in their passive cutaneous sensitivity tests.[17]

INSULIN LIPOATROPHY AND HYPERTROPHY

Although not an allergic manifestation to insulin, loss of subcutaneous tissue at the site of insulin injections is not an infrequent problem. Teuscher reported that 24 percent of 1096 consecutive diabetics of all ages treated with insulin developed some degree of lipoatrophy.[30] Hypertrophy of the subcutaneous tissue may also be present, but it is much less common than lipoatrophy.[31] Lipoatrophy is more prevalent in females and in patients under the age of 20.[30] It usually develops 3 to 6 months after initiation of insulin treatment. Histologically, there is no evidence of cellular infiltration, nor could insulin antibodies be demonstrated by immunofluorescence. Patients treated with only monocomponent insulin did not develop lipoatrophy. Furthermore, injection of single-peak or monocomponent insulin into the areas of lipoatrophy have caused return of the subcutaneous tissue.[3,10,30,32] Wentworth et al. treated 100 patients with single-peak insulin and 5 with monocomponent insulin. Marked improvement or complete disappearance of the lipoatrophy was noted in 85 percent of the patients. The average length of treatment until improvement was evident was 60 days. However, many patients were aware of some changes within 30 days. Five percent of the patients had slight improvement, which was than followed by recurrence. The remaining patients derived no benefit despite treatment for up to 1 year. Three of these had allergy to insulin, and some of the others were not injecting the insulin directly into the involved areas. Some of the patients who showed no improvement were treated with monocomponent insulin.

INSULIN RESISTANCE

Insulin resistance has been defined as the requirement of at least 200 U of insulin per day.[33] This definition was based on the erroneous assumption that the normal human pancreas produced this much insulin daily. Since Goldner and Clark[34] postulated that the daily insulin production rate in the human is about 40–50 U, patients requiring more than this amount probably also demonstrate some insensitivity to the hypoglycemic effects of the hormone. Insulin insensitivity can be established in several ways in addition to the criteria based on daily insulin requirement. Himsworth[35] characterized insulin-insensitive diabetics as those whose arteriovenous glucose difference did not increase following glucose and insulin administration. An inadequate reduction of the blood glucose following intravenous administration of 0.1 U of insulin per kilogram also indicates some degree of insulin insensitivity. The magnitude and timing of the blood glucose response in the diabetic may be modified by the presence of insulin antibodies. Under certain circumstances, an exaggerated plasma insulin response to various stimuli without a commensurate reduction in blood glucose also signifies insulin insensitivity.

CHRONIC INSULIN RESISTANCE

Chronic insulin resistance exists when the daily dose exceeds 200 U for several days in the absence of diabetic ketoacidosis, infections, or associated endocrinologic diseases.[33] Several reviews have considered various aspects of chronic insulin resistance.[36–41] Most of the patients have been adults, but Guthrie et al.[38] reviewed 23 patients under the age of 19. Sixteen of them were age 16 or less. There has not been any sex predilection.[20,40] Chronic insulin resistance may develop anytime during the course of insulin treatment, but it is unusual for it to be present at the onset of insulin therapy. Three of the 41 patients described by Oakley et al. appeared to be resistant within a few weeks of the initiation of insulin therapy.[20] Twelve of the 21 patients who developed insulin resistance during the first year of therapy became resistant during the initial 6 months of insulin treatment. The longest interval between initiation of insulin treatment and development of resistance was 19 years. Four of the 34 cases described by Shipp et al. had a rather abrupt onset of insulin resistance.[40] As in insulin allergy, a history of interrupted administration of insulin was very common. Although insulin resistance and allergy may coexist in the same patient,[16,18–20,24] this is usually not the case. None of the 41 cases reported by Oakley et al. had generalized allergic reactions to insulin. In that series, localized reactions were no more common than in patients without insulin resistance,[20] while 10 of the 34 insulin-resistant patients reported by Shipp et al. had allergic reactions to insulin.[40] Two-thirds of the patients in one series remained resistant for less than 6 months, while about 25 percent were resistant for over a year, and in 1 patient it persisted for 14 years.[40] Most of the resistant patients received less than 500 U/day, while almost one-third required more than 1000 U/day.[40] The duration and severity of the insulin resistance did not correlate with the patients' insulin requirement prior to the resistance.

ROLE OF INSULIN ANTIBODIES

Most patients with chronic insulin resistance have increased insulin antibodies in the plasma. Oakley et al. demonstrated increasing insulin antibodies in the plasma of a patient several weeks before the clinical appearance of insulin resistance.[20] The mean insulin-binding capacity was 2.8 ± 0.27 mU/ml serum in 50 randomly selected diabetics requiring insulin[8] and was less than 10 mU/ml in almost all insulin-treated diabetic patients.[4,42] The insulin-binding capacity ranged from 60 to 1500 mU/ml in the majority of patients with insulin resistance.[4,42] There was not always a good correlation between insulin dosage and the concentration of insulin antibody.[20,42–46] Although only 29 of the 41 patients in one series had insulin antibodies measured by passive cutaneous anaphy-

laxis,[20] this method is less sensitive than utilization of ^{131}I-insulin binding by gamma globulins. Steinke and Soeldner[42] concluded that the factor responsible for some cases of chronic insulin resistance behaved differently from insulin antibody. However, the large amounts of insulin that such patients had in their plasma could have markedly decreased the amount of antibody available for binding ^{131}I-insulin.

Insulin-neutralizing antibodies in patients with chronic insulin resistance are found in the gamma globulins,[18,23,47] and have variable cross-reactivity with insulins from different species, including human and fish.[3,19,38,48–50] Although chronic insulin resistance has been observed in patients with a variety of other diseases, only hemochromatosis and other types of liver disease have been etiologically implicated.[36,51–53] The role of insulin antibodies in the insulin resistance in such patients is not completely clear, since some,[53] but not all,[20,52,54] of these patients had increased levels of insulin antibody as measured by passive cutaneous anaphylaxis. The relative insensitivity of this method is indicated by the observation that a patient with negative passive cutaneous anaphylaxis had excessive amounts of an insulin-neutralizing material in her plasma.[55]

PERIPHERAL TISSUE UNRESPONSIVENESS AS A CAUSE OF INSULIN RESISTANCE

Peripheral tissue unresponsiveness to insulin has been implicated as a cause of insulin resistance in some patients whose plasma contained excessive amounts of insulin but not insulin antibodies. In some of the early cases, however, it is probable that the insulin represented exogenous hormone that the patient was receiving.[56–59] However, in 1961, Field et al. reported severe insulin resistance in a young female patient whose plasma did not have excess insulin antibody but did contain very large amounts of biologically active insulin many months after her last known injection of insulin.[60] She also had acanthosis nigricans and amenorrhea. Similar patients have subsequently been reported by Tucker et al.[61] and Flier et al.[62] The latter group of investigators has demonstrated that insulin binding to monocytes from such patients is markedly decreased, indicating an abnormality at the insulin receptor as a cause for the resistance. Kahn et al. have described two apparent subtypes of the syndrome of insulin resistance associated with acanthosis nigricans.[63] The patients with type A were younger females who had signs of virilization or accelerated growth. In these patients the defect appeared to be a reduction in the number of insulin receptors of the cell. Type B patients were older females who had additional findings suggestive of an immunologic disease. These included arthalgia, an elevated sedimentation rate, proteinuria, the presence of antinuclear and anti-DNA antibodies, decreased compliment, leukopenia, and increased plasma globulins. In such patients the number of receptors was normal, but there was a reduction in the affinity of insulin for its receptors. Plasma of patients with the type B syndrome inhibited binding of insulin to its receptors. It has been postulated that such activity, which is contained in the gamma globulin fraction, is an antibody to the insulin receptor.[64] The titer of the antibody correlated reasonably well with the degree of insulin resistance in type B patients. In addition to inhibiting the binding of insulin to the receptor and its biologic effect on rat fat cells, the antibody also reproduced some of the actions of insulin on this tissue. ^{125}I-labeled antibody was bound to several tissues containing insulin receptors in a parallel fashion to ^{125}I-insulin. Insulin and several of its analogues competed for binding of the antibody in direct proportion to their affinity for the insulin receptor. Despite the marked insulin resistance of some of these patients, symptoms of diabetes have usually been mild, and ketonuria has usually been minimal or absent. The patient described by Field et al. has been unique, since she had complete remission of her insulin resistance, diabetes mellitus, and acanthosis nigricans.

At least two other clinical entities have been described with diabetes mellitus and severe insulin resistance with or without acanthosis nigricans. One of these includes patients with lipoatrophic diabetes[65-68] (see Chapter 89). In addition to the absence of subcutaneous fat, patients with the congenital form of total lipodystrophy have hepatosplenomegaly, hypertrichosis, acanthosis nigricans, genital hypertrophy, increased growth rate, elevated basal metabolic rate, elevated blood lipids, and neurological, cardiac, and renal abnormalities.[65,66,68] Patients with the acquired form of lipoatrophic diabetes mellitus also have acanthosis nigricans, hepatosplenomegaly, and elevated blood lipids, but the condition does not begin until adolescence or early adult life. Increased subcutaneous fat in the lower extremities is usually present in progressive partial lipodystrophy, and there are elevated blood lipids and renal involvement. Patients with lipoatrophic diabetes have not had excessive insulin antibodies[66] but have had elevated levels of plasma insulin.[66,68] A factor has been isolated from the urine of patients with lipoatrophic diabetes that has lipid-mobilizing and insulin-neutralizing activities.[67,69] This material may be identical to that which has been obtained from bovine and human pituitary glands.[70] Patients with some similar features but without evidence of lipoatrophy have been found to have abnormalities of the pineal gland.[71-73] They have also had increased plasma insulin levels, acanthosis nigricans, genital hypertrophy, and multiple somatic abnormalities. Excess insulin antibodies have not been found, and the entity seems to have some genetic basis, since several siblings have been afflicted.

TREATMENT OF CHRONIC INSULIN RESISTANCE ASSOCIATED WITH EXCESS ANTIBODIES

The antibodies in patients with chronic insulin resistance may be species-specific and neutralize only the species of insulin injected. If the patient has some endogenous insulin that does not cross-react with the insulin antibodies, discontinuation of insulin treatment may cause no adverse effects, and the diabetes may be adequately regulated by diet alone.[74,75] Depending on the specificity of the insulin antibody, patients may be successfully treated by changing the species of the insulin. Berson and Yalow reported that about 50 percent of patients with chronic insulin resistance benefit from a change in the species of the insulin.[76] The use of pork insulin has frequently been beneficial, but not all patients respond to this maneuver.[48,75] The results using human insulin have been variable,[75,77] as have those using fish insulin.[3,50] Acute insulin tolerance tests or measurements of insulin-binding capacities using insulin from different species have not always had any predictive value.[75] Single-peak or monocomponent insulins have not been very useful in treating chronic insulin resistance.[3,8,10]

Chemical modification of the insulin molecule has been beneficial in the treatment of chronic insulin resistance. Sulfated[49,78,79] and phenylated insulin[28] have been effective in some patients. The results with immunosuppressive therapy have been variable.[40,80,81] Some patients have responded to the oral antidiabetic agents, both sulfonylureas[40,46,82-84] and phenformin.[46,85] However, it was not always apparent that this did not represent a spontaneous remission, since it often required 1 to 4 weeks of treatment, and maximum insulin reduction was not realized until 10 to 12 weeks.[82] This was excluded in 3 patients, since withdrawal of tolbutamide was associated with exacerbation of the diabetes.

Adrenocorticosteroids have been most consistent in amelio-rating chronic insulin resistance associated with excess insulin antibodies.[20,40,44,86] Significant effects occurred as early as the second day of treatment, and most of the patients had some reduction in insulin dosage during the first 2 weeks of therapy.[20,40,44] A significant reduction in insulin antibody titer usually accompanies the reduction in insulin dosage.[20,44] The dosage of prednisone should be 60 mg/day in divided doses. Initially, steroids may exacerbate the diabetes and increase the insulin requirement,[46] but more prolonged administration will usually then result in reduction of the insulin dosage. At this point, the dosage should be tapered to the least amount that will maintain a remission of the insulin resistance. After an initial beneficial effect, steroids may be responsible for an increased insulin requirement which will fall when the steroid dosage is further reduced.[20] Insulin resistance may actually develop while the patient is receiving steroids for another condition.[20] Increasing the steriod dose caused amelioration of the resistance. Steroids have not been uniformly successful, especially in patients with negative passive cutaneous anaphylaxis.[20,87-89] The mechanism of the steroid effect is not fully understood. Decreased antibody production,[53] acceleration of dissociation of the insulin–insulin antibody complexes, or altered tissue responsiveness to such complexes[86] have all been suggested. However, data exist indicating that the effects cannot be attributed to decreased antibody formation or modification of the half-life of circulating insulin–insulin antibody complexes.[44,86,90]

REFERENCES

1. Berson, S. A., Yalow, R.S., Bauman, A., et al: Insulin-I[131] metabolism in human subjects: Demonstration of insulin binding globulin in the circulation of insulin treated subjects. *J Clin Invest 35:* 170, 1956.
2. Andersen, O.: Insulin antibody formation. *Acta Endocrinol 71:* 126, 1972.
3. Tantillo, J., Karam, J., Burrill, K., et al: Immunogenicity of single peak beef-pork insulin in diabetic subjects. *Diabetes 23:* 276, 1974.
4. Berson, S., Yalow, R.: The present status of insulin antagonists in plasma. *Diabetes 13:* 247, 1964.
5. Lockwood, D., Prout, T.: Antigenicity of heterologous and homologous insulin. *Metabolism 14:* 530, 1965.
6. Root, M. A., Chance, R. E., Galloway, J.: Immunogenicity of insulin. *Diabetes 21 (Suppl 2):* 657, 1972.
7. Schlichtkrull, D., Brange, J., Christiansen, H., et al: Clinical aspects of insulin-antigenicity. *Diabetes 21:* 649, 1972.
8. Yue, D., Turtle, J.: Antigenicity of "monocomponent" insulins. *Lancet 2:* 1022, 1974.
9. Czyzyk, A., Lawecki, J., Rogala, H.: Serum levels of insulin-binding antibodies in diabetic patients treated with monocomponent insulin. *Diabetologia 10:* 233, 1974.
10. Andreani, D., Iavicoli, M., Tamburrano, G., et al: Comparative trials with monocomponent (MC) and monospecies (MS) pork insulins in the treatment of diabetes mellitus. Influence on antibody levels, on insulin requirement and on some complications. *Horm Metab Res 6:* 447, 1974.
11. Andersen, O.: Insulin antibody formation. *Acta Endocrinol 72:* 33, 1973.
12. Andreani, G., Corti, L.: Allergy to insulin: Statistical study of 1500 diabetics. *Diabetes 4:* 406, 1955.
13. Paley, R., Tunbridge, R.: Dermal reactions to insulin therapy. *Diabetes 1:* 22, 1952.
14. Kreines, K.: The use of various insulins in insulin allergy. *Arch Intern Med 116:* 167, 1965.
15. Hanauer, L., Batson, J.: Anaphylactic shock following insulin injection. *Diabetes 10:* 105, 1961.
16. Goldner, M., Ricketts, H.: Insulin allergy. *J Clin Endocrinol Metab 2:* 595, 1942.
17. Lieberman, P., Patterson, R., Metz, R., et al: Allergic reactions to insulin. *JAMA 215:* 1106, 1971.
18. Dolovich, J., Schnatz, J., Reisman, R., et al: Insulin allergy and insulin resistance. *J Allergy 46:* 127, 1970.
19. Lowell, F. L.: Immunologic studies in insulin resistance: II The

presence of a neutralizing factor in the blood exhibiting some characteristics of an antibody. *J Clin Invest 23:* 233, 1944.

20. Oakley, W., Jones, V., Cunliffe, A.: Insulin resistance. *Br Med J 2:* 134, 1967.
21. Constam, G.: Thrombocytopenic purpura as a probable manifestation of insulin allergy. *Diabetes 5:* 121, 1956.
22. Arkins, J., Engbring, N., Lennon, E.: The incidence of skin reactivity to insulin in diabetic patients. *J Allergy 33:* 69, 1962.
23. Yagi, Y., Maier, P., Pressman, D., et al: Multiplicity of insulin binding antibodies in human sera. *J Immunol 90:* 760, 1963.
24. Sherman, W.: A case of coexisting insulin allergy and insulin resistance. *J Allergy 21:* 49, 1950.
25. Poliakoff, H.: Rapid treatment of severe diabetic ketosis associated with severe insulin allergy. *NY State J Med 58:* 243, 1958.
26. Cockel, R., Mann, S.: Insulin allergy treated with low dosage hydrocortisone. *Br Med J 3:* 722, 1967.
27. Dolger, H.: Denatured insulin. A simplified, rapid means of treatment of allergy to insulin complicating diabetic ketosis. *NY State J Med 52:* 2023, 1952.
28. Katsilambros, L.: Treatment of insulin allergy and insulin resistance with phenylated insulin. *Israel J Med Sci 8:* 893, 1972.
29. Davidson, J. A., Galloway, J. A., Petersen, B. H., et al: The use of purified insulins in insulin allergy. Personal communication.
30. Teuscher, A.: Treatment of insulin lipoatrophy with monocomponent insulin. *Diabetologia 10:* 211, 1974.
31. Robbins, L. R., Odom, D. D., Dobson, H. L.: Cutaneous alterations from injected insulin. *Tex Med 64:* 85, 1968.
32. Wentworth, S., Galloway, J., Haunz, E., et al: The use of purified insulins in the treatment of patients with insulin lipoatrophy. *Diabetes 22:* 290, 1973.
33. Martin, W. P., Martin, H. E., Lyster, R. W., et al: Insulin resistance. *J Clin Endocrinol Metab 1:* 387, 1941.
34. Goldner, M. G., Clark, D. E.: The insulin requirement of man after total pancreatectomy. *J Clin Endocrinol Metab 4:* 194, 1944.
35. Himsworth, H. P.: Diabetes mellitus. Its differentiation into insulin-sensitive and insulin-insensitive types. *Lancet 1:* 127, 1936.
36. Smelo, L. S.: Insulin resistance. *Proc Am Diabetes Assoc 8:* 77, 1948.
37. Field, J. B.: Insulin resistance in diabetes. *Annu Rev Med 13:* 249, 1962.
38. Guthrie, R. A., Murphy, D. Y. N., Wolmack, W.: Insulin resistance in diabetes in juveniles: A case report in a child and a review of the literature. *Pediatrics 40:* 642, 1967.
39. Oakley, W. G., Jones, V. E., Cunliffe, A. C.: Insulin resistance. *Br Med J 2:* 134, 1967.
40. Shipp, J. C., Cunningham, R. W., Russel, R.O., et al: Insulin resistance: Clinical features, natural course and effects of adrenal steroid treatment. *Medicine (Baltimore) 44:* 165, 1965.
41. Field, J. B.: Chronic insulin resistance. *Acta Diabetol Lat 7:* 220, 1970.
42. Steinke, J., Soeldner, S.: Insulin resistance. Differentiation into two types by measurement of serum insulin-like activity in vitro. *Diabetes 14:* 432, 1965.
43. Arquilla, E. R., Stavitsky, A. B.: The production and identification of antibodies to insulin and their use in assaying insulin. *J Clin Invest 35:* 458, 1956.
44. Field, J. B.: Studies on steroid treatment of chronic insulin resistance. *Diabetes 11:* 165, 1962.
45. Field, J. B., Woodson, M. L.: Studies on the circulating insulin inhibitor found in some diabetic patients exhibiting chronic insulin resistance. *J Clin Invest 38:* 551, 1959.
46. Morse, J. H.: Correlation of insulin requirements with the concentration of insulin-binding antibody in two cases of insulin resistance. *J Clin Endocrinol Metab 21:* 533, 1961.
47. Faulk, W., Tomsovic, E., Fudenberg, H.: Insulin resistance in juvenile diabetes mellitus. *Am J Med 49:* 133, 1970.
48. Devlin, J. G., Brian, T. G.: Relationship between differential antibody binding capacity and clinical requirements of beef and pork insulin. *Metabolism 14:* 1034, 1965.
49. Feldman, R., Grodsky, G., Kohout, F. W., et al: Immunologic studies in a diabetic subject resistant to bovine insulin but sensitive to porcine insulin. *Am J Med 35:* 411, 1963.
50. Yalow, R. S., Berson, S. A.: Reaction of fish insulin with human insulin antiserums. *N Engl J Med 270:* 1171, 1964.
51. Axelrod, A., Lobe, S., Orten, J., et al: Insulin resistance. *Ann Intern Med 27:* 555, 1947.
52. Buchanan, J., Young, E. J.: Insulin resistance in haemochromatosis. *Postgrad Med J 42:* 551, 1966.
53. Colwell, A. R., Weiger, R. W.: Inhibition of insulin action by serum gamma globulin. *J Lab Clin Med 47:* 844, 1956.
54. Haunz, E. A.: Present status of insulin resistance: Report of a case with autopsy. *Arch Intern Med 83:* 515, 1949.
55. Oakley, W. G., Field, J. B., Sowton, G. E., et al: Action of prednisone in insulin-resistant diabetes. *Br Med J 1:* 1601, 1959.
56. Tyler, R., Beigelman, P.: Insulin-resistant diabetic coma. *Diabetes 9:* 97, 1960.
57. Davidson, J. K., III, Eddleman, E. E., Jr.: Insulin resistance. *Arch Intern Med 86:* 727, 1950.
58. Presland, J. R., Todd, C. M.: An investigation of prolonged insulin resistance in a case of diabetes mellitus. *Q J Med 25:* 275, 1956.
59. Shipp, J. C., Russel, R. O., Steinke, J., et al: Insulin resistance with high levels of circulating insulin-like activity demonstrable in vitro and in vivo. *Diabetes 10:* 1, 1961.
60. Field, J. B., Johnson, P., Herring, B.: Insulin-resistant diabetes associated with increased endogenous plasma insulin followed by complete remission. *J Clin Invest 40:* 1672, 1961.
61. Tucker, W. R., Klink, D., Goetz, F. C., et al: Insulin resistance and acanthosis nigricans. *Diabetes 13:* 395, 1964.
62. Flier, J. S., Kahn, C. R., Roth, J., et al: Circulating antibodies that impair insulin receptor binding in patients with an unusual diabetic syndrome and extreme insulin resistance. *Science 190:* 63, 1975.
63. Kahn, C. R., Flier, J. S., Bar, R. S., et al: The syndromes of insulin resistance and acanthosis nigricans. *N Engl J Med 294:* 739, 1976.
64. Flier, J. S., Kahn, C. R., Jarrett, D. B., et al: Characterization of antibodies to the insulin receptor. A cause of insulin-resistant diabetes in man. *J Clin Invest 58:* 1442, 1976.
65. Lawrence, R. D.: Lipodystrophy and hepatomegaly with diabetes, lipaemia, and other metabolic disturbances. *Lancet 1:* 724, 1946.
66. Schwartz, R., Schafer, I., Renold, A.: Generalized lipoatrophy, hepatic cirrhosis, disturbed carbohydrate metabolism and accelerated growth (Lipoatrophic diabetes). *Am J Med 28:* 973, 1960.
67. Taton, J., Malczewski, B., Wisniewska, A.: Studies on the pathogenesis of lipoatrophic diabetes: A case of congenital systemic absence of adipose tissue associated with insulin-resistant diabetes mellitus and hepatosplenomegaly. *Diabetologia 8:* 319, 1972.
68. Dunnigan, M., Cochrane, M., Kelly, A., et al: Familial lipoatrophic diabetes with dominant transmission. *Q J Med 43:* 33, 1974.
69. Louis, L. H.: Lipoatrophic diabetes: An improved procedure for the isolation and purification of a diabetogenic polypeptide from urine. *Metabolism 18:* 545, 1969.
70. Louis, L. H., Conn, J. W., Appelt, M. M.: Induction of hyperinsulinemia and hyperglycemia in dogs by administration of diabetogenic bovine pituitary peptide. *Metabolism 20:* 326, 1971.
71. Rabson, S. M., Mendenhall, E. N.: Familial hypertrophy of pineal body, hyperplasia of adrenal cortex and diabetes mellitus. Report of 3 cases. *Am J Clin Pathol 26:* 283, 1956.
72. West, R., Borin, H., Turner, M., et al: Familial insulin resistant diabetes mellitus. *Arch Dis Child 47:* 153, 1972.
73. Barnes, N., Palumbo, P., Hayles, A., et al: Insulin resistance, skin changes and virilization: A recessively inherited syndrome possibly due to pineal gland dysfunction. *Diabetologia 10:* 285, 1974.
74. Faludi, G., Mehbod, H.: Modified pork insulin in the treatment of insulin resistant diabetes. *J Am Med Wom Assoc 20:* 333, 1965.
75. Boshell, B. R., Barrett, J. C., Wolinsky, A. S., et al: Insulin resistance. Response to insulin from various animal sources, including human. *Diabetes 13:* 144, 1964.
76. Berson, S. A., Yalow, R. S.: Insulin in blood and insulin antibodies. *Am J Med 40:* 676, 1966.
77. Akre, P. R., Kirtley, W. R., Galloway, J. A.: Comparative hypoglycemia response of diabetic subjects to human insulin or structurally similar insulins of animal source. *Diabetes 13:* 135, 1964.
78. Little, J. A., Arnott, J. H.: Sulfated insulin in mild, moderate, severe and insulin-resistant diabetes mellitus. *Diabetes 15:* 457, 1966.
79. Menczel, J., Levy, M., Bentwich, Z.: Insulin resistant diabetes treated with sulfated insulin. *Israel J Med Sci 2:* 764, 1966.
80. Friedlander, E. O., Bryant, M. D., Jr.: Idiopathic insulin-resistant diabetes mellitus. *Am J Med 26:* 139, 1959.
81. Geller, W., Ladue, J. S., Glass, G. B., Jr.: Insulin-resistant diabetes precipitated by cortisone and reversed by nitrogen mustard. *Arch Intern Med 87:* 124, 1951.
82. Barrett, J. C., Boshell, B. R.: Tolbutamide in the therapy of insulin resistance. *Diabetes 11 (Suppl):* 35, 1962.
83. Friedlander, E. O.: Use of tolbutamide in insulin-resistant diabetes: Report of a case. *N Engl J Med 257:* 11, 1957.
84. Friedlander, E. O.: Use of ACTH and Adrenocortical steroids in

idiopathic insulin-resistant diabetes. *J Maine Med Assoc 51:* 229, 1960.

85. Molnar, G. D., Striebel, J. L., Goetz, F. L., et al: On the use of phenformin to reduce high insulin requirements in diabetes mellitus. *Proc Mayo Clin 37:* 455, 1962.

86. Palumbo, P. J., Molnar, G. D., Tauxe, W. N.: Adrenal steroid therapy in insulin resistance: A clinical and immunologic study. *Proc Mayo Clin 39:* 161, 1964.

87. Ezrin, C., Moloney, P. J.: Resistance to insulin due to neutralizing antibodies. *J Clin Endocrinol Metab 19:* 1055, 1959.

88. Kaye, M., McGarry, E., Rosenfeld, I.: Acquired insulin resistance. A case report. *Diabetes 4:* 133, 1955.

89. Loveless, M. H., Cann, J. R.: Distribution of blocking antibody in human serum proteins fractionated by electrophoresis convection. *J Immunol 74:* 329, 1955.

90. Kantor, F. S., Berkman, P. M.: Steroid amelioration of immunogenic insulin-resistant diabetes: A proposed mechanism. *Yale J Biol Med 40:* 46, 1967.

87

Diabetes in Pregnancy

Boyd E. Metzger
Richard L. Phelps
Norbert Freinkel

Pregnancy is the only physiological event of a diabetogenic nature. Particularly in late gestation, the insulin requirements of known diabetics increase, and latent diabetic propensities may become unmasked transitorily (i.e., ''gestational diabetes''). Frank diabetes is encountered in about 1 out of every 200 pregnancies. Life-threatening dangers to the mother have been virtually eliminated by improved obstetrical practices and insulin. However, the course of pregnancy and the survival of the progeny remain significantly affected. Toxemia occurs in about 25 percent of pregnant diabetics,[1] and the incidence of hydramnios is approximately 20 percent[2] vis-à-vis the normal 0.5 to 1 percent frequency. Despite some controversy, most concede that there is a two to fourfold increase in congenital malformations in the offspring of these mothers and that lethal malformations are four to five times more frequent.[3] Most importantly, even under optimal management, there remains 10 to 15 percent fetal wastage, which is equally apportioned between stillbirths in utero and neonatal deaths. In the offspring that survive, increased birth weight and stigmata of prematurity are frequent. Despite some earlier reports to the contrary, these phenomena do not occur when the father is the only

Supported in part by Research Grant AM-10699 and Training Grants AM-05071 and AM-07169, from the National Institutes of Health, Bethesda, Maryland, by a Research Grant from the Kroc Foundation, and by Research Grant 6-136 from the National Foundation-March of Dimes.

diabetic parent. Thus, in large measure, they appear to be distinct from the genetic aspects of diabetes and linked instead to the alterations in the maternal environment to which the developing fetus is exposed.

MATERNAL METABOLISM DURING GESTATION

ROLE OF THE CONCEPTUS IN GESTATIONAL DIABETOGENESIS

The metabolic alterations of pregnancy are not manifest with equal intensity throughout gestation. Rather, there is a characteristic temporal progression in which the increasing demands for insulin (and resistance to insulin action) parallel the growth of the conceptus. Indeed, in the immediate postpartum period, the exuberant insulinogenic response to secretory stimulation in normal subjects disappears, normoglycemia may supervene in gestational diabetics, and the therapeutic insulin requirements may precipitously decline in patients with established diabetes mellitus.

These clinical features and their temporal correlations have prompted efforts to link them with properties of the conceptus.[4-6] Three aspects have been implicated.

The Placenta as an Insulin-degrading Structure

Nearly two decades ago, Freinkel and Goodner first explored the possibility that maternal insulin turnover might be altered as a consequence of the interposition of a new site for insulin degradation. In 1959 they demonstrated that the placenta contains systems for degrading insulin into nonhypoglycemic cleavage products throughout gestation and that the added potential for insulinolysis parallels total placental mass.[7,8] It was shown with labeled insulin that fractional rates of insulin removal from the circulation in the rat near term were increased approximately 30 percent and reverted to nongravid levels following expulsion of the conceptus.[9,10] It was also demonstrated by equilibrium infusion that effects of the conceptus upon maternal insulin removal were confined to the placenta and that no meaningful transplacental passage of insulin occurs, although some insulin may be sequestered in the placenta.[10,11] Many of these results have been confirmed recently. Thus, insulin-binding[12,13] and degrading[14] mechanisms have now been characterized and partly purified in human placenta. Failure of insulin to cross the placenta has been corroborated in several other species,[6] including man.[15] Equilibrium infusion studies with *unlabeled* insulin have clearly shown that insulin turnover is indeed accelerated during late pregnancy in the rat, although this property is not shared by proinsulin or C-peptide[16] As yet, direct extraction ratios across the placenta have not been performed and the impact of placental sequestration and degradation upon net insulin economy within any single species may well depend upon the fraction of cardiac output that is accounted for by placental blood flow. In the rat, with multiple placentas and fetuses, the contributions may be appreciable. In human pregnancy, however, extra insulin losses via placental degradation may make relatively minor contributions to total insulin removal. Efforts to assess these contributions by the comparatively crude method of "single-shot" injections have failed to disclose significantly accelerated rates of insulin disappearance from the circulation.[17] Thus, precise quantitation of the effects of pregnancy on fractional rates of insulin turnover in gravid humans remains to be established as does the question of whether the placental capacity to degrade other peptide hormones such as ACTH and glucagon[8] influences other aspects of maternal endocrine economy significantly.

The Placenta as an Endocrine Structure

The placenta constitutes an added site for the biosynthesis of hormones. For some hormones, such as human placental lactogen (HPL) and progesterone, the elaboration parallels the growth and development of the placenta.[18] Their biological implications with regard to insulin action are well established. HPL can elicit lipolysis in vitro[19] and when infused overnight into normal subjects in amounts designed to approach the blood levels of late pregnancy, HPL can effect insulin resistance, as evidenced by the need for higher blood levels to sustain normal oral glucose tolerance.[20] Similarly, the intramuscular administration of progesterone to nongravid subjects in amounts simulating those of late pregnancy effects an increase in basal plasma insulin and in the insulinogenic response to oral glucose.[21] Thus, in addition to perhaps effecting a shorter biological survival for maternal insulin in late pregnancy, the placenta may compromise insulin action, especially in late pregnancy, by the elaboration of hormones with contrainsulin properties.[4,5] The early belief that placental hormonal release is unresponsive to excursions in maternal fuels has been challenged recently. Meaningful increments in plasma HPL have been elicited with prolonged maternal fasting[22] or insulin-induced hypoglycemia,[23] and substantial loading with intravenous (25 g)[23] or oral (100 g)[24] glucose has effected small, albeit significant, reduction in HPL titers.

The Placenta as a Site for Removing Maternal Fuels

The placenta is the conduit through which the conceptus continuously siphons maternal fuels for its metabolic and biosynthetic needs. Glucose is generally believed to serve as the major source of metabolic energy in the developing conceptus. In addition, glucose or 3-carbon intermediates serve as precursor molecules for the glycogen, glycoproteins, and glyceride-glycerol in the triglycerides and phospholipids of the conceptus. These synthetic and oxidative needs have been estimated to require a glucose utilization rate of 6 mg/kg/min in the human fetus at term,[25] in contrast to glucose turnover of 2–3 mg/kg/min in normal adult humans.[26] To sustain these fetal demands, glucose delivery across the placenta is achieved by facilitated diffusion. This step is augmented by the usual 10–20 mg/dl gradient from maternal to fetal plasma glucose.

It has been estimated that in the third trimester, growth of the human fetus requires the net transfer of 54 mM of nitrogen per day across the placenta.[27] Furthermore, at least in sheep, amino acids may be catabolized for oxidative energy needs of the conceptus.[28] Thus, although precise quantitative measurement of total nitrogen requirement for fetal growth is not available, it is clear that these requirements can exert an unremitting drain upon maternal nitrogen reserves.

Maternal triglyceride stores represent the largest reserve fuel depot. However, this reserve can support metabolic needs of the conceptus only to a limited extent. Triglycerides as such have not been shown to cross the placental barrier, and most evidence indicates that transfer of maternal free fatty acids to the human fetus may be quite limited. Glycerol can be transferred across the placenta readily, but its contribution in nonruminant mammalian species is probably negligible.

Ketones, derived via oxidation of fatty acids in maternal liver, can readily cross the placenta and are present in fetal circulation in concentrations equal to those of maternal blood.[29] The enzymes necessary for ketone oxidation are present in the human fetus[30] as well as in the rat and other species.[31,32] Furthermore, when fetal tissues, including brain, are incubated in vitro with concentrations of ketones that simulate those that obtain under fasting conditions in vivo, substantial oxidation of ketones is seen even in the presence of alternative metabolic fuels (i.e., fasting concentrations of glucose, lactate, and amino acids).[32] Indeed, the oxidation of ketones obtunds that of the other fuels and may "spare" them for biosynthetic disposition or other pathways in the fetus.[33] Thus, it is likely that ketones may subserve important metabolic functions within the fetus whenever ketonemia supervenes. However, this may not fully serve all key anabolic needs within the fetus and may even inhibit some. It has been reported that maternal ketonuria (and by implication fetal ketonemia), whatever the source, i.e., diabetes or starvation, may be associated with significant reduction of I.Q. in the offspring at age 4.[34] Similar results recently reported from an independent study of offspring tested at age 3 and 5[35] are the first to confirm these earlier uncontrolled epidemiologic observations.

MODIFICATIONS OF THE FASTED STATE AND "ACCELERATED STARVATION"

How does the mother alter her metabolism to cope with the needs of the conceptus as described above? In 1964, on the basis of theoretical[4] and clinical[36] considerations, it was postulated that the maternal response to dietary deprivation during late pregnancy could be characterized as "accelerated starvation." It was reasoned that maternal transition to endogenous fuels should be more rapid and exaggerated during fasting, since the mother would have to support not only her own oxidative needs but also the anabolic demands of the developing conceptus. It was emphasized that simple "accelerated" recall of potential 2-carbon fragments from maternal fat stores would not suffice. Formation of complex macromolecules during continuous fetal growth would also siphon less expendable maternal building blocks to which the placenta was permeable (see above). Thus the concept of "accelerated starvation" proposed that the fasting mother in late gestation should be unable to conserve critical endogenous stores with the same parsimony that characterizes starvation under nongravid conditions.[4] As a corollary, it was suggested that more rapid diversion by the mother to the oxidation of fat could importantly support fetal growth by "sparing" moieties such as glucose for transplacental transfer.[4]

As summarized elsewhere,[37] much substantive support for

this concept has accumulated. More rapid activation of lipolysis in gravid animals during fasting in late gestation has been corroborated with isolated fat pads[38-40] and direct estimates of FFA and glycerol in plasma and tissues.[40,41] Increased muscle breakdown has been demonstrated by reduction in muscle mass and augmented urinary excretion of nitrogen and appropriate electrolytes.[6,40,41] Exaggerated rises in plasma and urinary ketones attest to accelerated ketogenesis.[37,40,41] And, amidst all of this enhanced and more rapidly activated maternal catabolism during fasting, total fetal growth is relatively preserved in experimental animals,[37] although the development of certain structures such as the brain may be compromised.[42,43]

Reluctance to impose dietary deprivation upon gravid women has restricted the accumulation of comparable data in humans. However, manifest "accelerated starvation" with hyperketonemia, increased urinary nitrogen losses, hyperlipacidemia, and hypoglycemia has been documented by Felig and Lynch[44] and by Tyson et al.[45,48] in physically healthy women fasted for 84 to 90 hours prior to therapeutic abortion in midgestation. In late human pregnancy, all observers have noted lower values for plasma glucose and amino acids after an overnight fast. The two phenomena may be interrelated, since the frank hypoglycemia that supervenes as the fast is extended has been localized to limitations in the generation of gluconeogenic precursors from the periphery[46-48] rather than to limitations in intrahepatic gluconeogenic performance.[49] Higher plasma levels of FFA[36] and ketones[50] after an overnight fast have also been noted in late human pregnancy by most, but not all,[51] workers. Increased fatty acid turnover during late gestation is readily demonstrable with isolated human adipocytes (as with rat adipose tissue in vitro).[52] These properties of adipose tissue have been ascribed to a primary activation of lipolysis rather than to impaired esterification or resistance to insulin,[38] and it has been suggested that "the hormones of pregnancy" may be responsible, at least in part.[40] Although increased intake of food and heightened availability of insulin may offset the net lipolytic effects in the fed state, a heightened turnover of adipose stores is always present. Thus the pregnant animal appears better poised to mobilize her preformed fat whenever exogenous nutrients are withheld.[37,40] This would enable her to conserve glucose and gluconeogenic precursors under such circumstances and assure their availability for maternal brain and fetal tissues.

The increasing placental elaboration of metabolically active principles with contrainsulin as well as insulinogenic potentialities in parallel with the growth of the fetus would provide the right temporal juxtaposition "to make it all work." The "extra" insulin that is required in the fed state (i.e., for anabolism whenever the mother eats) may represent the overhead* that she must pay for her survival via "accelerated starvation" in the fasted state.[37,40]

MODIFICATIONS OF THE FED STATE AND "FACILITATED ANABOLISM"

Basically, when access to food is unrestricted, pregnancy is an anabolic event. Heightened maternal appetite may account for some of the net anabolism, and the pregnant subject with normal pancreatic reserve compensates for the prevailing insulin resistance*[54,55] by an enhanced elaboration of immunoreactive insulin.[36,56,57] The latter truly consists of insulin; the possibility of an

increased release of immunoreactive products with lesser biological reactivity, such as proinsulin, has been excluded.[58]

Certain aspects of postprandial fuel disposition are altered, however. Despite lower values for fasting blood sugar, the upper "normal" limits for the excursions in blood sugar during oral glucose tolerance (100 g glucose) are higher and more prolonged during pregnancy than under nongravid conditions[59] (Table 87-1). As pointed out by Freinkel and co-workers,[4,37,60] some of these changes during gestation may reflect antecedent "accelerated starvation." In the least, the concept of "accelerated starvation" suggests that the pregnant animal in late gestation should start off from a different metabolic baseline whenever she eats. Her tissues should contain more unesterified fatty acids, be burning more fat, and have experienced greater antecedent challenges to nitrogen reserves. Thus the "normal" gestational prolongation of postprandial hyperglycemia could reflect persistent maternal metabolism of fat with consequent "impedance" to glucose disposition.[61] The proposition is consistent with the correlation between basal plasma FFA after an overnight fast in late gestation and the integrated rise in plasma glucose levels for the 3 hours following the administration of oral glucose at this time.[61] Regardless of mediation, however, the net increase in the duration of postprandial hyperglycemia should prolong the heightened availability of ingested glucose to the fetus, since transplacental transfer of glucose is directly proportional to the prevailing concentrations of glucose in maternal blood.[62,63] Fetal anabolism would thereby be "facilitated." Small, albeit significant, acute increases in plasma triglyceride levels have also been observed in approximately 60 percent of normal pregnant subjects immediately following ingestion of 100 g glucose.[61,64] These transitory increments in triglyceride levels are primarily found in the VLDL fraction of plasma. The "carbohydrate-induced triglyceridemia" constitutes another mechanism for preempting ingested glucose from immediate oxidation by the mother. It could sequester some of the glucose as glyceride-glycerol for subsequent retrieval and transplacental passage as a 3-carbon moiety when endogenous maternal fuels are called upon again.

Certain other features of the fed state in pregnancy could "facilitate anabolism" in the mother or fetus. For example, as demonstrated by Daniel et al.[65] and confirmed by others,[66] oral glucose elicits greater and more prolonged decrements of plasma glucagon in pregnant than in nongravid subjects. The heightened suppression of glucagon in response to glucose feeding could interrupt glucagon contributions to ongoing maternal glycogenolysis, gluconeogenesis, and ketogenesis more promptly. Finally, following ingestion of "mixed meals" (i.e., meals containing protein and fat as well as carbohydrate), maternal anabolism from amino acids may be enhanced by the heightened outpouring of insulin, even though protein feeding elicits lesser rises in plasma

Table 87-1. Criteria for Normal 100 g Oral Glucose Tolerance When Pregnant and Nonpregnant

Status	Glucose Concentration (mg/dl)[a]			
	Fasting	1 Hour	2 Hour	3 Hour
Pregnant[b]	105	190	165	145
Nonpregnant[c]	125	195	140	125

From J. B. O'Sullivan and C. M. Mahan, *Diabetes* 13: 278–285, 1964.
[a]Original study measured whole blood. Since most laboratories now perform serum glucose determinations, corresponding values for serum or plasma have been calculated by adding 15% of whole blood value.
[b]Diagnostic of diabetes if any two values equal or exceed those indicated.
[c]Diagnostic of diabetes if any three values, or fasting and 3-hour value, equal or exceed those indicated.

---

*The basis for all the observed resistance to insulin has not yet been explained fully. Maternal insulin receptors have not been quantified, and it remains to be tested whether the total number of insulin receptors is reduced via "down regulation"[53] as a consequence of the prevailing maternal hyperinsulinemia.

amino acids during pregnancy.[60,67] Preliminary findings in humans[67] and corresponding animal studies[68,69] suggest that aminogenic stimulation of glucagon is well preserved in pregnancy. The combination of an enhanced beta-cell response to glucose and a preserved alpha-cell response to amino acids could "facilitate anabolism" during the disposition of "mixed meals" as follows: The "extra" insulin could blunt the gluconeogenic potential of glucagon during the immediate postprandial hyperglycemia and so "spare" ingested amino acids for maternal or fetal access. Contrariwise, after disposal of the carbohydrate, the responsiveness of the alpha cell to the persistent hyperaminoacidemia could initiate enough gluconeogenesis to prevent postprandial hypoglycemia in the mother.

SUMMARY OF THE RELATIONSHIPS BETWEEN THE FED AND FASTED STATE IN THE NORMAL MOTHER

As summarized above, a "profile" characteristic of normal maternal metabolism during pregnancy has now been delineated. In essence, metabolic adjustments in pregnancy are geared to adapt an intermittently eating host, the mother, to a continuously feeding (and, in part, independently regulated) new structure, the conceptus. The oscillations between the fed and the fasted state in the mother are characterized by greater amplitude than under nongravid conditions,[61] and some novel features are conferred via "accelerated starvation" and "facilitated anabolism." Demands for flexibility in insulin-secretory mechanisms are much greater. Appreciation of this metabolic lability has facilitated understanding of the pathogenesis of gestational impairments in carbohydrate metabolism and may provide a rational basis for the clinical management of diabetes in pregnancy.

CLINICAL FEATURES AND MANAGEMENT OF DIABETES IN PREGNANCY

Pregnancy occurring in previously diagnosed, insulin-treated diabetics accounts for approximately 0.5 percent of all gestations. An additional 2 to 3 percent of pregnant women have asymptomatic glucose intolerance, usually first detected during gestation ("gestational diabetes"). Such glucose intolerance may be transitory, reverting to normal shortly after delivery. The chance of successful pregnancy outcome in diabetes is related to duration of diabetes, and the degree of angiopathy. The widely used classification scheme of White[70] is based on these variables. In the discussion that follows, the White classification has been adopted with minor modification (Table 87-2). Diabetic pregnancy has also been classified on the basis of complications occurring during gestation that presage poorer prognosis.[71] Compared to overt diabetics (White classes B–F), perinatal risks appear to be smaller in patients with asymptomatic glucose intolerance (White class A). However, lack of uniform clinical criteria has complicated attempts to define prognostic expectations in the latter group. Accordingly, in the discussion that follows, classes B–F and class A will be considered separately.

INSULIN-DEPENDENT DIABETES (WHITE CLASSES B–F)

Historical Background

In the pre-insulin era, the occurrence of pregnancy in known diabetics was unusual due in part to the significant mortality occurring in the ketosis-prone juvenile diabetic before the repro-

Table 87-2. Classification of Diabetes in Pregnancy

Class	Description
A	Asymptomatic, abnormal OGTT, fasting plasma glucose (FPG) < 130 mg/dl
A$_1$	FPG < 105 mg/dl
A$_2$	FPG ≥ 105–129 mg/dl
B	Insulin-treated diabetic (prior to pregnancy) or untreated diabetic with diabetic symptoms or FPG ≥ 130 mg/dl. Duration 0 to 9 years, age at diagnosis > 19 years. No evident diabetic angiopathy.
C	Insulin-treated diabetic. Duration 10 to 19 years, age at diagnosis 10 to 19 years. No evident diabetic angiopathy.
D	Insulin-treated diabetic. Duration > 19 years, age at diagnosis 0 to 9 years, or background diabetic retinopathy.
F	Insulin-treated diabetic, with diabetic nephropathy and/or proliferative retinopathy.

Modified from P. White, in *Joslin's Diabetes Mellitus* (ed. 11), Lea and Febiger, Philadelphia, 1971, pp. 581–598.

ductive years, but also due to impaired fertility in the sexually mature diabetic female. Estimates of fertility ranged from 2 to 6 percent,[72] significantly below that for nondiabetic women.[73] When pregnancy did occur, it was associated with such grave prognosis for the mother and such doubtful fetal survival that therapeutic abortion was commonly instituted.[74]

After insulin became available, life expectancy for the juvenile-onset diabetic increased, and fertility was restored to near normal. Thus, increasing numbers of diabetic women reached physiological maturity with full reproductive potential. Although maternal mortality remained unacceptably high in the first insulin-treated patients (approximately 10 percent[75]), it was soon reduced to levels approaching the nondiabetic population. Unfortunately, these gratifying improvements for the diabetic woman were not accompanied by comparable reductions in fetal wastage. Thus, in series collected in the 1930s, perinatal loss averaged 40 percent[1] and a similar rate of loss was recorded in English teaching hospitals in the 1940s.[76]

General appreciation that fetal survival was linked to the diabetic control of the mother evolved gradually, and this association has been made frequently in the last two decades.[77–81] Particularly persuasive was the 10 percent perinatal mortality achieved by Pedersen[78] in a group of highly motivated pregnant diabetics in whom extraordinary measures were instituted for rigid control of the diabetes.

A prompt decline in fetal loss, from 24.3 to 13.1 percent, was also reported by Oakley,[82] using the management program pioneered by Pedersen[78] in which hospitalization of patients from week 32 onward was combined with tight outpatient regulation. Even better results have been obtained,[83–89] although reports of perinatal mortality ranging from 12 to 25 percent continue to appear.[90–95] The reasons for the improvement in fetal salvage are probably (1) more aggressive efforts to normalize maternal metabolism throughout gestation, (2) increasing sophistication of obstetric techniques for assessing fetal well being and maturation in utero, (3) pediatric advances in management of the neonate, and (4) ascendancy of the "team" and "center" concept for the management of this unique group of patients requiring specialized and experienced care.

The first factor is of paramount importance. That abnormalities in the maternal environment rather than genetic factors are responsible for the heightened perinatal mortality and morbidity is indicated by the failure to encounter similar problems when only the father is diabetic (see above). Moreover, phenomena such as polyhydramnios, stillbirths, and fetal macrosomia have been reduplicated in pregnant primates rendered insulinopenic by treatment with streptozotocin.[96]

Principles of Treatment

The primary treatment objecive is to achieve the best possible control of diabetes. To meet this goal, all pregnant diabetics should be managed by a skilled "team" including diabetologist, obstetrician, and neonatologist. Their efforts are pooled to carefully treat the mother, monitor fetal well-being, carry the pregnancy near to term, and deliver a viable infant at minimal risk for neonatal complications. Many treatment regimens have been advocated and success in terms of good perinatal survival has been reported with a variety of approaches to diet and insulin therapy, frequency and duration of hospitalization, and timing and technique of delivery. The plan of management described below is based for the most part on well-documented, widely accepted practices. Where uncertainty or controversy exists, we have drawn upon our own experiences at Northwestern University McGaw Medical Center.

Diet.   Pregnancy does not alter the basic principles of diet management of the diabetic. Because of the heightened propensity for "accelerated starvation" (see above), however, an evening snack is routinely included, and carbohydrate intake should not be restricted below 250 g. Protein intake of 1.5–2.0 g/kg is recommended as in the pregnant nondiabetic. We advocate the same weight gain of 24 to 25 pounds that has been recommended for normal pregnancy by the Committee on Maternal Nutrition of the National Research Council[97] and try to achieve this with a diet of 38 kcal/kg of ideal body weight, composed of approximately 18 percent protein, 45 percent carbohydrate, and 37 percent fat. However, these recommendations are based on few objective data, since protein and lipid metabolism in pregnant diabetics are just beginning to receive detailed inquiry.

Insulin.   Optimal therapy necessitates individualization. Because of the exaggerated metabolic oscillations that characterize normal metabolism in pregnancy (see previous section), combinations of intermediate and regular insulin are usually employed. Early in gestation, this can often be accomplished with injections twice daily. However, after 28 weeks of gestation, when the contrainsulin factors in pregnancy reach peak intensity (see above), most diabetics of long duration and severity, i.e., classes C–F, and some with diabetes of short duration, i.e., class B, are treated in our center with regular insulin three times daily prior to meals and additional smaller amounts of intermediate-acting insulin (at breakfast, supper, or bedtime) as necessary to minimize the excursions in plasma glucose. Control of diabetes at this time is monitored on the basis of glucosuria and by measuring plasma glucose four times per day. The therapeutic objective consists of maintaining premeal plasma glucose concentrations below 100 mg/dl.

Outpatient Management and Hospitalization.   Patients receiving insulin at the time of referral are hospitalized as soon as possible for 1 week of initial assessment of diabetic complications, patient reeducation, and establishment of "tight" diabetic regulation. Outpatients are followed every 2 weeks until week 30 of gestation and weekly thereafter. If the initial hospitalization occurs before 24 weeks of gestation, patients are hospitalized for another 4 to 7 days at 28 weeks. The more intensive program of insulin therapy is started at that time and continued until delivery. In the absence of complications, class B diabetics are hospitalized at 36 weeks of gestation, class C at 34 weeks, and classes D and F at 32 weeks. They then remain in the hospital until delivery.

Appearance of any of the following is considered an indication for immediate hospitalization at any time during gestation: (1) patient neglect of diabetic care and/or question of falsification of patient's assessments of diabetic regulation, (2) any acute illness jeopardizing diabetic control, (3) deterioration in diabetic control which within 1 week's time cannot be restored to a level present at the time of most recent hospital discharge, or (4) impending ketoacidosis.

Delivery.   The objective at our center is to permit pregnancy in the diabetic to be carried near to term (i.e., 38 to 40 weeks) unless fetal health becomes compromised. Fetal well-being is assessed by daily urinary estriol determinations during the final hospitalization (beginning at 32 to 36 weeks, depending on diabetic class), weekly nonstress testing beginning at 30 weeks in all patients, weekly contraction stress tests beginning at 34 to 37 weeks, depending on diabetic class, and amniocentesis at 34, 36, and 38 weeks in class D and F and 36 and 38 weeks in class B and C patients. The amniocentesis is designed to assess fetal pulmonary maturation on the basis of the ratio of lecithin/sphingomyelin (L/S ratio). An abnormal contraction stress test in conjunction with a meaningful decline in estriol excretion is considered sufficient evidence for uteroplacental insufficiency and constitutes an indication for intervention prior to 38 weeks.

Unless fetal well-being is in jeopardy or the mother has had prior cesarean section, vaginal delivery is attempted. For elective vaginal induction, pitocin administration is begun at 7 to 9 A.M.. On the day prior to induction the usual diet and insulin are given. The patient receives nothing by mouth after midnight, and plasma glucose is measured 1 hour before the start of induction and at 4-hour intervals throughout labor. Glucose (50 g every 6 hours) is administered intravenously, and sufficient regular insulin is administered to maintain plasma glucose between 80 and 120 mg/dl. When labor begins spontaneously, management is individualized on the basis of the time lapse since the preceding meal and insulin administration.

For delivery by elective cesarean section, the procedure is scheduled as the first morning case. The usual amounts of insulin and diet are given the day prior to delivery. The patient receives nothing by mouth after midnight, and her morning insulin is withheld until after delivery unless plasma glucose is above 140 mg/dl 1 hour prior to section. In the event the 1-hour predelivery plasma glucose is below 75 mg/dl, glucose is infused at a rate of 50 g every 6 hours. Following delivery, the insulin dose is initially reduced by one-half to two-thirds from antepartum levels.

GESTATIONAL DIABETES (WHITE CLASS A)

Complexities of Definition and Classification

Several factors have contributed to the confusion in the literature concerning the definition of "gestational diabetes," or "White class A," and the attendant prognostic expectations and therapeutic recommendations.

One major source of confusion has been the failure to apply a standard set of criteria uniformly in order to differentiate normal from abnormal glucose tolerance during pregnancy. The criteria for oral glucose tolerance proposed by O'Sullivan and Mahan[59] (see Table 87-1) are the best available because they are derived from tests in 752 unselected women during pregnancy using a 100 g glucose load. That these criteria can identify a population of women at high risk for permanent diabetes is borne out by the development of clinical diabetes within 15 years in approximately 60 percent of the women who tested abnormally during pregnancy.[98] Intravenous glucose tolerance tests have been proposed by some as more sensitive and reproducible for characterizing glucose metabolism in pregnancy. However, none of the recommended intravenous procedures[99] have received sufficient clinical trial to gain uniform acceptance.

Failure to standardize what is meant by "asymptomatic" has been another source of confusion. The original distinction between class A and B, as proposed by White, is vague, class A referring to an asymptomatic patient with an abnormal glucose tolerance test, but with "fasting values normal or near normal."[70] Some have used fasting glucose as the distinguishing criteria and have designated patients as class A only if fasting plasma glucose remains in the normal range for their laboratory.[87,100,101] Others do not consider fasting glucose values in differentiating between class A and class B. Thus, O'Sullivan et al.[102] exclude asymptomatic patients from their "gestational diabetic," i.e., class A, category if any blood glucose value (during a 100 g OGTT) equals or exceeds 300 mg/dl, and Stallone et al.[103] categorize patients class B if any postprandial plasma glucose equals or exceeds 160 mg/dl regardless of fasting values. Still others[2] distinguish class A from class B on the basis of whether or not insulin is used in management, without indicating how such decisions are made. Comparisons from the literature regarding pregnancy risk and optimal management for patients so designated are therefore hazardous at best.

In our hands, pregnant women are designated as class A, or "gestational diabetics," if they (1) exhibit abnormal oral glucose tolerance according to the criteria of O'Sullivan and Mahan,[59] (2) have fasting plasma glucose values less than 130 mg/dl, and (3) are clinically asymptomatic. Patients receiving oral hypoglycemic agents when first seen are evaluated and categorized in a similar fashion after the medications have been withdrawn for 1 to 2 weeks under careful observation. It is our practice to treat class A patients with insulin only if fasting plasma glucose exceeds normal (104 mg/dl) (Class A_2, see below). It is recognized that the diabetic class assigned may depend, in part, on when such patients come to medical attention. However, until the precise determinants of complications in the diabetic are better understood, all classifications must be arbitrary to a certain extent

O'Sullivan et al.[104] have suggested that maternal age and weight are two additional variables that may influence outcome of pregnancy in women with gestational glucose intolerance. They found that perinatal deaths are increased only when maternal age is greater than 25 years and that obesity may add further risk. Their findings indicate that variables such as age and weight should also be incorporated into any analysis of gestational diabetes.

Pathogenesis of Gestational Diabetes

The relative importance of contrainsulin factors vis-à-vis impaired insulin secretion in the pathogenesis of this form of early, potentially reversible diabetes has not been elucidated fully. Neither basal hyperglucagonemia[65,66,105] nor abnormal suppressibility of alpha-cell secretion of glucagon following glucose ingestion[65,66] appears to be implicated. Circulating basal levels of human placental lactogen (HPL), a contrainsulin hormone of pregnancy, are similar in normal pregnant women and in gestational diabetics, and HPL suppressions following oral glucose ingestion do not differ in the two groups.[24] Studies of proinsulin secretion in pregnancy by Phelps et al.[58] and Kuhl[106] indicate that gestational diabetes cannot be ascribed to the increased elaboration of components such as proinsulin or intermediates that possess insulinlike immunoreactivity but little biological activity. Measurements of early insulin release during OGTT by Metzger et al.[107] indicate that, as a group, gestational diabetics manifest "sluggish" early (15 min) insulin release. However, the population is not homogenous. In about 20

percent of cases, acute insulin responsiveness does not appear to be obtunded.

Principles of Treatment

Since pregnancy in this population may be attended by heightened incidence of perinatal complications, especially in mothers over 25 years of age,[104] careful medical and obstetric monitoring is indicated. Because the majority of gestational diabetics are obese, some investigators have advocated hypocaloric diets in the routine treatment of this group.[1,2,89] However, it has not been documented that such caloric restriction can be carried out without enhancing ketosis. Thus, we continue to recommed that calories should not be restricted in gestational diabetics. Instead, we advocate the same dietary program as in class B–F diabetics with the objective of achieving a 24- to 25-pound weight gain during pregnancy (see above).

On the basis of the reports by O'Sullivan[108] and others[84] of improved fetal salvage in gestational diabetics treated with insulin, some have advocated the use of insulin routinely in gestational diabetics over 25 years of age.[109] Until additional controlled studies can confirm these potentially important observations, we do not advocate the use of insulin routinely. We have limited the use of insulin in class A patients to those whose fasting plasma glucose exceeds 104 mg/dl on two successive determinations (class A_2); the remainder do not receive insulin therapy (class A_1). Because of the known hazard of severe neonatal hypoglycemia associated with their use and the inability to wholly exclude teratogenic potentialities, sulfonylureas are strictly avoided.

The progress of pregnancy is monitored by nonstress testing (weekly after 32 weeks gestation and 3 times weekly from 38 weeks until term) and amniocentesis at 36 and 38 weeks. Gestational diabetics are permitted to go to term and enter spontaneous labor unless evidence of fetal deterioration is observed. To avoid ketosis during labor, patients receive 50 g of glucose intravenously every 8 hours and plasma glucose levels are measured every 4 hours. This seldom results in plasma glucose levels exceeding 120 mg/dl. Patients who undergo cesarean section are managed in a similar fashion as class B–F diabetics.

THE INFANT OF THE DIABETIC MOTHER

Detailed description and analysis of the multiple neonatal problems that can confront the infant of a diabetic mother (IDM) are beyond the scope of this chapter. Several excellent reviews on the subject have been published recently.[2,109,110] Thus the comments below focus on those features that seem to relate most directly to maternal metabolism and diabetic control.

Although "good diabetic control" has been the common objective, in most recent publications this often has not been defined precisely, and efforts to document the degree of control achieved have been few. Implicit in any definition of good control is the absence of ketoacidosis, a complication resulting in fetal death in 37 to 83 percent of pregnancies.[2,111,114] Moreover, it has been reported that maternal acetonuria is associated with a lower I.Q. in later childhood[34,35] (see above). Beyond this, stated objectives have varied widely.[82,111,115,117] Recent measurements[89,118,119] indicate that mean blood glucose values throughout the day in normal pregnant women in the third trimester may be lower than has commonly been appreciated, with peak values rarely exceeding 110–120 mg/dl. In addition, data have been presented to suggest that perinatal mortality is considerably diminished when maternal blood sugar is kept below 100 mg/dl.[92,94,120] These observations, plus the commonly held belief that transient episodes of hypoglycemia in the mother have no deleterious effect on the fetus,[2,85] may be responsible for the recent trend toward more rigid control of maternal blood glucose. Such efforts have been associated with excellent results in terms of perinatal mortality.[84,87] However, further salutory benefits of "tight" regulation of maternal blood glucose cannot be gauged by improvements in fetal salvage alone because (1) perinatal losses may be approaching irreducible minima and (2) major contributions to survival may have been provided by newer pediatric and obstetric techniques.[121–124] Therefore, assessment of the effectiveness of medical management may necessitate more subtle parameters than simple estimates of neonatal survival. This highlights the other features that may distinguish the offspring of diabetic mothers from offspring of a normal pregnancy.

Many IDM display birth weights exceeding the expected normal levels for their period of gestation.[93,125] The macrosomia is accompanied by increased adiposity[2,125] and visceromegaly (affecting particularly the heart[126,127]). Hypocalcemia, hyperbilirubinemia, heart failure, polycythemia, hyperviscosity, and symptomatic neonatal hypoglycemia are encountered with increased frequency in IDM.[2,110,128] Hyaline membrane disease and respiratory distress syndrome[129] pose the most frequent life-threatening challenges, but less serious pulmonary problems of other etiologies such as the "wet lung syndrome" may also occur when hydramnios and intrauterine hypoxia coexist. In addition, congenital anomalies are two to four times more common, and cerebral dysfunction and a heightened propensity to later diabetes are also present. It is tempting to consider that some of these phenomena may be linked to the altered availability and delivery of maternal fuels to the IDM during fetal life. The prominent hyperplasia of the islets of Langerhans that is seen at birth in IDM is consistent with this proposition. Indeed, significant diminutions in the incidence of respiratory distress syndrome, hyperbilirubinemia, and congenital malformations have been reported in one series in which mean maternal glucose was maintained below 100 mg/dl throughout late gestation.[93]

REFERENCES

1. Kyle, G. C. Diabetes and pregnancy. *Ann. Intern. Med. 59 (Suppl 3):* 1–82, 1963.
2. Pedersen, J. The Pregnant Diabetic and Her Newborn (ed 2). Williams and Wilkins Company, Baltimore, 1977.
3. Pedersen, L. M., Tygstrup, I., and Pedersen, J. Congenital malformations in newborn infants of diabetic women. *Lancet 1:* 1124–1126, 1964.
4. Freinkel, N. Effects of the conceptus on maternal metabolism during pregnancy. *In* On the Nature and Treatment of Diabetes, B. S. Leibel and G. A. Wrenshall, eds. Excerpta Medica Foundation, Amsterdam, 1965, pp. 679–691.
5. Freinkel, N. Pregnancy and diabetes mellitus. *In* Diabetes Mellitus: Diagnosis and Treatment, vol. II., G. J. Hamwi and T. S. Danowski, eds. American Diabetes Association, Inc., New York, 1967, pp. 161–165.
6. Freinkel, N. Homeostatic factors in fetal carbohydrate metabolism. *In* Fetal Homeostasis, vol. 4, R. M. Wynn, ed. Appleton-Century-Crofts, New York, 1969, pp. 85–140.
7. Goodner, C. J., and Freinkel, N. Carbohydrate metabolism in pregnancy: The degradation of insulin by extracts of maternal and fetal structures in the pregnant rat. *Endocriology 65:* 957–967, 1959.
8. Freinkel, N., and Goodner, C. J. Carbohydrate metabolism in pregnancy. I. The metabolism of insulin by human placental tissue. *J. Clin. Invest. 39:* 116–131, 1960.
9. Goodner, C. J. and Freinkel, N. Carbohydrate metabolism in pregnancy: The turnover of ^{131}I insulin in the pregnant rat. *Endocrinology 67:* 862–872, 1960.
10. Freinkel, N., and Goodner, C. J. The placenta as a center of carbohydrate regulation in pregnancy. *In* Proceedings of the Fourth Congress of the International Diabetes Federation. Medecine et Hygiene, Geneva, 1961, pp. 391–393.
11. Goodner, C. J., and Freinkel, N. Carbohydrate metabolism in pregnancy. IV. Studies in the permeability of the rat placenta to ^{131}I insulin. *Diabetes 10:* 383–392, 1961.
12. Marshall, R. N., Underwood, L. E., Voina, S. J., et al. Characterization of the insulin and somatomedin-C receptors in human placental cell membranes. *J. Clin. Endocrinol. Metab. 39:* 283–292, 1974.
13. Posner, B. I. Insulin receptors in human and animal placental tissue. *Diabetes 23:* 209–217, 1974.
14. Posner, B. I. Insulin metabolizing enzyme activities in human placental tissue. *Diabetes 22:* 552–563, 1973.
15. Buse, M. G., Roberts, W. J., and Buse, J. The role of the human placenta in the transfer and metabolism of insulin. *J. Clin. Invest. 41:* 29–41, 1962.
16. Katz, A. I., Lindheimer, M. D., Mako, M. E., et al. Peripheral metabolism of insulin, proinsulin, and C-peptide in the pregnant rat. *J. Clin. Invest. 56:* 1608–1614, 1975.
17. Bellman, O., and Hartmann, E. Influence of pregnancy on the kinetics of insulin. *Am. J. Obstet. Gynecol. 122:* 829–833, 1975.
18. Hytten, F. E., and Leitch, I. Hormones. *In* The Physiology of Human Pregnancy (ed 2). Blackwell Scientific Publications, Oxford, 1971, chap. 6, pp. 179–233.
19. Turtle, J. R., and Kipnis, D. M. The lipolytic action of human placental lactogen on isolated fat cells. *Biochim. Biophys. Acta 144:* 583–593, 1967.
20. Beck, P., and Daughaday, W. H. Human placental lactogen: Studies of its acute metabolic effects and disposition in normal man. *J. Clin. Invest. 46:* 103–110, 1967.
21. Kalkhoff, R. K., Jacobson, M., and Lemper, D. Progesterone, pregnancy and the augmented plasma insulin response. *J. Clin. Endocrinol. Metab. 31:* 24–28, 1970.
22. Kim, Y. J., and Felig, P. Plasma chorionic somatomammotropin levels during starvation in mid-pregnancy. *J. Clin. Endocrinol. Metab. 32:* 864–867, 1971.
23. Spellacy, W. N., Buhi, W. C., Schram, J. D., et al. Control of human chorionic somatomammotropin levels during pregnancy. *Obstet. Gynecol. 37:* 567–573, 1971.
24. Surmaczynska, B., Nitzan, M., Metzger, B. E., et al. Carbohydrate metabolism in pregnancy. XII. The effect of oral glucose on plasma concentrations of human placental lactogen and chorionic gonadotropin during late pregnancy in normal subjects and gestational diabetics. *Isr. J. Med. Sci. 10:* 1481–1486, 1974.
25. Page, E. W. Human fetal nutrition and growth. *Am. J. Obstet. Gynecol. 104:* 378–387, 1969.
26. Cahill, G. F. Jr., and Owen, O. E. Some observations on carbohydrate metabolism in man. *In* Carbohydrate Metabolism and Its Disorders, vol. I, F. Dickens, P. J. Randle, and W. J. Whelan, eds. Academic Press, New York, 1968, chap. 16, pp. 497–522.
27. Young, M. Placental transfer of glucose and amino acids. *In* Early Diabetes in Early Life, R. A. Camerini-Davalos and H. S. Cole, eds. Academic Press, New York, 1975, pp. 237–242.
28. Gresham, E. L., James, E. J., Raye, J. R., et al. Production and excretion of urea by the fetal lamb. *Pediatrics 50:* 372–379, 1972.
29. Scow, R. O., Chernick, S. S., and Smith, B. B. Ketosis in the rat fetus. *Proc. Soc. Exp. Biol. Med. 98:* 833–835, 1958.
30. Adam, P. A. J., Raiha, N., Rahiala, E. L., et al. Oxidation of glucose and D-B-OH-butyrate by the early human foetal brain. *Acta Paediatr. Scand. 64:* 17–24, 1975.
31. Dierks-Ventling, C., and Cone, A. L. Aceto-acetyl-coenzyme A thiolase in brain, liver, and kidney during maturation of the rat. *Science 172:* 380–382, 1971.
32. Shambaugh, G. E., Mrozak, S. C., and Freinkel, N. Fetal fuels. I. Utilization of ketones by isolated tissues at various stages of maturation and maternal nutrition during late gestation. *Metabolism 26:* 623–635, 1977.
33. Shambaugh, G. E., Koehler, R. A., and Freinkel, N. Fetal fuels. II. Contributions of selected carbon fuels to oxidative metabolism in the rat conceptus. *Am. J. Physiol.* (in press).
34. Churchill, J. A., and Berendes, H. W. Intelligence of children whose mothers had acetonuria during pregnancy. *In* Perinatal Factors Affecting Human Development. Sci. Pub. 185, Pan American Health Organization, Washington, D.C., 1969, p. 30.

35. Stehbens, J. A., Baker, G. L., and Kitchell, M. Outcome at ages 1, 3, and 5 years of children born to diabetic women. *Am. J. Obstet. Gynecol. 127:* 408–413, 1977.

36. Bleicher, S. J., O'Sullivan, J. B., and Freinkel, N. Carbohydrate metabolism in pregnancy. V. The interrelations of glucose, insulin, and free fatty acids in late pregnancy and postpartum. *N. Engl. J. Med. 271:* 866–872, 1964.

37. Freinkel, N., Metzger, B. E., Herrera, E., et al. The effect of pregnancy on metabolic fuels. *In* Proceedings of the VII Congress of the International Diabetes Federation. Excerpta Medica International Congress Series No. 231, Amsterdam, 1971, pp. 656–666.

38. Knopp, R. H., Herrera, E., and Freinkel, N. Carbohydrate metabolism in pregnancy. VIII. Metabolism of adipose tissue isolated from fed and fasted pregnant rats during late gestation. *J. Clin. Invest. 49:* 1438–1446, 1970.

39. Herrera, E., Knopp, R. H., and Freinkel, N.: Estudio metabólico del tejido adiposo en la rata prenada. *In* Actas de la XII Reunión Nacional de la Sociedad Española de Ciencias Fisiológicas, G. Torroba, ed., 1971, pp. 361–363.

40. Freinkel, N., Herrera, E., Knopp, R. H., et al. Metabolic realignments in late pregnancy: A clue to diabetogenesis? *In* Early Diabetes, R. A. Camerini-Davalos and H. S. Cole, eds. Academic Press, New York, 1970, pp. 205–219.

41. Herrera, E., Knopp, R. H., and Freinkel, N. Carbohydrate metabolism in pregnancy. VI. Plasma fuels, insulin, liver composition, gluconeogenesis, and nitrogen metabolism during late gestation in the fed and fasted rat. *J. Clin. Invest. 48:* 2260–2272, 1969.

42. Shambaugh, G. E., Mrozak, S. C., Metzger, B. E., et al. Glutamine-dependent carbamyl phosphate synthetase during fetal and neonatal life in the rat. *Dev. Biol. 37:* 171–185, 1974.

43. Winick, M. *In* Malnutrition and Brain Development. London, Oxford University Press, 1976.

44. Felig, P., and Lynch, V. Starvation in human pregnancy: Hypoglycemia, hypoinsulinemia, and hyperketonemia. *Science 170:* 990–992, 1970.

45. Tyson, J. E., Austin, K. L., and Farinholt, J. W. Prolonged nutritional deprivation in pregnancy: Changes in human chorionic somatomammotropin and growth hormone secretion. *Am. J. Obstet. Gynecol. 109:* 1080–1082, 1971.

46. Metzger, B. E., Hare, J. W., and Freinkel, N. Carbohydrate metabolism in pregnancy. IX. Plasma levels of gluconeogenic fuels during fasting in the rat. *J. Clin. Endocrinol. Metab. 33:* 869–873, 1971.

47. Felig, P., Kim, Y. J., Lynch, V., et al. Amino acid metabolism during starvation in human pregnancy. *J. Clin. Invest. 51:* 1195–1202, 1972.

48. Tyson, J. E., Austin, K., Farinholt, J., et al. Endocrine-metabolic response to acute starvation in human gestation. *Am. J. Obstet. Gynecol. 125:* 1073–1084, 1976.

49. Metzger, B. E., Agnoli, F., Hare, J. W., et al. Carbohydrate metabolism in pregnancy. X. Metabolic disposition of alanine by the perfused liver of the fasting pregnant rat. *Diabetes 22:* 601–608, 1973.

50. Williamson, D. H. Regulation of the utilization of glucose and ketone bodies by brain in the perinatal period. *In* Early Diabetes in Early Life, R. A. Camerini-Davalos and H. S. Cole, eds. Academic Press, New York, 1975, pp. 195–202.

51. Persson, B. Treatment of diabetic pregnancy. *Isr. J. Med. Sci. 11:* 609–616, 1975.

52. Elliott, J. A. The effect of pregnancy on the control of lipolysis in fat cells isolated from human adipose tissue. *Europ. J. Clin. Invest. 5:* 159–163, 1975.

53. DeMeyts, P., Kahn, C. R., Roth, J., et al. Hormonal regulation of the affinity and concentration of hormone receptors in target cells. *Metabolism 25:* 1365–1370, 1976.

54. Burt, R. L. Peripheral utilization of glucose in pregnancy; insulin tolerance. *Obstet. Gynecol. 7:* 658–664, 1956.

55. Knopp, R. H., Ruder, H. J., Herrera, E., et al. Carbohydrate metabolism in pregnancy. VII. Insulin tolerance during late pregnancy in the fed and fasted rat. *Acta Endocrinol. 65:* 352–360, 1970.

56. Spellacy, W. N., and Goetz, F. C. Plasma insulin in normal late pregnancy. *N. Engl. J. Med. 268:* 988–991, 1963.

57. Kalkhoff, R., Schalch, D. S., Walker, J. L., et al. Diabetogenic factors associated with pregnancy. *Trans. Assoc. Am. Physicians 77:* 270–280, 1964.

58. Phelps, R. L., Bergenstal, R., Freinkel, N., et al. Carbohydrate metabolism in pregnancy. XIII. Relationships between plasma insulin and proinsulin during late pregnancy in normal and diabetic subjects. *J. Clin. Endocrinol. Metab. 41:* 1085–1091, 1975.

59. O'Sullivan, J. B., and Mahan, C. M. Criteria for the oral glucose tolerance test in pregnancy. *Diabetes 13:* 278–285, 1964.

60. Freinkel, N., Metzger, B. E., Nitzan, M., et al. "Accelerated starvation" and mechanisms for the conservation of maternal nitrogen during pregnancy. *Isr. J. Med. Sci. 8:* 426–439, 1972.

61. Freinkel, N., and Metzger, B. E. Some considerations of fuel economy in the fed state during late human pregnancy. *In* Early Diabetes in Early Life, R. A. Camerini-Davalos and H. S. Cole, eds. Academic Press, New York, 1975, pp. 289–301.

62. Pedersen, J. Diabetes and Pregnancy. Blood Sugar of Newborn Infants. Danish Science Press, Copenhagen, 1952.

63. Coltart, T. M., Beard, R. W., and Turner, R. C., et al. Blood glucose and insulin relationships in the human mother and fetus before onset of labor. *Br. Med. J. 4:* 17–19, 1969.

64. Freinkel, N., Metzger, B. E., Nitzan, M., et al. Facilitated anabolism in late pregnancy: Some novel maternal compensations for accelerated starvation. *In* Proceedings of the VIIIth Congress of the International Diabetes Federation, W. Malaisse and J. Pirart, eds. *Excerpta Medica International Congress Series No. 312,* Amsterdam, 1974, pp. 474–488.

65. Daniel, R. R., Metzger, B. E., Freinkel, N., et al. Carbohydrate metabolism in pregnancy. XI. Response of plasma glucagon to overnight fast and oral glucose during normal pregnancy and in gestational diabetes. *Diabetes 23:* 771–776, 1974.

66. Kuhl, C., and Holst, J. J. Plasma glucagon and the insulin: glucagon ratio in gestational diabetes. *Diabetes 25:* 16–23, 1976.

67. Metzger, B. E., Unger, R. G., and Freinkel, N. Carbohydrate metabolism in pregnancy. XIV. Relationships between circulating glucagon, insulin, glucose, and amino acids in response to "mixed meal" in late pregnancy. *Metabolism 26:* 151–156, 1977.

68. Saudek, C. D., Finkowski, M., and Knopp, R. H. Plasma glucagon and insulin in rat pregnancy: Roles in glucose homeostasis. *J. Clin. Invest. 55:* 180–187, 1975.

69. Kalkhoff, R. K., and Kim, H. J. Islet insulin and glucagon secretion in pregnancy. *Clin. Res. 23:* 536, 1975 (abstract).

70. White, P. Pregnancy and diabetes. *In* Joslin's Diabetes Mellitus (ed 11). Lea and Febiger, Philadelphia, 1971, pp. 581–598.

71. Pedersen, J., and Pedersen, L. M. Prognosis of the outcome of pregnancies in diabetics. *Acta Endocrinol. 50:* 70–78, 1965.

72. Gellis, S. S., and Hsia, D. Y. The infant of the diabetic mother. *Am. J. Dis. Child. 97:* 1–41, 1959.

73. Hamblen, E. C. Sterility-incidence and cause. *In* Endocrinology of Woman, Charles C. Thomas, Springfield, 1945, chap. 47, pp. 490–497.

74. Williams, J. W. The clinical significance of glycosuria in pregnant women. *Am. J. Med. Sci. 137:* 1–26, 1909.

75. Skipper, E. Diabetes mellitus and pregnancy; clinical and analytical study, with special observations upon 33 cases. *Q. J. Med. 2:* 353–380, 1933.

76. Peel, J. H., and Oakley, W. G. *In* Trans. XII Brit. Cong. of Ob. Gyn., London, 1950, p. 161.

77. Oakley, W. Prognosis in diabetic pregnancy. *Br. Med. J. 1:* 1413–1415, 1953.

78. Pedersen, J., and Brandstrup, E. Foetal mortality in pregnant diabetics. Strict control of diabetes with conservative obstetric management. *Lancet 1:* 607–610, 1956.

79. Harley, J. M. G., and Montgomery, D. A. D. Management of pregnancy complicated by diabetes. *Br. Med. J. 1:* 14–18, 1965.

80. Delaney, J. J., and Ptacek, J. Three decades of experience with diabetic pregnancies. *Am. J. Obstet. Gynecol. 106:* 550–556, 1970.

81. Bibergeil, H., Godel, E., and Amendt, P. Diabetes and pregnancy: Early and late prognosis of children of diabetic mothers. *In* Early Diabetes in Early Life, R. A. Camerini-Davalos and H. Cole, eds., Academic Press, New York, 1975, pp. 427–434.

82. Oakley, W. The treatment of pregnancy in diabetes mellitus. *In* On the Nature and Treatment of Diabetes, B. S. Leibel and G. A. Wrenshall, eds., Excerpta Medica Foundation, Amsterdam, 1965, pp. 673–678.

83. Pedersen, J., Mølsted-Pedersen, L., and Andersen, B. Assessors of fetal perinatal mortality in diabetic pregnancy. *Diabetes 23:* 302–305, 1974.

84. Roversi, G. D., Canussio, V., and Gargiulo, M. Insulin in gestational diabetes. *In* Early Diabetes in Early Life, R. A. Camerini-Davalos and H. Cole, eds. Academic Press, New York, 1975, pp. 469–475.

85. Essex, N. L., Pyke, D. A., Watkins, P. J., et al. Diabetic pregnancy. *Br. Med. J. 4:* 89–93, 1973.

86. Tyson, J. E., and Hock, R. A. Gestational and pregestational diabe-

tes: An approach to therapy. *Am. J. Obstet. Gynecol. 125:* 1009–1027, 1976.

87. Gugliucci, C. L., O'Sullivan, M. J., Opperman, W., et al. Intensive care of the pregnant diabetic. *Am. J. Obstet. Gynecol. 125:* 435–441, 1976.

88. White, P. Diabetes mellitus in pregnancy. *Clin. Perinatol. 1:* 331–347, 1974.

89. Persson, B. Assessment of metabolic control in diabetic pregnancy. *In* Size at Birth, K. Elliot and J. Knight, eds. CIBA Foundation Symposium 27 (New Series), 1974, pp. 247–267.

90. Shea, M. A., Garrison, D. L., and Tom, S. K. H. Diabetes in pregnancy. *Am. J. Obstet. Gynecol. 111:* 801–803, 1971.

91. Dundon, S., Murphy, A., Raftery, J., et al. Infants of diabetic mothers. *J. Isr. Med. Assoc. 67:* 371–375, 1974.

92. Haworth, J. C., and Dilling, L. A. Effect of abnormal glucose tolerance in pregnancy on infant mortality rate and morbidity. *Am. J. Obstet. Gynecol. 122:* 555–560, 1975.

93. Karlsson, K., and Kjellmer, I. The outcome of diabetic pregnancies in relation to the mother's blood sugar level. *Am. J. Obstet. Gynecol. 112:* 213–220, 1972.

94. Larsson, Y., and Ludvigsson, J. Perinatal dödlighet vid diabetesgraviditet. *Läkartidningen 71:* 155–157, 1974.

95. Bailey, P., Blake, M., Younger, B., et al. Amniotic fluid osmolality in pregnancies complicated by diabetes. *Am. J. Obstet. Gynecol. 124:* 257–262, 1976.

96. Mintz, D. H., Chez, R. A., and Hutchinson, D. L. Subhuman primate pregnancy complicated by streptozotocin-induced diabetes mellitus. *J. Clin. Invest. 51:* 837–847, 1972.

97. Maternal nutrition and the course of pregnancy. Summary Report, National Academy of Sciences, U.S. DHEW, Rockville, Md., 1970, p. 5.

98. O'Sullivan, J. B. Long term follow up of gestational diabetics. *In* Early Diabetes in Early Life, R. A. Camerini-Davalos and H. S. Cole, eds. Academic Press, New York, 1975, pp. 503–510.

99. Hadden, D. R. Glucose tolerance tests in pregnancy. *In* Carbohydrate Metabolism in Pregnancy and the Newborn. H. W. Sutherland and J. M. Stowers, eds. Churchill Livingstone, Edinburgh, London, and New York, 1975, pp. 19–41.

100. Posner, N. A., Silverstone, F. A., Pomerance, W., et al. The outcome of pregnancy in class A diabetes mellitus. *Am. J. Obstet. Gynecol. 111:* 886–895, 1971.

101. Gabbe, S. G., Mestman, J. H., Freeman, R. K., et al. Management and outcome of class A diabetes mellitus. *Am. J. Obstet. Gynecol. 127:* 465–469, 1977.

102. O'Sullivan, J. B., Mahan, C. M., Charles, D., et al. Medical treatment of the gestational diabetic. *Obstet. Gynecol. 43:* 817–821, 1974.

103. Stallone, L. A. and Ziel, H. K. Management of gestational diabetes. *Am. J. Obstet. Gynecol. 119:* 1091–1094, 1974.

104. O'Sullivan, J. B., Charles, D., Mahan, C. M., et al. Gestational diabetes and perinatal mortality rate. *Am. J. Obstet. Gynecol. 116:* 901–904, 1973.

105. Metzger, B. E., Pek, S., Hare, J., et al: Relationships between glucose, insulin and glucagon during fasting in late gestation in the rat. *Life Sci. 15:* 301–308, 1974.

106. Kuhl, C. Serum proinsulin in normal and gestational diabetic pregnancy. *Diabetologia 12:* 295–300, 1976.

107. Metzger, B. E., Nitzan, M., Phelps, R. L., et al. The beta cell in gestational diabetes: Victim or culprit? *Clin. Res. 23:* 445A, 1975 (abstract).

108. O'Sullivan, J. B. Insulin treatment for gestational diabetics. *In* Early Diabetes in Early Life, R. A. Camerini-Davalos and H. Cole, eds. Academic Press, New York, 1975, pp. 447–453.

109. Felig, P. Body fuel metabolism and diabetes mellitus in pregnancy. *Med. Clin. North Am. 61:* 43–66, 1977.

110. Cornblath, M., and Schwartz, R. Disorders of Carbohydrate Metabolism in Infancy (ed. 2). Vol. III in Major Problems in Clinical Pediatrics series. W. B. Saunders Co., Philadelphia, 1976, pp. 115–154.

111. Koller, O. Diabetes and pregnancy. *Acta Obstet. Gynecol. Scand. 32:* 80–103, 1953.

112. Jones, W. S. Management of the pregnant diabetic. *Diabetes 7:* 439–445, 1958.

113. Drury, M. I. Pregnancy in the diabetic. *Diabetes 15:* 830–835, 1968.

114. Biegelman, P. M. Severe diabetic ketoacidosis ("diabetic" coma). *Diabetes 20:* 490–500, 1971.

115. Given, W. P., and Tolstoi, E. Present day management of the pregnant diabetic: success or failure? *Surg. Clin. North Am. 37:* 369–378, 1957.

116. Hoet, J. P., Hoet, J. J., and Gommers, A. Endocrine disturbances of pregnancy and foetal pathology. *Proc. R. Soc. Med. 52:* 813–816, 1959.

117. Zarowitz, H., and Moltz, A. Management of diabetes in pregnancy. *Obstet. Gynecol. 27:* 820–826, 1966.

118. Victor, A. Normal blood sugar variation during pregnancy. *Acta Obstet. Gynecol. Scand. 53:* 37–40, 1974.

119. Gillmer, M. D. G., Beard, R. W., Brooke, F. M., et al. Carbohydrate metabolism in pregnancy. Part I: Diurnal plasma glucose profile in normal and diabetic women. *Br. Med. J. 3:* 399–402, 1975.

120. Moller, E. B. Studies in Diabetic Pregnancy. Studentlitterature, Lund, 1970.

121. Sabbagha, R. E., Turner, J. H., Rockette, H., et al. Sonar BPD and fetal age. Definition of the relationship. *Obstet. Gynecol. 43:* 7–14, 1974.

122. Goebelsmann, U., Freeman, R. K., and Mestman, J. H., et al. Estriol in pregnancy. II. Daily urinary estriol assays in the management of the pregnant diabetic woman. *Am. J. Obstet. Gynecol. 115:* 795–802, 1973.

123. Freeman, R. K. The use of the oxytocin challenge test for antepartum clinical evaluation of uteroplacental respiratory function. *Am. J. Obstet. Gynecol. 121:* 481–489, 1975.

124. Gluck, L., and Kulovich, M. V. Lecithin-sphingomyelin ratios in amniotic fluid in normal and abnormal pregnancy. *Am. J. Obstet. Gynecol. 115:* 539–546, 1973.

125. Osler, M. Structural and chemical changes in infants of diabetic and prediabetic mothers. *In* On the Nature and Treatment of Diabetes, B. S. Leibel and G. A. Wrenshall, eds. Excerpta Medica Foundation, Amsterdam, 1965, pp. 692–699.

126. Miller, H. C. Cardiac hypertrophy in newborn infants. *Yale J. Biol. Med. 16:* 509–518, 1944.

127. Naeye, R. L. Infants of diabetic mothers: A quantitative, morphological study. *Pediatrics 35:* 980–988, 1965.

128. Tsang, R. C., Chen, I., Friedman, M. A., et al. Parathyroid function in infants of diabetic mothers. *J. Pediatr. 86:* 399–404, 1975.

129. Robert, M. F., Neff, R. K., Hubbell, J. P., et al. Association between maternal diabetes and the respiratory-distress syndrome in the newborn. *N. Engl. J. Med. 294:* 357–360, 1976.

88

Diabetes in Acromegaly and Other Endocrine Disorders

Jeffrey S. Flier
Jesse Roth

Diabetes mellitus is a condition of unknown etiology, characterized by (1) impaired glucose tolerance and insulin secretion, (2) thickening of capillary basement membranes throughout the body, and (3) a specific group of late complications involving, most importantly, the retina, the glomerulus, and the peripheral nerves. Abnormalities of glucose tolerance and insulin secretion are commonly encountered in a variety of endocrinopathies other than diabetes, arising coincident with or subsequent to the onset of the endocrinopathy. It is these states of altered glucose tolerance that form the subject of this chapter.

GENERAL CONSIDERATIONS

The glucose intolerance occurring secondary to endocrine disorders is usually of moderate degree. Marked hyperglycemia and glycosuria are uncommon, and ketosis is rare. The nature of the link between these or other metabolic abnormalities and the late complications of diabetes remains an active subject for investigation and debate. It is important to stress, however, that whereas the metabolic abnormalities observed in these patients vary over a broad range of severity and duration, thus far late complications have been remarkably rare. Thus, whereas retinopathy, nephropathy, and neuropathy are common in diabetes mellitus, they are rarely encountered in patients with glucose intolerance secondary to endocrinopathies. In addition, the characteristic thickening of capillary basement membranes has not been demonstrated in these patients[1] with the exception of acromegalics with fasting hyperglycemia (see p. 1047).

The underlying endocrinopathy usually represents the chief cause of morbidity and mortality. For this reason, treatment of the underlying condition should be the primary therapeutic concern. Furthermore, successful treatment of the endocrinopathy is usually accompanied by a complete reversal of the carbohydrate disorder. It should be noted that some experimental animals treated with growth hormone or glucocorticoids can, under certain conditions, develop permanent glucose intolerance and destruction of beta cell function,[2] but this phenomenon has not been convincingly demonstrated in man. Thus, in treating the glucose intolerance, we seek only to keep the patient free of ketosis, polyuria, and dangerous levels of hyperglycemia. Since carbohydrate tolerance and insulin sensitivity are likely to change with the natural history of the underlying disease, excessively tight control of blood glucose may be particularly hazardous. Finally, such mainstays of diabetic care as meticulous foot care and frequent eye examinations are not required in these settings.

Endocrinopathies may alter glucose tolerance and insulin secretion by multiple interdependent mechanisms and at a number of loci in the processes of hormone synthesis, release, clearance, and action at the target cell. Although our knowledge of each of these aspects of hormone physiology continues to increase, we remain unable in most cases to predict accurately a particular clinical outcome from the integrated sum of our physiological observations. For this reason, we will try to balance what we know clinically and what we believe to be relevant at a molecular level.

Our discussion will be limited to the direct effects of hormones on carbohydrate homeostasis. However, endocrinopathies can affect glucose tolerance in a variety of indirect ways. Thus, endocrinopathies often produce marked changes in food intake, body weight, serum electrolytes, body composition (e.g. muscle wasting), and physical activity, which in turn can have substantial effects on carbohydrate tolerance. These should be viewed as important additional factors in the resultant glucose intolerance, but they will not be covered in this chapter.

GLUCOSE TOLERANCE WITH ACROMEGALY AND ISOLATED GROWTH HORMONE DEFICIENCY

Abnormalities of glucose tolerance and insulin secretion are common features of acromegaly and isolated growth hormone deficiency. We will first summarize our current understanding of the actions of growth hormone on relevant metabolic processes and then review the clinical aspects of the association.

METABOLIC EFFECTS OF GROWTH HORMONE

Growth hormone (GH) has multiple effects on many tissues, some of which are insulinlike and others of which oppose the action of insulin. The molecular mechanisms of these effects are largely unknown.

After intravenous injections of pharmacologic doses of GH into experimental animals and man, early (i.e., within minutes) insulinlike effects have been observed.[3,4] These include increased glucose disappearance rate and reduced FFA levels. Similar effects have been observed with extremely high concentrations of GH in vitro.[5] These effects of GH may simply be artifacts of the dose and preparations employed. Alternatively, the in vivo effects may be mediated by the GH-stimulated release of one or more "growth peptides," such as the somatomedins and NSILA-s.[6] These peptides have, in addition to potent growth-promoting properties, a weak but definite insulinlike activity, which is mediated by binding to the insulin receptor on insulin target tissues.[7,8]

The less immediate actions of GH have been somewhat better defined, and the data on this subject have been more uniform. Two important effects of GH on carbohydrate metabolism are an insulinotropic action and an effect to reduce tissue sensitivity to insulin. A direct effect of GH to promote insulin secretion is supported by in vitro and in vivo experiments. Isolated islets from hypophysectomized rats have decreased insulin content and impaired insulin release to numerous stimuli. This defect is corrected by treatment for several days with GH.[9] Growth hormone can acutely stimulate the release of insulin and glucagon from an isolated, perfused rat pancreas preparation at physiological as well as pharmacological concentrations.[10] In addition, GH pretreatment of normal subjects causes a profound increase in the amount of insulin released in response to insulin secretagogues prior to a measurable effect on the level of blood glucose.[3,11]

Growth hormone administration has been shown to reduce insulin sensitivity in both hypopituitary and normal subjects,[3] and this effect may be seen as early as several minutes after administration.[12] The effect of this reduced insulin sensitivity on glucose homeostasis depends, at least in part, on the adequacy of the compensatory increase in insulin secretion that is evoked.

Growth hormone administration also accelerates lipolysis, with a significant rise in nonesterified fatty acids within several hours of administration.[13,14] The hormone also has potent anabolic effects on protein synthesis in muscle, skeletal tissue, and connective tissue, as well as in other sites. While some of these effects have been seen in vitro with high concentrations of hormone,[15] the in vivo effects of GH on protein anabolism may be mediated largely by GH dependent growth peptides (vide supra).

Recent studies of the insulin receptors in acromegalic patients and animals with GH-secreting tumors provide new insights into the mechanisms of insulin resistance in states of growth hormone excess. Insulin receptors of acromegalic patients, measured on their circulating monocytes, may be abnormal in at least two respects.[16] First, the concentration of insulin receptors in these patients may be reduced. As in obesity, in which insulin resistance has been extensively studied, the concentration of insulin receptors in acromegaly is inversely related to the degree of basal hyperinsulinemia; patients with normal basal insulin levels have normal receptor concentration, and patients with marked hyperinsulinemia have the greatest receptor loss. It is likely that, as in obesity, the receptor loss is a direct cellular effect of the hyperinsulinism.

A second alteration in some patients with GH excess is that the receptor has an increased affinity for insulin but only at resting, physiological concentrations of insulin.[16] This increase in receptor affinity, first observed in obese hyperinsulinemic patients during a fast,[17] may represent some compensation in the postabsorptive period for the insulin-induced receptor loss.

Rats treated with growth hormone develop mild insulin resistance.[19] Insulin receptors on hepatic plasma membranes of these animals show changes analogous to those observed on the monocytes of acromegalic patients.[20] There is a small reduction in receptor number and a modest increase in receptor affinity at resting concentrations of insulin. The role of these receptor changes in the insulin resistance of acromegaly is far from clear. Specifically, the opposite effects on receptor number and receptor affinity may allow normal or nearly normal insulin binding at resting concentrations of insulin, making it likely that defects subsequent to receptor binding are major causes of insulin resistance both in these animal models and in acromegalic patients.

ROLE OF GROWTH HORMONE IN NORMAL CARBOHYDRATE METABOLISM

The precise role of growth hormone in the control of normal carbohydrate metabolism has not been defined. Growth hormone administration causes enhanced fat utilization, diminished carbohydrate consumption, and decreased protein catabolism.[22] This constellation of effects is similar to the changes observed during fasting and led to the suggestion that growth hormone might have a role in the metabolic adaptation to a prolonged fast. In fact, growth hormone levels rise acutely during induced hypoglycemia and in the early stages of fasting.[23,24] Growth hormone levels return to baseline, however, after 5 days of continuous fasting.

The best data on the role of GH in metabolic homeostasis come from studies of familial isolated growth hormone deficiency.[25] These studies indicate that GH plays a role in the regulation of glucose homeostasis during a fast but that GH is not important in the control of protein or fat metabolism under these conditions (vide infra). Similarly, GH administration is unable to reverse the protein catabolism that occurs when obese patients are fasted.[11]

GLUCOSE TOLERANCE IN ACROMEGALY

Acromegaly results from increased levels of growth hormone due to persistent hypersecretion of the hormone by the pituitary. Two effects of GH predominate among its many effects observed in vitro and in vivo. These are resistance to the glucose lowering effects of insulin and promotion of insulin secretion. As many as 60 percent of acromegalics have abnormal oral glucose tolerance.[26,27] About one-third of these patients have elevated levels of fasting glucose, of whom one-third may require insulin therapy; the dosage of insulin required to control blood glucose may be increased.

The prevalence of abnormal glucose tolerance in these subjects markedly underestimates the frequency and severity of the insulin resistance in this disease. With intravenous insulin tolerance tests, as many as 80 percent of patients are insulin-resistant.[27] Furthermore, measurements of insulin levels by immunoassay reveal basal as well as stimulated (glucose, arginine, tolbutamide, leucine) hyperinsulinemia in a similar or greater percentage[26-32] (Fig. 88-1). Some studies have demonstrated a diminished insulin secretory response to provocative stimuli in patients with the very severe glucose intolerance.[26]

Thus the defect in glucose tolerance in these patients may be divided into at least four groups, ranging from normality to severe diabetes. A small minority of affected patients have completely normal glucose tolerance, insulin secretion, and insulin sensitivity by all available tests. In a significantly larger group, insulin resis-

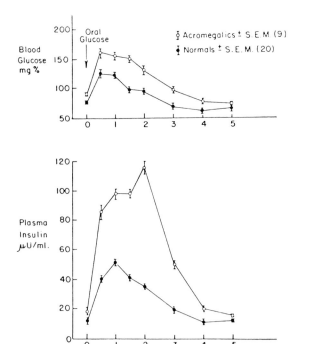

Fig. 88-1. Plasma concentrations of glucose and insulin after oral glucose (100 g) in normal and acromegalic patients (From P. Beck et al., *Journal of Laboratory and Clinical Medicine* 66:366–379, 1965.)

tance exists, but normal glucose tolerance is maintained by compensatory hyperinsulinemia. In the largest group of patients, abnormal glucose tolerance develops despite hyperinsulinemia. A smaller group develops serious degrees of hyperglycemia in some cases associated with failure of compensatory islet cell hyperfunction.

Attempts to relate absolute levels of GH in a group of acromegalics to their degree of glucose intolerance or insulin resistance have shown only a weak correlation, although a major reduction of GH levels associated with disease inactivity is clearly associated with improvement or normalization of blood glucose levels and sensitivity to intravenous insulin.[26,30,33] Despite high growth hormone concentration for as long as 9 years and glucose intolerance of substantial degree, we have not detected the retinal, renal, neuropathic or small vessel disease characteristic of genetic diabetes mellitus.*

ISOLATED GROWTH HORMONE DEFICIENCY

Systematic studies of carbohydrate tolerance and insulin secretion have been performed on groups of patients with inherited monotropic deficits in growth hormone secretion.[34,35] It is not known whether these studies are also representative of sporadic cases of isolated growth hormone deficiency, either congenital or acquired.

In the largest group of these patients, fasting glucose is normal, but glucose tolerance is impaired following both oral glucose and mixed meals. The plasma insulin at the start is normal or low,

---

*Siperstein and Raskin (in unpublished studies) found that acromegalics who have fasting hyperglycemia (but not other acromegalics) have thickened capillary basement membranes indistinguishable from those characteristic of diabetes. It is unclear whether the acromegalics with fasting hyperglycemia are independently afflicted with genetic diabetes or whether the basement membrane changes are a consequence of the long-standing hyperglycemia.

but it rises subnormally following all stimuli, despite prolonged hyperglycemia (Fig. 88-2). Standard intravenous insulin tolerance tests (0.1 U/kg) produce a prompt fall in glucose and FFA, but the return to normal is clearly delayed. After GH therapy for several days, insulin levels rise *(vide supra)*. Glucose tolerance may remain impaired, however, possibly secondary to GH-induced reduction in tissue sensitivity to insulin.[36] Prolonged fasting is associated with hypoglycemia despite diminished insulin levels. In addition, production of free fatty acids and ketones is accelerated when compared to controls.[25]

A smaller subset of these patients, with what appears to be a different mode of inheritance, have hyperglycemia with moderate hyperinsulinism, along with normal or subnormal responses to intravenous insulin.[34] Despite the long duration of significant glucose intolerance, none of these subjects has developed late complications of diabetes.

DIABETES AND CUSHING'S SYNDROME

Cushing's syndrome is caused by elevated concentrations of plasma glucocorticoids. These may be produced by the adrenals, either autonomously or under ACTH stimulation, or may result from the exogenous administration of glucocorticoids or ACTH. Although experimentally ACTH has many extra-adrenal effects, the clinical disturbances of carbohydrate metabolism in Cushing's syndrome can be ascribed completely to the effects of the elevated glucocorticoid concentrations.

EFFECTS OF GLUCOCORTICOIDS ON CARBOHYDRATE METABOLISM

Overall, the actions of glucocorticoids result in diminished glucose utilization, increased glucose production, and hyperglycemia.[37] Gluconeogenesis in liver and kidney is increased, as is synthesis of glycogen and urea in the liver. The enhanced gluconeogenesis is the result of induction of hepatic enzyme activity,[38] as well as an increased concentration of gluconeogenic precursors as a result of a catabolic action on muscle and fat.[39] *In vitro*,

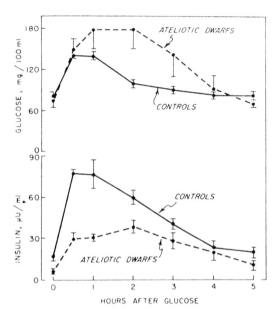

Fig. 88-2. Plasma concentrations of glucose and insulin after oral glucose (50 mg) in control and growth hormone deficient patients (ateliotic dwarfs). (From Merimee, T. J., et al. *Metabolism 17:* 1005–1011, 1968.)

glucocorticoids increase the release of free fatty acids from adipose tissue and enhance free fatty acid release in response to catecholamines, ACTH, and growth hormone.[40,41] This may be the result of impaired reesterification of FFA secondary to reduced glucose transport and metabolism and therefore to reduced levels of α-glycerol phosphate. Diminished glucose uptake after exposure to glucocorticoids has been demonstrated with adipocytes, fibroblasts, and lymphoid cells, and these cells have also shown reduced sensitivity to insulin. The mechanisms by which glucocorticoids may produce this insulin-resistant state are complex and involve several steps in the pathways for insulin action.

Glucocorticoid excess in rats, whether produced by exogenous administration of ACTH or dexamethasone, results in insulin resistance and a marked decrease in insulin binding to its receptors, both in liver and adipose tissue[20,21,42] (Fig. 88-3). In contrast to the decrease in insulin binding observed in obesity (and acromegaly), this decrease in binding appears to result from a marked decrease in the affinity of the insulin receptor for insulin.[21] Conversely, adrenalectomy produces an increase in insulin binding by increasing the affinity of the insulin receptor, which is consistent with the increase in insulin sensitivity that occurs in this state.[21] In addition, postreceptor abnormalities have been demonstrated after glucocorticoid treatment. Thus, there is a major inhibition of the glucose transport system.[43–45] Intracellular steps distal to glucose transport may also be affected, but their contribution to the glucocorticoid-induced insulin resistance is less clear.

EFFECTS OF EXOGENOUS GLUCOCORTICOIDS IN MAN

Administration of glucocorticoids to normal human subjects has been clearly shown to produce temporary abnormalities of glucose tolerance associated with resistance to endogenous and exogenous insulin[46] (Fig. 88-4). There are several variables that determine the extent of these effects. Glucose intolerance is observed in nearly all normals if studied in the first few days of treatment.[46,47] The duration of administration is important, be-

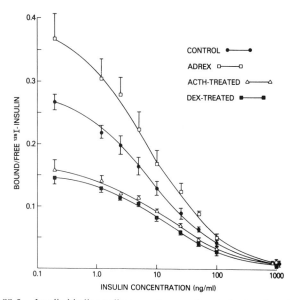

Fig. 88-3. Insulin binding to liver membranes of control rats, adrenalectomized rats, and rats with glucocorticoid excess caused by ACTH or dexamethasone (From Kahn et al., unpublished data.)

EFFECT OF STEROIDS ON INSULIN BINDING

CONTROL ●——●
ADREX □——□
ACTH-TREATED △——△
DEX-TREATED ■——■

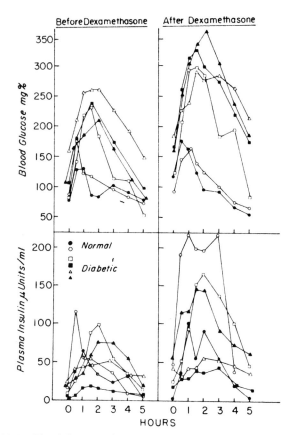

Fig. 88-4. Blood glucose and plasma insulin responses to oral glucose (100 g) in normal subjects and patients with mild diabetes before and after dexamethasone, 2 mg, four times a day for 3 days. (From Perley, N., et al. *New Eng. J. Med. 274:* 1237–1240, 1960.)

cause in most cases, the disturbance subsides to a significant degree during chronic therapy,[48] although the basis for this phenomenon is not clear. The incidence of abnormality will depend on the index used to determine the presence of a defect. Thus, fasting blood glucose is a less sensitive index of insulin resistance than is a GTT. The GTT is, in turn, less sensitive than determination of insulin levels, which are often elevated both basally and after stimulation by glucose or tolbutamide even in patients with normal glucose tolerance.[46] Individual susceptibility is an important factor, since steroids may exacerbate a previously latent diabetic state on the basis of genetic predisposition or obesity.

GLUCOSE TOLERANCE IN CUSHING'S SYNDROME

The prevalence of abnormal glucose tolerance in Cushing's syndrome is very high and may range up to 90 percent.[49] Severe fasting hyperglycemia and ketosis are uncommon and occur in less than 20 percent of cases. However, most patients have hyperinsulinemia, both basal and following stimulation by glucose or tolbutamide, irrespective of whether glucose tolerance is disturbed.[50,51] A few patients with severe glucose intolerance have subnormal insulin responses to several stimuli, suggesting failure of compensatory hyperinsulinemia as a factor contributing to their deterioration. The cause of the elevated insulin levels appears to be the tissue resistance to insulin, which leads to elevated blood glucose and a consequent insulin secretory response. Data suggesting a direct effect of steroids to produce islet hypertrophy most likely reflect such compensatory changes.

Despite some cases of prolonged glucose intolerance in association with Cushing's syndrome, specific late diabetic complications are rarely observed. The metabolic changes produced in these patients are entirely reversible after correction of the steroid excess.

GLUCOSE INTOLERANCE AND HYPERTHYROIDISM

Thyroid hormone may affect carbohydrate metabolism at many loci. As a result of its acceleration of nearly all metabolic processes, tissue utilization of glucose is enhanced, which would dampen any tendency to reduced glucose tolerance. Hepatic glycogen is diminished, and the glycemic response to glucagon is impaired.[52] On the other hand, many effects of thyroid hormone might be expected to decrease glucose tolerance. These include an increased rate of gastric emptying, increased rate of glucose absorption from the intestine, and elevated levels of nonesterified fatty acids which may interfere with glucose utilization.[53-55] Insulin degradation has been shown to be increased in rats made hyperthyroid with exogenous T_4. In addition, thyroid hormone excess causes a "hyperadrenergic state," which may in part be due to a thyroxine-induced increase in the concentration of beta-adrenergic receptor sites. One effect of this adrenergic overactivity may be to dampen insulin secretion via adrenergic receptor influence on beta-cell responsivity.[57] In this regard, guanethedine administration has been reported to improve glucose tolerance and improve insulin/glucose ratios in hyperthyroid subjects without altering the BMR, the PBI, or the level of nonesterified fatty acids.[58] While this and other data[59] suggest an impairment of insulin release in this disorder, other investigators have detected hyperinsulinemia and have postulated an insulin refractory state.[60]

Studies of oral glucose tolerance in thyrotoxic patients have not yielded consistent results. Fasting glucose is usually normal, but elevated levels have been seen with variable frequency after glucose ingestion; surprisingly, peak plasma levels of glucose may occur somewhat later than in normals. Hyperthyroidism has been reported to be associated with glucose intolerance in 2 to 57 percent of cases.[60-63] This wide range may be a consequence of the different criteria employed, as well as the numerous, often counterbalancing, effects of thyroid hormones on glucose tolerance.

In the experience of most workers when glucose intolerance occurs in hyperthyroidism, it is usually mild and does not require treatment; the severity of the glucose intolerance appears unrelated to the degree of hyperthyroidism. Occasional patients have marked hyperglycemia, glycosuria, and ketonuria, and insulin requirements in these patients vary widely. There are conflicting reports on the state of glucose tolerance after restoration of the euthyroid state. The study that reported a 57 percent incidence of glucose intolerance in hyperthyroid patients claimed that the defect persisted in half the patients after euthyroidism was attained.[63] These data, if confirmed, would indicate an increased prevalence of genetic diabetes mellitus in hyperthyroidism.

GLUCOSE INTOLERANCE AND PHEOCHROMOCYTOMA

The clinical manifestations of pheochromocytoma result from increased amounts of circulating catecholamines, primarily norepinephrine. Catecholamines have major effects on fuel disposition by influencing glucose generation, lipolysis, and the release and action of insulin.[64] The actions of catecholamines have been divided into two groups, alpha and beta, each of which is mediated by a specific cell membrane receptor. The second messenger for the alpha-adrenergic pathway is unknown, whereas the beta-adrenergic receptor is linked via adenylate cyclase to the second messenger cyclic AMP. Classic studies demonstrated that epinephrine both increased cyclic AMP and promoted glycogenolysis and gluconeogenesis in liver. However, recent studies indicate that in the liver, catecholamines (possibly by alpha-adrenergic pathways) stimulate gluconeogenesis and probably also glycogenolysis independently of their ability to stimulate beta-adrenergic pathways, adenylate cyclase, and cyclic AMP.[65,66] At physiological concentrations, epinephrine stimulates glycogenolysis in muscle and lipolysis in fat. A direct effect on hepatic glucose production at concentrations of epinephrine observed in vivo is a matter of controversy. Clinically, the most significant effect produced by catecholamines appears to be interference with insulin release by the pancreas. Both epinephrine and norepinephrine infusions cause a prompt rise in blood glucose in normal subjects coincident with a fall in plasma insulin levels.[57] Insulin release, provoked by glucose, tolbutamide, and glucagon, is inhibited by infusion of catecholamines. This effect appears to be mediated by alpha-adrenergic receptors, since alpha-adrenergic receptor blockers (i.e., phentolamine) completely block the catecholamine effect on insulin release.[57]

In patients with pheochromocytoma, fasting blood glucose is usually within the normal range.[67,68] Pheochromocytoma may give rise to either a persistent or paroxysmal hypertension; glucose intolerance can accompany either. Oral glucose tolerance is modestly impaired in most patients in association with a diminished and delayed insulin secretory response. Insulin treatment is characteristically not required. In several reported cases, the hypoglycemic response to intravenous insulin was mildly (and reversibly) blunted.[67] However, in the one patient of ours who required insulin, ketonuria and glycosuria responded well to small doses of insulin, suggesting that the inhibition of insulin output was the predominant effect of the catecholamines.

In some but not all patients, the administration of the alpha-adrenergic blocker phenoxybenzamine restores the secretory responses of insulin and improves glucose tolerance.[68] Phentolamine has similarly resulted in significantly increased plasma insulin levels.[67]

Curative surgery completely restores glucose tolerance in most of the reported cases.[67-69] The remainder show marked improvement, and it is rare to find no improvement in carbohydrate metabolism. Normal fasting blood sugar and improved glucose tolerance can be seen by 1 month after resection in association with an enhancement in insulin/glucose ratios. Insulin tolerance has been reported to become normal by 3 to 4 months, with concomitant improvement in the response to tolbutamide with both an increase in insulin output and in the magnitude of the hypoglycemic response.

In some patients, glucose intolerance can persist for many months after tumor resection before reverting to normal.[67,70] This is not attributable to residual impairment of insulin release, since the insulinogenic index is improved significantly in the early postoperative period. Glucose intolerance at this time may represent a state of relative insulin resistance, and this is consistent with the finding of a concomitantly decreased responsiveness to exogenous insulin. Subsequently, insulin responsiveness slowly improves.

Diabetic complications are not a feature of the glucose intolerance of pheochromocytoma.

GLUCOSE INTOLERANCE AND GLUCAGONOMA

The role of glucagon in both normal physiology and in diabetes mellitus is a subject of intense debate and is reviewed in detail elsewhere in the text. Administration of a pharmacologic dose of glucagon to normal man causes a prompt rise in blood glucose through an increase in hepatic glucose production, an accelerated rate of lipolysis, and enhanced hepatic utilization of amino acids (especially alanine) for gluconeogenesis. In addition, insulin secretion is directly stimulated. The role of physiological alterations in glucagon levels is much less clear, however, in large part as a result of the absence of a clear-cut disease of glucagon deficiency. Attempts to define the role of glucagon have relied heavily on the use of somatostatin, an agent that inhibits both glucagon and insulin secretion. These studies indicate that glucagon probably plays a role in the maintenance of basal hepatic glucose production in normal man.[71,72] Although glucagon secretion may be instrumental in the prevention of insulin-induced hypoglycemia after protein ingestion,[73,74] changes in glucagon levels are probably not important for the normal disposal of a glucose load.

The role of glucagon in the diabetic state has received much attention because diabetes is characterized by absolute or relative hyperglucagonemia.[75] Hyperglucagonemia has been implicated in the pathogenesis of diabetes, in the development of diabetic ketoacidosis, and in the glucose intolerance associated with a variety of diseases, including severe infection, trauma, cirrhosis, uremia, and pancreatitis. Most studies show that hyperglucagonemia (at levels obtained in disease states) has only minor effects on the blood glucose level unless insulin is deficient, in which case glucagon can promote marked increases in blood glucose levels as well as ketonemia.[14,76] Thus, hyperglucagonemia may contribute importantly to the diabetic state. In the past several years, an increasing number of cases have been described in which glucagon-secreting tumors of the pancreatic islets are associated with a distinct clinical syndrome, of which glucose intolerance is a predominant feature.[77–79]

In some cases, glucagon has been shown to respond appropriately to a variety of stimuli, although with much higher blood levels than normal. In one case, 60 to 90 percent of circulating immunoreactive glucagon was associated with a higher (10,000) molecular weight pro-glucagon-like species, which possessed 30 percent of the biologic activity of normal pancreatic glucagon.[80]

The clinical glucose intolerance that occurs in most of these subjects has been mild, but in some cases, large doses of insulin failed to effect good control. Other clinical features are a female preponderance, age generally over 45 years, anemia, weight loss, and a characteristic skin lesion termed necrolytic migratory erythema. The skin lesion is often widespread, is most severe on the lower abdomen, groin, perineum, and mouth and begins as an erythematous area with central blistering, weeping, and crusting. There is usually central healing and hyperpigmentation. The pancreatic tumors, which are composed of alpha-cells by histochemical, electron-microscopic, immunofluorescence, and bioassay criteria, are commonly malignant (>50 percent) but may be quite slow growing. Several cases have responded to streptozotocin therapy.[80]

GLUCOSE INTOLERANCE AND THE CARCINOID SYNDROME

Patients with metastatic carcinoid tumors and the carcinoid syndrome have been reported to have an increased incidence of glucose intolerance and impaired insulin secretion.[81] In one study,

50 percent of the patients with carcinoid syndrome and elevated serotonin levels had frankly abnormal glucose disposal rates after intravenous glucose administration associated with impaired insulin secretory responses. Fasting glucose and insulin levels were abnormal in 10 percent of cases. Patients with carcinoid tumors without clinical evidence of the carcinoid syndrome or elevated levels of serotonin had normal intravenous glucose tolerance. Studies with the serotonin antagonist cyproheptadine and the serotonin synthesis blocker p-chlorophenylalanine suggest a role for serotonin in the glucose intolerance of the carcinoid syndrome. Such a role is further supported by *in vitro* evidence that serotonin may directly inhibit insulin secretion.

DIABETES MELLITUS COMPLICATED BY ENDOCRINOPATHY

The development of an endocrinopathy in a patient with preexisting diabetes may be heralded by substantial alterations in diabetic control. Acromegaly, Cushing's disease, pheochromocytoma, and hyperthyroidism can produce a marked increase in hyperglycemia, ketonuria, and insulin requirement. Alternatively, loss of growth hormone, thyroid, or adrenal function may cause a marked reduction in blood glucose, insulin requirement, and propensity to hyperketonemia. More importantly, these patients may suddenly develop bouts of severe hypoglycemia on small or trivial doses of insulin. Correction of the endocrinopathy usually restores the premorbid state.

The concurrence of genetic diabetes mellitus and another endocrinopathy would be expected for a variety of reasons. These include the usual risk for diabetes occurring independently in any patient, the fact that these patients are very likely to undergo careful metabolic scrutiny as part of their evaluation, and the ability of several endocrine conditions to bring out latent diabetes by specific hormonal effects. Further, the diabetic state and other endocrinopathies may be linked by common etiologies, such as polyglandular immune destruction or immune-mediated hormone resistance.[82,83] On occasion, it will not be possible to distinguish the glucose intolerance caused by an endocrinopathy from coexistent diabetes mellitus. Our ability to make this distinction with assurance must await discovery of a marker (or markers) of the diabetic state independent of the abnormality in glucose tolerance.

REFERENCES

1. Siperstein, M. D., Unger, R. H., Madison, L. L.: Studies of muscle capillary basement membranes in normal subjects, diabetic and prediabetic patients. *J. Clin. Invest.* 47: 1973–1999, 1968.
2. Houssay, B. A., Andersen, E.: Diabetogenic action of purified anterior pituitary hormones. *Endocrinology* 45: 627–629, 1949.
3. Daughaday, W. H., Kipnis, D. M.: The growth promoting and anti-insulin action of somatotropin. *Rec. Prog. Horm. Res.* 22: 49–93, 1966.
4. Zahnd, G. R., Steinke, J., Renold, A. E.: Early metabolic effects of human growth hormone. *Proc. Soc. Exp. Biol. Med.* 105: 455–470, 1960.
5. Goodman, H. M.: Growth hormone and the metabolism of carbohydrate and lipid in adipose tissue. *Ann. N.Y. Acad. Sci.* 148: 419–424, 1968.
6. Daughaday, W. H.: In Luft R., Hall, K. (eds.): Advances in Metabolic Disorders, vol. 8. New York, Academic Press, 1975, p. 159.
7. Megyesi, K., Kahn, C. R., Roth, J., et al.: The NSILA-s receptor in liver plasma membranes: Characterization and comparison with the insulin receptor. *J. Biol. Chem.* 250: 8990–8998, 1976.
8. Rechler, M. M., Nissley, S. P., Podskalny, J. M., et al.: Identification of a receptor for somatomedin-like polypeptides in human fibroblasts. *J. Clin. Endocrinol. Metab.* 44: 820–830, 1977.

89

Lipoatrophic Diabetes

Aldo A. Rossini

George F. Cahill, Jr.

INTRODUCTION

Although the syndrome of lipoatrophic diabetes is characterized by diabetes mellitus and the absence of adipose tissue, the etiology (or etiologies) still remains an enigma. The association of these findings was first observed by Ziegler in 1928[1] and Hansen and McQuarrie in the 1940s,[2] but it was not until 1946 that Lawrence[3] established the classical criteria. Following these initial reports various observations of patients with similar findings were reported, and finally two apparently separate types of lipoatrophic diabetes were delineated, although some patients may present with mixed features of the two types (Table 89-1). The congenital type of this disease is probably transmitted by autosomal recessive inheritance, in which the lipoatrophy, present at birth, precedes the onset of diabetes by an average of 12 years. In the acquired type, the diabetes may even precede the lipoatrophy by a variable amount of time. The acquired type of the syndrome may follow an illness (e.g., pertussis, varicella, rubeola), and this correlation may be important for a further understanding of the pathophysiology of both forms of the disease.

The major clinical findings of this syndrome are shown in Table 89-2. A common clinical difficulty, that of overdiagnosing this syndrome, is apparent. The thin brittle underweight juvenile diabetic who often may have hyperlipidemia and hepatomegaly shares many similar findings, and confusion in diagnosis may be present. However, the elevated BMR, which averages approximately +64% in the postabsorptive state, the absence of clinical ketosis, the marked insulin resistance (as much as thousands of units of insulin per day without the presence of insulin antibodies without appreciably altering blood sugar) may be helpful clues in differentiating the diagnosis of this syndrome from the thin brittle diabetic.

Of all the cases of lipoatrophic diabetes, a statistical analysis of the causes of death is lacking. The most common reason has been the complications of liver disease, i.e., hepatic coma and esophageal bleeding. Interesting reported findings[4-6] have been the presence of neuropathy, nephropathy, and retinopathy, which suggests that the elevated glucose milieu may be an important constituent to the complications of the diabetic syndrome.

HORMONES

INSULIN

Various studies have shown that the basal immunoreactive insulin levels are increased without clinical signs of hyperinsulinism. The percentage of proinsulin present at baseline and following perturbations, such as with glucagon and tolbutamide tolerance, remained at between 4 and 6 percent of the total immunoreactive insulin activity.[7] Similarly, after these perturbations or after amino acid infusion there is a brisk insulin release to levels as high as 1000 μU/ml; however, occasionally the insulin release has been found delayed and suboptimal.[5,6] The insulin activity has also been measured by biological assay (rat diaphragm and epididymal fat pad) and has been found to be normal.[8] Anti-insulin and insulin-neutralized antibodies have not been found.[9,10]

Insulin disappearance rate using ^{131}I has been found normal[6] with a half-life of 12 min, and this was unchanged in both the fed and fasted states.[9] Also noteworthy is the presence in one studied instance of normal insulin receptors on mononuclear cells.[9] In a few cases where autopsies have been performed, hypertrophy of the islets was found whereas fibrosis of pancreas parenchyma has also been observed.[11,12]

THYROID

Since the original observations by Lawrence that elevated basal metabolic rates were present, although there was no other clinical evidence of hyperthyroidism, this finding has been confirmed by various laboratories, and numerous thyroid function studies have been found to be normal. The thyromegaly, which has been frequently noted, has been interpreted as secondary to the absence of surrounding fat tissue. Thyroidectomy has been performed, which produced a marked fall of the BMR to the normal range, but because of the severely clinical hypothyroid state which ensued, thyroid replacement was necessary, and the hypermetabolism returned to the pretreatment state. Spontaneous hypothy-

Table 89-1. Lipoatrophic Diabetes

Type	Congenital	Acquired
Eponym	Berardinelli–Seip	Lawrence
Heredity	Autosomal recessive	Not noted
Onset	Infancy	Childhood or adulthood
Cases reported (1974)	37	30
Consanguinity	Very high	None noted
Preceded by an illness	None	Often
Sex distribution	Equal	Female > male 2:1
Onset of lipoatrophy	At birth	Childhood or later life
Onset of diabetes	Usually childhood onset (12 years)	Often precedes the lipoatrophy
Maturation and growth	Accelerated	Depending on age of onset
Muscle hypertrophy	Marked	Mild
Liver cirrhosis	Mild–moderate	Severe
Acanthosis nigricans	Mild	Severe
Associated congenital defects	Often	Rare
Cerebral pathology	Frequent	Rare

roidism has been reported and has been histologically confirmed to be due to Hashimoto's thyroiditis.[9]

GROWTH HORMONE

The clinical appearance of the patient with lipoatrophic diabetes, namely the acromegaloid features, organomegaly, thickened skin, increased muscle mass, insulin resistance, and accelerated bone age and growth, has been a tantalizing rationale for a putative hypersecretion of growth hormone. Various differences in the response of growth hormone release have been reported. Intermittently elevated basal levels and even hypersecretion after arginine infusion have been noted.[13] However, in various other patients studied with this syndrome, a lack of response following intravenous arginine stimulation and a lack of growth hormone response during slow-wave sleep have also been characterized.[9–14] The discrepancies may be due to the great degree of heterogeneity.

Other explanations could be the presence of an abnormal regulation of growth hormone secretion which is intermittently expressed, or the production of an abnormal growth hormone which is measured by some immunoreactive assays but not others, or a variability of the expression of the syndrome itself.

GLUCAGON

Although the measurement of this hormone is recent, the level in one reported case has been normal.[15] However, another report reveals a markedly increased level in both the fed state and following a 110-h fast, both being greater than 500pg/ml.[9]

CORTISOL

The response of the adrenal gland is variable but most cases reveal that in the basal state and after ACTH stimulation there is a normal response.[16,17] Similarly, a normal diurnal response and an increase during the rapid eye movement state of sleep have also been observed.[9] The marked elevation of biologically measured cortisol-releasing factor which has been found in a few cases of this syndrome[18,19] is difficult to interpret in view of the intact normal physiologic feedback. However, a few cases have been shown to have a poor response to metapyrone, thus suggesting again that there may be much heterogeneity within this syndrome.

GONADOTROPINS

In the males with this syndrome, few data are available with the exception of the genitomegaly in childhood. In the female, menstrual disturbances and the concomitant presence of the polycystic ovaries (Stein–Leventhal syndrome) have often been described.[1,12,20] Urinary estrogens and pregnanediol are reported to be appropriate for the degree of maturity and time of cycle, while FSH levels are normal.[21] In other cases slight elevations were found.[20] A recent study in one subject of the congenital form revealed a normal oscillation of FSH and LH levels during frequent sampling throughout a day.[9] It is noteworthy that this case with the normal diurnal variations was a female who 2 years previously had a wedge resection for polycystic ovaries which was diagnosed by amenorrhea of 1-year duration, and an ovarian mass which was clinically apparent.

FUELS

CARBOHYDRATES

The glucose intolerance is present to a variable degree, depending on whether the syndrome is of the congenital or acquired type. In the congenital group the elevated blood sugar is usually not present for the first decade, although some variability exists. On the other hand, in the acquired type, the glucose abnormality may be present before the lipoatrophy. The failure to control glucose levels with large doses of insulin (thousands of units in 24 h) reveals the great insulin insensitivity that is present.[9]

A sedentary 50-kg female was observed to eat an average of 3200 cal, of which 52 percent was carbohydrate, without any change in weight, explainable by her hypermetabolism and an average daily excretion of 250 g of glucose in her urine. The large chronic urinary volume which is present with the excretion of such a large quantity of carbohydrate may produce the dilated ureters frequently observed in both these patients and in patients with diabetes insipidus.[9] Along with the large quantity of carbohydrate ingested is the marked increase of protein intake with elevated glucagon levels which will further increase the carbohydrate pool by augmenting hepatic gluconeogenesis. The postabsorptive fasting nonprotein respiratory quotient performed on another patient was compatible with the metabolizing of a mixture of 0.5 parts carbohydrate and 1 part fat.[10] With the administration of insulin, the quotient increased, which indicated an increased carbohydrate utilization. Utilizing [^{14}C]glucose it has been shown that the rate of

Table 89-2. Lipoatrophic Diabetes

1. Absence of clinically apparent adipose tissue
2. Insulin-resistant diabetes mellitus
3. Markedly diminished capacity to develop ketoacidosis
4. Elevated basal metabolic rate (BMR)
5. Hyperlipidemia and hepatomegaly

Common associated findings
Muscular hypertrophy ("Herculean")
Thick curly hair
Acromegaloid features
Acanthosis nigricans
Phlebomegaly
Genitomegaly
Splenomegaly
Sclerotic and thickened bone
Cystic angiomatous lesions in bones

oxidation of glucose to CO_2 was within normal limits, but the rate of CO_2 production was increased, suggesting oxidation of fat.[11] During a fast of 110 h in one studied subject, the blood glucose level decreased to 110 mg/100 ml. In this subject caloric restriction or a diet primarily of medium chain triglycerides decreased fasting glucose levels as well.[9] The effect of glycogen formation by insulin appears to be intact with a normal to increased glycogen content as evidenced by biopsies of both liver and muscle.[21] Similarly, following the administration of glucagon a rapid elevation of blood glucose is noted, which suggests an intact and responsive glycogen store.[22]

PROTEIN

The increase of the muscle mass as clinically represented by the "Herculean" appearance is confirmed by both body composition studies using radioisotopes and by the elevated daily excretion of creatinine.

Biopsy of the muscles previously failed to reveal any histologic abnormality.[23] Recently, high resolution light microscopy and electron microscopy of muscle biopsies in congenital lipoatrophic diabetes showed variation in fiber size and various degrees of fiber degeneration and fragmentation, with accumulation of glycogen, aggregations of mitochondria, streaming of Z line, myofilamentous inclusions, and dilation of sarcoplasmic reticulum profiles.[24] Similarly, normal enzyme contents of phosphorylase and phosphorylase kinase have been determined.[25] In evaluating the amino acid content in the postabsorptive state, increased levels of alanine and glutamine are present while the branched-chain amino acids (valine, isoleucine, and leucine) are normal. Following the administration of insulin at 0.1 μU/kg or 0.5 μU/kg to one studied subject a slight fall of the glucogenic and branched-chain amino acids occurred. This finding may suggest that the insulin effect on the glucose levels is very minimal; however, there is a response of the amino acid pool to insulin administration. Similarly, there is a fall of certain amino acids during fasting similar to the decrease found in normals; however, the level of alanine, which fell 50 percent, is still well above the normal. The urinary nitrogen during the fed state in a case extensively studied was found to average approximately 22 g in a 24-h period, in agreement with her marked hyperphagia. However, during a fast, urinary nitrogen fell to 12 g daily which represents a persistent breakdown of approximately 80 g of muscle protein during the fast, again within the rate of that found in normals. The glucagon levels in the 110-h fast were only slightly decreased from the >500-pg/ml level during the postabsorptive state.

LIPIDS

Of all the fuels in this syndrome, lipids have been the most extensively studied. The marked hyperlipemia which belongs to the type V classification, the frequent observation of eruptive xanthomatosis, and hyperlipemia retinalis are clinical signs which confirm the biochemical observations of triglyceride levels of 2–3000 mg/100 ml. Deposition of this excessive amount of circulating triglycerides into the liver, spleen, and other reticuloendothelial tissues has been confirmed by histologic examination.[1] Interesting is the fall of the triglyceride levels during the fast of 110 h in which a halving of the liver size was documented.[9] The finding that the triglyceride levels are higher following a carbohydrate meal compared to a high fat diet has also been demonstrated.[6] The basal postabsorptive plasma nonesterified free fatty acids are usually within normal levels and do not increase during a fast. However, the glycerol levels are reported to be slightly elevated to as much

as three to six times the normal value during the fast, suggesting a turnover of adipose triglycerides greater than normal. In radioisotopic studies, [^{14}C]acetate was found to be incorporated into triglycerides and cholesterol at a more rapid rate and in increased amounts.[10] Interestingly, the rate of disappearance of the activity from the lipid fractions was also decreased. There has been much variability in assays of postheparin lipoprotein lipase activity in serum, ranging from normal to markedly decreased values.[6,15,26]

The lack of ketosis which is characteristic of this syndrome has been considered to be due to a paucity of mobilizable fat. In a few reports low levels of ketone bodies were found present after severe stress or infection.[10] Following brief fasts of 24 or 48 h there has been no evidence of ketones.[27] However, after a 110-h fast in one intensively studied subject there was a significant and measurable increase of the ketone bodies, while the nonesterified (free) fatty acids failed to increase. It is noteworthy that insulin levels decreased during the fast, and when insulin was administered a 50 percent fall of the ketone levels occurred. Thus not only the availability of fatty acid but the effect of insulin appears to be critical for the development of ketone production.

OTHER LABORATORY TESTS

ELEVATED OXYGEN CONSUMPTION

The elevated BMR, which is one of the important and significant findings in this syndrome in the absence of hyperthyroidism or the Luft–Ernster syndrome (hypertrophy of mitochondria), has been difficult to explain. The lack of adipose tissue may falsely elevate the calculated BMR and may account for an increase of 10 to 20 percent above baseline. The interesting finding that the diet of 3000 cal/day causes no change in weight and that approximately 36,000 cal/month are not accountable even when the calories lost in the urine and stool are subtracted from the intake, has suggested that the excess caloric intake and metabolic rate may be related. Following the balanced intake of a meal (1500 cal) and measurement of oxygen consumption, as well as skin and oral temperatures, a dramatic increase in these parameters has been found. The oxygen consumption is found to increase markedly following the meal while there are great fluctuations of the skin temperatures (34–38 °C) associated with shivering and sweating. Thus during a meal, the increased oxygen utilization and the dissipation of this energy as heat are observed. Similarly, during a fast, the oxygen consumption falls to normal. Thus the disposal of excess calories by oxidation instead of storing in the fat depots could account for the caloric expenditure, a true example of "luxus consumption."[28]

The recent histologic finding of a marked increase of mitochondria may reflect the state of increased metabolic activity as described in the Luft–Ernster syndrome.[29] Thus the possibility of increasing the utilization of dietary fuels by increasing metabolic expenditure through a futile cycle could be invoked as a possible mechanism of dietary-induced thermogenesis.[30]

LIPID MOBILIZING FACTOR

In a heterogenous group of cases of lipoatrophic diabetes the finding of a "diabetogenic" peptide in the urine has been demonstrated.[31] Following the extraction of this peptide and then its administration into various animal models including man, the production of hyperglycemia and an insulin insensitivity is manifested. This peptide has also been shown to have lipid-mobilizing effects on fat cells as well. The peptide is not unique for lipoatrophic diabetes since it has also been observed in the urine of diabetics with proteinuria.[32] A substance with similar activity has also been found in the pituitary gland of various animals.[33]

The possibility that this peptide causes a rapid turnover of fat stores so that lipolysis occurs as rapidly as triglyceride is synthesized has been postulated as the mechanism in this syndrome.[31] The inability of demonstrating this substance in all the studied cases as well as the inability of finding the peptide in the urine unless proteinuria is present is a puzzling observation. Similarly, the ability of so small an area of the hypothalamic or pituitary region to produce such a large quantity as can be recovered in the urine is difficult to ascertain.

RELEASING FACTORS

The recent observation of an elevation of the activity of hypothalamic–pituitary releasing factors in lipoatrophic diabetes has been found using in vivo bioassays. Elevated levels of corticotropin releasing factor (CRF), follicle-stimulating hormone-releasing factor (FRF), and melanocyte-stimulating hormone-releasing factor (MRF) have been found in approximately 6 patients with this syndrome.[34] Upton, Corbin, and colleagues have hypothesized that in lipoatrophic diabetes there is a defect in the hypothalamus of the enzyme, dopamine β-hydroxylase, which causes an accumulation of dopamine and thus a decrease in norepinephrine levels. According to the hypothesis, dopamine produces stimulation of the releasing factors whereas norepinephrine decreases this effect. Hence the end result is a continuous stimulation of the releasing factors with the absence of normal inhibition. Furthermore, the administration of pimozide, a narcoleptic which apparently has a direct inhibiting effect on the stimulatory effect of dopamine on releasing factors, has produced ameliorization of this syndrome in at least one case. Not only was there a decrease in the measurable levels of the releasing factors but clinical changes such as decreases of the curly hair, acanthosis nigricans, and hepatomegaly have been described.[35] However, with other clinical trials, the administration of pimozide has been unrewarding. Also, in a metabolic study in one patient administration of the drug for a 2-week period failed to alter several biochemical parameters such as oxygen consumption, insulin insensitivity, and levels of various fuels. Further investigation in examining the effectiveness of this medication, possibly in some cases of lipoatrophic diabetes, may be worthwhile, and the variable effect may be related to the possible differences in etiology.

ETIOLOGY

The etiology of lipoatrophic diabetes is still unknown (Table 89-3). The absolute absence of the fat cell has been disputed since histologically typical signet cells or even immature fat cells are evident. However, the paucity of these cells remains a hallmark of this syndrome. The next possible defect is in the fat cell itself. The lack of effect of exogenous or endogenous insulin in lowering free

Table 89-3. Etiology of Lipoatrophic Diabetes

1. Congenital absence of adipose cells
2. Rapid turnover of adipose triglyceride
    Autonomic nervous system defect
    Hypothalamic defect—anatomic
    Excess hypothalamic releasing factors
    Excess lipid-mobilizing factors
3. Receptor defects
    Adipose tissue receptor abnormality
    Adipose tissue post-receptor abnormality
    Hormone receptor abnormalities in other tissues

fatty acids in either the fed or fasted state may provide evidence that the fat cell receptor for insulin may be deficient. The presence of normal insulin receptors has been shown in the mononuclear cells of one patient with this syndrome, and this finding may be important since it has been suggested in animal models that the mononuclear cell insulin receptor may mirror the insulin receptor in both the liver and fat cell.[36] In one reported case of progressive partial lipoatrophy an autotransplantation of adipose tissue from a normal site to the lipoatrophic area was unsuccessful due to the atrophy of the transplanted tissue.[37] Similarly, when tissue removed from a lipoatrophic area was transplanted to a nonaffected area there was growth and viability of the fat cells. A third and more tenable theory is that a lipoatrophic substance may be released into the circulation, and another theory may be an altered state of the central nervous system. In the latter instance the insulin-insensitive state, lipolysis, and hypermetabolism are conditions which may be analogous to that seen with excess stimulation of the sympathetic nervous system, such as those in subjects with pheochromocytoma. The hypothalamus has also been implicated in other syndromes which affect adipose tissue, e.g., the diencephalic syndrome of emaciation.[38] It is noteworthy that in a number of cases of lipoatrophic diabetes there have been congenital abnormalities of the third ventricle, and the findings of tumors in this region as well.[39] Thus releasing factors or the lipid-mobilizing factors, which may be the same material, may be inappropriately released into the circulation, causing an effect on other tissues. The observation that a transient improvement of the lipoatrophic diabetes syndrome with a decrease of the acanthosis nigricans, liver size, and insulin resistance occurred during a hypophysectomy[40] may illustrate the importance of this anatomical area in the etiology of this disease. Although the finding with pimozide appears to be helpful in selected cases the possibility that the effect of this compound may be a key to resolving the enigma associated with this syndrome awaits further investigation.

Finally, a hypothesis can be presented which postulates that there may be alterations in the various intracellular signals elicited by insulin in tissues of the lipoatrophic. The amino acid decrease after near-physiologic levels of insulin and the hypertrophic muscles, the increased organ sizes, and dermal elements all suggest adequate insulinization. Likewise, the marked antiketogenesis in the syndrome also suggests an increased insulin effect on liver, if anything. The same could be said for the levels of liver and muscle glycogen. In contrast, the hyperglycemia, elevated glycerol levels, lack of decreases in levels of glucose, free fatty acids, and glycerol after insulin suggest deficient insulin effectiveness. Thus a differential deletion of certain of insulin's intracellular and cell membrane effects is suggested. If this be congenital in the hereditary form of the disease, it would be expected to be expressed in infancy by diabetes as well as by the lipoatrophy, which is usually not the case. Hence the pathophysiology remains inexplicable in view of present knowledge.

Although mentioned previously that in one case of lipoatrophic diabetes insulin receptors were normal, more recent observations have shown a decreased binding of insulin to its receptor in a series of patients with generalized lipoatrophic diabetes, and when fasted for 60 h, the insulin binding increased.[41] The decreased insulin binding may be related to a circulating receptor antibody similar to that described in patients with acanthosis nigricans, glucose intolerance, hyperinsulinemia, and marked resistance to exogenous insulin without evidence of lipoatrophy.[42] Further studies will be needed to resolve the relationship of insulin receptor deficiency to the other hormones which may result in many of the clinical and laboratory findings observed in lipoatrophic diabetes.

ACKNOWLEDGMENTS

This work was supported in part by U.S.P.H.S. Grants No. AM-05077 and AM-15191, and the Capps Fund, Harvard University.

REFERENCES

1. Ziegler, L. H.: Lipodystrophies: Report of seven cases. *Brain 51:* 147, 1928.
2. Hansen, A. E., and McQuarrie, I.: Serum and tissue lipids in peculiar type of generalized lipodystrophy (lipohistiodiaresis). *Am. J. Dis. Child. 60:* 754, 1940.
3. Lawrence, R. D.: Lipodystrophy and hepatomegaly with diabetes, lipaemia, and other metabolic disturbances. A case throwing new light on the action of insulin. *Lancet 1:* 724, 733, 1946.
4. Marcus, R.: Retinopathy, nephropathy and neuropathy in lipoatrophic diabetes. Case report and discussion. *Diabetes 15:* 351, 1966.
5. Tourniare, J., Guinet, P., Marnex, R., Veyrat, A., and Magniem, J. M.: Diabetic lipoatrophique. Etude clinique et biologique d'un cas atypique. *Sem. Hop. Paris 44:* 3289, 1968.
6. Hamwi, G. J., Kruger, F. A., Eymontt, M. J., Scarpelli, D. G., Gwinup, G., and Byron, R.: Lipoatrophic diabetes. *Diabetes 15:* 262, 1966.
7. Sovik, O., Oseid, S., and Oyasaeter, S.: Studies in congenital generalized lipodystrophy. V. Circulating insulin and pro-insulin. *Acta Endocrinol. 73:* 731, 1973.
8. Sovik, O., and Oseid, S.: Studies in congenital generalized lipodystrophy. I. The effects of patients' plasma on glycogen synthesis in rat diaphragm and adipose tissue in vivo. *Acta Endocrinol. 72:* 495, 1973.
9. Rossini, A. A., Self, J., Aoki, T. T., Goldman, R., Newmark, S. R., Meguid, M. M., Soeldner, J. S., and Cahill, G. F., Jr.: Metabolic and endocrine studies in a case of lipoatrophic diabetes. *Metabolism 26:* 637, 1977.
10. Schwartz, R., Schafer, I. A., and Renold, A. E.: Generalized lipoatrophy, hepatic cirrhosis, disturbed carbohydrate metabolism and accelerated growth (lipoatrophic diabetes): Longitudinal observations and metabolic studies. *Am. J. Med. 28:* 973, 1960
11. Craig, J. W., and Miller, M.: Lipoatrophic diabetes. In R. H. Williams (ed.): Diabetes, New York. Paul B. Noeber, Inc., 1960, pp. 700–707.
12. Brunzell, J. D., Shankle, S. W., and Bethune, J. E.: Congenital generalized lipodystrophy accompanied by cystic angiomatosis. *Ann. Intern. Med. 69:* 501, 1968.
13. Tzagournis, M., and George, J.: Increased growth hormone in partial and total lipoatrophy. *Diabetes 22:* 388, 1973.
14. Oseid, S.: Studies in congenital generalized lipodystrophy. III. Growth hormone levels. *Acta Endocrinol. 73:* 427, 1973.
15. Kem, D., Collin, D., and Martin, C.: Immunoreactive glucagon in total lipodystrophy. *Clin. Res. 18:* 122, 1970.
16. Ruvalcaba, R. H., Somals, E., and Kelley, V. C.: Lipoatrophic diabetes. I. Studies concerning endocrine function and carbohydrate metabolism. *Am. J. Dis. Child 109:* 279, 1965.
17. Reed, W. B., Dexter, R., Corley, C., and Fish, C.: Congenital lipodystrophic diabetes with acanthosis nigricans. *Arch. Dermatol. 91:* 326, 1965.
18. Seip, M., and Trygstad, O.: Generalized lipodystrophy. *Arch. Dis. Child. 38:* 447, 1963.
19. Brubaker, M. M., Levan, N. E., and Kaplan, S. A.: Acanthosis nigricans with lipodystrophy and growth abnormalities. *Arch. Dermatol. 89:* 292, 1964.
20. DeGennes, J. L., Saltiel, H., Tremoberes, J., Apfelbaum, M., and Landat, B.: Revision de l'exploration metabolique et endocrinienne d'un cas de diabete lipo-atrophique. *Presse Med. 75:* 2605, 1967.
21. Seip, M.: Lipodystrophy and gigantism with associated endocrine manifestations: A new diencephalic syndrome? *Acta Paediatr. 48:* 555, 1959.
22. Seip, M.: Generalized Lipodystrophy. *Ergeb. I. Med. Kinder. 31:* 59, 1971.
23. Taton, J., Malczewski, B., and Wisniewska, A.: Studies on the pathogenesis of lipoatrophic diabetes: A case of congenital systemic absence of adipose tissue associated with insulin-resistant diabetes mellitus and hepatosplenomegaly. *Diabetologia 8:* 319, 1972.
24. Afifi, A. K., Mire-Salman, J., and Najjar, S.: The myopathology of congenital generalized lipodystrophy light and electron microscopic observations. *Johns Hopkins Med. J. 139 (Suppl.):* 61, 1976.
25. Ruvalcaba, R. H., and Kelley, V. C.: Lipoatrophic diabetes. II. Metabolic studies concerning mechanism of lipemia. *Am. J. Dis. Child. 109:* 287, 1965.
26. Havel, R. J., Basso, L. V., and Kane, J. P.: Mobilization and storage of fat in congenital and late-onset forms of total lipodystrophy. *J. Clin. Invest. 47:* 1068, 1967.
27. Kikkawa, R., Hoshi, M., Shigeta, Y., and Izumi, K.: Lack of ketosis in lipoatrophic diabetes. *Diabetes 21:* 827, 1972.
28. Neumann, R. O.: Experimentelle Beitrage zur Lehre von dem Taglichen Nahrungsbedarf des Menschen unter besonderer Berucksichtigung der notwendigen Eiweifsmenge (Selbstyersuche). *Arch. Hyg. 45:* 1–87, 1902.
29. Luft, R., et al.: A case of severe hypermetabolism of nonthyroid origin with a defect in the maintenance of mitochondrial respiratory control. A correlated clinical, biochemical and morphological study. *J. Clin. Invest. 41:* 1776, 1962.
30. Sims, E. A. H.: Experimental obesity, dietary-induced thermogenesis, and their clinical implications. *Clin. Endocrinol. Metab. 5:* 377, 1976.
31. Louis, L. H., Conn, J. W., and Minich, M. C.: Lipoatrophic diabetes. Isolation and characterization of an insulin antagonist from the urine. *Metabolism 12:* 867, 1963.
32. Louis, L. H., and Conn, J. W.: A urinary diabetogenic polypeptide in proteinuric diabetic patients. *Metabolism 18:* 556, 1969.
33. Louis, L. H., and Conn, J. W.: Diabetogenic polypeptide from hog and sheep andenohypophysis similar to that found in lipoatrophic diabetes. *Metabolism 17:* 475, 1968.
34. Mabry, C. C., Hollingsworth, D. R., Upton, G. V., and Corbin, A.: Pituitary-hypothalamic dysfunction in generalized lipodystrophy. *J. Pediatr. 82:* 625, 1973.
35. Corbin, A., Upton, G. V., Mabry, C. C., and Hollingsworth, D. R.: Diencephalic involvement in generalized lipodystrophy: Rationale and treatment with the neuroleptic agent, pimozide. *Acta Endocrinol. 77:* 209, 1974.
36. Soll, A. H., Goldfine, I. D., Roth, J., and Kahn, C. R.: Thymic lymphocytes in obese (ob/ob) mice. *J. Biol. Chem. 249:* 4127, 1974.
37. Langhof, H., and Zabel, R.: Uber lipodystrophia progressiva. *Arck. Klin. Exp. Dermatol. 210:* 313, 1960.
38. Torrey, E. F., and Uyeda, C. I.: Diencephalic syndrome of infancy. *Am. J. Dis. Child. 110:* 689, 1965.
39. Berardinelli, W.: An undiagnosed endocrinometabolic syndrome: Report of 2 cases. *J. Clin. Endocrinol. 14:* 193, 1954.
40. Mabry, C. C., and Hollingsworth, D. R.: Failure of hypophysectomy in generalized lipodystrophy. *J. Pediatr. 81:* 990, 1972.
41. Oseid, S., Beck-Nielsen, H., Pedersen, O., and Sovik, O.: Decreased binding of insulin to its receptor in patients with congenital generalized lipodystrophy. *N. Engl. J. Med. 296:* 245, 1977.
42. Kahn, C. R., Flier, J. S., Bar, R. S., Archer, J. A., Gordon, P., Martin, M. M., and Roth, J.: The syndromes of insulin resistance and acanthosis nigricans. Insulin receptor disorders in man. *N. Engl. J. Med. 294:* 739, 1976.

Hypoglycemia

Ronald A. Arky

Normal man maintains a circulating plasma glucose that fluctuates between 60 and 160 mg/dl (3.3–8.8 mM) during the fasted and fed states. This striking constancy of plasma glucose results from the integration of the hormonal and neural factors that affect plasma glucose at any point in time. When the circulating glucose level declines to a concentration at which the central nervous system is deprived of glucose, a characteristic set of symptoms evolve.[1,2] These symptoms of hypoglycemia or neuroglycopenia usually appear when plasma glucose levels are below 50 mg/dl or when whole blood glucose levels are below 40 mg/dl. Specific levels of glucose at which symptoms are noted vary greatly, and in some individuals little correlation exists between circulating levels of glucose and symptomatology. Symptoms from neuroglycopenia are dependent upon the status of the cerebral circulation, the functional and structural integrity of cerebral tissue, the rapidity of fall and prolongation of the depressed glucose, and the availability

to the brain,[3,4] as well as to other tissues, of fuels other than glucose.

Symptomatic hypoglycemia reflects an abnormality of glucose homeostasis and occurs in a wide variety of clinical settings. To understand the pathogenesis of any episode of neuroglycopenia, the clinician must evaluate each of the several factors that influence glucose homeostasis at the time of the symptoms.

This review attempts to analyze and classify the various clinical hypoglycemic states from the standpoint of their pathophysiology. Specific aspects of normal physiology are summarized to provide a background, while diagnostic and therapeutic principles are included in the clinical discussions.

PHYSIOLOGIC CONSIDERATIONS

The storage of nutrient to provide substrate for periods of food deprivation begins immediately in the postprandial period. In our Western culture, most adults consume approximately 45 percent of their calories as carbohydrate.[5] Of the 200–400 g of carbohydrate ingested daily, 60 percent is starch or complex carbohydrate, 30 percent is sucrose, and the remainder is milk lactose. Within the intestinal lumen and the intestinal brush borders, all complex carbohydrates are hydrolyzed to monosaccharides—primarily glucose, fructose, and galactose.[6] The alimentation process is accompanied by a series of events that culminate in the secretion of insulin from the beta cells of the islets of Langerhans. During the digestive process, enteric factors are released into the circulation from the duodenum and jejunum and serve as insulin secretogogues.[7] Current views favor gastric inhibitory polypeptide (GIP) as the most likely "gut hormone" influential in the release of insulin after the ingestion of carbohydrate.[8] Circulating glucose itself plays a major role not only in the release of insulin from the beta cell but also as a stimulant of insulin biosynthesis.[9]

Plasma glucose rises within minutes of a carbohydrate-containing meal. In normal subjects, plasma levels usually peak between 1 and 2 hours after eating and rarely exceed 160 mg/dl (8.8 mM). A parallel exists between increments in plasma glucose and those in immunoreactive insulin. Factors that determine the magnitude and the time sequence of the increments in plasma glucose in the postprandial period are described by Freinkel and Metzger.[10] These include the amount and type of carbohydrate ingested, the rates of gastric emptying and intestinal absorption (often determined by noncarbohydrate constituents of the meal), the impedence of glucose outflow from the liver, and the rate of glucose distribution in body tissues.

The liver is freely permeable to glucose and extracts approximately 50 percent of the absorbed monosaccharide.[11] Within the hepatocyte, glucose is immediately phosphorylated via the catalytic action of glucokinase, an enzyme whose availability is insulin-dependent.[12] In the postabsorptive state, the phosphorylated glucose is readily converted to glycogen under the aegis of glycogen synthetase, an enzyme regulated by insulin. Hepatic concentrations of glycogen in the postabsorptive period range from 1.4 to 8.0 g/100 g wet weight.[13] During the postabsorptive period, while hepatic glycogenesis occurs, glycogenolysis and gluconeogenesis are impaired and hepatic glucose output ceases.[14] Glucose not sequestered in the liver is distributed throughout the body; approximately 25 to 30 percent is utilized by noninsulin-dependent structures (brain and erythrocytes); the remaining 15 to 20 percent of glucose is taken up by insulin-dependent structures as adipose tissue and muscle.[15] The latter provides not only a source for immediate energy needs but also building blocks for muscle glycogen and adipose tissue triglyceride. Overall, the fuel stores of carbohydrate as muscle and hepatic glycogen provide miniscule energy reserves[16] (Table 90-1).

In certain pathological situations, the orderly process by which carbohydrates are absorbed and assimilated during the "fed state" is distorted. Diabetes and insulin-deficient states are obvious examples. Diseases of the gastrointestinal tract may alter the absorptive phase of the "fed state" pattern. Endocrine disorders characterized by excessive circulating glucocorticoids or insufficient quantities of growth hormone affect the distribution steps of the process.

Energy is stored in adipose tissue and muscle as well as in the liver (Table 90-1). Triglyceride stores in adipose tissue represent the primary and most efficient reservoir. Glycogen is a relatively inefficient form to store energy, since each gram of glycogen within hepatic or muscle cells requires the presence of 1–2 g of intracellular water.[13,17] Hence, 1 g of stored hepatic glycogen yields only a half to a quarter of the theoretical 4 cal per gram. Similarly, protein stores are bathed in intracellular water, so that muscle and other protein-rich tissues represent only a quarter to a fifth protein by weight. Lipid is stored within cells in a relatively water-free environment. Of the 15 kg of adipose tissue present in a 70-kg adult, 90 percent is triglyceride. Thus adipose tissue yields very close to the theoretical 9.4 cal per gram.

GLYCOGENOLYSIS

Hepatic stores of glycogen synthesized during the immediate postabsorptive state become a resource for plasma glucose within 2 to 3 hours after a meal. Glycogen is a macromolecule whose glucose moieties are joined by 1,4 as well as 1,6 linkages. The highly branched glycogen molecule has greater solubility than the plant starches. The process of glycogenolysis is regulated by several enzymes. Liver phosphorylases initiate glycogenolysis and catalyze the stepwise cleavage of glucosyl units from the nonre-

ducing end of a 1,4-glucosyl chain of glycogen and liberate glucose-1-P. (Fig. 90-1) Liver phosphorylase exists in an active (a) and an inactive (b) form; activation is accomplished by a highly specific phosphokinase which requires ATP and Mg^{2+}. Inactivation of liver phosphorylase is effected by a specific phosphatase. Liver phosphorylase is activated by both glucagon and epinephrine through their stimulatory effects on phosphorylase kinase; only epinephrine activates skeletal muscle phosphorylase.[18] Glucagon activates the phosphorylase kinase by increasing tissue concentrations of cyclic AMP.[19]

Phosphorylase attacks the glycogen molecule from the nonreducing terminus of each chain and releases successive glucose residues as glucose-1-P until four glucose residues remain on each branch. To further degrade the glycogen, the three end glucose groups remaining after the action of phosphorylase are transferred from the side to the main chain of glycogen by the enzyme oligo-1,4-1,4 glucantransferase.[20] The exposed a-1,6 bond is hydrolyzed by amylo-1,6-glucosidase to release free glucose (Fig. 90-1). When the whole side chain is removed, phosphorylase action resumes. Both glucantranferase and glucosidase activities seem to reside in a single protein, whose molecular weight is 270,000.[20]

Glucose-1-P provided by the phosphorylase activity undergoes transformation to glucose-6-P under the action of phosphoglucomutase. Glucose-6 phosphatase, a microsomal enzyme, is present in liver, kidney, and intestinal mucosa and is vital for both glycogenolysis and gluconeogenesis. It is the enzyme that readily supplies free glucose. Activity of this hepatic enzyme is increased by the administration of glucocorticoids, by starvation, and in diabetes.[21–23] Insulin administration decreases the activity of the enzyme in the diabetic and in normal individuals.

Hepatic stores of glycogen in the postprandial period are variable and range from 14 to 80 g of glycogen per kilogram wet weight of liver. Nilsson and Hultman showed with serial liver

Table 90-1. Fuel Reserves in a Fed 70-kg Man

Fuel	Calories
Carbohydrate	
Glycogen–muscle	600
Glycogen–hepatic	300
Protein	
Muscle	24,000
Fat	
Adipose tissue	141,000
	165,900

From Cahill, G. F., Jr.: Starvation in man. N. Engl. J. Med. *282:* 668, 1970.

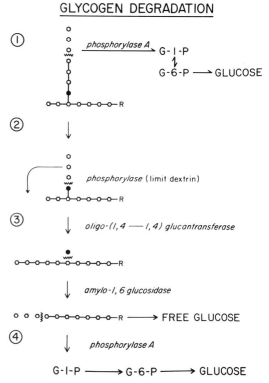

Fig. 90-1. Glycogen degradation. The steps in the clearance of glycogen are detailed in the text. Liver phosphorylase is activated via a phosphokinase system.

biopsies that during a 2 to 4-hour period of starvation following an overnight fast, glycogenolysis occurs at the mean rate of 51.6 ±5.09 mg of glycogen per minute per kilogram of liver in 19 normal individuals.[28] Prolonged starvation or carbohydrate-poor normocaloric diet decreases the liver glycogen from a mean of 38 g/kg wet weight to 4–9 g during 24 hours. When the subjects were fasted or were fed the carbohydrate-poor diets for another 8 days, there was little change in hepatic glycogen content. In spite of the marked depletion of glycogen stores, blood glucose levels do not significantly change.

A finely balanced regulatory mechanism initiates glycogenolysis through activation of phosphorylase. This intricate system became apparent with the discovery of glycogen synthetase and recognition that glycogen phosphorylase plays solely a catabolic role. Increments in plasma insulin and in intrahepatic concentrations of G-6-phosphate after the ingestion of carbohydrate lead to the conversion of the inactive (b) form of glycogen synthetase to the active (a) form. In a reciprocal fashion, as glucose is assimilated and plasma levels of insulin and intracellular levels of glucose-6 phosphate decrease, inactivation of glycogen synthetase occurs and activation of the phosphorylase system ensues (Fig. 90-2).

Control of hepatic glycogen metabolism is modulated by balance in activities of the enzymes of glycogen synthesis and breakdown, which are under both substrate and hormonal control. Not only is phosphorylase activated by a rise in the concentration of cyclic AMP, but glycogen synthetase is simultaneously converted to its inactive form. Coordination of activities occurs because both pathways are responsive to cyclic AMP in a reciprocal fashion.[29] Fluxes in insulin and glucagon levels play a dominant role in this balanced system.

GLUCONEOGENESIS

As hepatic stores of glycogen wane several hours into the postabsorptive state, there is need to draw upon other sources to maintain levels of circulating glucose.[28] Gluconeogenesis, the formation of glucose from noncarbohydrate precursors, provides that means (Fig. 90-3). Gluconeogenesis is dependent upon (1) the supply and availability of endogenous gluconeogenic precursors—amino acids, glycerol, and lactate; (2) an intact, functional, and specific enzyme system; and (3) availability of the "gluconeogenic hormones" that modulate the processes.[30] Each of these factors warrants consideration, since deficiencies at any level affect glucose homeostasis and may eventuate in clinical hypoglycemia.

SUBSTRATE AVAILABILITY

Both in man and in laboratory animals, the rate-limiting factor for gluconeogenesis is the availability of substrate.[31,32] Saturation of the gluconeogenic capacity of the liver is not exceeded when amino acids are supplied in concentrations 20 to 30-fold greater than physiological levels.[31] In vivo and in vitro studies indicate that amino acids play the dominant role as precursors of new glucose.[33,34] In the steady state after an overnight fast, glycogen degradation accounts for approximately 75 percent of the glucose released by the liver, while gluconeogenesis is responsible for the remainder. Alanine provides the carbon skeleton for 25 to 30 percent of the glucose produced via gluconeogenesis during the steady state. The contributions of the other precursors are listed in Table 90-2.[35–37]

Alanine is the most important amino acid precursor of glucose.[38] While almost all amino acids are potentially glucogenic, studies in fasted man indicate that about 50 percent of glucose derived from amino acids is formed from alanine.[35] Correspondingly, after 12 to 24 hours of fasting, approximately 30 percent of the total amino acid efflux from muscle[39] is in the form of alanine, although alanine accounts for only 7 to 10 percent of the amino acid residue in muscle.[40] A proposal to account for this disproportionate output of alanine by skeletal muscle contends that alanine is an essential component of a metabolic cycle—the alanine–glucose cycle.[35,38] Alanine conveys amino groups and a carbon skeleton from muscle to the liver for conversion to urea and glucose, respectively. Glucose released by the liver is taken up by muscle and converted to pyruvate, which is then transaminated to alanine. Alanine thus produced is released by muscle to complete the cycle. Others point out that alanine production by muscle may be independent of glycolysis and the presence of pyruvate but may

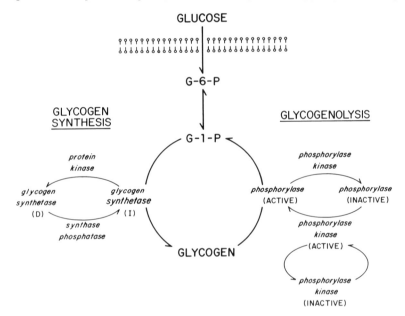

Fig. 90-2. Glycogen synthesis versus glycogenolysis. A reciprocal relation exists between glycogen synthesis and glycogenolysis. Factors that activate the glycogen synthetic system directly or indirectly inactivate the phosphorylase system. The glycogen synthetase system is suppressed when phosphorylase is activated.

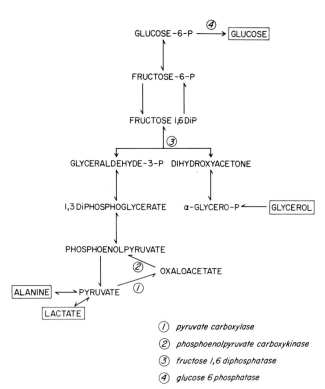

1 pyruvate carboxylase
2 phosphoenolpyruvate carboxykinase
3 fructose 1,6 diphosphatase
4 glucose 6 phosphatase

Fig. 90-3. Gluconeogenesis. The three major substrates and the four gluconeogenic enzymes are depicted to demonstrate the "entrance" point of the precursors and the relationship to the unidirectional reactions that the enzymes govern.

reflect de novo synthesis of an amino acid.[41-43] The branched chain amino acids are a prime source for intramuscular protein synthesis;[44] these amino acids, in contrast to others, are oxidized primarily in muscle and not in the liver.[45] Undoubtedly, the alanine released from muscle during the steady state reflects that derived from the transamination of glucose-derived pyruvate as well as that synthetized de novo.

In the basal or steady state, amino acids other than alanine show a significant arteriohepatic vein differential. Among those that account for a portion of the glucose produced during gluconeogenesis are phenylalanine; tyrosine, serine, threonine, and glycine. Plasma levels of the latter three amino acids rise progressively with starvation.[32] Glycerol plays only a minor role as a source for glucose in the basal state[46] but has a more substantial role during prolonged starvation.[47] Similarly, while lactate and pyruvate provide only 10 to 15 percent of the skeleton for glucose in the basal state, their relative contribution to total glucose production after prolonged periods of food deprivation increases to 45 to 50 percent.[47] Most of the lactate emanates from cellular blood elements that derive their energy from glycolysis.

When starvation or glucose deprivation is continued for 72 hours, plasma glucose levels fall rapidly. This decline is more

Table 90-2. Sources of Splanchnic Glucose in Subjects Fasted Overnight

Rate of glucose release by splanchnic bed	160–350 g/ 24 hr
Glycogen degradation	75%
Gluconeogenesis	25%
From pyruvate and lactate	10–15%
From alanine	5–10%
From amino acids other than alanine	5%
From glycerol	2%

From Felig, P.: The glucose-alanine cycle. Metabolism 22: 179, 1973.

marked in women than in men[48] (Table 90-3) and is accompanied by a fall in insulin, a rise in glucagon levels, and an increased extraction of alanine by the liver.[32] After 72 hours of starvation, plasma glucose levels tend to stabilize in spite of a progressive fall in total glucose production. Following 5 to 6 weeks of starvation, total glucose production falls to about 90 g/day; the liver is responsible for only 55 percent of this amount, and the kidney is responsible for the remainder. After such fasts, plasma alanine levels fall (300 uM/L basal to 110 μM/liter after prolonged starvation), and splanchnic extraction of alanine diminishes. Renal gluconeogenesis utilizes glutamine as a major source for glucose production.[47]

ENZYMES

Each of the gluconeogenic precursors except glycerol must be converted to either pyruvate and/or oxaloacetate prior to formation of glucose. Since several steps in the glycolytic pathway, including the final step (phosphoenolpyruvate → pyruvate), are irreversible, the liver and kidney contain specific enzymes to circumvent these thermodynamic barriers. A brief summary of these "gluconeogenic" enzymes is included, since deficiencies or interference with their activity can lead to clinical hypoglycemia. Most of the kinetic information about these enzymes derives from animal studies.

Gluconeogenic enzymes have the following characteristics: (1) they catalyse one-way reactions; (2) they are absent in cells that rely upon glycolysis and require rapid glucose utilization; (3) they are present only in tissues (liver and kidney) where gluconeogenesis occurs; (4) their amounts and activities correlate with the intensity of gluconeogenesis.[49]

The four gluconeogenic enzymes are listed below.

1. *Pyruvate carboxylase:* This mitochondrial enzyme catalyzes the carboxylation of pyruvate to oxaloacetate:

pyruvate + CO_2 + ATP → oxaloacetate + ADP + Pi

The enzyme has an absolute requirment for divalent cations such as Mg^{2+}, Mn^{2+}, Co^{2+} and for acetyl CoA.

2. *Phosphoenolpyruvate carboxykinase:* This enzyme is present in both the cytosol and intramitochondrial space and catalyzes the conversion of oxalacetate to phosphoenolpyruvate:

oxalacetate + GTP → phosphoenolpyruvate + GDP + CO_2

It requires Mg^{2+} or Mn^{2+} for activity.

Table 90-3. Plasma Glucose Concentrations During Brief Starvation— Men Versus Women

Basal:
Women (12)*: 84. ± 2.4
Men (12): 89.0 ± 3.5
24 Hour:
Women (44)**: 57.7 ± 11.6
Men (12) 79.1 ± 12.9
48 Hour:
Women (35) 49.6 ± 6.4
Men (12) 74.6 ± 12.3
72 Hour:
Women (45) 41.3 ± 13.4
Men (12) 67.5 ± 8.6

Merimee, T. J. and Tyson, J. E.: Stabilization of plasma glucose during fasting. Normal variation in two separate studies. N. Engl. J. Med. 291: 1275, 1974.
*Figures in parentheses denote number of subjects. Glucose values in mg/dl expressed as mean ± SEM.
**Menstrual cycle had no influence on these values.

3. *Fructose-1, 6-diphosphatase:* This enzyme catalyses the hydrolysis of fructose 1,6 diphosphate to fructose 6-phosphate and inorganic phosphate

fructose 1,6 diphosphate + H_2O → fructose 6 phosphate + Pi

4. *Glucose-6-phosphatase:* This microsomal enzyme, which catalyzes the hydrolysis of glucose 6-phosphate to glucose and inorganic phosphate, is vital to both glycogenolysis and glyconeogenesis. No cations are required for its activity.

glucose 6-phosphate + H_2O → glucose + Pi

The activity of this enzyme is inhibited by glucose.

The quantity of the enzymes and activity of the enzymes in this group are affected in situations where increased glucose production occurs. Thus, following the administration of glucocorticoids, in diabetes and starvation, enzyme activity is increased.

HORMONAL FACTORS IN GLUCOSE HOMEOSTASIS

Several components of the endocrine system are cohesively integrated to provide for the relative constancy of blood glucose both during periods of caloric deprivation and in those instances when the blood glucose is acutely lowered. These hormones play an essential role in the provision of substrate needed to synthesize glucose and glycogen, facilitate the uptake of substrate by the liver, and augment the activities of those enzymes that are vital both for the process of glucose production and for the release of free glucose from the liver. Acute challenge to glucose homeostasis readily calls forth those hormones that protect circulating glucose or assist in the counterregulation of the glucopenic state. Following the acute lowering of circulating glucose, the counterregulatory hormones function to (1) provide circulating glucose via facilitation of glycogenolysis and gluconeogenesis; (2) alter the utilization of substrates by peripheral tissues so that glucose is available for the tissues in the central nervous system; (3) provide alternate substrate such as free fatty acids and ketones for energy needs of non-glucose-requiring tissues; and (4) prevent the endogenous secretion of insulin and prolongation of hypoglycemia (Fig. 90-4).

The glucoregulatory hormones (glucocorticoids, catecholamines, glucagon, and growth hormone) and their actions are reviewed to provide a background for the later discussion of the clinical states of hypoglycemia. The role of each of the hormones will be considered both in the setting of the diurnal fluctuations of plasma glucose and in circumstances when glucose homeostasis is acutely challenged.

Insulin certainly has glucoregulatory actions and most of its effects oppose those of the counterregulatory hormones. While thyroidal, gonadal, and other hormonal factors such as prolactin

	INCREASE HEPATIC GLUCOSE OUTPUT	ALTER GLUCOSE UTILIZATION	PROVIDE ALTERNATIVE SUBSTRATE	SUPPRESS ENDOGENOUS INSULIN
CATECHOLAMINE	+ +	+ +	+ +	+ + +
GLUCOCORTICOID	+ +	+ + +	+	—
GLUCAGON	+ + + +	—	+ + +	—
GROWTH HORMONE	—	+ + +	+ + +	

Fig. 90-4. Effects of the counterregulatory hormones. The * indicates hepatic glucose output from both glycogenolysis and gluconeogenesis. The + marks indicate the intensity of the effect.

and somatostatin may modulate carbohydrate homeostasis, the complete effects of these factors require further elucidation.

Cortisol and the Glucocorticoids

Adrenalectomized animals have diminished stores of hepatic glycogen, low fasting blood glucose, and excrete reduced quantities of urinary nitrogen.[50] Replacement therapy with cortisol or other glucocorticoids reverses these derangements.[51] Thus, glucocorticoids promote the conversion of protein to carbohydrate and the storage of carbohydrate as glycogen. These two actions of the glucocorticoids may be independent. In the conversion of protein to carbohydrate, glucocorticoids facilitate the mobilization of amino acids from muscle,[52,53] the uptake of amino acids by the liver,[54] and the activation of the several hepatic enzymes essential for gluconeogenesis.[55] Glucocorticoids promote the formation of glycogen from glucose either by partially blocking the movement of pyruvate to pathways other than glycogen synthesis or by interfering with the release of glucose from the liver.[56] In addition, glucocorticoids depress the oxidation of glucose by muscle and adipose tissue. Adrenalectomized animals cannot break down endogenous protein at an adequate rate, and if deprived of exogenous amino acids, hypoglycemia develops.[57]

Through their "permissive action," glucocorticoids also influence metabolic events within adipocytes. The mobilization of stored lipid as free fatty acids is modulated by cortisol, a hormone that seems to be vital for the full expression of the adipokinetic effect of epinephrine.[58]

Glucocorticoids affect all the hepatic enzymes vital for gluconeogenesis.[30,49,55,59] Increased activities of phosphoenolpyruvate carboxykinase and pyruvate carboxylase are present in steroid-treated animals. The actual levels of phosphoenolpyruvate are increased by glucocorticoids, whereas in the case of pyruvate carboxylase the effect may be on activation of the enzyme. While augmented activity of fructose-1,6-diphosphatase is reported, the physiological significance of this finding is questioned. Glucocorticoids do not augment the activity of the enzymes involved in the glycolytic or phosphogluconate pathways but do increase the activity of glucose-6-phosphatase, an enzyme instrumental to both glycogenolysis and gluconeogenesis. Tryptophan pyrrolase is directly induced by cortisol, while the activity of transaminases such as tyrosine-a-ketoglutarate and alanine-a-ketoglutarate are augmented by the "permissive action" of the steroid.[60]

Diurnal fluctuations in cortisol may affect circulating glucose. Bursts of cortisol activity are greatest during the last 3 hours of sleep and the first waking hour[61] and may regulate that component of the fasting blood sugar attributable to gluconeogenesis. Starvation per se reduces the rate of cortisol secretion, but circulating levels remain within the normal range.[62] Cortisol levels increase significantly 30 minutes following the acute induction of hypoglycemia[63] and may be instrumental in the increased incorporation of alanine into glucose in the posthypoglycemic period.[64] On the other hand, some contend that glucocorticoids play only a "permissive" role in glucose homeostasis.[65]

Catecholamines: Epinephrine and Norepinephrine

Catecholamines play little or no role in the maintenance of a stable plasma glucose level in healthy adults unless hypoglycemia supervenes. While the release of insulin and glucagon is altered by direct stimulation of the sympathetic and parasympathetic nerves of the pancreas, and sympathetic agonists and antagonists modify the response of these hormones in pharmacological experiments,[66] patients with complete transection of the cervical cord and without sympathetic innervation maintain normal basal glucose levels.[67,68] Moreover, animal studies indicate a reduction in sympathetic activity with starvation.[69]

When plasma glucose falls acutely to 50 mg/dl or less, epinephrine and norepinephrine levels rise progressively. Glucopenia stimulates glucoreceptors in either the ventromedial nucleus or other centers within the hypothalamus, activating sympathetic discharges that eventuate in the secretion of epinephrine from the adrenal medulla.[70] Plasma epinephrine levels rise almost 10-fold by 25 minutes after an insulin injection induces hypoglycemia.[64] The small rise in norepinephrine in the posthypoglycemic period represents only that fraction of the total released from sympathetic postganglionic neurons that escapes axonal reuptake and local metabolism.[71] However, the adrenal medulla may be responsible for the changes in plasma levels of both catecholamines.[72]

Catecholamines released after glucopenia activate glycogenolysis and immediately increase hepatic glucose output.[64] While these plasma levels of epinephrine may be insufficient to produce glycogenolysis in an in vitro system,[73] it is thought that sufficient catecholamines are released by sympathetic nerve endings near glycogen-laden cells to effect glycogen degradation.[74] Norepinephrine probably has little effect on blood glucose concentration. Epinephrine in the face of hypoglycemia may inhibit glucose uptake by skeletal muscle and simultaneously augment glycogenolysis in muscles so that lactate is produced and released into the circulation.[75,76] This lactate readily becomes available for hepatic gluconeogenesis.

Catecholamines activate triglyceride lipase and in part account for the increased release of free fatty acids and glycerol from adipose tissue following hypoglycemia.

Free fatty acids provide an alternate substrate for muscle and serve as a source for hepatic production of ketones. The glycerol released serves as a gluconeogenic precursor. Finally, the posthypoglycemic increments in catecholamines may impede the pancreatic beta cells from releasing insulin as the blood sugar returns to the euglycemic range.[77]

Thus, while the catecholamines exert little influence over the diurnal fluctuations in plasma glucose, they serve as major counterregulatory forces to hypoglycemic challenge. Figure 90-4 summarizes their role as well as that of the other glucoregulatory hormones.

Glucagon

The hyperglycemic activity of pancreatic extracts has been recognized for many years,[78] and yet the physiological importance of this "hyperglycemic factor," glucagon, has only been appreciated in the last decade.[79] Pancreatic glucagon has been difficult to assay in plasma because of the presence of a glucagonlike substance produced by the gut and other circulating factors produced by the pancreas that cross-react with "true" pancreatic glucagon antibody. Overnight fasted values in normal subjects are approximately 70–100 pg/ml as determined with a highly specific antibody.[80]

Starvation[81,82] and acutely induced hypoglycemia[83] lead to increases in the secretion of pancreatic glucagon. Other stimulants are high-protein feedings, exercise, trauma, hemorrhage, and other stressful stimuli. Catecholamines may directly induce increments in glucagon.[84]

It is uncertain how the alpha cell senses fluxes in circulating glucose. Tissue perfusion studies indicate an inherent ability of the alpha cell to respond to stimulants,[85] and yet other studies indicate that there is no intrinsic glucose-sensing capacity in the alpha cell.[86] Unger and Orci stress the relationship of the alpha cell to

other cell type of the islets and suggest that the D cells and B cells may exert regulatory effects.[87] Multiple studies using adrenergic agonists and antagonists and neural stimulation strongly imply that glucagon secretion is modulated via the sympathoadrenal system. However, when hypoglycemia was induced with insulin in subjects with complete transection of the cervical cord, the glucagon response was normal.[68] Thus the importance of neural regulation in the control of glucagon secretion during acute stress seems questionable. Distortion of the system that regulates the alpha cell is apparent in diabetes mellitus: normal glucagon levels are observed in the basal state in diabetics in spite of hyperglycemia, and conversely some diabetics fail to secrete increased quantities of glucagon following hypoglycemia.[88,89]

Isolated defects of the alpha cells in man are unknown, and hence it is difficult to define precisely the physiological role of glucagon. Glucagon at physiological levels stimulates hepatic glycogenolysis.[90,91] In perfused liver preparations, the hormone enhances gluconeogenesis by augmenting the incorporation of amino acids and lactate into glucose;[92,93] similar observations pertain to man.[82] Glucagon interacts with membrane-bound adenyl cylase in the hepatocyte[94] and induces elevated intracellular levels of cyclic AMP, which in turn activate the phosphorylase system and the process of glycogenolysis.[91] Also enhanced is the conversion of pyruvate to glucose, or the process of gluconeogenesis. In the adipocyte, lipolysis is activated by glucagon, and free fatty acids and glycerol are released into the circulation.[95] Another important action of glucagon in the liver involves the stimulation of ketogenesis by diversion of fatty acids into the mitochondria via the carnitine acyltransferase pathway.[96] While some have proposed a prime role for glucagon in the control of fasting glucose levels,[97] the major evidence indicates that insulin is more important in the control of hepatic glucose output.[98] Glucagon at physiological concentrations modulates glucose availability in times of need and simultaneously provides alternate fuel for those tissues able to oxidize fatty acids and ketones. Its effects are short-lived and in most cases easily suppressed by insulin.[99]

Growth Hormone

In man, growth hormone plays a role in glucose homeostasis. Individuals with an isolated deficiency of growth hormone have lower fasting glucose levels and experience more profound falls in blood glucose during starvation than do control subjects. Both these phenomena are corrected with small amounts (2 mg/m²) of human growth hormone.[100] In addition, individuals with isolated growth hormone deficiency manifest marked sensitivity to insulin-induced hypoglycemia, a defect reversed by treatment with small quantities of growth hormone.[101]

Administration of growth hormone to normal subjects has a biphasic effect on blood glucose: the initial response, a decline in blood glucose, occurs within 30 minutes, while the later hyperglycemic effect is evident after several hours.[102] Several mechanisms have been postulated for the initial "insulinlike" actions of growth hormone. Of note is the similarity between somatomedin and the nonsuppressible insulinlike activity (NSILA) of plasma.[103] The hyperglycemic effect of growth hormone relates to the antagonistic effects of the peptide on insulin's actions. When growth hormone is administered to man or is secreted in excess, as in acromegaly, resistance to insulin at the cellular level develops.[104,105] Patients with an isolated deficiency of growth hormone demonstrate impaired insulin secretion that is corrected by growth hormone therapy.[106] Peake and colleagues showed an increase in the number and size of pancreatic beta cells in rats with growth-hormone-secreting tumors; the islets of such animals contain increased amounts of insulin.[107] Hence, growth hormone influences insulin production by the beta cell as well as by insulin's effectiveness on peripheral tissue.

Administered growth hormone has a biphasic effect on adipose cells, too. Initially, the hormone enhances glucose utilization and lipogenesis but after several hours of exposure to the hormone, glucose utilization is depressed and lipolysis ensues. This latter effect is dependent upon the synthesis of new proteins within adipocytes, since they are inhibited by actinomycin D and puromycin. Growth hormone significantly inhibits the metabolism of glucose, fructose, and pyruvate by adipose tissue in vitro when administered to animals 3.5 hours prior to sacrifice.[108]

Acute hypoglycemia stimulates the release of growth hormone. Peak plasma growth hormone levels appear 20 to 60 minutes following nadir blood glucose. The threshold for growth hormone release is a decline of glucose by 20–30 mg/dl below basal values.[109,110] A circadian rhythm of human growth hormone (HGH) response to hypoglycemia exists; the rise in HGH is greater in the morning than at night.[111] Hypoglycemic-induced release of HGH is mediated through the hypothalamus and median eminence. Lesions of the median eminence, sectioning of the pituitary stalk, or microinfusions of glucose into the median eminence prevent the posthypoglycemic rise in growth hormone. Greenwood and associates demonstrated that in normal subjects the maximal levels of HGH after acute hypoglycemia (36.2–34.5 ng/ml) and maximal increments (33.1–32.7 ng/ml) did not relate to the profoundness of the hypoglycemia.[63] Prepubertal subjects have lower HGH responses to hypoglycemia than adults. Alpha-adrenergic blockade suppresses[112] and beta-adreneric blockage augments the HGH response to insulin-induced hypoglycemia.

Growth hormone levels increase during periods of brief starvation, but the pattern of increase is variable; some normal subjects show no increment, while others show a marked increment.[109,113] Obese individuals have insignificant elevation of growth hormone during starvation. While the role of growth hormone per se in glucose homeostasis defies precise definition, it is apparent that the hormone, via its interaction with other glucoregulatory hormones (e.g., insulin and cortisol), does influence the status of circulating glucose.

CEREBRAL METABOLISM AND HYPOGLYCEMIA

Substrates

Observations of the effects of hypoglycemia on cerebral function were possible after the discovery of insulin; the classical descriptions are those made in schizophrenic patients undergoing insulin shock therapy. Himwich has "staged" the sequence of progressive, deepening hypoglycemia with regard to the cortical "layers" involved (Table 90-4).[1] Clinical signs and symptoms accompanying neuroglycopenia reflect a progressive rostralcaudal deterioration of CNS function, with many analogies to the patterns of anoxic and toxic encephalopathies.[114] Parenteral administration of glucose rapidly reverses the neurological dysfunction. When the brain has been deprived of glucose for prolonged periods or when the hypoglycemia has been very severe, however, glucose may not reverse the signs of neuroglycopenia. Seizure activity occurring during hypoglycemia may contribute to irreversibility of the neuroglycopenia.[115]

Readily reversible hypoglycemia is not associated with structural damage of nervous tissue. However, neuropathological changes occur after severe hypoglycemia and in individuals with irreversible neurological dysfunction. In the adult human brain, the neuropathological changes include laminar and pseudolaminar necrosis of cerebral cortex, degenerative changes of neurons in subcortical nuclei, and gliosis. Rarely does the white matter of the cerebrum degenerate. Such changes are similar to those observed after severe hypoxia.[116] In the neonate, hypoglycemia produces necrotic changes in the cerebral cortex with loss of white matter, dilatation of lateral ventricles, and microcephaly. Calcium deposits and status spongiosis are often observed in the areas of neurons.[117]

The biochemical alterations that accompany the clinical and neuropathological changes of several hypoglycemia are not completely understood.[114] The concept that hypoglycemia produces cerebral dysfunction through depletion of high-energy phosphate compounds is attractive, since most of the high-energy phosphate bonds in the CNS are produced via oxidative metabolism of glucose. However, studies to confirm this point produce conflicting results. Discrepancies in such studies relate to differences in the animal models used, to the degree of hypoglycemia produced, and to technical problems in securing and processing cerebral tissue rapidly so as to prevent biochemical change (Table 90-5). Current consensus based upon animal studies indicates that cerebral tissue stores of high-energy phosphates (ATP and phosphocreatine) are not depleted until blood glucose is reduced so severely (<1 mM/liter or 18 mg/dl) that the EEG is isoelectric. At the time hypoglycemia is of lesser severity (1–2 mM/liter) so as to induce slow-wave patterns or polyspike convulsive activity on the EEG, the energy status of the cerebral cortex, as evaluated by ATP, ADP, AMP, and phosphocreatine levels, is unaltered from control animals. However, prolonged convulsive activity leads to depletion of cerebral ATP and progressive coma, with an isoelectric

Table 90-4. Himwich's Classification of Hypoglycemia

Phase	Signs and Symptoms	A-VO₂ Difference	EEG
1. Cortical	Disorientation, incoherent speech, vague perception, deepening somnolence, loss of contact with environment	6.8	Increased slow-wave activity, Alpha-band rhythm (8–13 cps)
2. Subcortical-diencephalic	Inability to discriminate sensations and response appropriately to specific stimuli, uncontrolled motor behavior. Sympathetic overdischarge with tachycardia and pupillary dilatation		Slower wave activity in the theta band
3. Mesencephalic	Tonic spasticity. Inconjugate deviation of eyes. Plantar reflexes are abnormal	2.6	Delta rhythms of 1–4 cps
4. Premyencephalic	Extensor spasms of extremities induced by rotation of head		
5. Myencephalic	Coma with shallow respirations and bradycardia. Pupils are fixed and miotic. Hypothermia and hypoflexia are present.	1.8	Very slow to flat record

Table 90-5. Studies of Labile Phosphates in Brain During Hypoglycemia

Reduced	No Change
Kerr and Ghantus, 1936[118]	Tarr et al., 1962[123]
Olsen and Klein, 1947[119]	King et al., 1967[124]
Tews et al., 1965[120]	Mayman and Tijerina, 1971[125]
Goldberg et al., 1966[121]	Ferrendell and Chang, 1973[126]
Hinzen and Müller, 1971[122]	Lewis et al., 1974[115]

EEG. It seems unlikely that energy failure within the CNS contributes to the clinical signs of neuroglycopenia.

The decreased glucose consumption by human brain during hypoglycemia is proportionally greater than the decrease in oxygen utilization.[127,128] Hence, with the induction of hypoglycemia, the human brain must oxidize endogenous substrate. Animal studies reveal that when blood glucose falls below 2 mM/liter, cerebral tissue levels of alanine, glutamine, gamma-aminobutyric acid (GABA), and glutamate fall. These changes are preceded by decreased concentrations of glycogen, G-6-P, pyruvate, and citrate.[129] Lewis and colleague postulate that depletion of carbohydrate stores in cerebral tissue leads to depletion of NADH and explains the lower levels of tissue amino acids.[129]

A tentative formulation of the relationship between the clinical manifestations of hypoglycemia and substrate oxidation by the brain can be developed from studies on cerebral metabolism of hypoglycemic animals and the few available studies of man. Early neurological signs associated with hypoglycemia occur when intracellular glucose is diminished and when endogenous substrate is being utilized while oxidative metabolism and the level of high energy phosphates are unchanged. The depletion of endogenous substrate coincides with a reduction in oxidative processes and diminished quantities of high-energy phosphates. This latter state predisposes to an abnormal EEG and pathological changes that forebode irreversibility of the clinical picture.

Electroencephalography

A deficient supply of glucose to the central nervous system causes appearance of slow waves on the EEG. The more severe the hypoglycemia, the slower is the frequency of waves that appear, until a rhythm of 2–3 cycles per second predominate. When normal subjects are given insulin and the blood glucose falls, the first change observed on the electroencephalogram is a slowing of the dominant frequency, and yet the rhythm remains in the alpha band (8–13 cps). As the glucose level continues to fall, theta (4–7 cps) and finally delta (1–4 cps) rhythms predominate.[128]

The blood glucose level at which EEG activity slows is variable. Davis showed in a group of students that changes begin to occur with whole blood glucose levels between 53 and 85 mg/dl.[129] Slow rhythm activity occurs at relatively high blood glucose levels if there is evidence of slow activity prior to the induction of hypoglycemia. Individuals are consistent in the level at which they demonstrate slow-wave activity. Hypoglycemia aggravates preexisting EEG abnormalities.

Himwich, in his study of schizophrenics undergoing hypoglycemic therapy, showed that alpha-wave activity vanishes at approximately the same time that the functions of the cerebral cortex are completely suppressed and contact with the environment is lost. When glucose is administered to terminate coma, the alpha waves reappear with restoration of consciousness.[130]

Sympathoadrenomedullary Axis and Hypoglycemia

While the integrity of the sympathetic nervous system is essential for the hyperglycemic rebound to induced hypoglycemia, the relative importance of the several components of the system is being assessed. Glucopenia directly stimulates the hypothalamus, most likely through the cells of the ventromedial nucleus.[131] Sympathetic fibers originate in the hypothalamus, are activated by neuroglycopenia, and transmit impulses through the entire sympathetic chain. Fibers to the adrenal medulla derive from the coeliac and renal plexuses, traverse the adrenal cortex, and terminate as encirclements around the cells of the medulla. Disruption of the sympathetic system, as occurs in individuals with complete transection of the cervical cord, impairs catecholamine discharge after induced hypoglycemia.

Cannon and his co-workers stressed the role of the adrenal medulla as a mediator of neural-induced hyperglycemia.[132] Recent studies challenge this classical concept. Stress hyperglycemia is not absent after adrenalectomy.[133] Stimulation of the sympathetic fibers of the splanchnic nerve induces activation of glycogenolytic enzymes and glycogenolysis more rapidly than can be accounted for by epinephrine release.[134,135] Adrenalectomized man exhibits some rebound to hypoglycemia that can be attributed to activation of hepatic sympathetic nerve endings.[136] In the rat, electric stimulation of the ventromedial hypothalamus induces a rapid rise in plasma glucose that is unaltered by adrenalectomy.[137]

The sympathoadrenomedullary axis plays a multifaceted role in the counterregulation to induced hypoglycemia. Neuroglycopenia is interpreted by the hypothalamus, which responds via the sympathetic nervous system to stimulate directly the process of hepatic glycogenolysis and the release of epinephrine from the adrenal medulla. The latter augments the action of norepinephrine released by the sympathetic nerve endings in the liver. An integrated neurohumoral response to acute hypoglycemia occurs, provided there is no disruption of the sympathetic chain above the level of the liver. Such an integrated response results in rapid increases in the glucose output of the liver and relief of neuroglycopenia.

PATHOLOGICAL CONSIDERATIONS

CLASSIFICATION OF HYPOGLYCEMIC STATES

A variety of approaches are used to classify the hypoglycemic states. A categorization of the entities according to physiological defects affords the best insight into pathogenesis and the best basis for therapy. Often, however, such a classification is not feasible for clinical assessment, and consequently a popular method of classifying the hypoglycemic states emphasizes the manner of clinical presentation. Such a classification divides the hypoglycemic states into those that occur spontaneously in the fasted state without the influence of external agents such as drugs or toxins and those that are induced in the postprandial state by factors such as diet, exercise, or medication. Any system used for classification must acknowledge that in any individual several factors may combine to produce hypoglycemia, although one factor may be the prime culprit. Thus the patient with diminished adrenocortical reserve is more sensitive to the hypoglycemic action of ethanol.

From the physiological standpoint all hypoglycemic states are considered from the view that

circulating level of glucose available at any time =
the input of glucose into the circulation − quantity of glucose being utilized

In the steady state, the input of glucose into the circulation is dependent upon the availability of glucose precursors and the capability of the liver to manufacture and release glucose. Obviously, inadequate precursor or defective machinery to manufacture will result in hypoglycemia if utilization continues. When utilization is excessive or in any way exceeds production rate, glucopenia ensues (Fig. 90-5).

A classification of the hypoglycemic states based upon these simple physiological principles appears in Table 90-6A. Table 90-6B classifies the hypoglycemic states from the clinical standpoint.

DIAGNOSIS OF HYPOGLYCEMIC STATES

Glucopenia can often be diagnosed by a thorough history of the patient's illness and a complete physical examination. While the astute physician is frequently able to differentiate between psychosomatic and organic symptoms, this is not always possible. Any suspicion of hypoglycemia compels the physician to inquire: (1) whether symptoms occur immediately after meals or during periods of fasting (in excess of 6 hours postprandially); (2) whether the patient takes any medication; and (3) whether there are symptoms of systemic disease. All patients with complaints referrable to neuroglycopenia must be thoroughly examined. Such varied findings as evidence of recent weight loss or gain, needle puncture marks, hyperpigmentation, or abdominal masses are major diagnostic hints.

Since plasma glucose levels obtained sporadically even when the patient complains of neuroglycopenic symptoms may be normal, a systematic diagnostic approach should be initiated as soon as is feasible. A timetable for diagnostic tests should be outlined and each test evaluated before proceeding to a more complex or invasive procedure. Metabolic parameters used to diagnose the hypoglycemic states vary from day to day and often depend on the nutritional and emotional status of the subject. All carbohydrate tolerance tests require that the subject ingest 300 g of a carbohydrate daily for a minimum of 3 days before testing.

Each patient must be assessed according to the history and observations on physical examination. The factors listed below serve as guides for study. If symptoms appear in the fasting state, consideration should be given to the following:

1. *Fasting glucose and insulin levels.* Repeated simultaneous measurements of both should be obtained; a C-peptide measurement, if available, is helpful especially if an insulin-secreting tumor or factitious hypoglycemia is a diagnostic possibility. Insulin response to tolbutamide, leucine, and glucagon is useful in specific instances.

2. *Endocrine function studies.* Basal cortisol levels are helpful, but often stimulation studies with ACTH or Cortrosyn are necessary. Rarely are measurements of thyroid function helpful. Likewise, growth hormone values are seldom helpful in the adult with fasting-state glucopenia.

3. *Liver function tests.* Hepatic disease is usually apparent on physical examination, although these tests may be useful in patients with low glucose levels who have hepatitis. Liver biopsies may be required for the definitive diagnosis of children with inborn enzyme deficiencies.

If symptoms appear in the immediate postprandial state, the following tests warrant consideration:

1. *Oral glucose tolerance test.* A 6-hour test with samples for glucose and insulin obtained at least every 30 minutes and at the time of neuroglycopenic or adrenergic symptoms should be administered. To correlate symptoms and signs with glucopenia, blood pressure and pulse rate should be monitored throughout the test.

2. *Tests of gastrointestinal mobility.* These are most helpful when the oral glucose tolerance curve reveals a rapid early rise and precipitous fall in patients with or without gastric surgery.

3. *Personality profile.* Many of the individuals with functional hypoglycemia tend to be "emotionally unstable, tense, anxious and compulsive in personality."[65]

DEFICIENT SUBSTRATE AVAILABILITY

Ketotic Hypoglycemia of Childhood

Ketotic hypoglycemia is the most common form of hypoglycemia of childhood and usually manifests itself between the ages of 18 months and 5 years and then remits spontaneously before age 8 or 9 (Table 90-7). The disorder presents with the triad of convulsions, hypoglycemia, and acetonuria, which occur after an over-

CARBOHYDRATE HOMEOSTASIS OF FASTING

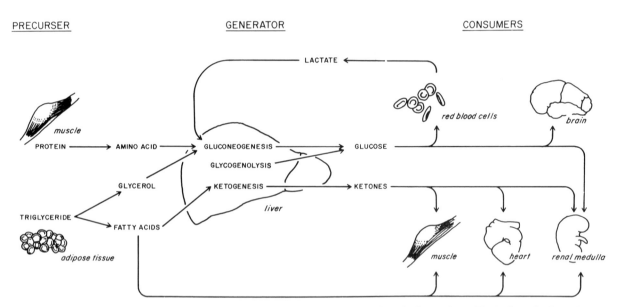

Fig. 90-5. Carbohydrate homeostasis of fasting. Precursors of glucose are derived from muscle and adipose tissue. The brain, red cells, and renal medulla require glucose at all times, while skeletal and cardiac muscle derive energy from fatty acids and ketones.

Table 90-6A. Physiological Classification of the Hypoglycemic States

I. Deficiency in availability of substrate
   A. Ketotic hypoglycemia of childhood
   B. Chronic renal insufficiency
   C. Adrenocortical insufficiency
   D. Starvation: pregnancy
II. Generator failure
   A. Structural incompetency, toxin induced
      1. Severe liver disease: necrosis, hepatitis
      2. Congestive heart failure: infiltrative diseases.
   B. Enzyme deficiencies
      1. Glycogenolytic enzymes
      2. Gluconeogenic enzymes
   C. Altered intrahepatic metabolism: inhibitors of gluconeogenesis
      1. Ethanol
      2. Hypoglycin
III. Consumer overutilization
   A. Endogenous hyperinsulinism
      1. Insulin-secreting tumors
      2. Alimentary hypoglycemia
      3. Leucine sensitivity
      4. Hypoglycemia of early diabetes
      5. Erythroblastosis fetalis
      6. Infants of diabetic mother
   B. Exogenous hyperinsulinism: hypoglycemic agents other than insulin
      1. Hypoglycemia in the diabetic
         a. Insulin
         b. Oral hypoglycemic agents
      2. Factitious hypoglycemia
      3. Reactive hypoglycemias
   C. Extrapancreatic tumors
   D. Increased sensitivity to insulin
      1. Hypopituitarism
      2. Exercise
      3. Pharmacological agents

Table 90-6B. Clinical Classification of the Hypoglycemic States

I. Fed-state hypoglycemias
   A. Alimentary hypoglycemia (postgastrectomy or pyloroplasty)
   B. Functional or reactive hypoglycemia
   C. Hypoglycemia of early diabetes mellitus (chemical stage)
   D. Neonatal hypoglycemia in children of diabetic mothers
   E. Erythroblastosis fetalis
   F. Leucine sensitivity
   G. Hereditary fructose intolerance
   H. Galactosemia
II. Fasted-state hypoglycemias
   A. Hepatic dysfunction
      1. Severe liver disease: hepatic necrosis, infiltrative disease, congestive heart failure
      2. Inborn errors of glucogenesis
   B. Adrenocortical insufficiency: primary and secondary
   C. Growth hormone deficiency
   D. Insulin-secreting tumors: adenoma, nesidioblastosis, beta cell hyperplasia
   E. Extrapancreatic neoplasms
   F. Ketotic hypoglycemia of infancy
   G. Impairment of gluconeogenesis
      1. Ethanol
      2. Hypoglycin
III. Variable without relationship to feeding.
   A. Factitious or iatrogenic hypoglycemia
      1. Insulin-induced
      2. Oral hypoglycemic agents
      3. Other pharmacological agents
   B. Artifactual hypoglycemia
      1. Leukocytosis: leukemia, leukemoid reaction
      2. Interfering agents: hyperlipidemia

Table 90-7. Characteristics of Ketotic Hypoglycemia

1. Age at onset rarely less than 18 months
2. Dietary irregularity or vomiting prior to convulsion
3. Acetonuria during and following the convulsion
4. Blood and spinal fluid glucose low at time of convulsion
5. Convulsion responds to intravenous glucose
6. Patient characteristics:
   a. Males three times more common than females
   b. Mildly retarded weight and height
   c. Birth weight below 2500 g; birth weight low for gestational age
   d. Outgrow by age 8 or 9

night fast or during the course of an acute illness. The entity is more common in males and in children with lower than normal birth weights.[138,139] Hypoglycemia associated with ketonemia may occur in a variety of conditions; however, the alanine-deficiency form will be considered here.

Extensive studies of children with this entity reveal no deficiency in the hepatic enzyme required for gluconeogenesis or glycogenolysis. Responses to glucagon and epinephrine are normal, and plasma insulin levels are concordant with the level of circulating glucose.

Pagliara and colleagues have found that susceptible children have significantly lower basal alanine levels than normal children and that alanine levels fall even further when susceptible youngsters are given hypocaloric ketogenic diets. When these children are infused with alanine (250 mg/kg of body weight), plasma glucose rises rapidly.[140,141] The reason for the lower basal alanine level remains an enigma; pituitary and adrenal dysfunction cannot be implicated. However, possible defects in protein metabolism have not been thoroughly investigated, nor has the possibility of a decreased muscle mass been adequately evaluated. Most pediatricians accept the premise that the underlying defect is present at birth but does not become manifest until the child is stressed by infection or other conditions that cause a reduced caloric intake. As the supply of endogenous substrate increases with age and with the relative decrease in glucose demand, spontaneous remission occurs. Treatment consists of frequent feedings of a high-protein, high-caloric diet. Testing the urine for ketones in susceptible children during episodes of infection or other stressful situations is a cautionary method of avoiding hypoglycemia, since ketonuria precedes hypoglycemia. Glucose should be administered orally or parenterally as soon as ketones are detected.

Chronic Renal Insufficiency

Glucose intolerance is a frequent concomitant of renal failure.[142] On the other hand, clinical amelioration of diabetes has been associated with progressive deterioration of renal function.[143,143a] Spontaneous hypoglycemia in the presence of chronic renal failure occurs in diabetics and nondiabetics.[144–147] No correlation exists between the severity of the renal failure and hypoglycemia. Patients present in a comatose or lethargic state and respond immediately to intravenous glucose.[148] Hypoglycemic agents cannot be implicated, since none of these patients received such agents at the time of their hypoglycemic episodes. Hepatic, adrenal, and thyroid functions are normal. While patients with chronic renal failure may have a deficiency in growth hormone, this is not thought to be the cause of spontaneous hypoglycemia. Hyperglucogonemia is often present in chronic renal failure.

Garber and his colleagues studied a hypoglycemic patient with chronic renal insufficiency and demonstrated an exaggerated fall in plasma alanine with starvation. Alanine turnover in this patient was approximately 50 percent of that in normal controls (241 ± 10.7 mmol/kg/hr versus 488 ± 48 in controls), and correspondingly, the absolute rate of glucose production from alanine was markedly depressed.[149] Although the metabolic derangements in chronic renal failure are complex, there is indication that decreased gluconeogenesis due to substrate limitation is an important factor in the development of hypoglycemia. Perhaps a deficiency in alanine delivery relates to the reduced protein intake usually prescribed for patients with renal failure.

Adrenocortical Insufficiency

Patients with adrenocortical insufficiency tend to have fasting glucose values in the range of 60 mg/dl.[51,150,151] Symptoms of neuroglycopenia are rare but occur after minimal periods of starvation or during illnesses that impair chronic intake. Rarely are hypoglycemia and neuroglycopenia the presenting clinical manifestations of adrenal insufficiency. The threshold for hypoglycemic symptoms is reduced in patients with Addison's disease, a circumstance that is normalized with the administration of glucocorticoids. Neuroglycopenic symptoms in Addisonians clear after hydrocortisone therapy without significant increases in circulating glucose.[152] Individuals with glucocorticoid deficiency are extremely sensitive to the hypoglycemic effects of insulin, sulfonylureas, and ethanol.[153–155]

While several mechanisms might be implicated to explain hypoglycemia in the presence of adrenal insufficiency, a deficit in circulating glucogenic amino acids is the major cause of the diminished gluconeogenesis and resulting glucopenia. Glucocorticoids are vital for the egress of amino acids from muscle into the circulation.[156] Although substantial evidence from human studies is lacking, extrapolation from animal studies indicates that in individuals with glucocorticoid deficiency, starvation causes insufficient mobilization from muscle of alanine and other glucogenic amino acids to provide substrate for needed glucose formation.[50,57] Concomitantly, the diminished availability of both substrate and glucocorticoids lower the activity of gluconeogenic enzymes within the liver. Glucocorticoids regulate the activity of pyruvate carboxylase, the enzyme vital for the initial incorporation of pyruvate into the gluconeogenic cycle, and via this function also modulate the process of gluconeogenesis.[30,157] In addition, hepatic uptake of amino acids may be curtailed in the absence of adequate glucocorticoids.[54]

The incidence of symptomatic hypoglycemia in patients with adrenal insufficiency varies with different observers. Dunlop claims that 20 of 47 patients with Addison's disease followed in his clinic had signs and symptoms of hypoglycemia, especially in the early morning.[150] On the other hand, in a study of Addisonian crises, only 8 of 61 episodes were accompanied by a blood sugar of less than 70 mg/dl.[158] Most authors agree that symptomatic hypoglycemia is a rarity in the Addisonian.[61] Neuroglycopenia has been observed in all forms of adrenal insufficiency and in patients of all ages. Primary and secondary adrenal insufficiency both result in inappropriate low levels of plasma cortisol. Secondary forms of insufficiency are due to total pituitary dysfunction or isolated defects[159] in the elaboration of adrenocorticotropin. Infants with the adrenogenital syndrome may have defective cortisol synthesis and manifest hypoglycemia as well as all the signs of glucocorticoid deficiency.[160]

Treatment with hydrocortisone readily reverses the lower fasting plasma glucose of patients with adrenal insufficiency. In acute situations, parenteral glucose will correct the glucopenia and reverse any symptoms of neuroglycopenia.

Pregnancy: Starvation

Basal levels of plasma glucose fall progressively during the course of normal pregnancy. This decline is exaggerated when healthy pregnant women are starved for prolonged periods (Table 90-8).[161] This decrement in plasma glucose exceeds that observed when nonpregnant individuals are fasted for similar periods. Normal pregnancy is characterized by low levels of circulating alanine. Starvation further aggravates this hypoalaninemia.[162] It is the lack of this key glucogenic substrate rather than any altered intrahepatic process that limits hepatic gluconeogenesis and contributes to gestational hypoglycemia. In spite of maternal hypoglycemia, the free outflow of glucose across the placenta to provide a prime substrate for fetal metabolism continues. Lower alanine levels also characterize pregnancy in the baboon and rat.[163]

Diminished availability of glucogenic amino acids is a constant concomitant of the glucopenia that accompanies starvation during pregnancy. The basis for the hypoaminoacidemia of normal pregnancy is unknown. Alterations in insulin[164] and glucagon[165] that accompany pregnancy cannot be implicated. Renal and placental losses of alanine and other glucogenic amino acids should not exceed the capacity of skeletal muscle efflux. Whether de novo synthesis of alanine[42,43] in muscle is influenced by the altered hormonal milieu[166] of pregnancy requires clarification.

Symptomatic neuroglycopenia during pregnancy is unusual and occurs only in the setting of prolonged starvation. It is often difficult to define the cause of such symptoms as headache and fatigue when they occur in a pregnancy individual with intercurrent illness. If there is any question of hypoglycemia, a glucose measurement should be obtained and parenteral glucose administered, particularly if the patient has been vomiting.

Pregnancy or lactating ruminants often exhibit evidence of marked hypoglycemia accompanied by ketonemia. Ruminants such as cows and ewes derive all of their circulating glucose from glucogenic amino acids and proprionic acid absorbed from the intestine. Glucose and other carbohydrates are not absorbed from the gut in ruminants. During pregnancy or lactation,* glucose is siphoned from the maternal circulation across the placenta or into the mammary gland at rates that exceed the ability of the ruminant to manufacture new glucose. The ketotic hypoglycemia observed during pregnancy or lactation in the ruminant represents another example of inadequate availability of glucose percursors.[167]

GENERATOR FAILURE

Structural Incompetency

Although the liver is essential to maintain circulating glucose levels both in the basal state and during short-term fasts, common hepatic diseases are rarely associated with glucose levels below 50 mg/dl. The classical studies of Mann and Magath indicate that removal or destruction of 80 percent of the liver's mass is necessary before disturbances in glucose homeostasis are evident.[168–170] In man, fasting glucopenia occurs only when there is widespread injury or damage to the liver's parenchyma. Patients with portal cirrhosis, toxic hepatitis, or metastatic liver disease rarely experi-

---

*In the highly bred dairy cow, more than half the carbohydrate produced each day is extracted by the mammary glands, often leaving insufficient glucose to maintain cerebral metabolism.

Table 90-8. Effect of Starvation on Glucose Levels During Pregnancy

	12 Hours	36 Hours	60 Hours	84 Hours
Nonpregnant (6)*	76.2 ± 1.9	69.5 ± 4.2	65.0 ± 3.2	60.7 ± 2.7
Pregnant (12)†	66.7 ± 1.4	50.7 ± 1.7	47.6 ± 1.9	46.8 ± 2.5
p	<.001	<.001	<.001	<.005

From Felig, P. and Lynch, V.: Starvation in human pregnancy: Hypoglycemia, hypoinsulinemia, and hyperketonemia. Science *170:* 990, 1970.
*Age 19–23 female volunteers
†16–22 weeks of gestation and scheduled to undergo therapeutic abortion

ence fasting hypoglycemia.[171] No correlation exists between the degree of hepatic dysfunction, as judged by standard laboratory tests, and the level of fasting glucose.

Fulminant hepatitis due to an infectious agent[172] or encountered in the third trimester of pregnancy may be associated with hypoglycemia. The hypoglycemia may aggravate the encephalopathy caused by the liver disease and necessitate constant infusions of glucose. Toxic agents such as carbon tetrachloride, chloroform, halothane, phosphorus, and glycol can cause widespread hepatic necrosis and consequent glucopenia.[173] Infiltrative diseases such as metastatic carcinomas, amyloidosis, sarcoidosis, and hemochromatosis rarely replace sufficient parenchymal tissue to curtail the glucose-producing capacity of the liver. Acute hypoglycemia resulting from fatty infiltration of the liver occurs in countries where kwashiorkor is prevalent; hypoglycemia is a common cause of death in individuals suffering from this form of chronic malignant malnutrition. Hypoglycemia has been cited in instances of ascending cholangitis, hepatic abscesses, and empyema of the gallbladder.[174]

Severe congestive heart failure in both children[175] and adults may be associated with glucopenia.[176,177] All forms of heart disease are reported as the basis for the congestive failure and hepatomegaly. Most of the patients exhibit muscle wasting and evidence of cardiac cachexia. The hypoglycemia responds to therapy for congestive heart failure and does not recur unless cardiac decompensation ensues.

Hypoglycemia that accompanies widespread destruction of hepatic parenchyma results from decreased hepatic output of glucose. Both glycogenolysis and gluconeogenesis are reduced in this setting. As an example, children with congestive heart failure and glucopenia have markedly reduced stores of glycogen and yet have normal levels of phosphorylase and glucose-6-phosphatase. The impaired ability of the liver to form glycogen or release glucose is reflected by fasting glucopenia and elevated postprandial glucose levels that decline gradually to low levels within 4 to 5 hours of eating. Hepatocellular disease is diagnosed from both clinical and laboratory features. Treatment of fulminant hepatic dysfunction necessitates maintenance of glucose levels until liver regeneration can occur.

Enzyme Deficiencies

Glycogen-Storage Diseases (Table 90-9).

Glucose-6-Phosphatase Deficiency. Glucose-6-phosphatase deficiency is the most commonly encountered glycogen-storage disorder. While the enzyme is essential for both the processes of glycogenolysis and gluconeogenesis, the degree of hypoglycemia observed in the absence of the enzyme is variable. In the most flagrant cases, profound hypoglycemia and acidosis may be present during the first days of life, and death may ensue if the

diagnosis is not rapidly made. On the other hand, infants may be asymptomatic even in the presence of severe hypoglycemia. This lack of symptoms has been attributed to the ability of the brain of the newborn to utilize ketones.[178,179]

Youngsters with this autosomal recessive disorder are short-statured and have protuberant abdomens caused by massive hepatic enlargement. Splenomegaly and cardiomegaly are not part of this syndrome. Easy bruisability, a hemorrhagic tendency, and prominent venules are common features. Exudative xanthomata and lipemia retinalis are reflections of the hypertriglyceridemia that often accompanies glucose-6-phosphatase deficiency. Muscular development is poor and yet adiposity involving the buttocks and facial fat pads is commonplace; the latter gives rise to the "doll-like facies" that characterizes this entity. Renal enlargement is apparent on radiological studies. The IQ is usually normal, and mental retardation is uncommon, although motor development and growth are slow.[180]

The fasting glucose is in the low-normal or frankly low level. Ketonuria and metabolic acidosis develop after brief fasts. High plasma concentrations of lactate and pyruvate reflect the backlogging of three-carbon fragments secondary to the impairment of glycogenesis and gluconeogenesis. Circulating levels of phospholipids and cholesterol are also elevated.[18] Uric acid values tend to be high, and acute gouty arthritis may occur.[181] The levels of serum enzymes such as glutamic oxaloacetic transaminase (SGOT), glutamine pyruvic transaminase (SGPT), fructose-1, 6-diphosphate aldolase (ALD), and ornithine carbamoyl transferase (OCT) may be elevated. The glucose tolerance test is usually of a diabetic type.

The diagnosis is best established by biochemical analysis of liver biopsy material. A biopsy should not be taken until the possibility of a bleeding disorder is ruled out. Biopsy specimens must be frozen immediately and analyzed for glycogen and for activities of the enzymes of the glycogen cycle. Absent or minimal (<10 percent) enzyme activity strongly suggests a deficiency of glucose-6-phosphatase. A glycogen content of greater than 5 percent of wet tissue supports the diagnosis.[182] Glucagon and epinephrine tolerance tests are useful to confirm the diagnosis; however, these tests are not specific, since similar results can be obtained in patients with amylo-1,6-glucosidase and phosphorylase deficiencies.

Prognosis in early infancy is guarded because of the high incidence of infection. Survival beyond adolescence is associated with adaptation to the disease and improvement of symptoms.[178] Individuals with a partial deficiency of hepatic glucose-6-phosphatase may have mild manifestations during childhood but develop tophaceous gout and urate nephropathy in adult life.[183]

Therapy is directed toward the maintenance of glucose levels that will prevent the secondary consequences of hypoglycemia and acidosis. In severe cases, feedings must be given every 3 to 4 hours continuously. To combat high blood lactate levels, supplementary oral sodium bicarbonate is indicated. The many forms of hormonal

Table 90-9. Glycogen-Storage Diseases Associated with Hypoglycemia

Enzyme Defect	Organs Involved	Severity of Hypoclycemia	Clinical Picture
Glucose-6-phosphatase	Liver, kidney	+++	Onset early in life, massive hepatomegaly; hypertriglyceridemia with xanthomata; lactate and pyruvate elevated
Amylo-1,6-glucosidase	Liver, muscle, heart, erythrocytes	++	Less severe than G-6-Pase deficiency; lactate levels are normal; glycogen has abnormal structure
Phosphorylase	Liver, kidney, erythrocytes, leukocytes	+	Triglycerides elevated; lactate is normal-high

therapy that include long-acting zinc glucagon, corticosteroids, androgens, and thyroid have not been consistently efficacious. Prolonged intravenous hyperalimentation and portal shunt procedures are currently being employed.

Amylo-1,6-Glucosidase Deficiency (Debrancher Enzyme). This disorder is clinically and physiologically similar to that of glucose-6-phosphatase deficiency.[184] Patients with the disorder tend to have a milder disease. Hepatomegaly and hypoglycemia are present, but the latter is usually not as severe as in glucose-6-phosphatase deficiency.[185] Lactic acidemia is less common, although ketonemia occurs with starvation. This enzyme deficiency is frequently unsuspected until a protuberant abdomen is noted. A low fasting glucose and mild elevation of cholesterol may be the only hints of the diagnosis. Responses to epinephrine and glucagon are variable. Specific diagnosis is possible by the analysis of erythrocytes[186] or leukocytes[187] for debrancher enzyme. Muscle and hepatic tissue also reveal a deficiency of amylo-1,6-glucosidase, which accounts for their high content of glycogen with abnormal structure having short outer chains (Fig. 90-1).[20,188]

Therapy aims to maintain euglycemia and prevent progressive hepatic enlargement. Fasting should be avoided and nighttime feedings encouraged. Survival to adulthood is usual, and after that time, the liver recedes in size.

Phosphorylase Deficiency (Hepatic). This entity is clinically and physiologically related to the two deficiency states just described. Fasting hypoglycemia is a variable, and subjects with this defect are less symptomatic than those with glucose-6-phosphatase and amylo-1,6-glucosidase deficiency. Hepatomegaly is present because of the accumulation of glycogen; the structure of the excessive glycogen is normal in contrast to that in subjects with amylo-1,6-glucosidase deficiency.[188] In addition to hepatic tissue, leukocytes are also deficient in phosphorylase.[189] The degree of the deficiency in hepatic tissue varies greatly, and hence the responses to glucagon and epinephrine are variable. The course and long-term prognosis of patients with hepatic phosphorylase defect requires clarification.

Gluconeogenic Enzyme Deficiencies.

Fructose-1,6-Diphosphatase Deficiency. Children with a deficiency of the gluconeogenic enzyme fructose-1,6-diphosphatase present with hypoglycemia and lactic acidemia as well as with ketonemia. Since the entity was first described in 1970, more than 10 children have been reported, ranging in age from 6 months to 5½ years.[190–194] The deficiency seemingly is transmitted as an autosomal recessive trait. Hypoglycemia and acidosis are precipitated by fasting, ingesting a diet high in fat content, or by any stressful event that induces hypercatabolism. Foods containing fructose or sorbitol may induce hypoglycemia.

The diagnosis is established by demonstrating a deficiency of fructose-1,6-diphosphatase in liver,[190,192] leukocytes,[195] or jejunal mucosa.[193] The degree of the deficiency is variable. Infusions of fructose, glycerol, or alanine will not produce the normal increments in glucose but may, in fact, induce hypoglycemia. Although the precise mechanism for this effect is unclear, it is postulated that the phosphorylated intermediates of these substrates may inhibit glycogenolysis at the phosphorylase step.[139] Hepatomegaly secondary to fat infiltration may be present.

Management requires that the family and physician maintain an alertness for any catabolic event that may set off hypoglycemia. When such an event occurs, intravenous glucose should be given immediately, as hypoglycemia and lactic acidosis develop rapidly.

Deficiency States of Other Hepatic Gluconeogenic Enzymes. Within the last several years, there have been reported cases of youngsters with hypoglycemia in the fasted state and suggestions that hepatic gluconeogenic enzymes other than glucose-6-phosphatase and fructose-1,6-diphosphatase are deficient. One 9-month-old female with episodic hypoglycemia had normal glycogenolytic and gluconeogenic enzymes except for reduced pyruvate carboxylase and markedly low phosphoenolpyruvate carboxykinase.[196] While reports of pyruvate carboxylase deficiency do not cite hypoglycemia as a feature of that defect,[197,198] hepatic phosphoenolpyruvate carboxykinase deficiency is accompanied by glucopenia.[199]

Altered Intrahepatic Metabolism: Inhibitors of Gluconeogenesis

Hepatic gluconeogenesis is vital for glucose homeostasis after a short period of fasting. While the process requires the integration of metabolic substrate, enzymatic components, and circulating hormonal factors, it is apparent that certain exogenous agents can disrupt the process. Among those agents that impede the process are ethanol and hypoglycin.

Ethanol-Induced Hypoglycemia. Ethanol, when ingested in the fasted state, may induce hypoglycemia. Chronic alcoholics are most vulnerable; however, youngsters and nonalcoholic adults may manifest symptomatic hypoglycemia after the ingestion of large quantities of ethanol. No correlation exists between blood ethanol levels and the degree of hypoglycemia, since hypoglycemia often occurs while blood ethanol levels are declining.[200,201]

During the oxidation of ethanol to acetaldehyde and acetate within hepatic cytoplasm, diphosphopyridine nucleotide (NAD) is reduced to NADH. The increased NADH/NAD ratio that results from the oxidation of ethanol provides an unfavorable intracellular environment for the oxidation of such substrate as lactate and glutamate to pyruvate and a-ketogluturate, respectively.[202,203] These and other (Fig. 90-6) gluconeogenic precursors accumulate, and the process of gluconeogenesis is stymied. When lactate is not oxidized to pyruvate, levels of pyruvate fall below the Km for pyruvate carboxylase (0.4 mM) and oxaloacetate and phosphoenolpyruvate are not formed. Hypoglycemia may result whenever

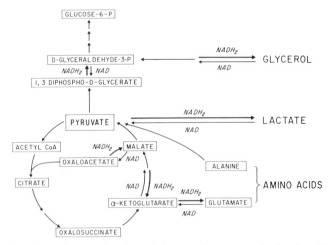

Fig. 90-6. Effect of ethanol metabolism on gluconeogenesis. As ethanol is oxidized to acetaldehyde and acetate, NADH₂ levels increase within hepatic cytosol, and the NADH₂/NAD ratio increases. All reactions that are affected by this redox alteration are diverted as shown. Ethanol inhibits gluconeogenesis by impeding the entrance of specific substrate into the gluconeogenic cycle.

hepatic glycogen stores are depleted and ethanol is being metabolized and gluconeogenesis impeded. Starved subjects, decompensated diabetics, and patients with thyroxicosis and adrenal insufficiency are especially vulnerable to the hypoglycemic action of ethanol.[204,205] Some chronic alcoholics, infants, and children[206,207] demonstrate susceptibility to ethanol-induced hypoglycemia after very brief periods of food deprivation. On the other hand, obese individuals are resistant to the hypoglycemia induced by ethanol.[204]

In addition to the alteration of intracellular processes, ethanol inhibits gluconeogenesis at two other sites (Table 90-10). Lactate,[208] alanine,[201] and glycerol[209] uptake by hepatic tissue is decreased in the presence of elevated levels of ethanol. Moreover, ethanol influences the availability of alanine for the formation of new glucose. Ethanol acutely lowers circulating alanine levels, purportedly by inhibiting influx from muscle stores.[210]

Clinically, the hypoglycemia of ethanol abuse is indistinguishable from that of other causes. Often the patients are considered to be severely inebriated. Rarely are the symptoms associated with increased sympathoadrenomedullary discharge present; often the "adrenergic response" to hypoglycemia is absent,[205] since repeated exposure to ethanol may deplete catecholamine stores.[211] Most of the patients are comatose and manifest hypothermia, conjugate deviation of the eyes, extensor rigidity of the extremities, unilateral or bilateral Babinski reflexes, trismus, or convulsions.[212,213] The clinical picture suggests a cerebral vascular accident or other insults to the cerebrum; focal neurological signs may be present if the patient has had previous cerebral vascular disease.

Glucose values as low as 5 mg/dl have been noted. Response to intravenous glucose is usually immediate; however, coma may recur if adequate carbohydrate is not administered. Glucagon and epinephrine are not effective therapeutic measures, since hepatic glycogen stores are depleted. Prompt diagnosis and initiation of therapy is mandatory in light of a reported 11 percent mortality in adults and 25 percent in children.[200] These rates may be even higher, since it is likely that some deaths attributed to severe alcoholism may, in fact, be due to ethanol-induced hypoglycemia. Susceptible individuals who ingested ethanol-containing beverages experience repeated episodes of hypoglycemia.

Ethanol will potentiate the hypoglycemia effects of other agents such as insulin.[214] Moreover, ethanol per se has a "priming effect" on the pancreatic beta cell, so that they secrete more insulin than normal in response to oral or intravenous glucose.[215,216] In some individuals, the augmented insulin response induced by "priming" doses of ethanol leads to increased peripheral uptake of glucose and may result in reactive hypoglycemia and neuroglycopenia.

Hypoglycin: Jamaican Vomiting Sickness. As early as 1916, it was suspected that an acute disorder seen only in Jamaican children and characterized by vomiting, prostration, tachycardia, hypotension, and profound hypoglycemia was related to the ingestion of unripe ackee fruit *(Blighia sapida).*[216a] In the mid-1960s, two Ninhydrin-positive substances, hypoglycin A and B, were extracted from the ackee fruit and found to be potent hypoglycemic agents. Hypoglycin is methylene cyclopropyl alanine, a compound

that inhibits oxidative phosphorylation in liver mitochondria. Species susceptibility is variable: cats and dogs are not vulnerable but primates are.[216b,216c]

An analogue of methylene cyclopropyl alanine, 4-pentenoic acid, has been extensively studied. In a manner similar to long-chain fatty acids, this compound is activated to its acyl CoA derivative at an extramitochondrial site. The acyl CoA derivative serves as a substrate for the enzyme carnitine acyltransferase and thereby depresses the availability of free carnitine and coenzyme A. This sequence results in a decrease of both the transport and the oxidation of long-chain fatty acids and hence limits formation of acetyl CoA, a substance critical for gluconeogenesis.[216d]

Hypoglycine or its experimental analogue 4-pentenoic acid preempts available coenzyme A and carnitine; consequently, they are able to inhibit fatty acid oxidation. Normally, oxidation of long-chain fatty acids results in the production of acetyl CoA, NADH, and ATP. Acetyl CoA is an absolute prerequisite for the activity of pyruvic carboxylase, the rate-limiting enzyme of gluconeogenesis. Hence, as hepatic mitochondria are busily oxidizing hypoglycin or 4-pentenoic acid, gluconeogenesis is inhibited. This inhibition can be overcome in vitro by provision of additional free carnitine and coenzyme A.

Symptoms occur several hours after ingestion of unripe fruit, and vomiting precedes the prostration, convulsions, and coma. Blood glucose as low as 3 mg/dl are reported. Acidosis without ketosis, presumably lactic acidosis, is present. Hepatic glycogen stores are depleted. Most children affected are chronically malnourished and range between the ages of 2 and 5, although many are between 5 and 10 years of age. If intravenous glucose is administered early, irreversible changes are prevented. Education of the susceptible population and improvement in the general nutritional status should eliminate this hypoglycemic disorder.

CONSUMER OVERUTILIZATION

Endogenous Hyperinsulinism

Insulin-Secreting Tumors. Insulin-producing tumors often provide a diagnostic challenge. These tumors can occur in all age groups but appear most commonly in the fourth to sixth decades. They show no sex predilection. Hypoglycemia is insidious in onset and may mimic a wide variety of neurological or psychiatric disorders. Exercise and fasting may precipitate a hypoglycemic episode. Adrenergic symptoms associated with hypoglycemia, such as hunger and sweating, are unusual but may occur; more often the neuroglycopenic or "cerebral" picture of hypoglycemia predominates. Most episodes occur in the morning before breakfast, but occasionally if the noon meal is missed, afternoon attacks appear. Patient's protect against hypoglycemic attacks by eating, although obesity is not common among patients with insulinomas.[217,218]

About 80 percent of insulinomas are benign and consist of a single lesion; 10 percent are multiple and consist of scattered microadenomas interspersed with normal islet tissue. The remaining 10 percent of insulinomas are malignant and often metastasize by the time of diagnosis. Malignant insulinomas often arise in the tail of the pancreas and have been associated with the secretion of such peptide hormones as gastrin, glucagon, ACTH, and serotonin. Benign isolated tumors are usually 0.5–3.0 cm in diameter, but lesions as large as 15.0 cm have been reported.[219,220] In adults, in contrast to infants, diffuse hyperplasia of the islets, or nesidioblastosis, is rarely the cause of hyperinsulinism.[221]

Fasting hypoglycemia is the hallmark of the insulin-secreting

Table 90-10. Mechanisms by Which Ethanol and Its Metabolism Induce Hypoglycemia

1. Disrupt gluconeogenic pathway by altering NADH/NAD ratio
2. Inhibit uptake of alanine, lactate, and glycerol by the liver

tumor. The diagnosis is confirmed by (1) the demonstration of a level of immunoreactive insulin (IRI) that is inappropriately high for the blood glucose and (2) identification of the pancreatic tumor. Prolonging an overnight fast for 4 hours will exaggerate the dichotomy between IRI and glucose.[219] Exercise in the fasted state is another method that exaggerates the fall in circulating glucose without an appropriate decline in the IRI level.

Should the diagnosis not be evident after the above maneuvers are completed, other studies as outlined in Table 90-11 should be pursued. Proinsulin or proinsulinlike components are still measured only as a research procedure.[222,223] The tolbutamide test should be performed with caution and not initiated if the fasting plasma glucose in 45 mg/dl or less.[224] Finally, when the diagnosis of an insulin-secreting tumor is certain, selective arteriography of the celiac and superior mesenteric artery is suggested so that the position of the tumor may be defined, and the possibility of multiple tumors or metastatic disease is ascertained prior to surgery.

Surgical resection is the definitive therapy for benign functioning tumors. In about 25 percent of the cases, however, no tumor is visualized or palpated during the initial exploration. In such cases, a partial pancreatectomy is performed. If hypoglycemia persists, reexploration is necessary, and further excision of pancreatic tissue becomes mandatory. In elderly debilitated patients, surgical exploration may be contraindicated.

Symptomatic medical therapy consisting of multiple feedings or constant glucose infusions. The latter may be necessary while the patient is being prepared for surgery. Glucocorticoids, growth hormone, and long-acting glucagon should be reserved for inoperable patients or those with metastic disease; these agents are only transiently effective. Diazoxide, a benzothiadiazene, suppresses insulin secretion and alleviates hypoglycemia in patients with metastatic disease as well as in those with inoperable benign disease. The sodium-retaining effects of this medication may be troublesome, especially in elderly patients. Streptozotocin, a naturally occurring N-methyl-nitrosourea-glucosamine isolated from cultures of *Streptomyces achromogenes*, alters the function of beta cells by depressing the pyridine nucleotides, NAD and NADH. This antibiotic has been effective in the treatment of metastatic insulinomas and is the treatment of choice at the present time. (The renal tubular damage that results from streptozotocin therapy should be appreciated.)[224]

Alimentary Hypoglycemia. Patients who have undergone gastrectomy, gastrojejunostomy, or vagotomy and pyloroplasty ex-hibit an abrupt, abnormally high rise in plasma glucose within 35 to 65 minutes after a glucose challenge.[225-227] Glucose levels fall precipitiously so that by 95 to 215 minutes after the challenge, values of less than 50 mg/dl are not unusual. A minority of these individuals experience adrenergic and neuroglycogenic symptoms that coincide with the lowest plasma glucose and are labeled as symptomatic alimentary hypoglycemics. While almost everyone who has undergone gastric surgery may manifest chemical hypoglycemia after an oral glucose load, the proportion with neuroglycopenic symptoms ranges from 5 to 50 percent, and the characteristics that predispose an individual to have symptoms are poorly defined. Plasma insulin values also rise excessively, and that rise parallels the increment in plasma glucose. A correlation exists between the height of the early insulin rise and depth of the later fall in glucose.[228,229]

Alimentary hypoglycemia is caused by the rapid gastric emptying that occurs after gastric surgery.[230] When the pylorus is removed, gastric emptying time is accelerated, and ingested carbohydrate is presented to and absorbed rapidly from the small intestine. The ensuing hyperglycemia and hyperinsulinemia lead to the hypoglycemia. Surgical procedures on the pylorus per se may modify glucose absorption and insulin secretion.

Alimentary hypoglycemia is not always a benign disorder. In addition to the annoying adrenergic symptoms, neuropsychiatric disease may be manifest.[231] Seizures, coma, and other neurological signs that occur in these patients may be unrelated to the glucopenia, and if neurological events cannot be temporally related to the hypoglycemia, other causes should be sought.[232] In many patients who have had a gastrectomy or pyloroplasty, symptoms of epigastric fullness, nausea, and weakness occur 30 to 60 minutes after meals (the "dumping syndrome") and are indistinguishable from the adrenergic symptoms of alimentary hypoglycemia.[233]

Alimentary hypoglycemia occurs in the absence of gastrointestinal surgery.[234,235] Individuals with this entity demonstrate rapid absorption of glucose and hyperinsulinemia for reasons not defined, although accelerated gastric emptying or an excessive release of the "gut hormones" that stimulate insulin release are postulated. In such individuals with intact gastrointestinal tracts, hypoglycemia occurs 90 to 120 minutes after a meal and is accompanied by adrenergic and neuroglycopenic symptoms.

The diagnosis of alimentary hypoglycemia should be suspected in symptomatic individuals who have had previous gastric surgery. Confirmation is based upon the precipitious rise in plasma glucose and insulin and subsequent rapid fall in glucose that fol-

Table 90-11. Diagnosis of Insulin-secreting Tumor

1. Thorough history and physical examination: documentation of hypoglycemia in the fasted state
2. Fasting plasma glucose and insulin levels: inappropriate IRI for corresponding glucose level
   a. At least 5 daily determinations after overnight fast
   b. Extend overnight fast for 4 hours
   c. Terminate an overnight fast with 20-minute period of exercise
3. Proinsulin or proinsulinlike component: determine the percentage of total IRI; if greater than 20%, suggestive of diagnosis
4. Stimulation tests
   a. Sodium tolbutamide (1.0 g) iv: blood samples for glucose and IRI every 15 minutes for first hour, every 30 minutes during second and third hours; may terminate after 30 minutes and measure IRI; if $195\mu U/ml$ at 15 minutes and $50\mu U/ml$ at 30 minutes, diagnosis suggestive
   b. Glucagon (1.0 mg) iv: blood samples at 15, 30, 45, and 60 minutes for IRI: positive if increments above pretest are $160\mu U/ml$ at 15, $60\mu U/ml$ at 30, $40\mu U/ml$ at 40, and $20\mu U/ml$ at 60 minutes
   c. Leucine (150 mg/kg) orally in water: blood samples for glucose and IRI at 15-minute intervals for 1 hour; a positive test is a fall of glucose 40% of basal
5. Suppression tests
   a. Fish insulin: (0.2 U) im every 45 minutes until hypoglycemic symptoms appear; samples for glucose and IRI every 10 minutes; observe for failure of endogenous insulin suppression
   b. Diazoxide (100 mg every 8 hours) orally
6. Angiography: selective celiac and superior mesenteric artery study to locate tumor, define number, and visualize possible hepatic lesions

lows an oral challenge with glucose.[236] Frequently, these individuals cannot consume concentrated glucose solutions without experiencing dumping. As with other "fed state" glucopenias, glucose measurements should be monitored frequently during the tests. Clinical observations should be recorded frequently to correlate glucopenia with adrenergic and neuroglycopenic symptoms.

Symptomatic patients should be treated. In the past, diets low in carbohydrate were prescribed with varying success. Anticholinergic agents such as propantheline given 30 to 45 minutes before meals may be effective.[230,234] Propranolol in 10-mg doses before meals prevents profound dips in postprandial glucose, but its effectiveness stems from inhibition of adrenergic symptoms and is presently the treatment of choice.[237] Oral hypoglycemia agents have little usefulness in the treatment of alimentary hypoglycemia.

Leucine Sensitivity. While attempting to define the pathogenesis of hypoglycemia in a group of infants, Cochrane and colleagues observed that leucine caused a marked fall in the glucose levels of these children.[238] Subsequently, other infants previously thought to have "idiopathic hypoglycemia" were shown to be sensitive to leucine. Leucine-induced hypoglycemia occurs in the first 6 months of life, and often infants with the deficit suffer mental retardation and neurological deficits because of inordinate delays in diagnosis.

Signs and symptoms appear shortly after a protein-containing feeding. However, these infants also have low fasting plasma glucoses. Lethargy and convulsions are common signs. Ketonuria is usually not present. After the intravenous administration of leucine (75 mg/kg), the plasma glucose decreases to at least 50 percent of the basal level within 20 to 45 minutes. Insulin levels rise as glucose values fall. Parenteral glucose must be administered as soon as symptoms occur. When infants with the defect are deprived of calories, hypoglycemia and seizures occur. By the time children with leucine sensitivity reach 5 to 6 years of age, fasting glucose levels spontaneously return to normal and sensitivity to protein feeding disappears.[239]

Neither the origin nor the molecular defect in leucine-sensitive hypoglycemia is known. There is a high family incidence of the defect.[240] Hypoglycemia results from excessive secretion of insulin. Hyperplasia of the beta cells of the islets of Langerhans has been observed in several instances. Some feel that the defect merely represents a marked exaggeration of the physiological response to leucine.[241] Whether the hyperplasia is the result of or the cause for the leucine sensitivity remains to be clarified.

Immediate therapy is directed toward correction of the hypoglycemia with glucose. Long-term therapy provides a diet with minimal amounts of leucine and yet one that assures normal growth. Cochrane suggests that a high-carbohydrate feeding be given at least three times a day. Glucocorticoids such as prednisone ameliorate the hypoglycemia but may adversely affect growth. Diazoxide effectively controls the hypoglycemia.[242]

Postprandial Hypoglycemia as an Early Manifestation of Diabetes Mellitus. In the early phase of maturity-onset diabetes, some patients experience neuroglycopenic symptoms 3 to 5 hours after meals.[243,244] These individuals tend to be obese and to have a strong family history of diabetes. The portion of newly uncovered diabetics that experience these symptoms is unknown, although Seltzer et al. observed 110 such patients over a 6-year period.[245] Fasting glucose levels are normal or only slightly elevated, but after a meal, glucose levels ascend slowly, achieve a zenith that may persist for ½ to 1 hour and then gradually descend to hypoglycemic levels. Insulin levels rise sluggishly but are excessive by 2 to 4 hours. Formerly, the glucopenia was attributed to the inappro-

priately high insulin values, but recent studies show no difference in insulin secretion in early diabetics with neuroglycopenia and in those without.[232,246]

It is postulated that with time, the degree of glucose intolerance worsens and the hypoglycemic pattern disappears.[245] Yet few quantitative data on the natural history of this form of postprandial hypoglycemia are available.[230] Since insulin secretion patterns in newly discovered diabetics with glucopenia do not differ from those without glucopenia, the reason for the hypoglycemia is presently not apparent. Whether differences in tissue sensitivity to insulin or to other hormones as catecholamines account for glucopenia remains to be elucidated.[232]

Erythroblastosis Fetalis. Neonates with moderate to severe erythroblastosis may manifest clinical signs of neuroglycopenia shortly after birth or immediately after an exchange transfusion.[247,248] Approximately 18 percent of newborns with a cord hemoglobin of less than 10 g/dl have hypoglycemia.[249] The hypoglycemia of erythroblastosis results from absolute or relative hyperinsulinism.[248] Both fasted and stimulated insulin levels are inappropriately elevated. An example of the latter is the hypoglycemia observed after the cessation of the hyperglycemic solutions (ACD) used for exchange transfusions.[250]

The prevention of Rh erythroblastosis fetalis with Rho GAM diminishes the hyperinsulinism and resultant hypoglycemia. Infants with severe erythroblastosis should have blood glucose measurements at regular intervals and especially following exchange transfusions. When hypoglycemia is detected, treatment with parenteral glucose must be initiated immediately.

Neonatal Hypoglycemia in Infants of Diabetic Mothers. Infants born to diabetic mothers may have profound hypoglycemia for the first few days of life.[179] Approximately 60 percent of babies of insulin-dependent mothers have glucose levels below 30 mg/dl in the first few hours of life, while only 15 percent of the infants born to gestational diabetics have such low values.[251] The severity of the hypoglycemia relates to the magnitude of maternal hyperglycemia during pregnancy. Glucose passes freely across the placenta, and hence maternal hyperglycemia induces beta-cell hypertrophy in the fetus. Increased circulating insulin levels and an increased pancreatic content of insulin reflect this consequence of maternal hyperglycemia. The elevated insulin levels suppress gluconeogenesis in addition to enhancing glucose utilization. A temporary deficiency of glucagon may aggravate the suppressive effect of insulin on gluconeogenesis.[65]

Most infants of diabetic mothers have a transient, asymptomatic period of hypoglycemia that lasts from 1 to 4 hours and abates spontaneously. Some have severe hypoglycemia (glucose less than 15 mg/dl) with symptoms that require immediate therapy with parenteral glucose. A third, small group experience a benign initial phase but then develop symptoms 12 to 24 hours after birth.[252] Infants of diabetic mothers are given frequent glucose-containing feedings during the first few days of life to maintain euglycemia. Symptomatic neonates require parenteral therapy. Some recommend that fructose, which does not stimulate insulin release, be given to diabetic mothers 2 to 3 hours before delivery to prevent neonatal hypoglycemia.[253]

Exogenous Hyperinsulinism

Hypoglycemia in the Insulin-dependent Diabetic. Clinically, hypoglycemia is most commonly encountered in the insulin-dependent diabetic. Factors that warrant consideration when hypoglycemia occurs in such patients are listed in Table 90-12.[254] When the

Table 90-12. Hypoglycemia in the Insulin-dependent Diabetic

Excessive dosage:
Inadvertent: poor vision; inadequate instruction and knowledge—mismatching potency of insulin and syringe; poor injection technique—inappropriate site of injection
Deliberate: to seek attention; to satisfy the physician
Reduced need for insulin:
Inadequate or diminished caloric intake: skipped or delayed meals, increased exercise or activity
Onset of a concomitant disorder:
Endocrinologic: hypopituitarism, hydroadrenocorticalism, hypothyroidism, termination of pregnancy
Systemic: severe renal or hepatic failure.
Recovery from "stress states" that necessitated added insulin:
Medical: infections, ketoacidosis, pancreatitis, myocardial infarction, etc.
Surgical
Psychic
Use of other hypoglycemic agents or agents that have hypoglycemic potential.

diabetic has excessive quantities of circulating insulin, peripheral utilization of glucose is enhanced and gluconeogenesis is suppressed. Concurrently, certain counterregulatory mechanisms may be deficient.[89]

Diabetics with ocular failure may self-administer excessive quantities of insulin because of an inability to visualize the numerical scale on the syringe or the amount of insulin contained in the syringe. Mismatching of syringe and insulin (i.e., use of U-100 insulin in a U-40 syringe) is often evidence of insufficient instruction by the physician. Insulin administered inappropriately or at specific sites may be absorbed irregularly and cause hypoglycemia. Diabetics have been known to intentionally administer extra insulin to induce hypoglycemia in order to gain attention or to impress the physician and gain approbation for the conscientiousness for control of glycemia.

Among insulin-dependent diabetics, the failure to eat on a regular schedule is the most frequent cause of "reactions." A missed meal, particularly in the setting of increased physical activity, is a common tale. Endocrinologic and systemic disorders that ameliorate diabetes and diminish insulin needs are summarized in Table 90-12. Often during an acute illness, the diabetic requires increasing amounts of insulin to control hyperglycemia. When the acute illness subsides, insulin dosage usually diminishes. Failure to appreciate the lesser demand for insulin may result in neuroglycopenic symptoms. Similiarly, if the diabetic receives pharmacological agents that have hypoglycemic potential, insulin needs may diminish (Table 90-13).[255]

Non-insulin-dependent diabetics receiving sulfonylureas may experience hypoglycemia and neuroglycopenia. All available sulfonylureas can cause hypoglycemia, but specific agents are common culprits. Chlorpropamide has a half-life of 35 hours and is excreted by the kidneys, as are several of the hypoglycemic by-products of acetohexamide. Hence, these agents induce hypoglycemia in patients with renal disease. Table 90-13 lists other agents known to potentiate the hypoglycemic action of the sulfonylureas.

Factitious Hypoglycemia. Self-induction of hypoglycemia by insulin or oral hypoglycemic agents is observed most frequently in nurses and other paramedical personnel or their relatives. Reasons for such behavior vary; some patients suffer from psychiatric illness, others seek attention or sympathy. Often the diagnosis is difficult because the individual has a medical background and deliberately hinders the clinician. The history resembles that of a patient with insulinoma, although the hypoglycemia bears no relationship to meals, exercise, etc., since the hypoglycemic agent is administered at irregular intervals. These patients often have multiple hospital admissions, undergo laparatomy, and fulfill many of the characteristics of the Munchausen syndrome. Even under close surveillance, these individuals display extreme audacity and ingenuity in hiding the hypoglycemic agent.[256–258]

Individuals who self-induce glucopenia as a result of insulin injections will have high plasma levels of immunoreactive insulin and low levels of C-peptide immunoreactivity when hypoglycemic.[259] The latter differentiates these patients from those with insulinomas.[260] Measurement of circulating insulin antibodies is a helpful diagnostic aid, provided the individuals is not an insulin-requiring diabetic or an example of the rare instance in which insulin antibodies arise on an autoimmune basis. An intensive search should be made for an insulin ampule or syringe in the suspected individual's personal belongings; the addition of iodide 131 to the ampule of insulin, with detection of the radioisotope in the patient's thyroid or urine, helps confirm the diagnosis.

The management of patients with factitious hyperinsulinism involves psychiatric and social adjustments. Insulin has been used as both a suicidal and a homicidal weapon. Occasionally, individuals self-induce hypoglycemia with sulfonylureas such as chlorpropamide. If this is suspected, blood levels of the drug should be obtained.[261,262]

Idiopathic Postprandial Hypoglycemia (Functional, or Vagotonic)

In 1924, Harris described the occurrence of postprandial hypoglycemia in a group of nervous, emotionally labile individuals who had a variety of somatic complaints.[263] Others confirmed this report and attributed the hypoglycemia to hyperinsulinism "secondary to excessive vagal tone," and the disorder came to be known as functional, or vagotonic, hypoglycemia.[65,174] Few of the earlier investigators attempted to correlate glucose levels with symptomatology.[264]

Within the last decade, many individuals with such somatic complaints as chronic fatigue, anxiety, mental dullness, and lethargy have self-diagnosed themselves as "hypoglycemics"—in some geographical area, the numbers of such individuals are so large as to create "an epidemic condition."[265] Unfortunately, in

Table 90-13. Agents That Potentiate Hypoglycemic Drugs or Induce Hypoglycemia Independently

Potentiate Insulin	Potentiate Sulfonylureas	Independent of Other Agents
Ethanol	Sulfisoxazole	Para-aminobenzoic acid
Propranolol	Sulfaphenazole	Haloperidol
Oxytetracycline	Sulfadimidine	Propoxyphene
Ethylenediamine tetra-acetic acid	Bishydroxycoumarin	Chlorpromazine plus orphenadrine
Manganese	Phenylbutazone	
Mebanazine		

From Seltzer, H. S.: Drug-induced hypoglycemia. Diabetes *21:* 955, 1972.

many instances, physicians perpetuate this misconception and patients become victims of quacks and charlatans who prescribe a variety of hormonal potions for cure of this nonentity.

A diagnosis of idiopathic postprandial hypoglycemia requires that biochemical glycopenia correlate with the "true" neuroglycopenic symptoms of hunger, sweating, palpitations, piloerection, and irritability. Insulin-dependent diabetics and individuals with insulin-secreting tumors rarely complain of the fatigue and lethargy so commonly cited in individuals in the "nonhypoglycemic" epidemic. Oral glucose tolerance tests carried out for 5 to 6 hours are used to establish the diagnosis. However, it is often not appreciated that 23 percent of the normal population will exhibit blood glucose values below 50 mg/dl if sampling is done hourly between 2 and 5 hours after a glucose challenge. Occasionally, values below 35 mg/dl are seen in normal subjects without neuroglycopenic symptoms.[266]

Hyperinsulinism is not a constant feature in subjects with verified idiopathic postprandial hypoglycemia. In fact, the insulin-secretory patterns in these individuals are heterogeneous, although both obese and nonobese idiopathic hypoglycemics had a delay in insulin secretion compared to controls.[232,246,267] The reason for the glucopenia and neuroglycopenic symptoms remain an enigma. A suggestion that the neurological symptoms relate to shifts in electrolytes has been made.[268] Whether the glucopenia represents a hypersensitive response of tissue to normal quantities of insulin also requires clarification. Nevertheless, there are a group of anxious, compulsive individuals with intact gastrointestinal tracts and nondiabetic glucose tolerance curves who manifest symptomatic, chemically proven hypoglycemia during the postprandial period. Treatment with multiple feedings of high-protein, low-carbohydrate meals should be tried initially. If a dietary approach is unsuccessful, then small doses of propranolol should be considered to alleviate symptoms.

Extrapancreatic Tumors Inducing Hypoglycemia

Severe hypoglycemia has been reported in approximately 250 patients with extrapancreatic tumors of mesothelial, epithelial, or endothelial origin. Both benign and malignant tumors are included. The presentation of many of these patients with extrapancreatic tumors is indistinguishable from that of patients with insulin-producing tumors. A high percentage of these tumors are of mesothelial origin and include fibrosarcomas, leiomyosarcomas, and rhabdomyosarcomas. The tumors originate in the thorax, in the retroperitoneal space, or in the pelvis (Table 90-14). Primary hepatic carcinomas, carcinomas of the adrenal cortex, gastrointestinal carcinomas, and bronchogenic carcinomas are also included among the extrapancreatic neoplasms that are associated with hypoglycemia. Some of the mesenchymal tumors associated with

Table 90-14. Extrapancreatic Tumors Associated with Hypoglycemia

Origin	%
Mesenchymal	45
Hepatoma	23
Adrenal cortex	10
Gastrointestinal tract	8
Lymphoma	6
Miscellaneous (ovary, lung, kidney)	8

From Laurent, J., Debry, G., and Floquent, J.: Extrapancreatic tumours inducing hypoglycaemia, in Hypoglycaemic Tumours. Amsterdam, Excerpta Medica, 1961.

hypoglycemia are difficult to differentiate microscopically from metaplastic carcinoma of the islet cells. Characteristically, these tumors are extraordinarily large in size (2–20 kg) and slow-growing. Patients with these tumors are often elderly. Hypoglycemia is alleviated by resection or irradiation of the tumor mass[269] and recurs when metastatic disease appears.

The pathogenesis of the hypoglycemia that accompanies these extrapancreatic tumors is complex and multifactorial.[270] In the same patient, increased glucose utilization, decreased glucose production, defective glycogen synthesis and degradation, and defective mobilization of alternate metabolic substrate may coexist. Infrequently, the tumors have been shown to consume large quantities of glucose[271] and to possess high rates of anaerobic glycolysis and lactic acid production.[272] Some of the tumors contain nonsuppressible insulinlike activity (NSILA), which may account for increased peripheral utilization of glucose or restrained gluconeogenesis.[273] The latter has also been attributed to the tryptophan content of the tumor; tryptophan or its metabolites inhibit gluconeogenesis. Defective counterregulatory mechanisms have also been indicated as etiological factors in the hypoglycemia.[275]

Diagnosis is not difficult, since the tumor is readily discernible on physical examination or by roetgenography. Often the patient appears cachectic, with obvious loss of muscle and adipose tissue mass. Plasma immunoassayable insulin levels are commensurate with the level of glycemia. Fasting proinsulin and C-peptide levels are not elevated, and insulin secretogogues such as tolbutamide and leucine cause minimal or no increments in these levels. As contrasted to the patient with an islet-cell tumor, these patients demonstrate diminished endogenous insulin release with hypoglycemia.

Hypoglycemia is a rare concomitant of hepatomas, and only McFadzean and Yeung from Hong Kong report a substantial incidence (26 percent) among their patients with hepatoma.[276] Most of these patients show considerable deterioration from their disease prior to the onset of hypoglycemia, but occasionally fasting glucopenia and neuroglycopenia are early signs. The hypoglycemia is readily corrected by glucose. The mechanism or mechanisms of hypoglycemia in hepatoma patients are as variable as those for the other extrapancreatic tumors.

Hypoglycemia is alleviated when the tumor is resected or successfully irradiated. Often, however, total resection is not feasible because of the tumor's size. Patients with inoperable tumors represent a difficult challenge. Frequent oral feedings or constant infusions may be the only means to prevent neuroglycopenia. Diazoxide, streptozotocin, and other substances that alter beta-cell function are ineffective.

Increased Sensitivity to Insulin

Growth Hormone Deficiency. Children with an isolated deficiency of growth hormone exhibit fasting hypoglycemia and marked reactive glucopenia postprandially.[100,277] These dwarfed individuals have low-normal amounts of circulating insulin and are exquisitely sensitive to small quantities of exogenous insulin. Growth-hormone-deficient youngsters cannot withstand fasting for longer than 24 hours without hypoglycemia and ketonemia appearing.[278] When growth hormone deficiency is part of panhypopituitarism or secondary to a hypothalamic lesion, growth hormone therapy in addition to other hormonal replacement is essential to achieve glucose homeostasis.[279] Hence, in children with both growth hormone and ACTH deficiency, cortisone therapy alone only partially corrects the abnormality, while the addition of growth hormone completely normalizes glucose homeostasis and the sensitivity to insulin.[280,281] The exact manner by which growth hormone regulates the sensitivity of specific tissues to insulin is not known.

Adults with hypopituitarism caused by destructive neoplastic lesions, granulomata, or necrosis (Sheehan's syndrome) may have fasting glucopenia[282] and usually are sensitive to exogenous insulin. In addition to growth hormone deficiency, those individuals may have deficits of other tropic hormones. Adults with hypopituitarism and glucopenia are not given growth hormone replacement therapy.

Strenuous Exercise. Muscular exercise increases the assimilation of glucose by muscle, but this change is compensated by an increase in glucose output by the liver so that plasma glucose levels remain steady or even rise slightly after brief exercise. Extreme, prolonged muscular effort such as a marathon run may lead to declines in glucose to as low as 45 mg/dl.[283] Whether these glucopenic levels are responsible for the various symptoms complained of after a prolonged run is uncertain.[284]

During both forearm and leg exercise the uptake of glucose by working muscles increases 20 to 35-fold above the basal value.[285,286] This increment is a function of both the intensity and the duration of the work. The increased uptake of glucose occurs, while plasma insulin levels decline. During prolonged exercise at a low work intensity, blood glucose levels fall because hepatic glucose output fails to keep pace with the augmented utilization of glucose. Initially during exercise, hepatic glycogen stores are mobilized, but after 4 hours of exercise, these stores are almost depleted, and 45 percent of splanchnic glucose output derives from gluconeogenesis.[287] Glucagon levels rise over fivefold after 4 hours of continuous exercise, and glucagon seems to play a major role in the metabolic adaption to exercise.[288]

Symptomatic hypoglycemia rarely occurs with strenuous exercise but might be anticipated in situations where hepatic glycogen stores are diminished or glycogen mobilization is impeded. However, neuroglycopenia commonly occurs in the insulin-requiring diabetic who exercises strenuously. Insulin levels in such diabetics are regulated by exogenous injections and do not decline with exercise, so that the augmented uptake of glucose is further increased and hepatic glucose output is restrained.[289] Insulin-dependent diabetics must have available a ready source of carbohydrate before undertaking strenuous activity.

Artifactual Hypoglycemia

When blood that contains large numbers of leukocytes stands for any length of time, glycolysis occurs at a rapid rate and the glucose content falls. Hypoglycemia observed in subjects with leukemia or leukemoid reactions may be artifactual and related to the increased glycolysis.[290,291] The process continues even when fluoride is added to leukemic blood in amounts normally adequate to impede glucose utilization.

Since 1913 when the first techniques to measure blood sugar were introduced, many new methods have been developed. Most of these, with the exception of the glucose-oxidase and hexokinase methods, are nonspecific and measure sugars and reducing substances other than glucose. When glucose is measured by these nonspecific methods, non-glucose-reducing or chromogenic substances collectively known as "saccharoids" may obscure the presence of hypoglycemia. When specific enzyme methods such as glucose-oxidase and hexokinase are used to measure glucose, artifactually low values are reported if substances are present that interfere with the chromatogenic reactions coupled with the enzyme. Thus the presence of materials used to precipitate proteins

or drugs such as tolbutamide or tolazamide may interfere with the peroxide-peroxidase reaction employed in these methods and may account for falsely low glucose values.[292]

REFERENCES

1. Himwich, H. E.: The somatic division of the central nervous system: studied through the symptoms of hypoglycemia and acute anoxia, in Brain Metabolism and Cerebral Disorders. Baltimore, William & Wilkins, 1951, pp. 257.
2. Marks, V. and Rose, F. C.: Symptomatology, in Hypoglycaemia. Philadelphia, F. A. Davis Co., 1965, chap. 5, pp. 66–79.
3. Page, M. A. and Williamson, D. H.: Enzymes of ketone-body utilization in human brain. *Lancet 2:* 66, 1971.
4. Owen, O. E., Morgan, A. P., Kemp, H. G., Sullivan, J. M., Herrera, M. G. and Cahill, G. F., Jr.: Brain metabolism during fasting. *J. Clin. Invest. 46:* 1589, 1967.
5. LeBovit, C., Cofer, E., Murray, J., and Clark, F., Dietary evaluation of food used in households in United States. United States Department of Agriculture Household Food Consumption Survey Report No. 16, 1955.
6. Gray, G. M., Intestinal digestion and maldigestion of dietary carbohydrates. *Annu. Rev. Med. 22:* 391, 1971.
7. Fajans, S. S., Floyd, J. C., Jr.: Stimulation of islet cell secretion by nutrients and by gastrointestinal hormones released during digestion, Steiner, D. S. and Freinkel, N. (eds.): Handbook of Physiology. Endocrine Pancreas. Washington, D. C. American Physiological Society, 1972, p. 473.
8. Brown, J. C., Dryburgh, J. R., Ross, S. A. and Dupre, J.: Identification and actions of gastric inhibitory polypeptide. *Recent Prog. Horm. Res. 31:* 487, 1975.
9. Matschinsky, F. M., Landgraf, R., Elerman, J. and Kotler-Brajtburg, J.: Glucoreceptor mechanisms in islets of Langerhan. *Diabetes 21 (Suppl. 2):* 555, 1972.
10. Freinkel, N. and Metzger, B. E.: Oral glucose tolerance curve and hypoglycemia in the fed state. *N. Engl. J. Med. 280:* 820, 1969.
11. Felig, P., Wahren, J. and Hendler, R.: Influence of oral glucose ingestion on splanchnic glucose and gluconeogenic substrate metabolism. *Diabetes 24:* 4268, 1975.
12. Brown, J., Miller, D. M., Halloway, M. T. and Leve, G. D.: Hexokinase isoenzymes in liver and adipose tissue of man and dog. *Science 155:* 205, 1967.
13. Nilsson, L. H. S.: Liver glycogen content in man in the postabsorptive state. *Scand. J. Clin. Lab. Invest. 32:* 317, 1973.
14. Felig, P. and Wahren, J.: Influence of endogenous insulin secretion on splanchric glucose and amino acid metabolism in man. *J. Clin. Invest. 50:* 1702, 1971.
15. Felig, P.: Pathophysiology of diabetes, Sussman, K. E. and Metz, R. J. S. (eds): Diabetes Mellitus (ed 4). New York, American Diabetes Association Inc., 1975, chap. 1, p. 1.
16. Cahill, G. F., Jr.: Starvation in man. *N. Engl. J. Med. 282:* 668, 1970.
17. Fenn, W. O., Haege, L. F.: The disposition of glycogen with water in the livers of cat. *J. Biol. Chem. 136:* 87, 1940.
18. Howell, R. R.: The glycogen storage diseases, in Stanbury, J. B., Wyngaarden, J. B., and Frederickson, D. S. (eds.): Metabolic Basis of Inherited Diseases (ed 3). New York, McGraw-Hill, 1972, chap. 7, pp. 149–179.
19. Pohl, S. L., Birnbaumer, L. and Rodbell, M.: Glucagon-sensitive adenyl cylase in plasma membrane of hepatic parenchymal cells. *Science 164:* 566, 1969.
20. Brown, D. H. and Illingsworth, B.: The role of oligo-1,4 1,4-glucotransferase and amylo-1, 6-glucosidase in the debranching of glycogen, in Boston, Little, Brown, Control of Glycogen Metabolism. Whelan, W. J. (ed.): 1964, pp. 139–150
21. Arion, W. J. and Nordlie, R. C.: Liver glucose-6-phosphatase and pyrophosphate-glucose phosphotransferase: Effects of fasting. *Biochem. Biophys. Res. Commun. 20:* 606, 1965.
22. Langdon, R. G. and Weakley, D. R.: Influence of hormonal factors and diet upon hepatic glucose-6-phosphatase activity. *J. Biol. Chem. 214:* 167, 1955.
23. Fisher, C. J. and Stetten, M. R.: Parallel changes in vivo in microsomal inorganic pyrophosphate, pyrophosphate-glucose phosphotransfrase and glucose-6-phosphatase activities. *Biochem. Biophys. Acta 121:* 102, 1966.

24. Hildes, J. A., Sherlock, S. and Walsche, V.: Liver and muscle glycogen in normal subjects, in diabetes mellitus and in acute hepatitis. Part 1. Under basal conditions. *Clin. Sci. 7:* 287, 1949.

25. Dzúrik, R. and Brixovà, E.: Liver glycogen concentrations in patients with chronic uremia. *Experimentia (Basel) 24:* 552, 1968.

26. Vaishnava, H., Raju, T. R. S., Malik, G. B. and Gulati, P. D.: Hepatic glycogen studies in Indian diabetics. *Metabolism 20:* 657, 1971.

27. Bergström, J., Findor, J. and Hultman, E.: The contents of glycogen and potassium in human liver tissues obtained by needle biopsy. *Scand. J. Clin. Lab. Invest. 13:* 353, 1961.

28. Nilsson, L. H. S. and Hultman, E.: Liver glycogen in man-the effect of total starvation or a carbohydrate-poor diet followed by carbohydrate refeeding. *Scand. J. Clin. Lab. Invest. 32:* 325, 1973.

29. Hers, H. G., DeWulf, H., Stalmans, W. and van den Berghe, G.: The control of glycogen synthesis in the liver. *Adv. Enzyme Regul. 8:* 171, 1970.

30. Exton, J. H.: Gluconeogenesis. *Metabolism 21:* 945, 1972

31. Mallete, L. E., Exton, J. H. and Park, C. R.: Control of gluconeogenesis from amino acids in the perfused rat liver. *J. Biol. Chem. 244:* 5713, 1969.

32. Felig, P., Owen, O. E., Wahren, J. and Cahill, G. F., Jr.: Amino acid metabolism during prolonged starvation. *J. Clin. Invest. 48:* 584, 1969.

33. Ross, B. D., Hems, R. and Krebs, H. A.: The rate of gluconeogenesis from precursors in the perfused rat liver. *Biochem. J. 102:* 942, 1967.

34. Aikawa, T., Matsutaka, H., Takezawa, K. and Ishikawa, E.: Gluconeogenesis and amino acid metabolism. I. Comparison of various precursors for hepatic gluconeogenesis in vivo. *Biochem. Biophys. Acta 279:* 234, 1972.

35. Felig, P.: The glucose-alanine cycle. *Metabolism 22:* 179, 1973.

36. Felig, P. and Wahren, J.: Influence of endogenous insulin on splanchnic glucose and amino acid metabolism. *J. Clin. Invest. 50:* 1702, 1971.

37. Nilsson, L. H. S., Furst, P. and Hultman, E.: Carbohydrate metabolism of the liver in normal man under varying dietary conditions. *Scand. J. Clin. Lab. Invest. 32:* 331, 1973.

38. Felig, P., Pozefsky, T., Marliss, E. and Cahill, G. F., Jr.: Alanine: Key role in gluconeogenesis. *Science 167:* 1003, 1970.

39. London, D. R., Foley, T. H. and Webb, C. G.: Evidence for the release of individual amino acids from resting human forearm. *Nature 208:* 588, 1968.

40. Kominz, D. R., Hough, A., Symond, P. and Laki, K.: The amino acid composition of actin, myosin, tropomyosine and the meromyosins. *Arch. Biochem. Biophys. 50:* 148, 1954.

41. Odessey, R., Khairallah, E. A. and Goldberg, A. L.: Origin and possible significance of alanine production by skeletal muscle. *J. Biol. Chem. 249:* 7623, 1974.

42. Garber, A. J., Karl, I. E. and Kipnis, D. E.: Alanine and glutamine synthesis and release from skeletal muscle I. Glycolysis and amino acid release. *J. Biol. Chem. 251:* 826, 1976.

43. Garber, A. J., Karl, I. E. and Kipnis, D. E.: Alanine and glutamine synthesis and release from skeletal muscle II. The precursor role of amino acids and glutamine synthesis. *J. Biol. Chem. 251:* 836, 1976.

44. Buse, M. G. and Reid, S. S.: Leucine. A possible regulator of protein turnover in muscle. *J. Clin. Invest. 56:* 1250, 1975.

45. Buse, M. G., Biggers, J. F., Friderici, K. H. et al: Oxidation of branched chain amino acids by isolated hearts and diaphragms of the rat. *J. Biol. Chem. 247:* 8085, 1972.

46. Borchgrevink, C. F. and Havel, R. J.: Transport of glycerol in human blood. *Proc. Soc. Exp. Biol. Med. 133:* 946, 1963.

47. Owen, O. E., Felig, P., Morgan, A. P., Wahren, J. and Cahill, G. F., Jr.: Liver and kidney metabolism during prolonged starvation. *J. Clin. Invest. 48:* 574, 1969.

48. Merimee, T. J. and Tyson, J. E.: Stabilization of plasma glucose during fasting. Normal variation in two separate studies. *N. Engl. J. Med. 291:* 1275, 1974.

49. Pontremoli, S. and Grazi, E.: Gluconeogenesis, in Dickins, F., Randle, P. G., and Whelan, W. J. (eds.): Carbohydrate Metabolism and Its Disorders, vol. I. London, Academic Press, chap. 8, 1968, pp. 260–295.

50. Long, C. N. H., Katzin, B. and Fry, E. G.: The adrenal cortex and carbohydrate metabolism. *Endocrinology 26:* 309, 1940

51. Thorn, G. W., Koepf, G. F., Lewis, R. A. and Olsen, E. F.: Carbohydrate metabolism in Addison's disease. *J. Clin. Invest. 19:* 813, 1940.

52. Bondy, P. K.: The effect of adrenal and thyroid glands upon the rise of plasma amino acids in the eviscerated rat. *Endocrinology 45:* 605, 1949.

53. Ryan, W. L. and Carver, M. J.: Immediate and prolonged effects of hydrocortisone on free amino acids of rat skeletal muscle. *Proc. Soc. Exp. Biol. Med. 114:* 816, 1963.

54. Noall, M. W., Riggs, T. R., Walker, L. M. and Christensen, H. W.: Endocrine control of amino acid transport. *Science 126:* 1002, 1957.

55. Exton, J. H., Mallette, L. E., Jefferson, L. S. et al: The hormonal control of hepatic gluconeogenesis. *Recent Prog. Horm. Res. 26:* 411, 1970.

56. Lecoca, F. R., Mebane, D. and Madison, L. L.: The acute effect of hydrocortisone on hepatic glucose output and peripheral glucose utilization. *J. Clin. Invest. 43:* 237, 1964.

57. Bondy, P. K., Engel, F. L. and Farrar, B. W.: The metabolism of amino acids and protein in the adrenalectomized-nephrectomized rat. *Endocrinology 44:* 1476, 1949.

58. Shafrir, E. and Steinberg, D.: The essential role of the adrenal cortex in the response of plasma free fatty acids, cholesterol and phospholipids to epinephrine injections. *J. Clin. Invest. 39:* 310, 1960.

59. Weber, G., Banerjee, G. and Bronstein, S. B.: Role of enzymes in homeostasis III. Selective induction of increases of liver enzymes involved in carbohydrate metabolism. *J. Biol. Chem. 236:* 3106, 1961.

60. Ashmore, J. and Weber, G.: Hormonal control of carbohydrate metabolism in the liver, in Dicken, F., Randle, P. J., and Whelan, W. J. (eds.): Carbohydrate Metabolism and Its Disorders, vol. 1. London, Academic Press, 1968, chap. 10, p. 336.

61. Bondy, P. K.: The adrenal cortex, in Bondy, P. K., and Rosenberg, L. E. (eds.): Duncan's Diseases of Metabolism (eds.). Philadelphia, W. B. Saunders, 1974, p. 1105.

62. Garces, L. Y., Kenny, F. M., Drash, A., and Taylor, F. H.: Cortisol secretion rate during fasting of obese addescent subjects. *J. Clin. Endocrinol. 28:* 1843, 1968.

63. Greenwood, F. C., Landon, J. and Stamp, T. C. B.: The plasma sugar, free fatty acid, cortisol and growth hormone response to insulin I. In control subjects. *J, Clin. Invest. 45:* 429, 1966.

64. Garber, A. J., Cryer, P. E., Santiago, V. et al: The role of adrenergic mechanisms in the substrate and hormonal response to insulin-induced hypoglycemia in man. *J. Clin. Invest. 58:* 7, 1976.

65. Ensinck, J. W. and Williams, R. H.: Disorders causing hypoglycemia, in Williams, R. H. (ed.): Textbook of Endocrinology (ed 5). Philadelphia, W. B. Saunders, 1974, chap. 10, pp. 627–659.

66. Woods, S. C. and Porte, D., Jr.: Neural Control of the endocrine pancreas. *Physiol. Rev. 54:* 596, 1974.

67. Brodows, R. G., Pi-Sunyer, F. X. and Campbell, R. G.: Neural control of counter-regulatory events during glucopenia in man. *J. Clin. Invest. 52:* 1841, 1973.

68. Palmer, J. P., Henry, D. P., Benson, J. W., Johnson, D. G. and Ensinck, J. W.: Glucagon response to hypoglycemia in sympathectomized man. *J. Clin. Invest. 57:* 522, 1976.

69. Young, J. B. and Landsberg, L.: Suppression of sympathetic nervous system during fasting. *Science 196:* 1473, 1977.

70. Cantu, R. C., Wise, B. L., Goldfien, A., Gullixson, K. S., Fischer, N. and Ganong, W. F.: Neural pathways mediating the increase in adrenal medullary secretion produced by hypoglycemia. *Proc. Soc. Exp. Biol. 114:* 10, 1963.

71. Axelrod, J. and Weinschilboum, R.: Catecholamines. *N. Engl. J. Med. 287:* 237, 1972.

72. Bloom, S. R., Edwards, A. V., Hardy, R. N., Malinowska, K. W. and Silver, M.: Endocrine responses to insulin hypoglycemia in the young calf. *J. Physiol. 244:* 783, 1975.

73. Sokal, J. E., Sarcione, E. J. and Henderson, A. M.: Relative potency of glucagon and epinephrine as hepatic glycogenolytic agents: Studies with the isolated perfused rat liver. *Endocrinology 74:* 930, 1964.

74. Edwards, A. V. and Silver, M.: The glycogenolytic response to stimulation of the splanchnic nerves in adrenalectomized calves. *J. Physiol. 211:* 109, 1970.

75. Cori, C. F. and Cori, G. T.: The mechanism of epinephrine action. IV. The influence of epinephrine on lactic acid production and blood glucose utilization. *J. Biol. Chem. 84:* 683, 1929.

76. Abramson, E. A. and Arky, R. A.: Role of beta-adrenergic receptors in counter-regulation to insulin-induced hypoglycemia. *Diabetes 17:* 141, 1968.

77. Porte, D., Jr. and Williams, R. H.: Inhibition of insulin release by norepinephrine in man. *Science 152:* 1248, 1966.

78. Sutherland, E. W. and DeDuve, C.: Origin and distribution of hyperglycemic-glycogenolytic factor of the pancreas. *J. Biol. Chem. 175:* 663, 1948.

79. Park, C. R. and Exton, J. H.: Glucagon and the metabolism of glucose, in Lefebvre, P. J., and Unger, R. H. (eds.): Glucagon: Molecular Physiology, Clinical and Therapeutic Implications. Oxford, Pergamen Press, 1972, pp. 77–108.

80. Unger, R. H., Aguilor-Parada, E., Muller, W. A. et al: Studies of pancreatic alpha cell function in normal and diabetic subjects. *J. Clin. Invest. 49:* 837, 1970.

81. Aguilar-Parada, E., Eisentraut, A. M. and Unger, R. H.: Effects of starvation on plasma pancreatic glucagon in normal man. *Diabetes 18:* 717, 1969.

82. Marliss, E. B., Aoki, T. T., Unger, R. H., Soeldner, J. S. and Cahill, G. F., Jr.: Glucagon levels and metabolic effects in fasting man. *J. Clin. Invest. 49:* 2256, 1970.

83. Unger, R. H., Eisentraut, A. M., McCall, M. S. and Madison, L. L.: Measurement of endogenous glucagon in plasma and the influence of blood glucose concentration upon its secretion. *J. Clin. Invest. 41:* 682, 1962.

84. Gerich, J. E., Karam, J. H. and Forsham, P. H.: Stimulation of glucagon secretion by epinephrine in man. *J. Clin. Endocrinol. Metab. 37:* 479, 1973.

85. Pek, S., Tai, T-Y., Crowther, R. and Fajans, S. S.: Glucagon release precedes, insulin release in response to common secretogogues. *Diabetes 25:* 764, 1976.

86. Tiengo, A., Fedele, D., Marchiori, E. et al: Suppression and stimulation mechanisms controlling glucagon secretion in a case of islet cell tumor producing glucagon, insulin and gastrin. *Diabetes 25:* 408, 1976.

87. Orci, L. and Unger, R. H.: Hypothesis: Functional subdivisions of the islets of Langerhan and the possible role of insular D-cell. *Lancet 2:* 1243, 1975.

88. Unger, R. H.: Role of glucagon in diabetes. *Arch. Intern. Med. 137:* 482, 1977.

89. Gerich, J. E., Langlois, M., Noacco, C.: Lack of glucagon response to hypoglycemia in diabetes. Evidence for an intrinsic pancreatic alpha cell defect. *Science 182:* 171, 1973.

90. Sokal, J. E. and Ezdenli, E.: Basal plasma glucagon levels of man. *J. Clin. Invest. 46:* 778, 1967.

91. Sutherland, E. W. and Cori, C. F.: Effect of hyperglycemic-glycogenolytic factor and epinephrine on liver phosphorylase. *J. Biol. Chem. 188:* 531, 1951.

92. Miller, L. L.: Glucagon: a protein catabolic hormone in the isolated perfused rat liver. *Nature 185:* 248, 1960.

93. Mallette, L. E., Exton, J. H. and Park, C. A.: Effects of glucagon on amino acid transport and utilization in the perfused rat liver. *J. Biol. Chem. 244:* 5724, 1969.

93a. Chiasson, J. L., Liljenquist, J. E., Sinclair-Smith, B. C. and Lacy, W. W.: Gluconeogenesis from alanine in normal postabsorptive man. Intrahepatic stimulatory effect of glucagon. *Diabetes 24:* 574, 1975.

94. Rodbell, M., Krans, H. M., Pohl, S. L. and Bernbaumer, L.: The glucagon-sensitive adenyl cyclase system in plasma membranes of rat liver. III. Binding of glucagon: method of assay and specificity. *J. Biol. Chem. 246:* 1861, 1971.

95. Bjorntorp, B., Karlsson, M. and Horden, A.: Quantitative aspects of lipolysis and re-esterification in human adipose tissue in vitro. *Acta. Med. Scand. 185:* 85, 1969.

96. McGarry, J. D., Wright, P., and Foster, D.: Hormonal control of ketogenesis: rapid activation of hepatic ketogenic capacity in fed rats by anti-insulin serum and glucagon. *J. Clin. Invest. 55:* 1202, 1975.

97. Alford, F. P., Bloom, S. R., Nabarro, J. D. N. et al: Glucagon control of fasting glucose in man. *Lancet ii:* 974, 1974.

98. Felig, P., Wahren, J., Sherwin, R. and Hendler, R.: Insulin, glucagon and somatostatin in normal physiology and diabetes mellitus. *Diabetes 25:* 1091, 1976.

99. Alberti, K. G. M. M., and Nattrass, M.: The physiological function of glucagon. *Eur. J. Clin. Invest. 7:* 151, 1977.

100. Parader, A., Zackmann, M., Poley, J. R., Illig, R.: The metabolic effect of a small uniform dose of human growth hormone in hypopituitary dwarfs and in control children II. Blood glucose response to insulin-induced hypoglycemia. *Acta. Endocrinol. 57:* 129, 1968.

101. Brasel, J. A., Wright, J. C., Wilkins, L. and Blizzard, R. M.: An evaluation of seventy-five patients with hypopituitarism beginning in childhood. *Am. J. Med. 38:* 484, 1965.

102. Frohman, L. A., MacGillivray, M. H. and Aceto, T., Jr.: Acute effects of human growth hormone on insulin secretion and glucose utilization in normal and growth hormone deficient subjects. *J. Clin. Endocrinol. 27:* 561, 1967.

103. Chochinov, R. H. and Daughaday, W. H.: Current concepts of somatomedin and other related growth factors. *Diabetes 25:* 994, 1976.

104. Zierler, K. L. and Rabinowitz, D.: Roles of insulin and growth hormone based on studies of forearm metabolism in man. *Medicine 42:* 385, 1963.

105. Fineberg, S. E., Merimee, T. J., Rabinowitz, D. and Edgar, P. J.: Insulin secretion in acromegaly. *J. Clin. Endocrinol. 30:* 288, 1970.

106. Merimee, T. J., Burgess, J. A. and Rabinowitz, D.: Influence of growth-hormone in insulin secretion. Studies of growth-hormone deficient subjects. *Diabetes 16:* 478, 1967.

107. Peake, G. T., McKeel, D. W., Mariz, I. K. and Daughaday, W. H.: Insulin storage and release in rats bearing growth hormone secreting tumors. *Diabetes 18:* 619, 1969.

108. Root, A. W.: Chemical and biological properties of growth hormone, in Human Pituitary Growth Hormone. Springfield, Ill., Charles C. Thomas, 1972, chap. 1, pp. 3–34.

109. Glick, S. M., Roth, J., Yalow, R. S. and Berson, S. A.: The regulation of growth hormone secretion. *Recent Prog. Horm. Res. 21:* 241, 1965.

110. Glick, S. M.: Hypoglycemic threshold for human growth hormone release. *J. Clin. Endocrinol. 30:* 619, 1970.

111. Takebe, K., Kunita, H., Sawano, S. et al: Circadian rhythms of plasma growth hormone and cortisol after insulin. *J. Clin. Endocrinol. 29:* 1630, 1969.

112. Balckard, W. G. and Heindingsfelder, S. A.: Adrenergic receptor control mechanism for growth hormone secretion. *J. Clin. Invest. 47:* 1407, 1968.

113. Cahill, G. F., Jr., Herrera, M. G., Morgan, A. P. et al: Hormone-fuel interrelationships during fasting. *J. Clin. Invest. 45:* 1751, 1966.

114. Ferrendelli, J. A.: Hypoglycemia and the central nervous system, in Ingvar, D. H. and Lassen, N. A. (eds.): Brain Work. The Coupling of Function, Metabolism and Blood Flow in the Brain. Proceedings of the Alfred Benzon Symposium VIII. Copenhagen, Munksgaard, 1975, pp. 298–311.

115. Lewis, L. D., Ljunggren, B., Ratcheson, R. A., Siesjo, B. K.: Cerebral energy state in insulin-induced hypoglycemia, related to blood glucose and EEG. *J. Neurochem. 23:* 673, 1974.

116. Adams, R. D. and Sidman, R. L.: Introduction to Neuropathology. New York, McGraw-Hill, 1968, p. 248.

117. Banker, B. Q.: Neonatal anoxic and hypoglycemic encephalopathy. *Med. Child. Neurol. 9:* 544, 1967.

118. Kerr, S. E. and Ghantus, M.: The carbohydrate metabolism of brain. II. The effect of varying the carbohydrate and insulin supply on the glycogen, free sugar and lactic and in mammalian brain. *J. Biol. Chem. 116:* 9, 1936.

119. Olsen, N. S. and Klein, J. F.: Effect of insulin hypoglycemia on brain glucose, glycogen, lactate and phosphates. *Arch. Biochem 13:* 343, 1947.

120. Tews, J. K., Carter, S. H. and Stone, W. E.: Chemical changes in brain during insulin hypoglycemia and recovery. *J. Neurochem. 12:* 679, 1965.

121. Goldberg, N. D., Passonneau, J. V. and Lowry, O.: Effects of changes in brain metabolism on the levels of citric acid cycle intermediates. *J. Biol. Chem. 241:* 3997, 1966.

122. Hinzen, D. H. and Muller, V.: Energestoffwechsel und Funktion des Kaninchengehirns wahrend Insulin-hypoglykamic. *Pflugers Arch. Physiol. 322:* 47, 1971.

123. Tarr, M. Brada, D. and Sampson, F. E., Jr.: Cerebral high energy phosphates during insulin hypoglycemia. *Am. J. Physiol. 203:* 690, 1962.

124. King, L. J., Lowry, O. H., Passonneau, J. V. and Venson, V.: Effects on convulsants on energy reserves in the cerebral cortex. *J. Neurochem. 15:* 599, 1967.

125. Mayman, C. I. and Tyerina, M. L.: The effect of hypoglycemia on energy reserves in adult and newborn brain, in Brurly, J. B., Meldrum, B. S., and Polani, P. E. (eds.): Brain Hypoxia. Philadelphia, J. B. Lippincott, 1971, pp. 242–249.

126. Ferrendelli, J. A. and Chang, M.-M.: Brain metabolism during hypoglycemia. *Arch. Neurol. 28:* 173, 1973.

127. Eisenberg, S. and Seltzer, H. S.: The cerebral metabolic effects of

acutely induced hypoglycemia in human subjects. *Metabolism 11:* 1162, 1962.

128. Dawson, M. E. and Greville, G. D.: Biochemistry, in Hill, D., and Parr, G. (eds.): Electroencephalography. A Symposium on Its Various Aspects. London, MacDonald, 1963, chap. V, pp. 147–192.

129. Davis, P. A.: Effect on electroencephalogram of changing blood-sugar level. *Arch. Neurol. Psychiatry 49:* 186, 1943.

130. Himwich, H. E., Frostig, J. P., Fazekas, J. F., Hadidian, Z.: The mechanism of the symptoms of insulin hypoglycemia. *Am. J. Psychiatry 96:* 371, 1939.

131. Marshall, N. B., Barrnett, R. J. and Mayer, J.: Hypothalamic liaison in gold-thioglucose injected mice. *Proc. Soc. Exp. Bio. Med. 90:* 240, 1955.

132. Cannon, W. B., McIver, M. A. and Bliss, S. W.: Studies on the conditions of activity in endocrine glands. XIII. A sympathetic and adrenal mechanism for mobilizing sugar in hypoglycemia. *Am. J. Physiol. 69:* 46, 1924.

133. French, E. B. and Kilpatrick, R.: Role of adrenaline in hypoglycemic reactions in man. *Clin. Sci. 14:* 639, 1955.

134. Shimazu, T. and Amakawa, A.: Regulation of glycogen metabolism in liver by the autonomic nervous system. II. Neural control of glycogenolytic enzymes. *Biochem. Biophys. Acta 165:* 335, 1968.

135. Shimazu, T. and Amakawa, A.: Regulation of glycogen metabolism in liver by the autonomic nervous system. III. Differential effects of sympathetic-nerve stimulation and of catecholamines on liver phosphorylase. *Biochem. Biophys. Acta 165:* 349, 1968.

136. Brodows, R. G., Pi-Sunyer, F. X. and Campbell, R. G.: Sympathetic control of hepatic glycogenolysis during glucopenia in man. *Metab. Clin. Exp. 24:* 617, 1975.

137. Frokman, L. and Bernardis, L. L.: The effect of hypothalamic stimulation on plasma glucose, insulin and glucoagon levels. *Am. J. Physiol. 221:* 1596, 1971.

138. Colle, E. and Ulstrom, R. A.: Ketotic hypoglycemia. *J. Pediatr. 74:* 632, 1964.

139. Cornblath, M. and Schwartz, R.: Specific hypoglycemic syndromes, in Disorders of Carbohydrate Metabolism in Infancy. Philadelphia, W. B. Saunders, 1976, chap. 11, pp. 378–429.

140. Pagliara, A. S., Karl, I. E., DeVivo, D. C., Feigin, R. D. and Kipnis, D. M.: Hypoalaninemia: A concomitant of ketotic hypoglycemia. *J. Clin. Invest. 51:* 1440, 1972.

141. Haymond, M. W., Karl, I. E. and Pagliara, A. S.: Ketotic hypoglycemia: an amino acid substrate limited disorder. *J. Clin. Endocrinol. Metab. 38:* 52, 1974.

142. Cohen, B. D. and Horowitz, H. L.: Carbohydrate metabolism in uremia. *Am. J. Clin. Nutr. 21:* 407, 1968.

143. Runyan, J. W., Hurwitz, D. and Robbins, S. L.: Effect of K-W Syndrome on insulin requirements in diabetes. *N. Engl. J. Med. 252:* 385, 1955.

143a. Hatch, F. E., Watt, M. F., Kramer, N. C., Parrish, A. E. and Howe, J. S.: Remission of diabetes in renal failure. *Am. J. Med. 31:* 216, 1961.

144. Block, M. B. and Rubinstein, A. H.: Spontaneous hypoglycemia in diabetics with renal insufficiency. *J.A.M.A. 213:* 1863, 1970.

145. White, M. G. and Kutzman, N. A.: Hypoglycemia in non-diabetics with renal failure. *J.A.M.A. 215:* 117, 1971.

146. Rabau, M., Dor, J., Adar, R., Walden, R. and Mozes, M.: Spontaneous hypoglycemia in a diabetic patient with renal failure. *Israel J. Med. Sci. 9:* 1036, 1973.

147. Mataverde, A., El-Ravi, R. and Cohen, M.: Spontaneous hypoglycemia in chronic renal failure (abstract) *Clin. Res. 22:* 475A, 1974.

148. Frizzell, M., Larsen, P. R. and Field, J. B.: Spontaneous hypoglycemia associated with chronic renal failure. *Diabetes 22:* 493, 1973.

149. Garber, A. J., Bier, D. M., Cyrer, P. E. and Pagliara, A. S.: Hypoglycemia in conpensated chronic renal insufficiency. *Diabetes 23:* 982, 1974.

150. Dunlop, D.: Eighty-six cases of Addison's disease. *Lancet 2:* 887, 1963.

151. Porges, O.: Veber Hypoglykamie bei Merbus Addison sowie bei nebennierenlosen. *Hunden Z. Klin. Med. 69:* 341, 1910.

152. Frawley, T. F.: The role of the adrenal cortex in glucose and pyruvic acid metabolism in man including the use of intravenous hydrocortisone in acute hypoglycemia. *Ann. N.Y. Acad. Sci. 61:* 464, 1955.

153. Maranon, G.: Action de l'insuline dans l'insuffisance surrendale. *Presse Med. 33:* 1665, 1925.

154. Wajchenberg, B. L., Pierira, V. G., Pupo, A. A. et al: On the mechanism of insulin hypersensitivity in adrenocortical insufficiency. *Diabetes 13:* 169, 1964.

155. Arky, R. A. and Freinkel, N.: The response of plasma growth hormone to insulin and ethanol-induced hypoglycemia in two patients with isolated adrenocorticotropic defect. *Metabolism 13:* 547, 1964.

156. Bondy, P. K., Ingle, D. J. and Meeks, R. C.: Influence of adrenal cortical hormones upon the levels of plasma amino acids in eviscerated rats. *Endocrinology 55:* 354, 1954.

157. Baxter, J. D. and Forsham, P. H.: Tissue effects of glucocorticoids. *Am. J. Med. 53:* 573, 1972.

158. Knowlton, A. I.: Addison's disease, A review of its clinical course and management, in Christy, N. P. (ed): The Human Adrenal Cortex. New York, Harper and Row, 1971, chap. 12, pp. 329–358.

159. Odell, W. D., Green, G. and Williams, R. H.: Hypoadrenotropism. The isolated deficiency of adrenotropic hormone. *J. Clin. Endocrinol. 20:* 1017, 1960.

160. White, F. P. and Sutton, L. E.: Adrenogenital syndrome with associated episodes of hypoglycemia. *J. Clin. Endocrinol. 11:* 1395, 1951.

161. Felig, P. and Lynch, V.: Starvation in human pregnancy: Hypoglycemia, hypoinsulinemia and hyperketonemia. *Science 170:* 990, 1970.

162. Felig, P. Kim, Y. J., Lynch, V. and Hendler, R.: Amino acid metabolism during starvation in human pregnancy. *J. Clin. Invest. 51:* 1195, 1972.

163. Metzger, B. E. and Freinkel, N.: Regulation of maternal protein metabolism and gluconeogenesis in the fast state, in Camerini-Davalos, R. A. and Cole, H. S. (eds.): Early Diabetes in Early Life. New York, Academic Press, 1975, pp. 303–312.

164. Bleicher, S. J., O'Sullivan, J. B. and Freinkel, N.: Carbohydrate metabolism in pregnancy v. The interrelations of glucose, insulin and free fatty acids in late pregnancy and postpartum. *N. Engl. J. Med. 271:* 866, 1964.

165. Kuhl, C. and Holst, J. J.: Plasma glucagon and the insulin: Glucagon ratio in gestational diabetes. *Diabetes 25:* 16, 1976.

166. Kalkhoff, R., Schalch, D., Walker, J. L. et al, Diabetogenic factors associated with pregnancy. *Trans. Assoc. Am. Physicians 77:* 270, 1964.

167. Widmark, E. M. P.: On lactation hypoglycaemias. *Acta Med. Scand. Suppl. 26:* 164, 1928.

168. Mann, F. C. and Magath, T. B.: Studies on the physiology of the liver. II. The effect of the removal of the liver on the blood sugar level. *Arch. Intern. Med. 30:* 73, 1922.

169. Mann, F. C. and Magath, T. B.: Studies on the physiology of the liver. IV. Effect of total removal of liver, after pancreatectomy on blood sugar level. *Arch. Intern. Med. 31:* 797, 1923.

170. Mann, F. C.: Effects of complete and partial removal of the liver. *Medicine 6:* 419, 1927

171. Zimmerman, H. J., Thomas, L. J. and Scherr, E. H.: Fasting blood sugar in hepatic disease with reference to infrequency of hypoglycemia. *Arch. Intern. Med. 91:* 577, 1953.

172. Samson, R. I., Trey, C., Timme, A. H. and Saunders, S. J.: Fulminating hepatitis with recurrent hypoglycemia and hemorrhage. *Gastroenterology 53:* 291, 1967.

173. Marks, V. and Rose, F. C.: Hepatogenous hypoglycaemia, in Marks, V. and Rose, F. C. (eds.): Hypoglycaemia. Philadelphia, F. A. Davis, 1965, chap. 9, pp. 166–172.

174. Conn, J. W.: The diagnosis and management of spontaneous hypoglycemia. *J.A.M.A. 134:* 130, 1947.

175. Benzing, G., Schubert, W., Hug, G., Kaplan, S.: Simultaneous hypoglycemia and acute congestive heart failure. *Circulation 40:* 209, 1969.

176. Mellinkoff, S. M. and Tumulty, P. A.: Hepatic hypoglycemia. Its occurrence in congestive heart failure. *N. Engl. J. Med. 247:* 745, 1952.

176a. Tumulty, P. A. and Mellinkoff, S. M.: Hypoglycemia in congestive heart failure. *Diabetes 7:* 147, 1958.

177. Block, M. B., Resenkov, L., Gambetta, M. and Rubinstein, A.: Spontaneous hypoglycaemia in congestive heart failure. *Lancet ii* 736: 1972.

178. van Crevald, S.: Clinical course of glycogen storage disease. *Chem. Weekblad 57:* 445, 1961.

179. Pagliara, A. S., Karl, I. E., Haymond, M. and Kipnis, D. M.:

Hypoglycemia in infancy and childhood, pt. I. *J. Pediatr. 82:* 365, 1973.

180. Sidbury, J. B., Jr. and Heick, H. M. C.: Glycogen storage disease. A review with emphasis on gastrointestinal manifestations. *South. Med. J. 61:* 915, 1968.

181. Howell, R. R., Ashton, D. M. and Wyngaarden, J. B.: Glucose-6-phosphatase deficiency glycogen storage disease. Studies on the interrelationship of carbohydrate, lipid and purine abnormalities. *Pediatrics 29:* 553, 1962.

182. Steinitz, K.: Laboratory diagnosis of glycogen diseases. *Adv. Clin. Chem. 9:* 227, 1967.

183. Stamm, W. E. and Webb, D. I.: Partial deficiency of hepatic glucose-6-phosphatase in an adult patient. *Arch. Intern. Med. 135:* 1107, 1975.

184. Illingworth, B. and Cori, G. T.: Structure of glycogens and amylopectins. III. Normal and abnormal human glycogen. *J. Biol. Chem. 199:* 653, 1942.

185. van Creveld, S.: The Blackader Lecture 1962: the clinical course of glycogen disease. *Can. Med. Assoc. J. 88:* 1, 1963.

186. Sidbury, J. B., Cornblath, M., Fisher, J. and House, E.: Glycogen in erythrocytes of patients with glycogen storage disease. *Pediatrics 27:* 103, 1961.

187. Williams, H. E., Kendig, E. M. and Field, J. B.: Leukocyte debranching enzyme in glycogen storage disease. *J. Clin. Invest. 42:* 656, 1963.

188. Illingworth, B., Cori, G. T., and Cori, C. F.: Amylo-1, 6-glucosidase in muscle tissue in generalized glycogen storage disease. *J. Biol. Chem. 218:* 123, 1956.

189. Hers, H. G.: Etudes enzymatiques sur pagments hépatiques; application à la classification des glycogénoses. *Rev. Int. Hepatol. 9:* 35, 1959.

190. Williams, H. E. and Field, J. B.: Low leukocyte phosphorylase in hepatic phosphorylase deficient glycogen storage disease. *J. Clin. Invest. 40:* 1841, 1961.

191. Hülsmann, W. C. and Fernandes, J.: A child with lactic-acidemia and fructose diphosphatase deficiency in liver. *Pediatr. Res. 5:* 633, 1971.

192. Pagliara, A. S., Karl, I. E., Keating, J. P., Brown, B. I. and Kipnis, D. M.: Hepatic fructose-1, 6 diphosphatase deficiency. A cause of lactic acidosis and hypoglycemia in infancy. *J. Clin. Invest. 51:* 2115, 1972.

193. Greene, H. L., Stifel, F. B. and Herman, R. H.: Ketotic hypoglycemia due to hepatic fructose-1, 6-diphosphatase deficiency. Treatment with folic acid. *Am. J. Dis. Child. 124:* 415, 1972.

194. Melancon, S. B., Khachadurian, A. K., Nadler, H. L. and Brown, B. I.: Metabolic biochemical studies in fructose-1, 6 diphosphatase deficiency. *J. Pediatr. 82:* 560, 1973.

195. Melancon, S. B. and Nadler, H. L.: Detection of fructose-1, 6-diphosphatase deficiency with use of white blood cells. *N. Engl. J. Med. 286:* 731, 1972.

196. Fiser, R. H., Melsher, H. L. and Fischer, D. A.: Hepatic phosphoenolpyruvate carboxykinase deficiency: A new cause of hypoglycemia in childhood. *Pediatr. Res. 8:* 432, 1974.

197. Saudubray, J. M., Marsac, C., Charpentier, C. et al: Neonatal congenital lactic acidosis with pyruvate carboxylase deficiency in two siblings. *Acta Pediatr. Scand. 65:* 717, 1976.

198. Hommes, F. A., Polman, H. A., and Reerink, J. D.: Leigh's encephalopathy: an inborn error of gluconeogenesis. *Arch. Dis. Child. 43:* 423, 1968.

199. Hommes, F. A., Bendien, K., Clema, J. D., Bremer, H. J., and Lombeck, L.: Two cases of phosphoenolxyruvate carboxykinase deficiency. *Acta Paediatr. Scand. 65:* 233, 1976.

200. Madison, L. L.: Ethanol-induced hypoglycemia. *Adv. Metab. Dis. 3:* 85, 1968.

201. Arky, R. A.: The effect of alcohol on carbohydrate metabolism: Carbohydrate metabolism in alcoholics, in Kessen, B. and Begleiter, H. (eds.): The Biology of Alcoholism. New York, Plenum Press, 1971, chap. 6, pp. 197–227.

202. Krebs, H. A., Freedland, R. A., Hems, R. and Stubbs, M.: Inhibition of hepatic gluconeogenesis by ethanol. *Biochem. J. 112:* 117, 1969.

203. Madison, L. L., Lochner, A., Wueff, J.: Ethanol-induced hypoglycemia. *Diabetes 16:* 252, 1967.

204. Arky, R. A. and Freinkel, N.: Alcohol hypoglycemia. V. Alcohol infusion to test gluconeogenesis in starvation with special reference to obesity. *N. Engl. J. Med. 274:* 426, 1966.

205. Freinkel, N., Singer, D. L., Arky, R. A. et al: Alcohol hypoglycemia. I. Carbohydrate metabolism in patients with clinical alcohol hypoglycemia and the experimental reproduction of the syndrome with pure ethanol. *J. Clin. Invest. 42:* 1112, 1963.

206. Cummins, L. H.: Hypoglycemia and convulsions in children following alcohol ingestion. *J. Pediatr. 58:* 23, 1961.

207. Tolis, A. D.: Hypoglycemic convulsions in children after alcohol ingestion. *Pediatr. Clin. North Am. 12:* 423, 1965.

208. Kreisberg, R. A., Siegal, A. M. and Owen, W. G.: Glucose-lactate interrelationships: effect of ethanol. *J. Clin. Invest. 50:* 175, 1970.

209. Lundquist, F. Tygstrup, N., Winkler, K. and Birger Jensen, K.: Glycerol metabolism in the human liver: inhibition by ethanol. *Science 150:* 616, 1965.

210. Siegel, F. L., Roach, M. K. and Pomeroy, L. R.: Plasma amino acid patterns with alcoholism: the effects of ethanol loading. *Proc. Natl. Acad. Sci. 51:* 605, 1964.

211. Perman, E. S.: The effect of ethyl alcohol on the secretion from the adrenal medulla in man. *Acta Physiol. Scand. 44:* 241, 1958.

212. DeMoura, M. C., Correlia, J. P. and Madeira, F.: Clinical alcohol hypoglycemia. *Ann. Intern Med. 66:* 893, 1967.

213. Freinkel, N. and Arky, R. A.: Effects of alcohol on carbohydrate metabolism in man. *Psychosomatic Med. 27:* 551, 1966.

214. Arky, R. A., Veverbrants, E. and Abramson, E. A.: Irreversible hypoglycemia. A complication of alcohol and insulin. *J.A.M.A. 206:* 575, 1968.

215. Metz, R. Berger, S. and Mako, M.: Potentiation of the plasma insulin response to glucose by prior administration of alcohol. *Diabetes 18:* 517, 1969.

216. Nikkila, E. A. and Taskinen, M. R.: Ethanol-induced alterations of glucose tolerance, postglucose hypoglycemia and insulin secretion in normal, obese and diabetic subjects. *Diabetes 24:* 933, 1975.

216a. Jelliffe, D. B. and Stuart, K. L.: Acute toxic hypoglycemia in the vomiting sickness of Jamaica. *Br. Med. J. 1:* 75, 1954.

216b. Bressler, R. Corredor, C. and Brendel, K.: Hypoglycin and hypoglycin-like compounds. *Pharmacol. Rev. 21:* 105, 1969.

216c. von Holt, C. von Holt, M. and Böhm, H.: Metabolic effects of hypoglycin and methylenecyclopropaneacetic acid. *Biochim. Biophys. Acta. 125:* 11, 1966.

216d. Brendel, K. and Bressler, R.: Mechanism of inhibition of gluconeogenesis by 4-pentenoic acid. *Am. J. Clin. Nutr. 23:* 972, 1970.

217. Scholtz, D. A. Re Mine, W. H., and Priestley, J. T.: Clinics in endocrine and metabolic diseases. Hyperinsulinism: review of 95 cases of functioning pancreatic islet cell tumors. *Proc. Staff Meeting Mayo Clin. 35:* 545, 1960.

218. Larouche, G. P., Ferris, D. O., Priestley, J. T. et al: Hyperinsulinism: Surgical results and management of occult functioning islet cell tumors: Review of 154 cases. *Arch. Surg. 96:* 763, 1968.

219. Schein, P. S., DeLellis, R. A., Kahn, C. R., Gorden, P. and Kraft, A. R.: Islet cell tumors: Current concepts and management. *Ann. Intern. Med. 79:* 239, 1973.

220. Broder, L. E. and Carter, S. K.: Pancreatic islet cell carcinoma. I. Clinical features of 52 patients. *Ann. Intern. Med. 79:* 101, 1973.

221. Yakovac, W. C., Baker, L., Hummeler, K.: Beta cell nesidioblastosis in idiopathic hypoglycemia in infancy. *J. Pediatr. 79:* 226, 1971.

222. Gorden, P., Sherman, B., and Roth, J.: Proinsulin-like component of circulating insulin in the basal state and in patients and hamsters with islet cell tumors. *J. Clin. Invest. 50:* 2113, 1971.

223. Melani, F., Ryan, W. G., Rubenstein, A. H. et al: Proinsulin secretion by pancreatic beta-cell adenoma. *N. Engl. J. Med. 283:* 713, 1970.

224. Broder, L. E. and Carter, S. K.: Pancreatic islet cell carcinoma. II. Results of therapy with streptozotocin in 52 patients. *Ann. Intern. Med. 79:* 108, 1973.

225. Gilbert, J. A. L. and Dunlop, D. M.: Hypoglycaemia following partial gastrectomy. *Br. Med. J. 2:* 330, 1947.

226. Akiya, Y., Hirota, M. and Matsuhashi, T.: Hypoglycemic symptoms following gastrectomy. *Yokohama Med. Bull. 11:* 471, 1960.

227. Wiznitzer, T., Shapiro, N., Stadler, J. et al: Late hypoglycemia in patients following vagotomy and pyloroplasty. *Int. Surg. 59:* 229, 1974.

228. Breuer, R. I., Moses, H. III, Hagan, T. C. and Zuckerman, L.: Gastric operations and glucose homeostasis. *Gastroenterology 62:* 1109, 1972.

229. Cameron, A. J., Ellis, J. P., McGill, J. I. and LeQuesne, L. P.:

Insulin response to carbohydrate ingestion after gastric surgery with special reference to hypoglycemia. *Gut 10:* 825, 1969.

230. Permutt, M. A.: Postprandial hypoglycemia. *Diabetes 25:* 719, 1976.

231. Hafken, L., Leichter, S., and Reich, T.: Organic brain dysfunction as a possible consequence of postgastrectomy hypoglycemia. *Am. J. Psychiatry 132:* 1321, 1975.

232. Hofeldt, F. D., Lufkin, E. G., Hagler, L. et al: Are abnormalities in insulin secretion responsible for reactive hypoglycemia? *Diabetes 23:* 589, 1974.

233. Machella, T. E.: The mechanism of the post-gastrectomy dumping syndrome. *Ann. Surg. 130:* 145, 1949.

234. Veverbrants, E., Olsen, W. and Arky, R. A.: Role of gastrointestinal factors in reactive hypoglycemia. *Metabolism 18:* 6, 1969.

235. Permutt, M. A., Kelly, J., Bernstein, R., Alpers, D. H., Siegel, B. A. and Kipnis, D. M.: Alimentary hypoglycemia in the absence of gastrointestinal surgery. *N. Engl. J. Med. 288:* 1206, 1973.

236. Cole, R. A., Benedict, G. W., Margolis, S. and Kowarski, A.: Blood glucose monitoring in symptomatic hypoglycemia. *Diabetes 25:* 984, 1976.

237. Leichter, S. B. and Permutt, M. A.: Effect of adrenergic agents on postgastrectomy hypoglycemia. *Diabetes 24:* 1005, 1975.

238. Cochrane, W. A., Payne, W. W., Simpkiss, M. J. and Woolf, L. I.: Familial hypoglycemia precipitated by amino acids. *J. Clin. Invest. 35:* 411, 1956.

239. Mabry, C. C., DiGeorge, A. M. and Auerbach, V. H.: Leucine-induced hypoglycemia. I. Clinical observations and diagnostic considerations. *J. Pediatr. 57:* 526, 1960.

240. Cornblath, M.: Hypoglycemia, in Dicken, F., Randle, P. J., and Whelan, W. J. (eds.): Carbohydrate Metabolism and Its Disorders, vol. 2. New York, Academic Press. 1967, p. 51.

241. Fajans, S. S., Knopf, R. F., Floyd, J. C., Jr. et al: The experimental induction in man of sensitivity to leucine hypoglycemia. *J. Clin. Invest. 42:* 216, 1963.

242. Bower, B. D., Rayner, P. H. W. and Stimmler, L.: Leucine-sensitive hypoglycemia treated with diazoxide. *Arch. Dis. Child. 42:* 410, 1967.

243. Skillern, P. G. and Rynearson, E. H.: Medical aspects of hypoglycemia. *J. Clin. Endocrinol. Metab. 13:* 587, 1953.

244. Allen, O. P.: Stymptoms suggesting prodromal stage of diabetes mellitus. *Ohio State Med. J. 49:* 213, 1953.

245. Seltzer, H. S., Fajans, S. S. and Conn, J. W.: Spontaneous hypoglycemia as an early manifestation of diabetes mellitus. *Diabetes 5:* 437, 1956.

246. Luyckx, A. S. and Lefebvre, P. J.: Plasma insulin in reactive hypoglycemia. *Diabetes 20:* 435, 1971.

247. Barrett, C. T. and Oliver, T. K., Jr.: Hypoglycemia and hyperinsulinism in erythroblastosis fetalis. *N. Engl. J. Med. 278:* 1260, 1968.

248. From, G. L. A., Driscoll, S. G. and Steinke, J.: Serum insulin in newborn infants with erythroblastosis fetalis. *Pediatrics 44:* 549, 1969.

249. Raivio, K. O. and Osterlund, K.: Hypoglycemia and hyperinsulinemia associated with erythroblastosis fetalis. *Pediatrics 43:* 217, 1969.

250. Schiff, D., Aranda, J. V., Colle, E. and Stern, L.: Metabolic effects of exchange transfusion. II. Delayed hypoglycemia following exchange transfusion with citrated blood. *J. Pediatr. 79:* 589, 1971.

251. Cornblath, M., Nicolopoulos, D., Ganzin, A. F. et al: Studies of carbohydrate metabolism in the newborn infant. IV. The effect of glucagon on the capillary blood sugar in infants of diabetic mothers. *Pediatrics 28:* 592, 1961.

252. Cornblath, M. and Schwartz, R.: Infant of the diabetic mother, in Disorders of Carbohydrate Metabolism in Infancy. (ed 2). Philadelphia, W. B. Saunders, 1976, chap. 4, pp. 115–154.

253. McCann, M. L. Chen, C. H., Katigbak, E. B. et al: The effect of fructose on hypoglucosemia in infants of diabetic mothers. *N. Engl. J. Med. 275:* 1, 1966.

254. Arky, R. A. and Arons, D. L.: Hypoglycemia in diabetes mellitus. *Med. Clin. North Am. 55:* 919, 1971.

255. Seltzer, H. S.: Drug-induced hypoglycemia. *Diabetes 21:* 955, 1972.

256. Rynearson, E. H.: Hyperinsulinism among malingerers. *Med. Clin. North Am. 31:* 477, 1947.

257. Burnim, J. J., Federman, D. D., Black, R. L. et al: Factitious diseases: Clinical staff conference at the National Institutes of Health. *Ann. Intern. Med. 48:* 1328, 1958.

258. Berkowitz, S., Parrish, J. E. and Field, J. B.: Factitious hypoglyce-

259. Couropmitree, C., Freinkel, N. Nagel, T. C. et al: Plasma C-peptide and diagnosis of factitious hyperinsulinism: Study of an insulin-dependent diabetic patient with 'spontaneous' hypoglycemia. *Ann. Intern. Med. 82:* 201, 1975.

260. Service, F. J., Rubinstein, A. H. and Horowitz, D. L.: C-peptide analysis in diagnosis of factitial hypoglycemia in an insulin-dependent diabetic. *Mayo Clin. Proc. 50:* 697, 1975.

261. Duncan, G. G., Jenson, W. and Eberly, R. J.: Factitious hypoglycemia due to chlorpropramide: Report of a case, with clinical similiarty to an islet cell tumor of the pancreas. *J.A.M.A. 175:* 904, 1961.

262. Forman, B. H., Feeny, E. and Boas, L.: Drug-induced hypoglycemia. *J.A.M.A. 229:* 522, 1974.

263. Harris, S.: Hyperinsulinism and dysinsulinism. *J.A.M.A. 83:* 729, 1924.

264. Fabrykant, M.: The problem of functional hyperinsulinism or functional hypoglycemia attributed to nervous causes. I. Laboratory and clinical correlations. *Metabolism 4:* 469, 1955.

265. Yager, J. and Young, R. T.: Now-hypoglycemia is an epidemic condition. *N. Engl. J. Med. 291:* 907, 1974.

266. Cahill, G. F., Jr. and Soeldner, J. S.: A non-editorial on non-hypoglycemia. *N. Engl. J. Med. 291:* 905, 1974.

267. Sussman, K. E., Stimmler, L., Birenboim, H.: Plasma insulin levels during reactive hypoglycemia. *Diabetes 15:* 1, 1966.

268. Arieff, A. I., Doerner, T., Zelig, H. et al: Mechanisms of seizures and coma in hypoglycemia: Evidence for a direct effect of insulin on electrolyte transport in brain. *J. Clin. Invest. 54:* 654, 1973.

269. Laurent, J., Debry, G., and Floquent, J.: Extrapancreatic tumours inducing hypoglycaemia, in Hyoglycaemic Tumours. Amsterdam, Excerpta Medica, 1961, chaps. 10–18.

270. Unger, R. H.: The riddle of tumor hypoglycemia. *Am. J. Med. 40:* 325, 1966.

271. Chandalia, H. B. and Boshell, B. R.: Hypoglycemia associated with extrapancreatic tumors. *Arch. Intern. Med. 129:* 447, 1972.

272. August, J. T. and Hiatt, H. H.: Severe hypoglycemia secondary to a non-pancreatic fibrosarcoma with insulin activity. *N. Engl. J. Med. 258:* 17, 1958.

273. Megyesi, K., Kahn, C. R. and Roth, J.: Hypoglycemia in association with extrapancreatic tumors: demonstration of elevated plasma NSILA-s by a radioreceptor assay. *J. Clin. Endocrinol. Metab. 38:* 931, 1974.

274. Silverstein, M. N., Wakim, K. C., Bahn, R. C. and Decker, R. H.: Role of tryptophan metabolites in the hypoglycemia associated with neoplasia. *Cancer 19:* 127, 1966.

275. Silbert, C. K., Rossini, A. A., Ghazvinian, S. et al: Tumor hypoglycemia: deficient splanchnic glucose output and deficient glucagon secretion. *Diabetes 25:* 202, 1976.

276. McFadzean, A. J. S. and Euyng, R. T. T.: Further observations on hypoglycaemia in hepatocellular cardinoma. *Am. J. Med. 47:* 220, 1969.

277. Nadler, H. L., Neumann, L. L., and Gershberg, H.: Hypoglycemia growth retardation and probable isolated growth hormone deficiency in a one-year old child. *J. Pediatr. 63:* 977, 1963.

278. Roe, T. F., and Kogut, M. D.: Hypopituitarism and ketotic hypoglycemia. *Am. J. Dis. Child. 121:* 296, 1971.

279. Goodman, H. G., Grumbach, M. M. and Kaplan, S. L.: Growth and growth hormone. II. A comparison of isolated growth-hormone deficiency and multiple pituitary-hormone deficiencies in 35 patients with idiopathic hypopituitary dwarfism. *N. Engl. J. Med. 278:* 57, 1968.

280. Hopewood, N. J., Forsman, P. J., Kenny, F. M. and Drash, A. L.: Hypoglycemia in hypopituitary children. *Am. J. Dis. Child. 129:* 918, 1975.

281. Haymond, M. W., Karl, I., Weldon, V. V. and Pagliara, A. S.: The role of growth hormone and cortisone on glucose and gluconeogenic substrate regulation in fasted hypopituitary children. *J. Clin. Endocrinol. Metab. 42:* 846, 1976.

282. Clark, E. C., Franklin, M. and Saks, A. L.: Post-partum atrophy of the adenohypophysis with hypoglycemic convulsions. *Arch. Neurol. Psych. 65:* 724, 1951.

283. Levine, S. A., Gordon, B. and Derick, C. L.: Some changes in the chemical constituents of the blood following a marathon race, with special reference to the development of hypoglycemia. *J.A.M.A. 82:* 1778, 1924.

284. Best, C. H. and Partridge, R. C.: Observations on olympic athletes. *Proc. R. Soc. (Lond) B. 105:* 323, 1930.

285. Jorfeldt, L. and Wahren, J.: Human forearm muscle metabolism during exercise. V. Quantitative aspects of glucose uptake and lactate production during prolonged exercise. *Scand. J. Clin. Lab. Invest. 26:* 73, 1970.

286. Wahren, J., Felig, P., Ahlborg, G. and Jorfeldt, L.: Glucose metabolism during leg exercise in man. *J. Clin. Invest. 50:* 2715, 1971.

287. Ahlborg, G., Felig, P., Hagenfeldt, L., Hendler, R. and Wahren, J.: Substrate turnover during prolonged exercise in man. Splanchnic and leg metabolism of glucose, free fatty acids and amino acids. *J. Clin. Invest. 53:* 1080, 1974.

288. Felig, P., Wahren, J., Hendler, R. and Ahlborg, G.: Plasma glucagon levels in exercising man. *N. Engl. J. Med. 287:* 184, 1972.

289. Sanders, C. A., Levinson, G. E., Abelmann, W. H. and Freinkel, N.: Effect of exercise on the peripheral utilization of glucose in man. *N. Engl. J. Med. 271:* 220, 1964.

290. Field, J. B. and Vilhams, H. E.: Artifactual hypoglycemia associated with leukemia. *N. Engl. J. Med. 79:* 946, 1961.

291. Hanrahan, J. B., Sax, S. M. and Cillo, A.: Factitions hypoglycemia in patients with leukemia. *Am. J. Clin. Pathol. 40:* 43, 1963.

292. Sharp, P., Riley, C., Cook, J. G. H. and Pink, P. J. F.: Effect of two sulphonylureas on glucon determinations by enzyme methods. *Clin. Chem. Acta 36:* 93, 1972.

Adrenal Cortex

Anatomy of the Adrenal Cortex

James C. Melby

EMBRYOLOGY, GENERAL MORPHOLOGY, AND VASCULATURE

EMBRYOLOGY

The adrenal gland consists of two principal parts, the cortex and the medulla. These are derived from embryologically different structures and are really two separate functional and morphological structures within a single capsule. The intimate proximity of the cortex and medulla in an encapsulated organ is only observed in mammals. The cortex develops from celomic epithelium and is of mesodermal origin. The medulla is derived from sympathogonia, which migrate from the neural crest and are, therefore, of ectodermal origin. In amphibians, reptiles, and birds, the chromatin cells are distributed widely throughout the cortical tissue. In mammals the medulla is surrounded by the cortex and then encapsulated. The medullary tissue is concentrated medially in the right adrenal gland and in the lower pole of the left adrenal gland. As a result of the migration of both chromaffin and cortical cells, accessory adrenal tissue is often found distributed among the retroperitoneal structures. Accessory adrenocortical tissue is usually distributed in the celiac plexus and adjacent fatty tissue, or along the path of the spermatic cord. The cortical portion of the adrenal is first recognized between the fourth and sixth weeks of fetal life. The cortical structures grow rapidly and exceed the kidney in size at about the fourth month of fetal life and are about a third of the size of the kidney at birth. By contrast, in the adult human, the size of the adrenal is only about one-thirtieth of the size of the kidneys. The fetal adrenal cortex regresses during the last month of gestation.[1]

GENERAL MORPHOLOGY

Each adrenal gland tops the superior-medial pole of its corresponding kidney. There are considerable differences in the morphology and relationships of the right and left glands. The right gland is triangular in shape with slightly concave margins located anteriorly and superiorly to the right kidney and in close proximity to the bare area of the liver. The left adrenal gland is larger, more flattened, and elongated and rounded or crescenteric in shape, and is closely related to the superior-medial border of the left kidney. The right adrenal appears narrow in profile, whereas the left appears more triangular when observed by radioangiography. The left adrenal gland is generally larger than the right and, in the adult, each adrenal gland weighs between 3 and 5 g and has dimensions of about 2.5×0.5 cm.[2]

VASCULATURE

The adrenal cortex is supplied predominantly by three arterial vessels and numerous small twigs which enter the gland at a radiating spokelike manner over its entire surface. The superior adrenal artery arises from the inferior phrenic artery, the middle adrenal artery arises directly from the abdominal aorta medially, and the inferior adrenal artery arises from the renal artery. The superior and inferior adrenal arteries supply most of the right adrenal gland, while the middle and inferior arteries supply most of the left adrenal gland. Great variation exists. The venous drainage of the adrenals is much simpler since all of the veins channel into a large central vein in the substance of the gland. The right adrenal vein is about 1 cm in length and empties directly into the inferior vena cava. The left adrenal vein is between 2 and 4 cm in length and drains into the upper surface of the renal vein. The left adrenal vein is larger than the right. Occasionally, the left adrenal vein may empty into the inferior phrenic vein, but rarely it does cross the aorta to enter the inferior vena cava directly.[3]

HISTOLOGICAL ORGANIZATION OF THE ADRENAL CORTEX—ZONATION

The adrenal cortex constitutes approximately 80 percent of the weight and volume of the whole adrenal gland and is composed of three clearly definable concentric zones—zona glomerulosa, zona fasciculata, and zona reticularis. These three zones of the adrenal cortex exhibit unique light microscopic and electron microscopic appearances and also exhibit differences in steroidogenic patterns and responsiveness to regulatory peptides.

ZONA GLOMERULOSA

The narrow zone glomerulosa is directly adjacent to the capsule of the adrenal gland and consists of small epithelioid cells when examined by light microscopy. Electron microscopy reveals numerous and elongated mitochondria that possess lamellar cristae which differ strikingly from the appearance of mitochondria of the other cortical zones. These transverse infoldings of the cristae of the mitochondria are the distinguishing characteristics of the zona glomerulosa cell by electron microscopy. Aldosterone is specifically and exclusively elaborated by the cells of the zona glomerulosa of the adrenal cortex in most mammalian species, and only the zona glomerulosa is responsive to alterations in the physiologic concentrations of angiotensin II and potassium.[4]

ZONA FASCICULATA

The columnar cells of the largest zone of the adrenal cortex are contiguous with the cell groups of the zona glomerulosa. These cells are polygonal, forming long cords radiating from the subcapsular zona glomerulosa. The zona fasciculata is the widest zone. Its cells contain large numbers of lipid droplets and the cytoplasm of these cells appears to be highly vacuolated. Electron microscopy of the cells of the zona fasciculata reveals an extensive network of agranular endoplasmic reticulum. The mitochondria vary in size but are usually much larger than the mitochondria of the zona reticularis or the zona glomerulosa. Cristae exist as short tubular vesicular invaginations of the inner mitochondrial membrane or as vesicles lying free in the mitochondrial matrix. Functionally, the zona fasciculata is more versatile than the zona glomerulosa and is the exclusive source of cortisol.

ZONA RETICULARIS

The innermost zone of the adrenal cortex adjacent to the adrenal medulla consists of networks of interconnecting cells which vary enormously in size, shape, and density ("light" or "dark"). There are much smaller numbers of lipid droplets in these cells. The mitochondria are remarkably similar to the mitochondria of the cells of the zona fasciculata. Although the mitochondria are slightly more elongated, they contain "flattened" cristae. Functionally, the cells of the zona reticularis appear to produce predominantly C-19 and C-18 steroids, and predominantly C-19 steroids of the androst-5-ene structure.

RADIOGRAPHIC ANATOMY

GENERAL

Although traditional radiographic methods have been useful in demonstrating large adrenal tumors, small adenomas such as those causing primary aldosteronism are rarely shown. These methods include adrenal tomography, alone or in combination with retroperitoneal pneumography, aortography, and intravenous urography. Retroperitoneal pneumography demonstrates the adrenal gland with its fatty envelope, making recognition of tumors less than 2 cm in diameter unlikely. Even with the most careful performance of adrenal tomography in association with pneumography, one or more borders of the adrenal gland is frequently not outlined by the gas. Aortography without selective adrenal arteriography is useful in demonstrating highly vascular tumors, such as pheochromocytomas and cortisol-secreting adenomas. Abdominal aortography without selective catheterization of the adrenal arteries usually does not identify the normal adrenal structure because the faint vascular blush is usually obscured by overlying structures such as the kidneys, the bowel, inferior vena cava, and splenic artery and vein. This virtually precludes the aortographic detection of small avascular tumors such as aldosterone-producing adenomas. In carcinoma of the adrenal cortex, and in a significant percentage of pheochromocytomas the tumors are large and may be supplied by markedly hypertrophied vessels. Adrenal artery and the kidneys are often displaced inferolaterally and the remainder of the adrenal gland is displaced upward. These alterations can easily be recognized by abdominal aortography and adrenal tomog-

raphy associated with intravenous urography. The aortographic appearance of a large adrenocortical carcinoma specifically exhibits parasitization of vascularity from every adjacent structure including that of the kidney lumbar vessels, pancreatic and splenic, as well as hepatic vessels. In an increasing number of pheochromocytomas, cortisol-producing adrenocortical adenomas, and most aldosterone-producing adenomas, these radiographic techniques will not suffice and selective adrenal radioangiography must be undertaken.

SELECTIVE ADRENAL RADIOANGIOGRAPHY

Adrenal Venography

Bilateral percutaneous adrenal vein catheterization by the Seldinger technique is primarily undertaken to obtain blood samples from the two adrenal veins for comparison of steroid hormone or catecholamine levels in the adrenal venous effluent of the two adrenal glands. Adrenal venography is not undertaken to obtain visual detail of the adrenal glands, although more than 80 percent of adrenal neoplasms can be recognized by this procedure (Fig. 91-1). Selective adrenal arteriography is used for radiographic diagnosis of adrenal neoplasms or other structural abnormalities. In functional tumors of the adrenal, analysis of hormone content in the adrenal venous effluent is unambiguous and invaluable in localizing the lesion. The placement of catheters for sampling of the venous effluent of the two adrenals is usually without hazard and is accomplished with serial doses of contrast medium by immediate prior selective adrenal radioarteriography. Clinically significant intraadrenal hemorrhage resulting from rupture of the corticomedullary venous system by contrast medium injected too rapidly, or in too great a volume, occurs in about 10 percent of patients in which adrenal venography is performed for the purpose of visualizing the adrenals. In patients with Cushing's disease and bilateral adrenocortical hyperplasia, even the placement of catheters for sampling of the adrenal venous effluent is accompanied by

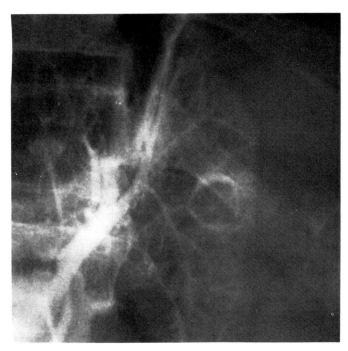

Fig. 91-1. Venogram of the left adrenal in a 41-year-old male with severe hypertension. An aldosterone-secreting tumor is clearly demonstrated in the gland.

significant hazard because the cortical medullary plexus is already overdistended and friable. Adrenal venous sampling for aldosterone measurement, on the other hand, is ordinarily safe and produces definitive information.[5]

Selective Adrenal Arteriography

Selective catheterization of the adrenal arteries is currently the most useful method for the detailed radiographic visualization of adrenal tissue. The inferior phrenic arteries supplying the upper poles of the adrenal gland are catheterized with relative ease. The middle adrenal arteries are more difficult to enter, though this can be done over 90 percent of the time (Fig. 91-2). Inferior adrenal arteries can be seen with selective renal arterial injections.[6] The adrenal arteries are end vessels and an anastomotic ring often exists around the periphery of the gland, especially between the superior and middle adrenal branches. It is, therefore, often sufficient to catheterize the superior and inferior adrenal artery to get a satisfactory picture of the gland. With selective adrenal arteriography, aldosterone-producing adenomas appear as sharply defined avascular areas in a region of dense cortical blush. In Cushing's disease with bilateral adrenocortical hyperplasia, both glands can be shown to be enlarged, as can their feeding artery. Cushing's syndrome due to a cortisol-secreting adenoma can be easily determined because these adenomas are sharply defined, exhibit tumor vessels and have a parenchymal blush. Because the adjacent normal adrenal cortex is atrophic, no cortical blush is seen either in this tissue or in the contralateral gland. Adrenocortical carcinomas are often highly and irregularly vascular and usually need only abdominal aortography to indicate their presence (Fig. 91-3). Pheochromocytomas that are highly vascular with a distinct parenchymal blush are in sharp contrast to the normally hypovascular

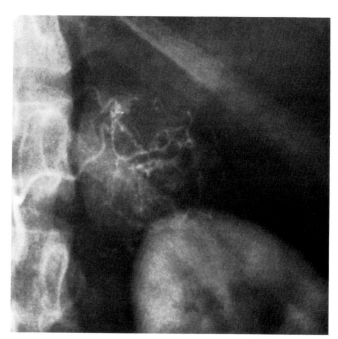

Fig. 91-3. A vascular tumor of the adrenal seen on arteriogram. Although the radiographic appearance suggested malignancy the tumor was found to be benign.

adrenal medullary tissue. Pheochromocytomas are less well circumscribed than cortical adenomas but lack the neovascularity of carcinomas.

ADRENAL IMAGING WITH RADIOCHOLESTEROL

Following the intravenous injection of 2 mCi of radiocholesterol as [19-^{131}I]iodocholesterol or [6β-^{131}I]iodomethyl-19-norcholesterol, adrenal imaging by scintiscans can be performed within 1–14 days. This procedure has been used to localize functional adrenocortical tumors and to establish the presence of bilateral macro- or micronodular hyperplasia in patients with hyperaldosteronism. An iodine solution is given to suppress thyroidal ^{131}I uptake. Adrenal scintography with radiocholesterol appears to be safe and is not associated with discomfort. In patients with aldosteronism, the additional suppression of ACTH is accomplished by the administration of dexamethasone; this increases the sensitivity of the procedure. The application of this technique is inhibited only by the strategic problems of radiochemical availability and necessity of repeating scintiscans at intervals.[7,8]

The application of ultrasound technology to the diagnosis and localization of adrenocortical disease is just beginning. Larger adrenocortical tumors can be easily outlined by ultrasound technology but the more frequent smaller functional tumors and hyperplasias are less well defined at this writing.

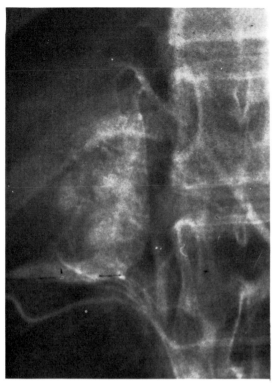

Fig. 91-2. Selective adrenal arteriography with injection of 4 ml contrast material into the right middle adrenal artery demonstrated a large right adrenal gland with a suggestion of a rounded mass in the lower pole. A benign adenoma was found at surgery.

REFERENCES

1. Arey, L. B.: Developmental Anatomy. Philadelphia, Saunders, 1965, pp 516–519.
2. Bourne, G. H.: In Moon, H. D. (ed): The Adrenal Cortex. New York, Paul B. Hoeber, 1961, p 20.
3. Dobbie, J. W., Symington, T.: The human adrenal gland with special reference to the vasculature. *J Endocrinol 34:* 479, 1966.
4. Melby, J. C.: Intermediary metabolism of aldosterone. In Page, I. H., Bumpus, F. M. (eds): *Angiotensin Handbook of Pharmacology, vol 37.* New York, Springer-Verlag, 1974, pp 298–322.

5. Melby, J. C.: Solving the adrenal lesion(s) of primary aldosteronism. *N Engl J Med 294:* 441–442, 1976.

6. Kahn, P. C., Kelleher, M. D., Melby, J. C., et al: Adrenal arteriography and venography in primary aldosteronism. *Radiology 101:* 71–78, 1971.

7. Seabold, J. E., Cohen, E. L., Beierwaltes, W. H., et al: Adrenal imaging with [131]I-19-iodocholesterol in the diagnostic evaluation of patients with aldosteronism. *J Clin Endocrinol Metab 42:* 41–52, 1976.

8. Sarkar, S. D., Beierwaltes, W. H., Lee, R. D., Basmadjiam, G. P., Hetzel, K. R., Kennedy, W. P., Mason, M. M.: A new and superior adrenal scanning agent: NP-59. *J Nucl Med 16:* 1038–1042, 1975.

92

Synthesis of Adrenal Cortical Steroids and Mechanism of ACTH Effects

Boyd W. Harding

PLASMA MEMBRANE RECEPTORS FOR ACTH

The metabolism of the cells of the adrenal cortical fasciculata and reticularis is controlled by ACTH binding to external plasma membrane receptors. Formation of the ACTH–receptor complex activates adenylate cyclase and increases the synthesis of cAMP which, in turn, activates adrenal cellular phosphoprotein kinases. These events are temporally associated with an increased rate of secretion and biosynthesis of the corticosteroids. ACTH was one of the first polypeptide hormones to be shown to act by binding plasma membrane receptors. This was accomplished by linking the polypeptide to large agarose polymers too large to enter the adrenal cell and showing that this complex could, nevertheless, stimulate corticosteroidogenesis as readily as free ACTH.[1] The adrenal ACTH receptor has a high degree of specificity and affinity ($K_a = 9 \times 10^{11}$ liters/mol).[2] Adrenal cortical cells have receptors for substances other than ACTH. *Escherichia coli* and cholera enterotoxins bind to adrenal cortical tumor cells and activate steroidogenesis.[3] Certain rat adrenal tumor cells have receptors for TSH, FSH, and epinephrine in addition to ACTH.[4]

Studies of isolated receptor preparations, isolated intact cells, and tumor cells in culture have demonstrated that the corticotropin$_{1-20}$ fragment of ACTH contains both the binding and biological activity of the entire ACTH molecule. Unlike a number of other polypeptide hormones, binding can be dissociated from biological activity since corticotropin$_{11-20}$ containing the highly charged amino acid sequence Lys·Lys·Arg·Arg readily displaces [^{125}I]ACTH, but is unable to activate adenylate cyclase.[5] The ACTH receptor is destroyed by trypsin, phospholipase, and neuraminidase,[2,6] and therefore is assumed to be a protein containing a carbohydrate moiety in covalent linkage with sialic acid. The ACTH receptor is apparently dependent for its structural integrity on its phospholipid environment. While the mechanism of activation of adenylate cyclase by ACTH binding to its membrane receptor is not known, it appears to be dependent on the Ca^{2+} ion.[7]

Presumably, the hormone–receptor complex is complementary to the membrane-bound adenylate cyclase; migration of the complex and inactive cyclase in the plane of the phospholipid bilayer results in the formation of a new hormone–receptor–cyclase complex which has catalytic activity.

Better understanding of adrenal receptors promises new insights into both the etiology and rational therapy of certain adrenal disorders. For example, synthesis of biologically inactive peptide analogs with the capacity for binding the ACTH receptor and thus preventing ACTH binding could provide effective means for medical treatment of bilateral adrenal cortical hyperplasia. Although data are not yet available for human adrenal tumors, the demonstration of multiple receptors in rat adrenal carcinoma cells for hormones which are under no feedback control by glucocorticoids[4] suggests a possible etiology not only for these adrenal tumors but for certain human tumors and nodular hyperplasias as well.

CYCLIC NUCLEOTIDES AND PHOSPHOPROTEIN KINASE

While the weight of evidence supports the hypothesis that immediate control of corticosteroidogenesis as well as long-term control of trophic changes in the adrenal cortex is mediated by cAMP,[8-10] a number of recent studies have reported a partial or complete dissociation between ACTH stimulation of steroidogenesis and activation of adenylate cyclase.[11,12] Consequently, the hypothesis that cAMP mediates all the effects of ACTH in the adrenal cortex must be held with reservations.

cAMP binds a specific high-affinity ($K_d = 3 \times 10^{-8}$ M) adrenal receptor protein which has been identified as the regulatory subunit for adrenal cortical phosphoprotein kinase. Upon binding cAMP, the regulatory subunit dissociates from the catalytic subunit which becomes fully active.[13]

Studies of phosphoprotein kinases in other tissues indicate that modulation of the regulatory subunit interaction with cAMP may be achieved by a number of agents, including ATP, Mg^{2+}, a heat-stable protein, and the catalytically active phosphoprotein kinase subunit itself. In adrenal cortical tissue, the cAMP-activated phosphoprotein kinase catalyzes the phosphorylation of several ribosomal proteins.[13] Since cAMP stimulation of steroidogenesis is inhibited by cycloheximide,[14] it has been postulated that cAMP-activated phosphorylation of adrenal ribosomal proteins may control the translation of a labile regulatory protein from a stable mRNA which is somehow involved in stimulating corticosteroidogenesis.[13] However, in view of the foregoing remarks, and the observation that significant stimulation of steroidogenesis by

ACTH can occur without activation of phosphoprotein kinase in isolated adrenal cortical cells,[15] this postulated sequence of events may be oversimplified.

CONTROL OF PROTEIN SYNTHESIS

As mentioned previously, steroidogenesis is blocked by protein biosynthetic inhibitors such as puromycin and cycloheximide and is reportedly insensitive to actinomycin D inhibition of RNA synthesis.[16] Inhibition of steroidogenesis by inhibitors of mRNA translation has been repeatedly confirmed both in vivo and in vitro in a variety of animal and adrenal preparations. Because the onset of inhibition of ACTH-stimulated steroidogenesis by cycloheximide is very rapid, reaching half-maximal inhibition within approximately 10 min after administration, and because this inhibition appears to affect only the rate-limiting conversion of cholesterol to pregnenolone, it has been assumed that ACTH stimulates ribosomal translation of a relatively stable mRNA for some regulatory protein(s) which controls cholesterol side chain cleavage (scc).[15] There are at least two criticisms of this assumption. First, it is known that cycloheximide and puromycin have other effects on cellular metabolism besides inhibition of translation of mRNA, and consequently, their effects on steroidogenesis may not be wholly secondary to their inhibition of protein synthesis.[17,18] Second, more recent studies of the effects of actinomycin D on steroidogenesis show diverse results ranging from inhibition through no effect to potentiation of ACTH stimulation of steroidogenesis, depending on the cell preparation employed and the dosage and time of exposure.[19,20] Consequently, not only the function of new protein synthesis but that of new RNA synthesis in the mechanism of ACTH regulation of steroidogenesis must be considered unsettled.

Although the possible existence of a regulatory labile protein functioning to control steroidogenesis has been under consideration for over 12 years, identification and characterization of such protein(s) have yet to be accomplished. Evidence for a rapid ACTH-stimulated incorporation of ^{14}C-labeled amino acids into several adrenal protein fractions[21] and for two crude adrenal cortical fractions, one inhibiting and the other stimulating steroidogenesis,[22] has been reported, but these observations remain unconfirmed. It has been postulated that the putative regulatory protein(s) may function as cholesterol carriers facilitating cholesterol transport from vacuoles or other cytoplasmic compartments into the mitochondria, the site of the $P450_{scc}$ enzyme system. Carrier proteins have been isolated from the adrenal cortex which accelerate cholesterol SCC,[23] and certain studies have demonstrated that ACTH stimulation results in an accumulation of intramitochondrial cholesterol.[24] However, direct measurements of the concentrations of cholesterol bound to its SCC enzyme fail to show mitochondrial accumulation of cholesterol following ACTH stimulation[25] unless the animal is pretreated with cycloheximide. Since cholesterol transport to the mitochondria is unaffected under these circumstances where steroidogenesis and protein synthesis are inhibited, it would not appear that the putative regulatory protein functions in cholesterol transport. Apparently, cycloheximide either blocks the synthesis of a protein which is somehow concerned with activating cholesterol or its $P450_{scc}$ oxygenase or inhibits the oxygenase in some other fashion.

Although ACTH is known to regulate adrenal cytochrome P450 synthesis in intact animals and cell cultures,[26–29] control of the concentration of P450 itself does not appear to be the primary regulator of corticosteroidogenesis since the half-life of this family of enzymes following hypophysectomy is approximately 3½

days,[26] and since the return of corticosteroid biosynthesis following hypophysectomy appears before changes in mitochondrial P450 concentration are observed.[28]

ADRENAL CYTOCHROME P450s

The adrenal cytochrome P450s are a family of hemoprotein oxygenases having a characteristic spectral absorption maximum at 450 nm in the reduced carbon monoxide-bound state. They are hydrophobic proteins that are intimately integrated into the lipophilic membranes of the smooth endoplasmic reticulum and intramitochondrial cristae. Their functional integrity appears to be dependent on this hydrophobic environment, and agents that alter this environment markedly influence the activity of these enzymes. They are members of a class of hydroxylases known as mixed function oxygenases which employ molecular oxygen and reducing equivalents to catalyze the formation of equimolar amounts of hydroxylated product and H_2O.[30]

Attempts to isolate and purify the adrenal P450s have met with varying degrees of success. It has been difficult to achieve major increases in the ratio of P450 to protein over the original starting material, suggesting either a lack of significant purification or a continuous degradation of the enzyme to an inactive protein which is not readily separated from the active form, or both. As purification proceeds, the loss of phospholipid and possibly other components in the membranous preparation is associated with decreasing enzyme activity; in addition, it has not always been possible to obtain one hydroxylase activity separate from another.[31,32] One laboratory has claimed a purification to homogeneity of $P450_{scc}$ (which, nevertheless, still retains significant 11β-hydroxylase activity) with a molecular weight of 500,000–600,000 daltons.[31] The enzyme is reported to exist in a polymeric form which can be dissociated to monomers of 50,000–60,000 daltons by high salt concentrations.

The absolute absorption spectrum of one of the more purified preparations of cytochrome P450 from bovine adrenal cortical mitochondria is shown in Figure 92-1.[32] This preparation still retains considerable bound cholesterol as indicated by its characteristic oxidized high spin hemoprotein absorption spectrum. Incubation of the preparation with purified adrenodoxin reductase, adrenodoxin, and TPNH, followed by reisolation of the enzyme permits removal of this cholesterol and its product, pregnenolone, and results in an enzyme with a low spin hemoprotein spectrum with absorption maxima at 418, 535, and 565 nm (not shown). Conclusions drawn from such visible absorption spectra have been corroborated by studies of the EPR spectra of mitochondrial P450s. The substrate-free form of the enzyme has strong absorption values around $g = 2.0$ which are markedly decreased upon binding with substrate, whereas the substrate-bound enzyme shows absorption values around $g = 8.0$ in the low field spectrum. These spectral changes reflect electronic rearrangements in the d orbitals of the heme iron of P450 as it changes from a low spin s = ½ (coordinate covalent binding) to a high spin s = 5/2 (ionic binding) state upon binding substrate.[33]

Although the significance of the spin state changes in cytochrome P450 has not yet been fully assessed, it seems likely that steroid substrate binding induces a conformational change in the P450s which alters the binding of heme iron to one of its internal ligands. The net effect may be to lower the redox potential of the P450, allowing an accelerated rate of reduction, and consequently an accelerated hydroxylation rate.[34] Although it is not believed that the steroid substrates form heme iron ligands directly, a large

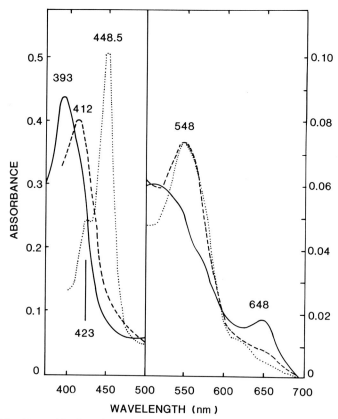

Fig. 92-1. Absolute absorption spectrum of bovine adrenal cortical mitochondrial P450. The oxidized enzyme (solid lines) has absorption maxima at 393, 510, and 648 nm. The reduced enzyme (dashed lines) has absorption maxima at 412 and 598 nm, and the reduced carbon monoxide-bound enzyme (dotted lines) shows a major absorption band in the Soret region near 450 nm at 448.5 nm and a minor absorption band at 423 nm.

number of nitrogenous agents, as well as carbon monoxide and cyanide, do form heme iron ligands. Many inhibitors of steroid hydroxylation including aminoglutethimide and metyrapone are capable of interfering with the ligand field of the heme iron, altering its electronic properties as well as its catalytic capacity.[35] The demonstration that spironolactone and certain of its metabolites inhibit 11β- and 18-hydroxylation by the adrenal cortical P450s[36] emphasizes the possibility that many therapeutic agents, particularly those with steroid-like structures, may react with the adrenal hydroxylases to alter steroid biosynthesis.

All of the hydroxylation reactions concerned with corticosteroid biosynthesis from cholesterol appear to have the properties of mixed function oxygenases. However, conclusive evidence for the involvement of cytochrome P450 has been obtained for only four of the adrenal hydroxylases: the cholesterol SCC system,[37] 21-hydroxylase,[38] 11β-hydroxylase,[39] and 18-hydroxylase.[40]

REDUCTIVE ENERGY REQUIREMENTS FOR HYDROXYLATION

Activation of molecular oxygen for steroid hydroxylation by cytochrome P450 requires two reducing equivalents for each hydroxylated intermediate or product formed. This energy is supplied by electron transport over two or three pathways in the adrenal cell.[41] In the mitochondrion, TPNH is oxidized by a flavoprotein dehydrogenase (F_{p_T}) called adrenodoxin reductase which is oxidized by an iron–sulfur protein (ISP) called adrenodoxin. This,

in turn, reduces cytochrome P450. While TPNH is the immediate source of reducing equivalents for this electron transport system, an active mitochondrial pyridine nucleotide transhydrogenase (DPNH → TPN⁺) makes available reducing equivalents from DPN⁺-linked dehydrogenases as well. In the smooth endoplasmic reticulum, two electron transport systems may exist for providing reducing equivalents to the oxygenases. The first is composed of a TPN⁺-linked flavoprotein dehydrogenase (F_{p_T}) which is linked to the reduction of P450 by an unidentified carrier (X), and the second, postulated from studies of liver smooth endoplasmic reticulum, is composed of a DPN⁺-linked flavoprotein dehydrogenase (F_{p_D}) which transports electrons via cytochrome b_5 to P450. The DPN- and TPN-linked pathways may be connected as noted by the dashed arrows. The enzyme systems, their compartmentalization, and relationship to the respiratory enzymes are illustrated in Figure 92-2.

Apparently, the high demand of the adrenal hydroxylases for reducing energy is met by a multiplicity of enzyme systems.[42,43] While debate continues over the relative contribution of the various electron donors, reducing equivalents for the hydroxylases bound to the inner mitochondrial membrane such as P450₁₁βOH, P450₁₈OH, and P450scc apparently can be derived from almost all of the known substrates for mitochondrial dehydrogenases.

The cyclic mechanism by which cytochrome P450 binds steroid substrates and oxygen and catalyzes the formation of 1 mol each of hydroxylated product and water is not completely established, but the evidence supports the scheme in Figure 92-3 for the mitochondrial hydroxylases.[41]

The process begins with the binding of steroid substrates (S), ①, for example, 11-deoxycortisol or cholesterol. This initiates a shift in the type of ligand binding of the heme iron from low spin to high spin. Although it has not been established for mammalian P450, it is believed that this spin state change may alter the redox properties of the cytochrome, resulting in electron transport in the adrenodoxin system with reduction of P450Fe³⁺ to P450Fe²⁺, ②. The reduced ferrous heme iron may now bind O_2 or CO, ③, one competing with the other. The CO-bound enzyme (P450Fe²⁺–CO) has an intense spectral absorption at 450 nm and may be dissociated with light energy at this wavelength. One of the O_2-bound enzyme species also has a characteristic absorption at around 440 nm which can be observed only in the steady state since the cyclic process is initiated once O_2 is admitted in the presence of reducing equivalents.[41] Two electronic transitions in the heme iron–O_2 complex, one before and one after donation of a second electron from

SMOOTH ENDOPLASMIC RETICULUM

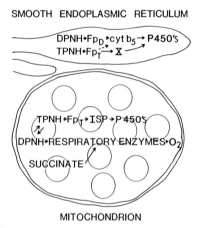

Fig. 92-2. Electron transport pathways for steroid hydroxylation reactions in the adrenal cortical microsomes and mitochondria. See text for explanation.

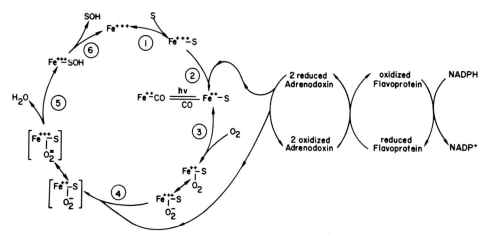

Fig. 92-3. Schematic representation of the role of cytochrome P450 and adrenodoxin in adrenal cortex mitochondrial steroid hydroxylation. See text for description.

reduced adrenodoxin, ④, are postulated to form the unstable ferric enzyme–hydroperoxo complex

$$Fe^{3+}-S$$
$$|$$
$$O_2^{2-}$$

which is believed to decompose to H_2O, ⑤, and a highly reactive ferric enzyme–monooxygen species which is in resonance with the ferryl ion complex (not shown). This reactive species rapidly hydroxylates substrate by a two-electron oxidation to form hydroxylated product (SOH), ⑥, and regenerates the ferric enzyme (Fe^{3+}).

BIOSYNTHETIC PATHWAYS

The adrenal cortical hormones are normally synthesized solely from cholesterol derived either from circulating plasma cholesterol or from acetyl CoA via mevalonate and squalene.[45] The relative contributions of these two cholesterol sources to corticoid biosynthesis are variable, species dependent, and probably related to the extent of adrenal cortical stimulation.[46] The biosynthesis of cholesterol in the adrenal occurs by the same pathway as in other tissues. Acetyl CoA is first converted to mevalonate which is pyrophosphorylated and decarboxylated to 3,3-dimethylallyl pyrophosphate and isopentyl pyrophosphate. Geranyl pyrophosphate is formed from condensation of these two intermediates and, in turn, condenses with another molecule of isopentyl pyrophosphate to form farnesyl pyrophosphate. Two molecules of farnesyl pyrophosphate condense to form presqualene pyrophosphate which is reduced to squalene in the presence of NADPH. Finally, squalene is cyclized to the 30-carbon sterol lanosterol which is successively oxidatively demethylated to desmosterol. Reduction of the C_{24-25} double bond of desmosterol produces cholesterol.

COLESTEROL STORAGE

Except under conditions of prolonged stimulation of the adrenal by ACTH, free cholesterol apparently passes through a pool of cholesterol esters stored in cytoplasmic vacuoles. The cholesterol is esterified to long chain C_{16}, C_{18}, and C_{20} saturated and unsaturated fatty acids. Hydrolysis of the cholesterol ester is achieved by a cAMP-activated esterase apparently similar to the adipocyte hormone-sensitive lipase.[47] Movement of free cholesterol to the

intramitochondrial $P450_{scc}$ may be facilitated by carrier proteins[24] or by a direct fusion of the vacuolar membrane with the mitochondrion. ACTH stimulation, therefore, results in mobilization of its own cholesterol ester store, increases the rate of synthesis of cholesterol by the mevalonate–squalene pathway, and increases transport from the plasma into the adrenal cell, the quantitative importance of each source being dependent on the species, the degree of stimulation, and unknown factors.

FORMATION OF Δ^5-PREGNENOLONE

Cholesterol is oxidatively cleaved by successive hydroxylations to Δ^5-pregnenolone and isocaproylaldehyde. These hydroxylations are accomplished by an enzyme complex called the cholesterol side chain cleaving (SCC) enzyme or desmolase which resides in the inner membrane of the mitochondrial cristae.[45] As noted earlier, this enzyme complex has the properties of a cytochrome P450. The hydróxylated cholesterol intermediates in this SCC reaction have been difficult to identify apparently because of their very high affinity for the enzyme complex. Hydroxylation poceeds sequentially with negligible liberation of the intermediates from their enzyme sites. Recent studies support the following order of hydroxylations, shown in Figure 92-4.[48]

As discussed earlier, considerable interest is directed to the possible existence of additional activator proteins whose synthesis is controlled by ACTH and which either bind and activate cholesterol itself or the $P450_{scc}$. SCC is efficiently inhibited by aminoglu-

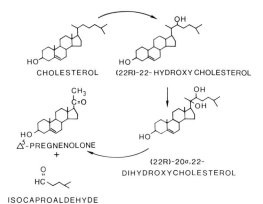

Fig. 92-4. Biosynthetic intermediates in the synthesis of Δ^5-pregnenolone from cholesterol.

tethimide.[49] Administration of this agent results in accumulation of cholesterol and inhibition of corticoid secretion in a manner that mimics the lipoid hyperplastic form of congenital adrenal hyperplasia. Aminoglutethimide forms either a heme ligand or otherwise alters the heme ligand field of $P450_{scc}$, producing an abnormal spectral shift and noncompetitive inhibition of cholesterol SCC.[50]

CONVERSION OF Δ^5-PREGNENOLONE TO GLUCOCORTICOIDS, ANDROGENS, AND ALDOSTERONE

The C_{21} carbon skeleton of Δ^5-pregnenolone is the precursor for all mammalian steroid hormones. Pregnenolone formed in the intramitochondrial cristae structure moves out of the mitochondria where, under normal circumstances, it becomes the precursor for the major corticoids secreted by the human adrenal: the glucocorticoid, cortisol, the mineralocorticoid, aldosterone, and the androgen, dehydroepiandrosterone (DHEA). While small amounts of other C_{19} and C_{18} steroids (e.g., androstenedione, testosterone, estrone, and possibly estradiol-17β) are normally secreted by the adrenal, they are quantitatively insignificant in comparison to the levels of DHEA sulfate secreted. The function of this adrenal androgen in adult life is unclear. DHEA is formed from Δ^5-pregnenolone by the consecutive action of 17α-hydroxylase and 17-20-lyase enzyme complexes having the characteristics of cytochrome P450s but not proven to be such. Both of these enzymes are located in the smooth endoplasmic reticulum. This pathway for DHEA and ultimately androstenedione is shown as the right-hand branch of the main glucocorticoid pathway in Figure 92-5.

The central glucocorticoid pathway proceeds from pregnenolone via formation of 17α-hydroxypregnenolone in the smooth endoplasmic reticulum of the human adrenal. 17α-Hydroxypregnenolone is further metabolized by two additional enzymes of the smooth endoplasmic reticulum, 3β-hydroxy steroid dehydrogenase and Δ^5-Δ^4-isomerase. The dehydrogenase with NAD$^+$ as cofactor forms the keto derivative of 17-hydroxypregnenolone, 17-hydroxypregn-5-ene-3,20-dione, which is subsequently converted to 17-hydroxyprogesterone by the Δ^5-Δ^4-isomerase.[45] The remaining reactions leading to the formation of cortisol are two hydroxylations, the first at C_{21} catalyzed by a cytochrome P450 located in the smooth endoplasmic reticulum, and the second at C_{11} catalyzed by a cytochrome P450 located in the intramitochondrial cristae. Both cortisol and DHEA are products of the cells of the fasciculata and reticular zones of the adrenal.

The mineralocorticoid pathway leading to the biosynthesis of aldosterone shown in the left-hand column of Figure 92-5 is restricted to the glomerulosal cells of the cortex. These cells, while also partly controlled by ACTH, are regulated by control mechanisms different from those in the remaining cortical cells. They also differ in their complement of steroid biosynthetic enzymes. The smooth endoplasmic 17α-hydroxylase is replaced by a mitochondrial 18-hydroxylase which normally catalyzes the formation of 18-hydroxycorticosterone and an 18-hydroxydehydrogenase which oxidizes the 18-alcohol to an aldehyde, thus forming aldosterone. It is not believed that the corticoid intermediates or final products normally accumulate in the adrenal cells nor that they diffuse extensively between different adrenal cell types.

The foregoing discussion emphasizes the extensive subcellular compartmentalization of the corticoid biosynthetic enzymes which is illustrated in Figure 92-6. Little is known regarding the factors controlling the circulation of intermediates among these compartments. Carrier proteins and permeability barriers for cer-

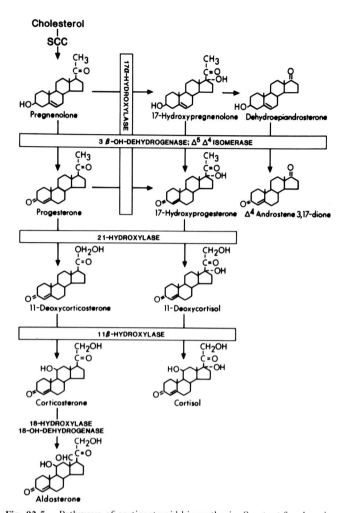

Fig. 92-5. Pathways of corticosteroid biosynthesis. See text for description.

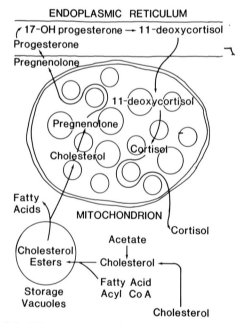

Fig. 92-6. Subcellular compartmentalization of the corticosteroid biosynthetic enzymes and the flow of biosynthetic intermediates. See text for explanation.

tain intermediates have been postulated and some evidence obtained which supports their existence and function in controlling the biosynthetic process. However, the physical properties of the intermediates, their affinities for the various biosynthetic enzymes, and the concentrations of these enzymes may be the primary factors in determining the complex flow of intermediates.

REFERENCES

1. Schimmer, B. P., Ueda, K., Sato G. H.: Site of action of adrenocorticotropic hormone (ACTH) in adrenal cell cultures. *Biochem Biophys Res Commun 32:* 806–810, 1968.
2. Lefkowitz, R. J., Roth, J., Pastan, I.: ACTH-receptor interaction in the adrenal: A model for the initial step in the action of hormones that stimulate adenyl cyclase. *Ann NY Acad Sci 185:* 195–209, 1971.
3. Donta, S. T.: Differentiation between the steroidogenic effects of cholera enterotoxin and ACTH through use of a mutant adrenal cell line. *J Infect Dis 129:* 728–731, 1974.
4. Schorr, I., Rathnam, P., Saxena, B. B., et al: Multiple specific hormone receptors in the adenylate cyclase of an adrenocortical carcinoma. *J Biol Chem 246:* 5806–5811, 1971.
5. Hofmann, K., Wingender, W., Finn, F. M.: Correlation of adrenocorticotropic activity of ACTH analogs with degree of binding to an adrenal cortical particulate preparation. *Proc Natl Acad Sci USA 67:* 829–836, 1970.
6. Haksar, A., Baniukiewicz, S., Peron, F. G.: Inhibition of ACTH-stimulated steroidogenesis in isolated rat adrenal cells treated with neuraminidase. *Biochem Biophys Res Commun 52:* 959–966, 1973.
7. Lefkowitz, R. J., Roth, J., Pastan, I.: Effects of calcium on ACTH stimulation of the adrenal: Separation of hormone binding from adenyl cyclase activation. *Nature 228:* 864–866, 1970.
8. Haynes, R. C., Koritz, S. B., Peron, F. G.: Influence of adenosine 3',5'-monophosphate on cortical production by rat adrenal gland. *J Biol Chem 234:* 1421–1423, 1959.
9. Grahame-Smith, D. G., Butcher, R. W., Ney, R. L., et al: Adenosine 3',5'-monophosphate as the intracellular mediator of the action of adrenocorticotropic hormone on the adrenal cortex. *J Biol Chem 242:* 5535–5541, 1967.
10. Ney, R. L.: Effects of dibutyryl cyclic AMP on adrenal growth and steroidogenic capacity. *Endocrinology 84:* 168–170, 1969.
11. Beall, R. J., Sayers, G: Isolated adrenal cells: Steroidogenesis and cyclic AMP accumulation in response to ACTH. *Arch Biochem Biophys 148:* 70–76, 1972.
12. Mackie, C., Richardson, M. C., Schulster, D.: Kinetics and dose–response characteristic of adenosine 3',5'-monophosphate production by isolated rat adrenal cells stimulated with adrenocorticotropic hormone. *FEBS Lett 23:* 345–348, 1972.
13. Gill, G. N.: Mechanism of ACTH action. *Metabolism 21:* 571–588, 1972.
14. Ferguson, J. J., Jr.: Protein synthesis and adrenocorticotropin responsiveness. *J Biol Chem 238:* 2754–2759, 1963.
15. Richardson, M. C., Schulster, D.: The role of protein kinase activation in the control of steroidogenesis by adrenocorticotrophic hormone in the adrenal cortex. *Biochem J 136:* 993–998, 1973.
16. Ferguson, J. J., Jr., Morita, Y.: RNA synthesis and adrenocorticotropin responsiveness. *Biochim Biophys Acta 87:* 348–350, 1964.
17. Hofert, J., Boutwell, R. K.: Puromycin-induced glycogenolysis as an event independent from inhibited protein synthesis in mouse liver; effects of puromycin analogs. *Arch Biochem Biophys 103:* 338–344, 1963.
18. Appleman, M. M., Kemp, R. G.: Puromycin: A potent metabolic effect independent of protein synthesis. *Biochem Biophys Res Commun 24:* 564–568, 1966.
19. Bransom, E. D.: Actinomycin D in vivo: Paradoxical and nonspecific effects on adrenal cortex. *Endocrinology 85:* 1114–1128, 1969.
20. Mostafapour, M. K., Tchen, T. T.: Effects of actinomycin D on hormone-induced steroidogenesis by superfused rat adrenal glands. *Biochem Biophys Res Commun 48:* 491–495, 1972.
21. Grower, M. F., Bransom, E. D.: Adenosine 3',5'-monophosphate adrenocorticotropic hormone and adrenocortical cytosol protein synthesis. *Science 168:* 483–485, 1970.
22. Farese, R. V.: Adrenocorticotropin-induced changes in the steroido-

23. Kan, K. W., Ritter, M. C., Ungar, F., et al: The role of a carrier protein in cholesterol and steroid hormone synthesis by adrenal enzymes. *Biochem Biophys Res Commun 48:* 423–429, 1972.
24. Mahaffee, D., Reitz, R. C., Ney, R. L.: The mechanism of action of adrenocorticotropic hormone. The role of mitochondrial cholesterol accumulation in the regulation of steroidogenesis. *J Biol Chem 249:* 227–233, 1974.
25. Bell, J. J., Cheng, S. C., Harding, B. W.: Control of substrate flux and adrenal cytochrome P-450. *Ann NY Acad Sci 212:* 290–306, 1973.
26. Pfeiffer, D. R., Chu, J. W., Kuo, T. H., et al: Changes in some biochemical parameters including cytochrome P-450 after hypophysectomy and their restoration by ACTH administration in rats four months posthypophysectomy. *Biochem Biophys Res Commun 48:* 486–490, 1972.
27. Kowal, J., Simpson, E. R., Estabrook, R. W.: Adrenal cells in tissue culture. V. On the specificity of the stimulation of 11β-hydroxylation by adrenocorticotropin. *J Biol Chem 245:* 2438–2443, 1970.
28. Ruhmann-Wennhold, A., Nelson, D. H.: Corticosteroidogenesis and its relation to ACTH-dependence of mitochondrial components. *Endocrinology 93:* 977–982, 1973.
29. Purvis, J. L., Canick, J. A., Mason, J. I.: Lifetime of adrenal cytochrome P-450 as influenced by ACTH. *Ann NY Acad Sci 212:* 319–343, 1973.
30. Gunsalus, I. C., Pederson, T. C., Sligar, S. G.: Oxygenase-catalyzed biological hydroxylations. *Annu Rev Biochem 44:* 377–407, 1975.
31. Shikita, M., Hall, P. F.: Cytochrome P-450 from bovine adrenocortical mitochondria: An enzyme for the side chain cleavage of cholesterol. *J Biol Chem 248:* 5598–5604, 1973.
32. Horie, S., Watanabe, I.: Properties of high spin type P-450 preparations from bovine adrenal cortex mitochondria. *J Steroid Biochem 6:* 401–409, 1975.
33. Whysner, J. A., Ramseyer, J., Harding, B. W.: Substrate-induced changes in visible absorption and electron spin resonance properties of adrenal cortex mitochondrial P450. *J Biol Chem 245:* 5441–5449, 1970.
34. Cheng, S. C., Harding, B. W.: Substrate-induced difference spectral, electron paramagnetic resonance, and enzymatic properties of cholesterol-depleted mitochondrial cytochrome P-450 of bovine adrenal cortex. *J Biol Chem 248:* 7263–7271, 1973.
35. Wilson, L. D., Oldham, S. B., Harding, B. W.: Studies on adrenal cortical cytochrome P-450. II. Effects of inhibitors of 11β hydroxylation on its optical and magnetic properties. *Biochemistry 8:* 2975–2981, 1969.
36. Cheng, S. C., Suzuki, K., Sadee, W., et al: Effects of spironolactone, canrenone and canrenoate-K on cytochrome P450, and 11β- and 18-hydroxylation in bovine and human adrenal cortical mitochondria. *Endocrinology 99:* 1097–1106, 1976.
37. Simpson, E. R., Boyd, G. S.: The cholesterol side-chain cleavage system of bovine adrenal cortex. *Eur J Biochem 2:* 275–285, 1967.
38. Estabrook, R. W., Cooper, D. Y., Rosenthal, O.: The light reversible carbon monoxide inhibition of the steroid C21-hydroxylase system of the adrenal cortex. *Biochem Z 338:* 741–755, 1963.
39. Wilson, L. D., Harding, B. W.: Studies on adrenal cortical cytochrome P-450. III. Effects of carbon monoxide and light on steroid 11β hydroxylation. *Biochemistry 9:* 1615–1620, 1970.
40. Greengard, P., Psychoyos, S., Tallan, H. H., et al: Aldosterone synthesis by adrenal mitochondria. III. Participation of cytochrome P-450. *Arch Biochem Biophys 121:* 298–303, 1967.
41. Estabrook, R. W., Mason, I. J., Baron, J., et al: Drugs, alcohol and sex hormones. A molecular perspective of the receptivity of cytochrome P450. *Ann NY Acad Sci 212:* 27–49, 1973.
42. Harding, B. W., Bell, J. J., Oldham, S. B., et al: Corticosteroid biosynthesis in adrenal cortical mitochondria. In McKerns K. W. (ed): Functions of the Adrenal Cortex. New York, Appleton, 1968, p. 831.
43. Simpson, E. R., Estabrook, R. W.: Mitochondrial malic enzyme: The source of reduced nicotinamide adenine dinucleotide phosphate for steroid hydroxylation in bovine adrenal cortex mitochondria. *Arch Biochem Biophys 129:* 384–395, 1969.
44. Hrycay, E. G., Gustafsson, J., Ingelman-Sundbert, M., Ernster, L: The involvement of Cytochrome P-450 in hepatic microsomal steroid hydroxylation reactions supported by sodium periodate, sodium chlorite, and organic hydroperoxides. *Eur J Biochem 61:* 43–52, 1976.

45. Samuels, L. T., Nelson, D. H.: Biosynthesis of the corticosteroids. In Handbook of Physiology, Section 7: Endocrinology; vol VI, Adrenal Gland. Washington, D.C., *Am Physiol Soc,* 1975, p 55.

46. Ichii, S., Kobayashi, S.: Studies on the biosynthesis of sterol and corticosterone in rat adrenal gland. *Endocrinol Jap 13:* 39–45, 1966.

47. Boyd, G. S., Trzeciak, W. H.: Cholesterol metabolism in the adrenal cortex: Studies of the mode of acton of ACTH. *Ann NY Acad Sci 212:* 361–377, 1973.

48. Burstein, S., Gut, M., Han, G.: Kinetics and mechanism of the conversion of cholesterol to pregnenolone in bovine adrenal cortex. Program of the 57th Annual Meeting of the Endocrine Society, New York, 1975, p 56.

49. Kahn, F. W., Neher, R.: Adrenal steroid biosynthesis in vitro. 3. Selective inhibition of adrenal cortical function. *Helv Chim Acta 49:* 725–732, 1966.

50. Wilson, L. D., Harding, B. W.: Oxidation of 20α-hydroxycholesterol by adrenal cortex mitochondria. *J Biol Chem 248:* 9–14, 1973.

93

Plasma ACTH and Corticosteroids

Dorothy T. Krieger

PLASMA ACTH

ACTH STRUCTURE

Human ACTH consists of a single peptide chain of 39 amino acid residues. The N-terminal 1–24 amino acid sequence has a steroidogenic potency[1] and adrenal receptor affinity[2] similar to those of the complete molecule. However, studies in the human indicate that the duration of action following intravenous injection of ACTH[1-24] is shorter than that of highly purified ACTH[1-39], suggesting that the larger amino acid sequence of the natural hormone delays its intravascular inactivation.[3] Size heterogeneity of ACTH, with the presence of immunoreactive ACTH components of larger molecular size than ACTH[1-39], "big" ACTH, has been reported in plasma samples from patients with Nelson's syndrome, "ectopic ACTH syndrome," or from patients postbilateral adrenalectomy for Cushing's disease.[4,5] Excesses of extreme N-terminal[1-13] and C-terminal immunoreactive ACTH have been described in plasma from patients with the ectopic ACTH syndrome and those with Cushing's disease.[6] There are no reports of such heterogeneity in normal subjects under basal conditions, although "big" ACTH has been noted in a few instances when normal subjects were stimulated with either 2-deoxyglucose or metyrapone.[3,4] It should be noted that "big" ACTH, using an in

vitro rat bioassay system, has less than 4 percent of the biological activity of ACTH[1-39].[7] Shortening of the N-terminal[1-24] amino acid sequence is associated with progressive loss of biological activity, although some steroidogenic activity is still manifest in isolated adrenal cell preparations that are exposed to ACTH[4-10].[8]

It is generally considered that peptide hormones exist in an unbound form in plasma. An ACTH-binding factor in plasma has been described,[9] however, with no characterization of its specificity.

METHODS OF MEASUREMENT OF PLASMA ACTH

Definition of the ACTH Unit

At present ACTH potency is defined in terms of the Third International Standard for Corticotropin,[10] which is a highly purified extract of porcine pituitaries. One international unit is considered to be equivalent to 10 μg of ACTH[1-39] as measured by the rat adrenal ascorbic acid depletion assay, in response to the subcutaneous administration of ACTH. Similar potencies were obtained when assayed using as an endpoint the effect on plasma corticosteroid levels.[9] Potency of a given ACTH preparation as assayed by the intravenous route yields results approximately one-third of those obtained by subcutaneous administration.

Bioassay

Historically this was the first type of assay employed,[11] but, as originally described, was relatively insensitive and not suitable for measurement of physiological, nonstimulated plasma ACTH levels. Even with subsequent bioassays,[12] relatively large plasma volumes were required, making impractical studies in which frequent sampling was desired to document the dynamics of ACTH response. Recently three different types of bioassay have been introduced with marked increases in sensitivity.

Steroidogenic Response of Isolated Dispersed Adrenal Cells. In 1971, Sayers et al.[13] introduced an assay based upon the steroidogenic response of dispersed rat adrenal cells (obtained following tryptic digestion and mechanical agitation). This type of assay can detect between 2 and 5 pg of ACTH[1-39] per incubation vial.[14] Attempts to utilize this technique for measurement of plasma ACTH concentrations were unsuccessful, due apparently to the presence in plasma of one or more substances which inhibit the response of the cells to ACTH.[15] An extraction technique has recently been devised[16] which removes such inhibitory substances, so that concentrations of 2 pg ACTH[1-39] can be detected. Twenty-five samples can be processed in one working day. In such a bioassay, ACTH fragments[17-39,11-24], and β-MSH are ineffective in stimulating steroidogenesis and ACTH[1-10,4-10], and α-MSH are effective only in amounts 10^6-fold greater than effective concentrations of ACTH[1-39].

Binding of ACTH to Adrenal Receptors. There have been two reports of specific binding of labeled ACTH to receptors obtained from homogenates prepared from mouse ACTH-sensitive adrenal tumors[2] or from rat, rabbit, or bovine adrenal glands.[17] Obtaining active adrenal extracts requires extreme methodological care. Extraction of plasma is not required and 1 pg of ACTH can be detected. To date there have been no systematic reports of applicability to physiological or clinical situations. Using a particulate fraction from beef adrenal, a significant correlation between binding and *in vivo* adrenocorticotrophic activity has been reported.[18] However, the inactive 11–20 NH_2 derivative also binds significantly, suggesting that the Lys–Lys–Arg–Arg 15–18 sequence is involved in binding, and that fragments may be present in plasma which could bind in a receptor assay and not be biologically active.

Cytochemical "Redox" Bioassay. This assay is based on changes in the extent of reduction of ferricyanide to ferrocyanide, presumably due to ascorbic acid depletion, produced by exposing guinea pig adrenal sections to ACTH. Such reduction is quantitated by microdensitometry scanning of the zona reticularis.[19] Extraction of plasma is not necessary, very small amounts of plasma are required, and a sensitivity of 50 fg/ml can be attained. There is no cross-reactivity with LH, prolactin, α-MSH or β-MSH, or α-ACTH[18–39]. α-ACTH[1–18] is fully potent as is α-ACTH[1–39]. At present a maximum of 50 samples per week can be processed.[20,21] (To date, there have been no studies to determine whether other peptides or nonpeptide substances are also capable of altering the reducing potency of adrenal sections in this cytochemical assay, as has been reported using the *in vivo* ascorbic acid depletion assay.)

Comparison of ACTH Concentrations as Determined by Various Bioassay Methods. There have been no comparisons of plasma ACTH concentrations from given subjects assayed by different bioassays, except for one study[20] in which plasma samples with high ACTH concentrations were compared using the cytochemical and the in vivo Lipscomb–Nelson assay, where good agreement was found. Table 93-1 lists ACTH concentrations reported by several laboratories in various clinical states and testing conditions utilizing the recently developed as well as the older bioassay methodology. Although the data are limited, there is generally good agreement between all cited methods, save for the greatly increased levels in Cushing's disease reported by the adrenal tumor receptor assay and in one instance by *in vivo* bioassay, and the wide range reported in the patients with Addison's disease. Since plasma ACTH concentrations undergo a well-defined circadian variation in untreated patients with primary Addison's disease,[27] ACTH concentrations reported in such patients can only be compared if they are obtained at similar times of day.

Immunoassay

A number of radioimmunoassay procedures have been described for the determination of plasma ACTH concentrations. Problems have been encountered in part secondary to (a) the low concentrations of ACTH present in human plasma, in contrast to those of other peptide hormones; (b) the binding of ACTH to glass surfaces; (c) the susceptibility of ACTH to inactivation (presumably by proteolytic enzymes) upon relatively short exposure to room temperature; (d) the presence in plasma of substances which either "damage" ACTH or alter the antigen–antibody reaction leading to erroneously high bound/free (B/F) ratios[28]; and (e) the difficulty of obtaining appropriate high affinity antisera, as well as the heterogeneity of the antisera available, i.e., the site of the

ACTH molecule to which the antibody is directed. In one radioimmunoassay system[29] advantage has been taken of the phenomenon of paradoxical binding, i.e., the occurrence of an *increase* in binding of labeled ACTH to antibody with increasing concentrations of unlabeled ACTH.

Numerous methods have been devised for the production of antisera by varying the antigen employed (use of either porcine or human ACTH[1–39], or ACTH[1–24] alone or conjugated to various proteins) the dose, route and number of sites of administration of antigen, and the choice of either guinea pigs, rabbits, or sheep for immunization. As stated by Orth,[30] "It is probable that these factors have no major influence on antibody production, the development of useful antisera may have been more serendipity than science." It would obviously be desirable that antisera employed have high enough affinity for antigen to enable the use of unextracted plasma, and recognize only the biologically active portion of the ACTH molecule. In evaluating reports of immunoassayable ACTH concentrations in various clinical and physiological states it is important to be aware of the specificity of the antisera employed. Of those antisera for which there is available clinical data, that of Berson and Yalow[31] can be used with unextracted plasma and apparently recognizes the major portion of the ACTH molecule including at least the 1–25 sequence, as well as "big" ACTH[5]; that of Landon and Greenwood[32] (extracted plasma) apparently recognizes the 14–24 sequence; three reported by Orth (unextracted plasma) recognize the 1–24, both 1–24 and 25–39, and the 25–39 sequence, respectively. The first of these does not react with fragments up to 1–16 (see Figure 93-1). The antiserum employed by Matsukura et al.[29] (unextracted plasma) apparently recognizes the C-terminal (beyond 1–24), whereas the Kendall antiserum[34] supplied by the National Pituitary Agency requires the use of extracted plasma and recognizes the N-terminal 1–24, as well as the 1–13 (α-MSH) fragment. The West antiserum, also currently supplied by the National Pituitary Agency, requires extracted plasma, recognizes the ACTH[1–39], ACTH[1–24], and ACTH[11–24] on an approximately equimolar basis. This antiserum does not react with the [1–13] fragment or with C-terminal fragments. Although the actual volume required for assay is a function both of antibody sensitivity and the level of ACTH present, plasma volumes of only 100–200 μl are usually employed for assays utilizing unextracted plasma, whereas volumes of 1–5 ml may be required for those requiring extraction. The sensitivity of reported assays varies from 5 to 25 pg/ml.

Correlation of ACTH Concentrations as
Determined by Bioassay and
Immunoassay

It should be emphasized that such correlations must be interpreted in the light of the portion of the ACTH molecule being recognized in the different assays. Bioassayable and immunoassayable ACTH concentrations will be most similar when the steroidogenic and immunologic determinants most closely coincide. Therefore, close parallelism would not be expected between results obtained on a given plasma analyzed by bioassay and an immunoassay where the antibody recognizes a C-terminal sequence. Furthermore, in dynamic studies of ACTH secretion, the possibility exists that, during the course of study, the ACTH molecule may be degraded to smaller fragments, which, while biologically inactive, may not only be immunologically reactive, but have longer half-lives than that of the intact molecule. Alternatively (especially in the case in which a C-terminal antibody is employed), cleavage of the terminal portion of the ACTH molecule could occur so that biologically active components remain, al-

Table 93-1. Human Plasma ACTH Levels in Various Clinical States as Determined by Different Bioassays

Clinical Condition	Dispersed Adrenal Cell* n	pg/ml	Receptor Adrenal Tumor[2] (pg/ml) n	Range	Mean	Normal Adrenal[17] (pg/ml) n	Range	Mean	Cytochemical (pg/ml) n	Range	Mean	In Vivo Bioassay[12] (mU/100 ml†) n	Range	Mean
Normal adult														
06:00	2	8.0										6	0.10–0.59[23]	0.25
		14.0										7	Not sig.[24]	
08:00–10:00			7	ND‡–88		18	30–100	75	14	35–105[22]	69.8	8	0.40–0.80[23]	
												4	ND[24]‡	
09:00–10:00	14	66.0 (range 22–90)												
15:30						11	10–100	54						
17:00–18:00	13	29.5 (range 25–62)							13	5–45[22]	23.8			
20:00	5		3	200–500					12	50–250[22]	140.0			
Normal		168												
max. level		132												
p̄ insulin-induced		168												
hypoglycemia		71												
p̄ metyrapone		52	6	100–300§										
Hypopituitarism (adrenal insufficiency)			3	ND‡					8	0.017–0.96[26]	0.35			
Corticosteroid-suppressed subjects			2	ND										
Chronic						4	4–10ǁ		1	5[22]¶				
Acute									1	38				
1° Addison's disease		223#					2000**					8	2–36[24]#	
		1028††					200‡‡							
Cushing's disease		199	6	200–7000		1	50,160					7	0.6–0.8[24]	
		312										5	0.34–1.81[22]	
		162										3	ND‡	
		145										11	2120 pg/ml[6]	
Nelson's syndrome		755										17	2–400[25]	63
"Ectopic" ACTH		391												
		138												
		145												
		208	31	200–10,000								6	0–3.9[25]	

*Unpublished observations.
†1 mU/100 ml = ≈100 pg/ml.
‡ND = not detectable.
§08:00 (conc. p̄ 2 g po at 23:00).
ǁ08:00 (conc. p̄ 2 mg dexamethasone po at 23:00).
¶Conc. 60 min p̄ i.v. cortisol (5 mg) or 0.5 mg dexamethasone.
#Untreated 15:15 PM.
**24 h p̄ discontinuance of replacement medication (time of day not specified).
††9 AM (12 h p̄ discontinuance of replacement medication).
‡‡8 h p̄ discontinuance of replacement medication (time of day not specified).

though immunoreactivity would disappear. However, until methodology for direct analysis of various portions of the ACTH molecule is available, such immunoassay–bioassay comparisons should give some insight as to the nature of the ACTH secreted under various clinical and physiological conditions, and supplement that obtained by other methods such as gel filtration which is feasible only with specimens having relatively high ACTH concentrations.

Until recently, because of the relative insensitivity of available bioassays, such bioassay–immunoassay correlations were reported only with regard to plasma samples having elevated plasma ACTH concentrations. Such studies, therefore, could be performed only on subjects in whom ACTH half-lives were measured

following elevation of ACTH concentration by infusion of ACTH (vide infra) or in patients with disease conditions associated with high endogenous ACTH levels. In these disease conditions the possibility also remains that the forms of ACTH secreted may be different from that seen in the normal subject, forms with steroidogenic and immunogenic properties different from those of hACTH[1–39].

Multiple samples obtained in two normal subjects over separate 3–4 h spans of the 24-h period have revealed highly significant correlation between immunoassayable and bioassayable ACTH concentrations (Table 93-2)[35] employing an N-terminal antibody (also reacting with α-MSH). Additional studies on single speci-

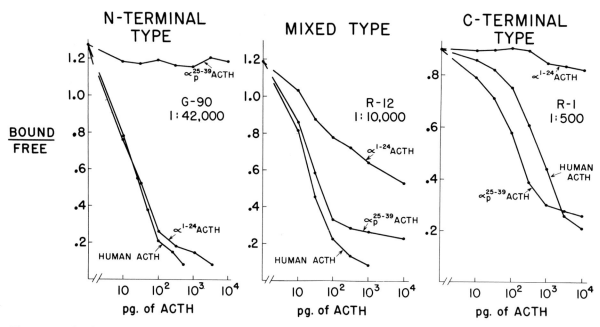

Fig. 93-1. Three types of antisera developed in response to ACTH immunization. G-90 apparently developed in response to an antigenic locus in the N-terminal 1–24 portion of the ACTH molecule. R-12 contained antibodies directed to both the N- and C-terminal fragments, although neither was as effective as the whole molecule. R-1 was apparently directed to a C-terminal site.[33]

mens obtained from different subjects between 09:00–10:00 and 17:00–18:00 reveal essentially similar correlations.

Following induction of insulin hypoglycemia, in a limited number of studies, we have observed increased ratios of plasma immunoassayable–bioassayable ACTH in specimens obtained in the course of such testing, when compared to ratios seen in basal specimens (vide infra). Similar observations have been noted when I/B ratios have been followed during the course of insulin-induced hypoglycemia, using the redox assay for measurement of bioassayable ACTH concentrations.[37] Further study is necessary to assess the significance of such observations. Marked variability of such ratios is also reported following metyrapone administration (Table 93-2).[36]

In untreated subjects with Cushing's disease limited data indicate no abnormality in immunoassayable/bioassayable ACTH ratios. In a limited number of samples assayed, these ratios also did not appear to be significantly altered following remission induced by bilateral adrenalectomy.

In patients with the ectopic ACTH syndrome (all but one 2^0 to carcinoma of the lung) marked variability of I/B ratios is noted. Data are too limited to comment on respective correlations with plasma cortisol concentrations.

Following a single intravenous injection of either porcine (natural or synthetic) or natural human ACTH, immunoassayable and bioassayable ACTH concentrations were essentially similar in a given normal subject 10 min after injection. With continued sampling, there were marked discrepancies in immunoassayable (N-terminal antibody) and bioassayable ACTH concentrations, so that at 120 min following injection I/B ratios were approximately 10:1.[41] C-terminal fragments were present, so that if a C-terminal antibody had been used, such ratios would have been even greater, in view of the markedly longer half-life of such C-terminal fragments.

HALF-LIFE OF PLASMA ACTH

In judging the values reported for the half-life of plasma ACTH, several factors have to be considered: (a) whether such values are based upon the disappearance of endogenously secreted

"physiological" levels of ACTH or of exogenously administered ACTH, either as a pulse injection or as a prolonged infusion—and in this instance the nature of the ACTH preparation employed (human, porcine, or synthetic $ACTH^{1-24}$ or $ACTH^{1-39}$); (b) whether such disappearance has been studied under normal conditions or in dexamethasone-suppressed subjects; (c) the frequency of sampling employed; (d) the method employed in calculating such half-lives—i.e., disappearance of radioactivity following administration of labeled ACTH; determination of ACTH concentrations by immunoassay (and the type of antibody employed) or by bioassay.

Early studies of ACTH half-life in humans utilized relatively crude preparations. In more recent studies, reported values for the half-life of immunoassayable ACTH have been as follows:

1. 8 min: derived from the fall of endogenous ACTH concentrations during spontaneous peaks of secretion[39] (nature of ACTH antibody not stated), and 7–12 min in similar studies in which an N-terminal antibody was employed.[35]
2. 13–44 min (C- or N-terminal antibody),[40] not greater than 10–15 min (antibody recognizing entire molecule, not N- or C-terminal),[41] and 22–28 min (N-terminal antibody).[27] These observations were all based on studies in which the rate of decline of the elevated plasma ACTH concentrations seen in patients postadrenalectomy for Cushing's disease[30] or in patients with Addison's disease was measured following either a pulse injection[27,29] or prolonged infusion[27,41] of corticosteroid. (The reason for the difference in the observed half-times of disappearance of endogenous immunoassayable ACTH in normal subjects, 7–12 min, and Addisonian subjects, 15–30 min,[27] is not clear, and will have to await studies of half-life of bioassayable ACTH in patients with Addison's disease.)
3. Values of 11–28 min (mean 18 min) have been reported in studies in which the decline in plasma ACTH concentrations was measured following the pulse or continuous administration to normal subjects of human or porcine ACTH in amounts comparable to those reported to cause maximal adrenocortical secretion.[38] In this latter study,

Table 93-2. Reported Correlations of Immunoassayable and Bioassayable Plasma ACTH Concentrations

Clinical Category*	Plasma Immunoreactive ACTH Concentration (pg/ml)			Plasma Bioassayable ACTH Concentration (pg/ml)	I/B*	Comments
	Extreme N-terminal Antibody (1–13)	N-terminal Antibody (1–23 or 1–16)	C-terminal Antibody (17–39, 25–39)			
Normal adult subjects						
06:40–07:30 $\overline{(11)}$		116.3 ± 13.4[35]†		91.5 ± 11.9	1.37	Bioassay[16]
$\overline{(8)}$		112.5 ± 19.9		87.0 ± 18.9	1.36	
10:00–13:00 $\overline{(37)}$		55.8 ± 3.0		44.5 ± 4.8	1.42	
16:00–20:00 $\overline{(48)}$		22.0 ± 1.5		15.1 ± 1.0	1.49	
09:00–10:00 $\overline{(14)}$		90.8 ± 9.1‡		66.0 ± 4.9	1.37	
17:00–18:00 $\overline{(13)}$		40.8 ± 6.4‡		29.5 ± 5.1	1.41	
p̄ metyrapone§		(15)	1.20–1450[36]	115–673	0.45–4.9 2.8 (mean)	Bioassay[12]
Addison's disease						
			2480[36]	805	3.10	Bioassay[12] Pt. at least 24 h. p̄ steroid withdrawal
		337‡		223	1.50	Bioassay[6] Pt. untreated (15:00)
		1226‡		1028	1.10	No Rx for 12 h (09:00)
Cushing's disease		1840[6]	7080	2120		Bioassay[12]
Untreated $\overline{(37)}$	207.4 ± 9.3[35]			162.7 ± 5.1	1.27	Bioassay[16]
Remission postpituitary irradiation (0900)		64‡		47.8	1.33	Bioassay[12]
		85‡		35.0	2.80	No replacement medication
Remission p̄ bilateral adrenalectomy			2100[36]	1669	1.30	Bioassay[12]
			2160	954	2.30	No steroid replacement for 24 h
			655	660	1.00	
			429	237	1.80	
Nelson's syndrome		1217‡		755	1.60	2 h p̄ replacement cortisone 25 mg po
		760‡		387	1.90	3 h p̄ replacement cortisone 25 mg. po
"Ectopic" ACTH syndrome	6740	3295	12,800[6]	2900		Bioassay[12]
		835‡		674	1.20	Bioassay[16]
		627‡		391	1.60	
		185‡		138	1.30	
		362‡		145	2.50	
		911‡		208	4.40	

$\overline{(\ )}$ Number of specimens obtained every 5 min over indicated time period in a given subject.

$(\ )$ Number of specimens from different subjects.

*Ratio of immunoassayable ACTH concentration to bioassayable ACTH concentration.

†SE.

‡Unpublished observations.

§Clinical condition not specified. Specimens obtained 4 h after last of 6 po doses of 750 mg/4 h.

an N-terminal antibody was employed. (When the C-terminal antibody was used to follow the disappearance of ACTH added to thawed plasma, a fourfold greater half-time of disappearance was noted than that seen with the N-terminal antibody.) The number of observations in this study were not sufficient to state if there were significant differences in the disappearance of synthetic porcine verses native porcine ACTH, human versus porcine ACTH, larger or smaller concentrations of administered ACTH, or following pulse or prolonged infusion. In this same study ACTH half-life as calculated by bioassay ranged between 4.9 and 18.2 min (mean 9 min), and discrepancies between bioassayable and immunoassayable ACTH levels were present within 15–30 min following pulse ACTH injection (15 min) being the first sampling time after injection). In other studies in which comparison of bioassayable and immunoassayable ACTH half-lives was based on the fall of endogenous ACTH concentrations during spontaneous peaks of secretion (samples were obtained at 5-min intervals), these were 3–9 and 7–12 min, respectively.[35]

Finally, a value of 7 min has been reported for ^{131}I-labeled ACTH[1-24], with a single slope of disappearance.[42] In contrast, in the study in which immunoassayable and bioassayable half-lives were calculated following exogenous ACTH[1-39] administration,[38] plasma ACTH disappearance curves appeared to be multiphasic, with an initial fast phase followed by a slow phase. This slow phase was also noted in an earlier study in which the half-life of bioassayable ACTH was measured following injection of a relatively crude porcine ACTH preparation.[43]

All of these studies cannot be compared to each other for

several reasons. At present, there is insufficient information to be sure the molecular species of ACTH seen in normal subjects is the same as that found in patients with Addison's or Cushing's disease (type 2 versus type 1 studies just listed). There are also differences of distribution that are seen following a pulse of exogenous ACTH and following the constant infusion of ACTH. Studies utilizing steroid suppression of endogenously elevated levels may overestimate half-life if such suppression is not complete and instantaneous. There is also evidence that $ACTH^{1-24}$ is more rapidly inactivated in vivo than the native hormone,[3] thereby shortening its biological, if not immunological, half-life.

In view of these considerations the cited half-lives can only be considered as an approximation. Until further information is obtained, it would appear reasonable to consider that the half-life of biologically active ACTH in normal subjects is less than 8 min, and somewhat more than 3 min.

RELATIONSHIP OF PLASMA ACTH CONCENTRATION TO PITUITARY ACTH SECRETION

In studies which utilized an ACTH half-life in plasma of 10 min and a volume of distribution for ACTH of 40 percent of body weight,[42] the metabolic clearance rate of ACTH has been calculated to be 2 liters/min.[44] In such calculations, it has been assumed that the metabolic clearance rate is independent of the ACTH plasma concentration. (This may have to be modified if there is additional support for the preliminary evidence that ACTH may be bound to plasma proteins.[28,45]) Assuming a linear, single-compartment system, the rate of ACTH secretion can then be calculated from the product of the metabolic clearance rate and the steady state plasma ACTH concentration. Assuming a steady state, Urquhart has calculated an ACTH secretion rate of 0.12 U ($\approx$1.2 μg)/h in the late afternoon, corresponding to a plasma level of approximately 10 pg/ml; morning rates of secretion would therefore be expected to be approximately tenfold higher (i.e., 1.2 U or 12 μg/h),[44] in view of the higher plasma ACTH concentrations at this time of day (Table 93-2).

While such calculations may be valid (using late afternoon plasma ACTH concentrations, which show least ultraradian fluctuations—see Fig. 93-2 and Table 93-2), they may not accurately describe ACTH secretion during episodes of rapid changes in plasma ACTH concentration, when no steady state exists. In calculations based on a single subject,[39] and taking samples at 5-min intervals, ACTH secretion was calculated from the formula

$$\text{amount of hormone secretion} = V(C_t - C_0) + \frac{C_0 + C_t}{2} \cdot \frac{\Delta t}{\overline{T}}$$

where V is volume of distribution, C_0 initial concentration of ACTH hormone in plasma (at start of a secretory episode), C_t peak concentration of the hormone in plasma (during that secretory episode), Δt (min) duration of the secretory episode, and $\overline{T}$ mean life of the hormone (1.44 $\times$ $t_{1/2}$, where $t_{1/2}$ is half-life of the hormone). Then using an ACTH half-life of 7 min and a 43 percent volume of distribution, the amount of ACTH secreted during the time of maximum secretory activity and highest ACTH concentrations (6:35 AM–7:45 AM, maximum ACTH concentration 160 pg/ml) was 14.1 μg (86 IU = 1 mg), which represents observed secretion during 35 min of this hour. This figure is in rather good agreement with the 12 μg/h calculated earlier from steady state assumptions. (ACTH concentrations were determined by immunoassay which, as noted previously, may overestimate actual plasma ACTH concentrations. A conversion factor of 100 IU = 1 mg was employed.)

Calculations based on similar data from our laboratory on two subjects studied at 5-min intervals over different time spans of the 24-h period[35] indicated that total amounts (μg/h) of immunoassayable ACTH secreted were highest in the hour preceding awakening (6:30–7:30 AM, 12.9 and 12.2 μg/h), 5.3 and 4.0 μg/h between 10:00 and 11:00 AM, and 1.4 and 1.7 μg/h between 9:00 and 10:00 PM. During the early morning period of active secretion there was no major difference between the calculated amounts of secretion of immunoassayable and bioassayable ACTH. Approximation of the total amount of immunoassayable ACTH secreted in one normal subject over a 24-h period yielded a value of 73 μg. Berson and Yalow[31] calculated an ACTH turnover in normal subjects of 7.24 μg/day. In these calculations, however, a turnover time of 25 min and a distribution volume of only the extracellular space was employed. Since the calculations in the present data (and those of Urquhart) employed a turnover time of 10 min and a 43 percent volume of distribution, it would be expected that these calculations would vary at least by a fivefold factor.

In 3 patients with clinically active Cushing's disease, calculated immunoassayable ACTH secretion varied from 19.2 to 34.3 μg/h, the magnitude of the ACTH secretion appearing to be positively correlated with the magnitude of the 24-h corticosteroid excretion. Since plasma ACTH concentrations do not undergo a circadian variation in such patients this would indicate an apparent ACTH secretion varying from 480 to 840 μg/day.

Assayable pituitary content of ACTH in the human adult is estimated to be no more than 250 μg.[46] This would indicate a considerable secretory reserve if one assumes that major ACTH secretion occurs only over a limited portion of the 24-h period. When ACTH was infused to normal subjects at a rate of 4 U/h, plasma ACTH concentrations equivalent to approximately 500 pg/ml were attained.[47] These same investigators had previously shown that plasma levels of 3 mU/100 ml (approximately 300 pg/ml)[48] were sufficient to stimulate maximal adrenal cortical activity. By extrapolation, therefore, such maximal activity could be achieved with a steady state secretion of approximately 2.5 U (25 μg)/h.

PLASMA CORTISOL

METHODS OF ASSAY

Cortisol is the major glucocorticoid secreted by the adrenal cortex. It is currently measured clinically by either a fluorometric method,[49] competitive protein binding assay,[50] or radioimmunoassay.[51] Volume requirements vary from 1 ml to as little as 10–50 μl of plasma for the two latter types of assay. All of these methods as currently performed measure "total corticosteroid," i.e., both free and protein bound. Thus far, none of these methods is completely specific for cortisol, in that other corticosteroids and synthetic steroids exhibit various degrees of cross-reactivity.

In the fluorometric assay (of the steroids that are extracted in the procedure commonly employed), corticosterone (depending on the conditions of analysis) exhibits an equal or greater percentage of fluorescence when compared to equivalent amounts of cortisol. 20-Hydroxycortisol (a metabolite of cortisol, presumably produced in negligible quantities) and 21-deoxycortisol (a possible cortisol precursor) also exhibit significant fluorescence.[52] In addition, a variable amount of "nonspecific" fluorescence ($\approx$1–2 μg/100 ml) is seen in plasma from dexamethasone-suppressed subjects.[52] The presence of an 11-hydroxyl group and a 2–4 unsaturated ketone group in ring A has a strong positive influence on the extent of fluorescence, whereas a 17-hydroxyl group has minor influence on the development of fluorescence.

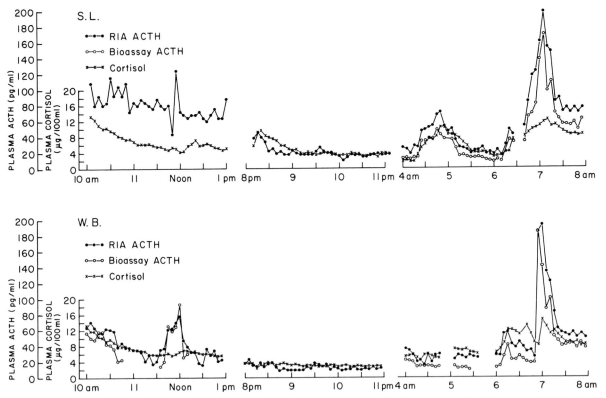

Fig. 93-2. Plasma concentrations of immunoassayable ACTH, bioassayable ACTH, and cortisol in two normal subjects sampled at 5-min intervals at different times of day. (Studies depicted in different segments were performed on different days.) Note concordance of immunoassayable and bioassayable ACTH concentrations, and periods (especially between 6:30 and 7:30 A.M.) where increments in plasma ACTH concentrations were associated with no or markedly diminished increments in plasma cortisol concentrations.

In the competitive protein binding assay, corticosteroid binding globulins (CBG; the ligand employed) obtained from different species have different affinities for different corticosteroids; i.e., monkey, rat, and mouse CBG have a greater affinity for corticosterone than for cortisol, whereas the opposite is true for dog and human CBG. Of the synthetic steroids, prednisone and 6-methylprednisolone exhibit significant binding.

In the radioimmunoassay, cross-reaction varies with the nature of the antibody employed. Table 93-3 indicates the extent of such cross-reactivity in two antibody systems as compared with the competitive protein binding method.

Of these cited cross-reacting steroids, only corticosterone is present in the plasma of normal human subjects in any significant concentration (less than 4 percent of that of cortisol). It has been demonstrated that the concentration of corticosterone varies in parallel with that of cortisol, as determined by studies of circadian periodicity, dexamethasone suppressibility, and ACTH stimulation.[55] Furthermore, no significant variation in corticosteroid binding globulin has been reported under normal physiological conditions, although definitive studies have not yet been reported. Therefore, for routine purposes, measurement of "plasma corticosteroids" by any of these methods would be valid, although the limits of the normal range would vary with the method employed (Table 93-4). No significant sex differences have been noted in the plasma concentration of samples obtained at different times of day[56] (fluorometric method) or in the 24-h integrated concentration of plasma corticosteroids as obtained by blood collection over 20-min periods over a 24-h span, using a nonthrombogenic catheter and a small portable withdrawal pump[57] (competitive protein binding method). Normal subjects studied under ambulatory conditions tend to have slightly higher plasma concentrations than similar

subjects who are studied after several days of hospitalization.[56] Over the 15–90 year age range, there are no significant age-associated differences in circadian plasma corticosteroid concentrations.[59]

Table 93-3. Cross-Reactions in Percentage of the Cortisol Antibodies and of the Human Plasma Specimen Used for the Protein-Binding Method

	Vecsei et al.*	Ruder et al.†	Murphy et al.‡
Cortisol	100	100	100
Compound S	10	100	89
21-Deoxycortisol		100	
17-OH-Progesterone		56	47
Corticosterone	1.4	46	61
18-OH-Corticosterone	0		
Deoxycorticosterone	0	46	
18-OH-Deoxycorticosterone	0.42		
Progesterone	5.5	28	20
Prednisone		16	
Testosterone		13	4
Dexamethasone		2.0	
Spironolactone		1	
Aldadiene	0.36		
11-OH-Progesterone	0.4		
Aldosterone	0.36	0.01	3
Dehydroepiandrosterone		0.01	
17-OH-Pregnenolone		0.01	
Estradiol	0	0.01	
Cholesterol		0.01	

*Antigen, cortisol-21–hemisuccinate–bovine serum albumin complex.
†Antigen, cortisol-21–hemisuccinate–bovine serum albumin complex.
‡Protein-binding assay.
Source: From Vecsei.[51]

Table 93-4. Plasma "Corticosteroid" Concentration in Normal Subjects (μg/100 ml) as Reported Utilizing Different Methods

Sampling Time	Fluorometric Determinations		Competitive Protein Binding Assay		Radioimmunoassay	
	n	Mean $\pm$ SD	n	Mean $\pm$ SD	n	Mean $\pm$ SD
7:00 AM	18*	21.4 $\pm$ 5.6[52]				
8:00 AM	13*	26.1 + 7.5[56]	10†	10 $\pm$ 4.0[57]	30	12.8 $\pm$ 4.1[54]
	19†	22.1 $\pm$ 5.9[56]				
	673†	22.3 $\pm$ 0.30[58]‡				
				Range		
9:00 AM	8*	13.0 $\pm$ 3.3[52]		6–18[50]§		
	30†	19.5 $\pm$ 0.8[58]		8–24‖		
Noon	13*	15.7 $\pm$ 5.5[45]				
	19†	13.0 $\pm$ 5.2[56]				
	30†	12.3 $\pm$ 0.25[58]				
4:00 PM	13*	13.2 $\pm$ 2.9[56]				
	19†	10.3 $\pm$ 2.6[56]				
8:00 PM	13*	10.8 $\pm$ 4.5[56]	10†	4.5 $\pm$ 2.5[57]		
	19†	7.4 $\pm$ 1.8[56]				
	36†	11.9 $\pm$ 1.2[59]				

*Ambulatory subjects.
†Hospitalized normal subjects.
‡SE.
§Cortisol.
‖"Corticoids" (compounds F, B, S).

HALF-LIFE OF PLASMA CORTISOL

The half-life of plasma cortisol is considered to be approximately 70 min,[60] in contrast to the half-life of plasma ACTH of 3–8 min noted earlier. These differing half-lives are of importance when attempting to define plasma ACTH and cortisol interrelations, and the response of the pituitary–adrenal axis to different stimuli.

INTERRELATIONSHIP OF PLASMA ACTH AND CORTISOL CONCENTRATIONS

In considering such interrelationships several points should be stressed:

1. As noted earlier, ACTH and cortisol have different half-lives.
2. The corticosteroid response to the administration of ACTH is evident within 5 min.
3. The duration of such a response is dependent on the dose of ACTH administered.
4. The magnitude of the corticosteroid response is in part dependent on the recent history of prior adrenal exposure to ACTH.
5. The volume of distribution of ACTH is calculated at approximately 43 percent of body weight[42] which is greater than that of cortisol (calculated to be equivalent to that of the thiocyanate space, or approximately 25 percent of body weight).
6. Corticosteroids exert a negative feedback on ACTH, the duration of which may depend more on the prevailing pituitary or central nervous system concentration of corticosteroid than on plasma corticosteroid concentrations. The dose and type of corticosteroid, and the phase of the circadian cycle in which such steroid is secreted or administered, also affect the nature of the ACTH response.

In view of these and other possible considerations, a temporal point-for-point comparison of plasma ACTH and cortisol concentrations (even if corrected for the time lag of onset of ACTH action) will not necessarily indicate the dose–response characteristics of the pituitary–adrenal system. For example, it had been suggested that the circadian rise in adrenal corticosteroid was consequent to release of ACTH provoked by low corticosteroid concentrations in the immediately preceding hours. The invalidity of this observation could be seen when circadian variation of plasma ACTH concentrations was demonstrated in the presence of continually low plasma corticosteroid concentrations, as seen in subjects with Addison's disease (vide infra).

Despite these reservations it is evident that characterization of normal ACTH–cortisol interrelationships would be of value in delineating responses secondary to physiological perturbation and the alterations of these interrelationships in disease. These interrelationships will be considered separately with regard to factors governing the adrenal response to ACTH and studies of the effect of variation of corticosteroid concentrations on ACTH concentrations.

FACTORS GOVERNING THE ADRENAL RESPONSE TO ACTH

The adrenal corticosteroid response to ACTH is governed by a number of variables. Although the effects of some of these may be dissected by studying them as independent variables, in some instances the adrenal response may be a resultant of the interaction of these variables, which may lead to an effect different than the sum of the individual effects.

The variables most thoroughly studied have been the concentration of ACTH and the rate at which it is presented to the adrenal. Such studies have utilized in the main either measurement of corticosteroid secretory rate following arterial perfusion of the isolated adrenal in the hypophysectomzed dog, measurement of plasma cortisol or urinary 17-hydroxycorticosteroid concentration following ACTH infusion to human subjects, or measurement of corticosteroid production by isolated adrenal cells or superfused adrenals. In studies on isolated glands, the effect of resultant steroidogenesis on the adrenal response to continued ACTH infusion is obviated, which is not the case in human infusion studies. Superfusion and isolated adrenal cell studies, in addition, pose the problem that a microcirculation to the adrenal is absent, so that contact of ACTH with cells depends on the accessibility of these cells to ACTH by means other than the circulatory delivery of such ACTH. In most of these studies, ACTH infusion was at a constant rate, unlike the intermittent secretion to which the adrenal is normally exposed.

In addition to possible differences in adrenal response to ACTH secondary to the use of different techniques, additional local factors have to be considered, which may modify the dose–response (magnitude and time course) seen with a given ACTH concentration. It has been suggested[61] that the number and affinity of receptors in a target tissue decrease with increasing concentrations of the agent specifically binding to such receptors. Furthermore, if fragments of ACTH are formed following ACTH secretion or infusion, the half-lives of these fragments and the availability and affinity of the receptors to such fragments also have to be considered. There is also a question as to whether or not adrenal cells can continue to respond to bound hormone after ACTH administration has been discontinued. Recent studies in dexamethasone-pretreated conscious trained sheep with cervical adrenal autotransplants have demonstrated an apparently limited, but significant difference in arteriovenous immunoassayable ACTH concentrations at 5 and 10 min following initiation of ACTH administration, with evidence indicating a positive correlation between cortisol output and adrenal uptake of ACTH.[62] In view of the different half-lives of ACTH and cortisol, correlation of simultaneously obtained plasma ACTH and cortisol concentrations should consider that the latter reflect not only newly secreted cortisol but that still present from prior stimulation. Finally, cognizance should be taken of the well-known observation that the corticosteroid response of the adrenal to a given concentration of ACTH is dependent on the extent of prior exposure of the gland to ACTH. Such prior exposure enhances the response to a given ACTH concentration (which is in the physiological range) as compared to the response to the same concentration administered without prior ACTH exposure.

ACTH Concentrations

The adrenal response to ACTH has been related to the expression[7] $B/B_{max} = A/(A + A_{50})$, where B is the rate of corticosteroid production, B_{max} the maximum rate of corticosteroid production, A the dose of ACTH, and A_{50} the dose required to induce half of B_{max}. (A_{50} can then be considered to be related to the affinity of hormone for its receptor, in that the lower the A_{50} the greater the affinity.) It would therefore be expected that the rate of corticosteroid production be proportional to the dose of ACTH (and hence its plasma concentration), and until the point where receptor saturation is reached, that corticosteroid concentration (reflecting rate of steroidogenesis) be proportional to the dose of ACTH. In these calculations it is only the dose of ACTH that is being considered, not the duration of exposure to such a dose.

Studies in humans in which different amounts of ACTH were injected intravenously[63] have demonstrated that both the *magnitude* and *duration* of the adrenal response do vary directly with the dose employed. It should be observed that the initial rate of rise in plasma cortisol concentrations in response to varying doses of ACTH is the same. It should also be noted in this study that a given dose of ACTH (0.5 U) produced similar responses at 08:00 and 14:00, so that no circadian variation in the response of the adrenal to ACTH was apparent.

One should not relate absolute amounts of ACTH employed in these studies with correlations of a given plasma ACTH and cortisol concentration. First, although the volume of distribution of ACTH may be calculated, as noted previously, to be 43 percent, within the first few minutes following ACTH administration (when binding to receptors would be critical for onset of hormone action), most of the ACTH is within the vascular compartment. Second, the amount of ACTH received by the subject may not be equal to that infused, in view of the well-known property of ACTH to adhere to glass surfaces.

When plasma ACTH concentrations (either those of endogenous ACTH obtained by sampling of normal subjects, or of exogenous ACTH as attained after infusion of ACTH) are plotted against simultaneously obtained plasma corticosteroid concentrations, an approximately linear relationship is seen between the plasma corticosteroid concentration and that of the logarithm of plasma ACTH concentration from 0.05 to 3.0 mU/100 ml (approximately 5–300 pg/ml).[18] (See Figure 93-3.) The plasma corticosteroid concentration at this upper ACTH concentration was approximately 50 μg/100 ml (Porter–Silber chromogens). Some inherent error, however, exists in such determinations.

Adrenal Blood Flow

When the plasma ACTH concentration perfusing isolated adrenal glands was held constant within the physiological range, the adrenal blood flow was doubled, and the cortisol secretion rate was also approximately doubled.[65] Such blood flow effects were

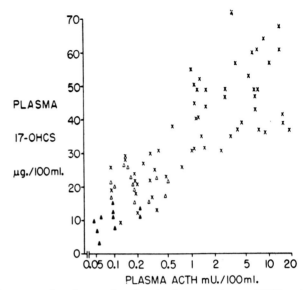

Fig. 93-3. Coordinate values for simultaneous plasma ACTH and 17-OHCS concentrations in normal subjects. ▲, 6 PM; △, 6 AM in normal subjects; ×, values of normal subjects receiving ATH infusions. Plasma corticosteroid concentrations appear to be rectilinear functions of the logarithm of plasma ACTH concentration for all values of the latter less than 3 mU/100 ml. Above this concentration, additional increments of plasma ACTH concentration produce no further increment in plasma corticosteroid concentration.[23]

not apparent when ACTH concentrations were employed that exceeded the physiological range. Therefore, since adrenal blood flow is relatively constant, except in instances where arterial blood pressure varies, or vasodilators or vasoconstrictors are employed, ACTH concentration rather than its presentation rate (i.e., the blood flow times ACTH concentration) can be considered to be an appropriate measure of stimulus strength.

Duration of Exposure of the Adrenal to ACTH

Saffran and Rowell[66] using adrenal superfusion have reported that the same amount of corticosterone is produced when a given dose of ACTH is administered over a short time interval or a longer one (varying from 62,500 μU/ml for 5 min to 3875 μU/ml for 80 min). Urquhart[44] obtained similar data in the calculated simulated adrenocortical response to a constant total quantity of ACTH, using a mathematical model[64] based on the Koritz–Hall hypothesis for ACTH action on steroidogenesis.[67] There was an equal quantity of cortisol secreted over 90 min with exposure of adrenals to 2 μU/ml for 60 min or 64 μU/ml for 1.9 min. Studies in humans have reported[68] that the plasma corticosteroid response to a given dose of ACTH does vary directly with the duration of time over which this dose is administered. This may merely reflect the contribution of previously secreted cortisol (with its 70 min half-life) to the final corticosteroid concentration observed at the end of each of the time spans studied.

Summary

It may be concluded that if the duration of ACTH administration (either as a single pulse or a continuous infusion) is kept constant, then the magnitude and duration of the resultant corticosteroid response is proportional to the concentration of ACTH reaching the adrenal, until maximum steroidogenesis is attained. If *mean* ACTH concentration is kept constant within a relatively small range, but the frequency over a given time span at which it is presented to the adrenal varies, the magnitude of the corticosteroid response will vary, with greater secretion occurring at the lower frequency. When ACTH concentration is kept constant but the duration of administration of this concentration is varied, the total amount of corticosteroid secreted in the different time spans is the same, although plasma corticosteroid concentrations may vary directly with duration.

FEEDBACK CONTROL OF ACTH SECRETION

Methodological Considerations

The principle of feedback (both negative and positive) of a target gland hormone on its trophic hormone is well accepted. It is also obvious that the major stimulus to adrenal corticosteroid secretion is ACTH. If one attempts to correlate point for point plasma ACTH and cortisol concentrations (which may not be a completely meaningful physiological exercise (see the section on the half-life of plasma ACTH), such correlations also have to consider the effect of the stimulated corticosteroid secretion on ensuing pituitary ACTH secretion. In attempting to assess studies investigating such interaction there are numerous methodological considerations.

1. The effect of administration of a synthetic corticosteroid on pituitary ACTH secretion may be different than that of a naturally occurring corticosteroid.
2. The effect of exogenously administered corticosteroid may be different in an adrenalectomized subject than in a normal one.
3. The effect of corticosteroid feedback may be different on basal ACTH secretion than on stress-stimulated or circadian ACTH secretion.
4. The effect of a "pharmacological" dose of exogenously administered corticosteroid may be different than that of physiological concentrations.
5. The effect of chronically elevated corticosteroid concentrations on ACTH responsiveness may be different from that of acute elevation.
6. The point in time at which such interrelations are studied is of importance. Many studies have investigated feedback effect hours, not minutes, after elevation of plasma corticosteroid concentrations.
7. The suppression of ACTH release may be marked long after the induced plasma corticosteroid increment has subsided.[70] The effect, mechanism, and time course of a decrease in plasma corticosteroid concentration on plasma ACTH concentration may differ from those seen in response to an increase in plasma corticosteroid concentration.[71]
8. When plasma ACTH concentrations are being used as the endpoint in measuring corticosteroid–ACTH interactions, it may be of importance to distinguish between such concentrations as measured by bioassay and immunoassay.
9. Finally, it should be stressed that most studies have been on animals, with little extrapolation to the human.

Site of Feedback

Over the past four decades there has been considerable controversy as to the site of corticosteroid feedback control of ACTH secretion.[72] Emphasis has varied from favoring a pituitary locus to a hypothalamic (or more properly a central nervous system, CNS) locus.[73] It may well be that both areas may represent feedback sites under different conditions, and that pituitary feedback may affect ACTH release, whereas hypothalamic feedback may regulate ACTH synthesis as well as release. Although it has been axiomatically accepted that an increase or decrease in pituitary ACTH and plasma ACTH concentrations reflects a simultaneous increase or decrease in hypothalamic corticotrophic-releasing factor (CRF), this has not been subjected to rigorous proof, CRF has not yet been isolated, and the specificity of any CRF-like action detected in various assay systems has not been definitively demonstrated. Usually there is virtually no time lag between stimuli believed to activate CRF and the resultant ACTH–corticosteroid response. Electrical[74] or chemical[75] stimulation of the hypothalamus results in increases in plasma ACTH concentrations within 1.5 min, and of plasma cortisol concentrations within 5 min. (It has previously been noted that stimulation of corticoidogenesis by ACTH occurs within 3–5 min.) The time course of CRF suppression has not been so discreetly studied. In view of these considerations, the following sections consider "feedback" in a nonspecific anatomical sense and describe the relationship of increases and decreases in plasma cortisol concentrations and those of plasma ACTH irrespective of the mechanism(s) involved.

Effect of Acute Increase in Corticosteroid Concentration

In most of these studies the endpoint measured has been plasma corticosteroid, and changes in plasma ACTH concentrations have been inferred.

On Basal Secretion.   Acute elevation of plasma corticosteroid concentrations (by exogenous administration to patients with Addison's disease) to the range encountered under physiological stress conditions is followed by a subsequent decrease (within 30–60 min) of ACTH to very low levels as measured by bioassay.[76] In vitro release of ACTH from bovine pituitary glands was noted to be inhibited following 1 h of incubation with corticosteroids.[77] Other time periods were not tested. Intravenous administration of hydrocortisone produced discernible decrements within 5 min in the elevated plasma ACTH concentrations seen in an untreated patient with Addison's disease.[27]

On Circadian Release.   In both the experimental animal[78] and the human[79] administration of synthetic corticosteroids will suppress the subsequent circadian peak of plasma corticosteroid concentrations.

On Stress-Induced Release.   Corticosteroid responses to stress have been characterized as being "steroid suppressible" or "insuppressible".[80] In both humans[81] and animals[82,83] the suppressive effect of a single dose of dexamethasone (administered orally or intraperitoneally) on vasopressin or a "steroid suppressible" stress-induced ACTH release is a function of the time of pretreatment with the synthetic steroid. In these studies the time interval necessary for corticosteroid pretreatment to produce inhibition of ACTH release varied with the stress employed (from 35 min to 4 h). The time of onset of such suppression is apparently not a function of the dose of dexamethasone employed, although the duration of such suppression appears to be dose related.

More rapid suppression of stress responsiveness (within 2.5 min) has been reported in animals receiving intravenous injections or intraperitoneal infusion of corticosterone.[71] These findings have led to the suggestion[70] that steroid feedback encompasses a *rate-sensitive* period (effective only over a 5-min period following rapid changes in corticosteroid concentration) and a subsequent delayed response, which occurs approximately 2 h after corticosteroid administration and is *proportional* to the extent of elevation of plasma corticosteroid concentration. These latter studies, besides differing from the earlier ones cited with regard to type of steroid employed and route of administration, also employed anesthetized animals. It remains to be seen whether rate-sensitive and proportional responses really exist and reflect different feedback mechanisms and loci, or whether they are apparent only because of the use of anesthesia or related to the different types of steroids employed. The physiological implications of these observations are also unclear. What is being measured in all of these cited studies is the effect of a dose of corticosteroid given prior to a stress on the subsequent adrenal corticosteroid response to the stress. In clinical situations one is actually more concerned with the effect of an increase in corticosteroid concentrations, engendered physiologically, on the *subsequent* functioning of the CNS–pituitary–adrenal system. Studies in which the effect of endogenously elevated corticosteroid concentrations (produced by stress) on the ACTH release produced by a subsequent stress was measured, did not display either the delayed inhibitory effect or the rate-sensitive feedback effect. (Again these studies were performed on anesthetized animals.[84]

Effect of Acute Decrease in Corticosteroid Concentration

Two studies reporting the pituitary and plasma ACTH response to adrenalectomy in the rat, reveal an acute rise in bioassayable plasma ACTH concentrations (as measured in a hypophysectomized rat assay[85] or by the redox method[86]) within 2.5 min following adrenalectomy. (The magnitude of the rise in the two studies varied—the higher concentration, $\approx$1500 pg/ml, noted with the redox method than with the hypophysectomized rat assay, $\approx$400 pg/ml, perhaps reflects the use of continuously anesthetized animals in the latter protocol.) This rise was then followed by a gradual decline in plasma ACTH concentrations so that a plateau was reached, at 40 min[86] or at 12 h,[85] which persisted until 4 days following adrenalectomy, at which time persistently elevated levels were seen. The increase in plasma ACTH concentrations was accompanied by an increase in pituitary ACTH concentrations, which attained greater than normal concentrations by 3[85] to 8[86] days following adrenalectomy.

Matsuyama *et al.* found that adrenalectomy resulted in only a limited immediate increase in plasma ACTH which they ascribed to the stress of the operation. Plasma ACTH levels were not greatly elevated for 24 h following adrenalectomy but then rose progressively over the next 2 weeks to attain the very high levels found in adrenalectomized animals. These authors suggest that a decrease in corticosteroid blood levels (at least following the stress of adrenalectomy) does not produce an immediate marked increase in ACTH output.[87]

There have been no studies in humans following adrenalectomy. Markedly elevated plasma ACTH concentrations have been noted in Addisonian subjects sampled 12 h after they had received their last dose of replacement corticosteroid.[76,27] Such subjects also show a circadian variation in plasma ACTH concentrations (in the face of continually low plasma corticosteroid concentrations), indicating that the circadian rise in plasma ACTH concentrations is not secondary to a decrease in plasma cortisol concentrations.

The time course of the response of immunoassayable ACTH concentrations in response to a decrease in plasma corticosteroid concentrations brought about by metyrapone administration is quite variable following oral administration of the drug, with inconstant elevation first noted 3–8 h following the onset of drug administration (on a 750 mg/4 h basis).[31,88] In the latter study, plasma cortisol concentrations were significantly decreased within 2 h of drug administration. Studies with intravenous metyrapone infusion demonstrated a greater magnitude of ACTH release when such infusion was performed between midnight and 4:00 AM than when performed between 8:00 AM and noon, although the degree of elevation of plasma desoxycortisol was equivalent in both regimens, and the extent of elevation of plasma metyrapone concentration was greater in the 8:00 AM to noon study. The time course of ACTH response, however, was similar in both infusion regimens, with increments noted at 4 h following the start of infusion (the earliest time sampled) and peak ACTH concentrations 6 h after the start of infusion.

Effect of Chronic Elevation of Corticosteroid

Such observations are purely pharmacological ones, obtained in patients receiving exogenous corticosteroids or those with autonomously functioning adrenal tumors. (These observations do not pertain to plasma ACTH–cortisol interactions in bilateral adrenocortical hyperplasia, where the pathophysiology is secondary to increased ACTH production.) Serial measurements of plasma 17-hydroxycorticosteroid and ACTH concentrations obtained following discontinuance of long-term exogenous corticosteroid treatment or removal of an adrenal adenoma, revealed initially decreased plasma ACTH and corticosteroid concentrations, a subsequent increase to supernormal plasma ACTH concentrations within 2–5 months (still accompanied by decreased plasma corticosteroid concentrations), and finally normal plasma ACTH and corticosteroid concentrations within 9 months.[89] The circadian rhythm of plasma ACTH concentrations (based on two-point sampling over the 24-h period) was apparently present within 5 months after discontinuance of excess corticosteroids (with no apparent rhythm in plasma corticosteroid concentrations). Considerable individual variation may be noted in the rate of recovery of pituitary–adrenal function, dependent in part on the dose and duration of preceding corticosteroid elevation.

Summary

From the foregoing it would appear that plasma ACTH concentrations respond rapidly to increments and less rapidly to decrements in plasma corticosteroid concentration, and that plasma cortisol concentrations respond rapidly to increases and decreases in plasma ACTH concentration. An additional variable that may modulate such responses (and hence make for lesser significant correlation between plasma ACTH and cortisol concentrations) is the prolonged retention of corticosteroid within the CNS, which may affect plasma ACTH concentrations long after changes in peripheral corticosteroid concentrations have disappeared.

Under physiological conditions, it would appear that the effect of plasma ACTH on plasma cortisol concentrations is the paramount one, as exemplified in the correlations seen in the episodic release, circadian rise, and stress-activated release of both hormones (see the following sections). The major role of steroid feedback may be in terminating a stress-provoked increment in plasma ACTH concentration (which might be deleterious if unchecked) as well as a possible direct CNS effect of such stress-provoked corticosteroid release in modulating behavioral responses to a future similar stress.[91]

RELATIONSHIP OF PLASMA ACTH AND CORTISOL CONCENTRATIONS IN BASAL AND STIMULATED STATES

RESPONSE TO EXOGENOUS STIMULI

Insulin Hypoglycemia

In this, as in most other studies to be considered, most reported ACTH concentrations are measured by immunoassay. Figure 93-4 depicts the relationship seen among plasma cortisol, plasma ACTH, and blood glucose concentrations. Plasma cortisol concentrations remain elevated during the time that plasma ACTH concentrations are decreasing, this discrepancy in part reflecting the discrepant half-lives of the two hormones. The range of elevation of plasma immunoassayable ACTH concentrations noted is similar to that reported in other studies.[31,92-94] Maximum ACTH levels as determined by bioassay tend to be somewhat lower (see Table 93-1). From inspection of a representative study depicted in Figure 93-5, it may be seen that bioassayable (dispersed adrenal cell) and immunoassayable ACTH concentrations tend to follow a similar course, with immunoassayable concentrations being consistently higher than bioassayable concentrations and with greater discrepancies present during the course of the insulin tolerance test than that seen in the baseline values. Such discrepancies are reflected by altered ratios of immunoassayable/bioassayable

ACTH concentration. Whereas such ratios ranged from 1.10 to 1.42 in baseline specimens,[95] ratios of 1.77–4.13 were seen in normal subjects at times between 30 and 120 min following insulin administration (unpublished observations). This may represent the longer persistence in the circulation of immunologically active fragments than of biologically active ones.

Vasopressin

Results of immunoassay studies only will be considered because of the variability noted in previous reports employing a relatively insensitive bioassay. The largest series[94] reports peak ACTH concentrations of 49–141 pg/ml, with a mean of 94 pg/ml which is within the range noted in smaller reported series.[31,95] Such ACTH concentrations tend to peak somewhat earlier than those achieved following insulin hypoglycemia.

Pyrogen

The administration of pyrogen causes a more prolonged and greater rise in plasma immunoassayable ACTH concentrations (Fig. 93-6), and the time of peak concentration of plasma cortisol occurs later (i.e., at 3 h) than following insulin hypoglycemia.[29,94,96] As noted in Figure 93-7, the magnitude of the rise in plasma cortisol concentration following pyrogen administration is not significantly different from that occasioned by other stimuli of ACTH release. This may be related to the previously cited observation that maximal adrenal stimulation is seen at plasma ACTH concentrations of 300 pg/ml, or it may be that the nature of the ACTH secreted in response to this stimulus is different and is biologically less active. Limited data on the response of bioassayable ACTH concentrations to pyrogen administration report maximal concentrations of only 50–250 pg/ml.[94,96]

Surgical Stress

Immunoassayable plasma ACTH concentrations displayed marked fluctuation during the course of major surgery, with elevation evident within 15 min following incision (earliest time sam-

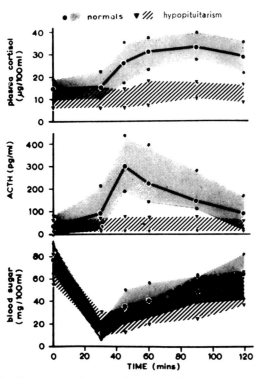

Fig. 93-4. Blood sugar, plasma cortisol, and ACTH responses to insulin in normal subjects and patients with hypopituitarism. The insulin was given at 0 min. The mean responses in normal subjects are given by the continuous lines. The shaded areas give the range of the observed responses.[91]

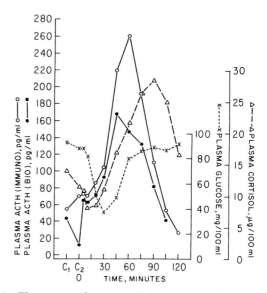

Fig. 93-5. Time course of response of plasma ACTH (immunoassayable, bioassayable) and plasma cortisol concentrations to insulin-induced hypoglycemia in a normal subject.

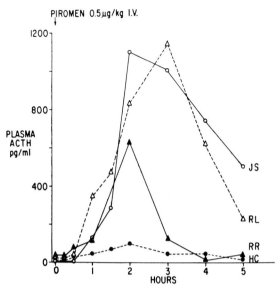

Fig. 93-6. Plasma ACTH and cortisol responses to the intravenous injection of a bacterial pyrogen in normal subjects. Injection was given at 4 PM.[29]

pled).[97] The maximum concentrations noted varied from 110 to 1100 pg/ml. Another study[36] in which plasma ACTH concentrations were determined during open heart surgery revealed bioassayable concentrations varying from 238 to 940 pg/ml, and immunoassayable concentrations varying from 325 to 1300 pg/ml, with immunoassayable/bioassayable ACTH ratios varying from 0.35 to 3.2.

CIRCADIAN VARIATION

A circadian variation in immunoassayable[31] and bioassayable[35] ACTH concentrations has been demonstrated, similar in time course to that described for the circadian variation of plasma corticosteroid concentration.

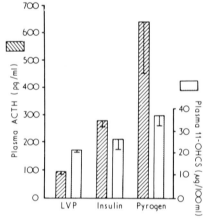

Fig. 93-7. Peak plasma immunoreactive ACTH (hatched) and corticosteroid (stippled) levels after LVP, insulin hypoglycemia, and pyrogen tests in seven subjects. Mean values are shown as columns and the standard error of the mean as vertical bars. Note disparity between extent of plasma cortisol increment and that of plasma ACTH in response to the various stimuli.[94]

EPISODIC VARIATION

In view of the time course of ACTH–cortisol interaction and the half-life of ACTH, only studies in which a blood sampling frequency of a maximum of 5-min intervals between samples was employed might be expected to give some insight into plasma ACTH–cortisol interrelationships under "normal" nonstress conditions. One recent study[38] in which samples were obtained on one subject between the hours of 01:00 and 09:00 demonstrated excellent qualitative but not quantitative relationship between immunoassayable plasma ACTH and cortisol concentrations. This was confirmed in another study[35] in which samples were obtained in two subjects during 3–4 h segments comprising 14 h of the 24-h day (between 10:00 AM to the subsequent 8:00 AM). Both immunoassayable (I-ACTH) and bioassayable (B-ACTH) as well as cortisol concentrations were determined (see Fig. 93-2). Although in general these studies demonstrated significant correlation between I-ACTH or B-ACTH concentrations and those of plasma cortisol, in both subjects there were time periods during which marked rises in both I- and B-ACTH concentrations occurred with concomitant or markedly diminished increments in plasma cortisol concentrations. These findings cannot be explained by biological inactivity of the ACTH since highly significant correlations were present between I- and B-ACTH concentrations at all times. The basis for such a finding is unclear at present—it does not appear to be secondary to any of the factors governing the adrenal response to ACTH discussed earlier (i.e., differences in the rate of change of plasma ACTH concentrations, extent of previous exposure to ACTH, or the presence of maximal ACTH concentrations).

CLINICAL RELEVANCE

Heretofore determinations of either urinary or plasma corticosteroid concentrations and their response to stimulation or suppression have been used to characterize various states of adrenocortical function, and have also served as an indirect assessment of plasma ACTH concentrations. The increased availability of simultaneous plasma corticosteroid and plasma ACTH determinations (both immunoassayable and bioassayable) can now more readily characterize the nature of adrenocortical as well as pituitary pathophysiology.

ADRENAL RESERVE

Customary testing of adrenal cortical responsiveness has been performed by assessing the response of plasma or urinary corticosteroids to the intramuscular administration of porcine ACTH[1–39] or intravenous or subcutaneous administration of synthetic ACTH[1–24] (amounts equivalent to 25 U ACTH) or to prolonged (6–8 h) infusion of the equivalent of approximately 5 U/h. Such modes of testing utilize supramaximal amounts of ACTH, and moderate degrees of decrease in adrenocortical reserve cannot be detected with such testing. To do so, a more accurate delineation of the normal response to submaximal doses of ACTH will have to be obtained, with concomitant monitoring of plasma ACTH concentrations.

For example, following acute intravenous ACTH (25 U ACTH[1–39], 0.25 mg ACTH[1–24]) plasma ACTH concentrations of approximately 18,000 pg/ml (ACTH[1–39]) or 12,000 pg/ml (ACTH[1–24]) are attained within 1 min of administration, and plasma ACTH concentrations are maintained at levels greater than

300 pg/ml (see earlier) for the hour following such administration. Prolonged intravenous ACTH infusion[41] at the rate of only 1 U/h results in steady state plasma ACTH concentrations of 500–1500 pg/ml. It is apparent that these levels are in excess of the concentration of 300 pg/ml noted to produce maximal adrenocortical stimulation.

PITUITARY ACTH RESERVE

Currently employed tests utilizing metyrapone usually measure such reserve indirectly, either by following the response of plasma compound S or urinary 17-hydroxycorticosteroid concentration (Fig. 93-8). By substituting measurement of plasma ACTH for that of compound S[99] a more direct assessment of pituitary reserve is possible, with complete discrimination between normal subjects and those with pituitary insufficiency.

DIAGNOSIS OF ADRENOCORTICAL HYPERFUNCTION (Cushing's Disease and Syndrome)

One of the hallmarks of these conditions is absence of the normal circadian variation of plasma corticosteroid concentrations. Such a difference from the normal may be more readily apparent when late afternoon plasma corticosteroid concentrations are determined, in view of the marked circadian decline in such concentrations in normal subjects. It is generally recognized that even if morning plasma corticosteroid concentrations are within, or only slightly above the normal range, in a patient suspected of adrenal cortical hyperfunction, the presence of similar concentrations in an afternoon specimen is highly suspicious of such a disorder.

Such information, however, does not characterize the etiology of the adrenal cortical hyperfunction. Determination of plasma ACTH concentrations may provide such characterization without the necessity for prolonged suppression studies. In cases of adrenal adenoma or carcinoma (Table 93-5) plasma ACTH concentrations will be markedly lower than those seen in a normal subject for a given time of day. Distinguishing patients with Cushing's syndrome secondary to a documented *primary* pituitary ACTH-producing tumor from those secondary to nontumorous adrenocor-

tical hyperfunction (Cushing's disease) may be accomplished by sellar microtomography. There is limited information available with regard to plasma ACTH concentration in patients with a primary pituitary ACTH-producing tumor. In 3 cases that we have followed, plasma ACTH concentrations have been within the range of those seen in nontumorous adrenocortical hyperfunction (Table 93-2). Patients with primary pituitary tumors may also be differentiated from those with nontumorous adrenal cortical hyperfunction by the lack of dexamethasone suppressibility (8 mg daily for 2 days) and the lack of response of plasma ACTH and cortisol concentrations to pitressin administration in the patients with pituitary tumors. Patients with adrenocortical hyperfunction secondary to "ectopic" ACTH production, in addition to differences in clinical presentation (see Chapter 95) also manifest the highest plasma ACTH concentrations seen in any etiology of Cushing's syndrome, although there may be some overlap with levels seen in cases of nontumorous adrenocortical hyperfunction. Responses to dexamethasone suppression and pitressin administration in patients with ectopic ACTH production are usually similar to those described for primary pituitary tumors.

Data currently available comparing immunoassayable and bioassayable ACTH concentrations in untreated patients with Cushing's disease indicate that immunoassayable/bioassayable ACTH ratios are similar to those seen in normal subjects (Table 93-2).[35] This would indicate that the form in which ACTH is secreted in these patients is similar to that seen in normals. There is insufficient data currently available with regard to the reported presence of "big" ACTH in some patients with Cushing's disease[5] to invalidate this conclusion.

Patients with "ectopic" ACTH production and evidence of hypercortisolism may have normal or markedly increased immunoassayable/bioassayable ACTH ratios (Table 93-2). Two patients with clinically evident "ectopic" ACTH production have been reported[5] as having only "big" ACTH in plasma. (Some conversion to "little" ACTH[1–39] must occur in these patients, since in vitro "big" ACTH has less than 4 percent of the biological activity of ACTH[1–39].[7])

ADRENAL INSUFFICIENCY

Plasma ACTH concentrations can readily distinguish between primary and secondary adrenal insufficiency. It has already been noted that plasma ACTH concentrations undergo a circadian variation in untreated patients with primary adrenal insufficiency. Such patients will have plasma ACTH concentrations that are markedly increased at any given time of day when compared to those seen at similar times in normal subjects. The nature of plasma ACTH in patients with Addison's disease appears to be similar to that seen in normal subjects from the limited information available from comparison of immunoassayable/bioassayable ACTH ratios (Table 93-2) and from Sephadex gel filtration patterns.[5]

Immunoassayable plasma ACTH concentrations at any time of day are either immeasurable or decreased (less than 20 pg/ml) in patients with hypopituitarism manifesting evidence of adrenocortical failure.[29,31] Using the cytochemical assay (which is more sensitive than the immunoassay) plasma ACTH concentrations ranging from 0.017 to 0.96 pg/ml were detected in hypopituitary patients whose plasma corticosteroid levels were undetectable by a fluorometric assay.[26] Significant, although small, absolute increases in such levels were seen in such patients following insulin-induced hypoglycemia.

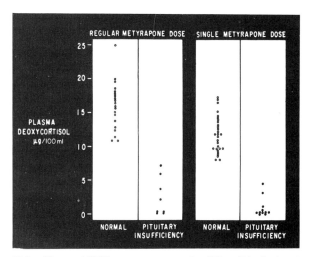

Fig. 93-8. Plasma ACTH responses to regular (750mg/4 h six times) and single (2–3 g at midnight) orally given metyrapone test in the same normal subjects and patients with pituitary insufficiency. Dots represent individual values at 8 AM.[99]

Table 93-5. Plasma ACTH and Cortisol Concentrations in Cushing's Disease or Syndrome

Clinical Condition	8:00 AM–9:00 AM		5:00 PM–6:00 PM	
	Plasma Cortisol (CBG Method)	Plasma ACTH (Immunoassay)	Plasma Cortisol	Plasma ACTH
Normal	8–20 μg/100 ml	20–140 pg/ml[91]*	4.4–11 μg/100 ml	10–88 pg/ml[43]*
Nontumorous adrenocortical hyperfunction	Normal or ↑	Usually moderately ↑	↑	↑
Adrenal adenoma	Normal or ↑	↓	↑	↓
Adrenal carcinoma	↑ ↑	↓	↑	↓
1° pituitary tumor	Normal or ↑	↑	↑	↑
"Ectopic" ACTH	↑ ↑	↑ ↑	↑ ↑	↑ ↑

*Mean.

PLASMA ACTH AS A POSSIBLE MARKER FOR MALIGNANCY (Asymptomatic "Ectopic" ACTH Production)

In 1968[100] it was noted that approximately one-third of patients with carcinoma of the lung (oat cell, squamous cell, or adenocarcinoma) and without evidence of endocrinopathy, had either elevated plasma corticosteroid levels, lack of normal suppressibility of such levels following dexamethasone administration, or elevated plasma ACTH concentrations. Insufficient detail was given to characterize the nature of the ACTH determined, and no control patients were studied. Later studies questioned whether these findings could be considered as simply being secondary to stress, since similar corticosteroid findings were present in chronically ill patients with malignancy of other etiologies. Subsequently, however, studies utilizing N-terminal, mixed, and C-terminal type ACTH antisera (see Fig. 93-1) as well as ACTH bioassay, reported increased immunoassayable and bioassayable ACTH concentrations in tumors from 14 patients with malignancy, who had no evidence of endocrinopathy.[101] The majority of these patients had carcinoma of the lung, either oat cell, squamous cell, or adenocarcinoma. All the levels were greater than those found in nontumorous tissue from patients dying suddenly from nonmalignant disease or in muscle tissue from a patient with malignant disease. Elevated tumor ACTH was also noted in single cases of pheochromocytoma, pleural mesothelioma, pancreatic, renal, or gastric carcinoma, and ileal carcinoid. Plasma ACTH concentrations were inadequately studied in this report.

Since "big" ACTH has been reported in the plasma of patients with the ectopic ACTH syndrome,[5] and this form of ACTH has minimal in vitro biologic activity,[7] it was considered possible that cases of tumor production of immunoreactive ("big") ACTH would be found in the absence of clinical manifestations of Cushing's syndrome. When this was looked for,[102] 53 percent of 83 patients with carcinoma of the lung had elevated afternoon plasma ACTH concentrations (greater than 150 pg/ml). Simultaneous plasma cortisol concentrations in 39 of 45 of these patients were noted to be less than 20 μg/100 ml (CBG method, normal 4–11 μg/ 100 ml). Elevated plasma ACTH concentrations were also found in 31 percent of patients with chronic obstructive pulmonary disease and in 28 percent of patients with other severe lung disease, as well as in 6 percent of control subjects. In the patients with carcinoma of the lung and chronic obstructive pulmonary disease, it was stated that 40 to 90 percent of the ACTH present in plasma was in the "big" form. Plasma from patients with other types of carcinoma was not studied. Immunoreactive ACTH was found in almost all tissue extracts of lung carcinoma in these patients, the predominant form being "big" ACTH. Tumor ACTH was also detected in one of seven insulinomas, and one of two non-beta-cell pancreatic tumors.

Increased immunoassayable and bioassayable plasma ACTH concentrations as well as increased immunoassayable/bioassayable plasma ACTH ratios have been noted, respectively, in 77, 55, and 78 percent of afternoon preoperative plasma specimens obtained in 13 patients with carcinoma of the lung without clinical manifestations of hypercortisolism (unpublished observations). Of these patients, 54 percent also had significant elevation of afternoon plasma cortisol concentrations. ACTH was detected in all of the eight tumors assayed. In these tumors, immunoreactive ACTH concentrations were higher than those of bioassayable ACTH, and controlled (10 sec) trypsinization of the tumor led to the finding of increased bioassayable ACTH concentrations, suggesting conversion from a "big" form.[7] It should also be noted, however, that we have seen elevated plasma ACTH levels and increased immunoassayable/bioassayable ratios in patients with gastrointestinal tumors, whose tumors contained no ACTH on assay. One might therefore speculate with regard to the role of chronic disease or "stress" in determining the nature of ACTH secretion.

The finding of increased and "abnormal" forms of ACTH in tumors and plasma specimens of patients with carcinoma and without clinical evidence of Cushing's syndrome is obviously of great theoretical interest. It may well be that such patients would eventually have developed the "ectopic" ACTH syndrome and are being detected at an earlier stage in their clinical course when the extent of the induced hypercortisolism is insufficient to produce clinical manifestations. The use of plasma ACTH determinations per se (without further characterization of an "abnormal" form by either gel filtration or comparison of immunoassayable and bioassayable ACTH concentrations) cannot be considered as a specific marker for neoplasm since ACTH is the product of a normal endocrine gland, and the stress of chronic illness or proposed operative procedures may be sufficient to cause elevation of plasma concentrations. There is no available information as to the effect of stress per se on the chemical forms of secreted ACTH. If abnormal forms of ACTH are found in screening of populations with pulmonary disease, it may be valid to follow plasma concentrations as evidence of the effectiveness of therapy or for evidence of recurrence. The presence of placental hormones in the serum of patients with carcinoma would serve as a better marker for neoplasia, since such hormones are never detected in the serum of normal individuals without malignant disease. However, the incidence of detection of such hormones (placental alkaline phosphatase, human placental lactogen, and human chorionic gonadotropin) is only 6 percent in patients with inoperable bronchogenic carcinoma,[103] which is far lower than that noted for the presence of "abnormal" forms of ACTH in such patients. Therefore, at the present time, determination and characterization of plasma ACTH offers a "marker" which identifies a higher percentage of patients with malignant disease than other available indices.

REFERENCES

1. Schuler, V. W., Schar, B., Desaulles, P.: Zur pharmakologie eines ACTH-wirksamen, vollsynthetischen polypeptids, des β^{1-24} cortico-tropins, Ciba 30920-Ba, synacthen. *Schweiz Med. Wochenschr. 93:* 1027–1030, 1963.

2. Lefkowitz, R. J., Roth, J.: Radioreceptor assay of adrenocortico-tropic hormone: New approach to assay of polypeptide hormones in plasma. *Science 170:* 663–635, 1970.

3. Landon, J., James, V. H. T., Cryer, R. J., et al: Adrenocorticotropic effects of a synthetic polypeptide-β^{1-24}-corticotropin in man. *J Clin Endocrinol 24:* 1206–1213, 1964.

4. Yalow, R. S., Berson, S. A.: Size heterogeneity of immunoreactive human ACTH in plasma and in extracts of pituitary glands and ACTH-producing thymoma. *Biochem Biophys Res Commun 44:* 439–445, 1971.

5. Yalow, R. S., Berson, S. A.: Characteristics of "big ACTH" in human plasma and pituitary extracts. *J Clin Endocrinol Metab 36:* 415–423, 1973.

6. Orth, D. N., Nicholson, W. E., Mitchell, W. M., et al: Biologic and immunologic characterization and physical separation of ACTH and ACTH fragments in the ectopic ACTH syndrome. *J Clin Invest 52:* 1756–1769, 1973.

7. Gewirtz, G., Schneider, B., Krieger, D., et al: Big ACTH: conversion to biologically active ACTH by trypsin. *J Clin Endocrinol Metab 38:* 227–230, 1974.

8. Schwyzer, R., Schiller, P., Seelig, S., et al: Isolated adrenal cells: Log dose response curves for steroidogenesis induced by ACTH$_{1-24}$, ACTH$_{1-10}$, ACTH$_{4-10}$ and ACTH$_{5-10}$. *FEBS Lett 19:* 229–231, 1971.

9. Fehm, H. L., Voigt, K. H., Lang, R., et al: Influence of plasma on ACTH stimulated corticosterone production of isolated adrenal cells. *FEBS Lett 36:* 109–112, 1973.

10. Bangham, D. R., Mussett, M. V., Stack-Dunne, M. P.: The third international standard for corticotropin. *Bull Org Mond Sante 27:* 395–408, 1962.

11. Sayers, M. A., Sayers, G., Woodbury, L. A.: The assay of adreno-corticotrophic hormone by the adrenal ascorbic acid-depletion method. *Endocrinology 42:* 379–393, 1948.

12. Lipscomb, H. S., Nelson, D. H.: A sensitive biologic assay for ACTH. *Endocrinology 71:* 13–23, 1962.

13. Sayers, G., Swallow, R. L., Giordano, N. D.: An improved technique for the preparation of isolated rat adrenal cells: A sensitive, accurate and specific method for the assay of ACTH. *Endocrinology 88:* 1063–1068, 1971.

14. Sayers, G., Beall, R. J.: Isolated adrenal cortex cells: Hypersensitivity to adrenocorticotropic hormone after hypophysectomy. *Science 179:* 1330–1331, 1973.

15. Sayers, G., Giordano, N. D.: Adrenal ascorbic acid depletion and isolated rat adrenal cell methods. In Berson, S. (general editor): Methods in Investigative and Diagnostic Endocrinology, vol IIA. American Elsevier, New York, 1973, p 359.

16. Liotta, A., Krieger, D. T.: A sensitive bioassay for the determination of human plasma ACTH levels. *J Clin Endocrinol Metab 40:* 268–277, 1975.

17. Wolfsen, A. R., McIntyre, H. B., Odell, W. D.: Adrenocorticotropin measurement by competitive binding receptor assay, *J Clin Endocrinol 34:* 684–689, 1972.

18. Hofman, K., Wingender, W., Finn, F. M.: Correlation of adrenocorticotropic activity of ACTH analogs with degree of binding to an adrenal cortical particulate preparation. *Proc Natl Acad Sci USA 67:* 829–836, 1970.

19. Daly, J. R., Loveridge, N., Bitensky, L., et al: The cytochemical bioassay of corticotrophin. *Clin Endocrinol 3:* 311–318, 1974.

20. Holdaway, I. M., Rees, L. H., Ratcliffe, J. G., et al: Validation of the redox cytochemical assay for corticotropin. *Clin Endocrinol 3:* 329–334, 1974.

21. Alaghband-zadeh, J., Daly, J. R., Bitensky, L., et al: The cytochemical section assay for corticotrophin. *Clin Endocrinol 3:* 319–327, 1974.

22. Daly, J. R., Fleisher, M. R., Chambers, D. J., et al: Application of the cytochemical bioassay for corticotrophin to clinical and physiological studies in man. *Clin Endocrinol 3:* 335–345, 1974.

23. Ney, R. L., Shimuzu, N., Nicholson, W. E., et al: Correlation of plasma ACTH concentration with adrenocortical response in normal human subjects, surgical patients, and patients with Cushing's disease. *J Clin Invest 42:* 1669–1677, 1963.

24. Vance, V. K., Reddy, W. J., Nelson, D. H., et al: Adrenocorticotropic hormone in human plasma. *J Clin Invest 41:* 20–28, 1962.

25. Nelson, D. H., Sprunt, G., Mims, R. B.: Plasma ACTH determinations in 58 patients before or after adrenalectomy for Cushing's syndrome. *J Clin Endocrinol 26:* 722–728, 1966.

26. Holdaway, I. M., Rees, L. H., Landon, J.: Circulating corticotrophin levels in severe hypopituitarism and in the neonate. *Lancet ii:* 1170–1171, Nov 24, 1973.

27. Krieger, D. T., Gewirtz, G.: The nature of the circadian periodicity and suppressibility of immunoreactive ACTH levels in Addison's disease. *J Clin Endocrinol Metab 39:* 46–52, 1974.

28. Fehm, H. L., Voigt, K. H., Pfeiffer, E. F.: Problems and artifacts in ACTH assay. *Horm Metab Res 4:* 477–481, 1972.

29. Matsukura, S., West, C. D., Ichikawa, Y., et al: A new phenomenon of usefulness in the radioimmunoassay of plasma adrenocortico-tropic hormone. *J Lab Clin Med 77:* 490–499, 1971.

30. Orth, D. N.: Adrenocorticotrophic hormone and melanocyte stimulating hormone. in Jaffe, B. M., Behrman, H. R. (eds): *Methods of Hormone Radioimmunoassay*. Academic Press, New York, 1974, pp 125–159.

31. Berson, S. A., Yalow, R. S.: Radioimmunoassay of ACTH in plasma. *J Clin Invest 47:* 2725–2751, 1968.

32. Landon, J., Greenwood, F. C.: Homologous Radioimmunoassay for plasma-levels of corticotrophin in man. *Lancet Feb 10:* 273–276, 1968.

33. Orth, D. N., Island, D. P., Nicholson, W. E., et al: ACTH radioimmunoassay: Interpretation, comparison with bioassay and clinical application. In Hayes, R. L., Goswitz, F. A., Murphy, B. E. P. (eds): Radioisotopes in Medicine. U.S. Atomic Energy Commission, 1968, pp 251–272.

34. Rees, L. H., Cook, D. M., Kendall, J. W., et al: A radioimmunoassay for rat plasma ACTH. *Endocrinology 89:* 254–261, 1971.

35. Krieger, D. T., Allen, W.: Relationship of bioassayable and immunoassayable plasma ACTH and cortisol concentrations in normal subjects and in patients with Cushing's disease. *J Clin Endocrinol Metab. 40:* 675–687, 1975.

36. Matsuyama, H., Harada, G., Ruhmann-Wennhold, A., et al: A comparison of bioassay and radiommunoassay for plasma cortico-tropin in man. *J Clin Endocrinol 34:* 713–717, 1972.

37. Chaye, J., Bitensky, L., Daly, J. R.: Cytochemical bioassay of hormones. *Life Sci 15:* 191–201, 1974.

38. Besser, G., Orth, D. N., Nicolson, W. E., et al: Dissociation of the disappearance of bioactive and radioimmunoreactive ACTH from plasma in man. *J Clin Endocrinol 32:* 595–603, 1971.

39. Gallagher, T. F., Yoshida, K., Roffwarg, J. D., et al: ACTH and cortisol secretory patterns in man. *J Clin Endocrinol Metab 36:* 1058–1068, 1973.

40. Besser, G. M., Cullen, D. R., Irvine, W. J., et al: Immunoreactive corticotrophin levels in adrenocortical insufficiency. *Br Med J 1:* 374–376, 1971.

41. Yalow, R. S., Glick, S. M., Roth, J., et al: Radioimmunoassay of plasma ACTH. *J Clin Endocrinol Metab 24:* 1219–1223, 1964.

42. Wolf, R. L., Mendlowitz, M., Soffer, L. J., et al: Metabolism of corticotropin in man. *Proc Soc Exp Biol Med 119:* 244–248, 1965.

43. Meakin, J. W., Bethune, J. E., Despointes, R. H., et al: Rate of disappearance of ACTH activity from blood. *J Clin Endocrinol Metab 19:* 1491–1494, 1959.

44. Urquhart, J.: Physiological actions of adrenocorticotrophic hormone, in Handbook of Physiology. American Physiological Society, Washington, D.C., 1974, pp. 133–158.

45. Upton, V. G., Hollinsworth, D. R., Lande, S., et al: Comparison of purified human and porcine ACTH in man. *J Clin Endocrinol 30:* 190–195, 1970.

46. Daughaday, W.: The adenohypophysis. In Williams, R. H. (ed): *Textbook of Endocrinology*. Saunders, Philadelphia, 1974, p 38.

47. Liddle, G. W., Island, D., Meador, C. K.: Normal and abnormal regulation of corticotropin secretion in man. *Rec Prog Horm Res 18:* 125–153, 1962.

48. Ney, R. L., Shimizu, N., Nicholson, W. E., et al: Correlation of

plasma ACTH concentration with adrenocortical response in normal human subjects, surgical patients, and patients with Cushing's disease. *J Clin Invest 42:* 1669–1677, 1963.

49. Braunsberg, H., James, V. H. T.: The fluorometric determination of adrenocortical steroids. *Anal Biochem 1:* 452–468, 1960.

50. Murphy, B. E. P.: Some studies of the protein-binding of steroids and their application to the routine micro and ultramicro measurement of various steroids in body fluids by competitive protein-binding radioassay. *J Clin Endocrinol 27:* 973–990, 1967.

51. Vecsei, P.: Glucocorticoids: cortisol, corticosterone and compound C. In Jaffe, B. M., Behrman, H. R. (eds): Methods of Hormone Radioimmunoassay. Academic Press, New York, 1974, pp 393–415.

52. Nielsen, E., Asfeldt, V. H.: Studies on the specificity of fluorimetric determination of plasma corticosteroids ad Modum De Moor and Steeno. *Scand J Clin Lab Invest 20:* 185–194, 1967.

53. Vecsei, P., Penke, B., Katzy, R., and Baek, L.: Radioimmunoassay of plasma cortisol. *Experientia 28:* 1104–1105, 1972.

54. Ruder, H. J., Guy, R. L., Lipsett, M. B.: A radioimmunoassay for cortisol in plasma and urine. *J Clin Endocrinol 35:* 219–224, 1972.

55. Nabors, C. J., Jr., West, C. D., Mahajan, D. K., et al: Radioimmunoassay of human plasma corticosterone: Method, measurement of episodic secretion and adrenal suppression and stimulation. *Steroids 23:* 363–378, 1974.

56. Krieger, D. T., Allen, W., Rizzo, F., et al: Characterization of the normal temporal pattern of plasma corticosteroid levels. *J Clin Endocrinol Metab 32:* 266–284, 1971.

57. de Lacerda, L., Kowarski, A., Migeon, C. J.: Integrated concentration and diurnal variation of plasma cortisol. *J Clin Endocrinol Metab 36:* 227–248, 1973.

58. de Moor, P., Osinski, P., Deckx, R., et al: The specificity of fluorometric corticoid determinations. *Clin Chim Acta 7:* 475–480, 1962.

59. Silverberg, A., Rizzo, F., Krieger, D. T.: Nyctohemeral periodicity of plasma 17-OHCS levels in elderly subjects. *J Clin Endocrinol Metab 28:* 1661–1663, 1968.

60. Peterson, R. E., Wyngaarden, J. B., Guerra, S. L., et al: The physiological disposition and metabolic fate of hydrocortisone in man. *J Clin Invest 34:* 1779–1785, 1955.

61. Roth, J.: Recent Progress in Hormone Research, vol 30. Academic Press, New York, 1974.

62. Espiner, E. A., Donald, R. A., Hart, D. S., et al: Evidence for adrenocortical uptake of ACTH in vivo. *Am J Physiol 226:* 96–104, 1974.

63. McDonald, R. K., Sollberger, A. R., Mueller, P. S., et al: The effect of small doses of human ACTH on serum corticosteroid levels in man. *Proc Exp Biol Med 131:* 1091–1094, 1969.

64. Urquhart, J.: Blood-borne signals: The measuring and modeling of humoral communication and control. *Physiologist 13:* 7–39, 1970.

65. Urquhart, J.: Adrenal blood flow and the adrenocortical response to corticotropin. *Am J Physiol 209:* 1162–1168, 1965.

66. Saffran, M., Rowell, P.: Response of rat adrenal tissue to ACTH in a flowing system. *Endocrinology 85:* 652–656, 1969.

67. Koritz, S. B., Hall, P. F.: End product inhibition of the conversion of cholesterol to pregnenolone in an adrenal extract. *Biochemistry 3:* 1298–1304, 1964.

68. Eik-Nes, K., Sandberg, A. A., Nelson, D. H., et al: Changes in plasma levels of 17-hydroxycorticosteroids during the intravenous administration of ACTH. I. A test of adrenocortical capacity in the human. *J Clin Invest 33:* 1502–1508, 1954.

69. Urquhart, J., Li, C. C.: The dynamics of adrenocortical secretion. *Am J Physiol 214:* 73–85, 1968.

70. Hodges, J. R., Sadow, J.: Impairment of pituitary adrenocorticotrophic function by corticosterone in the blood. *Br J Pharmacol Chemother 30:* 385–391, 1967.

71. Dallman, M. F., Yates, F. E.: Dynamic asymmetries in the corticosteroid feedback path and distribution-metabolism-binding elements of the adrenocortical system. *N.Y. Acad Sci 156:* 696–721, 1969.

72. Yates, F. E., Maran, J. W., Cryer, G. L., et al: The pituitary adrenal cortical system: stimulation and inhibition of secretion of corticotropin. In Handbook of Physiology. American Physiological Society, Washington, D.C., pp 367–404.

73. Kendall, J. W.: Feedback control of ACTH secretion. In Martini, L., Ganong, W. F. (eds): Frontiers in Neuroendocrinology. Oxford University Press, New York, 1971, pp 177–207.

74. Grizzle, W. E., Dallman, M. F., Schramm, L. P., et al: Inhibitory and facilitatory hypothalamic areas mediating ACTH release in the cat. *Endocrinology 95:* 1450–1461, 1974.

75. Krieger, H. P., Krieger, D. T.: Chemical stimulation of the brain: Effect on adrenal corticoid release. *Am J Physiol 218:* 1632–1641, 1970.

76. Bethune, J. E., Nelson, D. H., Thorn, G. W.: Plasma adrenocorticotrophic hormone in Addison's disease and its modification by the administration of adrenal steroids. *J Clin Invest 36:* 1701–1707, 1957.

77. Pollock, J. J, Labella, F. S.: Inhibition by cortisol of ACTH release from anterior pituitary tissue in vitro. *Can J Physiol Pharmacol 44:* 549–555, 1966.

78. Zimmerman, E., Critchlow, V.: Negative feedback and pituitary-adrenal function in female cats. *Am J Physiol 216:* 148–155, 1969.

79. Krieger, D. T., Allen, W., Rizzo, F., et al: Characterization of the normal temporal pattern of plasma corticosteroid levels. *J Clin Endocrinol Metab 32:* 266–284, 1971.

80. James, V. H. T., Landon, J.: The investigation of hypothalamic-pituitary-adrenal function. *Mem. Soc Endocrinol 17:* 39–72, 1968.

81. Takebe, K., Kunita, H., Sakakura, M., et al: Effect of dexamethasone on ACTH release induced by lysine vasopressin in man; time interval between dexamethasone and vasopressin inspection. *J Clin Endocrinol 28:* 644–650, 1968.

82. Takebe, K., Kunita, H., Sakakura, M., et al: Suppressive effect of dexamethasone on the rise of CRF activity in the median eminence induced by stress. *Endocrinology 89:* 1014–1019, 1971.

83. Sirett, N. E., Gibbs, F. P.: Dexamethasone suppression of ACTH release: Effect of the interval between steroid administration and the application of stimuli known to release ACTH. *Endocrinology 85:* 355–359, 1969.

84. Dallman, M. F., Jones, M. T.: Corticosteroid feedback control of ACTH secretion: Effect of stress-induced corticosterone secretion on subsequent stress responses in the rat. *Endocrinology 92:* 1367–1375, 1973.

85. Dallman, M. F., Jones, M. T., Vernikos-Danellis, J., et al: Corticosteroid feedback control of ACTH secretion: Rapid effects of bilateral adrenalectomy on plasma ACTH in the rat. *Endocrinology 91:* 961–968, 1972.

86. Buckingham, J. C., Hodges, J. R.: Interrelationships of pituitary and plasma corticotrophin and plasma corticosterone in adrenalectomized and stressed, adrenalectomized rats. *J Endocrinol 63:* 213–222, 1974.

87. Matsuyama, H., Mims, R. B., Ruhmann-Wennhold, A., Nelson, D. H. Bioassay and radioimmunoassay of plasma ACTH in adrenalectomized rats. *Endocrinology 88:* 696–701, 1971.

88. Jubiz, W., Matsukura, S., Meikle, A. W., et al: Plasma metyrapone, adrenocorticotropic hormone, cortisol and deoxycortisol levels. *Arch Intern Med 125:* 468–471, 1970.

89. Graber, A. L., Ney, R. L., Nicholson, W. E., et al: Natural history of pituitary-adrenal recovery following long-term suppression with corticosteroids. *J Clin Endocrinol 25:* 11–16, 1965.

90. Bohus, B.: Central nervous structure and the effect of ACTH and corticosteroids on avoidance behavior. In De Weid, D., Weijnen, J. A. W. M. (eds): Progress in Brain Research, vol 32. Elsevier, Amsterdam, 1970, pp 170–185.

91. Donald, R. A.: Plasma immunoreactive corticotrophin and cortisol response to insulin hypoglycemia in normal subjects and patients with pituitary disease. *J Clin Endocrinol 32:* 225–231, 1971.

92. Ichikawa, Y., Nishikai, M., Kawagow, M., et al: Plasma corticotropin, cortisol and growth hormone responses to hypoglycemia in the morning and evening. *J Clin Endocrinol 34:* 895–898, 1972.

93. Demura, R., Demura, H., Nunokawa, T., et al: Responses of plasma ACTH, GH, LH and 11-hydroxycorticosteroids to various stimuli in patients with Cushing's syndrome. *J Clin Endocrinol 34:* 852–859, 1972.

94. Staub, J. J., Jenkins, J. S., Ratcliffe, J. G., et al: Comparison of corticotrophin and corticosteroid response to lysine vasopressin, insulin and pyrogen in man. *Br Med J 1:* 267–269, 1973.

95. Strott, C. A., Nankin, H., Nugent, C. A.: A phenylalanine-lysine-vasopressin test of ACTH release. *J Clin Invest 27:* 448–451, 1967.

96. Takebe, K., Setaishi, C., Hirama, M., et al: Effects of a bacterial pyrogen on the pitituitary adrenal axis at various times in the 24 hours. *J Clin Endocrinol 26:* 437–442, 1966.

97. Ichikawa, Y., Kawagoe, M., Nishikai, M., et al: Plasma corticotropin (ACTH), growth hormone (GH), and 11-OHCS (hydroxycorticosteroid) response during surgery. *J Lab Clin Med 78:* 882–890, 1971.

98. Krieger, D. T., Gewirtz, G. P.: Recovery of hypothalamic-pituitary-

adrenal function, growth hormone responsiveness and sleep EEG pattern in an adrenal cortical adenoma. *J Clin Endocrinol Metab 38:* 1075–1082, 1974.

99. Jubiz, W., Meikle, A. W., West, C. D., et al: Single-dose metyrapone test. *Arch Intern Med 125:* 472–474, 1970.

100. Hauger-Klevene, J. H.: Asymptomatic production of ACTH: Radio immunoassay in squamous cell, oat cell and adenocarcinoma of the lung. *Cancer 22:* 1262–1267, 1968.

101. Ratcliffe, J. G., Knight, R. A., Besser, G. M., et al: Tumour and plasma ACTH concentrations in patients with and without the ectopic ACTH syndrome. *J Clin Endocrinol 1:* 27–44, 1972.

102. Gewirtz, G., Yalow, R. S.: Ectopic ACTH production in carcinoma of the lung. *J Clin Invest 53:* 1022–1032, 1974.

103. Rosen, S. W., Weintraub, B. D., Vaitukaitis, J. L., et al: Placental proteins and their subunits as tumor markers. *Ann Intern Med 82:* 71–83, 1975.

Laboratory Tests for the Diagnosis of Cushing's Syndrome and Adrenal Insufficiency and Factors Affecting Those Tests

Charles D. West
A. Wayne Meikle

INTRODUCTION

Suitable laboratory methods for measuring adrenocortical steroids and related hormones in patients have been developed only during the past 25 years. Prior to that time physicians were almost totally dependent on their clinical skills for the diagnosis of adrenal insufficiency and Cushing's syndrome. At the present time many laboratory tests are available for this purpose. Unfortunately, none of these laboratory tests are absolutely reliable; they all have their advantages and disadvantages.

This chapter was written to help physicians select the best and most appropriate adrenal function tests for their purposes. An understanding of the basic physiology and pathophysiology involved in adrenal function testing is absolutely essential to accomplish this goal, and will be reviewed. Most of the adrenal function tests in use today will be critically evaluated using practical clinical criteria such as diagnostic reliability, availability, cost, and patient welfare. Finally, recommendations will be given as to which laboratory tests should be used for specific problems in the diagnosis of adrenal insufficiency and Cushing's syndrome. (See Chapter 99.)

BASIC PHYSIOLOGICAL PRINCIPLES IN TESTING ADRENOCORTICAL FUNCTION

STEROID HORMONES SECRETED BY THE ADRENAL CORTEX

The adrenal cortex secretes all classes of biologically active steroids: glucocorticoids, mineralocorticoids, androgens, and estrogens. All of these hormones may be overproduced in Cushing's syndrome and underproduced in adrenal insufficiency, but adrenal function tests for the diagnosis of these diseases are concerned primarily with cortisol production and metabolism. From the standpoint of laboratory diagnosis, Cushing's syndrome may be equated with hypercortisolism and adrenal insufficiency to hypocortisolism. Other steroids may have an effect in some adrenal function tests and will be discussed for this reason.

Most methods used to measure cortisol and its metabolites are nonspecific and measure other steroids as well. To interpret many adrenal function tests correctly it is important to know what steroids are being measured and which ones are produced by the adrenal cortex in what amounts.

Methods used to measure cortisol and its metabolites may also measure corticosterone, cortisone, and their metabolites to a greater or lesser degree, depending on the methods used. The amounts of these three glucocorticoids produced daily by normal subjects, their concentration in plasma at 8 A.M., and their relative biological potencies are given in Table 94-1.

In man the normal adrenal cortex secretes much more cortisol per day (10–30 mg) than any other steroid except dehydroepiandrosterone sulfate (DHEAS). The concentration of cortisol in plasma (5–25 μg/dl) also far exceeds that of any other steroid except DHEAS (100–250 μg/dl). In man cortisol is primarily responsible for maintaining life. Corticosterone performs this function in many animals. On a weight basis corticosterone has about half as much glucocorticoid activity as cortisol and about 1.5 times as much mineralocorticoid activity. Man produces substantial amounts of corticosterone (about one-fifth as much as cortisol) and plasma concentrations are fairly high (about 1/20th as high as cortisol), but it is uncertain whether corticosterone has a specific physiological function in man.

Among the glucocorticoids, cortisone is second only to cortisol in terms of plasma concentration (about 1/10th as high as cortisol). Most of the cortisone in blood is not secreted by the adrenal cortex but is derived from the metabolism of cortisol by peripheral tissues.[1-3] Probably less than 20 percent of the cortisone in blood is actually secreted by the adrenal. Accurate measurements of the amount of cortisone secreted or produced per day are not available because of methodological difficulties.

The normal adrenal cortex secretes little androgen directly into the bloodstream but does secrete relatively inactive C-19 precursor steroids that are converted to testosterone by the liver and other peripheral tissues.[4-10] These precursor steroids include Δ^4-androstenedione, DHEA, and DHEAS. Forty to sixty percent of the testosterone in the blood of women arises from the peripheral conversion of Δ^4-androstenedione. Another 4 to 15 percent comes from the metabolism of DHEA and DHEAS. The remaining fraction ($\approx$25 percent) is probably secreted by the adrenal cortex and the ovaries. In men most of the blood testosterone is secreted by the testes. Although androgen production may be abnormal in adrenal insufficiency and Cushing's syndrome, androgens are seldom measured for the diagnosis of these disorders. Androgen determinations are important in the diagnosis of virilizing syndromes which may be of adrenal origin (see Chapter 97).

11-Deoxycortisol (S) is the immediate precursor of cortisol and is not normally an important secretory product of the adrenal cortex. However, in the metyrapone adrenal function test large amounts of S are secreted and plasma concentrations rise to very high levels if both the adrenal cortex and anterior pituitary are functionally intact. Plasma S determinations can be used in this way to assess both adrenal and pituitary function with a high degree of reliability.[11]

An inadequate production of aldosterone by the adrenal cortex is very important in the pathogenesis of many of the clinical findings in adrenal insufficiency. However, aldosterone determinations are not commonly used in the laboratory diagnosis of adrenal insufficiency, primarily because of methodological difficulties. In the laboratory diagnosis of Cushing's syndrome, aldosterone determinations are not useful because they are usually normal.

The normal adrenal cortex unquestionably secretes small amounts of estrogens, and in Cushing's syndrome urinary estrogens are modestly increased. The effect of adrenal insufficiency on

Table 94-1. Major Adrenal Glucocorticoids

Steroid	Relative Glucocorticoid Activity	Relative Mineralocorticoid Activity	8 AM Plasma Concentration (Mean ± SD)	Production Rate (mg/day)
Cortisol	1.0	1.0	13.5 ± 3.5	10–30
Cortisone	0.8	0.8	2.6 ± 0.5	—
Corticosterone	0.5	1.5	0.5 ± 0.3	1.5–44

total body estrogen production is not known. No adrenal function tests for adrenal insufficiency or Cushing's syndrome based on estrogen measurements have been developed. Estrogen determinations are useful in the diagnosis of the feminizing adrenogenital syndrome.

CORTISOL IS SECRETED EPISODICALLY IN A DIURNAL RHYTHM

For a long time it was thought that cortisol was secreted more or less continuously by the adrenal cortex and that plasma cortisol levels increased and decreased slowly over a 24-h period, with maximum levels occurring during sleep in the early morning hours and minimum levels occurring late at night just prior to sleep. This diurnal variation has been referred to as the normal nyctohemeral rhythm for adrenal function. It has also been known for some time that single plasma cortisol determinations are not very reliable in the diagnosis of either Cushing's syndrome or adrenal insufficiency. Normal subjects and eucorticoid patients frequently have plasma cortisol values that are high and consistent with Cushing's syndrome or low and suggestive of adrenal insufficiency. Furthermore, patients with established Cushing's syndrome or adrenal insufficiency often have normal plasma cortisol levels.

The explanation for these apparently paradoxical findings was made clear by the demonstration by Weitzman et al.[12] that cortisol is not secreted continuously but is secreted intermittently throughout the day for short periods of time lasting only a few minutes. Between these short bursts of secretion the adrenal cortex may not secrete any cortisol for several minutes to hours. This secretory process has been called "episodic secretion." Most secretory episodes occur at night during sleep and the fewest before midnight, which explains the nyctohemeral rhythm observed previously.

Episodic secretion (coupled with a rapid clearance of cortisol from the bloodstream) results in rapid and wide fluctuations in plasma cortisol concentrations and accounts for the overlap in plasma cortisol levels that have been observed between normal subjects and patients with Cushing's syndrome or adrenal insufficiency.

NEGATIVE FEEDBACK REGULATION OF CORTISOL AND ACTH SECRETION

An understanding of how the normal negative feedback mechanism operates to regulate the secretion of cortisol by the adrenal cortex and ACTH by the anterior pituitary is essential for using adrenal function tests appropriately and for interpreting the results correctly. The normal negative feedback mechanism has been discussed in detail elsewhere in this book (see Chapter 93). In primary adrenal insufficiency (caused by a destruction of the adrenal cortex) there is a striking increase in ACTH production resulting in plasma ACTH concentrations that are sustained at very high levels in an attempt to compensate for the cortisol deficiency. One of the best ways to test for adrenal insufficiency is to measure ACTH and cortisol levels in the same plasma sample. A very high plasma ACTH associated with a low plasma cortisol level makes the diagnosis of primary adrenal insufficiency highly probable. No other interpretation is likely. On the other hand, a low plasma ACTH coupled with a low cortisol indicates that the adrenal insufficiency is secondary to or caused by an insufficiency in ACTH production by the pituitary.

In Cushing's syndrome the simultaneous measurement of plasma ACTH and cortisol is primarily useful in the differentiation between adrenal hyperplasia and adrenal tumors as the cause of Cushing's syndrome. In patients with adrenal tumors the autonomous overproduction of cortisol causes a suppression in ACTH production and plasma ACTH concentrations are very low (usually immeasurable). On the other hand, the overproduction of cortisol in patients with adrenal hyperplasia is caused by an overproduction of ACTH by the pituitary.

CORTISOL TRANSPORT IN BLOOD: CORTISOL BINDING BY PLASMA PROTEINS

Cortisol is relatively insoluble in water, and is solubilized for transport in blood by binding to two plasma proteins, an α-2 globulin called cortisol binding globulin (CBG) and albumin. CBG has a molecular weight of approximately 52,000 and binds cortisol strongly with an affinity constant (K_a) on the order of 10^8 liters/mol. The concentration of CBG in plasma is relatively low (30 mg/dl) and CBG has only one cortisol receptor site per molecule. Consequently, CBG has a low capacity for binding cortisol even though it binds strongly. The binding sites on CBG are saturated by plasma cortisol concentrations of approximately 20 μg/dl.[13–15]

Albumin has a much greater capacity for binding cortisol (since there is so much more of it in plasma), but its binding is much weaker (K_a 10^3 liters/mol or 100,000 times less than CBG). Under normal conditions the high affinity binding prevails and most of the cortisol in blood (75 percent) is bound to CBG. Approximately 15 percent is bound to albumin, and the remaining 10 percent is unbound or "free" cortisol.

Free or unbound cortisol in plasma is the biologically active form at the tissue and cellular level. Since it is not bound to plasma proteins it is able to move out of the bloodstream into tissue cells where it acts. It is really the concentration of free cortisol in plasma that determines the physiological adrenal status of the patient. As free cortisol moves out of the blood into tissues, it is rapidly replenished from the bound fraction. In this way CBG acts as a reservoir that maintains a constant level of free cortisol for tissues in spite of wide fluctuations in cortisol secretion and metabolism.

Since free cortisol is the biologically active fraction of the total cortisol in plasma, the measurement of plasma free cortisol levels constitutes an excellent test of adrenal function. Unfortunately, methods for measuring plasma free cortisol are difficult and impractical for clinical use. The total amount (both bound and free) of cortisol in plasma is usually measured in patients.

CBG is important in assessing adrenal function for two practical reasons: (1) The total plasma cortisol level is dependent on the plasma CBG level and directly proportional to it, and (2) excellent methods for measuring not only cortisol but many other steroids have been developed using CBG as the binding protein in radioassays. Fluctuations in plasma CBG levels may be responsible for very low or very high plasma cortisol concentrations in eucorticoid patients that may be erroneously interpreted to indicate adrenal disease. Estrogen excess is the single most important factor that increases plasma CBG and cortisol concentrations in eucorticoid patients. CBG is synthesized by the liver and estrogens stimulate CBG production.[16–18] High plasma cortisol levels in eucorticoid patients are encountered frequently in practice because of the large number of women taking estrogen-containing oral contraceptive medications.

Low plasma cortisol levels secondary to a CBG insufficiency are encountered most often in patients with severe liver disease who are unable to synthesize adequate amounts of CBG, or in patients with plasma-protein-losing diseases such as nephrosis, exudative enteropathies, or multiple myeloma.[18-21] A rare inherited defect in CBG synthesis that causes low plasma cortisol in eucorticoid patients has also been reported.[22]

CBG binds steroids other than cortisol and can be used in radioassays to measure these steroids. Steroids that can be assayed in this manner are listed in Table 94-2 along with the strength of their binding relative to cortisol. The principles of radioassay methods are discussed later.

THE REMOVAL OF CORTISOL FROM THE BLOODSTREAM

Alterations in the rate at which cortisol is cleared from the bloodstream can obviously have a profound effect on adrenal function tests. The kinetics of cortisol removal from the bloodstream has been investigated intensively by many investigators with general agreement on the following conclusions: (1) Compared to other hormones the rate of cortisol turnover in the body occupies an intermediate position. The half-time of cortisol clearance from blood in normal subjects averages about 80 min. Many peptide hormones and other steroids are cleared much more rapidly, with half-times in the range of 15–30 min. On the other hand, thyroid hormones are cleared much more slowly, with half-times of several days. (2) The liver is primarily responsible for regulating the rate at which cortisol is removed from the bloodstream. Hepatic cells bind cortisol by means of high affinity protein receptors and metabolize it irreversibly to excretory products. Thus, a gradient is established that favors the flow of cortisol out of the bloodstream into hepatic cells. The magnitude of this gradient and the rate of liver blood flow are the major factors that control the rate at which cortisol is removed from the bloodstream. (3) Target tissues for cortisol action do not greatly influence cortisol clearance rates even though they have high affinity receptor sites that bind cortisol strongly. Presumably, the reason for this is that target cells do not metabolize cortisol and it reenters the circulation unaltered after it has acted. In addition, blood flow through most target tissues is relatively small compared to the liver.

The concentration of cortisol in plasma is controlled by the balance between the rate at which it leaves the circulation and the rate at which it enters. The entry rate is determined primarily by the rate of cortisol secretion by the adrenal cortex although a small fraction of the cortisol is derived from the peripheral conversion of cortisone. There are no other known sources for cortisol in blood. As discussed earlier, the rate at which cortisol leaves blood is determined primarily by the liver. Consequently, diseases that alter the capacity of the liver to concentrate and metabolize cortisol can cause abnormal adrenal function tests in patients without adrenal disease.

Table 94-2. Relative Binding of Steroids by CBG

Steroid	Relative CBG Binding (%)
Cortisol	100
Cortisone	25
Corticosterone	100
Aldosterone	10
11-Deoxycortisol	70
17-OHP	60
DOC	50

Source: From Murphy et al.[28]

CORTISOL METABOLISM BY THE LIVER AND OTHER PERIPHERAL TISSUES

Urinary metabolites of cortisol are frequently measured to assess adrenal function. The breakdown of cortisol to excretory products occurs primarily in liver by the enzymatic pathways shown in Figure 94-1. The reduction of the A ring is most important in the inactivation of cortisol. This reduction is accomplished in two sequential steps by two hepatic enzymes, a 5α-reductase that reduces the double bond between C4 and C5 and a 3β-ol dehydrogenase that converts the C3 ketone to a hydroxyl. The product of the first step is dihydrocortisol. Very little dihydrocortisol is secreted because it is rapidly converted to tetrahydrocortisol (THF). Part of the THF is reduced at C-20 to form cortols.

In the periphery, cortisol and cortisone are interconvertible, with the equilibrium favoring cortisol by a ratio of about 10:1. This interconversion is carried out by an 11β-ol dehydrogenase that is found in the liver, kidney, and other peripheral tissues. Recent evidence suggests that the kidney may be the most important site of this interconversion.[1] Because of this interconversion cortisol and cortisone share metabolic pathways. Consequently, THF, THE, cortols, and cortolones are major excretory products of both cortisol and cortisone. Together these excretory products account for approximately 80 percent of the cortisol produced, with 50 percent in THF and THE and 30 percent in the cortols and cortolones.

Five to ten percent of the cortisol produced is metabolized to 11-oxygenated 17-ketosteroids by the pathway shown in Figure 94-1 (11-β-OH-androstenedione and 11β-OH-etiocholanolone). Other steroids secreted by the adrenal cortex are metabolized to 17-ketosteroids, so that urinary 17-ketosteroid determinations are useful in certain selected situations. Roughly two-thirds of the urinary 17-ketosteroids in men (and over three-quarters in women) arise from the peripheral metabolism of C-19 steroids secreted by the adrenal cortex: Δ^4-androstenedione, dehydroepiandrosterone (DHEA), and DHEAS. In men most of the remaining one-third of the urinary 17-ketosteroids are derived from the metabolism of testosterone which is secreted by the testes.

There are other pathways for cortisol metabolism but at the present time the metabolites formed are not measured in the assessment of adrenal function.

Most of the major cortisol metabolites are rendered water soluble by conjugation with glucuronic acid. Only a small fraction of the cortisol metabolites is sulfated.

FUNDAMENTAL METHODOLOGICAL CONSIDERATIONS IN THE MEASUREMENT OF ADRENOCORTICAL HORMONES (CHEMISTRY, SPECIFICITY, RELIABILITY, SENSITIVITY, ACCURACY)

In recent years tremendous advances have been made in the development of methods for measuring cortisol and its metabolites in blood and urine. Less than 30 years ago only a few bioassays were available for measuring glucocorticoid activity. These were too insensitive and impractical for clinical use. Today we have highly specific methods that can measure less than 10^{-12} g of hormone reliably and easily. A brief chronological review of these advances in laboratory methodology seems appropriate for this chapter.

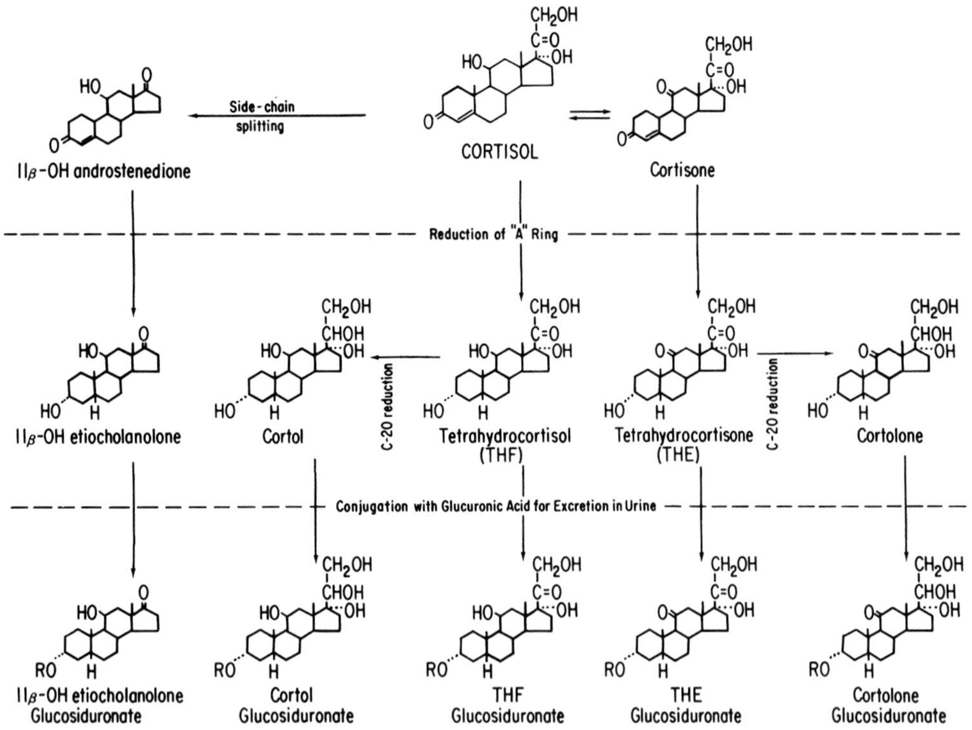

Fig. 94-1. Metabolism of cortisol by the liver.

17-KETOSTEROID DETERMINATIONS

In 1935 Zimmermann reported that 17-ketosteroids in urine could be measured colorimetrically by reacting crude urinary extracts with m-dinitrobenzene in alkali to form a pink derivative.[23] It was then observed that urinary 17-ketosteroids were frequently low in adrenal insufficiency and high in Cushing's syndrome. Unfortunately, with more experience urinary 17-ketosteroids proved to be unreliable in the diagnosis of adrenal hypo- and hyperfunction. The reasons for this unreliability are that less than 10 percent of the cortisol produced daily is metabolized to 17-ketosteroids, and most of the 17-ketosteroids are derived from biologically inactive C-19 steroids secreted by the adrenal and from testosterone which is secreted primarily by the testes.

Today, urinary 17-ketosteroid determinations should not be used as screening tests for adrenal insufficiency or Cushing's syndrome. As will be discussed later, better methods are available for diagnosing these diseases. Nevertheless, 17-ketosteroid determinations are still useful in special situations. One of these is in the diagnosis of adrenal tumors. Patients who have Cushing's syndrome or the virilizing or feminizing adrenogenital syndrome caused by an adrenal tumor (especially a carcinoma) will frequently excrete very large amounts of 17-ketosteroids in their urine. 17-ketosteroid measurements are not absolutely diagnostic in these adrenal diseases but they help in the diagnosis. 17-Ketosteroids are also useful in the diagnosis of congenital adrenal hyperplasia and in monitoring therapy.

Methods in which formaldehyde and acetaldehyde were generated from metabolites of cortisol and other glucocorticoids were developed next. They were capable of measuring milligram amounts of these steroids in urine, but they were not very useful clinically, primarily because of insensitivity and lack of specificity. Soon thereafter, sensitive photometric and fluorometric methods that could measure microgram amounts of cortisol and its metabolites in both plasma and urine were developed. These methods represented a real improvement in specificity and sensitivity and are still widely used today.

PORTER–SILBER STEROID ASSAYS

One of these photometric methods utilized the so-called Porter–Silber reaction, named after the investigators who first applied the reaction to the assay of corticosteroids.[24] Nelson and Samuels developed the first reliable "Porter–Silber" method for measuring cortisol in plasma.[25] In this assay C-21 steroids possessing a 17,21-dihydroxy, 20 keto configuration in the side chain react with phenylhydrazine in an acid solution to form a yellow derivative that can be measured colorimetrically. Compared with other steroid group assays, the Porter–Silber reaction is quite specific. It measures primarily cortisol and cortisone in plasma and tetrahydrocortisol and tetrahydrocortisone in urine. The latter urinary steroids are referred to most often as urinary 17-OH corticosteroids (17-OHCS) or occasionally as Porter–Silber urinary chromogens. It has been estimated that the Porter–Silber reaction measures about one-third of the urinary metabolites of cortisol.

The Porter–Silber reaction is not absolutely specific for these steroids. In CAH and with the urinary metyrapone test tetrahydro-S may be excreted in large amounts and measured by the Porter–Silber reaction. Naturally occurring nonsteroidal ketones (such as acetone) react with Porter–Silber reagents to give falsely elevated values. From a practical viewpoint these ketones are rarely a serious problem and should not cause confusion in the assessment of adrenal function. Certain drugs may also interfere, including commonly used ones such as antihypertensives (spironolactone), tranquilizers (Atarax, Vistaril, Librium), and antidepressants (Monase). For reliable results these drugs should be discontinued several days before Porter–Silber assays are done.

Over the years a greater clinical experience has been built up with the use of the Porter–Silber reaction than with any other assay for cortisol and its metabolites. In general the Porter–Silber assay has given satisfactory results and is still widely used.

FLUOROMETRIC ASSAYS FOR 11-OH CORTICOSTEROIDS

Any steroid possessing a Δ^4, α, β-unsaturated A ring and a 20-keto, 11β, 21-dihydroxy configuration will fluoresce in a mixture of sulfuric acid and alcohol and can be measured fluorometrically. Cortisol and corticosterone are the major steroids with this chemical configuration, and fluorometry is used primarily to measure these two steroids in plasma and urine. Steroids measured fluorometrically in this fashion are customarily called 11-OH corticosteroids (11-OHCS). Tetrahydro metabolites of cortisol, cortisone, and corticosterone and the cortols and cortolones cannot be measured in urine by fluorometry since they lack the appropriate A ring and side chain configuration.

Although fluorometric methods are quite specific for steroids, there are several nonsteroidal materials that interfere seriously with the assay, and limit its clinical usefulness. There are many drugs that fluoresce under the conditions of the assay, including quinine, quinidine, niacin, spironolactone, benzoyl alcohol, among others. In addition, unidentified fluorescent substances are often encountered in extracts of plasma and urine from patients with severe liver and kidney disease, severe malnutrition, and other diseases. Nonspecific fluorescence is also encountered frequently in extracts of normal plasma and urine. This nonspecific fluorescence causes high blanks in fluorometric methods that seriously limit their sensitivity and usefulness in measuring low amounts of 11-OHCS. Therefore, fluometric 11-OHCS determinations are not recommended for the diagnosis of adrenal insufficiency. If precautions are taken to eliminate interfering drugs, fluorometry is very useful in tests for Cushing's syndrome.

ASSAY FOR 17-KETOGENIC STEROIDS

When C-21 steroids with hydroxyl groups on C-17 and C-20 are reacted with periodate, the side chain is split off by oxidative cleavage between C-17 and C-20 and the corresponding 17-ketosteroid is formed. The quantity of 17-ketosteroids formed is measured by means of the Zimmermann reaction, giving rise to the name "17-ketogenic steroids." Cortols and cortolones are the major urinary metabolites of cortisol and cortisone that have the prerequisite side chain configuration and are measured as urinary 17-KGS. It is customary to reduce urinary extracts with borohydride prior to periodate oxidation for two reasons: (1) to eliminate endogenous 17-ketosteroids that are not derived primarily from cortisol by reducing the C-17 ketone to a hydroxyl, and (2) to convert THF and THE to cortol and cortolone (by reducing the C-20 ketone) so that they will also be measured.

Because the 17-KGS assay (with prior reduction) measures THF and THE as well as cortols and cortolones, a much larger fraction of the total urinary metabolites of cortisol is measured by the 17-KGS method than by the Porter–Silber method. Consequently, the 17-KGS method would appear to have a real advantage over the Porter–Silber method. However, the 17-KGS method also has disadvantages, one of which is that it measures steroids not derived from cortisol. 21-Deoxy, 20-keto, 17-OH steroids (such as pregnanetriol) which are not metabolites of cortisol are measured by the 17-KGS method and not by the Porter–Silber reaction. Glucose carried over into plasma and urine extracts can seriously suppress 17-KGS values. Several commonly used drugs, i.e., penicillin, meprobamate, and radioopaque dyes, may also interfere. From a practical standpoint interference from drugs and other materials does not often cause a serious problem, and 17-KGS determinations are widely used today to assess adrenal function.

RADIOASSAYS FOR ADRENAL STEROIDS AND ACTH: RADIOIMMUNOASSAYS, COMPETITIVE PROTEIN BINDING RADIOASSAYS, AND RADIORECEPTOR ASSAYS

With colorimetry and fluorometry, endocrine methodology advanced from the "milligram era" into the "microgram era" in which micrograms of hormones could be measured. Our ability to diagnose adrenal hypo- and hyperfunction improved greatly with the development of these photometric methods. However, they were inadequate for measuring many hormones that were known to be involved in adrenal function, such as ACTH and other adrenal steroids. Many of these hormones were measured in plasma and urine by gas chromatography and radioisotope dilution. These methods have not been used extensively in clinical medicine because of technical difficulties.

The routine measurement of picogram quantities of hormones in plasma and urine was made possible by the development of hormone "radioassays." Radioassay is a term used to cover all those methods that utilize protein binding and displacement of radioactve substrate, and includes radioimmunoassay (RIA), competitive protein binding (CPB), and radioreceptor assay (RRA). In 1959 Berson and Yalow developed the first hormone radioassay which was a radioimmunoassay for plasma insulin.[26] This assay was based on the displacement of radioactive insulin from insulin antibodies by unlabeled insulin. Since 1959 radioimmunoassays have been developed for several nonantigenic hormones as well as antigenic peptide hormones. In 1957 Erlanger and co-workers[27] prepared the way for developing steroid RIAs by demonstrating that antibodies could be produced to nonantigenic steroids by injecting animals with steroids conjugated to foreign proteins. However, the development of steroid RIAs was preceded by the development of steroid CPB radioassays that utilize plasma proteins (such as CBG) for the binding protein in radioassays instead of antibodies. In 1967 Murphy et al.[28] developed the first CPB radioassay for measuring plasma corticosteroids. Since then RIAs and CPB radioassays have been developed for virtually every adrenal steroid. Most recently, radioreceptor assays in which receptor proteins from target tissues are used have been developed.[29–31] Radioreceptor assays have not been widely used so far, primarily because of the instability of most receptor protein preparations. In the future RRAs may prove to have real advantages over RIA and CPB radioassays in terms of specificity and sensitivity.

It is beyond the scope of this chapter to discuss the methodology of radioassays in detail. Several monographs and books are available for more detailed information on methodology.[32–35] Most radioassays utilize the same basic principles and procedures, which are outlined briefly in the following.

A radioactive trace of the hormone being measured is added to a dilute solution of the hormone binding protein (antibody, plasma protein, or tissue receptor protein) to form a soluble protein–hormone complex. When "cold" or nonradioactive hormone is added, there is competition between the "cold" and radioactive hormone for the limited number of binding sites on the protein. In effect, the cold hormone "displaces" the labeled hormone from the protein binding solution. Quantitation results from the fact that the amount of radioactivity "displaced" from the protein is proportional to the amount of "cold" hormone added. This can be measured simply by separating the free hormone from the protein-bound hormone and counting the radioactivity.

Radioassays have several distinct advantages over other methods for measuring hormones. No other method is as sensitive yet as specific and convenient. Of all the hormones known to be produced by the adrenal cortex only cortisol was measured routinely in plasma for clinical diagnosis prior to the development of radioassays. With radioassays it is now possible to measure plasma concentrations of nearly every hormone produced by the adrenal cortex. In addition the peptide hormones that regulate adrenal function (ACTH and renin) can also be measured in plasma by radioassay. The availability of these radioassays has made possible many investigations that have given us a better understanding of adrenal physiology and pathophysiology.

Radioassays have been put to two practical uses: (1) They have displaced other methods for measuring hormones in established adrenal function tests. For example, plasma and urinary cortisol can be measured by radioassay instead of by the Porter–Silber reaction or fluorometry. Radioassay has also substituted for gas chromatography and radioisotope dilution methods in the measurement of aldosterone in plasma and urine. (2) Radioassays have made it possible to develop new laboratory tests for assessing different aspects of adrenal function. For example, plasma 17-OH-progesterone, Δ^5-17-OH-pregnenolone, progesterone, and DOC concentrations can be measured by radioassay for the diagnosis of congenital adrenal hyperplasia.[36–38] In the metyrapone test for adrenal and pituitary ACTH function plasma S responses can be measured instead of urinary 17-OH corticosteroids.[11]

Radioassays are not without disadvantages. Antisera for most RIAs are quite expensive at present because of the high cost of production, and may be difficult to obtain. In the future antisera should become more available and less expensive. The cost of CPB radioassays is already very reasonable because plasma proteins are readily available and inexpensive. The instability of tissue receptor proteins limits the clinical usefulness of RRAs at the present time.

In general radioassays are less precise than chemical methods, but this is not a serious problem. Coefficients of variation of 5 percent or less for assay precision are not unusual for chemical methods. Most radioassays have coefficients of variation in the 5 to 10 percent range. For most clinical purposes this precision is more than adequate.

METHODS FOR MEASURING CORTISOL PRODUCTION RATES AND METABOLIC CLEARANCE RATES

The amount of cortisol produced daily can be measured in patients using the principles of radioisotope dilution. To determine CPR a known amount of radioactive cortisol is injected intravenously and the rate of dilution with unlabeled cortisol produced endogenously is determined either by serial measurements of the specific activity of the cortisol in blood or from the dilution in specific activity of a urinary metabolite of cortisol. The former method is referred to as a "blood production rate" and the latter as a "urine production rate." From the rate of dilution of the labeled cortisol in blood the metabolic clearance rate can be calculated (conventionally expressed in terms of the milliliters of blood that are completely cleared of cortisol per minute, ml/min). The blood method also allows for calculation of other metabolic parameters, such as volume of distribution, turnover rate, half-time in blood, and removal rate constants. Recently a nonisotopic method in which cortisol production rates were calculated from episodic secretion data has also been reported.[12] For details of methods for measuring cortisol production rates the reader is referred to reviews and original publications.[39–41]

It seems reasonable to expect that the adrenocortical status of the body would be determined by the rate of cortisol production,

and that the measurement of CPR would accurately reflect adrenal function. That this expectation is well founded has been established by a wide experience with CPR determinations in patients with adrenal insufficiency and Cushing's syndrome. However, CPR determinations have serious disadvantages and are seldom done in patients except by research laboratories. Perhaps the main reason for this is that potentially hazardous radioactive hormones must be administered to patients. In addition, all CPR methods are complex, expensive, and time-consuming. There are also technical problems in measuring CPR. One of the basic tenets of the urine method is that the urinary metabolite used to measure radioisotope dilution must be derived exclusively from the hormone being measured. There appears to be no such unique urinary metabolite for cortisol. Recently it has been demonstrated that the simultaneous measurement of radioisotope dilution in different cortisol urinary metabolites resulted in CPR determinations that varied considerably.[42,43] This observation might account in part for the large normal range in CPR values and the overlap observed between normal subjects and some patients with adrenal dysfunction.

A potential problem in the measurement of CPR by blood methods has recently come to light. In the blood CPR method it is assumed that the metabolic clearance rate (MCR) for cortisol does not vary during the experimental period. The assumption is critical to blood CPR calculations. Recently it has been shown that the MCR for cortisol varies considerably throughout the day.[44] It has long been known that blood CPRs do not ordinarily agree with urine CPRs measured simultaneously in the same patient. Whether the MCR for cortisol varies enough during the experimental period to alter blood production rate calculations seriously is a problem that has not yet been resolved.

ALTERATIONS IN ADRENAL FUNCTION TESTS BY EXTRAADRENAL FACTORS

There are many extraadrenal factors that may alter adrenal function tests and cause errors in the diagnosis of Cushing's syndrome and adrenal insufficiency.

EFFECTS OF AGE

Age has a serious effect on adrenal function only in the very young and the very old. This effect of age has practical importance since both Cushing's syndrome and adrenal insufficiency occur in both extremes in age.

During the newborn period it may be very difficult to differentiate between normal eucorticoid infants and those with adrenal insufficiency. In contrast to the adult the newborn produces cortisone in preference to cortisol and low plasma cortisol levels by adult standards are normal in newborn infants.[45] Cortisone and cortisol are also metabolized differently and the major urinary excretory products are different. The newborn liver is deficient in adult enzymes that reduce the A ring in steroids and those that conjugate steroids with glucuronic acid.[46–48] Consequently, relatively little THE, THF, cortol, and cortolone (the most important metabolites in adults) is formed and excreted in the urine.[47,49] Clinical laboratory methods that measure these metabolites yield low values. Both urinary 17-OH corticosteroids (measured by the Porter–Silber reaction) and urinary 17-ketogenic steroids may be decreased to levels that can be mistaken for adrenal insufficiency.

To inactivate cortisol and cortisone and convert them to water-soluble excretory products, the newborn liver hydroxylates these steroids in the C-6 position.[46] Large amounts of C-6 hydroxylated steroids are excreted in the urine by newborns, and theoreti-

Table 94-3.   Summary of Laboratory Test Results in Adrenal Insufficiency

Test	Time	Treatment	Dose	Normal	1°	2°
Baseline	8 AM plasma cortisol (μg/dl)	None		5–28	N or ↓	N or ↓
	Plasma ACTH (pg/ml)	None		20–150	↑	N or ↓
Metyrapone	8 AM plasma S (μg/dl)	Metyrapone	30 mg/kg body wt. midnight	7–22	↓	↓
	Plasma cortisol (μg/dl)	ACTH	25 U 8 AM–2 PM	30–50	↓	N or ↓
Hypoglycemia	Plasma cortisol	0.1–0.4 U/kg body wt. iv		↑ >7 μg/dl	↓	↓
ACTH Stimulation		ACTH	40 U b.i.d. im × 3 day		↓	N
			Then 25 U 8 AM–2 PM	30–50		

cally they could be measured to assess adrenal function in the newborn. Unfortunately, there is no practical clinical method available for measuring C-6 hydroxylated steroids.

Adrenal steroid production and metabolism usually convert to the adult pattern within a few days after birth and adrenal function tests used in adults become reliable. By adult standards urinary 17-OHCS and 17-KGS values appear to be low during childhood but usually fall into the normal adult range if they are corrected for the difference in body weight and surface area. Urinary 17-ketosteroids are low during childhood but rise to adult levels beginning with adrenarche and increasing progressively through puberty. Prior to adrenarche (at about 8 years) urinary 17-ketosteroid values in milligrams per 24 h are usually less than half the chronological age of the patient.

Plasma cortisol concentrations and cortisol production rates usually rise to normal adult ranges within 1 week after birth. Plasma cortisol concentrations may not vary in the normal adult nyctohemeral pattern during the first year of life.[50]

Old age is associated with a modest decrease in cortisol production and metabolism that is occasionally of sufficient magnitude to be mistaken for adrenal insufficiency.

EFFECT OF NUTRITION

In massvely obese patients cortisol production may be increased, resulting in elevated urinary 17-OHCS, 17-KGS, and 17-KS and a possible erroneous diagnosis of Cushing's syndrome.[51–56] Plasma and urinary cortisols are not abnormal in obesity and can be used reliably to differentiate Cushing's syndrome from obesity.

In severe inanition the rate of both cortisol production and metabolism may decrease.[57–60] Conventional urinary corticosteroid determinations are often low. Paradoxically, plasma cortisol concentrations are either normal or high. Values in the Cushing's range may be encountered presumably because of a disproportionately greater decrease in cortisol clearance and metabolism than in production.

EFFECT OF PREGNANCY AND ESTROGENS[18,61,62]

During pregnancy plasma cortisol levels rise progressively into the Cushing's range because of an estrogen-induced increase in plasma CBG concentration. Plasma free cortisol is high normal or slightly increased as is urinary free cortisol. In contrast to the high levels in Cushing's syndrome, urinary 17-OHCS and 17-KGS values are decreased in pregnancy probably due to estrogen-induced hepatic enzymes that metabolize cortisol by different routes.

The administration of estrogens is associated with changes in cortisol metabolism that are quite similar to those occurring in pregnancy. Estrogen therapy in the form of oral contraceptives is by far the commonest cause of elevated plasma cortisol concentrations in our society today.

EFFECT OF LIVER DISEASE[63–67]

In patients with hepatic failure there is a decrease in the rate of cortisol removal from blood and an alteration in enzymatic inactivation by the liver. In hepatic failure 20α reduction of cortisone is favored over A ring reduction which is normally more important. Consequently, tetrahydrocortisone formation is decreased and 20α-cortolone is increased. Cortisol inactivation is not similarly affected. Tetrahydrocortisol and cortol formation is unchanged. Glucosiduronate conjugation is also reduced. These enzymatic alterations in liver failure result in (1) a decrease in urinary 17-OHCS measured by the Porter–Silber reaction, (2) an increase in urinary 17-KGS, and (3) a decrease in urinary 17-KS. The cortisol production rate is either low normal or slightly depressed.

In actual practice liver failure seldom causes problems in the diagnosis of adrenal diseases. Liver failure must be fairly far advanced to alter adrenal laboratory tests sufficiently to cause confusion. Plasma and urinary free cortisol values are not usually abnormal in liver failure and may help to exclude adrenal disease in the occasional problem case.

EFFECT OF RENAL DISEASE[53,68,69]

Since steroid glucuronides and sulfates are excreted by the renal glomerulus, it is not surprising that the excretion of commonly measured steroids in the urine is impaired in patients with renal failure in proportion to the reduction in glomerular filtration. Urinary steroid assays are often low and unreliable in patients with creatinine clearances of less than 50 ml/min. The excretion of unconjugated steroids is affected much later in the course of renal failure, probably because free steroids are strongly bound to plasma proteins and are reabsorbed in the renal tubule. Cortisol production rates and plasma cortisol concentrations usually remain within the normal range in renal failure.

EFFECT OF THYROID DYSFUNCTION[70–74]

Hyperthyroidism accelerates cortisol metabolism whereas hypothyroidism depresses it. Cortisol blood clearance and production rates are accelerated in hyperthyroidism and the excretion of all urinary metabolites is increased. Just the opposite occurs in hypothyroidism. Plasma cortisol levels are unaffected and are usually in the normal range.

EFFECT OF STRESS[75-80]

Of all the extraadrenal factors that interfere in laboratory tests for Cushing's syndrome, stress is probably most important because of its frequency. In addition, adrenal hyperfunction is a normal physiological response to stress and to differentiate this from the pathological hyperfunction in Cushing's syndrome by laboratory tests may be difficult or impossible depending on the severity of the stress. Cortisol production rates, plasma levels, and urinary metabolites may be increased to comparable levels in both stress and Cushing's syndrome. Adrenal stimulation and suppression tests are also frequently invalidated by stress. It is a good rule to delay adrenal function tests for Cushing's syndrome until after the stressful episode has passed.

Usually the stress must be acute and severe to result in Cushingoid values on laboratory testing, i.e., high fever, surgery, trauma, burns, and so on. Ordinarily, emotional stress is not severe enough to interfere with most adrenal function tests. Dexamethasone suppression tests are rarely invalidated by emotional stress. The diurnal variation in plasma cortisol concentrations may be disturbed at times. Abnormal adrenal function tests have been reported in patients with severe mental illnesses, especially those with chronic depression.

The stress of chronic diseases (such as rheumatoid arthritis, chronic pulmonary insufficiency) does not ordinarily alter cortisol metabolism as assessed by the usual clinical laboratory tests.

EFFECT OF DRUGS[81-86]

Drugs that are inducers of hepatic mixed function oxidases (such as diphenylhydantoin, phenobarbital, and o,p-DDD) modify the metabolism of cortisol and related glucocorticoids. 6-Hydroxylated steroids and probably other hydroxylated metabolites are increased in urine. As a consequence urinary 17-OHCS and 17-ketogenic determinations may be low in eucorticoid patients treated with these drugs. These medications also interfere greatly in dexamethasone suppression tests and metyrapone tests since they induce enzymes which inactivate dexamethasone and metyrapone and render them ineffective. As a consequence, Cushing's syndrome may be erroneously diagnosed in patients treated with these drugs because of a lack of normal suppression with dexamethasone. Similarly, pituitary or adrenocortical insufficiency may be diagnosed erroneously because of an apparent lack of response to metyrapone.

GENERAL CONSIDERATIONS IN LABORATORY TESTS FOR EVALUATING HYPOTHALAMIC–PITUITARY–ADRENAL FUNCTION

In many clinical situations, it is most useful to know whether a patient has normal, subnormal, or supranormal pituitary–adrenal secretory function. Normally ACTH and adrenal steroidal hormones are secreted episodically and also fluctuate in a diurnal pattern (see Chapter 93). Thus, baseline hormonal values are generally unsatisfactory for confirmation of pituitary–adrenal pathophysiology because values from normal individuals frequently overlap into the abnormal range. Tests designed to manipulate the normal adrenal physiology have proven more satisfactory because of less overlap between normals and abnormals. The results of these tests are highly reliable in the diagnosis of pituitary–adrenal disorders when they and the corresponding assays are properly performed. There are many potential pitfalls that produce erroneous results and consequently incorrect diagnoses. Many of these problems can be avoided (while maintaining excellent diagnostic accuracy) by utilizing the same tests while administering unconventional doses of the test drug or by using specialized laboratory assays.

LABORATORY TESTS RECOMMENDED FOR THE DIAGNOSIS OF HYPOFUNCTION OF THE HPA SYSTEM AS A WHOLE (PRIMARY AND SECONDARY ADRENAL INSUFFICIENCY)

Cortisol deficiency may result from insufficient ACTH secretion by the pituitary, secondary adrenal insufficiency, or from primary disorders of the adrenal gland. The etiology of adrenal insufficiency, either primary or secondary, is diverse and the laboratory approach to diagnosis is different for these two types but does not depend in most cases on the specific etiology. Secondary adrenal insufficiency may be due to tumors,[87-91] vascular insufficiency,[92,93] or numerous other etiologies[94-114] (see Chapter 18). Primary adrenal insufficiency also has multiple etiologies[115-119] (see Chapter 96). The factors to be considered in selecting an appropriate test are safety to the patient, convenience of its performance, and the availability of satisfactory assays. Evidence is lacking that any one of the following tests: metyrapone, insulin-induced hypoglycemia, pyrogen, or lysine vasopressin test, is more reliable than any other in the diagnosis of adrenal insufficiency. When properly performed, all of them test the functional integrity of the HPA axis.[91,120-126] Evidence that any of these specifically confirms a disorder of CRF or ACTH release is minimal at the present time, despite some claims that LVP selectively stimulates ACTH release.[125,127-129] There is some evidence that it may stimulate release of CRF as well.[129] A subnormal response to the test stimuli is considered as evidence of hypofunction. However, a severe stress such as surgery may produce a normal response. Most investigators have felt it desirable to err on the side of overdiagnosis of adrenal insufficiency rather than underdiagnosis. Thus, the metyrapone test has gained widespread popularity.

OVERNIGHT SINGLE DOSE METYRAPONE TEST

Rationale: Metyrapone inhibits the formation of cortisol by blocking 11β-hydroxylation. The negative feedback mechanism of the normal hypothalamic–pituitary system responds to the low plasma cortisol concentrations and ACTH is released. ACTH stimulates the adrenal cortex which then produces large quantities of the low potency glucocorticoid, S, because of the block in 11β-hydroxylation. Plasma S concentrations in normal subjects increase from less than 1 μg/dl to 7–22 μg/dl at 8 A.M. following a single dose of metyrapone at midnight. Its metabolite, tetrahydro-11-deoxycortisol (THS), a 17-OHCS measured as a Porter–Silber chromogen or as 17-KGS, is also excreted in larger quantities in the urine.[85,120,121]

Procedure[130-132]: Metyrapone, 30 mg/kg body weight, is given as a single oral dose at midnight with a small snack. An 8 A.M. plasma sample is collected in which the concentration of plasma S is measured by CPB radioassay after differential solvent extraction[11] or by a specific RIA.[133] A normal plasma S response to metyrapone is 7–22 μg/dl (Figure 94-2).

We have found the test to be safe in patients with both primary and secondary adrenal insufficiency, and have observed no cases with adrenal insufficiency in which the test produced acute adrenal crisis. The test should not be performed in patients with acute adrenal insufficiency. Instead, we recommend obtaining a plasma cortisol and then treating the patient for acute adrenal crisis.

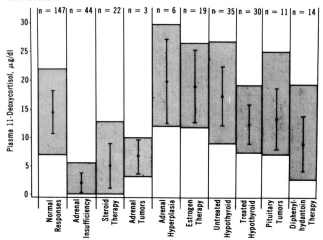

Plasma 11-deoxycortisol responses to single-dose metyrapone test in several groups of patients. Stippled areas represent ranges, dots represent means, and vertical lines are standard deviation.

Fig. 94-2. Single dose metyrapone test. (Spiger, M., et al: *Arch Intern Med 135:* 699, 1975.)

Interpretation: The metyrapone test was introduced by Liddle and associates[120] as a test of the pituitary's ability to secrete ACTH under stimulation through the normal negative feedback mechanism. It is now recognized as an excellent test of function for the entire HPA axis. A normal response indicates a normal function of the axis, and no additional tests of HPA function are indicated. An abnormal response to metyrapone indicates a defect somewhere in the HPA axis. The metyrapone test with steroid determinations only cannot be used to determine whether the adrenal, pituitary, or hypothalamus is defective. To determine the site of the defect other tests are required (as described later). Plasma ACTH determinations in association with the metyrapone test help distinguish between a defect of the adrenal and one of the pituitary. In primary adrenal disease plasma ACTH is high and in pituitary disease it is low (Figs. 94-3 and 94-4).

False positives (also see factors that may invalidate metyra-

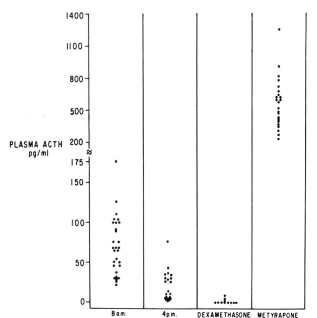

Fig. 94-3. Basal plasma ACTH levels in normal subjects at 8 AM, at 4 PM, and at 8 AM after dexamethasone or metyrapone administration. (Matsukura, S., et al: *J Lab Clin Med 77:* 496, 1971.)

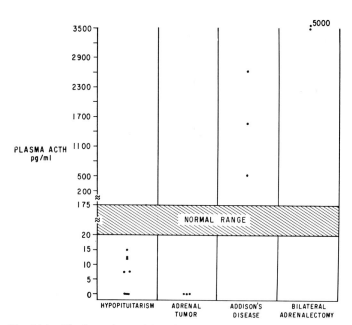

Fig. 94-4. The 8 AM plasma ACTH levels in those patients with hypopituitarism, adrenal tumors, Addison's disease, and postbilateral adrenalectomy for Cushing's syndrome with adrenal hyperplasia. (Matsukura, S., et al: *J Lab Clin Med 77:* 496, 1971.)

pone tests): Apparently because of rapid clearance of metyrapone and reduced metyrapone from plasma, approximately 4 percent of normal individuals fail to have a normal rise of plasma S with the single dose test.[132] To determine whether this has happened, cortisol should be measured in the postmetyrapone samples. Cortisol values greater than 20 µg/dl indicate inadequate suppression by metyrapone and an unsatisfactory test that cannot be interpreted. We recommend routinely measuring cortisol levels in all postmetyrapone samples with a low plasma S value.[132]

TWO-DAY MULTIPLE DOSE METYRAPONE TEST[11,85,120]

The rationale is the same as with the overnight single dose metyrapone test.

Procedure: Beginning at 8 A.M., 750 mg of metyrapone is ingested every 4 h for 6 doses.

Plasma S test: A plasma sample is collected at 8 A.M. or 4 h after the last dose. Normal subjects have plasma S levels of 10–30 µg/dl.

Urine test: Beginning at 8 A.M. 24-h urine collections are made for 3 days: the baseline (the day before), the day of metyrapone administration, and the day following. An increment of more than 6 mg of 17-OHCS or THS or 10 mg of 17-KGS (baseline versus the day after metyrapone) indicates normal HPA function.

The interpretation is the same as with the overnight dose metyrapone test.

False positives: Interfering chromogens from drugs are a problem with the urinary methods but not with the plasma methods. These problems are discussed in the section on factors that may invalidate metyrapone tests.

INSULIN-INDUCED HYPOGLYCEMIA TESTS

Rationale: Acute hypoglycemia is a potent stress that stimulates the release of ACTH from the pituitary.[91]

Procedure: Regular insulin, 0.1 U/kg body weight, is injected intravenously to reduce the plasma glucose to less than 40 mg/dl.[91] (An initial test with 0.05 U/kg may be desirable if hypopituitarism is suspected.) Plasma samples are collected at 0, 30, 60, 90, and 120 m for measurement of cortisol by CPB, RIA, or a fluorometric assay. An increment of greater than 7 μg/dl is considered normal. Caution: Patient must be observed throughout test for treatment of life-threatening hypoglycemia.

Interpretation: A normal response also excludes HPA dysfunction. If subnormal, it indicates adrenal insufficiency. As with the metyrapone test, simultaneous measurement of plasma ACTH values or performance of the ACTH stimulation test is also needed to differentiate between primary and secondary adrenal insufficiency.

Interference: Inhibitors of serotonin inhibit ACTH release induced by hypoglycemia.[134] Drugs producing fluorescence in plasma might be a problem in some individuals, if cortisol is measured with a fluorometric assay. We prefer the metyrapone test because it is simple, safe, and also highly reliable.

URINARY FREE CORTISOL
DETERMINATIONS[135,136]

Rationale: Urinary free cortisol is an index of the biologically active cortisol in plasma. As the free level increases or decreases in plasma, its excretion in the urine also changes. Data in patients with adrenal insufficiency are limited. Cortisol excretion appears to be an exponential function of the cortisol production rate.

Procedure: A baseline 24-h urine is collected for 24 h and then ACTH is infused at a rate of 4–6 U/h for 6–8 h. Normal subjects show large increases following ACTH (Fig. 94-5).

Interpretation: Patients with primary insufficiency have subnormal rises in response to ACTH. Those with secondary adrenal insufficiency will show normal increases if appropriately stimulated. If urinary free cortisol is specifically assayed after paper chromatography, preliminary data suggest it will establish adrenal hypofunction if assayed in baseline samples.

FACTORS THAT MAY INVALIDATE METYRAPONE TESTS—DETECTION AND CORRECTION OF FALSE TESTS

EFFECT OF DRUGS (ANTICONVULSANTS, ETC.) THAT CAUSE A RAPID INACTIVATION OF METYRAPONE BY INDUCING CATABOLIC HEPATIC ENZYMES

Rationale: Anticonvulsants increase the metabolism of metyrapone and reduce metyrapone by enhancing the activity of hepatic microsomal mixed oxidases. Therefore, metyrapone levels are low, 11β-hydroxylase inhibition is inadequate, and the response of the HPA axis is subnormal. The plasma concentration of metyrapone can be increased sufficiently in patients receiving anticonvulsants to stimulate a normal response of the pituitary–adrenal axis.[85] This is accomplished by administering 750 mg of metyrapone orally every 2 h for 12 doses (double dose test) instead of the usual dose of 750 mg every 4 h for 6 doses.[85] There is no evidence that anticonvulsants impair the HPA response to metyrapone except through their effect on the metabolism of metyrapone. Further, other stimuli including pyrogen and surgery produce normal responses in anticonvulsant-treated individuals.[85]

Procedure: Beginning at 8 A.M., 750 mg of metyrapone is given orally every 2 h for 12 doses.[85] Patients with an enhanced rate of metabolism of metyrapone as a result of anticonvulsant therapy tolerate this dose well, whereas it is poorly tolerated in

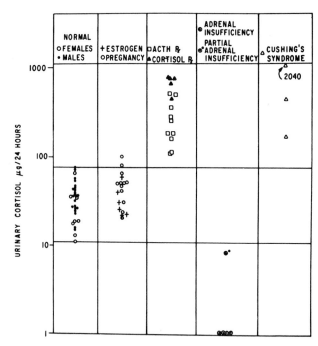

Fig. 94-5. Urinary cortisol excretion in various clinical conditions. The normal range is shown by the horizontal lines. (Meikle, A. W., et al: *J Lab Clin Med* 74: 807, 1969.)

those not receiving anticonvulsants. Plasma S is measured in the sample obtained 2 h after the last dose. A normal response is indicated by a plasma S of greater than 10 μg/dl or an increment of urinary THS or 17-OHCS of greater than 6 mg/day.

Interpretation: Normal responsiveness excludes HPA disease. In those with subnormal results, an ACTH stimulation test in addition to the metyrapone test will confirm primary or secondary adrenal hypofunction.

MULTIFACTORIAL EFFECTS OF ESTROGEN THERAPY

Rationale: Urinary steroid increases in response to metyrapone are frequently subnormal in estrogen-treated patients, although rises in ACTH and plasma S are in the normal or supranormal range. The effects of estrogens on steroid and metyrapone metabolism are complex. An alteration in the rate of production and excretion of THS appears to explain the difference between the responses based on plasma and urinary methods. Although it also slightly enhances the metabolism of metyrapone, the effect is minimal as compared to that of anticonvulsants. The metyrapone test with measurement of plasma S is the test of choice in estrogen-treated patients (and in pregnancy).

Procedure: Either the single dose or the regular dose metyrapone test with measurement of plasma S is satisfactory.[145] Urinary metyrapone tests give false results and are not recommended.

SUPPRESSIVE EFFECT OF PRIOR GLUCOCORTICOID THERAPY

Rationale: Administration of hydrocortisone or its potent synthetic analogs suppresses the release of ACTH induced by multiple stimuli including the stress of surgery.

Procedure: Single or standard dose metyrapone test.

Interpretation: The degree of the impaired responsiveness is directly related to the duration of therapy and to the dose administered. The responsiveness is generally in the normal range following the daily administration of 5.0 mg of prednisone or its biological equivalence for several years. Chronic doses of 7.5–10 mg daily produce significant impairment in about half of the individuals, and doses of 15 mg or greater produce marked unresponsiveness.[89] The recovery of the HPA axis following prolonged high dose therapy with glucocorticoid has been studied and found to take several months to return to normal in most patients.[110] The implication is that during the recovery period patients may tolerate stress poorly. Thus, the functional integrity of the HPA following chronic administration of 5–10 mg of prednisone is either unimpaired or normal within a few weeks, whereas after larger doses it frequently requires months to become normal.

EFFECT OF HYPOTHYROIDISM AND CERTAIN NONENDOCRINE DISEASES

Hypothyroidism,[146,147] cirrhosis of the liver, renal failure,[148] and malnutrition[90,149] have all been reported to cause subnormal responsiveness to metyrapone as determined with a urinary steroid index. In contrast, the plasma S index has been normal.[60,130,132] Urinary steroid metabolism and excretion are altered in these diseases and appear to explain the discrepancy. Thus, tests utilizing plasma assays are recommended for evaluation of these patients to eliminate false positive responses.

LABORATORY TESTS RECOMMENDED FOR DIFFERENTIATING BETWEEN PRIMARY AND SECONDARY ADRENAL INSUFFICIENCY (HYPOPITUITARISM)

ACTH STIMULATION TESTS

Rationale: Patients with primary adrenal insufficiency are unable to respond to ACTH stimulation, whereas those with secondary insufficiency will respond.[137–140]

Procedure: One milligram of dexamethasone is given at midnight and 0.5 mg at 8 AM. An infusion of 25 U of ACTH in 250 ml of saline is given over 6 h and the plasma samples are collected at 0 and 360 min for assay of cortisol.[137] At 6 h the plasma cortisol concentration is between 30 and 50 μg/dl in normal individuals.

Interpretation: In primary adrenal insufficiency, values are less than 14 μg/dl, and generally less than 5 μg/dl. Most patients with secondary adrenal insufficiency have increments greater than 15 μg/dl.[139,140] In those with values less than 15 μg/dl, 0.5 mg of dexamethasone is given every 6 h and 40 U of ACTH gel is injected intramuscularly twice a day for 3 days. This will cause responsiveness of adrenal glands in those with secondary adrenal hypofunction but not in those with primary disease. The ACTH infusion test, as described earlier, is repeated on the fourth day and a normal response is observed in secondary but not in primary adrenal hypofunction.

Commercial ACTH preparations are reliable and biologically active if handled as directed by the instructions. Other investigators have found urinary responses to an 8-h intravenous infusion of ACTH to produce satisfactory separation of primary and secondary adrenal insufficiency. Intramuscular ACTH tests are generally considered to be unsatisfactory apparently because the absorption of IM ACTH is unpredictable.

PLASMA ACTH DETERMINATIONS

Rationale: Although ACTH is secreted episodically and fluctuates in a diurnal pattern with high values in the early AM and low values in the PM, plasma ACTH concentrations respond to the negative feedback mechanism. Individuals with cortisol deficiency caused by primary adrenal disorders have elevated concentrations of ACTH, and those with hypothalamic or pituitary dysfunction have decreased levels.[141–144] It also increases in response to metyrapone and to insulin-induced hypoglycemia.[141,142]

Procedure: An 8 AM plasma sample is collected for assay of ACTH by RIA.[141–144] Normal individuals have values from 20 to 150 pg/ml (Fig. 94-3).

Interpretation: From the data available it appears that the 8 AM plasma contents of both ACTH and cortisol would be diagnostic of primary adrenal insufficiency. Baseline cortisol values of less than 10 μg/dl and an ACTH level of greater than 250 pg/ml are diagnostic of primary adrenal insufficiency (Fig. 94-3). A stimulation test appears to be required for the diagnosis of secondary adrenal hypofunction. Following a single or standard dose of metyrapone, a subnormal concentration of both plasma ACTH and S is diagnostic of secondary adrenal insufficiency. An ACTH assay combined with a steroidal assay eliminates the need to perform the ACTH stimulation test for the diagnosis of secondary adrenal insufficiency.

PROCEDURES RECOMMENDED FOR THE LABORATORY DIAGNOSIS OF ACUTE ADRENAL INSUFFICIENCY

Rationale: Acute stress results in activation of the HPA axis in normal individuals. In individuals with an abnormality of the axis, the production of cortisol by the adrenal cortex is subnormal and the consequence may be adrenal crisis.

Procedure: A plasma sample is obtained for a cortisol measurement and then the patient is treated appropriately for adrenal insufficiency. During acute stress, normal subjects have plasma cortisol values of greater than 15 μg/dl.[150]

Interpretation: When the patient is acutely stressed from a life-threatening illness, the possibility of adrenal insufficiency can be excluded by observing a high plasma concentration of cortisol. During such stress, a plasma level of less than 15 μg/dl is compatible with adrenal insufficiency. The patient can be treated until the clinical course is stable and then tested with the ACTH stimulation test (as described earlier). A normal response would then establish the diagnosis of secondary adrenal insufficiency; and a subnormal one, primary adrenal insufficiency.

LABORATORY TESTS OF LIMITED VALUE IN THE DIAGNOSIS OF ADRENAL INSUFFICIENCY

24-H BASELINE URINARY STEROID DETERMINATIONS (17-OHCS, 17-KGS, 17-KS) AND BASELINE PLASMA STEROID DETERMINATIONS (Cortisol, 17-OHCS, and 11-OHCS)

Rationale: Urinary 17-OHCS and 17-KGS methods primarily measure metabolites of cortisol. Thus, these steroids and the plasma level of cortisol reflect the production rate of cortisol. Their correlation with the cortisol production rate is significant.[151] 17-KS measures steroids and their metabolites produced by the adrenal but also some that are excreted by the gonads.

Procedure: Baseline urine is collected for 24 h and assayed for adrenal steroid metabolites, or a plasma sample is obtained for measurement of cortisol. The normal range is 4–12 mg/day for 17-

Table 94-4. Causes of False Positive Dexamethasone Suppression Tests

	Frequency of Occurrence	Reference
A. Failure to take proper dose	Uncommon	
B. Stress	Common	
1. Acute—emotional		159
2. Acute—physical		90
3. Chronic	Rare	161
a. Malnutrition		161
b. Diabetes mellitus—juvenile type		160
C. Intrasellar tumors (non-ACTH producing)	Rare	90
D. Pregnancy	Rare	
E. Drugs	Uncommon	
1. Alcoholism		61
2. Estrogens		162
3. Anticonvulsants, diphenylhydantoin, phenobarbital, particularly		86

OHCS, 3–25 mg/day for 17-KGS, and 7–20 mg/day for 17-KS. Depending on the time of sample collection the plasma concentration of cortisol might vary from 0 to 28 μg/dl in normal individuals.

Interpretation: Baseline values of any of these steroids are of limited diagnostic accuracy. They may suggest adrenal insufficiency but do not confirm it unless appropriate stimulation tests are also performed. The explanation for their limited diagnostic accuracy in adrenal insufficiency is that most methods have blank values that approach values in the low range of normal. It is therefore useless to use baseline urinary 17-OHCS, 17-KGS, 17-KS, or plasma cortisol for the diagnosis of adrenal insufficiency.

WATER-LOADING TESTS FOR ADRENAL INSUFFICIENCY[152]

It is well recognized that patients with adrenal insufficiency have an abnormal excretion of a water load. The test becomes normal after administration of hydrocortisone to the patient with adrenal insufficiency. Water loading may be poorly tolerated by patients with secondary adrenal insufficiency because it results in water intoxication. In contrast, those with acute primary adrenal insufficiency may tolerate the test because they already have volume depletion but also have a renal defect in water excretion due to the absence of corticosteroid. This test has been superceded by others more specific and safer diagnostic tests of adrenal hypofunction.

LABORATORY TESTS RECOMMENDED FOR THE DIAGNOSIS OF CUSHING'S SYNDROME (WITHOUT DIFFERENTIATING ETIOLOGY)

In this section we will consider the etiology of excess secretion of cortisol by the adrenal cortex, or "hypercortisolism." Causes include excess secretion of ACTH by the pituitary either from a small pituitary tumor or possibly from a hypothalamic driving force with excess secretion of CRF. Nonpituitary etiology of Cushing's syndrome includes adrenal adenomas and carcinomas and excess secretion of ACTH or corticotropin releasing factor from nonendocrine tumors. The major criteria for establishing Cushing's syndrome are (1) clinical evidence of hypercortisolism, (2) abnormal feedback of the HPA axis, and (3) biochemical evidence of hypercortisolism. It should be recognized that there have been no absolute criteria established for the diagnosis of Cushing's syndrome. Although the diagnosis can be made with ease in most cases, it can be very difficult in others, because the results of some tests may be equivocal whereas others are distinctly abnormal. Table 94-5 lists the results of laboratory tests that are used for the diagnosis of Cushing's syndrome. (Refer to Chapters 95 and 99 for recommended procedures for diagnosis of Cushing's syndrome.)

OVERNIGHT SINGLE DOSE DEXAMETHASONE SUPPRESSION TEST[155]

Rationale: The rationale of the dexamethasone suppression test is based on the observation that glucocorticoids participate in negative feedback by inhibiting either the release of ACTH directly from the pituitary or the secretion of CRF from the hypothalamus. The potent glucocorticoid, dexamethasone, behaves like cortisol in participating in this feedback mechanism. Since it is more potent

Table 94-5. Summary of Laboratory Test Results in Cushing's Syndrome[141,174–178]

	R_x	Normal	Pituitary Dependent	Adrenal Tumors	Nodular Hyperplasia	Nonendocrine ACTH Secretion
Baseline 8 AM cortisol (μg/dl)	None	5–25	N or ↑	N or ↑	N or ↑	N or ↑
Diurnal rhythm	None	Present (usually)	Absent	Absent	Absent	Absent
Baseline plasma ACTH (pg/ml)	None	20–150	N or ↑	↓	↓	N or ↑
8 AM cortisol after dexamethasone	1 mg at midnight	<5	↑	↑	↑	↑
	0.5 mg q 6 h × 8	<5	↑	↑	↑	↑
Urinary 17-OHCS	mg/g creatinine	<3.5	↑	↑	↑	↑
8 AM cortisol after dexamethasone	2.0 mg q 6 h × 8	<2	50% ↓	↑	↑	↑
Urinary 17-OHCS		<3.5	50% ↓	↑	↑	↑
Single oral dose Metyrapone test with determination of plasma 11-deoxycortisol (μg/dl)	30 mg/kg body wt. at midnight	7–22	N or ↑	↓	↓	N or ↓
ACTH test with determination of plasma cortisol (μg/dl)	25 U over 6 h iv	30–50	N or ↑	N or ↓	↓	N or ↑

than cortisol, a smaller dose of dexamethasone is required to produce marked suppression of the HPA axis. This steroid, therefore, is not measured with the various cortisol assays in plasma or with the urinary measurements to be discussed subsequently. Following dexamethasone therapy, the feedback mechanism is abnormal in the various types of Cushing's syndrome except in those receiving exogenous corticosteroids.

Procedure: One milligram of dexamethasone is administered between 11 PM and 12 PM and an 8 AM plasma sample is obtained for measurement of plasma cortisol. The cortisol level decreases to less than 5 μg/dl in patients without Cushing's syndrome.

Interpretation: A plasma cortisol level of greater than 5 μg/dl after the 1 mg overnight dexamethasone suppression test is presumptive evidence that the patient has Cushing's syndrome, and additional diagnostic tests are indicated in the evaluation of the patient. This test has few false negatives and therefore is highly reliable in excluding the diagnosis of Cushing's syndrome. False positives are frequently obtained with the fluorometric determination of cortisol because of the high blank and low sensitivity of this method. In some laboratories, as many as 50 percent of the patients have false positive tests, whereas this is not observed in patients using more specific and sensitive methods for measuring cortisol.[155–158] The blank values with the fluorometric test vary from 0 to 7 μg/dl. It would appear, therefore, that in patients with a high blank value combined with a cortisol level of 4–5 μg/100 ml, this would result in an abnormally high level of cortisol and therefore a false positive test. False negative tests are not a problem with the fluorometric determination.

The various causes of false positive dexamethasone suppression tests are listed in Table 94-4.

MULTIPLE LOW DOSE DEXAMETHASONE SUPPRESSION TEST[167]

Rationale: The rationale of this procedure is similar to that described for the overnight dexamethasone suppression test.

Procedure: After a screening test is performed (either the 1 mg overnight dexamethasone suppression test or urinary free cortisol determination), patients with positive tests are hospitalized for confirmatory tests and to differentiate the cause of the Cushing's syndrome. The low dose dexamethasone suppression test is performed. It appears that comparable satisfactory results can be obtained with either the 1 mg dexamethasone suppression test (as described earlier) or the low dose dexamethasone suppression test. The 1 mg overnight suppression test is repeated or 0.5 mg of dexamethasone is administered every 6 h for 8 doses. With either test, 8 AM plasma cortisol measured at the end of the test[168] is less than 5 μg/dl in normal subjects. Urinary 17-OHCS is normally less than 3.5 mg/day/g of creatinine on the second day of the multiple dose test, and 17-KGS is less than 5.0 mg/day.[136,167]

Interpretation: Patients with Cushing's syndrome regardless of etiology fail to exhibit normal suppression to one of these tests. Many of these patients show some responsiveness to low dose dexamethasone suppression but it is usually abnormal. However, in some patients with so-called suppressible Cushing's syndrome, the low dose dexamethasone suppression test produced false negative results.[156,165,169–173] (These are discussed later under plasma cortisol–dexamethasone nomogram.)

The causes of false positive tests are listed in Table 94-4. It is very important to exclude the possibilities listed, particularly the problem of drug interference with the dexamethasone suppression test. The reliability of these tests when properly performed is greater than 90 percent[157]

URINARY CORTISOL DETERMINATIONS[135]

Rationale: It is well recognized that as the plasma cortisol level increases the non-protein-bound fraction also increases. As the cortisol concentration exceeds the binding capacity of corticosteroid binding globulin, the increase of the free fraction is greater than the rise of total steroid concentration. The free fraction of cortisol in plasma is filtered by the glomerulus and excreted in the urine. Its excretion appears to be an exponential function of the cortisol production rate (Fig. 94-6). Therefore, as the cortisol production rate exceeds normal there is a disproportionately greater increase in the urinary excretion of free cortisol. With hypercortisolism the increase in urinary free cortisol secretion generally exceeds that observed for excretion of urinary metabolites of cortisol, urinary 17-OHCS, 17-KGS, and also the cortisol production rate.

Procedure: A total 24-h urine collection is made, generally beginning at 8 AM. The free fraction of cortisol is extracted from the urine and measured by competitive protein binding assays, radioimmunoassays, or fluorometry. In most laboratories normals excrete less than 100 μg/day.[136,163–165]

Interpretation: A urinary free cortisol determination is an excellent screening test for the diagnosis of Cushing's syndrome. In patients with Cushing's syndrome of various etiologies, urinary free cortisol is elevated. Eucorticoid obese individuals have normal urinary free cortisol. The diagnostic accuracy of this test when properly performed is above 90 percent and parallels the reliability of the dexamethasone suppression test.[157]

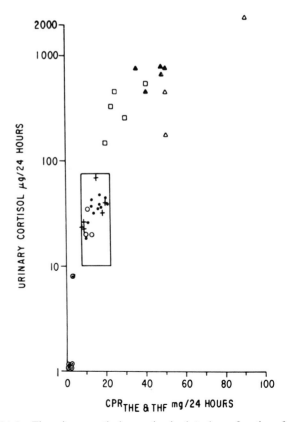

Fig. 94-6. The urinary cortisol excretion is plotted as a function of mean of CPR_{THE} and CPR_{THF}. ⊙, Adrenal insufficiency; ⊙*, partial adrenal insufficiency; ●, normal male subjects; ○, normal female subjects; +, estrogen-treated males; □, normal subjects after a 6-h ACTH infusion; ▲, normal subjects after a 6-h cortisol infusion; Δ, Cushing's syndrome caused by adrenal cortical tumor. (Meikle, A. W., et al: *J Lab Clin Med* 74: 809, 1969.)

False positives: There appear to be few false positives with this test. Concomitant diuretic administration or a high salt diet may cause increased urinary free cortisol excretion, and therefore erroneous results may be obtained in these situations.[166] Urinary free cortisol determinations need to be standardized for normal subjects and the laboratory regardless of the method of determination for cortisol. The competitive protein binding techniques and fluorometric methods may not be specific for measurement of urinary cortisol. It appears, however, that the noncortisol materials that are measured with these procedures reflect steroidal secretion by the adrenal gland, and therefore chromatographic isolation and specific measurement of urinary free cortisol is not always necessary.[135,156]

CORTISOL PRODUCTION RATE DETERMINATIONS

Rationale: Cortisol secretion rate is elevated in patients with hypercortisolism as compared to normals.

Procedure: Isotopically labeled cortisol is administerd, and a subsequent 24-h collection of urine is made in which the specific activity of a metabolite of cortisol is estimated. The constant effusion technique reported by DeLacerda et al.[44] can also be used to determine the production rate. The rate of cortisol production in normal subjects varies from 10 to 35 mg/day.

Interpretation: Excessive elevation in cortisol production rates would appear to establish the diagnosis of hypercortisolism.[165,171] However, there are limitations of the test. Many obese patients may also have an elevation of their cortisol production rate without having hypercortisolism. Therefore, this has not been an enormously useful test. It is also a difficult test to perform, and cannot be used on a routine basis. If the cortisol production rate is expressed as a function of urinary creatinine excretion, it has been shown by Streeten and associates[165] to be a reliable test for differentiating between simple obesity and hypercortisolism.

LABORATORY TESTS RECOMMENDED FOR DIFFERENTIATING THE SPECIFIC ETIOLOGY OF CUSHING'S SYNDROME (PITUITARY-DEPENDENT ADRENAL HYPERPLASIA, ADRENAL TUMORS, OR ACTH-PRODUCING ECTOPIC TUMORS)

MULTIPLE HIGH DOSE DEXAMETHASONE SUPPRESSION TEST[167]

Rationale: In patients with pituitary-dependent Cushing's syndrome the feedback mechanism is responsive to glucocorticoids, but it is limited. It is absent, with few exceptions, in those with adrenal tumors or those with nonendocrine ACTH-secreting tumors.

Procedure: Dexamethasone, 2 mg, is administered orally every 6 h for 8 doses beginning at 8 A.M.. At the conclusion of the test, a plasma level of cortisol is measured and/or urine is collected daily for measurement of urinary 17-OHCS or 17-KGS. The plasma cortisol concentration is generally undetectable and urinary 17-OHCS and 17-KGS are, respectively, less than 3.5 mg/day/g creatinine and 5 mg/day in patients without Cushing's syndrome. With pituitary-dependent Cushing's syndrome, suppression of greater than 50 percent is observed for either plasma cortisol or urinary 17-OHCS or 17-KGS.

Interpretation: A reduction of either plasma cortisol or urinary 17-OHCS of greater than 50 percent, but occasionally only about 25 percent, in a patient with known Cushing's syndrome is evidence that it is pituitary dependent. Patients with adrenal tumors or nonendocrine ACTH-secreting tumors usually fail to show suppression of either the plasma cortisol concentration or urinary 17-OHCS, or 17-KGS to the high dose dexamethasone. Therefore, this is a convenient means of separating those with pituitary-dependent Cushing's syndrome from those with other causes of Cushing's syndrome. It should be recognized that some patients with pituitary-dependent Cushing's syndrome will not show adequate suppression with the high dose test. Therefore, it is our policy when patients fail to exhibit suppression to high dose dexamethasone to increase the dose to 4–8 mg every 4 h for 8 doses. This will suppress ACTH secretion in those with pituitary-dependent Cushing's syndrome. It generally will not cause suppression in those with adrenal tumors or those with nonendocrine formation of ACTH. The high dose suppression test is not absolutely accurate in differentiating patients with pituitary-dependent Cushing's syndrome from those with other causes. The metyrapone and/or ACTH stimulation tests may be useful in establishing the correct diagnosis.

METYRAPONE TEST

Rationale: In patients with pituitary-dependent Cushing's syndrome the responsiveness of the feedback mechanism is diminished. However, when the plasma cortisol level is decreased, these patients will release ACTH, often in excessive amounts. Cortisol deficiency fails to enhance release of ACTH in patients with nonendocrine causes of ACTH secretion. In patients with adrenal tumors, the pituitary has been subjected to chronic high cortisol levels and therefore is unresponsive to a low plasma cortisol concentration. Furthermore, the contralateral adrenal gland is atrophic and any ACTH administered acutely generally fails to produce substantial stimulation of that adrenal gland.

Procedure: The single dose metyrapone test or the standard oral dose of metyrapone.[11,90,120,121,132]

Interpretation: Once a diagnosis of Cushing's syndrome has been established a metyrapone test is extremely valuable in confirming whether the patient has pituitary-dependent Cushing's syndrome or Cushing's syndrome of other etiologies. Following metyrapone, in the pituitary-dependent type, the combined production rate of S and cortisol is increased as compared to the basal secretion rate of cortisol, but it is essentially unchanged in those with adrenal tumors or those with ACTH-secreting tumors. Those with a pituitary-dependent form exhibit normal to high normal responsiveness of plasma S, and in those with adrenal tumors, responsiveness is invariably subnormal. It is generally subnormal in those with nonendocrine ACTH-secreting tumors; however, there are a few patients in whom the rate of cortisol secretion is very high. In these patients, although there is marked reduction in plasma cortisol levels following metyrapone, the plasma S concentration is in the normal range. The apparent explanation for this is that cortisol secretion is inhibited but the adrenal glands are under marked stimulation by ACTH; therefore, the adrenals have a capacity to make large quantities of plasma S. In these patients, the plasma S levels are much less than the baseline plasma cortisol values. Interferences with the metyrapone test include those previously considered.

ACTH STIMULATION TESTS[139,140]

Rationale: Patients with bilateral adrenal hyperplasia of the pituitary-dependent form usually have excessive responsiveness to the infusion. Those with adrenal tumors show inconsistent responsiveness to ACTH; and in patients with ectopic ACTH syndrome the responsiveness varies, depending on whether their baseline stimulation is approaching maximum.

Procedure: The standard ACTH stimulation test was described earlier.

Interpretation: Documentation of adrenal hyperplasia with this test is good, and therefore, taking into consideration the other laboratory tests performed, it is further evidence that the patient has pituitary-dependent Cushing's syndrome. It is not a particularly good test for differentiation between adrenal carcinoma and adenoma, for some patients with carcinoma also respond to the ACTH stimulation test. Some patients with adrenal tumors have exaggerated responses to ACTH that are indistinguishable from those observed in patients with adrenal hyperplasia.[157]

URINARY 17-KETOSTEROID DETERMINATIONS AFTER DEXAMETHASONE SUPPRESSION[136,157]

Rationale: In patients with adrenal carcinomas 90 percent of patients have elevated 17-KS. This is apparently because the adrenal carcinoma is less efficient in producing cortisol and makes other 17-KS precursors. This test is indicated in virilized patients who are also suspected of having Cushing's syndrome.

Procedure: Baseline 24-h urines are collected for 4 days for measurement of 17-KS. Dexamethasone, 0.5 mg, is administered orally every 6 h for 3 days. Baseline urinary 17-KS levels vary from 7–20 mg/day in normal adult subjects, and decrease to less than 5 mg after dexamethasone suppression for 3 days.

Interpretation: A fourfold elevation is suggestive of adrenal carcinoma. Only 15 percent of patients with nonendocrine ACTH-secreting tumors and only 3 percent of those with bilateral adrenal hyperplasia have elevations of this magnitude. By way of contrast urinary 17-KS levels are normal or subnormal in about 70 percent of patients with adrenal adenomas, and only 10 percent of patients with adrenal carcinomas have normal levels. When combined with the dexamethasone suppression test it can also be a highly useful test for separation of patients with congenital or acquired adrenogenital syndromes from those with adrenal or ovarian tumors. In the latter, dexamethasone fails to inhibit secretion of 17-KS, but in the former it does inhibit secretion.

FACTORS THAT MAY INVALIDATE DEXAMETHASONE SUPPRESSION TESTS— DETECTION AND CORRECTION OF FALSE TESTS

EFFECT OF HEPATIC ENZYME-INDUCING DRUGS

It is well documented that chronic diphenylhydantoin therapy accelerates the clearance rate of dexamethasone from plasma.[86] A false positive test result is observed frequently following either the 1 mg overnight or multiple low dose dexamethasone suppression test in patients receiving the anticonvulsant. Following the multiple high dose dexamethasone suppression test, adrenal function is suppressed; thus, the results might be interpreted erroneously to indicate pituitary-dependent Cushing's syndrome (refer to the hydrocortisone suppression test). Other anticonvulsants also enhance the rate of disposal of dexamethasone and produce apparent failure of suppression.[168] Other drugs also produce hepatic enzyme induction, but their effects on the result of the test have not been well documented.

SIMULTANEOUS MEASUREMENT OF PLASMA CORTISOL AND DEXAMETHASONE CONCENTRATIONS (Plasma Cortisol–Dexamethasone Nomogram)

There have been many reports of patients with so-called suppressible Cushing's syndrome. It has been unclear why a usual low dose of dexamethasone produced a normal response in them.[156,165,169–173]

Rationale: There is a variable rate of dexamethasone metabolism among patients. It is reasoned that in those with slow rates of metabolism of dexamethasone a usual dose would produce a high level of dexamethasone and might cause greater suppression of ACTH in the pituitary-dependent type of Cushing's syndrome. Patients with more rapid metabolism of dexamethasone can also be identified because usual doses of dexamethasone would produce low plasma levels of the steroid. Therefore, by relating the dexamethasone level to the simultaneous plasma value of cortisol, more accurate interpretation of the dexamethasone suppression test would be obtained.

Procedure: Measurement of plasma levels of cortisol and simultaneous determination of dexamethasone by radioimmunoassay. The relation of the 8 AM plasma cortisol level to the plasma dexamethasone level is observed in the nomogram (Fig. 94-7).

Interpretation: A nomogram is used for the interpretation of the dexamethasone suppression test (Fig. 94-7). Patients with high levels of dexamethasone for the dose can be identified and their metabolism of dexamethasone can be studied. In those with low levels of dexamethasone, appropriate interpretation of the data can be made by relating the plasma dexamethasone level to the plasma concentration of cortisol. Although this test has not had widespread experience, in our laboratory we have found it to be most useful in interpreting some otherwise confusing data. We have documented one patient with "suppressible" Cushing's syndrome in whom the apparent explanation for this anomalous response was slow metabolism of dexamethasone. When the nomogram was used for interpretation of the test, it was apparent that this patient did exhibit resistance to the suppressive effect of the steroid. This nomogram interpretation, however, does not compensate for factors such as stress. It has a particular application in evaluation of patients treated with drugs that increase the rate of metabolism of dexamethasone, such as anticonvulsant agents.

SUBSTITUTION OF THE HYDROCORTISONE SUPPRESSION TEST FOR THE DEXAMETHASONE SUPPRESSION TEST IN PATIENTS ON HEPATIC ENZYME-INDUCING DRUGS[179]

Rationale: Anticonvulsants increase the rate of metabolism of dexamethasone and therefore erroneous laboratory results are obtained in patients so treated. However, the rate of clearance of cortisol from plasma is minimally affected by the anticonvulsants. It has been possible to substitute hydrocortisone for dexamethasone and perform the suppression test.

Procedure: Baseline 8 AM plasma is obtained for measurement of corticosterone, and then the following midnight 50 mg of hydrocortisone is given orally and an 8 AM plasma sample is obtained for measurement of corticosterone.

Interpretation: Following hydrocortisone, anticonvulsant-treated patients without Cushing's syndrome have plasma corticosterone levels of less than 270 ng/dl and less than 50 percent of the baseline value. In those not receiving anticonvulsants, the corticosterone values are less than 120 ng/dl and also less than 50 percent

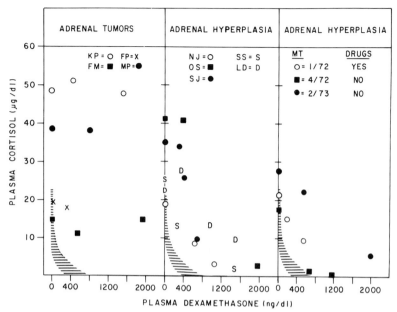

Fig. 94-7. Plasma dexamethasone and cortisol values at 8 A.M. following oral dexamethasone in patients with Cushing's syndrome. The baseline levels of cortisol are shown on the left of each panel. Patients with adrenal tumors (KP and FM had adrenal carcinomas and FP and MP adrenal adenomas) are shown in the left (A). Those with bilateral adrenal hyperplasia in the center (B), and MT, also with bilateral hyperplasia, on the right (C). Most patients with Cushing's syndrome received 1 mg of dexamethasone the previous midnight and 0.5 and 2.0 mg every 6 h for 8 doses (the last dose was given 6 h before the plasma was obtained for assay of the concentration of the steroids). The normal range is crosshatched. Data on FP and MP are shown following 0.5 and 2.0 mg every 6 h for 8 doses, respectively. NJ, who had delayed clearance rate of dexamethasone and pituitary-dependent Cushing's syndrome, received 0.5 and 1.0 mg doses the previous midnight. MT in panel C was tested on three occasions. On one she received drugs which appeared to increase the rate of clearance of dexamethasone from plasma. No suppression of plasma cortisol was observed in patients with adrenal tumors (A). In contrast, plasma cortisol decreased as the dexamethasone concentration was increased by oral dexamethasone in patients with pituitary-dependent Cushing's syndrome (B and C). However, their plasma cortisol concentrations were also abnormally high when compared to the plasma level of dexamethasone. (From Ref. 169.)

of the baseline level. This test appears to be an excellent test for exclusion of the diagnosis of Cushing's syndrome in anticonvulsant-treated patients. It also has application in patients receiving other drugs that are known to increase the activity of microsomal enzymes and to increase the clearance of dexamethasone from plasma.

MULTIFACTORIAL EFFECTS OF ESTROGEN THERAPY[145,162]

Rationale: The clearance rate of cortisol is delayed in patients receiving estrogen or during pregnancy with the excess production of estrogen. With an increase in corticosteroid binding globulin, the cortisol levels are higher and clearance from plasma is slower than normal. Therefore, the more prolonged tests allow for clearance of the cortisol from the plasma, and more reliable interpretation of the data would appear to be obtained with these tests. Estrogen does not interfere with utilization of plasma 11-deoxycortisol but may, in large doses, suppress the inhibition of 11β-hydroxylation.

Procedure: Low dose (multiple dose) and high dose dexamethasone suppression tests, and the single or standard oral dose metyrapone test with measurement of plasma 11-deoxycortisol are performed as already described.

Interpretation: Normal responses exclude Cushing's syndrome. If the tests are abnormal, they should be repeated if possible after withdrawal of estrogen for 4 weeks.

PERIODIC HORMONOGENESIS[180,181]

Rationale: Some patients receiving dexamethasone appear to have stimulation of ACTH release instead of the typical suppression after dexamethasone. The explanation for this paradoxical responsiveness to dexamethasone has been unclear.

Procedure: A 24 h collection of urine is made over several consecutive days for measurement of metabolites of cortisol or cortisol itself.

Interpretation: A case was recently reported by Brown and associates[180] in which a possible explanation for this abnormal responsiveness to dexamethasone was discussed. It appeared that this patient had a cycle of high secretion of cortisol followed by normal secretion rates of cortisol. Therefore, if one were performing the dexamethasone suppression test during the low levels, normal results might be observed. On the other hand, if one were doing dexamethasone suppression tests during the phase of increased secretion, it might appear that the patient had paradoxical response to the dexamethasone. The exact incidence of periodic hormonogenesis in patients with Cushing's syndrome is unknown.

OTHER LABORATORY TESTS IN THE DIAGNOSIS OF CUSHING'S SYNDROME

24-H BASELINE URINARY STEROID DETERMINATIONS (17-OHCS, 17-KGS, 17-KS) AND BASELINE PLASMA STEROID DETERMINATIONS (CORTISOL, 17-OHCS, AND 11-OHCS)

Rationale: These steroids reflect the production of cortisol and therefore are a rough approximation of the absolute production rate of cortisol in patients.

Procedure: Baseline plasma cortisol and urinary 17-KGS, 17-KS, 17-OHCS are measured with conventional methods.

Interpretation: As discussed earlier, the cortisol production rate in obese subjects and in patients with Cushing's syndrome may overlap. Also there is overlap between the excretion of these steroids in the urine in patients with documented Cushing's syndrome and in obese subjects. However, the tests may be useful in documenting hypercortisolism if they are markedly elevated. This would confirm the excessive cortisol production rate that is observed in the patients with Cushing's syndrome. Baseline levels of these steroids are useful but not diagnostic of Cushing's syndrome unless they are utilized with physiologic manipulation tests.

MEASUREMENT OF THE DIURNAL VARIATION IN PLASMA CORTISOL CONCENTRATIONS[136,156]

Rationale: Most patients with Cushing's syndrome have lost their diurnal variation of cortisol secretion.

Procedure: Plasma levels of cortisol are measured between 8 and 9 AM and between 4 and 6 PM. Most normal subjects have values in the afternoon that are much lower than those in the morning.

Interpretation: An abnormal diurnal variation is suggestive but not diagnostic of Cushing's syndrome.

DETERMINATION OF CORTISOL EPISODIC SECRETION PATTERN[182]

Rationale: It was presumed that patients with autonomous tumors would have smooth secretion of hormone from the tumor, and there would not be a fluctuation in blood level. Those with pituitary-dependent Cushing's syndrome might exhibit some fluctuation.

Procedure: Multiple plasma samples are obtained at 10–20 min intervals over a 24-h period. Normal subjects exhibit episodic secretion and a diurnal variation in cortisol and ACTH secretion.

Interpretation: Although the data are relatively limited, episodic secretion in patients with Cushing's syndrome demonstrates that it is not possible to differentiate the etiology with the study. At the present time this test certainly is most difficult, although it would be an excellent research technique for further investigation. It does, however, distinguish between normal subjects and patients with Cushing's syndrome. Patients with Cushing's syndrome have much higher levels of the steroid than normal individuals, and they also have abnormal diurnal variations.

GUIDELINES FOR THE LABORATORY WORKUP OF PATIENTS SUSPECTED OF ADRENAL DYSFUNCTION

For the convenience of practicing physicians who need a "ready reference" for the selection of appropriate adrenal function tests, a practical guide for the laboratory workup of patients suspected of having adrenal insufficiency or Cushing's syndrome has been prepared (see Chapter 99). This guide is written in the form of a brief outline in which the recommended laboratory workup is given in sequential steps for each specific adrenal problem. It is intended that this guide should be used by the physician only to orient himself as to which adrenal function tests should be used in each individual situation. For details on the performance of the tests and the correct interpretation of the results, the physician should refer to the appropriate section in this chapter which has been referenced for easy accessibility.

REFERENCES

1. Srivastova, L. S., Werk, E. E., Thrasher, K., et al: Plasma cortisone concentration as measured by radioimmunoassay. *J Clin Endocrinol Metab 36:* 937–943, 1973.
2. Bailey, E., West, H. F.: The secretion, interconversion and catabolism of cortisol, cortisone and some of the metabolites in man. *Acta Endocrinol 62:* 339–359, 1969.
3. Kowarski, A., Lawrence, B., Hung, W., et al: Interconversion of cortisol and cortisone in man and its effect on the measurement of cortisol secretion rate. *J Clin Endocrinol Metab 29:* 377–381, 1969.
4. Horton, R., Tait, J. F.: In vivo conversion of DHEA to plasma androstenedione and testosterone in man. *J Clin Endocrinol Metab 27:* 79–88, 1967.
5. Horton, R., Tait, J. F.: Androstenedione production and interconversion rates measured in peripheral blood and studies on the possible site of its conversion to testosterone. *J Clin Invest 45:* 301–313, 1966.
6. Migeon, C. J., Kirschner, M. A., Bardin, C. W.: Physiologic basis of disorders of androgen metabolism. *Ann Intern Med 68:* 1327–1344, 1968.
7. Rivalola, M. A., Singleton, R. I., Migeon, C. J.: Splanchnic extraction and interconversion of testosterone and Δ-androstenedione in man. *J Clin Invest 46:* 2095–2100, 1967.
8. Gandy, H. M., Peterson, R. E.: Measurement of testosterone and 17-ketosteroids in plasma by the double isotope dilution derivative technique. *J Clin Endocrinol Metab 28:* 949–977, 1968.
9. Lipsett, M. B., Wilson, H., Kirschner, M. A., et al: Studies on Leydig cell physiology and pathology: Secretion and metabolism of testosterone. *Recent Prog Horm Res 22:* 245–281, 1966.
10. Siiteri, P. K., Vande Wiele, R. L., Lieberman, S.: Occurrence of DHEA glucoronoside in normal human urine. *J Clin Endocrinol Metab 23:* 588–594, 1963.
11. Meikle, A. W., Jubiz, W., Hutchings, M. P., et al: A simplified metyrapone test with determination of plasma 11-deoxycortisol (metyrapone test with plasma S). *J Clin Endocrinol Metab 29:* 985–987, 1969.
12. Weitzman, E. D., Fukushima, D., Nogeine, C., et al: Twenty-four hour pattern of the episodic secretion of cortisol in normal subjects. *J Clin Endocrinol Metab 33:* 14–22, 1971.
13. Seal, U. S., Doe, R. P.: Purification and properties of transcortin, the cortisol binding globulin, from patients with cancer of the prostate. *Cancer Chemother Rep 16:* 329–334, 1962.
14. Slaunwhite, W. R., Schneuler, S., Wissler, F. C., et al: Transcortin: A corticosteroid-binding protein of plasma. IX. Isolation and characterization. *Biochemistry 5:* 3527–3532, 1966.
15. Muldoon, T. G., Westphal, U.: Steroid–protein interactions. XV. Isolation and characterization of corticosteroid-binding globulin from human plasma. *J Biol Chem 242:* 5636–5643, 1967.
16. Slaunwhite, W. R., Jr., Sandberg, A. A.: Transcortin: A corticosteroid-binding protein in plasma. *J Clin Invest 38:* 384–391, 1959.
17. Doe, R. P., Zinneman, H. H., Flink, E. B., et al: Significance of nonprotein bound plasma cortisol in normal subjects, Cushing's syndrome, pregnancy, and during estrogen therapy. *J Clin Endocrinol Metab 20:* 1484–1492, 1960.
18. Musa, B. U., Seal, U. S., Doe, R.: Excretion of CBG and TBG and total protein in adult males with nephrosis: Effect of sex hormones. *J Clin Endocrinol Metab 27:* 768–774, 1967.
19. Daughaday, W. H., Adler, R. F., Mariz, I. K., et al: Measurement of the binding capacity of CBG in human plasma. *J Clin Endocrinol Metab 22:* 704–710, 1962.
20. Daughaday, W. H.: Binding of corticosteroids by plasma proteins: V. CBG activity in normal human beings and in certain disease states. *Arch Intern Med 101:* 286–290, 1958.
21. Doe, R. P., Fernandez, R., Seal, U. S.: Measurement of CBG in men. *J Clin Endocrinol Metab 24:* 1029–1039, 1964.
22. Doe, R. P., Lahrenz, F., Seal, U. S.: Familial decrease in corticosteroid-binding globulin. *Metab Clin Exp 14:* 940–943, 1965.
23. Zimmermann, W.: Eine farbreaktion der sexualhormone und ihre anwendung zur quantitoven colorimetrischen bestimmung. *Hoppe Segler Z Physiol Chem 233:* 257–264, 1935.
24. Porter, C. C., Silber, R. H.: A quantitative color reaction for cortisone and related 17, 21-dihydroxy-20-ketosteroids. *J Biol Chem 185:* 201–207, 1950.
25. Nelson, D. H., Samuels, L. T.: A method for the determination of

17-hydroxycorticosteroids in blood; 17-hydroxycorticosterone in the peripheral circulation. *J Clin Endocrinol Metab 12:* 519–526, 1952.

26. Berson, S. A., Yalow, R. S.: Recent studies on insulin-binding antibodies. *Ann NY Acad Sci 82:* 338–344, 1959.

27. Erlanger, B. F., Borch, F., Lieberman, S.: Steroid-protein conjugates. I. Preparation and characterization of conjugates of bovine serum albumin with testosterone and cortisone. *J Biol Chem 228:* 713–727, 1957.

28. Murphy, B. R., Engelberg, W., Pattee, C. J.: Simple method for the determination of plasma corticoids. *J Clin Endocrinol Metab 23:* 293–300, 1963.

29. Korenman, S. G., Tulchinsky, D., Eaton, L. W., Jr.: Radioligand procedures for estrogen assay in normal and pregnancy plasma. Proceedings of the Second Symposium. Steroid assay by protein-binding. Karolinska Institutet, Stockholm, 1970, pp 291–304.

30. Corker, C. S., Erdez, D., Naftolin, F.: Assay of 17β-estradiol by competitive protein binding methods. Proceedings of the Second Symposium. Steroid assay by protein binding. Karolinska Institutet, Stockholm, 1970, pp 305–319.

31. Wolfsen, A. R., McIntyre, H. B., Odell, W. D.: ACTH measurement by competitive binding receptor assay. *J Clin Endocrinol Metab 34:* 684–689, 1972.

32. Peron, F. G., Caldwell, B. V. (eds): Immunologic Methods in Steroid Determinations. Appleton, New York, 1970.

33. Kirkham, K. E., Hunter, W. M. (eds): Radioimmunoassay Methods. Churchill Livingstone, London, 1971.

34. Jaffe, B. M., Behrman, H. R. (eds): Methods of Hormone Radioimmunoassay. Academic Press, New York, 1974.

35. Odell, W. D., Daughaday, W. H. (eds): Principles of Competitive Protein-Binding Assays. Lippincott, Philadelphia, 1971.

36. Strott, C. A., Yoshimi, T., Lipsett, M. B.: Plasma progesterone and 17-OH progesterone in normal men and children with CAH. *J Clin Invest 48:* 930–939, 1969.

37. Barnes, N. D., Atherden, S. M.: Diagnosis of CAH by measurement of plasma 17-OH progesterone. *Arch Dis Child 47:* 62–65, 1972.

38. West, C. D., Stanchfield, J. B., Atcheson, J. B., et al: Circadian variations in plasma ACTH and cortisol and its precursors in CAH. *Clin Res 21:* 190, 1973.

39. Cope, C. L., Black, E. G.: The behavior of ¹⁴C cortisol and estimation of cortisol production rate in man. *Clin Sci 17:* 147–163, 1958.

40. Peterson, R. E., Wyngaarden, J. B.: The miscible pool and turnover rate of cortisol in man. *J Clin Invest 35:* 552–561, 1956.

41. Tait, J. F.: Review: The use of isotopic steroids for the measurement of production rates in vivo. *J Clin Endocrinol Metab 23:* 1285–1297, 1963.

42. Fukushima, D. K., Bradlow, H. L., Hellman, L., et al: Further studies of cortisol secretion rates. *J Clin Endocrinol Metab 29:* 1042–1045, 1969.

43. Gallagher, T. F., Fukushima, D. K., Hellman, L.: Clarification of discrepancies in cortisol secretion rate. *J Clin Endocrinol Metab 31:* 625–631, 1970.

44. DeLacerda, L., Kowarski, A., Migeon, C. J.: Diurnal variation of the metabolic clearance rate of cortisol. Effect on measurement of cortisol production rate. *J Clin Endocrinol Metab 36:* 1043–1049, 1973.

45. Hellman, D. A., Geroud, C. J. P.: Plasma cortisone and cortisol levels at birth and during the neonatal period. *J Clin Endocrinol Metab 25:* 243–248, 1965.

46. Reynolds, J. W., Colle, E., Ulstrom, R. A.: Adrenocortical steroid metabolism in newborn infants. *J Clin Endocrinol Metab 22:* 245–254, 1962.

47. Bertrand, J., Gilly, R., Loros, B.: Neonatal adrenal function. In The Human Adrenal Cortex. Curvie, A. R., Symington, T., Grant, J. K. (eds). Livingstone, Edinburgh, 1962, p. 608.

48. Aarskog, D.: Cortisol in the newborn infant. *Acta Paediatr Scand Suppl 158,* 1965.

49. Migeon, C. J.: Cortisol production and metabolism in the neonate. *J Pediatr 55:* 280–295, 1959.

50. Franks, R. C.: Diurnal variation of plasma 17-OHCS in children. *J Clin Endocrinol Metab 27:* 75–78, 1967.

51. Garces, L. Y., Kenng, F. M., Drash, A., et al: Cortisol secretion rate during fasting of obese adolescent subjects. *J Clin Endocrinol Metab 28:* 1843–1847, 1968.

52. DeMoor, P., Steeno, O., Meulepas, E. et al: Influence of body size and of sex on urinary corticoid excretion. *J Clin Endocrinol Metab 23:* 677–683, 1963.

53. Burke, C. W.: Hormones in urine: Uses and misuses. *J Roy Coll Physicians Lond 8:* 335–354, 1974.

54. Migeon, C. J.: Study of adrenocortical function in obesity. *Metabolism 12:* 718–739, 1963.

55. Dunkelman, S. S., Fairhurst, B., Plager, J., et al: Cortisol metabolism in obesity. *J Clin Endocrinol Metab 24:* 832–841, 1964.

56. Prezio, J. A., Carreon, G., Clerkin, E., et al: Influence of body composition on adrenal function in obesity. *J Clin Endocrinol Metab 24:* 481–485, 1964.

57. Cooke, J. N. C., James, V. H. T., Landon, J., et al: Adrenocortical function in chronic malnutrition. *Br Med J 1:* 662–666, 1964.

58. Bliss, E. J., Migeon, C. J.: Endocrinology of anorexia nervosa. *J Clin Endocrinol Metab 17:* 766–776, 1957.

59. Husely, R. A., Reed, F. C., Smith, T. E.: Effects of semistarvation and water deprivation on adrenal cortical function and corticosteroid metabolism. *J Appl Physiol 14:* 31–36, 1959.

60. Smith, S. R., Bledsoe, T., Chhetri, M. K.: Cortisol metabolism and the pituitary-adrenal axis in adults with protein-calorie malnutrition. *J Clin Endocrinol Metab 40:* 43–52, 1975.

61. Peterson, R. E., Nokes, G., Chen, P. S., Jr., et al: Estrogens and adrenocortical function in man. *J Clin Endocrinol Metab 20:* 495–514, 1960.

62. Plager, J. E., Schmidt, K. G., Staubitz, W. J.: Increased unbound cortisol in the plasma of estrogen-treated subjects. *J Clin Invest 43:* 1066–1072, 1964.

63. Peterson, R. E.: Adrenocortical steroid metabolism and adrenal cortical function in liver disease. *J Clin Invest 39:* 320–331, 1960.

64. Zumoff, B., Bradlow, H. L., Gallagher, T. F., et al: Cortisol metabolism in cirrhosis. *J Clin Invest 46:* 1735–1743, 1967.

65. Peterson, R. E., Wyngaarden, J. B., Guerra, S. L., et al: The physiological disposition and metabolic fate of hydrocortisone in man. *J Clin Invest 34:* 1779–1794, 1955.

66. Tucci, J. R., Albocete R. A., Martin, M. M.: Effect of liver disease upon steroid circadian rhythms in man. *Gastroenterology 50:* 637–644, 1966.

67. McCann, V. J., Fullon, T. T.: Cortisol metabolism in chronic liver disease. *J Clin Endocrinol Metab 40:* 1038–1044, 1975.

68. Englert, E., Brown, H., Willardson, D. G., et al: Metabolism of free and conjugated 17-OHCS in subjects with uremia. *J Clin Endocrinol Metab 18:* 36–48, 1958.

69. Pekkarinen, A., Kasansen, A.: Plasma levels, urinary excretion, and clearance of 17-OHCS in renal patients after intravenous cortisol. *Acta Endocrinol 38:* 13–21, 1961.

70. Peterson, R. E.: The influence of the thyroid on adrenal cortical function. *J Clin Invest 37:* 736–743, 1958.

71. Yates, F. E., Urguhart, J., Herbst, A. L.: Effects of thyroid hormones on ring A reduction of cortisone by liver. *Am J Physiol 195:* 373–380, 1958.

72. Brown, H., Englert, E., Wallack, S.: Metabolism of free and conjugated 17-hydroxycorticosteroids in subjects with thyroid disease. *J Clin Endocrinol Metab 18:* 167–179, 1958.

73. Hellman, K., Bradlow, H. L., Zumoff, B., et al: The influence of thyroid hormone on hydrocortisone production and metabolism. *J Clin Endocrinol Metab 21:* 1231–1247, 1961.

74. Gallagher, T. F., Hellman, L., Finklestein, J., et al: Hyperthyroidism and cortisol secretion in man. *J Clin Endocrinol Metab 34:* 919–927, 1972.

75. Emerth, Y., Hedner, P., Wiklander, O.: Corticoid concentration in plasma in shock and after ACTH. *Acta Chir Scand 130:* 411–423, 1965.

76. Bliss, E. L., Migeon, C. J., Branch, C. H. H., et al: Reaction of adrenal cortex to emotional stress. *Psychosom Med 18:* 56–76, 1956.

77. Lingjaerde, P. S.: Plasma hydrocortisone in mental disease. *Br J Psychiatry 110:* 423–432, 1964.

78. Persky, H., Zucherman, M., Curtis, G. C.: Endocrine function in emotionally disturbed and normal men. *J Nerv Ment Dis 146:* 488–497, 1968.

79. West, H. F.: Corticosteroid metabolism and rheumatoid arthritis. *Ann Rheum Dis 16:* 173–182, 1957.

80. Winter, J. A., Sundberg, A. A., Slaunwhite, W. R., Jr.: Cortisol binding in plasma and synovial fluid in rheumatoid arthritis. *Arthritis Rheum 9:* 389–393, 1966.

81. Bledsoe, T., Island, D. R., Neg, R. L., et al: An effect of o,p-DDD in the extra-adrenal metabolism of cortisol in man. *J Clin Endocrinol Metab 24:* 1303–1311, 1964.

82. Southren, A. L., Tochimoto, S., Isuruge, K., et al: The effect of *o,p*-DDD on the metabolism of infused cortisol. *Steroids 7:* 11–79, 1960.

83. Burstein, S., Klaiber, E. L.: Phenobarbital-induced increase in 6β-OH cortisol excretion. *J Clin Endocrinol Metab 25:* 293–296, 1965.

84. Werk, E. E., Jr., Macbee, J., Skoleton, L. J.: Effect of diphenylhydantoin on cortisol metabolism in man. *J Clin Invest 43:* 1824–1835, 1964.

85. Meikle, A. W., Jubiz, W., Matsukura, S., et al: Effect of diphenylhydantoin on the metabolism of metyrapone and the release of ACTH in man. *J Clin Endocrinol Metab 29:* 1553–1558, 1969.

86. Jubiz, W., Meikle, A. W., Levinson, R. A., et al: Effect of diphenylhydantoin on the metabolism of dexamethasone: Mechanism of the abnormal dexamethasone suppression tests in humans. *N Engl J Med 283:* 11–14, 1970.

87. Jenkins, J. S.: Pituitary Tumors: Appleton, New York, 1973, pp 22–37.

88. Kahana, L., Kahana, S., McPherson, H. T.: Endocrine manifestations of intracranial extrasellar lesions. In An Introduction to Clinical Endocrinology. Eörs Bajusz (ed). Williams & Wilkins, Baltimore, 1971, pp 254–272.

89. Arnoldsson, H.: Pituitary-adrenocortical function after steroid therapy: Significance of dosage and responsiveness to stress. In An Introduction to Clinical Endocrinology. Eörs Bajusz (ed), Williams & Wilkins, Baltimore, 1971, pp 201–215.

90. Liddle, G. W., Island, D., Meador, C. K.: Normal and abnormal regulation of corticotropin secretion in man. *Recent Prog Horm Res 18:* 125–164, 1962.

91. Faglia, G., Ambrosia, B., Beck-Percoz, P., et al: Hypothalamic-pituitary-adrenal function in patients with pituitary tumors. *Acta Endocrinol 73:* 223–232, 1973.

92. Haddock, L., Vega, L. A., Aguilo, F., et al: Adrenocortical, thyroidal and human growth hormone reserve in Sheehan's syndrome. *Johns Hopkins Med J 131:* 80–99, 1972.

93. Sheehan, H. L., Summers, V. K.: The syndrome of hypopituitarism. *Q J Med 18:* 319–378, 1949.

94. Pearson, O. H., Ray, B. S.: Results of hypophysectomy in the treatment of metastatic mammary carcinoma. *Cancer 12:* 85–92, 1959.

95. Rand, R. W., Daske, A. M., Paglia, D. E., et al: Stereotaxic cryohypophysectomy. *JAMA 189:* 255–259, 1964.

96. Lawrence, J. H., Tobias, C. A., Linfoat, J. A., et al: Heavy particles, the Bragg curve and suppression of pituitary function in diabetic retinopathy. *Diabetes 12:* 490–501, 1963.

97. Martin, L. G., Martrel, P., Connors, T. B., et al: Hypothalamic origin of idiopathic hypopituitarism. *Metabolism 21:* 143–149, 1972.

98. Jenkins, J. S., Buckell, M., Carter, A. B., et al: Hypothalamic-pituitary-adrenal function after subarachnoidal haemorrhage. *Br Med J 4:*707–709, 1969.

99. Waxman, A. D., Berk, P. D., Schaleh, D., et al: Isolated adrenocorticotrophic hormone deficiency in acute intermittent porphyria. *Ann Intern Med 70:* 317–323, 1969.

100. Stocks, A. E., Martin, F. I. R.: Pituitary function in haemochromatosia. *Am J Med 45:* 839–845, 1968.

101. Hayek, A., Driscoll, S. G., Warshaw, J. B.: Endocrine studies in anencephaly. *J Clin Invest 52:* 1636–1641, 1973.

102. Kornblaum, R. N., Fischer, R.: Pituitary lesions in craniofascial injuries. *Arch Pathol 88:* 242–248, 1969.

103. Hoff, J. T., Patterson, R. H.: Craneopharyngiomas in children and adults. *J Neurosurg 36:* 299–302, 1972.

104. Gilroy, J., Meyer, J. S.: Cerebral vascular disease and endocrine disorders. In An Introduction to Clinical Endocrinology. Eörs Bajusz (ed). Williams & Wilkins, Baltimore, 1971, pp 340–355.

105. Green, W. L., Ingbar, S. H.: Decreased corticotropin reserve in isolated pituitary defect. *Arch Intern Med 108:* 945–952, 1961.

106. Carter, M. E., James, V. H. T.: Effect of corticotrophin therapy on pituitary-adrenal function. *Ann Rheum Dis 29:* 73–80, 1970.

107. Carter, M. E., James, V. H. T.: Pituitary-adrenal response to surgical stress in patients receiving corticotrophin treatment. *Lancet 1:* 328–330, 1970.

108. Danowski, T. S., Bonessi, J. V., Sabeh, G., et al: Probabilities of pituitary-adrenal responsiveness after steroid therapy. *Ann Intern Med 61:* 11–26, 1964.

109. Treadwell, B. L. J., Savage, O., Sever, E. D., et al: Pituitary-adrenal function during corticosteroid therapy. *Lancet 1:* 355–358, 1963.

110. Graber, A. L., Ney, R. L., Nicholson, W. E., et al: Natural history of pituitary-adrenal recovery following long-term suppression with corticosteroids. *J Clin Endocrinol Metab 25:* 11–16, 1965.

111. Malone, D. N. S., Grant, I. W. B., Percy-Robb, J. W.: Hypothalamopituitary-adrenal function in asthmatic patients receiving long-term corticosteroid therapy. *Lancet 2:* 733–735, 1970.

112. Martin, M. M., Gaboardi, F., Podolsky S., et al: Intermittent steroid therapy: Its effect on hypothalamic-pituitary-adrenal function and the response of plasma growth hormone and insulin to stimulation. *N Engl J Med 279:* 273–278, 1968.

113. Ackerman, G. L., Nolan, C. M.: Adrenocortical responsiveness after alternate day corticostroid therapy. *N Engl J Med 278:* 405–409, 1968.

114. Meakin, J. W., Tamtongco, M. S., Crabbe, J., et al: Pituitary-adrenal function following long-term steroid therapy. *Am J Med 29:* 459–464, 1960.

115. Symington, T.: Functional Pathology of the Human Adrenal Gland. Williams & Wilkins, 1969, pp 78–82.

116. McDonald, F. D., Myers, A. R., Pardo, R.: Adrenal hemorrhage during anticoagulant therapy. *JAMA 198:* 1052–1056, 1966.

117. O'Connell, T. X., Aston, S. J.: Acute adrenal hemorrhage complicating anticoagulant therapy. *Surg Gynecol Obstet 139:* 355–357, 1974.

118. Kelch, R. P., Kaplan, S. L., Biglieri, E. G., et al: Hereditary adrenocortical unresponsiveness to adrenocorticotrophic hormone. *J Pediatr 81:* 726–736, 1972.

119. Sperling, M. A., Wolfsen, A. R., Fisher, D. A.: Congenital adrenal hypoplasia: An isolated defect of organogenesis. *J Pediatr 82:* 444–449, 1973.

120. Liddle, G. W., Estep, H. L., Kendall, J. M., Jr., et al: Clinical application of a new test of pituitary reserve. *J Clin Endocrinol 19:* 875–894, 1959.

121. Gold, E. M., Kent, J. R., Forsham, P. H.: Clinical use of a new diagnostic agent, methopyrapone (SU-4885), in pituitary and adrenocortical disorders. *Ann Intern Med 54:* 175–188, 1961.

122. Eddy, R. L.: Aqueous vasopressin provocative test of anterior pituitary function. *J Clin Endocrinol Metab 28:* 1836–1839, 1968.

123. Kohler, P. O., O'Malley, B. W., Rayford, P. L., et al: Effect of pyrogen on blood levels of pituitary trophic hormones. Observations on the usefulness of the growth hormone response in the detection of pituitary disease. *J Clin Endocrinol Metab 27:* 219–226, 1967.

124. Hiner, B., Hedner, P., Karlefos, T.: Adrenocortical activity during induced hypoglycemia: An experimental study in man. *Acta Endocrinol (Kbhn) 40:* 421–429, 1962.

125. Yates, F. E., Russell, S. M., Maran, J. W.: Brain-adenohypophyseal. Communication in mammals. *Annu Rev Physiol 33:* 393–444, 1971.

126. Farmer, T. H., Hill, S. R., Pittman, J. A., et al: The plasma 17-hydroxycorticosteroid response to corticotropin, SU-4885 and lipopolysaccharide pyrogen. *J Clin Endocrinol Metab 21:* 433–455, 1961.

127. McCann, S. M., Antunes-Rodriquez, J., Nallan, R., et al: Pituitary-adrenal function in the absence of vasopressin. *Endocrinology 79:* 1058–1064, 1966.

128. Yates, F. E., Russell, S. M., Dallman, M. F., et al: Potentiation by vasopressin of corticotropin release induced by corticotropin-releasing factor. *Endocrinology 88:* 3–15, 1971.

129. Hedge, G. A., Yates, M. B., Marcus, R., et al: Site of action of vasopressin in causing corticotropin release. *Endocrinology 79:* 328–340, 1966.

130. Jubiz, W., Meikle, A. W., West, C. D.: Single-dose metyrapone test. *Arch Intern Med 125:* 472–474, 1970.

131. Meikle, A. W., West, S. C., Weed, A. J., et al: Single dose metyrapone test: 11β-hydroxylase inhibition by metyrapone and reduced metyrapone assayed by radioimmunoassay. *J Clin Endocrinol 40:* 298–303, 1975.

132. Spiger, M., Jubiz, W., Meikle, A. W., et al: Single-dose metyrapone test. Review of a four-year experience. *Arch Intern Med 135:* 698–700, 1975.

133. Mahajan, D. K., Wahlen, J. D., Tyler, F. H., et al: Plasma 11-deoxycortisol radioimmunoassay for metyrapone test. *Steroids 20:* 609–620, 1972.

134. Plonk, J. W., Bivens, C. H., Feldman, J. M.: Inhibition of hypoglycemia-induced cortisol secretion by the serotonin antagonist cyproheptadine. *J Clin Endocrinol 38:* 836–840, 1974.

135. Meikle, A. W., Takiguchi, H., Mizutani, S., et al: Urinary cortisol excretion determined by competitive protein-binding radioassay: A test of adrenal cortical function. *J Lab Clin Med 74:* 803–812, 1969.

136. Tyler, F. H., West, C. D.: Laboratory evaluation of disorders of the adrenal cortex. *Am J Med 53:* 664–672, 1972.

137. Nugent, C. A., MacDiarmid, W. D., Nelson, A. R., et al: Rate of

adrenal cortisol production in response to maximal stimulation with ACTH. *J Clin Endocrinol Metab 23:* 684–693, 1963.

138. Renold, A. E., Jenkins, D., Forsham, P. H., et al: The use of intravenous ACTH: A study in quantitative adrenocortical stimulation. *J Clin Endocrinol Metab 12:* 763–797, 1952.

139. Eik-Nes, K., Sandberg, A. A., Migeon, C. L., et al: Change in plasma levels of 17-hydroxycorticosteroids during the intravenous administration of ACTH. II. Response under various clinical conditions. *J Clin Endocrinol Metab 15:* 13–21, 1955.

140. Christy, N. P., Wallace, E. Z., Jailer, J. W.: The effect of intravenously administered ACTH on plasma 17,21-dihydroxy 20-ketosteroids in normal individuals and in patients with disorders of the adrenal cortex. *J Clin Invest 34:* 899–906, 1955.

141. Matsukura, S., West, C. D., Ichikawa, Y., et al: A new phenomenon of usefulness in the radioimmunoassay of plasma adrenocorticotrophic hormone. *J Lab Clin Med 77:* 490–500, 1971.

142. Berson, S. A., Yalow, R. S.: Radioimmunoassay of ACTH in plasma. *J Clin Invest 47:* 2725–2751, 1968.

143. Krieger, D. T., Gerwitz, G. P.: The nature of the circadian pattern and suppressibility of immunoreactive ACTH levels in Addison's disease. *J Clin Endocrinol 39:* 46–52, 1974.

144. Liotta, A., Krieger, D. T.: A sensitive bioassay for the determination of human plasma ACTH levels. *J Clin Endocrinol Metab 40:* 268–277, 1975.

145. Meikle, A. W., Jubiz, W., Matsukura, S., et al: The effect of estrogen on the metabolism of metyrapone and release of ACTH. *J Clin Endocrinol 30:* 259–263, 1970.

146. Brownie, A. C., Sprunt, J. G.: Metopirone in the assessment of pituitary-adrenal function. *Lancet 1:* 772–778, 1962.

147. Kaplan, N. M.: Assessment of pituitary ACTH secretory capacity with metopirone: 1. Interpretation. *J Clin Endocrinol 23:* 945–952, 1963.

148. Henke, W. J., Doe, R. P.: Plasma and urinary 11-deoxycorticosteroids (11-DOC S) response to metyrapone in pituitary, renal, and hepatic disease. *J Clin Endocrinol 27:* 1565–1572, 1967.

149. Mecklenburg, R. S., Loriaux, D. L., Thompson, R. H., et al: Hypothalamic dysfunction in patients with anorexia nervosa. *Medicine 53:* 147–159, 1974.

150. Jacobs, J. S., Nabarro, J. D. N.: Plasma 11-hydroxycorticosteroids and growth hormone levels in acute medial illnesses. *Br Med J 2:* 595–598, 1969.

151. Juseleius, R. E., Kenny, F. M.: Urinary free cortisol excretion during growth and aging: Correlation with cortisol production rate and 17-hydroxycorticosteroid excretion. *Metabolism 23:* 84–852, 1974.

152. Soffer, L. J., Gabrilove, J. L.: A simplified water-loading test for the diagnosis of Addison's disease. *Metabolism 1:* 504–510, 1952.

153. Frawley, T. F.: The Thorn test. *Triangle 2:* 146–155, 1956.

154. Thorn, G. W., Forsham, P. H., Prunty, F. T. G., et al: A test for adrenocortical insufficiency. The response to pituitary adrenocorticotrophic hormone. *JAMA 137:* 1005–1009, 1948.

155. Nugent, C. A., Nichols, T., Tyler, F. H.: Diagnosis of Cushing's syndrome. Single dose dexamethasone suppression test. *Arch Intern Med 116:* 172–176, 1965.

156. Eddy, R. L., Jones, A. L., Gilliland, P. F., et al: Cushing's syndrome: A prospective study of diagnostic methods. *Am J Med 55:* 621–630, 1973.

157. Nichols, T., Nugent, C. A., Tyler, F. H.: Steroid laboratory tests in the diagnosis of Cushing's syndrome. *Am J Med 45:* 116–128, 1968.

158. Connolly, C. K., Gore, M. B. R., Stanley, N., et al: Single-dose dexamethasone suppression in normal subjects and hospital patients. *Br Med J 2:* 665–667, 1968.

159. Blumenfield, M.: Dexamethasone suppression in basic trainees under stress. *Arch Gen Psychiatry 23:* 299–304, 1970.

160. Asfeldt, V. H.: Hypophyseo-adrenocortical function in diabetes mellitus. *Acta Med Scand 191:* 349–354, 1972.

161. Stokes, P. E.: Adrenocortical activation in alcoholics during chronic drinking. *Ann NY Acad Sci 215:* 77–83, 1973.

162. Grant, S. D., Pavlatos, F., Forsham, P. H.: Effects of estrogen therapy on cortisol metabolism. *J Clin Endocrinol Metab 25:* 1057–1066, 1965.

163. Burke, C. W., Beardwell, C. G.: Cushing's syndrome: An evaluation of the clinical usefulness of urinary free cortisol and other steroid measurements. *Q J Med 42:* 195–204, 1973.

164. Murphy, B. E. P.: Clinical evaluation of urinary cortisol determinations by competitive protein-binding radioassay. *J Clin Endocrinol Metab 28:* 343–348, 1968.

165. Streeten, D. H. P., Stevenson, C. T., Dalakos, T. G., et al: The diagnosis of hypercortisolism. Biochemical criteria differentiating patients from lean and obese normal subjects and from females on oral contraceptives. *J Clin Endocrinol Metab 29:* 1191–1211, 1969.

166. Ehrlich, E. N.: Reciprocal variations in urinary cortisol and aldosterone in response to sodium depleting influence of hydrochlorothiazide and ethacrynic acid in humans. *J Clin Endocrinol Metab 27:* 836–842, 1967.

167. Liddle, G. W.: Tests of pituitary-adrenal suppressibility in the diagnosis of Cushing's syndrome. *J Clin Endocrinol Metab 20:* 1539–1559, 1960.

168. West, C. D., Meikle, A. W., Tyler, F. H.: Unpublished observation.

169. Meikle, A. W., Lagerquist, L. G., Tyler, F. H.: Apparently normal pituitary-adrenal suppressibility in Cushing's syndrome: Dexamethasone metabolism and plasma levels. *J Lab Clin Med 86:* 472–478, 1975.

170. Braverman, L. E., Woeber, K. A., Ingbar, S. H.: An unusual case of Cushing's syndrome. *N Engl J Med 273:* 101–1020, 1965.

171. Schteingart, D. E., Gregerman, R. I., Conn, J. W.: A comparison of the characteristics of increased adrenocortical function in obesity and in Cushing's syndrome. *Metabolism 12:* 484–497, 1963.

172. Cassidy, C. E., Rosenfeld, P. S., Bokat, M. A.: Suppression of activity of the adrenal cortex by dexamethasone in Cushing's syndrome. *J Clin Endocrinol Metab 26:* 1181–1184, 1966.

173. Schletter, F. E., Cliff, G. V., Meyers, R., et al: Cushing's syndrome in childhood: Report of two cases with bilateral adrenocortical hyperplasia, showing distinctive clinical features. *J Clin Endocrinol Metab 27:* 22–28, 1967.

174. Besser, G. M., Landon, J.: Plasma levels of immunoreactive corticotrophin in patients with Cushing's syndrome. *Br Med J 4:* 552–554, 1968.

175. Croughs, R. J. M., Tops, C. E., DeJong, F. H.: Radioimmunoassay of plasma adrenocorticotrophin in Cushing's syndrome. *J Endocrinol 59:* 439–449, 1973.

176. Raux, M. C., Binoux, M., Lupton, J. P., et al: Studies of ACTH secretion control in 116 cases of Cushing's syndrome. *J Clin Endocrinol Metab 40:* 186–197, 1975.

177. Nelson, D. H., Sprunt, J. G., Grims, R. B.: Plasma ACTH determinations in 58 patients before and after adrenalectomy for Cushing's syndrome. *J Clin Endocrinol Metab 26:* 722–728, 1966.

178. Amatruda, T. T., Upton, G. V.: Hyperadrenocorticism and ACTH-releasing factor. *Ann NY Acad Sci 230:* 168–180, 1974.

179. Meikle, A. W., Stanchfield, J. B., West, C. D., et al: Hydrocortisone suppression test for Cushing's syndrome: Therapy with anticonvulsants. *Arch Intern Med 134:* 1068–1071, 1974.

180. Brown, R. D., Van Loon, G. R., Orth, D. N., et al: Cushing's syndrome with paradoxical hormogenesis: One explanation for paradoxical response to dexamethasone. *J Clin Endocrinol Metab 36:* 445–451, 1973.

181. Bailey, R. E.: Periodic hormogenesis—A new phenomenon: Periodicity in function of a hormone-producing tumor in man. *J Clin Endocrinol Metab 32:* 317–327, 1971.

182. Soderberg-Olsen, P., Binder, C., Kehlet, H., et al: Episodic variation in plasma corticosteroids in subjects with Cushing's syndrome of differing etiology. *J Clin Endocrinol Metab 36:* 906–910, 1973.

95

Cushing's Syndrome

Don H. Nelson

INTRODUCTION

Cushing's syndrome is a general term used to refer to patients who have increased secretion of cortisol by the adrenal cortex. Corticosterone, aldosterone, desoxycorticosterone, substance S, and dehydroepiandrosterone are often increased along with cortisol, with variations dependent upon the pathology producing Cushing's syndrome. Increased secretion of specific adrenal hormones other than cortisol produces syndromes such as hyperaldosteronism and the adrenogenital syndrome (Chapters 97 and 98). As will be described in greater detail below, patients with Cushing's syndrome may have increased secretion of aldosterone, androgens, and all the normal secretory products if the gland is hyperplastic secondary to production of ACTH. A general increase in secretion of a number of hormones is also characteristic of, but not uniformly found in, patients with adrenal carcinomas that produce Cushing's syndrome.

For the purposes of this discussion, Cushing's disease will refer to those patients who have adrenal hyperfunction secondary to an increase in ACTH secretion by the pituitary gland. A general discussion of this condition will be presented, followed by specific discussions of other etiologies for Cushing's syndrome, such as adrenal tumors or ectopic tumors that produce ACTH. In these later discussions, emphasis will be placed upon those findings that differ from those seen in Cushing's disease in order to avoid repetition of the basic findings of the syndrome, which are best reviewed in discussing the condition of pituitary etiology, which is most common. Since an understanding of basic physiology and biochemistry is essential to a clear understanding of Cushing's syndrome, it is suggested that the reader refer to specific sections on ACTH control of cortisol secretion (Chapter 93), corticosteroid synthesis (Chapter 92), and/or tests of adrenal function (Chapter 94) when a better in-depth knowledge of the area being discussed is desired.

Cushing described most of the important clinical features in his monograph published in 1912.[1] As the condition was first reported in the Soviet Union by Dr. N. M. Itsenko, the condition is referred to in that area of the world as Itsenko-Cushing syndrome. Although the syndrome carries the name of Cushing, he refers to five earlier reports in which the "precisely same syndrome" is described. However, Cushing is credited with recognizing the association between the pituitary gland and adrenal hyperactivity and with giving us a clear description of the clinical features of the disease in a number of patients. Although studies by many other workers have clarified the multiple etiologic factors in the production of Cushing's syndrome, it remains a fact that approximately 75 percent of patients with the condition (if one excludes nonendocrine carcinomas that may secrete ACTH) have a pituitary-related etiology for their disease.

CUSHING'S DISEASE

CLINICAL PRESENTATION

The typical clinical presentation of the patient with Cushing's disease is a middle-aged female, less often a male, who presents with truncal obesity, hirsutism, plethora, and moderate hypertension. Glucose intolerance is often, but not always, present. Prominent symptoms include weakness, fatigue, a history of increased bruisability, and not uncommonly emotional disturbances. An increase in weight and appearance of the typical red striae may also be noted. Amenorrhea is frequently, but not always, present. The striae should not be confused with those that occur in adolescents who gain considerable weight during their teens or early twenties. The striae developed during this period also are often violaceous, while the well-known "stretch marks" occurring during pregnancy and often recognizable thereafter seldom develop this coloration (see Fig. 95-1). A change in appearance to the typical plethoric "moon facies" may not be readily apparent to patient or physician, but pictures of the patient taken over a period of years may point out the changes that have occurred. Table 95-1 lists the most common signs seen in two series of patients and in a group collected from the literature. Figure 95-2 illustrates the marked

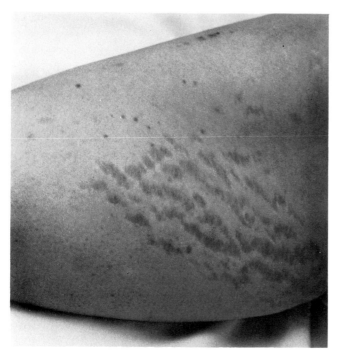

Fig. 95-1. Typical stria of Cushing's disease. Those shown are on the upper arm, but they may also be present on the thigh and most commonly on the abdomen.

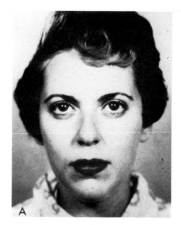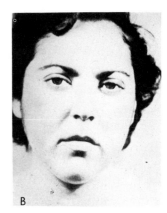

Fig. 95-2. A patient with Cushing's syndrome as first seen (a), and the remarkable change in appearance that occurred following cure of the condition (b).

change in facial appearance that Cushing's syndrome may produce.

The challenge to the clinician is to identify those patients with any combination of the above symptoms who require further laboratory examination in order to make the diagnosis. The benefits of proper therapy are so great that the application of reasonable screening tests to a patient with a combination of the above symptoms to rule out the diagnosis would appear to be a good utilization of the "health dollar."

EFFECTS OF INCREASED CORTISOL

Cortisol Effects on Fat and Fat Distribution

The obesity of Cushing's syndrome is classically described as truncal in nature. The limbs are not as heavily obese as one might

Table 95-1. Comparison of Percentage Incidence of Clinical Signs in Mount Sinai Hospital Series, Presbyterian Hospital Series, and Cases Collected From Literature*

Sign	Mount Sinai Series (50 cases) %	Columbia Series (33 cases) %	Collected from Literature (189 cases) %
Amenorrhea	72	86	71
Obesity	86	97	97
Virilism	84	73	69
Hypertension	88	84	85
Edema of lower extremities	66	60	28
Hemorrhagic manifestations	68	60	23
Plethora	78	89	50
Asthenia	58	83	50

*Mount Sinai series is from Soffer et al.[111] Columbia series and cases collected from literature came from review by Plotz et al.[23]

expect to see in patients of similar weight. It should be emphasized, however, that the obesity of Cushing's syndrome is generally of a moderate nature, and thus patients having great obesity rarely have the syndrome, although most patients weigh more than their ideal weight. Some of the apparent sparing of the limbs may be due to muscular atrophy, which in severe cases may be pronounced. Although there may be increased superclavicular fat pads as well as a "buffalo hump" (an accentuation of normal fat pad over the upper back), these findings are not diagnostic but may be considered useful additional clinical findings in the individual with the disease. A special prominence of fat tissue in the patients' cheeks contributes to the typical "moon face" that is often seen in these patients (see Fig. 95-2).

In a metabolic study, Kyle was able to demonstrate an increase in body fat without an increase in whole body weight in a patient given cortisol while maintained on a constant food intake.[2] Animals treated with large doses of corticosteroids lose weight, but the loss of protein is more rapid than that of fat. It is of interest that "brown fat" is particularly affected by corticosteroid therapy and may increase markedly in response to treatment with cortisone.[3] It has been suggested that the adiposity results not from a direct action of the glucocorticoids but rather as a secondary consequence of the increased secretion of insulin that accompanies increased gluconeogenesis produced by the corticosteroids.[4] The increased levels of insulin stimulate lipogenesis and contribute to, but are probably not the total cause of, the obesity. Fat-mobilizing substances such as epinephrine fail to act in the adrenalectomized animal, and glucocorticoids administered to intact or adrenalectomized animals do not result in mobilization of fat as determined by fat in the liver. Corticoids thus play a permissive role in allowing other hormones to affect fatty tissues. All patients with Cushing's syndrome will not be obese. Patients with carcinomas may have enough inanition to lose not only their typical truncal obesity but also their characteristic areas of fat deposition.

Cortisol Effects on Muscle

The effect of large doses of cortisol upon the muscles of the patient with Cushing's syndrome varies from slight to very marked. The patients may have so much muscle wasting that they simulate muscular dystrophy or may have little that can be identified. The presence or absence of increased androgens may be important in determining the extent of muscular disease. The anabolic action of the androgens appears to at least partially counteract the catabolic effect of the glucocorticoids. Muscular weakness is not always clearly associated with the extent of muscle wasting. Weakness may be due to hypokalemia which can occasionally be severe, but patients with a normal serum potassium and little apparent muscle wasting may also have weakness.

There is biochemical evidence of loss of amino acids from muscle and a decrease in the incorporation of labeled amino acids into muscle proteins in adrenal insufficiency, thus indicating both catabolic and antianabolic effects of corticosteroids.[5] The breakdown of protein makes available increased levels of amino acids to the liver, contributing to the increased gluconeogenesis that is characteristic of corticosteroid action.[6] Treatment of animals with glucocorticoids causes changes in both ribosomal and mitochondrial function of the muscles.[7] The actions of corticoids in the production of muscular weakness and wasting are multiple or at least affect multiple systems.

Cortisol Effects on Carbohydrate Metabolism

The ability of glucocorticoids to induce a "steroid diabetes" with decreased glucose tolerance, fasting hyperglycemia, and glucosuria is well known. There is considerable variation in the extent to which diabetes is seen in patients with Cushing's disease. It seems likely that those with a genetic predisposition to the condition are the patients who most quickly develop a severe form of diabetes. Cushing's disease may exist, however, with only mild variation in the glucose tolerance or indeed with none at all.

Glucocorticoids have such widespread effects that it is unlikely that the diabetes of the Cushing's patient can be explained wholly by an increase in gluconeogenesis. The effect of glucocorticoids to inhibit lipogenesis, noted above, results in decreased glucose uptake by the fat cell and in this sense is contributory to a hyperglycemic state. Similarly, muscle shows a decreased glucose uptake when exposed to excessive glucocorticoids and becomes relatively insulin-insensitive. The effect of glucocorticoids to stimulate gluconeogenesis both by its effect on the amino acid metabolizing enzymes tryptophan oxygenase and tyrosine transaminase and by its effect on the glycolytic rate-limiting enzymes have been extensively studied. The problem at present is, not to demonstrate an effect of glucocorticoids to bring about changes in glucose metabolism, but to sort out those specific points of action that may initiate their extensive and widespread actions. Thus the ability of the glucocorticoids to produce diabetes in the patient with Cushing's disease is probably a combination of increased gluconeogenesis with increased glucose formation from protein and a relative anti-insulin effect with decreased glucose uptake by both fat and muscle.[8]

Cortisol Effects on Bone

The patient with Cushing's disease of long duration will almost always demonstrate demineralization of bone. In severe cases, this may lead to pathologic fractures but more commonly results in radiologic evidence without obvious physical findings. The effects of corticosteroids are multifactorial and have been shown to entail inhibition of formation of the protein matrix of the bone, a decrease in the absorption of calcium by inhibiting the action of vitamin D, an increase in urinary calcium loss, and possibly other factors.[9,10] The rate of synthesis of the extracellular bone collagen matrix is undoubtedly influenced by many factors, but the ability of corticosteroids to suppress collagen synthesis is an important factor in their action on bone. Occasionally, patients with Cushing's syndrome may demonstrate the avascular necrosis of bone that is seen more commonly in patients receiving large doses of exogenous corticosteroids.[11] Although demineralization of bone demonstrable by x-ray may persist indefinitely in the adult,

in growing children normal bone will be laid down following cure of the Cushing's disease, and the bones will gradually return to near-normal mineralization.

Cortisol Effects on Growth

The young patient who develops Cushing's disease or who receives corticosteroids in excessive doses exhibits definite growth retardation. Skeletal maturation is delayed as well, and once again, explanation of the mechanisms responsible will require further investigation.[12] It is likely that the effects on protein metabolism are important, and it has been suggested that the ability of corticosteroids to inhibit growth hormone secretion may also have an effect.[13] The effects of corticosteroids on bone referred to above may also be of importance, and the loss of the anabolic and growth stimulatory effects of the adrenal androgens may play a role as well. It is of interest that growth often resumes with a rapid rate when the excess corticosteroids are removed, although permanent stunting in height can occur. An effect of the corticoids to inhibit collagen formation and incorporation of proline into cartilage may be important in their effects on decreasing the bony matrix, on healing, and on growth.[14] Studies in children have noted the frequency with which these patients are obese and of short stature and the difficulty that may be encountered in recognizing and making the diagnosis.[15] Response to growth hormone with increased growth may be seen.[16]

Cortisol Effects on the Gastric Mucosa

An extensive literature has suggested the importance of corticosteroids in producing ulcers. Although the incidence of ulcer is not high in patients with Cushing's syndrome, the possibility should be considered. Spiro and Miles have emphasized the importance of aspirin given in conjunction with corticosteroids in producing gastric irritation.[17] It would seem reasonable, therefore, to limit the use of aspirin in patients who are exposed to excessive corticosteroids.

Cortisol Effects on the Central Nervous System and Emotional Lability

Patients with Cushing's syndrome are characteristically subject to emotional instability. Symptoms range from hypomanic behavior to depression. The latter is particularly common in patients following adrenalectomy and may require considerable support and/or therapy with antidepressants.[18] Patients may complain of increased activity or increased somnolence. The corticosteroids are known to affect a number of enzymes that are located in cerebral cells, including glycerol phosphate dehydrogenase, tryptophan hydroxylase, and a mitochondrial NADH oxidase.[19–21]

Cortisol Effects on Blood Pressure

Almost all patients with Cushing's disease present with an increase in blood pressure. The hypertension is usually moderate in character, although malignant hypertension in association with Cushing's disease has been described, albeit rarely. These patients usually have hypertension of the "low renin" type, which is indicative of extracellular fluid expansion related to sodium retention. As cortisol has some sodium-retaining activity and these patients also have increased secretion of 11-desoxycortisol (substance S), corticosterone, and desoxycorticosterone, steroids that are increased in response to ACTH stimulation of the adrenal cortex, it is consistent that they develop this type of hypertension. The other cardiovascular complications of Cushing's disease, namely congestive failure and cerebrovascular accidents, are predominantly secondary to the hypertension. In addition to the effects on total volume, it has been suggested that corticoids increase the sodium and water content of the arterioles with a decrease in the lumen and thus an increase in peripheral vascular resistance.[22] Plotz et al[23] found that 40 percent of patients dying of their disease did so as a result of complications related to hypertension and/or arteriosclerosis.

Cortisol Effects on Leukocytes and Susceptibility to Infection

Corticosteroids have many effects on leukocytes that are associated with the clinical picture. They cause a decrease in peripheral levels of lymphocytes and eosinophils and acutely produce an increase in the granulocytic series. The decrease in lymphcytes is probably due to increased destruction of the cells, whereas an increase in granulocytes results from increased release of the cells from the bone marrow as well as a decrease in their migration from the blood.[24,25] Polycythemia is a common finding in the patient with Cushing's disease and has been related to an increase in both erythrocyte volume and hemoglobin mass chiefly as the result of increased androgen effect.

In the untreated patient with Cushing's disease, death occurs in approximately half of the patients from intercurrent infections.[23] Demonstration of the importance of the corticosteroids in influencing bactericidal killing may account for the relative susceptibility of these patients to infection. Since corticosteroids were first demonstrated to inhibit the NADH oxidase of granulocytes, a number of studies have been formulated to more clearly define their role in these reactions. It appears clear that superoxide anion produced in response to an NADH oxidase of leukocytes plays an important role in the killing process.[26] It is also well demonstrated that corticosteroids both in vitro and in vivo can inhibit the production of this anion and its products and thus markedly decrease leukocyte bactericidal activity.[27] Although it has been suggested that some of the sensitivity to infection is due to decreased antibody responses, rather high doses of corticosteroids are required to inhibit antibody production, and it has been easier to inhibit a primary response than an anamnestic response.[28] Glucocorticoids suppress delayed hypersensitivity reactions, which probably accounts in part for the increased susceptibility to tuberculosis in corticosteroid-treated patients.[29]

Cortisol Effects on Wound Healing and Scar Tissue

There is a considerable increase in bruisability in the patient with full-blown Cushing's disease. The poor wound healing that is seen in these patients is a problem not only during the course of the disease but particularly at the time of surgery. The problem can be so great that some surgeons prefer a course of adrenal suppressive therapy, with substances such as aminoglutethimide, for a few weeks prior to the surgery in order to allow normal wound healing to return. There is a definite inhibition of collagen formation with corticosteroid therapy.[30] The latter is responsible for the frequency of wound breakdown in postsurgical patients.

EFFECTS OF INCREASED ANDROGENS

The effects of increased adrenal androgens are covered more fully in Chapters 97, 113, and 121. However, some mention should be made here of their action in Cushing's disease.

Moderate hirsutism is a common clinical sign of Cushing's disease in the female and results from the increased production of adrenal androgens by the stimulated adrenal cortex. Although the hirsutism is not usually as severe as that seen with purely androgen-producing tumors, it can range from very mild to moderately severe. As levels of plasma testosterone or urinary 17-ketosteroids do not necessarily correlate with the extent of the hirsutism, it is thought that "end-organ sensitivity" of the hair follicle may influence the degree to which hirsutism is apparent. This may be due, at least in part, to the metabolism of testosterone to dihydrotestosterone or other metabolites by the end-organ.

Amenorrhea or oligomenorrhea was present in 86 percent of the cases of Cushing's syndrome described by Plotz et al.[23] (see Table 95-1). The mechanism for amenorrhea is probably a combination of suppression of gonadotropin production by the increased levels of androgens and a direct effect of the androgens on the uterine endometrium with an "antiestrogen" effect. Patients with secretion of only cortisol, as from an adenoma, are more likely to have normal menstrual periods than are those with Cushing's disease who produce increased androgens.

EFFECTS OF INCREASED ALDOSTERONE

Aldosterone contributes little to the sodium retention, hypertension, and potassium deficiency of the patient with Cushing's disease. The effects of this hormone are described in detail in Chapter 98.

LABORATORY FINDINGS IN CUSHING'S DISEASE

Laboratory findings in the patient with Cushing's disease result largely from the effects of cortisol described above, with varying modifications by androgens and aldosterone. Serum potassium may be decreased, and as a result, a hypokalemic alkalosis may be present. Total leukocyte count may be increased with a relative preponderance of neutrophils and a decrease in lymphocytes and eosinophils. Polycythemia is occasionally seen. A diabetic glucose tolerance and, in more severe cases, an elevated fasting blood sugar may be present.

X-ray examination may demonstrate demineralization of bone and cardiac enlargement secondary to the hypertension. An enlarged sella turcica may be present, although relatively rarely. Although various radiological studies may demonstrate an adrenal tumor, these should be reserved for localization after the chemical diagnosis has been made (see Chapter 91).

The essential laboratory findings in the diagnosis of Cushing's disease are those measurements of pituitary ACTH and plasma and urinary corticosteroids that demonstrate both increased levels and a relative resistance to suppression by exogenous corticosteroids. These will be described briefly here. The details by which the tests are performed and errors in interpretation are presented in Chapter 94 (see also synopsis of tests in diagnosis of adrenal disorders, Chapter 99).

Plasma Cortisol and Diurnal Variation

Plasma cortisol is usually elevated, but as a result of the episodic variation in levels of these hormones, single determinations may or may not be elevated. Since most patients with Cushing's disease have lost the normal diurnal variation in secretion of the corticoids, measurement of an early morning and a late evening plasma cortisol will demonstrate loss of this variation. Demonstration of such loss of diurnal variation in the absence of stress may be taken as suggestive evidence of the presence of adrenal hyperactivity, but more definitive testing is necessary to establish the diagnosis.

Single-Dose Suppression Test

This is probably the simplest and easiest to perform screening test for Cushing's disease.[31] Almost all normal patients will have a lower morning plasma cortisol value following administration of 1 mg dexamethasone at 11 PM the night before than they will have on a control day. The test appears to be particularly useful in the obese patient who may have high total urinary excretion of corticosteroids but will have normal suppression of corticoid secretion when this test is employed. This is not an absolute diagnostic test, but it is a good screening test. False-positives and false-negatives have been described.

Free Urinary Cortisol

The estimation of total free cortisol in a 24-hr urine collection is also a useful method for the estimation of adrenal hyperactivity.[32–34] These determinations have the disadvantage of necessitating a 24-hr urine collection, which requires an intelligent patient or better than average paramedical personnel for inpatient collection.

Urinary 17-Ketogenic and 17-Hydroxycorticosteroids (Porter–Silber Chromagens)

The measurement of either urinary 17-ketogenic or 17-hydroxycorticosteroids is also an accurate method for estimating adrenal hyperactivity but has the disadvantage of requiring 24-hr urine collections. Obese patients may have high values. Since many laboratories are now doing cortisol by radioimmunoassay, there is a trend for supplanting these determinations with free urinary cortisol determination. Twenty-four-hour urinary determinations have the advantage that they give an estimate of a whole day's secretion and are not subject to the diurnal and episodic variations typical of plasma determinations. These tests alone are suggestive but not diagnostic of the disease.

Urinary 17-Ketosteroids

Urinary 17-ketosteroids are usually increased in Cushing's disease, as they are chiefly an estimate of urinary androgens (dehydroisoandrosterone and androstendione). They are responsive to ACTH stimulation and are increased by its administration. Their determination is not nearly as important as is that of cortisol and its chief metabolites but does give useful information in demonstrating an increase in androgen or androgen precursor secretion.

Urinary Aldosterone

Urinary aldosterone is not generally elevated in patients with Cushing's disease. It is not important to make this measurement, as the cortisol estimation gives the required information. Measurement of only urinary aldosterone might give the clinician a mistaken impression in some adrenal carcinomas that hyperaldosteronism rather than Cushing's disease is present.

Suppression of Urinary Corticosteroids with Dexamethasone

This test, which was originally carried out with the use of fluorohydrocortisone, is generally now done using the approach of Liddle et al., i.e., giving either 0.5 mg every 6 hours for 48 hours or 2.0 mg every 6 hours for 48 hours.[35] The lower dosage causes suppression of almost all normal patients, whereas the higher dosage is generally required to bring about suppression of patients with Cushing's disease. Occasionally, this test is not consistent with the final diagnosis, since patients with Cushing's disease who have suppressed with the low dosage or failed to suppress with the high dosage have been described.[36]

Metyrapone

The use of the inhibitor of adrenal (chiefly) 11-β-hydroxylation is of considerable use in the diagnosis of the etiology of Cushing's syndrome.[37,38] Patients with Cushing's disease almost always show an increase in substance S (17 hydroxy-11-desoxycorticosterone) production and in plasma ACTH when metyrapone is administered, while patients with tumors are much less likely to show such an increase (see Chapter 94). The single-dose metyrapone test is easiest to perform, but the multiple-dose test performed over 24 hours with measurement of urinary rather than plasma steroids is also useful. Substance S and its metablites are measured either as urinary 17-ketogenic steroids or 17-hydroxycorticosteroids, so it is possible to use either of these determinations in the diagnosis of Cushing's disease. An increasing number of laboratories prefer plasma determination of cortisol and substance S.

Plasma ACTH

Estimation of plasma ACTH by radioimmunoassay in Cushing's disease will usually demonstrate a moderately elevated plasma ACTH value.[39,40] In those patients who have had the disease for long periods of time or who have demonstrable pituitary tumors, the levels may be considerably elevated.[41] ACTH levels in Cushing's disease are generally suppressible by the administration of corticosteroids in fairly large doses, but those patients with pituitary tumors in the later stages of the disease are relatively resistant to suppressibility. Very high plasma ACTH values are likely to be seen in patients with tumors of nonendocrine origin producing ACTH. Normal plasma ACTH levels vary between 20 and 180 pg/ml of plasma. Patients with Cushing's disease are likely to have levels of 200–500 pg/ml, although levels as high as 10,000 pg/ml or more have been seen in patients with Nelson's syndrome.[41,42] Of interest is the occasional patient who has an increase rather than a decrease in plasma ACTH following dexamethasone administration.[43] We hypothesize that the pituitary receptor in such patients is occupied by the dexamethasone molecule and excludes cortisol but does not fit well enough to function as a cortisol-receptor complex. The resultant signal suggests a decrease in cortisol with resulting increased stimulus to ACTH secretion.

DIFFERENTIAL DIAGNOSIS

The main problem in differential diagnosis of Cushing's disease is in distinguishing the patient with mild diabetes and moderate hypertension, who is often obese and may show mild hirsutism, from the patient who has true adrenal hyperactivity. This must be done by careful measurement of the hormones in plasma or urine. The single-dose dexamethasone test is a good screening exam for making this diagnosis, but elevated urinary corticosteroid excretion and demonstration of increased plasma levels of ACTH are confirmatory of the diagnosis. The obese patient may represent a problem in diagnosis. These patients suppress secretion relatively easily, although baseline urinary steroids may be elevated. The increased secretion of corticosteroids and their metabolic products in obese patients has been explained by rapid turnover rates of injected cortisol. The total production of cortisol is therefore increased, but the plasma levels are maintained at physiologic levels.[44] Diagnosis in children or in the older patient may be somewhat difficult as a result of a less florid appearance. The child having a carcinoma may have very high levels of corticoids with or without the florid presentation.

THERAPY OF CUSHING'S DISEASE

As this condition, by definition, is the result of increased secretion of ACTH by the pituitary gland, it would seem reasonable to direct therapy at this organ. Although choice may be influenced by the availability of highly specialized facilities and personnel for carrying out either irradiation or surgery directed to the pituitary gland, there appears to be enough evidence available to suggest a rational approach to this condition.[45,46]

Irradiation of the Pituitary Gland

Administration of approximately 5,000 roentgens to the pituitary gland with a high-energy linear accelerator has been found to produce cures of Cushing's disease in one third of adult patients and the majority of childhood Cushing's disease.[46a] Those who have failed to respond have generally been subjected to total adrenalectomy. The use of a proton beam which will more completely destroy pituitary tissue has also been advocated.[47] This form of therapy is available only in a few highly specialzed centers, and it is questionable whether it offers enough to the patient to justify transportation to a distant city for treatment. It should be noted that irradiation with lower voltage machines gives a lower rate of remission than has been observed with the linear accelera-

tor.[45,48,49] It is important to note that this form of irradiation does not generally cause harm to normal pituitary tissue, so these patients are usually left with essentially normal endocrine function if the remission is complete. The proton beam, on the other hand, causes destruction of normal as well as "pathologic" tissue. Those patients with apparent total cure following irradiation appear to lend support to the concept of single small adenomas as the major etiologic factor in the condition. Destruction of the pituitary by implantation of radon seeds, colloidal ^{198}Au or ^{90}Y, has been advocated. Athough this approach has been successful in some instances, it has not been widely adopted.[50]

Hypophysectomy

Hypophysectomy for Cushing's disease has, in the past, been reserved for those patients who have large pituitary tumors that may be impinging upon the optic nerves or causing neurologic damage from pressure on surrounding structures. The disadvantages to total hypophysectomy by the conventional frontal approach are the magnitude of the operation and the loss of other pituitary functions that accompanies removal of the gland.[51] The sphenoidal approach decreases the morbidity of the operation, and the success in removing an adenoma without total removal of normal pituitary tissue has resulted in cure of the Cushing's syndrome without loss of other pituitary function.[52,53] There is much to be said for this approach if proper facilities and personnel are available (see Fig. 95-3).[53a,53b]

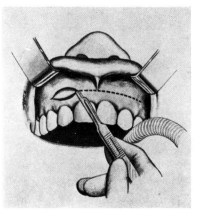
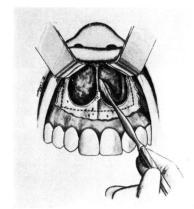
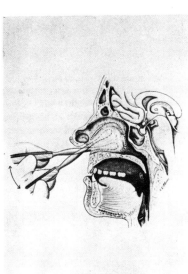
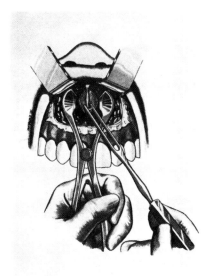

Fig. 95-3. Procedure of Hardy for the transphenoidal removal of a pituitary adenoma producing excess ACTH and Cushing's disease. (Reproduced by permission of J. Hardy.[52])

Total Adrenalectomy for Cushing's
Disease

In those patients in whom pituitary irradiation and/or surgery is not successful in returning corticosteroid secretion to normal, bilateral adrenalectomy is necessary.[54] Although in past years partial adrenalectomy has sometimes been advocated, this has not proven a useful approach to Cushing's syndrome, and thus bilateral removal of the glands should be considered. It has often been stated that adrenalectomy is the treatment of choice in those patients who have very severe Cushing's syndrome, as the effects of irradiation generally take 4 to 8 months to be complete. It has been thought that patients with severe disease should not be allowed to wait this period of time prior to having definitive therapy. With the availability of pharmacologic agents such as aminoglutethimide, which can markedly reduce adrenal function while the physician is waiting for the effects of irradiation to become apparent, fewer patients now require total adrenalectomy than did a few years ago.[55] The use of o,p'DDD or of aminoglutethimide as preparation for adrenalectomy or with pituitary irradiation has been advocated.[56] The medical treatment of the patient undergoing surgery is very important. An intravenous infusion of 100 mg of cortisol each 8 hours through the surgery and the first 24 hours thereafter is usually sufficient. Reduction of total cortisol to 150, 125, 100, and 75 mg given on successive days has generally been found satisfactory. Patients developing infections, to which these patients are especially prone, or other stressful complications may require an increase in steroid dosage. Patients often complain of arthralgias, desquamation of the skin, and occasionally have severe emotional disturbances as the cortisol is reduced. In such cases, a more gradual decrease in cortisol dosage is indicated. Continuance of cortisol dosage at the 75-mg level for a

week or more is likely to decrease withdrawal symptoms. When cortisol is reduced below 75 mg/day, addition of 0.1–0.2 mg fluorohydrocortisone is indicated. Therapy thereafter is as described for the patient with chronic Addison's disease (see Chapter 96).

Pharmacologic Agents in the Treatment
of Cushing's Syndrome

The use of cyproheptadine, a serotonin antagonist, has been advocated in the treatment of Cushing's disease. Administration of 24 mg daily for 3 to 6 months was associated with an apparently complete remission.[57] Plasma ACTH values fell from elevated to near-normal levels, and both cortisol secretion and responsiveness to dexamethasone suppression returned to normal. Although this has been interpreted to represent evidence to support a central nervous system cause for Cushing's disease, other pharmacologic effects of cyproheptadine must be considered. Further experience with this drug will have to be obtained, but its use at this time appears promising.

The effect of bromocriptine on plasma ACTH levels in patients with pituitary dependent Cushing's syndrome has also been studied. In 6 of 7 patients, this agent suppressed ACTH secretion. No long-term results with its use are available.[57a]

Both aminoglutethimide and o,p'DDD have been found successful in reducing corticosteroid secretion in Cushing's disease. Treatment with these drugs has been reported to be successful in many patients.[58–60] A distinct disadvantage of o,p'DDD is that the effect is not immediate and may require 4 to 6 months to lower the corticosteroid levels to normal (see Fig. 95-4). Aminoglutethimide, on the other hand, although acting more quickly, blocks the conversion of cholesterol to pregnenolone in other tissues and also blocks the concentration of iodine by the thyroid.[59] Therefore, it is

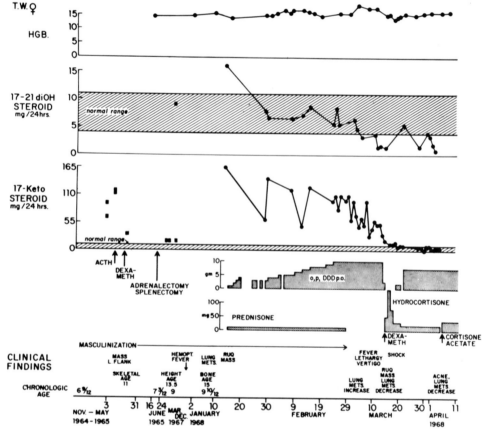

Fig. 95-4. Effect of o,p'DDD in reducing corticosteroid secretion in a patient with Cushing's syndrome. (Reproduced by permission of L. Helson, Clin. Chem. *17:* 1191, 1971.)

not a good drug for long-term therapy. In selective cases o,p'DDD has been given for as long as 5 years with cure of Cushing's syndrome, although nausea is a frequent accompaniment of such therapy. Aminoglutethimide, on the other hand, has been given for long periods only to patients with carcinoma but with success once again in suppressing adrenal secretion. Aminoglutethimide has the additional drawback that the increased ACTH secretion which accompanies its use may act to stimulate secretion of cortisol by the portion of the pathway that is not completely blocked. In order to overcome this, patients have been given dexamethasone with the aminoglutethimide so as to block ACTH secretion. Under these circumstances, total cortisol effect is not reduced, but it is possible to reduce mineralocorticoid, estrogen, and androgen secretion from the adrenal gland.

PROGNOSIS

Although spontaneous remissions have been described,[61,62] the general prognosis in Cushing's disease is one of gradually increasing pituitary ACTH secretion with concomitant increase in adrenal secretion. Although the common history at diagnosis is of only a year or two, patients who have had the disease for 10 or more years have been described. The finding of patients who have had the appearance of pituitary tumors following adrenalectomy for their disease suggests continued growth of small pituitary adenomas that were not recognized prior to adrenalectomy. Data is not conclusive, however, to rule out the possibility that some "abnormal stimulus" by CRH acting on the pituitary gland may have resulted in development of some of these tumors. Patients with postadrenalectomy enlargement of their sella turcica, intense pigmentation, and high plasma levels of ACTH have been described as having "Nelson's syndrome."[41,42,63] These patients usually have had progressive sellar enlargement during the course of their disease, with increasing pigmentation.[41,63,64] ACTH levels are usually not easily suppressible by the administration of corticosteroid, and high MSH activity has been reported.[65] These pituitary tumors are usually benign, although a rare carcinoma has been described.[66] Some have been responsive to pituitary irradiation, but hypophysectomy is generally indicated to prevent increase in size and impingement upon the optic nerves.

Any of the various modes of therapy referred to above that successfully reduce cortisol secretion to the normal range will adequately reverse most of the signs and symptoms of Cushing's disease. As noted under cortisol effects on bone, however, bony demineralization does not reverse except in the young patient. Although development of pituitary tumors postoperatively may occur in approximately 10 percent of patients, this is not a contraindication to adrenalectomy in those patients in whom a pituitary approach proves unsuccessful.

Pregnancy

The outcome of pregnancy in patients having Cushing's syndrome has been reported to be both favorable and unfavorable.[67,68] In the first report, removal of a benign adenoma in the second trimester was followed by a normal delivery. In the second report, 2 patients with adrenal adenomata gave birth to stillborn infants. A similar high incidence of stillborns has been reported by others.[69] A review of 27 pregnancies associated with Cushing's syndrome revealed 9 fetal deaths and 12 deliveries of term infants; adrenal adenoma was reported in 6 of 23 cases.[69a]

PATHOLOGY

Adrenal

The adrenal glands are consistently hyperplastic, the zona fasciculata almost always appears hyperplastic, and the zona glom-

erulosa is affected only slightly, if at all. The weight of the glands may vary from essentially normal (6 g total) to 10 times this size. In those patients with normal-sized adrenal glands, it may not be possible to make the diagnosis of Cushing's disease from histology of the organs.

Pituitary Tumors in Cushing's Disease

The association of tumors of the pituitary gland with Cushing's disease was well documented by Cushing in his classic monograph. Cushing remarked upon the collections of basophil cells that may be seen in many of these patients, but those tumors that have been examined have more often been chromophobic rather than basophilic in character. Although atrophy of the paraventricular nuclei or hyalin basophil changes were at one time thought to represent changes possibly responsible for increased ACTH secretion in these patients, later studies have demonstrated similar lesions following ACTH or cortisone administration. Thus they are thought to be secondary to the secretion of the adrenal gland, not responsible for it.[70] The majority of patients seen then and now, however, have not had tumors of the gland, but more recent evidence has suggested the frequency of microadenomas. Previous estimates of frequency of pituitary tumors associated with Cushing's disease have generally been approximately 10 percent.[64] These tumors are most frequently chromophobes, although basophilic tumors, of the type originally described by Cushing, are also seen. Figure 95-5 illustrates the most frequent location of such tumors in Hardy's series. With the introduction of transsphenoidal microsurgery, some investigators would place this figure higher. The former figure represents those patients who have had sufficient enlargement of the adenoma to be demonstrable by conventional means, i.e., disturbance of the bony sella turcica and/or evidence of growth outside the sella.

The demonstration that patients with Cushing's disease fail to respond to the stimulus of hypoglycemia[71] could also be interpreted to mean that the pituitary tumor is not under normal hypothalamic control. Loss of circadian rhythm of secretion is also consistent with this etiology, although neither finding rules out a "block with hyperactivity" at the hypothalamic level.

The occasional paradoxical response to dexamethasone in Cushing's disease also suggests a primary pituitary etiology.[72]

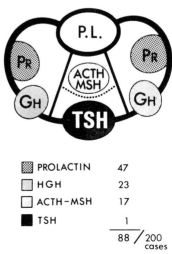

PROLACTIN	47
HGH	23
ACTH-MSH	17
TSH	1
	88 / 200 cases

Fig. 95-5. Localization of pituitary microadenomas. (Reproduced by permission of J. Hardy.[52])

Pituitary Tumors After Adrenalectomy with Marked Pigmentation (Nelson's Syndrome)

Although the frequency of demonstrable tumors of the pituitary gland associated with Cushing's disease preoperatively is not very large, a number of patients have also been described to have had continuing enlargement of the pituitary following bilateral adrenalectomy.[63,64] These patients have been demonstrated to have pituitary tumors producing high plasma levels of ACTH and MSH[64,65] and usually have extreme pigmentation. (see Figs. 95-6 and 95-7) The tumors rarely have been malignant. With the increasing demonstration of microadenomas of the pituitary gland, the concept that these small tumors have continued to grow following adrenalectomy appears to be a likely explanation of the occurrence of this syndrome. A review of 120 patients who had been adrenalectomized for bilateral adrenal hyperplasia for periods of 2 to 20 years demonstrated the development of pituitary tumors in 9 for an incidence of 8 percent. The tumors appeared from 6 months to 16 years after adrenalectomy, and of 20 patients who had received pituitary irradiation, 2 developed the pituitary tumor.[65a]

Although ACTH has some melanocyte-stimulating activity, high levels of MSH have been reported.[65,73] Recent evidence indicates that the substance measured is not β-MSH, however, but β-lipotropin.[73a]

The occurrence of exophthalmos in patients with Cushing's disease has been explained on the basis of an "exophthalmos-producing substance" being elaborated by the tumor.[74] Whether such a substance or some other etiology is responsible, 5 to 10 percent of patients in various series have been reported to have some degree of exophthalmos.

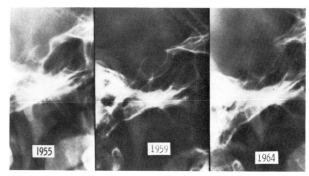

Fig. 95-7. Progressive enlargement of the sella turcica in a patient following adrenalectomy for Cushing's disease. There was a corresponding increase in skin pigmentation and in plasma ACTH levels.

BENIGN ADENOMAS OF THE ADRENAL CORTEX PRODUCING CUSHING'S SYNDROME

The clinical presentation of patients with Cushing's syndrome due to benign adenomas is very similar to that of Cushing's disease but may differ in a few characteristics. This form of Cushing's syndrome is variously reported to be produced by adenomas of the adrenal cortex in 10 to 30 percent of patients. It is seen much more frequently in women than in men, with the ratio being 4 or 5:1. The clinical picture is more likely to be that of production of cortisol alone, without increased levels of aldosterone or androgens, than is the case in either Cushing's disease or adrenal carcinoma. Additional findings suggestive of adenoma are failure of cortisol secretion to be suppressed by dexamethasone administration and failure to respond to metyrapone.

One note of caution should be added if the metyrapone test is used as a differential between hyperplasia and adenoma. With increasing determination of plasma levels of substance S with the metyrapone test, it becomes important to establish that one is not just measuring a block of 11-hydroxylation of the cortisol that is being secreted at a high and constant level by the tumor, which would then result in a marked increase in substance S production. This may be avoided either by making certain that the total of cortisol and substance S is increased after metyrapone administration or by performing a simultaneous plasma ACTH determination. The author has seen only 1 patient with an adrenal tumor that demonstrated an increase in plasma ACTH and substance S following the administration of metyrapone. The metyrapone test employed was the 2-day test with measurement of 17-ketosteroids and 17-ketogenic steroids in the urine. Further study of this patient demonstrated that the tumor was producing, chiefly, large quantities of substance S (17-hydroxy 11-desoxy corticosterone). As this substance does not suppress ACTH secretion, the normal adrenal tissue still present continued to produce cortisol. Thus, when metyrapone was given, cortisol secretion was suppressed, ACTH production increased, and this stimulated the adrenal to secrete increased quantities of 11-desoxycorticosteroids which were measured as ketogenic steroids in the urine. A rare case of a corticosterone-secreting carcinoma of the adrenal has been described.[75] This patient had a picture chiefly suggestive of primary hyperaldosteronism with a low serum potassium level and hypertension. Plasma levels of cortisol were normal. Neither 17-hydroxycorticosteroids nor 17-ketogenic steroids would be elevated in such cases as a result of the lack of a 17-hydroxyl group on corticosterone.

The diagnosis of an adenoma is suggested by finding the

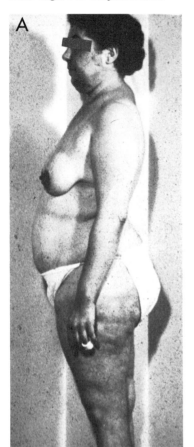
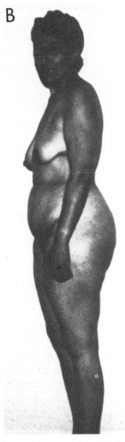

Fig. 95-6. A patient with Cushing's disease (*a*) and 3 years later (*b*) after the development of a pituitary tumor and intense pigmentation of Nelson's syndrome.

typical clinical picture of increased cortisol production, demonstrating failure to suppress plasma cortisol when the 1-mg overnight dexamethasone test is employed and failure to respond to the overnight metyrapone test. As adrenal rest tissue has been found in ovaries or testes,[76] an occasional patient has not been cured by bilateral adrenalectomy, and further studies have demonstrated an ectopic site for the tumor.[77] With tests available today, the probability that a tumor is present should prevent total adrenalectomy in such cases. The possibility of an ectopic location, however, increases the importance of tests to localize the tumor after the diagnosis is made and prior to surgery. Final diagnosis is usually made radiologically and then at surgery. It is reasonable that procedures to locate a tumor not be carried out until the diagnosis of a probable adenoma has been made chemically so as to avoid unnecessary isotopic or radiologic procedures that are often not definitive.

Localization studies usually depend upon the facilities and techniques, as well as on the expertise to use these techniques, that are available in a particular center. Intravenous pyelograms with tomograms have been successful in demonstrating the presence of a considerable number of these tumors. The use of [131]I 19-iodocholesterol may be of value not only in demonstrating the adenoma but also in finding occasional adrenal remnants from "subtotal" adrenalectomy.[78,79] Venous angiography has also proven to be of value and is a generally benign procedure, although it has been associated with adrenal hemorrhage and, rarely, even permanent adrenal insufficiency[80,81] (see Chapter 91 for a discussion of these techniques).

Definitive therapy for adrenal adenomas is, of course, surgical removal of the tumor. Because of the difficulties of differentiating a tumor from benign nodular hyperplasia, as well as the special technical skills employed in adrenal surgery, the author believes that a few surgeons should gain experience and be allowed to do adrenal surgery in a given geographical area. This surgery is sufficiently uncommon that it should not be performed by every general surgeon. Adenomas producing cortisol will characteristically cause atrophy of normal adrenal tissue through suppression of ACTH secretion by the pituitary gland. It is important, therefore, to administer cortisol in sufficient quantities to maintain the patient following removal of the adrenal gland. This requires administration of cortisol intravenously in a continuous drip beginning with the removal of the tumor and continuing through surgery and until oral medication can be given. Most patients can be taken off supplemental cortisol within a few days, but suboptimal doses of cortisol, 10–15 mg/day, may be necessary for a few weeks or, rarely, months to allow the remaining tissue to hypertrophy and to reestablish normal pituitary control of cortisol secretion.

Although there is a difference of opinion as to whether the primary defect in cortisol secretion following long-term suppression is in the adrenal or the control of ACTH secretion by the pituitary,[82–84] the available data suggest an abnormality of adrenal responsivity and of ACTH secretion following long-term exposure to increased levels of corticosteroid. Although the pituitary has been shown to be capable of secreting ACTH following an appropriate stress (such as metyrapone), these patients may continue to have adrenal atrophy for long periods of time. Administration of cortisol in low doses will relieve some of the symptoms of fatigue and weakness often experienced by these patients, but if more than about 15 mg of cortisol is given daily, the recovery of normal ACTH secretion may be delayed. The administration of ACTH has not been found useful in speeding recovery of normal function, as such therapy produces high levels of corticosteroids that continue the central suppression of endogenous ACTH.[85,86]

ACTH PRODUCTION BY NONPITUITARY TUMORS PRODUCING CUSHING'S SYNDROME (ECTOPIC ACTH SYNDROME)

The association between tumors of the lung, pancreas, and thymus and Cushing's syndrome has long been recognized.[23,87] Although the exact incidence has not been clearly delineated, in one series, approximately 20 percent of patients with Cushing's syndrome were found to have such nonpituitary origin of increased ACTH production.[88] ACTH may also be produced by tumors of the thyroid, adrenal medulla, testis, ovary, various sites in the GI tract, prostate, and parotid.[89] Both benign and malignant carcinoids, which may or may not produce increased calcitonin, have also been found to produce excessive ACTH.[90–93] It is well demonstrated that these tumors produce ACTH and that this ACTH is relatively nonsuppressible by the administration of corticosteroids. This represents an abnormality of ACTH production which may be due to derepression of DNA, which codes for production of this peptide in a tissue in which such coding would be normally suppressed.

The type of cell that produces ectopic hormones is generally thought to be of neuroectodermal origin. This general group of cells have been referred to as APUD cells (for amine precursor uptake and decarboxylation) and tumors of the cells have sometimes been called "apudomas."[93a] Such tumors may often produce increased quantities of big ACTH and also biologically inactive ACTH-like fragments (corticotropinlike intermediate lobe peptide, CLIP). Ability to measure these various types of ACTH may be helpful in the differentiation of the ectopic tumors from other types of Cushing's syndrome. Selective venous sampling for ACTH determination may also be found useful.[93b,93c,93d] It has been suggested that some of these tumors may also produce corticotropin-releasing factorlike activity.[93e]

These tumors have been reported to produce increased quantities of MSH, as well as ACTH, and thus the patient may become pigmented.[94,95] Ectopic production of hormones is not limited to ACTH and MSH, as numerous peptide hormones have been shown to be produced by tumors arising in tissue that would not normally produce them (see Chapter 139).

A number of patients have been recognized to have ACTH-producing tumors of other than pituitary origin months or years following initial therapy for Cushing's syndrome.[96] In other cases, the syndrome has been cured following removal of the peptide-producing tumor. It becomes important, therefore, to consider the possibility of such a tumor whenever Cushing's syndrome is diagnosed. Although the tumor may be readily apparent, this is not always the case. Such tumors generally fail to suppress when dexamethasone is given, and thus the possibility of a primary adrenal tumor may be considered. The finding of an elevated plasma ACTH in such a case will rule out adrenal cortical adenoma and suggest the ectopic ACTH-producing tumor. If the ACTH level is markedly elevated, greater than 1000 pg/ml in the absence of signs of a pituitary tumor, this should also suggest the presence of an ectopic tumor. As a result of the high ACTH levels that may be produced, the clinical picture is often pronounced in these patients, and the frequent association of severe hypokalemic alkalosis has been noted.[97]

Therapy should be directed toward resection of the primary tumor where feasible. Although adrenalectomy will reduce the high levels of corticosteroids that are being secreted, it is not usually indicated. Therapy with aminoglutethimide may be employed to temporarily reduce corticosteroid secretion and prepare the patient for surgery directed toward the ectopic ACTH-producing tumor.

NODULAR ADRENAL CORTICAL HYPERPLASIA

A number of patients have been described who have multiple adrenal cortical nodules in both adrenal glands.[98,99] As nodules are relatively common in the adrenal and are frequently seen in patients with "essential hypertension," it has been difficult to conclude whether nodular hyperplasia represents multiple benign adenomas that are occurring at the same time in one or more adrenal glands and are not under ACTH control or whether they represent nodular hyperplasia in patients with Cushing's disease and increased pituitary ACTH production. These patients have been described to have both no response and excessive response to the administration of ACTH and metyrapone.[99,100] Such patients have uniformly failed to suppress when given 2 mg of dexamethasone per day but often showed suppression on 8 mg of dexamethasone per day. The finding of low plasma ACTH levels in some cases, which have failed to increase with metyrapone or stress, also suggests that the lesion is primary in the adrenal cortex. As the pathologic lesion is not a totally distinctive one, it may be that some patients who have been described with normal plasma levels of ACTH do not have the syndrome. Until a more distinctive description of this group of patients can be made, this author would prefer to believe that they represent patients with Cushing's disease who happen to have more apparent nodular hyperplasia of their glands than is customary and possibly another group of patients with multiple benign adenomas.

ADRENAL CORTICAL CARCINOMAS PRODUCING CUSHING'S SYNDROME

These carcinomas are often large, rapidly growing, and usually produce all the chief secretory products of the adrenal cortex, i.e., cortisol, corticosterone, aldosterone, and the adrenal androgens. An inability to hydroxylate at the 11 position has been noted as a characteristic of many such tumors. Nine of 10 cases were found in one series to have deficient 11-β-hydroxylation and increased excretion of tetrahydro substance S.[101] Pregnanediol excretion was increased in the 4 cases studied, and 1 patient had decreased 3-β-hydroxysteroid dehydrogenase. It is of interest that although 11-β-hydroxylation of substance S was decreased, 11-β-hydroxyandrosterone was found to be increased along with the other C-19 steroids, dehydroepiandrosterone, etiocholanolone, and androsterone. Increased production of desoxycorticosterone has been noted in adrenal carcinoma (but also in adrenal hyperplasia).[102] Rapid growth with early metastasis is the rule.

Cushing's syndrome in children has a high incidence of carcinoma.[103] It has been suggested that the late diagnosis of patients with adrenal carcinoma is due to the low rate of production of steroids by the carcinoma. Thus the tumor must be fairly large and is palpable in as many as 50 percent of cases before the hormonal secretion reaches the level that produces clinical features of Cushing's syndrome. Fifty percent of patients were noted to die within 2 years of the onset of symptoms in one series and 13 of a group of 55 survived for 3 years in another.[104,105]

Although corticosteroid secretion may be temporarily reduced by surgery to remove the main tumor mass or by administration of o,p'DDD and aminoglutethimide, these are generally palliative, and cures are uncommon.[106] It should be noted, however, that adrenal carcinomas producing androgens but not cortisol may have a longer and more benign course (see Chapter 97). When o,p'DDD was given in a collaborative study to 138 patients, a greater than 50 percent reduction in steroid excretion was seen in 69 percent of patients. The mean duration of steroid response was only 4.8 months and of tumor regression, 7 months. There did not appear to be a difference in the response of patients with functioning or nonfunctioning tumors.[107] In 1 patient a positive [131]I-19-iodocholesterol scan was reported to demonstrate both a cortisol-secreting adrenal carcinoma and its hepatic metastases.[107a]

FEMINIZING ADRENOCORTICAL CARCINOMAS

Of 52 tumors of the adrenal in one review, 4 were found to have feminizing characteristics.[108] Most of these patients have been shown to have elevated urinary estrogens. In one instance, a decrease in androsterone with a concomitant increase in etiocholanolone secretion was thought to enhance the estrogenic effect.[109] Patients with a positive "chorioniclike" gonadotropin test have been reported, as well as others with positive "pituitary gonadotropin" tests.[110] These carcinomas are generally not responsive to ACTH, although occasionally some response may be seen. Universally, they fail to suppress when dexamethasone is given.

Prognosis in this group of carcinomas has been uniformly poor, although some temporary relief has been obtained with the use of chemotherapy.

REFERENCES

1. Cushing, H. The pituitary body and its disorders, Philadelphia, Lippincott, 1912.
2. Kyle, L. H., Meyer, R. J., Schaaf, M., and Werdein, E. J. The effect of compound A (11 dehydrocorticosterone) and compound F (17-hydroxycorticosterone) on total body fat. *J. Clin. Invest. 35:* 1045, 1956.
3. Aronson, S. M., Teodorn, C. V., Adler, M., and Schwartzman, G. Influence of cortisone upon brown fat of hamsters and mice. *Proc. Soc. Exp. Biol. Med. 85:* 214, 1954.
4. Hausberger, F. X., and Hausberger, B. C. Effect of insulin and cortisone on weight gain, protein and fat content of rats. *Amer. J. Physiol. 193:* 455, 1958.
5. Smith, O. K., and Long, C. N. H. Effect of cortisol on plasma amino nitrogen of eviscerated adrenalectomized-diabetic rat. *Endocrinology 80:* 561, 1967.
6. Wool, I. G., and Weinshelbaum, E. I. Incorporation of C-14 amino acids into protein of isolated diaphragms: Role of the adrenal steroids. *Amer. J. Physiol. 197:* 1089, 1959.
7. Bullock, G. R., Carter, E. E., Eliot, P., Peters, R. F., Simpson, P., and White, A. M. Relative changes in the function of muscle ribosomes and mitochondria during the early phase of steroid-induced catabolism. *Biochem. J. 127:* 881, 1972.
8. Steele, R. Influences of corticosteroids on protein and carbohydrate metabolism. In Greep, R. O., and Astwood, E. B. (ed): Handbook of Physiology, Section 7, Endocrinology, Vol. VI. Adrenal Gland, Washington D.C., Am. Physiological Society, 1975, p. 135.
9. Kimberg, D. V. Effects of vitamin D and steroid hormones on the active transport of calcium by the intestine. *N. Engl. J. Med. 280:* 1369, 1969.
10. Avioli, L. V., Birge, S. J., and Lee, S. W. Effects of prednisone on vitamin D metabolism in man. *J. Clin. Endocrinol. Metab. 28:* 1341, 1968.
11. Heimann, W., and Freiberger, R. Avascular necrosis of the femoral and humeral heads after high dosage corticosteroid therapy. *N. Engl. J. Med. 263:* 673, 1960.
12. Sobel, E. H. The influence of testosterone and cortisone on growth. In Gardner, L. I. (ed): Adrenal Function in Infants and Children. New York, Grune and Stratton, 1956, p. 137.
13. Frantz, A. G., Rabkin, M. T. Human growth hormone: Clinical measurement of response to hypoglycemia and suppression by corticosteroids. *N. Engl. J. Med. 271:* 1375, 1964.

14. Daughaday, W. H., and Mariz, I. K. Conversion of proline-U-C¹⁴ to labelled hydroxyproline by rat cartilage *in vitro:* Effects of hypophysectomy, growth hormone, and cortisol. *J. Lab. Clin. Med. 59:* 741, 1962.

15. McArthur, R. G., Cloutier, M. D., Hayles, A. B., and Sprague, R. G. Cushing's disease in children. *Mayo Clin. Proc. 47:* 318, 1972.

16. Melvin, K. E. W., Wright, A. D., Hartog, M. et al. Acute metabolic response to growth hormone in different types of dwarfism. *Brit. Med. J. 3:* 196, 1967.

17. Spiro, H. M., and Miles, S. S. Clinical and physiologic implications of the steroid induced peptic ulcer. *N. Engl. J. Med. 263:* 286, 1960.

18. Fawcett, J. A., and Bunney, W. E., Jr. Pituitary adrenal function and depression. *Arch. Gen. Psychiat. 16:* 517, 1967.

19. Woodbury, D. M., Thomas, P. S., and Vernadakis, A. Influence of adrenocorticol steroids on brain function and metabolism. In Hormones, Brain Function and Behavior. New York, Academic Press, 1957.

20. DeVellis, J., English, D. Hormonal control of glycerol phosphate dehydrogenase in the rat brain. *J. Neurochem. 15:* 1061, 1958.

21. Roosevelt, T. S., Ruhmann-Wennhold, A., and Nelson, D. H. Adrenal corticosteroid effects upon rat brain mitochondrial metabolism. *Endocrinology 93:* 619, 1973.

22. Tobian, L. Interrelationship of electrolytes, juxtaglomerular cells and hypertension. *Physiol. Rev. 40:* 280, 1960.

23. Plotz, C. M., Knowlton, A. I., and Ragan, C. The natural history of Cushing's syndrome. *Amer. J. Med. 13:* 597, 1952.

24. Dougherty, T. F., and White, A. Influence of hormones on lymphoid tissue structure and function. *Endocrinology 35:* 1, 1944.

25. Bishop, C. R., Athens, J. W., Boggs, D. R., Warner, H. R., Cartwright, G. E., and Wintrobe, M. M. Leukokinetic studies XIII. A non-steady-state kinetic evaluation of the mechanism of cortisone-induced granulocytosis. *J. Clin. Invest. 47:* 249, 1968.

26. Fridovich, I. Superoxide radical and the bactericidal action of phagocytes. (Editorial) *N. Engl. J. Med. 290:* 624, 1974.

27. Mandell, G. L., Rubin, W., and Hook, E. W. The effect of an NADH oxidase inhibitor (hydrocortisone) on polymorphonuclear leukocyte bactericidal activity. *J. Clin. Invest. 49:* 1381, 1970.

28. Bergland, K. Studies on factors which condition the effect of cortisone on antibody production. 1. The significance of time or hormone administration in primary hemolysin response. *Acta Path. Microbiol. Scand. 38:* 311, 1956.

29. Casey, W. J., and McCall, C. E. Suppression of the cellular interactions of delayed hypersensitivity by corticosteroid. *Immunology 21:* 225, 1971.

30. Uitto, J., and Mustakallio, K. K. Effect of hydrocortisone acetate, fluocinolone acetonide, fluclorolone acetonide, betamethasone-17-valerate and fluprednyliden-21-acetate on collagen biosynthesis. *Biochem. Pharmacol. 20:* 2495, 1971.

31. Nugent, C. A., Nichols, T., and Tyler, F. H. Diagnosis of Cushing's syndrome. Single dose dexamethasone suppression test. *Arch. Intern. Med. 116:* 172, 1965.

32. Ross, E. J. Urinary excretion of cortisol in Cushing's syndrome: Effect of corticotropin. *J. Clin. Endocrinol. 20:* 1360, 1960.

33. Mattingly, D. Rapid screening test for adrenal cortical function. *Lancet ii:* 1046, 1964.

34. Burke, C. W., and Beardwell, C. G. Cushing's syndrome: An evaluation of the clinical usefulness of urinary free cortisol and other steroid measurements. *Q. J. Med. 42:* 195, 1973.

35. Liddle, G. W. Tests of pituitary-adrenal suppressability in the diagnosis of Cushing's syndrome. *J. Clin. Endocrinol. Metab. 20:* 1539, 1960.

36. Silverman, S. R., Marnell, R. T., Sholiton, L. J., Werk, E. E., Jr. Failure of dexamethasone suppression test to indicate bilateral adrenocortical hyperplasia in Cushing's syndrome. *J. Clin. Endocrinol. Metab. 23:* 167, 1963.

37. Liddle, G. W., Estep, H. L., Kendall, J. W., et al. Clinical application of a new test of pituitary reserve. *J. Clin. Endocrinol. Metab. 19:* 875, 1959.

38. Weiss, E. R., Rayyis, S. S., Nelson, D. H., et al. Evaluation of stimulation and suppression tests in the etiological diagnosis of Cushing's syndrome. *Ann. Intern. Med. 71:* 941, 1969.

39. Nelson, D. H., Sprunt, J. G., and Mims, R. B. Plasma ACTH determinations in 58 patients before or after adrenalectomy for Cushing's syndrome. *J. Clin. Endocrinol. Metab. 26:* 722, 1966.

40. Besser, G. M., and Landon, J. Plasma levels of immunoreactive corticotrophin in patients with Cushing's syndrome. *Brit. Med. J. IV:* 552, 1968.

41. Nelson, D. H., Meakin, J. W., and Thorn, G. W. ACTH-producing pituitary tumors following adrenalectomy for Cushing's syndrome. *Ann. Intern. Med. 52:* 560, 1960.

42. Liddle, G. W., Island, D., Meador, C. K. Regulation of corticotropin secretion in man. *Recent Prog. Horm. Res. 18:* 125, 1962.

43. Rayyis, S. S., and Bethune, J. E. Radioimmunoassayable ACTH in dexamethasone nonsuppressible Cushing's syndrome. *J. Clin. Endocrinol. Metab. 29:* 1231, 1969.

44. Dunkelman, S. S., Pairhurst, B., and Plager, J. Cortisol metabolism in obesity. *J. Clin Endocrinol. Metab. 24:* 832, 1964.

45. Orth, D. N., and Liddle, G. W. Result of treatment in 108 patients with Cushing's syndrome. *N. Engl. J. Med. 285:* 243, 1971.

46. Hardy, J. Transsphenoidal hypophysectomy. *J. Neurosurg. 34:* 581, 1971.

46a. Jennings, A. S., Liddle, G. W., Orth, D. N. Results of treating childhood Cushing's disease with pituitary irradiation. *N. Engl. J. Med. 297:* 957, 1977.

47. Lawrence, J. H., Tobias, C. A., Linfoot, J. A., et al. Heavy particle therapy in acromegaly and Cushing's disease. *J.A.M.A. 235:* 2307, 1976.

48. Sosman, M. C. Cushing's disease-pituitary basophilism. *Amer. J. Roentgenol. 62:* 1, 1949.

49. Linfoot, J. A., Lawrence, J. H., Tobias, C A., et al. Progress report on the treatment of Cushing's disease. *Trans. Am. Clin. Climatol. Assoc. 81:* 196, 1970.

50. Molinatti, G. M., Camanni, F., and Tedeschi, M. Implantation of the pituitary with yttrium⁹⁰ in a case of Cushing's syndrome. *J. Clin. Endocrinol. Metab. 19:* 1144, 1959.

51. Luft, R., Olivecrona, H., Ikkos, D., et al. Treatment of Cushing's disease by pituitary surgery. Report of two cases. *Acta Endocrinol. 24:* 1, 1957.

52. Hardy, J. Transphenoidal surgery of hypersecreting pituitary tumors. In Diagnosis and Treatment of Pituitary Tumors. Amsterdam, Exerpta Medica, 1973, p. 179.

53. Lagerquist, L. G., Meikle, A. W., West, C. D., et al. Cushing's disease with cure by resection of a pituitary adenoma. *Amer. J. Med. 57:* 826, 1974.

53a. Salassa, R. M., Laws, E. R., Jr., Carpenter, P. C., Northcutt, R. C. Transsphenoidal removal of pituitary microadenoma in Cushing's disease. *Mayo Clin. Proc. 53:* 24, 1978.

53b. Tyrrell, J. B., Brooks, R. M., Fitzgerald, P. A., et al. Cushing's disease selective trans-sphenoidal resection of pituitary microadenomas. *N. Engl. J. Med. 298:* 753, 1978.

54. Welbourn, R. B., Montgomery, D. A. D., and Kennedy, T. L. The natural history of treated Cushing's syndrome. *Brit. J. Surg. 58:* 1, 1971.

55. Fishman, L. M., Liddle, G. W., Island, D. P., et al. Effects of amino-glutethimide on adrenal function in man. *J. Clin. Endocrinol. Metab. 27:* 481, 1967.

56. Hunter, P. R., Ross, W., Hall, R., et al. Treatment of Cushing's disease with adrenal blocking drugs and megavoltage therapy to the pituitary. *Proc. R. Soc. Med. 67:* 1225, 1974.

57. Kreiger, D. T., Amorosa, L., Linick, F. Cyproheptadine-induced remission of Cushing's disease. *N. Engl. J. Med. 293:* 893, 1975.

57a. Lamberts, S. W. J., and Birkenhager, J. C. Effect of bromocriptine in pituitary-dependent Cushing's syndrome. *J. Endocrinol. 70:* 315, 1976.

58. Smilo, R. P., Earll, J. M., Forsham, P. H. Suppression of tumorous adrenal hyperfunction by aminoglutethimide. *Metabolism 16:* 374, 1967.

59. Cash, R., Brough, A. J., Cohen, M. N. P., et al. Aminoglutethimide as an inhibitor of adrenal steroidogenesis: Mechanism of action and therapeutic trial. *J. Clin. Endocrinol. 27:* 1239, 1967.

60. Santen, R. J., Lipton, A., and Kendall, J. Successful medical adrenalectomy with amino-glutethimide. *J.A.M.A. 230:* 1661, 1974.

61. Pasqualini, R. Q., Gurevich, N. Spontaneous remission in a case of Cushing's syndrome. *J. Clin. Endocrinol. 16:* 406, 1956.

62. Hayslett, J. P., and Cohn, G. L. Spontaneous remission of Cushing's disease. Report of a case. *N. Engl. J. Med. 276:* 968, 1967.

63. Nelson, D. H., Meakin, J. W., Dealy, J. B., et al. ACTH-producing tumor of the pituitary gland. *N. Engl. J. Med. 259:* 161, 1958.

64. Salassa, R. M., Kearns, T. P., Kernohan, J. W., Sprague, R. G., and McCarty, C. S. Pituitary tumors in patients with Cushing's syndrome. *J. Clin Endocrinol. 19:* 1523, 1959.

65. Abe, K., Nicholson, W. E., Liddle, G. W., et al. Radioimmunoassay of β-MSH in human plasma and tissues. *J. Clin Invest. 46:* 1609, 1967.

65a. Moore, T. J., Dluhy, R. G., Williams, G. H., and Cain, J. P. Nelson's syndrome: Frequency, prognosis, and effect of prior pituitary irradiation. *Ann. Intern. Med. 85:* 731, 1976.

66. Queiroz, L. de S., Facure, N. O., Facure, J. J., et al. Pituitary carcinoma with liver metastases and Cushing's syndrome. *Arch. Path. 99:* 32, 1975.

67. Eisenstein, A. B., Karsch, R., and Gall, I. Occurrences of pregnancy in Cushing's syndrome. *J. Clin. Endocrinol. Metab. 23:* 971, 1963.

68. Kreines, K., Perin, E., and Salzer, R. Pregnancy in Cushing's syndrome. *J. Clin Endocrinol. 24:* 75, 1964.

69. Grimes, E. M., Fayez, J. A., and Miller, G. L. Cushing's syndrome and pregnancy. *Obstet. Gynecol. 42:* 550, 1973.

69a. Anevlavis, E. S., and Schletter, F. E. Normal infant delivered of woman with Cushing syndrome. *J.A.M.A. 236:* 589, 1976.

70. Golden, A., and Bondy, P. K. Cytologic changes in rat adenohypophysis following administration of adrenocorticotrophin or cortisone. *Proc. Soc. Exp. Biol. Med. 79:* 252, 1952.

71. James, V. H. T., Landon, J., Wynn, V., et al. A fundamental defect of adrenocortical control in Cushing's disease. *J. Endocrinol. 40:* 15, 1968.

72. French, F. S., Macfie, J. A., Baggett, B., et al. Cushing's syndrome with a paradoxical response to dexamethasone. *Amer. J. Med. 47:* 619, 1969.

73. Lerner, A. B., and McGuire, J. S. Melanocyte-stimulating hormone and adrenocorticotropic hormone. Their relation to pigmentation. *N. Engl. J. Med. 270:* 539, 1964.

73a. Bachelot, I., Wolfsen, A. R., Odell, W. D. Pituitary and plasma lipotropins: demonstration of the artificial nature of βMSH. *J. Clin. Endocrinol. Metab. 44:* 939, 1977.

74. Schwarz, F., Der Kinderen, P. J., and Houstra-Lanz, M. Exophthalmos-producing activity in the serum and in the pituitary of patients with Cushing's syndrome and acromegaly. *J. Clin. Endocrinol. 22:* 718, 1962.

75. Fraser, R., James, V. H. T., Landon, J., et al. Clinical and biochemical studies of a patient with a corticosterone-secreting adrenocortical tumour. *Lancet 2:* 1116, 1968.

76. Hamwi, G. J., Gwinup, G., Mostow, J. H., et al. Activation of testicular adrenal rest tissue by prolonged excessive ACTH production. *J. Clin Endocrinol. Metab. 23:* 861, 1963.

77. Ney, R. L., Hammond, W., Wright, L., et al. Studies in a patient with an ectopic adrenocortical tumor. *J. Clin. Endocrinol. 26:* 299, 1966.

78. Herwig, K. R., Schteingart, D. E. Successful removal of adrenal remnant localized by ^{131}I-19-iodocholesterol. *J. Urol. 111:* 713, 1974.

79. Moses, D. C., Schteingart, D. E., Sturman, M. F., et al. Efficacy of radiocholesterol imaging of the adrenal glands in Cushing's syndrome. *Surg. Gynecol. Obstet. 139:* 201, 1974.

80. Reuter, S. R., Blair, A. J., Schteingart, D. E., et al. Adrenal venography. *Radiology 89:* 805, 1967.

81. Mitty, H. A., Nicolis, G. L., and Gabrilove, J. L. Adrenal venography: Clinical roentgenographic correlation in 80 patients. *Am. J. Roentgen. Rad. Ther. Nucl. Med. 119:* 564, 1973.

82. Graber, A. L., Ney, R. L., Nicholson, W. E., et al. Natural history of pituitary-adrenal recovery following long-term suppression with corticosteroids. *J. Clin. Endocrinol. Metab. 25:* 11, 1965.

83. Nelson, D. H. Present status of the problem of iatrogenic adrenal cortical insufficiency. *Anesthesiology 24:* 457, 1963.

84. Nelson, D. H. Regulation of glucocorticoid release. *Am. J. Med. 53:* 590, 1972.

85. Plager, J. E., Cushman, P. Suppression of the pituitary-ACTH response in man by administration of ACTH or cortisol. *J. Clin. Endocrinol. Metab. 22:* 147, 1962.

86. Tucci, J. R., Meloni, C. R., Carreon, G. G., et al. Pituitary adrenal functional abnormalities in corticogenic adrenal atrophy. *J. Clin. Endocrinol. Metab. 25:* 823, 1965.

87. Brown, W. H. A case of pluriglandular syndrome: Diabetes of bearded women. *Lancet 2:* 1022, 1928.

88. O'Neal, L. W. Correlation between clinical pattern and pathological findings in Cushing's syndrome. *Med. Clin. N. Amer. 52:* 313, 1968.

89. O'Riordan, J. L. H., Blanshard, G. P., Moxham, A., et al. Corticotrophin-secreting carcinomas. *Q. J. Med. 35:* 137, 1966.

90. Morse, W. I., Kerenyi, N., and Nelson, D. H. Prolonged hyperadrenocorticotrophism and pigmentation associated with bronchial carcinoid tumour. *Canad. Med. Assoc. J. 96:* 104, 1967.

91. Steel, K., Baerg, R. D., Adams, D. O. Cushings syndrome in association with a carcinoid tumor of the lung. *J. Clin. Endocrinol. Metab. 27:* 1285, 1967.

92. Olurin, E. O., Sofowora, E. O., Afonja, A. O., et al. Cushing's syndrome and bronchial carcinoid tumor. *Cancer 31:* 1514, 1973.

93. Strott, C. A., Nugent, C. A., and Tyler, F. H. Cushing's syndrome caused by bronchial adenomas. *Am. J. Med. 44:* 97, 1968.

93a. Tischler, A. S., Dichter, M. A., Biales, B., and Greene, L. A. Neuroendocrine neoplasms and their cells of origin. *N. Engl. J. Med. 296:* 919, 1977.

93b. Berenyi, M. R., Singh, G., Gloster, E. S., Davidson, M. I., and Woldenberg, D. H. ACTH-producing pheochromocytoma. *Arch. Pathol. Lab. Med. 101:* 31, 1977.

93c. Rees, L. H. ACTH, lipotrophin and MSH in health and disease. *Clin. Endocrinol. Metab. 6:* 137, 1977.

93d. Corrigan, D. F., Schaaf, M., Whaley, R. A., Czerwinski, C. L., and Earll, J. M. Selective venous sampling to differentiate ectopic ACTH secretion from pituitary Cushing's syndrome. *N. Engl. J. Med. 296:* 861, 1977.

93e. Suda, T., Demura, H., Demura, R., Wakabayashi, I., Nomura, K., Odagiri, E., and Shizume, K. Corticotropin-releasing factorlike activity in ACTH producing tumors. *J. Clin. Endocrinol. Metab. 44:* 440, 1977.

94. Schimizu, N., Ogata, E., Nicholson, W. E., et al. Studies on the melanotropic activity of human plasma and tissues. *J. Clin. Endocrinol. Metab. 25:* 984, 1965.

95. Hallwright, G. P., North, K. A. K., and Reid, J. D. Pigmentation and Cushing's syndrome due to malignant tumor of the pancreas. *J. Clin. Endocrinol. Metab. 24:* 496, 1964.

96. Flint, L. D., and Jacobs, E. C. Belated recognition of adrenocorticotropic hormone-producing tumors in post-adrenalectomized Cushing's syndrome. *J. Urol. 112;* 688, 1974.

97. Bagshawe, K. D. Hypokalemia carcinoma and Cushing's syndrome. *Lancet 2:* 284, 1960.

98. Kirshner, M. A., Powell, R. D., and Lipsett, M. B. Cushing's syndrome: Nodular cortical hyperplasia of adrenal glands with clinical and pathological features suggesting adrenocortical tumor. *J. Clin. Endocrinol. Metab. 24:* 947, 1964.

99. Meador, C. K., Bowdoin, B., Owen, W. C., Jr., et al. Primary adrenocortical nodular dysplasia: a rare cause of Cushing's syndrome. *J. Clin. Endocrinol. Metab. 27:* 1255, 1967.

100. Choi, Y., Werk, E. E., and Sholiton, L. J. Cushing's syndrome with dual pituitary-adrenal control. *Arch. Intern. Med. 125:* 1045, 1970.

101. Lipsett, M. B., and Wilson, H. Adrenocortical cancer: Steroid biosynthesis and metabolism evaluated by urinary metabolites. *J. Clin. Endocrinol. Metab. 22:* 906, 1962.

102. Crane, M. G., and Harris, J. J. Desoxycorticosterone secretion rates in hyperadrenocorticism. *J. Clin. Endocrinol. Metab. 26:* 1135, 1966.

103. Sprague, R. G., Randall, R. V., Salassa, R. M., et al. Cushing's syndrome a progressive and often fatal disease: a review of 100 cases seen between July 1945 and July 1954. *Arch. Intern. Med. 98:* 389, 1956.

104. Lipsett, M. B., Hertz, R., and Ross, G. T. Clinical and pathophysiologic aspects of adrenocortical carcinoma. *Am. J. Med. 35:* 374, 1963.

105. Hutter, A. M., and Kayhoe, D. E. Adrenal cortical carcinoma. Clinical features of 138 patients. *Am. J. Med. 41:* 572, 1966.

106. Egdahl, R. H. Surgery of the adrenal gland. *N. Engl. J. Med. 278:* 939, 1968.

107. Hutter, A. M., and Kayhoe, D. E. Adrenal cortical carcinoma. Results of treatment with o,p'DDD in 138 patients. *Am. J. Med. 41,* 581, 1966.

107a. Chatal, J. F., Charbonnel, B., Le Mevel, B. P., and Guihard, D. Uptake of ^{131}I-19-iodocholesterol by an adrenal cortical carcinoma and its metastases. *J. Clin. Endocrinol. Metab. 43:* 248, 1976.

108. Gabrilove, J. L., Sharma, D. C., Wotiz, H. H., et al. Feminizing adrenocortical tumors in the male. A review of 52 cases including a case report. *Medicine 44:* 37, 1965.

109. Okano, K., Matsomoto, K., Matsuda, A., et al. Adrenocortical carcinoma causing feminization in an adult male. *Acta Path. Japon. 12:* 431, 1962.

110. Rose, L. I., Williams, G. H., Jagger, P. I., et al. Feminizing tumor of the adrenal gland with positive chorionic-like gonadotropin test. *J. Clin. Endocrinol. Metab. 28:* 903, 1968.

111. Soffer, L. J., Iannacone, A., and Gabrilove, J. L. Cushing's syndrome—a study of fifty patients. *Am. J. Med. 30:* 129, 1961.

96

Diagnosis and Treatment of Addison's Disease

Don H. Nelson

HISTORY

The earliest description of primary adrenal insufficiency was that published by Thomas Addison in 1855 in which he described 11 cases with autopsy findings.[1] Previously in 1849 he had published a short note in which the anemia of Addison's disease was not clearly differentiated from that of pernicious anemia. In his scholarly report on this disease, Addison noted those findings that are commonly seen in the condition: "anemia, general languor and debility, remarkable feebleness of the heart's action, irritability of the stomach, and a peculiar change of color in the skin." The lithographs clearly demonstrated the characteristic pigmentation of the condition, and the autopsy findings included what was probably tuberculous destruction of the cortex, atrophic adrenals, and metastases to the adrenals from cancer of the breast (metastases to the adrenals can, but seldom do, produce clinically significant adrenal insufficiency).

Although Addison had, with remarkable clarity for the times, described the clinical and pathological picture of primary adrenal insufficiency, it was many years before the significance of his description was recognized and a century before adequate therapeutic measures for the condition were available. At the time Addison was doing his clinical work, Brown-Séquard confirmed that adrenalectomy caused death in experimental animals.[2] Although some of his findings were challenged, it soon became apparent that the adrenal gland was necessary for life. It was another three quarters of a century before studies demonstrated that it was the cortex and not the medulla that contained the life-maintaining substance.[3]

With the preparation in 1929–1930 by Rogoff and Stewart and by Swingle and Pfiffner of crude lipid cortical extracts that would maintain adrenalectomized cats indefinitely, the stage was set for the rapid increase in knowledge concerning what the gland secretes, how it is controlled, and its significance in maintaining the activity of numerous biochemical and physiological functions in the organism.[4,5]

Clinical trials of these crude extracts were made by Rogoff and Stewart in 1929.[4] They described the recovery and maintenance of patients with Addison's disease and a marked increase in appetite and strength. Shortly thereafter, Loeb demonstrated that the primary deficiency of the addisonian patient, loss of sodium chloride, could be restored with oral or rectal saline solutions with a beneficial effect upon the patient.[6] It was apparent also that although salt was beneficial, it could not maintain life in the totally adrenalectomized animal with the exception of the rat.

During this same period in the 1930s, Winterstiner and Pfiffner, Reichstein, and Kendall and their collaborators were actively isolating a large number of corticosteroids from the adrenal cortex. A thousand pounds of beef glands yielded 333 mg of corticosterone and 34 mg of 17-hydroxycorticosterone, and 600 mg of steroid were isolated from 1000 lb of porcine adrenal glands. Although an amorphous fraction remained, the chemical nature of which was yet to be determined, it was recognized that it possessed potent physiologic activity.[7]

These substances obtained from expensive and laborious isolations could not be made available for clinical use. Synthesis of 11-deoxycorticosterone, and demonstration by Thorn and co-workers of its efficacy in preventing sodium loss in the addisonian patient, made it the major therapeutic substance for the treatment of Addison's disease on a chronic basis.[8] This substance did not protect against the "effects of stress," and thus various adrenal extracts of low hormonal potency were given sporadically to severely ill patients with occasional success but frequent failure.

With the discovery of means of synthesizing the 11-hydroxylated compounds (cortisone and cortisol), a new era arrived in which the patient with adrenal insufficiency could be treated adequately on either an acute or a chronic basis.

It was demonstrated that 17-hydroxycorticosterone (cortisol) was the major corticosteroid secreted by the dog[9] and that it, corticosterone, and androgens were the major compounds secreted in man and a variety of animals.[10–12] This information led to the development of objective methods for the measurement of adrenal steroids and the diagnosis of disorders of secretion of the adrenal cortex.[10] An understanding of most of the pathophysiology of the gland has resulted in recent years.

The final historical note of importance in the delineation of the function of the gland was the isolation by Simpson and Tait, with the collaboration of Riechstein and Wettstein, of aldosterone and then the synthesis of this most potent and important mineralocorticoid produced by the adrenal cortex.[13,14]

The past two decades have produced much information concerning the control of secretion of these hormones and have made inroads toward understanding the mechanism by which they produce their widespread effects on many tissues. Further information concerning the effects of the adrenal cortical hormones on various tissues and enzyme systems can be found in Chapter 95.

CLINICAL PICTURE OF ADDISON'S DISEASE

All patients with Addison's disease complain of weakness[15] (see Table 96-1) The patient may also be aware of increased pigmentation and postural hypotension. Gastrointestinal symptoms are common, with nausea and vomiting occurring most frequently. Patients are anorectic, have lost weight, and in the most severe cases may complain of chronic diarrhea. Because of the frequency of such gastrointestinal complaints, which may also include abdominal pain in acute insufficiency, patients are often studied for gastrointestinal disease prior to the diagnosis of adrenal insufficiency.

On questioning, the patient will often indicate that he wakes up feeling fairly good but that activity or exertion is unusually tiring. (This in contradistinction to the patient with asthenia who wakes up tired and who in time "gets going.") Inquiry concerning pigmentation often results in responses such as "My suntan doesn't fade in the winter but now stays with me all year." An occasional patient develops "salt craving" in response to the sodium depletion that may occur. A rare patient has discovered the sodium-retaining effects of excessive licorice ingestion and gives a history of large intake of this substance.[16]

In the patient who presents at the operating table or in the emergency room with the picture of adrenal crisis (see below) but no observable pigmentation, a history of previous intake of corticosteroids that may have caused adrenal atrophy and/or signs suggestive of hypopituitarism may explain acute adrenal insufficiency in the absence of pigmentation.

Amenorrhea may occur in the more severe case. This may be secondary to general debility but is also often secondary to autoimmune disease of the ovary along with similar involvement of the adrenal.

PHYSICAL FINDINGS

The most striking physical finding in the patient with Addison's disease is the increased pigmentation of the skin and the mucous membranes. (Fig. 96-1) This may vary in the light-skinned subject from a slight tan or a few "black freckles" to an intense generalized pigmentation which has resulted in patients being mistakenly considered to be of a darker skinned race. Most commonly pigmentation is visible over extensor surfaces such as the back of the hands (phalangeal and metacarpal-phalangeal joints), elbows, knees, in the creases of the hands, at the dental gingival margin, on the lips, or on the buccal mucosa. Increased pigmentation of scars is common. The pigmentation of scars formed after the onset of the disease is generally more pronounced than that of scars preceding onset of adrenal insufficiency. It should be noted, however, that a number of patients have no significant increase in pigmentation, even with well-documented primary adrenal insufficiency. Members of the black races have pigmentation in the areas described

Table 96-1. Major Symptoms and Signs of Addison's Disease in 108 Patients*

Findings	% of Patients
Weakness and fatigability	100
Weight loss	100
Hyperpigmentation	92
Hypotension	88
Hyponatremia	88
Hyperkalemia	64
Gastrointestinal symptoms	56
Postural dizziness	12
Adrenal calcification	9
Hypercalcemia	6
Muscle and joint pains	6
Vitiligo	4

*Adapted from J. Nerup, Acta Endocrinol. 76:127, 1974.

but may give a history of accentuation of such pigmentation with the onset of the disease. Vitiligo is often seen in association with the pigmentation and has been ascribed to autoimmune destruction of the melanocytes. This has been shown to occur in 10 to 20 percent of patients with Addison's disease and usually occurs in hyperpigmented areas (Fig. 96-1). In the dark-skinned races, the vitiligo may be much more of a cosmetic problem than is the hyperpigmentation.

The cardiovascular findings of low blood pressure and a small heart are not early manifestations of the disease and are usually accompanied by the other signs and symptoms noted. Certainly the finding of a normal blood pressure and heart size[17] does not rule out the possibility of Addison's disease being present.

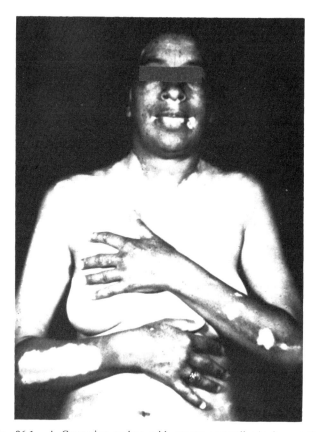

Fig. 96-1. A Caucasian patient with severe generalized pigmentation associated with Addison's disease. There are large areas of vitiligo accompanying the hyperpigmentation.

Decreased body hair is a common finding in the female patient. This is the result of decreased production of the adrenal androgens, the chief source of androgens in the female patient. In the male the preponderance of testicular androgen secretion makes the absence of the adrenal androgen go unnoticed. Calcification of cartilage with hardening of the ears, sometimes to a stonelike consistency, adds an uncommon but interesting physical finding in some patients with Addison's disease. Increased calcification of costal cartilage may also be noted. Such increased calcification is more of a physical curiosity than a diagnostic sign and has been described in other conditions such as sarcoidosis, acromegaly, and ochronosis.[18]

LABORATORY FINDINGS IN ADDISON'S DISEASE

SERUM ELECTROLYTES

The typical serum changes in patients with Addison's disease include an elevation of the serum potassium level with a depressed serum sodium level and a moderately elevated BUN or creatinine level. The electrolyte changes result from corticoid effects upon renal function and also the shift of electrolytes between the intracellular and extracellular spaces. Aldosterone has a major effect on reabsorption of sodium and excretion of potassium by the renal tubule (see Chapter 98). The patient with adrenal insufficiency loses varying quantities of sodium through the kidneys. In the mildly diseased patients, this loss may be compensated by increased salt intake, but in the severely ill patient, it may result in a serum sodium level as low as 110 mEq/100 ml. The serum sodium level also is affected by the action of cortisol, and to a lesser extent aldosterone, on maintenance of the normal gradient between intracellular and extracellular sodium and potassium.[19] It has been suggested that this action is largely secondary to effects upon the sodium-potassium pump. In the absence of cortisol, this gradient is not normally maintained and potassium moves out of the cell and sodium into it, with a resultant increase in extracellular potassium and a decrease in serum sodium levels. Potassium levels in the serum are therefore affected by both the action of aldosterone on the renal tubule and the effects of cortisol on shifts of electrolytes between the intracellular and extracellular spaces. The uncommon finding of an increased serum calcium level in adrenal insufficiency has been difficult to explain. Elevated calcium levels have been found both in idiopathic Addison's disease and following adrenalectomy. The prompt reduction of the calcium to normal levels following cortisol administration makes clear the causative role of deficiency of this hormone.[20,21]

ADH AND H$_2$O BALANCE

Another factor of importance in determining the level of serum sodium is antidiuretic hormone (ADH), which is secreted by the posterior pituitary gland. One of the protective mechanisms against loss of volume is the secretion of ADH, with its resultant antidiuretic effect upon the renal collecting tubules and a decrease in urinary water loss. The effect of excess sodium loss to increase urinary water loss is counterbalanced by the action of ADH to retain water. This mechanism causes retention of water and dilution of serum sodium in the early stages of the disease in which the patient is well hydrated. An additional factor that may accentuate ADH secretion is the decrease in cardiac output with a fall in effective circulating volume; this also will act as a stimulus to ADH secretion.[22]

RENAL FUNCTION

Most patients with untreated Addison's disease have an elevated BUN and/or creatinine levels. Cortisol is known to be necessary for the maintenance of normal renal hemodynamics. In its absence there is a decrease in the glomerular filtration rate (GFR) and renal blood flow even in the absence of sodium depletion.[23] This reduction in the glomerular filtration rate reduces sodium loss in the adrenal-insufficient patient. Non-sodium-retaining glucocorticoids, such as prednisone or dexamethasone, given to adrenal-deficient patients increase the glomerular filtration rate and urinary sodium loss if some sodium-retaining hormone is not present to counteract the subsequent tendency to increased excretion of sodium.[24]

The patient is usually mildly acidotic as a result of the decreased secretion of ammonia and hydrogen ion. This can be demonstrated by the administration of an acid load, which is cleared less readily than in the normal subject. The correction of the acidifying defect by the administration of desoxycorticosterone or aldosterone suggests that the defect is largely a result of the effect of the sodium-retaining hormones upon hydrogen ion secretion by the renal tubule.

The inability of the patient with adrenocortical insufficiency to normally excrete a water load was formerly used as a diagnostic test. With the availability of more definitive measurements of corticosteroids, such indirect tests are not of sufficient value to justify their use. Although it has been reported that there is a return to normal free water clearance following restoration of the extracellular fluid volume, other studies have shown that in the absence of cortisol, neither a normal extracellular fluid volume nor mineralocorticoid therapy is sufficient to return free water clearance to normal. In the patient with hypopituitarism who secretes aldosterone but not cortisol from the adrenal cortex in the absence of ACTH, there is a definite defect in excretion of a water load.[25] The administration of cortisol in a single large dose is followed by a water diuresis. In this case, cortisol is probably acting on multiple sites. Thus the effect of cortisol to increase cardiac output and effective circulating volume undoubtedly produces an increase in the GFR and effective circulating volume, a reduction in antidiuretic hormone, and also appears to affect the renal tubule and its ability to excrete water. Kleeman et al. have demonstrated that the impaired excretion of water in these patients is not due to the effects on ADH.[26]

HYPOGLYCEMIA

Hypoglycemia with a low serum glucose level may be seen in the patient with Addison's disease. That the hypoglycemia is largely due to defects in gluconeogenesis is made apparent by the infrequency with which such hypoglycemia occurs in the fed patient. The adrenal-insufficient patient is extremely sensitive to fasting, however, and when the patient is deprived of food for any length of time, blood sugar may fall to low symptomatic levels.

BLOOD

Eosinophilia of a moderate degree is a common finding in Addison's disease. A decrease in the eosinophils following the administration of ACTH, or epinephrine, was once used as a diagnostic test for adrenal insufficiency, but it, like the water excretion test, has been superseded by measurements of corticosteroids. Anemia is usually found following rehydration of the dehydrated patient, and a relative lymphocytosis is often present.

PATHOGENESIS

BACTERIAL AND FUNGAL INFECTION

Addison's disease results from destruction of the total adrenal cortex, in contradistinction to the atrophy of the fasciculata and reticularis with maintenance of the zonae glomerulosa seen in patients with decreased ACTH secretion. The two chief etiologies are adrenal atrophy with destruction due to an autoimmune process and tuberculosis. The latter was the most common cause of destruction of the adrenals when tuberculosis infection was more common, but a recent review of 108 cases found 66 percent to be idiopathic, 17 percent to result from tuberculosis, and 17 percent of undetermined etiology.[15] Calcification of the adrenal glands is common in tuberculosis (see Fig. 96-2). Other less common etiologies include fungal infections such as coccidioidomycosis,[27] histoplasmosis,[28] and blastomycosis.[29] Adrenal hemorrhage may be associated with severe infection, particularly in meningococcemia (Waterhouse-Friderichsen syndrome).[30] This condition can probably occur in association with any severe sepsis with endotoxin release and shock. In one series of infants and children, 9 of 51 dying with septicemic adrenal hemorrhage had meningococcemia, but *P. aeruginosa* was isolated in 14 cases and was the predominant pathogen.[31] Thus the vascular collapse is a combination of the generalized effects of the endotoxin and the decrease in corticosteroid secretion following adrenal destruction.[32] Corticosteroids have been used in the treatment of gram-negative sepsis and endotoxin shock with variable success.[31a] The amounts that have been given, one to several grams a day of prednisone, are far more than replacement dosage. In some cases, this therapy may replace decreased secretion from the adrenal, but in most instances it must be considered pharmacologic therapy, the mechanism of action of which is still to be determined.

ANTICOAGULANT THERAPY

Over 50 patients who have experienced spontaneous adrenal hemorrage during anticoagulant therapy have been reported in the literature.[33] This is not an easy diagnosis to make, as most such patients have other possible etiologies for the hypotension which is likely to be the chief indication of acute adrenal insufficiency. Although it has been suggested that the combination of stress, with its accompanying increased adrenal blood flow, and anticoagulant therapy somehow function synergistically to produce adrenal he-

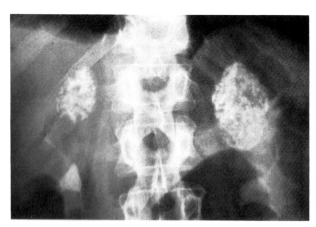

Fig. 96-2. Marked calcification of the adrenal glands in a patient with Addison's disease. The calcification was probably secondary to tuberculous destruction of the glands.

morrage, the absolute mechanism is not presently clear. Thus, in any patient on anticoagulant therapy in whom there is sudden onset of hypotension, nausea, vomiting, tachycardia, and/or hyperpyrexia, one should add to the differential diagnosis of pulmonary embolism, hemorrhage, and infection the possibility that acute adrenal apoplexy with resultant adrenal insufficiency may have occurred.

ADRENAL INSUFFICIENCY FOLLOWING LONG-TERM CORTICOSTEROID THERAPY

The occurrence of adrenal atrophy in the patient who has received large dose corticosteroid therapy for a nonendocrine condition is well known. Although the incidence of such adrenal suppression is not known, there have been numerous reports of patients who, following discontinuance of corticosteroid therapy, have developed adrenal insufficiency when exposed to some stressful situation. This has resulted, in many instances, in a fatal outcome. Such patients are found to have marked adrenal atrophy. The adrenals are unable to produce sufficient quantities of corticosteroid to maintain the patient during the stressful situation, even though the pituitary gland has some residual capacity to produce ACTH during stress.[34] In this situation, the adrenal has not been stimulated sufficiently during nonstressed periods, so that it can respond normally during periods of increased ACTH secretion.

The mechanism for this defect has not been finally proven. It has been suggested that the adrenal cortex is relatively unresponsive to ACTH and that there may be moderately elevated levels of ACTH in these patients.[35] Others have attributed the defect to long-term suppression of the hypothalamic-pituitary centers that control ACTH secretion.[36] In this instance the defect is thought to be one of insufficient ACTH secretion, such that the adrenal cortex atrophies and is not properly responsive to ACTH secreted during periods of stress. Investigation of this problem is difficult as a result of the great variability in the response of patients to suppressive therapy and the relative unlikelihood of developing long-term adrenal atrophy following discontinuance of the steroid.

A few general rules can be formed concerning the likelihood of the condition and the need for therapy.

1. All patients receiving corticosteroid therapy will have some degree of adrenal atrophy. Those receiving lower doses, i.e., less than 30 mg of cortisol equivalent per day, will likely continue to have some secretion from their own glands. All such patients however, will benefit from increased corticosteroid therapy when exposed to trauma or some stressful situation. The use of alternate day corticosteroid therapy will reduce the likelihood of severe adrenal atrophy.[37,38]

2. Although the length of time necessary to produce adrenal atrophy is not known for the individual patient, it is known that suppression of ACTH secretion in animals for only 24 to 48 hours causes significant adrenal atrophy, and thus patients who have received corticosteroids for only a few days will have some adrenal atrophy. In almost all such cases the adrenal quickly returns to normal size when corticosteroid therapy is discontinued. In patients who receive corticosteroid therapy for longer periods, i.e., months or years, the possibility increases that the adrenal atrophy will continue when corticosteroid therapy is discontinued. All such patients potentially have adrenal insufficiency, particularly when exposed to a stressful situation.

3. The administration of ACTH with the corticosteroids, in the hope of either maintaining adrenal size and responsiveness or returning the adrenal to normal function, is not likely to be of benefit. Studies have demonstrated a relative lack of adrenal responsiveness in patients who have been on long-term ACTH therapy, similar to that in patients who have been on long-term corticosteroids therapy.[39] The adrenals of such patients are responsive to ACTH, but these studies suggest that the adrenals will again atrophy following discontinuance of any course of ACTH. This view has been questioned by other workers,[40] and it has also been confirmed.[41]

4. As a result of the widespread use of corticosteroids, it is probably not practical to study every patient who has received corticosteroids in order to determine if a defect is present. Even if such a defect is demonstrated, the period of time required for it to be corrected, if indeed the patient does spontaneously correct the defect, is not known.

A practical approach to the problem is as follows: (1) A high index of suspicion must be maintained for any patient who has received corticosteroid therapy in any significant quantity over any period of weeks or months. If the patient undergoes a stressful procedure, the occurrence of signs or symptoms of adrenal insufficiency should be treated with corticosteroids. (2) If time allows, such patients may be tested with metyrapone prior to a surgical procedure in order to determine the status of their pituitary adrenal axis. (3) When in doubt, such patients should receive corticosteroids. A fatal outcome of adrenal insufficiency can easily occur while awaiting laboratory results that would prove or disprove the diagnosis.

FAMILIAL UNRESPONSIVENESS TO ACTH

A number of children have been described who have decreased cortisol responsiveness to ACTH administration but normal aldosterone secretion.[42] These children have presented typically with hypoglycemia, hyperpigmentation, and feeding problems. They are not thought to have a specific defect in steroid hydroxylation as is seen in congenital adrenocortical hyperplasia, since they do not overproduce precursors of cortisol (see Chapter 97). The condition may be inherited as a recessive trait. These patients fail to increase cortisol secretion on prolonged stimulation with ACTH and in a few cases have been found to have adrenal atrophy at autopsy.

AUTOIMMUNE DISEASE AND ADRENAL INSUFFICIENCY

The most common cause of adrenal insufficiency at present is autoimmune destruction of the adrenal glands. There is a loss of the normal architecture of the cortex, and often only islets of cells surrounded by fibrous tissue and lymphocytic infiltration are present. Although the adrenal glands are generally atrophic, there may be sufficient lymphocytic infiltration for them to appear near normal in size.[43] Although the specific antigens produced have not been identified, complement fixation and immunofluorescent techniques carried out by a number of workers have demonstrated adrenal antibodies. Irvine and Barnes found a higher incidence of adrenal antibodies among females than males, with 109 of 174 sera from patients with idiopathic Addison's disease demonstrating antibodies, while none was found in 46 sera from 4 patients with tuberculosis as the cause of the disease and only 1 in 224 control

sera.[44] Nerup and Bendixen reported organ-specific antiadrenal cell-mediated hypersensitivity in 8 of 11 males and 6 of 19 females with idiopathic Addison's disease.[45]

The occurrence with idiopathic Addison's disease of a number of other autoimmune disorders has been frequently noted. Schmidt described 2 patients with chronic lymphocytic thyroiditis and nontuberculous Addison's disease.[46] The term "Schmidt's syndrome" has since been used to describe the association of adrenal and thyroid insufficiency. McHardy-Young et al. studied thyroid function in 33 patients with Addison's disease. Of 27 of these patients who were thought to have the idiopathic type of adrenal disease, 13 had thyroid microsomal antibodies. Ten of these 13 also had elevated TSH levels.[47]

There is also a suprisingly high incidence of pernicious anemia associated with idiopathic Addison's disease. Of 174 patients studied in one series, 10 had pernicious anemia with malabsorption of vitamin B_{12}, while 16 of these subjects had antibodies to intrinsic factor. An increase in subclinical atrophic gastritis was also noted in this series.[44]

An increased incidence of diabetes in patients with idiopathic Addison's disease has been described.[48] A study of 883 diabetics showed an increased incidence of thyroid cytoplasmic and gastric parietal cell antibodies in young insulin-dependent diabetics. Although an autoimmune mechanism for the production of diabetes mellitus has not been demonstrated, this association with an autoimmune disease deserves further investigation.[49]

The association of hypoparathyroidism with Addison's disease is well known. Blizzard et al. found parathyroid antibodies by immunofluorescence in 26 percent of 92 patients with idiopathic Addison's disease and in 38 percent of 74 patients with idiopathic hypoparathyroidism.[50] Such antibodies were found in 12 percent of 49 patients with Hashimoto's thyroiditis and in only 6 percent of 245 control subjects. The antibody used did not react with parathyroid hormone or with a number of other tissues. These workers found that patients with idiopathic hypoparathyroidism also had an increased incidence of antibodies to gastric, thyroid, and adrenal tissue.

Gonadal failure in patients with Addison's disease has generally been attributed to the debility that may accompany advanced stages of the disease. Anderson et al., however, has described antibodies that react with cells of both the ovary and the testis in patients with idiopathic Addison's disease,[51] and Irvine et al. found antibodies that reacted with "steroid-producing cells of the gonads" in a number of such patients, as well as low estrogen levels and high levels of gonadotropins.[52] Although some of the patients with "steroid cell antibodies" had normal menstrual function, there appeared to be a strong association between ovarian failure and Addison's disease. Other conditions that have occasionally been associated with Addison's disease and that may have an autoimmune basis include Schilder's disease, vitiligo, and asthma.

FAMILIAL

A familial basis for Addison's disease has been noted in a number of studies of siblings found to have the disease, and in these, pairs of identical twins were involved.[44,53,54] These patients are notable for the frequent association of other autoimmune diseases, such as hypothyroidism, idiopathic hypoparathyroidism, and pernicious anemia. A number of these patients have been found to have a rare familial disorder, which has been called adrenoleukodystrophy. This condition, which has an X-linked transmission, leads to destruction of human cerebral white matter and the adrenal cortex. Pathologically there are large areas of cerebral demyelination and accumulation of a specific lipidlike material in the adrenal cortical cells.[54a,54b]

POSTMATURE NEONATES

Postmaturity is one of several conditions that has been noted to subject the fetus to increased distress during labor. It has been suggested that one of the defects in these infants leading to increased mortality is a relative adrenocortical insufficiency.[54c] Term infants double peripheral plasma cortisols in response to labor, but the postmature infant appears unable to raise the cortisol level even to normal.

DIFFERENTIAL DIAGNOSIS OF ADDISON'S DISEASE

The conditions to be considered in the differential diagnosis of Addison's disease are all those that are likely to produce pigmentation, chronic gastrointestinal disturbance, or chronic fatigue. The diagnosis must therefore be considered frequently, although the condition itself is infrequent, with estimates of its prevalence ranging from 30 to 60 per million population.

PIGMENTATION

The classical pigmentation is characteristic but not diagnostic. The pigmentation of hemochromatosis is not likely to involve the mucous membranes. Pigmentation in this condition is usually grayish brown and is characterized by hemosiderin in the sweat glands. Porphyria cutanea tarda may also be characterized by a generalized brown color of the skin but should be easily recognized by the large amount of uroporphyrin in the urine, stools, and plasma and by features such as bullae and scars on the face and hands. Patients suffering from severe nutritional deficiencies may have increased pigmentation. Those with sprue may have rather generalized hypermelanosis, whereas in pellagra those areas exposed to light or to irritation may become pigmented. The chloasma of pregnancy or that seen in patients taking oral progestational agents can cause patchy areas of pigmentation, particularly on the face. Those conditions causing spotty brown macules or "café au lait spots," such as neurofibromatosis and polyostotic fibrous dysplasia, do not have characteristic pigmentation but none the less have the brown spots that should not be confused with those caused by Addison's disease. Similarly, patients with Peutz-Jeghers syndrome may present with abdominal pain and well-circumscribed dark brown macules around the lips, eyes, and nostrils as well as intraorally. Pigmentation of Addison's disease, on the other hand, is chiefly on the buccal mucosa, although it may also occur on the palate and along the gingival margin. A number of heavy metals such as zinc, lead, and mercury may also cause a blue-black pigmented line along the gingival margin but do not cause buccal pigmentation.

FATIGUE

Differential diagnosis of the fatigue of Addison's disease can include an almost endless list of conditions. The fatigue of Addison's disease is characteristically accentuated by activity and improved by rest. A surprising amount of activity may be maintained in some patients. The author has seen 1 patient with severe pigmentation and little remaining adrenal function who continued to play competitive tennis but who noted that he tired more easily

than before the onset of the disease. In the presence of pigmentation and fatigue, it is necessary to carry out laboratory tests as noted below to determine whether adrenal function is normal.

GASTROINTESTINAL SYMPTOMS

The frequency of nausea, vomiting, anorexia, and occasionally diarrhea has already been referred to in patients with Addison's disease. Such patients should always be examined for the possible presence of pigmentation and, particularly if fatigue is a prominent symptom, should have examination of adrenal function. Rarely, patients with severe hyperkalemia may undergo near total paralysis as part of the picture of untreated adrenal insufficiency.[55]

LABORATORY DIAGNOSIS OF ADDISON'S DISEASE

Although changes in serum electrolytes and cellular components of the blood may be suggestive of adrenal insufficiency, the final diagnosis depends on measurement of the corticosteroids in plasma and urine. Plasma ACTH may be useful in the nonstressed patient. The methodology and application of these tests are described in detail in Chapter 94. A single plasma cortisol determination may be useful for ruling out the condition if found to be greater than 25 μg/dl, but levels in the 5–20 μg/dl range may be seen in patients whose adrenals are functioning at maximal capacity to produce these levels but who have no reserve in times of stress. Likewise, urinary levels of corticosteroids may be in the normal range in association with a high plasma ACTH level, so baseline levels of plasma or urinary corticosteroids are not sufficient to make the diagnosis of Addison's disease. An elevation in the baseline ACTH plasma level in an unstressed patient with a clinical picture of adrenal insufficiency is usually diagnostic of the disease, but patients with other disturbances of adrenal function, such as congenital adrenal hyperplasia, may have moderate increases in plasma ACTH as well.

Preference for screening tests to be used are largely dependent upon the laboratory facilities available. As noted in Chapter 94, if serum substance S and ACTH measurements are available, the single-dose methyrapone test may be found very useful. Although continued administration of metyrapone may accentuate adrenal insufficiency, a single-dose test functions very well as a screening test. If ACTH measurements are available, measurement of an early morning plasma ACTH and cortisol will give considerable information, although it will not be totally diagnostic. Most endocrinologists still prefer to administer ACTH intravenously on a 1- or 2-day basis with measurement of plasma cortisol or urinary 17-ketogenic steroids and/or urinary free cortisol to determine whether the adrenal gland is responsive to ACTH stimulation. A failure to respond to ACTH stimulation can be considered diagnostic of Addison's disease, while a significant response rules out the condition.

The diagnosis of secondary adrenal insufficiency due to lack of ACTH is discussed in Chapters 18 and 94. These patients have low plasma ACTH values as well as low plasma corticosteroids in association with a low T4 and TSH and lack of response of pituitary hormones to administration of the hypothalamic hormones TRH and GRH. It should be noted that such patients will have adrenal responsiveness with prolonged ACTH administration, i.e., 2 to 3 days, but generally will not have an increase in corticosteroid secretion when ACTH is initially given.

ADRENAL CRISIS

Acute adrenal insufficiency, usually associated with stress, is characterized by nausea, vomiting, severe hypotension, and the picture of shock and dehydration. The onset of acute adrenocortical insufficiency may vary from a gradual course over a period of days in the individual who is not acutely stressed to a sudden fall in blood pressure associated with acute trauma or surgery inadvertently performed on a patient with Addison's disease who is not receiving replacement therapy.[55a] The known addisonian patient who develops acute insufficiency usually does so as a result of intercurrent infection or trauma.

The patient presenting for the first time with such a picture should be examined for the presence of characteristic pigmentation, but the diagnosis should not be ruled out if this is not found. Characteristically the laboratory will show low serum sodium levels, elevated serum potassium and BUN levels, and other findings associated with dehydration and shock. Plasma corticosteroid determination should be obtained immediately, but therapy should not be delayed awaiting laboratory results.

THERAPY OF ACUTE ADRENAL INSUFFICIENCY

If the diagnosis appears likely, 100 mg of a soluble corticosteroid preparation such as Solucortef should be immediately given intravenously, followed by a rapid infusion of 5% glucose in saline containing another 100 mg of a soluble cortisol preparation. Patients may be hypoglycemic, particularly if they have not eaten for some time, and almost certainly will be dehydrated and sodium-deficient. Although the serum sodium level may be very low, restoration of volume is more important than restoration of sodium, so the administration of hypertonic saline is not indicated except perhaps in the rare instance where extreme hyperkalemia is present. With the administration of cortisol, there is usually a fairly rapid fall in serum potassium levels with passage of potassium into the intracellular space. As therapy progresses, there may be a tendency to develop hypokalemia, as many of these patients have a total body deficit of potassium. Hyperkalemia and volume depletion are the most immediate dangers, however, and no potassium should be given until true hypokalemia has been demonstrated.

Continued administration of isotonic saline (in amounts varying from 2–4 liters over a 24-hour period), with a total of 300–400 mg of cortisol given in the first 24 hours with this fluid, will usually totally correct the water and sodium disturbance. In the typical patient with acute adrenal insufficiency, cortisol will have a dramatic effect on restoration of blood pressure. The author has seen response from a nonobtainable diastolic blood pressure to one over 80 within 15 minutes of administration of the initial dose of cortisol. Although the adrenal medulla, as well as the cortex, may be destroyed in patients with tuberculous or other infectious destruction of the glands, there is no place for catecholamines or other vasoconstrictors in the treatment of adrenal insufficiency. As acute adrenal insufficiency is often precipitated by other factors, these should be identified and treated appropriately. The severe gastrointestinal symptoms associated with the onset of the condition may mistakenly direct attention to this organ system. Fever is usually present and again, may or may not be associated with infection.

If the initiating event is controlled, the response to therapy is dramatic, and the patient can generally be placed on oral fluids and medication within 24 hours. A convenient approach is to administer approximately 100–150 mg of cortisol on the second day and half of this on the third day, with a maintenance dose thereafter.

There is no need to give supplemental sodium-retaining hormone while the patient is receiving 100 or more milligrams of cortisol per 24 hours, but as the dose of cortisol is reduced below these levels, it is advantageous to begin therapy with sodium-retaining hormone.

THERAPY OF CHRONIC ADRENAL INSUFFICIENCY

The usual chronic replacement dose of cortisol is 30–40 mg of cortisol a day with approximately two thirds being given on arising in the morning and one third in the late afternoon. Large doses given at bedtime may produce insomnia, and most patients find it difficult to get up and function normally without their early morning dose of corticosteroid. Patients should be advised to increase corticoid intake in response to any stressful situation. The regular dose should be doubled for a day or two with a mild upper respiratory infection. Any severe infection or gastrointestinal disturbance requires immediate medical consultation and follow-up, as these patients are particularly prone to severe water and electrolyte losses and of course must receive corticosteroids parenterally if they are unable to take them by mouth. The patient whose calcified adrenals are shown in Figure 96-2 died suddenly 36 hours after the onset of moderate intestinal flu. He failed to contact his physician until quite weak and died prior to the arrival of an ambulance, which was immediately dispatched upon notification of his physician of the illness.

The usual dose of mineralocorticoid is 0.1–0.2 mg of fluorohydrocortisone by mouth per day. It should be noted that the patient who has not produced sodium-retaining hormone for some time may demonstrate extreme sensitivity to its administration. Thus, as little as 0.1 mg may produce marked sodium and water retention with clinical edema when initially given. Discontinuance of the drug for a few days followed by administration every other day for a few days after the edema has cleared will result in increased tolerance for the drug. It may then be given on a daily basis and may require increased dosage. This increased sensitivity may result from an increase in hormone receptors during a period of mineralocorticoid deficiency.

Adjustment of the dosage of the drug is generally done on an empirical basis within the general ranges noted above. Too little cortisol will result in loss of appetite, decreased weight, and a general return of fatigue. Too much, however, is likely to produce increase in appetite, with excessive weight gain, excessive euphoria, and insomnia. With continued increased dosage, any of the signs and symptoms of Cushing's syndrome, as described in Chapter 95, may occur. Too much sodium-retaining hormone may produce excessive sodium retention and edema, an increase in blood pressure, excessive loss of potassium, and the picture of hyperaldosteronism as described in Chapter 98. A moderate increase in fluorohydrocortisone is indicated for the patient exposed to excessive heat with accompanying perspiration and loss of fluid and electrolytes. An occasional patient who is prone to gastric hyperacidity may have some accentuation of this complaint when placed on corticosteroids.[56] A moderate increase in fluorohydrocortisone and a decrease in cortisone may be beneficial in this situation.

All patients with adrenal insufficiency should wear some type of warning bracelet or necklace and carry a card in their wallet or purse indicating the presence of the disease and the need for immediate medical attention if found unresponsive or if severely injured. Patients traveling in areas where medical care may not be immediately available should be furnished with a needle, syringe, and a soluble corticoid preparation so that they or an accompanying individual may be able to administer parenteral cortisol if it cannot be taken orally.

SURGERY IN PATIENTS WITH ADDISON'S DISEASE

Patients undergoing surgical procedures with general anesthesia require intravenous corticosteroids. Infusion of 100 mg of a soluble cortisol preparation throughout the operation and during the immediate postoperative period is required. The amount of cortisol given and the length of time of administration is dependent upon the duration and severity of the surgical procedue. It is certainly advisable to maintain a corticosteroid drip until the patient is fully awake, and a slow rate intravenous administration or intramuscular cortisol must be maintained until the patient is able to resume taking corticosteroids by mouth. Some surgeons prefer to give intramuscular cortisol prior to the operation in doses of 50–100 mg so as to ensure proper coverage. If 200 mg of cortisol has been administered on the day of operation, it is usual to give 100 mg on the first postoperative day, 50 mg on the second postoperative day, and then return to the maintenance dose if the patient is making a rapid recovery.

PREGNANCY IN ADDISON'S DISEASE

Most addisonian patients are able to go through pregnancy uneventfully.[57] Care must be taken that the nausea and vomiting of early pregnancy does not prevent normal daily intake of cortisol, and in some cases, it may be necessary to administer the hormone intramuscularly. The management of delivery is similar to that for the patient coming to surgery with administration of intravenous cortisol during the period of stress. A decreased responsiveness to the sodium-retaining actions of aldosterone during late pregnancy has been attributed to the high levels of progesterone that are present, which have a "sodium-losing effect."[58] The observed increase in aldosterone levels during pregnancy may, at least in part, be due to the high levels of progesterone that are also present.

PROGNOSIS

With early diagnosis and adequate replacement therapy, the prognosis in Addison's disease is good. Although the patient is not able to increase corticosteroid output during periods of increased need (stress), these needs can be easily supplied if the patient is adequately instructed and seeks medical help. The chief danger to the patient is failure to seek and obtain medical aid during stressful periods. If adequate maintenance therapy is maintained, with additional corticosteroids available when needed, a normal, fully active life can be enjoyed by the patient with Addison's disease.

REFERENCES

1. Addison, T.: On the constitutional and local effects of disease of the supra-renal capsules. London, Highley, 1855.
2. Brown-Sequard, E.: Les capsules surrenales. *Arch Gen Med 8:* 385, 1856.
3. Thorn, G. W.: The adrenal cortex: 1. Historical aspects. *Johns Hopkins Med J 123:* 49, 1968.
4. Rogoff, J. M., Stewart, G. N.: Suprarenal cortical extracts in suprarenal insufficiency (Addison's disease). *JAMA 92:* 1569, 1929.
5. Swingle, W. W., Pfiffner, J. J.: An aqueous extract of the suprarenal cortex which maintains the life of bilaterally adrenalectomized cats. *Science 71:* 321, 1930.
6. Loeb, R. F.: The effect of sodium chloride on the treatment of a patient with Addison's disease. *Proc Soc Exp Biol Med 30:* 808, 1933.
7. Kendall, E. C.: A chemical and physiological investigation of the suprarenal cortex. *Cold Spring Harbor Symp Quant Biol 5:* 299, 1937.
8. Thorn, G. W., Dorrance, S. S., Day, E.: Addison's disease: Evaluation of synthetic desoxycorticosterone acetate therapy in 158 patients. *Ann Intern Med 16:* 1053, 1942.
9. Nelson, D. H., Reich, H., Samuels, L. T.: Isolation of a steroid hormone from the adrenal-vein blood of dogs. Science 111: 578, 1950.
10. Nelson, D. H., Samues, L. T.: A method for the determination of 17-hydroxycorticosteroids in blood: 17-hydroxycorticosterone in the peripheral circulation. *J Clin Endocrinol Metab 12:* 519, 1952.
11. Bush, I. E.: Species differences in adrenocortical secretion. *J Endocrinol 9:* 95, 1953.
12. Romanoff, E. B., Hudson, P., Pincus, G.: Isolation of hydrocortisone and corticosterone from human adrenal vein blood. *J Clin Endocrinol 13:* 1546, 1953.
13. Simpson, S. A., Tait, J. F., Bush, I. E.: Secretion of a salt-retaining hormone by the mammalian adrenal cortex. *Lancet 2: 226, 1952.*
14. Simpson, S. A., Tait, J. F., Wettstein, A., et al: Constitution of aldosterone, a new mineralocorticoid. *Experentia 10:* 132, 1954.
15. Nerup, J.: Addison's disease—clinical studies. A report of 108 cases. *Acta Endocrinol 76:* 127, 1974.
16. Cotterill, J. A., Cunliffe, W. J.: Self medication with liquorice in a patient with Addison's disease. *Lancet 1:* 294, 1973.
17. Jarvis, J. L., Jenkins, D., Sosman, M. C., et al: Roentgenologic observations in Addison's disease. A review of 120 cases. *Radiology 62:* 16 1954.
18. Batson, J. M.: Calcification of the ear cartilage associated with the hypercalcemia of Sarcoidosis. *N Engl J Med 265:* 876, 1961.
19. Swingle, W. W., Da Vango, J. P., Glenister, D., et al: Role of gluco- and mineralo-corticoids in salt and water metabolism of adrenalectomized dogs. *Am J Physiol 196:* 283, 1959.
20. Walser, M., Robinson, B. H. B., Duckett, J. W., Jr.: The hypercalcemia of adrenal insufficiency. *J Clin Invest 42:* 456, 1963.
21. Jorgensen, H.: Hypercalcemia in adrenocortical insufficiency. *Act Med Scand 193:* 175, 1973.
22. Bartter, F. C., Schwartz, W. B.: The syndrome of inappropriate secretion of antidiuretic hormone. *Am J Med 42:* 790, 1967.
23. Garrod, O., Davis, S. A., Cahill, G. Jr.: The action of cortisone and desoxycorticosterone acetate on glomerular filtration rate and sodium-water exchange in the adrenalectomized dog. *J Clin Invest 34:* 761, 1955.
24. Crabbe, J., Reddy, W. J., Ross, E. J., et al: The role of the adrenal cortex in the normal adaptation to dietary sodium deprivation. *J Clin Endocrinol Metab 18:* 1147, 1958.
25. Moses, A. M., Gabrilove, J. L., Soffer, L. J.: Simplified water loading test in hypoadrenocorticism and hypothyroidism. *J Clin Endocrinol Metab 18:* 1413, 1958.
26. Kleeman, C. R., Czackes, J. W., Cutler, R.: Mechanism of impaired water excretion in adrenal and pituitary insufficiency. *J Clin Invest 37:* 1799, 1958.
27. Maloney, P. J.: Addison's disease due to chronic disseminated coccidiodomycosis. *Arch Intern Med 90:* 869, 1952.
28. Crispell, E. R., Parson, W., Hamlin, J., et al: Addison's disease associated with histoplasmosis: Report of four cases and review of the literature. *Am J Med 20:* 23, 1956.
29. Abernathy, R. S., Melby, J. C.: Addison's disease in North American blastomycosis. *N Engl J Med 54:* 189, 1961.
30. D'Agati, V. C., Marangoni, B. A.: The Waterhouse-Fridericksen syndrome. *N Engl J Med 232:* 1, 1945.
31. Margaretten, W., Hisayo, N., Landing, B. H.: Septicemic adrenal hemorrhage. *Am J Dis Child 105:* 346, 1963.
31a. Schumer, W.: Steroids in the treatment of clinical septic shock. *Ann Surg 184:* 333, 1976.

32. Levin, J., Cluff, L. E.: Endotoxemia and adrenal hemorrhage. A mechanism for the Waterhouse-Fridericksen syndrome. *J Exp Med 121:* 247, 1965.

33. O'Connell, T. X., Ashton, S. J.: Acute adrenal hemorrhage complicating anticoagulant therapy. *Surg Gynecol Obstet 139:* 355, 1974.

34. Meakin, J. W., Tantongco, M. S., Crabbé, J., et al: Pituitary-adrenal function following long-term steroid therapy. *Am J Med 29:* 459, 1960.

35. Graber, A. L., Ney, R. L., Nicholson, W. E., et al: Natural history of pituitary-adrenal recovery following long-term suppression with corticosteroids. *J Clin Endocrinol Metab 25:* 11, 1965.

36. Nelson, D. H.: Regulation of glucocorticoid release. *Am J Med 53:* 590, 1972.

37. Harter, J. G., Reddy, W. J., Thorn, G. W.: Studies on intermittent corticosteroid dosage regimen. *N Engl J Med 269:* 591, 1963.

38. Ackerman, G. L., Nolan, C. M.: Adrenocortical responsiveness after alternate-day corticosteroid therapy. *N Engl J Med 278:* 405, 1968.

39. Plager, J E., Cushman, P. Jr.: Suppression of the pituitary-ACTH response in man by administration of ACTH or cortisol. *J Clin Endocrinol 22:* 147, 1962.

40. Carter, M. E., James, V. H. T.: Effect of corticotrophin on pituitary-adrenal function. *Ann Rheum Dis 29:* 73, 1970.

41. Donald, R. A., Espiner, E. A.: The plasma cortisol and corticotrophin response to hypoglycemia following adrenal steroid and ACTH administration. *J Clin Endocrinol Metab 41:* 1, 1975.

42. Migeon, C. J., Kenny, F. M., Kowarski, A., et al: The syndrome of congenital adrenocortical unresponsiveness to ACTH. Report of six cases. *Pediatr Res 2:* 501, 1968.

43. Irvine, W. J., Stewart, A. G., Scarth, L.: A clinical and immunological study of adrenocortical insufficiency (Addison's Disease). *Clin Exp Immunol 2:* 31, 1967.

44. Irvine, W. J., Barnes, E. W.: Adrenocortical insufficiency. *Clin Endocrinol Metab 1:* 549, 1972.

45. Nerup, J., Bendixen, G.: Anti-adrenal cellular hypersensitivity in Addison's disease. *Clin Exp Immunol 5:* 341, 1969.

46. Schmidt, M. B.: Eine biglandulare erkrankung (Nebennieren und Schilddruse) bei morbus Addisonii. *Verh Dtsch Pathol 21:* 212, 1926.

47. McHardy-Young, S., Lessof, M. H., Maisey, M. N.: Serum TSH and thyroid antibody studies in Addison's disease. *Clin Endocrinol 1:* 45, 1972.

48. Beaven, D. W., Nelson, D. H., Renold, A. E., et al: Diabetes mellitus and Addison's disease: A report on 8 patients and a review of 55 cases in the literature. *N Engl J Med 261:* 443, 1959.

49. Irvine, W. J.: Thyroid and gastric autoimmunity in patients with diabetes mellitus. *Lancet 2:* 163, 1970.

50. Blizzard, R. M., Chee, D., Davis, W.: The incidence of adrenal and other antibodies in the sera of patients with idiopathic adrenal insufficiency. *Clin Exp Immunol 2:* 19, 1967.

51. Anderson, J. R.: Immunological features of idiopathic Addison's disease: an antibody to cells producing steroid hormones. *Clin Exp Imunol 3:* 107, 1968.

52. Irvine, W. J., Chan, M. M. W., Scarth, L.: The further characterization of auto-antibodies reactive with extra-adrenal steroid-producing cells in patients with adrenal disorders. *Clin Exp Immunol 4:* 489, 1969.

53. Meakin, J. W., Nelson, D. H., Thorn, G. W.: Addison's disease in two brothers. *J Clin Endocrinol Metab 19:* 726, 1959.

54. Heggarty, H.: Addison's disease in identical twins. *Br Med J 1:* 559, 1968.

54a. Schaumburg, H. H., Powers, J. M., Raine, C. S., Suzuki, K., Richardson, E. P.: Adrenoleukodystrophy. A clinical and pathological study of 17 cases. *Arch Neurol 32:* 577, 1975.

54b. Johnson, A. B., Schaumburg, H. H., Powers, J. M.: Histochemical characteristics of the striated inclusions of adrenoleukodystrophy. *J Histochem Cytochem 24:* 725, 1976.

54c. Nwosu, U. C., Wallach, E. E., Boggs, T. R., Bongiovanni, A. M.: Possible adrenocortical insufficiency in postmature neonates. *Am J Obstet Gynecol 122:* 969, 1975.

55. Van Dellen, R. G., Purnell, D. C.: Hyperkalemic paralysis in Addison's disease. *Mayo Clin Proc 44:* 904, 1969.

55a. Hubay, C. A., Weckesser, E. C., Levy, R. P.: Occult adrenal insufficiency in surgical patients. *Ann Surg 181:* 325, 1975.

56. Gray, S. J., Ramsey, C. G., Thorn, G. W.: Adrenal influences on the stomach: peptic ulcer in Addison's disease during adrenal steroid therapy. *Ann Intern Med 45:* 73, 1956.

57. Osler, M.: Addison's disease and pregnancy. *Acta Endocrinol 41:* 67, 1962.

58. Drucker, W. D., Hendrikx, A., Laragh, J. H.: Effect of administered aldosterone upon electrolyte excretion during and after pregnancy in two women with adrenal cortical insufficiency. *J Clin Endocrinol 23:* 1247, 1963.

97

Diagnosis and Treatment of Adrenogenital Disorders

Claude J. Migeon

Adrenogenital disorders represent a group of syndromes characterized by abnormalities of the secretion of adrenocortical steroids resulting in genital symptoms of virilism or feminization. These disorders are part of the group of diseases due to hyperadrenocorticism. Depending upon the predominance of a specific adrenal steroid, hyperadrenocorticism can be classified as follows:

1. *Cushing's syndrome,* which is characterized by an increased secretion of *cortisol.*
2. The *adrenogenital syndrome,* which is related to an elevated output of *androgens.* It can be due either to virilizing adrenal tumors or to congenital adrenal hyperplasia.
3. *Feminizing syndromes,* which are due to tumors secreting large amounts of *estrogens.*
4. *Hyperaldosteronism,* which is due to an abnormal production of *aldosterone.*

In this chapter we specifically consider the diagnosis and treatment of congenital adrenal hyperplasia, virilizing adrenal tumors, and feminizing adrenal tumors (Table 97-1).

Although cases of the adrenogenital syndrome resulting from virilizing adrenal tumors or adrenal hypertrophy were reported early in the literature, DeCrecchio[1] in 1865 gave the first detailed description of a patient with female pseudohermaphroditism due to congenital adrenal hyperplasia. Later, Apert[2] and Gallais[3] attempted to classify patients presenting various types of hirsutism associated or not associated with obesity. However, a great deal of confusion remained until 1932 when Cushing[4] described the syndrome that bears his name and that is now known to be due to a hypersecretion of cortisol. Ten years later, Albright[5] clearly distinguished Cushing's syndrome, which he attributed to excessive secretion of a sugar or "S" hormone from virilizing congenital adrenal hyperplasia which he related to abnormal production of an "N" hormone (hormone producing a positive nitrogen balance). A few years later, Wilkins et al.[6] and Bartter et al.[7] demonstrated the therapeutic effects of cortisone in congenital adrenal hyperplasia, whereas Gardner and Migeon[8] showed its lack of beneficial effects in virilizing adrenal tumors. Many workers contributed to our present understanding of the pathogenesis of congenital adrenal hyperplasia, but the work of Bongiovanni and Eberlein,[9–11] Prader and Gurtner,[12,13] and Biglieri et al.[14] made possible the elucidation of the various enzymatic deficiencies in the syndrome.

CONGENITAL ADRENAL HYPERPLASIA (CAH)

This form of the adrenogenital syndrome is now well recognized as an inherited inborn error of metabolism and is due to specific enzymatic deficiencies in the biosynthesis of cortisol by the adrenal cortex (Table 97-1). The adrenal hyperplasia that results from such enzymatic deficiencies is related to a compensatory secretion of ACTH by the pituitary gland. This hyperplasia is responsible for the name given to the syndrome. It must be noted that some enzymatic systems are common to the adrenal glands and the gonads, and a deficiency of these enzymes results in abnormal secretion of both adrenal and gonadal steroids.

Although all the forms listed in Table 97-1 have been observed, by far the most frequent ones are the *simple virilizing* and *salt-losing forms* (Table 97-2).

SIMPLE VIRILIZING FORM

Abnormal Steroidogenesis

In this form of the syndrome there is a partial 21-hydroxylase deficiency that is well compensated for by an increase in ACTH output, so that the cortisol secretion is close to normal (Fig. 97-1). At the same time, the increased ACTH secretion produces a massive elevation of androgens and cortisol precursors (Fig. 97-2). Some of them, such as progesterone and 17-hydroxyprogesterone, have a salt-losing tendency. These steroids appear to block the sodium-retaining activity of aldosterone at the level of the renal tubule. This tendency, however, is well compensated for by an increase in plasma renin activity and consequently an increase in aldosterone secretion (Fig. 97-3).

As part of the overall homeostatic response to the 21-hydroxylase deficiency, large amounts of androgens are secreted by the adrenal cortex. Among them is, in particular, androstenedione, which is found in large amounts in blood. Although this steroid has little biological activity of its own, it can be metabolized peripherally to testosterone, which is the virilizing steroid in the syndrome. Androgens with an oxygen on carbon-11 are also secreted in large amounts, so that the ratio of 11-desoxy to 11-oxy-17-ketosteroids in urine is close to 1:1, whereas this ratio is 4:1 in favor of the 11-desoxy-17-ketosteroids in normal adult subjects.

Table 97-1.   Adrenogenital Syndrome with Respective Enzyme Deficiency and Resulting Steroid Pattern

	Enzyme Deficiency	Cortisol	Androgens	Estrogens	Aldosterone	Renin Activity
Congenital adrenal hyperplasia						
Simple virilizing	Partial 21-OH	N	2+ to 3+	1+	2+	2+
Salt-losing	More complete 21-OH	−	2+ to 3+	1+	−	2+
Hypertensive	11-hydroxylase	− (S++)	2+ to 3+	1+	− (Doc+)	−
17-OH deficiency	17-hydroxylase	− (B++)	−	−	− (Doc+)	−
3β-ol deficiency	3β-ol dehydrogenase	−	3+ (DHA+)	−	−	2+
Lipid hyperplasia	Prior to Δ⁵-pregnenolone	−	−	−	−	2+
Virilizing adrenal tumor	?	N	3+ (DHA)	N to 1+	N	N
Feminizing adrenal tumor	?	N	1+	1+ to 2+	N	N

N = normal secretion; − = lower than normal; 1+ to 3+ = higher than normal; S = compound S; B = corticosterone; Doc = desoxycorticosterone; DHA = dehydroisoandrosterone.

Table 97-2.   Relative Incidence of the Different Types of Congenital Adrenal Hyperplasia

	Simple Virilizing			Salt-losing			Hypertensive			3β-ol Deficiency			Total		
Authors	M	F	Total	M	F	Total	M	F	Total	M	F	Total	M	F	Total
Wilkins	14	64	78	10	35	45	2	5	7	1	−	1	27	104	131
Prader et al.	26	37	63	22	33	55	−	2	2	1	1	2	49	73	122
Raiti, Newns	13	16	29	11	17	28	1	0	1	−	−	−	25	33	58
Total	53	117	170	43	85	128	3	7	10	2	1	3	101	210	311

Note: One must also add 2 females with lipoid adrenal hyperplasia in Prader's series.

The precursors of cortisol with 21 carbons are metabolized by the liver and appear in the urine in large amounts. One of these is pregnanetriol which is the main metabolite of 17-hydroxyprogesterone; its excretion is used as a diagnostic test. Dehydroisoandrosterone and its sulfate are also secreted in abnormally large amounts; however, its proportion to the total urinary 17-ketosteroids remains normal (Table 97-3). Physiologically, the adrenal glands secrete small amounts of estrogens. In addition, androgens are metabolized peripherally to estrogens, and patients with congenital adrenal hyperplasia also have an increased level of estrogenic steroids.

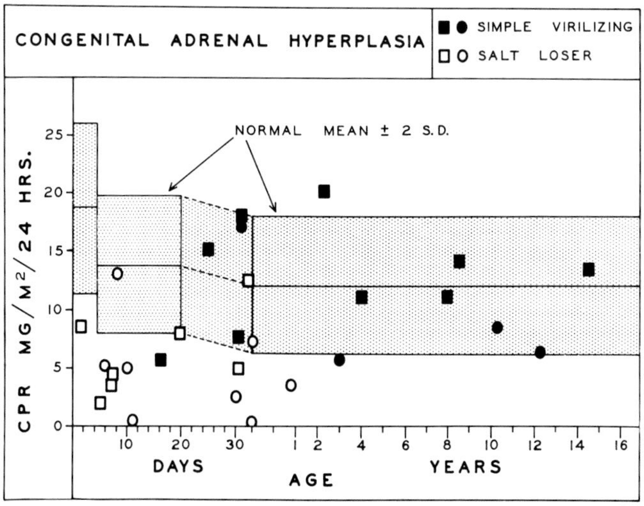

Clinical Manifestations as Related to Hormonal Abnormalities

This is a congenital disorder, and the deficient 21-hydroxylase is manifested early during fetal life. As a consequence, excessive secretion of adrenal androgens in the female fetus causes masculinization of the external genitalia with enlargement of the clitoris and a variable degree of labioscrotal fusion (Fig. 97-4). In some cases the fusion may be so extensive that the external genitalia are mistaken for those of a cryptorchid male with or without hypospadias (Fig. 97-5). However, the genital ducts and gonads of these female fetuses remain perfectly normal. In the male, the increased secretion of fetal adrenal androgens is of little significance in relation to the fetal production of testicular androgens. Usually, no abnormality of the external genitalia is observed at birth. In some boys, slight enlargement of the phallus and increased pigmentation of the scrotum are seen.

Later on in life, progressive virilization occurs in both sexes, with early appearance of pubic and axillary hair, followed somewhat later by facial hair, increased total body hair, deepening of the voice, and acne. There is also some degree of phallic enlargement with frequent erections. Simultaneously, rapid somatic growth, accelerated osseous development, and increased musculature are noted. Although the patients are taller than normal during early childhood, abnormally short adult stature results because of

Fig. 97-1.   Cortisol production rate in the simple virilizing and the salt-losing forms of congenital adrenal hyperplasia. The shaded area represents the value of the mean ± 2 standard deviations in normal infants and children. (From Migeon, C J., and Kenny, F. M., J. Pediatr. 6: 779, 1969.)

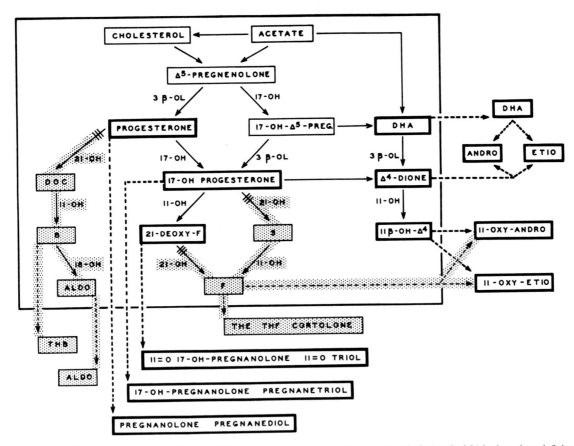

Fig. 97-2. Biosynthesis of adrenocorticosteroids in the salt-losing form of congenital adrenal hyperplasia (marked 21-hydroxylase deficiency). Steroids situated inside large rectangle represent adrenal biosynthesis, while compounds situated outside rectangle represent urinary metabolites. The secretion of steroids that are situated after the enzymatic deficiency is decreased or absent (shaded boxes), while that of steroids prior to block is increased (heavy boxes). Decrease in cortisol secretion results in increased output of ACTH and, as a consequence, elevated secretion of androgens and cortisol precursors. There is also a decrease or absence of aldosterone secretion, which explains the salt loss. (From Migeon, C. J. In R. E. Cooke (ed), The Biological Basis of Pediatric Practice. Copyright 1968 by McGraw-Hill Book Company.)

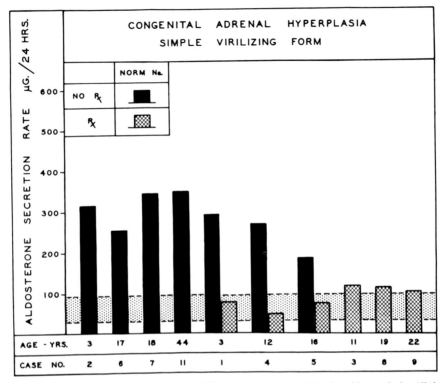

Fig. 97-3. Aldosterone secretion rate in 10 patients with the simple virilizing form of congenital adrenal hyperplasia. All the patients were on a normal sodium diet, and they were either untreated or had been treated for at least 7 days. The shaded area represents the range of variation of aldosterone secretion rate in normal adults on a normal sodium diet. When the patients were untreated, the secretion rates were greater than normal, whereas they came to the normal range after a week of treatment. (From Kowarski, A., Finkelstein, J. W., Spaulding, J. S., Holman, G. H., and Migeon, C. J., J. Clin. Invest. *44:* 1505, 1965.)

Table 97-3. Excretion of Urinary 17-KS in the Adrenogenital Syndrome

	Androsterone Etiocholanolone	DHA-S	11-Oxygenated 17-KS	Suppression of 17-KS in Suppression Test
Congenital adrenal hyperplasia				
Simple virilizing form	3+	In proportion to total 17-KS	2+	Yes
Salt-losing form	3+	Same	2+	Yes
Hypertensive form	3+*	Same	−	Yes
3-β-ol-dehydrogenase deficiency	−	3+	−	Yes
Lipoid hyperplasia	−	−	−	Low control 17-KS
17-hydroxylase deficiency	−	−	−	Low control 17-KS
Virilizing adrenal tumor	1+	3+	N	No
Feminizing adrenal tumor	N to 2+	N to 2+	N	No

N = normal levels; − = lower than normal; 1+ to 3+ = higher than normal.
*Etiocholanolone, mostly.

premature closure of the epiphyseal discs. At the time of puberty, the normal increase of pituitary gonadotropin secretion does not occur because of the negative feedback resulting from the increased secretion of adrenal androgens. This results in absence of menses in girls and small size of the testes in boys. However, there are some exceptions, menses and spermatogenesis being present in a few untreated patients. In adulthood the subjects are quite short, with strong musculature and heavy facial and body hair (Fig. 97-6). In this form of CAH, patients do not show problems with electrolytes and water balance. Their blood pressure is normal despite the increased secretion of aldosterone. The elevated aldosterone level is related to the salt-losing tendency created by the hypersecretion of progesterone, 17-hydroxyprogesterone, and possibly 16-hydroxyprogesterone.

Diagnostic Laboratory Tests

The measurement of total urinary 17-ketosteroids remains an important diagnostic test (Table 97-4). However, because normal infants and prepubertal children excrete small amounts of 17-ketosteroids and because their urine contains nonspecific pigments, it is important to read the Zimmermann color reaction at three different wave lengths (440,520,600 mμ) in order to carry out an Allen correction.

The urinary 17-ketosteroids can be fractionated; as shown in Table 97-3, the proportion of the various steroids is fairly characteristic. An important function test is the suppression of urinary 17-ketosteroids (Fig. 97-7). This can be carried out by administration of fairly large amounts of cortisol. However, it must be remembered that up to 10 percent of the administered cortisol may be excreted as part of total urinary 17-ketosteroids. For this reason the more potent synthetic glucocorticoid dexamethasone is preferred, given in the daily dose of 1.25 mg/m²/24 hr for 7 days. It must be noted that this test will differentiate congenital adrenal hyperplasia from virilizing adrenal tumors (Table 97-3).

Androgens can also be measured in plasma. There is a characteristic increase in androstenedione and, to a smaller extent, in testosterone. As mentioned earlier, the testosterone arises from the peripheral metabolism of androstenedione rather than from direct secretion by the adrenal glands.

There is also increased secretion of urinary pregnanetriol (Fig. 97-8) and, to a lesser degree, of urinary pregnanediol. However, low urinary pregnanetriol is sometimes found very early in life. This is because newborns have low glucuronyl-transferase activity, and laboratory methods for urinary pregnanetriol measure only glucuronide conjugates. In order to avoid this problem, it is now possible to measure plasma 17-hydroxyprogesterone, the precursor of urinary pregnanetriol. However, it must be noted that the concentration of this steroid is physiologically elevated in cord blood (Table 97-5). 17-Hydroxyprogesterone levels in plasma can also fluctuate rapidly in normal subjects, particularly under conditions of stress. Patients with the simple virilizing form of CAH have extremely elevated levels of 17-hydroxyprogesterone.

Baseline levels of plasma cortisol and urinary 17-hydroxycorticosteroids are in the normal range, but their increment under ACTH stimulation is smaller than normal. Plasma renin activity and aldosterone secretion rate are moderately elevated, but their diagnostic value is not well established.

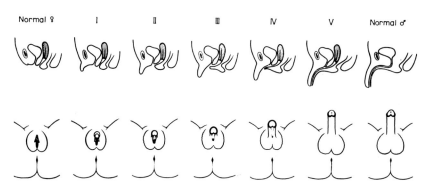

Fig. 97-4. Genital configuration in female pseudohermaphroditism due to congenital adrenal hyperplasia as compared to normal males and females. In type I the only abnormality is enlargement of the clitoris, while in type II, partial labioscrotal fusion is found. In type III, there is a funnel-shaped urogenital sinus at the posterior end of a shallow vulva, while in type IV, a very small urogenital sinus is situated at the base of the enlarged phallus. In type V, a penile urethra is present. (From Prader, A., Helv. Paediatr. Acta *13:* 5, 1958.)

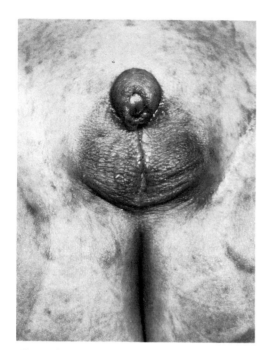

Fig. 97-5. External genitalia of a female infant. The urethra opens at the tip of the phallus. The labioscrotal folds are completely fused mimicking a male scrotum. However, no gonads can be palpated.

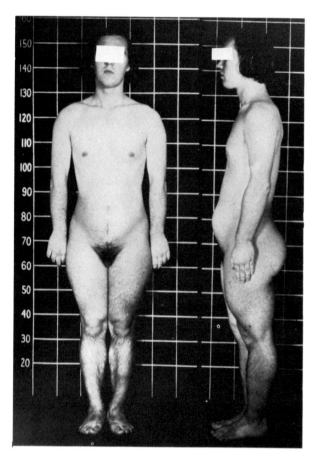

Fig. 97-6. Results of the progressive virilization and hirsutism in a 16-year-old girl with untreated congenital adrenal hyperplasia. The subject had coarse hair on the trunk and extremities and shaved her face daily. Also note the male habitus and short stature.

Table 97-4. Measurement of Total Urinary 17-Ketosteroids

Hormones measured:	Unconjugated and conjugated neutral C_{19}-steroids with a 17-ketone (Zimmermann reaction).
Limitations:	Does not measure biologically active androgenic hormones but their metabolites. Only a fraction of the metabolites are excreted as urinary 17-ketosteroids (about $\frac{1}{3}$ for testosterone).
Normal values: (mg/24 hr)	First few weeks of life = up to 2 mg
	1 month to 5 years = 0.5 mg or less
	5 to 8 years = 1.0–2.0 mg
	Puberty = progressive increase to adult levels
	Normal adult males = 7–17 mg
	Normal adult females = 5–15 mg

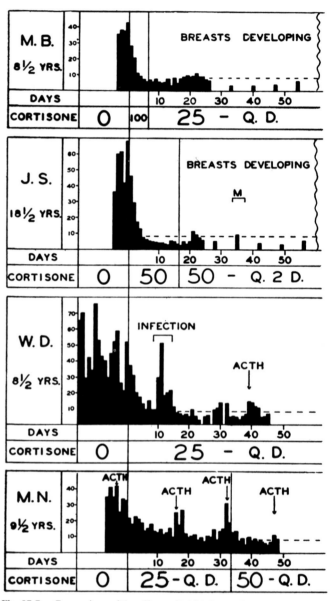

Fig. 97-7. Comparison of the effects of initial doses of 100 mg, 50 mg, and 25 mg of cortisone on the suppression of urinary 17-ketosteroids of 4 female pseudohermaphrodites. Note the response of urinary 17-ketosteroids to infection and to exogenous ACTH. (From Wilkins, L., Gardner, L. I., Crigler, J. R., Jr. Silverman, S. H., and Migeon, C. J., J. Clin. Endocrinol Metab. *12:* 257, 1952)

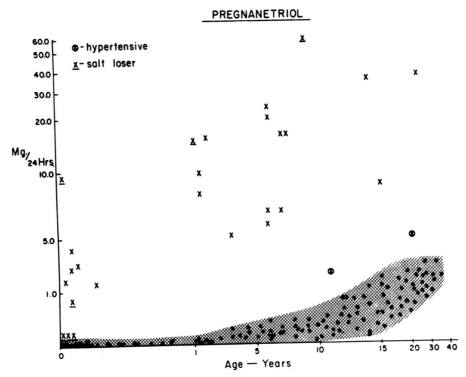

Fig. 97-8. Urinary excretion of pregnanetriol in normal subjects (black dots in the shaded area) and in patients with congenital adrenal hyperplasia (x). (From Bongiovanni, A. M., and Eberlein, W. R., Metabolism, *10:* 917, 1961.)

Pathological Findings

Most pathological studies have been made in the salt-losing form, since all these patients used to die of the disorder prior to the availability of cortisone. However, evidence suggests that pathological findings are similar in both the simple virilizing and salt-losing forms. The main finding in all cases is the marked enlargement of the adrenal glands, which can be 4 to 10 times greater than normal for the age of the patient. On gross examination, the glands have a light tan or gold color, their surface being irregular. In older subjects adenomatous formations can often be observed. On microscopic examination it is evident that there is a marked hyperplasia of the zona reticularis, which makes up to 90 percent of the cortex. There is also hyperplasia of the zona fasciculata, but the distinction between the two zones is not clear.[15] Although the zona glomerulosa is atrophic in salt-losing cases, it seems fairly normal in non-salt-losing patients.

The adrenal cells appear to be hyperplastic. Their cytosol is eosinophilic, and their nuclei are vesicular with a large nucleolus. Between these richly pigmented cells is another type of cell with granular cytoplasm and large vacuoles rich in lipids. This second type of cells often forms cordlike arrangements.

The presence of hyperplastic adrenal tissue in the testes of male patients has been observed in a number of cases and represents a hyperplasia of ectopic tissue. Such ectopic tissue has also been observed on occasion in the broad ligaments of females.

Prior to puberty the genital ducts are perfectly normal. In particular, there is normal ovarian follicle development. However, at puberty the internal sex organs remain infantile because of the lack of gonadotropin stimulation. In adult females the ovaries can appear polycystic, with a thick albuginea resembling that observed in the Stein-Leventhal syndrome. It also seems that with advanced age there is less and less follicular activity with disappearance of primordial follicles. In the postpubertal male the germinal epithelium remains infantile, occasionally with primary spermatocytes, while the interstitial cells appear atrophic. Following glucocorticoid therapy, both testes and ovaries recover their normal adult appearance. In rare instances, the development of adrenal tumor has been reported in subjects with adrenal hyperplasia. They all occurred in untreated patients, and one could speculate that the tumors were the result of prolonged ACTH stimulation.

Positive and Differential Diagnosis

In view of the great effectiveness of glucocorticoid therapy in correcting the anomalies of the syndrome, it is of extreme impor-

Table 97-5. Mean (± S.D.) Concentrations of Androgens and 17-Hydroxyprogesterone in Plasma of Normal Subjects (ng/100 ml)

	Adult Males	Adult Females	Pregnant Females	Females at Delivery	Cord	Prepubertal Children < 7 yr
Testosterone	560 ± 150	50 ± 15	115 ± 40	135 ± 70	45 ± 25	12 ± 5
Androstenedione	115 ± 20	180 ± 60	250 ± 80	390 ± 175	125 ± 60	20 ± 15
Dehydroisoandrosterone	555 ± 180	535 ± 160	365 ± 235	1015 ± 805	205 ± 140	40 ± 30
Dehydroisoandrosterone sulfate (μg/100 ml)	125 ± 35	115 ± 30	—	40 ± 20	90 ± 40	6 ± 5
17-OH-progesterone	95 ± 30	60 ± 20	230 ± 30*	660 ± 60*	2220 ± 280* (vein)	35 ± 25
		270 ± 60			1400 ± 230* (artery)	

*Tulchinsky and Simmer, J. Clin. Endocrinol. Metab. 35: 799, 1972.

Table 97-7. Treatment of Congenital Adrenal Hyperplasia at Time of Surgery

Days to Surgery	Elective Surgery		Emergency Surgery		
	IM Cortisol (mg/M²/day)	IM Doca (mg/day)*	IM Cortisol (mg/M²/day)	IV Solu-Cortef (mg/day)	(IM Doca (mg/day)*
		PO Florinef			
−2	37.5 to 50	0.05 to 0.10			
−1	37.5 to 50	0.05 to 0.10			
Preanesthesia	37.5 to 50	IM Doca 1	37.5 to 50		1
During surgery				50 (stat) 50 to 100 (continuous infusion during surgery and recovery)	
+1	37.5 to 50	1	37.5 to 50		1
+2	37.5 to 50	1	37.5 to 50		1
+3	37.5 to 50	1	37.5 to 50		1
+4	25 to 37.5	1	25 to 37.5		1
+5	Resume replacement therapy		Resume replacement therapy		

*If pellets, no additional Doca necessary.

it is of great importance to adjust therapy during stress, it is also of importance to return to maintenance levels as soon as possible in order to avoid problems of overtreatment resulting in poor growth and symptoms of Cushing's syndrome.

Preparation of Patients for Surgery. When possible, the patient should be hospitalized 2 days prior to surgery in order to start IM cortisol at three to four times maintenance levels (Table 97-7). This is continued on the day of surgery and for the next 3 days. In general, by the fourth day it is possible to reduce the dosage and to resume replacement therapy on the fifth day. However, if there is any intercurrent complication, it might be necessary to continue the "stress" therapy.

At the time of an emergency such as surgery, IM cortisol therapy is started simultaneously with immediate iv administration of 50 mg of hydrocortisone. This is followed by a continuous infusion of 50–100 mg of hydrocortisone added to the intravenous fluid and given during surgery and recovery. After that time, therapy is similar to that outlined for elective surgery.

A number of general principles must be followed in the overall treatment of congenital adrenal hyperplasia:

1. Therapy should be started as early as possible because of the influence of the untreated syndrome on growth and on psychological adjustments of patients.

2. Cortisol (or cortisone) remains the drug of choice for glucocorticoid replacement therapy. There are various reasons for this, including the fact that it is the major physiologic steroid secreted by the adrenal cortex. Also it contributes to sodium retention, while a number of synthetic preparations do not have such an effect. However, prednisolone or prednisone (5 mg and 6 mg/m²/24 hours, respectively) can be successfully used; one advantage of this preparation is that it can often be obtained for a lower price. Other synthetic compounds such as triamcinolone are not recommended. Overtreatment with any glucocorticoid may result in pseudotumor cerebri. It seems, however, that the synthetic products may have a greater tendency to bring about this side effect. Finally, the great potency of synthetic products such as dexamethasone makes it more difficult to find the optimal dosage, particularly in childhood.

3. The maintenance dosage must be adjusted to the requirement of each patient. Careful follow-up of 17-ketosteroids and pregnanetriol excretion, of growth curves and bone age, and of blood pressure are necessary (Fig. 97-10).

4. Patients and their parents must be properly educated so that they will understand the need of treatment for a lifetime. They also must understand the importance of adjusting therapy during Stress. It is advised that patients wear a bracelet indicating that they are receiving cortisol therapy so that in case of accident with loss of consciousness they may continue to receive treatment.

SALT-LOSING FORM

Pathogenesis of Salt Loss

Such patients have been shown to have an almost complete deficiency of 21-hydroxylase.[18,19] Under such conditions and despite an increase in ACTH, there is no proper compensation (Fig. 97-1), and the plasma cortisol levels are well below normal. As in the simple virilizing form, the enzyme deficiency results in hyperproduction of cortisol precursors including compounds that produce a salt-losing tendency. In addition, the 21-hydroxylase enzyme is also necessary for the formation of aldosterone. The inability to secrete aldosterone (Fig. 97-11), combined with the hyperproduction of salt-losing steroids, results in the acute adrenal crisis characteristic of this form of the syndrome.

Finally, as in the simple virilizing form, the increased ACTH secretion results in a hyperproduction of adrenal androgens. Such androgens are similar to those observed in the non-salt-losing form. However, there is evidence that the hypersecretion might be greater, resulting in a more complete virilization of the external genitalia of female patients during fetal life. Indeed, in patients with the salt-losing form of CAH, one most often finds the formation of a phallus, penile urethra, and complete fusion of the labioscrotal folds.

Clinical Manifestations

In general, an *acute adrenal crisis* occurs at the fifth to eighth day of life. Early descriptions of such patients are probably those of Phillips[20] and Fibiger,[21] who reported several siblings with female pseudohermaphroditism who died shortly after birth. As already mentioned, symptoms are not present at birth. An early sign is an increase in serum potassium levels. Such infants have a poor appetite and lose more weight than is physiologic. This is due to an excessive sodium loss which eventually results in a severe water loss and marked dehydration. There is also apathy, vomiting, diarrhea, and abdominal pain. These symptoms have often led

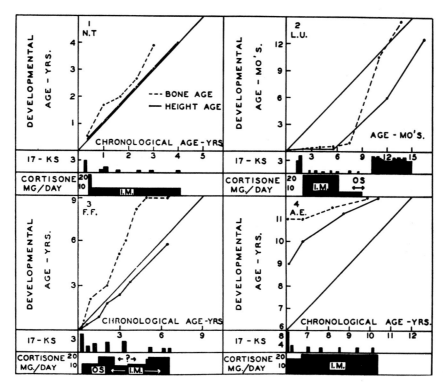

Fig. 97-10. *Rates of growth and osseous development as guides to optimal cortisone therapy.* Case 1: Satisfactory treatment. Normal growth and development. Case 2: Excessive treatment. Suppression of growth and development during the first 6 months. Case 3: Inadequate therapy. Excessive skeletal maturation. Case 4: Excessive osseous development was inhibited for 5 years, during which period growth proceeded at a normal rate. (From Wilkins, L., Postgrad. Med., *29:* 31, 1961.)

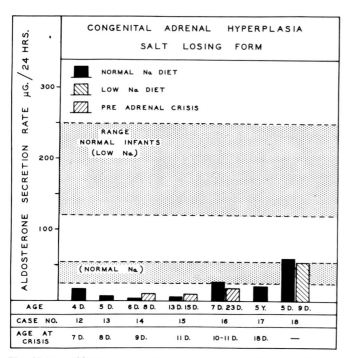

Fig. 97-11. *Aldosterone secretion rate in patients with the salt-losing form of congenital adrenal hyperplasia.* The 7 patients presented in this figure had no therapy and were receiving a normal sodium diet at the time of the study. A second study was carried out on patients 14, 15, and 16 just before an adrenal crisis and on patient 18 when on a low-sodium diet. The patients are arranged according to the severity of their salt-losing tendency as determined by their age at the time of the first spontaneous adrenal crisis; patient 18 did not go into crisis even when put on a low-sodium diet for 4 days. (From Kowarski A., Finkelstein, J. W., Spaulding, J. S., Holman, G. H., and Migeon, C. J., J. Clin. Invest. *44:* 1505, 1965.)

to an incorrect diagnosis of pyloric stenosis. If not treated, the features of the infant become pinched and sunken, and the skin assumes a dusky color. Cardiovascular collapse occurs, and in some cases, sudden cardiac arrest due to hyperkalemia is the cause of death. The low levels of serum sodium, chloride, and CO_2, along with the elevated potassium of the salt-losing form, contrast with the hypokalemic alkalosis characteristic of pyloric stenosis. In order to survive, the patients require administration of large amounts of NaCl and water. However, despite such treatment, dehydration persists, demonstrating the need for salt-retaining hormone. During the period of fluid and electrolyte therapy, a 24-hour urine collection should be initiated in order to demonstrate the increase in urinary 17-ketosteroids and pregnanetriol. The measurement of plasma 17-hydroxyprogesterone is also extremely useful in diagnosis.

The abnormalities of the external genitalia in girls attract the attention of the physician at birth. Male-appearing external genitalia, but with nonpalpable testes in the scrotum, should suggest the possibility of congenital adrenal hyperplasia and the need for buccal smear, chromosome analysis, and determination of urinary and plasma steroids. In infant boys, the lack of abnormality of the external genitalia makes the diagnosis more difficult. The history of neonatal death of previous siblings with a similar syndrome of dehydration should suggest the need for steroid determinations.

The tendency toward sodium loss appears to be less marked after the first 2 or 3 years of life, and a number of adult patients may even stop salt-retaining hormone therapy. However, the salt-losing tendency does not disappear, as the patient cannot adequately sustain a prolonged low-sodium diet. In some patients, the salt-losing tendency is discovered only later on in life. Such patients probably represent mild forms of the syndrome. They often have a normal aldosterone secretion rate but are unable to increase it adequately during low sodium diet.

Diagnostic Laboratory Tests

As mentioned above, the study of serum electrolytes will make the diagnosis of adrenal insufficiency. In addition, the increase in urinary 17-ketosteroids and pregnanetriol demonstrates the increased secretion of adrenal androgens and cortisol precursors. It is also possible to demonstrate a marked increase in plasma 17-hydroxyprogesterone and androstenedione.

A normal or low aldosterone secretion rate, combined with markedly elevated plasma renin activity, will further demonstrate the adrenal insufficiency. However, such assays are not practical at the early age at which the diagnosis must be made. Such comments also apply to the demonstration of very low plasma cortisol levels and markedly decreased cortisol secretion rate.

Treatment

The Acute Adrenal Crisis. It is usually possible to maintain the infant by salt and fluid replacement while the appropriate 24-hour urine specimen is collected for diagnostic purposes. In the presence of acute dehydration, the first hour of therapy will consist of 20 ml/kg of body weight of 0.9% NaCl in 5% glucose. However, this fluid therapy will not correct the acidosis and therefore the following mixture is preferable:

One third	⅙ m sodium lactate
Two thirds	0.85% sodium chloride
Addition of glucose to make a 5% solution	

At the end of the first hour, if the vital signs of the patient are satisfactory, the intravenous solution should be continued to deliver a total of 60 ml/kg over the next 24-hour period.

If at the end of the first hour the status of the infant and its blood chemistry have not improved, the administration of 1 mg IM desoxycorticosterone acetate is indicated. This steroid will not interfere with the measurement of urinary 17-ketosteroids or pregnanetriol. This type of regimen will usually be sufficient for satisfactory maintenance. In some cases, however, it is necessary to add glucocorticoid replacement given as IV hydrocortisone, 50 mg stat, and another 25 mg being placed in the intravenous solution. The 24-hour fluid requirement is from 80 to 120 ml/kg of body weight.

Sedatives such as morphine and barbiturates are contraindicated; potassium should not be added to the intravenous fluids. Sympathomimetic agents such as Levophed are rarely used in the neonatal period. There is also danger in administering too much intravenous fluid and/or NaCl along with large amounts of Doca, as it can result in pulmonary edema, cardiac failure, and hypernatremia. Hence, serum electrolytes, hematocrit, and body weight must be monitored carefully throughout the acute crisis.

Maintenance Therapy. Once the acute adrenal crisis is controlled, plans should be made for long-range maintenance. The need for replacement of mineralocorticoid (Fig. 97-12) is covered by a daily dose of 1 mg (sometimes 2 mg) of Doca im. Alternatively, 9α-fluorocortisol acetate (0.05–0.10 mg, orally, as a single daily dose) can be substituted for the im Doca. However, the therapy of choice is implantation of two 125-mg Doca pellets. These pellets are reabsorbed slowly and provide a constant level of mineralocorticoid activity. Following the initial implantation, there may be variable absorption. The patient may need 1 mg of Doca im on the day following implantation. Other patients may have rapid reabsorption with salt and water retention, which can best be handled by a low-sodium diet. Implants are usually reabsorbed in 9 to 10 months and can then be replaced. When the patient is 18 to 20 months of age, therapy is shifted to oral preparations. The implants are more practical than a daily im injection and safer than an oral preparation in an infant, who can easily regurgitate.

It is of interest to note that there is no need for adjustment of the replacement of mineralocorticoid therapy in relation to body size. This is probably related to the fact that the secretion rate of aldosterone in children after 2 weeks of age is not significantly different from that of older children and adults.[22]

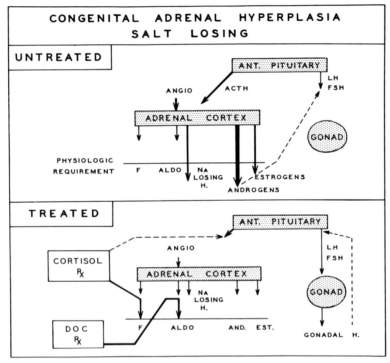

Fig. 97-12. Therapy in patients with the salt-losing form of congenital adrenal hyperplasia. Aldosterone replacement must be added to the cortisol treatment.

The maintenance therapy also includes glucocorticoid replacement (Fig. 97-12). This is carried out exactly as indicated for the simple virilizing form of the syndrome. All the various rules related to cortisol therapy also apply to the salt-losing patients.

HYPERTENSIVE FORM

Pathogenesis of Hypertension

In this form of the syndrome there is a defect of the 11-β-hydroxylase enzyme,[11,23] resulting in deficient cortisol secretion and leading to hypersecretion of ACTH. The ACTH causes excessive production of cortisol precursors, such as compound S (Fig. 97-13). The glucuronide conjugates of its tetrahydro derivatives are excreted in urine and measured as Porter-Silber chromogens. Therefore, an increased urinary excretion of 17-hydroxycorticosteroids is characteristic of this form of the syndrome. The secretion of 17-hydroxyprogesterone is also increased, although its elevation is usually not as great as in the simple virilizing form of CAH. In addition, the ACTH hypersecretion leads to increased desoxycorticosterone secretion, which is responsible for the hypertension. Its tetrahydro derivative can be determined in urinary specimens. Finally, there is hypersecretion of androgens, and therefore this form of the syndrome, like the simple virilizing form and salt-losing form, is characterized by masculinization and increased virilism.

Clinical Manifestations and Differential Diagnosis

This form of congenital adrenal hyperplasia is quite rare and represents not more than 3 percent of the total cases. The hypertension is usually moderate, although in a few patients the blood pressure may reach high levels. The hypertension is not permanent but disappears upon institution of cortisol therapy even though it may have existed for some time prior to treatment.

Female patients with this disorder show variable degrees of masculinization of the external genitalia at birth and have progressive virilization just as in the simple virilizing form. In male infants the external genitalia are normal; rapid somatic growth and early appearance of pubic hair attract attention and suggest the possibility of the syndrome.

As mentioned above, the hypertension is related to the hypersecretion of desoxycorticosterone. However, several patients without hypertension have been shown to have an 11-β-hydroxylase defect. It has been speculated that in such cases the enzymatic defect was partial and that the small amounts of desoxycorticosterone secreted were compensated by an appropriate decrease in aldosterone secretion.

A few patients have been described as having congenital adrenal hyperplasia with hypertension as well as sodium loss. It is probable that some of them were of the salt-losing type and had been overtreated with salt-retaining hormones.

In this form of congenital adrenal hyperplasia, differential diagnosis involves conditions causing virilism and hypertension. Suppression of the elevated urinary 17-ketosteroids and pregnanetriol during a dexamethasone suppression test is very helpful. In this test, suppression of elevated urinary 17-hydroxycorticosteroids (mainly tetrahydro derivatives of compound S) is pathognomonic. Characteristically, these patients also have low plasma renin activity and low aldosterone secretion rates.

Treatment

From what has been described of the pathogenesis of this form of adrenal hyperplasia, it is clear that glucocorticoid replace-

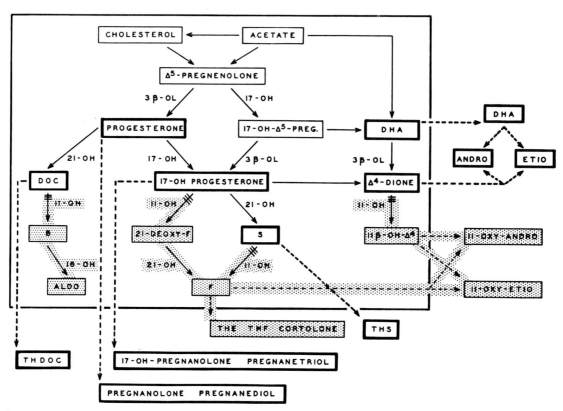

Fig. 97-13. Biosynthesis of adrenocortical steroids in patients with congenital adrenal hyperplasia due to 11-hydroxylase deficiency (hypertensive form). The metabolites found in increased amount in urine (outside the large rectangle) are THS, tetrahydrodeoxycorticosterone (THDOC), the derivatives of progesterone and 17α-hydroxyprogesterone, and the 11-deoxy-17-ketosteroids. (From Migeon, C. J. In R. E. Cooke (ed.), The Biological Basis of Pediatric Practice. Copyright 1968 by McGraw-Hill Book Company.)

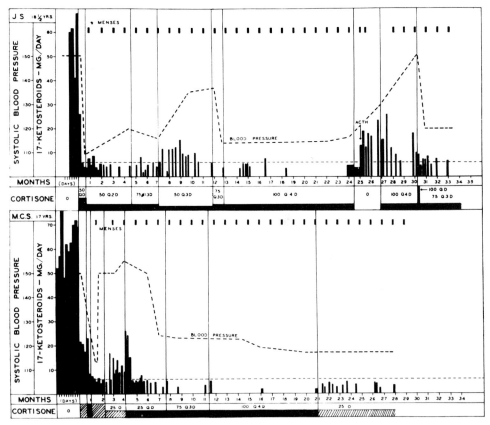

Fig. 97-14. Effect of cortisone therapy on the urinary 17-ketosteroids and the blood pressure in 2 sisters with female pseudohermaphrodism due to congenital adrenal hyperplasia. (From Wilkins, L., Crigler, J. F., Jr., Silverman, S. H., Gardner, L. I., and Migeon, C. J., J. Clin. Edocrinol. Metab. *12:* 1015, 1952.)

ment will correct the abnormal steroid secretion by suppressing the abnormal ACTH output.[24] The desoxycorticosterone secretion is brought back to normal, and hypertension disappears. Similarly, the increased secretion of androgens is suppressed (Fig. 97-14). It must be noted that treated patients who are submitted to a prolonged low-sodium diet may run into difficulty with sodium loss. Because of their enzymatic defect, they are unable to compensate by an increased aldosterone secretion, and because of the cortisol therapy, they are unable to increase their desoxycorticosterone output.[25]

DEFICIENCY OF (3β-HYDROXYSTEROID) DEHYDROGENASE

In 1961, Bongiovanni described 6 patients[46] with congenital adrenal hyperplasia whose main defect appeared to be in the transformation of 3β-hydroxy-Δ5-steroids to 3-keto-Δ1-steroid (Fig. 97-15). The steroids isolated from the urine of the patients included 16α-, 17-, and 21-hydroxylated 3β-hydroxy-Δ5-steroids. In vitro studies have confirmed the lack of 3β-hydroxysteroid dehydrogenase activity in the adrenals of such patients. This deficiency impairs the formation of both cortisol and aldosterone. In addition, the only androgen synthesized is dehydroisoandrosterone and its hydroxylated derivatives.

The 3 female patients reported by Bongiovanni had minimal hypertrophy of the clitoris and slight labial fusion, whereas the 3 male infants had incomplete masculinization of their external genitalia with perineal hypospadias. The 3β-hydroxy-Δ5-androgens have little histological activity, and only a very small fraction of dehydroisoandrosterone and its sulfate is transformed peripherally

to testosterone; this could account for the mild virilization of the external genitalia of the female that occurs during fetal life. Since masculinization of the external genitalia in the male is due to secretion of a testicular androgen in fetal life, it would appear that the testis of patients with the 3β-hydroxysteroid dehydrogenase deficiency present a similar defect.

In 5 patients there was a marked salt loss, and 4 died in early infancy. The only case without salt loss probably represented a partial defect, since tetrahydrocortisone was detected in urine.

Despite appropriate replacement therapy, most of these patients died in early infancy. It has been suggested that the enzyme deficiency of this form of the syndrome resulted in impaired liver function, which would cause the death of patients with complete deficiency.

CONGENITAL LIPOID HYPERPLASIA OF THE ADRENALS

Prader, Gurtner, and Siebenmann[12,13] described 2 patients with congenital lipoid hyperplasia of the adrenals and collected 5 other cases considered to have the same disorder. All 7 patients died before the eighth month of life with typical adrenal insufficiency. Prior to death, symptoms included weight loss, anorexia, vomiting, diarrhea, and marked skin pigmentation. The 17-ketosteroids and 17-hydroxycorticosteroids were low. Treatment with cortisone and Doca improved the patients, but they did not survive.

Of the 7 cases, 4 were males and 3 females, although in all patients the external genitalia appeared to be completely or almost completely female. In males, the testes were present in the abdo-

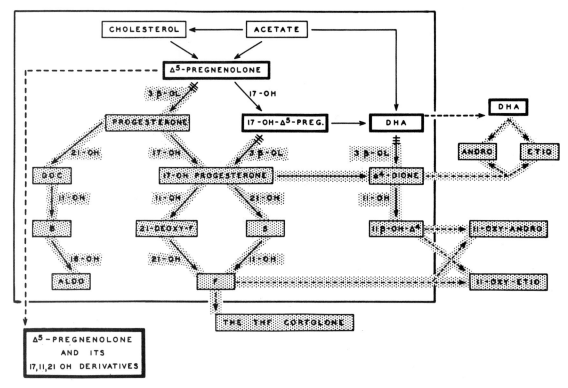

Fig. 97-15. Biosynthesis of adrenocorticosteroids in the form of CAH due to a deficiency of 3-β-hydroxysteroid dehydrogenase. In this form of the syndrome, aldosterone and cortisol secretions are decreased markedly and only Δ5-steroids are produced in large amounts. (From Migeon, C. J. In R. E. Cooke (ed.), The Biological Basis of Pediatric Practice. Copyright 1968 by McGraw-Hill Book Company).

men or in the inguinal canal. The adrenals were grossly hyperplastic, and the adrenal cells were filled with lipoid material. Little information is available concerning steroid biosynthesis in these patients. It has been suggested that there is a defect in one of the enzymes necessary for the formation of pregnenolone from cholesterol; it could involve either the 20-hydroxylase, or the 22-hydroxylase, or the 20,22-desmolase.

17-HYDROXYLASE DEFICIENCY

Clinical Manifestation and Abnormal Steroidogenesis

This disorder was first recognized by Biglieri et al.[14] and New et al.[27] A partial or complete deficiency of 17-hydroxylase results in a partial or complete inability to synthesize cortisol. As in the other forms of congenital adrenal hyperplasia, this results in a compensatory hypersecretion of ACTH. In the normal adrenal gland, desoxycorticosterone is secreted in very small amounts and is mainly the precursor of corticosterone (Fig. 97-16). However, there appear to be two separate metabolic pools of deoxycorticosterone in the adrenal, one in the zona glomerulosa, under the control of angiotensin, and another in the zona fasciculata-reticularis, under ACTH control. In the 17-hydroxylase deficiency, the desoxycorticosterone secretion controlled by ACTH is markedly increased, resulting in mild hypertension. At the same time, the increased corticosterone production compensates almost entirely for the decreased cortisol synthesis. As in 11-hydroxylase deficiency, the elevated blood desoxycorticosterone levels tend to decrease the formation of renin-angiotensin and hence decrease aldosterone secretion. Finally the 17-hydroxylation is a necessary step for the formation of steroids with 19 carbons. Therefore, in 17-hydroxylase deficiency the formation of adrenal androgens is impaired. Since androgens are the precursors of estrogens, this form

of the syndrome also results in impaired formation of estrogenic steroids. The same enzyme deficiency is present in the gonad, and patients with this form of the syndrome are unable to secrete gonadal hormones.

The clinical manifestations are directly related to the abnormal secretion of steroids. Although corticosterone does not have as much glucocorticoid activity as cortisol, its markedly increased secretion compensates adequately. On the other hand, corticosterone has a fair amount of mineralocorticoid activity. In combination with the increased desoxycorticosterone secretion, it results in hypertension and hypokalemia. It also explains the decreased secretion of aldosterone and low level of plasma renin activity.

An appropriate secretion of androgen by the fetal testes is necessary for the proper masculinization of the external genitalia of the male fetus. In 17-hydroxylase deficiency, as in the 3β-hydroxysteroid dehydrogenase deficiency and the deficiency of the enzymes prior to pregnenolone, male infants are born with external genitalia that might appear entirely female, the gonads being intra-abdominal or in the inguinal area. At puberty, in both male and female, there is no secretion of gonadal hormones and the patients remain entirely infantile.

Diagnosis

In males the diagnosis is made on the basis of the male pseudohermaphroditism, including negative buccal smear, XY sex chromosome complement, and external genitalia, which may appear completely female or partially masculinized. Laboratory tests indicate increased secretion of corticosterone with decreased cortisol secretion and show that the decreased aldosterone secretion has been compensated by an increased desoxycorticosterone output.

In females, the diagnosis is difficult early in life, since the genitalia appear entirely normal and since the clinical manifesta-

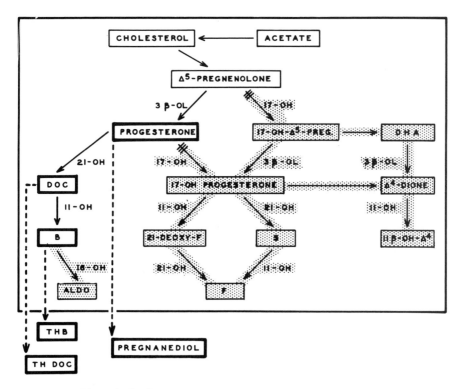

Fig. 97-16. Biosynthesis of adrenocorticoids in 17 hydroxylose deficiency.

tions will be those of hypertension and possibly hypokalemia. Later on in life the absence of sexual maturation at puberty makes one think of this type of enzymatic deficiency.

Treatment

Replacement therapy with cortisol suppresses the hypersecretion of ACTH. This, in turn, results in decreased secretion of corticosterone and desoxycorticosterone with return of the blood pressure to normal levels. At puberty, both males and females require replacement therapy with sex hormones. In the case of male patients, marked abnormality of the external genitalia may have resulted in those patients having been raised as females. Removal of the abdominal testes will be necessary to avoid the possibility of tumor formation. Such individuals require replacement therapy with female hormones.

GENETICS OF CONGENITAL ADRENAL
HYPERPLASIA

Congenital adrenal hyperplasia occurs frequently in siblings, but the parents show no evidence of endocrine dysfunction. Despite a few reports to the contrary, it appears that an affected sibship presents only one form of the disease and often with the same degree of severity. On the basis of this type of inheritance, Childs et al.[28] deduced that the syndrome is due to a non-sex-linked recessive mutant gene, which expresses itself clinically only in homozygous offspring. The detection of the syndrome in twins, first cousins, and half-sisters is in accordance with this mode of inheritance. Although the number of female patients tends to be greater than that of male subjects, the study of affected sibs shows that the apparent difference in frequency is probably due to the greater difficulty in recognizing the disorder in males. This statement, of course, applies only to the 21-hydroxylase and 11-hydroxylase deficiencies. In the other forms (3β-hydroxysteroid dehydro-

genase deficiency, deficiency of enzymes prior to pregnenolone, and 17-hydroxylase deficiency) the incomplete masculinization of the males would reverse the bias.

Childs et al.[27] reported that there was at least 1 affected child per 62,500 births, and the incidence of the gene in the general population was at least 1 per 128 individuals. Studies in Switzerland by Prader[29] reported an incidence of the disease of about 1 in 5000 births, with a gene frequency of about 1 in 35. These studies were related only to the 21-hydroxylase deficiency, whatever its degree, and therefore involved both the simple virilizing form and the salt-losing form. A more recent study in the midwestern United States[30] suggested a frequency of the gene of 1 in 50.

In the past, attempts to detect the heterozygote trait in the parents of patients by studying their response to ACTH or metapyrone were unsuccessful. Recently, an acute ACTH test was used (iv injection of 1 mg of synthetic 1-24 ACTH with blood collection 30 and 60 minutes after injection). Under such conditions, it is possible to demonstrate a greater increase in plasma levels of 17-hydroxyprogesterone in obligate heterozygotes than in individuals taken at random.

GENERAL EVOLUTION UNDER TREATMENT

Medical Treatment

The treatment is basically replacement therapy, cortisol being given in a dose corresponding to the secretion rate of this steroid and salt-retaining hormone being given as replacement for deficient aldosterone production. The major goals of long-range treatment include:

1. Correction of the salt-losing tendency (deficiencies in 21-hydroxylase, and 3β-hydroxysteroid dehydrogenase) and of the hypertension (deficiencies of 11β-hydroxylase and 17-hydroxylase),
2. Attainment of normal adult height,

3. Suppression of prepubertal virilism in both sexes,
4. Normal gonadal maturation and normal fertility in adults.

Correction of Salt-losing Tendency. The administration of salt-retaining hormone corrects the sodium loss. Such therapy is absolutely required in infancy and childhood. Later in life, the requirement seems to be less complete.

A normal adult (body surface area = 1.8 m²) secretes 22.5 mg of cortisol and 50 μg of aldosterone per 24 hours or salt-retaining equivalent of 2.125 mg of desoxycorticosterone (1 mg desoxycorticosterone = 20 mg cortisol = 50 μg aldosterone), while a newborn (surface area 0.2 m²) secretes 2.5 mg of cortisol and 50 μg of aldosterone or the equivalent of 1.125 mg of desoxycorticosterone. When patients receive only cortisol replacement, the percentage of salt-retaining replacement is 53 percent in the adult and 11 percent in the newborn. This might, in large part, explain this "improvement" of the salt-losing tendency with age. However, as mentioned previously, prolonged sodium restriction in an adult patient can result in a salt-losing crisis, and administration of Florinef should be maintained throughout life.

Correction of Hypertension. Cortisol therapy usually results in a prompt return of the blood pressure to normal in subjects with either 11β-hydroxylase or 17-α-hydroxylase deficiency. In a few instances, the blood pressure may remain elevated and normal levels are obtained only after a short period of low-sodium diet.

Adult Height. Since cortisol therapy started a quarter of a century ago, the number of patients who have reached adulthood and who have received treatment from birth is still small. In our experience,[31] 42 female patients treated prior to 1 year of age and who completed their linear growth had a mean ± 1 S.D. height of 158.2 ± 7.2 cm, approximating the 25th percentile curve for normal women. Girls who had started therapy between 1 and 6 years of age had a significantly lower height of 156.0 ± 5.2 cm, whereas 28 females not treated prior to bony fusion were even shorter, 150.9 ± 4.3 cm.[31] The data suggest that early and proper treatment will result in normal statural growth.

Suppression of Prepubertal Virilism. The age at the time of appearance of coarse, pigmented pubic hair in normal girls is 11.69 ± 1.21 years (mean ± 1 S.D.). In our experience, untreated girls showed conspicuous pubic hair at 4.01 ± 1.61 years, whereas girls who started treatment between 1 and 6 years and those who started before 1 year, had pubic hair at 8.19 ± 3.25 and 10.25 ± 2.05 years, respectively.[31]

Gonadal Maturation. The development of puberty is more easily followed in girls than in boys; hence the data available on gonadal maturation are mainly for females. Early "breast budding" occurs normally at 11.15 ± 1.05 years and was observed at a similar age in early and adequately treated patients. These same 34 patients, however, had their menarche at 13.77 ± 1.71 years[31] as compared to a normal age of 12.90 ± 1.70 years.[32]

In order to maintain regular menses, adrenal secretion must be well suppressed, menarchial girls having a mean urinary 17-ketosteroid excretion of 6 mg/24 hr. The prompt onset of menses in patients initially treated after the age of bony fusion suggests that in adolescents inadequately treated, menses should begin within 6 to 12 months of the initiation of adequate replacement therapy. However, patients untreated until 20 years of age often have anovulatory cycles, raising the concern that inadequate control during adolescence may impair future fertility.

With few exceptions, testicular maturation occurs only after cortisone therapy has been initiated. In adequately treated patients, puberty occurs at a fairly normal age. Boys who start treatment late in life show full testicular maturation shortly after beginning therapy if their bone age has reached 13 to 14 years.[33]

Isolated reports have demonstrated that women with treated CAH can conceive and carry a normal pregnancy. However, to date, no information is available on the fertility rate in CAH. The young age of the majority of patients on follow-up treatment prevents adequate evaluation. In our limited experience of 17 women exposed to unprotected intercourse, 10 became pregnant (60 percent fertility rate) for a total of 15 pregnancies. Two pregnancies were terminated by elective abortion, and 9 resulted in normal living infants. The 4 unsuccessful pregnancies were due to 3 spontaneous abortions and 1 child born with meningomyelocele.[31] Not enough information is available to determine the causes of infertility in the patients unable to conceive. However, the time required for conception (5.6 months) in those women able to conceive is well within the normal range, suggesting that there may be two groups of patients: one group with normal fertility and another unable to conceive. Whether the infertility is a result of chronic postnatal androgen exposure or merely androgen exposure during the period of attempted pregnancy is not clear.

In managing the pregnant patient, the prepregnant glucocorticoid dose was found adequate to maintain the pregnancy. This is consistent with the finding that the cortisol secretory rate does not change during normal pregnancy.[34]

Surgical Treatment

In females, it is advisable, for psychological reasons, to carry out surgical correction of the external genitalia between the ages of 1 and 3 years. Surgery should take place after the start of treatment and consist of incision of the fused labioscrotal folds. If the enlargement of the clitoris is conspicuous, the phallus will be extirpated almost completely in order to avoid painful erections of the stump.[35] This type of surgery leaves a small part of the corpora, which attaches to the pubis so that erotic feeling may remain.

The correction in cases of complete masculinization with penile urethra is more difficult. In a first stage the phallus is removed with partial opening of the scrotal folds. Later in life, further correction is needed to exteriorize the vaginal opening. In a few patients, constriction of the vaginal orifice may be a problem.

Prior to the use of cortisol, female patients with marked masculinization of the external genitalia, including the rare instances of penile urethra, were raised as males. Cortisone treatment in such patients at the time of puberty resulted in the development of female secondary sexual characteristics and the appearance of menses. Hysterectomy and ovariectomy had to be carried out prior to puberty. It was also necessary to administer testosterone, as would be done in agonadal males. At present, the true sex of these patients is determined early in life, and since they have perfectly female internal sexual organs, medical treatment will bring about normal feminization at puberty, while surgical correction will result in female external genitalia, despite some of the problems mentioned above.

Male patients present malformation of the external genitalia in cases of 3β-hydroxysteroid dehydrogenase deficiency and lipoid adrenal hyperplasia. Most subjects with these forms of the disease have died in early infancy despite medical treatment. In one instance of partial 3β-hydroxysteroid dehydrogenase deficiency with survival, there was enough masculinization of the external genitalia to permit a repair along masculine lines. The same problems are encountered in male patients with 17-hydroxylase deficiency.

Psychological Problems

In untreated children, psychological development is related to chronological age rather than to somatic development. For this reason, they may appear childish and awkward in relation to their physical appearance. Similarly, sexual behavior is related to chronological age rather than to physical development. Despite occurrence of erections, boys are usually not sexually delinquent. A minimal amount of psychological counseling for the patients and a good understanding of the situation by the parents will, in most cases, bring satisfactory results. Untreated adults, particularly females, on the other hand, often develop psychological problems and are sexually maladjusted. These problems may not be solved if therapy is started late. Sexual problems secondary to traumatic transmission of information concerning the defect at birth and the corrective surgery require counseling and long-term therapy by a person trained in psychoendocrinology.[36]

Compliance is always a problem when daily therapy is required for a lifetime. Indoctrination of the parents and progressive education of the patients are helpful. However, it is still difficult to reach a proper balance between the concept of the necessity of therapy and the problems that might arise from overemphasis of the fact that the patient is *different* from his or her contemporaries. A particularly difficult period is adolescence, when the usual conflicts or confrontations between parents and children may find their expression in neglect or refusal of therapy. Patients from families characterized by parental discord or absence are at particular risk for noncompliance. Such neglect might be particularly unfortunate in girls, as it might result in masculinization (facial hair, deepening of the voice) that will not regress even after resuming therapy and in delayed feminization (lack of breast development, menses). These somatic problems may have major repercussions on the overall psychology of the patients. In some girls, the appearance of symptoms of virilism can create a climate in which the patients become unsure of their gender identity. Incomplete surgical correction of the external genitalia may have similar effects. Salt-losing patients have used therapy withdrawal as a conscious suicidal threat. In both males and females, inadequate therapy during childhood results in short stature, which in itself brings about a certain set of problems. All these examples illustrate the importance of psychological guidance for these patients at various stages of their development.

Sexual behavior is not only influenced by the genetic sex but also by other factors, the most important being sex of rearing. Properly handled, female pseudohermaphrodites who have been raised as males have generally made an excellent adjustment. It has been shown that there are great psychological risks in changing the sex after the age of 2 to 4 years. However, in view of the complete feminization, including fertility, which can result from cortisone therapy, a change of sex can be considered even in late childhood. Such changes should be undertaken only after intensive psychological study of both the patient and his or her parents reveals that the gender identity has differentiated in such a way as to be flexible and ambiguous enough to tolerate the change. Then the prognosis may be favorable.

VIRILIZING ADRENAL TUMORS

These tumors are rare even though they are the most frequent type of adrenal tumors. The fact that the number of cases occur-

ring in women[37] is twice that reported in men probably is related to the fact that the clinical manifestations are more obvious in female subjects.

Virilizing tumors of the adrenals can develop at any period of life; a few have been reported to occur as early as the first year. However, there are no reports of tumors arising during fetal life and almost none occurring immediately after birth. This is of help in differentiating them from congenital adrenal hyperplasia.

CLINICAL MANIFESTATIONS

In *prepubertal* girls, the appearance of pubic hair is often the first sign. Clitoral enlargement also may attract attention initially. However, in contrast to patients with CAH, those with virilizing tumors have no labial fusion. Usually no breast development takes place, and menses do not appear at the usual pubertal age.

Virilizing adrenal tumor in the *prepubertal boy* produces macrogenitosomia praecox and hirsutism without testicular maturation (Fig. 97-17). The penis and prostate can be enlarged to adult size, and pubic and axillary hair are present. In almost all patients,

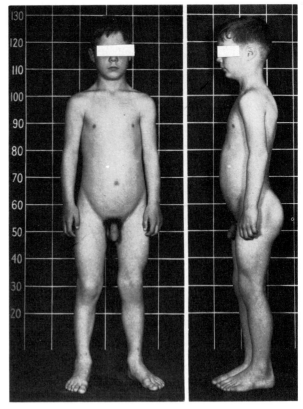

Fig. 97-17. Virilizing adrenal tumor in a boy. Age, 4¾ years; height age, 8 years; bone age, 12 years; 17-KS (mg/24 hr), 106-504 (more than 90 percent as DHA).

Case History: At 3 years of age, enlargement of the penis was noted; a few months later, pubic hair and acne appeared. Intravenous pyelogram showed a mass depressing the left kidney. During the following year, rapid growth and virilization continued as the voice became deeper and axillary hair appeared. Administration of cortisone (100 mg/day for 8 days) had no effect on urinary excretion of 17-KS and DHA (Gardner, L. I., and Migeon, C. J. Helv. Pediatr. Acta 6: 465, 1951; J. CLIN. Endocrinol. Metab. 9: 1117, 1952). There was also some increase in urinary excretion of estrogens (Migeon, C. J. J. Clin. Endocrinol. Metab. 13; 3674, 1953). At 4¾ years of age, an adrenal tumor, 7 cm in diameter, was removed. A thick capsule was present; cells were of uniform appearance, but a few large and multinucleated cells also were seen. Patient is in excellent health 18 years after surgery.

the testes remain small and immature, contrasting with the obvious signs of virilism. This lack of testicular development is similar to that seen in CAH but is in contrast to the gonadal maturation found in isosexual precocious puberty of idiopathic origin. However, it must be noted that in a few patients with virilizing adrenal tumor, the testes were larger than expected for the age.

In both girls and boys, muscles are extremely well developed, and there is rapid statural growth with marked advance in osseous maturation. This results in early closure of the epiphyses, and the patient does not achieve full growth. The mental age is usually at the level of the chronologic age.

In *adult women,* these tumors usually occur between 30 and 40 years of age, but they can also arise after menopause. In most cases, hirsutism is the first clinical sign. Coarse, dark hair appears on legs, arms, chest, and back, with an increase in pubic hair extending up to the umbilicus. Facial hair also appears, while there is often thinning of scalp hair and bitemporal regression of the hairline. The skin becomes oily with acne. Menstrual disorders are constant. Oligomenorrhea appears first and can be followed by amenorrhea. Clitoral hypertrophy is frequent, and there is often hypertrophy and hyperpigmentation of the labia majora. Muscular hypertrophy with loss of characteristic female fat deposits may give the body a masculine appearance, and the voice may also become masculine. Atrophy of the breasts and the uterus may be observed. In most cases, there is a marked increase in libido. On rare occasions, hirsutism is the only manifestation of the tumor, and there is no disturbance of menstruation. It is of interest that a few patients have become pregnant.

In the *adult male,* virilism does not attract attention. In all cases of virilizing tumors, the tumor has been discovered by chance, an excessive excretion of androgen confirming the diagnosis.

HORMONAL ABNORMALITIES

In almost all patients the *total neutral 17-ketosteroids* (17-KS) in urine are greatly elevated (Table 97-3), but it must be remembered that there can be variability of levels from day to day. The elevation of the urinary 17-KS is due in great part to a marked *increase of dehydroepiandrosterone* (DHA); this steroid repre-

sents 50 percent or more of the total urinary 17-KS. DHA is excreted mostly as the ester sulfate. In addition, 7- and 16α-hydroxy derivatives of DHA are also excreted in large amounts. Among 21-carbon steroids, great quantities of compounds with a 5-6 double bond (pregnenolone, 17-hydroxypregnenolone, and their derivatives) are found in urinary extracts.

The *plasma concentration of DHA sulfate* in virilizing adrenal tumor can be extremely elevated, reaching values of 1–3 mg/100 ml of plasma. Unconjugated DHA also is found in increased concentrations. However, the concentration of unconjugated DHA is 1000 times less than that of its sulfate. The study of the simultaneous concentrations of androgens in peripheral and adrenal vein plasma has permitted the conclusion that DHA and its sulfates are secreted by adrenal tumors (Fig. 97-18).

In contrast with CAH, virilizing adrenal tumors show *no suppression of plasma androgens* or urinary 17-KS during a dexamethasone suppression test.[8] Furthermore, ACTH administration has no effect on the steroid output of the tumor, demonstrating that tumoral secretion is not ACTH-dependent. The large secretion of sulfate conjugates could be related to a decreased cholesterolesterase activity. It must also be noted that patients with virilizing tumors and normal subjects metabolize DHA differently, a much larger amount of DHA-sulfate being excreted in the urine of the patients.

In patients with virilizing adrenal tumors the urinary excretion of cortisol metabolites is normal despite the marked increase in DHA sulfate. In rare cases, a slight elevation of urinary 17-OHCS has been reported; this increase is due mainly to the tetrahydro derivatives of compound S.

Patients with virilizing adrenal tumors have never shown any abnormality of serum electrolytes, and aldosterone secretion has been reported to be normal in the few cases in which it was determined.

PATHOLOGY

When tumors are examined macroscopically, it often is hard to decide whether one is dealing with a carcinoma or an adenoma. Furthermore, the clinical evolution does not always parallel the pathologic appearance of the tumor. Adrenocortical carcinomas tend to be larger and to have greater vascularization. In advanced cases, malignancy is evidenced by local invasion of the kidney or by metastasis to the lung, liver, or other organs. The tumors are often heterogeneous, presenting areas of cystic formation, hemorrhage, necrosis, and sometimes calcification.

The microscopic appearance of the cells of the tumor rarely resembles that of the normal cells of the adrenal cortex. The signs of malignancy to look for are those characteristic of most carcinomas. In practice, however, it is often difficult to distinguish between an adenoma and a malignant tumor.

DIAGNOSIS

The diagnosis of virilizing adrenal tumors is made on clinical signs and symptoms along with markedly increased urinary 17-KS (50 percent or more DHA) which does not suppress during dexamethasone administration.

The tumor is rarely palpable, but often one can find a kidney pushed downward by the adrenal adenoma or carcinoma. The tumor often may be visualized by radiologic examination, particularly when combined with retroperitoneal CO_2 insufflation and/or intravenous pyelogram. Tumors can also arise in ectopic adrenal tissue; in one instance, the adrenocarcinoma was located in the liver of a 3-year-old boy.

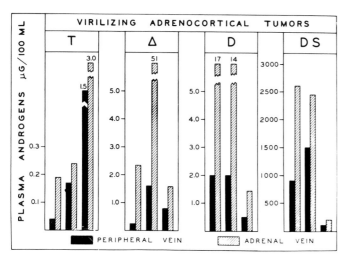

Fig. 97-18. Plasma androgens in virilizing adrenocortical tumors. In the 3 patients, the concentrations of testosterone (T), androstenedione (Δ), dehydroisoandrosterone (D), and its sulfate (DS) were greater in adrenal vein blood than in peripheral vein blood. (From Lipsett, M. B., Migeon, C. J., Kirschner, M. A., Bardin, C. A., Ann. Intern. Med. *68:* 1327, 1968.)

In the differential diagnosis, virilization due to androgens of either adrenal or gonadal origin must be considered.

In young girls with congenital adrenal hyperplasia, the labial fusion characteristic of the masculinization of the external genitalia will contrast with the absence of fusion in adrenal tumors. In boys, virilism due to CAH may not become evident until some time after birth and in some instances not until the age of 3 or 4 years. In both, the great excess of urinary pregnanetriol and 17-KS, which return to normal levels during a dexamethasone suppression test, help in making this diagnosis.

Certain ovarian tumors (arrhenoblastoma, hilus cell tumors, adrenal-rest tumors) can produce virilizing symptoms. These tumors are usually observed after puberty, at which time a careful gynecologic examination will reveal their presence. The urinary 17-KS are usually moderately increased.

In boys, a *Leydig cell tumor* of the testis may produce symptoms of masculinization. The testicular tumor and the small size of the contralateral testis will help in making the diagnosis. Urinary 17-KS can be quite elevated and are not suppressed during a dexamethasone test.

A few *hepatomas* have been observed to produce large amounts of gonadotropins, which in turn activate testicular function; this results in virilization of a prepubertal boy, but few symptoms will be found after puberty. An enlarged liver and high gonadotropin titers are characteristic of this condition. Such hepatomas are highly malignant.

Idiopathic sexual precocity in boys is due to an early maturation of the hypothalamus-pituitary. The finding of serum gonadotropins and steroid excretion, which are normal for a pubertal child, is in contrast to the low gonadotropins and elevated steroid excretion of virilizing adrenal tumors.

Premature pubarche in boys or girls will also be easily diagnosed on the basis of low gonadotropins, low plasma androgens (except for an increase in DHA-sulfate toward adult levels), and low urinary steroid excretion.

In *Cushing's syndrome,* especially when due to an adrenal carcinoma, the excretion of urinary 17-KS can be markedly elevated. In the late stage of development of such tumors, DHA may constitute a large proportion of the androgens. Neither the 17-KS nor the urinary DHA is suppressed in the dexamethasone suppression test. In such patients, the clinical symptoms of increased cortisol secretion along with the increased excretion of urinary 17-OHCS will help in the differentiation from purely virilizing adrenal tumors.

TREATMENT

The tumor should be excised carefully without cutting the capsule. When metastases are present, efforts should be made to remove them as completely as possible, since this may prolong the patient's life. When metastases are widespread and cannot be removed surgically, radiotherapy and chemotherapy should be used. There is no consensus as to the effectiveness of radiotherapy, but since adrenal tumors with metastases are extremely malignant, it seems justified to use x-ray. Chemotherapy (aminoglutethimide, o,p'-DDD) can also be attempted.

Virilizing adrenal tumors do not produce excessive amounts of cortisol, and for this reason the contralateral gland secretes cortisol normally. While it seems unnecessary to administer glucocorticoids prior to, during, and after ablation of such tumors, it is probably safer to give it. Adrenal carcinomas producing Cushing's syndrome have a great tendency to recur and metastasize, but tumors producing pure virilism generally grow more slowly, have less tendency to recur, and often have a very good prognosis. After surgery, patients should be checked frequently by thorough clinical examination and steroid determinations. A reappearance of symptoms or increased urinary 17-KS will suggest local recurrence.

FEMINIZING ADRENAL TUMORS

These tumors are very rare; not more than a dozen cases have been reported in children and only about 50 cases in adult males. It is of interest that no case has been reported in an adult female, probably because an increase in feminization could not be recognized.

CLINICAL MANIFESTATIONS

Most feminizing tumors occur in *adult males* between 25 and 45 years of age, although several patients between 50 and 60 years of age have been reported.[38] The frequency of certain symptoms is shown in Table 97-8. Gynecomastia was a constant early symptom in most cases. Many patients experience painful tension in the breast prior to development of gynecomastia, which is usually bilateral but sometimes is more pronounced on one side. In some cases, pigmentation of the areola and superficial venous dilatation occur, and a few patients have secretion from the nipple. Atrophy of the testes occurs in more than half of the patients, but usually the prostate and the penis remain of normal size. A decrease or total loss of libido and potency is also observed in half the patients. Oligospermia has been reported in several cases. In most subjects, pubic hair remains unchanged, but in a few patients it is decreased, with formation of a female escutcheon. Rare manifestations include diffuse pigmentation and arterial hypertension.

In boys, gynecomastia is also an early symptom. In addition, there is rapid growth: height age and bone age are markedly advanced. The penis and testes are of normal size for the age of the patient, while pubic hair may or may not be present.

Feminizing tumors *in girls* result in manifestations similar to those found in isosexual precocious puberty; these include enlargement of the breast, appearance of pubic hair, estrogenization of the labia minora and of the vaginal smear, vaginal bleeding, and advanced bone age and height age (Fig. 97-19). In some patients, a concomitant increase in androgen secretion can also result in slight enlargement of the clitoris as well as increased muscular development.

Table 97-8. Incidence of Signs and Symptoms of Feminizing Tumors in the Male (52 Patients)

Sign or Symptom	Percent
Gynecomastia	98
Palpable tumor	58
Atrophy of testis	52
Diminished libido and/or potency	48
Pain at site of tumor	44
Tenderness of breast	42
Pigmentation of areolae	27
Obesity	27
Feminizing hair change	23
Atrophy of the penis	20
Elevation of the blood pressure	16
Increasing skin pigmentation	12
Varicocele	11
Acne	8

From J. L. Gabrilove, D. C. Sharma, H. H. Wotiz, and R. I. Dorfman, Medicine 44: 37, 1965.

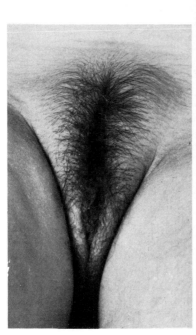
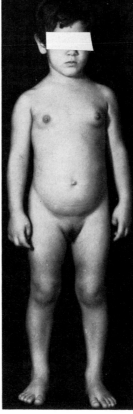
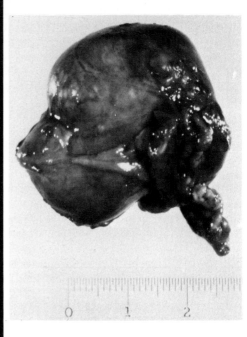

Fig. 97-19. Feminizing and masculinizing adrenal tumor in a girl. Labia and vagina are feminized. Pubic hair is present, but there is no clitoral enlargement. There is an encapsulated right adrenal tumor. Age, 3¼ yr; height age, 4 yr; bone age, 6 yr; 17-KS (mg/24 hr), 21-38.
Case History: At 3 years of age, the patient began to feminize with increased vaginal secretion and development of breasts and labia minora. Two months later, there was vaginal bleeding and growth of pubic hair. In addition to the manifestations of feminization, patient also had marked muscular development and a great deal of muscular strength.
Urinary 17-KS were elevated and consisted primarily of DHA. Urinary estrogens were also elevated for age of patient. Neither urinary 17-KS nor estrogens were changed during a suppression test.
Right adrenal tumor was not palpable but was revealed following presacral CO_2 insufflation. Following surgical removal of tumor, 17-KS dropped to 0.7 mg/24 hr, the pubic hair decreased markedly, and only a small amount of breast tissue remained. Patient has been well for over 10 years following surgery. (From Wilkins, L. The Diagnosis and Treatment of Endocrine Disorders in Childhood and Adolescence, 3rd ed. Springfield, Ill., Charles C. Thomas, 1965.)

HORMONAL ABNORMALITIES

Estrogens

Whether determined by bioassay or chemical technique, urinary estrogens are elevated in all patients as compared to norms for age and sex. However, in most patients the proportions of estrone, estradiol, and estriol are similar to those found in adult women.

Androgens

Although the main characteristic of feminizing adrenal tumors is an increase in estrogen production, there is also, in most patients, an increase in androgen secretion. In some patients, DHA represents more than 50 percent of the total 17-KS excreted. Furthermore, there is no decrease of urinary 17-KS or DHA during a dexamethasone suppression test.

Steroids with 21-carbons

In feminizing adrenal tumors, the urinary excretion of 17-OHCS is normal, as is aldosterone secretion. However, a few adult patients had increased urinary 17-OHCS along with symptoms of Cushing's syndrome, including impaired glucose tolerance, truncal

obesity, and hypertension. Although in most patients the urinary excretion of pregnanetriol is normal, there can be a moderate elevation in pregnanediol excretion.

PATHOLOGY

The feminizing tumors can be either an adenoma or a carcinoma. Their general appearance and histology is similar to that of the virilizing tumors. The testes of some patients have demonstrated atrophy of the seminiferous tubules and a decreased number of Leydig cells. These changes are probably due to the high level of circulating estrogen.

DIAGNOSIS

Feminizing adrenal tumors are large enough to be palpated in more than 50 percent of patients and sometimes are so large that compression of abdominal organs is evident. In general, adenomas are smaller than carcinomas, but in either case the tumors are easily detected by radiological examination. Calcification of the tumor has been observed.

The differential diagnosis of feminizing adenal tumors in adult males is easy. *Testicular tumors* have been reported to produce feminizing symptoms, but these are rare and the presence of an enlarged testis helps make the diagnosis. The gynecomastia of *Klinefelter's syndrome* will also easily be differentiated from that of an adrenal tumor by study of the sex chromatin and chromosomes and the increase of urinary gonadotropins. Gynecomastia may appear following *administration of certain drugs* (reserpine, meprobamate, digitalis). It can occur in patients with *malnutrition or liver disease,* but these disorders usually can be diagnosed easily. It also has been reported to occasionally occur in patients with *diabetes or thyrotoxicosis;* again, the clinical manifestations of these endocrinopathies usually are obvious.

In prepubertal boys, the differential diagnosis is mainly that of gynecomastia. *Transient gynecomastia* of moderate degree often occurs physiologically at the time of puberty. Since puberty is accompanied by a certain increase in excretion of urinary 17-KS and sometimes urinary estrogens, the differentiation from feminizing tumors which present with only moderately increased steroid excretion can be very difficult. In contrast to boys undergoing pubertal development, whether at the proper age or precociously, patients with feminizing adrenal tumors have no testicular enlargement. A normal suppression of urinary 17-KS during a suppression test also helps to rule out an adrenal tumor. Gynecomastia may appear following inadvertent *ingestion of estrogen-containing products.* A diligent search for a history of ingestion of such compounds will help in making this differential diagnosis.

The diagnosis of feminizing adrenal tumors can be difficult in prepubertal girls. The finding of increased urinary estrogen excretion along with increased urinary excretion of 17-KS and DHA, which does not respond to a dexamethasone suppression test, is the key to the diagnosis. *Premature thelarche* (early breast development without menstruation or pubic hair) and *idiopathic isosexual precocity* must be ruled out. The fact that these two conditions occur much more frequently than feminizing adrenal tumors should not result in failure to recognize a tumor. Elevated excretion of 17-KS and low levels of gonadotropins favor the presence of an adrenal tumor, while normal pubertal excretion of 17-KS with an elevation of LH levels, as observed at the time of adolescence, suggests idiopathic sexual precocity. In premature thelarche, both 17-KS and LH levels are low.

The lack of cases of feminizing adrenal tumors in females is probably the result of their diagnosis as Cushing's syndrome when the urinary 17-hydroxycorticosteroids are elevated, as virilizing adrenal tumors with low androgenicity if the 17-ketosteroids are increased, or as nonfunctioning tumors if there is little or no change in steroid excretion.

TREATMENT

The tumor should be removed as soon as the diagnosis is established. Pure feminizing tumors, like virilizing adrenal tumors, do not significantly alter cortisol secretion; however, it is safer to protect the patient from acute adrenal crisis by glucocorticoid administration during surgery. Of 52 cases of feminizing tumors in adult males, 41 were carcinomas, 7 were adenomas, and in 4 it could not be determined whether the tumor was malignant or benign.[38] It would seem that the rare tumors occurring in children are less malignant than those observed in adults, since most patients have survived surgery more than 5 years. Following surgery, gynecomastia regresses and libido usually returns to normal, as does spermatogenesis. Unfortunately, in most cases, metastases appear in a short time with or without a return of urinary steroids to the preoperative levels. Death often occurs within 1 year of surgery. In instances of adenoma, cures have been obtained.

REFERENCES

1. DeCrecchio, L. Sopra un caso di apparenze virili in una donna. *Il Morgagni 7:* 151, 1865.
2. Apert, E. Dystrophies en relation avec des lésions des capsules surrénales. *Bull. Soc. Pediatr. Paris 12:* 501, 1910.
3. Gallais, A. Le Syndrome Adréno-génital. Thèse, Paris,1912.
4. Cushing, H. Basophil adenomas of the pituitary body. *Bull Hopkins Hosp. 50:* 137, 1932.
5. Albright, F. Cushing's syndrome. *Harvey Lect. 38:* 123, 1942–43.
6. Wilkins, L., Lewis, R. A., Klein, R., and Rosemberg, E. The suppression of androgen excretion by cortisone in a case of congenital adrenal hyperplasia. *Bul. Hopkins Hosp. 86:* 249, 1950.
7. Bartter, F. C., Albright, F., Forbes, A. P., Leaf, A., Dempsey, E., and Carroll, E. Effects of adrenocorticotropic hormone and cortisone in adrenogenital syndrome associated with congenital adrenal hyperplasia: Attempt to explain and correct its disordered hormonal pattern. *J. Clin. Invest. 30:* 237, 1951.
8. Gardner, L. I., and Migeon, C. J. Le diagnostic des tumeurs virilisantes du cortex surrénalien: Effet de la cortisone sur les stéroides urinaires et utilisation d'une méthode colorimetrique pour le dosage de la dehydroisoandrosterone. *Helv. Paediatr. Acta 6:* 465, 1951.
9. Bongiovanni, A. M. Detection of pregnanediol and pregnanetriol in urine of patients with adrenal hyperplasia: Suppression with cortisone preliminary report. *Bull. Hopkins Hosp. 92:* 244, 1953.
10. Bongiovanni, A. M., and Root, A. W. The adrenogenital syndrome. *N. Engl. J. Med. 268:* 1283, 1342, 1391, 1963.
11. Eberlein, W. R., and Bongiovanni, A. M. Congenital adrenal hyperplasia with hypertension: An unusual steroid pattern in blood and urine. *J. Clin. Endocrinol. Metab. 15:* 1531, 1955.
12. Prader, A., and Gurtner, H. P. Das syndrom des pseudohermaphroditismus masculinus bei kongenitalennebennierenrinden-hyperplasie ohne androgenuberproduktion (adrenaler pseudohermaphroditismus masculinus). *Helv. Paediatr. Acta 10:* 397, 1955.
13. Prader, A., and Siebenmann, R E. Nebenniereninsuffizienz bei kongenitalenlipoidhyperplasie der nebennieren. *Helv. Paediatr. Acta 12:* 569, 1957.
14. Biglieri, E. G., Herron, M. A., and Brust, N. 17-hydroxylation deficiency in man. *J. Clin. Invest 45:* 1946, 1966.
15. Iversen,T. Congenital adrenocortical hyperplasia with disturbed electrolyte regulation. *Pediatrics 16:* 875, 1955.
16. Wilkins, L., Lewis, R. A., Klein, R., Gardner, L., Crigler, J. F., Rosemberg, E., and Migeon, C. J. Treatment of congenital adrenal hyperplasia with cortisone. *J. Clin. Endocrinol. Metab. 11:* 1, 1951.
17. Kenny, F. M., Preeyasombat, C., and Migeon, C. J. Cortisol production rate II Normal infants, children and adults. *Pediatrics 37:* 34, 1966.
18. Eberlein, W. R., and Bongiovanni, A. M. Steroid metabolism in "salt losing" form of congenital adrenal hyperplasia. *J. Clin. Invest. 37:* 889, 1958.
19. Migeon, C. J., and Kenny, F. M. Cortisol production rate V Congenital virilizing adrenal hyperplasia. *J. Pediatr. 69:* 779, 1966.
20. Phillips, J. Four cases of spurious hermaphrodism in one family. *Trans. Obstet. Soc. Lond. 28:* 158, 1887.
21. Fibiger, J. Beitrage zur kenntmis des weiblichen schweinzwitterkums. *Virchows Arch. [Pathol. Anat.] 181:* 1, 1905.
22. Weldon, V. V., Kowarski, A., and Migeon, C. J. Aldosterone secretion rates in normal subjects from infancy to adulthood. *Pediatrics 39:* 713, 1967.
23. Green, O. C., Migeon, C. J., and Wilkins, L. Urinary steroids in hypertensive form of congenital adrenal hyperplasia. *J. Clin. Endocrinol. Metab. 20:* 929, 1960.
24. Wilkins, L., Gardner, L. I., Crigler, J. F., Jr., Silverman, S. H., and Migeon, C. J. The control of hypertension with cortisone, with a discussion of variations in the type of congenital adrenal hyperplasia and report of a case with probable defect of carbohydrate regulating hormones. *J.Clin. Endocrinol. Metab. 12:* 1015, 1952.
25. Kowarski, A., Russell, A., and Migeon, C. J. Aldosterone secretion rate in the hypertensive form of congenital adrenal hyperplasia. *J. Clin. Endocrinol. Metab. 28:* 1445, 1968.
26. Bongiovanni, A. M. Adrenogenital syndrome with deficiency of 3β-hydroxysteroid dehydrogenase. *J. Clin. Invest. 41:* 2086, 1962.
27. New, M. I. Male pseudohermaphroditism due to 17α-hydroxylase deficiency. *J. Clin. Invest. 49:* 1930, 1970.
28. Childs, B., Grumbach, M. M., and Van Wyk, J. J. Virilizing adrenal

hyperplasia: A genetic and hormonal study. *J. Clin. Invest. 35:* 213, 1956.

29. Prader, A. Die haufigkeit der kongenitalen adrenogenitalen syndroms. *Helv. Paediatr. Acta 13:* 426, 1958.

30. Rosenbloom, A. L., and Smith, D. W. Congenital adrenal hyperplasia. *Lancet,* March 19, 1966, p. 660.

31. Klingensmith, G. J., Garcia, S. C., Jones, H. W., Jr., Migeon, C. J., and Blizzard, R. M. Twenty-five years experience with glucocorticoid treatment in girls with congenital adrenal hyperplasia. In Treatment of Congenital Adrenal Hyperplasia: A Quarter of a Century Later. P. A. Lee, L. P. Plotnick, A. A. Kowarski, and C. J. Migeon, Eds. Baltimore, University Park Press, 1976.

32. Root, A. W. Endocrinology of puberty. I. Normal sexual maturation. *J. Pediatr. 83:* 1, 1973.

33. Wilkins, L., and Cara, J. Further studies on the treatment of congeni-tal adrenal hyperplasia with cortisone. V. Effects of cortisone therapy on testicular development. *J. Clin. Endocrinol. Metab. 14:* 287, 1954.

34. Migeon, C. J., Kenny, F. M., and Taylor, F. H. Cortisol production rate: VIII. Pregnancy. *J. Clin. Endocrinol. Metab. 28:* 661, 1968.

35. Jones, H. W., Jr., and Scott, W. W. Hermaphroditism, Genital Anomalies and Related Endocrine Disorders. Baltimore, Williams and Wilks-ins Co., 1971, p. 197.

36. Money, J. Psychologic counseling: Hermaphroditism. In Endocrine and Genetic Diseases of Childhood and Adolescence, 2nd ed. L. I. Gardner, Ed. Philadelphia, W. B. Saunders, 1975, p. 609.

37. Overzier, C. Pseudohermaphroditism in Intersexuality. New York, Academic Press, 1963, p. 235.

38. Gabrilove, J. L., Sharma, D. C., Wotiz, H. H., and Dorfman, R. I. Feminizing adrenocortical tumors in the male: A review of 52 cases including a case report. *Medicine 44:* 37, 1965.

98

Diagnosis and Treatment of Hyperaldosteronism and Hypoaldosteronism

James C. Melby

SECONDARY ALDOSTERONISM (HYPERRENINEMIC HYPERALDOSTERONISM)

WITHOUT HYPERTENSION:

Secondary aldosteronism is the term used to describe excessive production of aldosterone by the cells of the adrenal glomerulosa activated by stimuli outside of the adrenal. With the exception of a single entity, the rare syndrome of glucocorticoid suppressible aldosteronism, secondary aldosteronism results from excessive prolonged stimulation by angiotensin II. In general, secondary aldosteronism is characterized by raised plasma renin activity (PRA), plasma angiotensin II levels, and plasma aldosterone concentrations. Aldosterone hypersecretion is appropriate for the degree of activation of the renin-angiotensin system. The heightened activity of the renin-angiotensin system in secondary aldosteronism is most often secondary to events reducing effective blood volume and extracellular fluid volume with increasingly negative sodium balance. Secondary aldosteronism must be viewed as a physiologic counterregulatory response to these events, although the manifestations of aldosterone overproduction are predominant. Disorders associated with secondary aldosteronism appear in Table 98-1.

Secondary aldosteronism is a concomitant of sodium depletion in pregnancy in healthy humans. With sodium depletion, there has been demonstrated both increased circulating levels of angiotensin II and increased adrenocortical sensitivity to angiotensin II in terms of aldosterone secretion.[1] During normal pregnancy, there is an increase in both PRA and aldosterone secretion. The latter reaches a maximum in the last trimester, attaining its peak just before delivery. The increased secretion of aldosterone is from 5- to 15-fold over the nonpregnant state. In pregnancy, increased renin secretion results in part from negative sodium balance accompanied by elevated levels of plasma renin substrate induced by raised estrogen levels. Thus, PRA and angiotensin II production are greater than would be anticipated in the nonpregnant condition.[2]

In pathological states, secondary aldosteronism leads to varying degrees of potassium depletion and, when edema is present, positive sodium balance. When healthy subjects are deprived of dietary sodium, potassium depletion does not ensue, since potassium excretion in tubular urine is dependent upon active sodium reabsorption. In pregnancy, progesterone is produced in abundance sufficient to compete with aldosterone for binding to its specific receptor protein in the cytoplasm of the renal tubular collecting duct epithelial cells. It is possible that the enormous overproduction of progesterone in the last trimester of pregnancy may have a primary role in the development of sodium depletion.

Edematous States and Secondary Aldosteronism (Hyperreninemic Hyperaldosteronism)

Nephrotic Syndrome. The fundamental abnormality in the nephrotic syndrome is an increased permeability of renal glomeruli to protein with loss of albumin in urine greater than 4 g/24 hr. Eventually, plasma albumin concentrations and oncotic pressure

Table 98-1. Classification of Hyperaldosteronism

I. Hyperaldosteronism associated with elevated plasma renin activity
   (Hyperreninemic or secondary hyperaldosteronism)
   A. Without hypertension
      1. Edematous states
         a. Nephrotic syndrome
         b. Hepatic cirrhosis with ascites
         c. Localized edema
         d. Idiopathic edema
         e. Congestive cardiac failure
      2. Nonedematous states
         a. Salt-losing nephritis
         b. Bartter's syndrome
         c. Renal tubular acidosis
   B. With hypertension
      1. Primary hyperreninism
         a. Juxtaglomerular cell tumor
         b. Wilms' tumor
      2. Secondary hyperreninism
         a. Accelerated hypertension
         b. Essential hypertension (10%)
         c. Hypertension treated with diuretics
         d. Oral contraceptive induced hypertension
         e. Pregnancy
II. Hyperaldosteronism associated with suppressed plasma renin activity (hyporeninemic or primary hyperaldosteronism)
   A. Aldosterone-producing adenoma (primary aldosteronism, Conn's syndrome)
   B. Idiopathic hyperaldosteronism—bilateral micronodular and/or macronodular adrenocortical hyperplasia
   C. Aldosterone-producing adrenocortical carcinoma
   D. Glucocorticoid-suppressible aldosteronism
   E. Congenital aldosteronism
   F. Facilitative hyperaldosteronism (? 16-α, 18-dihydroxy-11-deoxy-corticosterone excess)

may fall, with movement of extracellular fluid from the intravascular compartment to the interstitial space. The reduction of effective extracellular fluid volume (intravascular volume) activates the renin-angiotensin system and adrenal secretion of aldosterone. The nephrotic syndrome was first recognized as exhibiting hyperaldosteronism by J. A. Luetscher, who in 1954, discovered a sodium-retaining factor in the urine of children with this disorder.

Hepatic Cirrhosis with Ascites. The sequence of events in cirrhosis with ascites resembles that in nephrotic syndrome. The combination of increased portal pressure in the abdominal vasculature and diminished plasma oncotic pressure because of reduced albumin synthesis leads to edema with retranslocation of fluid to the abdomen. Because of the extravascular trapping of fluid and electrolytes in the ascitic compartment, there is reduced intravascular or effective extracellular fluid volume, which, when sensed by the kidney, leads to the hypersecretion of renin and production of angiotensin II and aldosterone. Aldosterone induces a marked positive sodium balance with further expansion of the ascitic compartment and eventual formation of anasarca. A clinically significant potassium depletion often occurs. Diuretic induced saliuresis in the treatment of this disorder often results in dangerous hypokalemia with worsening of the secondary aldosteronism. This response may be obviated by the concomitant administration of competitive antagonists of aldosterone.

Localized Edema. Dependent edema attributed to lymphatic or vascular obstruction provides the same milieu for the induction of secondary aldosteronism as does cirrhosis with ascites. Fluid moves into a local area, and ultimately the intravascular or effective extracellular fluid volume contracts.

Idiopathic Edema. Dependent edema developing in persons who are otherwise well is termed "idiopathic." It is observed primarily in premenopausal women and may be cyclic with fluctuations of body weight from 5 to 20 lbs, within 24- to 48-hour periods. Approximately 50 percent of these patients exhibit hyperreninemic hyperaldosteronism.[4] In these patients, secondary aldosteronism results from the abnormal loss of plasma volume when in the erect posture. This translocation of effective extracellular fluid volume (intravascular volume) sets the counterregulatory response of the renin-angiotensin-aldosterone system in motion.

Congestive Cardiac Failure. Congestive heart failure begins with the inefficient performance of the heart as a pump, so that cardiac output diminishes and systemic arterial vessels are inadequately filled. Volume receptors in the kidneys respond by retaining fluid, which enters the venous circulation. Persistence of increased venous blood volume is not transmitted to the arteries, and consequently, effective extracellular fluid volume (intra-arterial volume) remains low with continuing renal sodium and water retention. In those patients in whom there exists reduced intra-arterial blood volume or effective extracellular fluid volume, activation of the renin-angiotensin-aldosterone system occurs and promotes additional edema formation. However, PRA, plasma aldosterone concentrations, and aldosterone secretory activity are not increased in the majority of patients with untreated congestive heart failure.[5,6] Less than one third of patients with congestive cardiac failure exhibit secondary aldosteronism. It has been suggested that increased aldosterone secretion may not occur in congestive heart failure because the metabolic clearance rate of aldosterone is low; hence, plasma aldosterone levels would rise without an increase in secretion rate.[7] In most patients, reduction of the metabolic clearance rate of aldosterone is modest (10 to 20 percent) and markedly so (50 percent) in only a few seriously ill patients. Administration of massive doses of spironolactone to patients with untreated congestive heart failure has little effect on continued edema formation and renal sodium excretion in most instances.[8] Thus aldosterone does not consistently play a primary role in the production or maintenance of cardiac edema. Renal sodium retention in congestive cardiac failure can usually be adequately accounted for by nonaldosterone mechanisms, since increased proximal sodium reabsorption, which is independent of influence of aldosterone, appears to be the principal site of renal sodium retention.

Nonedematous, Nonhypertensive States
with Secondary Aldosteronism
(Hyperreninemic Hyperaldosteronism)

Salt-losing Nephritis. In chronic renal insufficiency, a transient or permanent salt-losing phase may develop in which sodium is lost in urine by osmotic diuresis through the reduced nephron population. Progressive sodium depletion and intense activity of the renin-angiotensin-aldosterone system is observed. In a significant proportion of patients, aldosterone action is limited because of destruction of a large population of the collecting ducts and distal tubules. Thus the effective extracellular fluid volume can only be restored by the administration of sodium.

Bartter's Syndrome. This syndrome was first described in children with proportional dwarfism, mental retardation, normal blood pressure, and hypokalemic alkalosis. These individuals have hyperplasia and hypertrophy of the juxtaglomerular apparatus in the kidney and marked hyperaldosteronism.[9] Patients do not respond to the pressor effects of infused angiotensin II, and increased plasma renin activity, angiotensin II levels, and plasma aldosterone concentrations have been regularly observed in these patients in all age groups, with and without dwarfism. Intravascular volume expansion restores pressor sensitivity to infused angiotensin. The lack of pressor sensitivity to infusions of angiotensin II observed in this syndrome does not differ from that observed in hyperreninemic hyperaldosteronism associated with severe sodium depletion and/or diminished intravascular volume. Renal sodium wastage has been thought to be the primary event in this syndrome, whereas renal potassium wastage has been completely ascribed to the severe hyperreninemic hyperaldosteronism.

Prostaglandins appear to be the mediators of renin release in Bartter's syndrome, and it is likely that negative sodium balance for any reason provokes increased prostaglandin discharge by the kidney.[9] Indomethacin and other potent inhibitors of prostaglandin synthetase are effective forms of therapy for this condition, especially in conjunction with potassium-sparing agents such as dyrenium or spironolactone.

Secondary aldosteronism probably does not account for a substantial portion of renal potassium wastage because chemical inhibition of aldosterone biogenesis, suppression of renin secretion by beta-adrenergic block (propranolol), neutralization of aldosterone activity by massive doses of aldosterone antagonists (spironolactone), and most convincingly, bilateral total adrenalectomy do not completely prevent renal potassium wastage. It has been suggested that the renal abnormality in Bartter's syndrome resides in the ascending loop of Henle and is due primarily to defective chloride transport, a situation that can be exactly mimicked by the prolonged administration of loop diuretics.[10] Increasingly, patients are observed who are chronic diuretic abusers, ingesting loop diuretics surreptitiously for rapid reduction in weight. The manifestations observed in these patients are indistinguishable from those of patients with Bartter's syndrome and can only be distinguished by screening for diuretics in urine.

Renal Tubular Acidosis. Renal tubular acidosis, whether due to impaired proximal tubular reabsorption of bicarbonate or to distal tubular failure of acidification of urine, is associated with renal sodium and potassium wastage. Potassium excretion in urine is determined in part by the same mechanism governing sodium loss and also by sodium depletion-induced hyperreninemic hyperaldosteronism.[11] Renal tubular acidosis is readily distinguishable from Bartter's syndrome in that patients with the former exhibit a metabolic acidosis, in contrast to the metabolic alkalosis regularly noted in Bartter's syndrome.

WITH HYPERTENSION:

When secondary aldosteronism accompanies certain hypertensive disorders in which volume contraction and negative sodium balance coexist, renin hypersecretion is reactive or secondary. On the other hand, the increased synthesis and release of renin by renin-producing tumors is primary and unresponsive to alterations in either extracellular fluid volume or sodium balance. Hypertension precipitated by administration of estrogen-containing oral contraceptives is frequently hyperreninemic, though not necessarily renin-dependent. Hyperreninemia is more often not as severe and manifestations of secondary aldosteronism not as intense as those observed in the nonhypertensive conditions with

secondary aldosteronism described above. It is estimated that in over 15 percent of the adult hypertensive population elevated plasma renin activity and hyperaldosteronism can be demonstrated. A majority of these patients have moderately severe or accelerated hypertension, the level of which is determined more by elevated peripheral arteriolar resistance than by any other determinant of blood pressure. Using a specific competitive antagonist to the vascular action of angiotensin II, Saralasin acetate (P-113) or Sar 1, ala[8] angiotensin II, it has been demonstrated that hypertensive patients with hyperreninemia respond with a significant reduction in blood pressure during angiotensin II blockade.[12]

Renin-producing Renal Tumors (Primary Reninism)

Renin hypersecretion, hypertension, and secondary aldosteronism have been demonstrated in patients with renal tumors, including juxtaglomerular cell and Wilms' tumors, and clear cell carcinoma of the kidney.[13] Fewer than 20 cases of renin-secreting tumors have been reported. Hypertension observed is due to the pressor effects of the angiotensin produced. Hyperaldosteronism is secondary and is responsible for the hypokalemic alkalosis, but aldosterone plays no major role in the development or perpetuation of hypertension. Hypertension and hyperaldosteronism disappear following nephrectomy. Hypertension is a common accompaniment of nephroblastoma (Wilms' tumor). Relief of the hypertension is obtained with nephrectomy in these patients.[14]

Severe, Accelerated, and Malignant Hypertension:

Progressive, severe hypertension, especially when characterized by hypertensive retinopathy and renal disease, is frequently associated with hyperproduction of renin and secondary aldosteronism. Renin hypersecretion is most often related to development of a necrotizing arteriolitis in the kidney.[15] Malignant hyperreninemic hypertension may supervene in any of the hypertensive disorders and may complicate renovascular disease. In renovascular disease, elevated peripheral plasma renin activity is not ordinarily observed unless the hypertension is accelerated. Intensive antihypertensive therapy can reverse the process of accelerated hypertension and renal ischemia and cause disappearance of hyperreninemia and hyperaldosteronism.

Diuretic Therapy or Hypertension Associated with Hyperreninemia and Secondary Aldosteronism:

Secondary aldosteronism associated with hypertension is most commonly observed in patients receiving thiazide diuretics. Assessment of the function of the renin-angiotensin-aldosterone system in hypertension should not be made unless diuretic agents have been discontinued for several weeks (3 or more) prior to testing.

Hypertension Induced by Estrogen-containing Oral Contraceptives

A small but significant number of women have become hypertensive while taking estrogen-containing oral contraceptives. Women who are already hypertensive experience an aggravation of hypertensive disease while receiving estrogens. Modest increments in systolic pressure are observed in practically all women on oral contraceptives, whereas 5 to 20 percent become frankly hypertensive. The estrogen moiety of the oral contraceptive stimulates hepatic synthesis of renin substrate. Plasma renin activity rises concurrently with increased plasma renin substrate, while renin secretion and renin concentrations are unchanged.[16] Correlation between plasma renin activity increments and appearance of hypertension is poor. The incidence of secondary aldosteronism is relatively low because of the modest increments in plasma renin activity. Whether or not oral contraceptive-induced hypertension is renin-dependent cannot be established with certainty. The oral contraceptive-induced hypertensive diathesis is frequently reversible on cessation of the use of the estrogen-containing preparation.

PRIMARY ALDOSTERONISM (HYPORENINEMIC HYPERALDOSTERONISM)

INTRODUCTION AND PATHOPHYSIOLOGY:

Aldosterone overproduction results in hypertension, potassium depletion, and suppression of plasma renin activity. Primary aldosteronism may be due to an aldosterone-producing solitary adenoma (Conn's syndrome), bilateral micronodular or macronodular hyperplasia of the adrenal cortex (idiopathic hyperaldosteronism), aldosterone-producing adrenocortical carcinoma, congenital aldosteronism (bilateral adrenocortical hyperplasia), and glucocorticoid remediable hyperaldosteronism (bilateral hyperplasia). Hypersecretion of aldosterone is autonomous or semiautonomous in primary aldosteronism except in patients with glucocorticoid remediable hyperaldosteronism. The clinical syndrome of primary aldosteronism results from the fundamental action of aldosterone on the kidney. Aldosterone stimulates active sodium transport by the distal convoluted tubule and collecting duct cells. With enhanced sodium reabsorption, there occurs a reciprocal movement of potassium and hydrogen ions into the tubular urine, leading to greater or lesser degrees of potassium depletion. Increased sodium reabsorption by the kidney leads to expansion of extracellular fluid volume and elevated total body sodium content. In man, expansion of the extracellular fluid volume and intravascular volume, induced by aldosterone or other mineralocorticoids, usually exceeds 2 liters and may expand by 4 liters. Expansion of the extracellular fluid volume is limited, however, by the renal counterregulatory mechanism of inhibition of proximal tubular sodium reabsorption. This phenomenon has been referred to as mineralocorticoid "escape."[17] Expansion of intravascular blood volume leads to the development of volume-dependent hypertension. Patients with primary aldosteronism exhibit hypervolemia, increased extracellular fluid volume, increased exchangeable sodium, and high cardiac output.[18] Hypervolemia, increased extracellular fluid volume, and exchangeable sodium directly suppress juxtaglomerular cell activity in the kidneys with resultant low PRA. Primary aldosteronism is a generic term for disorders in which chronic aldosterone excess is independent of the renin-angiotensin system and results in volume-dependent hypertension. Estimates of the incidence of primary aldosteronism vary from 0.5 to 2.0 percent of the hypertensive population with a prevalence of 115,000 to 460,000 cases in the United States at present.

CLINICAL FEATURES OF PRIMARY ALDOSTERONISM:

The peak age distribution for diagnosis is between the third and fifth decades, with more women affected than men by a ratio of 3:1. All the complications of severe long-standing hypertension have been observed in patients with primary aldosteronism. More than half of the patients have a persistent frontal headache, and there is no feature of hypertension that is distinctive. By and large,

the most obvious clinical manifestations of primary aldosteronism have been due to prolonged excessive renal potassium wastage. Spontaneous hypokalemia is observed in 80 percent of patients with primary aldosteronism. There are 20 percent of cases who have persistently normal serum potassium levels.[19] A substantial portion of patients with spontaneous hypokalemia admit to no symptoms, however. Nocturnal polyuria and polydipsia are common signs of the deficiency, and neuromuscular manifestations including weakness, paresthesias, intermittent paralysis, visual disturbances, and frank tetany may wax and wane with variations in potassium balance. Sodium restriction leads to potassium retention and improves hypokalemic manifestations. Demonstrably abnormal glucose-tolerance tests (in over half of the patients associated with insulinopenia) are due to potassium deficiency. Marked sensitivity to the thiazides, in terms of the production of hypokalemia, may be associated with the appearance of cardiac irregularity, paralyses, and tetany. Acute precipitation of potassium depletion by thiazide diuretics in the routine treatment of a hypertensive patient should immediately suggest the possibility of primary aldosteronism.

FORMS OF PRIMARY ALDOSTERONISM:

Solitary Aldosterone-producing Adenoma (Conn's Syndrome)

The most common adrenal lesion responsible for the syndrome of primary aldosteronism is a solitary adrenocortical adenoma, the first form of primary aldosteronism described.[20] It is estimated that between 60 and 70 percent of patients with the disorder have solitary aldosterone-producing adenomas. In general, the biochemical manifestations of Conn's syndrome are more pronounced than in other forms of primary aldosteronism. When the diagnosis of primary aldosteronism is made by the demonstration of inappropriately raised blood aldosterone concentrations in the presence of low or hyporesponsive plasma renin activity after acute induction of negative sodium balance, the adrenal lesion must be identified and, if unilateral, localized. It is important to distinguish between bilateral and unilateral adrenal disease because of the different therapeutic modalities. Unilateral adrenalectomy for the removal of a solitary adenoma results in the disappearance of hypertension for 1 or more years in 70 percent and permanently in half of the patients. Bilateral total adrenalectomy for micronodular or macronodular hyperplasia of the adrenals (idiopathic hyperaldosteronism) results in disappearance of hypertension in only one third of the patients so treated. Maneuvers to distinguish between bilateral and unilateral disease will be discussed under the section on Diagnosis. In Conn's syndrome, aldosterone biogenesis by the adenoma appears to be semiautonomous in that plasma aldosterone concentrations exhibit a circadian rhythm paralleling plasma cortisol and ACTH levels, whereas in idiopathic hyperaldosteronism, perturbations in plasma aldosterone concentrations are ACTH-independent.[21] In patients with adrenal nodular hyperplasia, plasma aldosterone levels rise during erect posture, presumably as a result of slight increments in plasma renin activity. In Conn's syndrome, postural change is without effect on plasma aldosterone.

Bilateral Macronodular and/or Micronodular Adrenocortical Hyperplasia (Idiopathic Hyperaldosteronism)

In this form of primary aldosteronism both adrenals are involved with diffuse micronodular or macronodular changes in the presence of hyperplasia of the zona glomerulosa. Nodules and hyperplastic tissue secrete excessive amounts of aldosterone, with resultant arterial hypertension, potassium depletion, and suppression of plasma renin activity.[22] Of patients with the syndrome of primary aldosteronism, between 15 and 30 percent have idiopathic hyperaldosteronism. Biochemical abnormalities of primary aldosteronism may not be as pronounced in these patients as in those with Conn's syndrome. The degree of hypokalemia may be less severe and suppression of plasma renin activity incomplete. Activation of aldosterone biogenesis by small increments in plasma renin activity is observed in these patients when they stand after prolonged recumbency, and no parallelism can be demonstrated between plasma aldosterone and cortisol concentrations.

Aldosterone-producing Adrenocortical Carcinoma

Adrenocortical carcinoma is a rare cause of primary aldosteronism. No more than 12 cases have been reported. The incidence in a large series was about 1 percent of patients with primary aldosteronism. Tumors are often large and are easily identifiable by excretory urography. Occasionally, other adrenocortical steroids are secreted by the tumor.[23]

Congenital or Juvenile Aldosteronism

Primary aldosteronism in the young is rare. It is usually associated with bilateral adrenal glomerulosa hyperplasia[24] and may have a familial occurrence.

Glucocorticoid-Remediable Hyperaldosteronism

This rare form of primary aldosteronism is associated with bilateral micronodular adrenocortical hyperplasia and is characterized by relief of hypertension and induction of positive potassium balance by the administration of glucocorticoids.[25,26] Dexamethasone-responsive hyperaldosteronism apparently is due to small but measurable increments in plasma ACTH levels without concomitant excessive cortisol secretion. Management involves long-term suppression of ACTH by the administration of small doses of dexamethasone or other long-acting glucocorticoids.

DIAGNOSIS

Primary aldosteronism should be suspected in the hypertensive patient who has had episodic or persistent spontaneous hypokalemia, who has become hypokalemic shortly after the initiation of thiazide or "loop" diuretic therapy, or who has become hypokalemic after ingestion of large amounts of sodium chloride. The salt-loading maneuver may be used as a provocative test for aldosteronism in hypertensive patients with persistently normal serum potassium levels. It has long been known that in primary aldosteronism, sodium loading intensifies potassium depletion and that sodium deprivation permits potassium repletion. When aldosterone secretion is suppressed by salt ingestion in healthy subjects, the distal tubular stimulus to sodium reabsorption is quickly dissipated, whereas patients with autonomous aldosterone secretion exhibit continued distal tubular sodium reabsorptive activity in response to a marked increase in the filtered sodium load. Ingestion of sodium in excess of 200 mEq/day (nine 1-g sodium chloride tablets per day) for 4 days does not influence the serum potassium in normal subjects or in hypertensive subjects who do not have aldosteronism. By contrast, hypertensive patients with aldosteronism on high-sodium intake for the same period exhibit a reduction of serum potassium to below 3.5 mEq/liter. Hypokalemia induced by sodium loading is strong indirect evidence for sustained excessive secretion of aldosterone.

Confirmation of Diagnosis

Diagnosis of primary aldosteronism rests on the demonstration of increased aldosterone secretion or plasma aldosterone concentration in the presence of low or hyporesponsive plasma renin activity.[27] The most simple and rewarding method for diagnosis is to obtain blood specimens simultaneously for plasma aldosterone concentration and plasma renin activity after maximal stimulation by acute volume depletion. The results of this maneuver are shown in Figure 98-1. The patient is given 80 mg of furosemide by mouth, and 3 hours later, specimens for plasma renin activity and plasma aldosterone are obtained. The patient is asked to remain upright during the test. Inappropriate elevation of plasma aldosterone for the level of suppressed renin activity is diagnostic for this syndrome. This test should be performed in patients ingesting normal amounts of sodium in their diet (100 ± 30 mEq/day) and in whom diuretic therapy has been discontinued for 3 weeks and other antihypertensive medications eliminated for 1 week. More cumbersome, but just as reliable, is the measurement of the 18-monoglucuronide of aldosterone excreted in urine over 24 hours or measurement of the secretion rate of aldosterone by the isotope dilution method.

Nonaldosterone Mineralocorticoid Suppression of Aldosterone Secretion

Administration of deoxycorticosterone acetate, 10 mg q 12 hours, or 400 μg of 9-α-fluorocortisol acetate for 3 days suppresses plasma aldosterone concentrations and urinary aldosterone metabolite excretion in patients with secondary aldosteronism but does not significantly reduce plasma aldosterone or aldosterone secretion in patients with primary aldosteronism.[28] Occasionally, patients with idiopathic hyperaldosteronism exhibit suppression of aldosterone secretion by exogenous mineralocorticoids, and in patients with aldosterone-producing adenoma, a significant suppression is rarely observed. If the finding of suppressed or hyporesponsive plasma renin activity in the presence of an inappropriately elevated plasma level of aldosterone or aldosterone secretion rate was unequivocal, there is no need to perform the suppression test. A suppression test may be used when ambiguity exists in the interpretation of the relationship of aldosterone secretion or plasma aldosterone to plasma renin activity.

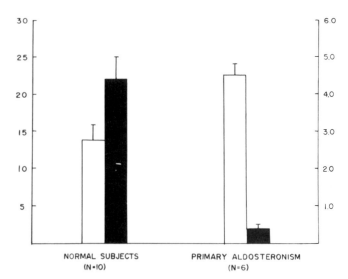

Fig. 98-1. Peripheral plasma aldosterone (ng/100 ml—open bars) and plasma renin activity (ng/ml/hr—solid bars) 3 hours after upright position—furosemide (80 mg PO) stimulation in normal subjects and patients with primary aldosteronism. Standard error of mean is indicated above bars.

HYPOTENSIVE RESPONSE TO SPIRONOLACTONE

Since overproduction of aldosterone is the proximate cause of hypertension in primary aldosteronism, neutralization of the action of aldosterone with spironolactone will completely relieve the hypertension in this disorder.[29] Spironolactone is a specific competitive antagonist of aldosterone. The molar concentrations required for inhibition of aldosterone activity, both in vivo and in vitro, range from 100 : 1 to 1000 : 1 (spironolactone to aldosterone). Administration of spironolactone in large doses (400 mg) for a protracted period (3 weeks) to patients with hypersecretion of aldosterone and hypertension reduces the blood pressure significantly in patients with primary aldosteronism. It does not affect the blood pressure in patients with secondary aldosteronism or in those in which hypertension is unresponsive to surgical removal of the adrenal. Significant reduction in blood pressure by spironolactone was observed in 90 percent of patients with primary aldosteronism in none of the hypertensive patients with secondary aldosteronism, and in 20 percent of patients with essential hypertension and normal aldosterone secretion.[30] Spironolactone nonresponders with primary aldosteronism are not relieved of hypertension by surgical management. The hypertensive response to spironolactone in primary aldosteronism is stereotyped. A weight loss of between 2 and 4 kg occurs within the first 7 to 10 days of therapy. Blood pressure declines slowly thereafter for the next 10 days. Spironolactone response test has prognostic rather than diagnostic importance.

Distinction Between Unilateral and Bilateral Adrenal Disease and Localization of Unilateral Aldosterone-producing Adenomas

Behavior of Aldosterone. Specimens of blood for aldosterone measurement should be obtained at 8:00 in the morning and again at 12:00 noon in patients who are up and about. Plasma aldosterone levels in Conn's syndrome are lower at 12:00 noon than at 8:00 A.M., and in idiopathic aldosteronism, they may be slightly above the 8:00 A.M. measurement.

Adrenal Venous Aldosterone Levels. Adrenal angiography, together with measurement of aldosterone in the adrenal venous effluent from both adrenals, obtained by percutaneous adrenal vein catheterization reliably distinguishes solitary aldosterone-producing adenoma from the bilateral involvement of idiopathic aldosteronism.[31,32] The accuracy of this procedure approaches 95 percent for unilateral and 90 percent for bilateral lesions. Radiographic appearance of the adrenals in primary aldosteronism is less accurate than adrenal venous aldosterone measurement, and recent uniform success in entering the right adrenal vein obviates extensive radiography and, particularly, adrenal venography. The complication of venography is intra-adrenal hemorrage resulting from rupture of the central venous system by contrast medium and is clinically significant in 10 percent of patients. Adrenal venous sampling for aldosterone measurement is carried out without venography and does not result in rupture of the corticomedullary system and hemorrhage. In idiopathic aldosteronism, concentrations of aldosterone in the venous effluent vary from 20 to 50 percent between the two adrenals. In Conn's syndrome, concentration of aldosterone in the adrenal venous effluent from the tumor-bearing gland is 20 to 50 times that in the venous effluent of the contralateral gland.

Adrenal Imaging with Radio-Iodocholesterol

Adrenal scintigraphy utilizing [131]I-29-iodocholesterol is a non-invasive and painless technique in which scintiscans are performed following the intravenous administration of 2 mCi of [131]I-19-iodocholesterol.[33] In this procedure, dexamethasone suppression of ACTH secretion is carried out concurrently with scintigraphy to differentiate adrenocortical hyperplasia (idiopathic aldosteronism) from Conn's syndrome (aldosterone-producing adenoma). The asymmetrical uptake between the two adrenals during suppression scintiscans is obvious at 5 days after the tracer is injected in patients with solitary aldosterone-producing adenomas. No lateralization of uptake is observed in patients with bilateral micronodular or macronodular hyperplasia. Correct identification of the nature of the adrenal lesion and its localization, when unilateral, is achieved in 80 percent of patients with adrenal scintigraphy. An even more useful agent, which appears to be superior to [131]I-19-iodocholesterol, is [131]I-6β-iodomethyl-19-norcholesterol (NP-59), which accumulates in the adrenals much more rapidly so as to permit diagnostic scintigraphy within 1 day of its administration.[34] NP-59 markedly intensifies imaging, while at the same time reducing radioactivity as background. It is likely that adrenal imaging with [131]I-6β-iodomethyl-19-norcholesterol will supplant adrenal vein catheterization for diagnosis and localization in a majority of patients with primary aldosteronism. Adrenal venous aldosterone measurements could then be obtained only when the results of scintigraphy were ambiguous.

MANAGEMENT OF PRIMARY ALDOSTERONISM

Aldosterone-producing Adenoma (Conn's Syndrome)

Unilateral adrenalectomy for an aldosterone-producing adenoma that has been identified and localized preoperatively results in significant lowering of blood pressure in all cases and remission of hypertension for years in 70 percent of cases. Fifty percent of patients are cured of hypertension. Preoperative preparation with spironolactone restores body potassium content and reactivates the renin-angiotensin-aldosterone system. This regimen is required because of the long suppression of the renin-angiotensin-aldosterone system. Postoperative, hypoaldosteronism is manifested by weakness, hyponatremia, and modest hyperkalemia. Its occurrence is markedly reduced by the preoperative preparation with spironolactone.

Idiopathic Hyperaldosteronism (Bilateral Micronodular and Macronodular Hyperplasia)

Bilateral total adrenalectomy for idiopathic hyperaldosteronism results in reduction of blood pressure in most patients. However, 68 percent remain hypertensive. Lifelong antihypertensive medication is required by a majority of patients after bilateral total adrenalectomy in addition to replacement for adrenal hypofunction. The hypertension of idiopathic hyperaldosteronism should be treated medically if antihypertensive drugs are effective. Spironolactone therapy is effective, especially in combination with other antihypertensive agents. The doses of spironolactone required may be substantial in order to maintain potassium balance and control of blood pressure. When spironolactone is administered in high doses for a prolonged period, it neutralizes the activity of secreted aldosterone, inhibits aldosterone biosynthesis, and diminishes the aldosterone secretion rate.[35] Because of the triple effect of this antialdosterone agent, it is possible to reduce its dosage, sometimes progressively, in patients receiving spironolactone for years. Spironolactone also possesses antiandrogenic properties that limit its application in the prolonged treatment of males with primary aldosteronism. Impotence and gynecomastia are frequently observed in patients receiving more than 100 mg of spironolactone per day for periods exceeding 3 months.

Other Forms of Primary Aldosteronism

Management of primary aldosteronism resulting from adrenocortical carcinomas involves surgical excision of the tumor and spironolactone therapy for persistent hypertension and potassium depletion when associated with functioning metastases. Limited experience with subtotal adrenalectomy for the treatment of congenital or juvenile hyperaldosteronism supports the efficacy of this approach.[24] Glucocorticoid-remediable hyperaldosteronism is dexamethasone-responsive and is best managed with this agent in a dose of 0.75 mg nightly.

NONALDOSTERONE MINERALOCORTICOID-HYPERTENSIVE SYNDROMES

PSEUDOMINERALOCORTICOID-HYPERTENSIVE SYNDROME

Glycyrrhizic Acid Derivative Ingestion

The ingestion of enormous quantities of licorice extracts which contain the ammonium salt of glycyrrhizic acid, may result in development of arterial hypertension, potassium depletion, and suppression of plasma renin activity indistinguishable from aldosterone excess. Glycyrrhizic acid stimulates distal tubule sodium reabsorption and reciprocal loss of potassium into tubular urine, similar to the activity of aldosterone. Licorice-induced hypertension and hypokalemic alkalosis was described before the isolation and identification of aldosterone.[36] Aldosterone secretion, plasma aldosterone levels, and aldosterone metabolite excretion in urine are negligible. The disappearance of this syndrome is complete within a few weeks after stopping licorice ingestion, which must exceed a pound a day to produce the syndrome in the first place. Spironolactone will promptly reverse the features of this syndrome.

A closely related substance, carbonoxolone sodium, which is a derivative of glycyrrhetinic acid, is prescribed for the treatment of peptic ulcer in the United Kingdom and may produce pseudoaldosteronism, arterial hypertension, and potassium depletion in the same manner as excessive ingestion of licorice.[37] Suppression of plasma renin activity and aldosterone secretion are also observed in this syndrome.

Inappropriate Excessive Renal Sodium Conservation (Liddle's Syndrome)

In this familial disorder, there is inappropriate and excessive renal tubular reabsorption of sodium with consequent development of hypertension, potassium depletion, plasma renin activity suppression, and inhibition of aldosterone secretion.[38]

DEOXYCORTICOSTERONE (DOC) EXCESS

Administration of deoxycorticosterone acetate (Doca) to laboratory animals and to man induces sodium retention, hypertension, and potassium loss in urine. In man, hypersecretion of DOC is apparently associated with the development of hypertension in certain inborn errors of cortisol biosyntheis distal to 21-hydroxylation, such as 17-α-hydroxylase and 11-β-hydroxylase deficiencies. In each of these conditions, DOC hypersecretion is associated with elevated plasma ACTH levels. Heightened DOC secretion is often observed in Cushing's syndrome, particularly when associated with ectopic production of ACTH by neoplastic tissue. Isolated DOC excess mimics the features of primary aldosteronism and may also be associated with excessive fluid retention.[39] Persistently elevated plasma DOC concentrations were observed in 25 percent of patients with low-renin "essential" hypertension.[40] These patients were also observed to have intermittent spontaneous hypokalemia. Remission of hypertension and hypokalemia followed the administration of spironolactone, and indirect evidence suggested that the adrenal lesions were most likely bilateral macronodular hyperplasia.

18-HYDROXY-11-DEOXYCORTICOSTERONE (18-OH-DOC) EXCESS

Excessive secretion of 18-OH-DOC has been demonstrated in four forms of hypertension, including 17-α-hydroxylase deficiency, Cushing's syndrome, primary aldosteronism, and in a small number of patients with essential hypertension and suppressed plasma renin activity.[41] In patients with suppressed renin activity and excessive 18-OH-DOC secretion, aldosterone secretion rate is diminished and spironolactone relieves hypertension. About half of these patients exhibit a significant reduction in diastolic blood pressure when given 1.5 mg of dexamethasone per day for 6 weeks. Isolated excessive secretion of 18-OH-DOC has also been found in some patients with essential hypertension and normally responsive plasma renin activity.[42] Elevated plasma concentrations of 18-OH-DOC more frequently are observed in patients with essential hypertension, with or without alterations in plasma renin activity, than any other group of patients thus far encountered. Significantly increased secretion of 18-OH-DOC, as reflected by urinary 18-OH-TH-DOC excretion, occurs in a proportion of patients with suppressed plasma renin activity and hypertension and also in other patients with essential hypertension who have normally responsive plasma renin activity. 18-OH-DOC excess may play a role in the genesis of hypertension in these patients.

16-β-HYDROXYDEHYDROEPIANDROSTERONE (16-β-OH-DHEA) EXCESS

Increased excretion in urine of the C-19 steroid, 16-β-OH-DHEA, has been observed in a significant number of patients with suppressed plasma renin activity and hypertension but not in patients with essential hypertension and normally responsive plasma renin activity.[43] It is not known whether secretion of 16-β-OH-DHEA or its precursor, DHEA, is altered in these patients. It is possible that the increased urinary excretion of this metabolite reflects increased hepatic metabolism of DHEA. It may be that 16-β-OH-DHEA functions as a biological marker for some more potent but as yet unidentified steroid, since 16-β-OH-DHEA has been shown to have only negligible affinity for mineralocorticoid receptors in vitro and negligible effect on induction of sodium retention in adrenalectomized animals.

DEHYDROEPIANDROSTERONE SULFATE (DHEA-S) EXCESS

Plasma concentrations of the principal C-19 steroid product of the adrenal cortex, DHEA-S, are significantly elevated in patients with essential hypertension.[44] The significance of these observations remains to be determined.

16-α, 18-DIHYDROXY-11-DEOXYCORTICOSTERONE (16-α, 18-DiOH-DOC) EXCESS

16-α, 18-DiOH-DOC, secreted by the human adrenal, is the product of 16-α-hydroxylation of 18-OH-DOC.[45] Biogenesis of this steroid is accelerated in some patients with low-renin essential hypertension. 16-α, 18-DiOH-DOC does not directly influence sodium metabolism and clearly enhances the activity of aldosterone in stimulating sodium reabsorption in the kidneys of adrenalectomized animals.[46] The significance of secretory excess of this steroid in hypertension remains to be evaluated.

LOW-RENIN "ESSENTIAL" HYPERTENSION

Numerous studies, beginning in 1967, have identified a subgroup of patients who seemingly have essential hypertension but who exhibit suppressed or hyporesponsive plasma renin activity when challenged by any maneuver that will acutely produce negative sodium balance.[47,48] This subpopulation of patients represents approximately 20 to 25 percent of the hypertensive population at large. Interestingly, the only other situation in which untreated patients with hypertension have suppressed plasma renin activity is in the mineralocorticoid-hypertensive syndrome. Demonstraion of increased exchangeable sodium, extracellular fluid, and plasma volume and also the hypotensive effects of sodium deprivation and diuretic therapy in both disorders suggest that increased renal sodium retention is an immediate cause of volume-dependent hypertension. Furthermore, compelling evidence has been obtained in support of the idea that adrenal mineralocorticoid excess has a primary role in the genesis of low-renin "essential" hypertension. The administration of inhibitors of adrenal steroidogenesis in patients with low-renin essential hypertension relieves hypertension but is without effect on blood pressure of patients with normally responsive renin activity and hypertension.[49] Patients with low-renin hypertension who undergo bilateral total adrenalectomy become normotensive, and the excised adrenals exhibit structural abnormalities, including micronodular and macronodular hyperplasia.[50] It is probable that a significant subpopulation of patients with low-renin "essential" hypertension is afflicted with the mineralocorticoid-hypertensive syndrome, but the mineralocorticoid(s) involved has yet to be characterized. This is strongly supported by the accumulating examples of altered steroidogenesis in the low-renin hypertensive population, as described above.

ISOLATED HYPOALDOSTERONISM

INTRODUCTION

Selective deficiency of aldosterone secretion without alterations in cortisol production results in persistent hyperkalemia, renal salt wastage (to a variable extent), and postural hypotension in some patients. Hyperkalemia may be associated with profound muscle weakness and cardiac arrhythmias. Isolated hypoaldosteronism was first described in 1957 by Hudson et al.[51] The clinical manifestations of isolated hypoaldosteronism are promptly reversed by the administration of exogenous mineralocorticoids, such as 9-α-fluorocortisol. Etiologies, including specific deficien-

Table 98-2. Isolated Hypoaldosteronism

A. Deficiencies of enzymes involved in aldosterone biosynthesis
   1. Corticosterone methyl oxidase type I deficiency—? 18-hydroxylase deficiency
   2. Corticosterone methyl oxidase type 2 deficiency—? 18-hydroxysteroid dehydrogenase deficiency
B. Failure of adrenal zona glomerulosa function
   1. Heparin and polysulfated glycosaminoglycan-induced adrenal glomerulosa failure
   2. ? Autoimmune glomerulosa insufficiency
      Isolated hypoaldosteronism associated with idiopathic hypoparathyroidism
C. Altered function of the renin-angiotensin system
   1. Postunilateral adrenalectomy for an aldosterone-producing adenoma
   2. Idiopathic hyporeninemic hypoaldosteronism
   3. Big renin hypersecretion, diabetes, renal disease, and hypoaldosteronism

cies of enzymes involved in aldosterone biosynthesis, selective destruction of the adrenal zona glomerulosa, and a variety of alterations in function of the renin-angiotensin system, are listed in Table 98-2. In the disorders of aldosterone biosynthesis and in those situations in which there appears to be failure of adrenal cortical zona glomerulosa function, plasma renin activity is usually elevated. By contrast, those disorders in which alterations in the function of the renin-angiotensin system are observed are generally characterized by low or unmeasurable plasma renin activity or by the presence of elevated levels of "big" renin.

Deficiencies of Enzymes Involved in Aldosterone Biosynthesis

The final steps in the biosynthesis of aldosterone involve the conversion of corticosterone to aldosterone. It had been assumed that the first step was a hydroxylation reaction at position 18 and that the second was a dehydrogenation at the same position. There is little evidence that 18-hydroxycorticosterone is an obligatory intermediate for the formation of aldosterone.[52] It is more likely that both steps involve mixed-function oxygenation and that the intermediate structure remains to be described. The reaction would involve a double hydroxylation of the angular methyl group at C-18, followed by a spontaneous dehydration to the aldehyde. Thus, corticosterone methyl oxidase deficiency type I could be characterized by overproduction of, corticosterone but without associated overproduction of 18-hydroxycorticosterone. Corticosterone methyl oxidase deficiency type II, on the other hand, could be associated with overproduction of both 18-hydroxycorticosterone and corticosterone. Corticosterone methyl oxidase deficiency type II is the more frequently observed defect. In this condition, there is marked renal salt wastage, growth retardation, and enormous overproduction of 18-hydroxycorticosterone and, to a lesser extent, corticosterone. The defect may be both hereditary and familial and has been observed in a number of Israeli children from families of Persian origin. Administration of exogenous mineralocorticoid restores normal growth rate and permits renal salt conservation.

FAILURE OF ADRENAL ZONA GLOMERULOSA TO FUNCTION

Heparin and related polysulfated glucosominoglycans (heparinoids), when given for a prolnged period, can produce continued suppression of aldosterone biosynthesis, aldosterone secretion, and generalized zona glomerulosa function.[53] These compounds actually reduce the width of the zona glomerulosa. There is but one case report in which the administration of heparin, 200 mg/day subcutaneously for 3½ years, produced severe aldosterone deficiency.[54]

The association of hypoaldosteronism and idiopathic hypoparathyroidism in a single patient led to the speculation that coexistence of these disorders may represent an autoimmune clustered disease, such as seen in idiopathic Addison's disease of childhood.[55]

ALTERED FUNCTION OF THE RENIN-ANGIOTENSIN SYSTEM

Postunilateral Adrenalectomy for an Aldosterone-producing Adenoma

Aldosterone deficiency, lasting from weeks to months, may occur after the removal of an adrenal bearing an aldosterone-secreting adenoma. Prolonged suppression of the renin-angiotensin system due to inappropriately elevated concentrations of aldosterone in plasma is responsible. Hyporesponsiveness of the renin-angiotensin system can be reduced by the preoperative administration of large doses of spironolactone.

Idiopathic Hyporeninemic Hypoaldosteronism

Hyporeninemic hypoaldosteronism is most often associated with mild renal insufficiency and is, undoubtedly, the most commonly observed variety of isolated hypoaldosteronism.[56,57] In patients with this variety of hypoaldosteronism, there is little or no increment in plasma renin activity or in plasma aldosterone in response to sodium depletion, but there may be normal or blunted responses to infused angiotensin II or ACTH. Hyperkalemia, a negative sodium balance, mild metabolic acidosis, and rapid deterioration with sodium restriction in elderly patients with mild azotemia characterize this condition. In large general hospital populations, there is increasing recognition of this syndrome, and it ranks high as a cause of hyperkalemia.

"Big" Renin Hypersecretion, Diabetes, Renal Disease, and Hypoaldosteronism

In certain patients with long-standing diabetes mellitus and mild to moderate chronic renal failure, selective hypoaldosteronism has been associated with markedly elevated plasma renin activity.[58] Gel filtration of plasma extracts from such patients may confirm the presence of so-called "big" renin or pro-renin, a relatively inactive form of renin with higher molecular weight than normal plasma renin. In this condition, elevated 18-hydroxycorticosterone secretion is likely in some patients because of increased excretion of 18-hydroxy-tetrahydro compound A in urine. The mechanism of this presumed corticosterone methyl oxidase type II deficiency is not understood.

REFERENCES

1. Boyd, G. W., Adamson, A. R., Arnold, M., James, V. H. T., and Peart, W. S.: The Role of Angiotensin in the Control of Aldosterone in Man. *Clin. Sci. 42:* 91, 1972.
2. Brown, J. J., Davies, D. L., Doak, P. B., Lever, A. F., and Robertson, J. I. S.: Plasma Renin in Normal Pregnancy. *Lancet II:* 900, 1963.
3. Luetscher, J. A., Jr., Johnson, B. B., Dowdy, A., Harvey, J., Lew, W., and Poo, L. J.: Observations on the Sodium-Retaining Corticoid (Aldosterone) in the Urine of Children and Adults in Relation to Sodium Balance and Edema. *J. Clin. Invest. 33:* 1441, 1954.

4. Luetscher, J. A., Dowdy, A. J., Arnstein, A. R., Lucas, C. P., and Murray, C. L.: Idiopathic Edema and Increased Aldosterone Excretion. In *Aldosterone,* edited by E. E. Baulieu and P. Robel. F. A. Davies Co., Philadelphia, 1964, pp. 487–498.
5. Sanders, L. L. and Melby, J. C.: Aldosterone and Edema of Congestive Failure. *Arch. Intern. Med. 113:* 331, 1964.
6. Hickie, J. B. and Lazarus, L.: Aldosterone Metabolism in Cardiac Failure. *Austral. Ann. Med. 15:* 289–300, 1966.
7. Tait, J. F., Bougas, J., Little, B., Tait, S. A. S. and Flood, C.: Splanchnic Extraction and Clearance of Aldosterone in Subjects with Minimal and Marked Cardiac Dysfunction. *J. Clin. Endocrinol. 25:* 219, 1965.
8. Sanders, L. L. and Melby, J. C.: Aldosterone and Edema of Congestive Heart Failure. *Arch. Intern. Med. 113:* 331, 1964.
9. Bartter, F. C., Pronove, P., Gill, J. R., Jr., and MacCardle, R. C.: Hyperplasia of the Juxtaglomerular Complex with Hyperaldosteronism and Hypokalemia Alkalosis: A New Syndrome. *Am. J. Med. 33:* 811–828, 1962.
9a. Taylor, A. A., Keiser, H. R., Seyberth, H. W., Gill, J. R., Jr., Frolich, J. C., Bowden, R. E., et al.: Bartter's Syndrome: A Disorder Characterized by High Urinary Prostaglandins and a Dependence of Hyperreninemia on Prostaglandin Synthesis. *Am. J. Med. 61:* 43, 1976.
10. Kurtzman, N. A. and Gutierrez, L. F.: The Pathophysiology of Bartter's Syndrome. *J. A. M. A. 134:* 758–759, 1975.
11. Gill, J. R., Bell, N. H., and Bartter, F. C.: Impaired Conservation of Sodium and Potassium in Renal Tubular Acidosis and Its Correction by Buffer Ion. *Clin. Sci. 33:* 577, 1967.
12. Berner, H. R., Gavras, H., and Laragh, J. A.: Angiotensin II Blockade in Man by Sar 1-ala⁸-Angiotensin II for Understanding and Treatment of High Blood Pressure. *Lancet II:* 1045–1048, 1973.
13. Robertson, P. W., Klidjian, A., Harding, L. K., Walters, G., Lee, M. R., and Robb-Smith, A. H. T.: Hypertension Due to a Resin-secreting Renal Tumor. *Am. J. Med. 43:* 963–976, 1967.
14. Mitchell, J. D., Baxter, T. J., Blair-West, J. R., and McCredie, D. A.: Renin Levels in Nephroblastoma (Wilms' Tumor): Report of a Renin-secreting Tumor. *Arch. Dis. Child. 45:* 376–384, 1970.
15. Laragh, J. H., Ulick, S., Januszewicz, V., Deming, Q. D., Kelly, W. G., and Lieberman, S.: Aldosterone Secretion in Primary and Malignant Hypertension. *J. Clin. Invest. 39:* 1091–1106, 1960.
16. Laragh, J. H., Sealey, J. E., Leadingham, J. G. G., Newton, M. A.: Oral Contraceptives: Renin, Aldosterone, and High Blood Pressure. *J. A. M. A. 201:* 918, 1967.
17. Relman, A. S., Stewart, W. K., and Schwartz, W. B.: A Study of the Adjustments to Sodium- and Water-retaining Hormones in Normal Subjects. *J. Clin. Invest. 37:* 924–925, 1958.
18. Safar, M., and Milliez, P.: Hemodynamic Findings in Human Arterial Hypertension. *Rev. Europ. Etudes Clin. Biol. 17:* 147–154, 1972.
19. Conn, J. W., Rovner, D. R., Cohen, E. L., and Nesbit, R. M.: Normokalemic Primary Aldosteronism. Its Masquerade as "Essential" Hypertension. *J. A. M. A. 195:* 21–26, 1966.
20. Conn, J. W.: Primary Aldosteronism: A New Clinical Syndrome. *J. Lab. Clin. Med. 45:* 3–6, 1955.
21. Ganguly, A., Melada, G. A., Luetscher, J. A., and Dowdy, A. J.: Control of Plasma Aldosterone in Primary Aldosteronism: Distinction Between Adenoma and Hyperplasia. *J. Clin. Endocrinol. Metab. 37:* 765–775, 1973.
22. Laragh, J. H., Leadingham, J. L. G., and Sommers, S. C.: Secondary Aldosteronism and Reduced Plasma Renin in Hypertensive Disease. *Trans. Assoc. Am. Phys. 80:* 168, 1967.
23. Foye, L. V., Jr., and Feichtmer, T. V.: Adrenocortical Carcinoma Producing Solely Mineralocorticoid Effect. *Am. J. Med. 19:* 966–973, 1955.
24. Moran, W., Goetz, F. C., Melby, J. C., Zimmermann, B., and Kennedy, B. J.: Primary Hyperaldosteronism Without Adrenal Tumor. *Am. J. Med. 28:* 638–647, 1960.
25. Sutherland, D. J. A., Ruse, J. L. and Laidlaw, J. C.: Hypertension, Increased Aldosterone Secretion and Low Plasma Renin Activity Relieved by Dexamethasone. *Canad. Med. Assoc. J. 95:* 1109, 1966.
26. New, M. I., and Peterson, R. E.: A New Form of Congenital Adrenal Hyperplasia. *J. Clin. Endocrinol. Metab. 27:* 300–305, 1967.
27. Conn, J. W., Cohen, E. L., and Rovner, D. R.: Suppression of Plasma Renin Activity in Primary Aldosteronism. Distinguishing Primary From Secondary Aldosteronism in Hypertensive Disease. *J. A. M. A. 190:* 213, 1964.
28. Biglieri, E. G., Stockigt, J. R., and Schambelan, M.: Preliminary

Evaluation for Primary Aldosteronism. *Arch. Inter. Med. 126:* 1004–1008, 1970.

29. Melby, J. C.: Aldosterone Inhibitors (Adrenal Cortex). In *Clinical Endocrinology, II,* edited by E. B. Astwood and C. Cassidy. Grune and Stratton, New York, 1968, chap. 5, pp. 477–488.

30. Spark, R. F. and Melby, J. C.: Aldosteronism in Hypertension: A Spironolactone Response Test. *Ann. Inter. Med. 69:* 685, 1968.

31. Melby, J. C., Spark, R. F., Dale, S. L., Egdahl, R. H., and Kahn, P. C.: The Diagnosis and Localization of Aldosterone-producing Adenomas by Adrenal-Vein Catheterization. *N. Engl. J. Med 277:* 1050–1056, 1967.

32. Melby, J. C.: Identifying the Adrenal Lesion in Primary Aldosteronism. *Ann. Intern. Med. 76:* 1039–1041, 1972.

33. Conn, J. W., Morita, R., Cohen, E. L., Beirwaltes, W. H., McDonald, W. J. and Herwig, K. R.: Primary Aldosteronism. Photo Scanning of Tumors After Administration of ^{131}I-19-Iodocholesterol. *Arch. Intern. Med. 129:* 417–425, 1971.

34. Sarkar, S. D., Beirwaltes, W. H., Lee, R. D., Basmadjian, G. P., Hetzel, K. R., Kennedy, W. P. and Mason, M. M.: A New and Superior Adrenal Scanning Agent: NP-59. *J. Nuclear Med 16:* 1038–1042, 1975.

35. Sundsfjord, J. A., Marton, P., Jorgensen, H., and Aakvaag, A.; Reduced Aldosterone Secretion During Spironolactone Treatment in Primary Aldosteronism. Report of a Case. *J. Clin. Endocrinol. Metab. 39:* 734–739, 1974.

36. Molhuysen, J. A., Gerbradney, J., DeVries et al: A Licorice Extract with a Deoxycortone-like Action. *Lancet II:* 381–386, 1950.

37. Mohammed, S. D., Chapman, R. S., and Crooks, J.: Hypokalemia, Flaccid Quadruparesis and Myoglobinuria with Carbenoxolone (Biogastrone). I (Sec. 2). *British Med. J. 5503:* 1581–1582, 1966.

38. Liddle, G. W., Bledsoe, T., and Coppage, W. S., Jr.: A Familial Renal Disorder Simulating Primary Aldosteronism but with Negligible Aldosterone Secretion. In *Aldosterone,* edited by E. E. Baulieu and E. Robel. F. A. Davies Co., Philadelphia, 1964, pp. 353–369.

39. Kahn, M., Melby, J. C., and Jacobs, D. R.: Isolated Deoxycrticosterone Excess: A Unique Syndrome Simulating Hyperaldosteronism with Marked Fluid Retention. *Clin. Res. 14:* 282, 1966.40.

40. Brown, J. J., Ferriss, J. B., Fraser, R., Lever, A.F., Love, D. R., Robertson, J. I. S., and Wilson, A.: Apparently Isolated Excess Deoxycorticosterone in Hypertension. *Lancet II:* 243–247, 1972.

41. Melby, J. C., Dale, S. L., Grekin, R. J., Gaunt, R., Wilson, T. E.: 18-Hydroxy-11-Deoxycorticosterone (18-OH-DOC) Secretion in Experimental and Human Hypertension. *Recent Progr. Horm. Res. 28:* 287–351, 1972.

42. Genest, J., Nowaczynski, W., Kuchel, O., and Sasaki C.: Plasma Progesterone Levels and 18-OH-DOC Secretion Rate in Benign Essential Hypertension in Humans. In *Hypertension,* edited by J. Genest and E. Koiw. Springer-Verlag, New York, 1972, pp. 293–298.

43. Liddle, G. W., Sennett, J. A.: New Mineralocorticoids in the Syndrome of Low-Renin Essential Hypertension *J Steroid Biochm. :* 751–753, 1974.

44. Sekihara, H., Ohsawa and Kosaka, K.: Serum Dehydroepiandrosterone Sulfate and Dehydroepiandrosterone Levels in Essential Hypertension. *J. Clin. Endocrinol. Metab. 40:* 156–157, 1975.

45. Dale, S. L., and Melby, J. C.: Isolation and Identification of 16α, 18-DiOH-DOC From Human Adrenal Gland Incubations. *Steroids 21:* 617–632, 1973.

46. Dale, S. L., and Melby, J. C.: Altered Adrenal Steroidogenesis in "Low-Renin" Essential Hypertension. *Trans. Assoc. Am. Phys. 87:* 248–257, 1974.

47. Kuchel, O., Fishman, L. N., Liddle, G. W., Michelakis, A. M.: Effect of Diazoxide on Plasma Renin Activity in Hypertensive Patients. *Ann. Intern. Med. 67:* 791–799, 1967.

48. Helmer, O. M., and Judson, W. E.: Metabolic Studies on Hypertension Patients with Suppressed Plasma Renin Activity Not Due to Hyperaldosteronism. *Circulation 38:* 965–976, 1968.

49. Woods, J. W., Liddle, G. W., Stant, E. G., Jr., Michelakis, A. M. and Brill, A. D.: Effect of an Adrenal Inhibitor in Hypertensive Patients with Suppressed Renin. *Arch. Intern. Med. 123:* 366–370, 1969.

50. Grim, C. E., Keitzer, W. F., Esterly, J. A., Longo, D. L.: Adrenalectomy in Low-Renin "Essential" Hypertension. *Clin. Res. 22:* 340A, 1974.

51. Hudson, J. B., Chobanian, A. V., Relman, A. S.: Hypoaldosteronism: A Clinical Study of a Patient with an Isolated Mineralocorticoid Deficiency, Resulting in Hyperkalemia and Stokes-Adams Attack. *N. Engl. J. Med. 257:* 529–536, 1957.

52. Ulick, S.: Diagnosis and Nomenclature of the Disorders of the Terminal Portion of the Aldosterone Biosynthetic Pathway. *J. Clin. Endocrinol. Metab. 43:* 92–96, 1976.

53. Laidlaw, J. C., Abbot, E. C., Sutherland, D. J. A., and Stiefel, M.: The Influence of Heparin-Like Compound on Hypertension, Electrolyses and Aldosterone in Man. *Trans. Am. Clin. Climatol. Assoc. 77:* 111–124, 1965.

54. Wilson, I. D., and Goetz, F. C.: Selected Hypoaldosteronism After Prolonged Heparin Administration. *Am. J. Med. 36:* 635–639, 1964.

55. Marieb, N. J., Melby, J. C. and Lyall, S. S.: Isolated Hypoaldosteronism Associated with Ediopathic Hypoparathyroidism. *Arch. Inter. Med. 134:* 424–429, 1974.

56. Weidmann, P., Reinhart, R., Maxwell, M. H., Rowe, P., Coburn, J. W. and Massry, S. G.: Syndrome of Hyporeninemic Hypoaldosteronism and Hypokalemia in Renal Disease. *J. Clin. Endocriol. Metab. 36:* 965–977, 1973.

57. Schambelan, M., Stockigt, J. R., and Biglieri, B. G.: Isolated Hypoaldosteronism in Adults—a Renin Deficiency Syndrome. *N. Engl. J. Med. 287:* 573–578, 1972.

58. DeLeiva, A., Christlieb, A. R., Melby, J. C., Graham, C. A., and Leutscher, J. A.: Big renin and biosynthetic defect of aldosterone in diabetes mellitus. *New Eng. J. Med. 295:* 639–643, 1976.

99

Synopsis of Diagnosis and Treatment of Diseases of the Adrenal Cortex

Don H. Nelson

This short chapter outlines an approach to the patient who may or may not have an abnormality of function of the adrenal cortex. Specifics of the assay method and normal values are given in greater detail in Chapters 94 and 95 for Cushing's syndrome, in Chapters 94 and 96 for adrenal insufficiency, in Chapter 97 for adrenogenital disorders, and in Chapter 98 for hyperaldosteronism and hypoaldosteronism.

DIAGNOSIS OF CUSHING'S SYNDROME

1. The initial procedure for the diagnosis of Cushing's syndrome is an adequate history and physical examination, with particular emphasis placed on change of physical appearance (as shown by photographs over the past few years), moon face, weakness, striae, hypertension, and psychological aberrations.
2. The simplest and easiest initial procedure is administration of 1 mg dexamethasone at midnight with estimation of plasma cortisol between 7:00 and 9:00 A.M. A normal suppression rules out Cushing's syndrome in 95 percent of cases. Failure to suppress normally requires further study.
3. Plasma cortisol and ACTH. If step 1 suggests Cushing's syndrome, repetition of the 1 mg dexamethasone suppression with estimation of plasma ACTH as well as plasma cortisol is indicated. (Simultaneous dexamethasone levels are useful if available.) Failure of ACTH as well as cortisol to suppress is highly indicative of Cushing's syndrome. Very high plasma ACTH levels in the absence of a pituitary tumor suggests a nonpituitary (ectopic) ACTH-producing tumor. Low to absent ACTH levels and a nonsuppressed cortisol level is suggestive of an autonomous adrenal adenoma.
4. Diurnal plasma cortisol determination. Failure to see a marked fall in the plasma cortisol late in the evening (9:00 to 12:00 P.M.) indicates lack of diurnal variation in plasma cortisol and may be used as additional evidence for continued stimulation of the adrenal cortex in an abnormal manner. In the absence of the availability of plasma cortisol and plasma ACTH determinations, urinary free cortisol, 17-ketogenic steroids, or 17-hydroxycorticosteroids may be employed. Elevation of any of these is once again suggestive of Cushing's syndrome. The obese patient may have levels higher than normal, but these suppress easily.
5. If a probable diagnosis of Cushing's syndrome has been made, standard practice would be to hospitalize the patient for further workup to determine the cause of the disease. This workup should include a metyrapone test and a low-dose/high-dose dexamethasone suppression test. Almost all patients with autonomous adrenal tumors will fail to respond to metyrapone, while patients with Cushing's disease are likely to exhibit hyperactive response. If plasma ACTH values are employed, the low-dose/high-dose dexamethasone suppression test is probably necessary only if the interpretation of the previously named tests is in doubt. In the interpretation of these values, however, it should be remembered that there is a marked diurnal as well as episodic variation in the secretion of the corticosteroids and ACTH (see Chapter 93) and thus two samples (A.M. and P.M.) are much better than single values.
6. Steps for the radiologic diagnosis of the etiology of the excess ACTH or cortisol are not indicated until a firm diagnosis of Cushing's syndrome has been made. All patients with Cushing's disease should have a careful study of the sella turcica, and all patients with probable adrenal cortical tumor should have a study to determine the location of that tumor. The choice of venography, iodocholesterol imaging, or arteriogram may depend upon the capability of the radiologist or radiology department available to the physician. Ectopic ACTH-secreting tumors producing the picture of Cushing's syndrome are usually readily demonstrable, but occasional exceptions

include pancreatic carcinomas or bronchial adenomas that are often difficult to locate.

TREATMENT OF CUSHING'S SYNDROME

1. Tumors are removed surgically. Inoperable carcinoma may respond to o,p' DDD and/or aminoglutethimide.
2. Cushing's disease may be treated by a number of approaches:
   a. Transsphenoidal surgery to remove pituitary adenoma has been very successful with experienced surgical help.
   b. Pituitary irradiation is successful in something less than half of cases and is noninvasive, but the disease may grow worse while waiting for full effects.
   c. Total adrenalectomy if approaches (a) and (b) are contraindicated or there is recurrent disease following these approaches.
   d. There is incomplete evidence that pharmacologic agents such as cyproheptadine or bromocriptine may be used chronically and thus obviate the need for surgery. These approaches are under investigation.

DIAGNOSIS OF ADDISON'S DISEASE

1. Clinical findings include increased pigmentation, weakness, loss of weight, and vascular collapse following exposure to stressful situations.
2. An elevated plasma ACTH with a low plasma cortisol is diagnostic of the disease. In practice the ACTH stimulation test is also usually carried out, as experience with the combination of plasma cortisol and ACTH is limited and one must be certain that the episodic secretion of ACTH with a single relatively high level is not interpreted to be abnormally elevated. Thus, values less than 250 pg/ml might not be diagnostic of elevation in the plasma ACTH level.
3. ACTH stimulation test. This is most conveniently done by the 6-hour test with measurement of plasma cortisol although urinary corticosteroids might be used.
4. The use of the single-dose metyrapone test with administration of metyrapone at midnight and measurement of an 8:00 A.M. plasma 11-desoxycortisol level has proven useful as an indication of adrenal secretion as well as pituitary responsiveness to a stimulus to ACTH secretion. Patients with either primary or secondary adrenal insufficiency will fail to respond to this test.
5. If secondary rather than primary adrenal insufficiency is considered, the measurement of serum thyroxine, testosterone (in the male), or other available reliable indices of pituitary function should be carried out.

DIAGNOSIS OF ACUTE ADRENAL INSUFFICIENCY

In the acutely ill patient in whom the diagnosis of adrenal insufficiency is considered, blood samples for plasma cortisol and ACTH determination should be obtained, but therapy should not be delayed while waiting for the results of these tests.

THERAPY OF ADRENAL INSUFFICIENCY

1. Acute, severe adrenal insufficiency should be treated by large amounts of intravenous cortisol, approximately 100 mg of cortisol every 8 hours. Glucose, saline, fluids, and other specific therapy such as antibiotics should be given as indicated by the patient's condition.
2. Chronic adrenal insufficiency may be treated adequately by the administration of cortisol orally in quantities of 20–30 mg immediately upon arising in the morning and 10–15 mg in the afternoon, usually 4:00 to 6:00 P.M. Supplementation with fluorohydrocortisome, 0.05–0.2 mg given once daily, is useful in maintaining sodium balance and also muscular strength. Excess cortisol may produce increased appetite (particularly in the early stages of therapy), insomnia (if too much is given prior to bedtime), and of course, cushingoid features if a continued excess is administered. Excess mineralocorticoid is likely to produce edema only in the early stages of therapy of a new Addisonian patient but may produce excess sodium retention and hypertension if given in excess over a period of weeks or months.

DIAGNOSIS OF ADRENOGENITAL DISORDERS

INFANTS AND YOUNG CHILDREN

1. These conditions may be recognized through clitoral enlargement and labioscrotal fusion in female infants and in male infants by slight phallic enlargement and scrotal pigmentation. Dehydration and shock occurs in some forms at the fifth to eighth days of life. Signs of virilism and/or hypertension occur in older patients.
2. If salt-losing, the patient will lose weight, be apathetic, have vomiting and diarrhea, and become markedly dehydrated. Elevated serum K, low serum Na, Cl, CO_2, low aldosterone, and elevated plasma renin levels are likely to be present.
3. Plasma androstenedione level is elevated.
4. Urinary pregnantriol is increased except in newborns.
5. Plasma 17-hydroxyprogesterone is increased (physiologically high in cord blood).
6. Increased urinary 17-ketosteroids are suppressed by dexamethasone.
7. Sex chromatin estimations should be carried out to establish genetic sex.
8. Intravenous pyelograms and vaginograms are useful for visualization of urogenital ducts.

ADULTS

1. A recent increase in hair growth, clitoral enlargement, or cessation of menses is suggestive of increased androgens in the female.
2. Increased plasma testosterone, androstenedione, dehydroisoandrosterone, dehydroisoandrosterone sulfate, or dihydrotestosterone is present. An increase in plasma 17-hydroxyprogestenone or urinary pregnantriol will be seen if a 21-hydroxylase defect is present.
3. Urinary 17-ketosteroids and 17-ketogenic steroids may be shown to be increased if above plasma determinations are not available.

4. Dexamethasone will suppress if condition 2 or 3 is due to hyperplasia, but no suppression is seen with most tumors.

TREATMENT OF ADRENOGENITAL DISORDERS IN INFANTS AND CHILDREN

1. Surgery if tumor is present.
2. Congenital adrenal hyperplasia
   a. If the patient is dehydrated, start 20 ml/kg 0.9% NaCl in 5% glucose solution. Switch to one third 1/6 M sodium lactate, two thirds 0.85% sodium chloride, and addition of glucose to make 5% solution if acidotic.
   b. After 1 hour, if not improved, give 1 mg desoxycorticosterone IM. If there is a question of acute glucocorticord insufficiency, give Solu-Cortef iv.
   c. Chronically, 2 pellets of 125 mg Doca implanted at approximately 9-month intervals 2 times. Then switch to oral 9-α-fluorocortisol, 0.05–0.1 mg daily.
   d. Infants receive 12 mg/m^2 body surface cortisol daily or 36 mg/m^2 im every third day (one third greater dosage if cortisone acetate used).
   e. If cortisol is given orally, approximately twice the dose is given fractionated into 8-hour doses.
   f. Patient education and medic alert bracelet are very important.

TREATMENT OF ADRENOGENITAL DISORDERS IN ADULTS

1. Surgery if tumor is present.
2. Dexamethasone, 0.2–0.5 mg at bedtime, will produce adequate suppression in most adult patients. Cortisol is preferred for congenital adrenal hyperplasia.
3. Patients with ovarian hyperandrogenism (Stein-Leventhal syndrome) may be treated with dexamethasone suppression of adrenal androgens (thus reducing total androgen secretion), or estrogen suppression of gonadotropins, or both. In some cases, partial oophorectomy (wedge resection) is indicated. (see Chapter 113).

DIAGNOSIS OF HYPERALDOSTERONISM

PRIMARY ALDOSTERONISM (LOW RENIN)

1. Patients present with hypertension and often with a low serum potassium level. The low serum potassium level may be associated with polyuria and polydipsia. Potassium may be lowered by salt loading if in normal range and the diagnosis is suspected.
2. An elevated plasma aldosterone and reduced plasma renin activity after the furosemide test is diagnostic of the disease.

3. Desoxycorticosterone or 9-α-fluorocortisol suppression test lowers aldosterone in secondary but not primary aldosteronism if the diagnosis is in doubt.
4. Cortisol therapy will suppress aldosterone secretion in a small percentage of cases with hyperplasia.
5. Spironolactone administration reduces blood pressure significantly in 90 percent of patients with primary aldosteronism but also in 20 percent of those with essential hypertension.
6. Adrenal venous aldosterone measurements for differentiating tumor from bilateral involvement.
7. Adrenal imaging with radio-iodocholesterol may be helpful in locating the tumor.
8. Rarely, hypertension, potassium depletion, and low plasma renin levels may be associated with low plasma aldosterone levels. Consider licorice or carbonoxolone ingestion, Liddle's syndrome, or increased desoxycorticosterone, corticosterone, or other mineralocorticoid.

SECONDARY ALDOSTERONISM (ELEVATED RENIN)

Without Hypertension

Plasma aldosterone, renin, and angiotension II levels are increased, and sodium retention, edema, and potassium depletion are often present. This type of secondary aldosteronism may be normally present in the last trimester of pregnancy. Rarely, it may be secondary to the sodium loss of salt-losing nephritis, and one should consider the surreptitious use of diuretics, Barrter's syndrome, or renal tubular acidosis.

With Hypertension

Plasma aldosterone, renin, and angiotension II levels are increased with renin-secreting tumors and in malignant hypertension with necrotizing arteriolitis of the kidney. Estrogen or oral contraceptive therapy may have increased plasma renin levels, but aldosterone level is usually not elevated.

THERAPY OF HYPERALDOSTERONISM

1. Unilateral adrenalectomy if tumor present.
2. Idiopathic hyperplasia may be treated with spironolactone.
3. Glucocorticoid-suppressible hyperaldosteronism can be treated with 0.75 mg dexamethasone at bedtime.

DIAGNOSIS AND THERAPY OF HYPOALDOSTERONISM

1. Increased serum potassium level with deficiency of aldosterone but normal cortisol secretion.
2. Correction of defect with 0.1–0.2 mg fluorocortisol per day is confirmatory of diagnosis and also therapeutic.

Catecholamines
and
Adrenal Medulla

100

Anatomy and Biochemistry of the Sympathetic Nervous System

Vincent DeQuattro
Mark R. Myers
Vito M. Campese

INTRODUCTION

THE ENDOCRINOLOGIST, THE SYMPATHETIC NERVOUS SYSTEM, AND THE PATIENT

The patient with malfunction of the sympathoadrenal system may eventually visit the endocrinologist. His visit may be early in the instance of a pronounced abnormality, or it may be late when subtle symptoms of a minor defect progress without recognition. Our experience with several patients serves to illustrate the scope of complaints that may be referable to the sympathoadrenal system.

A young woman in her 22nd week of pregnancy has the sudden onset of feelings of impending doom. Episodes of diaphoresis and palpitations are associated with findings of tachycardia and hypertension. The hypertension specialist, called in consultation, notes a pressor crisis when the patient assumes the supine position. He administers phentolamine intravenously, and the symptoms and pressure rise are abated. Urinary catecholamine excretion confirms the presumptive diagnosis of pheochromocytoma. During the 37th week, the mother gives birth to an infant with hyaline membrane disease. Thirty minutes later, the surgeon removes a 150-g right adrenal pheochromocytoma. However, 3 days later, after intermittent episodes of hypoglycemia, bradycardia, congestive failure, and diminished cardiac output, the baby dies of cardiorespiratory failure.

The counterpoint is a 21-year-old woman given to chronic drug abuse with amphetamines or "speed." She enters the hospital with a 3-week history of gradual onset of weakness and the inability to stand. She remembers giving herself an injection of some "bad-looking" amphetamines prior to her illness. After this, she develops malaise, sore throat, muscle aching, and fever for a few days. The physical examination reveals a marked fall in blood pressure upon standing without change in her pulse rate. Subsequently, her plasma norepinephrine (NE) and dopamine-beta-hydroxylase (DBH) levels are found to be low and nonresponsive to standing. She improves with fluohydrocortisone therapy.

A 28-year-old male drug addict is admitted in near thyrotoxic crisis. He has been extremely restless and agitated. He has refused surgical removal of a diffusely enlarged thyroid gland. He has been taking methimazole irregularly. His temperature is 101°, his pulse is 140, and his blood pressure is 160/80. His T-4 is 18 mg/100 ml, and his plasma NE level is low. He is started on propranolol, 10 mg p.o. q.i.d., and his symptoms begin to abate rapidly.

A 43-year-old man with maturity-onset diabetes self-administers 36 U of NPH subcutaneously each morning. Over the past 2 years he has developed, with increasing frequency, episodes of syncope late in the afternoon. Occasionally, he has nausea but no sweating or palpitations preceding these spells. If he eats candy, the faints will not occur. He is found unconscious on the ward on the day after admission. His skin is noted to be warm and dry prior to an intravenous infusion of 25 g of glucose. He is aroused immediately after the glucose infusion. His blood glucose during the crisis is 10 mg/100 ml, and his urinary epinephrine excretion is 0.75 μg per hour, unchanged from the excretion rate obtained when he was ambulatory and asymptomatic.

A 64-year-old seamstress is noted to be hypertensive on a

routine physical examination. Her only complaint is increasing fatigability with exertion. A hypertensive workup is unremarkable, although the plasma NE level is 650 ng/liter, greater than the normal means plus two standard deviations. The endocrinologist discovers that the patient has cold intolerance and a marked delay in relaxation of the deep tendon reflexes. The T-4 is 1.2 mg/100 ml, and the hypertension improves with thyroxine therapy.

An 81-year-old male hypertensive consults his urologist for problems with difficult micturition and inability to maintain erection during sexual intercourse. The urologist schedules the patient for a transurethral resection of the prostate. The patient is referred to the internist for preoperative evaluation. The latter finds that recently the patient's medication was changed from alpha-methyldopa to propranolol. When propranolol was discontinued and alpha-methyldopa reinstituted, all urogenital symptoms abated.

A 32-year-old woman develops exophthalmos and thyrotoxicosis 7 weeks after her husband leaves her and files for divorce. A 23-year-old male with familial dysautonomia has the body size and weight of a 13-year-old sibling.

These examples illustrate the wide range of symptoms and somatic effects that can be induced by hyperfunction or hypofunction of the sympathoadrenal system. In certain instances, the sympathetic nervous system involvement was obvious; in others, it was subtle and perhaps open to debate.

THE NEUROTRANSMITTERS

The sympathoadrenal system is basically the alarm system for flight or fight. Initially, it was thought that the pattern of response was generalized, as opposed to that of the parasympathetic nervous system. Recent findings suggest that there may exist selective central stimulation of one organ, i.e., the cardiac sympathetic nerves, without activation of the sudomotor nerves. The peripheral sympathetic nervous system is characterized as the thoracolumbar system, with cell bodies of the preganglionic myelinated fibers arising in the intermediolateral gray of that level of the spinal cord and being distributed via the anterior roots of the spinal nerves to the 22 pairs of vertebral ganglia and also the celiac and mesenteric ganglia via the white rami (Fig. 100-1). The gray rami arise from the ganglia and carry postganglionic fibers to the spinal nerves and then to the glands (sweat and lacrimal) and blood vessels (skin and muscle). The most cephalad cluster of ganglia is the cervical (superior, middle, and inferior), which innervate the pupils, the lacrimal and salivary glands, and the heart. The stellate is the next caudally of the paravertebral ganglia, which also innervates the cardiac muscles and other thoracic viscera. The most caudal paired ganglia are the sacral, which innervate blood vessels and glands of the legs. Many preganglionic fibers from the 5th to the 12th thoracic segment pass through the vertebral ganglia without synapsing and form the greater splanchnic nerves. These fibers synapse in the celiac ganglion. Postganglionic fibers from this ganglion innervate the liver, gallbladder, intestines, spleen, and kidney. Some of the preganglionic fibers in the splanchnic nerve end directly in the adrenal medulla, where they innervate chromaffin cells. Preganglionic fibers from the lumbosacral region pass directly to the superior and inferior mesenteric ganglia via the pelvic nerves, where they regulate function of the distal colon, rectum, bladder, and genitalia.

Nerve discharge releases acetylcholine from the preganglionic nerve endings. Subsequently, the postganglionic nerve is stimulated, and the terminals release NE in the region of the effector organ. The adrenal medulla is a specialized ganglion without axonal extentions. The chromaffin cells can synthesize, store, and

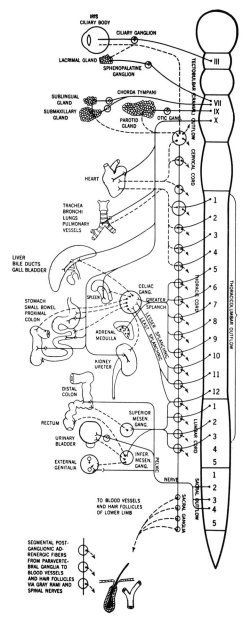

Fig. 100-1. The sympathetic nervous system: peripheral components of paired paravertebral nerves and ganglia. Parasympathetic nerves are cholinergic (solid lines) in nature, both preganglionic and postganglionic. Sympathetic nerves are cholinergic (solid lines) preganglionic and adrenergic (broken lines) postganglionic, (Adapted from ref. 40 with permission.)

release epinephrine as well as NE into the adrenal medullary effluent. While the adrenal medulla is an endocrine organ in the true sense, most of the NE present (80 percent) in the heart, spleen, and other sympathetically innervated organs is manufactured in situ, and the remainder reaches the tissue via circulation from other nerve endings.[1] However, little epinephrine passes unchanged through the capillary bed of the skeletal musculature or other sympathetically innervated organs.[2]

The adrenals (supra renals) were first described by Eustachius in the 16th century in his book *De Glandulis Quae Renibus Incumbent*. The adrenals were thought to be capsules filled with liquid because the medulla is subject to autolysis and is transformed into a viscous liquid if autopsies are not done in a few hours after death. In the 1860s, Henle observed that some granules in medullary cells developed a red–brown precipitate with potassium dichromate—the chromaffin reaction. At the turn of this century, Abel prepared epinephrine as the benzoylate salt of the pressor amines from adrenal extracts. Langly observed that the action of adrenal extracts and effluents of sympathetic nerve stimulation were similar. Later, Loewi and Cannon, in separate studies of isolated heart and hepatic nerves, respectively, characterized the liberated neurotransmitters as ''acceleran stuff'' and ''sympathin,'' respectively. Cannon tried to explain the dilating and constricting actions of epinephrine by the formation of sympathin I and E, respectively. It was not until 1946 that Alquist proposed the correct explanation for the dual actions of this compound. In 1946, von Euler identified NE as the sympathetic neurotransmitter in the spleen and heart.[3] Shortly thereafter, Carlson and Waldeck established the presence of dopamine, still another analogue, in brain tissue.[4] These three catecholamines remain the only proven active neurohumoral transmitters of the adrenal medulla or sympathetic neurone (Fig. 100-2A).

In 1960, Sutherland and Rall reported that these neurones act indirectly via stimulation of a second messenger system.[5] This system, when stimulated, results in the generation of the potent agonist and constrictor cyclic AMP or the antagonist and dilator cyclic GMP (Fig. 100-3).

The single link thus far omitted which transfers energy from aversive stimuli (i.e., a shark or a tax assessor) to dilated pupils, racing heart, and muscles, thus assisting attack or retreat, is the central component of the autonomic nervous system. While a great deal of work has been done by Haeusler, Doba, Reis, and others, there still remains no unifying hypothesis of central adrenergic control.[6,7] Although the histofluorescence studies of Fuxe and Dahlstrom have characterized dopamine-, noradrenergic-, and even epinephrine-synthesizing machinery in the central nervous system. the scheme we elaborate later is merely a ''crude hypothesis'' based upon these findings[8,9] (Fig. 100-4).

Autonomic reflexes can be elicited at the level of the spinal cord. Integration and central ramifications exist above the level of the spinal cord. The hypothalamus is the principal location of

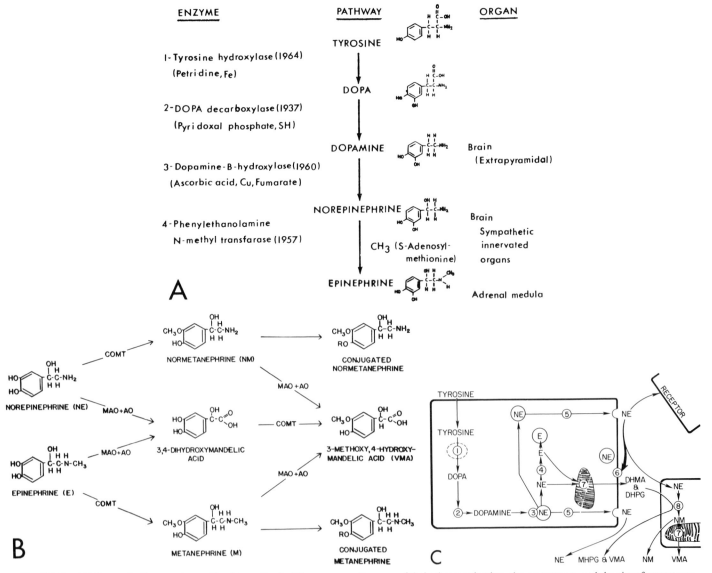

Fig. 100-2. (A) Sympathetic neurotransmitter biosynthesis. The enzymes, the year of their characterization, the coenzymes, and the site of neurotransmitter function are given for each step. (B) The major metabolic pathway for norepinephrine and epinephrine. COMT is catechol-O-methyltransferase. MAO + AO is monoamine oxidase and aldehyde oxidase. (C) Localization of catecholamine biosynthesis, storage, release, reuptake, and metabolism at a sympathetic neuroeffector junction. The N-methylation of norepinephrine primarily occurs in chromaffin cells of the adrenal medulla. Site Key: 1, tyrosine hydroxylase; 2, dopa decarboxylase; 3, dopamine-β-hydroxylase; 4, phenylethanolamine-N-methyltransferase; 5, release; 6, reuptake; 7, Monoamine oxidase and aldehyde oxidase; 8, Catechol-O-methyltransferase. Abbreviations are defined in the text.

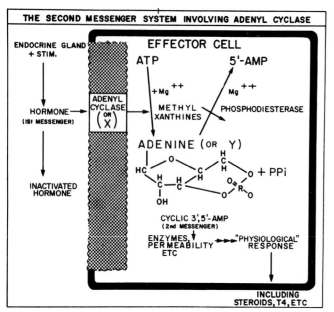

Fig. 100-3. The second messenger system: adenyl cyclase and cyclic AMP. (Reproduced with permission from R. W. Butcher, N Engl J Med 279: 1378–84, 1968.)

integration of the entire autonomic system. Posterior and lateral nuclei are mainly sympathetic, and stimulation results in massive discharge of the sympathoadrenal system. Two areas in the midbrain contain the epinephrine-synthesizing enzyme (PNMT) and are hyperactive in young animals who develop spontaneous hypertension.[10] When the sinoaortic nerves or the tractus solitarius, part of the corticobulbospinal pathway, is severed, hypertension ensues, which is associated with sympathetic hyperactivity and increased peripheral NE and E synthesis.[7,11] Antihypertensive drugs, such as clonidine and alpha-methyldopa, appear to exert their effects by stimulating the alpha-depressor system.[12]

The development of sensitive methods for measuring the neurotransmitters and the enzymes involved in their synthesis and metabolism was of great importance, leading to more rapid accumulation of knowledge of the sympathoadrenal system. Fluorimetric methods developed in the 1940s by Lund and co-workers replaced less sensitive bioassays of the 1930s.[13,14] Of the former techniques, the trihydroxyindole method was used to determine NE in urine,[15] in blood, and in spinal fluid until the 1970s.[16] The

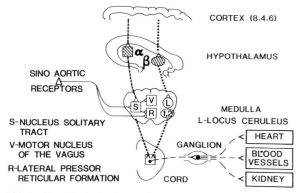

Fig. 100-4. Hypothetical schema of the sympathetic nervous system and its postulated role in neurogenic hypertension. The central inhibitory (bulbospinal) and excitatory (hypothalamic mesencephalic) pathways are postulated to be mediated by alpha- and beta-adrenergic receptors, respectively.

ethylene diamine condensation technique for plasma catecholamines did not achieve the same level of reproducibility and sensitivity in plasma as did the trihydroxyindole methods.[17] Enzymatic methods for estimation of NE and E in tissues, modified for application to plasma, were also introduced in the 1970s.[18] More recently, these have been further refined to enable measurements in small aliquots of tissue or biological fluids.[20,21]

Many innovative methods utilizing radiolabeled substrates or labeled donor groups have been developed to assess activities of the biosynthetic or degradative enzymes, as well as neurotransmitter content by separation and quantitation of the labeled products of their reactions mixtures. Table 100-1 gives a partial list of these assay procedures.

REGULATION AND INTERACTION

The major function of the sympathetic nervous system is the regulation of delivery of blood flow, depending on the action or dormancy of an organ. Thus, increased flow to skeletal muscles and simultaneously reduced splanchnic flow are prototypic changes induced by the sympathetic nervous system in an exercising athlete. The sympathetic nervous system mediates the facial pallor, the neck flush, and the sweat during fright. The short adrenergic system richly innervates the vasculature of the erectile tissue and the vas deferens. Thus, antiadrenergic drugs may produce impotence and retrograde ejaculation owing to interference with these functions. The parasympathetic nervous system, when activated via afferents from the baroreceptors, serves to decrease cardiac output and oppose sympathetic-nerve-induced increase in peripheral blood flow. Thus, increased cardiac rate in pathophysiologic states may be wrongfully assumed to be due to sympathetic excess when, in fact, deficient parasympathetic control is the cause.

Components of the sympathoadrenal system may be self-reinforcing in a variety of ways. Epinephrine released from the medulla may stimulate presynaptic beta-receptors at distant sites, enhancing further NE release from sympathetic neurones. Hypothalamic sympathetic stimulation of polypeptide secretion from both the anterior and posterior pituitary (ACTH and vasopressin) may produce the long-term effects of sympathoadrenal stimulation secondary to chronic stress. Peripheral sympathetic nerve stimulation of the JG cell results in renin-mediated formation of angiotensin II. This third polypeptide leads to sodium retention, which reduces sympathetic nerve vesicle storage of NE and E and sensitizes smooth muscle to the catecholamines. Angiotensin II further stimulates NE and E release via central excitation[22] and from peripheral sympathetic nerves[23] and the adrenal medulla, respectively.[24] Thus the sympathetic nervous system, by generating vasoactive pressor polypeptides, can exert an indirect reinforcement of the effects of directly released transmitter NE and E.

The sympathetic nervous system activates other inhibitory systems, either directly or indirectly, via altered circulation. The increased arterial pressure caused by angiotensin II and aldosterone release is modulated by increased kallikrein and prostaglandin synthesis. These substances are natriuretic, and some of their class, bradykinin, prostaglandin E, are vasodilatory. Thus, local and humoral effects of sympathoadrenal stimulation are reinforced or modulated by several systems resulting in acute or chronic changes in local or systemic arterial blood flow.

This section presents some of the work of men who studied sympathetic neurotransmitter biochemistry and pharmacology in earlier periods. Cannon, Selye, von Euler, Carlson, Axelrod, Udenfriend, Ahlquist, Sutherland, and Sjoersma are but a few who

Table 100-1. The Sensitivities of Various Assay Methods for
Catecholamines, Their Metabolites and Enzymes of Biosynthesis and Degradation

| | Sensitivity | | | |
Substance	Specimen-Amount	Amount of Substance Detectable	Method	First Author
Catecholamines				
NE, E	Urine—30 cc	10 ng	F	Crout[15]
	Tissue—30 mg			
	Plasma—10 ml	1 ng	F	Renzini[10]
DA	Urine—20 cc	10 ng	F	Drujan[43]
	Tissue—20 mg			
NE, E, DA	Plasma—50 μl	5 pg	RE	Passon[21]
	Tissue—1 μg			
NE	Plasma—50 μl	25 pg	RE	Henry[20]
	Tissue—1 μg			
Metabolites				
NMN, MN	Urine—2 cc	100 pg	F	Brunjes[44]
Total MMN + MN	Urine—10 cc	5 μg	P	Pisano[46]
VMA	Urine—5 cc	3 μg	P	Pisano[47]
VMA glycol	Urine—2 cc	2 μg	GLC	Wilk[48]
	CSF*—1–6 cc	5 ng	GLC	Karoum[45]
DOMA	Urine—2 cc	50 ng	RE	Sato[49]
	Plasma—20 ml	10 ng		
Biosynthetic enzymes				
TYH	Tissue—20 mg		RE	Nagatsu[50]
DDC	Tissue—10 mg		RE	Lovenberg[51]
DBH	Tissue—10 mg		P	Nagatsu[52]
	Plasma—0.5 cc		P	Nagatsu[52]
	Plasma—0.5 cc		RE	Weinshilboum[53]
PNMT	Tissue—1 mg		RE	Wurtman[34,54]
Metabolizing enzymes				
MAO	Tissue—1 mg (blood)		RE	Axelrod[55]
COMT	Tissue—1 mg (blood)		RE	Wurtman[56]

F = flurometric, RE = radioenzymatic, GLC = gas liquid chromatography,
P = photometric
*Cerebrospinal fluid
Substance abbreviations defined in text

have made valuable contributions to our understanding of the sympathoadrenal system via studies in animals and man. These principles were elaborated upon by a more recent generation, often their students—Spector, Oates, Nagatsu, Kopin, Wurtman, Kirshner, and many more. Further methodological developments by Fuxe, Dahlstrum, Engelman, Lovenberg, Winshilbaum, Lefkowitz, Robinson, and Reis have added to our understanding of the sympathetic nervous system in recent times and give us directions for the future.

ANATOMY

EMBRYOLOGY

The adrenal medulla and sympathetic nervous system are derived from the neural crest. It can be seen from the schema of the embryological development that the sympathogonia precursors of the sympathetic ganglion cells and chromaffin tissue have a common origin (Fig. 100-5). At about the sixth week, a block of celomic mesoderm cells condense into a small cluster of acidophilic cells between the root of the mesentery and the genital ridge. This structure, the precursor of the adrenal cortex, is invaded by

ectodermal neurogenic cells, sympathogonia, migrating down from the neural crest at 7 weeks. During the third and fourth months, the adrenals exceed the kidneys in size and are one-third as large at birth. There is a rapid involution of cortex in 1 year to reach the adult weight ratio of 1:28 for adrenal–kidney. At birth there are paraganglionic masses of chromaffin tissue which dominate the medulla. This extramedullary chromaffin tissue involutes after birth, but tumors may appear later from any of these cell types. There is an important distribution at the bifurcation of the aorta called the organ of Zuckerkandl. This is important for two reasons: they may proliferate and achieve a functional role if both adrenal medullas are removed or destroyed by disease, i.e., tuberculosis or neoplastic changes. They are frequently sites of pheochromocy-

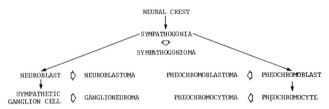

Fig. 100-5. The embryological derivation of neuroblastomas and pheochromocytomas from the neural crest precursor of the sympathetic ganglion and chromaffin cells.

toma, and this region must be explored carefully by the surgeon during the search for a chromaffin tumor.

The peripheral sympathetic nervous system and the adrenal medulla are operative at birth. Both norepinephrine and epinephrine are found in the plasma and urine of the newborn.[25] The development of the system is governed by the central release of nerve growth factor. This substance is a polypeptide with a molecular weight of about 44,000, whose actions have been characterized by Levi-Montalcini.[26] Immunosympathectomy is produced if the nerve growth factor is blocked by injection of its specific antiserum at birth in most animal species. Generally, this is not complete, and various regional sympathetic nerves (such as to the vas deferens and uterus in the rat) may be left intact. Administration of antinerve growth factor at 3 to 7 days after birth has markedly less effects on sympathetic nerve maturation.[27]

Functional features of the sympathetic nerves and pheochromocyte will be discussed in the remainder of this section. However, there are other cells that migrate from the neural crest which are of clinical importance but not generally considered to be related to sympathoadrenal function.

The melanocyte is functionally different in that it utilizes the substrate tyrosine to manufacture melanin via the enzyme tyrosine oxidase. This is a different enzyme species from the hydroxylase which converts tyrosine to dopa. Tumors of this species—melanoma—regain the functional ability to manufacture catecholamines and large amounts of the catecholamine metabolites—the catecholamine phenolic acids—may be found in the urine of these patients.[28] The embryological association of the melanocyte and pheochromocyte and sympathetic neurone is manifest in some patients with neurofibromatosis who have "café au lait" spots of melanin pigmentation, single or multiple pheochromocytomas, and singular and multiple neuromas of varying size or configuration (Fig. 100-6). Sipple's syndrome is a closely allied genetic disorder

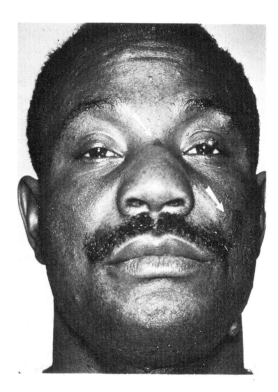

Fig. 100-6. Neurofibromata and cafe aú lait spots in a patient after removal of a right adrenal pheochromocytoma. The arrows indicate cafe aú lait spots. Neurofibromata are visible at the left eyebrow, eyelid, and jaw.

of multiple endocrine adenopathy type II, an autosomal dominant error with a high degree of penetrance. These patients usually have bilateral adrenal chromaffin tumors and multiple defects: medullary thyroid carcinoma, a neoplasm of the parafollicular C cell, and parathyroid adenoma.[29] During embryological development the C cell migrates from the neural crest to the region of the thyroid via the ultimo brachial body. When hyperplastic or neoplastic, these cells produce large amounts of calcitonin. The expression of this disorder may vary widely in affected individuals of any particular family. The thyroid carcinoma may precede the development and growth of the chromaffin tumors or vice versa. The occurrence of bilateral tumors may be separated by several years, and a preneoplastic change in adrenomedullary cells may occur.[30] The diagnosis of this disorder is confirmed by findings of increased plasma or urine catecholamines and plasma calcitonin. When family members are being screened for the presence of this disease, histamine stimulation of tumor catecholamines and calcium or pentagastrin stimulation of calcitonin release may be useful in early diagnosis.[31] A related genetic disorder is that of MEA type III (or IIB). These patients have peculiar facies, structural abnormalities of the lower extremities, i.e., pes cavus, and mucosal neuronomas. They usually do not have hyperparathyroidism.[32] Another family type is characterized by diarrhea, normotension, and prostaglandin production by the chromaffin tumor.[33]

ADRENAL MEDULLA

Structure

The weight of the human adrenal gland is normally 5–7 g. The right adrenal is triangular in shape, has legs 2–3 cm long, and sits on top of the kidney, whereas the left adrenal is crescent-shaped and lies more anterior and medial to the kidney. The medulla, surrounded by the cortex, usually comprises 8 to 10 percent of the gland. The right adrenal is in close approximation to the vena cava and the liver. The adrenals are at the level of the 12th thoracic vertebra and thus are located underneath the diaphragm in the retroperitoneal space. The surgeon removing the left adrenal must use caution in order to avoid injuring the spleen when proceeding via a transabdominal approach. Equal concern is required during removal of the right adrenal because of its proximity to the vena cava.

The arterial supply of the adrenals is rich and arises directly from the aorta and from branches of splenic, renal, intercostal, and diaphragmatic arteries. There are additional branches from the ovarian or internal spermatic arteries on the left. The adrenals are vascular organs receiving 6–7 cc of blood per gram per minute. The arteries form plexuses in the cortex. The plexuses are continuous with sinuses of the medulla which drain into the central vein of the latter. Because the medulla "lies in the arms of the cortex," the cortical venules bathe the medulla in steroid-rich blood. This relationship is thought necessary for the production of epinephrine in the human adrenal medulla.[34] The right adrenal vein has its connection with the vena cava at the level of T-12. The angle and size of this vessel in relation to the venae cavae makes it more difficult to catheterize than the left adrenal using Judkin's technique.

The left adrenal artery, as does the left spermatic, takes its origin from the left renal artery at approximately 3–4 cm from the origin of the latter. The venous return is analogous. The proximity of the adrenal venous effluent to the terminus of the spermatic vein is thought by some urologists to contribute to the increased incidence of spermatic vein varicosities of the left testes. Apparently, there are no untoward effects of this anatomical relationship of the left adrenal and left ovarian veins.

The cut surface of the adrenal medulla is brown and easily distinguished from the yellow cortical outer covering of the gland. The cells comprising the medulla are sympathetic ganglion cells and pheochromocytes. These are called "chromaffin" cells because they contain amines with catechol nucleus that precipitate chromium salts and stain brown with H+E (Fig. 100-7). Dense core vesicles containing norepinephrine and epinephrine can be seen more readily with electron microscopy (Fig. 100-8). The pathologist takes advantage of the reducing potential of these amines in identifying chromaffin tissue on surgical material using the chromaffin test. When a few drops of I_2 and a few drops of dichromate are placed successively on the cut tissue, a characteristic golden brown color is formed within 30 seconds.

Because of the effects of the catecholamines on lipolysis, a characteristic brown fat pad is formed in the region of the adrenal. This appearance is similar to the sympathetically innervated brown fat which is a feature of hibernating animals and is a source of fuel during their dormant periods.

Neurohumoral Control

Stimulation of the splanchnic nerve, the preganglionic sympathetic nerve fibers, results in exocytosis and secretion of the catecholamines, carrier protein, and dopamine-beta-hydroxylase from the adrenal medulla. The hypothalamus and brain stem control this innervation. Ganglionic blocking agents block, and nicotine stimulates, amine action. Transverse sectioning of the brain and brain stem serially from cephalad to rostrad interrupts this control when the level of the section is at the first cervical vertebra. This cervical cord center also functions to prevent reactive hypoglycemia after large meals or during the hypoglycemia of strenuous exercise. Epinephrine is released as determined by the blood glucose content or the rate of fall of blood glucose in this cord center. It is of utmost importance in the diabetic on insulin ther-

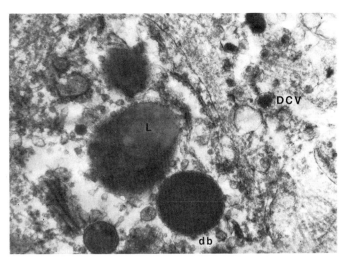

Fig. 100-8. Ultrastructure of a human pheochromocytoma. The relative size of the usual dense core vesicle (DCV) to the dense bodies (db) of the adrenal medulla is shown here. One of the dense bodies is partially replaced by a lipid-type body (L), a change considered to be characteristic of liofuscins. Other dense bodies are consistent with lysosomes, but enzymatic studies have not been done. Osmic acid fixation, uranyl acetate stain, 46,125X (Reproduced with permission from R. P. Sherwin, The adrenal medulla, paraganglia, and related tissues, in Endocrine Pathology. Baltimore, Williams & Wilkins, 1968.)

apy. Infants and children have been described with a defect in this regulatory mechanism and reduced epinephrine response to insulin-induced hypoglycemia.[35]

Epinephrine has been identified in the urine of some patients after bilateral adrenalectomy, suggesting that paraganglia rest cells in the sympathetic chain, perhaps in the area of Zuckerkandl, regain functional importance. However, steroids are the only replacement therapy required in patients after bilateral adrenalectomy.

SYMPATHETIC NERVES

The peripheral sympathetic nervous system is invaluable to the well-being of upright man. He cannot procreate or ambulate without it. Therefore, its vascular supply is of critical importance. Small arteries perfuse the larger peripheral nerve trunks and ganglia. These muscular vessels are susceptible to medial thickening and atherosclerosis. Thus, a kind of autosympathectomy may develop in some patients and tend to balance perfusion deficiencies of muscles and skin. The terminal neurons and central vasomotor centers are nourished by terminal arterioles that are susceptible to pathological changes of internal hypertrophy, collagen displacement, and lumen encroachment. The more common entities are arteriolosclerosis, diabetic vasculopathy, periarteritis nodosa, and amyloidosis. All of these may produce sympathetic nerve anoxia and degeneration. Although the sympathetic nervous system regulates venous tone, it is not known whether venous insufficiency and varicosities can produce sympathetic dysfunction. However, varicose veins are frequently an associated finding in patients with postural hypotension and autonomic insufficiency.[36]

Central Components

The sympathetic nervous system is comprised of central and peripheral components. The control centers are still a matter of intense investigation and debate. However, it is accepted that there are inhibitory and excitatory centers and tracts that regulate outflow to the peripheral sympathetic nerves. Afferent barorecep-

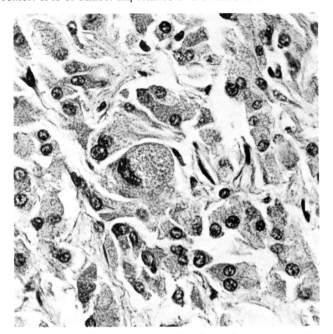

Fig. 100-7. Coarsely granular tumor cells of pheochromocytoma. Most of the tumor cells exhibit coarse, basophilic granules in the cytoplasm, some being as large as $2~\mu$ in diameter and most just within the limits of resolution of the microscope. The cytoplasm of the cell in the center is literally bulging with granules, and its enlarged nucleus appears to be displaced. Formalin fixation, H & E, 355X. (Reproduced with permission from R. P. Sherwin, The adrenal medulla, paraganglia, and related tissues, in Endocrine Pathology. Baltimore, Williams & Wilkins, 1968.)

tor fibers serve to tonically inhibit sympathetic outflow. Pressor receptors in the carotid sinuses and aorta, stimulated by the distending arterial pressure, serve to constantly bombard the vasomotor inhibitory center in the medulla. This center, in turn, inhibits sympathetic outflow.[6] The characteristics of the receptors of these inhibitory fibers are those of the alpha type. On the other hand, there are vasomotor centers in the medulla which when stimulated give rise to sympathetic hypertonicity.[37,38] The nature of these neurones and their receptors is not known. However, recently some areas described as A_1 and A_2 have been found to have high concentration of epinephrine-synthesizing enzyme, PNMT.[10] Because centrally acting beta-blockers and PNMT inhibitors can lower blood pressure, it is tempting to think that at least some stimulatory sympathetic pathways are beta-receptor-mediated.[10,39] *This hypothetical scheme* is shown in Fig. 100-4.

Peripheral Components

The peripheral organization of the sympathetic nervous system is generally accepted. The scheme in Fig. 100-1 is taken from Goodman and Gilman.[40] The main structures of the sympathetic nervous system are the sympathetic chains running parallel with and to either side of the vertebral column from the base of the cranium to the coccyx. They are comprised of a series of ganglia connected by longitudinal fibers. The white rami, restricted to the thoracolumbar outflow, carry myelinated preganglionic fibers from the spinal roots to the vertebral ganglia. The ganglia are swellings that accommodate the preganglionic-axonal–postganglionic-dendrite connection as well as the cell bodies of the postganglionic neurones. In addition, there are ganglion cells that do not participate directly in neuronal transmission. The postganglionic axonal extensions travel in unmyelinated nerves and are connected to the spinal nerves as gray rami. The spinal nerves are distributed to the tissues in target organs. In addition to NGF, other tropic factors, including cholinergic neurones within the spinal intermediolateral tracts, regulate development of peripheral adrenergic nerves.[41]

The storage of neurotransmitter-norepinephrine takes place in varicosities of the peripheral postganglionic nerve terminal. However, the enzyme machinery is manufactured in the cell bodies and shipped in packets down the axon to the terminal via a process called pinocytosis. Accumulation of enzymes proximal to a ligature and loss of dopamine-beta-hydroxylase distally can be demonstrated in the ligated splanchnic nerve during stimulation.[42]

BIOCHEMISTRY

BIOSYNTHESIS

The catecholamines—dopamine, norepinephrine, and epinephrine—are 3,4-dihydroxy derivatives of phenylethylamine. The biosynthesis of these amines occurs in the chromaffin cells of the adrenal medulla, in the central nervous system, and in the adrenergic neurones of postganglionic sympathetic fibers. Biosynthesis is regulated by end-product inhibition. The structural resemblance of phenylalanine and tyrosine to epinephrine suggested to early researchers that these amino acids were precursors on the biosynthetic pathway. The conversion of tyrosine to epinephrine involves four steps: (1) ring hydroxylation, (2) side-chain hydroxylation, (3) decarboxylation, and (4) N-methylation. The pathway considered to be quantitatively important of 24 possible sequences of these reactions was proposed by Blaschko[57] in 1939 (Fig. 100-2A and 100-2C).

The major support for this pathway came from isotope tracer studies. Gurin and Delluva were able to isolate radioactive epinephrine from rat adrenal glands after administering ^{3}H and ^{14}C-labeled phenylalanine, thereby demonstrating a ^{14}C-phenylalanine → ^{14}C-tyrosine → ^{14}C-epinephrine pathway.[58] Demis proved 3,4-dihydroxy-L-phenylalanine (Dopa) was a precursor when he found that ^{14}C-Dopa added to bovine adrenal glands homogenate was rapidly decarboxylated, with 2 to 3 percent of the radioactivity appearing as norepinephrine.[59] The pathway was further elucidated by the in vivo study of Leeper and Udenfriend.[60] They found five to ten times the specific activity in ^{14}C-norepinephrine isolated from rat adrenals when ^{14}C-dopamine was administered rather than ^{14}C-dopa. This evidence strongly suggested that dopamine was the more immediate precursor. Goodall and Kirshner incubated ^{14}C-tyrosine and ^{14}C-dopa with bovine adrenal slices.[61] Maximum isotope appeared in dopamine at 2 hours, in norepinephrine at 6 hours, and in epinephrine only very slowly, suggesting that norepinephrine was the immediate precursor to epinephrine. The name, norepinephrine, stems from the compound's proximal relationship to epinephrine, "nor-" standing for the initials of the German "*N-Ohne Radikal*" (without a radical on the nitrogen). Final acceptance of this pathway came in 1964 with the discovery of tyrosine hydroxylase.[50]

Tyrosine Hydroxylase

Characterization. Tyrosine hydroxylase (EC 1.14.3.a) is a soluble and particulate bound oxygen oxidoreductase (3-hydroxylating) found in the adrenal medulla, brain, and sympathetically innervated tissues.[50] Tyrosine hydroxylase (TH) is active in cytoplasm where it catalyzes the conversion of L-tyrosine to L-dopa according to reaction 1:

$$\text{Tyrosine} + \text{tetrahydropteridine} + O_2 \rightarrow \text{3,4-dihydroxy-L-phenyl-alanine} + \text{dihydrobiopterin} + H_2O \quad (1)$$

The enzyme requires tetrahydropteridine as cofactor.[62] The Michaelis constant, K_m, for tyrosine and tetrahydropteridine was not affected by Fe^{2+}, but the V_{max} *in vitro* was increased twofold by the inclusion of 0.5 mM Fe^{2+}.[63] Purified tyrosine hydroxylase is sensitive to H_2O_2 generated during the nonenzymatic oxidation of tetrahydropterin. In the presence of catalase, which protects tyrosine hydroxylase from peroxide-mediated inactivation, Fe^{++} does not stimulate the reaction.[64] It appears that the ability of Fe^{2+} to decompose H_2O_2 is responsible for the observed increase in tyrosine hydroxylase activity.

Packets of tyrosine hydroxylase are propagated via axonal flow to the nerve terminal. Some tyrosine hydroxylase may be synthesized in the peripheral nerve ending.

Rate-limiting Step. A model of end-product feedback regulation of catecholamine synthesis has been formulated on the basis of in vivo and in vitro studies which showed inhibition of adrenal tyrosine hydroxylase by tyrosine analogues and catechol derivatives.[50] The evidence supporting tyrosine hydroxylase as the rate-limiting step was convincing: (1) dopamine was a better precursor of norepinephrine in beef adrenal slices than tyrosine;[61] (2) the K_m for tyrosine → norepinephrine, 0.055 mM, was the same as for tyrosine → dopa in the isolated guinea pig heart preparation;[50] (3) the activity of tyrosine hydroxylase in adrenal medulla slices was 20–40 mμM/g/hr, while the activities of dopamine-β-hydroxylase and dopa decarboxylase were greater than 10,000 mμM/g/hr;[50] and (4) the tissue concentration of tyrosine is 10^{-4}M, while dopa and dopamine are normally undetectable.[50] These findings indicated that the tyrosine → dopa reaction was the rate-determining step in catecholamine synthesis. The concentration of tyrosine in human blood is 10–15 μg/ml, and it is the biologically important precursor of the catecholamines.

Inhibition. The hydroxylation of phenylalanine to tyrosine in the adrenal gland may be nonenzymatic, casting further doubt on the physiologic significance of phenylalanine as a precursor.[65] In phenylketonuria, however, the accumulation of phenylalanine metabolites may result in some inhibition of norepinephrine synthesis and depression of norepinephrine excretion.[66]

Tyrosine hydroxylase activity may be inhibited by a variety of compounds (Fig. 100-2C and Table 100-2). Competitive inhibitors are mainly tyrosine derivatives. Alpha-methyltyrosine is effective in the therapy of pheochromocytoma, causing a reduction of excretion and turnover of norepinephrine and its metabolites.[67] Although alpha-methyltyrosine reduces neurotransmitter synthesis and excretion in primary hypertension, it is less effective than

alpha-methyldopa as an antihypertensive for this disorder. The side effects of alpha-methyltyrosine in decreasing order are sedation (with insomnia on withdrawal), anxiety, tremor, diarrhea, and galactorrhea. Crystalluria occurred in animals given 50 mg/kg per day but not in patients receiving between 11 and 73 mg/kg per day.[67] Parkinsonlike features have occurred in patients after long-term use of alpha-methyltyrosine.[68] These effects, although generally reversible, may be due to reduction of dopamine content in basal ganglia.

The halogenated tyrosines, especially the iodinated series, also have inhibitory properties.[69,70] Thus, thyroxinelike analogues, precursors (3-iodotyrosine), and metabolites may account for some degree of tyrosine hydroxylase inhibition *in vivo*. Interestingly, and perhaps bearing on this point, plasma norepinephrine content is reduced in hyperthyroidism and increased in hypothyroidism.[71] Although these changes may be attributable to reflex decrease and increase of sympathetic nerve tonicity, respectively,

Table 100-2. Pharmacologic and Physiologic Effectors of Catecholamine Synthesis and Degradation

Action	Mechanism	Effector	Site*
Biosynthesis enhanced	Sympathetic stimulation (enzyme induction)	Exercise Hypothermia Mental stress	1> 3> 4
	Presynaptic α-receptor blockade	Phentolamine Phenoxybenzamine	
	Precursor supplementation	L-dopa	2
	Enzyme activation	Corticosteroids	1> 3> 4
		Chlorpromazine	1,2
		Reserpine	1
	Reducion of NE content (feedback inhibition by NE, NE degradation by MAO)	Reserpine	7
Reduced	Feedback inhibition	Epinephrine Norepinephrine Dopamine Dopa	1
	Degradation inhibition	Pargyline	7
	TH inhibition	α-Methyl-p-tyrosine 3-Iodotyrosine 3,4-Dihydroxyphenylpropylacetamide	1
	DDC inhibition	α-Methyldopa α-Methyldopa hydrazine (MK-485)	2
	DBH inhibition ($\uparrow$ dopamine, $\downarrow$ NE)	Benzylhydrazines Disulfiram Benzyloxyamines Picolinic acid derivatives Tropolone Tyramine**	3
	PNMT inhibition	Tranylcypromine SKF 7698 Pargyline (weakly) Nialamide (weakly)	4
Metabolism enhanced	Slow amine displacement (degraded by MAO)	Reserpine Guanethidine	7
	Rapid amine displacement (sympathomimetics)	Tyramine Ephedrine Amphetamine	5,8
	Interference with reuptake at nerve terminals	Cocaine Imipramine Chlorpromazine	6
Reduced	MAO inhibitors	Debrisoquine Pargyline Tranylcypromine Nialamide	7
	COMT inhibitors	Pyrogallol	8

*Refer to Fig. 2C, which illustrates sites.
**Storage displacement and competitive inhibition.

possibilities for control of norepinephrine synthesis by thyroxine and its analogues exist.

Another class of tyrosine hydroxylase inhibitors chelate iron and thus reduce the content of bioavailable cofactor. One of these is alpha-dipyridyl.[66] Thus the quantitation of tyrosine hydroxylase activity via *in vitro* techniques may not reflect *in vivo* synthesis rates, since iron is added in excess to the test tube assay. The experiments with iron are complicated by the nonenzymatic conversion of tyrosine to dopa by iron.

The third major series of inhibitors are those that compete for the pteridine cofactor. Most of these are catechol compounds including a catechol isostere, 4-isopropyltropolone.[111] Norepinephrine, epinephrine, and dopamine are thought to exert their "feedback inhibition" by competing for cofactor. Complexes of the Schiff base type are formed, thus removing the pteridine from the active enzyme site. None of these latter two classes of compounds is used clinically for their tyrosine hydroxylase inhibiting properties.

It has been suggested that the tyrosine hydroxylase of chromaffin tumors is not bound by the usual product inhibition. Nagatsu has described an increased tyrosine hydroxylase activity of chromaffin tumors and its relative lack of inhibition by norepinephrine and epinephrine.[72] Increased tyrosine hydroxylase activities have also been reported in hearts and adrenals of a neurogenic model of hypertension, the SAD rabbit. Similarly, vas deferens specimens of man with elevated systolic blood pressure have increased tyrosine hydroxylase content as compared with normotensive controls and men with increased diastolic blood pressure (see Chapter 104).

Adrenal and neuronal tyrosine hydroxylase activities were increased in animals treated with ganglionic blocking agents and reserpine, respectively. Tyrosine hydroxylase deficiency has been identified in immunosympathetomized animals and in patients and animals with congestive heart failure.[73,74] The reduction in tyrosine hydroxylase content is thought to be secondary to neuronal degeneration and impaired protein synthesis. Thus, tyrosine hydroxylase activity is a reliable tissue marker of intact sympathetic nerve function and neurotransmitter synthesis. It may be a better marker of sympathetic nerve activity than norepinephrine content per se, since defective norepinephrine storage may occur in association with increased tyrosine hydroxylase synthesis.

Dopa Decarboxylase

Characterization. Dopa decarboxylase (L-3,4-dihydroxyphenylalanine decarboxylyase) (EC 4.1.1.26) catalyzes the decarboxylation of Dopa to 3,4-dihydroxyphenylethylamine (dopamine) according to reaction 2:

3,4-dihydroxy-L-phenylalanine →

$$\text{3,4-dihydroxyphenylethylamine} + CO_2 \quad (2)$$

This soluble enzyme is tightly bound to pyridoxal phosphate, which activates the reaction.[75] Dopa decarboxylase is found in all tissues, the highest concentration in humans being in the liver, kidneys, brain, and vas deferens. It was the first enzyme of the series to be characterized.[76] There are a number of decarboxylases in various species which have slightly different substrate specificities, i.e., phenylalanine decarboxylase and dihydroxyphenylalanine decarboxylase. The enzyme dopa decarboxylase from the guinea pig will decarboxylate tryptophan but at two-thirds the rate at which it decarboxylates tyrosine or dopa. Dopa decarboxylase is also known as "aromatic L-amino acid decarboxylase" because of this broad specificity.

Inhibition. Inhibitors of dopa decarboxylase fall into two categories, competitive inhibitors whose structures resemble dopa, i.e., alpha-methyldopa, and halogenated compounds which form Schiff bases with cofactor. These amines, metabolites of alpha-methyldopa, are then taken up into central and peripheral nerves, stored, and subsequently released in place of norepinephrine. These products were called false transmitters because they were less potent than norepinephrine. It was thought that this was the major mechanism of antihypertensive action. However, at the present time alpha-methyldopa metabolites are thought to stimulate alpha-receptors of the inhibitory corticobulbar system in the central nervous system, thus reducing peripheral sympathetic nerve discharge and decreasing blood pressure.

Alpha-methyldopa and other decarboxylase inhibitors have been administered to patients with pheochromocytoma to reduce tumor norepinephrine biosynthesis without clinical success. Evidently, insufficient concentration of the enzyme inhibitors can be attained to overcome the K_m and content of the intraneuronal enzymes. The inhibitors play a role in the therapy of Parkinson's disease. Carbidopa does not cross the blood-brain barrier, but it exerts its peripheral decarboxylase inhibition and prevents peripheral degradation of 1-dopa with which it is coadministered. Thus, higher 1-dopa levels are available at central sites where 1-dopa is converted to dopamine and replenishes deficient basal ganglia stores.

Dopamine-Beta-Hydroxylase

Characterization. The aerobic hydroxylation of dopamine to norepinephrine is catalyzed by dopamine-beta-hydroxylase (DBH) (EC 1.14.2.1). Its requirement for oxygen and an external electron donor classify it as a mixed function oxidase. An external reducing agent donates a pair of electrons. The substrate donates the second pair to reduce O_2 to a hydroxyl group. Dopamine-beta-hydroxylase is released from the vesicles of the nerve ending or adrenal medulla with norepinephrine discharge. Although there is a reuptake mechanism for norepinephrine, none is known to be available for DBH. DBH reaches the venous system via the lymph. An enzyme of 290,000 mol wt, it has been purified, and antibodies to it have been manufactured for use in its quantitative analysis in biological fluids[77] and tissues via immunofluorescense.[78–81] The enzyme does not occur in tissues outside the neurone.

The requirement of DBH for copper has been investigated by Friedman and Kaufman.[82] They have found copper present in a concentration of 0.65–1.0 μg/mg enzyme (4–7 mol Cu/mol protein). The copper may be removed using potassium cyanide, resulting in enzyme inactivation which can only be reactivated 40 percent with the addition of Cu^{2+}. While the cuprous content of a given preparation may vary, the cupric content was shown to remain constant at 2 mol/mol enzyme.

Given ascorbate as the electron donor, Cu^{2+} as part of the active site, and fumarate as a modulator of activity, DBH can catalyze the conversion of 1000 mol dopamine per mol enzyme per minute at 25° C according to reaction 3:[85]

Dopamine + ascorbate + O_2 →

$$\text{1-noradrenaline} + \text{dehydroascorbate} + H_2O \quad (3)$$

Fumarate decreases the K_m but does not affect the V_{max}.[83] By shifting the O_2 binding equilibrium, fumarate may facilitate the formation of the reduced enzyme-oxygen complex.

An elegant kinetic analysis of the dopamine-β-hydroxylation reaction has been made by Goldstein et al.[83] Their analysis of the initial velocity patterns indicates a ping-pong mechanism (in the nomenclature of Cleland[84]), where the enzymatic binding of the first substrate, ascorbate, is followed by the release of the product, dehydroascorbate, before a second substrate can react. Subsequent substrates, dopamine and O_2, form a central ternary complex with the enzyme in the rate-limiting step of the β-hydroxylation reaction.

DBH substrates require a benzene ring with a two- or three-carbon atom side chain and terminal amine. *Meta*-hydroxyl or *para*-hydroxyl substitutions, or both, will increase hydroxylation while *ortho*-hydroxyl groups will eliminate activity.[85] This broad specificity of DBH is consistent with two alternative pathways for norepinephrine or epinephrine synthesis: (1) tyrosine → tyramine → norsynephrine → norepinephrine, and (2) tyrosine → dopa → dopamine → epinine → epinephrine. The dopamine to epinine reaction is catalyzed by a nonspecific N-methyltransferase. Neither alternative pathway has been shown to have clinical significance.

The preference that DBH shows for the reaction utilizing dopamine may be due to compartmentalization of this enzyme. Indeed, DBH is found in the particulate fraction of adrenal homogenates,[86] while dopa decarboxylase is present in the soluble portion. Gagnon et al.[87] pulse-labeled DBH with 50 μCi/ml ^{3}H-leucine and followed the time course of the appearance of newly synthesized DBH in the various subcellular compartments of adrenal medulla cells. Their findings suggest that newly synthesized DBH is incorporated directly into storage vesicles.

Traditional staining methods show intensely dark staining granules containing norepinephrine and lighter staining granules containing epinephrine. More recently, the vesicles have been observed as small intensely fluorescent (SIF) cells using immunofluorescent techniques.[78-80] The multiplicity of functions that these vesicles are now known to be involved in include uptake, biosynthesis, storage, and secretion of catecholamines. Chromaffin vesicle membranes contain DBH, ATPase (EC 3.6.1.3), cytochrome b561 and cytochrome b561:NADH reductase (EC 1.6.99.3).[88] Catalytic sites of DBH are available to substrate only from the interior of the intact vesicle.[89] The stimulatory effects of Mg^{2+}-ATP on substrate uptake by the vesicle membrane and the inhibitory effect on uptake caused by reserpine indicate an ATPase-mediated active transport of substrates.[89] The function of cytochrome b561 and its reductase is unknown.

Inhibition. Disulfiram (Antabuse) inhibits DBH activity by binding copper ions. Large doses in rats reduce cardiac norepinephrine and increase tissue dopamine.[90,91] The chelating properties of disulfiram also inhibit the Fe^{2+}-dependent tyrosine hydroxylase reaction. There are additional potent inhibitors—picolinic acid and its derivatives whose actions are noncompetitive and do not involve chelation of copper.[60] The drug fusaric acid (5-butyl picolinic acid) inhibits DBH in both animals and man.[113] DBH inhibition by disulfiram is probably of no clinical importance.

Phenylethanolamine-N-
Methyltransferase

Characterization. Phenylethanolamine-N-methyltransferase (PNMT) (EC 2.1.1.f) is the enzyme that catalyzes the N-methylation of norepinephrine to form epinephrine. Because PNMT is highly localized in the soluble fraction of the adrenal medulla,[54] it is believed that norepinephrine is converted to epinephrine in the cytosol. In vivo and in vitro studies show that the methyl group of methionine[92] or S-adenosylmethionine[93] may be used by PNMT in the N-methylation reaction. PNMT will also methylate the nor-

mally occurring phenylethanolamine derivatives normetanephrine, octopamine, synephrine, metanephrine, and epinephrine (N,N-dimethyl derivative). PNMT is strongly inhibited by physiologic concentrations of epinephrine, providing feedback regulation of its synthesis.

Steroid Dependence. The first evidence of a hormonal role in the regulation of catecholamine biosynthesis came when Coupland[94] observed that chromaffin cells store noradrenalin when they are not in contact with adrenal cortical tissue. Wurtman et al.[95] found that glucocorticoids have no effect on PNMT activity in vitro, but in vivo dexamethasone caused an increase in PNMT activity. The dexamethasone effect took many hours or even days to reach a plateau and could be blocked by actinomycin D or puromycin. These results implied a glucocorticoid-induced synthesis of PNMT enzyme. This was confirmed by measurement of ^{3}H-tyrosine incorporation into dog adrenal medulla PNMT protein; hypophysectomized dogs accumulated less ^{3}H-PNMT that did control dogs or hypophysectomized dogs treated with ACTH.[95] Thus, hormonal factors are involved in the control of PNMT synthesis.

Only in the mammalian embryo is an adrenal medulla, composed largely of chromaffin cells, surrounded by a cortex of steroid-secreting tissue.[96] This peculiar arrangement allows for preferential delivery of glucocorticoid hormones to the medulla via an intra-adrenal portal vascular system; glucocorticoids in this vascular system are 100 times the concentration of systemic arterial blood.[97] This explains why simple replacement dosages of dexamethasone fail to induce PNMT in hypophysectomized dogs. The delivery of lower concentrations of glucocorticoids via systemic arterial blood alone would result in decreased synthesis[97] and secretion[98] of catecholamines as well as a reduction in the mass of medullary chromaffin cells.[96] These effects are not entirely due to PNMT induction. Hydrocortisone is known to cause an increase in the number of chromaffin cells *in vivo*[78,79] and *in vitro*.[80] Nerve growth factor is also known to enhance the growth and differentiation of sympathetic neurons. A selective induction of TH and DBH is observed in newborn rats treated with nerve growth factor for 10 days.[99] This induction is not accounted for simply on the basis of increases in ganglia volume. It appears that hormones play an integral role in catecholamine biosynthesis through enzyme induction and formation of adrenergic structures.

Inhibition. The clinical value of reducing PNMT activity was suggested by animal studies using the PNMT inhibitor [3-methyl-1,2,3,4-tetrahydro[1]benzo thiono-(3,2-C)] pyridine hydrochloride (SKF 7698).[100] The lowering of PNMT activity in A_1 and A_2 areas of the brain stem in Doca-salt hypertensive rats and in spontaneous hypertension was associated with normalization of blood pressure.

Neurogenic Induction of Enzyme Activity

Catecholamine biosynthesis and tyrosine hydroxylase activity are increased after prolonged psychosocial stimulus.[101] This response to chronic sympathetic nerve activity is due to formation of new TH.[104] Although norepinephrine synthesis is increased after short periods of nerve stimulation,[114] the content of tyrosine hydroxylase is not increased. This suggests that conformational changes may take place which activate the enzyme; as the level of norepinephrine is reduced in the cytosol, feedback inhibition is also reduced. Induction of TH is linked to the physiologic demand for catecholamines from the stored supply. For example, the blocking agent, phenoxybenzamine, decreases adrenal catecholamine levels by 70 percent and increases TH activity and norepinephrine biosynthesis, while another alpha blocking agent, phentolamine, has no effect on catecholamine content, biosynthesis, or TH activity.[105]

A neuronally mediated induction of DBH has also been reported.[106] When reserpine is given to rats for 6 days, there is an increase in the DBH of sympathetic stellate ganglia and nerve terminals of the heart[106] and adrenal gland.[107] If the preganglionic nerve to the superior cervical ganglia is cut unilaterally before administration of reserpine, the increase in DBH is observed only in the innervated ganglia. Cycloheximide blocks the reserpine-induced increase in stellate ganglia DBH. These results indicate a transsynaptic induction of DBH synthesis.

The influence of neural and endocrine factors differs in the biosynthesis of catecholamine-synthesizing enzymes. Thus, while denervation will abolish increases in activity of TH and DBH, the stress-induced increases in PNMT persist. Hypophysectomy abolishes these increases in PNMT activity, slightly reduces DBH activity, and leaves TH activity unchanged. Thus, TH activity depends largely upon the neural component. DBH activity is mainly dependent upon the neural component but may depend to some extent on the endocrine component for maintenance. PNMT is largely under endocrine control.

The net and total formation of catecholamines are dependent upon a large set of variables. They include (1) the amount and activities of biosynthetic enzymes; (2) the kinetics of uptake processes: tyrosine → chromaffin cell, dopamine → chromaffin vesicles; (3) the rate of catecholamine release; and (4) the rate of uptake into mitochondria where monoamine oxidase can degrade the amine.

In cases where new enzyme protein is induced, it generally constitutes an adaptive mechanism to maintain homeostasis in response to some physiologic stress. This response could profoundly contribute to the symptoms associated with many metabolic disorders. Lower glucocorticoid levels in the blood, such as that seen after hypophysectomy or in idiopathic Addison's disease, would result in depressed epinephrine synthesis. The decrease in epinephrine synthesis, and thereby release, leads to decreased activation of target tissues. This is the case in pituitary insufficiency where postprandial hypoglycemia is associated with a diminished epinephrine response, creating an insulin sensitivity. Inappropriate catecholamine synthesis may be associated with Parkinson's disease, idiopathic orthostatic hypotension (Chapter 103),[108] primary hypertension (Chapter 104), pheochromocytoma (Chapter 102), and familial dysautonomia (Chapter 103).[109]

STORAGE, RELEASE, AND UPTAKE OF CATECHOLAMINES

Catecholamines are found in various sympathetically innervated organs: highest in the adrenal medulla (0.5–1 mg/g); less in the spleen, vas deferens, parts of the brain, and the spinal cord (1–5 μg/g); and least in the liver, gut, and skeletal muscles (0.1–0.5 μg/g).

Storage

Adrenal Medulla. In 1953, Blaschko and Welch and Hillarp et al. demonstrated that catecholamines of the adrenal medulla were stored in dense granules which can be separated by density-gradient centrifugation.[115,116] Electron-microscopic studies have shown that these granules are approximately 1μ in diameter. The granules are multifunctional organelles designed for uptake, storage, biosynthesis, and secretion of catecholamines. The granules contain catecholamines, lipids, adenine nucleotides, Ca^{2+} and

Mg^{2+}, and water-soluble proteins, chromogranins. The primary component of the latter is chromogranin A. Catecholamines are bound to ATP in a ratio of 4:1 (0.55 M catecholamines and 0.13 M adenine nucleotides). The ratio of catecholamines to ATP in granules isolated from pheochromocytoma is much higher.[117] Catecholamines and ATP are present with proteins in a ratio approaching electrical equivalence, thereby maintaining the amines in a nondiffusible complex. The interior surface of the membrane of the chromaffin granules contains dopamine-beta-hydroxylase and ATPase. The latter regulates catecholamine transport into the vesicle.

The high concentration of catecholamines within the granules requires an ATP-dependent membrane transport mechanism.[118] In fact, the ATP-Mg^{2+} complex increases the uptake of norepinephrine, epinephrine, and dopamine into the granules and inhibits their release. Reserpine and prenylamine inhibit the effects of ATP-Mg^{2+}.[119] Storage vesicle uptake is important in maintaining catecholamine stores. Norepinephrine leaves the granules, is N-methylated in the cytoplasm to epinephrine, and then reenters a different group of granules where it is stored. Epinephrine accounts for approximately 80 percent of the catecholamines (CA) of the human adrenal medulla. The remaining 20 percent is norepinephrine. On the other hand, the urinary excretion pattern of epinephrine to norepinephrine is reversed, with 80 to 90 percent present as norepinephrine. Small amounts of dopamine have been found in the granules isolated from the adrenal medulla of sheep.[119]

Nerve stimulation of the adrenal medulla stimulates catecholamines secretion by exocytosis. Vesicles fuse with the membrane of the adrenal chromaffin cell, and their contents are extruded into the extracellular space. There is influx of calcium ions, release of ATP, chromogranin, and DBH simultaneously with catecholamine secretion.[120] There is a proportional release of catecholamines and ATP from the perfused cat adrenal gland.[121] The ratio of DBH/CA released in the perfusate, however, was only a small fraction of the ratio in the soluble lysate of purified chromaffin vesicles. Furthermore, secretion of catecholamines was reduced after reserpine, while DBH secretion remained unchanged, suggesting an independence of release of DBH and catecholamines.[122] Incubation of adrenal medulla in a suspension medium produces a spontaneous release of catecholamines that is dependent on temperature and pH. A pH below 6 enhances the release of catecholamines. At 0° C the catecholamine content of the isolated adrenal medulla vesicles is stable, whereas it decreases rapidly at temperatures above 10° C.

Sympathetic Nerves. In 1956, von Euler and Hillarp demonstrated norepinephrine storage within particles in the peripheral sympathetic nerves of bovine and rat spleens.[123] From 80 to 90 percent of nerve noradrenaline is present in the storage vesicles, and the remainder is in the cytosol in equilibrium with the granules. Norepinephrine in the cytosol appears to regulate synthesis through feedback inhibition of tyrosine hydroxylase. Granules have been identified in nonterminal axons and terminal varicosities of sympathetic nerves by density gradient and by electron microscopy. The nerve granules participate actively in the synthesis of norepinephrine. The hydroxylation of tyrosine to dopa occurs during the passage of the former through the axonal membrane, whereas the decarboxylation of dopa to dopamine takes place in the cytoplasm. Dopamine then enters the granules where it is converted to norepinephrine by the action of dopamine-beta-hydroxylase.

Three types of norepinephrine-storing particles have been found in sympathetic nervous fibers: large dense-cored vesicles having a diameter of 800–1200 Å, small dense-core vesicles, and small clear vesicles having a diameter of 300–600 Å. The large dense-core vesicles of splenic nerve axons contain norepinephrine, ATP, chromogranin A, and dopamine-beta-hydroxylase. The norepinephrine content of these granules is much less than that of chromaffin granules of the adrenal medulla (10–100 nM of norepinephrine versus 2500 nM/mg protein). However, the content of dopamine-beta-hydroxylase is much higher in sympathetic nerve granules. The low concentration of norepinephrine in axonal nerve vesicles may be due to immaturity. The vesicles probably reach their maximum norepinephrine content in nerve terminals.[124] It has been suggested that the large granules are relatively deficient in norepinephrine in preterminal axons, but they take up more norepinephrine in the terminal. The molar ratio of CA/ATP in the nerve vesicles has generally been assumed to be 4:1 as in the adrenal granules. However, Lagercrantz et al. have recently estimated the ratio of NE/ATP to be about 12:1 and 18:1 in the proximal and distal nerve vesicles, respectively.[125] Less is known about the composition of small, dense-cored vesicles that contain norepinephrine and ATP in a molar ratio ranging from 2.2 to 3.7. Dopamine-beta-hydroxylase is present in small vesicles of nerve terminals of vas deferens.[126]

Granules storing norepinephrine have also been found in the sympathetic ganglia, which are similar to although less numerous than the heavy type of noradrenergic vesicle found in nerve axons and terminals.

Central Sympathetic Nerves. Norepinephrine is present in the mammalian brain and spinal cord, mainly in the hypothalamus, the central gray matter of the mesencephalon, and the area postrema. The amount of epinephrine in most regions, except the brain stem, is thought to be negligible. From 60 to 80 percent of norepinephrine is present in synaptosomes and particles within nerve endings. However, there is no hard evidence that nerve endings contain more than one type of granule. Dopamine represents more than 50 percent of the total catecholamine content in the brain and spinal cord of many species. Approximately 80 percent of the total cerebral dopamine is present within the basal ganglia complex, the corpus striatum content being particularly abundant.[127] Dopamine within the brain seems to be stored within dense-core vesicles in the synaptosomes.

Release

The release of norepinephrine from the terminal varicosities of a sympathetic neurone is initiated by the arrival of action potentials. Calcium ions enter into the terminal, and subsequently norepinephrine is released by exocytosis. Norepinephrine is released from the large noradrenergic vesicles; the function of small vesicles is less clear. Small vesicles containing DBH may derive from the residual membrane of larger ones. A spontaneous release of catecholamines from vesicles isolated from the splenic nerve can take place. This release is higher than that from vesicles of the adrenal medulla and is dependent on temperature.

Reserpine inhibits the spontaneous release of noradrenaline from noradrenergic vesicles of the splenic nerves but not that of ATP, leading to a change of the molar ratio amine/ATP.[117,128] Tyramine releases norepinephrine from nerve terminals, primarily from the free store in the cytosol, whereas the nerve impulse releases norepinephrine mostly from the large granules by exocytosis. Cocaine prevents and MAO inhibitors increase the amount of norepinephrine released by tyramine, whereas these drugs do not affect the release of norepinephrine by impulses. Ca^{2+} is obligatory for the release of norepinephrine by nerve impulses but not by tyramine. Prostaglandin E_2 inhibits and angiotensin II potentiates the release of norepinephrine by nerve impulses but do not affect the amount released by tyramine.[129] Furthermore, tyramine does not release DBH. Phenoxybenzamine, an alpha-adrenergic blocking agent, increases the release of amines from nerve vesicles via blockade of alpha-presynaptic receptor. These aspects of release and others involving prostaglandins and angiotensin will be discussed in Chapter 101.

Uptake

Uptake 1. After release of norepinephrine from the nerve terminals, approximately 75 to 80 percent of the amount released is transported from the extracellular space across the axonal membranes of adrenergic nerves into the free catecholamine pool in the cytosol. Subsequently, catecholamines are actively taken up into the granules to reestablish the equilibrium between the free and bound pools. This process is called "uptake 1." A similar process exists in the central nervous system both for norepinephrine and for dopamine. Whitby et al. demonstrated in 1961 that reuptake 1 of catecholamines is an important mechanism for the inactivation of these amines.[130] Uptake 1 results from an active membrane carrier system requiring metabolic energy. This process is inhibited by many sympathomimetic amines such as metaraminol and levorotatory amphetamine, which act as competitive substrates for uptake 1.[131,132] Other drugs inhibit uptake 1. The most potent among these are amitriptiline, imipramine, and desipramine. The latter is the most potent of all known inhibitors of uptake 1. Bretylium, guanethidine, cocaine, phenoxybenzamine, chlorpromazine, dischloroisoprenaline, and the monoamine-oxidase inhibitors harmine, tranylcypromine, and phenelzine also inhibit uptake 1. Reserpine and prenylamine have no effect on uptake 1. Neuronal uptake has an absolute requirement for Na^+; a low concentration of K^+ stimulates and high concentrations of K^+ inhibit uptake 1. Neither Ca^{2+} nor Mg^{2+} has any effect on uptake 1.

Dopamine Uptake. An uptake process for dopamine has been recognized for dopamine-containing neurones in the central nervous system. This process can be inhibited by both stereoisomers of amphetamine and by many anticholinergic and antihistaminic drugs. Dopamine uptake is, however, not inhibited by desipramine and other tricyclic antidepressants.

Uptake 2. Extraneuronal peripheral tissues, such as cardiac muscle cells, vascular smooth muscle, collagen, or elastin, and certain glandular tissues may bind catecholamines. Extraneuronal uptake comprises two major mechanisms: intracellular uptake and binding to connective tissue. Although uptake 1 is most effective at low concentrations of catecholamines, higher concentrations of catecholamines are taken up more rapidly by the cardiac muscle or smooth muscle cells by uptake 2. This process is different from uptake 1 in that it has a higher affinity for isoprenaline followed by epinephrine and, finally, norepinephrine. Uptake 2 is not highly specific; in fact, 5-hydroxytryptamine and histamine can also be transported. Uptake of catecholamines by this process is rapidly followed by intracellular catabolism and not by storage. The uptake 2 process is a saturable process and is inhibited by steroids, phenoxybenzamine and other alkylamines, normetanephrine, metanephrine, anti-MAO, anti-COMT, and by cold. Uptake 2 is not affected by cocaine, metaraminol, and desmethylimipramine, which inhibit neuronal uptake. Connective tissue binding, in contrast, is insensitive to all the drugs that inhibit uptake 1 or smooth muscle uptake and is inhibited only by oxytetracycline. The function of uptake 2 seems to be that of terminating the action of norepinephrine. This role is probably of less physiologic importance than that of uptake 1, but it could become the primary factor in the inactivation of catecholamines in conditions that inhibit the uptake 1 process. Connective tissue uptake has been regarded as being of little importance. However, when this process is blocked after oxytetracycline, it can be shown that it is a major mechanism of inactivation in some tissues.

Effects on Metabolism. Neuronal reuptake (uptake 1) is the major mode of inactivating NE at nerve endings with narrow synaptic clefts.[223] The fate of this NE is more likely intraneuronal oxidative deamination to DOMA than metabolic degradation via COMT, which is active in extraneuronal sites. NE is initially inactivated via O-methylation when the uptake process is blocked, efflux is rapid, the synaptic cleft is wide, and NE is taken up into target or extraneuronal cells by uptake 2. Thus, in this way, cocaine inhibits deamination,[224] and cortisone inhibits O-methylation.[225] Therefore, the balance achieved by uptakes 1 and 2 and the presynaptic receptors modulating the rate of neuronal NE release serve to regulate the eventual metabolic pathway.

METABOLISM

Pathways

Catechol-O-methyltransferase (COMT: EC 2.1.1.6) and monoamine oxidase (MAO: EC 1.4.3.4) generate O-methylated and deaminated compounds from endogenous dopamine, norepinephrine, and epinephrine (Fig. 2B).

Inactivation of the catecholamines by deamination was described by Blaschko et al.[133] They found that epinephrine was a substrate for an "amine oxidase." Subsequently, another degradative step was suggested after finding 4-hydroxy-3-methoxymandelic acid in human urine.[134] After parenteral administration of norepinephrine or the ingestion of 3,4-dihydroxymandelic acid (DOMA), the urinary excretion of the O-methylated deaminated metabolite 4-hydroxy-3-methoxymandelic acid (vanillylmandelic acid, VMA) increased: VMA concentrations were also found to be higher in the urine of patients with the catecholamine-secreting tumor pheochromocytoma.[135] Axelrod and his co-workers[136,138] demonstrated that O-methylated metabolites of dopamine, norepinephrine, and epinephrine in tissues and urine were intermediates in the formation of VMA.

COMT introduces a methyl group, usually at the 3 position of the benzene ring, to form methoxy derivatives: 4-hydroxy-3-methoxyphenylethylamine (methoxytyramine, MT) from dopamine, 4-hydroxy-3-methoxyphenylacetic acid (homovanillic acid, HVA) from 3,4-dihydroxyphenylacetic acid (DOPAC), 1-(4-hydroxy-3-methoxyphenyl)-2-aminoethanol (normetanephrine, NMN) from norepinephrine, and 1-(4-hydroxy-3-methoxyphenyl)-2-methylaminoethanol (metanephrine, MN) from epinephrine.

Oxidative deamination by MAO gives rise to an aldehyde: 3,4-dihydroxyphenylglycoaldehyde from norepinephrine and 4-hydroxy-3-methoxyphenylglycoaldehyde from epinephrine. These metabolites are usually not detected in tissues or urine but have been observed in in vitro experiments.[139]

The combined action of MAO and COMT results in deaminated O-methylated metabolites: 4-hydroxy-3-methoxyphenylglycoaldehyde from norepinephrine and 4-hydroxy-3-methoxyphenylacetaldehyde from dopamine. These compounds and the catecholaldehydes formed by MAO alone will react further with aldehyde dehydrogenase (EC 1.2.1.3) to produce an acid metabolite or with aldehyde reductase (EC 1.1.1.1) to produce an alcohol metabolite. Thus, following deamination by MAO, the dopamine catecholaldehyde becomes DOPAC or 3,4-dihydroxyphenyl-

ethanol (DOPET); the norepinephrine catecholaldehyde can form DOMA and 3,4-dihydroxyphenylglycol (DOPEG). If either COMT or aldehyde dehydrogenase is inhibited, increased amounts of DOPET and DOPEG are excreted.[140,141] Following the actions of COMT and MAO, the dopamine methoxycatecholaldehyde can form HVA or 4-hydroxy-3-methoxyphenylethanol (MOPET); the norepinephrine methoxycatecholaldehyde can form VMA or 4-hydroxy-3-methoxyphenylglycol (MOPEG).

The quantitative importance of these pathways in man has been determined by examination of the metabolites formed following the infusion of physiologic amounts of radioactive catecholamines. After injecting L-epinephrine-7-H[3] and L-metanephrine-methoxy-C[14], Kopin[142] found that approximately 70 percent of the circulating epinephrine in man is methoxylated, with about 24 percent also being deaminated. Other studies confirm that the essential metabolic products of endogenous dopamine, norepinephrine, and epinephrine are both O-methylated and deaminated in man to HVA,[134] MOPEG,[143] and VMA,[135] respectively. The intermediary products are 3-methoxytyramine,[136] NMN, and MN.[137] These O-methoxylated catecholamine derivatives are further metabolized by conjugation with glucuronic acid or sulfuric acid. In man, these are usually conjugated with sulfuric acid at the 4 position of the benzene ring. Intravenous infusion of norepinephrine and epinephrine in man results in the excretion of ethereal sulfates of NMN, MN,[147,148] and MOPEG.[143] The importance of the inactivation of circulating catecholamines by conjugation is suggested by reports that parkinsonian patients receiving L-dopa therapy have high levels of conjugated dopamine 3-0-sulfate in their plasma and urine.[149–151]

The acid metabolites of dopamine, norepinephrine and epinephrine, DOMA, DOPAC, VMA, and HVA, can be quantitated in urine.[134,144–146] Of these, VMA is the O-methylated acid metabolite of norepinephrine and epinephrine, and HVA is the analogous metabolite of dopamine.

Catechol-O-Methyltransferase

Characterization. Catechol-O-methyltransferase catalyzes the enzymatic O-methylation of catecholamines according to reaction 4:

$$A\ catechol\ +\ S\text{-}adenosylmethionine\ \xrightleftharpoons{Mg\,2+}\ a\ guiacol$$
$$+\ S\text{-}adenosylhomocysteine \qquad (4)$$

The conversion requires a divalent cation and S-adenosylmethionine as the methyl donor.[138] Methylation is predominantly at the *meta* position in vivo.[137] Normally occurring catechol substrates for COMT include dopa, dopamine, norepinephrine, epinephrine, DOMA, DOPAC, DOPET, and DOPEG.[138] The amino acid L-dopa, given for the treatment of Parkinson's disease, is primarily metabolized by COMT to form 3-methoxydopa.[152,153] It has been suggested that metabolism of large doses of dopa could cause a depletion of the methyl donor S-adenosylmethionine, since the demand for methionine in the reaction may exceed the average daily intake of methionine.[154]

Localization. COMT is an intracellular enzyme localized in the cytosol.[138] It is present in homogenates of cultured astrocytoma cells[155] and gliomas,[156] which may partially explain the finding of COMT activity throughout the central nervous system.[157] Although COMT is localized in nerve terminals with about 50 percent of the activity from brain homogenates found in synaptosomes,[158,159] there is an uneven distribution in the brain; the highest activity is in the area postrema, the lowest in the cerebellar cortex.[160] Surgical sympathectomy in tissues with dense sympathetic innervation leads to a decrease in COMT activity which parallels the decrease of endogenous norepinephrine.[161] Although this suggests localization in sympathetic nerve terminals, 50 to 60 percent of the COMT activity remains, indicating an extraneuronal localization as well. Activity has been found in the pineal and pituitary glands,[162] the liver, kidneys, intestine, spleen, salivary gland, aorta, vena cava,[138] the uterus,[163] neuroblastoma,[164] adipose tissue,[165] and red blood cells.[166]

Activity in Clinical States. The activity of COMT in different organs is known to change in association with some natural and morbid conditions. Activity remains constant in the brain but increases in the liver and decreases in the kidney of the aging rat.[167] During pregnancy, there is a twofold increase in COMT activity in the rat uterus.[163] Hypophysectomy and large doses of thyroxine will reduce rat liver COMT.[168] Patients with congestive heart failure have an increase in total COMT in the heart.[169,170] A significant reduction of COMT in red blood cells is associated with depression in females[171] (cf. reduction of MAO in affective disorders discussed below). COMT is elevated in the heart, liver, and kidneys of spontaneously hypertensive rats during the development of hypertension.[172]

Weak Agonist Products. Normetanephrine has only 1/1000 the effect of its precursor, norepinephrine, on beta-adrenoceptors of cardiac muscle,[173] and yet these congeners have a similar potency on the alpha-adrenoceptors of nictitating membrane.[174] The O-methylated deaminated metabolite of norepinephrine, VMA, has no such action. It appears, then, that detoxification of norepinephrine utilizes both COMT and MAO. The predominant pathway is reflected in the ratio of the excretion rate of products from O-methylation (metanephrines) to the excretion rate of products from both O-methylation and deamination (VMA). In normal humans the ratio is 1:10,[175] indicating the importance of both COMT and MAO. Because normetanephrine has a higher affinity for MAO than does norepinephrine,[176] O-methylation would more efficiently precede deamination. Abnormal excretion patterns of metanephrines and VMA are described in Chapter 104.

Monoamine Oxidase

Characterization. Monoamine oxidase is an oxidoreductase that deaminates monoamines according to reaction 5:

$$R \cdot CH_2 \cdot NH_2 + O_2 + H_2O \rightleftharpoons RCHO + NH_3 + H_2O_2 \qquad (5)$$

The normal endogenous substrates for this reaction are thought to be derivatives of phenylethylamine and indolethylamine. The enzyme is associated with flavin fluorescence (FAD) in the human brain that is at least partially reduced by the presence of substrate.[177] Although MAO is inhibited by chelating agents,[177,178] highly purified preparations with very little metal content have been shown to have high activity.[179] The involvement of metal ions in the deamination reaction may be confined to maintaining the structure of MAO-containing particles.[180]

Localization. Monoamine oxidase is widely distributed in mammalian species, but there are great differences in activities and specificities between the same organs from different species.[181] Liver, kidney, stomach, and intestines have the highest activities among human tissues; this indicates a role for MAO in the metabolism of ingested monoamines. The enzyme has also been found in nervous tissue, smooth muscle,[181] gonads, heart muscle, aorta, blood platelets,[182] adrenal cortex and medulla,[183] and throughout the brain.[184,185] Some of the MAO activity in the brain is present in glial cells[155] and synaptosomes;[186] there is an increase in human brain MAO and a decrease in norepinephrine levels[191] with aging. It has also been demonstrated in low concentrations in skeletal muscle and plasma.[181]

Histochemical and denervation studies provided evidence for both an intraneuronal and an extraneuronal distribution in innervated tissues. The majority appears to be extraneuronal in parenchymal tissue,[187] vas deferens,[188] rat heart,[189] and adrenergically innervated organs.[190]

There is strong evidence which indicates that MAO activity is localized in the outer membrane fraction of the mitochondrion.[192,193] The apparent microsomal localization of some MAO activity in rat liver[194,195] has been suggested to be an artifact of the fractionation procedure.[192] This suggestion is supported by the findings of Jarrot and Iversen.[196] MAO activity in the adrenal medulla is mainly mitochondrial; little activity is associated with the chromaffin granules.[197]

Isoenzymes. Isozymes of MAO have been found in electrophoretic studies of the human brain[198] and placenta.[199] The multiple forms of MAO were abolished when chaotropic agents were used to treat a soluble preparation from the brain,[200] suggesting that the membrane environment may confer allotropic properties upon a single enzyme species. However, two isozymes have been identified in vivo in the brain by using species selective inhibitors.[201,202] Johnston introduced the concept of MAO-A and MAO-B on the basis of differences in substrate preference and susceptibility to inhibition by clorgyline (N-methyl-N-propargyl-3-[2,4-dichlorophenoxyl] propylamine).[203] MAO-A is the neuronal species of the enzyme. It preferentially deaminates serotonin, epinephrine, and norepinephrine while being sensitive to inhibition by clorgyline, harmine, Lilly 51641 (N-[2(O-chlorophenexyl)-ethyl]-cyclopropylamine),[204] and P.C.O. [5-phenyl-3-(N-cyclopropyl)-ethylamine 1,-2,4-oxidiazole].[205] MAO-B, the extraneuronal species, preferentially deaminates benzylamine and 2-phenylethylamine while being inhibited by deprenyl (phenylisopropylmethyl-propinylamine)[206] and, to a lesser extent, by pargyline.[207] Dopamine and tyramine are substrates for both enzyme species.

The presence of two forms of MAO with distinctive pharmacologic properties is a finding of great clinical importance. Depressed patients have higher platelet MAO (type B) than do normal controls.[208] Furthermore, there is a higher incidence of depression in females and the aged, both groups having higher levels of MAO-B. Progesterone increases the level of MAO in women and promotes depression, while estrogens inhibit MAO and often act as antidepressants.[209,210] Other affective disorders have MAO involvement; platelet MAO activity is decreased in the bipolar depressed patient[211] and in the chronic schizophrenic.[212] Recently, the antidepressant properties of deprenyl (MAO-B inhibitor) were contrasted to those of clorgyline (MAO-A inhibitor) in rats.[213] The antidepressant properties of deprenyl were independent of catecholamine deamination, these neurotransmitters being metabolized by MAO-A. Deprenyl potentiated the stereotyped sniffing behavior induced by the MAO-B-specific substrate 2-phenylethylamine, whereas clorgyline did not. The involvement of phenylethylamine in affective disorders has been reviewed elsewhere.[214]

Monoamine oxidase inhibitors (MAOI) have been used in the treatment of depression and hypertension. There are two theories on the mechanism of their action: (1) false neurotransmitters may be produced as the accumulated tyramine is beta-hydroxylated to octopamine,[215] and/or (2) there may be selective depression of sympathetic nerve transmission.[216] The practical uses of MAO inhibitors are strictly limited by adverse reactions with certain foods[213] and other drugs.[201,218] Most interdictions stem from the hypertensive crisis that occurs when an indirect sympathomimetic amine is ingested. Agents that precipitate crises include cold capsules; asthma tablets; high-tyramine-content foods, such as wines, cheeses, and herring; methyldopa; L-dopa; narcotics; tricyclic antidepressants; and oral hypoglycemic agents. The hypertensive crisis may closely resemble that occurring in patients with pheochromocytoma. The clinical features are those of sympathetic hyperactivity: palpitations, flushing, increased perspiration, throbbing headaches. The peak effect is reached within 2 to 4 hours and recedes over the next 2 to 6 hours. Subarachnoid hemorrhage with hemiplegia, coma, and death are the most serious potential sequelae. Patients should be treated with intravenous phentolamine. Patients receiving MAO inhibitors must be warned of foods and drugs to avoid and of the symptoms that may occur and should carry phentolamine tablets as a prophylactic measure. Pargyline (Eutonyl) does not exert the indirect sympathomimetic activity discussed above, making it the only MAO inhibitor available for the treatment of hypertension.[219] However, because of their potential dangers, MAO inhibitors are used rarely in the treatment of hypertensive patients.

Clinical Value of Metabolite Excretion

Urinary excretion of HVA and VMA, as well as the metanephrines, is a useful index of total endogenous catecholamine production. Determinations of urinary VMA and HVA have been of clinical value in the early diagnosis of neuroblastoma, in elucidating treatment response, and in formulating the prognosis.[220–222]

In pheochromocytoma, 95 to 99 percent of the patients have catecholamine excretion greater than 10 μg/hr and metanephrine excretion greater than 30 μg/hr; 80 percent have VMA excretion greater than 500 μg/hr (12 mg/day). Measurement of catecholamine metabolites is usually required in the evaluation of patients with tumors derived from the sympathetic nervous system (Chapter 102). Importantly, alpha-methyldopa is not metabolized to VMA or to the metanephrines, and this drug does not falsely elevate these values in urine of patients. On the other hand, alpha-methyldopa and its metabolites may increase urine catecholamines for 1 week after its administration. The apparent catecholamine pattern after methyldopa, as determined by Crout's method, is 80 percent NE and 20 percent E.

ACKNOWLEDGMENT FOR CHAPTERS 100 to 104

We greatly appreciate the assistance with various phases of preparation of these chapters by Jan Saito, Grace Fung, Nancy Stowell, and Eiko DeQuattro. We are indebted to the artistic talents of Krista Osterberg and to the library research, graphic presentations, and general legwork by Mark R. Myers. Finally, I personally and affectionately thank my wife, Eiko, for the encouragement and "push" that made it all possible.

REFERENCES

1. Kopin, I. J., Gordon, E. K., Horst, W. D.: Studies on tissue uptake of l-norepinephrine-C[14]. *Biochem Pharmacol 14:* 753–758, 1965.
2. Mangan, G. F., Jr., Mason, J. W.: Fluorometric measurement of exogenous and endogenous epinephrine and norepinephrine in peripheral blood. *J Lab Clin Med 51:* 484–493, 1958.
3. von Euler, U. S.: A specific sympathomimetic ergone in adrenergic nerve fibres (sympathin) relations to adrenaline and nor-adrenaline. *Acta Physiol Scand 12:* 73, 1946.
4. Carlsson, A., Waldeck, B.: Dopmaine and norepinephrine in the brain. *Acta Physiol Scand 44:* 293, 1958.
5. Sutherland, E. W., Rall, T. W.: The relations of adenosine 3'-5' phosphate and phosphorylase to the actions of catecholamines and other hormones. *Pharmacol Rev 12:* 265–299, 1960.
6. Hausler, G.: Adrenergic neurone and control of blood pressure, in Usdin, E., Snyder, S., (eds): Frontiers in Catecholamine Research. Oxford, Pergamon Press, 1973, pp. 879–881.
7. Doba, N., Reis, D. J.: Acute fulminating neurogenic hypertension produced by brainstem lesions in the rat. *Circ Res 32:* 584–593, 1973.
8. Fuxe, K., Hokflet, T., Ungerstedt, U.: Localization of indolealkylamines in CNS. *Adv Pharmacol 6A:* 235–251, 1968.
9. Dahlstrom, A., Fuxe, K.: Evidence for the existence of monoamine neurones in the central nervous system: II. Experimentally induced changes in the intraneuronal amine levels of bulbospinal neurone systems. *Acta Physiol Scan 64 (Suppl 247):* 1–37, 1965.
10. Saavedra, J. M., Grobecker, N., Axelrod, J.: Adrenaline-forming enzyme in brainstem: Elevation in genetic and experimental hypertension. *Science 191:* 483–484, 1976.
11. DeQuattro, V., Nagatsu, T., Maronde, R., Alexander, N.: Catecholamine synthesis in rabbits with neurogenic hypertension. *Circ Res 24:* 545–555, 1969.
12. Schmitt, H., Schmitt, H. Bossier, J. R., Giudicelli, J. F., Fichelle, J.: Cardiovascular effects of 2-(2,6-dichloro phenylamino-2-1 imidazoline hydrochloride 1 st 155) II. Central sympathetic structures. *Eur J Pharmacol 2:* 340, 1968.
13. Lund, A.: Fluorimetric determination of adrenaline in blood. I. Isolation of the fluorescent oxidation product in adrenaline. *Acta Pharmacol Toxicol 5:* 75–94, 1949A.
14. Barsoum, G. S., Gaddum, J. H.: The pharmacologic estimation of adenosine and histamine in blood. *J Physiol 85:* 1, 1935.
15. Crout, J. R.: Catecholamines in urine, in Seligson, D., (ed): Standard Methods of Clinical Chemistry, vol 3. New York, Academic Press, 1961, pp 62–80.
16. Renzini, V., Brunori, C. A., Valori, C.: A sensitive and specific fluorimetric method for the determination of noradrenalin and adrenalin in human plasma. *Clin Chem Acta 30:* 587–594, 1970.
17. Weil-Malherbe, H., Bone, A. D.: Chemical estimation of adrenaline like substances in blood. *Biochem J 51:* 311–318, 1952.
18. Engelman, K., Portnoy, B., Lovenberg, W.: A sensitive and specific double-isotope derivative method for the determination of catecholamines in biological specimens. *Am J Med Sci 255:* 259–268, 1968.
19. Engelman, K., Portnoy, B.: A sensitive double isotope derivative assay for norepinephrine and epinephrine-normal resting human levels. *Circ Res 26:* 53–57, 1970.
20. Henry, D. P., Starman, B. J., Johnson, D. G.: A sensitive radioenzymatic assay for norepinephrine in tissues and plasma. *Life Sci 16:* 375–384, 1975.
21. Passon, P. G., Peuler, J. D.: A simplified radiometric assay for plasma norepinephrine and epinephrine. *Anal Biochem 51:* 618–631, 1973.
22. Ferrario, C. M., Gildenberg, P. L., McCubbin, J. W.: Cardiovascular effects of angiotensin mediated by the central nervous system. *Circ Res 12:* 553, 1963.
23. Benelli, G., Bella, D. D., Gandini, A.: Angiotensin and peripheral sympathetic nerve activity. *Br J Pharmacol 22:* 211, 1964.
24. Feldberg, W., Lewis, G. P.: The action of peptides on adrenal medulla: Release of adrenaline by bradykinin and angiotensin. *J Physiol 171:* 98, 1964.
25. Zeisel, H., Kuschke, H. J.: Die catechinamine adrenalin und noradrenalin im harn des kindes. *Klin Wochenschr 37:* 1168, 1959.
26. Levi-Montalcini, R., Angeletti, P. U.: The nerve growth factor. *Physiol Rev 48:* 534–569, 1968.
27. Levi-Montalcini, R., Angeletti, P. U.: Immuno-sympathectomy. *Pharmacol Rev 18:* 619–628, 1966.
28. Takahashi, H., Fitzpatrick, T. B.: Catecholamine metabolism in melanoma. *J Invest Dermatol 42:* 161, 1964.
29. Sipple, J. H.: Association of pheochromocytoma with carcinoma of thyroid gland. *Am J Med 31:* 163, 1964.
30. Carney, J. A., Sizemore, G. W., Sheps, S. G.: Adrenal medullary disease in multiple endocrine neoplasia, type II, pheochromocytoma and its precursors. *Am J Clin Pathol 66:* 279–290, 1976.
31. Hennessy, J. F., Gray, T. K., Cooper, C. W., Ontjes, D. A.:

Stimulation of thyrocalcitonin secretion by pentagastrin and calcium in two patients with medullary carcinoma of the thyroid. *J Clin Endocrinol Metab 36:* 200, 1973.

32. Schimke, R. N., Hartmann, W. H., Prout, T. E., Rimoin, D. L.: Syndrome of bilateral pheochromocytoma, medullary thyroid carcinoma and multiple neuromas: A possible regulatory defect in the differentiation of chromaffin tissue. *N Engl J Med 279:* 1, 1968.

33. Bernier, J. J., Ramboud, J. C., Cahan, D., Prost, A.: Diarrhea associated with medullary carcinoma of the thyroid. *Gut 10:* 980, 1969.

34. Wurtman, R. J., Axelrod, J.: Adrenalin synthesis: Control by the pituitary gland and adrenal glucocorticoids. *Science 150:* 1464–1465, 1965.

35. Brobergoer, O., Zetterstrom, R.: Hypoglycemia with an inability to increase the epinephrine secretion in insulin-induced hypoglycemia. *J Pediatr 59:* 215, 1961.

36. Sheperd, J. T.: Role of the veins in the circulation. *Circulation 33:* 484, 1966.

37. Day, M. D., Roach, A. G.: Beta adrenergic receptors in the CNS of the cat concerned with control of arterial pressure and heart rate. *Nature (New Biol) 242:* 30, 31, 1973.

38. Day, M. D., Roach, A. G.: Central α and β adrenoceptors—modifying arterial blood pressure and heart rate in conscious cats. *Br J Pharmacol 51:* 325–333, 1974.

39. Bhargava, K. P.: Central α and β adrenoceptors in cardiovascular regulation, in Milyez, P., Safar, M., (eds): Recent Advances in Hypertension, vol II. Paris, Labratories Boehringer Ingelheim, 1975, pp 109–129.

40. Goodman, L., Gilman, A.: The Pharmacologic Basis of Therapeutics. New York, MacMillan, 1975, p 406.

41. Black, I. B., Mytilinbou, G.: Trans-synaptic regulation of end organ and organ innervation by sympathetic neurones. *Brain Res 101:* 503–521, 1976B.

42. Brimijohn, S.: Transport and turnover of dopamine β hydroxylase in sympathetic nerves of the rat. *J Neurochem 19:* 2183–2193, 1972.

43. Drujan, B. D., Sourkes, T. L., Layne, D. S., Murphy, G. F.: The differential determination of catecholamines in urine. *Can J Biochem 37:* 1153–1159, 1959.

44. Brunjes, S., Wybenga, D., Johns, V.: Fluorimetric determination of urinary metanephrine and normetanephrine. *Clin Chem 10:* 1–12, 1964.

45. Karoum, F., Ruthven, C. R. J., Sandler, M.: Gas chromatographic assay of phenolic alcohols in biological material using electron capture detection. *Biochem Med 5:* 505–514, 1971.

46. Pisano, J. J.: A simple, analysis for normetanephrine and metanephrine in urine. *Clin Chem Acta 5:* 406–414, 1960.

47. Pisano, J. J., Crout, R., Abraham, D.: Determination of 3-methoxy-4 hydroxy mandelic acid in urine. *Clin Chem Acta 7:* 285–291, 1962.

48. Wilk, S., Gitlow, S., Clarke, D., Paley, D.: Determination of urinary 3-methoxy-4 hydroxyphenyl etheline glycol by gas-liquid chromatography and electron capture detection. *Clin Chem Acta 16:* 403–403, 1967.

49. Sato, T., DeQuattro, V.: Enzymatic assay for 3, 4-dihydroxymandelic acid (DOMA) in human urine, plasma and tissues. *J Lab Clin Med 74:* 672–681, 1969.

50. Nagatsu, T., Levitt, M., Udenfriend, S.: Tyrosine hydroxylase. *J Biol Chem 239:* 2910–2917, 1964.

51. Lovenberg, W., Weissbach, H., Udenfriend, S.: Aromatic L-amino acid decarboxylase. *J Biol Chem 237:* 89–93, 1962.

52. Nagatsu, T., Udenfriend, S.: Photometric assay of dopamine-beta hydroxylase activity in human blood. *Clin Chem 18:* 980–983, 1972.

53. Weinshilboum, R., Axelrod, J.: Serum dopamine-beta-hydroxylase activity. *Circ Res 28:* 307–315, 1971.

54. Axelrod, J.: Purification and properies of phenylethanolamine-N-methyl transferase. *J Biol Chem 237:* 1657–1660, 1962.

55. Axelrod, J., Tomchick, R.: Enzymatic O-methylation of epinephrine and other catechols. *J Biol Chem 233:* 702–705, 1958.

56. Wurtman, R. J., Axelrod, J.: A sensitive and specific assay for the estimation of monoamine oxidase. *Biochem Pharmacol 12:* 1439–1441, 1963.

57. Blaschko, H.: The specific action of L-dopa decarboxylase. *J Physiol 96:* 50P–51P, 1939.

58. Gurin, S., Delluva, A. M.: The biological synthesis of radioactive adrenaline from phenylalanine. *J Biol Chem 170:* 545–550, 1947.

59. Demis, O., Blaschko, H., Welch, A. D.: The conversion of dihy-

droxyphenylalanine-2-C^{14}(dopa) to norepinephrine by bovine adrenal medullary homogenates. *J Pharmacol 117:* 208–212, 1956.

60. Leeper, L., Udenfriend, S.: Dihydroxyphenylethylamine as precursor of adrenal epinephrine in the intact rat. *Fed Proc 15:* 298, 1956.

61. Goodall, McC., Kirshner, N.: Biosynthesis of adrenaline and noradrenaline in vitro. *J Biol Chem 226:* 213–221, 1957.

62. Lloyd, T., Mori, T., Kaufman, S.: 6-Methyltetrahydropterin: Isolation and identification as the highly active hydroxylase cofactor from tetrahydrofolate. *Biochemistry 10:* 2330–2336, 1971.

63. Pollion, W. N.: Kinetic properties of brain tyrosine hydroxylase and its partial purification by affinity chromatography. *Biochem Biophys Res Comm 44:* 64–70, 1971.

64. Shiman, R., Miki, A., Kaufman, S.: Solubilization and partial purification of tyrosine hydroxylase from bovine adrenal medulla. *J Biol Chem 246(5):* 1330–1340, 1971.

65. Fellman, J. H., Delvin, M. K.: Concentration and hydroxylation of free phenylalanine in adrenal glands. *Biochim Biophys Acta 28:* 328–332, 1958. Cited in Kaufman, S., Friedman, S.: Dopamine-β-hydroxylase. *Pharmacol Rev 17:* 71–100, 1965.

66. Nagatsu, R., Levitt, M., Udenfriend, U. S.: Tyrosine hydroxylase. The initial step in norepinephrine biosynthesis. *J Biol Chem 239:* 2910–2917, 1964.

67. Engelman, K., Horowitz, D., Jequier, E., Sjoerdsma, A.: Biochemical and pharmacological effects of α-methyltyrosine in man. *J Clin Invest 47:* 577–594, 1968.

68. Gitlow, S. E., Pertsemlidis, D., Bertani, L.: Management of patients with pheochromocytoma. *Am Heart J 82:* 557–567, 1971.

69. McGeer, E. G., McGeer, P. L., et al: Inhibition of brain tyrosine hydroxylase by 5-hydroxytryptophans. *Life Sci 6:* 2221–2232, 1967.

70. Spector, S.: Inhibition of endogenous catecholamine biosynthesis. *Pharmacol Rev 18:* 599–609, 1966.

71. Christensen, N. J.: Plasma noradrenaline and adrenaline in patients with thyrotoxicosis and myxoedema. *Clin Sci Mol Med 45:* 163–171, 1973.

72. Nagatsu, T., Mizutani, K., Sudo, Y., et al.: Tyrosine hydroxylase in human adrenal glands and human pheochromocytoma. *Clin Chim Acta 39:* 417–424, 1972.

73. DeQuattro, V., Nagatsu, T., Mendez, A., Verska, J.: Determinants of cardiac noradrenaline depletion in human congestive failure. *Cardiovasc Res 7:* 344–350, 1973.

74. Pool, P. E., Covell, J. W., Levitt, M., Gibb, J, Braunwald, E.: Reduction of cardiac tyrosine hydroxylase activity in experimental congestive heart failure. *Circ Res 20:* 349–353, 1967.

75. Christenson, J. G., Dairman, W., Udenfriend, S.: Preparation and properties of a homogeneous aromatic L-amino acid decarboxylase from hog kidney. *Arch Biochem Biophys 141:* 356–367, 1970.

76. Holtz, P., Heise, R., Ludtke, K.: Fermentativer abbau von 1-dioxyphylalanin (dopa) durch niere. *Arch Exp Pathol Pharmakol 191:* 87–118, 1939.

77. Rush, R. A., Thomas, P. E., Udenfriend, S.: Measurement of human dopamine-β-hydroxylase in serum by homologous radioimmunoassay. *Proc Natl Acad Sci 72:* 750–752, 1975.

78. Eränkö, O., Eränkö, L.: Small, intensely fluorescent granule-containing cells in the sympathetic ganglion of the rat. *Prog Brain Res 34:* 39–51, 1971.

79. Eränkö, L., Eränkö, O.: Effects of hydrocortisone on histochemically demonstrable catecholamines in the sympathetic ganglia and extra-adrenal chromaffin tissue of the rat. *Acta Physiol Scand 84:* 125–133, 1972.

80. Eränkö, O., Eränkö, L., Hill, C. E., Bumstock, G.: Hydrocortisone-induced increase in the number of small intensely fluorescent cells and their histochemically demonstrable catecholamine content in cultures of sympathetic ganglia of the newborn rat. *Histochem J 4:* 49–58, 1972.

81. Fuxe, K., Goldstein, M., Hökfelt, T., Hyub, Joh T.: Cellular localization of dopamine-β-hydroxylase and phenylethanolamine-N-methyl transferase as revealed by immunochemistry. *Prog Brain Res 34:* 127–138, 1971.

82. Friedman, S., Kaufman, S.: 3,4-Dihydroxyphenylethylamine-β-hydroxylase: A copper protein. *J Biol Chem 240:* PC552–554, 1965.

83. Goldstein, M., Joh, T. H., Garvey, T. Q.: Kinetic studies of the enzymatic dopamine-β-hydroxylation reaction. *Biochemistry 7:* 2724–2730, 1968.

84. Cleland, W. W.: The kinetics of enzyme-catalyzed reactions with two or more substrates or products. *Biochim Biophys Acta 67:* 104, 1963.

85. Creveling, C. R., Daly, J. W., Witkop, B., Udenfriend, S.: Substrates and inhibitors of dopamine-β-oxidase. *Biochim Biophys Acta* 64: 125–134, 1962.

86. Kirschner, N.: Pathway of noradrenaline formation from dopa. *J Biol Chem* 226: 821–825, 1957.

87. Gagnon, C., Otten, H., Thoenen, H.: Dopamine-β-hydroxylase in organ culture of rat adrenal medulla: Synthesis, storage release and trans-synaptic induction, in Usdin, E., (ed): Catecholamines and Stress. Oxford, Pergamon Press, 1976, pp 305–312.

88. Hillarp, N. A.: Adenosinephosphates and inorganic phosphate in the adrenaline and noradrenaline containing granules of the adrenal medulla. *Acta Physiol Scand* 42: 321–332, 1958.

89. Kirshner, N.: Uptake of catecholamines by a particulate fraction of the adrenal medulla. *J Biol Chem* 237: 2311–2317, 1962.

90. Musacchio, J. M., Goldstein, M., Anagnoste, B., Poch, G., Kopin, I. J.: Inhibition of dopamine-β-hydroxylase by disulfiram in vivo. *J Pharmacol Exp Ther* 152: 56–61, 1966.

91. Goldstein, M., Nakajima, K.: The effects of disulfiram on the repletion of brain catecholamine stores. *Life Sci* 5: 1133–1138, 1966.

92. Keller, E. B., Boissonnas, R. A., duVigneaud, V.: The origin of the methyl group of epinephrine. *J Biol Chem* 183: 627–732, 1950.

93. Kirshner, N., Goodall, McC.: The formation of adrenaline from noradrenaline. *Biochim Biophys Acta* 24: 658–659, 1957.

94. Coupland, R. E.: On the morphology and adrenaline-noradrenaline content of chromaffin tissue. *J Endocrinol* 9: 194–203, 1953.

95. Wurtman, R. J., Pohorecky, L. A., Baliga, B. S.: Adrenocortical control of the biosynthesis of epinephrine and proteins in the adrenal medulla. *Pharmacol Rev* 24(2): 411–426.

96. Wurtman, R. J., Pohorecky, L. A.: Adrenocortical control of epinephrine synthesis in health and disease. *Adv Metab Disord* 5: 53–76, 1971.

97. Wurtman, R. J., Axelrod, J.: Adrenaline synthesis: Control by the pituitary gland and adrenal glucocorticoids. *Science* 150: 1464–1465, 1965.

98. Wurtman, R. J., Casper, A., Pohorecky, L. A., Bartter, F. C.: Impaired secretion of epinephrine in response to insulin among hypophysectomized dogs. *Proc Natl Acad Sci USA* 61: 522–528, 1968.

99. Thoenen, H., Angeletti, P. U., Levi-Montalcini, R., Kettler, R.: Selective induction of tyrosine hydroxylase and dopamine-β-hydroxylase in the rat superior cervical ganglia by nerve growth factor. *Proc Natl Acad Sci USA* 68: 1598–1602, 1971.

100. Saavedra, J. M., Horst, G., Axelrod, J.: Adrenaline-forming enzyme in brainstem: Elevation in genetic and experimental hypertension. *Science* 191: 483, 1976.

101. Axelrod, J., Mueller, R. A., Henry, J. P., Stephens, P. M.: Changes in enzymes involved in the biosynthesis and metabolism of noradrenaline and adrenaline after psychosocial stimulation. *Nature (London)* 225: 1050–1060, 1970.

102. Thoenen, H.: Induction of tyrosine hydroxylase in peripheral and central adrenergic neurones by cold exposure of rats. *Nature (London)* 228: 861–862, 1970.

103. Kevetnansky, R., Weise, V. K., Kopin, I.: Elevation of adrenal tyrosine hydroxylase and phenylethanolamine-N-methyltransferase by repeated immobilization of rats. *Endocrinology* 87: 744–749, 1970.

104. Joh, T. H., Gegman, C., Reis, D. J.: Immunochemical demonstration of increased accumulation of tyrosine hydroxylase protein in sympathetic ganglia and adrenal medulla elicited by reserpine. *Proc Natl Acad Sci USA* 70: 2767, 1973.

105. Bhagat, B.: Role of catecholamines in induction of adrenal tyrosine hydroxylase, In Usdin, E., Snyder, S., (eds): Frontiers in Catecholamine Research. Oxford, Pergamon Press, 1974.

106. Molinoff, P. B., Brimijoin, W. S., Weinshilboum, R. M., Axelrod, J.: Neurally mediated increase in dopamine-B-hydroxylase activity. *Proc Natl Acad Sci USA* 66: 453–458, 1970.

107. Brimijohn, S., Molinoff, P. B.: Effects of 6-hydroxydopamine on the activity of tyrosine hydroxylase and dopamine-β-hydroxylase in sympathetic ganglia of the rat. *J Pharmacol Exp Ther* 178: 417–425, 1971.

108. Black, I. B., Petito, C. K.: Catecholamine enzymes in the degenerative neurological disease idiopathic orthostatic hypotension. *Science* 192: 910–912, 1976.

109. Weinshilboum, R. M., Axelrod, J.: Reduced plasma dopamine-β-hydroxylase activity in familial dysautonomia. *N Engl J Med* 285: 938–942, 1971.

110. Nagatsu, T., Levitt, M., Udenfriend, S.: Tyrosine hydroxylase—the initial step in NE biosynthesis. *J Biol Chem* 239: 2910–2917, 1964.

111. Udenfriend, S., Zaltsman-Nirenberg, P., Nagatsu, T.: Inhibitors of purified beef adrenal tyrosine hydroxylase. *Biochem Pharmacol* 14: 837–845, 1965.

112. Bevan, J. A., Bevan, R. D., Duckles, S. P.: Adrenergic regulation of vascular smooth muscle, in Handbook of Physiology of the American Physiological Society, 1977 (in press).

113. Matta, R. D., Wooten, G. F.: The pharmacology of fusaric acid in man. *Clin Pharmacol Ther* 14: 541–546, 1973.

114. Sedvall, G. C., Kopin, I. J.: Influence of sympathetic denervation and nerve impulse activity of tyrosine hydroxylase in the rat submaxillary gland. *Biochem Pharmacol* 16: 39–46, 1967B.

115. Blaschko, H., Welch, A. D.: Localization of adrenaline and cytoplasmic particles of the bovine adrenal medulla. *Arch Exp Pathol Pharmacol* 219: 17–22, 1953.

116. Hillarp, N. A., Lagerstedt, S., Nilson, B.: The isolation of a granular fraction from the suprarenal medulla containing the sympathomimetic catecholamines. *Acta Physiol Scand* 29: 251–263, 1953.

117. Stjarne, L.: Studies of catecholamine uptake storage and release mechanisms. *Acta Physiol Scand* 62 (Suppl 228): 1–60, 1964.

118. Kirshner, N.: The role of the membrane of chromaffin granules isolated from the adrenal medulla. Proceedings of Second International Pharmacological Meeting, vol 3. New York, Pergamon Press, 1963, pp 225–233.

119. Lishajko, F.: Studies on catecholamine release and uptake in adreno-medullary storage granules. *Acta Physiol Scand Suppl* 362: 1–60, 1971.

120. Douglas, W. W., Rubin, R. P.: The role of calcium in the secretory response of the adrenal medulla to acetylcholine. *J Physiol* 159: 40–57, 1961.

121. Douglas, W. W., Poisner, A. M.: On the relations between ATP splitting and secretion in the adrenal chromaffin cell: Extrusion of ATP (unhydrolyzed) during release of catecholamines. *J Physiol* 183: 249–256, 1966.

122. Dixon, W. R., Garcia, A. G., Kirpekar, S. M.: Release of catecholamines and dopamine-beta-hydroxylase from the perfused adrenal gland of the cat. *J Physiol* 244: 805–824, 1975.

123. von Euler, U. S., Hillarp, N. A.: Evidence for the presence of noradrenaline in submicroscopic structures of adrenergic axons. *Nature (London)* 177: 43–45, 1956.

124. von Euler, U. S.: The presence of the adrenergic neurotransmittor in intraaxonal structures. *Acta Physiol Scand* 43: 155–166, 1958.

125. Lagercrantz, H., Fried, G., Dahlin, I.: An attempt to estimate the in vivo concentrations of noradrenaline and ATP in sympathetic large dense core nerve vesicles. *Acta Physiol Scand* 94: 136–138, 1975.

126. Richardson, K. C.: Electron microscopic identification of autonomic nerve endings. *Nature* 210: 756, 1966.

127. Hornykiewicz, O.: Dopamine in the basal ganglia. *Br Med Bull* 29: 172–178, 1973.

128. von Euler, U. S., Lishajko, F.: Effect of reserpine on the release of catecholamines from isolated nerve and chromaffin cell granules. *Acta Physiol Scand* 52: 137–145, 1961.

129. Smith, A. D.: Mechanisms involved in the release of noradrenaline from sympathetic nerves. *Br Med Bull* 29: 123–129, 1973.

130. Whitby, L. G., Axelrod, J., Weil-Malherbe, H.: The fate of H³-norepinephrine in animals. *J Pharmacol Exp Ther* 132: 193–201, 1961.

131. Iversen, L. L.: The Uptake and Storage of Noradrenaline in Sympathetic Nerves. London, Cambridge University Press, 1967.

132. Iversen, L. L.: Catecholamine uptake processes. *Br Med Bull* 29: 130–135, 1973.

133. Blaschko, H. D., Richter, D., Schlossman, H.: The oxidation of adrenaline and other amines. *Biochem J* 31: 2187–2196, 1937.

134. Armstrong, M. D., Shaw, K. N. F., Wall, P. E.: The phenolic acids of human urine. *J Biol Chem* 218: 293–303, 1956.

135. Armstrong, M. D., McMillan, A., Shaw, K. N. F.: 3-Methoxy-4-hyroxy-d-mandelic acid, a urinary metabolite of norepinephrine. *Biochem Biophys Acta* 25: 422–425, 1957.

136. Axelrod, J.: O-methylation of epinephrine and other catechols in vitro and in vivo. *Science* 126: 400–401, 1957.

137. Axelrod, J., Senoh, S., Witkop, B.: O-methylation of catecholamines in vivo. *J Biol Chem* 233: 697–701, 1958.

138. Axelrod, J., Tomchick, R.: Enzymatic O-methylation of epinephrine and other catechols. *J Biol Chem* 233: 702–705, 1958.

139. Leeper, L. C., Weissbech, H., Udenfriend, S.: Studies on the

metabolism of norepinephrine, epinephrine and their O-methyl analogs by partially purified enzyme preparations. *Arch Biochem Biophys 77:* 417–427, 1958.

140. Goldstein, M., Friedhoff, A. J., Pomerantz, S., Contrera, J. F.: The formation of 3,4-dihydroxyphenylethanol and 3-methyoxy-4-hydroxyphenylethanol from 3,4-dihydroxyphenylethylamine in the rat. *J Biol Chem 236:* 1816–1821, 1961.

141. Kopin, I. J., Axelrod, J.: 3,4-Dihydroxyphenylglycol, a metabolite of epinephrine. *Arch Biochem Biophys 89:* 148, 1960.

142. Kopin, I. J.: Technique for the study of alternate pathways: epinephrine metabolism in man. *Science 131:* 1372–1374, 1960.

143. Axelrod, J., Kopin, I. J., Mann, J. D.: 3-Methoxy-4-hydroxyphenylglycol sulfate, a new metabolite of epinephrine and norepinephrine. *Biochim Biophys Acta 36:* 576–577, 1959.

144. von Euler, U.: Distribution and metabolism of catechol hormones in tissues and axones. *Recent Prog Horm Res 14:* 483–512, 1958.

145. von Euler, U. S., Floding, I., Lishajko, F.: The presence of free and conjugated 3,4-dihydroxyphenylacetic acid (DOPAC) in urine and blood plasma. *Acta Soc Med Upsalien 64:* 217–225, 1959.

146. Shaw, K. N. F., McMillan, A., Armstrong, M. D.: The metabolism of 3,4-dihydroxyphenylalanine. *J Biol Chem 226:* 255–266, 1957.

147. Goodall, M. C., Alton, H., Henry, M.: Noradrenaline and normetadrenaline metabolism in portal cirrhosis. *Am J Physiol 207:* 1087–1094, 1964.

148. LaBrosse, E. H., Axelrod, J., Kopin, I. J., Kety, S. S.: Metabolism of 7-H³-epinephrine-d-bitartrate in normal young men. *J Clin Invest 40:* 253–259, 1961.

149. Tyce, G. M., Sharpless, N. S., Muenter, M.: Free and conjugated dopamine in plasma during levodopa therapy. *Clin Pharmacol Ther 16:* 782–788, 1974.

150. Jenner, W. N., Rose, F. A.: Dopamine 3-O-sulfate, an end product of L-dopa metabolism in Parkinsonian patients. *Nature 252:* 237, 1974.

151. Bronaugh, R. L., Hattox, S. E., Hoehn, M. N., et al: The separation and identification of dopamine 3-O-sulfate and dopamine 4-O sulfate in urine of parkinsonian patients. *J Pharmacol Exp Ther 195:* 441–452, 1975.

152. Bartholini, G., Kuruma, I., Pletscher, A.: Distribution and metabolism of L-3-O-methyldopa in rats. *Br J Pharmacol 40:* 461–467, 1970.

153. Calne, D. B., Karoum, F., Ruthven, C. R. J., Sandler, M.: The metabolism of orally administered L-dopa in parkinsonism. *Br J Pharmacol 37:* 57–68, 1969.

154. Wurtman, R. J., Chou, C., Rose, C.: The fate of C¹⁴ dihydroxyphenylalamine (C¹⁴-dopa) in the whole mouse. *J Pharmacol Exp Ther 174:* 351–356, 1970.

155. Silberstein, S. D., Shein, H. M., Berv, K. R.: Catechol-O-methyltransferase and monoamine oxidase activity in cultured rodent astrocytoma cells. *Brain Res 41:* 245–248, 1972.

156. Katz, R. I., Goodwin, J. S., Kopin, I. J.: Disposition of neurotransmitters in experimental mouse glioma. *Life Sci 8:* 561–569, 1969.

157. Axelrod, J., Albers, W., Clemente, C. D.: Distribution of catechol-O-methyltransferase in the nervous system and other tissues. *J Neurochem 5:* 68–72, 1959.

158. Alberici, M., Rodriguez, G., De Robertis, E.: Catechol-O-methyltransferase in nerve endings of the rat brain. *Life Sci 4:* 1951–1960, 1965.

159. Broch, O. J., Jr., Fonnum, F.: The regional and subcellular distribution of catechol-O-methyltransferase in the rat brain. *J Neurochem 19:* 2049–2055, 1972.

160. Daly, J. W., Axelrod, J., Witkop, B.: Dynamic aspects of enzymatic O-methylation and demethylation of catechols in vitro and in vivo. *J Biol Chem 235:* 1155–1159, 1960.

161. Jarrott, B., Iversen, L. L.: Noradrenaline metabolizing enzymes in normal and sympathetically denervated vas deferens. *J Neurochem 18:* 1–6, 1971.

162. Axelrod, J., Maclean, P. D., Albers, R. W., Weissbach, H.: Regional distribution of methyl transferase enzymes in the nervous system and glandular tissues, in Kety, S. S., Elkes, J., (eds): Regional Neurochemistry. Oxford, Permagon Press, 1961, pp 307.

163. Wurtman, R. J., Axelrod, J., Potter, L. T.: The disposition of catecholamines in the rat uterus and the effect of drugs and hormones. *J Pharmacol Exp Ther 144:* 150–155, 1964.

164. Labrosse, E. H., Karen, M.: Catechol-O-methyltransferase activity in neuroblastoma tumor. *Nature 196:* 1222, 1962.

165. Traiger, G. J., Calvert, D. N.: O-methylation of ³H-norepinephrine by epididymal adipose tissue. *Biochem Pharmacol 18:* 109–117, 1969.

166. Axelrod, J., Cohn, C. K.: Methyl transferase enzymes in red blood cells. *J Pharmacol Exp Ther 176:* 650–654, 1971.

167. Prange, A. J., Jr., White, J. E., Lipton, M. A., Kinkead, A. M.: Influence of age on monoamine oxidase and catecholmethyl transferase in rat tissue. *Life Sci 6:* 581–586, 1967.

168. Landsberg, L., DeChamplain, J., Axelrod, J.: Increased biosynthesis of cardiac norepinephrine after hypophysectomy. *J Pharmacol Exp Ther 165:* 102–107, 1969.

169. Krakoff, L. R., Buccino, R. A., Spann, J. F., DeChamplain, J.: Cardiac catechol-O-methyltransferase and monoamine oxidase activity in congestive heart failure. *Am J Physiol 215:* 549–552, 1968.

170. DeQuattro, V., Nagatsu, T., Mendez, A., Verska, J.: Determinants of cardiac noradrenaline depletion in human congestive failure. *Cardiovasc Res 7:* 344–350, 1973.

171. Cohn, C. K., Dunner, D. L., Axelrod, J.: Reduced catechol-O-methyltransferase activity in red blood cells of women with primary affective disorder. *Science 170:* 1323–1324, 1970.

172. Creveling, C. R., Dalgard, N., Nikodejevic, B. V.: Elevated catechol-O-methyltransferase activity in spontaneously hypertensive rats. *Fed Proc 23:* 416, 1969.

173. Kukovetz, W. R., Hess, M. E., Shanfeld, J., Haugaard, N.: The action of sympathomimetic amines on isomatic contraction and phosphorylase activity of the isolated rat heart. *J Pharmacol Exp Ther 127:* 122–127, 1959.

174. Langer, S. Z., Rubio, M. C.: Effects of the noradrenaline metabolites on the adrenergic receptors. *Naunyn Schmiedebergs Arch Pharmacol 276:* 71–88, 1973.

175. DeQuattro, V., Miura, Y.: Neurogenic factors in human hypertension. Mechanism or myth? *Am J Med 55:* 362, 1973.

176. Tipton, K. F., Youdim, M. B. H., Spires, I. P. C.: Beef adrenal medulla monoamine oxidase. *Biochem Pharmac 21:* 2197–2204, 1972.

177. Nagatsu, T., Yamamoto, T., Harada, M.: Purification and properties of human brain mitochondrial monoamine oxidase. *Enzymologia 39:* 15–25, 1969.

178. Lagnado, J. R., Sourkes, T. L.: Inhibition of amine oxidase by metal ions and by sulphydryl compounds. *Can J Biochem Physiol 35:* 1185–1194, 1956.

179. Yasunobu, K. T., Igaue, I., Gomes, B.: The purification and properties of beef liver mitochondrial monoamine oxidase. *Adv Pharmacol 6A:* 43–59, 1968.

180. Veryovkina, I. V., Gorkin, V. Z., Mityushin, V. M., Elpiner, I. E.: On the effect of ultrasonic waves on monoamine oxidase connected with the submicroscopial structures of mitochondria. *Biophysics 9:* 503–506, 1964.

181. Davison, A. N.: Physiological role of monoamine oxidase. *Physiol Rev 38:* 729–747, 1958.

182. Collins, G. G. S., Sandler, M.: Human blood platelet monoamine oxidase: Purification and characterization. *Biochem Pharmacol 20:* 289–296, 1971.

183. Blaschko, H., Hagen, J. M., Hagen, P.: Mitochondrial enzymes and chromaffin granules of the adrenal medulla. *J Physiol (London) 139:* 316–322, 1957.

184. Bogdanski, D. F., Weissbach, H., Udenfriend, S.: The distribution of serotonin, 5-hydroxytryptophan decarboxylase, and monoamine oxidase in brain. *J Neurochem 1:* 272–278, 1957.

185. Weiner, N.: The distribution of monoamine oxidase and succinic oxidase in brain. *J Neurochem 6:* 79–86, 1960.

186. Arnaiz, G. R., deL., DeRobertis, E. D. P.: Cholinergic and noncholinergic nerve endings in the rat. II. Subcellular localization of monoamine oxidase and succinate dehydrogenase. *J Neurochem 9:* 503–508, 1962.

187. Jonason, J.: Metabolism of catecholamines in the central and peripheral nervous system. *Acta Physiol Scan Suppl 320:* 1–50, 1969.

188. Jarrott, B., Iversen, L. L.: Noradrenaline metabolizing enzymes in normal and sympathetically denervated vas deferens. *J Neurochem 18:* 1–6, 1971.

189. Horita, A., Lowe, M. C.: On the extraneuronal nature of cardiac monoamine oxidase in the rat. *Adv Biochem Psychopharmacol 5:* 227–242, 1972.

190. Klingman, G. I.: Monoamine oxidase activity of peripheral organs and sympathetic ganglia of the rat after immunosympathectomy. *Biochem Pharmacol 15:* 1729–1736, 1966.

191. Robinson, D. S., Nies, A., et al: Ageing, monoamines, and mono-amine-oxidase levels. *Lancet 1:* 290, 1972.

192. Schnaitman, L., Erwin, V. G., Greenawalt, J. W.: The submito-chondrial localization of monoamine oxidase. *J Cell Biol 32:* 719–735, 1967.

193. Tipton, K. F.: The submitochondrial localization of monoamine oxidase in rat liver and brain. *Biochim Biophys Acta 135:* 910–920, 1967.

194. Hawkins, J.: The localization of amine oxidase in the liver cell. *Biochem J 50:* 577–581, 1952.

195. Oswald, E. O., Strittmatter, C. F.: Comparative studies in the characterization of monoamine oxidase. *Proc Soc Exp Biol Med 114:* 668–673, 1963.

196. Jarrott, B., Inversen, L. L.: Subcellular distribution of monoamine oxidase activity in rat liver and vas deferens. *Biochem Pharmacol 17:* 1619–1625, 1968.

197. Laduron, P., Belpaire, F.: Tissue fractionation and catecholamines. II. Intracellular distribution patterns of tyrosine hydroxylase, dopa decarboxylase, dopamine-β-hydroxylase, phenylethanolamine N-methyl transferase, and monoamine oxidase in adrenal medulla. *Biochem Pharmacol 17:* 1127–1140, 1968.

198. Youdim, M. B. H.: Multiple forms of monoamine oxidase and their properties. *Adv Biochem Psychopharmacol 5:* 67077, 1972.

199. Youdim, M. B. H., Collins, G. G. S., Sandler, M.: Isoenzymes of soluble mitochondrial monoamine oxidase, in Shugar, D., (ed): Enzymes and Isoenzymes. Structure, Properties and Function. New York, Academic Press, 1970, pp 281–289.

200. Tipton, K. F., Housley, M. D., Garrett, N. J.: Allotopic properties of human brain monoamine oxidase. *Nature 246:* 213–214, 1973.

201. Fuller, R. W.: Selective inhibition of monoamine oxidase. *Adv Biochem Psychopharmacol 5:* 339–354, 1972.

202. Yang, H-Y. T., Neff, N. H.: The monoamine oxidases of brain: Selective inhibition with drugs and the consequences for the metabolism of the biogenic amines. *J Pharmacol Exp Ther 189:* 733–740, 1974.

203. Johnston, J. P.: Some observations upon a new inhibitor of monoamine oxidase in brain tissue. *Biochem Pharmacol 17:* 1285–1297, 1968.

204. Fuller, R. W.: Kinetic studies and effects *in vivo* of a new monoamine oxidase inhibitor, N-(2-[O-chlorophenoxy]-ethyl)-cyclopropylamine. *Biochem Pharmacol 17:* 2097–2106, 1968.

205. Mantle, T. J., Wilson, K., Long, R. F.: Studies on the selective inhibition of membrane-bound rat liver monoamine oxidase, *Biochem Pharmacol 24:* 2031–2038, 1975.

206. Knoll, J., Magyar, K.: Some puzzling pharmacological effects of monoamine oxidase inhibitors. *Adv Biochem Psychopharmacol 5:* 393–408, 1972.

207. Fuller, R. W., Warren, B. J., Molloy, B. B.: Selective inhibition of monoamine oxidase in rat brain mitochondria. *Biochem Pharmacol 19:* 2934–2936, 1970.

208. Nies, A., Robinson, D. S., Harris, L. S., Lamborn, K. R.: Neuro-psychopharmacology of monoamine and their regulatory enzymes, in Usdin, E., (ed): Advances in Biochemistry and Psychopharmacology, vol 12. New York, Raven Press, 1974, pp 59–70.

209. Grant, E. C. G., Davies, J. P.: Effect of oral contraceptives on depressive mood changes and on endometrial monoamine oxidase and phosphatases. *Br Med J 28:* 777–780, 1968.

210. Youdim, M. B. H., Holzbauer, M., Woods, H. F.: Neuropsycho-pharmacology of monoamine and their regulatory enzymes, in Usdin, E., (ed): Advances in Biochemistry and Psychopharmacology. New York, Raven Press, 1974, pp 11–28.

211. Murphy, D. L., Weiss, R.: Reduced monoamine oxidase activity in blood platelets from bipolar depressed patients. *Am J Psychiatry 128:* 1351–1357, 1972.

212. Murphy, D. L., Wyatt, R. J.: Reduced monoamine oxidase activity in blood platelets from schizophrenic patients. *Nature (London) 238:* 225–226, 1972.

213. Braestrup, C., Andersen, H., Randrup, A.: The monoamine oxidase B inhibitor deprenyl potentiates phenylethylamine behavior in rats without inhibition of catecholamine metabolite formation. *Eur J Pharmacol 34:* 181–187, 1975.

214. Sabelli, H. C., Mosnaim, A. D.: Phenylethylamine hypothesis of affective behavior. *Am J Psychiatry 131:* 695, 1974.

215. Kopin, I. J.: False adrenergic transmitters. *Annu Rev Pharmacol 8:* 277, 1968.

216. Puig, N., Waked, A. R., Kiskepan, S. M.: Effect on the sympathetic nervous system-chronic treatment with pargyline and L-dopa. *J Pharmacol Exp Ther 182:* 130, 1972.

217. Blackwell, B., Marley, E., Price, E. J., Taylor, D.: Hypertensive interactions between monoamine oxidase inhibitors and food-stuffs. *Br J Psychiatry 113:* 349, 1967.

218. Goldberg, L. I.: Monoamine oxidase inhibitors: Adverse reactions and possible mechanisms. *JAMA 190:* 456, 1964.

219. Sutnick, A. L., Femell, J. W., Eshenshade, J. H.: Pargyline hydrochloride, a new antihypertensive agent. *Clin Pharmacol Ther 5:* 167, 1964.

220. Gitlow, S. E., Bertani, L. M., Rausen, A., Gritbetz, D., Dziedzic, S. W.: Diagnosis of neuroblastoma by qualitative and quantitative determination of catecholamine metabolites in urine. *Cancer 25:* 1377, 1970.

221. Liebner, E. J., Rosenthal, I. M.: Serial catecholamines in the radiation management of children with neuroblastoma. *Cancer 32:* 623, 1973.

222. Bond, J. V.: Clinical significance of catecholamine excretion levels in diagnosis and treatment of neuroblastoma. *Arch Dis Child 50:* 691, 1975.

223. Bevan, J. A., Bevan, R. D., Duckles, S. P.: Adrenergic regulation of vascular smooth muscle, in Handbook of Physiology of the American Physiological Society, 1977 (in press).

224. Langer, S. Z., Enero, M. A.: The potentiation of responses to adrenergic nerve stimulation in the presence of cocaine: Its relationship to the metabolic fate of released norepinephrine. *J Pharmacol Exp Ther 191:* 431–443, 1974.

225. Luchelli-Fortis, M. A., and Langer, S. Z.: Selective inhibition by hydrocortisone of ³H-normetanephrine formation during ³H-transmitter release elicited by nerve stimulation in the isolated nerve-muscle preparation of the cat nictitating membrane. Nauyn Schmiedebergs *Arch Pharmacol 287:* 261–275, 1975.

101

Functional Components of the Sympathetic Nervous System: Regulation of Organ Systems

Vincent DeQuattro
Vito M. Campese

NEUROTRANSMITTER PROPERTIES

FIRST MESSENGER

The neurotransmitters are catecholamines comprised of a catechol nucleus (benzene ring with two adjacent hydroxyls) and an ethyl amine side chain (Table 101-1). The amino acid tyrosine is the natural precursor for all the biologically occurring catecholamines (see Fig. 100-1, Chapter 100).

Dopamine

Of the series of agonists given in Table 101-1, the first listed, dopamine, is a central nervous system (CNS) neurotransmitter, especially in the corpus striatum, basal ganglia, and substantia nigra. It is believed that in the peripheral sympathetic nervous system, dopamine serves chiefly as a precursor of norepinephrine. When dopamine is utilized as a pharmacologic agent via intravenous infusion, however, it has both constrictor and dilator properties. Its action on vascular smooth muscle is dependent on both alpha and beta stimulation. These effects can be blocked, using alpha and beta blocking agents respectively. Dopamine also stimulates specific receptors in the kidney, resulting in renal vasodilation and natriuresis. This apparent action on dopamine-specific receptors can be blocked by haloperidol.

Norepinephrine

The addition of the OH group to the β carbon of the ethyl amine side chain results in the agonist, norepinephrine, which has potent alpha receptor agonistic properties. The substitution of a methyl group for a hydrogen of the amine then confers beta-stimulating as well as alpha-stimulating properties to the basic catecholamines. Neo-Synephrine, a congener of norepinephrine, is also a potent alpha stimulator. The deletion of a hydroxyl group from the ring confers greater stability and a longer duration of action than norepinephrine.

Epinephrine

N-methyl norepinephrine or epinephrine (adrenaline) is the predominant adrenal medullary pressor amine synthesized from norepinephrine via PNMT. Epinephrine is released with norepinephrine in a 3 or 4:1 ratio from the adrenal medulla following splanchnic nerve discharge. Epinephrine stimulates both beta$_1$ (cardiac and vascular) and beta$_2$ receptors (bronchi) and is a weak alpha receptor stimulator as compared with norepinephrine. Thus, its chief cardiovascular action is chronotropic and inotropic to the heart and vasodilatory to skin and skeletal muscles. Epinephrine is thermogenic and increases the basal metabolic rate by stimulating lipolysis and gluconeogenesis via its actions on the pancreatic alpha cell to stimulate glucagon and on the beta cell to suppress insulin release. In some adrenalectomized animal models treated with steroids and exposed to severe cold and stress, there is deficient heat production due to lack of epinephrine and an increased morbidity and mortality. Although the metabolic effects of norepinephrine are less in this regard, patients with pheochromo-

Table 101-1. Chemical Structures and Actions of the Catecholamines and Some Agonists and Antagonists

					EFFECTOR	
					Receptor	Actions
Dopamine	3OH, 4OH	H	H	H	Alpha, $Beta_1$ Dopaminergic	Pressor
Tyramine*	4OH	H	H	H	Alpha, $Beta_1$ (Indirect)	Pressor via NE release
Norepinephrine	3OH, 4OH	OH	H	H	Alpha, $Beta_1$ (Cardiac)	Pressor
Phenylephrine*	3OH	OH	H	CH_3	Beta	Pressor
Epinephrine	3OH, 4OH	OH	H	CH_3	Alpha, $Beta_{1\ \&\ 2}$	Pressor, Bronchodilation, Cardiac stimulation
Isoproterenol	3OH, 4OH	OH	H	$CH(CH_3)_2$	$Beta_{1\ \&\ 2}$	Pressor, Bronchodilation, Cardiac stimulation
Isoxuprine*	4OH	OH	CH_3	$CHCH_2O\text{-}\phi$ CH_3	$Beta_1$	Muscle vessel dilatation
Terbutaline	3OH, 5OH	OH	H	$C(CH_3)_3$	$Beta_2$	Bronchodilation
Amphetamine*		H	CH_3	H	Alpha, $Beta_{1\ \&\ 2}$ (Indirect, weak peripheral and strong central	CNS stimulation, pressor
Ephedrine*		OH	CH_3	CH_3	Alpha, $Beta_{1\ \&\ 2}$	Pressor, Bronchodilation, Cardiac stimulation
Alpha Methyl Norepinephrine*	3OH, 4OH	OH	CH_3	H	False transmittor, Central alpha agonist	Antihypertensive (metabolite of alpha methyl dopa)

Clonidine*		Central alpha	Antihypertensive
Phentolamine		Alpha	Transient competitive blockade
Phenoxybenzamine		Alpha	Non equilibrium blockade (competitive)
Propranolol		$Beta_{1\ \&\ 2}$	Competitive blockade
Practolol		$Beta_1$	Competitive blockade
Haloperidol		Dopaminergic	Competitive blockade, Antipsychotic
Guanethidine		Alpha (Inhibits NE release)	Antihypertensive

* Indicates Agonists

cytoma with either norepinephrine or epinephrine excess may have profound metabolic abnormalities. There are several more important actions of epinephrine: it relaxes bronchial smooth muscle (an aid to 0_2 consumption), dilates the pupil (to aid distal accommodation), and enhances platelet adhesiveness to prevent blood loss. The synthetic isopropyl substituted catecholamine (isoproterenol) is a much more potent $beta_2$ stimulant than epinephrine

and has less $beta_1$ stimulatory properties (see below). A subgroup of hypertensive patients with clinical features of beta-adrenergic stimulation—restlessness, tachycardia, sweating—have been found to be exquisitely sensitive to isoproterenol infusion.[1] Although these hypertensive patients have some clinical resemblance to patients with pheochromocytoma, they have normal urinary catecholamine excretion and increased pressor responses to isoproterenol. On the other hand, we have described patients with clinical evidence of sympathoadrenal excess who have raised plasma norepinephrine and renin levels.[2] Some of these patients have increased urinary excretion of norepinephrine and evidence of enhanced release of newly synthesized norepinephrine.

Agonists

Studies of the structural/activity relationship of the catecholamines have led to synthesis of related agonists in order to produce desired physiologic effects. Some of these agonists and their major pharmacologic actions are listed in Table 101-1 along with some of their antagonists and indications for clinical use.

ADRENERGIC RECEPTORS

Alpha

The concept of adrenergic receptors was introduced by Alquist in 1948[3] after his comparative pharmacologic study of the structure/activity relationship of five sympathomimetic amines. Alquist classified these receptor sites as alpha and beta.[3] The alpha receptors are more responsive to norepinephrine and epinephrine and least responsive to isoproterenol. The alpha-receptor-mediated effects are antagonized by alpha-adrenergic antagonists such as phentolamine and phenoxybenzamine. By contrast, beta receptors are more responsive to isoproterenol and less responsive to epinephrine and norepinephrine. The beta-receptor-mediated effects can be inhibited by competitive antagonists such as propranolol. The activation of alpha receptors in smooth muscle is usually excitatory and results in vasoconstriction and contraction of uterine musculature and other types of smooth muscle contraction.

Beta

The stimulation of beta-adrenergic receptors usually results in inhibition of contraction of smooth muscle, such as vascular and uterine smooth muscles. Beta-adrenergic receptors, on the other hand, mediate excitatory effects of catecholamines on the heart, on lipolysis in fat cells, and on glycogenolysis in hepatic and skeletal muscle tissue.

Activation of both alpha and beta receptors produces inhibition of intestinal smooth muscle. The inhibitory effect of alpha receptors on the intestine is thought to be related to an inhibition of parasympathetic ganglion cells of Auerbach's plexus. To completely prevent the inhibitory effect of epinephrine on the intestine, the presence of both an alpha and a beta blocking agent is required.[4]

The distribution of alpha and beta receptors differs in different organs. Smooth muscle of blood vessels supplying skeletal muscles have both alpha and beta receptors. At low concentrations of epinephrine the activation of beta receptors predominates, leading to vasodilatation. At higher concentrations the effect on alpha receptors predominates. Thus the threshold concentration for activation of beta receptors is probably lower. Lands et al., on the basis of comparative agonistic structure/activity relationship of isoproterenol derivatives, proposed the subdivision of the beta receptors into beta$_1$ and beta$_2$.[5]

This concept has been confirmed by the discovery of specific blocking agents for each of these receptors. Beta$_1$ receptors are present in cardiac, small intestine, and adipose tissue; beta$_2$ receptors are present in bronchi, vascular beds, uterus, and skeletal muscle and mediate hepatic glycogenolysis.

Drugs that selectively activate beta$_2$ receptors, such as salbutamol, relax bronchial smooth muscle with little accompanying cardiac stimulation.[6] Norepinephrine, on the other hand, is quite potent at beta$_1$ receptor sites, being approximately one-third to one-fourth as potent as isoproterenol, whereas it is much less effective at beta$_2$-adrenergic receptors, being 1/100th as potent as isoproterenol.

Dopaminergic

More recently a third type of adrenergic receptor has been defined. These receptors have been termed dopaminergic because they are more responsive to dopamine than to other catecholamines. Dopaminergic receptors have been found in certain regions of the brain and in the renal vasculature, where they cause vasodilatation. The dopaminergic-mediated effects are not antagonized by alpha- or beta-adrenergic antagonists; instead, they are specifically and competitively antagonized by haloperidol.[7] It is well established that the function of the pituitary is modulated by the hypothalamus. It has been found that norepinephrine and epinephrine in relatively higher doses (5–100 μg) and dopamine in lower doses (approximately 1 μg) had a stimulatory effect in release of LH and FSH and an inhibitory effect on prolactin and growth hormone secretion.[194] Drugs like reserpine, which deplete CNS dopamine, cause increased prolactin release and plasma prolactin concentrations. Lysergic acid derivatives such as bromocriptine and lergotrile are potent inhibitors of prolactin secretion as a result of their dopamine agonist properties.[195] These compounds have been used in the therapy of galactorrhea, acromegaly, and parkinsonism. Recent studies in humans suggest that increased serum prolactin content of some hypertensive patients is related to defective central dopaminergic activity.[196]

Several studies suggest that alpha and beta receptors are not immutable structures. Studies with frog hearts have shown that the adrenoreceptors that mediate inotropic responses are altered qualitatively by ambient temperature. The characteristics of these receptors changes from beta to alpha when the temperature of the isolated hearts is reduced, suggesting that alpha and beta receptors probably represent allosteric conformations of the same structure.[8] Hypothyroidism can also induce in frog hearts the presence of alpha adrenoceptors that are absent or unreactive in euthyroid animals.[9] Atria from rats pretreated with propylthiouracil show increased sensitivity to phenylephrine and decreased sensitivity to isoproterenol.[10] The blocking potency of propranolol is reduced in hearts of hypothyroid rats.[11]

Presynaptic

Presynaptic receptors modulate the release of neurotransmitter in response to nerve impulses. Several types are arranged on the terminal membrane and reinforce or inhibit norepinephrine (NE) release. The presynaptic alpha$_2$ receptor plays an important role in feedback regulation of NE when a critical concentration of NE is reached within the synaptic cleft.[270] The antagonists, phenoxybenzamine or phentolamine, block this inhibition in concentrations 30 times that required to block the alpha receptors of the effector organ.[271] It is of interest that feedback regulation of NE release does not occur after release by tyramine. Apparently, inhibition of NE release is calcium-dependent, since nerve stimulation and potassium, but not tyramine, require calcium for NE release.[272] Dopamine activates a different presynaptic receptor to inhibit NE release, which is blocked by chlorpromazine but not by phentolamine.[273] Dopamine receptors are probably not of physiological importance, since chlorpromazine did not increase NE release in the nictitating membranes of cats.

Feedback modulation is operative whether the effector receptor is alpha or beta. Presynaptic inhibition is increased by cocaine because the latter increases the NE concentration in the neuronal cleft by interfering with reuptake. Normally, there is little NE overflow, since the content of NE from the region of the cleft inhibits further NE release. Most is taken up into the nerve ending, and the remainder is metabolized intraneuronally via MAO and the rest by COMT at the postsynaptic site. The larger the width of the synaptic cleft, the greater the NE efflux and overflow to the venous effluent (Fig. 101-1).

Clonidine, an alpha-receptor agonist, inhibits NE release by alpha₂ stimulation of peripheral nerves. Additionally, the antihypertensive effect is mediated via inhibitory alpha receptors of the central nervous system. Haloperidol may increase dopamine turnover in the central nervous system by blocking the regulatory receptors.[274] At least three or four other substances, prostaglandin E, LSD, purines, and acetylcholine (mediated via muscarinic receptors), serve to inhibit NE release (Fig. 101-2).[273] Prostaglandins, synthesized in the nerve terminal or at the effector site, are released with neuronal discharge. Blockade of prostaglandin synthesis increases NE release[276] but does not alter the effects of alpha-receptor blockade on NE release.[277] Other less well characterized substances,[178] metenkephalin (an opiate analogue) and substance P, derived from peptidergic neurones, may inhibit the release of NE.[279]

Presynaptic beta receptors modulate NE release by a positive feedback system. Thus, neuronal NE release is reinforced by epinephrine from the adrenal medulla.[275] It is possible that beta blocking drugs are effective in hypertension due in part to their antagonistic effects at this site.

Angiotensin II enhances neuroeffector transmission by both presynaptic and postsynaptic actions, increasing NE per pulse and enhancing effector responses to NE.[280]

SECOND MESSENGER

Sutherland et al. developed the theory that the link between receptor binding and biological response is a "second messenger."[12] Most evidence suggests that nearly all beta-adrenergic effects are mediated through the stimulation of the membrane-bound enzyme adenylate cyclase with the subsequent formation of 3′,5′-cyclic AMP, the second messenger.[13] After adenylcyclase is activated, the rate of 3′,5′-cyclic AMP production increases; the latter presumably mediates the particular beta-adrenergic effects

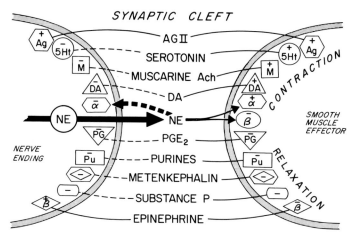

Fig. 101-2. Presynaptic regulation of neurotransmitter release by various pressor and depressor substances. Solid lines indicate activation and broken lines indicate inhibition of norepinephrine (NE) release. These substances activate relaxation or contraction at the neuroeffector as indicated. NE facilitates contraction at β_1 receptors of the heart. AGII, angiotensin II; DA, dopamine; PGE₂, prostaglandin E₂.

through interaction with specific cyclic-AMP-dependent protein kinase and phosphorylation of specific proteins.[14]

Membrane phospholipids are involved in coupling the beta-adrenergic receptors to the catalytic unit of adenylate cyclase. More recently, it has been shown that guanyl nucleotides such as GTP and, even more strikingly, the GTP analogue 5′-guanylyl imidodiphosphate regulate both basal and catecholamine-sensitive adenylcyclase.[15]

Alpha-adrenergic effects may be associated with increased tissue levels of cyclic 3′,5′-guanosine monophosphate (GMP). This cyclic nucleotide is thought to stimulate a distinct class of protein kinases.[16] Whereas cyclic AMP mediates cardiac stimulation and arteriolar muscle constriction, cyclic GMP has the opposite effects. As with beta adrenoceptors, the second messenger for dopaminergic effects appears to be 3′,5′-cyclic AMP[17] (see Fig. 100-3, Chapter 100).

CATECHOLAMINERGIC CONTROL MECHANISMS

CARDIOVASCULAR SYSTEM

Phenylephrine is the prototype of an alpha agonist which increases systolic, diastolic, and mean arterial pressures and reduces heart rate. This drug produces vasoconstriction in most vascular beds, especially in those with high concentrations of alpha receptors: kidney, skin, and connective tissue. Vasoconstriction is less pronounced in skeletal muscles and absent in the coronary and cerebral vasculature. Phenylephrine does not stimulate the heart. Prior administration of an alpha-receptor blocking agent, such as phenoxybenzamine or phentolamine, abolishes the activity of phenylephrine.

The intravenous administration of isoproterenol to an anesthetized dog increases heart rate, cardiac output, and systolic blood pressure but decreases diastolic blood pressure. The pulse pressure widens, and the mean arterial pressure falls. Vasodilation is greatest in skeletal muscle vessels. The prior administration of a beta blocking agent, such as propranolol, prevents all the cardiovascular effects of isoproterenol.

The effects of norepinephrine resemble those of phenylephrine, although only norepinephrine has a profound direct action

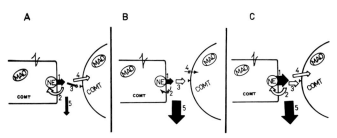

Fig. 101-1. Schematic representation of transmitter release and transmitter overflow during nerve stimulation. (A) Normal; (B) increase in overflow due to inhibition of sites of loss, no change in transmitter release; (C) increase in overflow due to an actual increase in transmitter release, sites of loss unaffected. 1, Total amount of transmitter released by nerve stimulation; 2, norepinephrine recaptured by neuronal uptake, subsequently deaminated or stored in the vesicles; 3, fraction of the transmitter released available for activation of the receptors of the effector organ; 4, norepinephrine taken up at extraneuronal sites, subsequently metabolized mostly by COMT; 5, overflow: norepinephrine collected during and after the period of nerve stimulation. NE, norepinephrine; MAO, monoamine oxidase; COMT, catechol-O-methyltransferase (Reproduced from reference 273 with permission.)

on the heart. The hemodynamic effects of therapeutic doses of epinephrine are similar to those produced by isoproterenol. A major difference is that epinephrine causes a fall in total peripheral resistance despite increased resistance of skin and renal vessels. Blood flow to the skeletal muscle is increased because the action on beta₂ receptors predominates and is only partially counteracted by the constrictive action on the alpha receptors. Higher doses of epinephrine produce vasoconstriction in the skeletal muscles and lead to increased total peripheral resistance and increased diastolic blood pressure. After the initial rise, blood pressure falls below the control level and then, finally, reaches the steady state. This biphasic response is due to the longer action of epinephrine on beta receptors than on alpha receptors. Epinephrine has no vasoconstrictor action on cerebral arterioles. Pressor doses in humans (20–70 μg/min) increase cerebral blood flow and oxygen uptake without any significant change in vascular resistance.[17] Epinephrine reduces renal blood flow even at subpressor doses. The glomerular filtration rate is unchanged, and the filtration fraction is increased. Excretion of sodium, potassium, and chloride is decreased. The effect on urinary volume is variable; it can be either increased or decreased. Tubular reabsorptive and excretory functions are unchanged. Renin release is increased.

The net effect of epinephrine on coronary circulation is increased coronary blood flow. The direct effect on coronary vessels in humans is constriction.[18] However, this effect is largely counteracted by a metabolic dilatory effect mediated by the release of locally produced metabolites, such as adenosine. The concentration of adenosine in coronary circulation increases rapidly after cardiac sympathetic stimulation as a consequence of a relative myocardial hypoxia.[19] Epinephrine directly stimulates the beta₁ receptors of the myocardium, cardiac pacemaker, and conducting system. As a result of this stimulation, heart rate and cardiac output increase, cardiac systole is shortened, and oxygen consumption increases. Cardiac efficiency, that is, the amount of work done in relation to oxygen consumption, is reduced. Cardiac arrhythmias frequently arise.

LIPID METABOLISM

Fatty acids are a major metabolic source of energy for tissues during fasting and exercise and account for much of the basal metabolic rate in the resting as well as in the fed state. Lipolysis is a major pathway for the supply of fatty acids to the bloodstream and is regulated by catecholamines. The administration of epinephrine in humans leads to increased lipolysis and, consequently, to higher serum concentrations of free fatty acids (FFA) and glycerol.[20] This increase is generally attributed to a direct action on adipose tissue, although a contributory factor could be the inhibition of insulin secretion.[21] The lipolytic activity in vitro is pH-dependent, being more pronounced at pH 8.4 than at pH 7.4.[22] Growth hormone seems to antagonize the lipolytic action of epinephrine.[23] The effects of epinephrine on adipose tissue, although similar, present striking differences. Epinephrine in dogs produces a transitory rise in the serum concentration of FFA, which returns to normal even during the infusion.[24] The infusion of norepinephrine, on the other hand, generates a persistent rise of FFA and glycerol.[24] This difference is thought to be dependent upon the more marked hyperglycemia induced by epinephrine as compared with norepinephrine. The elevated glucose concentration presumably increases the reesterification of fatty acids in the adipose tissue. In fact, despite the early decrease of plasma FFA concentration with epinephrine, the glycerol concentration persists and remains elevated for a longer period of time.[25] On the other hand,

in isolated canine adipose tissue, epinephrine is 10 times more potent than norepinephrine in releasing FFA, further supporting the hypothesis that in vivo the hyperglycemic and/or lactacidemic effect of epinephrine decreases plasma FFA.[26]

The first step in the activation of lipolysis by catecholamines is the combination of the hormone with a stereospecific receptor on the plasma membrane of the adipocyte,[27] probably a beta-adrenergic receptor. Thus, propranolol in fact, blocks the lipolytic activity of epinephrine, whereas phentolamine potentiates the effects of norepinephrine. The adipocyte membrane probably contains beta and alpha receptors which mediate opposite actions on lipolysis,[27,28] stimulatory and inhibitory, respectively. The interaction of catecholamines with beta receptors activates a membrane-bound enzyme, adenylcyclase. The effects of norepinephrine and epinephrine on lipid metabolism may be due to their *direct effect* on adenylcyclase. The activation of this enzyme leads to the formation of 3′,5′-cyclic AMP, which is believed to activate a protein kinase.[29] The latter phosphorylates the inactive triglyceride lipase to an active form which results in the breakdown of triglycerides to fatty acids and glycerol. This chain of events seems likely in view of the increased levels of free fatty acids, glycerol, and cyclic AMP after the addition of catecholamines to adipose tissue in vitro[29,30] (Fig. 101-3).

An *indirect effect* through inhibition of insulin release has been suggested but does not seem to play a major role. Insulin reduces the lipolytic effect of epinephrine, probably by inhibiting adenylcyclase.[31,32]

The lipases which are activated by norepinephrine and epinephrine include a specific monoglyceride, a diglyceride, a lipoprotein, a triglyceride, and possibly a triglyceride-monoglyceride fatty acyltransferase.[33] Epinephrine and norepinephrine increase the activity of the enzyme catalyzing the first step in triglyceride breakdown, which is normally the rate-limiting one.

Norepinephrine and epinephrine also increase the plasma concentration of lipids other than FFA, including triglycerides, phospholipids, and cholesterol. The increase of plasma triglycerides occurs only 24 hours after the infusion of norepinephrine in dogs, although the increase in cholesterol and phospholipids may occur earlier.[34] It is possible that the elevated concentration of FFA in the blood leads to increased uptake in the liver, which incorporates FFA into triglycerides and, to a lesser extent, into phospholipids.[35] Triglycerides accumulate in the liver and are not released for the first few hours after infusion, probably because norepinephrine inhibits the secretion of VLDLP from the liver. Prolonged infusion of norepinephrine may result in accumulation of triglycerides not only in the liver but also in skeletal muscle and heart. The increase of plasma and tissue triglycerides after infusion of epinephrine is

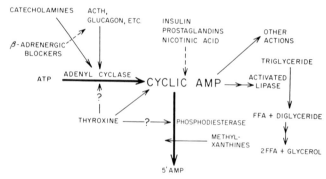

Fig. 101-3. Relationship of catecholamines to free fatty acid synthesis (Reproduced with permission from R. W. Butcher, *N Engl J Med* 279: 1378–84, 1968.)

not as marked as a result of the transitory increase in plasma FFA. The synthesis of triglycerides in adipose tissue is also increased by epinephrine and norepinephrine, secondarily to the increased concentration of FFA. Epinephrine also stimulates the synthesis of cholesterol by the liver. This effect may be related to the increased supply of free fatty acids or to a direct effect on 3-hydroxy-3-methylglutaryl coenzyme,[36] a reductase; this enzyme is believed to be the rate-limiting enzyme of rat hepatic cholesterol synthesis.[37,38] The catecholamine-induced stimulation of this reductase does not appear to be mediated through cyclic AMP levels, whereas the fatty acid synthesis does seem to be mediated through cyclic AMP[37] (Fig. 101-3). Epinephrine, but not norepinephrine, causes sustained increase of plasma cholesterol concentrations in the dog.[39] The oxidation of FFA by adipose tissue, heart, liver, and skeletal muscle is increased as well.[33,40–42] This effect is mostly dependent on the increased concentration of FFA; in fact, the oxidation of FFA is proportional to the concentration in the tissues. Whether epinephrine and norepinephrine have a direct effect on fatty acid oxidation is not clear. As a consequence of this increased fatty acid oxidation, the production of ketone bodies is increased.[33]

CARBOHYDRATE METABOLISM

Direct actions of epinephrine and norepinephrine have been demonstrated in vitro in striated muscle, heart, smooth muscle, liver, and adipose tissue. These actions are mediated through increased 3′,5′-cyclic AMP. The glygogenolytic effect of epinephrine in most tissues is mediated by beta receptors, while the receptor type responsible for hepatic gluconeogenesis is less clear.[43] Propranolol has no effect on gluconeogenesis induced by epinephrine but does block the catecholamine-induced increase in cyclic AMP in isolated rat liver cells. Isoproterenol is ineffective in enhancing gluconeogenesis, although it increases cyclic AMP. Phentolamine has no effect on catecholamine stimulation of gluconeogenesis.[43]

Epinephrine produces an increase of glycogen phosphorylase and a decrease of glycogen synthetase in skeletal muscle. Epinephrine, through an increase in 3′,5′-cyclic AMP, accelerates the conversion of inactive phosphorylase b to the active form a, thus accelerating glycogenolysis. Epinephrine decreases the proportion of glycogen synthetase in the I versus the D form, thus leading to an inhibition of glycogen synthesis and a decrease of muscle glycogen. Epinephrine inhibits the uptake of glucose by muscle; this effect depends upon the glycogen content of the tissue, being higher when the glycogen content is low. Epinephrine increases the amount of hexose phosphates in the incubation medium without changing the rate of glycolysis. The amount of lactate increases, not as a consequence of changes of the regulation of glycolysis, but because elevated FFA concentration inhibits pyruvate metabolism and diverts pyruvate to lactate.[44,45]

The infusion of epinephrine into a perfused heart causes an increase in the concentrations of 3′,5′-cyclic AMP and of phosphorylase activity. In contrast to skeletal muscle, epinephrine increases the proportion of the more active form I of glycogen synthetase. The overall change in carbohydrate metabolism due to epinephrine is also entirely different in the heart as compared to skeletal muscle. ATP and creatine phosphate decrease in the heart, whereas ADP, AMP, and phosphate concentration are increased. The rate of glycolysis increases, whereas in skeletal muscle it does not change. The source of the hexose phosphate used in glycolysis is mostly glucose from the medium at low concentrations of epinephrine. Glycogenolysis takes place at higher concentrations as well. Under these conditions the amount of lactate produced is

equal to the amount of glycogen disappearing. The increased activity of glycogen synthetase I indicates an increased synthesis of glycogen despite the net breakdown. The inotropic effect of epinephrine seems to be correlated with the increase in concentration of 3′,5′-cyclic AMP.[13] It is possible, however, that 3′,5′-cyclic AMP may trigger another change, such as an increase of ionized calcium. It must be remembered that between 60 and 80 percent of the energy requirement of the heart stimulated by epinephrine is obtained from the oxidation of lipids, the contribution of glucose being approximately 15 percent.[46]

Epinephrine produces an increase in 3′,5′-cyclic AMP and relaxation in smooth muscles. Subsequently, the amount of phosphorylase activity increases.[47] Lactate production also increases. Epinephrine increases the proportion of the active form of glycogen phosphorylase in the liver, leading to an increase of glycogenolysis and of the output of glucose from the cells.[48] Epinephrine also stimulates gluconeogenesis from lactate.

Intravenous infusion of epinephrine causes a persistent rise in blood glucose as long as the infusion continues. Norepinephrine, on the contrary, causes only a transient increase in blood glucose, and the increase lasts only 1 hour, even if the infusion is continued for as long as 24 hours.[49] The hyperglycemic effect of epinephrine is the result of at least five different actions:

1. After infusion of epinephrine, 0.05 μg/kg/min, plasma glucose level rises very rapidly as a result of increased hepatic glucose output.[50] The increase in lactate turnover is more gradual. Epinephrine activates phorphorylase in the liver, thereby causing increased glycogenolysis. At physiological concentrations, epinephrine may not have a glycogenolytic effect.

2. Epinephrine increases gluconeogenesis from lactate in the liver.[51,52] The increased lactate turnover is accompanied by a proportional increase in the rate of conversion of lactate to glucose. Thus, epinephrine in vivo seems to have no specific effect on gluconeogenesis other than to cause considerable increase in the substrate supply. Therefore, the gluconeogenic effect of epinephrine seems primarily the result of increased lactate turnover and, consequently, depends on the rate of glycolysis in peripheral tissues.[53]

3. Epinephrine inhibits the action of glucose in stimulating the secretion of insulin by the pancreas both in vivo and in vitro.[21,25] The inhibitory effect of epinephrine on insulin release seems to be due to a glucose-independent facilitation of both the outward transport and the vascular uptake of calcium from the beta cells.[54]

4. Epinephrine increases the concentration of FFA, which in turn can modify glucose tolerance.[55,56] The hyperglycemia produced by epinephrine, however, is not significantly related to the rise of FFA, since inhibition of the rise of FFA does not alter the hyperglycemic effect.

5. Epinephrine stimulates the secretion of ACTH and, consequently, of glucocorticoids by the adrenal cortex.[57] Glucocorticoids accelerate gluconeogenesis by the liver. This process is not a rapid one and is involved in the prolonged hyperglycemia caused by infusion of epinephrine for several hours. Glucocorticoids potentiate the metabolic effects of epinephrine, probably by decreasing the activity of phosphodiesterase and therefore leading to a greater accumulation of intracellular 3′,5′-cyclic AMP.[58] This may explain why patients with elevated plasma levels of glucocorticoids after physical or physiological stress may have extreme changes in carbohydrate metabolism. Epi-

nephrine increases the secretion of growth hormone in rats,[59] but not in humans.[60] Norepinephrine has a lesser hyperglycemic effect than epinephrine. Norepinephrine does not exert glycogenolytic action in muscle, nor does it increase the blood lactate concentration.[61] As a consequence, gluconeogenesis will not be increased.[50] Norepinephrine, therefore, must be considered a lipid-mobilizing hormone with little effect on glucose production or lactate turnover. Epinephrine, by contrast, causes only a transient increase in FFA, and in steady state its effect is restricted to carbohydrate metabolism. Epinephrine inhibits the incorporation of amino acids or other precursors into protein.[62]

SKELETAL MUSCLE

Skeletal muscle fibers do not receive direct sympathetic innervation.[63] Sympathetic nerves stimulate skeletal muscle via diffusion of adrenergic transmitters from the vascular sympathetic fibers or from the circulation. Epinephrine acts on mammalian muscle fibers via beta$_2$ receptors. Epinephrine prolongs the active state of white, fast-contracting muscles and curtails the active state of red, slow-contracting muscles. The direct effects on skeletal muscles seem to be mediated through activation of the adenylcyclase/3',5'-cyclic AMP system, which leads to an increase in the rates of uptake of Ca^{2+} by the sarcoplasmic reticulum.[63]

Epinephrine facilitates neuromuscular transmission in all muscles via the activation of alpha receptors located in the prejunctional motor nerve endings. The activation causes hyperpolarization of motor nerve endings and increased acetylcholine release by the nerve impulse. Epinephrine exerts a temporary defatiguing action in mammalian fast-contracting muscles. This action is mainly due to stimulation of prejunctional alpha receptors, but the direct action on fast-contracting fibers is also a contributing factor. Epinephrine has no defatiguing effect in red, slow-contracting muscles.

Epinephrine increases motor power in the injected limb of patients with myasthenia gravis for approximately 30 minutes after intra-arterial administration. Amphetamines and ephedrine given orally produce the same effects. Hypocalcemia increases the sensitivity of the skeletal muscle to this stimulatory effect of epinephrine. Tetany is produced after intra-arterial injection of epinephrine in patients with hypocalcemia. The physiological role for epinephrine on skeletal muscles is not clear. It appears that only the action on slow-contracting red muscle fibers has any significance. This action may enhance physiological and parkinsonian tremor produced in humans and may cause the tremor often associated with pheochromocytoma.[63]

GASTROINTESTINAL TRACT

Epinephrine relaxes the gastrointestinal smooth muscle, leading to an inhibition of frequency and amplitude of spontaneous contractions. Pyloric and ileocecal sphincters are usually contracted unless the preexisting tone is already high, in which case epinephrine causes relaxation.

REGULATION AND MODULATION OF OTHER ORGANS

ADRENAL CORTEX

The adrenal cortex influences the formation of epinephrine in the adrenal medulla. Hypophysectomy in rats reduces tyrosine hydroxylase,[65] dopamine-beta-hydroxylase (DBH),[66] phenylethanolamine-N-methyltransferase (PNMT),[67] and epinephrine in the adrenal medulla. The administration of ACTH or dexamethasone to those animals restores the activity of these enzymes in the gland. ACTH and glucocorticoids do not affect adrenal monamine oxidase or catechol-O-methyltransferase activities.[68] These data suggest that glucocorticoids stimulate the synthesis of new enzymes molecules in the adrenal medulla, thus influencing the synthesis of hormones. ACTH and corticosterone have also been shown to be involved in the methylation of norepinephrine in extra-adrenal chromaffin tissues.[69]

Adrenocortical steroids seem to play a permissive role in the actions of catecholamines. Injection of epinephrine in adrenalectomized rats does not elevate plasma FFA and produces only a slight increase in plasma glucose. Administration of glucocorticoids to these rats restores normal lipolytic and glycogenolytic responses. Adrenalectomized rats, on exposure to cold, show no sign of shivering, piloerection, or vasoconstriction and are unable to mobilize FFA or glucose. Their resistance to the effects of low temperature and strenuous exercise is reduced. Pretreatment of adrenalectomized rats with steroids restores a normal sympathetic response to cold exposure and to physical exercise, whereas infusion of epinephrine alone fails to restore the lipolytic and glycogenolytic responses. These abnormalities are thought to be related to poor responsiveness of adrenergic receptors to catecholamines in the absence of adrenocortical steroids.[70] Electrolyte imbalance may be a primary factor in these abnormal sympathetic responses, however.

Epinephrine does not convert phosphorylase b to the active form in the skeletal muscle of adrenalectomized rats. When these animals are pretreated with cortisone or aldosterone, they show a normal activating process.[70] The effects of mineralocorticoids in restoring normal phosphorylase activation suggest that for epinephrine to be effective, a critical electrolyte environment is required. In contrast, the activation of phosphorylase by 3',5'-cyclic AMP is not dependent on the ionic environment, suggesting that in adrenalectomized rats the lesion lies at the step between the release of catecholamines and the activation of adenylcyclase. It is possible that corticoids act on cell membranes, enabling the catecholamines to reach the enzyme.[71]

Glucocorticoids, when applied locally, produce a slowly developing vasoconstriction of cutaneous vessels.[72] This effect has been attributed to enhanced response to adrenergic stimuli. Hydrocortisone potentiates the response of isolated aortic strip to both epinephrine and norepinephrine.[73] The pressor responses to epinephrine, norepinephrine, and isoproterenol were reduced in adrenalectomized dogs and rats and in dogs with methyrapone-induced cortical insufficiency.[74,75] Other workers have not found significant changes in response to norepinephrine and epinephrine in adrenalectomized dogs.[76] Both mineralocorticoid and glucocorticoid properties of steroids are required to restore a normal response.[74] Hydrocortisone and aldosterone seem to potentiate the vasoconstrictor response to epinephrine but not to norepinephrine and other sypathomimetic amines when administered to anesthetized dogs or cats.[77] Ginsburg and Duff in 1958 infused the brachial arteries of normal people with cortisol alone, epinephrine and norepinephrine alone, and cortisol followed by epinephrine or norepinephrine. They found that cortisol followed by epinephrine caused a more marked reduction in flow than that seen with epinephrine alone. Cortisol alone did not alter blood flow and did not potentiate the vasoconstrictor activity of norepinephrine.[78] These data suggest that steroids do not increase the ability of arteriolar smooth muscle to contract, but they quite specifically increase the affinity of epinephrine to adrenergic receptors.[77] The action of corticoids seems to be mediated through a membrane effect which facilitates access of catecholamines to the intracellu-

lar enzymes. Adrenalectomy inhibits the step between the release of adrenergic neurohormone and the formation of 3',5'-cyclic AMP.[70] Pretreatment with pharmacologic doses of synthetic corticosteroids profoundly decreases catecholamine release in endotoxin shock.[79]

Catecholamines are probably inhibitory neurotransmitters for the physiologic steady-state discharge of corticotropin-releasing factor (CRF) from the neuronal terminals in the median eminence of the hypothalamus. Administration of reserpine, in fact, causes a hypersecretion of CRF and ACTH.[80,81]

PANCREAS

Catecholamines inhibit insulin release by stimulation of a pancreatic alpha receptor. This inhibition has been attributed to a decrease in intracellular cyclic AMP concentration.[82] The inhibition of insulin release, however, is probably related to some direct inhibitory effect independent of the intracellular concentration of cyclic AMP.[83,84]

Pancreatic islet cells are also supplied with an adrenergic receptor which responds to stimulation with an elevation of intracellular cyclic AMP and an increase in insulin secretion. More recently, with frequent and earlier time sampling,[84] Porte and Robertson demonstrated that insulin levels drop sharply after infusion of epinephrine, reaching the maximum inhibitory effect after 10 minutes. This phase is followed by a recovery phase during which insulin levels return and eventually surpass the basal levels. The early phase is prevented by phentolamine, indicating that it is mediated by alpha-receptor stimulation. Propranolol, on the other hand, can delay the recovery phase, suggesting that it is mediated by beta receptors. The same findings have been observed during acute stress states. Insulin levels are usually slightly lowered during the acute stress state but may become normal or elevated if the stress is prolonged.

In 1971, Frohman and Bernandis[85] established the hypothalamic control of the pancreatic alpha and beta receptors. Stimulation of the ventromedial nucleus causes glucagon release. Sympathetic nerve stimulation of mixed autonomic nerves of the pancreas,[86] as well as catecholamine infusion, stimulated glucagon release via beta-adrenergic stimulation that can be blocked by propranolol.[87] This response is not altered by atropine.[86] The effects of catecholamines on insulin and glucagon may be explained by the hypothesis proposed by Unger.[88] According to Unger, the insulin/glucagon ratio varies inversely with the need for endogenous glucose production, and the juxtaposed alpha, beta cell pair may be viewed as a single bicellular functional unit.[89] In conditions of stress, where sympathetic nerve activity is increased, the amount of glucose needed as oxidative fuel is increased. Thus, inhibition of insulin and stimulation of glucagon provides increased availability of glucose.

THYROID

Most clinical and laboratory data indicate that thyroid hormones modulate the effects of catecholamines. Many symptoms of hyperthyroid states, such as tachycardia, palpitations, tremor, sweating, CNS hyperactivity, increased oxygen consumption, and elevated BMR, mimic adrenergic hyperactivity. On the other hand, many of the symptoms of hypothyroidism mimic those of depressed sympathetic tone.

Cardiovascular System

Increased heart rate, cardiac output, ventricular stroke work, and cardiac oxygen consumption are observed in hyperthyroidism and are thought to be mediated by catecholamines rather than by a direct effect of thyroid hormone. Thyrotoxicosis increases the susceptibility to epinephrine-induced arrhythmias.[90] The concept is supported by the observation that many drugs that deplete or block the action of catecholamines, such as reserpine, guanethidine, or propranolol, improve many of the symptoms of thyrotoxic patients.[91–93] Some findings, however, suggested that sensitivity of the cardiac pacemaker to catecholamines in hyperthyroid animals or humans was not increased. They indicated that the major cause of the resting tachycardia was related to a direct effect of thyroxine on the intrinsic rate of the pacemaker.[94–98] Furthermore, the reduction in heart rate produced by propranolol in humans was not greater in hyperthyroid than in euthroid subjects, suggesting that increased adrenergic input to the pacemaker was not a contributory factor to the tachycardia.[99] On the other hand, in 1969 Wiener et al. showed that propranolol altered the hemodynamic exercise response of hyperthyroid patients in a manner different from that reported in euthyroid subjects.[93] The exercise increment in cardiac output, left ventricular tension time, and left ventricular work in hyperthyroid patients was in excess of that seen in euthyroid subjects. Cardiac efficiency, expressed as the ratio of left ventricular work and tension time index, was improved after propranolol administration in hyperthyroid patients, suggesting that beta blockade reduces the exaggerated myocardial oxygen requirements of thyrotoxicosis. Wiener believes that his data support the concept that the cardiac effects of thyroid hormone are mediated, at least in part, via the sympathetic nervous system.[93] Wildenthal and Wakeland have shown in vitro that triiodothyronine can act directly on the fetal mouse heart to enhance sensitivity to norepinephrine.[100]

Heimbach and Crout observed that the increase in heart rate produced by full doses of atropine is less in hyperthyroid than in euthyroid subjects, suggesting that the tachycardia of hyperthyroidism could be partially dependent upon an impairment of vagal inhibition of heart rate.[101] The therapeutic effect of reserpine was interpreted as resulting from stimulation of cholinergic function rather than from an inhibition of sympathetic tone.

Thyroid hormones potentiate the pressor response to catecholamines. Arteries isolated from thyrotoxic animals are sensitized to the constricting effects of epinephrine.[102]

Metabolism

The serum concentration of free fatty acids is increased in hyperthyroidism and decreased in hypothyroidism.[103] Hyperthyroidism potentiates, whereas hypothyroidism inhibits the lipolytic effect of epinephrine.[104,105] The response of adipose tissue to all lipolytic agents is reduced after thyroidectomy and increased by treatment with thyroid hormone.[104] The thyroid hormones probably modify the effects of cyclic AMP in adipose tissue.

The concentration of cardiac glycogen and the activation of myocardial phosphorylase are also influenced by the thyroid status. The mobilization of glycogen from the heart muscle induced by catecholamines is accelerated by treatment with thyroid. On the other hand, the mobilization of glycogen is reduced in hypothyroidism.[106] Thyroid hormones increase the amount of active phosphorylase and shift the dose-response curve for activation of phosphorylase by norepinephrine to the left. Since the activation of phosphorylase in muscle and liver is mediated by cyclic AMP, it is conceivable that the action of thyroid hormones is also mediated by cyclic AMP.[107] As a result of liver and muscle glycogenolysis, thyroid hormone excess enhances the hyperglycemic and glycosuric effect of epinephrine.[108] The calorigenic effects of epinephrine are inhibited by thyroidectomy and potentiated by treatment with thyroxine.[109,110]

Neuromuscular Responses

Excessive amounts of thyroid hormones exaggerate the tremor induced by epinephrine. Blepharoptosis is a common sign of myxedema and is caused by diminished noradrenergic tone of Müller's superior palpebral muscle. Instillation of phenylephrine will overcome the ptosis. Conversely, lid retraction in hyperthyroidism can be reduced by instillation of phentolamine into the conjunctival sac.[111]

Plasma, Urinary, and Tissue Catecholamines

Plasma catecholamines, in particular norepinephrine, are depressed in hyperthyroidism and increased in hypothyroidism.[112–114] Urinary excretion of norepinephrine after tilting at 70° was increased only twofold in hyperthyroidism, significantly less than the response in normal subjects.[115] Coulombe et al., on the other hand, did not find any difference in plasma and urinary concentrations of epinephrine between hyperthyroid, hypothyroid, and euthyroid subjects.[116]

The concentration of epinephrine in the adrenal medulla of rats, sheep, and guinea pigs was reduced significantly by treatment with thyroid hormones, whereas the concentration was increased in hypothyroidism.[117,118] These apparent paradoxes suggest that catecholamine responses are influenced by the concentration of circulating thyroid hormones and that the altered sensitivity probably leads to a reflex inhibition or stimulation of adrenergic nervous system in hyperthyroidism and hypothyroidism, respectively. Plasma dopamine-beta-hydroxylase concentration was reduced in patients with hyperthyroidism[119] and elevated in those with hypothyroidism. A very low level was observed in one case of thyrotoxic crisis.[120]

Mechanism of Interaction

Thyroid and sympathetic nervous system interrelationships are difficult to assess, since the respective hormones have some similar direct actions. From our previous analysis, however, it seems clear that thyroxine potentiates the action of catecholamines. Many hypotheses have been advanced to explain such interactions. Levey and Epstein in 1969 showed in vitro that independently of glucagon or beta-adrenergic activation, the rate of conversion of ATP to cyclic AMP increases 50 percent in hearts from cats treated with thyroxine or triiodothyronine.[121] Hardman et al. have shown reduced urinary excretion of cyclic AMP in thyroparathyroidectomized rats.[122] Urinary cyclic AMP is elevated in hyperthyroid humans, although some thought this resulted from depressed creatinine excretion in thyrotoxicosis rather than from a real increase in cyclic AMP production.[123,124] More recently, Guttler et al. have shown that although basal urinary cyclic AMP excretion is not increased in hyperthyroid humans, the infusion of epinephrine, parathyroid hormone, and glucagon causes augmented urinary cyclic AMP excretion in hyperthyroidism and diminished excretion in hypothyroidism when compared to a control group.[125,126] These data suggest that thyroxine modulates the response of multiple hormonal effects mediated by cyclic AMP.

Many studies have been performed on the effects of catecholamines on thyroid hormone synthesis and release, as well as on the effects of thyroid hormones on catecholamine synthesis, storage, release, metabolic degradation, and adrenoceptor properties. The human thyroid is supplied with vascular and interfollicular adrenergic fibers, which is evidence for direct sympathetic control of cells producing thyroid hormones. Sympathetic stimulation causes endocytosis and release of thyroid hormones.[127] Catecholamines stimulate the synthesis of thyroid hormones in isolated calf thyroid cells, which is further evidence that the sympathetic nervous system participates in the modulation of thyroid hormone secretion in response to appropriate physiologic stimulation.[128] This effect is inhibited by phentolamine and therefore seems to be mediated by alpha receptors. More importantly, the thyroid hormones affect sympathetic nerve function. Storage, synthesis, and turnover of norepinephrine are depressed in hyperthyroidism.[129] Norepinephrine turnover and H^3-NE efflux are increased in hearts and adrenal glands of hypothyroid rats.[130]

Recently, Dratman et al. have shown that uptakes of T_3 and T_4 are greater in innervated than in denervated salivary glands, thus suggesting that iodotyrosine amino acids may interfere with adrenergic nerves in a way similar to that of alpha methyl tyrosine. In fact, thyroxine inhibits the uptake of tyrosine C^{14} and the synthesis of NE in cultured superior cervical ganglia. The possibility thus exists that thyroxine molecules might enter adrenergic nerves and form false neurotransmitters.[131]

Abnormal monoamine oxidase activity has been found in both hyperthyroidism and hypothyroidism.[132] Large doses of thyroxine increase the activity of monoamine oxidase in mitochondrial preparations. The activity of monoamine oxidase of intestinal mucosa is inversely related to the excretion rate of monoamines. The activity of monoamine oxidase was decreased in biopsies of intestinal mucosa from hyperthyroid patients, whereas the excretion of two monoamines, tryptamine and tyramine, was increased.[133] The activity of catechol-O-methyltransferase in the liver of animals was reduced after large doses of thyroxine.[134]

More recently, the possibility has been suggested that thyroid hormone alters the number of adrenergic receptors or even produces an interconversion of alpha and beta receptors. After incubation of isolated myocardial cell nuclei of newborn rats with T_3 for 24 hours, the concentration of beta-adrenergic receptors in myocardial cells was increased in a dose-dependent fashion.[135] Infusion of T_3 in rats induced an increase in the number of myocardial beta-adrenergic receptors. No changes in the affinity of these receptors for isoproterenol or for the antagonist dihydroalprenol were found.[136] The increase in number of beta-adrenergic receptors in hearts from hyperthyroid animals was associated with an increased sensitivity of beta-adrenergic stimulation of myocardial cyclic AMP levels, phosphorylase activity, and contractility.

In hearts from hypothyroid rats, alpha receptors are absent or unreactive in comparison to euthyroid animals, suggesting the possibility of interconversion of myocardial alpha and beta adrenoceptors produced by altered thyroid hormone levels.[137] This interconversion could explain the decreased blocking potency of propranolol in the hearts of hypothyroid subjects[127] the increased sensitivity to phenylephrine and decreased sensitivity to isoproterenol of atria from hypothyroid rats,[138] the decreased vasoconstriction in the hind limbs of hyperthyroid dogs,[139] the diminished lipolytic response to norepinephrine, and many other signs of altered sympathetic response.

SEXUAL FUNCTION

Female

Ovulation. Sympathetic nerve function influences female sexual activity at various levels. Ovarian denervation produces disturbances of the estrous cycle in the rat, mouse, and guinea pig but not in the baboon.[140,141] It has been suggested that, at least in certain species, adrenergic stimulation produces contraction of muscle fibers which lie in the ovarian stroma to facilitate ovum

ejection. These stromal muscle fibers in the cat are excited by alpha-adrenergic agonists and depressed by beta-adrenergic agents.[142] Dibenzyline, an alpha-adrenergic antagonist, depresses ovulation in the rabbit and chicken.[143,144] Adrenergic innervation might also contribute to the secretory function of the ovarian interstitial cells.[145]

Ovum Transport. Adrenergic innervation is important for the movement of the ovum along the fallopian tube. The thick circular musculature of the isthmus has a rich adrenergic innervation. Alpha-receptor stimulation produces contraction of this muscle, whereas beta receptors produce inhibitory responses obtainable only in the presence of high concentrations of progesterone.[146,147] It has been suggested that the function of the isthmic sphincter is to allow retention of the ovum in the ampulla for a certain time after its release into the infundibulum. This delay seems to be very important for successful implantation of the ovum. In the rabbit the contraction of the smooth muscle cells of the isthmus during estrus seems to depend upon the ability of estrogens to enhance the alpha-stimulating effect of catecholamines.[148] This effect is antagonized by alpha-adrenergic blocking agents.[149] The activity of catecholamines on the longitudinal musculature of the ampulla is also modified by the estrogen–progesterone balance in a manner similar to that of the isthmic musculature.[150] The importance of estrogen–progesterone balance for the response of ampulla musculature to adrenergic stimuli has also been shown in humans.[151] The beta-inhibitory responses are pronounced when progesterone dominates, whereas alpha-stimulatory responses are pronounced during estrus. Autonomic dysfunction can alter the normal passage of the ovum. A correlation has been found between habitual tubal pregnancies and emotional stress.[152] Alpha-adrenergic blocking agents have been found useful in cases of infertility due to tubal spasm.[153]

Uterus. The uterus is furnished with a rich adrenergic innervation which increases from the body to the cervix.[154,155] The functional importance of this sympathetic innervation is not completely clear. Both alpha and beta receptors are present with a variable concentration or sensitivity depending upon the estrogen–progesterone balance. The hormonal state of the uterus thus modulates the response of the uterine myometrium to adrenergic agents.[156] Pregnancy or progesterone treatment enhances uterine sensitivity to beta stimulation in rabbit, rats, and women.[155,157] On the other hand, pregnancy or progesterone induces a relative dominance of alpha receptors.[158] Administration of beta-blocking agents to rat uteri with a predominance of beta receptors produces contraction. This contractile action has been interpreted by some as being mediated by a release of prostaglandins rather than dependent upon the direct effect of catecholamines on alpha receptors.[159] Variation in the estrogen–progesterone balance can also change the uterine stores of norepinephrine.[160] Estrogens inhibit the storage and uptake of catecholamines in the uterus, although the significance of this interference is unknown. Chronic administration of estrogens increases the uterine content and uptake of catecholamines, whereas acute administration of estrogens decreases the content of catecholamines.[161–163] Ovariectomy decreases the uterine catecholamine content.[164] Progesterone also reduces norepinephrine stores.[160] Epinephrine produces a marked increase in both cyclic AMP and glycogen phosphorylase in rat uteri. The magnitude of the responses is greater in uteri pretreated with estrogen. The magnitude of both the cyclic AMP and phosphorylase responses is significantly reduced by withdrawing estrogens but adding progesterone to the estrogen treatment or by

changing to progesterone from estrogens.[165] A resting adrenergic excitation has been found in the uterus of the estrogen-primed rabbit.[166]

The pregnant or nonpregnant human uterus is excited by norepinephrine or by beta-blocking agents and is inhibited by beta agonists or alpha-adrenergic blocking agents.[167] These results indicate that there is present in the human uterus a resting inhibitory sympathetic tone resulting from beta-receptor stimulation.

Pregnancy. In pregnant rats, rabbits, and dogs prior to term, uterine motility was enhanced by reserpinization or by systemic administration of beta-adrenergic blocking agents. In the rabbit during labor, administration of phenoxybenzamine can produce prolonged uterine inertia.[168]

The body of the uterus remains relaxed during gestation, whereas the cervix remains closed throughout pregnancy. At parturition, the body of the uterus must contract, whereas the cervix dilates. The dilator responses of the cervix seem to be mediated via beta-adrenergic receptors.[169] The role of the sympathetic nervous system in human labor has not been defined. Some investigators have reported increased excretion of catecholamines during labor; however, the functional significance of this increase is uncertain.[170] Many investigators have studied the role of the sympathetic nervous system in the reproductive processes of female rats. Svetlov and Korsalva showed that if sympathectomy was performed on the day of conception, implantation was normal, whereas sympathectomy on the fourth day impaired implantation in 90 percent of the animals.[171] Cervical gangliectomy plus sympathectomy in female rats alter the regularity of estrous cycles in about 30 percent of the animals. If cervical gangliectomy is performed 1 month before mating, it does not prevent impregnation or nidation but does interfere with normal fetal development. Only 2 out of 22 matings were followed by successful pregnancies.[172]

Uterine Blood Flow. Electrical stimulation of the uterine sympathetic nerve fibers or infusion of norepinephrine and epinephrine produce vasoconstriction.[173–175] Estrogens, on the other hand, produce vasodilatation and an increase in blood flow which does not seem to be mediated by the effects of this hormone on uterine catecholamine content.[176] In fact, uterine denervation or destruction of adrenergic neurones with 6-hydroxydopamine does not interfere with the normal physiological action of estrogens.[178] Stimulation of alpha-adrenergic receptors of uterine arteries supplying the placenta leads to reduction of uterine blood flow and consequent fetal hypoxemia. Constriction of these vessels probably plays a role in restricting hemorrhage at parturition.[179] Constriction of uterine arteries seems also to limit menstrual bleeding. In fact, sympathetic denervation of the human uterus increases the volume and time course of menstrual bleeding and the regularity of the menstrual cycle.[180,181]

Male

Thoracolumbar sympathectomy produces ejaculatory and, less frequently, erectile failure.[182,183] The ejaculatory failure has been attributed to denervation of the internal vesicular sphincter, which normally closes the bladder from the urethra during ejaculation, leading to retrograde ejaculation. The processes of emission and orgasm are not affected.[182] Antihypertensive drugs which affect the autonomic nervous system, such as reserpine, guanethidine, alpha-methyldopa, monoamine oxidase inhibitors, imipramine, ganglionic blocking agents, phenoxybenzamine, propranolol, and clonidine, produce ejaculatory or erectile failure or dysfunction, that is, paresis of the internal vesicular muscle.

Among these antihypertensive drugs, guanethidine more frequently produces sexual dysfunction, although ejaculatory failure is the more common symptom reported.[184] Occasionally, orgasmic failure may be present and may persist even after cessation of therapy. The cause of the prolonged persistence of this side effect has been interpreted as dependent upon a more pronounced and persistent reduction of catecholamines in the hypogastric neurones as compared with other organs.[185] Chronic guanethidine treatment of rats destroys neuronal mitochondria with subsequent permanent cellular degeneration.[186]

These clinical observations emphasize the importance of the interrelationships between sympathetic nervous system and male sexual function. The sympathetic nervous system may not regulate spermatogenesis directly, although there is histochemical and ultrastructural evidence for adrenergic innervation of Leydig cells in man.[187] Scrotal sweating, which seems to be important in the thermoregulatory control of spermatogenesis, is eliminated by sympathectomy.[188] Sympathetic function is important in spermatic movement at all extratesticular levels[189,190] and therefore in the process of emission and ejaculation. Emission consists of spermatic movement along the vas deferens to the pelvic urethra and then to the penile urethra after it mixes with secretions from the accessory glands. The human vas deferens is furnished with both alpha and beta receptors. The excitatory response seems to be mediated via alpha receptors. The beta receptors seem to be responsible for the quiescence of the vas deferens.[191] The role of the sympathetic nervous system in accomplishing penile erection is not clear. It is generally believed that the pelvic parasympathetic nerves are primarily responsible for erection. There is evidence that the sympathetic nervous system might also participate,[192] however, perhaps through a diminution of the resting vasoconstrictor tone or through a contraction of a muscle sphincter in the wall of the base of the human dorsal penile vein.[193]

RENIN–ANGIOTENSIN SYSTEM

There exist several endocrinological disorders that result in direct or indirect changes in the renin–angiotensin system. Some are mediated by the sympathetic nervous system. Patients with pheochromocytoma have increased renin during periods when the tumor is secreting norepinephrine.[270] Patients with hyperthyroidism also have hyperreninemia.[271] Patients with aldosteronoma have a depression of the renin axis. Patients with Cushing's disease have increased renin, which is a primary factor in their angiotensinogenic high blood pressure.[272]

Sympathoadrenal Control

Green[197] suggested that overactivity of the sympathetic nervous system results in the release of a vasoconstrictor from the kidney. Scornik[198] showed that intravenous infusion of norepinephrine produced a small increase in plasma angiotensin. Wathen et al.[199] and Vander[200] demonstrated that infusion of norepinephrine into the renal artery or into the peripheral vein caused marked renin release. Subsequently, Gordon et al.[201] showed that physiologic stimulation of the sympathetic nervous system by cold, upright posture or sodium deprivation resulted in increased urinary catecholamine, aldosterone, and plasma renin activity. In patients with autonomic dysfunction and postural hypotension, however, assuming the upright position did not result in an increase in plasma renin activity or in catecholamine excretion. Kotchen et al.[202] found parallel increments in urinary catecholamines and in plasma renin activity to graded exercise.

Dustan et al.[203] found that cardiac index and left ventricular ejection rate were directly related to renin activity in patients with essential hypertension and renal arterial and parenchymal diseases. Venous return and the shift of blood to the central circulation which determines cardiac output and left ventricular ejection rate were regulated by sympathetic vasomotor activity. Thus, these hemodynamic–renin relationships give further support for neurogenic control of renin release.

Bunag et al.[204] showed that increased sympathoadrenal discharge induced by hemorrhage in dogs stimulated renin release in the absence of measurable change in either renal blood pressure or flow. This renin release was prevented by ganglionic blockade or local anesthesia of the renal nerves. The response of renin release stimulated by hemorrhage in rats was also blunted by pretreatment with reserpine or dibenamine.[205] Various hypotensive agents—diazoxide,[206] sodium nitroprusside,[207] hydralazine,[208]—are potent stimuli of renin release, mediated by reflex sympathoadrenal stimulation.

Renal Nerve Control

The contribution of the renal nerves to the renin-releasing mechanisms has been proved; electrical stimulation of the renal nerves caused essentially the same effects on renin liberation as the intravenous infusion of norepinephrine.[200] Denervation of the renal nerves delayed the renin response to sodium depletion[209–211] and caused a decrease in renin content of the renal nerves.[214] Ganglionic blockade reduced the response of renin induced by sodium nitroprusside.[215]

The renal nerves or circulating catecholamines can amplify renin release by various stimuli (1) to the juxtaglomerular stretch receptor by affecting afferent arteriolar constriction, or (2) to the macula densa chemoreceptor by decreasing the glomerular filtration rate and changing the sodium load in the distal tubule, or (3) they might act directly on the production or release of renin in the juxtaglomerular cells, since a rich adrenergic innervation has been observed.[211,213,216]

These observations indicate the importance of the renal nerves in renin release. However, ganglionic blockade cannot completely prevent the renin response to sodium depletion[209,210] or to sodium nitroprusside-induced hypotension.[215] It has been reported that the renin–angiotensin–aldosterone system functioned normally in patients with renal homotransplant and, presumably, a denervated kidney. The transplanted kidney maintained excretory functions and an unimpaired response of renin release to high or low salt load[217,218] and to upright posture,[217] although there was the possibility for renal nerve regeneration. In anephric patients without detectable plasma renin activity, renin activity appeared in peripheral venous blood immediately after the kidney was transplanted with relatively large daily variations.[219] This renin originated from the transplanted kidney.

Vandongen et al.,[220] using the isolated rat kidney, demonstrated that there was a direct intrarenal stimulatory effect of norepinephrine, isoproterenol, and glucagon on renin secretion. Such catecholamine effects can be reproduced in vitro; the renin production in the incubation medium of renal cortical cell suspension[221] and renal slices[222] was stimulated by catecholamines but was inhibited by angiotensin.[222] Thus, it seems that the renin-releasing mechanism does not necessarily require renal innervation. In this situation it is possible that circulating catecholamines mediate in part the response of renin liberation to various stimuli through a direct chemical action on the juxtaglomerular cells.

Adrenergic Receptor Blockade

Winer and his co-workers[223] found that renin secretion in normal subjects was uniformly suppressed by adrenergic blockade, regardless of the stimulus. Renin secretion provoked by

upright posture or administration of diazoxide, ethacrynic acid, or theophyllin was markedly decreased after infusion of either alpha (phentolamine) or beta (propranolol) adrenergic blocking drugs. The enhancement of renin secretion by intravenous infusion of the sympathomimetic agents norepinephrine, isoproterenol, and cyclic AMP, adrenalectomy, hemorrhage, renal artery constriction, and sodium depletion was also blocked by both phentolamine and propranolol.[224,225]

Subsequent studies performed by other groups consistently supported the concept that the beta-adrenergic receptor is involved in the sympathetic control of renin secretion. However, alpha-adrenergic blockade (phenoxybenzamine or Dibenzyline) had no effect on the renin response to norepinephrine infusion[220,226] or to upright posture.[227] Ganong et al.[228] reported that insulin-induced hypoglycemia in anesthetized dogs, associated with the elevation of plasma epinephrine, increased plasma renin activity; after these animals were adrenalectomized, exogenous epinephrine, but not norepinephrine, enhanced renin secretion. Further, renin release stimulated by epinephrine was slightly potentiated by phenoxybenzamine, whereas it was abolished by propranolol.[229] It remains inconclusive whether or not the discrepancies regarding the alpha-adrenergic blockade of renin release were due to different experimental procedures or to the different alpha-adrenergic blocking agents used. It seems likely that the beta-adrenergic receptor plays a predominant role in the neurogenic control of the renin-releasing mechanism.

Recently, Laragh et al.[230] described a direct relationship of the propranolol-induced inhibition of renin secretion to its antihypertensive effect. The antihypertensive effectiveness of propranolol was related closely to both the preexisting level of plasma renin activity and to the extent of renin reduction induced by the drug. Patients with high renin hypertension—either malignant, renovascular, or essential—showed the greatest falls in both blood pressure and renin activity with propranolol. Conversely, little or no blood pressure response and a smaller decline in renin activity were observed in patients with low renin hypertension. The antihypertensive effect of propranolol has been confirmed by many investigators.[231–234] These findings further support the possibility of an associated neurogenic mechanism in patients with high renin hypertension.[236]

Sympathetic Nervous System and Renin– Catecholamine Interrelationships in Hypertension

Increased plasma renin activity is often observed in patients with pheochromocytoma.[235] Six of 12 patients with pheochromocytoma on a regular hospital diet had raised plasma renin activity. Normal renin activity was found in 5 of 6 patients in the attack-free period and in 3 of 10 patients in the attack period. These findings suggested that renin release was related closely to catecholamine secretion from the tumor. Further, urinary catecholamine excretion in patients with high renin activity was significantly greater than respective values in patients with normal renin activity. Alpha- and beta-adrenergic blocking agents prevented hypertensive attacks and reduced the enhanced renin release.

Determination of simultaneous plasma renin activity and plasma catecholamines in patients with primary hypertension are shown in Fig. 101-4. No patient had evidence of heart or renal failure, endocrine disorders, or any other complication that might influence renin secretion. All patients were studied in the outpatient clinic and received a regular diet with liberal sodium intake. All medications were withdrawn at least 2 weeks prior to study.

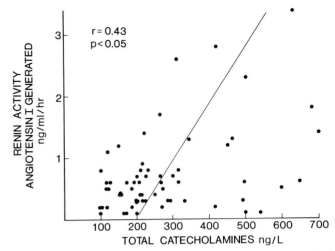

Fig. 101-4. Correlation of plasma catecholamines with renin activity in supine patients with primary hypertension (Reproduced from reference 236 with permission.)

Blood specimens were obtained from the antecubital vein of each patient after 30 minutes in the supine position during the hours of 8 to 10 AM after an overnight fast. There was a significant correlation between total plasma catecholamines and renin activities.[237] This relationship supported earlier findings in a smaller group in whom the regression line was defined by $y = 625x-75$; y = concentration of plasma catecholamines (nanograms per liter), x = plasma renin activity (nanograms per milliliter per hour) ($r = 0.491$, $p < 0.05$). These observations also suggested that sympathoadrenal activity and circulating catecholamines were causally related to renin-releasing mechanisms in some patients with hypertension.[177]

Renin–Sympathetic Nervous System Interaction: A Positive Feedback System

The elevated arterial pressure of rats with unilateral renal artery stenosis in the chronic phase was not alleviated after removal of the affected kidney.[238] In animals with renal hypertension, renin activity is usually increased in the acute phase only, not in the chronic phase.[239] In patients with renovascular hypertension 30 percent have a normal resting peripheral plasma renin activity.[240,241] Active immunization of animals with angiotensin II does not prevent the development or maintenance of renal hypertension.[242–244] These facts indicate that renal hypertension may be caused and maintained by mechanisms other than the renin–angiotensin system. Increased sympathetic nerve function has been described in human hypertensive subjects with renal artery stenosis.[245,246] These patients frequently have postural hypotension reflecting receptor insensitivity. Similar insensitivity is characteristic of patients with pheochromocytoma.[247] There are several ways in which the sympathetic nervous system may contribute to renal hypertension.

Angiotensin on Sinoaortic Buffer Nerves. McCubbin and his co-workers[248,249] demonstrated that the sensitivity of the sinoaortic baroreceptor was reduced in dogs with uninephrectomy and chronic perinephritic hypertension. Using an electroneurographic technique, they clarified that both the range and the threshold of the response of the carotid sinus reflexes are shifted upward, adapting or resetting to the higher pressure levels of chronic hypertension. Those functions act at the higher level and thus maintain rather than oppose pressure. These observations have been confirmed in humans as well as in dogs. A percutaneous

application of a small amount of epinephrine temporarily lowered the arterial pressure.[250] Since the blood pressure can often be restored to normal by repairing the renovascular lesions, the sinoaortic baroreceptor mechanism may not play a leading role in the origin of this hypertension. However, normalization of blood pressure in a patient with renovascular hypertension may take from 3 to 4 weeks after successful surgical correction of the renal artery lesion.[251] This indicates that extrarenal mechanisms such as the resetting of the sinoaortic baroreceptor may in part account for maintenance of the hypertension.

Angiotensin II Action on the Sympathoadrenal System. The cardiovascular action of angiotensin II, which is mediated by the central nervous system, was demonstrated using cross-circulation experiments in dogs. Injection of angiotensin into an isolated head caused a systemic pressor response in its body, although the two parts were connected only by the spinal cord.[252] It has now been recognized that angiotensin has a central vasomotor action resulting in increased sympathetic nerve discharge and an elevation of arterial blood pressure.[253] Intact sympathetic innervation is necessary for the full peripheral actions of angiotensin.[254-257] Pressor responses to tyramine are enhanced by the infusion of angiotensin II and also during the chronic phase of renal hypertension.[255,259] Angiotensin inhibited norepinephrine inactivation and reuptake in the sympathetic nerve ending.[260] Infusion of angiotensin I and II into the adrenal artery or peripheral vein stimulates the release of endogenous catecholamines from the adrenal medulla[261-264]. Feldberg and Lewis[264] pointed out that angiotensin does not act through release of acetylcholine from cholinergic nerve endings but acts directly on the medullary cells. Peach[265] held that angiotensin and its analogues were interacting with a common adrenal medullary receptor to alter chromaffin cell permeability to calcium and complete the link stimulating catecholamine secretion.

Renovascular Hypertension on Catecholamine Biosynthesis and Metabolism. To determine the pathogenesis of renovascular hypertension, it seems important to define variations in the biosynthesis and metabolism of the adrenergic neurotransmitter. Some of these findings in experimental models with various types of renovascular hypertension[266-269] suggest increased NE synthesis and release. These will be detailed in Chapter 104. However, no elevation of urinary norepinephrine or its metabolites have been reported in human renovascular hypertension. The measurements of total excretion of catecholamines reflect a summation of overall sympathetic nerve activity. Catecholamine excretion rate and plasma concentration are influenced not only by rates of NE biosynthesis and metabolism but also by the rate of reincorporation of liberated NE into nerve endings. Therefore, significant localized alterations of sympathetic nerve activity may be undetected. Recently, we found normal plasma catecholamines in a small number of patients with renovascular hypertension.[266]

REFERENCES

1. Frohlich, E. D., Tarazi, R. C., Dustan, H. P.: Hyperdynamic beta-adrenergic circulatory state. Increased beta receptor responsiveness. *Arch Intern Med 123;* 1 1969.
2. DeQuattro, V., Campese, V., Miura, Y. et al: Sympathotonia in primary hypertension and in a caricature resembling dysautonomia. *Clin Sci Mol Med 51:* 435–438, 1976.
3. Ahlquist, R.P.: A study of the adrenotropic receptors. *Am J Physiol 153;* 586–600, 1948.
4. Ahlquist, R. P., Levy, B.: Adrenergic receptive mechanism of canine ileum. *J Pharmacol Exp Ther 127:* 146–149, 1959.
5. Lands, A. M., Arnold, A., McAuliff, J. P. et al: Differentiation of receptor systems activated by sympathomimetic amines. *Nature 214:* 597–598, 1967.
6. Choo-Kang, Y. F. J., Parker, S. S., Grant, I. W. B: Response of asthmatics to isoprenaline and salbutamol aerosols administered by intermittent positive-pressure ventilation. *Br Med J 4:* 465–468, 1970.
7. Iversen, L. L.: Dopamine receptors in the brain: A dopamine-sensitive adenylate-cyclase models synaptic receptors, illuminating antipsychotic drug action. *Science 188:* 1084–1089, 1975.
8. Kunos, G., Yong, M. S., Nickerson, M.: Transformation of adrenergic receptors in the myocardium. *Nature New Biol 241:* 119–120, 1973.
9. Kunos, G., Vermes-Kunos, I., Nickerson, M.: Effects of thyroid state on adrenoceptor properties. *Nature 250:* 779–781, 1974.
10. Nakashima, M., Hagino, Y.: Evidence for the existence of alpha adrenergic receptor in isolated rat atria. *Jpn J Pharmacol 22:* 227–233, 1972.
11. Hirvonen, L., Paavilainen, T. O. A.: Response of rat atrium to propranolol and catecholamines in various states of thyroid action. *Acta Physiol Scand 69:* 284–294, 1967.
12. Sutherland, E. W., Rall, T. W.: The relations of adenosine 3'-5' phosphate and phosphorylase to the actions of catecholamines and other hormones. *Pharmacol Rev 12:* 265–299, 1960.
13. Robinson, G. A., Butcher, R. W., Øye, I. et al: The effect of epinephrine on adenosine 3'-5' phosphate levels in the isolated perfused rat heart. *Mol Pharmacol 1:* 168–177, 1965.
14. Langer, A., Hung, C. T., McA'nulty, J. A., et al: Adrenergic blockade. New approach to hyperthyroidism during pregnancy. *Obstet Gynecol 44:* 181–186, 1974.
15. Lefkowitz, R. J.: Biochemistry of beta adrenergic receptors and adenylate cyclase, in Wollemann, M. (ed): Properties of Purified Cholinergic and Adrenergic Receptors. Amsterdam, Holland, 1975, pp. 69–83.
16. Goldberg, N., O'Dea, R. F., Haddox, M. K.: Cyclic GMP, in Drummond, G. I., Greengard, P., Robinson, G. A. (eds): Advances in Cyclic Nucleotide Research, vol. 3. New York, Raven Press, 1975, pp. 155–224.
17. King, B. D., Sokoloff, L., Wechsler, R. L.: The effects of 1-epinephrine and 1-norephinephrine upon cerebral circulation and metabolism in man. *J Clin Invest 31:* 273–279, 1952.
18. Andersson, R., Holmberg, S. et al: Adrenergic alpha and beta receptors in coronary vessels in man: An in vitro study. *Acta Med Scand 191:* 241–244, 1972.
19. Berne, R. M., Rubio, R., Dobson, J. G. et al: Adenosine and adenine nucleotides as possible mediators of cardiac and skeletal muscle blood flow regulation. *Circ Res 28 (Suppl I):* 115–119, 1971.
20. Mueller, P. S., Horwitz, D.: Plasma free fatty acid and blood glucose responses to analogues of norepinephrine in man. *J Lipid Res 3:* 251–255, 1962.
21. Malaisse, W., Malaisse-Lagae, F., Wright, P. H. et al: Effects of adrenergic and cholinergic agents upon insulin secretion in vitro. *Endocrinology 80:* 975–978, 1967.
22. Ashley, B. C. E., Goldrick, R. B.: Lipolysis, esterification and glucose oxidation by human omental isolated adipose cells: The effects of pH1 buffer and epinephrine. *Lipids 5:* 498–500, 1970.
23. Goodman, H. M.: Antilipolytic effects of growth hormone. *Metabolism 19:* 849–855, 1970.
24. Havel, R. J., Goldfien, A.: The role of the sympathetic nervous system in the metabolism of free fatty acids. *J Lipid Res 1:* 102–108, 1959.
25. Porte, D. Jr., Graber, A. L., Kuzuya, J. et al: The effect of epinephrine on immunoreactive insulin levels in man. *J Clin Invest 45:* 228–236, 1966.
26. Rudman, D.: The mobilization of fatty acids from adipose tissue by pituitary peptides and catecholamines. *Ann NY Acad Sci 131:* 102, 1965.
27. Galton, D. J.: Plasma fatty acids and the control of lipolysis by catecholamines. *S Afr Med J 49:* 465–468, 1975.
28. Östman, J., Efendić, S.: Catecholamines and metabolism of human adipose tissue. *Acta Med Scand 187:* 471–476, 1970.
29. Butcher, R. W., Ho, R. J., Meng, H. C. et al: Adenosine 3'-5' monophosphate in biological materials. II. The measurement of adenosine 3'-5' monophosphate in tissues and the role of the cyclic nucleotide in the lipolytic responses of fat to epinephrine. *J Biol Chem 240:* 4515–4523, 1965.
30. LeBoeuf, B., Flinn, R. B., Cahill, G. F. Jr.: Effect of epinephrine on

glucose uptake and glycerol release by adipose tissue in vitro. *Proc Soc Exp Biol Med 102*: 527–529, 1959.

31. Butcher, R. W., Sneyd, J. G. T., Park, C. T. et al: Effect of insulin on adenosine 3'-5' monophosphate in the rat epididymal fat pad. *J Biol Chem 241*: 1651–1653, 1966.

32. Jungas, R. L.: Role of cyclic 3'-5' AMP in the response of adipose tissue to insulin. *Proc Natl Acad Sci USA 56*: 757–763, 1966.

33. Steinberg, D.: Catecholamine stimulation of fat mobilization and its metabolic consequences. *Pharmacol Rev 18*: 217–235, 1966.

34. Carlson, L. A., Liljedahl, S. O., Wirsén, C.: Blood and tissue changes in the dog during and after excessive free fatty acid mobilization. A biochemical and morphological study. *Acta Med Scand 178*: 81–102, 1965.

35. Spitzer, J. J., Gold, M., Branson, B. J.: Oxidation of free fatty acids by dog liver. *Proc Soc Exp Biol Med 118*: 149–150, 1965.

36. Bortz, W.: On the control of cholesterol synthesis. *Metabolism 22*: 1507–1524, 1973.

37. Edwards, P. A.: The influence of catecholamines and cyclic AMP on 3-hydroxy-3-methylglutaryl coenzyme a reductase activity and lipid biosynthesis in isolated rat hepatocytes. *Arch Biochem Biophys 170*: 188–203, 1975.

38. White, L. W., Rudney, H.: Regulation of 3-hydroxy-3-methylglutarate and mevalonate biosynthesis by rat liver homogenates. Effects of fasting, cholesterol feeding and triton administration. *Biochemistry 9*: 2725–2731, 1970.

39. Gans, J. H., Cater, M. R.: The effects of catecholamines on the distribution of ^{14}C-cholesterol in dogs. *Lipids 4*: 533–538, 1969.

40. Bally, P. R., Cahill, G. F., Leboeuf, B. et al: Studies on rat adipose tissue in vitro V. The effects of glucose and insulin on the metabolism of palmitate C^{14}. *J Biol Chem 235*: 333–336, 1960.

41. Gold, M., Attar, H. J., Spitzer, J. J. et al: Effect of norepinephrine on myocardial free fatty acid uptake and oxidation. *Proc Soc Exp Biol Med 118*: 876–879, 1965.

42. Nestel, P. J., Steinberg, D.: Fate of palmitate and of linoleate perfused through the isolated rat liver at high concentrations. *J Lipid Res 4*: 461–469, 1963.

43. Tolbert, M. E. M., Butcher, F. R., Fain, J. N.: Lack of correlation between catecholamines. Effects of cyclic adenosine 3'-5' monophosphate and gluconeogenesis in isolated rat liver cells. *J Biol Chem 248*: 5686–5692, 1973.

44. Ellis, S.: Relation of biochemical effects of epinephrine to its muscular effects. *Pharmacol Rev 11*: 469–479, 1959.

45. Garland, P. G., Newsholme, E. A., Randle, P. J.: Regulation of glucose uptake by muscle. 9 Effects of fatty acids and ketone bodies and of alloxan-diabetes and starvation on pyruvate metabolism and on lactate/pyruvate and L-glycero-3-phosphate/dihydroxyacetone phosphate concentration ratios in rat heart and rat diaphragm muscles. *Biochem J 93*: 665–678, 1964.

46. Kreisberg, R. A.: Effect of epinephrine on myocardial triglyceride and free fatty acid utilization. *Am J Physiol 210*: 385–89, 1966.

47. Diamond, J., Brody, T. M.: Effect of catecholamines on smooth muscle motility and phosphorylase activity. *J Pharmacol Exp Ther 152*: 202–211, 1966.

48. Himms-Hagen, J.: Sympathetic regulation of metabolism. *Pharmacol Rev 19*: 367–461, 1967.

49. Feigelson, E. G., Pfaff, W. W., Karmen, A. et al: The role of plasma free fatty acids in development of fatty liver. *J Clin Invest 40*: 2171–2179, 1961.

50. Issekutz, B. Jr., Allen, M.: Effect of catecholamines and methylprednisolone on carbohydrate metabolism of dogs. *Metabolism 21*: 48–59, 1972.

51. Exton, J. H., Park, C. R.: The stimulation of gluconeogenesis from lactate by epinephrine, glucagon and cyclic-3'-5' adenylate in the perfused rat liver. *Pharmacol Rev 18*: 181–188, 1966.

52. Fain, J. N., Tolbert, M. E. M., Pointer, R. H. et al: Cyclic nucleotides and gluconeogenesis by rat liver cells. *Metabolism 24*: 395–407, 1975.

53. Campbell, J., Rastogi, K. S.: Effects of glucagon and epinephrine on serum insulin and insulin secretion in dogs. *Endocrinology 79*: 830–835, 1966.

54. Brisson, G. R., Malaisse, W. J.: The stimulus-secretion coupling of glucose-induced insulin release. XI. Effects of theophylline and epinephrine on ^{45}Ca efflux from perfused islets. *Metabolism 22*: 455–465, 1973.

55. Nestel, P. J., Carroll, K. F., Silverstein, M. S.: Influence of free fatty acid metabolism on glucose tolerance. *Lancet II*: 115–117, 1964.

56. Paul, P., Issekutz, B. Jr., Miller, H. I.: Interrelationship of free fatty acids and glucose metabolism in the dog. *Am J Physiol 211*: 1313–1320, 1966.

57. Grana, E., Lilla, L.: On the adrenocorticotrophic activity of some sympathomimetic amines. *Arch Int Pharmacodyn Ther 126*: 203–213, 1960.

58. Senft, G., Schultz, G., Munske, K. et al: Effects of glucocorticoids and insulin on 3'-5' AMP phosphodiesterase activity in adrenalectomized rats. *Diabetologica 4*: 330–335, 1968.

59. Krulich, L., McCann, S. M.: Effect of alterations in blood sugar on pituitary growth hormone content in the rat. *Endocrinology 78*: 759–764, 1966.

60. Luft, R., Cerasi, E., Madison, L. L. et al: Effect of a small decrease in blood glucose on plasma growth hormone and urinary excretion of catecholamines in man. *Lancet II*: 254–256, 1966.

61. Bloom, W. L., Russell, J. A.: Effects of epinephrine and of norepinephrine on carbohydrate metabolism in the rat. *Am J Physiol 183*: 356–364, 1955.

62. Wool, I. G.: Incorporation of C^{14}-amino acids into protein of isolated diaphram: Effect of epinephrine and norepinephrine. *Am J Physiol 198*: 54–56, 1960.

63. Bowman, W. C., Nott, M. W.: Actions of sympathomimetic amines and their antagonists on skeletal muscle. *Pharmacol Rev 21*: 27–72, 1969.

64. Reid, J. L., Dargiehj, Franklin, S. S., Fraser, B.: Plasma noradrenaline and renovascular hypertension in the rat. *Clin Sci Mol Med 51*: 4395–4425, 1976.

65. Mueller, R. A., Thoenen, H., Axelrod, J.: Effect of pituitary and ACTH on the maintenance of basal tyrosine hydroxylase activity in the rat adrenal gland. *Endocrinology 86*: 751–755, 1970.

66. Weinshilboum, R., Axelrod, J.: Dopamine-beta-hydroxylase activity in the rat after hypophysectomy. *Endocrinology 87*: 894–899, 1970.

67. Axelrod, J.: Relationship between catecholamines and other hormones. *Recent Prog Hormone Res 31*: 1–35, 1975.

68. Wurtman, R. J., Axelrod, J.: Control of enzymatic synthesis of adrenaline in the adrenal medulla by adrenal cortical steroids. *J Biol Chem 241*: 2301–2305, 1966.

69. Ciaranello, R. D., Jacobowitz, D., Axelrod, J.: Effect of dexamethasone on phenylethanolamine n-methyltransferase in chromaffin tissue of the neonatal rat. *J Neurochem 20*: 799–805, 1973.

70. Brodie, B. B., Davies, J. I., Hynie, S. et al: Interrelationships of catecholamines with other endocrine systems. *Pharmacol Rev 18*: 273–289, 1966.

71. Murad, F., Chi, Y. M., Rall, T. W. et al: Adenyl cyclase III. The effect of catecholamines and choline esters on the formation of adenosine 3'-5' phosphate by preparations from cardiac muscle and liver. *J Biol Chem 237*: 1233–1238, 1962.

72. McKenzie, A. W., Stoughton, R. B.: Method for comparing percutaneous absorption of steroids. *Arch Dermatol 86*: 608–610, 1962.

73. Besse, J. C., Bass, A. D.: Potentiation by hydrocortisone of responses to catecholamines in vascular smooth muscle. *J Pharmacol Exp Ther 154*: 224–238, 1966.

74. Chopae, C. T., Brahmankar, D. M., Sheorey, R. V. et al: The effect of acute bilateral adrenalectomy on vasopressor responses to catecholamines in dogs. *J Pharm Pharmacol 27*: 262–267, 1975.

75. Ramey, E. R., Goldstein, M.: The adrenal cortex and the sympathetic nervous system. *Physiol Rev 37*: 155–195, 1957.

76. Salmoiraghi, G. C., McCubbin, J. W.: Effect of adrenalectomy on pressor responsiveness to angiotonin and renin. *Circ Res 2*: 280–284, 1954.

77. Yard, A. C., Kadowitz, P. J.: Studies on the mechanism of hydrocortisone potentiation of vasoconstrictor responses to epinephrine in the anesthethized animal. *Eur J Pharmacol 20*: 1–9, 1972.

78. Ginsburg, J., Duff, R. S.: Influence of intra-arterial hydrocortisone on adrenergic responses in the hand. *Br Med J 2*: 424–427, 1958.

79. Prager, R. L., Dunn, E. L., Seaton, J. F.: Increased adrenal secretion of norepinephrine and epinephrine after endotoxin and its reversal with corticosteroids. *J Surg Res 18*: 371–375, 1975.

80. Bhattacharya, A. N., Marks, B. H.: Reserpine and chlorpromazine induced changes in hypothalamo-hypophyseal adrenal system in rats in the presence and absence of hypothermia. *J Pharmacol Exp Ther 165*: 108–116, 1969.

81. Hodges, J. R., Vellucci, S. V.: The effect of reserpine on hypothalamo-pituitary-adrenocortical function in the rat. *Br J Pharmacol 53*: 555–561, 1975.

82. Robinson, G. A., Butcher, R. W., Sutherland, E. W.: Adenyl cy-

clase as an adrenergic receptor. *Ann NY Acad Sci 139:* 703–723, 1967.

83. Porte, D. Jr., Bagdade, J. D.: Human insulin secretion: An integrated approach. *Annu Rev Med 21:* 219–235, 1970.

84. Porte, D. Jr., Robertson, R. P.: Control of insulin secretion by catecholamines, stress, and the sympathetic nervous system. *Fed Proc 32:* 1792–1796, 1973.

85. Frohman, L. A., Bernardis, L. L.: Effect of hypothalamic stimulation on plasma glucose, insulin and glucagon levels. *Am J Physiol 221:* 1596–1603, 1971.

86. Marliss, E. B., Girardier, L., Seydoux, J. et al: Glucagon release induced by pancreatic nerve stimulation in the dog. *J Clin Invest 52:* 1246–1259, 1973.

87. Iversen, J.: Adrenergic receptors and the secretion of glucagon and insulin from the isolated, perfused canine pancreas. *J Clin Invest 52:* 2102–2116, 1973.

88. Unger, R. H.: Glucagon and the insulin: Glucagon ratio in diabetes and other catabolic illnesses. *Diabetes 20:* 834–838, 1971.

89. Unger, R. H.: Glucagon physiology and pathophysiology. *N Eng J Med 285:* 443–448, 1971.

90. Murray, J. F., Kelly, J. J. Jr.: The relation of thyroidal hormone level to epinephrine response: A diagnostic test for hyperthyroidism. *Ann Intern Med 51:* 309–321, 1959.

91. Canary, J. J., Schaaf, M., Duffy, B. J. et al: Effects of oral and intramuscular administration of reserpine in thyrotoxicosis. *New Engl J Med 257:* 435–442, 1957.

92. Howitt, G., Rowlands, D. J.: Beta sympathetic blockade in hyperthyroidism. *Lancet 1:* 628–631, 1966.

93. Wiener, L., Stout, B. D., Cox, J. W.: Influence of beta sympathetic blockade (propranolol) on the hemodynamics of hyperthyroidism. *Am J Med 46:* 227–233, 1969.

94. Benfey, B. G., Varma, D. R.: Cardiac and vascular effects of sympathomimetic drugs after administration of triiodothyronine and reserpine. *Br J Pharmacol Chemother 21:* 174–181, 1963.

95. Cairoli, V. J., Crout, J. R.: Role of the autonomic nervous system in the resting tachycardia of experimental hyperthyroidism. *J Pharmacol Exp Ther 158:* 55–65, 1967.

96. Aoki, V. S., Wilson, W. R., Theilen, E. O. et al: The effects of triiodothyronine on hemodynamic responses to epinephrine and norepinephrine in man. *J Pharmacal Exp Ther 157:* 62–68, 1967.

97. Aoki, V. S., Wilson, W. R., Theilen, E. O.: Studies of the reputed augmentation of the cardiovascular effects of catecholamines in patients with spontaneous hyperthyroidism. *J Pharmacal Exp Ther 181:* 362–368, 1972.

98. Levey, G. S.: Catecholamine sensivity, thyroid hormone and the heart—A re-evaluation. *Am J Med 50:* 413–420, 1971.

99. Wilson, W. R., Theilen, E. O., Hege, J. H., Valenla, M. R.: Effects of beta adrenergic receptor blockage in normal subjects before, during and after triiodothyronine induced hypermetabolism. *J Clin Invest 45:* 1159–1160, 1966.

100. Wildenthal, K., Wakeland, J. R.: Studies of isolated fetal mouse hearts in organ culture: Evidence for a direct effect of triiodothyronine in enhancing cardiac responsiveness to norepinephrine. *J Clin Invest 51:* 2702–2709, 1972.

101. Heimbach, D. M., Crout, J. R.: Effect of atropine on the tachycardia of hyperthyroidism. *Arch Intern Med 129:* 430–432, 1972.

102. Smith, D. J.: Immediate sensitization of isolated swine arteries and their vasa vasorum to epinephrine, acetylcholine and histamine by thyroxine. *Am J Physiol 177:* 7–12, 1954.

103. Rich, C., Bierman, E. L., Schwartz, I. L.: Plasma nonesterified fatty acids in hyperthyroid states. *J Clin Invest 38:* 275–278, 1959.

104. Goodman, H. M., Bray, G. A.: Role of thyroid hormones in lipolysis, *Am J Physiol 210:* 1053–1058, 1966.

105. Vaughan, M.: An in vitro effect of triiodothyronine on rat adipose tissue. *J Clin Invest 46:* 1482–1491, 1967.

106. Bray, G. A., Goodman, H. M.: Effect of epinephrine on glucose transport and metabolism in adipose tissue of normal and hypothyroid rats. *J Lipid Res 9:* 714–719, 1968.

107. McNeill, J. H.: Amine-induced cardiac phosphorylase A after reserpine-triiodothyronine pretreatment. *Eur J Pharmacol 7:* 235–238, 1969.

108. Comsa, J.: Adrenaline-thyroxine interaction in guinea pigs. *Am J Physiol 161:* 550–553, 1950.

109. Swanson, H. E.: Interrelation between thyroxine and adrenaline in the regulation of oxygen consumption in the albino rat. *Endocrinology 59:* 217–225, 1956.

110. Svedmyr, N.: Studies on the relationship between some metabolic

111. Lee, W. Y., Morimoto, P. K., Bronsky, D. et al: Studies on thyroid and sympathetic nervous system interrelationships. I. The blepharoptosis of myxedema. *J Clin Endocrinol 21:* 1402–12, 1961.

112. Christensen, N. J.: Plasma noradrenaline and adrenaline in patients with thyrotoxicosis and myxoedema. *Clin Sci Mol Med 45:* 163–171, 1973.

113. Stoffer, S. S., Jiang, N. S., Gorman, C. A. et al: Plasma catecholamines in hypothyroidism and hyperthyroidism. *J Clin Endocrinal Metab 36:* 587–589, 1973.

114. Ghione, S., Pellegrini, M., Buzzigoli, G. et al: Plasma and urinary catecholamine levels and thyroid activity in relation to cardiovascular changes in hyper- and hypothyroidism. *Hormone Metab Res 6:* 93, 1974.

115. Harrison, T. S.: Reflex liberation of catecholhormones in hyperthyroidism. *J Surg Res I:* 77–81, 1961.

116. Coulombe, P., Dussault, J. H., Letarte, J. et al: Catecholamines metabolism in thyroid disease-I. Epinephrine secretion rate in hyperthyroidism and hypothyroidism. *J Clin Endocrinol Metab 42:* 125–131, 1976.

117. Leak, D.: The Thyroid and the Autonomic Nervous System. *London, William Heinemann Medical Books,* 1970.

118. Hökfelt, B.: Noradrenaline and adrenaline in mammalian tissues. *Acta Physiol Scand Suppl:* 92, 1951.

119. Noth, R. H., Spaulding, S. W.: Decreased serum dopamine-beta-hydroxylase activity in hyperthyroidism. *Clin Res 22:* 344A, 1974.

120. Nishizawa, Y., Hamada, N., Fujii, S. et al: Serum dopamine-beta-hydroxylase activity in thyroid disorders. *J Clin Endocrinol Metab 39:* 599–602, 1974.

121. Levey, G. S., Epstein, S. E.: Myocardial adenyl cyclase: Activation by thyroid hormones and evidence for two adenyl cyclase systems. *J Clin Invest 48:* 1663–1669, 1969.

122. Hardman, J. G., Davis, J. W., Sutherland, E. W.: Measurement of guanosine 3′-5′ monophosphate and other cyclic nucleotides. *J Biol Chem 241:* 4812–4815, 1966.

123. Rosen, O. M.: Urinary cyclic AMP in Grave's disease. *New Engl J Med 287:* 670–671, 1972.

124. Lin, T., Kopp, L. E., Tucci, J. R.: Urinary excretion of cyclic 3′-5′ adenosine monophosphate in hyperthyroidism. *J Clin Endocrinol Metab 36:* 1033–1036, 1973.

125. Guttler, R. B., Shaw, J. W., Otis, C. L. et al: Epinephrine-induced alterations in urinary cyclic AMP in hyper- and hypothyroidism. *J Clin Endocrinol Metab 41:* 707–711, 1975.

126. Guttler, R. B., Croxson, M. S., DeQuattro, V. L. et al: The effects of thyroid hormone on plasma adenosine 3′-5′ monophosphate production in man. *Metabolism 1977 (in press).*

127. Melander, A., Ericson, L. E., Ljunggren, J. G. et al: Sympathetic innervation of the normal human thyroid. *J Clin Endocrinol Metab 39:* 713–718, 1974.

128. Maayan, M. L., Ingbar, S. H.: Epinephrine: Effect on uptake of iodine by dispersed cells of calf thyroid gland. *Science 162:* 124–125, 1968.

129. Axelrod, J.: Relationship between catecholamines and other hormones. *Recent Prog Hormone Res 31:* 1–35. 1975.

130. Tv, T., Nash, C. W.: The influence of prolonged hyper- and hypothyroid states on the noradrenaline content of rat tissues and on the accumulation and efflux rates of tritiated noradrenaline. *Can J Physiol Pharmacol 53:* 74–80, 1975.

131. Dratman, M. B.: On the mechanism of action of thyroxin, an amino acid analog of tyrosine. *J Theor Biol 46:* 255–270, 1974.

132. Levine, R. J., Oates, J. A., Vendsalu, A. et al: Studies on the metabolism of aromatic amines in relation to altered thyroid function in man. *J Clin Endocrinol 22:* 1242–1250, 1962.

133. Bray, G. A., Jacobs, H. S.: Thyroid activity and other endocrine glands, in Greep, R. O., Astwood, E. B. (eds): Handbook of Physiology. Section 7: Endocrinology. Vol III: Thyroid. Washington, D. C., American Physiological Society, 1974, pp. 413–433.

134. Bray, G. A.: Clinical and experimental aspects of the interrelations between thyroid and catecholamines, in Astwood, E. B., Cassidy, C. E. (eds): Clinical Endocrinology, vol. II. New York, Grune & Stratton, 1968, pp. 177–194.

135. Tsai, J. S., Chen, A.: L-triiodothyronine increases the level of beta-adrenergic receptor in cultured myocardial cells. *Clin Res 25:* 303A, 1977.

136. Williams, L. T., Lefkowitz, R. J., Watanabe, A. M. et al: Thyroid hormone regulation of beta-adrenergic receptor number: Possible

biochemical basis for the hyperadrenergic state in hyperthyroidism. *Clin Res 25:* 458A, 1977.

137. Kunos, G., Vermes-Kunos, I., Nickerson, M.: Effects of thyroid state on adrenoceptor properties. *Nature 250:* 779–781, 1973.

138. Nakashima, M., Maeda, K., Sekiya, A., Hagino, Y.: Effect of hypothyroid status on myocardial responses to sympathomimetic drugs. *Jpn J Pharmacol 21:* 819–825, 1971.

139. Zsoter, R., Tom, H., Chappel, C.: Effect of thyroid hormones on vascular response. *J Lab Clin Med 64:* 433–441, 1964.

140. Towner-Hill, R.: Paradoxical effects of ovarian secretion, in Zuckerman, S. et al (eds): The Ovary, Vol. III, New York, *Academic Press,* 1961, pp 231–262.

141. Lepere, R. H., Benoit, P. E., Hardy, R. C. et al: The origin and function of the ovarian nerve supply in the baboon. *Fertil Steril 17:* 68–75, 1966.

142. Rocereto, R., Jacobowitz, D., Wallach, E. E.: Observations of spontaneous contractions of the cat ovary in vitro. *Endocrinology 84:* 1336–1341, 1969.

143. Virutamesen, P., Hickok, R. L., Wallach, E. E.: Local ovarian effects of catecholamines on human chorionic gonadotropin induced ovulation in the rabbit. *Fertil Steril 22:* 235–243, 1971.

144. Bahr, J., Kao, L., Nalbandov, A. V.: The role of catecholamines and nerves in ovulation. *Biol Reprod 10:* 273–290, 1974.

145. Vogt, M.: The secretion of the denervated adrenal medulla of the cat. *Br J Pharmacol 7:* 325–330, 1952.

146. Nakanishi, H., Wansbrough, H., Wood, C.: Postganglionic sympathetic nerves innervating human fallopian tube. *Am J Physiol 213:* 613–619, 1967.

147. Seitchik, J., Goldberg, E., Goldsmith, J. P. et al: Pharmacodynamic studies of the human fallopian tube in vitro. *Am J Obstet Gynecol 102:* 727–735, 1968.

148. Davids, A. M., Bender, M. B.: Effects of adrenaline on tubal contractions of the rabbit in relation to the sex hormones. *Am J Physiol 129:* 259–263, 1940.

149. Pauerstein, C. J., Fremming, B. D., Martin, J. E.: Estrogen-induced tubal arrest of ovum: Antagonism by alpha-adrenergic blockade. *Obstet Gynecol 35:* 671–675, 1970.

150. Coutinho, E. M., Mattos, C. E. R., DaSilva, A. R.: The effect of ovarian hormones on the adrenergic stimulation of the rabbit fallopian tube. *Fertil Steril 22:* 311–317, 1971.

151. Coutinho, E. M., Maia, H., Filo, J. A.: Response of the human fallopian tube to adrenergic stimulation. *Fertil Steril 21:* 590–594, 1970.

152. Asherman, J. G.: Etiology of ectopic pregnancy: A new concept. *Obstet Gynecol 6:* 619–624, 1955.

153. Sandler, B.: The mechanism of tubal spasm. *Proc Soc Study Fertil 5:* 59–65, 1953.

154. Owman, C., Rosengren, E., Sjöberg, N. O.: Adrenergic innervation of the human female reproductive organs: A histochemical and chemical investigation. *Obstet Gynecol 30:* 763–773, 1967.

155. Nakamshi, H., McLean, J., Wood, C. et al: The role of sympathetic nerves in control of the nonpregnant and pregnant human uterus. *J Reprod Med 2:* 20–33, 1969.

156. Miller, J. W.: Adrenergic receptors in the myometrium. *Ann NY Acad Sci 139:* 788–798, 1966.

157. Pauerstein, C. J., Zauder, H. L.: Autonomic innervation, sex steroids and uterine contractility. *Obstet Gynecol Surv 25:* 617–630, 1970.

158. Tsai, T. H., Fleming, W. W.: The adrenotropic receptors of the cat uterus. *J Pharmacol Exp Ther 143:* 268–272, 1964.

159. Tothill, A., Rathbone, L., Willman, E.: Relation between prostaglandin E$_2$ and adrenaline reversal in the rat uterus. *Nature 233:* 56–57, 1971.

160. Sjöberg, N. O.: The adrenergic transmitter of the female reproductive tract: Distribution and functional changes. *Acta Physiol Scand 72:* Suppl 305, 1–89, 1967.

161. Adham, N., Schenk, E. A.: Autonomic innervation of the rat vagina, cervix and uterus and its cyclic variation. *Am J Obstet Gynecol 104:* 508–516, 1969.

162. Wurtman, R. J., Chu, E. W., Axelrod, J.: Relation between the oestrous cycle and the binding of catecholamines in the rat uterus. *Nature 198:* 547–548, 1963.

163. McKercher, T. C., Van Orden III, L. S., Bhatnagar, R. K. et al: Estrogen-induced biogenic amine reduction in the rat uterus. *J Pharmacol Exp Ther 185:* 514–522, 1973.

164. Oskarsson, V.: Influence of ovarian hormones and denervation on

the catecholamines of the rat uterus. *Acta Endocrinol 34:* 38–44, 1960.

165. Rinard, G. A., Chew, C. S.: Interacting effects of estrogens, progesterone and catecholamines on rat uterine cyclic AMP and glycogen phosphorylase. *Life Sci 16:* 1507–1512, 1975.

166. Setekleiv, J.: Uterine motility of the estrogenized rabbit. IV. Reflex excitation and inhibition. *Acta Physiol Scand 62:* 304–312, 1964.

167. Wansbrough, H., Nakaniski, H., Wood, C.: The effect of adrenergic receptor blocking drugs on the human uterus. *J Obstet Gynaecol Br Commonw 75:* 189–198, 1968.

168. Shabanah, E. H., Toth, A., Omay, Y. et al: The role of the autonomic nervous system in uterine contractility and blood flow. V. Interrelationship of estrogen, progesterone, and the pituitary trophic hormones in the control of myometrial function. *Am J Obstet Gynecol 100:* 981–986, 1968.

169. Barnes, A. B.: Chronic propranolol administration during pregnancy. *J Reprod Med 5:* 179–180, 1970.

170. Goodall, McC., Diddle, A. W.: Epinephrine and norepinephrine in pregnancy. *Am J Obstet Gynecol III:* 896–904, 1971.

171. Svetlov, P. G., Korsakova, G. F.: Influence of denervation of the uterus in rats upon the course of implantation. *Bull Exp Biol Med 43:* 78–82, 1957.

172. Barnea, A., Shelesnyak, M. C.: Studies on the mechanism of nidation. XV. The effect of cervical ganglionectomy. *J Endocrinol 32:* 199–204, 1965.

173. Ryan, M. J., Clark, K. E., Brody, M. J.: Neurogenic and mechanical control of canine uterine vascular resistance. *Am J Physiol 227:* 547–555, 1974.

174. Robson, J. M., Schild, H. O.: Effect of drugs on the blood flow and activity of the uterus. *J Physiol 92:* 9–19, 1938.

175. Bell, C.: Dual vasoconstrictor and vasodilator innervation of the uterine arterial supply in the guinea pig. *Circ Res 23:* 279–289, 1968.

176. Spaziani, E.: Accessory reproductive organs in mammals: Control of cell and tissue transport by sex hormones. *Pharmacol Rev 27:* 207–286, 1975.

177. DeQuattro, V., Miura, Y.: Neurogenic factors in hypertension: Mechanism or Myth? *Am J Med 55:* 362–378, 1973.

178. Brody, M. J., Edvinsson, L., Sjöberg, N. O.: Preservation of estrogen-induced increase of uterine blood volume following catecholamine and mast cell histamine depletion. *Proc Soc Exp Biol Med 149:* 120–123, 1975.

179. Carter, A. M., Göthlin, J., Olin, T.: An angiographic study of the structure and function of the uterine and maternal placental vasculature in the rabbit. *J Reprod Fertil 25:* 201–210, 1971.

180. Davis, A.: The present position of neurosurgery in gynaecology. *Br Med J 2:* 585–590, 1948.

181. Maughan, G. B., Shabanah, E. H., Toth, A.: Experiments with pharmacologic sympatholysis in the gravid. *Am J Obstet Gynecol 97:* 764–776, 1967.

182. Abramovici, H., Weisz, G. M., Timor-Tritsch, I. et al: Male infertility following aortic surgery. *Int J Fertil 16:* 144–146, 1971.

183. Whitelaw, G. P., Smithwick, R. H.: Some secondary effects of sympathectomy with particular reference to disturbance of sexual function. *New Engl J Med 245:* 121–130, 1951.

184. Rosenbloom, S. E., Shapera, R. P., Goldbloom, R. S. et al: Technic of controlled drug assay. III. Comparison of guanethidine, mecamylamine and a placebo in the hypertensive patient. *New Engl J Med 268:* 797–803, 1963.

185. Gannon, B. J., Iwayama, T., Burnstock, G.: Prolonged effects of chronic guanethidine treatment on the sympathetic innervation of the genitalia of male rats. *Med J Aust 2:* 207–208, 1971.

186. Burnstock, G., Evans, B., Gannon, B. J.et al: A new method of destroying adrenergic nerves in adult animals using guanethidine. *Br J Pharmacol 43:* 295–301, 1971.

187. Baumgarten, H. G., Holstein, A. F.: Ultrastructure, innervation, and noradrenaline content of smooth muscle layers of the human epididymis and ductus deferens. *J Anat 109:* 348–349, 1971.

188. Monro, P. A. G.: Sympathectomy. London, Oxford University, 1959.

189. Wakade, A. R., Kirpekak, S. M.: Chemical and histochemical studies on the sympathetic innervation of the vas deferens and seminal vesicle of the guinea pig. *J Pharmacol Exp Ther 178:* 432–441, 1971.

190. Bell, C.: Autonomic nervous control of reproduction: Circulatory and other factors. *Pharmacol Rev 24:* 657–736, 1972.

191. Baumgarten, H. G., Holstein, A. F., Rosengren, E.: Arrangement.

ultrastructure and adrenergic innervation of smooth musculature of the ductuli efferentes, ductus epididymis and ductus deferens of man. *Z Zellforsch Mikroskop Anat 120:* 37–79, 1971.

192. Root, W. S., Bard, P.: The mediation of feline erection through sympathetic pathways with some remarks on sexual behavior after deafferentation of the genitalia. *Am J Physiol 151:* 80–90, 1947.

193. Haines, R. W.: An unstriped sphincter of the dorsal vein of the penis. *J Anat 107:* 385, 1970.

194. Kamberi, I. A.: Hypothalamic catecholamines and the secretion of gonadotropins and gonadotropin releasing hormones, in: Frontiers in Catecholamine Research. London, Pergammon Press, 1973, pp 849–852.

195. Del Pozo, E., Brun del Re, R., Varga, L., Friesen, H.: The inhibition of prolactin secretion in man by CB-154 (2-Br-Alpha-ergocryptine). *J Clin Endocrinol Metab 35:* 768–771, 1972.

196. Stumpe, K. O., Kolloch, R., Higuchi, M. et al: Hyperprolactiaemia and antihypertensive effect of bromocriptine in essential hypertension. *Lancet ii:* 211, 1977.

197. Green, H. D.: Pharmacology of antihypertensive drugs *Am J Med 17:* 70, 1954.

198. Scornik, O. A., Paladini, A. C.: Significance of blood angiotensin levels in different experimental conditions. *Can Med Assoc J 90:* 269, 1964.

199. Wathen, R. L., Kingbury, W. S., Stouder, D. A., Schneider, E. G., Rostorfer, H. H.: Effects of infusion of catecholamines and angiotensin II on renin release in anesthetized dogs. *Am J Physiol 209:* 1012, 1965.

200. Yander, A. J.: Effect of catecholamines and the renal nerves on renin secretion in anesthetized dogs. *Am J Physiol 209:* 659, 1965.

201. Gordon, R. D., Kuchel, O., Liddle, G. W., Island, D. P.: Role of the sympathetic nervous system in regulating renin and aldosterone production in man. *J Clin Invest 46:* 599, 1967.

202. Kotchen, T. A., Hartley, L. H., Rice, T. W. et al: Renin, norepinephrine, and epinephrine responses to graded exercise. *J Appl Physiol 31:* 178, 1971.

203. Dustan, H. P., Tarazi, R. C., Frohlich, E. D.: Functional correlates of plasma renin activity in hypertensive patients. *Circulation 41:* 555, 1970.

204. Bunag, R. D., Page, I. H., McCubbin, J. W.: Neural stimulation of release of renin. *Circ Res 19:* 851, 1966.

205. Birbari, A.: Effect of sympathetic nervous system on renin release. *Am J Physiol 220:* 16, 1971.

206. Kuchel, O., Fishman, L. M., Liddle, G. W., Michelakis, A.: Effect of diazoxide on plasma renin activity in hypertensive patients. *Ann Intern Med 67:* 791, 1967.

207. Kaneko, Y., Ikeda, T., Takeda, T. et al: Renin release in patients with benign essential hypertension. *Circulation 38:* 353, 1968.

208. Ueda, H., Kaneko, Y., Takeda, T. et al: Observations on the mechanism of renin release by hydralazine in hypertensive patients. *Circ Res 26, 27 (Suppl II):* 201, 1970.

209. Vander, A. J., Luciano, J. R.: Neural and humoral control of renin release in salt depletion, *Circ Res 20, 21 (Suppl II):* 69, 1967.

210. Brubacher, E. S., Vander, A. J.: Sodium deprivation and renin secretion in unanesthetized dogs. *Am J Physiol 214:* 15, 1968.

211. Mogil, R. A., Itskovitz, H. D., Russell, J. H., Murphy, J. J.: Renal innervation and renin activity in salt metabolism and hypertension. *Am J Physiol 216:* 693, 1969.

212. Taquini, A. C., Blaquier, P., Taquini, A. C. Jr.: On the production and role of renin. *Can Med Assoc J 90:* 210, 1964.

213. Tobian, L. Braden, M., Maney, J.: The effect of unilateral renal denervation on the secretion of renin (abstract). *J Lab Clin Med 64:* 1011, 1964.

214. Ueda, H., Yasuda, H., Takabatake, Y. et al: Increased renin release evoked by mesencephalic stimulation in the dog. *Jpn Heart J 8:* 498, 1967.

215. Kaneko, Y., Takeda, T., Ikeda, T. et al: Effect of ganglion-blocking agents on renin release in hypertensive patients. *Circ Res 27:* 97, 1970.

216. Bunag, R. D., Vander, A. V., Kaneko, Y., McCubbin, J. W.: Control of renin release, in Page, I. H., McCubbin, J. W., (eds): Renal Hypertension. Chicago, Year Book Medical Publishers, 1968, p. 100.

217. Greene, J. A. Jr., Vander, A. J., Kowalczyk, R. S.: Plasma renin activity and aldosterone excretion after renal hemotransplantation. *J Lab Clin Med 71:* 586, 1968.

218. Blaufox, M. D., Lewis, E. J., Jagger, P. et al: Physiologic responses

of the transplanted human kidney: sodium regulation and renin secretion. *N Engl J Med 280:* 62, 1969.

219. Miura, Y., Yoshinaga, K., Taguchi, K., Abo, S.: Plasma renin activity in patient with renal homotransplatation (abstract). *Jpn J Nephrol 13:* 160, 1971.

220. Vandongen, R., Peart, W. S., Boyd, G. W.: Adrenergic stimulation of renin secretion in the isolated perfused rat kidney. *Circ Res 32:* 290, 1973.

221. Michelakis, A. M., Caudie, J., Liddle, G. W.: In vitro stimulation of renin production by epinephrine, norepinephrine, and cyclic AMP. *Proc Soc Exp Biol Med 130:* 748, 1969.

222. Veyrat, R., Rossett, E.: In vitro renin release by human kidney slices: Effect of norepinephrine, angiotensin II and I, and aldosterone in Genest, J., Koiw, E., (eds): Hypertension '72. New York, Springer-Verlag, 1972, p. 44.

223. Winer, N., Chokshi, D. S., Yoon, M. S., Freedman, A. D.: Adrenergic receptor mediation of renin secretion. *J Clin Endocrinol 29:* 1168, 1969.

224. Winer, N., Chokshi, D. S., Walkenhorst, W. G.: Effects of cyclic AMP, sympathomimetic amines, and adrenergic receptor antagonists on renin secretion. *Circ Res 29:* 239, 1971.

225. Winer, N.: Mechanism of increased renin secretion associated with adrenalectomy, hemorrhage, renal artery constriction and sodium depletion, in Genest, J., Koiw, E., (eds): Hypertension '72. New York, Springer-Verlag, 1972, p. 25.

226. Ueda, H., Yasuda, H., Takabatake, Y. et al: Observations on the mechanism of renin release by catecholamines. *Circ Res 26, 27 (Suppl II):* 195, 1970.

227. Michelakis, A. M., McAllister, R. G.: The effect of chronic adrenergic receptor blockade on plasma renin activity in man. *J Clin Endocrinol 34:* 386, 1972.

228. Otsuka, K., Assaykeen, T. A., Goldfien, A., Ganong, W. F.: Effect of hypoglycemia on plasma renin activity in dogs. *Endocrinology 87:* 1306, 1970.

229. Assaykeen, T. A., Clayton, P. L., Goldfien, A., Ganong, W. F.: Effect of alpha- and beta-adrenergic blocking agents on the renin response to hypoglycemia and epinephrine in dogs. *Endocrinology 87:* 1318, 1970.

230. Buhler, F. R., Laragh, J. H., Baer, L. et al: Propranolol inhibition of renin secretion: a specific approach to diagnosis and treatment of renin-dependent hypertensive disease. *N Engl J Med 287:* 1209, 1972.

231. Prichard, B. N. C., Gillam, P. M. S.: Treatment of hypertension with propranolol. *Br Med J 1:* 7, 1969.

232. Zacharias, F. J., Cowen, K. J.: Controlled trial of propranolol in hypertension. *Br Med J 1:* 471, 1970.

233. Beilin, L. J., Juel-Jensen, B. E.: Alpha and beta adrenergic blockade in hypertension. *Lancet 1:* 979, 1972.

234. Lydtin, H., Kusus, T., Daniel, W. et al: Propranolol therapy in essential hypertension. *Am Heart J 83:* 589, 1972.

235. Maebashi, M., Miura, Y., Yoshinaga, K.: Plasma renin activity in pheochromocytoma. *Jpn Circ J 32:* 1427, 1968.

236. DeQuattro, V., Campese, V., Miura, Y., Meijer, D.: Increased plasma catecholamines in high renin hypertension. *Am J Cardiol 38:* 801, 1976.

237. DeQuattro, V., Campese, V., Miura, Y., Meijer, D.: Biochemical markers of sympathetic nerve activity and renin in primary hypertension, in Berglund, G., Hansson, L., Werko, L., (eds): Pathophysiology and Management of Arterial Hypertension. Molndal, Sweden, Lindgren and Soner, 1975, pp 23–31.

238. Floyer, M. A.: The effect of nephrectomy and adrenalectomy upon the blood pressure in hypertensive and normotensive rats. *Clin Sci 10:* 405, 1951.

239. Koletsky, S., Pritchard, W. H.: Vasopressor material in experimental renal hypertension. *Circ Res 13:* 552, 1963.

240. Brown, J. J., Davies, D. L., Lever, A. F., Robertson, J. I. S.: Plasma renin concentration in human hypertension. II. Renin in relation to aetiology. *Br Med J 2:* 1215, 1965.

241. Miura, Y., Sato, T., Abe, K. et al: Plasma renin activity in renovascular hypertension. *Jpn Circ J 35:* 1357, 1971.

242. Eide, I., Aara, H.: Renal hypertension in rabbits immunized with angiotensin. *Nature (London) 222:* 571, 1969.

243. Louis, W. J., MacDonald, G. J., Renzini, V. et al: Renal-clip hypertension in rabbits immunized against angiotensin II. *Lancet 1:* 333, 1970.

244. MacDonald, G. J., Louis, W. J., Renzini, V. et al: Renal-clip hyper-

tension in rabbits immunized against angiotensin II. *Circ Res 27:* 197, 1970.

245. Frohlich, E. D., Ulrych, M., Tarazi, R. C. et al: A hemodynamic comparison of essential and renovascular hypertension. Cardiac output and total peripheral resistance supine and tilted patients. *Circulation 35:* 289, 1967.

246. Frohlich, E. D., Tarazi, R. C., Ulrych, M. et al: Tilt test for investigating a neural component in hypertension: its correlation with clinical characteristics. *Circulation 36:* 387, 1967.

247. Goldenberg, M., Aranow, H. Jr., Smith, A. A., Faber, M.: Pheochromocytoma and essential hypertensive vascular disease. *Arch Intern Med (Chicago) 86:* 823, 1950.

248. McCubbin, J. W., Green, J. H., Page, I. H.: Baroceptor function in chronic renal hypertension. *Circ Res 4:* 205, 1956.

249. McCubbin, J. W.: Carotid sinus participation in experimental renal hypertension. *Circulation 17:* 791, 1958.

250. Kezdi, P., Hilker, R.: Local application of epinephrine to carotid sinus: lowering blood pressure and modification of hyper-reactor response in hypertensive patients. *Arch Intern Med (Chicago) 95:* 720, 1955.

251. Miura, Y., Sato, T., Abe, K. et al: Studies on plasma renin activity in patients with renovascular hypertension. *Jpn Circ J 36:* 617, 1972.

252. Bickerton, R. K., Buckley, J. P.: Evidence for a central mechanism in angiotensin induced hypertension. *Proc Soc Exp Biol Med 106:* 834, 1961.

253. Ferrario, C. M., Gildenberg, P. L., McCubbin, J. W.: Cardiovascular effects of angiotensin mediated by the central nervous system. *Circ res 30:* 257, 1972.

254. McCubbin, J. W., Page, I. H.: Renal pressor system and neurogenic control of arterial pressure. *Circ Res 12:* 553, 1963.

255. Benelli, G., Bella, D. D., Gandini, A.: Angiotensin and peripheral sympathetic nerve activity. *Br J Pharmacol 22:* 211, 1964.

256. Zimmerman, B. G.: Effect of acute sympathectomy on responses to angiotensin and norepinephrine. *Circ Res 11:* 780, 1962.

257. Zimmerman, B. G.: Evaluation of peripheral and central components of action of angiotensin on the sympathetic nervous system. *J Pharmacol Exp Ther 158:* 1, 1967.

258. McCubbin, J. W., Page, I. H.: Neurogenic component of chronic renal hypertension. *Science 139:* 210, 1963.

259. Page, I. H., Kaneko, Y., McCubbin, J. W.: Cardiovascular reactivity in acute and chronic renal hypertensive dogs. *Circ Res 18:* 379, 1966.

260. Peach, M. J., Bumpus, F. M., Khairallah, P. A.: Inhibition of norepinephrine uptake in hearts by angiotensin II and analogs. *J Pharmacol Exp Ther 167:* 291, 1969.

261. Feldberg, W., Lewis, G. P.: The action of peptides on the adrenal medulla: release of adrenaline by bradykinin and angiotensin. *J Physiol 171:* 98, 1964.

262. Peach, M. J., Cline, W. H. Jr., Watts, D. T.: Release of adrenal catecholamines by angiotensin II: *Circ Res 19:* 571, 1966.

263. White, F. N., Ross, G.: Adrenal-dependent circulatory responses to angiotensin in the cat. *Am J Physiol 210:* 1118, 1966.

264. Feldberg, W., Lewis, G. P.: Further studies on the effects of peptides on the suprarenal medulla of cats. *J Physiol 178:* 239, 1965.

265. Peach, M. J.: Adrenal medullary stimulation induced by angiotensin I, angiotensin II, and analogues. *Circ Res 28, 29 (Suppl II):* 107, 1971.

266. DeQuattro, V., Barbour, B. H., Campese, V. et al: Sympathetic nerve hyperactivity in "high" renin hypertension: effects of saralasin infusion. *Mayo Clin Proc 52 (6):* 369–373, 1977.

267. Volicer, L., Scheer, E., Hilse, H., Visweswaram, D.: The turnover of norepinephrine in the heart during experimental hypertension in rats. *Life Sci 7:* 525, 1968.

268. Henning, M.: Noradrenaline turnover in renal hypertensive rats. *J Pharm Pharmacol 21:* 61, 1969.

269. DeChamplain, J., Mueller, R. A., Axelrod, J.: Turnover and synthesis of norepinephrine in experimental hypertension in rats. *Circ Res 25:* 285, 1969.

270. Haggendal, J.: Some further aspects of the release of the adrenergic neurotransmitter, in Schumann, H. J., Kroneberg, G. (eds): New Aspects of Storage and Release Mechanisms of Catecholamines. Bayer Symposium II, Berlin, Springer-Verlag, 1970, pp. 100–109.

271. Starke, K.: Influence of extracellular noradrenaline on the stimulation-evoked secretion of noradrenaline from sympathetic nerves: Evidence for an α-receptor mediated feedback inhibition of noradrenaline release. *Naunyn Schmiedebergs Arch Pharmacol 275:* 11–23, 1972.

272. Trendelenberg, U.: Classification of sympathomimetic amines, in Blaschko, H., Muscholl, E. (eds): Handbook of Experimental Pharmacology, vol. 33. Berlin, Springer-Verlag, 1972, pp. 336–357.

273. Langer, S. Z.: Presynaptic regulation of catecholamine release. *Biochem Pharmacol 23:* 1793–1800, 1974.

274. O'Keefe, R., Sharman, D. F., Vogt, M.: Effects of drugs used in psychoses on cerebral dopamine metabolism. *Br J Pharmacol 38:* 287–304, 1970.

275. Stjarne, L.: Adrenoceptor mediated positive and negative feedback control of noradrenaline secretion from human vasoconstrictor nerves. *Acta Physiol Scand 95:* 18A–19A, 1975.

276. Hedqvist, P.: Modulating effect of prostaglandin E, or noradrenaline release from the isolated cat spleen. *Acta Physiol Scand 75:* 511–512, 1969.

277. Stjarne, L.: Role of α-adrenoceptors in prostaglandin E mediated negative feedback control of the secretion of noradrenaline from the sympathetic nerves of the guinea-pig vas deferens. *Prostaglandins 4:* 845–851, 1973.

278. Henderson, G., Hughes, J., Kosterlitz, H. W.: The effects of morphine on the release of noradrenaline from the cat isolated nictitating membrane and the guinea-pig ileum mesenteric plexus-longitudinal muscle preparation. *Br J Pharmacol 53:* 505–512, 1972.

279. Stjarne, L.: Substance P inhibits neurogenic tone in human omental vein by a postjunctional action. *Acta Physiol Scand, 1977 (in press).*

280. Amer, M. S.: Mechanism of action of β-blockers in hypertension. *Biochem Pharmacol 26:* 171–175, 1977.

281. Stjarne, L.: Angiotensin II enhances neurogenic tone on human omental vein by pre and post junctional actions. *Acta Physiol Scand, 1977 (in press).*

102

Pheochromocytoma: Diagnosis and Therapy

Vincent DeQuattro
Vito M. Campese

INTRODUCTION

A pheochromocytoma is a tumor that can cause spectacular cardiovascular disturbances. It is potentially fatal but is usually resectable, providing a cure. As a natural experiment in neurogenic hypertension, it has provided a better understanding of sympathetic nervous system function.

Since this is an era of emphasis on drug therapy for patients with hypertension, there is an increasing tendency to limit diagnostic studies. We are often asked, "Should every patient with significant hypertension (mean diastolic above 105 mm) be tested for pheochromocytoma?" Our answer, notwithstanding economic considerations, is "Yes." There is no classic picture, no stereotype for pheochromocytoma, although the history and physical signs are helpful. Patients come to the clinician in a variety of ways and settings. They may be brought to the emergency room with a transient ischemic attack or even a completed stroke. They may present with the signs and symptoms of diabetes mellitus, hyper-

thyroidism, hypercalcemia, congestive heart failure, myocardial infarction, shock, malignant hypertension, mental retardation, diarrhea, obstipation, or a variety of other conditions. They may have classic attacks of diaphoresis, headache, or feelings of impending doom, or they may have the identical symptoms and physical findings of patients with primary hypertension.

HISTORICAL BACKGROUND

In the 1920s the diagnosis of pheochromocytoma was made on the basis of symptomatic and physical findings. Mayo was the first to remove an adrenal pheochromocytoma and note the postoperative amelioration of the patient's hypertension. In the 1940s and 1950s, pharmacologic testing with histamine and phentolamine received attention.[1] In the late 1950s and early 1960s, bioassay and biochemical techniques were used to detect or confirm the presence of pheochromocytoma. Since that time, the concepts of preoperative therapy with alpha blocking agents to allow reexpansion of blood volume and the further replacement of volume after removal of the tumor have changed a formidable operative procedure with frequently horrendous results to one that can be performed sedately in any operating room with the proper monitoring devices.[2]

In the 1970s, pheochromocytoma continues to be the subject of basic research. The results of these endeavors may provide better understanding of the mechanism of both normal and abnormal biosynthesis, storage, and release of the catecholamines present in these tumors; the relationships of pheochromocytoma to medullary thyroid carcinoma and their embryological origin in the neural crest; and an insight into the role of other substances, such as prostaglandins and polypeptides, which are secreted by some pheochromocytomas.

INCIDENCE

It is estimated that about 1000 patients with pheochromocytoma are diagnosed annually, accounting for about 0.5 percent of patients with newly diagnosed hypertension.[3] If this statistic is correct, approximately 30 to 35 patients with pheochromocytoma should be discovered in Los Angeles County annually. We estimate that approximately one-half that number of patients are found here each year.

The tumor occurs with equal frequency in both sexes and at any age from childhood to the seventh decade, though it is most common in the third and fourth decades. In one Mayo Clinic study, the patients' ages ranged from 12 to 72 years, with a mean of 42.[4] Childhood pheochromocytomas are rare, but when they occur, they are frequently bilateral or multiple and are often associated with mottled skin, renal artery stenosis, polyuria, polydipsia, and obstructive uropathy.[5] There is a high familial incidence in children, inheritance being autosomal dominant with high penetration.

EMBRYOLOGICAL ORIGIN

Pheochromocytoma arises from chromaffin cells of the adrenal medulla. When other chromaffin cells of the paraganglia in other regions become neoplastic, they are often called phenochromocytoma, but a better term is functional paraganglioma.[6] They occur in the neck, in the posterior mediastinum, along the aorta, in the organs of Zuckerkandl, in the pelvis, and in the urinary bladder (see Fig. 102-1). Approximately 15 percent are multiple, and the most common location is the adrenal;[7] 10 to 12 percent are malignant. Familial tumors, although rare, usually show autosomal dominance, multiplicity of tumors, bilaterality, hypertension, and an association with medullary carcinoma of the thyroid gland.[8] Sipple's syndrome (multiple endocrine adenomata—type II) is an association of medullary carcinoma of the thyroid with amyloid stroma, parathyroid adenomas, and bilateral pheochromocytomas.[9] In other families the tumors are found in association with pes cavus and mucosal neuronoma[10] and in other kindreds, with abnormal facies and diarrhea.[11] Pheochromocytoma is also associated with other neuroectodermal syndromes: neurofibromatosis (5 percent of patients with neurofibromatosis are expected to develop a pheochromocytoma), von-Hippel-Lindau disease, Sturge-Weber disease, and tuberous sclerosis.[12,13]

NEUROBLASTOMA AND PARAGANGLIOMA

Neuroblastoma occurring in infancy and childhood is mentioned here for completeness. Deriving from the neuroblast of the neural crest, the tumor usually arises from the posterior mediastinum or retroperitoneum and commonly presents as an abdominal mass. Usually there are no physiological effects, although "functional" histologically "proven" neuroblastomas have been reported. In neuroblastoma, norepinephrine and epinephrine may be elevated and vanillylmandelic acid is usually increased. Increased excretion of dopamine and homovanillic acid is most specific for the diagnosis.

Paragangliomas are chromaffin tumors originating from sympathetic ganglia or cell rests outside the adrenal. These may have the same functional characteristics as tumors arising from the adrenal medulla. Those arising from the chest are usually easily found in the posterior mediastinum on the chest x-ray,[14] but others in the middle ear[15] or urinary bladder[16] may be more difficult to locate. Pheochromocytomas arise from the carotid body and may also be functional.[17] Functional chromaffin tumors from these and other extra-adrenal locations may have increased malignant potential (38 percent) and are more likely to metastasize to bone, lymph nodes, liver, and lung.[18]

ADRENOMEDULLARY HYPERPLASIA

This entity has remained mysterious and controversial since it was first described over 40 years ago.[19] The normal adrenal has a weight of 6–6.5 g, a medullary/cortical ratio of 1:10, and thus, a medullary weight of approximately 0.6–0.7 g. There have been reports, however, that this medullary weight has approached 1.5 to 2.0 g spontaneously in a patient without familial chromaffin tumors[20] and in patients with familial pheochromocytoma[21] in association with hypertensive crises and attacks similar to pheochromocytoma. In the patients with MEA II, it has been suggested that hyperplasia is a preneoplastic state in relation to pheochromocytoma, just as C-cell hyperplasia has been thought to precede medullary thyroid carcinoma.[22] It is thought that the presence of medullary tissue in the "tail" of the adrenal is diagnostic of medullary hyperplasia whether or not there is an increased proportion of medulla to cortex.[23] If this condition of hyperplasia exists at

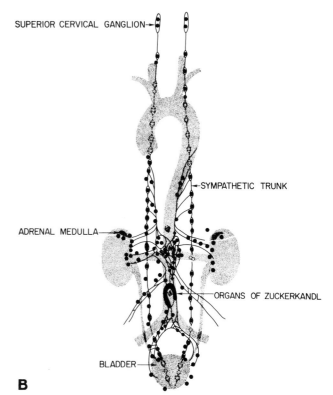

Fig. 102-1A. Sites of branchiomeric and intravagal paraganglia. This diagram represents the branchiomeric and intravagal paraganglia and their anatomic relationships. Less than 2 percent of functional paragangliomas occur in this region. (Adapted from reference 6 with permission.) **Fig. 102-1B.** Sites of aortico-sympathetic paraganglia. This is a diagrammatic representation of the distribution of aortico-sympathetic paraganglia (extramedullary chromaffin tissue) in a newborn child. Most functional paragangliomas occur below the diaphram. (Adapted from reference 6 with permission.)

all, it must be quite rare. Only a handful of well-documented instances have been published.[24-26] In only 1 patient has the removal of such an adrenal been followed by the cure of the hypertension.[27]

CLINICAL DIAGNOSIS AND PATHOPHYSIOLOGY

Pheochromocytoma was first diagnosed in a living patient in 1923.[28] The hypertension in a patient with pheochromocytoma may resemble that in "primary" hypertension without other signs or symptoms, but usually other signs or symptoms are present. The signs and symptoms are due to increased secretion of epinephrine or norepinephrine or both. Tumors of the adrenal medulla commonly secrete norepinephrine or a mixture of the two catecholamines. Tumors producing epinephrine alone are rare. Extraadrenal pheochromocytomas usually secrete only norepinephrine. Norepinephrine is less potent than epinephrine in causing hypermetabolism and glycogenolysis, but these "epinephrine" effects may be seen with tumors secreting only norepinephrine.

The symptoms are of two patterns: persistent and paroxysmal, probably related to the constant or pulsatile release of catecholamines. In a study of 76 consecutive cases at the Mayo Clinic, 39 presented with persistent hypertension and 37 with paroxysmal hypertension.[4] The symptoms of both groups in decreasing incidence were headache, sweating, palpitations, pallor, nervousness, tremor, nausea, weakness, abdominal pain, dyspnea, and warmth or flushing. Dizziness, paresthesias, and heat tolerance were also present. Attacks occurred from once every 2 months to 25 per day and lasted from 30 seconds to 1 week, with an average time of about 15 minutes. In this series, paroxysmal attacks were rarely associated with malignancy. Headaches were more common in paraoxysmal attacks and were usually severe and abrupt, bilateral, and of short duration. In the Mayo Clinic series described above, over half the patients with persistent hypertension had grade 3-4 K-W retinopathy. Patients with pheochromocytoma may be normotensive, moderately hypertensive, or markedly hypertensive. Marked lability of blood pressure is present in some but not all pheochromocytoma patients and occurs in many hypertensive patients without pheochromocytoma. Acute episodes of various types may occur in pheochromocytoma patients. Most commonly these consist of sweating, tachycardia, and hypertension. Anxiety is a common symptom. Although facial or even digital flushing may occur, the extremities are often pale. Vasospasm may be so severe that peripheral pulses are undetectable, and gangrene may be present, even though the blood pressure is markedly elevated. Attacks may be precipitated by smoking, induction of anesthesia, ganglionic blocking agents, hydralazine, and with large or extraadrenal tumors, massage of the tumor or changes in position. (see Tables 102-1A and 102-1B).

Patients with pheochromocytoma are hypermetabolic, having

Table 102-1A. Manifestations of Pheochromocytoma

Paroxysmal hypertension
Sustained hypertension with
 Paroxysmal attacks: palpitation, headache, sweating
 Headache
 Sweating and palpitations
 Diabetes
 Postural hypotension or tachycardia
 Hypermetabolism
 Weight loss
 Psychic change

Table 102-1B. Features Suggestive of Pheochromocytoma

- Paroxysmal hypertension
- Progressive hypertension
- Stable hypertension plus diabetes, hypermetabolism
- Hypertension in children
- Hypertensive response to induction of anesthesia or to histamine during gastric analysis
- Neurocutaneous lesions
- Family history of pheochromocytoma, medullary carcinoma of the thyroid, or hyperparathyroidism
- Hypertensive crisis during renal angiogram
- Unexplained post-operative shock
- Paradoxical response to antihypertensive drugs

the characteristics of thyrotoxicosis. The basal metabolic rate is elevated, but the PBI and ^{131}I uptake are normal. Hypermetabolism may be seen with pure norepinephrine-secreting tumors. Weight loss may be marked. Pheochromocytoma occurs less often in obese patients, but no type of body habitus is spared. Elevated blood sugars and glycosuria are common in pheochromocytoma patients, including those with pure norepinephrine-secreting tumors. Such patients may appear to be diabetics who are difficult to control, since they have frequent "insulin reactions." The combination of "diabetes" and hypermetabolism and hypertension is highly suggestive of a pheochromocytoma. Some patients develop severe diabetic retinopathy and neuropathy which is reversible after the tumor is removed. We and others[29] have seen patients with thyrotoxicosis in pheochromocytoma. In our patient, Graves' disease developed after the onset of symptoms due to pheochromocytoma. Perhaps agonist stimulation of the thyroid was involved.[30,31]

Postural hypotension is not unusual in pheochromocytoma. This may be related to decreased plasma volume,[7] to decreased sensitivity of receptors to neurotransmitters released with standing, to false transmitter effects of norepinephrine metabolites, or to the formation of vasodilator substances by the tumor. Sweating may be severe, with drenching night sweats or even dehydration. Sweating may be subtle, producing sticky skin and hair or the need for frequent showers. The cold pressor response may be reduced in pheochromocytoma patients compared with patients with primary hypertension.

Abnormalities of red cell distribution are common in pheochromocytoma patients. The packed cell volume (PCV) is often elevated, although the red cell mass is normal or reduced.[43] The pheochromocytomas may elaborate an erythrocyte-stimulating material, leading to an absolute increase in RBC mass.[33] The reduction in plasma volume is thought to be secondary to skimming of plasma in the constricted arteriolar bed, so that the peripheral hematocrit is greater than that centrally. The findings are similar to those in patients with chronic norepinephrine infusion.[32] The shock following removal of a pheochromocytoma is due to reexpansion of the vascular compartment and may be prevented by blood volume expansion using oral pheoxybenzamine preoperatively and administration of blood or plasma expanders immediately after the tumor vessels are ligated. As an example, the average blood loss of 200–300 cc is replaced using 1 liter of albumisol and 500 cc fluids.

In 20 to 30 percent of patients there is a catecholamine myocarditis which manifests itself in arrhythmias, congestive heart failure, and nonspecific EKG changes.[34] The congestive failure is due, in part, to the increased afterload presented to a heart with damaged myofibrils in varying stages of repair. The muscle injury is due to both direct inflammatory effects of the catecholamines and the indirect results of intense arteriolar constriction.[35] Thus, it is important to continue alpha blockade and digoxin therapy for sufficient time preoperatively to allow the muscle to heal. Dibenzyline is not given after the tumor removal. It seems prudent to discontinue digoxin 4 to 6 weeks postoperatively.[36]

Twenty percent of the patients with pheochromocytoma are thin with signs of weight loss, but some are obese. Some patients will have evidence of neurocutaneous involvement with cafe au lait spots, generalized hyper pigmentation, axillary freckling, and neurofibromas. Tremor, sweating, flushing, blanching, pallor, and signs of hypermetabolism may occur during a paroxysm. Intense arterial constriction may result in a falsely low brachial artery pressure. Frequently, the veins on the dorsum of the hand are inapparent as a result of intense venoconstriction. Central nervous system findings are diverse: from anxiety to frank psychosis and from transient ischemic attacks to completed strokes due to cerebral hemorrhages. The tumor itself is palpable very rarely, but when it is large or extra-adrenal, palpation of the area near the tumor may induce a paroxysm, which has great diagnostic value. It should be emphasized that a patient with a paroxysmally functioning pheochromocytoma may have a completely normal physical examination during a quiescent period.

PHARMACOLOGIC DIAGNOSIS

PROVOCATIVE TESTS

The provocative tests for diagnosis of pheochromocytoma are not without hazard (Fig. 102-2). Fatalities following administration of these drugs have been associated with hypertensive crises and cerebrovascular accidents. The tests should be performed only with an iv running and with the alpha-adrenergic blocking agent, phentolamine, available. The tests are most useful in patients of kindreds with familial pheochromocytoma who have MEA II or MEA II B syndromes without a documented increase in catecholamine excretion. It is important to exclude pheochromocytoma in these patients when they require surgery for the thyroid and parathyroid neoplasms.

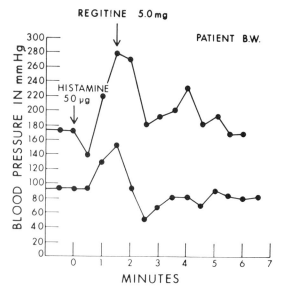

Fig. 102-2. Pressor response to histamine in a patient with pheochromocytoma. Typical blood pressure fall is noted after histamine intravenously. The pronounced blood pressure rise is reversed with phentolamine, 5.0 mg intravenously.

Tyramine Test

Tyramine increases the blood pressure in pheochromocytoma patients by releasing catecholamines from peripheral stores: an increase of greater than 20 mm Hg systolic pressure after a 1.0 mg dose iv indicates pheochromocytoma. False-negative tests are not uncommon (10 to 30 percent).[38] A marked pressor response may occur in patients receiving MAO inhibitor drugs, such as pargyline hydrochloride. There are anecdotal reports of pressor crises after ingestion of orange juice, which contains norsynephrine.

Glucagon Test

The glucagon test elicits pressor responses in pheochromocytoma in doses of 0.5–1.0 mg iv.[39] The mechanism is not known. Patients with primary hypertension are said not to have pressor responses. However, we have seen positive glucagon tests in primary hypertension as well as negative responses in pheochromocytoma patients.

Histamine Test

The histamine test should be done only when the laboratory data are equivocal and when the blood pressure is normal or only slightly elevated.[57] Histamine, 0.025–0.05 mg, is given intravenously. Following the normal drop in blood pressure, a secondary rise is seen in a positive test. Plasma and urinary catecholamines are increased by histamine in pheochromocytoma patients, suggesting that the pressor response is due to their release from the tumor. To be significant, the rise must be greater than that of a control cold pressor test. False-positive and false-negative tests are common, and the test is of limited value.

DEPRESSOR OR PHENTOLAMINE TEST

The most reliable pharmacologic test is the phentolamine test (Regitine). Phentolamine will lower elevated blood pressures of patients with pheochromocytoma in almost every instance. A dose of 5 mg iv should produce a drop of at least 35/35 and usually greater than 50/35 mm Hg systolic and diastolic pressure, respectively, in pheochromocytoma patients. Such a drop may occur in pheochromocytoma patients even when the initial pressure is normal or slightly elevated. False-positive tests are very common and are often due to reserpine or antiadrenergic drugs taken within 2 or 3 weeks, barbiturates, or an elevated BUN, or they may occur without any apparent cause. False-negative results are rare, however. A modification measuring the change in blood sugar after phentolamine has been described.[37] Since the catecholamines impair insulin release from the pancreas via the *alpha* receptors, the blood sugar is elevated in patients with pheochromocytoma receiving a glucose infusion. After the administration of phentolamine, there is a release of insulin and a sudden lowering of blood sugar. This has little clinical application, however.

BIOCHEMICAL DIAGNOSIS

The determination of the urinary catecholamines and their metabolites confirms the diagnosis of pheochromocytoma. The term "catecholamines" as used clinically refers to the sum of epinephrine (E) and norepinephrine (NE). Normal values are indicated for NE and E, metanephrine, and vanillylmandelic acid (VMA) (Table 102-2). These values, based on our own methods, are similar to those of commercial laboratories. Variations in

Table 102-2. The Excretion Rates of Catecholamines and Catecholamine Metabolites in Normal Subjects and in Patients with Pheochromocytoma

	Normal	Pheochromocytoma
Catecholamines (Free epinephrine plus norepinephrine)	2.5 ± 0.8	11 − 120
Metanephrine plus normetanephrine (Free plus conjugated)	16 ± 5	60 − 420
Vanillylmandelic acid (VMA)	240 ± 120	500 − 3,500

Note: Normal values were obtained in ambulatory subjects. Values are means ± SD in micrograms per hour.

normal values are due to differences both in the procedure used and in the activity of the patient during the period of collection.

URINARY CATECHOLAMINES

We prefer to assay total free catecholamines for the screening test for pheochromocytoma, although any of the procedures can be used. If the concentration of catecholamines is determined on an untimed specimen, a very dilute urine may lead to a false-negative value. When the patient has sustained hypertension, a 24-hour or a 2- or 3-hour single voiding specimen for catecholamines is recommended. When the hypertension is labile, urine should be collected during the period of an "attack" and this timed "attack" specimen compared with baseline catecholamine values. Urinary catecholamine assays can be performed with great accuracy and can be fractioned into E and NE to help localize the tumor. The tumor is usually in the adrenal glands or in the organs of Zuckerkandl when 20 percent or more of the elevated total catecholamines is epinephrine. Plasma catecholamine assays, while more expensive, are available in some laboratories. They may be useful in the localization of the pheochromocytoma. Catecholamine excretion may be increased with severe physical or mental stress after myocardial infarction, after surgery, or after infusion of isoproterenol and epinephrine or norepinephrine. Tetracycline drugs, quinine, dopa, and alpha-methyldopa will yield false-positive values.

CATECHOLAMINE METABOLITES

Urine metanephrine may be measured by the GLC, photometric, or fluorometric assays. The latter allows for fractionation of normetanephrine and metanephrine. Metanephrine may be elevated in patients taking monoamine oxidase inhibitors. It will not be elevated falsely after Aldomet. The VMA assay is least specific. In some laboratories there are up to 10 to 15 percent false-positive tests caused by food and beverages high in vanillin, such as bananas, coffee, nuts, and other fruits. VMA assay procedures are sensitive to phenolic acids in the diet.

If the Pisano assay is used as recommended, using an unoxidized blank and reading at 333 and 347 μ, the effects of parahydroxymandelic and other acids, which account for the diet-induced elevation, are eliminated.[40] Plasma catecholamine assays (Chapter 100), while slightly more expensive, are of value in episodic crises when urine collections are not possible or are unreliable and after histamine challenge. Fivefold or greater increases in plasma catecholamines after histamine indicates pheochromocytoma. MAO inhibitors and clofibrate may lower VMA values. Aldomet does not falsely increase VMA but may reduce endogenous VMA secretion slightly. We found normal VMA excretion in 15 to 20 percent

of patients with pheochromocytoma when the catecholamines and metanephrines were elevated (Fig. 102-3).

PLASMA CATECHOLAMINES

The total plasma catecholamines as determined in normotensive subjects are in the range of 100–500 ng/liter.[42] An infusion of norepinephrine, sufficient to raise these values to 2000–3000 ng/liter, will raise blood pressure levels to 190/120 mm Hg. It is remarkable that patients with pheochromocytoma can survive with plasma catecholamines 10 to 50 times normal. However, some patients with pheochromocytoma have catecholamine elevations in the range of 600–1000 ng/liter, values that overlap those of patients in various stressful states.

LOCALIZATION OF TUMOR(S)

Localization of the tumor(s) in a patient with pheochromocytoma may provide a valuable service to the patient and surgeon by decreasing the operating time and the incidence of cardiovascular accident, averting unnecessary adrenalectomy, or locating otherwise hidden tumors. The history of "attacks" occurring when bending to one side, when wearing a tight girdle, or when the bladder is full may help to localize the tumors. Careful quadrant by quadrant abdominal massage (with intravenous phentolamine available) is a useful localizing technique in 10 to 20 percent of patients with pheochromocytoma.

INTRAVENOUS PYELOGRAM

Usually the diagnosis of pheochromocytoma is suggested by the finding of a suprarenal mass on an intravenous pyelogram (IVP). The pyelogram with nephrotomogram localizes the tumors in at least 60 to 70 percent of patients with proven pheochromocytoma. The procedure of retroperitoneal CO_2 insufflation, in combination with an IVP and nephrotomogram, was successful in the past in locating suprarenal masses. Some investigators would advise no further attempt at localization after the IVP because 95 percent of these tumors occur within the abdomen.[43]

In our experience, vena cava sampling of blood for catecholamines locates tumors even when the IVP is negative, since tumors may be extra-adrenal. We advise that patients with negative pyelograms have catheterization for purposes of obtaining blood specimens from the vena cava and, if possible, from the adrenal veins.

ANGIOGRAPHY

Some investigators prefer angiography for localizing tumors when the IVP is negative. Angiography may be performed as a substitute for vena cava sampling and adrenal venography but only after adequate blocking therapy, for fatalities have occurred in unprepared patients. Our own practice is to routinely perform vena cava catheterization and angiography simultaneously. In 1 patient, lymphangiography was helpful in providing a cure of pelvic metastasis from a bladder pheochromocytoma (Fig. 102-4).

IODO SCANNING

A recent report describes localizing both cortical and medullary tumors in the adrenal by use of a scintiscanning technique after administration of radioactive substrates which are distributed to and concentrated in the adrenal glands.[44]

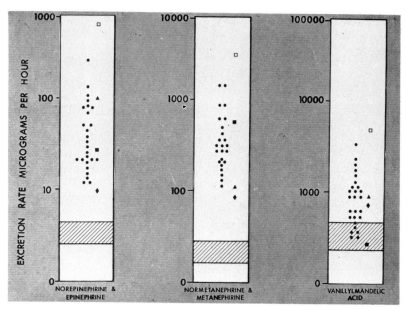

Fig. 102-3. Excretion rates of catecholamines and catecholamine metabolites in pheochromocytoma. Twenty-three of the collections were for 24 hours, and seven were timed 2- to 4-hour samples. One patient (□) was treated with guanethidine for several hours prior to the collection. One patient (△) had minimal increase in normetanephrine (fourfold) and VMA (twofold) with a 40-fold increase in catecholamine excretion. One patient (■), with the lowest VMA excretion, had 80 percent epinephrine excretion. The lowest catecholamine excretion rates were exhibited by a 10-year-old child (♦). (Reproduced with permission from V. DeQuattro, Calif. Med. 117: 53–62, 1972.)

VENOGRAPHY

Adrenal venography may be performed, and blood specimens for catecholamines must be obtained before the rapid injection of contrast media. We have encountered no special problems infusing contrast media into or near the site of tumors in patients with pheochromocytoma. These tumors are usually 3–4 cm or more in diameter and, when present in the adrenal gland, distort the adrenal venous system and become apparent on adrenal venograms. Catheterization of the left adrenal vein is usually done with ease, but that of the right adrenal veins is often not done because of technical difficulty.

VENA CAVA CATHETERIZATION AND VENOUS SAMPLING

Our technique for estimating the tumor location via catheterization is to obtain samples in rapid succession from the right atrium, region of the right adrenal, and at and below the renal veins in the vena cava. Additional samples may then be collected from

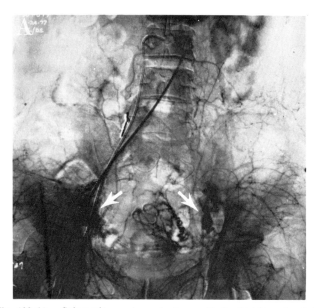

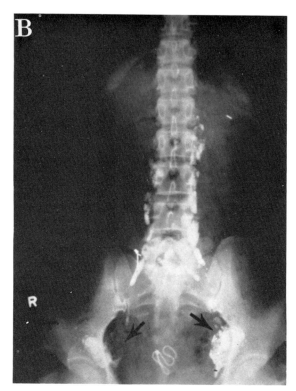

Fig. 102-4A. Subtraction angiography in a patient with bilateral pelvic node metastases. Arrows indicate bilateral vascular pelvic tumors. Fig. 102-4B. Pelvic and vertebral lymph angiography in a patient with pelvic metastases from bladder pheochromocytoma. Irregularly shaped pelvic nodes (arrows) contain pehochromocytomas. The other nodes were negative at surgical exploration.

the left and right adrenal veins. The diagram in Fig. 102-5 shows the catecholamines in the plasma from a patient with a right adrenal pheochromocytoma. Although the left adrenal vein values are elevated, the percentage of epinephrine is very high. However, the percentage in the right adrenal vein epinephrine is similar to that of the urinary excretion. The right adrenal contained a chromaffin tumor.

CT SCANS AND NEWER METHODS

We have encountered patients in whom the IVP, angiogram, and venograms have not localized the tumors. In 3 patients, vena cava and adrenal vein sampling of blood for estimation of catecholamine was performed before and after stimulation with intravenous histamine, using 50 μg base. Phentolamine, 5 mg, was administered intravenously a few seconds after the histamine to obviate any pressure response. Results with this method have localized tumors in 3 patients (Table 102-3). Of additional value in a patient challenged with histamine was the presence of a right supraadrenal mass on CT scan (Fig. 102-6).

THERAPY

MEDICAL CONTROL

The first successful surgical removal of this tumor was reported in 1927.[45] It was not until the late 1950s and the advent of preoperative therapy with blocking agents, however, that the operation was performed with a high degree of success.

Preparation for Surgery

Patients are treated with the alpha blocking agents phenoxybenzamine and phentolamine. These drugs block the pressor effect of circulating norepinephrine and can therefore be used to lower the blood pressure and increase the blood volume in pheochromocytoma patients. They are used for at least 1 to 2 weeks or longer if patients have catecholamine-induced myocarditis. For patients

Table 102-3. Modified* Histamine Test and Plasma Catecholamines from Various Vena Cava Sites and an Adrenal Vein for Localization of Pheochromoctyoma

	Prehistamine		Posthistamine	
	NE	E	NE	E
Above diaphragm	0.2	0.1	1.5	0.5
At right adrenal vein	0.3	0.1	5.4†	3.3
At renal veins	0.2	0.1	1.3	0.4
Below renal veins	0.4	0.1	1.2	0.2
In left adrenal vein	—	—	nil	11.2‡

Note: Values of catecholamine in micrograms per liter. Range of normal peripheral values. Total NE + E, 0.2 to 0.7. Right adrenal: tumor 9.8 NE + 0.9E mg/g (see tumor in Fig. 102-6). tissue 0.2 NE + 1.8E mg/g.
*50 μg of histamine base is given iv. Phentolamine 5.0 is given iv after initial BP drop as BP begins to rise.
†NE response from tumor.
‡E response from normal left adrenal.

with tumors secreting epinephrine primarily, particularly if tachycardia and ventricular arrhythmias are present, propranolol may be added in low doses (40 mg/day), after alpha blocking therapy is begun (phenoxybenzamino 20–40 mg/day). Propranolol blocks the beta agonist actions of epinephrine and the cardiac stimulating effects.

Medical Therapy

For malignancies, inoperable tumors, or patients who cannot tolerate a surgical procedure, there are two modes of therapy, neither of which is entirely satisfactory. Alpha- and beta-adrenergic blocking agents will prevent the effects of the increased plasma catecholamines. Alpha-methylparatyrosine, a drug that inhibits the rate-limiting tyrosine hydroxylase step in catechol synthesis, will lower tumor, plasma, and urinary catecholamines and normalize blood pressure in patients with pheochromocytoma (1–2 G/day).[46] Long-term use of the drug, however, has led to symptoms of parkinsonism.[17] Other enzymatic blocking agents have either proved ineffective or await further trials. Alpha-methyltyrosine can control the blood pressure and all other symptoms in patients with pheochromocytoma who are unresponsive to phenoxybenzamine. Streptozotocin, effective for other APUD neoplasm, has been tried with mixed success in malignant pheochromocytoma.[48]

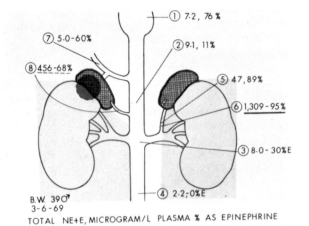

Fig. 102-5. Total catecholamines and percentage of epinephrine found in the blood from the vena cava and adrenal veins of a patient with right adrenal pheochromocytoma. Values at sites 5 and 6 are values before and after contrast media for venography. The percentage of epinephrine found in the elevated values of site 8 before contrast media was similar to that found in the urine. In this patient, site 3 was elevated as compared with site 4. Usually, patients with right adrenal tumors have a step-up in values at site 2, and patients with left adrenal tumors have a step-up at site 3. In this patient, however, tumor collateral venous circulation involved the right renal vein as well as the hepatic vein, site 7.

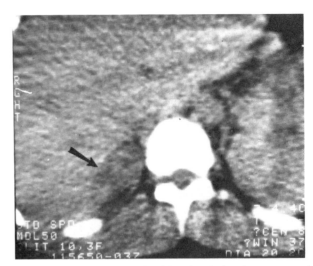

Fig. 102-6. CT scan demonstrating right adrenal pheochromocytoma in a patient with increased venous catecholamines after histamine (see Table 102-3). Arrow points dorsally and medially to retroperitoneal mass adjacent to vertebral column.

The infrequency of this disorder and the long course of even malignant pheochromocytoma may make its efficacy difficult to evaluate, however. Chemotherapy with other agents and radiotherapy are not effective. Radiotherapy usually arrests pheochromocytoma bone metastasis. We have had limited success in reducing symptoms and drug requirement in 1 patient treated with streptozotocin.

SURGICAL REMOVAL

Therapy During Surgery

We recommend that all patients have an EKG and that central venous pressure and intra-arterial pressure be monitored at all times during surgery. Meperidine and a short-acting barbiturate are good choices for preanesthetic medications. Just before induction of anesthesia, 5 mg iv of phentolamine are given to prevent the rise in blood pressure that usually accompanies intubation. We recommend thiopental and succinylcholine for induction and nitrous oxide and meperidine or fentamyl as anesthetic agents. Halothane, while not directly releasing catecholamines, may sensitize the heart to arrhythmias. Other halogenated hydrocarbons, e.g., methoxyflurane,[58] may be safer in this regard. Phentolamine is administered in 5-mg boluses for attacks of hypertension or supraventricular arrhythmias associated with hypertension. Xylocaine, in doses of 50 mg iv, or propranolol, in doses of 1–3 mg iv, can be given for ventricular arrhythmias. These agents will be required more often in patients with a high tumor secretion of epinephrine and during anesthesia with halothane.[43] Sodium nitroprusside, infused in amounts of 1 μg/kg/min, is also effective in management of the blood pressure during surgery in patients with chromaffin tumors.

An anterior abdominal incision, usually vertical, permits the surgeon to explore the entire abdomen for multiple tumors. By slowly exploring and manipulating areas of the abdomen, the surgeon can often find extra-adrenal tumors by the subsequent rise in blood pressure (Fig. 102-7). Whenever a tumor mass is found, its venous drainage should be clamped and ligated promptly to prevent additional catecholamines from entering the blood. Usually patients become hypotensive immediately after the tumor is removed, despite preoperative medical management, but they respond readily to restoration of fluid volume with 1 or 2 liters of plasma expanders.

IN PREGNANCY

Pheochromocytoma associated with pregnancy is life-threatening for the mother and fetus. Schenker and Chowers reported in their review of 89 cases that when pheochromocytoma in pregnancy remained undiagnosed, the maternal mortality was 48 percent and the fetal mortality, 54 percent.[49] On the other hand, when the disease was diagnosed before term, the maternal mortality decreased to 17 percent. The fetal mortality, however, remained high at 50 percent. No maternal deaths have been reported in the recently published cases of pheochromocytoma diagnosed before term. The fetal mortality remains high, however.

Pregnant women with pheochromocytoma may die from cerebrovascular accidents, acute pulmonary edema, cardiac arrhythmias, shock, or malignancy. The fetal mortality can be due to spontaneous abortion. Most of the deaths, however, occur during or just after labor.

Raised catecholamines in maternal blood may harm the fetus secondary to uterine arterial vasoconstriction and uterine contractions and the resultant fetal hypoxia. Catecholamines probably do not damage the fetus directly. Less than 10 percent of norepinephrine administered to the mother crosses the placenta; most is metabolized by COMT and MAO in the placenta. The concentration of VMA is higher in the umbilical veins than in the mother.[50]

The morbidity and mortality data stress the importance of an early diagnosis. A high degree of suspicion is required, since no single clinical pattern is characteristic of the disease. Patients with pheochromocytoma may present with the symptoms of headache, nausea, vomiting, blurred vision, tightness of the chest, vasomotor phenomena, sweating, and anxiety. These symptoms are frequently ascribed to neurosis or thyrotoxicosis. Occasionally, patients without previous symptoms suddenly develop shock during or immediately after delivery. Because of these different clinical patterns, the possibility of pheochromocytoma must be considered in all pregnant women with hypertension and in cases of unsuspected shock during or after delivery.

The clinical symptoms and signs of pheochromocytoma in pregnancy are similar to those of other patients with this disease. Occasionally, hypertensive crisis can be elicited when patients lie on their backs, probably because of the compression exerted by the uterus on the tumor. Some hypotheses have been formulated to explain why many patients with a silent pheochromocytoma develop signs and symptoms during pregnancy, including stimulatory effects of estrogens on tumor cells or increased blood flow to the adrenal glands as well as all tissues during pregnancy.

The diagnosis is made on the basis of urinary catecholamines and metabolites. Therapy should be initiated with alpha blocking agents (phenoxybenzamine). Beta blocking agents should be used only in the event of tachycardia or arrhythmias. The pregnancy may be interrupted if the diagnosis is made before 20 to 25 weeks. After that time the pregnancy should probably be continued until the fetus has achieved maturity.[52,53] Diagnostic attempts to localize the tumor before delivery by an arteriogram should be avoided because of the risk of radiation to the fetus. However, localization may be attempted using ultrasound and CAT scanning to minimize radiation exposures. These techniques should be performed by expert radiologists. Vena cava catheterization and venous sam-

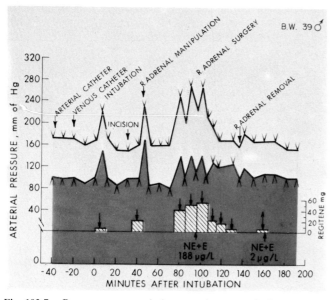

Fig. 102-7. Pressor responses during operative removal of adrenal chromaffin tumor. Pressor responses were manged by bolus injections of phentolamine (Regitine). Time and amount administered are given by arrows and hatched columns, respectively. (NE and E = plasma norepinephrine and epinephrine.)

pling for plasma catecholamine assay under fluoroscopic control may be performed a few days before the cesarean section in order to attempt to localize the tumor.

After delivery by cesarean section, an abdominal exploration is performed to localize and resect the tumor. Vaginal delivery should be avoided, because exposure of the patient to the stress of childbirth may provoke an acute hypertensive crisis. Particular attention should be given to the preoperative preparation and to the management of the patient during anesthesia as described.

Hypertensive crisis during the intervention can be managed with phentolamine or nitroprusside. After removal of the pheochromocytoma, hypotension responds rapidly to intravenous administration of fluids, colloid solutions, or blood. Only rarely is the administration of phenylephrine required.

Particular caution should be observed in the use of propranolol during pregnancy. This drug has been successfully used in the symptomatic treatment of pregnant women with hyperthyroidism and occasionally used in patients with pheochromocytoma accompanied by severe tachycardia.[54] This beta-adrenergic blocking agent can, in fact, produce many perinatal problems, including impaired response to anoxic stress, depression at birth, small placenta, intrauterine growth retardation, postnatal bradycardia, and postnatal hypoglycemia.[55,56]

REFERENCES

1. Chapman, W., Signg, M.: Evaluation of tests used in the diagnosis of pheochromocytoma. *Mod Concepts Cardiovasc Dis 23:* 221–224, 1954.
2. Brunjes, S., Johns, V., Crane, M.: Pheochromocytoma: Post-operative shock and blood volume. *N Engl J Med 262:* 393–396, 1960.
3. Barbeau, A.: Le pheochromocytoma. *Union Med Can 86:* 1045–1051, 1957.
4. Gifford, R., Dvale, W., Maher, F., et al: Clinical features, diagnosis and treatment of pheochromocytoma: A review of 76 cases. *Mayo Clin Proc 39:* 281–302, 1964.
5. Stackpole, R., Meyer, M., Uson, A.: Pheochromocytoma in children. *J Pediatr 63:* 315–330, 1963.
6. Glenner, G., Grimbley, P.: Tumors of the extraadrenal paraganglion system. *Ann Tumor Pathol Ser 2,* fasc 9, Wash DC, AF IP, 1974.
7. Sjoerdsma, A., Engelman, K., Waldmann, T. A., et al: Pheochromocytoma: Current concepts of diagnosis and treatment. *Ann Intern Med 65:* 1302–1326, 1966.
8. Moorhead, E. L. Jr., Brenner, M. J., Caldwell, J. R., et al: Pheochromocytoma: A familial tumor. A study of 11 families. *Henry Ford Hosp Med Bull 13:* 467–478, 1965.
9. Sipple, J.: The association of pheochromocytoma with carcinoma of the thyroid gland. *Am J Med 31:* 163–166, 1961.
10. Williams, E., Pollack, D.: Multiple mucosal neuromata with endocrine tumors: A syndrome allied to von Recklinghausen's disease. *J Pathol Bacteriol 91:* 71–80, 1966.
11. Bernier, J., Rambaud, J., Cattan, D., et al: Diarrhea associated with medullary carcinoma of the thyroid. *Gut 10:* 980–985, 1969.
12. Glushien, A., Mansuy, M., Littman, D.: Pheochromocytoma: Its relationship to the neurocutaneous syndromes. *Am J Med 14:* 318–327, 1953.
13. Mulholland, S. G., Atuk, N. O., Walzak, M. P.: Familial pheochromocytoma associated with cerebellar hemangioblastoma. A case history and review of the literature. *JAMA 207:* 1709–1711, 1969.
14. McNeill, A. D., Groden, B. M., Neville, A. M.: Intrathroacic pheochromocytoma. *Br J Surg 57(6):* 457–462, 1970.
15. Duke, W. W., Boshell, B. R., Soteres, P., Carr, J. H. A.: A norepinephrine-secreting glomus jugulare tumor presenting as a pheochromocytoma. *Ann Intern Med 60:* 1040, 1964.
16. Zimmerman, I. J., Biron, R. E., MacMahon, H. E.: Pheochromocytoma of urinary bladder. *N Engl J Med 25:* 249, 1953.
17. Glenner, G. G., Crout, J. R., Roberts, W. C.: A functional carotid-body-like tumor secreting levaterenol. *Arch Pathol 73:* 230, 1962.
18. Remine, W. H., Chong, G. C., Van Heerden, J. A., Sheps, S. G.,
19. Harrison, E. G.: Current management of pheochromocytoma. *Ann Surg 179(5):* 740–748, 1974.
20. Quinan, C., Berger, A. A.: Observations on human adrenals with especial reference to the relative weight of the normal medulla. *Ann Intern Med 6:* 1180–1192, 1933.
21. Visser, J. W., Axt, R.: Bilateral adrenal medullary hyperplasia: A clinicopathological entity. *J Clin Pathol 28:* 298–304, 1975.
22. Carney, J. A., Sizemore, G. W., Sheps, S. G.: Adrenal medullary disease in multiple endocrine neoplasia, type II, pheochromocytoma and its precursors. *Am J Clin Pathol 66:* 279–290, 1976.
23. Wolfe, H. J., Melvin, K. E. W., Cervi-Skinner, S. J., Al Saadi, A. A., et al: C-cell hyperplasia preceding medullary thyroid carcinoma. *N Engl J Med 289:* 437, 1973.
24. Visser, J., Axt, R.: Adrenomedullary disease in multiple endocrine neoplasia, type 2. *Am J Clin Pathol 67:* 610–611, 1977.
25. Rowntree, L. G., Ball, R. G.: Diseases of the suprarenal glands. *Endocrinology 17:* 263–294, 1933.
26. Schwab, R., Denninger, K.: Uber bezienhungen swischen paroxysmaler hypertonie und nebennierenmark. *A Ges Inn Med 7:* 592–594, 1952.
27. Drukker, W., Formijne, P., van der Schoot, J. B.: Hyperplasia of the adrenal medulla. *Br Med J 1:* 186–189, 1957.
28. Montalbano, F. P., Baronofsky, I. D., Ball. H.: Hyperplasia of the adrenal medulla. *JAMA 182:* 264, 1962.
29. Masson, P., Martin, J.: Paragangliome surrenal, etude d'un cas humain de tumeurs malignes de la medullo-surrenale. *Bull Assoc Franc Cancer 12:* 135–141, 1923.
30. Cryer, P. E., Kissane, J. M.: Metastatic catecholamine-secreting paraganglioma (extra-adrenal pheochromocytoma). *Am J Med 61:* 523–532, 1976.
31. Melander, A., Nilsson, E., Sundler, F.: Sympathetic activation of thyroid hormone secretion in mice. *Endocrinology 90:* 194, 1972.
32. Melander, A., Ranklev, E., Sundler, F., et al: Beta$_2$-adrenergic stimulation of thyroid hormone secretion. *Endocrinology 97:* 332, 1975.
33. Finnerty, F. A., Bucholz, H. J., Guilladean, R. L.: The blood volumes and plasma proteins during levarterenol-induced hypertension. *J Clin Invest 37:* 435, 1958.
34. Waldmann, T. A., Bradley, J. E.: Polycythemia secondary to a pheochromocytoma with production of an erythropoiesis stimulating factor by the tumor. *Proc Soc Exp Med Biol 108:* 425, 1961.
35. Engelman, K., Sjoerdsma, A.: Chronic medical therapy for pheochromocytoma. *Ann Intern Med 61:* 229–241, 1964.
36. Kline, I. K.: Myocardial alterations associated with pheochromocytoma. *Am J Pathol 38:* 539–551, 1961.
37. Robinson, R. G., DeQuattro, V., Grushkin, C. M., Lieberman, E.: Childhood pheochromocytoma treatment with alpha methyl tyrosine for resistant hypertension. *J Pediatr 91(1):* 143–147, 1977.
38. Spergel, G., Levy, L., Chowdhury, F., et al: A modified phentolamine test for the diagnosis of pheochromocytoma. *JAMA 211:* 266–269, 1970.
39. Engelman, K., Horwitz, D., Ambrose, I., et al: Further evaluation of the tyramine test for pheochromocytoma. *N Engl J Med 278:* 705–709, 1968.
40. Lawrence, A.: Glucagon provocative test for pheochromocytoma. *Ann Intern Med 66:* 1091–1096, 1967.
41. Pisano, J., Cout, R., Abraham, D.: Determination of 3-methoxy-4 hydroxymandelic acid in urine. *Clin Chim Acta 7:* 285–291, 1962.
42. DeQuattro, V.: Evaluation of increased norepinephrine excretion in hypertension using L-dopa-³H. *Circ Res 28:* 84–97, 1971.
43. DeQuattro, V., Chan, S.: Raised plasma-catecholamines in some patients with primary hypertension. *Lancet 1:* 806–809, 1972.
44. Sjoerdsma, A., Engleman, K., Waldmann, J., et al: Pheochromocytoma: Current concepts of diagnosis and treatment. *Ann Intern Med 65:* 1302, 1966.
45. Lieberman, L. M., Bejerwaltes, J. W., Conn, J. W., et al: Diagnosis of adrenal disease by visualization of human adrenal glands. *N Engl J Med 285:* 1387–1393, 1971.
46. Mayo, C.: Paroxysmal hypertension with tumors of retroperitoneal nerve: Report of a case. *JAMA 89:* 1047–1050, 1927.
47. Sjoerdsma, A., Engelman, K., Spector, S., Undenfriend, S.: Inhibition of catecholamines synthesis in man with alpha-methyl-tyrosine, an inhibitor of tyrosine hydroxylase. *Lancet,* November 1965, pp. 1092–1094.
48. Gitlow, S. E., Pertsemlidis, D., Bertani, L. M.: Management of patients with pheochromocytoma. *Am Heart J 82(4):* 557–567, 1971.
49. Hamilton, B. P. M., Cheikh, I. E., Rivera, L. E.: Attempted Treat-

ment of inoperable pheochromocytoma with streptozocin. *Arch Intern Med 137:* 762–765, 1977.

49. Schenker, J. G., Chowers, U.: Pheochromocytoma and pregnancy review of 89 cases. *Obstet Gynecol Surv 26:* 739–747, 1971.

50. Saarikoski, S.: Fate of noradrenaline in the human fetoplacental unit. *Acta Physiol Scand Suppl: 421,* 1974.

51. Sprague, A. D., Thelin, T. J., Dilts, P. V. Jr.: Pheochromocytoma associated with pregnancy, *Obstet Gynecol 39:* 887–891, 1972.

52. Smith, A. M.: Pheochromocytoma and pregnancy. *J Obstet Gynecol 80:* 848–851, 1973.

53. Griffith, M. I., Felts, J. H., James, F. M., et al: Successful control of pheochromocytoma in pregnancy. *JAMA 229:* 437–439, 1974.

54. Langer, A., Hung, C. T., McA'nulty, J. A., et al: Adrenergic blockade. A new approach to hyperthyroidism during pregnancy. *Obstet Gynecol 44:* 181–186, 1974.

55. Tunstall, M. E.: The effect of propranolol on the onset of breathing at birth. *Br J Anaesth 41:* 792, 1969.

56. Gladstone, G. R., Hordof, A., Gersony, W. M.: Propranolol administration during pregnancy: Effects on the fetus. *J Pediatr 86:* 962–964, 1975.

57. Amery, A., Conway, J.: A critical review of diagnostic tests for pheochromocytoma. *Am Heart J 73:* 129–133, 1967.

58. Crout, J., Brown, B.: Anesthetic management of pheochromocytoma: The value of phenoxybenzamine and methoxyfluorane. *Anesthesiology 30:* 29, 1969.

103

Orthostatic Hypotension: Causes and Therapy

Vito M. Campese
Vincent DeQuattro

Orthostatic hypotension is a clinical entity characterized by symptoms of impaired cerebral circulation due to a fall in blood pressure upon assuming the upright position. In normal people the gravitational shift of approximately 300–800 ml of blood to the lower extremities in the upright position tends to reduce venous return, stroke volume, cardiac output, and arterial pressure. Several adjustments normally intervene to counteract the hemodynamic effect of gravity (Fig. 103-1). The initial fall in blood pressure reduces baroreceptor drive via the carotid sinuses and aortic arch to the vasomotor center, leading to reflex sympathetic nerve stimulation. Arteriolar and venous constriction ensue, leading to increased peripheral resistance, increased venous return, and cardiac acceleration. Furthermore, increased tone and isotonic contractions of skeletal muscles in the lower extremities in the upright position enhance venous return. Orthostatic hyperventilation is also a result of increased venous tone. The result of these hemodynamic adjustments is a slightly lower systolic blood pressure and a mildly increased diastolic pressure. The mean blood pressure is unchanged. Numerous factors can alter these homeostatic mechanisms and lead to orthostatic hypotension (Table 103-1). Orthostatic hypotension is usually due to lower effective circulating blood volume.

CAUSES

HYPERBRADYKININISM

Patients with hyperbradykininism characteristically present with flushing of the face, neck, and anterior chest. Later, these changes cause ecchymosis and purple discoloration of the legs after standing. Systolic blood pressure drops markedly on standing, accompanied by severe tachycardia and increased diastolic blood pressure, leading to a very small pulse pressure. The syndrome occurs in two forms: one familial and one associated with the dumping syndrome. The familial syndrome appears to be related to impaired destruction of bradykinin. Plasma concentrations of bradykinin are always elevated, whereas the plasma concentrations of bradykininase I are commonly reduced. Treatment with propranolol, fluorocortisone, and cyprophetadine improves the symptoms.[1]

DYSAUTONOMIA

Dysautonomia is a frequent cause of orthostatic hypotension. It is characterized by an interruption of the baroreceptor reflex arc. Dysautonomia covers a wide variety of causes and conditions (see Table 103-1).

Drugs

The most frequent and overlooked drugs are antihypertensive agents, tranquilizers, sedatives, hypnotics, antidepressants, phenothiazines, and levodopa. Thus the history of prior use of these medications should be sought in patients who present with orthostatic hypotension.

Autonomic Neuropathy

Orthostatic hypotension may be a manifestation of the autonomic neuropathy of patients with diabetes,[2–4] alcoholism[5,6] and porphyria.[5,7] Approximately 10 percent of patients with amyloidosis develop orthostatic hypotension[8] and other symptoms of autonomic neuropathy: impotence, diarrhea, dyshydrosis, and urinary retention. Sensory and motor neuropathies are frequently present.[9] Signs of peripheral polyneuropathy, including postural hypotension, were present in 14 percent of a large series of primary amyloidosis.[10] The orthostatic hypotension of primary amyloidosis has been attributed to impairment of both the efferent sympathetic nerve pathway and the arteriolar wall.[7] Pathological studies show extensive deposition of amyloid material in vessels, interstitial tissue of the sympathetic ganglia, and the fibers of autonomic plexuses.[11–13]

Uremic patients frequently manifest peripheral neuropathy. Recently, evidence has accumulated which suggests the presence of autonomic insufficiency in some patients with chronic renal failure.[14,15] The autonomic dysfunction has been attributed to a generalized neuropathy and seems to play a role in non-volume-

Table 103-1. Orthostatic Hypotension Associated with Neurogenic Dysautonomia

Known Causes
1. Medications (antihypertensives, tranquilizers, sedatives, hypnotics, antidepressants, phenothiazines, levodopa)
2. Peripheral polyneuropathies: diabetes, uremia, amyloidosis, porphyria, alcoholism, B₁₂ deficiency, Guillain-Barré syndrome, etc.
3. Tabes dorsalis
4. Parkinson's disease
5. Cerebrovascular accident
6. Neoplastic infiltration of central autonomic nervous system
7. Syringomyelia
8. Amyotrophic lateral sclerosis
9. Disseminated sclerosis
10. Extensive sympathectomy
11. Spinal cord transection
12. Carcinomas of the bronchi, breast, pancreas, etc.

Unknown Causes
1. Idiopathic orthostatic hypotension (IOH)
   Type 1: without CNS involvement
      a. With no pressor response to tyramine
      b. With pressor response to tyramine
   Type 2: with CNS involvement (Shy-Drager syndrome)
2. Familial dysautonomia (Riley-Day syndrome)

responding hypotension during hemodialysis.[15] The evidence for autonomic dysfunction is indirect and includes abnormal response in heart rate during Valsalva maneuver, reduced increment in heart rate in response to amyl-nitrite-induced hypotension, and abnormal hand-grip response, fixed heart rate, and fall in peripheral resistances during hemodialysis-induced hypotension.[14,15] Plasma catecholamine concentrations have been found to be elevated in 29 regular hemodialysis patients and to respond normally to passive orthostasis.[16]

Patients with idiopathic parkinsonism have a normal recumbent arterial pressure but a significant fall on tilting,[17] the mechanism of which is unclear considering that these patients have a normal Valsalva response. Orthostatic hypotension due to neurogenic dysautonomia has been shown in patients with carcinomas of the bronchi,[18] breast,[5] and pancreas.[19] Dysautonomia may revert after radiotherapy[20] in patients with bronchial carcinoma.

MECHANISMS

The mechanism of orthostatic hypotension in neurogenic dysautonomia is an interruption of the baroreceptor reflex arc. The lesion may reside in the afferent limb, in the vasomotor center, in the efferent limb, or in the arteriolar wall. The site of dysfunction may be the afferent limb in tabes dorsalis and diabetes mellitus. The vasomotor center may be involved by degenerative diseases of the central nervous system, tumors near the vasomotor center, vascular lesions of the brain stem, drugs such as phenothiazines, antidepressants, sedatives, and antihypertensives, including methyldopa, clonidine, and propranolol. An involvement of the efferent adrenergic pathway is responsible for orthostatic hypotension in patients with spinal cord transection, extensive sympathectomy, porphyria, diabetes, antihypertensive drugs, especially the ganglionic blocking agents and guanethidine, and most cases of idiopathic orthostatic hypotension (Fig. 103-2).

IDIOPATHIC ORTHOSTATIC HYPOTENSION

Idiopathic orthostatic hypertension (IOH) is a separate clinical entity among the myriad of conditions causing orthostatic hypotension. The disease was first described by Bradbury and Eggleston in 1925 and was attributed to a primary failure of sympathetic control of blood pressure.[21] Subsequently, Shy and Drager recognized that the disease is characterized by disturbances of multiple somatic systems as well as of the autonomic nervous system.[22] These authors called attention to the primary degenera-

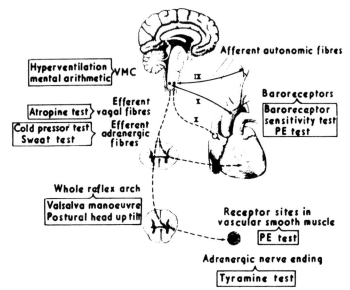

Fig. 103-2. Tests of autonomic cardiovascular reactivity. Various tests of autonomic function may be given to localize possible impairment in different components of the baroceptor arc. Responses to passive head-up tilt and the Valsalva maneuver[65] test integrity of the entire arc: efferent sympathetic fibers are investigated using the cold pressor test, stressful mental arithmetic, and the reflex sweat test. Vasomotor center (VMC) responsiveness is verified by reduction of arterial pressure after hyperventilation for 15 seconds.[66] Intravenous phenylephrine (PE) causes vasoconstriction and thereby increases systemic pressure if arteriolar smooth muscle receptors are intact; cardiac slowing indicates integrity of both the efferent cardiac vagal fibers and the afferent autonomic fibers from the baroreceptors. The heart rate response to atropine is a measure of the vagal component. The vasopressor response to tyramine is a measure of releasable intraneuronal norepinephrine. (Reproduced from reference 25 with permission.)

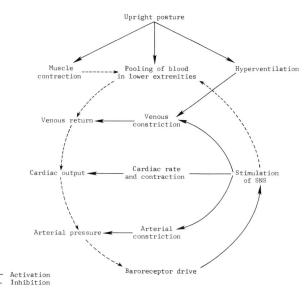

Fig. 103-1. Role of the sympathetic nervous system in hemodynamic adjustment to upright posture in humans.

tive change involving the autonomic as well as the central nervous system.

Many investigators classify IOH into two separate syndromes: IOH without other neurologic disorders (type I) and IOH combined with neurologic defects (type II or Shy-Drager syndrome).[23-25] Some investigators believe the somatic and neurologic symptoms to be a single syndrome[26,27] and that the two clinical entities represent either different clinical stages or anatomical diffusion of the same degenerative disorder of the central nervous system to the somatic system. It has been reported that in some patients, the disease starts exclusively with symptoms of autonomic nervous dysfunction and proceeds to affect multiple somatic neural structures.[28] The time interval between the appearance of symptoms of autonomic dysfunction and somatic neurologic manifestation ranges from 1 month to as long as 10 years, most commonly being 2 to 6 years. On the other hand, occasionally some patients can present with involvement of some somatic systems, followed months or years later by symptoms of autonomic nervous dysfunction. Idiopathic orthostatic hypotension is more common in the elderly. Males have twice the incidence of females. In a survey of 57 cases from the Mayo Clinic,[19] the ages of patients ranged from 42 to 76 years (mean 60); 21 were women and 36 were men. Occasionally the disease is familial.[29]

TYPE I

Patients with IOH may present with features of autonomic dysfunction of the bladder, bowel, sexual, or sweating system, but the cardinal symptom is bothersome hypotension with standing. There is usually a reduction of both systolic and diastolic arterial pressures of at least 25 mm Hg upon standing. The change in position is usually accompanied by light-headedness, faintness, weakness, unsteadiness of gait, slurring of speech, and dimness of vision. However, the fall in arterial pressure is not associated with pallor or coolness of skin, tachycardia, or increased sweating, all of which are common features in other types of syncopal episodes. Loss of sweating and, in men, loss of libido or impotence are frequent and often the presenting symptoms.

Autonomic dysfunction of the bladder includes urinary hesitancy, dribbling, retention, and nocturnal incontinence. Loss of rectal sphincter tone with rectal incontinence can also be present. Anisocoria, Horner's syndrome, and absence of pupil reaction can alternate from one side to the other. Impairment of tear formation, dryness of mouth, and rarely iris atrophy may be part of the syndrome. The symptoms of autonomic dysfunction are related mostly to sympathetic nervous system involvement and in part to parasympathetic nervous system control.

TYPE II

Some patients who develop postural hypotension may present with symptoms of the pyramidal, extrapyramidal, and cerebellar systems. These include gait and speech disturbances, incoordination, generalized weakness, impaired handwriting, atrophy of distal muscles, numbness of limbs, swallowing disturbances, and resting or intentional tremor. The neurologic examination may reveal involvement of pyramidal system with signs of hyperreflexia, extensor toe reflexes, and dysarthria. There may be extrapyramidal features such as rigidity, bradykinesia, masklike appearance, monotony of voice, and resting tremor of the limbs. There may be involvement of the cerebellar system with intentional tremor, ataxia, and ataxic-dysarthric speech. Intellectual and sensory deterioration may occur, but that is a rare occurrence. The cerebrospinal fluid and skull x-rays are normal. The electroenceph-

alogram may be normal or show diffuse dysrhythmia or slow wave activity. Pneumoencephalography is usually normal but can display diffuse atrophy. Electromyographic studies suggest peripheral neuropathy. The disease is progressive and irreversible, and the average survival time after the symptomatic onset of IOH is 7 to 8 years. The average survival after the onset of neurologic manifestation is 4 years.

HEMODYNAMIC STUDIES

There is evidence that suggests an interruption of the baroreceptor reflex arc in idiopathic orthostatic hypotension. In fact, patients with IOH have a marked reduction of arterial pressure without a significant increase in heart rate in response to passive head-up tilt. Furthermore, during the straining phase of the Valsalva maneuver, heart rate does not change in spite of a drop in arterial pressure. During the release phase of this maneuver, there is no overshoot of diastolic pressure. In patients with IOH, intravenous infusion of phenylephrine usually produces a pressor response and a reduction in heart rate, indicating that the receptor sites in the arteriolar wall, the afferent autonomic fibers from the baroreceptor, and the vagal efferent pathway are intact.[30] Hyperventilation produces a reduction of arterial pressure, indicating a normal response of the vasomotor center.

Patients with IOH have little or no blood pressure response to the cold pressor test and mental arithmetic. The reflex sweat test in response to hot environmental temperature is reduced, whereas the direct sweat test in response to iontophoresis is normal, indicating an alteration of the efferent sympathetic pathway. Acceleration of the heart after atropine infusion is reduced, suggesting some involvement of efferent cardiac vagal fibers.

Patients with IOH usually have a rapid resting heart rate but reduced response after head-up tilt or orthostatic position and reduced acceleration after atropine infusion. Heart rate can, however, be reduced by infusing a pressor agent. These data seem to indicate that the heart of patients with IOH is partially denervated. Although a vagal involvement seems clear by the diminished response after the administration of atropine, the reflex bradycardia after phenylephrine seems to indicate that the vagal denervation is only partial. The cardiac output is reduced as a result of a marked reduction of cardiac stroke volume and of left ventricular ejection. The ratio of stroke volume to cardiopulmonary volume is lower than in normal subjects, indicating that reduced plasma volume cannot account totally for the reduction of cardiac output, but other factors, such as a reduction of cardiac performance, are involved.[30] Paradoxically, total peripheral resistance is frequently increased.

Intra-arterial infusion of tyramine, an indirectly acting sympathomimetic amine, does not produce vasoconstriction, whereas intra-arterial administration of norepinephrine produces enhanced vasoconstrictor response in cases of type I IOH, suggesting norepinephrine depletion from the nerve endings and a denervation hypersensitivity of the arteriolar smooth muscle.[24] This hypersensitivity was present in adipose tissue of Type I patients.[31] A depletion of norepinephrine from sympathetic nerve endings has been confirmed histochemically by demonstrating the absence of catecholamine-specific fluorescence in sympathetic vasomotor nerves from the deltoid muscle.[24] Occasionally, patients without central nervous system involvement can manifest a pressor response to tyramine.[32] These patients probably have normal catecholamine stores at vasomotor endings, but for unknown reasons, catecholamines cannot be released by ordinary autonomic control. In these patients, a viral syndrome frequently precedes the onset of orthostatic hypotension. Patients with type II IOH seem to have a normal pressor response to tyramine and are not hyposensitive to norepinephrine infusion.[24] Hemodynamic studies performed in IOH seem to indicate that the disease is characterized by dysfunction of the autonomic nervous system.

BIOCHEMICAL FEATURES

The concept of dysautonomia is supported by the observation that the urinary excretion of catecholamines in IOH is reduced.[33–35] Resting plasma catecholamines may be lower or higher than normal. Catecholamines are reduced in patients with type I and normal in patients with type II IOH.[25,36] Furthermore, plasma norepinephrine and epinephrine fail to show any significant change after tilting in both type I and type II[25,36,37] (Fig. 103-3). The rate of metabolism of circulating norepinephrine is delayed in IOH.[38] Plasma dopamine-beta-hydroxylase was reduced in both groups.[25] The interrelationships between catecholamines, renin, and aldosterone in patients with postural hypotension have not been clarified. One patient with IOH failed to respond with normal elevation of urinary catecholamines, plasma renin activity, or urinary aldosterone in response to upright posture or sodium deprivation, despite a substantial fall in arterial pressure.[39] This observation was of particular physiologic interest, since it supported the hypothesis that plasma renin secretion is regulated by the activity of the sympathetic nervous system.[40,41] In contrast, other studies in patients with IOH have shown that normal or even exaggerated increases of plasma renin occur in response to tilting without changes in the excretion of plasma catecholamines.[35,42] Love and co-workers attempted an explanation of these contradictory results.[43] These authors suggested that patients with lesions of the afferent side of baroreceptor reflexes have a marked increase of plasma renin concentration after tilting, whereas no change occurred in patients thought to have a lesion of the efferent pathway.

PATHOLOGY

Autopsy findings in IOH revealed widespread degenerative lesions in the basal ganglia, substantia nigra, pons, olivae, cerebellum, spinal cord, and sympathetic ganglia.[22,44,45] The lesions were characterized by atrophy and gliosis. Occasionally, inclusions of the Lewy type or eosinophilic inclusions can be seen.[44] Eosinophilic bodies were present in sympathetic ganglia.[46] Cell loss in the substantia nigra, locus ceruleus, or cerebellar cortex were not found at autopsy of patients with type I IOH.[46]

The lesions frequently affect the pyramidal tracts and the interomediolateral columns in the spinal cord. The sympathetic ganglia often have hydropic degeneration and loss of Nissl substance. Histochemical studies have shown the absence of catecholamine-specific fluorescence in sympathetic vasomotor nerves from deltoid muscle.[24] Black et al. found that dopamine-beta-hydroxylase activity was reduced 85 percent in sympathetic ganglia and that tyrosine hydroxylase activity was reduced 98 percent in the pontine nucleus and locus ceruleus.[47] Thus, from the hemodynamic, biochemical, and pathologic standpoint, it appears that patients with idiopathic orthostatic hypotension can be divided into at least two types.

Type I

Patients without signs of central nervous system dysfunction have reduced plasma levels of catecholamines, reduced pressor response to indirectly acting sympathomimetic amines, hypersensitivity to exogenous norepinephrine, and absence of catecholamine-specific fluorescense in sympathetic vasomotor nerves. Limited studies have not found nerve growth factor antibodies.[64] An occasional patient may have a normal tyramine pressor response.

Type II

Patients with IOH and signs of central nervous system involvement were found to be normal with respect to recumbent plasma catecholamines, responses to tyramine and exogenous norepinephrine, and tissue levels of norepinephrine. Neither type has a postural increase in plasma catecholamines. Although this classification assists in understanding the pathophysiology of patients with IOH, it fails to explain why some patients evolve from type I to type II.

MANAGEMENT AND THERAPY

Patients with orthostatic hypotension should be systematically studied to identify and correct secondary causes of this disease (see Table 103-1). A careful history should exclude the possibility of drugs as a factor producing the orthostatic hypotension. The historian should search for other symptoms of autonomic neurologic dysfunction. Postural changes in heart rate and changes of blood pressure during a Valsalva maneuver should be investigated in order to separate patients with autonomic insufficiency from those with hypovolemia, adrenal insufficiency, pheochromocytoma, and hyperbradykininism. Tests should be performed to exclude the possibility of diabetes, syphilis, porphyria, and adrenocortical insufficiency. When clinically indicated, a complete

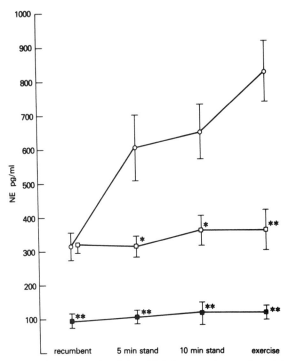

Fig. 103-3. Plasma norepinephrine (NE) in normal controls and in patients with orthostatic hypotension—recumbent, standing, and during exercise. NE concentrations (mean ± SEM) are shown for 10 control subjects (○), 6 patients with normal plasma norepinephrine while recumbent (□) who also had diffuse neurologic signs (Shy-Drager syndrome), and 4 patients with low plasma norepinephrine while recumbent (■) who did not have diffuse neurologic signs (idiopathic orthostatic hypotension). *Different from control subjects ($P < 0.01$ by student's t test). **($P < 0.001$). (Reproduced from reference 24 with permission.)

neurological workup should be performed to identify the cause of any neurological lesion.

Symptomatic treatment should be attempted after correctable causes of orthostatic hypotension are excluded. Patients should be instructed to avoid prolonged recumbency or sudden postural changes. They should exercise often. Patients should eat a diet rich in salt and avoid hypnotics, tranquilizers, and antidepressants. Mechanical appliances such as elastic stockings and abdominal binders have been useful.[48] Pressor agents have been used in the treatment of IOH with inconstant and unpredictable results. Vasopressin tannate in oil has been of value.[49,50] Sympathomimetic amine agents usually prove unsatisfactory. Mineralocorticoids have been used extensively with the best results.

Desoxycorticosterone acetate in oil was the first steroid to be used but was subsequently replaced by 9-alpha-fluorohydrocortisone because of the advantage of its oral administration.[49,51,52] This drug is effective in most of the patients with IOH, particularly in type I, even though the basic disturbance in the release of norepinephrine by the sympathetic nerve endings seems to be unaltered by this therapy. The mechanism of action is related to hypervolemia and increased cardiac output secondary to its sodium-retaining effect. Evidence suggests that steroids increase the responsiveness of vascular smooth muscle to norepinephrine.[52] Florinef should be started with low doses of 0.05 mg/day and subsequently gradually increased according to the therapeutic response. The usual doses range between 0.1 and 0.3 mg daily. Patients treated with Florinef and a high-sodium diet should be followed carefully because of the dangers of increased body weight and supine hypertension and the possibility of cardiac failure. More recently, therapy with a combination of monoamine oxidase (MAO) inhibitors and norepinephrine-releasing substances or foods containing tyramine, such as cheddar cheese or Chianti wine[42,53,54] has been proposed in patients with normal circulating catecholamines or type II IOH. The combination of a MAO inhibitor with a sympathomimetic amine is much more predictable and effective than the cheese therapy, probably because of different amounts of tyramine in individual batches.

These combinations are contraindicated in normal subjects because they may produce hypertensive crises. Amphetamines and tyramine release norepinephrine from the sympathetic nerve terminals, whereas MAO inhibitors potentiate the effect of amphetamines by reducing the rate of deamination of catecholamines at nerve endings. More recently, patients with Shy-Drager syndrome have been treated with a combination of levodopa and MAO inhibitors with encouraging results.[55,56] Patients with IOH presenting with profuse watery diarrhea benefit from the administration of aspirin. It is believed that diarrhea in IOH is the result of unopposed actions of prostaglandins on the gut.[57] The latest reports indicate that propranolol, a beta blocking agent, may alleviate postural hypotension in type I patients.[67]

FAMILIAL DYSAUTONOMIA

Familial dysautonomia is a syndrome characterized by symptoms of autonomic nervous dysfunction associated with neuromuscular, sensory, and mental disturbances. It occurs primarily in Eastern European Ashkenazi Jewish children and is inherited as an autosomal recessive trait. Both sexes are equally afflicted. Symptoms of autonomic nervous dysfunction can be present very early in life[58,59] and affect primarily the gastrointestinal tract. Infants have signs of incoordination of sucking and swallowing, such as spitting, drooling, choking, and aspiration which can lead to aspira-

tion pneumonia. Later in life, cyclic vomiting and bowel irregularities, with intermittent diarrhea, constipation, and sphincter incompetence become the most prominent features. The cardiovascular involvement of autonomic nervous dysfunction can lead to orthostatic hypotension without tachycardia, paroxysmal hypertension, skin blotching, acrocyanosis, or coldness of the extremities. Prolonged breath-holding spells and vacillation of temperature with bouts of fever can be present. The exocrine gland secretion is impaired, as manifested by reduced sweating and reduced or absent tears.

Neuromuscular dysfunction can be present: diminished deep tendon reflexes, hypotonia, poor muscular coordination, small stature, dysarthria, and kyphoscoliosis. Symptoms of central nervous system dysfunction include behavioral disturbance, motor-skill retardation, mental retardation, and convulsions. Decreased pain and temperature sensations can lead to mutilation secondary to injury. The fungiform papillae of the tongue are usually absent, and taste is impaired. Reduced lacrimation in conjunction with the corneal hypoesthesia may result in corneal abrasion or ulceration.

Abnormalities of catecholamine metabolism have been found in this syndrome. Increased urinary excretion of homovanillic acid (HVA), a product of dopamine metabolism, with decreased excretion of vanillylmandelic acid (VMA), a metabolite of norepinephrine and epinephrine, was reported by Smith.[60] Subsequently, Weinshilboum and Axelrod found that dopamine-beta-hydroxylase (DBH), the enzyme that converts dopamine to norepinephrine, was significantly decreased in some patients.[61] These metabolic abnormalities seem to indicate a block in the conversion of dopamine to norepinephrine. In patients with familial dysautonomia, the instillation of one drop of 3.5 percent of methacoline in the conjunctival sac results in marked constriction of the pupil. An intradermal injection of histamine produces a wheal 2–3 cm in diameter with a sharp red border without axon flare. These two methods are now used as screening tests in children of Jewish extraction who are hypotonic or who present feeding difficulties at birth. The measurements of HVA, VMA, and DBH are used to confirm the diagnosis. The prognosis of patients with Riley-Day syndrome has been improving, and large numbers of patients are entering adolescence and adulthood.

The pathology of familial dysautonomia is characterized by a marked reduction in the number of unmyelinated fibers in somatic peripheral nerves, which convey the sensation of pain, temperature, and taste, and a reduction of large myelinated fibers, which convey afferent impulses from muscle spindles.[62] These abnormalities may result from selective arrest of the development of these two types of fibers, which derive genetically from the same neuronal population. No reduction of autonomic fibers, which could explain the symptoms of sympathetic and parasympathetic denervation, has been demonstrated as yet. Pearson et al. have demonstrated depletion of dense-core-vesicle in sympathetic nerve terminals from the outer walls of blood vessels in skin and nerve biopsies from patients with familial dysautonomia.[63]

REFERENCES

1. Streeten, D. H. P., Kerr, L. P., Kerr, C. B., et al: Hyperbradykininism: A new orthostatic syndrome. *Lancet 2:* 1048–1053, 1972.
2. Rundles, R. W.: Diabetic neuropathy: General review with report of 125 cases. *Medicine 24:* 111–160, 1945.
3. Odel, H. M., Roth, G. M., Keating, F. R.: Autonomic neuropathy simulating the effects of sympathectomy as a complication of diabetes mellitus. *Diabetes 4:* 92–98, 1955.
4. Frank, H. J., Frewin, D. B., Robinson, S. M., et al: Cardiovascular responses in diabetic dysautonomia. *Aust NZ J Med 2:* 1–7, 1972.

5. Barraclough, M. A., Sharpey-Schafer, E. P.: Hypotension from absent circulatory reflexes. *Lancet 1:* 1121–1126, 1963.

6. Birchfield, R. I.: Postural hypotension in Wernicke's disease: A manifestation of autonomic nervous system involvement. *Am J Med 36:* 404–414, 1964.

7. Wagner, N. H. Jr: Orthostatic hypotension. *Bull Johns Hopkins Hosp 105:* 322–359, 1959.

8. Kyle, R. A., Kottke, B. A., Schirger, A.: Orthostatic hypotension as a clue to primary systemic amyloid. *Circulation 34:* 883, 1966.

9. Munsat, T. L., Poussaint, A. F.: Clinical manifestations and diagnosis of amyloid polyneuropathy. *Neurology 12:* 413–422, 1962.

10. Rukavina, J. G., Block, W. D., Jackson, C. E., et al: Primary systemic amyloidosis: A review and an experimental, genetic and clinical study of 29 cases with particular emphasis on the familiar form. *Medicine 35:* 239–334, 1956.

11. Gaan, D., Mahoney, M. P., Rowlands, D. J., et al: Postural hypotension in amyloid disease. *Am Heart J 84:* 395–400, 1972.

12. Fuidley, J. W. Jr., Adams, W.: Primary systemic amyloidosis simulating constrictive pericarditis with steatorrhea and hyperesthesia. *Arch Intern Med 81:* 342, 1948.

13. Fisher, H., Press, F. S.: Primary systemic amyloidosis with involvement of the nervous system. *Am J Clin Pathol 21:* 758, 1951.

14. Ewing, D. J., Winney, R.: Autonomic function in patients with chronic renal failure on intermittent hemodialysis. *Nephron 15:* 424–429, 1975.

15. Kersh, E. S., Kronfield, S. J., Unger, A., et al: Autonomic insufficiency in uremia as a cause of hemodialysis-induced hypotension. *N Engl J Med 290:* 650–653, 1974.

16. Brecht, H. M., Ernst, W., Koch, K. M.: Plasma noradrenaline levels in regular hemodialysis patients. *Proc Eur Dial Transplant Assoc 12:* 281–289, 1975.

17. Gross, M., Bannister, R., Godwin-Austen, R.: Orthostatic hypotension in Parkinson's disease. *Lancet 1:* 174–176, 1972.

18. Ivy, H. K.: Renal sodium loss and bronchogenic carcinoma. *Arch Intern Med 108:* 47–55, 1961.

19. Thomas, J. P., Shields, R.: Associated autonomic dysfunction and carcinoma of the pancreas. *Br Med J 4:* 32, 1970.

20. Park, D. M., Johnson, R. H., Crean, G. P., et al: Orthostatic hypotension in bronchial carcinoma. *Br Med J 3:* 510–511, 1972.

21. Bradbury, S., Eggleston, C.: Postural hypotension: Report of three cases. *Am Heart J 1:* 73–86, 1925.

22. Shy, G. M., Drager, G. A.: A neurological syndrome associated with orthostatic hypotension. *Arch Neurol 2:* 511–527, 1960.

23. Hughes, R. C., Cartlidge, N. E. F., Millac, P.: Primary neurogenic orthostatic hypotension. *J Neurol Neurosurg Psychiatry 33:* 363–371, 1970.

24. Kontos, H. A., Richardson, D. W., Norvell, J. E.: Norepinephrine depletion in idiopathic orthostatic hypotension. *Ann Intern Med 82:* 336–341, 1975.

25. Ziegler, M. G., Lake, C. R., Kopin, I. J.: The sympathetic-nervous-system defect in primary orthostatic hypotension. *N Engl J Med 296:* 293–297, 1977.

26. Ibrahim, M. M.: Localization of lesion in patients with idiopathic orthostatic hypotension. *Br Heart J 37:* 868–872, 1975.

27. Goodall, McC., Harlan, W. R. Jr., Alton H.: Decreased noradrenaline (norepinephrine) synthesis in neurogenic orthostatic hypotension. *Circulation 38:* 592–603, 1968.

28. Chokroverty, S., Barron, K. D., Katz, F. H., et al: The syndrome of primary orthostatic hypotension. *Brain 92:* 743–768, 1969.

29. Lewis, P.: Familial orthostatic hypotension. *Brain 87:* 719–728, 1964.

30. Ibrahim, M. M., Tarazi, R. C., Dustan, H. P., et al: Idiopathic orthostatic hypotension: Circulatory dynamics in chronic autonomic insufficiency. *Am J. Cardiol 34:* 288–294, 1974.

31. Engelman, K., Mueller, P. S., Horwitz, D., et al: Denervation hypersensitivity of adipose tissue in idiopathic orthostatic hypotension. *Lancet 2:* 927–929, 1964.

32. Nanda, R., Johnson, R., Keogh, H.: Treatment of neurogenic orthostatic hypotension with a monoamine oxidase inhibitor and tyramine. *Lancet 2:* 1164–1167, 1967.

33. Dobkin, B. H., Rosenthal, N. P.: Clinical assessment of autonomic dysfunction: An approach to the Shy-Drager syndrome. *Bull LA Neurol Soc 40:* 101–110, 1975.

34. Luft, R., von Euler, V. S.: Diminished excretion of norepinephrine and epinephrine in two cases of orthostatic postural hypotension. *J Clin Invest 32:* 1055–1059, 1955.

35. Hedeland, H., Dymling, J. F., Hökfelt, B.: Catecholamines, renin and aldosterone in postural hypotension. *Acta Endocrinol 62:* 399–410, 1969.

36. Hickler, R. B., Wells, R. E. Jr., Tyler, H. R., et al: Plasma catecholamine and electroencephalographic responses to acute postural change. *Am J Med 25:* 410–423, 1959b.

37. Adkins, T. R., Miller, T. I., Carter, T., et al: The hormonal mediation of neurovascular reflex adjustments: Catecholamine response to postural changes in man. *Am Surg 27:* 210–221, 1961.

38. Goodall, McC., Harlan W. R. Jr., Alton, H.: Noradrenaline release and metabolism in orthostatic (postural) hypotension. *Circulation 36:* 489–496, 1967.

39. Gordon, R. D., Kuchel, D., Liddle, G. W. et al: Role of the sympathetic nervous system in regulating renin and aldosterone production in man. *J Clin Invest 46:* 599–605, 1967.

40. Taquim, A. C., Blaquier, P., Taquini, A. C., Jr.: On the production and role of renin. *Can Med Assoc J 90:* 210–231, 1964.

41. Vander, A. J.: Effects of catecholamines and the renal nerves on renin secretion in anaesthetized dogs. *Am J Physiol 209:* 659–662, 1965.

42. Diamond, M. A., Murray, R. H., Schmid, P. G.: Idiopathic postural hypotension. Physiologic observations and report of a new mode of therapy. *J Clin Invest 49:* 1341–1348, 1970.

43. Love, D. R., Brown, J. J., Chinn, R. H., et al: Plasma renin in idiopathic orthostatic hypotension: Differential response in subjects with probable afferent and efferent autonomic failure. *Clin Sci 41:* 289–299, 1971.

44. Evans, D. J., Lewis, P. D., Malhotra, D., et al: Idiopathic orthostatic hypotension. Report of an autopsied case with histochemical and ultrastructural studies of the neuronal inclusion. *J Neurol Sci 17:* 209–218, 1972.

45. Graham, J. G., Oppenheimer, D. R.: Orthostatic hypotension and nicotine sensitivity in a case of multiple system atrophy. *J Neurol Neurosurg Psychiatry 32:* 28–34, 1969.

46. Roessmann, V., Van den Noort, S., McFarland, D. F.: Idiopathic orthostatic hypotension. *Arch Neurol 24:* 503–510, 1971.

47. Black, I. B., Petito, C. K.: Catecholamine enzymes in the degenerative neurological disease idiopathic orthostatic hypotension. *Science 192:* 910–912, 1976.

48. Sieker, H. O., Burnum, J. F., Hickam, J. B., et al: Treatment of postural hypotension with counter-pressure garment. *JAMA 161:* 132–135, 1956.

49. Hickler, R. B., Thompson, G. R., Fox, L. M., et al: Successful treatment of orthostatic hypotension with 9-alpha-fluoro-hydrocortisone. *N Engl J Med 261:* 788–791, 1959A.

50. Wagner, H. N. Jr., Braunwald, E.: Pressor effect of antidiuretic principle of posterior pituitary in orthostatic hypotension. *J Clin Invest 35:* 1412–1418, 1956.

51. Gregory, R.: Treatment of orthostatic hypotension with particular reference to use of desoxycorticosterone. *Am Heart J 29:* 246–252, 1945.

52. Hoehn, M. J.: Levodopa-induced postural hypotension. Treatment with fluorocortisone. *Arch Neurol 32:* 50, 51, 1975.

53. Seller, R. H.: Idiopathic orthostatic hypotension: Report of successful treatment with a new form of therapy. *Am J Cardiol 23:* 838–844, 1969.

54. Lewis, R. J., Cooper, G. H., Fricke, F. J., et al: Therapy of idiopathic postural hypotension. *Arch Intern Med 129:* 943–949, 1972.

55. Sharpe, J., Marquez-Julio, A., Ashby, P.: Idiopathic orthostatic hypotension treated with levodopa and MAO inhibitor: A preliminary report. *Can Med Assoc J 107:* 296–300, 1972.

56. Corder, C. N.: Orthostatic hypotension. *N Engl J Med 296:* 1175, 1977.

57. Smythies, J. R., Russell, R. O. Jr.: Possible role of prostaglandins in idiopathic postural hypotension. *Lancet II:* 963, 1974.

58. Riley, C. M., Day, R. L., Greeley, D. M., et al: Central autonomic dysfunction with defective lacrimation: Report of five cases. *Pediatrics 3:* 468–478, 1949.

59. Geltzer, A. I., Gluck, G., Talner, N. S., et al: Familial dysautonomia. *N Engl J Med 271:* 435–440, 1964.

60. Smith, A. A., Taylor, T., Wortis, S. B.: Abnormal catecholamine metabolism in familial dysautonomia. *N Engl J Med 268:* 705–707, 1963.

61. Weinshilboum, R. M., Axelrod, J.: Reduced plasma dopamine-beta-hydroxylase activity in familial dysautonomia. *N Engl J Med 285:* 938–942, 1971.

62. Aguayo, A. J., Nair, C. P. V., Bray, G. M.: Peripheral nerve abnormalities in the Riley-Day syndrome. Findings in a sural nerve biopsy. *Arch Neurol 24:* 106–115, 1971.

63. Pearson, J., Axelrod, F., Dancis, J.: Current concepts of dysauton-

omia: Neuropathological defects. *Ann NY Acad Sci 228:* 288–300, 1976.

64. Goedert, M., Buhler, F.: Nerve growth factor antibodies in idiopathic orthostatic hypotension? *N Engl J Med 297:* 336–337, 1977.

65. Sharpey-Schafer, E. P.: Effects of Valsalva's maneuver on the normal and failing circulation. *Br Med J 1:* 693–695, 1965.

66. Sharpey-Schafer, E. P., Taylor, P. J.: Absent circulatory reflexes in diabetic neuritis. *Lancet 1:* 559–562, 1960.

104

The Sympathetic Nervous System and Primary Hypertension in Man

Vincent DeQuattro
Mark R. Myers

INTRODUCTION

PHEOCHROMOCYTOMA—A REAL MODEL

Neurogenic hypertension exists in humans in the form of its natural experiment—pheochromocytoma. Secretion of norepinephrine and epinephrine from chromaffin tumors causes arteriolar constriction, increased cardiac output, and arterial hypertension. Sweating, pallor, flushing, tachycardia, and other characteristic manifestations of sympathetic nerve function excess are usually pronounced in these patients. These clinical signs are associated with biochemical evidence of increased production of norepinephrine and epinephrine and their metabolites. The hypertensive symptoms are remedied by extirpation of the tumor or following therapy with alpha- or beta-receptor blocking drugs.

A HYPOTHESIS UNDER FIRE

Antiadrenergic drugs and behavior modification reduce both sympathetic tone and arterial pressure, suggesting a causal relationship.[1,2] In the fright and flight response to stress, the normal increase in arterial pressure is mediated by the sympathetic nervous system. Stress is important in the maintenance of primary hypertension; the hypotensive effect of hospitalization or placebo on most patients with elevated blood pressure is legendary.

Von Euler characterized norepinephrine (NE) as the sympathetic neurotransmitter in 1946 and demonstrated that NE excretion reflects nerve tonicity.[3] Evidence of increased norepinephrine excretion, as reviewed by Brunjes,[4] enhanced vascular sensitivity,[5] and pressor responsiveness to norepinephrine,[6] sparked the neurogenic theory. Further findings of normal or reduced norepinephrine excretion[4] in other groups of hypertensives and a generalized sensitivity to pressor agents refuted the earlier work. The mapping of central adrenergic pathways by Dahlstrom and Fuxe,[8] studies of norepinephrine turnover in animal hypertension by Krakoff et al.,[9] and refined techniques for determination of plasma catecholamines by Engelman et al.[10] have refueled interest in research in neurogenic mechanisms.

CENTRAL NEUROGENIC REGULATION AND STRESS

Activation of the hypothalamic mesencephalic spinal pathway excites the peripheral system. Application of epinephrine to its hypothalamic or medullary receptors causes sympathetic nerve discharge and hypertension. On the other hand, activating the bulbospinal inhibitory system reduces peripheral sympathetic nerve tone and blood pressure. The two peripheral components are the afferent sinoaortic and the efferent thoracolumbar nerves. Normally, when arterial pressure increases, pressure receptors in the carotid sinus and aortic arch are stimulated, increasing sinoaortic and bulbospinal nerve traffic. In this manner, the blood pressure rise is buffered. When this inhibitory system is severed either in the sinoaortic afferent or in the tractus solitarius, there is unopposed sympathoadrenal stimulation and hypertension.[11] It is generally accepted that the central inhibitory system is mediated by alpha receptors. The exact nature of the nerve pathways for excitation and their transmitters and receptors are controversial subjects now under study (see Chapter 100, Fig. 100-4).

A dual control system of alpha-inhibitory and beta-excitatory pathways might explain the actions of clonidine and propranolol in lowering blood pressure. Both drugs concentrate in the brain. Clonidine is an alpha agonist that stimulates central alpha-inhibitory pathways; therefore, it diminishes sympathetic nerve outflow and lowers arterial pressure. Sudden cessation of clonidine therapy may result in a "pseudopheochromocytoma" syndrome of sweating, tachycardia, anxiety, tremor and hypertension, associated with increased plasma and urine catecholamines.[12]

Propranolol blocks both peripheral and central beta receptors; the latter action may be predominant, since oral propranolol lowers sympathetic tone and blood pressure in hypertensive patients.

The sympathetic nervous system regulates the renin-angiotensin system via its influence on the JG cell in the kidney. It is generally accepted that coarse adjustments of arterial pressure in humans are made by the renin-angiotensin-aldosterone system in response to salt and volume load or depletion but that fine adjustments are made via an interplay of the central inhibitory and excitatory aspects of the sympathetic nerves.

Recently, Saavedra et al. described increased adrenalin-forming enzymes in A_1 and A_2 regions of the medulla in spontaneously hypertensive rats before development of hypertension.[13] These regions may be part of the mesencephalic stimulatory pathway mediated by beta receptors.

NEUROGENIC FACTORS IN ANIMAL MODELS WITH HYPERTENSION

Animal models with various forms of hypertension have abnormal norepinephrine synthesis, storage, and metabolism. Norepinephrine synthesis rate is increased, turnover and release is increased, and storage is decreased in the heart and other innervated organs in the Doca-salt model.[9] Norepinephrine synthesis, turnover, and release are increased and storage is decreased in the SAD model[14] and in experimental renovascular hypertension.[15] Renovascular hypertension produced by kidney encapsulation and nephrectomy[72] or renal artery stenosis and contralateral nephrectomy (Goldblatt-1 kidney model)[73] have increased norepinephrine turnover in heart and brain.

Increased plasma catecholamines were found immediately after induction of hypertension in the 1 kidney model.[7] Renin is elevated only transiently in the 1 kidney model,[30] plasma catecholamines remained elevated at 1 month—the duration of the study.[7] No changes in plasma catecholamines were observed in the Goldblatt-2 kidney model,[7] although it has both an immediate and prolonged angiotensinogenic component.[30] Plasma catecholamines were also elevated in the Doca-salt rat with experimental hypertension.[52] Thus, plasma catecholamines were increased concomitantly with increased NE turnover in two models—Doca-salt and 1 kidney Goldblatt hypertension. It is of interest that plasma dopamine-beta-hydroxylase (DBH) was not increased in the latter model, casting doubt on the use of DBH in estimating sympathetic nervous system (SNS) function.[69]

The nature of the SNS involvement in both animal and human renovascular hypertension has not been clarified, although intracisternal 6 OH dopamine prevents the blood pressure rise in the 1 kidney animal,[69] and preliminary studies indicate deficient norepinephrine content in the hypothalamus and brain stem.[50] Other factors in addition to angiotension II generation are required to explain the genesis of hypertension, since plasma NE is increased when plasma renin activity is normal in the 1 kidney model[7] and plasma NE is normal when renin is high in the 2 kidney model and in humans with renovascular hypertension.[58]

After sinoaortic denervation in the rabbit, there was immediate hypertension concomitant with increased synthesis and release of norepinephrine from the heart and the adrenal medulla.[14] There was increased PNMT activity in the adrenal medulla of animals with neurogenic hypertension. Associated with the hypertension, biosynthesis of norepinephrine was increased in proximal mesenteric vessels and renal artery. At this time, the hypertension was characterized by increased cardiac output. Later, during chronic hypertension, cardiac output was normalized and peripheral vascular and splanchnic resistance, as well as NE synthesis in distal mesenteric vessels, was increased.[16] This biphasic hemodynamic pattern in an animal model with neurogenic hypertension resembles that reported by Eich in patients with primary hypertension.[17]

NEUROGENIC ASPECTS IN PRIMARY HYPERTENSION

CLINICAL AND HEMODYNAMIC MEASUREMENTS

Some clinical observations implicate autonomic dysfunction in hypertension. Hypertensive patients may display signs of sympathetic hyperactivity: pallor, sweating, flushing, blushing, evanescent rashes, piloerection, tachycardia, and palpitation.[18] However, these signs are absent in many patients with hypertension. Initially, only systolic blood pressure is elevated in some hypertensive patients; later, there may be labile elevations of both systolic and diastolic arterial pressures associated with findings of a vigorous active precordium and a functional systolic murmur. Resting cardiac outputs are frequently increased. Patients with this syndrome were formerly diagnosed as having "hyperkinetic heart syndrome."[19] Some patients with these problems were found to have increased vascular and central nervous system sensitivity to isoproterenol. They were described as having beta-adrenergic receptor hyperreactivity.[20]

Eich et al.[17] followed cardiac output and peripheral vascular resistance in patients with hypertension over a 4- to 5-year period. There was an initial increase in cardiac output in 20 to 30 percent of patients which reverted toward normal, while total peripheral vascular resistance increased. In patients with normal or low cardiac output initially, the tendency was to maintain an increased peripheral resistance and a normal or decreased cardiac output. Investigators have observed increased cardiac output in patients with borderline or labile hypertension and normal or decreased cardiac output in patients with sustained hypertension,[21–24] but these abnormal systemic hemodynamics may not be due to neurogenic influences.[25] The resting pulse rates of patients with labile hypertension are usually greater than those of normotensive subjects.[24] For this reason, it has been suggested that initially in some patients with hypertension, hyperfunction of the cardiac sympathetic nerves leads to increased cardiac output and systolic hypertension. Eventually, peripheral arteriolar constriction occurs and results in diastolic hypertension.[22] Finally, a gradual upward resetting of aortic and carotid baroreceptors may result in sustained hypertension. On the other hand, diastolic hypertension does not ensue in patients whose cardiac output is increased for other reasons, for example, thyrotoxicosis and Paget's disease.

There is some direct evidence for increased sympathetic nerve activity in patients with sustained hypertension.[26,27] Frohlich and co-workers[28] found the opposite, however, namely that sympathetic nerve responsiveness was inversely proportional to the severity and duration of the hypertension. Hypertensive patients have increased responsiveness and increased sensitivity of the digital and conjunctival vessels to infused norepinephrine.[26,29]

Although these various observations are subject to diverse interpretation, they raise the possibility that an alteration in the vascular neuroeffector mechanisms is responsible for the increased vascular resistance in primary hypertension.

BIOCHEMICAL EVALUATION OF TONICITY

Catecholamine Excretion

Many investigators found normal norepinephrine excretion rates in hypertensive patients,[4] but some[4,31,32] reported decreased excretion of catecholamines in hypertensive patients. These findings were explained by the postulation that in primary hypertension, blood pressure is maintained by an abnormal mechanism reducing the adrenergic requirements. This is compatible with the findings of decreased sympathetic nerve responsiveness after tilting in some hypertensive patients.[28] Nestel and Esler[33] found increased urinary excretion of norepinephrine in hypertensive subjects after stress and concluded that this was evidence of increased sympathetic nerve activity. In another study, increased catecholamine excretion was found in 5 percent of a group of patients with primary hypertension.[34] The clinical symptoms and the increase in norepinephrine excretion were suggestive of pheochromocytoma.

Dopamine, a neurotransmitter itself, is the immediate precursor of norepinephrine. The normal dopamine excretion rate is approximately 5 to 10 times that of norepinephrine. Dopamine excretion is abnormal in some hypertensive patients.[35,36] In one study, mean dopamine excretion in hypertensive patients was 50 percent of that in normal controls.[35] In another study, although the excretion rates of dopamine of labile hyperkinetic patients were similar to those of control subjects, the excretion of urinary norepinephrine was increased in the hypertensive patients. These investigators, impressed with the decreased ratio of dopamine to norepinephrine in hypertensive patients,[36] thought that the excessive norepinephrine in relation to dopamine might account for changes in regional blood flow resulting in hypertension.

Catecholamine Metabolite Excretion

The degree to which the various urinary norepinephrine metabolites reflect sympathetic activity in humans is not established. Stott and Robinson[37] found increased normetanephrine, while Brunjes[4] found decreased vanillylmandelic acid (VMA) in relation to unchanged normetanephrine in the urine of hypertensive patients. Enhanced norepinephrine excretion in some patients with hypertension was proposed to explain the former findings, and either defective oxidative-deamination or altered secretion of norepinephrine was the explanation proposed by Brunjes to explain his findings. Excretion of O-methylated catecholamines was increased in those patients with increased norepinephrine excretion, but VMA excretion was normal.[34] The excretion rate of dihydroxymandelic acid, the product of monoamine oxidase metabolism of norepinephrine, also reflects sympathetic nerve activity. Excretion rates of dihydroxymandelic acid were normal in the small number of hypertensive patients studied[38] (see Chapter 100, Metabolic Pathways).

Norepinephrine Turnover

Norepinephrine turnover studies in humans and animals indicated abnormal catecholamine metabolism in hypertension. Gitlow and his co-workers[39] demonstrated enhanced plasma norepinephrine clearance in patients with hypertension consistent with reduced norepinephrine storage. Later, they found a greater excretion of tritium after ³H-DL-norepinephrine infusion in patients with hypertension.[40]

Drugs that affect sympathetic nerve function and tissue norepinephrine in animals altered norepinephrine turnover in humans after ³H-dopa administration.[41] Chronic reserpine therapy did not change excretion of norepinephrine, dopamine, or VMA. However, it increased norepinephrine specific activity and turnover after administration of ³H-dopa. This suggested intact synthesis and reduced norepinephrine storage after reserpine. Parglyine, a monoamine oxidase inhibitor, decreased total catecholamine metabolite excretion in hypertensive patients but did not change total free catecholamine excretion. The half-life of norepinephrine turn-

over rate increased from 8 to 20 hours in pargyline-treated patients. Inhibition of intraneuronal norepinephrine degradation probably increased tissue norepinephrine, leading to feedback inhibition of tyrosine hydroxylase.

Norepinephrine turnover measured by the ³H-dopa technique was normal in most patients with primary hypertension,[41] although the method detected the increased sympathetic nerve activity during surgical stress and the alterations produced by antiadrenergic drugs. A subset of patients with increased norepinephrine excretion had increased norepinephrine turnover rates, however. The changes resembled those that occurred after reserpine, suggesting intact or enhanced norepinephrine synthesis but reduced norepinephrine storage.[34] Kopin et al.[71] demonstrated that norepinephrine released by tyramine was metabolized by COMT, whereas intraneuronal metabolism of norepinephrine was accomplished via monoamine oxidase. Excessive release of newly synthesized norepinephrine may have contributed to or perhaps initiated the hypertensive process in this small group of patients with increased norepinephrine excretion.[34]

Plasma Catecholamine and DBH Concentrations

Measurements of these substances as indices of sympathetic tone have been central to the investigation of the role of the sympathetic nervous system in hypertension. Norepinephrine is released with nerve discharge, and that which escapes reuptake, binding to receptors, and metabolism can be measured in plasma and urine. Louis et al.[1] found a concomitant reduction of catecholamines and blood pressure in hypertensives after ganglionic blockade, suggesting that increased sympathetic tone was a cause of their hypertension.(Fig. 104-1). Increased plasma catecholamines are evidence for increased sympathetic nerve tone, as in postural stress.[42] Reserpine, known to deplete tissue NE, also reduced plasma catecholamines.[43] Propranolol reduced plasma catecholamines at low doses but increased them at high doses.[44] Low plasma levels of norepinephrine occur in postural hypotension and dysautonomia.[45]

Norepinephrine is released from the nerve endings with DBH (Fig. 104-2). Dopamine-beta-hydroxylase, the final enzyme in norepinephrine biosynthesis, is expelled with nerve discharge and released into the synaptic cleft with norepinephrine and carrier protein. Information regarding release, reuptake, and disposition of DBH is still tentative, and the half-life in plasma is given

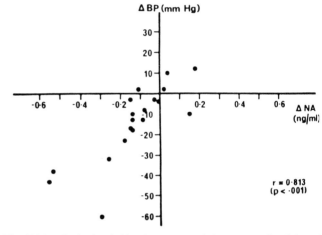

Fig. 104-1. Reduction in blood pressure and plasma norepinephrine after ganglionic blockade in patients with primary hypertension. Δ NA is the change in norepinephrine.

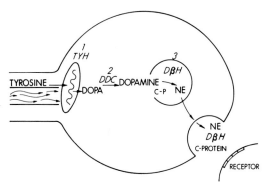

Fig. 104-2. Release of norepinephrine (NE) and dopamine-β-hydroxylase by exocytosis. Biosynthetic enzymes are tyrosine hydroxylase (TYH), dopa-decarboxylase (DDC) and dopamine-β-hydroxylase (DBH). C-protein represents carrier protein.

variously as from ½ to 3 hours, compared with 1 to 3 minutes for norepinephrine. After Weinshilboum and Axelrod[46] measured DBH in plasma, they presumed it would reflect sympathetic nerve tone. However, they and others have found a wide range of serum DBH activity in normal people. Many normal persons have no detectable DBH. Schanberg et al.[47] found increased DBH in young patients with labile hypertension. Other groups found slightly increased DBH in hypertensive patients, but the differences were not significant.[48] However, the changes in DBH after standing were related to those of norepinephrine in normotensives (Fig. 104-3). One study found impaired responsiveness of DBH to standing after furosemide in young patients with labile hypertension.[48]

Relation to Tissue Enzyme. Plasma catecholamines were raised in up to 30 percent of patients with primary hypertension, suggesting that their basal sympathetic nerve tone was increased.[1,10,42,49,51-53] In a group of men prior to vasectomy, plasma catecholamines were increased in 40 percent of those with both systolic and diastolic blood pressure elevation.[49] The increased plasma catecholamine content of patients prior to vasectomy was proportional to the tyrosine hydroxylase activity of their vas deferens tissue. This is evidence that the increased norepinephrine in plasma was related to enhanced synthesis of neurotransmitter.[49] Previously, studies of enhanced norepinephrine excretion in hypertension, using labeled dopa, led to findings of enhanced release of newly synthesized norepinephrine in these patients.[34] Men with elevated systolic blood pressure had both elevated plasma catecholamines and tissue tyrosine hydroxylase in their vas deferens.

On the other hand, men who had increased systolic and diastolic pressures had raised plasma catecholamines without increased tyrosine hydroxylase activity in their vas deferens. Patients with no detectable DBH in plasma had normal amounts of DBH in their vas deferens, thus further questioning the use of DBH as a marker of sympathetic nerve tone.

Relation to Renin Activity. The classification of hypertensives according to renin status, popularized by Brunner and co-workers,[54] provides a useful way to subdivide patients into groups. However, these groups are probably nonhomogeneous. Catecholamines and renin were measured during basal conditions and postural stress in two different populations of hypertensives, Californians[55] and Michiganders.[44] The former were men and women, ages 18 to 72; the latter were men, ages 18 to 35. None of the patients had sequelae of the elevated blood pressure, i.e., congestive failure, coronary artery disease, cerebrovascular accidents, or azotemia. Thirty percent of the Californians had "low" renin; 15 percent had "high" renin. The "low"-renin patients had higher blood pressure, more often of the sustained type (always above 90 mm Hg diastolic), and were older than the other two groups of patients. The "high"-renin patients were younger and frequently had more labile hypertension and clinical features of sympathetic nerve activity, such as flushing, sweating, and pallor. There was a greater incidence of raised catecholamines in the "high"-renin patients (70 percent) as compared with that of "low"- and "normal"-renin patients (14 percent) (Fig. 104-4). The individual hypertensive values were compared to normotensives by age and sex (Fig. 104-5). Whether these patients were treated with alpha blockade intravenously, (i.e., phentolamine) or chronic beta blockade with propranolol, they had marked reductions in mean arterial pressure. The reductions in blood pressure after beta blockade were accompanied by lowered plasma catecholamines.[56]

Esler and co-workers investigated the relation of hemodynamic status in the young hypertensives (Michiganders) to renin status. "High"-renin patients had features of sympathetic cardiac stimulation on both noninvasive[57] and invasive testing.[44] Heart rate was increased, and the cardiac preejection period index was shortened. With cardiac beta-adrenergic blockade (propranolol 0.2 mg/kg iv) heart rate, cardiac output, and preejection period index all returned to within normal limits[44] (Fig. 104-6A).

An increased level of neurogenic vasoconstriction, elevating

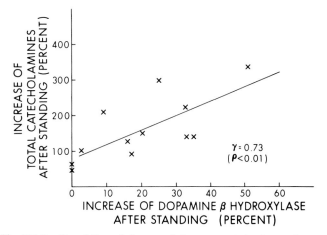

Fig. 104-3. Correlation of changes of plasma catecholamines and serum DBH after standing in normal volunteers. (Reproduced from reference 48 with permission.)

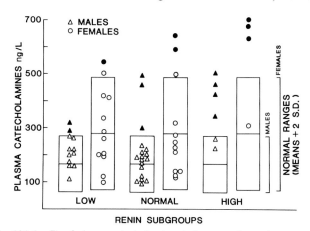

Fig. 104-4. Basal plasma catecholamines in hypertensive patients according to renin subgroupings. Solid triangles and circles (representing values for men and women, respectively) represent plasma catecholamine values greater than 2 standard deviations (SD) above the normal means. The two open circles shown above the 2 standard deviation boxes for women with low and normal renin hypertension show the normal values corrected for age. (Reproduced from reference 55 with permission.)

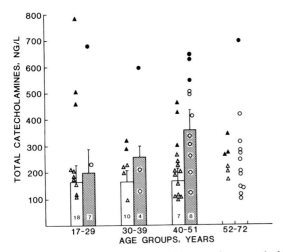

Fig. 104-5. Raised plasma catecholamines in age- and sex-matched hypertensives and normotensives. Open and shaded bars are means ±SD of male and female normotensives, respectively; the number of normotensives are given in the bars. Hypertensive males and females (triangles and circles, respectively) with total catecholamines greater than normotensive means ±2SD are shaded. There were no normotensive volunteers in the 50 to 72 age group.

total peripheral vascular resistance, was also demonstrable in the "high"-renin patients. With alpha-adrenergic blockade, using intravenous phentolamine, total peripheral resistance fell in the "high"-renin patients but not in the other renin subgroups or in normal subjects. With "total blockade," using atropine (for vagal blockade), propranolol, and phentolamine, blood pressure was

normalized in most (70 percent) of the patients with "high" plasma renin but not in the other hypertensives (Fig. 104-6B). "High"-renin hypertensives had increased plasma catecholamines when compared to "low"- and "normal"-renin patients and age-matched normotensive volunteers (Fig. 104-6C). Findings in Cali-

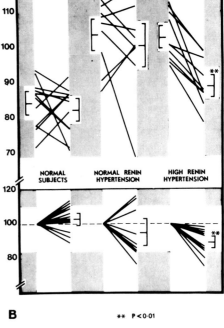

B   ** P < 0·01

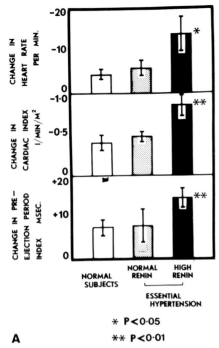

A   * P < 0·05
         ** P < 0·01

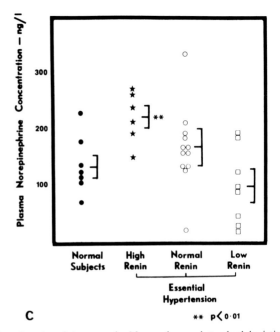

C   ** p < 0·01

Fig. 104-6A. Cardiac responses to beta-adrenergic blockade using propranolol, 0.2 mg/kg, given intravenously. Mean values and standard deviations are shown. The significance of the differences between normal subjects and hypertensive patients is indicated. (Reproduced from reference 44 with permission.) **Fig. 104-6B.** Hemodynamic response to pharmacologic autonomic blockade. The top panel shows the chance in mean arterial pressure (in millimeters of mercury) with "total" autonomic blockade (atropine, 0.04 mg/kg, given intravenously; propranolol, 0.2 mg/kg, given intravenously; and phentolamine, 15 mg/kg, given intravenously). The bottom panel shows the change (percent) in total peripheral vascular resistance with phentolamine after prior cardiac autonomic blockade. Mean values and standard deviations are indicated. Total peripheral resistance before phentolamine is shown as 100 percent. Significance levels of changes are indicated (paired t test). (Reproduced from reference 44 with permission.) **Fig. 104-6C.** Plasma norepinephrine concentrations in normal subjects and patients with essential hypertension. Mean values and standard deviations are shown. The significance of the differences between normal subjects and hypertensive patients is indicated. (Reproduced from reference 44 with permission.)

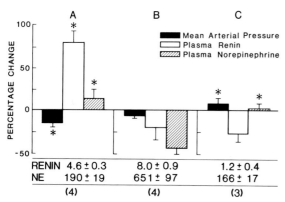

Fig. 104-7. Saralasin induced changes in mean arterial pressure, plasma renin activity, and norepinephrine. Renin status was determined by ambulatory renin/24-hour urine sodium nomograms; norepinephrine (NE) status was defined by supine pre saralasin values. A = high renin/normal NE; B = high renin/raised NE; C = normal renin/normal NE (designations depend on whether patient's values were in the range of the mean + 2 SD of 20 normotensive volunteers); ( ) = number of patients in each group; * = significantly different from values in group B. P < 0.05 for mean arterial pressure and P < 0.01 for plasma renin and NE.

fornia and Michigan indicated increased adrenergic tone in the "high"-renin patients.[44,55]

Sympathetic nerve tone, as reflected by raised plasma catecholamines, appeared to be increased in many patients with "high" renin hypertension. It may be causative in their hypertension in that the blood pressure, the clinical symptoms, and the plasma catecholamines were reduced by antiadrenergic drugs. On the other hand, there were differential responses of blood pressure, renin, and plasma norepinephrine to saralasin in three groups of patients: "high" renin normal norepinephrine, "high" renin raised norepinephrine, and normal renin normal norepinephrine[58] (Fig. 104-7. Patients with "high" renin normal norepinephrine have greater blood pressure reduction after saralasin, an angiotensin II blocker, than patients with "high" renin and raised norepinephrine or those with normal renin. These findings suggested that "high"-renin patients are heterogeneous. Those with positive saralasin tests have an important angiotensinogenic component contributing to the hypertension. Significant renovascular abnormalities were

identified in some of those patients. Mean arterial blood pressure was reduced 6 percent or less after angiotensin II blockade in the group with raised catecholamines. Patients with high renin in the group with raised catecholamines may have increased sympathetic nerve tone. Saralasin increased pressure in the "normal"- or "low"-renin patients, and in some of these there appeared to be a direct agonistic stimulus to norepinephrine release.[59] Saralasin has been associated with a pressor crises in patients with pheochromocytoma.[71]

Sympathetic nerve tone was related to blood pressure elevation in "normal"-renin patients and may have contributed to their hypertension.[60] On the other hand, tone was suppressed in some patients with "low" renin and did not appear to be a prominent factor in their blood pressure elevation.[61] A neurogenic stimulus in some patients with "high"-renin hypertension, perhaps unopposed central sympathetic stimulation, may contribute to the elevated renin.

Tissue Norepinephrine

Excretion rates of norepinephrine are not necessarily related to the tissue concentration of norepinephrine, as for example in the reserpine-treated patient.[41] Furthermore, although methods that measure norepinephrine turnover in humans may be of value in detecting in toto changes in sympathetic nerve function, as in patients after the administration of reserpine, they may not be sensitive enough to detect changes in norepinephrine turnover in specific organs or vascular beds. Tissue catecholamines are increased when metabolism or release of norepinephrine is prevented, as it is by monoamine oxadase inhibitors. Norepinephrine content was studied in human tissues directly by obtaining vas deferens specimens at the time of vasectomy.[49] The concentration of norepinephrine and the activities of its biosynthetic enzymes in vas deferens were correlated with each other and with the blood pressures and pulse rates of the men at vasectomy. Norepinephrine content was related directly to the activity of tyrosine hydroxylase. The means of norepinephrine content and tyrosine hydroxylase activities were greater in men with increased systolic pressure and pulse rates. This may indicate an enhanced systemic sympathetic nerve response to stress in the men with increased systolic pressure (Fig. 104-8).

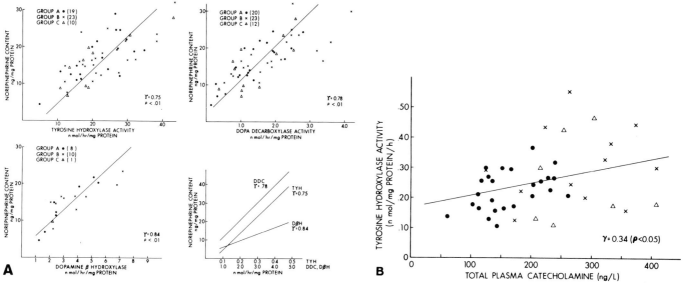

Fig. 104-8A. Norepinephrine content compared with the activities of the three biosynthetic enzymes in human vas deferens. Groups A, B, and C refer to men with normal, elevated systolic, and elevated systolic and diastolic blood pressures, respectively. **Fig. 104-8B.** Correlation of vas deferens TYH with plasma catecholamines just prior to vasectomy. Solid circles denote group A, X's group B, and triangles group C as in Fig. 104-8a.

AN OVERVIEW OF THE CONCEPT

PRIMARY SYMPATHOADRENAL HYPERACTIVITY

Hypertensive patients with primary "neurogenic" hypertension may be expected to have a greater increase in systolic than diastolic blood pressure initially with increased cardiac output and clinical features of sympathoadrenal hyperactivity. It may be that these protective and adaptive changes which occur in normal persons in response to real or imagined stress may persist to a pathologic degree. Perhaps learned behavior patterns persist as responses of continuous or pulsatile hypothalamic discharge. Finally, the increased sympathetic nerve activity results in a variety of functional changes.

There is no general consensus that "hard" biochemical evidence exists for neurogenic hypertension. Although several groups have reported increased plasma catecholamines in primary hypertension, there are a few who have found normal values in hypertensives.[62,63] These latter workers have called attention to an age-related increase in plasma catecholamines in normotension and hypertension.[63]

SECONDARY SYMPATHOADRENAL DYSFUNCTION

That patients with pheochromocytoma may have 10 times or more the catecholamine concentration in plasma or urine at blood pressure levels similar to that of patients with primary hypertension does not necessarily detract from a neurogenic concept. Patients harboring a pheochromocytoma may develop adaptive mechanisms and possibly a reduction in the number or sensitivity of vascular receptors. For example, blockade of beta receptors can result in a larger receptor population[64] (Fig. 104-9).

Secondary sympathetic nerve dysfunction may occur as a consequence of hypertension induced by other important mechanisms such as volume expansion and renal ischemia. Volume expansion hypertension, or low-renin hypertension,[65] may be a spectrum of disorders associated with excessive intravascular accumulation of sodium and water, as in patients with pyelonephritis or glomerulonephritis and in those with increased secretion or responsiveness to mineralocorticoids. The incidence of low-renin hypertension is in the range of 25 to 30 percent.[65] Increased vascular volume in these patients may secondarily inhibit both sympathetic nerve activity and renin secretion. Eventually, there might be abnormal norepinephrine metabolism and hypersensitivity of receptors to endogenously released transmitters. Indeed, urinary catecholamine excretion is either reduced or normal in these hypertensive patients with low plasma renin activity.[66,67] Esler et al.[68] found decreased plasma catecholamines in their low-renin patients.

Renin secretion and hypertension are accelerated in most patients with ischemic lesions of the kidney. There are several ways that the renin-angiotensin system may affect sympathoadrenal function and contribute to the hypertension. In the early stages, a relationship between plasma renin activity and plasma catecholamine content might be expected; later, stimulation of aldosterone secretion may contribute to a volume expansion component that diminishes sympathetic nerve activity by way of buffer mechanism.

INCIDENCE OF SYMPATHETIC NERVE DEFECTS IN HYPERTENSION

Increased plasma catecholamines occur in approximately 25 percent of patients with hypertension.[42] From these and other studies, an educated guess is that a primary neurogenic stimulus is present in 15 to 30 percent of hypertensive patients, in patients with high or normal renin. Secondary neurogenic factors may help maintain elevated blood pressure in at least 30 percent and perhaps as many as 50 percent of hypertensive (normal renin) patients. Fifteen to 20 percent of hypertensives may have blunted sympathetic tone (low renin).

Characterization of the primary and secondary neurogenic processes in individual patients may permit improved therapy. Antihypertensive agents could be matched to the underlying cause of the raised pressure. Patients with primary adrenergic dysfunction might be best treated by drugs that depress sympathetic outflow. Those with reflexly depressed sympathetic tone might be treated with drugs that are predominantly vasodilators. Specific therapy might then minimize adverse and secondary effects.[70]

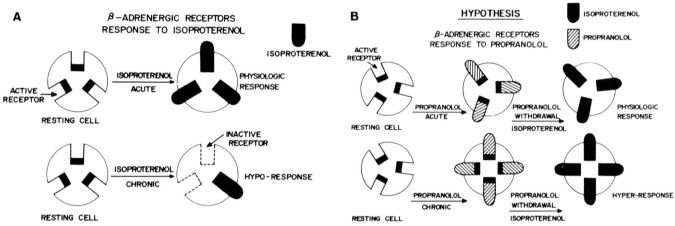

Fig. 104-9. Schematic representation of the effect of isoproterenol (A) and propranolol (B) on beta-adrenergic receptors. The activation of a resting cell by isoproterenol acutely leads to a physiologic response. With longer periods of exposure to isoproterenol, the number of beta-adrenergic receptors decreases, resulting in a blunted response to isoproterenol. The number of active beta-adrenergic receptors remains unchanged if a resting cell is blocked with propranolol acutely. This leads to physiologic response to isoproterenol after the disappearance of blockade. With longer periods of propranolol administration, however, the number of beta-adrenergic receptors increases, and this leads to a hypersensitivity to isoproterenol after the disappearance of blockade. (Reproduced from reference 64 with permission.)

REFERENCES

1. Louis, W. J., Doyle, A. E., Anavekar, S.: Plasma norepinephrine levels in essential hypertension. *N Engl J Med 288:* 599–601, 1973.
2. Stone, R. A., DeLeo, J.: Psychotherapeutic control of hypertension. *N Engl J Med 294:* 80–84, 1976.
3. von Euler, U.S.: Noradrenaline. Springfield, Ill, Charles C. Thomas, 1956.
4. Brunjes, S.: Catecholamine metabolism in essential hypertension. *N Engl J Med 271:* 120–124, 1964.
5. Doyle, A. E., Fraser, J. R. E.: Vascular reactivity in hypertension. *Circ Res 9:* 755, 1961.
6. Goldenberg, M., Aranow, H. Jr., Smith, A. A., Faber, M.: Pheochromocytoma and essential hypertensive vascular disease. *Arch Intern Med 86:* 823, 1950.
7. Reid, J. L., Dargie, H. J., Franklin, S. S., Fraser, B.: Plasma noradrenaline and renovascular hypertension in the rat. *Clin Sci Mol Med 51:* 4395–4425, 1976.
8. Dahlstrom, A., Fuxe, K.: Evidence for the existence of monoamine neurones in the central nervous system: II. Experimentally induced changes in the intraneuronal amine levels of bulbospinal neurone systems. *Acta Physiol Scand 64* (Suppl 247): 1–37, 1965.
9. Krakoff, L. R., deChamplain, J., Axelrod, J.: Abnormal storage of norepinephrine in experimental hypertension in the rat. *Circ Res 21:* 583, 1967.
10. Engelman, K., Portnoy, B., Sjoerdsma, A.: Plasma catecholamine concentrations in patients with hypertension. *Circ Res 27 (Suppl I):* 141–146, 1970.
11. Doba, N., Reis, D. J.: Acute fulminating neurogenic hypertension produced by brainstem lesions in the rat. *Circ Res 32:* 584–593, 1973.
12. Reid, J. L., Dargie, H. J., Davies, D. S., et al: Clonidine withdrawal in hypertension; Changes in blood pressure and plasma and urinary noradrenaline. *Lancet,* 1977, pp 1171–1173.
13. Saavedra, J. M., Grobecker, H., Axelrod, J.: Adrenaline-forming enzyme in brainstem: Elevation in genetic and experimental hypertension. *Science 191:* 483–484, 1976.
14. DeQuattro, V., Nagatsu, T., Maronde, R., Alexander, N.: Catecholamine synthesis in rabbits with neurogenic hypertension. *Circ Res 24:* 545–555, 1969.
15. Finch, L.: The neurogenic component in the experimental hypertensive rat. *Pharmacology 5:* 245–254, 1971.
16. DeQuattro, V., Alexander: Altered norepinephrine synthesis of splanchnic vessels in neurogenic hypertension. *Eur J Pharmacol 26:* 231, 1974.
17. Eich, R. H., Cuddy, R. P., Smulyan, H., Lyons, R. H.: Hemodynamics in labile hypertension. A follow-up study. *Circulation 34:* 299, 1966.
18. Page, I. H.: A syndrome simulating diencephalic stimulation occurring in patients with essential hypertension. *Am J Med Sci 190:* 9, 1935.
19. Gorlin, R., Brachfeld, N., Turner, J. D., et al: The idiopathic high cardiac output state. *J Clin Invest 38:* 2144, 1959.
20. Frohlich, E. D., Dustan, H. P., Page, I. H.: Hyperdynamic beta-adrenergic circulatory state. *Arch Intern Med 117:* 614, 1966.
21. Widimsky, J., Fejfarova, M. H., Fejfar, Z.: Changes of cardiac output in hypertensive disease. *Cardiologia 31:* 381, 1957.
22. Finkielman, S., Worcel, M., Agrest, A.: Hemodynamic patterns in essential hypertension. *Circulation 31:* 356, 1965.
23. Frohlich, E. D., Kozul, V. J., Tarazi, R. C., Dustan, H. P.: Physiological comparison of labile and essential hypertension. *Circ Res 26, 27* (Suppl I): 55, 1970.
24. Julius S., Pascual, A. V., Sannerstedt, R., Mitchell, C.: Relationship between cardiac output and peripheral resistance in borderline hypertension. *Circulation 43:* 382, 1971.
25. Sannerstedt, R., Julius, S.: Systemic hemodynamics in borderline arterial hypertension. Responses to static exercise before and under the influence of propranolol. *Cardiovasc Res 6:* 398, 1972.
26. Smirk, F. H.: The neurogenically maintained component in hypertension. *Circ Res 26, 27* (Suppl II): 55, 1970.
27. Walsh, J. A., Hyman, C., Maronde, R. F.: Venous distensibility in essential hypertension. *Cardiovasc Res 3:* 338, 1970.
28. Frohlich, E. D., Tarazi, R. C., Ulrych, M., et al: Tilt test for investigating a neural component in hypertension. Its correlation with clinical characteristics. *Circulation 36:* 387, 1967.
29. Silvertsson, R., Olander, R.: Aspects of the nature of the increased vascular resistance and increased "reactivity" to noradrenaline in hypertensive subjects. *Life Sci 7:* 1291, 1968.
30. Brunner, H. R., Kirschman, J. D., Sealey, J. E., Laragh, J. H.: Hypertension of renal origin: Evidence for two different mechanisms. *Science 174:* 1344–1346, 1971.
31. Sundin, I.: Influence of body posture on urinary excretion of adrenaline and noradrenaline. *Acta Med Scand 154* (Suppl 313): 1, 1956.
32. Birke, G., Duner, H., von Euler, U. S., Plantin, L. O.; Studies on adrenocortical, adreno-medullary and adrenergic nerve activity in essential hypertension. *Vitamin-Hormon-Fermentforsch 9:* 41, 1957–1958.
33. Nestel, P. J., Esler, M. D.: Patterns of catecholamine excretion in urine in hypertension. *Circ Res 26, 27* (Suppl II): 75, 1970.
34. DeQuattro, V.: Evaluation of increased norepinephrine excretion in hypertension using L-dopa³H. *Circ Res 28:* 84, 1971.
35. Serrano, P. A., Figueroa, G., Torres, M. Z., De Angel, A. R.: Adrenaline, noradrenaline and dopamine excretion in patients with essential hypertension. *Am J Cardiol 13:* 484, 1964.
36. Kuchel, L., Cuche, J. L., Hamet, P., et al: The relationship between adrenergic nervous system and renin in labile hyperkinetic hypertension, in Genest, J., Koiw, E., (eds): *Hypertension,* New York, McGraw-Hill, 1972, p. 118.
37. Stott, A. W., Robinson, R., Urinary normetadrenaline excretion in essential hypertension. *Clin Chim Acta 16:* 249, 1967.
38. Sato, T., DeQuattro, V.: Enzymatic assay for 3,4-dihydroxymandelic acid (DOMA) in human urine, plasma, and tissues. *J Lab Clin Med 74:* 672–681, 1969.
39. Gitlow, S. E., Mendlowitz, M., Wilk, E. K., et al: Plasma clearance of d, 1-B-³H norepine phrine in normal human subjects and patients with essential hypertension. *J Clin Invest 43:* 2009, 1964.
40. Gitlow, S. E., Mendlowitz, M., Bertani, L. M., et al: Tritium excretion of normotensive and hypertensive subjects after administration of tritiated norepinephrine. *J Lab Clin Med 73:* 129, 1969.
41. DeQuattro, V., Sjoerdsma, A.: Catecholamine turnover in normotensive and hypertensive man: Effects of antiadrenergic drugs. *J Clin Invest 47:* 2359–2373, 1968.
42. DeQuattro, V., Chan, S.: Raised plasma-catecholamines in some patients with primary hypertension. *Lancet 1:* 806–809, 1972.
43. DeQuattro, V., Miura, Y., Campese, V., Brunjes, S.: Catecholamine biosynthesis in man: Effects of hypertension and reserpine, in Milliez, P., Safar, M. (eds): Recent Advances in Hypertension, vol 1. Paris, Laboratories Boehringer Ingelheim, 1975, pp 13–26.
44. Esler, M., Julius, S., Zweifler, A., et al: Mild high-renin essential hypertension: A neurogenic human hypertension? *N Engl J Med 296:* 405–411, 1977.
45. Ziegler, M. G., Lake, C. R., Kopin, I. J.: The sympathetic-nervous-system defect in primary orthostatic hypotension. *N Engl J Med 296:* 293–297, 1977.
46. Weinshilboum, R., Axelrod, J.: Serum Dopamine-beta-hydroxylase activity. *Circ Res 28:* 307–315, 1971.
47. Schanberg, S. M., Stone, R. A., Kirshner, N., et al: Plasma dopamine-beta-hydroxylase: A possible aid in the study and evaluation of hypertension. *Science 183:* 523–525, 1974.
48. DeQuattro, V., Campese, V., Lurvey, A., et al: Low response of serum dopamine-beta-hydroxylase to stimuli in primary hypertension. *Biochem Med 15:* 1–9, 1976.
49. DeQuattro, V., Miura, Y., Lurvey, A., et al: Increased plasma catecholamines and vas deferens norepinephrine biosynthesis in men with elevated blood pressure. *Circ Res 36:* 118–126, 1975.
50. Petty, M. A., Reid, J. L.: Noradrenaline concentration in hypothalamic and brain stem nuclei of renovascular hypertensive rats. *Br J Pharm 59:* 483–484, 1977.
51. Jiang, N. S., Stoffer, S., Wadel, O., Sheps, S. G.: Laboratory and clinical observations with a two-column plasma catecholamine assay. *Mayo Clin Proc 48:* 47–49, 1973.
52. de Champlain, J., Farley, L., Cousineau, D., Ameringen, M.: Circulating catecholamine levels in human and experimental hypertension. *Circ Res 38:* 109–114, 1976.
53. Sever, P., Osikowska, B., Birch, M., Tunbridge, R. D. G.: Plasma-noradrenaline in essential hypertension. *Lancet 1:* 1078–1081, 1977.
54. Brunner, H., Laragh, J. H., Baer, L., et al: Essential hypertension: Renin and aldosterone, heart attack and stroke. *N Engl J Med 286 (9):* 441–449, 1972.
55. DeQuattro, V., Campese, V., Miura, Y., Meijer, D.: Increased plasma catecholamines in high renin hypertension. *Am J Cardiol 38:* 801–804, 1976.
56. DeQuattro, V., Campese, V., Miura, Y., Esler, M.: Sympathotonia in primary hypertension and in a caricature resembling dysautonomia. *Clin Sci Mol Med 51* (Suppl 3): 435–438, 1976.

57. Esler, M., Julius, S., Randall, O., et al: High-renin essential hypertension: Adrenergic cardiovascular correlates. *Clin Sci Mol Med* 51 (Suppl 3): 181–184, 1976.

58. DeQuattro, V., Barbour, B. H., Campese, V., et al: Sympathetic nerve hyperactivity in "high" renin hypertension: Effects of saralasin infusion. *Mayo Clin Proc 52:* 369–373, 1977.

59. Dunn, F. G., DeCarvalho, J. G. R., Kem, D. C., et al: Pheochromocytoma crisis induced by saralasin: Relation of angiotensin analogue to catecholamine release. *N Engl J Med 295:* 605–607, 1976.

60. DeQuattro, V., Campese, V., Miura, Y., Meijer, D.: Biochemical markers of sympathetic nerve activity and renin in primary hypertension, in Berglund, G., Hansson, L., Werko, L., (eds): Pathophysiology and Management of Arterial Hypertension, Molndal, Sweden, Lindgren & Soner, 1975, pp 23–31.

61. Esler, M., Zweifler, A., Randall, O., et al: Suppression of sympathetic nervous function in low-renin essential hypertension. *Lancet 2* (7977): 115, 1976.

62. Christensen, M. S., Christensen, N. J.: Plasma catecholamines in hypertension. *Scand J Clin Lab Invest 30:* 168, 1972.

63. Lake, C. R., Ziegler, M. G., Coleman, M. D., Kopin, I. J.: Age adjusted plasma norepinephrine levels are similar in normotensive and hypertensive subjects. *N Engl J Med 296:* 208–209, 1977.

64. Boudoulas, H., Lewis, R. P., Kates, R. E., Dalamangas, G.: Hypersensitivity to adrenergic stimulation after propranolol withdrawal in normal subjects. *Ann Intern Med 87:* 433–436, 1977.

65. Laragh, J. H., Baer, L., Brunner, H. R., et al: Renin, angiotensin and aldosterone system in pathogenesis and management of hypertensive vascular disease, in Laragh J. H. (ed): Symposium on Hypertension: Mechanisms and Management. *Am J Med 52:* 633, 1972.

66. Crane, M. G., Harris, J. J.: Hyporeninemic hypertension. *Am J Med 52:* 457, 1972.

67. Jose, A., Grout, J. R., Kaplan, N. M.: Suppressed plasma renin activity in essential hypertension: Roles of plasma volume, blood pressure and sympathetic nervous system. *Ann Intern Med 72:* 9, 1970.

68. Esler, M., Zweifler, A., Randall, O., et al: Suppression of sympathetic nervous function in low renin essential hypertension. *Lancet II:* 115–118, 1976.

69. Dargie, H. J., Franklin, S. S., Reid, J. L.: Plasma noradrenaline concentrations in experimental renovascular hypertension in the rat. *Clin Sci Mol Med 52:* 477–483, 1977.

70. Buhler, F. R., Laragh, J. H., Baer, L., et al: Propranolol inhibition of renin secretion: A specific approach to diagnosis and treatment of renin-dependent hypertensive disease. *N Engl J Med 287:* 1209, 1972.

71. Kopin, I. J., Gordon, E. K.: Metabolism of norepinephrine-3H released by tyramine and reserpine. *J Pharmacol Exp Ther 138:* 351, 1962.

72. Volicer, L., Scheer, E., Hilse, H., Visweswaram, D.: The turnover of norepinephrine in the heart during experimental hypertension in rats. *Life Sci 7:* 525, 1968.

73. Henning, M.: Noradrenaline turnover in renal hypertensive rats. *J Pharm Pharmacol 21:* 61, 1969.

Index